# Campbell's Psychiatric Dictionary

# Campbell's
# Psychiatric Dictionary

## Ninth Edition

## Robert Jean Campbell, M.D.

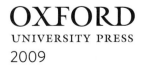

UNIVERSITY PRESS
2009

Oxford University Press, Inc., publishes works that further
Oxford University's objective of excellence
in research, scholarship, and education.

Oxford New York
Auckland Cape Town Dar es Salaam Hong Kong Karachi
Kuala Lumpur Madrid Melbourne Mexico City Nairobi
New Delhi Shanghai Taipei Toronto

With offices in
Argentina Austria Brazil Chile Czech Republic France Greece
Guatemala Hungary Italy Japan Poland Portugal Singapore
South Korea Switzerland Thailand Turkey Ukraine Vietnam

Copyright © 1940, 1953, 1960, 1970, 1981, 1989, 1996, 2004, 2009

By Oxford University Press, Inc.
Renewed 1968 by Leland E. Hinsie

The book was originally published under the title *Psychiatric Dictionary*, by Leland E. Hinsie and Jacob
Shatsky. The second and subsequent editions were written by Robert J. Campbell. The current book is a
revision of *Campbell's Psychiatric Dictionary, Eighth Edition* by Robert J. Campbell.

Published by Oxford University Press, Inc.
198 Madison Avenue, New York, New York 10016
www.oup.com

Oxford is a registered trademark of Oxford University Press

Library of Congress Cataloging-in-Publication Data

Campbell, Robert Jean, 1926-
 Campbell's psychiatric dictionary / Robert Jean Campbell.—9th ed.
 p. ; cm.
 ISBN: 978-0-19-534159-1
 1. Psychiatry—Dictionaries. I. Title. II. Title: Psychiatric dictionary.
 [DNLM: 1. Psychiatry—Dictionary—English.—WM 13 C189c 2009]
 RC437.H5 2009
 616.89003—dc22     2008035593

9 8 7 6 5 4 3 2 1
Printed in the United States of America
on acid-free paper

# Preface

To a large extent, psychiatry today is based on the clinical developments, technological advances, and research of the second half of the 20th century. The 4 major classes of psychopharmacologic agents—antipsychotics, antidepressants, anxiolytics, and lithium—were discovered between 1950 and 1960. In 1953 Watson and Crick presented their double helix model of DNA, and by 1966 the genetic code of nucleotide triplets had been broken. Advances in computer technology and brain imaging provided a basis for quantitative measurement of brain functioning. Together, these developments transformed our understanding of the brain and the functional roles of many of its regions; they spurred the growth of behavioral neurochemistry, cognitive neuroscience, and pharmacogenetics. They also raised hopes that disease-inducing genes would be identified and that more effective drugs, with faster onset, fewer side effects, and greater specificity, would be developed.

So far, those hopes have not been realized. The advances answered many questions, but raised as many new ones. Not all of them held up under longer-term scrunity, and many were not readily translatable into clinical practice. Compared with existing approaches, some of the technology developed produced marginal gains at premium costs. The "new" drugs turned out to be little different from the older ones, suggesting that researchers have been committed too long to a monoamine orientation in drug discovery. The search for a "schizophrenia gene," to cite but one example, has produced claims for association of more than 130 genes (on 21 of the 23 pairs of chromosomes) with the disease, but few of those claims have been replicated.

Those disappointments, however, have generated more research, in multiple areas. There has been an infusion of concepts and models derived from other branches of medicine and other fields of knowledge, and by cross-fertilization between many different disciplines, including the neurosciences, the behavioral and social sciences, epidemiology, economics, mathematics and computational models, and even political science. The language of the field of mental health has expanded to include that cross-fertilization, and one goal of this edition of the *Dictionary* is to make the major discoveries understandable to the reader of today's journals and textbooks of psychiatry and clinical psychology. No less important is making psychiatry and the behavioral sciences intelligble to lawmakers, judges, lawyers, economists, members of the clergy, the media, and the general public. Among the recent developments are the following.

*Neuroscience and Brain Imaging* In the 1970s, cognitive neuroscience research was focused on determining what parts of the brain were associated with perception, attention, memory, language, and emotion. Concurrent advances in brain imaging techniques—such as multiphoton microscopy, which is able to resolve the activity and structure of a single neuron; voltage-sensitive dyes and optical imaging, which provide simultaneous recordings from multiple cells in different networks; and photoactivable protein expression, which can trace individual neurons in the living brain—added immeasurably to our knowledge of neuronal activity in different neuronal networks and of the correlations and signaling between different networks. We now know that brain areas do not work in isolation; instead they belong to several intersection networks, and the neural computations that are implemented by an area will depend on the particular network(s) with which it is affiliated at the time. For the same reasons, cognition and affect are not readily separable in the brain; the "emotional" brain is also involved in cognition, and the "cognitive" brain is involved in emotion. Reseachers began to look at the different networks involved in more complicated mental activities, and social cognitive neuroscience and moral cognitive neuroscience were born. The social brain is engaged when a person is trying to understand others: Who are they? What do they want? What are they planning to do, etc.? A person's understanding of others reflects how others have treated that person in the past. A person's experiences with others, as well as the effects of a lifetime of learning to fit into a pattern of living that is acceptable to, or at least tolerated by, the culture within which the person operates has long-term effects—not only on how that person will act and feel when exposed to new and different people, but also how readily he or she can form an effective alliance with a therapist, and how likely it is that he or she can adhere to an outpatient medication regime. Moral cognitive neuroscience studies the cognitive and neural mechanisms that underlie moral behavior. Morality, in this sense, refers to the sets of customs and values endorsed by a cultural group to guide social conduct; it does not assume the existence of absolute moral values. Important to moral behavior are the brain processes involved in decision making and choice, and the later processing of self-regulation and volitional guidance. A moral judgment task that involves classic moral dilemmas (e.g., you kill an innocent person in order to save five other people?) has been found to activate the anterior prefrontal cortex. Decision difficulty is correlated with increased activity in anterior cingulate cortex. There is evidence that networks within prefrontal-temporal cortices and the limbic lobe may represent distinct moral emotions, including guilt, anger, and embarrassment.

*Genetics* Meantime, genetic studies continued to expose an increasing complexity in the path from genes to proteins to brain systems to behavior. By the 1980s it was recognized that many genes are found in two or more *normal* functional forms (polymorphism). The single nucleotide polymorphism (SNP) is the most common form of genetic variant.

The 22,000 genes in the human genome account for only 5% of the 3 billion base pairs that make up the DNA in the human genome. The other 95% is noncoding DNA, which contains a variety of types of regulatory DNA that turns genes on at the right time and in the right place or otherwise modulates their expression. Gene expression is also affected by epigenetic mechanisms, chemical modifications of the chromatin. The 22,000 genes code for about a million proteins; in the nervous system, they affect neural networks, not just a particular neuron, gyrus, or lobe of the brain. To understand how they are involved in disease, it is necessary to determine how multiple genes and proteins interact, how genes are turned on and off, how they are instructed to decrease or increase their activity, how that affects the proteins they encode, and how the multiple genes and proteins interact with the environment. Further, not only can a single gene and its products participate in multiple cognitive, affective, sensory, and motor processes, but mental functions involve the products of many different genes.

The result of such findings has been a shift in the direction of research. No longer are scientists looking for a single gene to explain a disease such as schizophrenia; they think it more likely that many rare structural changes, such as novel deletions or duplications that disrupt gene function, might contribute to the disorder. Attention has now turned to endophenotypes of heritable dysfunction that appear along the gene → behavior pathway (before the full clinical syndrome develops). The manifestations can take many forms, such as a physiological, biochemical, endocrinological, neuroanatomical abnormality or psychological trait; their importance is that they can be more precisely defined and quantified than can a psychiatric diagnosis. The hope is that they might also point the way to effective prevention.

Since the 1980s, more laws involving medicine an psychiatry have been introduced than in all of the preceding years of United States history. Laws such as the enunciation of patients' rights not only to receive treatment but also to refuse it when proffered, were followed by a corresponding increase in judicial decisions and regulations that directly affected training, research, and treatment programs. Mental health professionals deal with patients whose disorders are often expressed as distortions in social behavior and emotional relations. By its very nature, psychiatry deals with questions of guilt and conscience, soul and mind, attitude and values, freedom to think and to act, and the relationship of the individual to society. The psychiatrist deals not only with the patient's pain and distress, but also with the family's and society's attitudes and demands, including standards for employment and education, community expectations about social conformity and actions in public, and the definition of all of those in legal imperatives. In some cases, the psychiatrist is held responsible for the behavior of his or her patient, even while being accused of irresponsible interference with that patient's freedom. In the United States, designating undesirable conduct or even undesirable viewpoints as illness rather than as crime was an earmark of the 20th century. Psychiatrists find themselves in the dual role of helping patients to get better and at the same time helping society to run more smoothly.

In an age of consumerism and erosion of trust in social institutions, it was hardly a surprise that distrust of psychiatry blossomed. Those who might be designated "patients" faced as much suspicion and hostility as did those labeled "criminals." They feared that in the name of therapy, society would impose unwarranted controls with mind-altering drugs, electrode implantations, psychosurgery, operant conditioning, and the like.

All the foregoing were compounded when concern about spiraling health costs produced a shift from a funding backdrop of lavish abundance to one of parched frugality. Health care reform was launched and even today is directed largely to limiting access to care and controlling the duration and level of intensity of treatment. Managed care, utilization review, peer review, fee for service, and pay for performance were introduced, and even individual clinicians were forced to learn about cost shifting, case mix index, adverse selection, offset moral hazard, outliers, and the other jargon of insurance, accounting, and administration.

Denial of access to care was a special problem in the mental health field. Insurance programs typically discriminated against mental illness, and mental health professionals worried that their most severely ill patients might become major targets of plans to reduce the costs of health care. Psychiatry entered the field of public policy and pressed legislators for "parity" legislation to ensure that the mentally ill had the same access to care as did the physically ill. An essential part of that effort was educating legislators and public policy officials about mental illness and its treatments, and about the many advances in cross-disciplinary research and in the basic sciences that are reflected in this edition of the *Dictionary*.

*Ethics* As indicated above, there has always been concern that psychiatry might be used to help society run smoothly. Such " traditional" ethical issues continue: confidentiality, boundary violations, informed consent, conflicts of interest, double agentry, gene therapy, advance directives, dangerousness, commitment and involuntary treatment, assisted suicide, participating in court-ordered executions or torture. Some of the recent research described has fomented new concerns: the ability to predict the risk for mental disorder; the ability to manipulate the brain, use of cognition-enhancing pharmaceuticals, and the coercive use of interventions that alter brain function. It might be possible for example, to use "real time" fMRI to distinguish deliberate deceit from truthful answers (raising the issue of mind privacy). If studies of endophenotypes ultimately provide a list of risk factors for various diseases—autistic disorder, schizophrenia, depression, post-traumatic stress disorder, ADHD, for example—will this create a "genetically tainted" cohort of unadoptable children? Who should have control of the data? Under what conditions should the findings be released? To whom—the potential patient, the parents, school employers, insurance underwriters?

*Translational Research* It brings scientific discoveries and hypotheses into the clinical arena, bridges the time gap between scientific discovery and its application to clinical care settings, subjects clinical observations to objective scrutiny, and converts them into viable hypotheses and conclusions based on research evidence. Translational research seeks to improve quality by improving access, reorganizing and coordinating systems of care, helping clinicians and patients to change behaviors and make more informed choices, providing point-of-care decision support tools, and strengthening the patient–clinician relationship.

This edition of the *Dictionary* could not have been completed without the ongoing support, suggestions, and encouragement from my "core team," to whose members I shall forever be grateful: Cesare L. Santeramo, Marion Osmun, and my guides at Oxford University Press—Abby Gross, Shelley Reinhardt, and Mark O' Malley.

R.J.C., M.D.
January 2009

# Abbreviations and Acronyms

| | | | |
|---|---|---|---|
| AA | Alcoholics Anonymous; Achievement Age | AEDs | Antiepileptic drugs |
| AAMI | Age-associated memory impairment | AEP | Auditory evoked potential; average evoked potential |
| AANB | Alpha-amino-n-butyric acid | AFP | Alpha-fetoprotein |
| AAS | Anabolic-androgenic steroids; ascending activating system (reticular activating system) | AgCC | Agenesis of the corpus callosum |
| | | AGCT | Army General Classification Test |
| | | AgrP | Agouti-related peptide |
| | | AHP | Allied health professional |
| AAT | Animal-assisted therapy | AI | Artifical intelligence |
| ABEPP | American Board of Examiners in Professional Psychology | AID | Acute infectious disease(s); artificial insemination by donor; autoimmune disease(s) |
| ABL | Amyloid-beta-lipoproteinemia | | |
| AβP | Amyloid beta-protein | AIDS | Acquired immunodeficiency syndrome |
| ABPN | American Board of Psychiatry and Neurology, Inc. | AIMS | Abnormal Involuntary Movements Scale |
| ACA | Adult child of an alcoholic | AIP | Attention and information processing; acute intermittent porphyria |
| ACC | Anterior cingulate cortex | | |
| ACGME | Accreditation Council on Graduate Medical Education | | |
| | | AIS | Androgen insensitivity syndrome |
| Ach | Acetylcholine | | |
| AchE | Acetylcholinesterase | ALC | Alternate level of care |
| ACOA | Adult child of an alcoholic | ALDH | Aldehyde dehydrogenase |
| ACT | Assertive Community Treatment; Adaptive Control of Thought; atropine coma therapy | ALI | American Law Institute |
| | | ALS | Amyotrophic lateral sclerosis |
| | | AMA | Against medical advice; American Medical Association |
| ACTH | Adrenocorticotropic hormone | AMPA | α-amino-3-hydroxy-5 methyl-isoxazole-propionic acid |
| AD | Alzheimer disease; average deviation; antidepressant | | |
| ADAP | Alzheimer disease–associated protein | AMPT | Alpha-methyl-paratyrosine |
| | | ANI | Asymptomatic neurocognitive impairment |
| ADC | AIDS dementia complex | | |
| ADD | Attention deficit disorder; Administration on Developmental Disabilities | ANS | Autonomic nervous system |
| | | AOA | Ataxia with oculomotor apraxia |
| | | AOD | Alcohol and other drugs (of abuse) |
| ADDH | Attention deficit disorder with hyperactivity | | |
| | | AP | Anterior-posterior; antipsychotic drug |
| ADE | Adverse drug event | | |
| ADH | Alcohol dehydrogenase | APA | American Psychiatric Association; American Psychological Association |
| ADHD | Attention deficit hyperactivity disorder | | |
| ADI | Attention Deviance Index | | |
| ADIS | Anxiety Disorders Interview Schedule | APD | Antisocial personality disorder |
| | | aPFC | Anterior prefrontal cortex |
| ADL | Activities of daily living | Apo E | Apolipoprotein E |
| ADNFLE | Autosomal dominant nocturnal frontal lobe epilepsy | APP | Amyloid precursor protein |
| | | AQ | Accomplishment Quotient |
| | | Aqp | Aquaporin(s) |
| ADR | Adverse drug reaction | ARBD | Alcohol-related birth defect(s) |
| ADT | Antidepressant therapy | | |

| | | | |
|---|---|---|---|
| ARC | Arcuate nucleus of hypothalamus; AIDS-related complex | BLA | Basolateral nucleus of the amygdala |
| ARCOS | Automation of [controlled drug] Reports and Consolidated Orders System | BLM | Bucco-lingual-masticatory syndrome |
| | | BLS | Buccal-lingual syndrome; Blessed Rating Scales |
| ARJP | Autosomal recessive juvenile-onset Parkinson disease | BMPs | Bone morphogenic proteins |
| ARMS | At-risk mental state | BNCT | Boron neutron capture therapy |
| ARN | Appetite-regulating network (of hypothalamus) | BOLD | Blood oxygenation level-dependent |
| ARP | Argyll Robertson pupil | BPD | Borderline personality disorder; bipolar depression; bipolar disorder |
| ART | Assisted reproductive technologies | | |
| ASC | Altered states of consciousness | BPRS | Brief Psychiatric Rating Scale |
| ASD | Acute stress disorder; autism spectrum disorder | BPSD | Behavioral and psychological symptoms of dementia |
| | | BSEP | Brain stem evoked potential |
| ASDC | Association of Sleep Disorders Centers | BSR | Brain stimulation reward |
| | | BST | Brief stimulus therapy |
| ASL | American Sign Language | BTP | Breakthrough pain |
| ASPD | Antisocial personality disorder | BVRT | Benton Visual Retention Test |
| AT | Ataxia telangiectasia | BWAM | Brain wave activity measurement |
| ATM | Ataxia-teleangiectasia mutated | BWS | Battered wife syndrome |
| ATC | Alcoholism Treatment Center | BZRA | Benzodiazepine receptor antagonist |
| ATP | Adenosine triphosphate | | |
| AVED | Ataxia with isolated vitamin E deficiency | | |
| AVP | Arginine vasopressin | C-L | Consultation-liaison |
| AVT | Arginine vasotocin | CA | Chronological age; catecholamine; cancer |
| AZT | Azidothymidine (zidovudine) | | |
| | | CAA | Cerebral amyloid angiopathy |
| BAC | Blood alcohol concentration | CAC | Chemical aversive conditioning; certified alcoholism counselor |
| BACE1 | β-secretase | | |
| BAL | Blood alcohol level; British anti-Lewisite | CADASIL | Cerebral autosomal dominant arteriopathy with subcortical infarcts and leukoencephalopathy |
| BANC | Blink alpha neurocircuit | | |
| BASK | Behavior-affect-sensation-knowledge | CAE | Childhood absence epilepsy |
| | | CAH | Congenital adrenal hyperplasia |
| BCAA | Branched chain amino acid(s) | CAM | Cell adhesion molecule; complementary and alternative medicine |
| BDD | Body dysmorphic disorder | | |
| BDHI | Buss-Durkee Hostility Inventory | | |
| BDI | Beck Depression Inventory | cAMP | Cyclic adenosine monophosphate |
| BDNF | Brain-derived neurotrophic factor | CARE | Comprehensive Assessment and Referral Evaluation |
| BEAM | Brain electrical activity mapping | CARE-HD | Coenzyme Q10 and ramacemide evaluation in Huntington disease |
| BED | Binge eating disorder | | |
| BEP | Brief and emergency psychotherapy | | |
| | | cART | Combination antiretroviral therapy |
| BET | Benign essential tremor | | |
| BFPP | Bilateral frontoparietal polymicrogyria | CASH | Comprehensive Assessment of Symptoms and History |
| BFT | Behavioral family therapy | CAT | Choline acetyltransferase; computed axial tomograph (CT preferred) |
| BHMCO | Behavioral health managed care organization | | |

| | | | |
|---|---|---|---|
| CAVD | Completion, arithmetic, vocabulary, direction-following (tests of intelligence) | CME | Continuing medical education |
| | | CMHC | Community mental health center |
| CBA | Cost/benefit analysis | CMMS | Columbia Mental Maturity Scale |
| CBD | Corticobasal degeneration | CMP | Chronic mental patient; competitive medical plan(s) |
| CBS | Charles Bonnet syndrome | | |
| CBT | Cognitive behavior therapy | CMS | Centers for Medicare and Medicaid Services (formerly, HCFA) |
| CBZ | Carbamazepine | | |
| CCC | Citrated calcium carbamide | | |
| CCI | Calcium channel inhibitor | CMT | Chronic motor tics; Charcot-Marie-Tooth disease |
| CCK | Cholecystokinin | | |
| CCRT | Core conflictual relationship theme | CMV | Cytomegalovirus |
| | | CNS | Central nervous system |
| CDC | Centers for Disease Control | CNV | Contingent negative variation |
| CDD | Childhood disintegrative disorder | CO | Community organization or organizer |
| CDT | Clock-drawing test | COMT | Catechol O-methyltransferase |
| CEA | Cost-effectiveness analysis | CoQ | Ubiquinone |
| CeA | Central amygdala | CPP | Conditioned place preference |
| CED | Cell death abnormal (gene) | CPR | Cardiopulmonary resuscitation |
| CEEG | Computerized electroencephalography | CPT | Continuous performance test |
| | | CR | Conditional response; critical ratio |
| CeL/C | Lateral and capsular division of CeA | | |
| CeM | Medial part of CeA | CREB | cAMP response element binding protein |
| CEOP | Chronic external ophthalmoplegia plus | | |
| | | CRF | Corticotropin-releasing factor |
| CERAD | Consortium to Establish a Registry for Alzheimer Disease | CRH | Corticotropin-releasing hormone |
| | | CS | Conditional stimulus; consciousness |
| c.e.s. | Central excitatory state | | |
| CET | Cognitive enhancement therapy; computer electroencephalographic topography; cerebral electrotherapy | CSA | Childhood sexual abuse |
| | | CSD | Cortical spreading depression; critical stimulus duration |
| | | CSM | Chronic symptomatic maladjustment (= neuroses) |
| | | CSR | Continued stay review |
| CFF | Critical flicker fusion | CT | Computed tomography; conduction time |
| CFI | Camberwell Family Interview | | |
| CFS | Chronic fatigue syndrome | CTS | Carpal tunnel syndrome |
| CGI | Clinical global impression | CVA | Cerebrovascular accident |
| cGMP | Cyclic guanosine monophosphate | CVAH | Congenital virilizing adrenal hyperplasia |
| CGRP | Calcitonin gene-related peptide | CVS | Chorionic villus sampling |
| CHAMPUS | Civilian Health and Medical Program, Uniformed Services | CWF | Cornell Word Form |
| | | CYP | Cytochrome P450 isoenzyme system |
| CIDS | CNS injury–induced immunodepression | | |
| CIND | Cognitive impairment, no dementia | DA | Dopamine |
| | | DAF | Delayed auditory feedback |
| CIP | Caudal intraparietal area | DAG | Diacylglycerol |
| CIT | Crisis intervention team | DAH | Disordered action of the heart |
| CJD | Creutzfeldt-Jacob disease | DALY | Disability adjusted life year |
| CLAMS | Clinical Linguistic and Auditory Milestone Scale | DAP | Draw a person test |
| | | DAT | Dementia of the Alzheimer type; dopamine transporter |
| cM | Centimorgan | | |

| | | | |
|---|---|---|---|
| DAWN | Drug Abuse Warning Network | DSA | Digital subtraction angiography |
| DBH | Dopamine-β-hydroxylase | DSD | Depressive spectrum disorder; depression sine depression |
| DBS | Deep brain stimulation | | |
| DBT | Dialectical behavior therapy | DSH | Deliberate self-harm |
| DC | Dichorionic | DSIP | Delta sleep-inducing peptide |
| DD | Depersonalization disorder; dissociative disorder(s) | DSM | Diagnostic and statistical manual (APA) |
| DDIS | Dissociative Disorders Interview Schedule | DSPS | Delayed sleep phase syndrome |
| | | DST | Dexamethasone suppression test |
| DLPFC | Dorsolateral prefrontal cortex | DTI | Diffusion tissue imaging |
| DEEG | Depth EEG | DTs | Delirium tremens |
| DER | Disulfiram ethanol reaction | DUI | Driving under the influence (of alcohol or other drugs) |
| DES | Dissociative Experiences Scale; diethylstilbesterol | | |
| | | DWI | Driving while intoxicated; diffusion-weighted imaging |
| DESNOS | Disorder of extreme stress not otherwise specified | DZ | Dizygotic |
| DFA | Discriminant function analysis | EAA | Excitatory amino acid(s) |
| DFP | Diisopropylphosphorofluoridate | EAP | Employee assistance program |
| DG | Diacylglycerol | EBA | Extrastriate body area |
| DHA | Docosahexaenoic acid | EBL | Emotional body language |
| DI | Deterioration Index | EBM | Evidence-based medicine |
| DIB | Diagnostic Interview for Borderlines | EBV | Epstein-Barr virus |
| | | EC | Entorhinal cortex |
| DID | Dissociative identity disorder | ECA | Epidemiologic Catchment Area survey |
| DIMS | Disorders of initiating and maintaining sleep | | |
| | | ECB | Executive control battery |
| DIS | Diagnostic Interview Schedule | ECM | Extracellular matrix; external chemical messenger |
| DIVA | Digital intravenous angiography | | |
| | | EcoG | Electrocorticogram |
| DLB | Dementia with Lewy bodies | ECS | Electroconvulsive shock |
| DLPFC | Dorsolateral prefrontal cortex | ECT | Electroconvulsive therapy |
| DM | Myotonic dystrophy | EDR | Electrodermal response |
| DMD | Duchenne dystrophy | EDS | Excessive daytime sleepiness |
| DMPEA | 3,4-dimethoxyphenethylamine (pink spot) | EE | Expressed emotions |
| | | EEG | Electroencephalogram |
| dMRI | Diffusion magnetic-resonance imaging | EFAs | Essential fatty acids |
| | | EHR | Electronic health record system |
| DMT | Dimethyltryptamine | EIA | Enzyme immunoassay |
| DNA | Deoxyribonucleic acid | EID | Emotional intensity disorder |
| DO | Directive-organic (orientation or therapist) | ELISA | Enzyme-linked immunosorbent assay |
| DOES | Disorders of excessive somnolence | EMB | Extreme male brain |
| | | EMR | Educable mentally retarded |
| DRG | Diagnosis-related group; dorsal root ganglion | EMS | Emergency medical service(s); eosinophilia-myalgia syndrome |
| DRI | Differential reinforcement of incompatible behavior | EOG | Electro-oculograph |
| | | EOS | Early-onset schizophrenia |
| DRL | Differential reinforcement of low-rate behavior | EP | Evoked potential |
| | | EPA | Eicosapentaenoic acid |
| DRO | Differential reinforcement of other behavior | EPI | Echo-planar imaging; Eysenck Personality Inventory; extrapyramidal involvement |
| DRPLA | Dentatorubral-pallidoluysian atrophy | | |
| DS | Down syndrome | EPO | Erythropoietin |

| | | | |
|---|---|---|---|
| EPS | Extrapyramidal side effects, symptoms, syndrome, or system | FMRP | Fragile X mental retardation protein |
| EPSDT | Early and periodic screening, diagnosis, and treatment | FPDD | Familial pure depressive disease |
| EPSE | Extrapyramidal side effects | FR | Fixed ratio |
| EPSP | Excitatory postsynaptic potential | FRDA | Freidreich ataxia |
| ER | Endoplasmic reticulum; emergency room | FRET | Fluorescence-resonance energy transfer |
| ERISA | Employee Retirement Income Security Act of 1974 (U. S.) | FSPTFL | Fronto-striato-pallido-thalamo-frontal loop |
| ERP | Event-related potential; Exposure and Response Prevention | FSTC | Frontal-striatal-thalamic-cortical circuitry |
| ERSP | Event-related slow potential | FTA-ABS | Fluorescent treponemal antibody absorption test |
| ES | Embryonic stem cell | FTD | Fronto-temporal dementia |
| ESL | English is [the subject's] second language | FTM | Female-to-male (transsexual) |
| ESN | Educationally subnormal | FXTAS | Fragile X–associated tremor/ataxia syndrome |
| ESP | Extrasensory perception | | |
| EST | Electroshock therapy | GABA | γ-aminobutyric acid |
| est | Erhard seminar training | GABA-T | Gamma-aminobutryic acid transaminase |
| ETD | Eye tracking dysfunction | GAD | Glutamic acid decarboxylase; generalized anxiety disorder |
| ETOH | Ethanol (alcohol) | | |
| ETS | Electrical transcranial stimulation | GAF | Global Assessment of Functioning |
| EUCD | Emotionally unstable character disorder | GAI | Guided affective imagery |
| EWS | Early warning signs | GAS | Global Assessment Scale; general adaptation syndrome |
| EXIT | Executive Interview | | |
| | | GBMI | Guilty but mentally ill |
| FAB | Frontal Assessment Battery | Gc | Crystallized intelligence |
| FACS | Facial Action Coding System; Fellow, American College of Surgeons | GCSE | Generalized convulsive status epilepticus |
| | | GDNF | Glial cell line-derived neurotrophic factor |
| FAD | Familial Alzheimer disease | GDP | Guanosine diphosphate |
| FADD | Fas-associated death domain protein | GDS | Global deterioration scale |
| | | GERD | Gastroesophageal reflux disease |
| FAP | Fixed action pattern | Gf | Fluid intelligence |
| FAS | Fetal alcohol syndrome | GGT | γ-glutamyltransferase |
| FASPS | Familial advanced sleep-phase syndrome | GGTP | γ-glutamyltranspeptidase |
| | | GH | Growth hormone |
| FAST | Functional assessment stages | GHB | Gamma-hydroxybutyric acid |
| FDA | Food and Drug Administration (U.S.) | GHRH | Growth hormone–releasing factor |
| FFA | Fusiform face area | GHB | γ-hydroxybutyrate |
| FFI | Fatal familial insomnia | GLS | Generalized lymphadenopathy syndrome; glycolipid storage disease |
| FGA | First-generation (conventional) antipsychotic. | | |
| FHM | Familial hemiplegic migraine | GnRH | Gonadotropin-releasing hormone |
| FHN | Family history negative | | |
| FHP | Family history positive | GPCR | G protein–coupled receptor |
| FHRDC | Family History Research Diagnostic Criteria | GPI | General paralysis of the insane |
| FI | Fixed interval; fiscal intermediary | GRF | Growth hormone–releasing factor |
| fMRI | Functional magnetic-resonance imaging | | |

| GSR | Galvanic skin response |
| GSS | Gerstmann-Straussler-Scheinker syndrome |
| GSW | Gunshot wound(s) |
| GTP | Guanosine triphosphate |
| GTS | Gilles de la Tourette syndrome |
| HAART | Highly Active AntiRetroviral Therapy |
| HACS | Hyperactive child syndrome |
| HAD | HIV-associated dementia |
| HAND | HIV-associated neurocognitive disorders |
| HBMIs | Hybrid brain–machine interfaces |
| HBS | Homicidal behavior survey |
| HCA | Heterocyclic antidepressant drug |
| HCFA | Health Care Financing Administration of DHHS (now, CMS) |
| HD | Huntington disease (Huntington chorea); Hodgkin disease; Hansen disease |
| HGP | Human genome project |
| HGPRT | Hypoxanthine-guanine phosphoribosyltransferase |
| HGPS | Hutchinson-Gilford progeria syndrome |
| HHHO | Hypotonia, hypomentia, hypogonadism, obesity syndrome |
| HI | Hyperglycemic index |
| HIAA | Hydroxyindoleacetic acid |
| HIF | Higher intellectual function |
| HIV | Human immunodeficiency virus |
| HMO | Health maintenance organization |
| HNPP | Hereditary neuropathy with liability to pressure palsies |
| HPA | Hypothalamic-pituitary-adrenal axis |
| HPD | Histrionic (hysterical) personality disorder |
| HPT | Hypothalamic-pituitary-thyroid (axis) |
| HR | High-risk (proband or group) |
| HRB | Halstead-Reitan Battery |
| HRQoL | Health-related quality of life |
| HSCL | Hopkins Symptom Check List |
| HSV | Herpes simplex virus |
| HTLV-III | Human T-cell leukemia virus, type III |
| HTP | House-Tree-Person test |
| HYPAC | Hypothalamic-pituitary-adrenal cortex |
| Hz | Hertz (one cycle per second) |
| 5-HT | 5-hydroxytryptamine (serotonin) |

| 5-HTP | 5-hydroxytryptophan |
| 5-HTTLPR | Serotonin transporter gene promoter |
| I-R | Individual-response (specificity) |
| IADL | Instrumental activities of daily living |
| IAP | Inhibitor of apoptosis |
| IB | Index of body build |
| IBTA | Individualized Behavior Therapy for Alcoholics |
| ICD | International Classification of Diseases (WHO) |
| ICE | Interleukin-$1\beta$ |
| ICHD-II | International Classification of Headache Disorders, 2nd edition (2004) |
| ICSI | Intracytoplasmic sperm injection |
| ICSS | Intracranial self-stimulation |
| IED | Intermittent explosive disorder |
| IEED | Involuntary emotional expression disorder |
| IHS | International Headache Society |
| IHT | Interhemispheric transfer |
| IMEPS | Involuntary movement and extrapyramidal side effects scale |
| IMHV | Intermediate part of the medial hyperstriatum ventrale |
| INCL | Infantile neuronal ceroid lipofuscinosis |
| IP3 | Inositol triphosphate |
| IPSP | Inhibitory postsynaptic potential |
| IPSS | International Pilot Study of Schizophrenia |
| IPT | Integrated Psychological Therapy |
| IQ | Intelligence Quotient |
| IRB | Institutional Review Board |
| IRM | Inherited releasing mechanism |
| IS | Ischemic scale; index of sexuality |
| ISD | Inhibited sexual desire |
| ISI | Interstimulus interval |
| ITP | Interpersonal psychotherapy |
| ITPA | Illinois Test of Psycholinguistic Abilities |
| IVDU | Intravenous drug user |
| IVF | In vitro fertilization |
| IPV | Intimate partner violence |
| JCAHO | Joint Commission on the Accreditation of Healthcare Organizations |
| JND | Just noticeable difference |

| | | | |
|---|---|---|---|
| KIPS | Knowledge information processing systems | MCE | Medical Care Evaluation |
| KS | Kaposi sarcoma | MCH | Melanin-concentrating hormone |
| KSS | Kearns-Sayre syndrome | MCI | Mild cognitive impairment |
| | | MCMI | Millon Clinical Multiaxial Inventory |
| LA | Lateral nucleus of amygdala | MCR | Mother–child relationship |
| LAd | Dorsal subdivision of amygdala | MCS | Minimally conscious state; multiple chemical sensitivity |
| LAAM | Levo-α-acetylmethadol | | |
| LAS | Lymphadenopathy syndrome | MD | Mean deviation |
| LBD | Lewy body dementia | MDA | Methylenedioxyamphetamine |
| LD | Learning disabilities | MDD | Major depressive disorder |
| LHON | Leber hereditary optic neuropathy | MDI | Manic-depressive illness; major depressive illness |
| LI | Latent inhibition | MDMA | Methylenedioxymeth-amphetamine |
| LID | Levodopa-induced dyskinesia | | |
| LIP | Lateral intraparietal area | ME | Myalgic encephalitis |
| LIPS | Logical inferences per second | MEG | Magnetoencephalography |
| L-K | Linguistic-kinesic | MELAS | Mitochondrial myopathy, encephalopathy, lactic acidosis, strokelike episodes |
| LLI | Language-based learning impairment | | |
| LLP | Late-life psychosis | MERRF | Myoclonus epilepsy and ragged red fiber disease |
| LLPDD | Late luteal phase dysphoric disorder | MF | Multifactoral (model of inheritance) |
| LMT | Lowenfeld Mosaic Test | | |
| LNNB | Luria-Nebraska Neuropsychological Battery | MFB | Medial forebrain bundle |
| | | Mgm/PIN | Medial geniculate nucleus and adjacent thalamic posterior intralaminar nucleus |
| LOD | Logarithm of the odds (score) | | |
| LOS | Length of stay; late-onset schizophrenia | MHAOD | Mental health, alcohol, and other drugs |
| LP | Lumbar puncture | | |
| LPU | Least publishable unit | MHC | Major histocompatibility complex |
| LPW | Late positive wave | | |
| LQTS | Long QT syndrome | MHP | Mental health professional |
| LSD | Lysergic acid diethylamide; lysosomal storage disorder(s) | MHPG | 3-methoxy-4-hydroxyphenylglycol |
| LTB | Life-threatening behavior | MICA | Mentally ill chemical abuser |
| LTM | Long-term memory | MID | Multi-infarct dementia |
| LTP | Long-term potentiation | MIP | Medial intraparietal area |
| LVA | Low-voltage alpha brain wave | MIS | Medical Improvement Standard |
| | | MITN | Midline and intralaminar thalamic nuclei |
| MA | Mental age | | |
| MAC | Maximum allowable cost | MLD | Metachromatic leukodystrophy |
| MAG | Myelin-associated glycoprotein | MM | Moderation management |
| MAI | Mycobacterium avium intracellulare | MMC | Maternally inherited myopathy and cardiomyopathy |
| MAO-A | Monoamine oxidase A gene | MMECT | Multiple monitored electroconvulsive therapy |
| MAOI | Monoamine oxidase inhibitor | | |
| MAP | Microtubule-associated protein; member assistance program | MMPI | Minnesota Multiphasic Personality Inventory |
| MBD | Minimal brain dysfunction | MMSE | Mini-Mental State Examination |
| MC | Monochorionic | MMT | Multimodal therapy |
| MCAT | Medical College Admission Test | MMWR | Morbidity and Mortality Weekly Report (of the Centers for Disease Control) |
| MCDD | Multiple complex developmental disorder | | |

| | | | | |
|---|---|---|---|---|
| MN | Metanephrine | | NCA | Neurocirculatory asthenia; |
| MND | Mild neurocognitive disorder | | | National Council on Alcoholism |
| MOH | Medication overuse headache | | NCAM | Neural cellular adhesion |
| MPA | Minor physical anomaly; | | | molecule |
| | medroxyprogesterone acetate | | NCSE | Nonconvulsive status epilepticus |
| MPD | Multiple personality disorder; | | NDATUS | National Drug and Alcoholism |
| | myofascial pain dysfunction | | | Treatment Utilization Survey |
| MPH | Methylphenidate | | NDPH | New daily persistent headache |
| MPI | Maudsley Personality Inventory | | NDU | Nondominant unilateral (ECT) |
| MPPS | Massive parallel processing | | NE | Norepinephrine |
| | system | | NES | Night-eating syndrome; |
| MPTP | 1-methyl-4-phenyl-1,2,3, | | | nonepileptic seizures |
| | 6-tetrahydropyridine | | NFD | Neurofibrillary degeneration |
| MRI | Magnetic resonance imaging | | NFT | Neurofibrillary tangle(s) |
| MRS | Magnetic resonance spectroscopy | | NFTT | Nonorganic failure to thrive |
| MS | Multiple sclerosis | | NGF | Nerve growth factor |
| MSE | Mental status examination | | NGI, NGRI | Not guilty by reason of insanity |
| MSER | Mental Status Examination | | NGIC | Neurotransmitter-gated ion |
| | Report | | | channel |
| MSI | Magnetic source imaging | | NIAAA | National Institute on Alcohol |
| MSIS | Multi-State Information System | | | Abuse and Alcoholism |
| MSLT | Multiple sleep latency test | | NIC | Neuroleptic-induced catatonia |
| MSM | Men who have sex with men | | NIDS | Neuroleptic-induced deficit |
| msMRI | Magnetic-source magnetic- | | | syndrome |
| | resonance imaging | | NIH | National Institutes of Health |
| MSRPP | Multidimensional Scale for | | NIMD | Neuroleptic-induced movement |
| | Rating Psychiatric Patients (Lorr | | | disorder(s) |
| | scale) | | NIMH | National Institute of Mental |
| MST | Magnetic seizure therapy | | | Health |
| MSUD | Maple syrup urine disease | | NIP | Neuroleptic-induced |
| MSW | Master's degree in social work; | | | parkinsonism |
| | male sex worker | | NMDA | N-methyl-d-aspartate |
| mtDNA | Mitrochondrial DNA | | NLNC | Native language neural |
| MTF | Male-to-female (transsexual) | | | commitment |
| MTL | Medial temporal lobe | | NMN | Normetanephrine |
| MVP | Mitral valve prolapse | | NMR | Nuclear magnetic resonance |
| MZ | Monozygote, monozygotic | | | (imaging) |
| MZA | Monozygotic twins reared apart | | NMRS | Nuclear magnetic resonance |
| MZT | Monozygotic twins reared | | | spectroscopy |
| | together | | NMS | Neuroleptic malignant syndrome |
| | | | NO | Nitric oxide |
| N | Nerve (cranial) | | NPD | Narcissistic personality disorder |
| n | Number of subjects, size of | | NPH | Normal pressure hydrocephalus |
| | sample | | NPI | Neuropsychiatric Inventory |
| nAChR | Nicotinic acetylcholine receptor | | NPT | Nocturnal penile tumescence |
| NADH | Nicotinamide adenine | | NPY | Neuropeptide Y |
| | dinucleotide | | NREM | Non-rapid eye movement (sleep) |
| NAMH | National Association for Mental | | NRH | NMDA receptor hypofunction |
| | Health | | NRIs | Norepinephrine reuptake |
| NARP | Maternally inherited neurogenic | | | inhibitors |
| | muscle weakness, ataxia, and | | NRTs | Nicotine replacement therapies |
| | retinitis pigmentosa | | NS-XLMR | Nonsyndromic X-linked mental |
| NBIA | Neurodegeneration with brain | | | retardation |
| | iron accumulation | | NTD | Neural tube defect |

| | | | | |
|---|---|---|---|---|
| NTF | Neurotrophic factor(s) | | PCM | Patient care manager |
| NTR | Negative therapeutic reaction | | PCP | Phencyclidine; primary care physician; Pneumocystis carinii pneumonia |
| NT-3 | Neurotrophin-3 | | | |
| OAEs | Otoacoustic emissions | | pcpt | Perception |
| OAS | Overt aggression scale | | PCR | Polymerase chain reaction |
| OBE | Out-of-the-body experience | | PCSTF | Problem-centered Systems Therapy of the Family |
| OBOT | Office-based opioid agonist treatment | | PD | Parkinson disease; panic disorder; personality disorder; Paget disease |
| OBS | Organic brain syndrome; obstetrics; obsolete | | | |
| OCD | Obsessive-compulsive disorder | | PDA | Prescription drug abuse |
| OD | Overdose; every day; right eye | | PDD | Primary degenerative dementia; premenstrual dysphoric disorder; pervasive developmental disorder |
| OFC | Orbitofrontal cortex | | | |
| OFD | Orofacial dyskinesia; oro-facial-digital syndrome | | | |
| OGOD | One gene, one disorder | | PDE | Phosphodiester(s); Personality Disorder Examination |
| OH | Orthostatic hypotension | | PDI | Primary depressive illness |
| OI | Opportunistic infection | | PDP | Parallel distributed processing |
| OIT | Organic Integrity Test | | PE | Pneumoencephalogram; physical examination |
| OMPFC | Orbital and medial frontal cortex | | | |
| OR | Orienting response; operations research; operating room | | PEA-BD | Prepubertal and early adolescent onset bipolar disorder |
| OS | Left eye | | PEAQ | Personal Experience and Attitude Questionnaire |
| OT | Occupational therapy | | | |
| OXPHOS | Oxidative phosphorylation | | PEDF | Pigment epithelium-derived factor |
| PA | Physician's assistant; public affairs; psychoanalysis | | PER | Periodic Evaluation Record |
| PAC | Professional advisory committee; political action committee | | PERI | Psychiatric Epidemiology Research Interview |
| PACAP | Pituitary adenylyl cyclase activating protein | | PES | Psychiatric emergency service |
| | | | PET | Position emission tomography |
| PACE | Personal Assistance in Community Existence | | PFC | Prefrontal association cortex |
| | | | PGD | Preimplantation genetic diagnosis |
| PAD | Primary affect disorder | | PGR | Psychogalvanic reflex |
| PAF | Pure autonomic failure | | PHF | Paired helical filaments (of the neurofibrillary tangle) |
| PAG | Periaqueductal gray area | | | |
| PAH | Phenylalanine hydroxylase | | PHS | Public Health Service (U.S.) |
| PANDAS | Pediatric autoimmune neuropsychiatric disorders associated with streptococcal infection | | pHVA | Plasma homovanillic acid |
| | | | PI | Paradoxical intention; present illness |
| | | | PIP | Psychosis, intermittent hyponatremia, and polydipsia syndrome |
| PANSS | Positive and Negative Syndrome Scale | | | |
| PARs | Protease-activated receptors | | PKC | Protein kinase C |
| PAS | Physical Anhedonia Scale; parental alienation syndrome | | PKU | Phenylketonuria |
| | | | PMA | Primary mental abilities |
| PBC | Pregnancy and birth complication(s) | | PMDD | Premenstrual dysphoric disorder |
| | | | PME | Phosphomonoester(s) |
| PBD | Pediatric bipolar disorder | | PMG | Polymicrogyria |
| PBN | N-tert-butyl-α-phenyl nitrone | | PMI | Patient medication instructions |
| PCA | Principal components analysis | | PML | Progressive multifocal leukoencephalopathy |
| PCD | Programmed cell death | | | |

| | | | | |
|---|---|---|---|---|
| PMS | Premenstrual syndrome | | RAP | Rapid auditory processing |
| PNDs | Paraneoplastic neurological disorders | | RAS | Reticular activating system |
| | | | RBD | REM behavior disorder |
| PO | Postoperative; by mouth | | rCBF | Regional cerebral blood flow |
| POMC | Pro-opiomelanocortin | | RCT | Randomized controlled trial; randomized clinical trial; registered care technologist |
| POMR | Problem-oriented medical record | | | |
| POMS | Profile of Mood States | | RCZ | Rostral cingulate zone of posterior medial frontal cortex |
| POR | Problem-oriented record | | | |
| POSM | Patient-operated selected mechanism(s) | | RDC | Research diagnostic criteria |
| | | | REM | Rapid eye movement (sleep) |
| POW | Prisoner of war (syndrome) | | REST | Regressive electroshock therapy |
| PPA | Parahippocampal place area; preferred provider arrangements | | | |
| | | | RET | Rational emotive therapy |
| PPC | Patient placement criteria | | RFLP | Restriction fragment length polymorphism |
| PPI | Prepulse inhibition | | | |
| PPO | Preferred provider organization | | RI | Recombinant inbred (strain) |
| PrL | Prolactin | | RLS | Restless legs syndrome |
| PRP | Prion protein; program for relapse prevention | | RMT | Recovered memory therapy |
| | | | RNA | Ribonucleic acid |
| PRRs | Pattern recognition receptors | | RNAi | Ribonucleic acid interference |
| PSA | Proportion of survivors affected | | ROS | Reactive oxygen species |
| PSD | Postsynaptic density | | RS | Reiter syndrome; Rett syndrome; Reye syndrome |
| PSE | Present State Examination | | | |
| PSG | Polysomnography | | RSB | REM sleep behavior disorder(s) |
| PSM | Professional sexual misconduct; polysomnogram | | RSBT | Rhythmic sensory bombardment therapy |
| | | | | |
| PSN | Predominantly sensory neuropathy | | RT | Reaction time; recreation(al) therapy |
| | | | | |
| PSRO | Professional Standards Review Organization | | rTMS | Repetitive (rapid rate) transcranial magnetic stimulation |
| | | | | |
| PST | Prefrontal sonic treatment | | RUDAS | Rowland Universal Dementia Assessment Scale |
| PT | Planum temporale; physical therapy; Personal Therapy; physiotherapy; patient; part-time | | | |
| | | | S | Subject; stimulus |
| PTA | Post-traumatic amnesia; parent-teacher association | | SAD | Seasonal affective disorder; separation anxiety disorder; social anxiety disorder; schizoaffective disorder |
| PTPD | Post-traumatic personality disorder | | | |
| | | | | |
| PTSD | Post-traumatic stress disorder | | SADS-L | Schedule for Affective Disorders and Schizophrenia, Lifetime Version |
| PVN | Paraventricular nucleus of hypothalamus | | | |
| | | | SAF | Scrapie-associated fibril |
| PVS | Permanent vegetative state; persistent vegetative state | | SAH | Subarachnoid hemorrhage |
| | | | SAHS | Sleep apnea hypersomnolence syndrome |
| QA | Quality assurance | | | |
| QALY | Quality-adjusted life year | | SANS | Scale for the Assessment of Negative Symptoms |
| QB | Quantitative Electrophysiological Battery | | | |
| | | | SAPS | Scale for the Assessment of Positive Symptoms |
| QD | Daily | | | |
| QI | Quality improvement | | SBMA | Spinal and bulbar muscular atrophy |
| QID | Four times a day | | | |
| QNS | Quantity not sufficient | | SCAs | Spinocerebellar ataxias |
| QTL | Quantitative trait loci | | SCI | Spinal cord injury |

| | |
|---|---|
| SCID | Structured Clinical Interview for DSM-III |
| SCID-D | Structural Clinical Interview for DSM-III-R Dissociative Disorders |
| SCL | Skin conductance level |
| SCN | Suprachiasmatic nucleus of the anterior hypothalamus |
| SCOPE | Systematic, complete, objective, practical, and empirical set of diagnostic procedures |
| SCOR | Skin conductance orienting response |
| SCR | Skin conductance response |
| SDA | Serotonin-dopamine antagonist |
| SDAT | Senile dementia, Alzheimer type |
| SDD | Sporadic depressive disease |
| SDL/R | State-dependent learning and retrieval |
| SE | Spongiform encephalopathy |
| SEC | Structured event complex |
| SEG | Sonoencephalogram |
| SES | Socioeconomic status |
| SET | Self-instructional training |
| SHG | Self-help group(s) |
| SGA | Second-generation (atypical) antipsychotic. |
| SIADH | Secretion, inappropriate, of antidiuretic hormone |
| SIB | Self-injurious behavior; Schedule for Interviewing Borderline |
| SIDP | Structured Interview for DSM-III Personality Disorders |
| SIP | Special internal predisposition |
| SIS | Structured Interview for Schizotypy |
| SIV | Simian immunodeficiency virus |
| SIVD | Subcortical ischemic vascular disease |
| SLI | Specific language impairment |
| SMA | Supplementary motor area; sequential multichannel autoanalyzer |
| SMI | Severe mental illness |
| SML | Single major locus (model of inheritance) |
| SMR | Sensory motor rhythm |
| Snc | Substantia nigra pars compacta |
| SNE | Subacute necrotizing encephalomyelopathy |
| SNF | Skilled nursing facility |
| SNP | Single nucleotide polymorphism |
| Snr | Substantia nigra pars reticulata |

| | |
|---|---|
| SNRIs | Selective norepinephrine reuptake inhibitors |
| SNV | Selective neuronal vulnerability |
| SOA | Span of apprehension |
| SOD | Sexual orientation disturbance; superoxide dismutase |
| SPD | Schizotypal personality disorder |
| SPECT | Single photo emission computed tomography |
| SPEM | Smooth pursuit eye movements |
| SQUIDS | Superconducting quantum interference devices |
| SRIF | Somatotropin-release-inhibiting factor |
| SRO | Single-room occupancy |
| SRY | Sex-determining region of Y chromosome |
| SSLP | Simple sequence length polymorphism |
| SSPE | Subacute sclerosing panencephalitis |
| SSRI | Selective serotonin reuptake inhibitor |
| SSSM | Standard Social Science Model |
| SST | Social skills training; Self-Statement Training |
| STAPP | Short-term anxiety-provoking psychotherapy |
| STD | Sexually transmitted disease |
| STEPPS | Systems Training for Emotional Predictability and Problem Solving |
| STG | Superior temporal gyrus |
| STH | Somatotrophic hormone |
| STIs | Structured treatment interruptions |
| STM | Short-term memory |
| STN | Subthalamic nucleus |
| STR | Scientific-technical revolution |
| STS | Superior temporal sulcus |
| SUMO | Small ubiquitin-like modifier |
| SUNCT | Short-lasting unilateral neuralgiform headache attacks with conjunctival injection and tearing |
| SVD | Small-vessel disease |
| SWS | Slow-wave sleep |
| | |
| $T_4$ | Thyroxine |
| TA | Transactional analysis |
| TANs | Tonically active neurons |
| TAT | Thematic Apperception Test |
| TAU | Treatment as usual |
| TBI | Traumatic brain injury |

| | |
|---|---|
| TC | Therapeutic community |
| TCA | Tricyclic antidepressants |
| TCO | Threat-control-override |
| TD | Tardive dyskinesia |
| TEFRA | Tax Equity and Fiscal Responsibility Act (U.S.) |
| TEM | Treatment-emergent mania |
| THC | Tetrahydrocannabinol |
| TGA | Transient global amnesia |
| TGN | Trans-Golgi network |
| TIA | Transient ischemic attack |
| TID | Three times a day |
| TLE | Temporal lobe epilepsy |
| TLP | Time-limited psychotherapy |
| TM | Transcendental meditation |
| TME | Transmissible mink encephalopathy |
| TMJ | Temporomandibular joint syndrome |
| TMS | Transcranial magnetic stimulation |
| TNF | Tumor necrosis factor |
| ToM, TOM | Theory of mind (ToM preferred) |
| TOP | Temporal, occipital, parietal lobes association areas |
| TOTE | Test - Operate - Test - Exit |
| TPE | Therapeutic plasma exchange |
| TPI | Treponema pallidum immobilization test |
| TPN | Total parenteral nutrition |
| TRADD | TNF-associated death domain protein |
| TRD | Treatment-resistant depression |
| TRH | Thyrotropin-releasing hormone |
| TRHST | Thyrotropin-releasing hormone stimulation test |
| T3RU | T3 resin uptake |
| TS | (Gilles de la) Tourette syndrome; Turner syndrome; Tay-Sachs (disease) |
| TSD | Tay-Sachs disease |
| TSEs | Transmissible spongiform encephalopathies |
| TSF | Tyramine sensitivity factor |
| TSH | Thyroid-stimulating hormone |
| TTR | Type token ratio |
| TVD | Transmissible virus dementia |
| TTH | Tension-type headache |
| UAI | Unprotected anal intercourse |
| Ucs | Unconscious |
| UDD | Uniform determination of death |
| UFC | Urinary free cortisol |

| | |
|---|---|
| ULND | Unilateral nondominant (ECT) |
| UPS | Ubiquitin-proteasome system |
| UR | Utilization review |
| VaD | Vascular dementia |
| VBR | Ventricle-to-brain ratio |
| VCI | Vascular cognitive impairment |
| vCJD | Variant Creutzfeldt-Jacob disease |
| VDRL | Venereal Disease Research Laboratory test |
| VDT | Visual distortion test |
| VE | Virtual environment |
| VEOS | Very early onset schizophrenia |
| VEP | Visual evoked potential |
| VI | Variable interval |
| VIP | Vasoactive intestinal peptide; very important person |
| VLOS | Very late onset schizophrenia |
| VLPO | Ventrolateral preoptic areas |
| VLSIC | Very large scale integrated circuit(s) |
| VMA | 3-methoxy-4-hydroxymandelic acid |
| VMN | Ventromedial nucleus of hypothalamus |
| VNS | Vagus nerve stimulator; Visiting Nurse Service |
| VR | Variable ratio |
| VSDI | Voltage-sensitive dye imaging |
| VSNs | Vomeronasal sensory neurons |
| VTA | Ventral tegmental area of midbrain |
| WAIS | Wechsler Adult Intelligence Scale |
| WAIS-R | Wechsler Adult Intelligence Scale, Revised |
| WB | Western blot |
| WBS | Williams-Beuren syndrome |
| WCST | Wisconsin Card Sort Test |
| WFMH | World Federation for Mental Health |
| WHO | World Health Organization |
| WISC | Wechsler Intelligence Scale for Children; Wisconsin Card Sort Test (WCST preferred) |
| WMS | Wechsler memory subtest |
| WPA | World Psychiatric Association |
| WS | Werner syndrome |
| WSW | Women who have sex with women |
| YAVIS | Young, attractive, verbal, intelligent, and successful |

# Campbell's Psychiatric Dictionary

# A

**A type behavior**   See *type A.*

**A68**   A filament protein that is immunoreactive to ALZ-50, a monoclonal antibody to the homogenates of ventral forebrain from patients with Alzheimer disease. The A68 protein/antigen is not found in Guam-Parkinson dementia, dementia associated with Parkinson disease, Pick disease, or in neurologically normal controls. A68 is one of three ALZ-50 immunoreactive elements of *ADAP* (q.v.). See *tau.*

**A-71623**   A cholecystokinin (CCK) tetrapeptide with an affinity for CCK-A receptors that is more than 1000 times as strong as that of CCK; it demonstrates anorectic activity.

**AA**   Abbreviation for (1) *achievement age* (q.v.); (2) *Alcoholics Anonymous* (q.v.).

**AADD**   Adult attention deficit disorder. See *adult ADHD.*

**AAMI**   Age-associated memory impairment; *benign senescent forgetfulness*; considered to be a normal part of aging and not a sign of developing dementia.

**AAS**   *Anabolic-androgenic steroids* (q.v.).

**AAT**   *Animal assisted therapy* (q.v.); altered attention traits, seen in *attention deficit hyperactivity disorder* (q.v.).

**Aβ**   *β-amyloid peptide* (q.v.). See *amyloid.*

**Aβ immunotherapy**   Passive anti-β-amyloid peptide immunotherapy used experimentally in *Alzheimer disease* (q.v.) to reduce levels of Aβ, prevent and clear amyloid plaques, and improve cognitive behavior. Trials of the treatment were halted because of neuroinflammatory complications. It has been suggested that passive Aβ immunization increases the risk of cerebral hemorrhage by further weakening the wall of the amyloidotic vessel.

**Abadie sign**   (Jean Marie Abadie, French ophthalmologist, 1842–1932) An early sign in *tabes* (q.v.) in which there is loss of deep pain from pressure on the testes or Achilles tendon.

**abandonment**   Discontinuation of treatment by the physician before he has been dismissed by the patient, obtained the consent of the patient to withdraw, or furnished another doctor to continue treatment.

**abandonment depression**   A form of *dysphoric separation anxiety*, provoked by any movement toward separation or individuation; it includes a more primitive component related to the primal experience of impending loss of the *maternal stimulus barrier* against endopsychic and external stimulation. See *abandonment neurosis; depressive position; separation anxiety.*

Abandonment depression is particularly evident in borderline personality disorder and, to a somewhat lesser extent, in narcissistic personality disorder. It leads to self-defeating and self-destructive behavior (sometimes termed a lifelong *failure script*), and to feelings of emptiness of self and meaninglessness of the outside world (estrangement). See *borderline personality; borderline psychosis; empathic failure; personality disorders.*

**abandonment neurosis**   Crippling dependence on the idealized other, who is viewed as omnipotent, with the ability to create or abolish insecurity and helplessness. In therapy it is expressed in an idealizing self–object transference (Kohut) with the goal of sharing in the power and omnipotence of the therapist. One form of abandonment neurosis is *abandonment depression* (q.v.).

**abasia**   Inability to walk. See *astasia-abasia.*

**abderite**   *Obs.* Stupid person. Abdera was a town in Thrace, the birthplace of Democritus; its inhabitants were said to be more stupid than other people.

**abdominal reflex**   The upper (epigastric) and lower abdominal reflexes are superficial skin reflexes tested by stroking the skin of the abdomen. The abdominal muscles beneath the area stroked contract, and the umbilicus usually moves in the direction of the area stroked. The upper abdominal reflexes depend on $T_{7-10}$, the lower on $T_{10-12}$.

**abducens nerve**   The sixth cranial nerve. It arises in the lower portion of the pons and supplies the external rectus muscle of the eye. For symptoms of lesions of the abducens nerve, see *oculomotor nerve.*

**abecarnil**   A ligand for BZD receptors with anxiolytic and anticonvulsant action.

**ABEPP** American Board of Examiners in Professional Psychology.

**Aberdeen system** Day industrial feeding schools, used in the 19th century and associated with a social movement, spearheaded by Sheriff Watson, that gave priority to family ties, emphasized the rights of children, and advocated a day care system (rather than residential placement) to meet the needs of the whole child in his or her family and community setting.

**aberration, mental** Any deviation from normal thinking or behavior; the term ordinarily does not relate to deviations in intelligence, and it often implies a temporary condition.

**abetaliproteinemia** See *ABL*; *neuroacanthocytosis*.

**abient** See *avoidant*.

**abilities, primary mental** See *PMA test*.

**ability** Power to perform, whether physical, mental, moral, or legal, with the connotation that the act can be performed now, without further education or training. Aptitude refers to the level of competence to which a person can be brought by a specified level of training.

**ability, volitional** See *volition*.

**ability test** Any evaluation of presently existing potentiality or capacity to function; a test of maximal or optimal performance in any area.

**abiotrophy** Premature loss of vitality of cells or tissues. The concept of abiotrophy was used by Gowers as a possible explanation of dementia: precocious aging of the central nervous system was due to limited viability of the nerve cells concerned.

**ABL** Amyloid-beta-lipoproteinemia, characterized by lack of plasma lipoproteins containing apoB, fat malabsorption, acanthocytosis, pigmentary retinal degeneration, and progressive neurological disease with demyelination of the posterior columns and spinocerebellar tracts. ABL is due to a mutation of the microsomal triglyceride transfer protein (MTP), which prevents hepatic assembly and secretion of very-low-density lipoproteins, thereby impairing peripheral delivery of vitamin E and other fat-soluble substrates. *AVED* (q.v.) and ABL are believed to share a pathogenic mechanism of neurodegeneration that is linked to profound impairment of the antioxidant activity of vitamin E in both central and peripheral nervous systems.

**ablation** Removal or interruption of function of a bodily part or organ, especially by surgical means. See *prefrontal lobotomy*.

**ablemo-** Combining form meaning feeble, weak, less than normal, inadequate.

**ablutomania** Compulsion to wash or bathe, or incessant preoccupation with thoughts of washing or bathing; seen in *obsessive-compulsive disorder* (q.v.).

**abnormal psychology** That division of psychology devoted to the study of mental disorders and psychopathology.

**abnormality** Variant, disorder, *disease* (q.v.); any state or condition that is outside the usual statistical range. There has been a tendency in medicine to define a normal range for trait $x$ and thereby to have discovered two new diseases—hyper-$x$ and hypo-$x$.

**aboiement** *Obs.* Involuntary production of abnormal sounds, such as animalistic cries or grunts. See *Gilles de la Tourette syndrome*.

**aboriginal need** See *adaptational psychodynamics*.

**abortion, therapeutic** Interruption of pregnancy for medical reasons.

**aboulia** *Abulia* (q.v.).

**above and below** The Adlerian concept of man as above and woman as below, femininity being a position of inferiority to be avoided while masculinity is a goal of superiority to be attained.

**ABPN** American Board of Psychiatry and Neurology, Inc., established in 1934 as the official agency to examine and certify physicians as specialists (*diplomates*) in psychiatry, child psychiatry, neurology, neurology with special competence in child neurology, clinical neurophysiology, addiction psychiatry, and geriatric psychiatry. ABPN offered the first certification examination in psychosomatic medicine in 2005.

**Abraham, Karl** (1877–1925) First psychoanalyst in Germany; manic-depressive psychosis, pregenital stages, character types, symbolism.

**abreaction** The process of bringing to consciousness, and thus to adequate expression, material that has been unconscious (usually because of repression). Abreaction includes not only the recollection of forgotten memories and experiences but also reliving them with appropriate emotional display and discharge of affect. The method used to bring the repressed material into consciousness is called *catharsis* (q.v.); abreaction refers to the end result. *Abreaction of emotion* refers to the discharge of emotion in the course of psychotherapy.

**abreaction, motor** The living-out of an unconscious impulse through muscular or motor expression.

**abreactive drug** Any of the preparations, usually barbiturates, used in narcocatharsis. See *narcotherapy.*

**abscess, brain** *Purulent encephalitis; encephalopyosis;* an inflammation due to the invasion of pyogenic microorganisms resulting in a circumscribed collection of pus in any part of the brain.

**absence** 1. Loss of consciousness in a hysterical attack. 2. Petit mal. See *epilepsy.*

**absent state** The vacant, transfixed, dreamlike state characteristic of the patient with a temporal lobe seizure. Also characteristic of such seizures are hallucinations of smell or taste (the *uncinate fit,* q.v.), a feeling of dreamlike detachment, and the experience of panoramic memory, in which the patient may feel that he or she is rapidly reenacting long periods of his life. See *epilepsy; temporal lobe syndromes.*

**absentmindedness** Habitual inattention; a tendency to be occupied with one's own thoughts to such degree that inadequate attention is given to events that occur in external reality; consequently, memory may seem to be faulty, especially for routine and relatively insignificant happenings.

**absolute alcohol** *Ethyl alcohol* (q.v.) whose water content does not exceed one percent.

**absolute resistance** See *treatment resistance.*

**absorbed mania** Manic stupor. See *mania.*

**absorption** 1. Engrossment with one object or idea with inattention to others.

2. The extent to which an administered drug reaches the general circulation; also known as *bioavailability.*

**abstinence** Self-denial; forgoing the indulgence of one's appetite, craving, or desire. In the case of *alcoholism* and *addiction* (qq.v.), abstinence refers to the habitual cessation of and continuing avoidance of use of the psychoactive substance.

1. In relation to alcohol, abstinence generally means total abstention; *temperance* generally indicates moderate or controlled drinking. The phrase *temperance movement,* however, classically referred to a personal commitment to total abstinence as well as adherence to a national policy of prohibition of alcohol use.

More recently, temperance movement has come to refer to advocacy of a more consistent national policy favoring greater control over alcohol availability and consumption. Sobriety refers to maintenance of total abstinence from alcohol or other psychoactive substances; current abstainer is typically defined in population and follow-up surveys as a former user of alcohol who has maintained sobriety for the preceding 12 months.

2. In psychoanalytic therapy, the *rule of abstinence* does not refer to enjoining the patient to abstain from gratifications outside the treatment situation, so long as they are not harmful. Rather, it is the rule not to gratify the patient deliberately during the treatment process unless it is done for a very specific purpose—no matter how much the patient may plead for gratification. To break the rule is a *boundary violation* (q.v.) on the part of the therapist.

**abstinence, conditioned** See *withdrawal, conditioned.*

**abstinence delirium** The state of delirium, usually *delirium tremens* (q.v.), that follows the immediate withdrawal of alcohol from an alcoholic person. The syndrome may be observed in many forms of drug addiction.

**abstinence syndrome** *Withdrawal syndrome* (q.v.).

**abstinence-based methods** In the treatment of addictions, interventions whose goal is to eliminate the use of all alcohol and drugs of abuse. The methods typically include cognitive behavior therapy in group and individual settings and 12-step recovery programs, such as Alcoholics Anonymous and Narcotics Anonymous. See *relapse prevention.*

**abstract attitude** *Categorical attitude.* Goldstein noted that one characteristic of the patient with an *organic mental disorder* is a relative inability to assume the abstract attitude or to shift readily from the abstract to the *concrete* (where thinking is determined by and cannot proceed beyond some immediate experience) or vice versa. The *abstract* attitude includes the following abilities: assuming a mental set voluntarily; shifting voluntarily from one aspect of a situation to another; keeping in mind simultaneously various aspects of a situation; grasping the essentials of a whole, breaking the whole into its parts, and isolating these voluntarily; abstracting common properties; planning ahead ideationally; assuming an attitude to the merely possible; thinking or performing symbolically; and detaching the ego from the outer world. See *frontal lobe; organic syndrome.*

**abstract perceptions**    See *blank hallucination.*

**abstract thinking**    See *physiognomonic thinking.*

**abstracting disabilities**    Difficulties in organizing and understanding the inputs once information has been recorded in the brain.

**abstraction**    "The drawing out or isolation of a content (e.g., a meaning or general character, etc.) from a connection, containing other elements, whose combination as a totality is something unique or individual, and therefore inaccessible to comparison" (Jung, C. G. Psychological *Types*, 1923). Abstraction is an activity that belongs to psychological functions in general, and Jung differentiated between abstracting thinking, abstracting feeling, abstracting sensation, and abstracting intuition.

**abstractionism, systematic**    See *semantic dissociation.*

**abstractions, selective**    See *cognitive therapy.*

**absurdity**    In psychoanalysis, anything that is contradictory or incoherent or meaningless in a train of thought or a constellation of ideas.

**abulia**    Absence of willpower or wishpower; the term implies that the subject has a desire to do something, but the desire is without power or energy. Abulia itself is rare and occurs mainly in the schizophrenias. The more frequent disturbance in the will is a reduction or impairment (*hypobulia*) rather than a complete absence. Bleuler included abulia and hypobulia among the fundamental symptoms of the schizophrenias.

Social abulia means inactivity, focal or diffuse, of a person toward the environment, due to inability to settle on a plan of action. There may be a desire to contact the environment, but the desire has no power of action.

**abuse**    1. Illicit use of a substance, and especially the pathological and driven or "compulsive" use of a substance that leads to impaired social or occupational functioning. Abuse is closely related to substance dependence, which also leads to impaired social or occupational functioning but, in addition, includes signs of physiological tolerance or development of a withdrawal syndrome when intake of the drug is reduced or stopped.

2. Mistreatment; harming or injuring another. See battered child syndrome; violence; wife battering.

**abuse, alcohol**    See *alcoholism.*

**abuse, child**    See *battered child syndrome.*

**abuse potential**    The property of a substance that, by its physiological or psychological effects, or both, increases the likelihood that it will lead to dependence, abuse, or harmful or hazardous use.

**ACA**    *Adult child of an alcoholic* (q.v.).

**academic skills disorder**    In DSM-IV, *learning disorders* (q.v.).

**academic underachievement disorder**    A pattern of failing grades or inadequate school performance despite adequate (or even superior) intellectual potential and a supportive environment.

**academic (work) inhibition**    A form of performance anxiety concerning school or occupational tasks, manifested as examination anxiety, inability to write reports, or difficulty in concentration despite adequate intellectual or performance ability as demonstrated by previously adequate functioning.

**acalculia**    A type of *aphasia* (q.v.) characterized by inability to perform arithmetic operations, seen most commonly with parietal lobe (retrolandic) lesions. Various groups of acalculia are recognized: (1) *dyscalculia* of the spatial type in which disturbance of spatial organization of numbers predominates and is often associated with spatial dyslexia, spatial agnosia, sensorikinetic apraxia, somatospatial apractognosia, and directional and vestibular oculomotor disorders (typical of dominant parietal lobe dysfunction); (2) predominance of alexia or agraphia for numbers and figures; and (3) anarithmia, in which disturbances in the performance of arithmetic operations predominate. The second and third groups are often associated with speech disturbances and alterations in the process of verbalization.

**acamprosate**    *Calcium bis-acetyl homotaurinate,* a GABA agonist and structural analog that appears to reduce alcohol consumption in chronic alcoholics and may be useful in preventing relapse. It is generally used as an adjunct to a community-based alcohol rehabilitation program.

Acamprosate (marketed under the name Campral) increases (sedating) GABA activity (thereby decreasing the level of discomfort accompanying withdrawal) and inhibits excitatory amino acids such as glutamate, either directly or by inhibiting the NMDA receptor.

It is notable for its safety; it does not produce tolerance or a withdrawal syndrome, it does not increase the actions of alcohol (important in case of a "slip"), and it is not hepatotoxic. Its efficacy in controlled trials has been modest. See *relapse prevention*.

**acanthesthesia** A type of paresthesia in which the subject experiences a sensation of pinpricks.

**acarophobia** Fear of mites and, by extension, of a variety of small things, animate (e.g., worms) or inanimate (e.g., pins, needles). See *parasitophobia*.

**acatalepsia** Impairment of the reasoning faculty or comprehension.

**acatamathesia** *Obs.* Inability to understand language. This is the perceptive (sensory) aspect of aphasia. See *speech disorders*.

**acataphasia** Also, *akataphasia*. A form of disordered speech in which "the patients either do not find the expression appropriate to their thoughts, but only produce something with a similar sound ('displacement paralogia'), or they let their speech fall into quite another channel ('derailment paralogia'). A patient said he was 'wholly without head on the date' for 'he did not know the date'; another complained he 'lived under protected police' instead of 'under the protection of police'" (Kraepelin, E. *Dementia Praecox*, 1919). See *speech disorders*.

**acathexis** Lack of emotional charge or psychic energy with which an object would ordinarily be invested.

**acathisia** Also termed acathisia paraesthetica, acathisia psychasthenica, acathisia spastica. Inability to sit down because of the intense anxiety provoked by the thought of doing so. In acathisia spastica, the thought or act of sitting provokes convulsions.

Haase first applied the term (1955) to the inability to sit still and to other irritative, hyperkinetic symptoms that are sometimes seen as a complication of neuroleptic therapy. See *akathisia*.

**acault** Burmese term for a man who lives as a woman (*gynemimesis*); the belief is that a female spirit has bestowed a special spiritual quality on the acault.

**ACC** *Anterior cingulate cortex* (q.v.)

**acceleration, developmental** Precocious growth in any area—motor, perceptual, language, or social. An uneven growth pattern is often found in schizophrenia, with unusual sequences of retardation and acceleration. This has been interpreted by some as a disorder of timing and integration of neurological maturation.

**accelerative** In behavior therapy, techniques designed to strengthen behaviors that are incompatible with or replace the function of the targeted behavior being eliminated. Accelerative techniques include token economy, the related levels system, activity programming with the use of structured, supervised recreational activities within a treatment milieu, and *social skills training* (q.v.). *Differential reinforcement schedules* are designed to provide direct reinforcement for behaviors incompatible or competing with the targeted behavior(s), such as differential reinforcement of other behavior (*DRO*), differential reinforcement of low-rate behavior (*DRL*), providing reinforcement whenever the rate of the behavior being eliminated falls below a predetermined frequency; and differential reinforcement of incompatible behavior (*DRI*), providing reinforcement for behaviors that are impossible to perform simultaneously with the undesirable responses.

**accentuation, interface** See *network*.

**acceptance** See *tolerance, social*.

**acceptive phase** Copulatory phase; genital union. See *proceptive phase*.

**accessibility** Receptivity to external influences. Inaccessibility is characteristic of *withdrawal* (q.v.).

**accessory** Additional, contributory, or secondary as opposed to fundamental or primary. In psychiatry, the term is chiefly used in reference to the schizophrenias, whose symptoms were divided by Bleuler into (1) fundamental or primary and (2) accessory or secondary.

**accessory symptom** Bleuler differentiated between fundamental symptoms and accessory symptoms of the schizophrenias. The accessory, secondary symptoms include hallucinations, illusions, delusions, certain memory disturbances (e.g., déjà vu, déjà fait), some of the disturbances of the person (e.g., speaking of one's self in the second or third person and other pronominal reversals), speech and writing disturbances (e.g., coprolalia, verbigeration, neologisms, metonymy, asyndesis, interpenetration), and physical symptoms such as headache, paresthesiae, "will-o'-the-wisp" gait, weight loss, and general signs of metabolic asthenia. See *fundamental symptom*.

**accident, cerebrovascular**   See *cerebrovascular accident.*

**accident, intentional**   An accident that is psychologically determined. A resentful employee, following a threat of discharge, "accidentally" thrusts his hand between gears and thus gains instead many weeks of compensation and care.

**accident proneness**   Liability or tendency toward involvement in mishaps that cause some pain or injury to the subject; *accident habit.* In some instances, accident proneness can be traced to a specific emotional state existing prior to the injury. In many others, however, a tendency to repeated accidents appears to be an expression of deep-seated personality traits and unconscious conflicts.

The typical accident-prone person is a young male who is decisive or even impulsive; he concentrates upon immediate pleasures and satisfactions and acts on the spur of the moment. He likes excitement and adventure, eschewing planning and preparation. Often he will be found to have been reared strictly and harbors an unusual amount of resentment against authority; he is a rebel who cannot tolerate even self-discipline. At the same time he feels guilty about his rebellion, but in the unconsciously provoked accident he is able to express his resentment and to atone for his rebellion through the injury. See *traumatophilic diathesis; victimology.*

**accidental**   In psychoanalysis, accidental refers to that which is adventitious or of external origin, in contradistinction to that which is endowed or of inherent origin.

Accidental experiences are of two kinds: dispositional, when they occur early in life and strongly influence character development; and definitive, when they occur later and act as precipitating or provocative agents. Accidental-situational refers to sudden or unforeseen changes, such as a natural disaster or accident.

**accidental psychosis**   *Rare.* Organic psychosis.

**accidental stimuli**   Among the four general types of dream stimuli—which are (1) external sensory; (2) internal sensory (subjective); (3) internal physical (organic); (4) psychic—the group of accidental stimuli belongs to the first type, external sensory. Accidental stimuli are those chance happenings that seemingly precipitate dreams or become part of them. For example, the backfire of an automobile

passing in the street may emerge in the dream as the firing of a gun or as the "pop" of a champagne cork.

**accommodation**   1. Adjustment, especially of the eye for various distances. Absolute accommodation is the accommodation of either eye separately; binocular accommodation is like accommodation in both eyes in coordination with *convergence* (the accommodation reflex). Accommodation occurs on shift of far to near vision, which is followed by thickening of the lens, convergence of the eyes, and constriction of the pupils.

2. Nerve accommodation is the rise in threshold during the passage of a constant, direct electric current because of which only the make and break of the current stimulate the nerve.

3. Social accommodation refers to the functional changes in habits and customs occurring in persons and groups in response to other persons and groups and in response to the common environment. Such accommodation is typically made for the sake of social harmony. The concept of accommodation is used in analyzing attitudes in situations of superordination and subordination, as those of slavery, caste, class, status, and leadership. The social heritage, culture, and social organization are accommodations that are transmitted from generation to generation. See *equilibration.*

**accountability**   In group psychotherapy, the participant's responsibility for his or her behavior within the therapy group and for reporting the reasons for that behavior.

**accreditation**   Certification as being of a prescribed or desirable standard; credentialing; often a voluntary process in which a program or facility is reviewed by a professional organization responsible for setting standards of quality or competence. See *certification.*

**accretion**   Growth by simple addition of parts or coherence of elements. Used particularly in learning psychology to refer to the learning of responses through frequency of association rather than through any inherent relatedness.

**acculturated need**   *See adaptational psychodynamics.*

**acculturation**   Originally, a term of social anthropology—the transfer of one ethnic group's culture to another. By extension, the implanting in children of the customs, beliefs, and ideals held to be important by adults of the culture group: a process of cultural indoctrination of children, much of which is carried out by educators without a formal plan, as an unconscious attempt at disseminating their own beliefs.

Acculturation is also used to refer to the ability of a person to adapt to a new environment.

**accumulation**   See *soteria*.

**acebutolol**   A *beta blocker* (q.v.).

**acedia**   *Obs.* A syndrome characterized by carelessness, listlessness, apathy, and melancholia.

**acenesthesia**   Absence of the feeling of physical existence.

**acerophobia**   1. Fear of sourness. 2. Fear of criticism (of another's bitter tongue).

**acetaldehyde**   A toxic intermediate product in the metabolism of ethyl alcohol. In the body, under the influence of the catalyst alcohol dehydrogenase, oxidation of alcohol produces acetaldehyde, which itself is oxidized to acetate by aldehydre dehydrogenase. Alcohol-sensitizing drugs such as disulfiram interfere with the breakdown of acetaldehyde and produce the *alcohol flush reaction* (q.v.). See *Antabuse*.

**ACE test**   The American Council on Education intelligence test, designed for use with secondary school and college students.

**acetylaspartate**   One of the most abundant amino acids in the central nervous system; it is decreased in some degenerative dementias and is considered a surrogate marker of neuronal integrity. An occipital cortex *N*-acetylaspartate/creatine ratio of 1.61 or lower in patients with mild cognitive impairment predicts conversion to dementia within 3 years. See *GRM3*.

**acetylation**   A fundamental cell regulatory process in which acetyls are added to the histones. The acetyl groups lessen the attractiveness of histones to nearby DNA; this makes it possible for the proteins needed for gene activity to get close enough to interact with DNA. Conversely, removal of the acetyls closes the door on gene transcription by restoring histone's tight connections with DNA. N-acetyltransferase, a hepatic enzyme, is responsible for acetylation, which is genetically determined. A *rapid acetylator* often requires a higher dose of drug to attain the desired level of response, often responds unpredictably to the usual dose of a drug, and is likely to develp hepatotoxicity because of acetylhydrazine accumulation. About half the U.S. population falls into the *slow acetylator* class; such subjects demonstrate increased likelihood of adverse drug effects.

Phosphatases do the opposite of the kinases and remove phosphate groups from proteins. Upon *phosphorylation*, interactions occur that cause proteins to change their shape. Since a protein's function is highly dependent upon its conformation, phosphorylation produces significant changes in how the protein works. Post-translationally, phosphorylation of serine, threonine, or tyrosine residues by special protein kinases is probably the most common mechanism for altering the biochemical function of proteins in all cells. Phosphorylation is reversible. Another important post-translational modification is the addition of *ubiquitin*, which tags proteins for degradation by special proteases.

Proteins often need help to fold into, and then maintain, the three-dimensional structures necessary for them to function normally. Proteins that assist other proteins in folding to the correct final conformation are called *molecular chaperones*.

**acetylcholine (Ach)**   A reversible acetic acid ester that is synthesized from choline by the action of the enzyme choline acetyltransferase (CAT) and degraded enzymatically by *acetylcholinesterase* (AChE), which catalyzes the hydrolysis of acetylcholine. In the 1920s Otto Loewi showed that acetylcholine mediates transmission from the vagal nerve to the heart. Acetylcholine is a neurotransmitter of the biogenic amine class that is active in both the peripheral and the central nervous system; approximately 5% of central neurons use it as a neurotransmitter.

There are two types of cholinergic (acetylcholine) receptors, *nicotinic* and *muscarinic*. Nicotinic receptors are mimicked by nicotine and blocked by α-bungarotoxin; the effect of their activation is excitatory. Muscarinic synapses, the predominant type in the central nervous system, are both inhibitory and excitatory; they are mimicked by muscarine and blocked by atropine.

There is evidence that central cholinergic neurons play a critical role in memory, sleep, mood regulation, Alzheimer disease, Down syndrome, Parkinson disease, and perhaps in schizophrenia. See *cholinergic; cholinergic hypothesis*.

**ACGME** Accreditation Council on Graduate Medical Education (U.S.). As of January 2001, the ACGME required that all psychiatry residents demonstrate competence in the practice of brief therapy, cognitive-behavioral therapy, combined psychotherapy and psychopharmacology, psychodynamic therapy, and supportive psychotherapy.

**ACh** *Acetylcholine* (q.v.).

**achalasia** *Cardiospasm*; *GERD*; esophageal disorder of unknown etiology, characterized by impaired peristalsis, dysphagia, and, in about a third of cases, *nocturnal regurgitation* (*esophageal reflux*). Reflux of undigested food may cause aspiration and death.

**acheiria, achiria** Lacking hands; also, loss of sensation, total anesthesia, or a feeling of absence of the hands, sometimes a hysterical symptom.

**achievement age (AA)** The relationship between the chronological age and the age of achievement as established by standard achievement tests. The latter comprise a series of educational tests as distinguished from intelligence tests. Achievement age is synonymous with educational age and one speaks of educational or achievement quotient. When the latter is divided by the mental age (IQ), the result is expressed as *accomplishment quotient (AQ)*.

**achievement test** Any evaluation of what gains the subject has made in an area following training and instruction.

**Achilles reflex** Ankle jerk. Tapping the Achilles tendon results in plantar flexion at the ankle due to contraction of the soleus and gastrocnemius muscles; the tibial nerve is both afferent and efferent for this reflex, and its center is $S_{1-2}$.

**achluophobia** Fear of darkness.

**achromatopsia** The inability to perceive colors, usually due to damage to color-selective areas in the ventral occipitotemporal cortex. See *word blindness.*

**acme** In psychoanalysis the highest point of pleasure in sexual intercourse.

**acmesthesia** Perception of sharp points by touch rather than by pain; acuesthesia.

**ACOA** *Adult child of an alcoholic* (q.v.).

**acoasm** *Akoasm* (q.v.).

**acolasia** *Obs.* Morbid intemperance or lust.

**aconuresis** See *enuresis.*

**acoria** *Obs.* To Hippocrates it meant moderation in eating; but in Aretaeus it is used

in regard to drink in the sense of insatiable desire. See *bulimia.*

**acousma** See *akoasm.*

**acoustic nerve** See *auditory nerve.*

**acoustic neuroma** Vestibular schwannoma; *neurofibromatosis 2* (q.v.).

**acousticomotor epilepsy** See *reflex epilepsy.*

**acousticophobia** Fear of sounds.

**acquired immune deficiency syndrome** *AIDS* (q.v.).

**acquired immunity** Specific immunity that involves recognition of specific epitopes in invading pathogens (antigens) by cells (T and B lymphocytes) that have been genetically preprogrammed to respond to that antigen. See *innate immunity.*

**acquisitiveness** *Hoarding* (q.v.). See *soteria.*

**acrai** *Obs.* An Arabian term; nymphomania and satyriasis.

**acral lick dermatitis** Lick granuloma; an animal model of *obsessive-compulsive disorder* (q.v.), it is a disorder of grooming seen in a variety of mammalian species, in particular in large-breed canines. Characteristics are excessive licking or biting of the extremities, leading to localized alopecia and subsequent granulomatous lesions. The serotonin system may be involved in its development.

**acrasia, acrasy** *Obs.* Intemperance in anything; at one time it was synonymous with acratia, debility, impotence, inefficiency.

**acrescentism, emotional** Emotional deprivation.

**acro-** Combining form meaning pertaining to extremity or tip, from Gr. *akros,* highest, topmost.

**acrocephaly** See *craniosynostosis.*

**acrocinesia, acrocinesis** Excessive movements, such as those observed in the manic phase of bipolar disorder.

**acrocyanosis** Blueness of the extremities, extending usually to the wrists and ankles; in psychiatric subjects, it is seen most frequently among schizophrenics, perhaps because in persons with an asthenic habitus the venous bed typically preponderates over the arterial.

**acrodynia** *Pink disease; erythroedema polyneuropathy;* a form of chronic mercury poisoning that occurs in infants and young children, mainly in the winter. It is characterized by irritability, purplish cold edema of the skin of the hands and feet, albuminuria, hematuria, and, in advanced cases, peripheral neuropathy and signs of cerebral and cerebellar involvement. Mortality is 5%, and neurologic involvement indicates a poor prognosis for complete recovery.

**acroesthesia**  Increased sensitivity to pain in the extremities.

**acrohypothermy**  Abnormal coldness of the extremities, often associated with *acrocyanosis* (q.v.).

**acromania**  *Obs.* Chronic incurable insanity.

**acromegaly, acromegalia**  Hyperpituitarism produced usually by an acidophilic adenoma of the anterior lobe (epithelial portion) of the hypophysis; acromegaly is sometimes seen in subjects with no adenoma whose hypophysis shows an increase in number of eosinophilic cells in an otherwise normal gland. The disorder was first clearly defined by Pierre Marie in 1886 and hence is sometimes called *Marie disease*. Acromegaly occurs in adults after the epiphysial lines have closed; acidophilic adenomas arising prior to closure of the epiphysial lines in adolescence produce gigantism. Acromegaly consists of a localized increase in size of various structures (head, hands, feet, lips, jaw) resulting in a peculiar bodily configuration seen in no other disorder. Associated with this is profuse, offensive perspiration; bitemporal or frontal headache, excessive growth of hair, impotence, sterility, increase in basal metabolic rate, and glycosuria are also seen frequently. Bitemporal hemianopia develops with progression of the disorder. See *G protein; growth hormone*.

Acromegaly is regularly accompanied by striking alterations of personality: impulsiveness (about 90% of cases), moodiness and mood swings (60%), anger outbursts (50%), and often periodic or constant somnolence.

**acromicria**  Selective smallness and shortness of one or more extremities. Benda proposed the term *congenital acromicria* to replace *mongolism*, which he viewed as a form of pituitary hypofunction that to some extent is the opposite of acromegaly. See *Down syndrome*.

**acroparesthesia**  Numbness, tingling, and/or other abnormal sensations of the extremities; seen frequently in organic disorders, especially peripheral nerve lesions, but by some the term is used only to refer to such unpleasant sensations occurring without demonstrable organic basis. Still less commonly, the term refers to an extreme degree of paresthesia.

**acrophobia**  Fear of high places.

**acrotomorphilia**  A *paraphilia* (q.v.) in which sexual arousal is dependent on the sexual partner having an amputation stump.

**ACT**  1. Assertive Community Treatment; an outpatient program, used mainly for patients with schizophrenia, that provides for all the treatment, rehabilitation, and support services needed by the patient. Basic characteristics include assertive engagement, in vivo delivery of services, a multidisciplinary team approach, continuous responsibility and staff continuity over time, caseloads with high staff-to-client ratios, brief but frequent contacts (high service intensity), close liaison with the patient's support system, and a treatment focus on alternative activities.

Most studies have shown that ACT consistently reduces the rate and duration of psychiatric inpatient care. When it is intensive, *case management* (q.v.) also reduces inpatient utilization and increases the use of community-based services. Usually, though, case management provides a more limited array of direct services, delivered with less intensity, than does ACT.

2. Atropine coma therapy (q.v.)

3. In cognitive restructuring, adaptive control of thought, a general model of the architecture of cognition developed by Anderson in his work in artificial intelligence. See *behavior therapy; cognitive therapy*.

**act, unintentional**  See *symptomatic act*.

**act ending**  Termination of an act, such as eating, that was begun in order to relieve tension, once tension release or drive satiation has been reached; also termed "completion of the act." Childhood schizophrenics often show impairment of such act ending and will continue to eat, for example, without evidence of satiation.

**ACTH**  *Adrenocorticotropic hormone*; an anterior pituitary hormone and peptide *neuromodulator* (q.v.). See *brain peptide; DST; general adaptation syndrome; hypothalamic–pituitary–adrenal (HPA) axis*.

**act-habit**  Any personality trait, habitual mode of response, etc., that is an outgrowth of cultural-environmental attitudes, such as minimal attention, scientific rearing, oversolicitousness, overwarmth, or overprotectiveness.

**acting in**  A type of *acting out* (q.v.) that occurs during therapy sessions; the patient discharges drive tension through action rather than through words.

Particularly in the early phase of treatment, it may take the form of disruptive, inappropriate, provocative behavior designed to test the therapist's tolerance or to elicit regulatory controls, or to assess the therapist's trustworthiness and competence.

**acting out**  The partial discharge of drive tension that is achieved by responding to the present situation as if it were the situation that originally gave rise to the drive demand. Acting out is a displacement of behavioral response from one situation to another. See *alloplasticity*.

Transference is a type of acting out in which the attitude or behavior is in response to certain definite persons. Acting out is more than a single thought, expression, or movement; it is a real acting. Accordingly, compulsive acts and other symptoms that may involve a degree of acting are not considered to be acting out, for they are limited in extent and experienced as ego-alien. Acting out is an unrecognized repetition of earlier behavior in the analytic situation, a substitution of acting for remembering, and an attempt to escape awareness of the inner life. In addition, it may be an attempt to undermine the therapeutic process or to bring the competence of the therapist into question.

In psychoanalysis, the patient may act out memories, instead of recalling them. A young woman, for example, imagined herself pregnant from a much older man. It later became apparent that the woman was acting out her infantile incestuous desires for her father, which she was unable to verbalize under analysis. See *actualization*.

"Acting out" is used loosely in practice as an equivalent of misbehavior. Some writers use acting out to refer to behavior expressing unconscious conflict and *acting up* to refer to behavior stemming from impaired impulse control. See *episodic disorders*.

**acting up**  See *acting out*.

**action, automatic**  *Obs.* Tendencies or dispositions to the performance of an aggregate of coordinated movements that may be activated under the influence of appropriate precipitants.

**action, faulty**  See *symptomatic act*.

**action current**  *Action potential* (q.v.), which occurs when the intraneuronal electrical potential reaches its threshold. See *calcium channel; ion pump; synapse*.

**action guide**  *Principle* or *rule* (qq.v.).

**action interpretation**  "The non-verbal reaction of the therapist of the group to the statements or acts of the patient. Action interpretation is employed almost exclusively in activity group psychotherapy" (Slavson, S. R. *An Introduction to Group Therapy*, 1943).

**action pattern**  See *instinct*.

**action potential**  *Action current* (q.v.); the basic unit of information transmittal within the nervous system, consisting of a regular sequence of small electrical deflections accompanying physiological activity of muscle or nerve. Such changes in electrical potential are commonly measured by the cathode ray oscillograph. When the neuronal membrane is depolarized by the opening of sodium channels associated with excitatory receptors, the voltage difference across the membrane falls. This causes voltage-dependent sodium channels adjacent to the excitatory synapse to open, generating an action potential. The action potential is a self-limiting event in which rapid influx of sodium ions temporarily reverses the polarity of the membrane. In the action potential, a series of depolarizations moves along the membrane and down the axon like a line of falling dominoes.

In most nerve cells, action potentials are followed by a transient hyperpolarization, the hyperpolarizing *afterpotential*. This occurs because it takes a few milliseconds for all of the open channels to return to the closed state. See *resting membrane potential*.

**action potential, specific**  See *instinct*.

**action research**  Scientific study of ongoing process, aimed toward achieving some improvement in the methods of the operating program.

**action system**  A bodily system that enables the organism to take action in response to a desire: a desire to keep one's feet dry will cause one to walk around and not through a puddle. The means by which this action is taken is produced by the integration of receptor, coordinative, effector systems into a functioning unit or action system.

**action tremor**  *Intention tremor* (q.v.). See *tremor*.

**action understanding**  The capacity to achieve the internal description of an action and to use it to organize one's own behavior appropriately in the future. There are two theories about how action understanding occurs:

1. Visual hypothesis. Action understanding is based on a visual analysis of the

different elements that form an action; a description of motor events in visual terms is sufficient for action understanding. According to this hypothesis, the brain builds progressively more complex description of biological motion that culminate in the description of goal-directed actions.

2. Direct matching hypothesis. Action understanding requires the subject to map the visual representation of the observed action onto the subject's motor representation of that action; i.e., observation of the action causes the motor system of the observer to "resonate." Action understanding depends on *simulation* (q.v.) of the observed action and estimating the actor's intentions on the basis of a representation of one's own intentions. Monkeys as well as humans can infer the goal of an action even when the visual information about it is incomplete; data show that this inference might be mediated by *mirror neurons* (q.v.) in the absence of visual information (Rizzolatti, G. et al. *Nature Reviews Neuroscience 2*: 661–670, 2001). See *prediction*

**activated sleep**  See *dream.*

**activating RNA**  See *chromosome.*

**activating system**  An alerting system located in the brain stem (medulla, pons, and mesencephalon); its anatomic basis is the central reticular formation, and it acts on the cerebral cortex and the afferent pathways to the cortex to maintain the brain in a condition in which consciousness can occur. See *reticular formation.*

**activation value**  See *parallel distributed processing.*

**active**  When applied to homosexual behavior in males, insertion of the penis in anal intercourse or in fellatio; the one who inserts is termed active, the one who receives is termed passive. In some societies where male homosexuality per se was acceptable or tolerated, the passive role was considered unseemly, immoral, pathologic, or even punishable when adopted by adult males. By the first century A.D., terms came into being that differentiated between roles taken in homosexual behavior. Males who took the active role were called *exoleti, drauci, paedicatores,* and *glabri*; males who took the passive role were termed *calamiti, cinaedi, pathici, pueri* (Boswell, J. *Christianity, Social Tolerance, and Homosexuality,* 1980). In current gay slang, the male who takes the active role in anal intercourse is called a "top"; the male who takes the passive role is called a "bottom."

**active analysis**  A method of dream interpretation used in a technique in which the analyst does not confine himself to the mere passive elucidation of the subject's free associations but intervenes directly and actively, making revelations and giving advice suggested to him mainly by the manifest content of the dream. This method, introduced by Stekel, is also called "active analytical psychotherapy" (Stekel, W. *The Interpretation of Dreams,* 1943). See *direct analysis.*

**active mastery**  See *mastery.*

**active technique**  When applied to psychotherapy, anything that is not the classical expectant technique of psychoanalysis (i.e., maintaining neutrality throughout the analysis without recourse at any time to suggestion, exhortation, positive injunctions, or negative prohibitions); any more extensive interference on the part of the analyst than is usual in orthodox or classical psychoanalytic technique. Active techniques are associated particularly with the name of Ferenczi. Among the maneuvers utilized in active forms of therapy are injunctions or prohibitions aimed at habits, phobias, obsessions, psychosexual habits, etc. A major objection to the use of active techniques is that they encourage reenactment rather than memory work. See *brief psychotherapy; psychotherapy.*

Ferenczi's experiments with different analytic techniques incurred Freud's wrath; in mutual analysis he had tried ways of gratifying the analysand (e.g., with warmth, openness, responsiveness, empathy) and made no demands on the patient. Sometimes the warmth went as far as physically holding the patient, but Ferenczi was quite specific in prohibiting genital sexuality as part of mutual analysis.

**active therapy**  The psychoanalytical method in which the psychiatrist does not confine himself to the interpretation of psychic material, but goes further to force the patient to actions that are hindered by his neurosis. The patient has to be forced precisely into the situations he fears, in order to accustom him to these situations and consequently to enable him to overcome his fear.

**active zones**  See *vesicles.*

**activities, graded**  In occupational therapy, occupations and handicrafts classified according to the degree of mental and physical effort required for their accomplishment.

**activity group therapy**  A special technique of applying psychotherapy through group activity. "So that these [very shy] children might not feel threatened, a program of picnics and trips was arranged for them, and after some months of such therapy it was found that not only did they evidence gain in their social behavior, but that they had made general improvement in their personalities. From this inauspicious practice grew Slavson's activity group therapy" (Klapman, J. W. *Group Psychotherapy*, 1946). See *group psychotherapy.*

**activity hypothesis**  See *neurotrophic hypothesis.*

**activity quotient**  The ratio of the total number of verbs in a subject's speech or writing to the total number of adjectives; the activity quotient is said to be a measure of the subject's emotionality.

**activity theory of aging**  See *disengagement.*

**actograph**  An apparatus designed to record the movements of a sleeper, usually by means of connection with the spring mattress.

**actual neurosis**  In Freud's terminology, a true neurosis or *physioneurosis*, i.e., symptoms that develop as a result of actual, true, or real disturbances of the sexual economy. Forced abstinence, frustrated sexual excitement, incomplete or interrupted coitus, sexual efforts that exceed the psychical capacity, sexual outlet rendered inadequate by guilt feelings or other conflicts, the need to revert to more primitive and/or less satisfactory means of sexual expression—these are the common "present-day" disturbances of sexuality that give rise to actual neurosis. Psychoneurosis, on the other hand, is determined by infantile and childhood experiences, and present-day occurrences are significant only in that they represent or repeat earlier events. Freud considered neurasthenia (a form of which is hypochondriasis) and anxiety neurosis to be true or actual neuroses.

**actual self**  In Horney's terms, the whole person—as he or she really exists at any point in time. The *real self* is the person's potential for further growth and development. The person the neurotic believes himself to be (the result of identification with an idealized image of what he feels he should be) is the *idealized self*. The *neurotic process* includes all the behavior and mechanisms by which the person maintains his identification with the idealized image even though this alienates him from his real self and requires him to deny and reject his actual self.

**actualization**  1. Fulfilling or realizing one's potential, the goal of many self-help groups. 2. *Acting out* (q.v.). Actualization of the transference refers to acting out within the context of the therapeutic relationship, ususally manifested as early, intense reactions of an erotic, hostile, or contemptuously devaluating nature.

**actuarial**  Relating to the calculation of insurance premiums or risks. Actuarial factors that affect the costs of health care include age, sex, place of residence, previous episodes of illness, exposure to risk, etc.

**acuesthesia**  See *acmesthesia.*

**aculalia**  Nonsensical or jargon speech, such as is seen with Wernicke aphasia associated with lesions of the left angular gyrus (and usually also the base of the first and second temporal convolutions) in right-handed persons. The affected subject shows marked intellectual impairment, an inability to comprehend spoken or written language, and although the patient can speak, he or she is likely to talk nonsense. This corresponds to Head's *syntactical aphasia.*

**-acusia**  Combining form meaning hearing.

**acute**  In many classificatory systems, acute events are those of less than 6 months' duration. Sometimes acute also implies reversibility.

**acute affective reflex**  Kretschmer's term for the earliest indications of emotional discharge (usually, tremors) in response to great stress.

**acute brain disorders**  In *DSM-I* (q.v.), various psychiatric syndromes due to temporary, reversible, diffuse impairment of brain tissue function. These disorders are part of the group formerly designated *organic psychoses*; the term acute, as used in the revised nomenclature, refers primarily to the reversibility of the process, and an acute brain disorder is one from which the patient will ordinarily recover. See *brain disorder; organic mental disorders; organic syndrome; symptomatic.*

**acute confusional state**  See *confusional state, acute.*

**acute delusional psychoses**  See *reactive psychosis.*

**acute shock psychosis**  An acute psychiatric disturbance occurring during war. Its most prominent symptoms are a completely unconscious state (with flaccid limbs and closed eyes), lasting from minutes to hours; insensitivity to pain with no reaction to external stimuli; the eyelids flutter, the eyeballs are mobile and are rolled outward and upward. The condition occurs most commonly during active warfare, especially on forced marches and in active campaigns. See *traumatic neurosis; psychorrhexis.*

**acute stress disorder**    *ASD*; a form of *post-traumatic stress disorder* (q.v.) that develops in the immediate aftermath of a trauma. The traumatic event is one that threatens the person or significant other with death, injury, etc. and arouses intense fear, horror, or feelings of helplessness. ASD develops within 4 weeks of the traumatic event and lasts at least 4 days but not for more than 4 weeks. It consists of three or more of the following dissociative symptoms: subjective sense of numbing, detachment, or absence of emotional responsiveness; reduction in awareness of surroundings (such as the feeling of being in a daze); derealization; depersonalization; dissociative amnesia (inability to recall an important aspect of the trauma).

**AD**    *Alzheimer disease; antidepressant*; average deviation (qq.v.).

**Adam/Eve principle**    Embryologically, development of the human organism will follow the line of differentiation into a female, and induction of male differentiation requires that something be added (e.g., masculinizing hormone such as testosterone).

**ADAMs**    A disintegrin and *metalloproteinases* (q.v.).

**ADAP**    Alzheimer disease–associated protein; a large protein present in subjects with Alzheimer disease but not in adult, nondemented, normal controls. It has been detected before the appearance of senile plaques and neurofibrillary tangles and is markedly increased in the frontal and temporal cortex in Alzheimer disease; in consequence, it serves as a useful postmortem marker of the presence of Alzheimer disease.

ADAP contains three ALZ-50 immunoreactive elements, one of which is the filament protein *A68* (q.v.). *Tau* protein (q.v.) may also be recognized by ALZ-50, but it is different from A68 in that it is not destroyed by trypsin. ADAP may be an abnormal epitope of tau protein. Excessive or inappropriate phosphorylation of tau may transform it into A68. ApoE4 may be one factor that

contributes to the hyperphosphorylation of tau.

**adaptability, cultural**    According to Freud, a person's capacity to transform egoistic impulses into social drives.

**adaptability, homogeneous**    The capacity to adapt that is uniformly possessed by all members of the species, such as the adaptation to intensity of light entering the eye by means of the pupillary reflex. Homogeneous adaptability is differentiated from heterogeneous adaptability, which refers to genetic variability within the species or within a population (i.e., differences between individuals) in the capacity to adapt.

**adaptation**    1. Fitting or conforming to the environment, usually with the implication that advantageous change has taken place. Adaptation is typically achieved through a combination of alloplastic maneuvers (which involve alteration of the external environment) and autoplastic maneuvers (which involve a change in the self). The end result of successful adaptation is *adjustment*; unsuccessful attempts at adaptation are termed *maladjustment.*

A phenotypic trait is adaptive if possession of the trait gives an organism a reproductive advantage in its operating environment.

2. In occupational therapy, modification or alteration of an occupation to suit the specific need or disability of a patient.

3. In neurophysiology, the diminished rate of discharge shown by an end organ subjected over a period of time to a constant stimulus. Adaptation in this sense is comparable to the term tolerance when the latter is used in reference to a drug.

4. In sociobiology (q.v.), a phenotypic trait is called adaptive if possession of it gives an organism a reproductive advantage.

**adaptational psychodynamics**    Rado's system of psychoanalytic psychiatry, which views behavior disorders as disturbances of psychodynamic integration that interfere with the organism's adaptive life performance, its attainment of utility and pleasure. The integrative apparatus consists of four hierarchically ordered levels: (1) *hedonic*—the organism moves toward pleasure and away from pain; (2) *brute emotions*—integration is controlled by emotions based on present pain or the expectation of pain, such as fear, rage, retroflexed rage, guilty fear, and guilty rage;

(3) *emotional thought*—integration is controlled by the *welfare emotions*, based on present pleasure or the expectation of pleasure, such as pleasurable desire, affection, love, joy, self-respect, and pride; and (4) *unemotional thought*—at this level, thought, reason, common sense, and science prepare the ground for intelligent action and self-restraint.

The simplest forms of behavior disorder occur when the organism responds to danger with an overproduction of *emergency emotions*; such emergency dyscontrol is in itself a threat to the organism from within and leads to processes of miscarried prevention and miscarried repair. With emergency dyscontrol as a point of departure, Rado classified behavior disorders according to the increasing complexity of their patterns and mechanism: *moodcyclic disorders, schizotypal disorders, extractive disorders* (the ingratiating "smile and suck" and extortive "hit and grab" patterns of transgressive conduct), *lesional disorders, narcotic disorders,* and *disorders of war adaptation.*

Rado divided the methods of psychotherapy into (1) reconstructive (the adaptational technique of psychoanalytic therapy) and (2) reparative (less ambitious treatment methods with limited goals but in general also of shorter duration).

**adapted child**   In transactional analysis, that part of the child ego state that is subservient to parental influence: the constrained, compliant, dependent, inhibited, procrastinating, and withdrawing elements.

**adaptedness**   The state that results from appropriate adjustments to conditions, as distinguished from adaptation, which strictly speaking refers only to the process whereby the adjustments are brought about. In common usage, the term adaptation has both meanings.

**adaptor protein complex**   AP complex; a family of proteins that regulate formation of clathrin-coated vesicles and intracellular trafficking of membrane proteins. AP-3B is important in the regulation of GABA release and might underly the pathogenesis of some epilepsies.

**ADAS**   Alzheimer Disease Assessment Scale, consisting of an 11-item cognitive section that evaluates memory, praxis, and language, and a 10-item noncognitive section that assesses mood, vegetative symptoms, agitation, delusions, hallucinations, tremor, and concentration.

**ADAS-cog**   Alzheimer Disease Assessment Scale cognitive subscale.

**ADC**   *AIDS dementia complex* (q.v.).

**ADD**   *Attention deficit hyperactivity disorder* (q.v.); formerly called HACS (hyperactive child syndrome), hyperkinetic impulse disorder, or MBD (minimal brain dysfunction).

**ADDH**   Attention deficit disorder with hyperactivity; ADHD.

**addiction**   Loss of control over drug use (including alcohol), typically manifested as compulsive seeking and taking of drugs despite adverse consequences, with a high vulnerability to relapse. Addiction generally requires repeated drug exposure as well as a vulnerable brain. With some drugs, cessation of the drug produces an *abstinence syndrome* or *withdrawal syndrome*, but such signs of physiological *dependence* are not an invariable accompaniment of addiction (qq.v.). Cocaine, for example, is highly addictive but causes little withdrawal. Of more significance is the addict's continued engagement in self-destructive behavior despite adverse consequences. Addicts compulsively seek out and take drugs, even when they no longer provide pleasure and despite a strong will to quit.

Although often used interchangeably, addiction and dependency are not the same. Addiction is a behavioral disorder, whereas dependency is a physiological effect of a drug; often the two coexist. Addiction typically involves repeated drug exposure, the physiological effects of which may (particularly in a vulnerable brain) lead to dependence. Repeated exposures can produce tolerance to the drug(s), but they can also produce *sensitization* or reverse tolerance. Once dependence has developed, cessation of the drug (withdrawal) produces an abstinence syndrome.

There are three stages of addiction: (1) acute drug effects; (2) transition from recreational use to addictive patterns of use; (3) end-stage addiction, characterized by overwhelming desire to obtain the drugs, diminished ability to control drug seeking, and reduced pleasure from biological rewards. A cardinal feature is continued vulnerability to relapse, even after years of abstinence. Vulnerability arises from intense desire for the drug and reduced capacity to control that desire. The glutamatergic projection from prefrontal cortex to the accumbens provides motivational salience, and stimuli predicting drug availability intensely activate both PFC and glutamatergic drive to the accumbens. Dependence and withdrawal do not explain addiction, because they cannot explain persistence of relapse risk.

The rewarding effects of *acute* drug intake—the drug high and initiation of addiction—depend on increased dopamine release in the nucleus accumbens; increased dopamine transmission in the nucleus accumbens and the basal ganglia underlies the reinforcing responses to drugs of abuse. Many drugs of abuse also stimulate release of endogenous opioids in these regions. The dopamine increases are not directly related to reward (pleasure) per se, but to the prediction of reward and to salience (reflecting motivation, drive); dopamine increase motivates procurement of more drug regardless of whether the effects are pleasurable. The dopamine increase facilitates conditioned learning, so previously neutral stimuli (such as the house of the drug dealer, syringes) become salient.

Long-term drug use has effects on frontal lobe function and cognitive decision-making processes. Cocaine, amphetamine, methamphetamine, and ecstasy increase extracellular concentration of dopamine in limbic regions (including the nucleus accumbens in the ventral striatum) and prefrontal cortex (especially the orbitofrontal and anterior cingulate areas), some by inhibiting dopamine reuptake, others by promoting dopamine release through effects on dopamine transporters. Nicotine, alcohol, opiates, and marijuana work indirectly by stimulating GABA-mediated or glutamatergic neurons that modulate dopamine cell firing through their effects on nicotine, GABA, mu opiate, or cannabinoid CB1 receptors, respectively. Once addicted, the uncontrollable urge to obtain drugs and to relapse arise from a pathological form of the plasticity in excitatory transmission. Stress increases the propensity to relapse.

Genetic factors may account for 40%–60% of the vulnerability to addiction, but few genes have been identified with polymorphisms (alleles) that predispose to or protect from addiction. Substance use disorders have high comorbidity with mental illness: depression, conduct disorder, ADHD, and schizophrenia Volkow, N. D. & Li, T. -K. *Nature Reviews Neuroscience* 5: 963–970, 2004. See *dependence, drug; withdrawal syndrome.*

**addiction, sexual**    An inexact term that implies a reliance on sexual activity as a major defense against anxiety or other dysphoric feelings; sometimes used as equivalent to compulsive sexuality or hypersexuality.

**addiction medicine**    *Addictionology*; the branch of medicine that is concerned with the prevention, detection, treatment, and rehabilitation of persons with substance use disorders (alcoholism and other chemical dependencies or abuse). The practitioner is referred to as an addictionist. In parallel fashion, addiction psychiatry refers to the psychiatric aspects of those disorders, and the American Board of Psychiatry and Neurology grants a certificate of added qualification in addiction psychiatry. In Russia, the comparable terms are *narcology* and *narcologist.*

**addiction treatments**    There are two classes of pharmacological intervention in drug addiction. First are medications that interfere with the reinforcing effects of drugs of abuse (by interfering with the binding of the drug, with drug-induced dopamine increase, with postsynaptic responses, or with the drug's delivery to the brain, or by triggering aversive responses). Second are medications that decrease the prioritized motivational value of the drug, enhance the saliency value of natural reinforcers, interfere with conditioned responses, interfere with stress-induced relapse, or interfere with physical withdrawal.

Maintenance medications to prevent relapse are most effective in the context of psychotherapy or counseling. Medications in current use include methadone and buprenorphine (for heroin addiction), disulfiram, topiramate, modafinil, propranolol, and baclofen (for cocaine addiction), naltrexone, acamprosate, disulfiram, and topiramate (for alcohol addiction), and bupropion, nicotine replacement (with patch, nasal spray, or gun), and rimonabant (for nicotine addiction). Rimonabant has been reported to be of use in cocaine or alcohol addiction, and odansetron may be of use in alcohol addiction.

Heredity plays a role in all forms of drug addiction, and genes influence the pharmacological effects of the addicting substance and the subject's responsivity to any particular pharmacological agent. Thus no one drug is likely to be equally effective in all who are addicted to a particular drug.

**addictionist** Within the field of *addiction medicine* (q.v.) in the United States, including addiction psychiatry, the currently preferred term for the practitioner in that area. It replaces the older term, addictionologist, which is favored in many other countries (in Russia the comparable term is *narcologist*).

**addictionology** *Addiction medicine* (q.v.), including addiction psychiatry.

**Addisonian syndrome** (Thomas Addison, English physician, 1793–1860) *Addison disease; melasma suprarenale; adrenocortical insufficiency,* due usually to atrophy or destructive inflammatory lesions. Symptoms include weakness, anorexia, hypotension, cutaneous pigmentary changes (bronzed skin), hyponatremia, hyperkalemia, vomiting, diarrhea, irritability, periodic hypoglycemia, and decreased or absent secretion of α-ketosteroids and 11-oxysteroids. In some cases, paranoid reactions are seen.

**ADE** Adverse drug event; *medication error* (q.v.).

**ademonia** Agitated depression.

**adenylate cyclase, adenylyl cyclase** See *second messenger*.

**adephagia, addephagia** *Obs.* A morbidly voracious appetite. See *bulimia*.

**ADHD** *Attention deficit hyperactivity disorder* (q.v.).

**adhesion, cellular** Binding or linking of one cell to another, an important factor in *axon guidance* (q.v.) during neural migration. The three most important glycoproteins involved in neuradhesion are *NCAMs* (q.v.), members of the immunoglobulin group; the *cadherins*; and the *integrins*. Like NCAM, N-cadherin mediates cell adhesion by homophilic binding; both mediate adhesion between the surfaces of neural cells. The integrins, in contrast, mediate the adhesion of neural cells to glycoproteins in the extracellular matrix, and they use a *heterophilic* binding system.

**adhesion molecules** See *CAM*.

**adhibition** Attaching or affixing; the act of applying or allowing to enter. By extension, active engagement or accomplishment, the gaining of mastery or control, the opposite of inhibition. Examples of adhibitory coping maneuvers are rituals, orderliness, perseveration, and risk-taking.

**ADI** Attention Deviance Index, a battery of tests that includes the Continuous Performance Test, the Attention Span Test, and the Digit Span subtest from the WISC.

**adiadochokinesis** Loss of power to perform rapid alternating movements, indicative of disorder of the cerebellum or its tracts.

**Adie pupil** (William John Adie, British neurologist, 1885–1935) *Tonic pupil;* a unilateral condition in which the pupil responds poorly to light and very slowly to convergence.

**Adie syndrome** Pseudo-Argyll Robertson pupil; pupillotonic pseudotabes; a benign syndrome of unknown etiology characterized by enlarged pupil that shows the tonic pupillary reaction (when the patient is directed to gaze at a near object, the affected pupil slowly contracts to a size even smaller than the normal pupil) and by diminution or loss of tendon reflexes. The disorder occurs almost exclusively in females and usually has its onset in the third decade.

**adient** Positively oriented or moving toward. The adient drive or behavior or response is a situation that results in behavior acting toward the stimulus, increasing and perpetuating its action; it is the opposite of the avoidant drive.

**adiposogenital dystrophia** See *Frohlich syndrome; Laurence-Moon-Biedl syndrome*.

**ADIS** Anxiety Disorders Interview Schedule; a structured interview schedule that was designed (1) to distinguish between different anxiety disorders and (2) to diagnose major depression and psychosis. It incorporates the Hamilton Anxiety and Depression Scales and provides a way to quantify anxiety and depression.

**adjunctive therapy** Augmentation therapy, such as adding thyroid to an antidepressant regimen.

**adjustment** See *adaptation*.

**adjustment, social** Adaptation of the person to his or her social environment. Adjustment may take place by adapting one's self to the environment or by changing the environment.

**adjustment disorder** An imprecise term for a variety of symptoms (e.g., anxiety, depressed mood, disturbance of conduct, physical complaints, withdrawal, or work or academic inhibition) that develop in response to an identifiable stressor. Duration of the disorder is usually less than 6 months; if it extends beyond that time, it is usually specified as a persistent or chronic adjustment disorder (or is reevaluated as probably belonging to a different diagnostic category). See *transient situational disturbances*.

**adjustment reaction**   In the 1952 revision of psychiatric nomenclature (DSM-I), this term was used to refer to certain transient situational disturbances (q.v.) occurring in various periods of life.

**adjuvant therapy**   Subsidiary therapy; drugs, suggestion, hypnosis, and similar means to promote or consolidate the benefits of psychotherapy.

**ADL**   Activities of daily living such as bathing, dressing, toileting, continence, feeding, movement into and out of a chair, and other physical activities of self-care. One commonly used instrument to evaluate such basic self-maintenance behaviors is the Katz Activities of Daily Living Schedule. Other scales evaluate instrumental activities of daily living (*IADL*) such as ability to use the telephone, to cook, to keep house, to shop, travel, take medications, and handle finances. See *BEHAVE-ID*.

**Adler, Alfred**   (1870–1937) Austrian psychiatrist, founder of the school of Individual Psychology; inferiority complex; overcompensation. Adler believed that human behavior and actions must be explained teleologically, in terms of a final purpose ("guiding fiction"). The purpose, developed by the age of 5 years, was to move feelings of inferiority to those of superiority. Under the direction of the self-ideal, as a constellation of wishful thoughts of being strong and powerful; or, when overcompensation was present, in phantasies of godlike immutable supremacy.

Adler's rational and optimistic approach to interpersonal and social problems was in contrast with Freud's more pessimistic psychobiological one and with the mystical elements of Jung's theory. Adler later developed his concept of the "style of life," comprising both the person's "fictive" goal and the plans and schemes to achieve it, including self-evaluation. Adler's therapy emphasized prevention of adult maladjustment by early correction of the mistakes of the child. In 1927 he established 22 child guidance clinics in Austria (they had grown to 30 by the time they were closed down in 1933).

In 1935 Adler was appointed professor in medical psychology at the Long Island College of Medicine. He died in Aberdeen 2 years later, on the last day of a lecture series.

**administrative therapy**   Institutional treatment of psychologically disturbed people such as is employed in the *therapeutic community* (q.v.), in contrast to mere custodial care.

**admission certification**   See *review*.

**ADNFLE**   Autosomal dominant nocturnal frontal lobe epilepsy. See *frontal lobe seizures*.

**adolescence**   The state or period of growth from puberty to maturity. In normal subjects its beginning is marked by the appearance of secondary sexual characteristics, commonly at about age 12; its termination is at about age 20. Adolescence is the period in which sexual maturity is achieved in that for the first time both the sexual and reproductive instincts attain full maturity and unite into a single striving; it can further be considered the age of final establishment of a dominant positive ego identity, the age in which "tu-ism" replaces narcissism, the age in which sexual development dovetails into the development of object relationships leading to the mature, adult stage of impersonal object love (alloerotism) and unhampered orgastic sexuality.

According to Piaget, thinking changes in adolescence from the state of *concrete operations* to formal operational thinking, characterized by the ability to think abstractly, to construct hypotheses, and to use deductive reasoning.

**adolescent crisis**   The emotional changes that take place during adolescence; the psychological events during this period constitute a kind of crisis, the last battle fought by the individual before reaching maturity. The ego must achieve independence, the old emotional ties must be cast off and new attachments made. Biological development brings in its train great qualitative and quantitative changes, in both the physiologic and the psychologic fields, and as a result the adolescent ego is confronted with new difficulties. Because they are closely connected with instinctual life, the emotions are affected more than is any other part of the personality by the problems of growth and therefore represent a challenging problem for the adolescent.

**adolescent gynecomastia**   See *gynecomastia*.

**adolescent turmoil**   An inexact term describing what some observers believed to be an expected, normal phase of adolescence, consisting of rebelliousness, concern about identity and role, instability of mood, and changeable and unpredictable behavior. Studies of nonpatient adolescents do not support this concept of significant disruption in psychological equilibrium as being a typical phase of normal adolescence.

**adolescentilism** Impersonating an adolescent; sometimes a *paraphilia* (q.v.), in which orgasm depends upon being treated as an adolescent by the sexual partner.

**adopted child** According to Paulina Kernberg, the adopted child is at risk for development of narcissistic personality disorder: "rejection" by the biological parents undermines the child's self-image, while having been "chosen" by the adoptive parents fuels the *grandiose self* (q.v.). See *narcissistic personality disorder*.

**adoptees** See *cross-fostering*.

**adoption studies** Investigations of adopted children as a way to estimate the degree of heritability of a given trait or disorder; the Danish studies of adoption and rearing of the offspring of schizophrenic parents by Seymour Kety and David Rosenthal and their coworkers (1968) are now classic. Several techniques have been used:

1. *Adoptees family method.* The investigator selects as an index case a person who, adopted in childhood, by adulthood had been hospitalized with a diagnosis of schizophrenia; adoptees without psychiatric disorder serve as controls; the incidence of mental disorder in adoptive and biological parents, siblings, and half-siblings is compared in index cases and controls.

2. *Adoptees study method.* Biological parents of adoptees are divided into those with psychiatric disorder (index cases) and those without (controls); the adopted offspring are then studied for incidence of mental disorder.

3. *Adoptive parents method.* Schizophrenics who have been adopted are compared with schizophrenics who have been reared by their biological parents and the incidence of mental disorder in adoptive and biological parents is compared.

4. *Cross-fostering.* The offspring of parents who are not schizophrenic are reared by adoptive parents who are schizophrenic; the adopted offspring are then studied for incidence of schizophrenia.

**ADR** Adverse drug reaction; *medication error* (q.v.).

**adrenal hyperplasia** See *adrenogenital syndrome*.

**Adrenalin** A proprietary brand of *epinephrine* (q.v.).

**Adrenalin-Mecholyl test** *Funkenstein test*; first described by Funkenstein, Greenblatt, and Solomon in 1952 as a test of prognostic significance in relation to electroshock treatment (EST). Patients with a hypotensive response to intramuscular Mecholyl chloride (1) are benefited by EST; (2) also show a high rate of improvement when psychotherapy is the sole method of treatment; (3) have good abstraction ability and good personality organization; and (4) appear clinically to maintain an appropriate and adequate level of affect.

**adrenergic** Referring to neurons that are activated by or secrete epinephrine or norepinephrine, and to endogenous agents (such as neurotransmitters) or drugs that stimulate the action of sympathetic postganglionic nerves. In the latter sense, adrenergic is equivalent to *sympathomimetic*. (For parasympathomimetic agents, see *cholinergic*.)

Sympathomimetic agents include (1) α-adrenergic stimulants, such as dopamine, metaraminol, and phenylephrine and (2) β-adrenergic stimulants, such as albuterol, isoproterenol, and metaproterenol.

*Sympatholytic* (i.e., antiadrenergic) agents include (1) α-adrenergic blockers, such as dibenamine, phenoxybenzamine, phentolamine, and tolazoline hydrochloride and (2) β-adrenergic blockers, such as labetalol, metoprolol, oxyprenolol, pindolol, and propranolol.

**adrenergic circulatory state** Also, *hyperdynamic β-adrenergic circulatory state*; panic disorder or generalized anxiety disorder in which cardiac symptoms are the predominant complaints: chest pain, palpitations, breathlessness, a feeling of oppression, dizziness, sweating, fatigue, headache, tremor, and nervousness. Such symptoms are similar to what is also described as cardiac anxiety state, cardiac neurosis, da Costa syndrome, and effort syndrome.

**adrenergic receptor** There are three types of adrenergic receptor: the α-1 adrenergic receptor, which activates phospholipase C; the α-2 adrenergic receptor, which inhibits adenylate cyclase; and β-1 and β-2 adrenergic receptors, which activate adenylate cyclase. The binding of catecholamines to the β-adrenergic receptor within seconds activates adenylate cyclase and induces the intracellular formation of adenosine 3',5'-monophosphate (cAMP). The β-adrenergic receptor is a member of a family of receptors that activate an effector system through a G protein. This amplifies the reaction within the system approximately 10-fold, since one receptor can activate numerous G protein–cyclase molecules. See *catecholamine*.

**adrenochrome**   See *psychotomimetic*.

**adrenocortical insufficiency**   See *Addisonian syndrome*.

**adrenocorticotropic hormone (ACTH)**   One of the anterior pituitary hormones. See *general adaptation syndrome*.

**adrenogenital syndrome**   Congenital adrenal hyperplasia (CAH); congenital virilizing adrenal hyperplasia (CVAH); a recessive deficiency in cortisol and aldosterone synthesis, and excessive adrenal androgen and pituitary adrenocorticotropin that exert a profound masculinizing effect in both sexes. Although the female internal genitalia are differentiated, the external genitalia are profoundly altered—ranging from no more than clitoral enlargement in the least severe cases to external genitalia that closely resemble male genitalia except for lack of testes. In the male fetus, masculine differentiation is not altered but, if untreated, the male undergoes precocious puberty, sometimes as early as 18 months of age (the *infant Hercules syndrome*).

**adrenoleukodystrophy**   *X-ALD;* first described in 1923 as a rare and fatal neurodegenerative disorder that affected boys. It consists of a combination of primary adrenal insufficiency with an inflammatory demyelinating process that affects the cerebral hemispheres. Since its original description, it has been recognized to be X-linked; its incidence approximates that of phenylketonuria, and it presents in a wide range of phenotypic expression. At least half of patients with X-ALD are adults with milder manifestations, and women who are carriers may become symptomatic. It is often misdiagnosed as ADHD in boys and as multiple sclerosis in men and women. It often causes Addison disease.

In adults X-ALD is often manifested as a slowly progressive paraparesis, *adrenomyeloneuropathy (AMN)*, due to a noninflammatory distal axonopathy involving the long tracts of the spinal cord and, to a lesser extent, the spinal cord. About 20% of patients with AMN develop inflammatory cerebral involvement.

X-ALD is diagnosed by plasma VLCFA assay; in women and in fetuses, confirmation by DNA analysis is recommended. Although there is no known cure, prognosis is improved by adrenal replacement therapy, Lorenzo oil therapy (a 4:1 mixture of glyceryl-trioleate and glyceryl-trierucate), and, in the inflammatory cerebral forms of X-ALD, hematopoietic stem cell transplantation. (Moser, H. W., Raymond, G. V. & Dubey, P. *Journal of the American Medical Association 294*: 3131–3134, 2005).

**adrenomyeloneuropathy**   A slowly progressive, adult form of *adrenoleukodystrophy* (q.v.).

**Adrian, Edgar Douglas**   (1889–1977)   English neurologist and neurophysiologist who established the "all-or-none" character of the propagated nervous impulse; a pioneer in recording bioelectrical events in the nervous system; shared the Nobel prize in physiology or medicine with Sherrington in 1932.

**ADT**   *Antidepressant* treatment (q.v.).

**adult ADHD**   *Attention deficit hyperactivity disorder* (q.v.) in the adult, presumably a continuation of childhood ADHD. The DSM-IV criteria for ADHD are not based on testing of symptoms that are developmentally representative of adults; as a result, the criteria are overly restrictive and fail to identify significant numbers of adults with meaningful levels of dysfunction. The most consistent findings in ADHD neuropsychology are reduced performance on tasks of motor response inhibition and response variability, with frequent lapses of intention and attention and moment-to-moment inconsistency in performance. Evidence suggests that, over time, hyperactive-impulsive symptoms decrease more than inattentive symptoms.

Adults with ADHD demonstrate lower self-esteem, less educational achievement, poorer personal health choices, and greater driving risks than adults without ADHD. They also generally have a high rate of comorbid conditions, including mood disorders, anxiety disorders, and borderline personality disorder.

Typical symptoms include the following: often feeling "on edge"; difficulty relaxing or completing tasks; generally disorganized; poor concentration; anger and emotional lability, coupled with poor impulse control, leading to risky health behaviors, risky sexual behaviors, and poor driving habits and decision making; stress intolerance; and impulsivity, which may often take the form of socially inappropriate behavior such as interrupting or intruding on conversations. Comorbidities are frequent: mood disorders, anxiety disorders (including social phobia and OCD), antisocial personality, and alcohol or substance abuse.

**adult ego state**   See *transactional analysis*.

**adult neurogenesis**   Neuron renovation, an adaptive response to challenges imposed by an animal's environment or its internal states. The degree of postnatal neurogenesis decreases with increasing brain complexity; in mammals, it appears to be restricted to two regions: the subgranular zone of the hippocampal dentate gyrus and the subventricular zone, which contributes interneurons to the olfactory bulb.

**adult separation anxiety disorder**   See *separation anxiety*.

**adulthood**   Maturity. See *developmental levels*.

**adultomorphism**   *Enelicomorphism*; interpretation of the behavior of children in terms of adult behavior. See *anthropomorph*.

**adultomorphization**   Making into an adult, forcing into adulthood; said to be characteristic of the mothers of some subjects with narcissistic personality disorder: the mother insists on "grown-up" behavior and the child can please and obtain admiration from her by developing a facade of competency (and becoming a *pseudo-mature child*). See *empathic failure*.

**advance directive**   Also, health care advance directive; a combination of living will and power of attorney that allows a person to appoint someone to make medical decisions for him or her when the person himself is unable to do so. In an advance directive, the person can specify what he wants done—or not done—if he is unable to speak for himself. Every state in the United States allows some type of advance directive.

There are two major forms of advance directive, which may be used singly or together: (1) The *living will*. The person gives instructional directives for end-of-life care. (2) The *health care proxy* (also known as *durable power of attorney for health care, living will designee, medical power of attorney*). The person appoints a stand-in who is empowered to make decisions about which health care measures will be accepted and which will be refused in the event of the patient's incapacity. A specific form of health care proxy for psychiatric patients is the *Ulysses contract* (q.v.).

**advanced sleep-phase syndrome**   See *FASPS*.

**advantage by illness**   *Epinosic gain* (q.v.). "Every symptom must in some way comply with the demands of the ego which regulates repression, must offer some advantage, admit of some profitable utilization, or it would undergo the same fate as the original impulse itself which is being kept in check" (Freud, S. *Collected Papers*, 1924–25).

**adventitious motor overflow**   *Synkinesia* (q.v.).

**adventurousness**   Describing the child in the preschool period in which there is an urge to rough-and-tumble freedom and curiosity. See *wanderlust*.

**adverse drug event**   ADE; *medication error* (q.v.).

**adverse drug reaction**   ADR; any undesired or unintended response to a medication that itself requires treatment or requires a change in the treatment strategy; it includes unpleasant psychological or physical reactions to drug taking, such as a *bad trip* (q.v.). A side effect is one that is routinely anticipated; if it requires a change in treatment, it too is considered an adverse drug reaction.

**adverse selection**   In insurance terminology, accumulation of high-risk consumers within a given insurance plan; self-sorting of a population to which insurance plans are offered on the basis of how extensively they plan to use the services. Employees who use many health services, including psychiatric benefits, for example, will often gravitate toward the few carriers offering high benefit levels. As an increasingly higher percentage of the members of a plan use unusually high amounts of care, the premiums must rise to pay for it. Each premium increase to accommodate the cost of *high utilizers* results in a new wave of *low utilizers* opting out (i.e., deciding not to buy that plan), and as a result the selection process spirals higher and higher.

**adversity, adverse**   Negative outcome or response, hurtful or injurious environment. Adverse conditions during development, be they a reflection of inherent vulnerability, familial and other environmental factors, or interaction between the two, are of special significance in preventive psychiatry.

*Family adversity* is manifested in parental discord, inadequate parenting such as harsh, inconsistent, and rejecting attitudes or abuse, and parental mental disorder. Adverse environmental influences that increase a person's vulnerability to depression, as one example, include the following: parental affective disorder, particularly maternal depression, or depression of both parents; disturbances in parenting (e.g., affectionless control); severe marital discord; divorce; death of a parent in childhood; childhood physical abuse or neglect; separation or illness; and the experience of loss and failure.

*Protective factors* throughout life include high intelligence, having an easy temperament, having a good relationship with a supportive adult. An optimistic explanatory style—including learned optimism—may be protective; in contrast, negative explanatory styles such as learned pessimism may increase the risk of depression.

**advertising**  See *media*.

**adviser system**  An educational program for supervisory personnel (e.g., sergeants) used in the U.S. Armed Forces in World War II; by alerting such personnel to the emotional, domestic, and physical problems of trainees (inductees, draftees), and the ways in which they were likely to be expressed within their units, the program was able to reduce psychiatric disorders as well as behavior subject to disciplinary action.

**advocacy**  The act of pleading, defending, or interceding on behalf of another. A child advocacy system was recommended in the Report of the Joint Commission on Mental Health of Children (1969), largely in recognition of the fact that the organizational complexity of mental health services was of such degree that few parents had the ability effectively to engage the family and child with the system. Perhaps to a lesser degree, the same complexities render almost all human services relatively inaccessible to the people who need them most. See *expediter; community psychiatry*.

Legal advocacy refers to efforts to establish and enforce legal rights; in psychiatry (as in the rest of medicine), it includes consumer-oriented efforts to improve the quality and quantity of services (*consumerism*) and civil-rights-oriented efforts to protect the freedoms and fundamental rights of patients. See *consumerism*.

**adynamia**  Weakness; asthenia; lack of energy.

**AEDs**  *Antiepileptic drugs* (q.v.).

**AEP**  Average evoked potential. See *potential, evoked*.

**aero-**  Combining form meaning air, from Gr *aer*.

**aero-acrophobia**  Fear of open, high spaces—the morbid dread of being at a great height such as occurs when one is in an airplane. This malady should not be confused with airsickness, which is a disturbance of vertigo-type.

**aeroasthenia**  A form of *aeroneurosis* (q.v.).

**aeroneurosis**  A psychoneurosis or actual neurosis, said to occur among aviators; the symptoms are anxiety, restlessness, and various physical phenomena.

**aerophagia**  Swallowing of air, usually in such quantity as to produce abdominal distention and symptoms of hyperventilation (see *hyperventilation syndrome*). The symptom may be based on unconscious wishes or conflicts, such as pregnancy wishes or cannibalistic impulses.

**aerophobia**  Morbid dread of air, often ascribed to allegedly deleterious airborne influences; sometimes it also includes fear of one's own body odors.

**aeschromythesis**  *Obs*. Obscene language, as in telephone scatologia. See *psychosexual*.

**affect**  The feeling tone accompaniment of an idea or mental representation, representative of the various bodily changes by means of which the drives manifest themselves. The affects regularly attach themselves to ideas and other psychic formations to which they did not originally belong. If an affect is completely suppressed, it may appear not as an emotion but rather as physical changes of innervations, such as perspiration, tachycardia, or paresthesia.

Both "mood" and "affect" are abstractions, referring to a person's disposition to react emotionally in certain specific ways. Inferences about mood stem from present observations and past events, whereas inferences about affect usually stem from present observations only. Affect is the "feeling tone," the fluctuating, subjective aspect of emotion. See *mood*.

**affect, blunted**  See *affect disturbances*.

**affect block**  Inability to discharge emotions adequately or appropriately, seen typically in obsessive-compulsives, who often appear cold, unfeeling, and emotionally stiff and overcontrolled, and also in some schizophrenics. Freud termed this "isolation of affect."

**affect disturbances**  One of Bleuler's fundamental symptoms of the schizophrenias. Typical disturbances include indifference, blunted affect, shallowness, flatness, and constriction of the affects. Early in the course of the disorder there may be oversensitivity, overlability, or sanguineness. Mood is often inconsistent or exaggerated, with a lack of adaptability and of capacity for appropriate modulation of mood tone. Parathymia, paramimia, disharmony of mood, dissociation of affect and intellect, and contradictoriness of emotional expression are also among the schizophrenic disturbances of affectivity.

It is probably the incongruity between the affect displayed and the verbal productions of the patient that is more characteristic of schizophrenia than any other change in affect; lability of affect is seen in many organic brain disorders, and blunting or cooling of affect is particularly frequent in the presenile and senile mental disorders.

**affect hunger** Indiscriminate and insatiable demand for attention and affection, seen often in children who have suffered emotional deprivation. Affect hunger frequently takes the form of aggressive, hostile, antisocial behavior with an inability to accept limitations or recognize the needs of others. See *deprivation, emotional.*

**affect memory** A type of recall memory based on emotions experienced rather than on language. Infant research suggests that the infant is able to encode emotional experiences at least by the age of 7 months and long before the establishment of a language-based memory code. This is in accord with infantile amnesia, which refers to loss of memory for affect-laden experiences but does not involve amnesia for motor memories or semantic memories, because the subject does not forget how to walk or how to speak.

**affect phantasy** Jung's term for any phantasy that is strongly imbued with feelings.

**affectation** Artificiality of manner or behavior. Affectation is a form of simulation in that there is a crudely disguised effort to act as someone else, usually for purposes of gaining esteem.

**affection** A general term, implying feeling and emotion, as distinguished from cognition and volition. Also used to refer to love or positive feelings for another that are not sexual.

**affection, masked** Stekel's term for the kind actions and tender behavior adopted by one person to disguise his or her feelings of hatred for another. See *reaction formation.*

**affection, partial** Suggested by Hirschfield as a synonym for *fetishism.* See *fetish.*

**affectionless psychopath** See *antisocial personality disorder.*

**affective cathexis** See *cathexis.*

**affective dementia** See *affect disturbance; hebetude.*

**affect(ive) disorders** Mood disorders; a group of disorders characterized by a primary disturbance of mood, such as depression or elation. Included are depressive disorders, bipolar disorders, mood disorder caused by a general medical condition, and substance-induced mood disorders (associated with intoxication or withdrawal).

**affective epilepsy** Bratz's term to designate a form of *epilepsy* (q.v.) characterized by exaggerated emotional responses, which generally culminate in an epileptiform seizure. Bonhoeffer referred to such states as reactive epilepsies and Kraepelin classified many of them as epileptic swindlers.

**affective psychosis** A general term used to refer to any of those psychoses whose prominent feature is a disturbance in mood or emotion, viz. manic-depressive psychosis and involutional melancholia. See *affective disorders.*

**affective sensation** See *feeling sensation.*

**affective slumber** See *Alzheimer disease.*

**affective spectrum disorders** Included are major depression, bipolar disorder, schizoaffective disorder, attention deficit hyperactivity disorder, bulimia, cataplexy, irritable bowel syndrome, migraine, and panic disorder. In some classifications, pain disorders and posttraumatic stress disorder are also considered to be forms of affective spectrum disorder.

**affective vectors** The tags used to gain access to previous experience(s) of a currently pertinent nature.

**affective-motivational circuit** One of the networks of the *frontal-striatal system* (q.v.), consisting of projections from the paralimbic cortex (posteromedial orbitofrontal and anterior cingulate) to the *nucleus accumbens* of the striate and thence to the dorsomedial nucleus of the thalamus; this circuit plays a role in emotional or reward-based information processing. See *frontal-striatal system.*

**affectivity**   Susceptibility to affective stimuli: the affects, the emotions, and the feelings of pleasure and pain.

**affectomotor**   Characterized by intense mental excitement and muscular movements.

**affectomotor storms**   Mahler's term for the autonomic lability and overreactivity to shifting internal states characteristic of the *symbiotic stage* (q.v.) and pathologically retained in the borderline and narcissistic personality disorders. (See *borderline personality*, *narcissistic personality*.) In normal development, such storms are allayed by the mother, who takes the baby in her arms and brings it into contact with her body. The mother in such a relationship has been termed the *holding-soothing object*, the *good breast* (M. Klein, 1935), the *good enough mother* (Winnicott, 1965). Aspects and functions of the relationship between mother and infant have been termed *mutual cueing* (Mahler), the *average expectable environment* (Hartmann, 1939), the *facilitating environment* (Winnicott), *mirroring* (Kohut), and the *container-contained maternal function* (Bion, 1967).

**affectualizing**   In transactional analysis, pseudo-emotionality or playacting of feelings.

**Affenliebe**   See *monkey love*.

**afferent**   Moving toward; in neurophysiology, concerned with transmission of nerve impulse into the central nervous system, in contrast to *efferent*, concerned with transmission of nerve impulse away from the central nervous system. See *reflex*.

**affiliative need**   The desire to be associated with or allied with others in order to promote gratification of love, sexual desires, dependency, etc.

**affinal**   Related by marriage.

**affinity**   A marriage partner's relationship contracted with the other partner's (blood) kindred, by the act of marrying. See *kinship*.

**affinity hypothesis**   See *antagonism hypothesis*.

**affliction**   See *disease*.

**AFP**   Alpha-fetoprotein. See *neural tube defect*.

**aftercare**   Continuing treatment and rehabilitation services provided to a patient within the community to which he or she has gone following inpatient hospitalization.

**aftercontraction**   An involuntary movement occurring as a continuation of an original willed, voluntary movement; often utilized as a demonstration of suggestibility in the preinduction period of hypnosis by directing a subject to abduct his arm against a wall and after a few seconds telling him to step away from the wall. In many subjects, the previously abducted arm will then float upward involuntarily.

**afterdischarge**   Continuation of nerve impulse after cessation of the stimulus.

**afterexpulsion**   Secondary repression. See *repression*.

**afterpotential**   See *action potential*.

**aftersensation**   Continuation of sense impression after stimulation of the sense organ has ceased; afterimage.

**agapaxia**   Emotional hypersensitivity and hyperactivity to stimuli, as is seen particularly in persons of above-average intelligence.

**agapism**   The doctrine exalting the value of love, especially in its general, nonsexual sense.

**agastroneuria**   Neurasthenia of the stomach.

**AgCC**   Agenesis or hypogenesis of the *corpus callosum* (q.v.). Approximately 10% of cases have chromosomal abnormalities, and between 20% and 35% have recognizable genetic syndromes. Other cases are due to environmental influences on callosal development, as in the *fetal alcohol syndrome* (q.v.), in which alcohol exposure decreases gliogenesis and glial–interneuronal interactions in the fetus.

**AGCT**   Army General Classification Test of intelligence, used during World War II and after. It is designed for use with literate adults.

**age, basal**   In psychometrics, the highest age level of testing at which the subject passes all the subjects. See *scattering*.

**âge critique**   (F. "critical age") The menopausal or climacteric period. See *developmental levels*.

**âge de retour**   (F. "age of return") The period of old age or senility, when vital powers begin to be or are diminished. See *developmental levels*.

**ageing, aging**   *Senescence*; the natural changes in social, mental, and physical functioning associated with growing older. In medicine, aging denotes the gradual development of changes in body structures (and their functions) that are not due to preventable disease or trauma but are associated with an increased probability of death. Senescence, or *primary aging*, is intrinsic to the organism. Neuropsychiatry tends to focus on the cellular and molecular changes of normal aging that render neurons vulnerable to *neurodegeneration* (q.v.). Numerous genetic and environmental factors counteract or promote that vulnerability.

Brains of older adults have lower volumes of grey matter than younger adults, not because of cell death but because of lower synaptic densities. In healthy older adults, the largest declines in volume are in lateral regions of PFC (prefrontal cortex). Such changes are associated with poor performance on tasks of processing speed, immediate and delayed memory, and *executive function* (q.v.), but not with declines in general intelligence measures. Age-related memory impairment in humans is quite different from that seen even in early *Alzheimer disease* (q.v.). Decreased expression of NMDA receptors in the dentate gyrus has been proposed as one of the reasons for memory defects and for the long-term potentiation deficits that are detectable in healthy elders. After a delay, healthy elders retain new information, whereas patients with mild AD retain little new information.

*Senility*, or secondary aging, refers to defects and disabilities that are outside the range of normal aging, typically manifested as *neurodegenerative diseases* (q.v.). Even in subjects with no more than mild AD, there is extensive loss of neurons in the entorhinal cortex—as much as 50% of the neurons from layer II.

Most of the world sees age-related cognitive decline as a part of expected aging for many people. It has been suggested that *medicalization forces*, particularly Nobel-seeking, profit-making (through pharmaceutical interventions), and scientism in the wealthy countries have produced a search for a neural fountain of youth, ignoring the fact that many will die with cognitive impairment whatever the intervention, because the brain is the most fragile human organ.

**ageism** Stereotyping of elderly people, on the basis of their age alone, in such a way as to create negative expectations of them, discriminate against them, and avoid dealing with their social and physiologic problems. At least in part, ageism may be based on primitive fears of aging and death, but the specific recognized pathologic fear of old age or of aging is termed *gerontophobia*.

**agency** In *social cognitive neuroscience*, one's impression that the action of another is willful and goal-directed. See *theory of mind*.

**agency-centered consultation** See *consultant*.

**agenda, sexuoerotic** See *lovemap*.

**agenesis, agenisia** See *aplasia*.

**agenesis, callosal** Absent or inadequate development of the *corpus callosum* (q.v.). There have been reports that inadequacies in callosal development are more prominent in schizophrenic patients than in normal subjects.

**agenetic** Showing defective or absent development of some part or parts of the body.

**agent provocateur** (F. "instigating agent") Precipitating cause.

**ager naturae** (L. "the field of nature") The uterus.

**agerasia** A youthful appearance in an old person.

**ageusia, ageustia** Absence or impairment of the sense of taste; it may be due to disorder in the gustatory apparatus (i.e., the taste buds). Total ageusia is rare as an isolated neurological symptom; it has most frequently been reported in tumors and demyelination involving the nucleus of tractus solitarius (the gustatory nucleus) in the brain stem.

Ageusia is also seen in psychiatric conditions, particularly in depressed patients who complain that food is tasteless. Ageusia is sometimes a part of depersonalization syndromes, such as occur in hysteria and the schizophrenias.

**agglutination** Condensation of more than one word root or word into a single word. See *contamination; neologism*.

**aggregate field view** The belief that all regions of the brain participate in all mental functioning, a view that developed as a reaction against the localization view (especially as espoused by the 19th-century phrenologists) and against the materialistic philosophy that mind is totally biological. See *connectionism, cellular; equipotentiality*.

**aggregation** Summation; integration; synthesis. Bernard subdivided evolution into five periods, each of which is a result of aggregation such as occurred when unicellular organisms first colonized to produce multicellular organisms (physical aggregation). In the fifth period, in which humans emerge, the aggregation is psychical, occurring through the instinct of gregariousness and leading to the emergence of a "supermind."

**aggresomes** See *microsomes*.

**aggression** Overt behavior that has the intention of inflicting physical damage on another. Aggression is a complex social behavior that evolved in the context of defending or obtaining resources (in particular, food or mates) from competitors. The potential for aggressive behavior exists whenever the interests of two or more individuals conflict; it is motivated by anger, irritation, frustration, fear and, in some cases, pleasure.

In humans, two types of aggression are recognized: reactive and instrumental. Reactive or impulsive aggression is a response to an aversive stimulus, such as an insult, mistreatment, or what is perceived as deliberate provocation. Instrumental or controlled aggression is more purposeful and goal-oriented; it is aggressive behavior that is needed to achieve some other reward, such as money or social acceptance. The controlled-instrumental subtype is thought to be regulated by higher cortical systems and less dependent on the hypothalamic and limbic systems that are known to mediate impulsive aggression. See *instrumental aggression; reactive aggression.*

Mental disorders such as intermittent explosive disorder, PTSD, irritable aggression, and depression-linked aggression are associated with increased autonomic arousal, which can contribute to sudden and uncontrolled reactive aggression. Persons with borderline personality disorder tend to have high scores on measures of impulsive aggression. In contrast, people who are diagnosed with conduct disorder or antisocial personality disorder show unusually low autonomic responsiveness, which can contribute to increased instrumental aggression by blunting the typical emotional responses.

It has been suggested that aggressive behaviors are emergent properties of a *social behavior network* that includes the medial preoptic area, lateral septum, anterior and ventromedial hypothalamus, periaqueductal gray, medial amygdala, and bed nucleus of the stria terminalis (BNST). Many studies have reported a link between brain damage to the frontal cortex and increased aggressive behavior.

Circuits in the hypothalamus and amygdala that might promote aggression receive inhibitory input from the frontal cortex. Amygdala activation is positively correlated with scores on the LHA scale (Lifetime History of Aggression). Persons who rated highly for impulsive aggression had reduced activation of PFC, and SSRIs reduced their ratings of aggression.

Low 5-HT levels are associated with higher levels of impulsivity and aggressiveness. PET scans of humans have shown a negative correlation between LHA scores and 5-HT1A-binding potential, supporting the idea that it has an inhibitory influence on aggression. In general, it appears that 5-HT sets the tension of the 'trigger' for aggression, mainly by limiting impulsivity.

Aggression, aggressiveness, and aggressivity are often used interchangeably, and all have been used with different meanings, including the following: (1) destrudo, the energy of the death drive or *death instinct* (q.v.), as contrasted with libido; (2) ideas or behavior which is angry, hateful, or destructive; (3) activity or action carried out in a forceful way. While the terms "rage" and "hate" are often used interchangeably to indicate intensity of aggression, some would differentiate between them, using "rage" to describe a primitive reaction that occurs before the formation of stable object representations, and "hate" or "hatred" to describe a type of object-directed representation of aggression. Writers often fail to indicate which of the more than 200 definitions of aggression are included in their use of the term. Most agree, however, that an essential element is the intention to harm another, either physically or psychologically, and aggression is thereby differentiated from assertiveness, mastery, etc. See *violence; rage.*

The high level of violence characteristic of many television programs has been of concern to parents, educators, and physicians. The evidence so far available suggests that, far from providing a beneficial catharsis for pent-up feelings, fight scenes and similar aggressive presentations on the screen tend in both children and adults to activate ideas and feelings conducive to aggressive behavior.

**aggression, animal** The following types of aggressive behavior have been distinguished in animals:

1. *Predatory*—evoked by the presence of an object of prey; many workers do not consider this to be true aggression.

2. *Antipredatory*—defense of a territory against an intruder.

3. *Dominance*—evoked by a challenge to the animal's rank or desire for an object.

4. *Maternal*—evoked by the proximity of some threatening agent to the young of the particular female.

5. *Weaning*—evoked by the increased independence of the young when the parents will threaten or even gently attack their offspring.

6. *Parental disciplinary*—evoked by a variety of stimuli, such as unwelcome suckling, rough or overextended play, wandering.

7. *Sexual*—evoked in males by females for the purpose of mating or the establishment of a prolonged union.

8. *Sex-related*—evoked by the same stimuli that produce sexual behavior.

9. *Inter-male*—evoked by the presence of a male competitor of the same species.

10. *Fear-induced*—evoked by confinement or cornering and inability to escape, or by the presence of some threatening agent.

11. *Irritable*—evoked by the presence of an attackable organism or object.

12. *Instrumental*—any changes in environment in consequence of the above types of aggression which increase the probability that aggressive behavior will occur in similar situations.

**aggression panic**   See *homosexual panic.*

**aggressive conduct disorder**   See *conduct disorders.*

**aggressive drive**   In "Beyond the Pleasure Principle" (1920), Freud gave up the idea of ego instincts and divided the instincts into Eros, the libidinal or sexual instinct, and the death or aggressive instinct, which expressed the inertia of living matter. (The energy of the death instinct was called *destrudo* or *mortido* by some of his followers.) Although Melanie Klein is a prominent exception, most analysts today do not accept Freud's last theory of a primary death instinct. See *death instinct.*

In Fairbairn's view, aggression is not an instinct but a reaction to the frustration of libidinal drives. Kohut maintained that aggression is a breakdown product of the sense of self and that there is no primary aggressive drive.

**aging, theories of**   Numerous theories of aging have been proposed, but at best each of them explains only some of the phenomena of aging. Among the major hypotheses are the following:

1. *Genetic redundancy.* Life span is determined by the amount of DNA reserve within the genome that can be called upon to initiate and maintain vital functions.

2. *Watchspring theory.* The organism contains a fixed store of energy and when it is expended life ends.

3. *Free radical theory.* Free radicals are molecular entities that have an unpaired electron, and they have their highest concentration in the mitochondria. Some believe they may be destructive intermediate by-products and that aging is due to loss of ability to destroy them or otherwise defend against them. Others have suggested that free radicals themselves defend the body against invading microorganisms and that aging brings about a loss of their defensive activity.

4. *Accumulation of deleterious material.* An example is lipofuscin (an autooxidation product secondary to the increased degeneration of mitochondria that has been observed in brains of patients with Alzheimer disease); see *mtDNA.*

5. *Biologic programming.* The normal cell contains the memory and capability of ending the life of the cell, and after a determined number of doublings it stops reproducing itself.

6. *Immune system failure.* With aging, immune competence decreases and loss of control leads to the production of self-destructive autoantibodies.

7. *Cross-linkage* or *eversion theory.* The ester bonds that hold each interstitial collagen molecule together switch from within the molecule to between molecules of collagen. As the molecules of collagen become bound together connective tissue loses elasticity and can no longer maintain the structural integrity of tissue and organs.

8. *Aging clock theory.* The hypothalamus is the site of an aging clock, and loss of critical cells in the hypothalamus, whether genetically determined or due to trauma or disease, renders it unable to maintain homeostasis, for it can no longer respond appropriately to changes in the rest of the body.

9. *Cybernetic theory.* Aging is due to neuronal loss, reflected in increasing difficulty in handling information-transfer functions, from environmental inputs.

Various theories emphasize the psychosocial aspects of aging:

1. *Continuity theory.* A person's predispositions, an outgrowth of his or her experiences

in life that reflect the interaction between biological and psychological factors as well as socioeconomic opportunities, determine whether he or she disengages or remains active in old age.

2. *Life-event stress theory* Major life events are inevitable and they determine the person's attitudes toward and activities during old age.

3. *Disengagement theory.* Acceptance of the inevitability of diminishing social and personal interactions with increasing age is associated with a higher degree of satisfaction and better adjustment.

4. *Activity theory.* Continued activity and involvement are essential in order to maintain satisfaction, self-esteem, and health in old age.

**agitated depression** Any *depression* (q.v.) in which restlessness and increased psychomotor activity are a prominent part of the clinical picture; sometimes used interchangeably with involutional melancholia, where agitation rather than psychomotor retardation is the rule.

**agitation** A tension state in which anxiety is manifested in the psychomotor area with hyperactivity (such as handwringing or pacing) and general perturbation. Severe agitation is sometimes termed *jactation* or *jactitation.*

**agitolalia** *Agitophasia; cluttering; klazomania* (qq.v.).

**agitophasia** Cluttered speech due to excessive rapidity under stress of excitement. See *cluttering.*

**agnomenatio** See *homonym.*

**agnosia** Loss of ability to recognize or comprehend the meaning of sensory stimuli, a disturbance of higher-order sensory processing. *Apperceptive agnosia* is impaired ability to comprehend the meaning of an object, yielding a defective minimal object recognition unit. *Associative agnosia* is a dysfunction of postperceptual recognition; the object is correctly perceived but is not associated with its meaning.

*Visual agnosia*—inability to recognize images or visually presented objects—is the most common agnosia; in the language field, both visual and auditory agnosias are essentially aphasias. Other common agnosias are *astereognosia* (inability to perceive the shape and nature of an object and inability to identify it by tactile contact alone); *anosognosia* (ignorance of the existence of disease, especially hemiplegia, or

depersonalization in regard to paralyzed parts of the body); *autotopagnosia* or somatotopagnosia (impairment in ability to identify or orient the body or the relation of its individual parts); *ideational* or *sensory apraxia* is also essentially an agnosia (qq.v.).

*Finger agnosia*, the inability to tell which finger has been touched by the examiner, has been reported to occur in many childhood schizophrenics and in children with *attention deficit hyperactivity disorder.* See *parietal lobe; sensory neglect.*

**agnosia, pain** See *psychosocial dwarfism.*

**agonic social cohesion** See *hedonism.*

**agonist** An agent that stimulates a cell by occupying its receptor site.

**agonist, inverse** An active antagonist that in addition to occupying or blocking a receptor site exerts intrinsic activity.

**agoraphobia** Literally a dread of the marketplace; fear of open spaces. The term is currently applied to the severest form of *phobia* (q.v.), which usually is accompanied by panic attacks.

Agoraphobia is classified within the *anxiety disorders* (q.v.), where it appears as panic disorder with agoraphobia and agoraphobia without a history of panic disorder. Lifetime prevalence of agoraphobia is 5.3%, of full-blown panic disorder without agoraphobia, 3.5%.

The central feature is fear of being in embarrassing situations or in places or situations from which escape might be difficult or in which help may not be available in case of experiencing a *panic attack* (q.v.). Typically, in the late teens or early twenties the subject develops a fear of leaving the security of home following a series of unexpected panic attacks. Next appears anticipatory dread that panic and a feeling of helplessness or humiliation (*catagelophobia*) will return in certain settings or situations such as crowds, stores, elevators, buses, subways, airplanes, theaters, tunnels— any place from which there is no easy escape or access to help. Often the fears spread in time—as from the initial fear of being in a crowded department store, to a fear of taking the bus or crossing the bridge that would get one there, to going into the street in front of one's building, to entering the elevator in the building. The sufferer may finally become completely *homebound*, afraid even to leave the bedroom to go into other rooms of her house or apartment. (Between 65% and 95% of reported sufferers are women.)

It is sometimes easier for the agoraphobic if a specific person (the *phobic companion*) accompanies her; typically, such companionship becomes obligatory for the sufferer, whose demands are so insistent, unreasonable, and exacting that they provoke resentment and avoidance rather that the indulgent succoring that is sought. See *junctim*.

The most effective treatment appears to be a combination of antidepressant drug with behavior therapy (e.g., desensitization, flooding, or in vivo exposure). The antidepressant drug often controls or eliminates the spontaneous panic attacks, but directive or persuasive psychotherapy is usually required in addition to overcome the phobic-avoidant behavior. See *panic disorder*.

Many agoraphobics have been noted to be unusually sensitive to separation, often demonstrated from an early age as in school phobia. Some authorities believe agoraphobia to be a type of separation anxiety disorder. A pathologically lowered threshold for release of separation anxiety is posited by some to be based on a biological predisposition. Others emphasize unconscious conflicts over sexual or aggressive wishes (projected onto the proscribed territory), hostile-dependent conflicts as reenacted in the relationships between the agoraphobic and the phobic companion, object relation experiences with the childhood attachment-autonomy conflict, or pathologic family interactions.

About 80% of persons who develop panic attacks (with or without agoraphobia) have experienced a negative life event closely associated with the first attack: interpersonal conflict (marital or familial) in 34.5%; birth, miscarriage, or hysterectomy in 29%; death or illness of a significant other person in 15.5%; drug reaction in 12%; major surgery or illness in 3%; stress at work or school in 3%; and moving from an old household to a new one in 3%. There is accumulating evidence that panic disorder and agoraphobia are the expressions of a disorder with genetic vulnerability that is distinct from generalized anxiety.

**agrammaphasia**   Ungrammatical, incoherent speech.

**agrammatism**   Ungrammatical speech; a form of *aphasia* (q.v.), in which the patient forms words into a sentence without regard for grammatical rules of declension, conjugation, comparison of adjectives and adverbs, auxiliary verbs, prepositions, conjunctions, articles, etc. Agrammatism is seen most frequently in *Alzheimer disease* and in *Pick disease* (qq.v.).

With some authors, the term is synonymous with *syntactic aphasia*. See *speech disorders*.

**agraphia**   Loss of the ability to communicate (ideas) in writing; a subdivision of *aphasia* (q.v.). This is the motor (or expressive) aspect of the ailment of which the sensory (or perceptive) counterpart is *alexia* (q.v.). The inability may involve individual letters or syllables, words, or phrases, as in varieties of aphasia. Agraphia due to psychic or emotional factors is the graphic counterpart of *mutism* (q.v.). See *acalculia; speech disorders; word blindness*.

**agraphia, congenital**   Failure to acquire any writing ability. Total failure is rare, although varying degrees of difficulty (*dysgraphia*) may accompany other developmental disorders of language or reading.

**agraphognosia**   Inability to identify numbers or letters traced on the palm (or other parts of the body surface).

**agrin**   A protein secreted in different forms by neurons and muscle cells; muscle- and neuron-secreted forms of agrin work together to activate a clustering of receptors that will receive the neurotransmitters released by the presynaptic neuron.

**agriothymia**   *Obs.* Insane ferocity; maniacal furor; at one time synonymous with homicidal insanity.

**agriothymia ambitiosa**   *Obs.* The desire to destroy nations; *Alexanderism*.

**agriothymia hydrophobica**   *Obs.* Irresistible impulse to bite.

**agriothymia religiosa**   *Obs.* The desire to destroy other religions and those cultivating them, as in "holy wars."

**agromania**   Morbid desire to live in the open country, or in solitude or withdrawal.

**AgrP**   Agouti-related peptide, part of the orexigenic pathway in the *hypothalamus* (q.v.).

**agrypnia**   *Obs.* Insomnia.

**agrypnocoma**   *Coma vigil* (q.v.).

**agrypnotic**   Inducing wakefulness; somnifugous; relating to or characterized by insomnia.

**ague, leaping**   Dancing mania. See *choreomania*.

**agyiophobia**   Fear of streets. See *agoraphobia*.

**aha, ah-hah**   A term used to refer to a type of experience in which there is sudden insight into or solution of a problem; at a particular moment, the features of the problem suddenly fit together in a unitary pattern. See *brainstorm*.

**AHS**   *Ammon's horn sclerosis* (q.v.).

**ahypnia**   Insomnia.

**AI**   *Artificial intelligence* (q.v.).

**aichmophobia**   Fear or dread of pointed objects, such as knives, usually associated with the thought of using the feared object as an offensive weapon against someone, even though there is no conscious reason for doing so. The symptom often leads to peculiar eating habits, such as eating alone and without silverware, or to the selection of occupations in which dangerous implements or their symbolic equivalents are not likely to be encountered.

**AID**   Abbreviation for *acute infectious diseases* (usually of childhood); also, more recently, acronym for *artificial insemination by donor*, or for *autoimmune diseases*. See *autoimmunity*.

**aidoiomania**   *Erotomania* (q.v.).

**AIDS**   *Acquired immunodeficiency syndrome*; a cluster of disorders such as Kaposi sarcoma (KS) and opportunistic infections to which the subject is abnormally vulnerable because of the collapse of his or her immune defense system. The cause is a retrovirus, *HIV (human immunodeficiency virus)*, which infects and suppresses the $T_4$ lymphocyte or helper-inducer cell, the focal cell of the immune system. The virus not only reduces the number of $T_4$ cells, it also impairs their ability to propagate and synthesize immunoglobulins. In addition, the virus directly attacks specific types of cells, especially in the central nervous system and lungs. HIV enters the brain in infected monocytes and is stored in *microglia* (q.v.), which are a lifelong reservoir for HIV replication.

HIV enters the body via infected blood, semen, vaginal secretions, or urine and lodges itself in $T_4$ lymphocytes (accounting for its immunosuppressant effects) and in monocytes and macrophages (the source of HIV brain infection). *Seroconversion*, the point at which the blood test for the presence of HIV antibodies gives a positive result, usually occurs between 2 weeks and 3 months after infection, although it can be delayed until 12 to 14 months. The latency period or incubation period—the time from infection to the time of appearance of symptoms of AIDS—may be 3 to 10 years, or even longer.

Following the initial acute infection, the subject may remain well but infectious (i.e., he or she can transmit the virus, through blood, body fluids, and donation of organs, tissues, or sperm). After a variable period of latency, HIV infection may take several forms:

(1) development of lymphadenopathy and other signs of *ARC* (q.v.); (2) progression to classical AIDS, with development of AIDS-related disorders such as lymphoma and Kaposi sarcoma; (3) development of opportunistic diseases because of immune system inadequacy; (4) CNS involvement; and (5) combinations of the foregoing.

The global AIDS epidemic infected an estimated 5 million persons in 2003, bringing the world total of persons living with HIV and AIDS to 40 million. The disease claimed about 3 million lives, the highest toll ever for a single year. Sub-Saharan Africa accounts for about two-thirds of all infections and more than two-thirds of all deaths. One in five adults in southern Africa is infected with HIV.

HIV is also spreading rapidly in Eastern Europe; China, India, Indonesia, and Russia are threatened by a new wave of HIV, spread mostly through injecting drug use and unprotected sex. The most severely affected areas are the Russian Federation, Ukraine, and the Baltic states.

Between 70% and 90% of AIDS patients show histopathologic changes in the brain, and at least half of them have a clinical neurologic disorder during the course of the disease. See *HIV-associated neurocognitive disorders*. The most common CNS disorders are *AIDS dementia complex* (q.v.) and *progressive multifocal leukoencephalopathy (PML)*. Less commonly, the dysfunction is due to well-defined focal lesions, including opportunistic infection by *Toxoplasma gondii*, which may produce seizures or more subtle alterations in mentation and behavior. Myelopathy and peripheral neuropathy are other neurologic complications.

The brain of an AIDS patient typically is shrunken, with dilated ventricles—changes that can be detected in a living patient by CT scan. On microscopic examination, abnormalities are seen in the white matter and the subcortical and limbic areas rather than in the cortex. The white matter does not stain as darkly as normal (for unknown reasons), and in the spinal cord the white matter shows *vacuolar myelopathy*—a bubbly change in myelin tracts. The HIV virus infects macrophages, monocytes, and endothelial cells that line brain capillaries (but not endothelial cells elsewhere in the body). Neurons and glia are minimally affected and there is poor correlation between the severity of neurological symptoms and the degree to which the brain appears abnormal on histologic examination.

**AIDS dementia complex** *ADC*; *HIV-associated dementia (HAD)*; *HIV encephalopathy*; *HIV subacute encephalitis*; a generalized encephalopathy caused by direct attack on central nervous system cells by the human immunodeficiency virus (HIV). The dementia is of the subcortical type, similar to that found in Huntington and Parkinson diseases and in progressive supranuclear palsy. It is rarely confined to the brain; in the spinal cord it produces a characteristic vacuolar myelopathy.

AIDS dementia is the most common cause of chronic neurologic dysfunction in HIV-infected adults and the presenting picture in about 10% of cases. Initial symptoms are impaired concentration, impaired problem solving and reading, and poor control of fine movements. There may be mild memory loss, apathy, and heightened sensitivity to alcohol and other drugs.

In time, there is progression and deterioration in three areas: (1) cognitive—progression from difficulties in concentration to impaired memory, then to disorientation and a confusional state; (2) motor—tremors early, then slurring of speech, followed by gait disturbances, then paraplegia and incontinence; and (3) behavioral—initial withdrawal, followed by apathy and affective blunting, followed by agitation, then paranoid delusions, then hallucinations.

Other CNS manifestations may be the result of toxoplasmosis, lymphoma, herpes encephalitis, or progressive multifocal leukoencephalopathy. See *HIV lymphoma; HIV meningitis; HIV myelopathy; HIV neuropathy.*

**AIDS prodrome** See *ARC.*

**ailurophobia** Fear of cats; *galeophobia*; *gatophobia*. See *phobia.*

**aim** The activity in which an impulse or drive manifests itself and, more specifically, the activity by which the drive or impulse achieves gratification or discharge. The modes of pleasure during the infancy or pregenital period, that is, up to the latency period, chiefly center around the several erotogenic zones (oral, anal, phallic, dermal, muscular, etc.). During the latency period much of the energy and pleasure formerly identified with these zones is deflected by sublimations. The relinquishment of energy from the pregenital areas is called *aim-inhibited*. At puberty there is reanimation of the aim-inhibited tendencies and their somatic manifestations.

**aim of instinct** The aim of an instinct is the reestablishment of that state of relative total organismal balance that existed before the instinct was aroused, through either external or internal stimulation. Cannon coined the phrase *homeostatic equilibrium* for this state of relative harmony and balance, and used the term *homeostasis* for the multiplicity of forces that interact within the organism and react to internal or external stimulation in the direction of equilibrium.

The aim of an instinct must be distinguished from the *object* of that instinct. Water is the object of the instinct of thirst, while the aim of thirst is gratified through the imbibition and absorption of water by the tissues—namely, the disappearance of the unpleasurable state of thirstiness or "thirst."

**aim transference** The transfer of a person's objectives from one life situation to another. Transfer of early aims to the therapeutic situation constitutes the aim transference.

**AIMS** Abnormal Involuntary Movement Scale, for use by the clinician in detecting abnormal oral, facial, arm, leg, and trunk movements. Because the scale is easy to administer, it is often used for serial assessments of patients who develop, or are at risk of developing, dyskinesias as a side effect of treatment (e.g., with neuroleptics).

**Ainsworth Strange Situation** The standard paradigm for the assessment of attachment security; infants are observed as they negotiate a concentrated series of separations from and reunions with the caregiver.

**ainu**  A culture-specific syndrome described in Japanese women, consisting of easily provoked startle responses, automatic responses to commands, and utterances of obscenities.

**AIP**  1. Acute intermittent *porphyria* (q.v.).
2. *Attention and information processing* (q.v.).
3. Anterior intraparietal area; see *intraparietal sulcus*.

**air pollution syndrome**  Symptoms associated with exposure to air pollutants, such as headache, fatigue, irritability, depression, and impaired judgment.

**AIS**  *Androgen insensitivity syndrome* (q.v.).

**akataphasia**  See *acataphasia*.

**akathisia**  Akatisia; *acathisia* (q.v.); a neurologic side effect of treatment with neuroleptics consisting of motor restlessness, a feeling of muscular quivering, and an inability to sit, stand still, or remain inactive. In severe cases, patients pace constantly, forcefully and repeatedly stomping their legs. Those with milder cases show swinging of their crossed legs and foot jiggling, and their symptoms may be misinterpreted as an increase in anxiety. Akathisia tends to develop within the first week of treatment and it is more frequent in females. Some authorities consider it a variant of the *restless legs syndrome* of Ekbom (q.v.).

**Akerfeldt test**  A test for *ceruloplasmin* (q.v.).

**akinesia, akinesis**  Absence or diminution of voluntary motion; it may range from moderate inactivity to almost complete immobility. Ordinarily, it is accompanied by a parallel reduction in mental activity. In the stuporous phase of catatonic schizophrenia, for example, there is almost complete physical and mental immobility.

Akinesia may be circumscribed in the sense that the patient becomes immobile only in a given setting or while under the influence of a particular trend of thought; this is sometimes termed *selective akinesia*.

**akinesia algera**  *Obs.* General painfulness associated with any kind of movement.

**akinetic apraxia**  Inability to carry out spontaneous movements. See *apraxia*.

**akinetic epilepsy**  A type of *petit mal epilepsy* (q.v.).

**akinetic mania**  See *mania*.

**akinetic mutism**  First used by H. Cairns in 1941 (and hence also known as *Cairn stupor*) to describe a state of disturbed consciousness due to a tumor of the third ventricle. The patient lay inertly in bed, mute and almost totally unresponsive, although he followed the movements of people around him with his eyes. The syndrome is probably a result of interference with the reticular activating system, so that response to environmental stimuli is defective. The term has also been used to describe subjects with bilateral frontal lobe lesions who lack all drive and impulse to action, despite intact motor and sensory tracts.

A related condition is *coma vigil* (also known as the *deafferented state, "locked-in" syndrome*, and *pseudocoma*). The subject is conscious and aware but is unable to respond. The lesion is in the ventral pons with preservation of the dorsal tegmental area; the activating system is intact, but interruption of the corticobulbar and spinal pathways makes it impossible for the subject to move or speak.

**akinetic psychosis**  Wernicke's term for that extreme of catatonia marked by stupor, attonita, and cerea flexibilitas. Flexor action of the musculature predominates, and movement may be reduced almost to zero. At the other extreme of catatonia is the *hyperkinetic motor psychosis* (catatonic excitement).

**akinetic-abulic syndrome**  A group of symptoms that frequently appear in the course of treatment with neuroleptics: pseudoparkinsonism (tremor), bradykinesia, hypertonia, decreased mental drive, and lack of interest.

**akinetopsia**  The inability to perceive moving stimuli, usually a result of bilateral damage to the middle temporal area.

**akoasm**  Also akouasm, acoasm, acouasm; a nonverbal auditory hallucination, such as hearing buzzing, crackling, ringing, and the like. The more complicated hallucinations that are reported as "voices" by the patient are verbal auditory hallucinations or *phonemes* (q.v.).

**akoluthia**  Semon's term for a phase of engraphy corresponding to what others have termed *primary memory* or *memory in the making*.

**Alajouanine syndrome**  (Theophile Alajouanine, French neurologist, 1890–1980) A congenital neurological disorder with lesions of cranial nerves VI and VII, double facial paralysis, convergent strabismus, and double clubfoot.

**alalia**  Speechlessness; loss of ability to talk. It was used in the 18th and into the 19th century for what is now generally denoted by *aphasia*. At present the *-lalia* frequently used in constructions like *echolalia* and *bradylalia* connotes *talking* rather than *speaking*—saying, i.e., the exercise of the power of talking as contrasted with the faculty for significant or meaningful speech. See *speech disorders*.

**Al-Anon**  A self-help group fellowship of spouses, children, and relatives of alcoholics who are usually part of an AA group. Al-Anon was developed as a parallel but separate movement to *Alcoholics Anonymous* (q.v.) in the late 1940s. Since then, *Alateen* has developed as a similar network of voluntary support groups composed of the teenaged children of alcholics.

**alarm, learned**  See *interoceptive*.

**alarm reaction**  The first stage of the *general adaptation syndrome* (q.v.). The alarm reaction is a response to stress and as observed in experimental animals consists of adrenocortical enlargement with histologic signs of hyperactivity, thymicolymphatic involution, gastrointestinal ulcers, and often other manifestations of damage or shock.

**Alateen**  See *Al-Anon; Alcoholics Anonymous*.

**Albright disease**  A syndrome consisting of multiple pseudocysts in the skeleton, segmental pigment disorders of the skin, and *pubertas praecox* (q.v.); the disease is due to hypothalamic-hypophysial dysfunction.

**Albright osteodystrophy**  Pseudohypoparathyroidism. See *G protein*.

**albuterol**  A *beta blocker* (q.v.).

**ALC**  Alternate level of care; services provided by a hospital to a patient even though services at an inpatient level are not necessary. Most patients receiving such services are suitable for skilled nursing or health-related services, but they are retained in hospital because the other services are not locally available.

**alcohol**  Unless otherwise qualified, *ethanol* (ethyl alcohol), or beverages containing ethanol (*alcoholic beverages*), although the term in fact is a generic one for a group of organic chemical compounds that contain one or more hydroxyl (-OH) groups. The simplest alcohol is *methanol* (methyl alcohol, *wood alcohol*), used primarily as an industrial solvent. It is highly toxic and if ingested may produce blurred vision, blindness, coma, and death. See *alcoholic beverage*.

Alcohol is the most widely used psychoactive drug in Western countries; it is a central nervous system depressant similar to the *barbiturates* and other *sedatives/hypnotics* (q.v.). Up to a certain magnitude, an intake per time unit can be dealt with effectively by several metabolic degradation systems. Beyond that level, however, the capacity of those systems is exceeded and the pharmacological and toxic properties of alcohol become apparent in one or more organ systems. The extent of damage to those systems depends both on individual susceptibility and on the dosage, frequency, and persistence of drug use. In addition to central nervous system effects, the many possible physical complications include liver disease, gastritis, pancreatic disease, vitamin deficiencies and other nutritional disorders, cardiovascular abnormalities (including cerebrovascular accident), immune system disorders, endocrine abnormalities, various malignancies, and disorders of bone, muscle, skin, lungs, and blood-forming organs. See *alcoholism; BAL; dependence, drug*.

**alcohol abuse**  Ingestion of ethyl alcohol in a quantity and with a frequency that causes the user significant physiological, psychological, or social distress or impairment. Criteria include failure to fulfill major role obligations at work, school, or in the home; use in hazardous situation (e.g., driving while intoxicated); legal problems; and continued substance use despite persistent or recurrent related social or interpersonal problems in the absence of dependence. In the Collaborative Study on the Genetics of Alcoholism (Schuckit et al., *Alcoholism: Clinical and Experimental Research 26*: 980–987, 2002), more than three-quarters of subjects diagnosed with alcohol abuse without dependence endorsed only one criterion. The analysis also supported the high prevalence of hazardous use (92.0%), compared with interference with social functioning (23.1%), impaired role functioning (6.8%), and alcohol-related legal problems (1.6%).

**alcohol addiction**  Physiological and psychological dependence on alcohol; *alcoholism* (q.v.).

**alcohol dementia**  A gradually progressive dementing disorder manifested clinically by evidence of diffuse cerebral dysfunction: affecting not only memory (as in *Wernicke-Korsakoff syndrome*, q.v.), but also thinking, orientation, comprehension, calculation, learning capacity, language, judgment, emotional control, and social behavior. Some authorities doubt that alcoholic dementia occurs as a discrete syndrome and ascribe the dementia to other causes. See *dementia*; *alcoholic encephalopathy*.

**alcohol dependence** *Alcoholism* (q.v.); chronic loss of control over the consumption of alcoholic beverages, despite obvious psychological or physical harm to the person. Increasing amounts are required over time, and abrupt discontinuance may precipitate a withdrawal syndrome. Following abstinence, relapse is frequent.

**alcohol flush reaction** Flushing of the face, neck, and shoulders and often also nausea, tachycardia, and faintness following ingestion of alcohol. Such a reaction is provoked by *Antabuse* (q.v.), and it also occurs in half or more of some Asian groups as a result of a genetically determined aldehyde dehydrogenase insufficiency.

**alcohol idiosyncratic intoxication** In DSM-IV, this is not a separate entity but is considered, instead, a form of alcohol intoxication.

**alcohol use** Among youths aged 2 to 17, alcohol use was reported in 25% in 1990, in 18% in 1993. But more than 1.2 million young people reported having at least five alcoholic drinks on one occasion within a 2-week period in 1993, and alcohol use is believed to contribute significantly to other data: every day (in 1993) approximately 25 young people were infected with HIV, and over 1000 young females gave birth out of wedlock. In the same year, more than 18 million people in the United States needed treatment for alcohol or drug abuse.

**alcohol use, unhealthy** The spectrum of alcohol use disorders, including the following:

1. *Risky use*—for women and persons over 65 years of age, more than seven standard drinks per week or more than three drinks per occasion; for men under 65, more than 14 standard drinks per week or more than four drinks per occasion. A *standard drink* is defined as 12–14 grams of ethanol, corresponding to 12 ounces of beer, 5 ounces of wine, or 1.5 ounces of of 80-proof liquor. There is no evidence of dependence or other alcohol-related consequences, but there is risk of future physical, psychological, or social harm with increasing levels of consumption. *Binge drinking* (q.v.) is sometimes included within this category and is defined as prolonged use (more than 1 day) with cessation

of usual activities, or as drinking that exceeds the specified drinks per occasion.

2. *Problem drinking* (q.v.).

3. *Alcohol abuse, harmful use*—recurrence of any of the following impairments within 12 months: failure to fulfill major role obligations, use in hazardous situations, alcohol-related legal problems, or social or interpersonal problems caused or exacerbated by alcohol use.

4. *Alcohol dependence, alcoholism* (q.v.).

**alcohol use disorders** These are classified within the substance-related disorders; among the various syndromes associated with alcohol use are *alcohol abuse, alcohol dependence, alcohol intoxication, alcohol withdrawal* (qq.v.), alcohol delirium, alcohol persisting dementia, alcohol psychotic disorder (delusions, hallucinosis, etc.), alcohol-induced mood disorder, alcohol-induced anxiety disorder, alcohol-induced sleep disorder, and alcohol-induced sexual dysfunction. See *alcoholism; delirium tremens*.

**alcohol withdrawal** In a person with a pattern of heavy or prolonged drinking, symptoms develop within hours of cessation of drinking or of significant reduction in amount ingested: hand tremor and a variety of other signs and symptoms that may include nausea and vomiting; anxiety; autonomic hyperactivity manifested in sweating and increased pulse rate; agitation; insomnia; perceptual disturbances, such as transient visual, tactile, or auditory illusions or hallucinations with intact reality testing; and grand mal seizures. See *delirium tremens*.

**alcohol-Antabuse reaction** See *Antabuse*.

**alcoholic** Descriptive of a person who has experienced physical, psychological, social, or occupational impairment as a consequence of habitual, excessive consumption of alcohol. See *alcoholism*.

**alcoholic beverage** A liquid intended for consumption that contains ethanol. Nonbeverage alcohol refers to products containing alcohol that are not intended for consumption, such as mouthwashes and rubbing alcohol.

Fermentation of sugar by yeast yields ethanol. Under natural conditions, the conversion of sugar to alcohol stops when the alcohol concentration reaches 12%–14% (as in unfortified wines and beers). Distillation, introduced by the Arabs in the 9th century A.D., boils alcohol out of its mixture with sugar and recollects it in almost pure form. The distilled alcohol is then diluted with water to bring it to the desired strength, or "proof," which is twice the alcohol concentration (e.g., a beverage containing 50% alcohol by volume is 100 proof). Other chemicals (congeners) are added to give a distinctive color and taste.

Alcoholic beverages differ according to their source of sugar: grapes (wine, 24 to 28 proof), grain (beer and ale, 8 proof), grain and potatoes (vodka), rye or corn (whiskey), or sugar cane (rum). "Hard" liquors, such as whiskey, vodka, and gin, are 86 proof. Brandy is made by distillation of the fermented juice of grapes or other fruit; sherry is fermented grape juice fortified with brandy to bring it to approximately 40 proof.

**alcohol(ic) deterioration**   A complication of *alcoholism* (q.v.) characterized by emotional blunting, organic memory defect, and deterioration in the moral and ethical spheres.

**alcohol(ic) encephalopathy**   Any disturbance of brain function due to alcohol, including alcohol intoxication, alcohol idiosyncratic intoxication, alcohol withdrawal, alcohol withdrawal delirium, alcohol hallucinosis, alcohol amnestic disorder, and dementia associated with alcoholism. For many, the term implies a persisting disturbance such as Karsakoff disorder. Some writers use the term for miscellaneous organic mental syndromes due to alcohol that are not classified elsewhere. Others use the term to refer to more subtle cognitive deficits that appear in subjects who have been heavy drinkers for 10 years or more. See *alcoholism; alcohol intoxication; delirium tremens; Wernicke-Korsakoff syndrome.*

**alcoholic epilepsy**   A variety of manifestations associated with alcoholism and seizures. An alcoholic may experience an epileptiform seizure; or a person with epileptoid personality may try to solve his personality difficulties through alcohol; or the alcoholism and epilepsy may be more or less independent of each other. See *delirium tremens; epilepsy.*

**alcohol(ic) hallucinosis**   *Alcoholic withdrawal hallucinosis*; a form of acute hallucinosis seen in alcoholics following an unusual excess of alcohol intake or as part of an abstinence syndrome. The condition is relatively rare in the female. It consists of auditory hallucinations that appear in a clear intellectual field without confusion or intellectual impair-

ment. The hallucinations persist even when all other symptoms of withdrawal have disappeared. There is a slow return to normal within a period of weeks; however, recurrence is frequent,.

**alcohol(ic) intoxication**   Alcohol poisoning; the state resulting from excessive ingestion of alcohol; an acute brain syndrome that develops as a result of overdose of alcohol. This syndrome may be of two varieties: (1) acute intoxication, or (2) pathologic intoxication (also known as *mania à potu*).

*Acute intoxication*: Alcohol is a physiological depressant, but the release from higher control as a result of this depression leads to an initial heightening of physical and mental activities and to a greater psychomotor speed; during this initial period, organic tremors may be decreased. With increasing depression, however, there soon appear generalized muscular weakness, impairment of intellectual functions, and, because the cerebellar system is attacked early, ataxia, reeling gait, and coarse incoordination of the upper extremities. The marked loss of inhibition typically gives rise to many medico-legal problems. Walking a chalk line, repeating certain paradigmata, and chemical analysis of the breath, urine, and blood have all been used to determine the degree of intoxication, but none of these is completely valid because of the adaptation of the central nervous system to alcohol. Tolerance to alcohol varies greatly; the epileptic, the hysteric, many schizophrenics, and some psychopaths have a low tolerance, as do patients following a head injury. See *amethystic.*

*Pathologic (idiosyncratic) intoxication*: This occurs predominantly in people with a low tolerance to alcohol. Usually the syndrome lasts several hours, although it may continue for a whole day. It is characterized by extreme excitement ("alcoholic fury") with aggressive, dangerous, and even homicidal reactions. Persecutory ideas are common. The condition terminates with the patient falling into a deep sleep; there is usually complete amnesia for the episode.

**alcoholic Korsakoff psychosis**   When associated with alcoholism, the *Korsakoff psychosis* is also known as *chronic alcoholic delirium* and alcohol *amnestic disorder* (q.v.). Some authors also refer to it as chronic *delirium tremens*, because the syndrome frequently follows (acute) delirium tremens. Bleuler says that "the Korsakov psychosis in the majority of cases begins with a delirium tremens that recedes somewhat slowly and leaves behind the organic syndrome." The basic symptom picture includes memory defects, confabulations, impairment of apperception and attention, disorientation, ideational and affective disorders, in addition to such physical symptoms as are associated with general neuritis (pains, paralyses, atrophies, etc.) (*Textbook of Psychiatry*, 1930). See *Korsakoff psychosis; Wernicke-Korsakoff syndrome.*

**alcoholic melancholia** Delusional depression secondary to alcoholism, similar to that of major depression except that the delusions remain rudimentary and rarely last longer than 2 weeks.

**alcoholic paranoia** An inexact term, used by some writers as equivalent to *alcoholic hallucinosis* (q.v.), by others to refer to infidelity delusions that develop in alcoholics. Although alcoholics can develop any of the forms of *paranoia* (q.v.), they seem especially prone to jealousy delusions.

**alcoholic paranoid state** A chronic condition, presumed to be primarily of organic origin, consisting of persisting infidelity or jealousy delusions, that appears mainly in male alcoholics. The condition is very rare, and many doubt that it exists at all.

**alcoholic pseudoparesis** *Obs.* Alcoholic encephalopathy with *dementia* (q.v.), ideas of grandeur, hallucinations, delusions of jealousy, sometimes Argyll Robertson pupils, speech defect, tremors, and polyneuritis. Epileptiform attacks are frequent.

**alcoholic twilight state** A type of pathological intoxication, characterized by "sudden excitations or twilight states set free by alcohol, usually with mistaking of the situation, often also with illusions and hallucinations, and excessive affects, most of anxiety and rage. In individual cases the entire morbid process can transpire in hardly a minute, but it usually lasts longer, up to several hours" (Bleuler, E. *Textbook of Psychiatry*, 1930). See *alcoholic intoxication.*

**Alcoholics Anonymous (AA)** A nonprofessional organization of alcohol-dependent persons, formed in 1935 by an Akron physician and a New York broker, devoted to the achievement and maintenance of sobriety of its members through self-help and mutual support. Since its founding, Alcoholics Anonymous has expanded into an international movement. Its principles include (1) a belief in God or natural law, (2) frank self-appraisal, (3) a willingness to admit and correct wrongs done to others, (4) a trust in humankind, and (5) dedication to the rescue of those who sincerely desire to conquer alcoholism by making them members of the organization as successful abstainers.

No studies of more than 2 years have been conducted to assess the efficacy of AA or other treatments for alcoholism, even though it is generally agreed that a minimum of 5 years is needed to demonstrate success of a treatment program. Nonetheless, AA's approach is widely endorsed, because it combines four factors that have been found to be associated with relapse prevention: external supervision, encouragement of a competing dependency (such as food), development of a new love relationship, and increased spirituality (Vaillant, G. E. *Psychiatric Services* 55: 11–12, 2004).

**alcoholism** *Alcohol dependence.* See *dependence, drug.* In 1990, the American Society of Addiction Medicine defined alcoholism as a primary, chronic disease with genetic, psychosocial, and environmental factors influencing its development and manifestations. The disease is often progressive and fatal. It is characterized by continuous or periodic impaired control over alcohol drinking, preoccupation with the drug alcohol, use of alcohol despite adverse consequences, and distortions in thinking, most notably denial.

"Primary," in this context, underscores that alcoholism, as an *addiction* (q.v.), is not a symptom of an underlying disease state but is a disease (i.e., an involuntary disability) in its own right. *Impaired control* is the inability to limit alcohol use or to limit consistently on any drinking occasion the duration of the episode, the quantity consumed, or the behavioral consequences of drinking. Preoccupation indicates excessive, focused attention given to the drug, alcohol, its effects, or its use. Such relative overvaluation (*salience*) often leads to a diversion of energies away from life concerns that should be of importance to the subject. Denial is used not only in the psychoanalytic sense of a single psychological defense mechanism disavowing the significance of events, but also more broadly to include a range of psychological maneuvers designed to reduce awareness of the fact that alcohol use is the cause of the subject's problems rather than a solution to them.

Some workers maintain that physical dependence (as manifested by tolerance or withdrawal) is necessary to warrant the diagnosis of alcoholism; subjects who do not demonstrate physical dependence but show other patterns of compulsive use are given the diagnosis *alcohol abuse* (q.v.). Many writers avoid the word abuse on the grounds that it implies that the drinker could stop "if he really wanted to" or that it has the same pejorative implications as child abuse and self-abuse. As a result, *problem drinking* is sometimes used as an equivalent for alcohol abuse (see *alpha alcoholism*).

Because there are varieties of alcoholism, many theories of origin of the different varieties, and many ways in which those variants can affect the drinker or society, there is no agreed-upon, fixed terminology. The lines between "normal" social drinking, heavy drinking, problem drinking, and alcohol dependence are far from clear, and most workers in the field have been forced to construct ad hoc definitions of terms according to the focus of their investigations of *drinking behaviors* (q.v.).

Most investigators feel that alcoholism is a group of disorders. It is a genus with many species, according to Jellinek, who differentiated various forms phenomenologically: *alpha alcoholism, beta alcoholism, gamma alcoholism, delta alcoholism,* and *epsilon alcoholism* (qq.v.)

A more recent differentiation is based on the high prevalence of depression in alcoholics. Alcoholics have also been classified on the basis of time of onset of heavy or problem drinking.

Theories of the etiology of alcoholism abound. Psychodynamic explanations have been generally unsatisfactory. Early psychoanalytic studies implicated a specific oral craving in the genesis of alcoholism—frustration by an overindulgent mother, combined with an inconsistent or absent father, enforces a retreat to the earlier oral megalomaniacal phase of passive gratification.

In the United States, the family constellation of indulgent mother with inconsistent or absent father is considerably more common than alcoholism; no study has demonstrated that a particular personality type or a particular neurosis is characteristic of alcoholic persons. The psychologic factors adduced are not specific enough to indicate why alcoholism rather than some other disorder is their result or why particular social, racial, or economic groups are so susceptible to their influence. Various mental disorders may be associated with or result from alcohol ingestion and alcoholism. See *alcohol use disorders*.

Adoption studies clearly reveal a major genetic component in alcoholism, but it occurs in more than one genetic form (genetic heterogeneity). As of October 2006, 188 variants in genetic material located at 51 sites that may contribute to alcoholism have been identified. Three of the variants cluster on chromosome 7, near the area that codes for the neuropeptide S receptor; four of the variants on chromosome 3 lie within the gene that codes for the angiotensin II receptor. The genes with the strongest association with alcoholism are those that encode the major enzymes in alcohol metabolism, alcohol dehydrogenase genes (*ADH2* and *ADH3*, on chromosome 4), and *ALDH2*, an aldehyde dehydrogenase gene on chromosome 12. Three polymorphisms have been identified for *ADH2* (*1, *2, *3), two for *ADH3* (*1, *2), and two for *ALDH2* (*1,*2). The *ALDH2*2* polymorphism (which is very prevalent in Asian populations) has the strongest protective association with alcohol dependence, probably because the isoenzyme it encodes leads to impaired conversion of acetaldehyde to acetate, resulting in elevated levels of acetaldehyde, greater sensitivity to alcohol, and less alcohol consumption. *ADH2*2* and *ADH3*1* might also be associated with lower risk for alcohol dependence.

The hypothesis that a gene encoding a particular variant of the $D_2$ receptor for dopamine is related to the risk of alcoholism has not been substantiated. The genetic influences, which probably involve multiple genes, appear to be separate from a generic predisposition toward dependence on other drugs. Low level of response to alcohol at age 20 has been found to be predictive of alcoholism by the age of 35. Low responsivity may be one genetically influenced factor that contributes to 40% or more of the variance of alcoholism risk related to genetic factors.

**alcoholophilia, -mania**  *Rare.*  Craving for alcohol.

**alcohol-related deaths**  Automobile accidents related to alcohol use accounted for 9.8% per 100,000 deaths in 1990, for 6.8% in 1993.

**alcohol-sensitizing drugs**  See *acetaldehyde; Antabuse.*

**alcoolization**  See *delta alcoholism.*

**alector**  A person who is unable to sleep.

**alerting response**  See *alpha blocking.*

**alerting system**  See *reticular formation.*

**Alexander, Franz**  (1891–1964) Hungarian psychoanalyst; trained with Sachs and Abraham in Berlin; in 1929 appointed the first Professor of Psychoanalysis at the University of Chicago; chief contributions were in the areas of brief analytic therapy and psychosomatic medicine.

**Alexander disease**  A rare brain disorder characterized by macrocephaly and seizures, due to defects in the glial fibrillary acidic protein gene (GFAP), which appears as cytoplasmic inclusions in astrocytes. This is the first genetic brain disorder attributed to a defect in astrocytes.

**Alexanderism**  *Obs.* (From Alexander the Great) *Agriothymia ambitiosa* (q.v.).

**alexia**  An acquired disorder in reading ability, consisting of an inability to recognize words presented visually. It is often associated with lesions of the left medial temporo-occipital cortex, a region that in humans is distinct from areas activated during the processing of other visual features, such as faces and colored patterns. See *word blindness.*

Alexia is to be differentiated from *dyslexia*, which is a developmental problem in reading. (Strictly speaking, lexis and its derivatives refer to speech, not reading, because they are based on the Greek verb *legein*, to speak, and not on the Latin verb *legere*, to read. Current usage appears to reflect an etymologic error, so long accepted that to insist on correcting it would be useless.) See *acalculia; occipital lobe; reading disabilities; speech disorders; Potzl syndrome.*

**alexia, congenital**  Failure to acquire any reading ability; a rare disorder, usually associated with profound mental retardation. See *developmental disorders, specific; dyslexia.*

**alexithymia**  Difficulty in describing or recognizing one's emotions; suggested by P. Sifneos to describe those persons who define emotions only in terms of somatic sensations or

of behavioral reaction rather than relating them to accompanying thoughts. Characteristics are difficulties in identifying feelings and distinguishing between feelings and the bodily sensations of emotional arousal, and in describing feelings to other people; constricted imaginal processes (e.g., paucity of phantasies); and a stimulus-bound, externally oriented cognitive style. Alexithymia is sometimes described as the opposite of *creativity.*

Primary alexithymia is described as a personality trait, characterized by difficulty in identifying one's emotional state, with minimal phantasy life and inability to phantasize productively, and a focus on external and somatic concerns.

Secondary alexithymia is a "state" reaction to the effects of serious physical illness, perhaps a defense against depression or pain, or both. Some believe alexithymia reflects an absence of the ego functions that subserve affect and phantasy, but most writers explain it as due to primitive ego defenses that hide and distort the conscious experiences of affect and phantasy.

There is evidence that in some cases, a contributing factor is defective interhemispheric communication or inhibition of corpus callosum activity. It has also been suggested that alexithymia reflects a dysregulation of the anterior cingulate cortex that results in enhanced phenomenal awareness of positive affect and reduced awareness of the subject's current negative affect.

**alexithymic deficit model**  See *deficit model.*

**algedonic**  Characterized by or relating to pleasure and pain, or the agreeable and the disagreeable.

**-algesia**  Combining element meaning pain, from Gr. *algesis*, sense of threshold or limen of pain, the point at which pain registers in consciousness.

**algesimeter**  Same as *algometer* (q.v.).

**algolagnia**  Any psychosexual disorder in which physical or mental pain is an essential part; algolagnia may be active (*sadism*) or passive (*masochism*).

**algometer**  *Algesimeter*; an instrument that purports to measure sensitiveness to pain in terms of amount of pressure exerted on the skin by a blunt instrument.

**algophily**  *Rare.* A term coined by Féré (*L'Instinct Sexuel*), equivalent to masochism.

**algophobia**   Abnormal fear of pain.

**algopsychalia**   See *psychalgia*.

**algorithm, clinical**   *Flow chart* or *decision tree*; a graphic presentation of the sequential steps to be taken in making decisions about the diagnosis and treatment of a clinical problem.

**ALI**   American Law Institute; the ALI test or formulation is often used to establish an *insanity defense* (q.v.). See *criminal responsibility*.

**Alice in Wonderland effect**   *Metamorphopsia* (q.v.).

**alien hand sign**   A type of apraxia that may occur with lesions of the *corpus callosum* (q.v.): the hand (usually the left) performs actions independent of the subject's will.

**alienatio mentis**   (L. "alienation of the mind") Insanity.

**alienation**   1. A general term, now largely restricted to forensic psychiatry, indicating mental or psychiatric illness or insanity; when used in this way, alienation is ordinarily qualified by the adjective *mental*.

2. The repression, inhibition, blocking, or dissociation of one's feelings so that they no longer seem effective, familiar, or convincing to the subject. Such alienation of feelings is characteristic of obsessive-compulsive disorder; it may also be seen in the schizophrenias. Alienation may also reflect dysfunction of the dominant parieto-temporal lobe.

3. A mode of experience in which the person feels out of touch with himself; the syndrome often includes uncertainty about what role is expected of the person, doubt about his own decisions, loss of selfhood, dehumanization, and feelings of helplessness and futility. See *identity crisis*; *parietal lobe*; *sensory neglect*.

**alienist**   *Obs*. The specialist in psychiatry from the standpoint of law.

**alimentary orgasm**   Rado's term for the feeling of bliss and rapid reduction in tension experienced by the infant at the height of breast feeding; he related the wish to reexperience alimentary orgasm to mania, melancholia, and drug dependency.

**allachesthesia**   Referral of a tactile sensation to a point remote from the point of stimulation; *allesthesia*. Usually, the displacement of sensation is symmetrical; it suggests a temporal lobe lesion.

**allachesthesia, visual**   A rare phenomenon, suggesting a parietal lobe lesion, consisting of referral or transposition of visual images to an opposite point in space.

**Allan Dent disease**   *Arginosuccinic aciduria* (q.v.).

**allegoric interpretation**   "A view which interprets the symbolic expression as an intentional transcription or transformation of a known thing is allegoric" (Jung, C. G. *Psychological Types*, 1923). See *semiotic*.

**allele**   Also, allelomorph; one of several alternative forms of a gene. In a natural population, any gene at any locus will exist in a number of different although clearly related forms, called alleles. If a trait depends on a gene at a given locus, one allele may be dominant over the other (and the other is then recessive to the first).

Three or more genes occupying the same locus in homologous chromosomes in a species are called multiple alleles. The best known instance of multiple alleles in humans is in the blood groups.

Testing of *candidate alleles* is a relatively new approach in genetics that looks for a relation between the phenotype and a variant that alters gene structure and the function or expression of the gene product. It asks how a functional variant of a gene (the allele) is related to a phenotype. See *linkage*.

**allelic, allelomorphic**   Pertaining to or having the nature of an *allele* or *allelomorph*.

**allelic association**   See *recombination fraction*.

**allesthesia**   See *allachesthesia; sensory neglect*.

**alliance and splitting**   In a weak or ineffective parental coalition, the assumption of the dominant role by one (typically the mother), who forms a coalition with the children, thereby consigning the other parent to a marginal, split-off, and noninvolved role.

**allo-**   Combining form meaning different, other.

**alloch(e)iria**   A neurologic disorder in which the location of touch or pain sensations is transferred to a corresponding place on the part of the body opposite to that stimulated.

**allocortex**   *Rhinencephalon* (q.v.); a part of the olfactory and allied systems of the cerebral cortex. The term is used primarily in reference to the cytoarchitecture, or microscopic structure, of the cortex, in which case the allocortex is contrasted to the neocortex or *isocortex* (q.v.).

**allodynia**   Perception of a stimulus as painful when previously the same stimulus was reported to be nonpainful; characteristic of neuropathic pain. Long believed to be due to changes at the inflammation site(s) of the pain, hyperalgesia or *pain sensitization* is now recognized to be even more closely related to spinal cord changes. The α3 glycine receptor, which suppresses neuronal firing, is a key intermediate in transmitting pain signals from the spine to the brain. Prostaglandin E2 (PGE2) inhibits the glycine receptor, thereby facilitating transmission of pain signals to the brain and promoting pain sensitization.

**alloerotism, alloeroticism**   In classical psychoanalytic theory, the final phase in the development of object relationships, marked by a stable integration or fusion of the drives and their deflection into appropriate channels; also known as the phase of impersonal socialization, adult sexuality, and mature genitality. See *ontogeny, psychic; postambivalent stage.*

**alloesthesia**   *Allachesthesia* (q.v.).

**allokinesis**   A type of central sensitization for itch in which touch triggers the sensation of itch.

**allolalia**   Any unusual or abnormal form of speech.

**allometry**   In comparative biology, similarity based on physical accident rather than a common functioning background. See *analogy; homology.*

**allophasis**   *Obs.* Incoherent speech.

**alloplasticity**   *Acting out* (q.v.), often an expression of depression in children and adolescents.

**alloplasty**   Adaptation by means of altering the external environment; contrasted with *autoplasty* (q.v.).

**allopsyche**   The mind or psyche of another.

**allopsychic delusion**   See *autopsychic delusion.*

**all-or-none reaction**   In psychiatry the expression means that instinctive processes, when stimulated, respond with full force or not at all.

In neurophysiology, the all-or-none (or all-or-nothing) principle refers to the fact that individual neurons either transmit their messages maximally or not at all. Differences in intensity are conveyed by means of spatial and temporal summation of impulses.

**allostasis**   Biophysiological adaptation to acute stress, including all the changes in the internal milieu that are required to maintain homeostasis in order to protect the organism and ensure its survival. Once the acute stress has subsided, recovery requires other adaptive mechanisms to come into play to ensure that the organism does not remain in a state of acute stress

response. Failure to terminate the acute adaptive response appropriately has adverse consequences on both psychological and physiological functioning. Those adverse consequences are the "allostatic load" or burden borne by brain and body; they may manifest themselves in diverse ways, such as post-traumatic stress disorder, depression, immunosuppression, hypertension, cognitive impairment, abnormalities in motivation and reward mechanisms, cardiovascular events, etc.

**allosteric receptor**   See *neurotransmitter receptor; synapse.*

**allotriogeustia, -geusia**   1. Abnormal sense of taste.

2. Abnormal appetite.

**allotriophagy**   Impulse to eat unnatural foodstuffs; *pica* (q.v.).

**allotriorhexia**   Compulsive plucking out of threads of clothes; usually the threads are then swallowed (*allotriophagia*).

**allotropy**   Adolf Meyer's term for *allopsyche.*

**Allport, Gordon Willard**   (1897–1967) U.S. psychologist and educator; developed a holistic psychology of human behavior, the core concepts of which are the *proprium* (the nuclear self or self-concept, consisting of those habits, attitudes, and values that are deeply ego-involved) and the *personal disposition* (the hierarchy of perceptual-motivational-behavioral unities that characterize a person). Allport suggested that many therapeutic failures occur because the therapist keeps doggedly probing for infantile motivations in a personality that has been organized around adult roles and conflicts.

**allusive thinking**   *Loosening* (q.v.) of associations; ideas are transmitted by inference and suggestion rather than directly, concepts seem diffuse and amorphous, and argument is often by analogy that seems irrelevant to the matter at hand. Even though found in many schizophrenic subjects, it also occurs in a significant percentage of normal subjects; there is some evidence that this type of thinking is inherited.

**alogia**   1. Speechlessness usually due to intellectual deficiency or confusion. See *speech disorders.*

2. The lack of spontaneity and flow of conversation characteristic of the schizophrenic *deficit state* (q.v.).

**aloneness, autistic**   Kanner's term for the lack of desire for human contact that is a leading symptom of early infantile autism. See *autistic disorder*.

**Alpers disease** *Poliodystrophy, progressive infantile cerebral* (q.v.).

**alpha alcoholism** Psychological dependency on alcohol, which is used to relieve bodily or emotional pain; there is no loss of control, nor are there signs of progression to physiological dependence. Drinking is undisciplined, however, in regard to time, occasion, locale, amount, and behavioral effects. This type of alcoholism is sometimes called problem drinking, escape drinking, symptomatic or reactive alcoholism, dyssocial drinking (if effects are manifested chiefly in the family, social, or vocational sphere), or thymogenic drinking (if alcohol is used in a conscious effort to overcome social discomfort or to relieve emotional pain). See *alcoholism*.

**alpha arc** The sequence of a stimulus leading to motor behavior via a simple sensorimotor path. *Beta arc* refers to arousal of higher cortical paths by the functioning of an alpha arc (thus leading to a "sensation" rather than simple "awareness"), and not directly by an outside stimulus. The term alpha arc is approximately equivalent to *immediate response* in Watson's behavioristic psychology, while the term beta arc is roughly equivalent to Watson's *delayed response* or *implicit behavior*.

**alpha blocking** Also, *alerting response; arousal response; desynchronization*; the disappearance of alpha activity on the EEG when the subject is stimulated or when the eyes are opened. See *electroencephalogram*.

**alpha EEG activity** See *sleep*.

**alpha function** *Toilet-function; toilet-breast function*; Wilfred Bion's term for conversion of raw sense data (*beta elements*) into meaningful, integrated experiences. When alpha-function fails, raw sense data are undigested and unintegrated; beta elements are expelled by projective identification (q.v.) into the mother, who assimilates and converts them into alpha elements, which can then be taken back (introjected) by the infant. In therapy, the toilet-function of the analyst acts in similar fashion: the analyst assimilates, understands, and interprets material that can then be introjected by the analysand in a digested form. The analysand thereby comes to understand the meaning of the raw data, is helped to maintain the separation between self and

object, is supported in the capacity for reflection and ego structuring, and also gains an internal object onto which anxieties can be deposited.

**alpha rhythm, alpha wave** Oscillations of the electrical potential of the brain that occur at a frequency of 8–13 Hz. The alpha rhythm is the standby mode of the brain; *gamma rhythm* (q.v.) is the work mode. Standby activity over the cortex involved in movement and touch is sometimes called *mu*, or *motor alpha*; the standby rhythm for hearing is called *tau*, or *hearing alpha*. See *electroencephalogram*.

**alpha sleep** A *sleep disorder* (q.v.) of the DIMS class with atypical polysomnographic features, consisting of the superimposition of alpha (high voltage) waves on the sleep EEG. In normal *sleep* (q.v.), alpha activity is decreased, but in alpha sleep there is *riddling* of the NREM sleep EEG. REM sleep is usually spared. The patient complains of interrupted and nonrestorative sleep. Alpha sleep may be idiopathic, or it may occur for a long period following withdrawal from drugs or alcohol.

**alpha tests** A series of mental tests, first used in the United States military service (1917) to determine the relative mental ability of recruits. There were eight different types of test: for directions, arithmetical ability, practical judgment, synonyms and antonyms, correct arrangement of sentences, completion of series of digits, analogies, and information. The tests were designed particularly for group application and for rapid mechanical scoring.

**alpha wave training** A type of *biofeedback* (q.v.). Alpha brain waves (7.5–13.5 cps) are characteristic of relaxed and peaceful wakefulness (the alpha state). In alpha biofeedback training, the subject receives information on his EEG as a means of achieving the alpha state (relaxation). In one technique, a tone sounds in the absence of alpha waves and disappears when the subject produces alpha waves.

**alpha-adrenergic** See *adrenergic*.

**alpinism** A nonspecific term referring to neuropsychiatric syndromes appearing in relation to low atmospheric pressure, such as the asthenia syndrome of persons living in high altitudes.

**ALS** *Amyotrophic lateral sclerosis* (q.v.).

**alter** The other; the person in any social interaction with whom one interacts. See *dissociative identity disorder*.

**altered mind/body perception** Any of a group of altered states of consciousness that are

presumed to exist on a continuum ranging from ecstatic experiences of heightened
awareness to disorganizing episodes of psychotic decompensation with loss of identity.
Characteristic is a subjectively experienced
distortion of the normal spatial relationship
between body and mind. The term includes
out-of-body experiences, near-death experiences, body boundary disturbances, *autoscopy*,
and *depersonalization* (qq.v.).

**alter-ego transference**  *Twinship transference*; one
of the three major types of *self-object transference* described by Kohut (the other two are the
*mirroring* and the *idealizing* transferences).
Alter ego or twinship needs are expressed as a
need to feel that one is like other people; the
other person is experienced as a twin, exactly
like oneself. With development, this comes to
be a feeling of belonging. Lack of satisfactory
twinship self-objects in early life may result in
an intensified need for a twin in adulthood.
The person with an alter ego personality confirms his or her reality by forming a relationship with someone who shares his own values, interests, and convictions. Such twinship
needs are also expressed in the transference
relationship to the therapist. See *idealization;
mirroring; mirroring needs.*

**alter-egoism**  Altruistic feelings limited to others who are in the same situation as oneself.

**alternate care**  See *ALC.*

**alternating personality**  *Dual consciousness;* the
*split personality* seen in *dissociative identity
disorder* (q.v.); the subject lives now as one
person and then as another (as in the case of
Dr. Jeckyll and Mr. Hyde), but never as two
persons simultaneously.

**alternating psychosis**  Bipolar disorder in which
manic episodes alternate with depressive episodes in the same patient; originally described
by Falret, Jr., as *folie circulaire.* It is not as
common as either the recurrent depressive or
the recurrent manic type of *manic-depressive
psychosis* (q.v.).

**alternative group session**  A regularly scheduled
meeting of a therapy group that is held in the
absence of the therapist; often scheduled at
weekly intervals and sessions may be held in
the therapist's office or at the home of one of
the group's members.

**alternative medical therapies**  *Complementary
medicine; holistic medicine* (qq.v.).

**alternative psychologies**  Nontraditional approaches
to an understanding of human behavior

with emphasis on practical application,
consciousness raising, achievement of potential, and self-determination. They are based
on a variety of doctrines and philosophies,
including (1) elements from well-established
psychodynamic schemes, such as Jung's analytical psychology, Reich's orgone theories,
and Gestalt theory; (2) data from neurophysiological studies such as altered states
of consciousness, brain wave patterning, and
biofeedback; (3) mystical or Eastern philosophies, such as yoga, Zen Buddhism, Taoism,
astrology, the occult, parapsychology, psychical research; and (4) popular movements
such as est and sensitivity training. See *complementary therapy.*

**alternative splicing**  See *transcription.*

**alters**  Also known as alter personalities, personality states, subpersonalities, identities,
parts, disaggregate self states, and *ego states*
(q.v.), alters are fragmented parts of one person, expressing the structure, conflicts, deficits, and coping strategies of the mind of the
person with DID, *dissociative identity disorder*
(q.v.).

Alters have four characteristics that are not
intrinsic to the ego state: (1) they have their
own identities, involving a sense of self; (2)
they have a characteristic self-representation,
which may be discordant with how the subject is generally regarded; (3) they have their
own sense of autobiographic memory and
distinguish their own actions and experiences
from those of other alters; and (4) they have
a sense of ownership of their own experiences
and thoughts and may disavow ownership of
or responsibility for the actions and thoughts
of other alters.

Alters may be unaware of each other, but
more commonly there are varieties of asymmetric amnesia in which some alters know
about others but are not known by all of those
of whom they are aware. The alters often
interact in an "inner world" in which their
separate memories of "real world events" are
stored but typically severed from indicators
of their origin (*source amnesia*); events from
their inner world may be reported as occurrences in external reality. Some people with
DID create a protector or consoling friend
for each new trauma-based alter; others harbor rebirth phantasies and replace alters from
the "bad old days" with new, undamaged versions of themselves. Alters often regard the

host as simply another alter rather than as the core representation of the person.

Therapists who treat patients with DID feel that it is essential to work with alters; if individual alters are not dealt with, the mistreatments the patient suffered in childhood by the inattention and invalidation of the parent are recapitulated, reenacted, and legitimized.

The concept of multiple personalities and alters is a controversial one. Some deny that they exist at all as an independent presentation of a syndrome by a patient, claiming instead that such states are the responses of suggestible patients to the influence of the therapist. See *false memory*.

**altrigenderism**   The state of being attracted to the other gender. Beginning in the late infantile period the child takes an interest, to a greater or lesser extent, in members of the other gender, i.e., of the opposite sex. Altrigenderism refers to nonsexual relationships between persons of different genders. When the interests become amorous, though not overtly sexual, *heteroerotism* is the proper term. When the sexual element (without sexual congress) enters into these relations, the condition is called *heterosexuality*, while heterogenitality as a term is limited to sexual intercourse. None of these terms is in common use, and all of them are considered outmoded.

**altruism**   Regard for the interests and needs of others; a term coined by the French philosopher Auguste Comte (1798–1857), who maintained that the chief problem of existence is "vivre pour autrui" (to live for the sake of others). See *sociobiology*.

A behavioral trait is considered to be phenotypically *altruistic* if possession of that trait benefits the survival of some other organism, while the trait is phenotypically *selfish* if its possession benefits its owner's own personal survival. Similarly, a behavioral trait is genetically selfish if the effect of the behavior is to increase the likelihood of the organism's passing along copies of its own genotype to future generations, while the trait is genetically altruistic if its effect is to increase the likelihoood of genotypes different from its own being passed on.

**altruistic filicide**   See *infanticide*.

**altruistic suicide**   See *anomie*.

**alveolar hyperventilation syndrome**   See *pickwickian syndrome*.

**alveolar hypotension**   See *apnea, central*.

**alysm, alysmus**   *Obs*. Restlessness exhibited by a sick person.

**alysosis**   *Otiumosis*;   boredom,   sometimes appearing as a central phenomenon in the simple form of schizophrenia.

**Alzheimer disease**   (Alois Alzheimer, German neurologist, 1864–1915) In DSM-IV, a cognitive disorder termed *dementia of the Alzheimer type (DAT)*; Alzheimer disease (AD) now includes primary degenerative dementia (PDD) of both senile and presenile onset. It is also called *senile dementia, Alzheimer type (SDAT); dementia, Alzheimer type (DAT)*; and *simple senile deterioration*. AD is a genetically heterogeneous, progressive, neurodegenerative disorder of late-life onset characterized clinically by memory loss and other disorders of cognitive function.

Alzheimer disease is the predominant cause of dementia in late life and ranks fourth or fifth as the cause of death in the United States, accounting for about 100,000 deaths a year. Alzheimer disease affects between 17 and 20 million people worldwide. Average course of AD from onset to death is 5 years, with a range of one to 10 years.

Symptoms and signs progress through two phases, the early confusional or forgetfulness phase and the later phase of severe dementia. The major forms of neurodegeneration in AD are *amyloid plaques*, neurofibrillary tangles, and loss of synapses. Amyloid plaques arise from abnormal proteolytic processing of the amyloid precursor protein (APP), an integral membrane protein present in many cell types, including neurons and glia. Neurofibrillary tangles (*aygyrophilic dystrophy, paired helical filaments*) are the consequence of microtubule destabilization and aggregation of the microtubule-stabilizing protein tau. Plaques and tangles may be both causes and indicators of the neuronal malfunction that ultimately leads to synapse loss. The resulting reduction in neuronal connectivity is the most likely explanation for the memory loss and progressive dementia that are the classic clinical signs of AD.

PET provides greater diagnostic accuracy than standard clinical assessment methods. The characteristic parietal and temporal deficits observed on a PET scan can be recognized years prior to clinical confirmation, particularly when combined with genetic risk measures (APOE-4). Most of the studies have used PET to measure regional glucose metabolism, which reflects neuronal activity. More recently, methods have been developed for PET to provide measures reflecting the concentration of amyloid plaques and neurofibrillary tangles.

The most consistent neurotransmitter abnormality is decrease in brain choline acetyltransferase, the enzyme necessary for the synthesis of acetylcholine. Almost all studies have found abnormalities in multiple brain systems: monoaminergic (in the locus ceruleus and raphe complex) and glutamatergic (marked in the hippocampus and medial temporal lobe), and neuronal death in these areas leads ultimately to disconnection of the hippocampus and the neocortex), as well as in the cholinergic system (which innervates the amygdala, the hippocampus, and the neocortex). Treatments devised to replace acetylcholine have not been notably effective, however.

The neocortex and hippocampus are both affected by AD. The most vulnerable circuit in the cerebral cortex is the *perforant path*, which originates in layer II of the *entorhinal cortex* (EC) and terminates in the outer molecular layer of the *dentate gyrus*, thus providing the key interconnection between the neocortex and the hippocampus. The EC is a region of convergence of inputs from the association cortex; it funnels highly processed neocortical information into the dentate gyrus and plays a crucial role in memory.

Etiology of AD is unknown. Among the possible etiologic factors are brain inflammatory changes; deposition in the brain of a small neurotoxic protein, β-amyloid; excess phosphate addition to tau; possession of a particular variant of a cholesterol-carrying protein, apoE4 (which may inhibit the growth of the projections neurons use to communicate with one another); and mutation in presenilin genes 1 and 2.

Early-onset (familial) AD is associated with various mutations in different genes: five mutations of the APP gene (chromosome 21), and mutations of the presenilin genes PS1 (chromosome 14) and PS2 (chromosome 1). The known genetic alterations underlying familial AD increase the production or deposition (or both) of the Aβ in the brain. Late-onset AD is associated with the ApoE gene (chromosome 19) and, tentatively,

with mutations in the genes for *LRP-LDL receptor-related protein* (chromosome 12), $\alpha_2$-macroglobulin ($\alpha_2$M; chromosome 12), a third chromosome 12 gene product distinct from the preceding two, and *FE65* (chromosome 11), a cytoplasmic scaffold protein that interacts with the APP and LRP cytoplasmic domains. A mutation on chromosome 10 has been identified in a small group of AD patients. See $\alpha_2$-*macroglobulin ($A_2M$); apolipoprotein E*. Various other gene mutants are under investigation, such as *SORL1* and *VPS35*. Yet, despite decades of research, no key genetic factor has yet been identified. The e4 variant of the APOE gene on chromosome 19 is the best documented risk factor for AD. It accelerates the deposition of plaques, which are composed mostly of the β-amyloid protein; yet a *de*creased concentration of the protein in CSF is a diagnostic biomarker for established AD.

AD is not a single-gene disease. The available evidence favors a model of the disease in which diverse gene defects (some of which remain to be identified) lead to enhanced production, increased aggregation, or perhaps decreased clearance of Aβ peptides. These effects allow accumulation first of the highly self-aggregating $A\beta_{42}$ peptide and later the $A\beta_{40}$ peptide. The result is microglial and astrocytic activation, with concomitant release of cytokines and acute-phase proteins. Local neurons are damaged by such "inflammatory" changes or by direct Aβ neurotoxicity. Aβ is an early pathogenic factor in all known forms of familial AD, but it must be followed by many molecular and cellular changes before sufficient injury to limbic and association cortices results in symptoms of dementia.

Not all workers agree that beta amyloid deposition is the major cause of damage in Alzheimer disease. They believe instead that the disease is a chronic inflammatory disease involving the immune system, similar to arthritis. Both views may be correct, in that it is possible that beta amyloid is directly toxic to nerve cells and that it becomes even more so by activating the cell-killing complement proteins of the immune system. See *amyloid; apolipoprotein E; NFT*.

Esquirol first used the term demence senile in 1838. In 1907 Alzheimer described a type of presenile dementia accompanied by senile plaques and neurofibrillary tangles occurring in persons under 65. Arnold Pick had described presenile dementia in 1902. Until the 1960s, senile dementia was believed to be due to arteriosclerotic disease, but that is now recognized to be a relatively infrequent cause of senile or presenile dementia and is classified as a separate disorder, *vascular dementia* (see *cerebral arteriosclerosis*).

**α₂-macroglobulin (α₂M)** There is evidence that a common mutation in the gene encoding α₂-macroglobulin (A₂M) raises susceptibility to developing *Alzheimer disease* (q.v.) with increasing age. The number of AD cases that might be linked to the mutation is unknown, but it could be large, because an estimated 30% of the population carry the mutation. The normal A₂M protein binds to several potentially toxic proteins, rendering them harmless. Among those toxic proteins are the small protein β amyloid. The mutation may slow or eliminate the protective cleanup effect, leading to amyloid deposition and nerve cell death.

A₂M may prevent amyloid deposition by binding to the peptide and transporting it into cells for degradation, a step using the same receptor that apoE uses to enter cells. ApoE4 or excess amounts of other apoEs might block the A₂M-amyloid complex from binding to the receptor, preventing A₂M from removing the toxic amyloid. A₂M has paradoxical effects on one protease: it prevents the protease from degrading large proteins, but at the same time it triggers the protein to break down β-amyloid and thereby prevents toxic amyloid deposits from forming. The A₂M protein also interacts with a variety of cytokines, which influence immune activity; this suggests that A₂M might somehow dampen dangerous inflammatory reaction in the brain.

A₂M also binds to β-amyloid itself, preventing the formation of the insoluble amyloid fibrils that are most toxic to neurons, and by binding to LRP (low-density lipoprotein receptor-related protein) it allows the cells to take up and degrade the A₂M-amyloid complex.

**amantadine** An antiviral drug with antiparkinsonian activity, which is assumed to be due to dopamine augmentation.

**amathophobia** Fear of dust.

**amaurosis** Complete blindness. See *optic nerve*.

**amaurosis fugax** Fleeting blindness, which may be caused by transient ischemia of the retina.

**amaurotic family idiocy** See *Tay-Sachs disease*.

**amaxophobia** Fear of being in a vehicle.

**ambi-** Combining form meaning both.

**ambiguity, genital** *Hermaphroditism* (q.v.); intersexuality; failure to differentiate fully as either male or female: the newborn's sex cannot be determined on the basis of visual inspection.

**ambiguous loss** A situation in which the loved one is psychologically present but physically absent (such as the family of a person who might have been killed in the 9/11/01 attack on the World Trade Center in New York), or the loved one is physically present but psychologically absent (because of dementia or traumatic brain injury). The uncertainty of not knowing inflicts a state of suspension: how should the family cope with the swirl of emotions (anxiety, powerlessness, depression, guilt) that envelops them? Should they mourn, even though the loved one may not be dead? How can they find closure?

Pervasive cultural training exhorts people to control situations and find solutions. But in the case of ambiguous loss, there is no way to exert control. Instead of blaming themselves needlessly for failing to find a solution, persons in such a situation must learn to move beyond their cultural training, to realize they can live with ambiguity and temper their need for control. As a cynic once noted, "If there is no solution, there is no problem."

**ambilevous** Poor in manual dexterity with both hands; "doubly left-handed," clumsy.

**ambisexual** Having characteristics of both sexes, pertaining to anything that is shared by both sexes; bisexual. Strictly speaking, what is confined to males is masculine, what is confined to females is feminine, and everything that is sex-shared is ambisexual or bisexual. In practice, however, the terms refer not to what only men or only women do in fact, but to what they should (or should not) do according to the preferences and dictates of society. Thus bisexual is often used in a pejorative sense to indicate that something the speaker believes to be appropriate to one sex is manifested by a member of the other sex, who is therefore labeled as deviant or abnormal.

**ambitendency** Ambivalence in action. Bleuler equated ambivalence of the will with ambitendency. See *ambivalence*.

**ambition**  Psychodynamically, ambition represents a fight against *shame* (q.v.) by proving that there is no need to be ashamed anymore. Intense ambition is one of the major characteristics of subjects with *narcissistic personality disorder* (q.v.). See *aggression*.

**ambition, negative**  Reik's term used to describe the behavior of masochist who evades every possibility of achieving his goal: he seems to follow the line of greatest resistance against himself, instead of that of greatest advantage for himself. The negative ambition is a grim reversal of an originally strong and positive ambition, in such a way that every opportunity is missed, every chance of success is turned into failure, every competition is avoided.

**ambition, self-assertive**  See *cohesive self*.

**ambitious mania**  *Obs.* Delirium grandiosum; *megalomania* (q.v.); folie ambitieuse.

**ambitypic**  Belonging to both types; most frequently applied to the sexual bipotentiality of the mammalian (including the human) embryo. In the beginning, the gonads are undifferentiated and only during the course of development do they take form as testicles or ovaries. In accord with what has been termed the *principle of feminization*, the gonads will take the feminine form unless something is added to induce *masculinization*.

In the human, such masculinization is dependent upon two masculinizing hormones: (1) the müllerian-inhibiting hormone, which causes the embryonic müllerian ducts to atrophy and thus prevents them from developing into a uterus with bilateral fallopian tubes; and (2) *testosterone*, which actively induces the growth of masculine internal genitalia.

The external genitalia, by contrast, are *unitypic* rather than ambitypic: they cannot be both male and female simultaneously. Like the internal genitalia, the sexual centers and pathways of the brain are *dimorphic* or ambitypic, and the primary masculinizing hormone that acts upon them is testosterone.

**ambivalence, ambivalency**  *Bipolarity*; the coexistence of antithetic emotions, attitudes, ideas, or wishes toward a given object or situation. The term was coined by Bleuler, who differentiated among affective or emotional ambivalence, intellectual ambivalence, and ambivalence of the will. In current usage, the term ambivalence without further

qualification ordinarily refers to affective ambivalence.

Ambivalence is characteristic of the unconscious and of children. Its overt appearance in the adult implies the presence of definite pathology, such as obsessive-compulsive psychoneurosis, manic-depressive psychosis (bipolar disorder), or schizophrenia. See *splitting*. Ambivalence is one of the fundamental symptoms of schizophrenia (Bleuler), where it may appear in any one or more of its three forms.

In affective ambivalence, the very same concept is accompanied simultaneously by pleasant and unpleasant feelings; thus, a patient suffers the most intense anxiety that "they" will shoot her and yet constantly begs the doctor to shoot her. In ambivalence of the will, the desire to do a certain thing is accompanied by a desire not to do that thing. Thus a patient demands work only to become furious when something is given him to do. In ambivalence of the intellect, an idea appears simultaneously with the counter-idea. One schizophrenic patient complained that he had no face and yet asked for a razor to shave the beard off his face. Ambivalence of the will and intellect are often at the basis of what is considered to be obsessive doubting in schizophrenic patients.

**ambivalent**  Relating to the coexistence of antithetic emotions.

**ambiversion**  The balance of the two traits, introversion and extraversion.

**amblyopia**  Dimness or partial loss of vision without discoverable lesion in eye structures or optic nerve; often it appears to develop as a result of intoxication with drugs, including tobacco. See *optic nerve*.

**ambulatory insulin treatment**  A modification of insulin coma treatment consisting of intramuscular injection of relatively small doses of insulin, until hypoglycemia is reached. It has been observed that such subcoma treatment often relieves severe anxiety, tension, and anorexia; the mechanism of action is unknown. Also called *subshock* or *subcoma insulin treatment*.

**ambulatory schizophrenia**  *Obs.* The disease of the group of schizophrenics who, on the surface, appear normal, but can suddenly commit acts that reveal their abnormality. The puzzling aggressive, asocial acts committed by apparently sane persons have very often turned out to be acts of ambulatory schizophrenics.

**ambulatory treatment** Therapeutic measures carried out while the patient is up and about or is not hospitalized.

**amelectic** *Rare.* Indifferent, careless, apathetic.

**amenomania** *Obs.* The manic phase of bipolar disorder.

**amentia** *Obs.* Mental retardation; intellectual inadequacy. Amentia implies that the diminished intellectual capacity has been present from birth; in contrast, *dementia* (q.v.) implies that intellectual capacities were once intact but have since been dissipated, injured, or destroyed. Different degrees of amentia were often specified by those who used the terms *idiocy* for what would currently be labeled profound retardation (Wechsler IQ below 25), *imbecility* for severe to moderate retardation (IQ, 25–54), and *feeblemindedness* or *moron* for mild retardation (IQ, 55–69). See *retardation, mental.*

**amentia, developmental** Mental retardation that appears to be occasioned in part by genetic and in part by environmental factors, and particularly retardation with psychosocial (environmental) deprivation.

**American Law Institute test** See *insanity defense*; *criminal responsibility.*

**Ameslan** American Sign Language; see *sign language.*

**amethystic** Anti-intoxicant; sobering; protecting from drunkenness. Used particularly in relation to alcohol in the sense of a "sobering-up" drug. Many substances have been tried—among them acetylcholine, caffeine, GABA, analeptics, and cations—but none of them has been effective as an amethystic agent. To date, the most effective pharmacodynamic antagonist of intoxication has been *naloxone* (q.v.), but its use in such cases has been limited. See *alcohol intoxication*; *antidipsotropic.*

**ametropia** A refraction error in which parallel rays are focused not on the retina itself but in front of it (*myopia*) or behind it (*hyperopia*).

**amimia** A disorder of language, characterized by the inability to use gestures appropriately to conform with the idea to be expressed. The person with amimia may also be unable to imitate or reproduce by motion the facial expressions and gestures of others. He may likewise make the inappropriate or wrong gestures in endeavoring to convey his thoughts or feelings, e.g., shaking his head sideways when saying yes, and nodding his head when saying no. This is the motor (or expressive) aspect of amimia.

Its counterpart is sensory (or perceptive) amimia when the patient does not understand or assigns a wrong meaning to another's gesture, taking a sidewise shake of the head to mean consent, and a nod to mean disapproval. See *aprosodia; temporal lobe syndromes.*

**amine** An organic substance containing the radical group $NH_2$. Some biogenic amines work as neurotransmitters. They include the catecholamines (such as dopamine, norepinephrine, and epinephrine), the indoles (such as serotonin), *acetylcholine*, and *histamine* (qq.v.). See *catecholamine; indole.* The biogenic amine neurotransmitters are spread throughout major brain areas. The neurons in which they are synthesized usually have their cell bodies located in the reticular core within the brain stem. See *neurotransmitter.*

**amine oxidase** *Monoamine oxidase* (q.v.).

**aminergic pathways** There are three major aminergic systems: (1) the noradrenergic or ceruleospinal—see *locus ceruleus*; (2) the dopaminergic; there are about three or four times as many dopaminergic neurons as noradrenergic neurons in the brain—see *dopamine*; and (3) the serotonergic, the most extensive aminergic system in the brain stem; most of the neurons arise within the *raphe nuclei* (along the midline seam of the medulla, pons, and midbrain), and their projections to the hippocampus, neostriatum, and cerebral cortex exert mainly an inhibitory action.

**amino acids** Acids containing an amino group, typically in the form of $R$-$CH$(-$NH_2$)-$COOH$. Of the 20 amino acids that are incorporated into the proteins of all cells, some act as neurotransmitters: glutamate, aspartate, and glycine. Glycine is a transmitter in spinal cord inhibitory interneurons. Glutamate and aspartate are products of the Krebs cycle.

Glutamate is an excitatory neurotransmitter. GABA, which is synthesized from glutamate, is a major inhibitory neurotransmitter. Depending on the area of the brain involved, between 25% and 40% of neurons use GABA as a neurotransmitter. Between 25% and 30% of synapses in the brain stem and cord use glycine.

**Amish inbreeding & hereditary disorders** See *glutaric aciduria.*

**amixia** Restriction of marriage to one race, caste, etc., to prevent miscegenation.

**Ammon's horn sclerosis** *AHS*; a histopathological condition often associated with temporal lobe epilepsy, characterized by selective neuronal cell loss and reactive sclerosis in the CA1 and CA4 regions of the hippocampus.

**AMN** Adrenomyeloneuropathy. See *adrenoleukodystrophy.*

**amnemonic** Relating to loss of memory.

**amnesia** Inability to recall past experiences; loss of memory. *Anterograde amnesia* refers to inability to form new memories, either because of failure to consolidate what is perceived into permanent memory storage, or because of inability to retrieve memory from storage. *Retrograde amnesia* refers to loss of memory for events that occurred prior to the event or condition (toxin, trauma, vitamin deficiency, etc.) that is presumed to have caused the memory disturbance in the first place. See *amnestic syndrome; memory.*

Amnesia is associated with lesions of the *medial temporal region* (and, in particular, the *hippocampus*) and of the midline diencephalic region (and, in particular, the mediodorsal thalamic nucleus and the mammillary nuclei). Amnesic patients with damage to medial temporal areas have impairment of explicit memory, in the presence of normal implicit memory. There may be a *double dissociation* between subjects with damage to the medial temporal system and those with damage to the striatum. A double dissociation is demonstrated when amnesics fail explicit memory tasks and succeed at procedural tasks, and when subjects with Huntington disease (HD) or Parkinson disease (PD) fail procedural tasks but have preserved explicit memory. See *memory; MTL.*

Even small lesions in the inferomedial portions of the temporal lobes, and especially in the amygdala, hippocampus, fornix, mammillary bodies, and medical dorsal nucleus of the thalamus—the area that constitutes the *limbic lobe*—can produce a permanent dysmnesic syndrome with little disturbance in other aspects of mental functioning. The importance of this area is further attested by the symptom of *panoramic memory*, a well-recognized temporal lobe aura. Bilateral hippocampal lesions produce deficits in learning ability and in remote memory (or habit retention), but they do not have such a predictable effect on short-term memory.

In the usual form of amnesia due to brain deamage, *short-term memory* is intact but *long-term memory* (qq.v.) in the sense of the ability to form new permanent memories is impaired. Rarely, the reverse is found.

It is also recognized that learning occurs in both the cerebellar cortex and the deep cerebellar nuclei, which are critical for regulating the timing of movements. The cerebellum is involved in diverse cognitive and noncognitive neurobehavioral systems, including the attention and motor systems.

Amnesia may be psychogenic as well as organic in origin. Psychogenic amnesia is prominent in *multiple personality disorder* (q.v.), in which there is sudden inability to recall important personal information that is too great to be explained by ordinary forgetfulness. The subject may experience blank spells, memory lapses, blackouts (gaps in the experience of time) or gray-outs (partial or intermittent memory for a particular period), uncertainty about whether a specific activity has been carried out or has only been thought about, fugues (finding oneself in a place without knowing how one got there), or fragmentary recall of life history and sometimes complete amnesia for the first 9 or 10 years of life.

**amnesia, anterograde** See *retrograde amnesia.*

**amnesia, circumscribed** See *retrograde amnesia.*

**amnesia, continuous** Anterograde amnesia. See *retrograde amnesia.*

**amnesia, generalized** Total loss of autobiographical memory; particularly if it is of sudden onset, suggestive of a *dissociative disorder* (q.v.)

**amnesia, psychogenic** A dissociative disorder consisting of sudden onset of an episode of inability to recall important personal data. The amnesia may be *localized* (all memories for a period of hours or days surrounding a given event are lost), *generalized* (memory for the subject's entire lifetime is lost), *selective* (involving some memories but not all), or *continuous* (all memories subsequent to a specific time are lost, including the present, and the subject is unable to form new memories even though appearing to be alert and aware). See *amnesia; dissociative identity disorder.*

**amnesic syndrome** Profound loss of distant memory in a subject whose intelligence and recent memory are otherwise intact; related to bilateral lesions of the hippocampus and mammillary bodies. See *amnestic syndrome.*

**amnestic aphasia**  *Anomic aphasia* (q.v.).

**amnestic disorders**  In DSM-IV, a group of *cognitive disorders* that includes amnestic disorder due to a general medical condition and substance-induced persisting amnestic disorder. See *amnestic syndrome*.

**amnestic syndrome**  One of the forms of *organic mental disorders* (q.v.), consisting of impairment of *short-term memory* (i.e., unable to recall items 25 minutes after their presentation) but not of immediate memory (i.e., patient has a normal digit-span). Because of short-term memory impairment, memories are not consolidated and stored, or cannot be retrieved from storage; as a result, new memories cannot be formed (anterograde amnesia). Almost always there is some degree of retrograde amnesia, disorientation, apathy, inertia, and emotional blandness. *Confabulation* (q.v.) may occur. The amnestic syndrome is rare and usually occurs in association with alcoholism. See *Wernicke-Korsakoff sydrome*.

**amnestic syndrome, malignant**  See *Alzheimer disease*.

**amok**  Malayan for battling furiously (a variant spelling is *amuck*); a culture-specific syndrome of the Malayan peninsula consisting of an explosive outburst of homicidal fury, vented indiscriminately against anyone who happens to cross the subject's path. The outburst is often preceded by a period of mild depression, which is sometimes related to a recent loss or an experience that made the subject "lose face." Once the episode is over, the subject is amnesic for the episode and may commit suicide.

Another Malayan term for the attack is *matal elap* (darkened eye). The syndrome occurs almost exclusively in Malayan males; it has been reported on occasion in African and other tropical cultures.

**amor lesbicus**  Sapphism. See *homosexuality, female*.

**amorous paranoia**  *Obs.* By some, used to refer to the jealous or infidelity form of paranoia; by others, used to refer to the erotomaniacal form. The patient with amorous paranoia develops delusions of marital infidelity in relation to his spouse. According to Freud's analysis of the Schreber case, such delusions are based on a denial of unconscious homosexuality: "It is not I who love the man, it is she." See *jealousy, morbid*.

**amorphosynthesis**  Faulty perception of the form of objects; one type of amorphosynthesis is *metamorphopsia* (q.v.).

**amorphous communications**  See *communication, disordered*.

**amotivational syndrome**  Passivity, lack of interest, loss of drive; "dropping out," and difficulties in attention and concentration, described by some as the usual effect of long-term marijuana use. See *residual*.

Some use the phrase *amotivational states* to refer to *deficit symptoms* (q.v.) in schizophrenia. See *negative symptoms*.

**AMPA**  A glutamate agonist, α-amino-3–hydroxy-5–methyl-4–isoxazole propionic acid. It is bound by both the *kainate* and quisqualate *glutamate* (q.v.) receptors (hence they are referred to as AMPA receptors). The AMPA receptors are one subtype of *EAA receptors* (q.v.).

Like NMDA, AMPA is a glutamate-gated *ion channel* (q.v.); the channel opens and allows sodium ions to enter. An electrical current is thereby created which, if great enough, enhances the opening of other channels by neighboring NMDA receptors. One result is the long-term modification of the synapse characteristic of long-term potentiation (LTP). AMPA also activates many metabotropic receptors by way of G-protein. See *AMPAR*.

**ampakines**  Positive modulators of the AMPA receptor complex; by potentiating AMPA receptor-induced depolarization, they indirectly enhance *NMDAR* function (q.v.) They have been used experimentally in the treatment of schizophrenia. See *glutamate*.

**AMPAR**  AMPA receptor(s), vital mediators of hippocampal plasticity and modulators of inflammatory pain and of synaptic plasticity in the spinal nociceptive system. AMPARs in CNS contain subunits: GluRA,B, C, or D. Those containing the GluRB unit together with A, C, or D subunits have low permeability to $Ca^{2+}$, but receptors lacking the GluRB unit have much higher $Ca^{2+}$ permeability. The A and B subunits control the permeability of the receptors and also influence their trafficking and synaptic availability.

**amphetamine intoxication**  Symptoms of intoxication with amphetamine or similarly acting sympathomimetics include tachycardia, pupillary dilation, elevated blood pressure, hyperreflexia, sweating, chills, nausea or vomiting, and maladaptive behavior such as euphoria or grandiosity, enhanced vigor and alertness, hypervigilance, agitation, anger, repetitive behavior such as purposeless shining of shoes or dissembling of radios (*amphetamine stereotypy*), and impaired judgment. In some abusers, a delirium develops within 24 hours of use.

Probably dose-related are some life-threatening effects, including cardiac arrest; intracerebral hemorrhage; tetany, convulsions, coma, and death.

**amphetamine look**  Many patients on long-continued administration of amphetamine or its derivatives are said to show a characteristic facial appearance—a pale, pinched, serious facial expression with dark circles or hollows under the eyes.

**amphetamine stereotypy**  Repetitive and seemingly meaningless motor activity that occurs in a significant number of amphetamine abusers (and particularly in those who use intravenous amphetamines). The subject may spend an hour or more buffing the same pair of shoes, disassembling and reassembling a radio, or washing a plate. See *amphetamine intoxication*; *amphetamines*.

**amphetamine withdrawal**  Cessation of intake of amphetamine or related substances after prolonged or heavy use may produce a withdrawal reaction, with depressed mood and physiologic changes such as fatigue, intense drug craving, sleep disturbance, vivid and unpleasant dreams, increased appetite, and psychomotor agitation or retardation. A similar picture is observed in cocaine withdrawal.

**amphetamines**  *Amfetamines* (WHO-INN, List of International Nonproprietary Names); the generic name for a group of central nervous system stimulants, including the substituted phenylethylamines (e.g., amphetamine, dextroamphetamine, and methamphetamine) and related sympathomimetic amines, such as methylphenidate (MPH), phenmetrazine, and diethylpropion. The sympathomimetics function as direct and indirect agonists at the adrenergic receptor. They block the reuptake of dopamine and norepinephrine into the presynaptic neuron and increase their release into the extraneuronal space. They can act directly at the postsynaptic receptor.

The amphetamines produce a feeling of well-being and alertness, decreased need for sleep, and a decrease in hunger (probably because of their action on the lateral hypothalamic feeding center) with associated weight loss. Side effects include palpitation, dizziness, headache, dysphoria, apprehension, and vasomotor disturbances.

Use of the amphetamines in the treatment of narcolepsy and attention deficit hyperactivity disorder (ADD, ADHD) is rarely associated with abuse. Tolerance may develop if one drug is used for longer than a year. Also sometimes reported in hyperactive children is behavioral rebound: although symptoms are controlled during the school day, irritability, overtalkativeness, and motor hyperactivity reappear in the afternoon and evening.

Because of their generally high potential for abuse in many patients, amphetamines tend to be strictly controlled. Currently, if allowed at all, their use other than in narcolepsy and ADHD is typically limited to treatment of mild depression; as augmentors of treatment with tricyclic antidepressants and analgesics; and, under certain conditions, as anorectic agents in the short-term treatment of obesity disorders.

The usual route of administration in subjects who abuse amphetamines is by mouth or by intravenous injection. Oral administration brings self-confidence, exhilaration, an increase in phantasy, pressured thoughts, and rapid speech—all described by the user as a feeling of being "turned on." Intravenous administration produces a sudden, generalized, overwhelmingly pleasurable feeling (a "*flash*" or "*rush*"), and it is likely to lead to disorganization of thinking and speech, confusing and frightening perceptions and ideas, and perseverative, stereotyped behavior. Some users go on a "*run*," injecting the drug every 2 hours around the clock for 3 or more days, until they "fall out" and sleep for 12 to 18 hours. They awake lethargic and start a new run.

The street name, *speed*, originally referred to methamphetamine (users were called speed freaks). The name has been extended to include all amphetamines and related drugs. *Ice* is a pure preparation of methamphetamine that can be smoked; it is rapidly absorbed from the lungs and enters into the brain with effects comparable to intravenous administration.

Disorders associated with the use of amphetamines or related substances include abuse, dependence, intoxication, withdrawal, delirium, psychosis, mood disorder, anxiety disorder, sleep disorder, and sexual dysfunction. Chronic abuse commonly induces personality and behavior changes such as impulsivity, aggressivity, irritability, and suspiciousness. In some, this progresses to the development of an amphetamine psychosis with persecutory delusions that may be difficult to distinguish from a functional paranoid or schizophrenic episode. The delusions may be accompanied by auditory or tactile hallucinations, lability of mood, hyperactivity, hostility, and sometimes violence. See *abuse; dependence, drug.*

**amphierotism**    A term coined by Ferenczi to indicate the condition in which a person is able to conceive of himself as a male or female or both simultaneously.

**amphigenesis**    A form of sexual behavior in which a person, predominantly homosexual, is able also to have sexual relations with members of the opposite sex. Thus one speaks of amphigenic inversion in contradistinction to absolute inversion, in which sexuality is restricted to the members of the same sex only. Amphigenic males are also called double-gaited or metrosexual. See *swinging.*

**amphimixis**    1. A term used to indicate the fact that both parents contribute to the inheritance of their offspring. 2. Ferenczi's term for the union and integration of the component instincts (oral, anal, and urethral) into the genital function.

**AMPT**    α-Methylparatyrosine, a competitive inhibitor of the rate-limiting enzyme of catecholamine synthesis, tyrosine hydroxylase. It has no effect on mood in healthy persons or in drug-free depressed patients, but more than half of patients treated with norepinephrine reuptake inhibitors experience a transient return of depressive symptoms following AMPT administration.

**amputation doll**    A doll that can readily be taken apart; its use in play therapy with children was introduced by David Levy. The child often equates the doll with the mother. Sometimes a baby doll was added, or a brother or sister doll.

**Amsterdam retardation**    See *de Lange syndrome.*

**amuck**    *Amok* (q.v.).

**amurakh**    A culture-specific syndrome occurring in Siberian women; because the major

symptom is echopraxia, the syndrome is sometimes called *copying mania.*

**amusia**    Tone-deafness; inability to discriminate different musical notes. See *temporal lobe syndromes.*

**amychophobia**    Fear of being scratched.

**amygdala**    A small, almond-shaped structure, comprising 13 nuclei, buried in the anterior medial section of each temporal lobe, in front of the hippocampus. Along with hippocampus, cingulate cortex, fornix, septum, and mammillary bodies, it makes up the limbic system. It is the central structure associated with the learning of fear, fearful responding, and behavior responses. See *anxiety; stress.* The amygdala is involved not only in conditioned fear learning but also in the encoding, consolidation, and retrieval of emotional memories. The amygdala shapes behavior through the senses by detecting subtleties of emotional expression in others' eyes, faces, gaze, and social actions. It is activated when an observer tries to understand another person's feelings and intentions, to discern whether a stranger is friendly or hostile. See *theory of mind; ventromedial PFC.*

Anatomically, the amygdala is subdivided into various parts: *LA*, lateral nucleus; *BLA*, basolateral nucleus; *CeA*, central amygdala including *CeL/C*, the lateral and capsular division, and *CeM*, the medial part of CeA; *Lad*, dorsal division of amygdala. CeA expresses numerous neuropeptides and neuropeptide receptors, including high levels of receptors for vasopressin and oxytocin, which modulate activity in CeM neurons in opposite ways. Vasopressin enhances aggressiveness, anxiety, and stress levels and the consolidation of fear memory. Oxytocin decreases anxiety and stress and facilitates social encounters, maternal care, and the extinction of conditioned avoidance behavior. LA contains two genes, gastrin-related peptide (Grp) and *stathmin*. Mice lacking stathmin are relatively fearless; they seem not to have instinctive fear and venture bravely into potentially dangerous environments.

The amygdala plays an important role in anxiety and fear behavior. Fear learning involves its lateral and basolateral parts, which project to the central amygdala (CeA), whose efferents to the hypothalamus and brain stem trigger the autonomic expression of fear. When signals for aversive events no longer predict those events, fear to those signals subsides (*extinction*). Although the hippocampus is not the repository of extinction memories, it is involved in regulating when and where extinction memories are expressed. The amygdala facilitates memory storage in widespread areas of the brain.

The amygdala decodes the affective relevance of sensory inputs and initiates adaptive behavior via its connections to the motor systems. Lesions of the amygdala cause a lack of social inhibition, abolish characteristic fear behavior, and lead to excessive trust of others. Patients with amygdala lesions fail to focus on central gist information when their memory is tested for audiovisual narratives describing emotionally arousing events.

The amygdala is an essential part of two separate emotional circuits: (1) an automatic, reflexlike, predominantly subcortical circuit in the service of recognition and deliberations; this circuit sustains the rapid perception of emotional *body language* (EBL) and preparation of adaptive reflexes; and (2) a cortical network with reciprocal connections to the first circuit. The main role of the second circuit is to perceive EBL in detail and to compute the behavioral consequences of an emotion and decide on a course of action. The network includes the frontoparietal motor system and connections between the amygdala and the prefrontal and ventromedial prefrontal cortices.

**amygdaloidectomy, amygdolectomy** Ablation of the amygdaloid nucleus; a psychosurgical procedure that has been used particularly in hallucinating patients, in the belief that the amygdaloid nucleus is a mechanism for transforming thought processes into temporally patterned motor movements, either of the vocal musculature as in subjective auditory experiences, or of the still vaguer projections or representations experienced through vision, taste, or smell. Bilateral amygdaloidectomy in humans has been reported to produce hypersexuality and other gross expressions of biological needs, bulimia, polydipsia, and loss of social controls over behavior. See *Klüver-Bucy syndrome.*

**amyl nitrite** A volatile inhalant used medically to relieve the pain of angina pectoris and biliary colic. Its strong vasodilatant effects have led to its nonmedical use at or near the point of orgasm to enhance and prolong sexual pleasure; it is popularly termed a popper. See *inhalants.*

**amyloid** General term for a variety of protein aggregates that accumulate as extracellular fibrils of 7–10 mm. Their structural features include a hyaline gross structure, a β-pleated sheet conformation, and the ability to bind such dyes as Congo red and thioflavins S and T. Amyloid was used originally to refer only to the extracellular deposits characteristic of Alzheimer disease and systemic amyloid disorders; recently, its use has been extended to include some intracellular aggregates as well. The gene encoding amyloid precursor protein (APP), a membrane glycoprotein compound of fast axonal transport, has been mapped to chromosome 21. APP is a single gene; typically it consists of 770 amino acids, but it occurs in several isoforms depending upon where it is spliced.

The amyloid in *senile plaques* (q.v.) is β-amyloid peptide (Aβ), which is a product of the sequential cleavage of APP by β- and γ-secretases. β-secretase first cuts APP at a site just outside the membrane; then γ–secretase cuts at a location within the membrane. Depending on exactly where γ-secretase snips, it can produce a 40-amino-acid peptide, or a more pathogenic 42-amino form, which clumps into plaques inside and outside the neurons. The presenilin protein is essential for the γ-secretase cut.

Intraneuronal Aβ also occurs, when APP holoprotein is neither cleaved at the plasma membrane nor diverted into recycling endosomes by *SORL1* (sortilin-related receptor 1 gene). APP is then internalized by endocytosis into the multivesicular bodies (late endosomes), where Aβ is produced. Most intraneuronal Aβ ends at residue 42, not at residue 40. Within neurons, Aβ42 inhibits the ubiquitin-proteasome system, leading not only to higher Aβ42 levels but also to the buildup of *tau* (q.v.). Accumulation of intraneuronal Aβ is an early event in the progression of AD, preceding the formation of extracellular Aβ deposits. The brains of patients with early-stage AD might have more abundant intraneuronal Aβ, which becomes extracellular as the disease progresses and neuronal death and lysis occur.

Mutations in three genes—*APP, PS1,* and *PS2*—cause autosomal dominant AD, usually an early-onset form. One common mutation in APP is the Swedish mutation (APP$_{Swe}$), which leads to increased cleavage of APP by the β-secretase and higher levels of intracellular Aβ. The Arctic mutation (APP$_{Arc}$) increases aggregation of Aβ, leading to early onset, aggressive forms. Mutations in the presenilins increase levels of Aβ42, which aggregates more readily than Aβ40. Mutations in *SORL1* increase APP in the Aβ-producing endosomes. See *amyloid disorders; secretase.*

**amyloid angiopathy, cerebral** CAA; one of the *amyloid disorders* (q.v.). An autosomal dominant form of CAA is human hereditary cerebral hemorrhage with *amyloidosis, Dutch type (HCHWA-D)*, characterized by extensive amyloid deposition in the small leptomeningeal arteries and cortical arterioles, with recurrent intracerebral hemorrhages; it is typically fatal in the fifth or sixth decade. The APP gene (on chromosome 21) is tightly linked to HCWA-D; in consequence, and in contrast to familial *Alzheimer disease* (q.v.), it cannot be excluded as the site of mutation. The mutation is at codon 693, at position 22 of the AβP fragment. A cytosine-to-guanine transversion causes a single amino acid substitution (glutamine instead of glutamic acid).

**amyloid hypothesis** Also, *amyloid cascade hypothesis*: amyloid-β42 (Aβ42), a proteolytic derivative of the large transmembrane protein amyloid precursor protein (APP), has an early and vital role in Alzheimer disease (AD). In the first pathologic step in AD, overproduction, decreased clearance, or enhanced aggregation of Aβ42 leads to Aβ42 polymerization and deposition as diffuse plaques. In the next step, Aβ42 polymers affect synapses, leading to activation of microglia and astrocytes activation (involving complement and cytokines). This produces progressive synaptic and neuritic injury; the changed neuronal ionic homeostasis combines with oxidative injury to alter kinase/phosphatase activities and produce *neurofibrillary tangles.* The result is widespread neuronal/neuritic dysfunction and cell death with transmitter deficits, manifesting clinically as dementia. See *NFT.*

**amyloidotic polyneuropathy, familial** *FAP*; an autosomal dominant disorder that usually begins in the third decade with sensory loss and weakness in the distal extremities. Autonomic nervous system involvement is prominent, with postural hypotension, anhidrosis, impotence, and gastrointestinal dysfunction.

The cause is a single base pair mutation on chromosome 18 that encodes for transthretin (prealbumin), a carrier protein that transports thyroxine and retinoic acid (vitamin A). Amyloid fibrils (beta-pleated protein polymers) are deposited extracellularly in peripheral nerves, the heart, and the kidneys but not in brain or other tissues of CNS.

**amyostasia** Muscle tremor.

**amyosthenia** See *aphoria.*

**amyotony** See *aphoria.*

**amyotrophic lateral sclerosis** *ALS*; motor neuron disease; *chronic poliomyelitis; Charcot disease*; progressive bulbar palsy; progressive muscular atrophy; *Lou Gehrig disease.* ALS is a motor neuron degenerative disease involving both upper and lower motor neurons. Typically, it develops as a pure motor syndrome, characterized by progressive paralysis and death, usually within 5 years of onset of symptoms.

The pathology consists of degeneration of the large motor neurons of the brain and spinal cord. Typically, the disease begins insidiously. Mean age of onset is 55 years, and males are affected slightly more often than females. Prevalence is 4–6/100,000; incidence is 0.8–1.2/100,000; death rate is about 50/100,000. *Guamanina ALS* occurs among the Chamorros of Guam, who have an incidence 50 to 100 times that of the rest of the world.

Clinical manifestations include muscle weakness, spasticity, dysarthria, and dysphagia, with progression to total motor debilitation and death. Dementia occurs in about 5% of cases. Spread of the process to the tongue, palate, larynx, and pharynx produces *pseudobulbar palsy*, which resembles the effects of medullary lesions but is caused by bilateral disease of supranuclear corticobulbar fibers. Symptoms include dysarthria, dysphagia, and a nasal, slurred, and sometimes explosive speech with diminished volume. Because swallowing is impaired, the patient drools and chokes frequently on accumulated food and saliva. When severe, pseudobulbar palsy results in impaired voluntary control over emotional reactions, which may be exaggerated, explosive, and quite inappropriate.

Over 90% of ALS cases are sporadic and not linked to any identified chromosomal defect. The other cases are familial ALS (*FALS*); about 25% of them are associated with defects in the gene *superoxide dismutase* (CuZnSOD,

SOD, or SOD1), on chromosome 21. (The mutations were discovered in 1993.)

Mutant SOD1 (Cu/Zn superoxide dismutase) preferentially associates with membrane proteins in spinal cord mitochondria, but not in the mitochondria of unaffected tissues such as muscle or liver. This association initiates a cascade of damage, whereby SOD1 blocks the mitochondrial membranes, preventing import of necessary substances, and some even enters the mitochondria, disrupting their normal activity.

Mutant SOD1 interacts with the mitochondria by binding with BCL2, which in turn leads to accelerated cell death.

Thalidomide and its derivative, lenalidomide, have been found to extend the lives of some patients with the disease; it is believed that their effects are due to suppression of pro-inflammatory *cytokines* (q.v.).

In rare cases (probably < 5%) ALS arises concurrently with other neurodegenerative phenotypes such as frontotemporal dementia (FTD) or other extrapyramidal or cortical and subcortical syndromes. They have been found to be associated with defects on chromosomes 11, X, 9 (at two different locations), 2 (childhood onset, recessive ALS), or 15 (juvenile, recessive ALS) (Hosler, B. A. et al., *Journal of the American Medical Association*, 2000).

**Amytal interview**   See *narcotherapy.*

**anabolic**   1. Relating to the process of assimilating nutrients and converting them into protoplasm; the constructive side of metabolism.

2. *Obs.* In constitutional medicine, the anabolic biotype includes the *brachymorphic, megalosplanchnic, parasympathicotonic,* and *pyknic* types. See *pyknic type.*

**anabolic-androgenic steroids**   *AAS*; synthetic derivatives of testosterone, which has skeletal muscle-building (anabolic) and masculinizing (androgenic) effects. The AAS have legitimate medical uses, among them to promote protein anabolism and in the treatment of some anemias, hereditary angioedema, delays in growth, and osteoporosis. They are more frequently used (and abused) for nonmedical purposes, chiefly to aid in body building and to provide skeletal muscle enlargement or increased strength for persons in good health. Although the earlier literature (in the 1960s) denied that the AAS were effective, more recently it has been established that increases in skeletal muscle mass and strength do occur in users who are training intensively with weights and concomitantly maintain a high-protein, high-calorie diet. AAS use has spread from bodybuilders and weightlifters to football players, swimmers, track-and-field competitors, other athletes, and noncompetitors (such as fitness enthusiasts in health clubs and spas).

The doses used are typically 10 to as high as 1000 times those used for legitimate medical purposes. It is believed that most of the AAS used for nonmedical purposes are obtained through a well-organized black market, from athletes in other countries where such drugs are readily available, and by diversion from legitimate medical and veterinary supplies.

The effects, particularly long-term, of abuse of AAS have not been firmly established. Case studies and anecdotal reports indicate that long-term AAS abuse is likely to be associated with any of the following: impaired liver function, hepatitis, hepatic tumors; premature closing of epiphyses (producing permanent short stature) and premature development of secondary sexual characteristics in prepubertal children; testicular atrophy, gynecomastia, and lowered sperm count in males; menstrual irregularities, beard growth, and deepening of the voice in females; cardiovascular complications, such as coronary artery spasm, myocardial infarction, stroke, and premature atherogenesis. In some series, mood disorders or other psychotic syndromes have occurred in one-third of abusers. Violence and homicidal outbursts (*roid rage*) have also been reported.

**anabolic system**   In constitutional medicine, two large systems are described, anabolic and catabolic, which correspond with the megalosplanchnic (*pyknic*) and microsplanchnic (*asthenic*) habitus, respectively.

**anabolism**   Biochemical changes by which food is converted into living materials within a cell or the combination of cells forming an organism.

**anachoresis**   See *atelesis.*

**anaclinic**   See *anaclitic.*

**anaclisis**   A state of reclining; the infant's dependence on its mother or a substitute for well-being and sustenance. According to Jones, anaclisis is the process of a sexual drive becoming attached to and exploiting various nonsexual self-preservative trends, such as eating and defecation.

**anaclitic, anaclinic** Dependent on another or others; characterized by dependence of libido on another instinct, e.g., hunger.

**anaclitic depression** A term used by Spitz to refer to the syndrome shown by infants who are separated from their mothers for long periods of time. Initially, the infant gives indications of distress, but after 3 months of separation "the weepiness subsided, and stronger provocation became necessary to provoke it. These children would sit with wide open, expressionless eyes, frozen immobile face, and a faraway expression, as if in a daze, apparently not perceiving what went on in their environment.... Contact with children who arrived at this stage became increasingly difficult and finally impossible. At best, screaming was elicited" (*The Psychoanalytic Study of the Child*, 1946). See *maternal deprivation syndrome*.

In Spitz's series, the reaction occurred in children who were 6 to 8 months old at the time of separation, which continued for a practically unbroken period of 3 months. This reaction was seen in full form only in children who had left a "good" mother–child relationship; those with a "bad" relationship did not develop the syndrome.

Bakwin noted a similar syndrome, with listlessness, emaciation and pallor, relative immobility, quietness, unresponsiveness, indifferent appetite, failure to gain weight despite adequate diet, frequent stools, poor sleep, an appearance of unhappiness, proneness to febrile episodes, and absence of sucking habits. Bakwin and others refer to this syndrome as *hospitalism*.

Bowlby described a sequence of reactions in children deprived of their mothers: protest, followed by despair, followed in turn by detachment. The anaclitic depression is reversible if the mother is restored to the child within 3 months.

**anacusia** Total deafness.

**anaesthesia** See *anesthesia*.

**anagogic interpretation** H. Silberer's term for a form of dream interpretation. He says that every dream is capable of two different interpretations. The first he calls the *psychoanalytic*, referring particularly to interpretations from the standpoint of infantile sexuality; the second, the anagogic, referring to more serious or profound thoughts. Freud believed, however, that "The majority of dreams require no overinterpretation, and are especially insusceptible of an anagogic interpretation" (Freud, S. *The Interpretation of Dreams*, 1933).

**anagogic symbolism** Pertaining to or arising from the striving of the inner psychic forms toward progressive ideals; pertaining to the interpretation and psychotherapy of dreams, symptoms, etc., with emphasis on such striving (*anagogic methods*).

**anagogic tendency** See *katogogic tendency*.

**anagogy, anagoge** Psychic material that is expressive of ideals, e.g., dreams.

**anal castration anxiety** Fear of castration displaced, through regressive distortion, onto the anal area. Thus many "toilet phobias," such as fear of falling into the bowl or a fear that some monster will emerge from the toilet and crawl into one's anus, reveal themselves in analysis to refer to castration anxiety.

**anal character** *Compulsive character*; obsessive-compulsive personality disorder. The anal character is made up of three cardinal traits. The first is orderliness (reliability, conscientiousness, punctuality, etc.); the second is parsimony, which may be expressed as avarice; the third is obstinacy and its closely allied traits (defiance, vindictiveness, irascibility, etc.). See *anal erotism; character defense; anal phase; personality disorders*.

**anal eroticism** A psychoanalytic term for localization or concentration of libido in the anal zone. In psychoanalytic theory, the earliest concentration of libido is in the oral zone; with further development, most of it shifts to the anal region and, later, to the phallic area. Part of the libido originally connected with the anal zone becomes attached to the habits and disciplines identified with anal training (regularity of stool, control, cleanliness, etc.); the latter become incorporated into the personality as anal traits. Other portions of the original anal libido are invested in similar fashion in the results or products of anal activity.

"Thus the interest in feces is carried on partly as interest in money, partly as a wish for a child, in which latter an anal-erotic and a genital impulse ('penis-envy') coincide" (Freud, S. *Collected Papers*, 1924–25). See *anal character; character defense; coprolagnia; coprophilia; klismophilia*.

**anal impotence** Constipation in which the analogy to cases of neurotic genital sexual impotence in males is emphasized. In this type of constipation, anxiety concerning the injurious or filthy aspect of the fecal mass to be ejected or parted with is of central importance. This is analogous to the anxiety of many orgastically impotent men concerning the poisonous or sullying effect of the seminal ejaculation.

At military induction centers it is a frequent experience that many candidates cannot void (produce a urine specimen) in the presence of others. These symptoms can be thought of as the adult neurotic residues of conflicts between desires for cooperative regularity, giving, and cleanliness on the one hand, and desire for the maintenance of continued stubborn autonomy, spite, defiance, soiling, and direct stool pleasure on the other (Weiss, E. & English, O. S. *Psychosomatic Medicine*, 1949).

**anal phase**   In psychoanalytic psychology, the second stage of psychosexual development, immediately following the primary or oral stage. The anal phase (or stage) is subdivided into the early or first anal phase, commonly occurring in the third and fourth year of life, and the late or second anal phase, occurring between the ages of 4 and 6. See *ontogeny, psychic.*

The first anal phase is characterized by pleasure in expulsion of the fecal mass. The second anal phase occurs usually in the period between 4 and 6 years of age, marked by a predominant interest and pleasure in the retention, or holding back, of stool. The stool is treated as a possession of inordinately high value.

**anal rape phantasy**   The idea or fear of being raped per anum. Mouth, anus, and vagina are often equated unconsciously by both sexes, and such phantasies may occur in either male or female. See *anal erotism; anality; cloaca.*

**anal retention**   In psychoanalysis, the holding back of the fecal mass as part of toilet training and the characterologic or symptomatic carryovers of this in later life. Frugality, for example is considered to be a continuation of the anal habit of retention; stubbornness and obstinacy are related to the child's ability to spite parental efforts by tightening his sphincters.

Psychodynamically, anal retention is seen to contain two components, fear of loss of body contents or of control over instinctual impulses, and enjoyment of erogenous pleasure; and later

anal character traits represent an outgrowth of one or both of these components. See *anal character; anal eroticism.*

**anal sadism**   The aggression, destructiveness, negativism, and externally directed rage that are typical components of the anal stage of development; manifestations of the death instinct during the anal phase; the second portion of the anal stage of development, and its holdovers in later life. See *anal eroticism; anal phase; death instinct; oral sadism.*

**anal triad**   The three outstanding traits of the anal character: (1) obstinacy; (2) parsimony; (3) pedantic orderliness. In everyday language the connection between miserliness and the retention of stool, both having in common the tendency to hold on to something, or holding something back, is often clearly manifested. The folk saying "he's so tight he couldn't pass a raspberry seed," is an example of this (Sterba, R. *Introduction to the Psychoanalytic Theory of the Libido*, 1942). See *anal phase.*

**analeptic**   Psychostimulant. The term is generally limited to substances whose primary action is on the respiratory and cardiovascular centers of the brain, rather than on the cortex or limbic lobe. Analeptics are used in the treatment of coma; their chief drawback is the narrow range between the dosage required for therapeutic effect and the dosage that will produce convulsions or other serious side effects.

**analfabetia partialis**   *Obs.* Wolff's term (1916) for a type of *reading disability* (q.v.).

**analgesia, analgia**   Loss or absence of the sense of pain. Analgesia may be of somatic or psychic origin; the psychiatric conditions in which it is most frequently seen are schizophrenia, conversion hysteria, and hypnotic states.

**analgesic**   Any substance that reduces pain, such as aspirin, acetaminophen, and the opioids. See *non-dependence-producing substances.*

**anality**   A general term referring to the anal components of sexuality, to manifestations of instinctual conflict centering about the anal stage of sexual development, to manifestations of anal erogeneity which indicate fixation at the anal stage of development. Anality is prominent in obsessive-compulsive neurosis, hypochondriasis, and masochism. See *anal eroticism; anal phase.*

**analogies test**   A test of ability to comprehend relationships, usually by asking the subject to name the fourth term that bears the same relation to the third as the second does to the first. Example: Ship is to water as automobile is to what?

**analogous** See *homologous.*

**analogy** In comparative biology, similarity based on common function. See *allometry; homology.*

**analysand** The person who is being psychoanalyzed.

**analysis** *Psychoanalysis* (q.v.).

**analyst** One who analyzes, that is, resolves a whole into its parts. While the term psychoanalyst has its generic meaning, it is usually understood today to refer to those who adhere to the formulations of the psychoanalysis of Freud. Analysts who follow Jung's concepts are called analytical psychologists; those who use the concepts of Meyer are psychobiologists; those following Adler are individual psychologists. See *psychiatrist.*

**analytic group psychotherapy** See *group psychotherapy.*

**analytic mode** *Interpretive mode* (q.v.).

**analytic neurosis** A neurosis that develops subsequent to, and as a result of, interminable analysis. Stekel is of the opinion that after a too lengthy analysis, conducted over a period of many years, the patient, even if cured of his neurotic symptoms, "loses his natural attitude toward life, and what should have cured him becomes his illness." In this manner, after maintaining an emotional dependency for several years the patient develops toward analysis and analysts a special attitude that is called analytic neurosis. Similarly, the harmful effects upon psychic life produced by an analysis that is carried out without the necessary skill are also known as analytic, or postanalytic, neurosis (Stekel, W. *Compulsion and Doubt,* 1949).

**analytic psychology** Jung's system of psychology, some of whose major elements are as follows:

1. A personal unconscious as well as the *collective unconscious* (q.v.), containing prototypical or archetypal material and able to generate images prior to and independent of conscious experience. See *archetype.*

2. Within consciousness, the ego (the center of the conscious field, the experiencing "me") surrounded by the *persona* (q.v.), or mask, which is the face the subject presents to the world.

3. A 16-category personality typology derived from the various combinations of *attitudes* and psychological *functions*—the attitudes (introversion and extraversion) influence the direction of energy in the psyche, while the paired functions (the rational pair is thinking and feeling, the perceptual pair is sensation and intuition) describe the ways in which the subject relates to the world, perceives it, and evaluates it. See *feeling type, intuitive type, rational type; sensational type; thinking type.*

4. The first half of life (to approximately 40 years of age) is concerned with establishing one's position in the world, through the operation of the dominant attitude and the first function. Then there is a shift from finding one's way in the world to finding one's way out, and in the ultimate confrontation with mortality the previously neglected and less conscious portions of the personality, the opposite attitude and the fourth function (the polar opposite of the first function), are given expression.

5. Life proceeds toward an ultimate outcome, consisting of the achievement of selfhood, making the potential actual, reconciling opposites, and making all the functions and the nondominant attitude conscious and thus available for use. The process of achieving that outcome is *individuation* (q.v.).

**analytical therapy** Therapeutic application of the principles of analytic psychology (q.v.). According to Jung, the contents of consciousness are antithetic to those of the unconscious. One compensates for the others. "The aim of analytical therapy is to make the unconscious contents conscious in order that compensation may be established" (Jung, C. G. *Contributions to Analytical Psychology,* 1928). See *constructive; reductive.*

**analyzer** Pavlov's term for the functional neural unit that provides the basis for differential sensitivity; the analyzer consists of receptor, afferent nerves, and their central connections.

**anamnesis** Recollection; the historical account of a patient's illness antedating the period of illness. It is distinguished from catamnesis, which refers to the history of the patient following an illness.

**anamnesis, associative** A type of psychiatric history-taking developed by Deutsch (1939) that attempts to elicit the causal relationship between somatic symptoms and the patient's

58

psychic structure. Of consequence are not only the factual details but how they are said and when they are said in the interview. The patient is encouraged to give a detailed account of his complaints and his ideas about the illness. When he stops and does not continue spontaneously, the examiner repeats one of the points of his last sentence in interrogative form, using the patient's words. The patient then gives new information and is stimulated to further associations. References to others in his environment, present or past, appear. The person who appears first is usually the relevant person from a *psychosomatic* point of view.

During the associative anamnesis, which lasts from 1 to 2 hours, the examiner looks for three points in establishing the *psychosomatic* unity of the patient's complaints: the old conflict, the recent conflict, and the time factors involved.

**anamnestic analysis** Jung's term for his method of psychoanalytic investigation and treatment. The term emphasizes the importance of tracing the historical development of the patient's disorder and the desirability of supplementing the subject's own account with material gleaned from family members and associates.

**anamnestic apraxia** Inability to carry out a movement on command, owing to inability to remember a command—though there is the ability to perform that movement. See *apraxia.*

**anancasm** Any form of repetitious, recurrent, orderly, stereotyped behavior or thinking that if left unperformed will lead to an increase in anxiety and tension. Though including obsessive and compulsive traits, the term does not apply to repeated fulfillment of recurrent physiologically determined needs such as sleep and sex. Phobias might be considered anancasms, because they may drive the subject to seek protection through compulsions or obsessions.

**anancastia** *Compulsive personality (q.v.).*

**anancastic depression** Lion uses this term to refer to dejection or depression accompanied by tension, perplexity, anxiety, and obsessive and paranoid ideas occurring in persons whose premorbid personality was of the rigid, obsessive anancastic type. See *anancasm; involutional psychosis.*

**anandria** Absence of masculinity.

**anaphase** The third state of the division of a cell by mitosis, characterized by polar migration of the chromosomes.

**anaphia** Absence of sense of touch; commonly used to refer to a relative rather than an absolute loss of tactile sensibility.

**anaphrodisia** *Obs.* Absence of sexual feeling.

**anaphylaxis, psychic** Reactivation of earlier symptoms by an event similar to the one that initially produced the symptoms; it is often seen in *post-traumatic stress disorder* (q.v.).

**anarithmia** A type of *acalculia* (q.v.).

**anarthria** *Obs.* Complete inarticulateness; *aphasia* (q.v.). See *speech disorders.*

**anaudia** *Aphonia* (q.v.).

**anchorage dependence** Dependence of cell growth and survival on substrate attachment; i.e., attachment to other cells and to the fibrillar protein meshwork or *extracellular matrix* (*ECM*).

**anchoring symptoms** Kernberg's term for the cardinal or key symptoms of psychopathology that suggest a specific diagnosis; neurotic symptoms alone, for example, suggest a diagnosis of symptomatic neurosis, while defective reality testing indicates the presence of a borderline condition or functional psychosis and the dysmnesic syndrome points to the probability of an organic mental disorder.

**ancillary** Auxiliary, subordinate. In insurance terminology, ancillary costs or services are those related to diagnosis and treatment of the patient but not covered in the basic charge for the hospital bed or room, such as operating room, laboratory, and X-ray.

**androgen insensitivity syndrome** *AIS; testicular feminizing syndrome*; it is caused by an X-linked recessive gene that results in an inability of body cells to utilize testosterone. As a result, the body fails to masculinize.

Affected subjects are chromosomally male (46,XY) and gonadally male (testicular). The testicles have formed and secreted antimüllerian hormone, blocking the formation of uterus and fallopian tubes. No further masculinization occurs, however, so development continues along feminine lines but without female internal genitalia. Vaginal atresia and amenorrhea are manifested after birth. According to Money (1988), the cases studied were exclusively heterosexual as women, even though they lacked three of the criteria of female sex: 46,XX chromosomal pattern; ovarian gonads; and hormonal cyclicity.

Male hermaphroditism with incomplete masculine differentiation of the sex organs may also be caused by insensitivity of the tissues to androgen. The genital appearance is intersexual, with a small penis that is sometimes considered to be a clitoris. Hormonal feminization of such cases is usually preferred to masculinization, since the latter is unsatisfactory: it requires multiple surgical procedures in childhood, but the end result may be a deformed penis that is inadequate for copulation and often also for urination.

**androgenic steroids**   See *anabolic-androgenic steroids*.

**androgyne**   A person who displays a mixture of female and male roles; the condition itself is termed androgyneity, androgynism, or androgyny. Formerly, the term was used for a male pseudohermaphrodite; *gynandroid* was applied to a female pseudohermaphrodite.

The term has been more loosely applied in psychoanalysis, anthropology, and general literature to refer to bisexuality or to the capacity to develop characteristics of either sex. Such usage has not always kept pace with recent advances in knowledge about human sexuality, so the sense in which any author is using the term can only be inferred from context. It may mean any of the the following: (1) hermaphroditism, with physical features of both sexes; (2) confusion or uncertainty about one's *gender identity* (q.v.); (3) confusion or uncertainty about one's gender role, presenting a mixture of behaviors that will be labeled socially as both *masculine* and *feminine* (qq.v.). In this sense, the term is most commonly used to characterize a male as effeminate, often with the added implication that in sexual activity he prefers a partner of the same sex.

**androgynophilia**   *Bisexuality* (q.v.), but more specifically denoting sexual relationships with a man and a woman, either serially or concurrently (as in a "threesome"), by either a man or a woman.

**andromania**   *Nymphomania* (q.v.).

**andromimesis**   The state of a woman who lives full-time as a man. Unlike transvestic fetishism, in which cross-dressing appears episodically because it is required for erotic arousal and orgasm, the andromimetic adopts the male role and appearance full-time and may undergo hormonal masculinization, hysterectomy, breast removal, or full sex-reassignment

surgery. The counterpart of andromimesis in the male is *gynemimesis* (q.v.).

**andromimetophilia**   A *paraphilia* (q.v.) in which sexual arousal and orgasm are dependent on the subject being the partner of a male impersonator.

**andromonoecism**   See *hermaphroditism*.

**androphilia**   Sexual love of a man, by either a woman (female androphilia) or a man (male androphilia).

**androphobia**   Morbid fear of men.

**androphonomania**   *Obs.* Homicidal insanity.

**anemophobia**   Fear of wind.

**anencephaly**   A cranial malformation characterized by failure of the rostral portion of the neural tube to close, subjecting exposed cerebral or cerebellar tissues to erosion. The cerebral hemispheres may be reduced or absent, leaving only tangled blood vessels surrounding the basal ganglia and brain stem. The skeletal defects can extend to malformations of the skull floor and of the jaw and neck region.

**anergasia**   Loss of functional activity.

**anergia**   Lack of energy, passivity.

**anerotism**   See *negativism, sexual*.

**anesthesia, anaesthesia**   Absence of sensation.

**anesthesia, glove**   A disorder in the sensory field in which the patient has no sense of feeling in an area roughly corresponding to that covered by a glove; this form of anesthesia is usually psychogenic (hysterical).

**anesthesia, sexual**   *Frigidity, sexual* (q.v.).

**anesthesia, spiritua**   Amorality; lack of moral or ethical standards.

**anethopathy, anetopathy**   Absence of moral inhibitions; unethicalness; Karpman's term (1949) for primary, essential, genuine, idiopathic psychopathy or *psychopathic personality* (q.v.). This is the group from which so-called habitual criminals come. In such cases, usually no deep-seated psychic motivations can be elicited, and patients appear to be "disease fast" and unchanged by psychotherapy. The most conspicuous trait in their mental makeup is complete egocentricity, which is also reflected in narcissistic sexual behavior.

**aneuploidy**   A karyotype abnormality in which there is an abnormal number of chromosomes (i.e., not an exact multiple of the haploid number) or an abnormality of the chromosomes themselves. Among the best known examples of aneuploidy are D trisomy, E trisomy, G trisomy or Down syndrome, XXX (superfemale), XXY (Klinefelter syndrome), XO (Turner syndrome), XYY, and XXYY. See *chromosome*.

**aneuthanasia**   Painful death.

**angel dust**   *Phencyclidine* (q.v.).

**Angelman syndrome**   A developmental disorder caused by mutation or deletion of the UBE3A gene on the maternal chromosome 15q11–13. The same deletion in the paternal chromosome causes *Prader-Willi syndrome* (q.v.). Manifestations of Angelman syndrome are similar to both *autistic disorder* and *Rett syndrome* (qq.v.) and include developmental delay, movement disorder and clumsiness, tremulousness, hand-flapping, short attention span, slowed head growth, stereotypic mouthing behavior, increased sensitivity to heat, and fascination with water. Other symptoms are intractable seizures and affect dysregulation, with periodic bursts of unexpected and inappropriate laughter. See *imprinting, genomic*.

Mutations of the X-linked MeCP2 gene, the cause of the majority of cases of Rett syndrome, have caused some children to display an Angelman phenotype. It has been suggested that MeCP2 regulates the expression of UBE3A. Loss of function, duplications, and triplications of the UBE3A gene have been associated with autistic features in patients with 15q11–13 anomalies. Mutations in genes for neuroligin-3 and -4 (*NLGN*-3 on Xp22.3, and *NLGN*-4 on Xq13) can cause autistic disorder or *Asperger syndrome* (q.v.) in males; UBE3A, which is a ubiquitin ligase, might be involved in NLGN degradation.

**Anger Attacks Questionnaire**   A self-rating scale for the report of discrete spells of anger that are ego-dystonic, inappropriate to the situation, accompanied by irritability, associated with features resembling panic attack symptoms, followed by guilt or regret.

**anginophobia**   Fear of choking.

**angioblastoma**   See *intracranial tumor*.

**angiogram**   X-ray of an area following injection of an artery supplying the area with a suitable contrast medium. Internal carotid angiography is used to study the arterial vessels of the cerebral hemispheres; vertebral angiography (arteriography) is used to study the circulation of the posterior fossa and the posterior portions of the cerebral hemispheres. Angiography is useful in demonstrating intracranial aneurysms, vascular malformations, and tumors. Recent advances in MRI allow intracranial vessels to be imaged through a non-invasive technique, magnetic resonance angiography.

**angioma**   See *intracranial tumor*.

**angiomatosis, trigeminal cerebral**   *Sturge-Weber-Dimitri disease*; hemangioma over the meninges of the parietal and occipital lobes and underlying maldevelopment of the brain, resulting in mental retardation. See *Lindau disease*.

**angiophakomatosis**   See *von Hippel-Lindau disease*.

**angry woman syndrome**   A personality disorder described in housewives consisting of a morbidly critical attitude to others, perfectionism, obsessive neatness and punctuality, marital maladjustment, proneness to alcohol or drug abuse, periodic outbursts of unprovoked anger, and serious suicide attempts.

**anguish, existential**   See *ontological insecurity*.

**angular gyrus aphasia**   Lesions in the angular gyrus produce a fluent aphasia with excellent repetition, often associated with echolalaia (repetition of the last phrase of the questioner), or various types of nominal dysphasia (*amnesic dysphasia*): the patient insists that he knows what the object is and frequently tries to convey recognition by describing its use. He will usually totally reject the wrong name if offered it and accept the right one. Writing exhibits the same nominal defect, and there is much difficulty in comprehending spoken and written language. See *anomic aphasia*.

**angular gyrus syndrome**   A symptom complex associated with focal lesions of the dominant posterior hemisphere consisting of alexia with agraphia or *Gerstmann syndrome* (acalculia, agraphia, difficulty in differentiating left from right, finger agnosia, and constructional disturbances), in addition to fluent aphasia. Unlike Alzheimer disease, with which it is often confused, the angular gyrus syndrome begins abruptly, memory and topographic orientation are relatively well maintained, and affected subjects are aware of their language deficits and can be engaged in conversation. Neurologic examination may reveal right-sided defects, and both electroencephalography and CT scan may show left-sided abnormalities. Positron emission tomography typically shows a left posterior deficit, whereas bilateral hypometabolism is characteristic in Alzheimer disease.

**anhedonia**   Absence of pleasure in acts that are normally pleasurable. It is seen often in schizophrenia and depression. In behavioral terms, anhedonia is a state in which the reward value of usually reinforcing stimuli is blocked. As thus defined, anhedonia may be a side effect of neuroleptic agents, but whether this effect results from direct interference with the reward system or because of the interference with response patterns is not clear.

**anhidrosis**   Deficiency or absence of perspiration.

**aniconia**   Absence of mental imagery.

**anile**   To be in one's dotage; imbecilic.

**anilingus**   Stimulation of the anal zone by the tongue and lips, usually as a part of sexual foreplay; "rimming".

**anima**   In Jung's terminology, the soul, that part of the psyche that is directed inward and is in touch with the unconscious; the anima is contrasted with the *persona* (q.v.), which is the outer attitude or outer character. Because the outer attitude is often the opposite of the inner, Jung also uses *anima* to refer to the feminine soul of a very masculine man and animus to refer to the masculine soul of a very feminine woman. Everyone, male or female, has both animus and anima, and Jung's description of personality types reflects the balance that is struck between the two. See *analytic psychology*.

**animacy**   Aliveness, the state of being alive; attributions of animacy are part of one's social judgments that enable one to participate in social interactions. See *social cognitive neuroscience*; *theory of mind*.

**animal-assisted therapy**   *AAT*; goal-directed interactions between a patient, a therapist, and an animal. Dogs, horses, rabbits, cats, and birds have been used. Dogs are probably most frequently used because they are more easily trained and have fewer maintenance needs than most other animals. In addition, dogs are adept at reading body language and with training they can become predictable, reliable, and controllable. Data suggest that AAT may be of benefit in *BPSD* (q.v.), but results are confounded by the positive effects of pet interaction on caregivers.

**animastic**   Of or pertaining to the soul; psychic.

**animatism**   The ascription of psychic qualities to inanimate as well as animate objects; synonymous with *mentalism* (q.v.).

**animism**   The theory that all things in nature contain the so-called spirit or soul. See *animatism; mentalism*.

**animism, social**   The schizophrenic's selective interpretation of outer reality so as to conform to the emotion that possesses him at the moment. He feels inferior, unwanted, and unloved, sees every grouping of people in the street as a purposeful exclusion of him, and hears any question put to him as an affirmation of his worthlessness.

**animus**   See *anima*.

**anion channel**   See *ion channel*.

**aniracetam**   One of the ampakines, which enhance the activation of ion channels by *AMPA* (q.v.). Because of AMPA's role in the long-term potentiation that underlies learning and memory, the ampakines have been used experimentally in Alzheimer disease, but with little objective benefit.

**aniridia-ataxia syndrome**   A combination of absence of the iris in both eyes, cerebellar ataxia, and mental retardation. Because of the aniridia, visual acuity ranges between 20/100 and 20/200.

**anisocoria**   Inequality of the pupils in size.

**anisophrenia**   Depression.

**ankle clonus**   A rhythmical tremor of the foot elicited by placing the leg in simiflexion, holding the leg with one hand, grasping the foot with the other, and briskly dorsiflexing the foot one or more times. See *clonus*.

**ankle jerk**   *Achilles reflex* (q.v.).

**Anlage**   A particular genetic factor predisposing to a given trait or the entire *genotypical* structure of an individual. The term is an abbreviation of *Erbanlage*, or *hereditary predisposition*, and this is the sense in which it is used in American genetics. See *predisposition*.

**Anna O.**   A patient described by Freud, originally referred to Breuer at the age of 21 for "nervous" symptoms that had appeared following the death of her father. Breuer discovered that one symptom disappeared entirely after she had been able to recount the details of its first appearance. This was the origin of the "talking cure." Anna O (later identified as Bertha Pappenheim) had numerous conversion symptoms, among them hysterical pregnancy (which covered the phantasy that she was pregnant by Breuer) and paralysis of her arm (related to her father's death, at which time she was sitting at his bedside with her arm pressed against her chair).

**annexin** Calcium-binding protein(s) on the membrane of synaptic vesicles. $Ca^{2+}$ ions are involved in mobilization of vesicles from the synaptic terminal to the docking site at the synaptic membrane, and in fusion of the vesicle with the synaptic membrane during exocytosis of the transmitter into the synaptic cleft.

**anniversary excitement** Bleuler's term for episodes of agitation that appear on specific calendar dates and usually disappear after a few repetitions. He included anniversary excitements among the acute syndromes of the schizophrenias. Anniversary excitement is usually related to something that had happened to the patient on a certain day that had some connection with his or her complex or complexes.

**anniversary hypothesis** This hypothesis asserts the following: If a person has lost a parent by death in childhood, and that person subsequently marries and has children, and is later hospitalized for the first time for mental illness, the first hospitalization is likely to occur when the eldest child of that person is within I year of his own age when his parent died.

**anniversary reaction** Behavior, symptoms, dreams, etc. that occur on an anniversary of a significant experience; their time-specific relationship to the original experience is rarely recognized by the subject and they appear to be a type of *acting out*, i.e., an attempt to master through reliving rather than through remembering. See *Sunday neurosis*.

**annotation** In genomics, analysis of the sequence data of regions of the genome that is provided by computer tools. Annotation enables biologists to make sense of the billions of A's, T's, G's, and C's contained in databases such as those of the *Human Genome Project* (q.v.). The first priority of any annotation software is to pinpoint the genes. Only computers have the ability to scan billions of bases and pick out potential genes. They do this by looking for characteristic sequences at the beginnings and ends of genes, or by comparing new sequences to known genes or bits of genes. Additional computer programs translate those genes into proteins and, based on similarities to other proteins, attempt to assign a function to each one.

**annulment** A mental mechanism by which the patient annuls, i.e., renders nonexistent, certain specific events or ideas that are painful or disagreeable to him or her. In certain respects, this mechanism resembles repression. In annulment painful experiences are shifted into daydreams, while in repression painful experiences may be eliminated from consciousness.

**annulment, marriage** See *marriage, psychiatric aspects of.*

**anoesis** Absence of cognition or knowledge; a state of sheer feeling, having no reference to objects; noncognitive consciousness.

**anoikis** Homelessness; specifically, apoptosis secondary to the loss of integrin signalling that occurs when cells are detached from the extracellular matrix.

**anomaly** A deviation from the average. In medicine anomalies are distinguished from disease processes, although the clinical signs and symptoms may be similar in both. For example, an underdeveloped heart may be anomalous; it may be too small, organically and functionally, for the body in which it is located. The anomaly may be relative or absolute. See *disease*.

Personality may also be anomalous. The so-called *character neuroses* are of that order, in that the personalities are in the periphery of the normal or average personality circle. Schizoidism and cycloidism are also regarded as anomalies.

**anomia** 1. *Obs.* Rush's term for congenital defect of the moral sense. 2. In neurology, anomia is a type of aphasia with a disturbed capacity to name objects. See *motor aphasia*.

**anomic aphasia** Also called *angular gyrus aphasia, amnesic aphasia, amnestic aphasia, dysnomia, nominal aphasia.* A fluent aphasia characterized by an isolated defect in naming; there are frequent pauses in speaking while subject searches for words and frequent use of vague words such as "it" and "thing" and "you know." Some anomic patients can use concrete but not abstract nouns; others cannot name body parts, colors, living things, or proper names. Comprehension and repetition are intact. In its mildest form, anomic aphasia is a common disturbance and is seen following anxiety, fatigue, intoxication, or senility. When due to a focal cerebral lesion, amnestic aphasia usually indicates a lesion between the angular gyrus and the posterior part of the first temporal gyrus on the left side. See *aphasia*.

**anomie** Emile Durkheim (1858–1917) used this term to refer to lack of social control. He based his classification of suicide on the hypothesis of a relationship between suicide and social conditions. *Egotistic suicide* occurred in subjects who had lost their feelings of integration within their social group and were no longer subject to its controls. *Altruistic suicide* referred to sacrifice of one's life for the good of the social group. *Anomic suicide* occurs in a society that lacks "collective order" because it is in the midst of major social change; as a result, absence of regulation and control has permitted desires to grow beyond all hope of satisfaction.

**anonymous notification**   See *notification, anonymous*.

**anorexia**   Loss of appetite.

**anorexia, secondary mental**   Loss of appetite secondary to voluntary restriction of food intake in order to relieve digestive symptoms. Appetite tends to be lost whenever hunger goes unrelieved for a long time, no matter what the reason for the initial deprivation of food.

**anorexia, social**   Loss of appetite because of starvation or severe malnutrition, as seen in the poor, who cannot afford adequate food.

**anorexia nervosa**   An *eating disorder* characterized by failure to maintain body weight (typically, the maintained weight is 15%–25% below what would be normal), intense fear of gaining weight and a pronounced drive for thinness, faulty body image (e.g., denial of the degree and seriousness of weight loss, preoccupation with the thought that some part of the body is too large), and, in females, amenorrhea. Other symptoms include a pervasive sense of ineffectiveness and inability to achieve any degree of mastery or control, considerable increase in bodily activity (e.g., ritualized jogging or cycling), depression (in as many as 50%), and anxiety. Despite the name"anorexia," the affected person does not necessarily suffer a loss of appetite; the important feature is that, for some, reason, food is not taken in. Various rationalizations for this are offered, ranging from disgust for specific foods, fear of choking on food, or fear of vomiting after eating.

Some subjects, the bulimic type, engage in recurrent episodes of binge eating during episodes of anorexia; others, the nonbulimic or restricter type, do not.

Anorexia is much more frequent in women than in men (20:1). Its prevalence appears to have increased in the last quarter-century; in one study, incidence doubled during the period of 1970–76 when compared with the period of 1960–69. At greatest risk are those in highest social classes. Peaks of onset are at 14 years and 18 years; in probably only 5% is onset later than 25 years.

The syndrome has been known for centuries. In 1694 Richard Morton described a case of "self-starvation," with emaciation, refusal to gain weight, denial of illness, body image disturbance, hyperactivity, and a poor outcome. Sir William Gull described it as *apepsia hysterica* in 1874 and proposed the term anorexia nervosa in 1874.

Course is highly variable: between 5% and 9% die; at a 5- to 6-year follow-up, approximately 40% will be asymptomatic, 30% will be significicantly improved, and 20% will be unchanged or actively symptomatic.

Differentiation should be made between anorexia nervosa, as described above, and pituitary cachexia (Simmonds disease, panhypopituitarism). The 17-ketosteroids are reduced in Simmonds disease but normal in anorexia nervosa.

**anorgasmy**   Lack of sexual pleasure; inability to achieve orgasm (a side effect of some psychotropic agents).

**anorthosis**   Sexual impotence.

**anosmia**   Absence of sense of smell.

**anosognosia**   Unawareness of one's own physical illness or limitations. In persons with organic brain syndrome (first described by Anton in 1899), there is a tendency to suppress all knowledge of the disability. This is a protective mechanism that is particularly likely to occur when the incapacitation is total and so severe that the patient is unable to use the disturbed capacity at all. See *nonrecognition; organic syndrome; parietal lobe; sensory neglect*.

**anosphresia**   *Anosmia* (q.v.).

**anoxia, cerebral**   Inadequate supply of oxygen to the brain, generally divided into four types: *anoxic anoxia*, as in respiratory failure, asphyxia, or altitude sickness; *anemic anoxia*, as in severe anemia, blood loss, and carbon monoxide poisoning; *stagnant anoxia*, as in circulatory or cardiac failure, cardiac arrhythmias, cardiac arrest, and cerebral vascular disease; and *metabolic anoxia*, as in hypoglycemia or cyanide poisoning.

**ANS**   *Autonomic nervous system* (q.v.).

**Antabuse**   Trade name of a drug used in the treatment of alcoholism; chemically known as disulfiram and tetraethylthiuram disulfide. Antabuse interferes with the enzyme systems that normally break down alcohol in the organism. As a result, when alcohol is ingested by a subject with an adequate blood level of Antabuse, there occurs within a few minutes a characteristic response, the *alcohol-Antabuse* reaction (also, *alcohol flush reaction*; disulfiram-ethanol reaction or *DER*). This consists of flushing, injection of the conjunctivae, sweating, a sensation of warmth, and tachycardia; in 20 to 30 minutes, additional symptoms may appear—headache, dizziness, chest pain, palpitation, dyspnea, pallor, and nausea. With more severe reactions, vomiting, hypotension, vasomotor collapse, and sometimes convulsions may occur.

Disulfiram was approved by the FDA (U.S.) for use in treating alcoholism in 1951. Oral administration is most succcessful in patients who are older, well-motivated, with stable living conditions and in those in structured and closely monitored treatment programs. It is both a psychological deterrent and a pharmacological or metabolic deterrent to drinking. Its drawback is that the user can stop the drug at any point and within 24–48 hours resume drinking with impunity.

In France and Poland, particularly, *disulfiram implantation* is advocated; up to eight 100-mg trochars are implanted through a small incision in the lower abdomen. See *relapse prevention*.

**antacid abuse**   See *non-dependence-producing substances*.

**antagonism hypothesis**   The theory that the development of one specific disorder generally precludes the development of a specific second disorder, as in the belief that there is a mutual antagonism between epilepsy and schizophrenia. The *affinity hypothesis* is the opposite: the development of one specific illness puts the subject at higher than normal risk for the development of a second specific illness.

**antagonist**   In pharmacology, a drug that reduces or blocks the action of another drug. Naloxone, for example, blocks the action of morphine (the agonist) by competing with it for receptor sites in the brain and other tissues. By occupying those sites Naloxone prevents morphine from binding to the receptors and exerting its effect.

**antagonistic cooperation**   Alexander uses this term to describe the organizational nature of society. He says that in our "laissez-faire," competitive society we are at one and the same time both friends and rivals; we live in an antagonistic cooperation with our fellow men. This life pattern can lead to fears and hostility, frustrations and thwarted hopes, exaggerated ambitions and discouragement, all of which can cause disturbed human relations and can lead to mental and nervous symptoms (Alexander, F. & French, T. M. *Studies in Psychosomatic Medicine*, 1948).

**anterior cingular cortex**   *ACC.* The cingulate gyrus itself is an arched, crescent-shaped convolution on the medial surface of the cerebral hemispheres, lying immediately above the corpus callosum. The posterior cingulate extends backward to the parietal lobe. These connections enable ACC to act as a bridge between the limbic structures and the frontal lobe and provide it with the capacity to integrate cognitive activity with affective experience. The cingulate gyrus is involved in social, cognitive, sensory, and emotional functions.

The anterior cingular cortex is on the medial surface of the frontal lobe; anatomically, ACC is separated into the anterior division, midcingulate cortex, posterior cingulate cortex, and retrosplenial cortex, on the ventral bank of the posterior cingulate gyrus. Fear avoidance is associated mainly with activity in the anterior part of the midcingulate cortex, pain with activity in the posterior part of the midcingulate cortex, unpleasantness with the anterior division, and skeletomotor orientation of the body in response to noxious stimuli in the midcingulate and posterior cingulate cortices. ACC regulates selective attention and motivation, it detects malcoordinated intention and execution, it identifies times when the organism needs to be more strongly engaged in controlling its behavior, and overall it attends to the consequences of actions. Through its extensive connections with DLPFC it has access to the cognitive apparatus and plays a unique role in predicting error likelihood, performance monitoring, conflict monitoring, and response selection. ACC activity may also encode the degree of reward expectancy.

ACC has extended from attending to actions to attending to social *inter*actions; it deals with the attentive and selective aspects of a task, but it needs the working memory of DLPFC to direct and guide it. The perception of unfair treatment, especially by another human, activates the trio of DLPFC, ACC, and insula. ACC is more important for elaborating feelings of emotional distress, whereas PFC counteracts the painful feeling of being shunned and plays a self-regulatory role in mitigating the distressing effects of social exclusion. Moral dilemmas engage the ACC; it is activated, for instance when cooperative behavior is needed in playing a version of Prisoner's Dilemma. ACC is concerned with representations of mental states of the self; it provides access to feeling states related to past decisions when future decisions of a similar nature are being contemplated.

Overcoming inertia when initiating actions and curbing competing well-established or innate tendencies are two cornerstones of the willed control of behavior; lesions to the ACC interfere with both aspects. Bilateral lesions of the cingulate gyri may cause apathy, akinesia, and mutism. Abnormalities in the ACC have been implicated in several disorders, including depression, mania, OCD, and PTSD. See *DLPFC*; *paracingulate cortex*; *theory of mind*.

**anterograde amnesic syndrome** *Medial temporal lobe amnesia;* loss of recognition memory. Recognition memory is composed of at least two processes: (1) familiarity discrimination—"knowing" that I have seen you before but I do not remember a specific episode, and (2) recollective matching—remembering that I have seen you before because I can remember a specific episode, which automatically implies a successful familiarity judgment. Temporal lobe lesion studies indicate that familiarity discrimination depends on the perirhinal cortex, whereas a system centering on the hippocampus is concerned with recollective matching.

**anterograde memory** The ability to recall information consciously and deliberately after a given point in time or sentinel effect.

**anterograde transport** See *Golgi apparatus.*

**anthropo-** Combining form meaning human being.

**anthropocentrism** The doctrine or belief that humans are the center of the universe to which all else has reference.

**anthropology** The science of humankind in the widest sense; the history of human society; the branch of natural science that studies the developmental aspects of humans as a species, using archaeology as one of its main methods.

Anthropology is usually subdivided into (1) zoological anthropology, investigating the evolutionary conditions of humanity; (2) descriptive anthropology, or ethnology, describing the division of humankind into races and studying the origin, distribution, and relations of these racial groups; (3) general anthropology, dealing with the evolution of humankind as a human society.

The last division is anthropology proper and, according to Franz Boas (*General Anthropology*, 1938), includes the following main areas: (1) the reconstruction of human history; (2) the determination of types of historical phenomena and their sequences; (3) the dynamics of change. See *comparative psychiatry.*

**anthropology, medical** Study of the cultural aspects of providing and receiving health care.

**anthropology, psychological** The branch of anthropology that deals with the psychology of different civilizations and cultures and studies especially folklore, myths, and other expressions of the mentality of the people. Through comparisons the psychological investigations throw light on many observations made in children or in mentally sick persons in the culture. See *ethnology.*

**anthropometry** Used particularly in *anthropology* (q.v.), measurement of the human body for the description of the typical anatomical variability of a population. In anthropology, more attention must be given to the bony structure than to any other part of the body, since a comparison between present and past conditions can usually be based only on comparisons of skeletons.

**anthropomorphy** Interpretation of animal mental activities in terms of human adult logic; ascribing to nonhuman objects characteristics (motives, thoughts, feelings, etc.) of human beings.

**anthroponomy** W. Hunter's term for behavioristic psychology.

**anthropophobia** Fear of humans in general.

**anthropos** Primal man; one of Jung's archetypes. See *archetype*; *mother archetype.*

**anthroposcopy**   *Obs.* Various debatable procedures of character-reading from the features or other parts of the human body.

**anthroposophy**   A spiritual renewal movement associated with the name of Rudolf Steiner (1861–1925). In psychiatry, spiritually directed treatments include meditation, art, music, morning preview of what the day will bring, and evening retrospect of the day.

**anthrotype**   *Biotype* (q.v.); in constitutional medicine, classification into one or another group on the basis of morphological, physiological, immunological, and psychological characteristics.

**antiandrogen**   A drug that blocks or counteracts male hormones, such as medroxyprogesterone acetate (MPA, trade name Depo-Provera), used in the treatment of some paraphilias.

**antianxiety agents**   *Anxiolytic drugs*; sometimes called minor tranquilizers. *Sedatives/hypnotics* (q.v.) have also been used as anxiolytics. The other anxiolytics include the following: (1) antihistamine derivatives such as hydroxyzine and diphenhydramine; (2) *benzodiazepines* (q.v.); (3) *buspirone*: a non-benzodiazepine anxiolytic that has little sedative or hypnotic effect; it is also said to have significantly less abuse potential than the benzodiazepines; (4) *beta blockers* such as propranolol (acts centrally and peripherally), atenolol, and nadolol (act only peripherally); used to treat rage attacks and violent behavior in various neuropsychiatric conditions, and also for stage fright and the somatic symptoms of anxiety.

**antibody-barrier system**   See *blood–brain barrier.*

**anticathexis**   *Countercathexis; counterinvestment*; the energy that must be expended by the ego to maintain repression or otherwise block the entrance of id derivatives into consciousness.

**anticholinergic**   See *cholinergic.*

**anticholinergic syndrome**   See *central anticholinergic syndrome.*

**anticholinesterases**   *Cholinesterase inhibitors (CHEIs)*; drugs that counteract cholinesterase, the enzyme needed to metabolize acetylcholine, thereby preventing acetylcholine breakdown and enhancing its action. Because of that enhancing effect, anticholinesterases are also termed *cholinergic* (q.v.) or *parasympathomimetic* drugs. Among the anticholinesterases are physostigmine, neostigmine, organophosphates, and a group of newer drugs that are used to improve or maintain cognitive function in patients with Alzheimer disease: donepezil, galantamine, and rivastigmine.

**anticipation**   1. *Prediction*; the ability to foresee what is likely to happen on the basis of past experience. Anticipation allows danger to be avoided before it becomes a disaster and is an important element in planning. Anticipation is largely a frontal lobe function.

2. In heritable diseases, the appearance of the disease earlier or in increasing severity in successive generations; referred to as the *Sherman paradox* in the *fragile X syndrome* (q.v.). *Trinucleotide repeat* disorders (q.v.) are sometimes characterized as *dynamic mutations*, with a predilection for gaining repeat units when transmitted through subsequent mutations. The number of repeats is positively correlated with an increase either in disease severity (which may be manifested in earlier onset) or in penetrance. Genetic anticipation is considered a hallmark of such dynamic mutations.

**anticipatory anxiety**   Anxiety, fear, or panic that is triggered by the thought or threat of being exposed to the situation that has triggered such responses in the past. See *panic attack; panic disorder.*

**anticipatory autocastration**   See *autocastration; castration.*

**anticonvulsant**   *Antiepileptic*; controlling, inhibiting, or preventing seizures. See *antiepileptic drugs; epilepsy.*

**antidepressant**   Thymoleptic; referring to a drug that reverses or ameliorates clinical depression.

There are three major classes of antidepressants currently in use: (1) *heterocyclics* or *cyclics* (including bicyclics, tricyclics, tetracyclics, and others)—measured by the degree to which they inhibit reuptake of norepinephrine, even though it is known that most of them also affect other neurotransmitters, such as serotonin, dopamine, histamine, and acetylcholine. The best known members of this group are imipramine, desipramine, trimipramine, clomipramine, amitriptyline, nortriptyline, protriptyline, amoxapine, doxepin, and maprotiline; (2) *serotonergic* antidepressants such as trazodone, fluoxetine, paroxetine, sertraline, nefazodone, and venlafaxine, which inhibit serotonin reuptake; and (3) *monoamine oxidase inhibitors (MAOIs)* (q.v.)—isocarboxazid, phenelzine, and tranylcypromine. See *psychopharmacologic agents.*

*Psychostimulant* drugs are a fourth class of antidepressants; among them are *methylphenidate*, methamphetamine, *amphetamines*, and similar sympathomimetics (qq.v.). Bupropion is closer in structure to stimulants than to tricyclics and carries some potential for amphetamine-like abuse. All the other psychostimulants have a high potential for abuse and so are rarely prescribed as the primary or sole treatment for depression. In some states, their use is banned. Nonetheless, they may be useful adjuvants to other pharmacologic agents, and on occasion they may be a preferred short-term treatment.

Second-generation antidepressants are similar in their general effectiveness. Overall, 38% of patients did not respond favorably during 6–12 weeks of treatment with a second generation antidepressant, and 54% did not achieve remission. About 25%–50% of patients who fail on treatment with one SSRI will respond to a second, or to an antidepressant with a different mechanism (such as an SNRI or bupropion). If results are still unsatisfactory, augmentation with any of the following has sometimes been successful: lithium, L-triiodothyronine (T3), buspirone, mirtazapine, an atypical antipsychotic, or stimulants such as amphetamine or modafinil. The newer medications have the same mechanism of action as the older tricyclics; they must be administered for weeks or months, and side effects are a serious problem. The TCAs may produce atropine-like effects: postural hypotension; decrement in short-term memory; sedation; estrangement; and agitation. At higher doses they may introduce an anticholinergic delirium, characterized by misperceptions; impulsivity; impaired judgment; dry, warm skin; dilated, fixed pupils; fever; tachycardia; diminished peristalsis; and atonic bladder. TCAs are hazardous in overdose; desipramine may be more lethal than others in the class.

SSRIs appear much less lethal than TCAs, but they carry the risk of serotonin toxicity and SIADH (syndrome of inappropriate secretion of antidiuretic hormone). See *central anticholinergic syndrome; serotonin syndrome; SIADH.*

**antidipsotropic**   An antialcohol agent, such as acamprosate or *naltrexone* (q.v.), used to promote abstinence and prevent relapse. Sometimes drugs that trigger an aversive response to alcohol, such as disulfiram, are included within this category.

**antidiuretic hormone**   See *SIADH; vasopressin.*

**antiepileptic drugs**   *AEDs*; first-line AEDs include carbamazepine, lamotrigine, oxycarbazepine, and phenytoin. Other AEDs, generally used for adjunctive therapy only, include gabapentin, levetiracetam, tiagabine, topiramate, valproate, and zonisamide. See *psychopharmacological agents.*

To exert antiepileptic activity, a drug must act on one or more target molecules in the brain: ion channels, neurotranmitter transporters, neurotransmitter metabolic enzymes. AEDs act by (1) modulating voltage-gated ion channels, (2) enhancing synaptic inhibition, or (3) inhibiting synaptic excitation. Voltage-gated ion channels (including sodium, calcium, and potassium channels) shape the subthreshold electrical behavior of the neuron, allow it to fire action potentials, regulate its responsiveness to synaptic signals, contribute to the paroxysmal depolarization shift, and ultimately are integral to the generation of seizure discharge. In addition, they are crucial elements in neurotransmitter release, which is required for synaptic transmission. AEDs act by combinations of these mechanisms and in some cases by entirely different mechanisms. No two currently marketed drugs work in exactly the same way.

*Drugs that modulate voltage-gated sodium channels:* carbamazepine, lamotrigine, oxycarbazepine, phenytoin, zonisamide

*Drugs that inhibit calcium channels:* ethosuximide, gabapentin, lamotrigine, methsuximide, phenobarbital (and other barbiturates), valparoate, zonisamide

*GABAA receptor inhibitors:* felbamate, topiramate

*Others:* acetazolamide, clonazepam, clorazapate, diazepam, ethotoin, levetiracetam, mephenytoin, primidone, retigabine, tiagabin, trimethadione

AEDs are used primarily to prevent epileptic seizures. Missed medications are the leading identifiable factors that provoke seizures; other factors are alcohol withdrawal, fatigue, fever or illness, sleep deprivation, and stress.

AEDs have also been used in diverse nonepileptic conditions, including the following: alcohol dependence and withdrawal, anxiety disorders, bipolar disorder, PTSD, social phobia, dystonia, essential tremor, migraine, myotonia, neuropathic pain, and restless legs syndrome.

**antiexpectation technique** See *paradoxical therapy*.

**antifetishism** Hirschfeld's term for aversions that many latent homosexuals develop as a protection against conscious recognition of their homosexuality. "One man dislikes women with large feet, another is repelled by women with hair on their bodies. ...His search is endless because he is truly, though secretly, attracted by the male." (Stekel, W. *Bi-Sexual Love*, 1922).

**antihistamines** See *antianxiety agents*.

**anti-instinctual force** *Anticathexis* (q.v.).

**antikinesis** *Obs.* All forms of nervous response; those recurring regularly and in a definite manner in response to stimulation are termed reflexes, while all the volitional responses in which there is a variable factor due to the greater complexity and elaboration in the physiological mechanism are called *antiklises*.

**antilibidinal ego** See *libidinal ego*.

**antimanic agents** Psychopharmacologic agents used to treat manic episodes; among these are lithium, carbamazepine, valproate, and verapamil. Neuroleptics are also used to control the hyperactivity and agitation of manic episodes, but their action is not considered generally to be as specific as the action of antimanic agents.

**antimuscarinic** An anticholinergic, parasympatholytic drug that blocks muscarinic receptors for acetylcholine; the best known are atropine, homatropine, and scopolamine (hyoscine). See *cholinergic*.

*Muscarinic* receptors mediate the actions of acetylcholine in the central nervous system and in the smooth muscles of the heart and gut. In some cells, they activate the enzyme guanalate cyclase, which forms the second messenger cyclic guanalate monophosphate (cGMP). In other cells, muscarinic receptors are coupled to potassium channels; they cause the channels to close, preventing the escape of potassium from the cell and thereby enhancing the cell's excitability. See *ion channel; neurotransmitter receptor; second messenger*.

A second type of receptor—the *nicotinic receptor*—mediates acetylcholine action at the neuromuscular junctions in the rest of the parasympathetic nervous system.

**antinodal behavior** See *nodal behavior*.

**antioxidants** See *free radical*.

**antipathic sexual instinct** "Great diminution or complete absence of sexual feeling for the opposite sex, with substitution of sexual feeling and instinct for the same sex (homosexuality, or antipathic sexual instinct)" (Krafft-Ebing, R. v. *Psychopathia Sexualis*, 1908).

**antipsychiatry movement** A nonspecific term referring to a diversity of negative opinions about the theory or practice of psychiatry. In some cases, what is so designated is an extension of the antiintellectual, antiprofessional stance of the *consumerism* and *advocacy* movements (qq.v.) that assumed a prominent role in the United States beginning in the 1960s. In other cases, the term refers to organized attempts to interfere with the use of psychiatry, and particularly with the use of pharmacological or other physical agents in psychiatric treatment. Many critics of such treatment argue concretistically that if psychiatry is the science of the mind, no manipulation of the body will put things right and any such attempts are viewed as physical assaults. Other critics argue that psychiatry has become a tool of the state and is a social and political activity rather than a branch of medicine; *radical therapy* (q.v.) developed from such assumptions.

**antipsychotic** *AP; neuroleptic* (q.v.). Antipsychotic drugs are currently classified as follows:

First-generation (typical) antipsychotics — D2 antagonists; they include chlorpromazine, haloperidol, fluphenazine, thioridazine, loxapine, and perphenazine.

*Second-generation (atypical) antipsychotics*— D2 and 5-HT2 antagonists; they include clozapine, risperidone, olanzapine, quetiapine, ziprasidone, and amisulpride. With the exception of amisulpride, they are characterized pharmacologically by relatively more potent serotonin 2A (5-HT$_{2A}$) than dopamine D2 receptor antagonism. Second-generation APs are characterized by a relative lack of adverse extrapyramidal symptoms and, arguably, by an ability to improve cognition. But they provide little difference in efficacy in reducing positive and negative symptoms from conventional or typical APs. In addition, because of their side effects noncompliance remains a substantial problem.

*Third-generation (atypical) antipsychotics*— aripiprazole and bifeprunox. Aripiprazole acts as a functional antagonist at D2 receptors in hyperdopaminergic states and as a functional agonist in hypodopaminerigic stages. It is also a $5\text{-HT}_{1A}$ partial agonist and a $5\text{-HT}_{2A}$ antagonist. These dopamine-serotonin system stabilizer actions may provide efficacy against both manic and depressive symptoms. It has a low risk of adverse side effects. Aripiprazole was the first atypical antipsychotic to demonstrate this profile.

With atypical APs, hyperlipidemia tends to occur in parallel with weight gain. Patients treated with atypicals are more likely to develop diabetes than patients treated with typical antipsychotics. Clozapine and olanzapine are associated with the most weight gain and the highest occurrence of diabetes and dyslipidemia. See *psychopharmacologic agents.*

**antirisk factor**    See *risk factor.*

**antisocial activity, concealed**    The antisocial nature of certain types of behavior is sometimes concealed by the fact of its arising out of socially approved motivation. A. Kardiner refers to this as concealed antisocial activity. "Competitiveness must be regarded in our society as a normal manifestation of self-assertion, when it is governed by the super-ego system. But there are neurotic and criminal forms of self-assertion.

A neurotic self-assertion is an attempt to deny by force a deep feeling of inferiority or insecurity. There are some types of self-assertion that are injurious in intent, but that escape being criminal by a technicality. A good trader may misrepresent by omission, but not by commission. If he misrepresents by omitting damaging details, he is merely a sharp trader and is both condemned and applauded; if he deliberately misrepresents, he is lying and is therefore only condemned. It is by this route that much concealed antisocial activity passes for normal." (*The Psychological Frontiers of Society,* 1945)

**antisocial personality (disorder)**    *APD;* characteristics are onset before the age of 15 as evidenced by truancy, expulsion from school, delinquency, running away, persistent lying, casual or promiscuous sexual intercourse, substance abuse, vandalism, fighting, etc., and continuing social difficulties after the age of 18 (e.g., inconsistent or unsustained work or academic record, irresponsibility as a parent, conflict with the law or multiple arrests,

impulsivity, recklessness). See *psychopathic personality.*

O. Kernberg (1989) views antisocial personality as a *narcissistic personality* (q.v.) plus a specific pathology of internalized morality (superego functions) and a particular deterioration of internalized object relations. Persons with antisocial personality display characteristics of (1) narcissistic pathology—impersonal sex life, incapacity for love, unresponsiveness in interpersonal relations, poverty in affective reactions, egocentricity and (2) severe superegopathology—unreliability, insincerity, untruthfulness, lack of remorse, poor judgment, failure to learn by experience, failure to follow any life plan, manipulative behavior. See *personality disorders.*

Kernberg classifies personality with antisocial features on a gradient: antisocial personality disorder (the most severe), malignant narcissism, narcissistic personality with antisocial features, other severe personality disorders with antisocial features, neurotic personality with antisocial features, antisocial behavior in a symptomatic neurosis, and dyssocial reaction (the least severe).

There is an overlap between antisocial and narcissistic personality disorders, and between *antisocial* and *borderline* personalities (qq.v.). In common with the other forms of lower-level (borderline) personality organization as described by Kernberg (schizoid, paranoid, and hypomanic personalities), antisocial personalities show field-dependent reality testing, unstable self-identity, and a proclivity to use primitive defenses such as splitting, denial, omnipotent idealization, and projective identification.

In *affectionless psychopaths,* pervasive self-serving narcissism results from a failure to bond and develop the early mother-infant symbiosis that is the model for all later object relations.

**antisocial spectrum disorder**    A range of behaviors that have been interpreted as different manifestations of the same biological factors that predispose to conduct disorders and antisocial personality. Included are *alcoholism* and *somatization* disorder, based on the findings that the incidence of alcoholism is significantly above normal in the families of antisocial subjects, and that the incidence of somatization disorder is significantly above normal in the female relatives of antisocial subjects.

**antitechnology bias**    See *Frankenstein factor*.

**antlophobia**    Fear of floods.

**Anton syndrome**    A specific *anosognosia* (q.v.) consisting of absence of awareness of blindness, usually cortical. It is caused by lesions of occipito-parietal areas with or without involvement of occipito-temporal visual association areas (in addition to bilateral occipital regions if blindness is cortical).

**anxietas praesenilis**    Farrar describes three main forms of *involutional melancholia* (q.v.): anxietas praesenilis, with extreme anxiety and feelings of unreality; *melancholia vera*, resembling major depression; and *depressio apathetica*, the central symptom of which is apathy.

**anxietas tibiarum**    A nervous agitation, continually impelling the patient to change the position of his legs. See *akatizia*; *restless legs syndrome*; *tachyathetosis*.

**anxiety**    An affect that differs from other affects in its specific unpleasurable characteristics. Anxiety consists of a somatic, physiological side (disturbed breathing, increased heart activity, vasomotor changes, musculoskeletal disturbances such as trembling or paralysis, increased sweating, etc.) and of a psychological side. The latter includes "a specific conscious inner attitude and a peculiar feeling state characterized (1) by a physically as well as mentally painful awareness of being powerless to do anything about a personal matter; (2) by presentiment of an impending and almost inevitable danger; (3) by a tense and physically exhausting alertness as if facing an emergency; (4) by an apprehensive self-absorption which interferes with an effective and advantageous solution of reality-problems; and (5) by an irresolvable doubt concerning the nature of the threatening evil, concerning the probability of the actual appearance of the threat, concerning the best objective means of reducing or removing the evil, and concerning one's subjective capacity for making effective use of those means if and when the emergency arises" (Piotrowski, Z. *Perceptanalysis*, 1957). Anxiety is to be differentiated from *fear*, which lacks characteristics (4) and (5). Fear is a reaction to a real or threatened danger, whereas anxiety is more typically a reaction to an unreal or imagined danger. See *amygdala*.

Freud came to believe that anxiety arises automatically whenever the psyche is overwhelmed by an influx of stimuli too great to be mastered or discharged. Such automatic anxiety may arise in response to stimuli either of external or of internal origin, but most frequently it arises from the id, that is, from the drives (id anxiety). When anxiety develops automatically according to this pattern, the situation is called a traumatic one. See *stress*.

There is a second type of anxiety, characteristic of the psychoneuroses, which Freud called signal anxiety. In the course of development the child learns to anticipate the advent of a traumatic situation and reacts to this possibility with anxiety before the situation becomes traumatic. The unpleasure arising from this threat of a *danger situation* automatically sets into operation the pleasure principle. The latter acts by enabling the ego to check or inhibit whatever id impulses might be giving rise to the danger situation. There is a series of typical danger situations that occur in sequence in the child's life. The first of these dangers, characteristic of ego development up to about 1½ years, is separation (known also as loss of the love object and as primal anxiety); the second, seen at 1 to 2 years, is loss of love; the third, seen at 2½ to 3 years, is *castration* or other genital injury; and the fourth, which is seen after the age of 5 or 6 years, when the superego has been formed, is guilt (disapproval and punishment by the superego).

Some differentiate between state anxiety (anxiety felt at a moment in time) and trait anxiety (a habitual, and perhaps in part a genetically determined tendency to be anxious in general).

Twin studies have indicated that individual variation in measures of anxiety-related personal traits is 40%–60% heritable. The amount of neuroticism is influenced by two alleles (long and short) of a gene on chromosome 17 encoding a transporter for serotonin. The short allele is associated with more protein and more neuroticism.

**anxiety, discharge of**    The process by which unconscious anxiety (tension) is chronically and repetitively nullified through action and deed in the integral activity of everyday life. Sexual activity may be used to discharge anxiety of unconscious origin.

**anxiety, endogenous**    Uncued, spontaneous anxiety or *panic attack* (q.v.) that is not situationally bound.

**anxiety, exogenous**  Anxiety symptoms or *panic attack* (q.v.) that develops in response to an external trigger.

**anxiety, free-floating**  Anxiety that is neither attached to ideational content nor otherwise channeled into substitutive symptoms; it is characteristic of *anxiety neurosis* (q.v.).

**anxiety, ictal**  See *ictal emotions.*

**anxiety, primary**  The infant's passive experiencing of excitation that cannot be mastered but must be endured. As *mastery* (q.v.) and judgment develop, the ego declares that a certain situation might give rise to this primary anxiety, and instead of the original panic itself being experienced, a moderated, tamed fear is experienced that is anxiety in anticipation of what might happen. The first fear is of a recurrence of the primal anxiety, and from this develops the fear that the child's own instinctual demands, which gave rise to the overwhelming excitation beyond his capacity to master, are dangerous in themselves. This fear is complicated by animistic thinking (the belief that the external environment has the same instincts as the self), for if the desire to recapture the primary narcissism is to be achieved by eating the parents, the child feels that the deed will be undone by his being devoured himself (talion principle). This is how anxieties of physical destruction originate; the most important representative of this group is castration anxiety.

**anxiety depersonalization neurosis**  See *depersonalization.*

**anxiety depression**  *Reactive depression* (q.v.).

**anxiety disorder, generalized**  *Generalized anxiety disorder (GAD)* (q.v.).

**anxiety disorder, secondary**  Anxiety disorder due to a general medical condition, such as cardiac arrhythmias, collagen vascular disease, coronary insufficiency, Cushing syndrome, hyperparathyroidism, hyper- or hypothyroidism, hyperventilation syndrome, hypoglycemia, multiple sclerosis, obstructive pulmonary disease, pheochromocytoma, or temporal lobe epilepsy.

**anxiety disorders**  A group of disorders in which anxiety is the most prominent feature or in which anxiety appears when the affected person tries to resist his or her symptoms. Within this group are panic disorder with or without agoraphobia, agoraphobia without a history of panic disorder, specific (simple or isolated) phobia, social phobia, obses-sive-compulsive disorder, acute stress disorder, post-traumatic stress disorder, *GAD* (generalized anxiety disorder), anxiety disorder due to a general medical condition, and *substance-induced anxiety disorder* (in intoxication and withdrawal states) (qq.v.).

In the NIMH-ECA study, anxiety disorders had a higher prevalence (14.9%) of any mental disorder other than substance-related disorders (26.6%). The rates found in specific types of panic disorder are as follows: social phobia, 13.3%; simple phobia, 11.3%; agoraphobia, 5.3%; generalized anxiety disorder, 5.1%; full-blown panic disorder, 3.5% (but panic symptoms ca. 10%); obsessive-compulsive disorder, 2.56%. There is a hereditary element in anxiety disorders; in monozygotic twins, concordance rate is 41% but in dizygotic twins only 4%. Genetic vulnerability to panic disorder and agoraphobia appears to be distinct from the genetic vulnerability to other types of anxiety disorder.

Heritability of generalized anxiety disorder, phobias, or panic attacks is in the range of 30% to 40%. Some anxiety disorders may be due to an overactive amygdala (the accelerator), while others are due to an underactive prefrontal cortex (the brake). See *fear.*

**anxiety disorders of childhood**  A group of disorders in which anxiety is the central feature. In DSM-IV, the group is no longer kept separate from adult anxiety disorders; instead, the criteria for social phobia and generalized anxiety disorder have been revised to apply to children. As originally described, the group included (1) *separation anxiety disorder*—excessive anxiety about separation from significant others, such as worries that harm will befall attachment figures or the subject if separated, school phobia, and nightmares involving separation themes; (2) *avoidant disorder*—pathologic shyness that interferes with peer functioning, persistent shrinking from contact with strangers; (3) *overanxious disorder*—generalized persistent worrying about what the future holds or what humiliations the past contains, excessive need for reassurance, multiple unfounded somatic complaints.

**anxiety elation psychosis**  See *cycloid psychosis.*

**anxiety equivalent**  The physical symptoms often associated with manifest anxiety may alone constitute the anxiety attack. They appear in various forms; e.g., attacks of sudden diarrhea or attacks of sweating, often nocturnal.

**anxiety hysteria** Phobic neurosis; a primitive reaction type and the most frequent neurosis of childhood. The main symptom is a specific fear (see listings under *fear of*) that has usually arisen from the binding of primary diffuse anxiety to a specific content. The thing that is feared may be feared because it represents a temptation (especially a situation that would ordinarily call forth an aggressive or a sexual response), or it may be feared because it represents the punishment for the forbidden impulse either directly or indirectly through symbolism, or it may be feared because of a combination of these factors. Further, the phobia may be a fear that the anxiety will return; this is seen in some agoraphobics whose initial attacks occurred in the street. The phobia may not represent castration and punishment directly, but may be concerned mainly with a fear of loss of love. See *agoraphobia; phobia.*

The two most famous cases of phobia in psychoanalytic literature are those of little Hans (Freud 1902) and the Wolf-Man (Freud 1918).

**anxiety neurosis** In 1894, Freud detached the particular syndrome of anxiety neurosis from neurasthenia and described the clinical characteristics of anxiety neurosis as follows: general irritability, anxious expectation and pangs of conscience, the anxiety attack, and phobias. Freud considered that the etiology of the anxiety neurosis was a current or contemporary one, in which forced abstinence, frustrated sexual excitement, incomplete or interrupted coitus, sexual efforts that exceed the psychical capacity, etc., all unite in disturbing the equilibrium of psychical and somatic functions in sexual activity.

For the current conceptualization of this group, see *anxiety disorders.*

**anxiety object** The displacement of anxiety to an object that is a symbolic representation of the individual who originally caused the anxiety. For example, a child fears a horse. The horse elicits marked anxiety in the child because the horse is a symbolic representation of the father, who was the original focus for anxiety. See *anxiety hysteria.*

**anxiety preparedness** The increased sensory attention and motor tension that accompany anxiety and fear.

**anxiety reaction** In DSM-I (1952), *anxiety neurosis* (q.v.).

**anxiety resolution** The therapeutic process through which the unconscious roots of anxiety are brought into consciousness and there mastered. The key to the resolution of anxiety is the recovery, in consciousness, by the subject, of repressed, albeit "forgotten" infantile, instinctual, conflict-ridden experiences, which have been mastered or overcome, and which remain fixation and regression focal points in the pseudo-adult character. Full ego maturity, in the neurotic, cannot be achieved except through this arduous path. All the forces of defense and resistance combine and conspire to defeat this process.

**anxiety sensitivity** Fear of anxiety symptoms and a tendency to respond anxiously to sensations of arousal. It appears to be an enduring trait and is correlated with physiologic hyperarousal, hypervigilance, and temperamental fearfulness.

**anxiety tolerance** See *ego weakness.*

**anxiety typology** Description of different forms of the manifestations of anxiety. Most such typologies have been developed on an ad hoc basis and therefore have not been standardized on adequate population samples. Some consultation-liaison psychiatrists group surgical patients on the basis of preoperative anxiety into low-anxiety and high-anxiety groups. Low-anxiety patients have been called *repressors, avoiders*, or *deniers*; they typically have an external locus of control and see themselves as passive participants in their treatment. High-anxiety patients have been called *sensitizers* or *vigilant*; they typically have an internal locus of control and show more anticipatory anxiety. They ask more questions of the medical staff, demand more medication, report more pain, and have long hospital stays even after minor procedures.

**anxiolytic** Reducing or abolishing anxiety. See *antianxiety agents; GABA; psychotropic.*

**anypnia** *Obs.* Sleeplessness.

**AOA** Ataxia with oculomotor apraxia, one of the genomic instability syndromes. It has been described primarily in families from Portugal and Japan. Characteristics are early-onset cerebellar ataxia with choreoathetosis, cerebellar atrophy with severe loss of Purkinje cells, degeneration of posterior columns and spinocerebellar tracts of the spinal cord, marked loss of peripheral nerve fibers with peripheral neuropathy, mild mental retardation, and hypoalbuminuria.

AOA1 is associated with mutations in the *APTX* gene, which encodes aprataxin, a novel protein that interacts with PARP1, which has a central role in the repair of DNA strand breaks. AOA2 has been mapped to chromosome 9q34 in two families. It is characterized by cerebellar atrophy, axonal sensorimotor neuropathy, and oculomotor apraxia. It is distinguished from AOA1 by its later age of onset, elevated levels of α-fetoprotein, and normal serum albumin levels. AOA2 has also been called SCAR1 (spinocerebellar ataxia, recessive, non-Friedreich type 1). The AOA2 gene is *SETX* (senataxin). It is possible that SETX is part of a DNA repair pathway and that AOA2 is a spinocerebellar syndrome associated with disturbances of DNA maintenance or cell cycle (Taroni, F. & DiDonato, S. *Nature Reviews Neuroscience 5*: 641–655, 2004).

**AO-BD** Adolescent onset bipolar disorder. See *pediatric bipolar disorder.*

**AOD** Alcohol and other drugs that are used in addictive disorders.

**AOT** Assisted outpatient commitment. See *outpatient commitment.*

**AP** *Antipsychotic* (q.v.); anterior-posterior. See *neuroleptic; psychopharmacologic agents.*

**AP complex** *Adaptor protein complex* (q.v.).

**A-P psychiatrist** Analytic-psychological psychiatrist; referring to an approach that is essentially nondirective and utilizes a psychodynamic orientation with acceptance of such basic psychoanalytic concepts as unconscious mental activity, conflict, repression, and transference. See *D-O psychiatrist.*

**APA** American Psychiatric Association; also, American Psychological Association. The American Psychiatric Association was founded as the Association of Medical Superintendents of American Institutions for the Insane in 1844; its name was changed to American Medico-Psychological Association in 1891, and to American Psychiatric Association in 1921.

**Apaf** See *apoptotic pathway.*

**apallic syndrome** Kretschmer's term for a prolonged state of disturbed consciousness, generally following closed head trauma, characterized by mutism, akinesia, primitive mass reflex, oral reflex, contractions, and extrapyramidal disturbances.

**apandria** Aversion to men.

**apathetic** Without feeling; listless. See *hebetude.*

**apathetic syndrome** 1. A frontal lobe syndrome, associated with pathology in the mesial frontal neural system. See *orbitomedial syndrome.*

2. pathetic thyrotoxicosis—although hyperthyroidism often mimics an anxiety state, about 15% of patients manifest depression, with apathy and sluggishness.

**apathy** Loss of motivation, loss of interest in daily activities, loss of initiative, and a reduced affective response (lack of feeling). Apathy is frequent in neurodegenerative dementia, where it is manifested as loss of motivation, loss of interest in daily activities, loss of initiative, and reduced affective response. It has been correlated with a loss of brain activity in the anterior cingulate and orbitofrontal cortex. Apathy, more than depressed mood, is associated with deterioration in the quality of interpersonal, and especially spousal, relationships. See *hebetude.*

**apeirophobia** Fear of infinity. See *infinity neurosis.*

**aPFC** Anterior *prefrontal cortex* (q.v.); Brodmann area 10; frontal pole

**aphalgesia, haphalgesia** *Obs.* A rare type of psychogenic pain disorder; pain appears on contact with a substance that has some special significance for the subject, such as certain metals, liquids, or textures. For one subject, the mere thought of touching a peach skin produced a throbbing pain in his right forearm. See *somatoform disorders.*

**aphanisis** *Obs.* "Extinction of sexuality. The concept of "castration' should be reserved, as Freud pointed out, for the penis alone, and should not be confounded with that of 'extinction of sexuality' for which the term 'aphanisis' is proposed" (Jones, E. *Papers on Psycho-Analysis*, 1938).

**aphasia** More properly, *dysphasia*, any disturbance in the comprehension or expression of language due to brain lesion and not the result of faulty innervation of the speech muscles or disorders of articulation or mental retardation. The word *language*, as used in this definition, refers not only to the expression or communication of thought by word, writing, and gesture, but also to the reception and interpretation of such acts when carried out by others and also to the retention, recall, and visualization of the symbols involved. Thus aphasia would technically include the agnosias and the apraxias. Aphasia occurs in users of *sign language* (q.v.) as well as in persons who use spoken language.

The most common causes of aphasia are head trauma, which in the United States is responsible for about 200,000 cases each year, and stroke, which produces about 100,000 cases. In about 98% of aphasics, the damage is somewhere in the perisylvian region of the left cerebral hemisphere, the hemisphere that is specialized for *language* (q.v.). The anterior portion of this region, which contains the Broca area, is involved in the grammatical structure of language and not only the content of sentences.

Classification of the aphasias is confusing; some approaches are primarily anatomic, while others are primarily functional or physiologic. The different forms of aphasia are typically compared in terms of several prominent symptoms, such as fluency, intactness of repetition, comprehension, etc.

In *fluent aphasia* (approximately equivalent to the older term *receptive aphasia*), rate of speech is normal or rapid, and speech melody is preserved. Speech is lacking in informational content and paraphasias are prominent (see *paraphasia*). Among the fluent aphasias are Wernicke, anomic, conduction, and transcortical sensory aphasia.

In *nonfluent aphasia* (approximately equivalent to the older term *expressive aphasia*), verbal output is diminished. Dysarthria is present and great articulatory effort is required when the patient tries to speak. Speech melody is lost. Information content is preserved, but speech is filled with short phrases or single words and is agrammatic (*functor* words such as "an," "and," and "the" are missing). Paraphasias are not seen in the nonfluent aphasias. Among the nonfluent aphasias are Broca, global, transcortical motor, and mixed transcortical aphasia. See *frontotemporal lobar degeneration*.

The major types of aphasia are as follows:
1. Broca aphasia (q.v.)
2. Wernicke aphasia (q.v.)
3. Conduction aphasia (q.v.)
4. Global aphasia (q.v.)
5. Transcortical aphasias (q.v.)
6. Anomic aphasia (q.v.)
7. Subcortical aphasia (q.v.)

**aphasia, congenital** Inborn or constitutionally determined types of verbal or symbol-handling difficulty. The specific disability may appear in the fields of speaking, reading, writing, spelling, arithmetic, and even musical appreciation. The reading disability—*dyslexia* (q.v.), or congenital word-blindness—has received the most intensive study.

Specific reading, writing, and spelling difficulty is often found connected with a tendency to reverse letters and words in reading and writing. This condition has been named *strephosymbolia.*

Congenital word-deafness, a rare form of congenital aphasia, is characterized by the inability of otherwise intelligent children to comprehend the meaning of words heard. Deafness, in the ordinary sense, is not present. See *auditory aphasia.*

Certain forms of congenital aphasia, like *stuttering* (q.v.), seem connected with the whole question of handedness, eyedness, footedness, laterality, or the predominance, physiologically, of one cerebral hemisphere over the other in motor function.

**aphelxia** See *ecphronia.*

**aphemia** *Obs.* Speechlessness; loss of power of speech; *aphasia* (q.v.).

**aphephobia** Haptephobia; haphephobia; fear of being touched.

**aphonia, aphony** Voicelessness; muteness. Aphony may be due to organic or psychic causes, though the term is generally used today to indicate structural or organic changes.

**aphoria** *Obs.* Amyotony; asthenia and, particularly, the inability to increase energy or muscle tone through exercise (*amyosthenia*). Janet thought it characteristic of neurotics.

**aphoristic multiple sclerosis** A type of *multiple sclerosis* (q.v.) characterized by pyramidal signs in both lower extremities, with subjective symptoms limited to one extremity.

**aphrasia** Inability to utter or understand words connected in the form of phrases. A subdivision of *aphasia* (q.v.) that involves only the order of words in the phrase and goes a stage beyond individual words: the patient's power (1) *expressive* (motor), i.e., to utter, or (2) *perceptive* (sensory), i.e., to understand, *single words* may be unimpaired, whereas *groups* of words forming phrases may baffle the patient completely as far as using or understanding them is concerned. See *speech disorders.*

**aphrodisiac** Characterized by sexual excitation; also, any agent (e.g., odor) that stimulates sexual activity; entatic.

**aphthongia** A form of motor aphasia characterized by spasm of the speech muscles.

**apiphobia** Fear of bees.

**apistiatria**   Loss of faith in the physician.

**aplasia**   Complete or partial failure of tissue to grow or develop; arrested development; agenesis. It is to be distinguished from atrophy, that refers to the loss or diminution of structure that once had normal or average development. When tissue growth is partial, the term *hypoplasia* is used; when above average, *hyperplasia*.

**aplastic**   Without power to grow toward normal, healthy tissue.

**aplestia**   Greediness.

**apnea, central**   Cessation of breathing due to neurologic disturbances of ventilatoy drive and frequency (in contrast to the more usual obstructive apnea, which is due to abnormalities of the nasal, pharyngeal, or laryngeal passage). *Sleep apnea* and sleep hypopnea, the interruption of sleep by respiratory disturbances, may present only as complaints of sleepiness during the day, for the subject's breathing may be normal during waking hours and he or she does not remember the frequent awakenings that have occurred during the night because of the respiratory abnormality. See *sleep disorders.*

*Primary alveolar hypotension* is a result of defective chemoreceptors (which are sensitive to pH and carbon dioxide) or of damage to the pontine-medullary system that controls breathing during sleep. As a result, the subject fails to breathe during sleep and may, in fact, die during sleep (*Ondine curse*).

**Apo1**   *Fas* (q.v.).

**apocarteresis**   Suicide by hunger or starvation.

**apoclesis**   Aversion to, or absence of desire for, food.

**apolipoprotein E**   *Apo E*; a protein that mediates binding of lipoproteins to the low-density lipoprotein (LDL) receptor and to the LDL receptor–related protein (LRP). In the nervous system, apo E is synthesized primarily by the astrocytes and macrophages; its functions include maintaining homeostasis of plasma cholesterol and, probably, mobilization of lipids during normal development of the nervous system and in the regeneration of peripheral nerves after injury.

Genes that predispose their carriers to late-onset AD (after age 65) have products that interact with a class of cell-surface receptors known as the *low-density lipoprotein (LDL) receptor family*. All members of this multifunctional family are receptors for apolipoprotein E (Apo E, on chromosome 19), which in the brain is produced by glial cells (whereas its receptors are most abundantly expressed on neurons).

Apo E occurs in three major isoforms, Apo $\varepsilon2$, Apo $\varepsilon3$, and Apo $\varepsilon4$, which are products of three alleles at a single gene locus on chromosome 19. The most common isoform is Apo $\varepsilon3$. Apo $\varepsilon4$ is associated with familial late-onset and sporadic *Alzheimer disease* (q.v.). Subjects who inherit the Apo $\varepsilon4$ gene from both parents (Apo $\varepsilon4$/Apo $\varepsilon4$ combination) are nine times more likely to develop AD than subjects with the $\varepsilon3/\varepsilon3$ combination, and age of onset of the disorder in general reflects the concentration of the $\varepsilon4$ gene: age of onset is about 68 years in $\varepsilon4/$, 4 subjects, about 77 years in $\varepsilon4/\varepsilon3$ subjects, and about 85 years in $\varepsilon3/\varepsilon3$ subjects.

How Apo E enhances A$\beta$ deposition is unknown. Several pathways involving Apo E receptors may be involved in the pathogenesis of AD: (1) modulation of APP processing—APP interacts directly with Apo E; the interaction increases the rate at which the amyloid-$\beta$ peptide is released from APP;

(2) modulation of amyloid-$\beta$ removal—binding of Apo E to its receptors in CNS may promote the formation of lesions;

(3) modulation of tau phosphorylation—tau mutations have been identified as a cause for frontotemporal dementia in humans with parkinsonism (FTDP). A post-translational modification of tau that precedes tangle formation involves an abnormally high level of phosphorylation of tau. Tau phorphorylation is greatly increased in mouse brains harboring genetic defects in Apo E or in the reelin signalling pathway, which includes Apo E receptors.

**apoplectic type**   See *habitus apoplecticus.*

**apoplexy**   Stroke. See *cerebrovascular accident.*

**apopnixis**   *Globus hystericus* (q.v.).

**apoptosis**   (In Greek, *apoptosis* describes a flower losing its petals or a tree its leaves; "floral shedding") *Naturally occurring neuronal death, programmed cell death (PCD), cell pruning*; an active process that requires RNA and protein synthesis: cytoplasmic and nuclear condensation with shrinkage of the cell, cytoplasmic vacuolation, development of protuberances (blebs) on its membranes, and fragmentation of its DNA. (Degenerative cell death produced by injury, in contrast, consists of cell swelling and lysis.) Apoptosis is the outcome of a programmed intracellular cascade of genetically determined steps, first described by Kerr et al. in 1972. The cascade is centered on the activation of *caspases*, hence it is often called the *caspase cascade (q.v.)*. Cells that are programmed to die go through a predictable, well-choreographed series of events activated by a cell-intrinsic suicide program.

In many parts of the nervous system, more than half the neurons die before embryonic development is complete; this process of neuronal pruning is necessary if the brain is to form its multiple precise connections between nerve cells. Apoptosis is not limited to embryonic development (in the human, another massive pruning of neurons occurs at about the time of puberty), and it occurs in all tissues, not just in brain. It enables the immune system to rid itself of cells that attack the body's tissue in autoimmune diseases.

Apoptosis can be triggered by internal signals from within cells, such as DNA damage; by external signals from the cell surface, such as tumor necrosis factor α (TNF-α); and by reactive oxygen species. Two major groups of proteins in the *BCL2* (B-cell leukemia/lymphoma) family have pivotal roles in most types of apoptosis: proapoptotic proteins such as Bcl2-associated protein X (Bax) and Bcl-associated death promotor (Bad); and antiapoptotic proteins such as Bcl2, Bcl-xL, Bcl-w, and Boo. Bax and Bad increase mitochondrial membrane permeability and the release of apoptotic factors, whereas Bcl2 and Bcl-xL stabilize the membrane. The cell death pathway is initiated by the activation of proteolytic enzymes, the caspases (suitably named *executioner proteins)*. A high ratio of Bax to Bcl2 activates caspase family members to obliterate cellular proteins and DNA, leading to cell death. The reactive oxygen species activate apoptosis-inducing factor (ASF), which directly binds to targeting DNAs and degrades them.

In contrast to necrosis, apoptosis inflicts minimal damage on surrounding cells. Its physiological hallmarks are nuclear compaction, chromatin condensation, internucleosomal cleavage of DNA, blebbing of the plasma membrane, and disintegration of the cell into multiple vesicles. PCD is not the sole mediator of cell demise in neurodegenerative disorders, but it is an important member of the coalition of deleterious mechanisms that contribute to the degenerative process.

**apoptosis-related diseases**  Diseases associated with the inhibition of apoptosis include the following:

1. Cancer: folliclular lymphomas; carcinomas with p53 mutations; hormone-dependent tumors of the breast, prostate, and ovary.

2. Autoimmune disorders: systemic lupus, immune-mediated glomerlonephritis.

3. Viral infections: herpes viruses, poxviruses, adenoviruses

Diseases associated with increased apoptosis include the following:

1. AIDS

2. Neurodegenerative disorders: Alzheimer disease, Parkinson disease, amyotrophic lateral sclerosis, retinitis pigmentosa, cerebellar degeneration

3. Myelodysplastic syndromes: aplastic anemia

4. Ischemic injury: myocardial infarction, stroke

5. Toxin-induced liver disease: due to alcohol

**apoptotic pathway**  The different steps in *apoptosis* (q.v.). Proteases such as caspases and calpains trigger apoptosis by degrading various structural proteins. Two major groups of proteins in the Bcl2 (B-cell leukemia/lymphoma) family have central roles in apoptosis:

1. Pro-apoptotic proteins such as Bcl2-associated protein X (BAX) and Bcl-associated death promotor (BAD); BAX and BAD increase mitochondrial membrane permeability and the release of apoptotic factors.

2. Anti-apoptotic proteins such as Bcl2 and Bcl-X, which stabilize the membrane.

There are three categories of apoptotic stimuli: (1) those that engage the $Ca^{2+}$ gateway in the endoplasmic reticulum to release calcium; (2) those that depend upon the presence of Bax/Bad in the mitochondria; (3) those whose killing potency depends on both the reticular and mitochondrial pathways.

**apositia**  *Obs.* Loathing of food.

**apostle of the idiots**  Edouard Séguin (1812–1880), a French psychiatrist whose lifework was the care and welfare of the mentally retarded.

**apotemnophilia**  The wish to amputate one's own limb; it has been reported among some persons with *lata* (q.v.). The term is also used to refer to a *paraphilia* (q.v.) in which sexual arousal and orgasm are dependent upon the subject's being a self-amputee.

**APP** Amyloid precursor protein, which generates β-*amyloid peptide* (q.v.). APP processing is cholesterol dependent, and cholesterol depletion leads to reduced Aβ production. It is still unclear whether lowering cholesterol levels under physiological conditions will lead to significant changes in human brain Aβ metabolism.

**apparition** *Rare.* Visual hallucination or visual illusion, particularly when such phenomena occur as part of an organic delirium. Such visual illusions result from the visual distortion of an object and the interpretation of the object in terms of the (usually unconscious and morbid) impulses of the patient. In alcoholic delirium, for instance, any object may be regarded as a person who is about to kill the patient.

**apperception** Conscious realization; awareness of the significance of a percept and particularly interpretation of what is apprehended by relating it to similar, already existing knowledge. See *central integrative field factor.*

**apperception scheme** By this term Adler indicated that the person perceives what he wishes to perceive and selects from his whole experience what is useful in view of his directive fiction, forgetting or rejecting the rest of reality. See *fiction, directive.*

**apperceptions, gestalt** See *intelligence.*

**apperceptive dementia** *Obs.* Used by Weygandt to denote a type of dementia induced primarily by disorder in the volitional and intellectual spheres. Weygandt applied the term to dementia praecox (schizophrenia), conceiving the so-called deterioration in the light of "disintegration" of the will, which in turn interrupted the normal train of thought, the final effect appearing as dementia.

**apperceptive distortion** A subjective interpretation of a perception that is dynamically meaningful because it is influenced by memories of previous percepts. The various projective tests (Rorschach, TAT, etc.) deal with apperceptive distortions of different degrees.

**appersonification, appersonation** The act of embodiment or impersonation of another, typically on the basis of unconscious identification with another in part or in whole. See *depersonification; personality multiplication.*

**appetite** Desire for food or drink. See *arcuate nucleus.*

**appetite-regulating network** *ARN.* See *hypothalamus.*

**application groups** See *Group Relations Conferences, A. K. Rice.*

**apprehension** The simple or elementary intellectual act or process of becoming aware of some object or fact. *Misapprehension* is failure to understand or perceive correctly. Apprehension has also been used to refer to anxiety related to fear of some future event, but many prefer to call such anxiety *apprehensiveness.*

**apprehension, irresistible** Kraepelin's term for what is now termed *obsessive-compulsive disorder* (q.v.).

**apprehensiveness** See *apprehension.*

**apprentice complex** The time in a boy's life when he aims to be like his father and will act as a pupil or apprentice: in psychoanalytic terms, will have a penis like his father. To achieve this, he is submissive, passive, with the idea or phantasy that by this method, in the future, he will be prepared to be masculine and active, like his father.

**approach** Orientation, hypothesis, theory.

**approbative mirroring** See *empathic failure.*

**approval** Condonement; to be differentiated from social tolerance, in that what a society tolerates is not necessarily what a majority of its members personally approve of. See *tolerance, social.*

**approximate answers syndrome** A subject's tendency to answer questions with relevance to the general topic, but with glaring disregard for details—the so-called syndrome of approximate answers, also known in psychiatric literature as the *Ganser syndrome* (q.v.), the condition having been first described by him.

For instance, when shown a 25-cent piece the patient calls it a dollar or a dime. He writes three when asked to write two, raises the left arm when asked to raise the right, calls a match a cigarette; a comb is a brush or something to use for the hair. The syndrome usually occurs in persons facing criminal responsibility and may be an attempt to avoid trial and punishment.

**approximations, successive** *Shaping* (q.v.).

**apraxia** Impairment in executing learned skilled movements that cannot be explained by elementary sensory or motor deficits, lack of comprehension, inattention, weakness, ataxia, or basal ganglia disorder. Apraxia is usually a manifestation of a lesion of the frontal association area or the posterior parietal lobe. Apraxic patients are able to perform simple movements but not complex acts, such as combing the hair or brushing the teeth. They have difficulty in performing symbolic gestures and pantomimes, where movements must be guided by stored representations rather than by contextual cues. Parietal lesions can affect both motor production and ideation, because some patients with apraxia also have difficulty recognizing the meaning of gestures or in judging their accuracy. Various types of apraxia (or dyspraxia) have been described: *akinetic, constructional* (including *dressing apraxia*), *dynamic, ideational,* and *motor* (qq.v.). See *parietal lobe; parietal lobe dysfunction.*

**aprosexia**  Inability to maintain attention, common in organic states that affect the brain and in psychiatric conditions in which (1) there are present overwhelming emotions that constantly interfere with thought processes; (2) ideas are sparse, as in states of pronounced depression; (3) ideas are so abundant that the patient cannot fix attention on external objects, as in productive mania; (4) fixed ideas of the patient demand his constant attention. The patient may show excellent attentive capacity when his special interests are involved, that is, aprosexia may be selective for certain matters.

**aprosodia**  *Aprosody;* inability to inflect one's speech with affect or recognize emotional elements of another's speech. The aprosodias mirror the aphasias in that prosody and emotional gesturing are organized in the nondominant hemisphere just as the cognitive aspects of language are organized in the dominant hemisphere. Difficulty in expressing the emotional aspects of language (*motor aprosodia*) is an expression of nondominant frontal lobe disease; the affected subject's speech is bland, colorless, or blunted. Inappropriate emotional expression, on the other hand, and inability to understand the emotional aspects of another's speech (*sensory aprosodia*) suggests damage in the nondominant temporal area. See *frontal lobe; temporal lobe dysfunction.*

**apsychognosia**  Lack of awareness of one's own personality or mental state; used particularly to refer to the alcoholic's typical lack of awareness of the outside world's reaction to his or her drinking.

**apsychosis**  *Rare.* In F. M. Barnes's terminology, absence of mental functioning and particularly of thinking, as in stupor. Barnes also referred to *hyperpsychosis* (exaggeration of mental functioning), *hypopsychosis* (diminution of function), and *parapsychosis* (perversion of function) (*An Introduction to the Study of Mental Disorders,* 1923).

**aptitude**  In occupational therapy, the ability and natural skill of a patient in certain lines of endeavor.

**aptitude test**  A test of the probable level of future performance that will be reached following further maturation and/or training.

**APV**  See *NMDA receptor.*

**Aqp**  See *aquaporins.*

**aquaphobia**  Fear of going (to bathe or swim) into a body of water where one may drown.

**aquaporins**  Members of a family of specialized water channels that control rapid fluxes of water across cell membranes. Two subfamilies are differentiated: aquaporins, permeable only to water; and aquaglyceroporins, permeable also to glycerol and other solutes. Of the 11 members identified in mammals, the brain is known to contain three: Aqp1, restricted to the choroid plexus; Aqp4, in astrocytes and ependymal cells; and Aqp9, an aquaglyceroporin found in the ependymal lining of the third ventricle as well as in astrocytes and endothelial cells.

**aqueduct of Sylvius**  See *ventricle.*

**arachibutyrophobia**  Fear of peanut butter sticking to the roof of one's mouth.

**arachidonic acid**  One of the three second messenger systems (the others are cAMP and diacylglycerol-inositol); its metabolites can act directly on an ion channel. Arachidonic acid is involved in two intracellular pathways: (1) synthesis of prostaglandins and thromboxanes, involving the enzyme cyclooxygenase; and (2) synthesis of leukotrienes and lipoxins, which regulate cellular response in inflammation and immunity. See *omega-3 fatty acids.*

**arachnoid**  See *meninges.*

**arachnoiditis**  See *pseudotumor cerebri.*

**arachnophobia**  Fear of spiders.

**ARBD**  Alcohol-related birth defect(s), the best known of which is FAS, *fetal alcohol syndrome* (q.v.). Most workers believe that the adverse effects of alcohol on the fetus range on a continuum, with the most severe expression being FAS, the less severe demonstrating only some of the criteria for the diagnosis of FAS.

Sometimes, however, ARBD and FAS are used interchangeably.

**arbitrary inferences** See *cognitive therapy*.

**ARC** 1. AIDS-related complex, a clustering of certain symptoms that some clinicians consider to be the earliest indicators or premonitory signs of *AIDS* (q.v.), including lymph node enlargement, night sweats, persistent fevers, persistent cough, prolonged diarrhea, weight loss, and development of thrush. Other terms that have been used for such symptom clusters include *GLS* (generalized lymphadenopathy syndrome), *AIDS prodrome*, and *pre-AIDS*.

 2. *Arcuate nucleus* of the *hypothalamus* (qq.v.).

**arc, psychic reflex** Ferenczi's term for the primitive ontogenetic and phylogenetic stage of development in which adaptation is not achieved by a modification of the outer world, but instead by modifications of the organism itself, and particularly by simple motor discharge. Freud called this the *autoplastic* stage.

**arc de cercle** (F. "arc or segment of a circle") A pathological posture characterized by pronounced bending of the body, anteriorly or posteriorly (opisthotonus).

**archaeology** The science of antiquities, studies of the history, use, and meaning of prehistoric objects in different countries, in order to throw light on the remote past of humankind. See *anthropology*.

**archaic** Antiquated; stemming from a primitive or prehistoric age. Archaic modes of thinking and expression are seen frequently in the schizophrenias. See *paleologic*.

**archaic inheritance** The realization of racial influences operating in the development of the individual psyche. See *phylogenesis*.

**archaic-paralogical thinking** E. von Domarus (1924) classified thinking into (1) *prearchaic*; (2) *archaic-paralogical*; and (3) *paralogical-logical*. The latter two he considered to be typical of primitive savages, and common in schizophrenia, and the first as typical of the human's anthropoid progenitors and of schizophrenic stupor. In 1940, Osborne recommended changing the name of schizophrenia to palaeophrenia to emphasize the importance of regression to primitive subrational forms of thinking in the schizophrenic disorders.

 Primitive thinking, primordial thinking, anthropoid thinking—all are synonyms for archaic-paralogical thinking. They are all

characterized by impairment or deficiency of abstraction and generalization, with a tendency toward concrete rather than abstract thinking.

**archaism** In Jung's analytical psychology, the *ancient* character of psychic contents and functions, qualities that have the character of *survival* and correspond with the qualities of primitive mentality.

**archetype** In Jungian theory, an inherited idea or mode of thought, derived from the experience of the race, and present in the unconscious of the individual, controlling his ways of perceiving the world. See *analytic psychology*.

 The unconscious part of the mind is separated by Jung into two subdivisions, the personal unconscious and the collective unconscious. The *personal unconscious* lies directly beneath consciousness and contains psychic material that is not in consciousness, yet is subject to conscious recall. Constituting by far the largest area of the mind, and situated beneath the personal unconscious, is the *collective unconscious*. The material contained in this area is not derived from the lifeexperience of the person, but from the lifeexperience of the person's progenitors, all of them, and therefore of the entire human race. The record of this history and experience contains ideas, modes of thought, patterns of reaction that are fundamental and typical in all humanity: the archetypes are their representations in the collective unconscious.

 "In the language of the unconscious, which is a picture-language, the archetypes appear in personified or symbolized picture form.... We find them repeated in all mythologies, fairy tales, religious traditions, and mysteries.... Prometheus, the stealer of fire, Hercules, the slayer of dragons, the numerous myths of creation, the fall from Paradise, the sacrificial mysteries, the virgin birth, the treacherous betrayal of the hero, the dismembering of Osiris, and many other myths and tales portray psychic processes in symbolic-imaginary form. Likewise the forms of the snake, the fish, the sphinx, the helpful animals, the World Tree, the *Great Mother*, and otherwise the enchanted prince, the puer aeternus, the Magi, the Wise Man, Paradise, etc., stand for certain figures and contents of the collective unconscious. The sum of the archetypes signifies thus for Jung the sum of all the latent potentialities of the human psyche" (Jacobi, J. *The Psychology of C. G. Jung*, 1942).

**architecture of network**   The structure or design of the neural *network* (q.v.), particularly insofar as it imposes boundaries within which the network and brain can act. Connections between neurons are the essence of brain functioning, but they consume energy and occupy space. Neurons, circuits, and neural codes are designed to conserve space, material, time, and energy.

Gray matter, which accounts for slightly less than 60% of cerebral cortex, contains the synapses, dendrites, cell bodies, and local axons of neurons, and these structures form the neural circuits (wiring) that process information. Long-range connections between cortical areas constitute the white matter and occupy 44% of the cortical volume in humans. This wiring fraction minimizes local delays by striking the optimal balance between two opposing tendencies: transmission speed and component density.

About 50% of the brain's energy is used to drive signals along axons and across synapses. The remainder supports the maintenance of resting potentials and the vegetative function of neurons and glia. Cortical gray matter uses a higher proportion of total energy consumption for signaling, more than 75%, because it is so richly interconnected with axons and synapses. Several features of brain structure, in combination, conserve energy: (1) The convolutions of the human cortex allow the large cortical area to be packed in the skull but also allow cortical areas around the convolutions to minimize wire length. (2) Parallel columns—connectivity is much higher between neurons separated by less than 1 mm than between neurons farther apart. The probability of any two cortical neurons having a direct connection is around 1 in 100 for neurons in a vertical column 1 mm. in diameter, but only 1 in 1,000,00 for distant neurons. Use of cortical columns for rapid, local processing not only minimizes wire length, it also reduces the volume occupied by long-range connections. (3) In similar fashion, the layout of ganglia minimizes wire length (Laughlin, S. B. & Sejnowski, T. J., *Science 301*: 1870–1873, 2003). See *synchronization*.

**Arctic hysteria**   *Piblokto* (q.v.).

**arcuate fasciculus**   A neural pathway in the lower parietal lobe that connects the receptor and motor speech zones. If damaged, it produces the disconnection syndrome of conduction aphasia.

**arcuate nucleus**   The arcuate nucleus of the hypothalamus (ARH) contains two populations of neurons with opposing actions on food intake. One produces the orexigenic (appetite-stimulating) neuropeptides NPY (nucleopeptide Y) and AgRP (agouti-related protein). The second produces the anorexigenic (appetite-suppressing) neuropeptides POMC (proopiomelanocortin) and CART (cocaine- and amphetamine-regulated transcript). Increased NPY activity and reduced POMC activity appear to increase feeding and fat deposition, whereas reduced NPY activity and increased POMC activity decrease feeding and body mass. See *ghrelin*; *glucocorticoids*; *leptin*.

ARH projects to three other hypothalamic nuclei that are involved in food intake: the paraventricular nucleus (PVH), the dorsomedial hypothalamic nucleus (DMH), and the lateral hypothalamic area (LHA). See *hypothalamus*.

**area, delinquency**   A neighborhood or community with a disproportionately high rate of juvenile delinquents.

**area striata**   See *occipital lobe*.

**arecoline**   A parasympathomimetic drug; on occasion it has produced short-lived intervals of lucidity in schizophrenic subjects.

**argininosuccinic aciduria**   *Allan-Dent disease*; a metabolic defect characterized by a high quantity of argininosuccinic acid in the cerebrospinal fluid and urine; associated with this are epilepsy, EEG dysrhythmia, and mental retardation.

**Argyll Robertson pupil**   (Douglas Argyll Robertson, Scottish physician, 1837–1909) A pupil, usually miotic, that responds to accommodation but does not respond to light and reacts slowly to mydriatics. It is usually found in patients with neurosyphilis, although it may appear in other conditions (traumatic brain injury, brain tumor, infectious diseases of the brain, multiple sclerosis, etc.).

**argyrophilic dystrophy**   See *Alzheimer disease*.

**ARH**   *Arcuate nucleus* of hypothalamus (q.v.).

**aristogenic**   *Obs.* Best endowed eugenically. See *eugenics*.

**arithmetic disorder**   See *developmental disorders, specific*.

**arithmomania** Compulsion to count.

**ARJP** Autosomal recessive, juvenile-onset Parkinson disease. See *parkin*.

**ARMS** At-risk mental state; latent schizophrenia. See *schizophrenia prodrome*.

**Army mental tests** Tests devised during World War I to determine the intellectual status of recruits examined for the United States Army.

**ARN** Appetite-regulating network in the *hypothalamus* (q.v.).

**Arnold-Chiari malformation** (Friedrich Arnold, German anatomist, 1803–1890; and Hans Chiari, German physician, 1851–1916) A congenital abnormality of the central nervous system characterized by protrusion of the medulla and cerebellum into the spinal column. Hydrocephalus is usually present and, commonly, there is an associated meningomyelocele and lumbosacral spina bifida.

**arousal** Cortical vigilance or readiness; activation of the nervous system, alertness, wakefulness, usually with the implication that the subject is attentive and able to process information. See *reticular formation*.

The *hypocretins* (also known as *orexins*) constitute a neuropeptide system in the lateral hypothalamus that is central to the regulation of arousal states and energy metabolism. The densest projections outside the hypothalamus are to structures that regulate wakefulness, including the dorsal raphe nucleus and the locus coeruleus. Hypocretins increase wakefulness and suppress REM sleep. The hypocretin system links homeostatic needs and the level of arousal.

Arousal is a more general level of cortical readiness to respond than *attention* (q.v.). *Sexual arousal* refers to excitation or responsivity to erotic stimulation.

**arousal disorder, sexual** Inability to maintain an adequate lubrication-swelling response (in the female) or adequate erection (in the male) until completion of the sexual activity. Male sexual arousal disorder is also known as *erectile disorder*.

**arousal reconditioning** A behavioral technique used to reduce recidivism of paraphilic behavior: masturbatory pleasure and orgasm are paired with nondeviant fantasy. In those subjects who cannot be aroused by nondeviant fantasies, the subject masturbates to deviant stimuli first, and nondeviant stimuli are later introduced just before orgasm, and gradually earlier before orgasm is reached. See *reconditioning; satiation techniques*.

**arousal response** See *alpha blocking*.

**arousal theory** The hypothesis that diminution in personal space increases arousal, and that when personal space becomes inadequate arousal may be expressed in aggression.

**arrangement, neurotic** The construction and marshaling of erroneous ideas on the part of a neurotic patient in order to justify his neurosis with apparently logical reasons, by rearranging the events of his life to suit his neurosis (Stekel, W. *The Interpretation of Dreams*, 1943).

**arrhythmokinesis** Inability to maintain a desired or requested rhythmicity in the performance of an act.

**arson** Pathological or illegal fire-setting. See *pyromania*.

**arsphenamine hemorrhagic encephalitis** A toxic and probably idiosyncratic reaction (hence more correctly termed an encephalopathy) to the intravenous administration of arsphenamine. This is a rare complication and usually occurs 1 to 3 days after injection. Vomiting and headache are rapidly followed by restlessness and delirium, passing into coma with stertorous respiration and often generalized convulsions. In fatal cases, there is edema of the brain, capillary engorgement, and perivascular hemorrhage as well as nonhemorrhagic perivascular areas of necrosis and demyelination.

**ART** *Assisted reproductivetechnologies*, which began with *IVF* (q.v.), developed in England in 1977, and most recently *ICSI* (q.v.), developed in Belgium in 1992. Among the ethical and social questions raised by ICSI are as follows: (1) it enables sex predetermination, of inestimable benefit in individual instances but potentially disastrous if practiced widely in societies that greatly prefer male vs. female offspring; (2) it enables the sperm of a recently deceased man to be preserved, with the potential of generating a generation of instant orphans; and (3) it provides an opportunity for men who are genetically infertile to sire one or more children, but infertile men may carry other genetic defects (such as cystic fibrosis), and effective treatment of genetic infertility in such men may make the uninheritable heritable.

**arterenol** Norepinephrine. See *epinephrine*.

**arteriogram** *Angiogram* (q.v.).

**arthritis**   Inflammation of a joint, usually manifested by pain and stiffness in the joint. Of the various types of arthritis, the one of most interest to psychiatry is rheumatoid (atrophic) arthritis, consisting of a chronic proliferative inflammation of the synovial membrane, involving multiple joints but with a predilection for the smaller ones, and characterized by wide variations in severity and a tendency to inexplicable remissions and exacerbations. Some authorities have considered rheumatoid arthritis to be primarily a psychophysiological or psychosomatic disturbance. Alexander, for instance, believed that the specific dynamic pattern is repression of all hostile, competitive tendencies. If the aggressive attack in inhibited at the stage of psychological preparation, a migraine attack develops; if it is inhibited at the stage of vegetative preparation, essential hypertension develops; and if it is inhibited at the neuromuscular phase, an inclination toward arthritis may develop. See *hypertension, essential.*

**Arthur Point Scale test**   A nonverbal performance measure of intellectual ability, consisting of 10 subtests, mainly of the form-board variety. The test is most reliable within the 7- to 13-year age range and is of particular value when the subject's verbal capacity is compromised by foreign language handicap, speech or hearing defect, or personal and cultural factors.

**articulation**   The motor act of producing speech sounds.

**articulation disorder**   In DSM-IV, termed *phonological disorder.* See *developmental disorders, specific; speech disorders.*

**artificial intelligence**   *AI;* the science built around computer simulation, considered by many to be the central discipline in *cognitive science.* Its founding fathers were John McCarthy, Marvin Minsky, Allen Newell, and Herbert Simon. The Imitation Game, or the Turing Test, asserts that the existence of "thinking" is solely a matter of producing convincing responses to more or less arbitrary stimuli. Any "black box" that does a convincing job of imitating a human being in ordinary conversation would be deemed to possess genuine intelligence and could (and should) be thought of as a "thinking entity."

Artificial intelligence seeks to produce, on a computer, a pattern of output that would be considered intelligent if displayed by human beings. Computers can behave intelligently using two basic ingredients: (1) search, to find all the possibilities available, and (2) knowledge, which includes both factual data and heuristic knowledge (the rules of thumb built on previous experience that allow all the possibilities uncovered by the search to be reduced to manageable proportions). Such heuristic knowledge might be expressed in a number of logical propositions following the formula "*If* such conditions prevail, *then* proceed along path A." See *cognitive style; connectionism; parallel distributed processing.*

Although a microchip is much speedier than a neuron, the brain can make millions or billions of neuronal calculations simultaneously and in parallel, whereas most computers do their manipulations sequentially, in a one-step-at-a-time fashion. Artificial intelligence has demonstrated that the computer can be a useful tool for studying cognition and that it serves as a reasonable model for some human thought processes. But whether it is the best model for the most important processes is still very much an open question. No machine yet developed gives any indication of possessing common sense, which appears to depend on knowledge of a great number of facts that have yet to be codified into a form that can be manipulated by computers. Computers can imitate some aspects of human intelligence—in playing chess, for example—but they are no match for the human brain in others—such as recognizing a human face, understanding a nursery rhyme, or appreciating the humor of a play on words.

Many neuroscientists feel that the brain will provide the answers about its functioning in its own terms, without the need for an intervening computer model. There is, in other words, a split between the paradigms: thinking = the *way* the brain does it, and thinking = the *results* the brain gets. The split persists to this day, dividing the AI community into the "strong" and the "weak" schools of AI.

**artificialism**   Piaget's term for the child's tendency to believe that natural phenomena are caused by some human agency.

**artificial neurosis**   See *experimental neurosis.*

**arts therapies**   See *dance therapy.*

**arugamama**   See *Morita psychotherapy.*

**"as if"**   A term borrowed from the philosopher Vaihinger, used by Adler to indicate the fictitious and imaginary goal of complete superiority that some persons set for themselves.

"As if" also is used to refer to a personality type seen typically in schizophrenics before or between acute episodes.

**as-if performances** Sullivan's term for those dramatizations in which a person ordinarily assumes various roles in order to avoid punishment or elicit tenderness; also included are those preoccupations in which a child loses himself in order to combat anxiety.

**"as-if" personality** A prepsychotic condition indicative of loss of object cathexis; the subject's whole relation to life has something about it that is lacking in genuineness. The phenomenon is closely related to *depersonalization*, but, unlike the latter, the "as-if" personality is not perceived as a disturbance by the patient himself. The expressions of emotion in such patients are formal, and interpersonal relationships are devoid of any traces of warmth. The person gives the impression of a good adjustment to reality, but this is based on mimicry and identification with the environment and leads to a completely passive attitude toward the environment and a readiness to adopt whatever attitudes or reactions seem to be expected. Thus there is no single, integrated personality; instead, the person seems to shift with the tide of his or her surroundings. Similar to the narcissistic personality, the "as-if" personality shows inauthenticity, inordinate moral relativism, and a tendency to imitate idealized others; but such a person sequesters aggression to a greater degree than does the narcissist. See *narcissistic personality*.

According to Deutsch, the schizophrenic goes through an "as-if" stage before there is any delusional formation. She believes that the "as-if" personality represents a deep disturbance of the process of sublimation, which results in a failure to synthesize various infantile identifications into an integrated personality; this leads to an imperfect, one-sided, and purely intellectual sublimation of the instinctual strivings (*Psychiatric Quarterly II*, 1942).

M. Katan (*International Journal of Psycho-Analysis 39*, 1958), on the other hand, noting that this personality occurs almost exclusively in women, has suggested that the "as-if" personality arises as follows: while still in a stage of strong oral dependence, the little girl is

deprived of the mother figure and this, combined with another "loss" (the absence of a phallus), forces the ego to remain dependent and to "rely for its reactions completely upon the examples which it receives from the chance object to which it is attached at the moment. But this attachment never developed beyond a primary identification as it existed at the time the patient lost her mother." The nature of this primary identification is clearly revealed in the patient's reaction to dissolution of an object relationship; "A relinquished relationship is never followed up by an identification, but, contrary to such sequence, the identification disappears with the relationship" (ibid.).

Katan differentiates between the "as-if" personality and "*pseudo as-if*" (q.v.).

**ASAM-PPC** The American Society of Addiction Medicine *Patient Placement Criteria*, a model for addiction care that uses multidimensional needs assessment to match the patient to the service program most suitable to his or her needs. PPC matching is associated with less morbidity, better function, or less service utilization than mis-matching to a lower level of care.

**asapholalia** Indistinct or *mumbling* speech (q.v.).

**ASC** Altered states of consciousness. See *dissociation*; *dissociative disorders*.

**ascendance, ascendancy** Dominance; used especially to refer to character traits and interpersonal or group relationships. See *submissiveness*.

**ascertainment bias** A distortion of results based upon failure to consider the reasons that brought the subject into the experimental or observed group in the first place. One example is the synergistic effect of two conditions in bringing a subject to medical attention: studies have repeatedly shown that as many as 50% of children with Gilles de la Tourette syndrome are also diagnosed as having attention deficit hyperactivity disorder. This might suggest that the two disorders reflect similar or identical pathogenic mechanisms, yet family studies provide little evidence for a strong linkage between the two. The reason might be, instead, that both disorders disrupt social, academic, and vocational functioning and that both tend also to involve other people as well as the affected subject. When either disorder occurs alone, the disruption may not be severe enough to bring the subject to medical attention, but when they occur together the resultant disruption will almost certainly provoke engagement in the medical system.

**ascetic character**   A mode of life characterized by rigor, self-denial, and mortification of the flesh. Asceticism is seen typically as a phase in puberty, where it indicates a fear of sexuality and a simultaneous defense against sexuality. Asceticism is also seen as an extreme type of masochistic character disorder, where almost all activity is forbidden because it represents intolerable instinctual demands. In such cases, the very act of mortifying may become a distorted expression of the blocked sexuality and produce masochistic pleasure. An example of this is the eccentric who devotes his life to combating some particular evil that unconsciously represents his own instinctual demands.

**Aschner ocular phenomenon**   (Bernhardt Aschner, Viennese physician, 1883–1960) Pressure exerted over the eyeball produces a slowing of the pulse; also known as the *oculocardiac reflex.*

**Aschner treatment of schizophrenia**   *Obs.* A method of "constitutional" therapy employed by Bernhardt Aschner in the treatment of schizophrenia; the method included the use of cold baths, sweats, drastic purgatives, emmenagogues, emetics, blisters, and periodic bloodletting.

**ascorbic acid**   Vitamin C. See *vitamin C deficiency.*

**ASD**   *Autism spectrum disorder; acute stress disorder* (qq.v.).

**ASDC**   Association of Sleep Disorders Centers; their nosology of sleep disorders is generally recognized as the "official" one.

**asemia**   Loss of the ability, previously possessed, to make or understand any sign or token of communication, whether of organic or emotional origin; *asymbolia* (q.v.). See *speech disorders.*

**asitia**   Anorexia.

**ASL**   American Sign Language; see *sign language.*

**asocial**   Not social; indifferent to social values; without social meaning or significance.

**asomatognosia**   See *somatognosia.*

**asoticamania**   Self-destructive prodigality or squandering of money; profligate spending, which may constitute the outstanding behavioral feature of *mania* (q.v.).

**aspartate**   An *EAA;* like *glutamate,* it activates the *NMDA receptor* (qq.v.).

**Asperger disorder**   (Hans Asperger, Austrian physician, 1844–1954) First described as *autistic psychopathy* (q.v.) by the Austrian pediatrician Hans Asperger in 1944; also known as *right hemisphere deficit disorder;* characterized by high verbal IQ but low performance IQ.

Asperger disorder/syndrome has been used to denote different types of pervasive developmental disorder; some use it as equivalent to high-functioning autistic disorder, others as subthreshold pervasive developmental disorder not otherwise specified. It has also been used by workers of different disciplines to describe similar conditions, e.g, semantic-pragmatic processing disorder, right-hemisphere learning problems, and nonverbal learning disability.

Asperger syndrome is a neurological disorder of childhood manifested as a hypertrophy of intellect at the expense of feeling. Typical signs and symptoms include the following: lack of sensitivity, empathy, intuition, and normal human understanding; inappropriate one-sided social interaction; pedantic speech that is more a proclamation than a conversation (hence sometimes called "little professor syndrome"); inability to make friends; clumsiness and poor motor coordination; and poor visual spatial organization and integration skills. Unusual patterns of interest and behavior are common: obsessional interest in a highly selected topic (e.g., the giant squid), compulsive reiteration (e.g., of a page of a book—sometimes called *perseverative scripting*), and *auditory hyperacuity* (oversensitivity to sounds, such as irrational fears of a ticking clock).

Most children with Asperger syndrome usually have inattentive-subtype attention deficit disorder as well, with inattention, disorganization, and frequent daydreaming. Typical academic problems are dysgraphia, dyscalculia, and impairment in expressive written language.

During the first 3 years of life, children with Asperger syndrome are indistinguishable from those with *autistic disorder* (q.v.) because of their monotonic speech, social isolation, and lack of empathy. But after the age of 3, Asperger subjects become talkative and demonstrate their rigid, insular, fact-oriented speech. Children with Asperger disorder demonstrate much greater verbosity and higher verbal performance IQs than children with autistic disorder. Unlike autistic children, they make active social approaches to others but in a tactless and inappropriate way. Most authorities believe that autistic disorder and Asperger syndrome exist on a spectrum. Males are five or more times as frequently affected as females (Volkmar, F. R. et al. *American Journal of Psychiatry 157*: 262–267, 2000).

**aspermia, psychogenic**   See *impotence, psychic.*

**asphyxiation, autoerotic**   See *hypoxyphilia.*

**asphyxiophilia**   Self-strangulation; see *hypoxyphilia.*

**ASPM**   One of the genes (four others have been identified) that can cause *microcephaly* (q.v.). *ASPM* acts during fetal development to prescribe the number of cells in the future cerebral cortex.

**assemblies, neural**   Distributed local networks of neurons that are linked, transiently, by reciprocal dynamic connections. It is believed that a specific neuronal assembly underlies the operation of every cognitive act.

**assembly, cell**   *Engram* (q.v.); any group of neurons that has come to function as a unit by reason of repeated stimulation. See *memory.*

**assertiveness training**   See *behavior therapy.*

**assessment**   Diagnosis; evaluation. See *nosology.* Clinical assessment includes objective measures, but it is more than testing. It implies the use of judgment based on experience and the drawing of inferences about the individual subject's behavioral patterns and personality from all the information available (including psychometric testing results, historical and developmental information, mental status evaluation, and knowledge of how pathogenic factors might affect the subject).

**assessment of competence**   See *MacCAT-T.*

**assignment therapy**   In Moreno's system of sociometry, placement of the patient into a group in accord with his sociometric position in the community. It tries to give the individual the best opportunity for adjustment in the group in accordance with his abilities.

**assimilation**   In analytical psychology (Jung), "the absorption or joining up of a new conscious content to already prepared subjective material, whereby the similarity of the new content with the waiting subjective material is specially emphasized, even to the prejudice of the independent quality of the new content. Fundamentally, assimilation is a process of apperception…which, however, is distinguished from pure apperception by this element of adjustment to the subjective material." (Jung, C. G. *Psychological Types*, 1923).

In Fromm's theory of character, assimilation is one of two ways of relating to the world (the other is socialization). Assimilation types relate to material things rather than to people, and Fromm distinguishes five subtypes: (1) *receiving*—the person feels that the only way to get what he wants is to receive it passively from some outside source; (2) *exploiting*—the person feels that he can get what he wants only by stealing it or by using some artful, cunning scheme; (3) *hoarding*—the person doubts that he can ever get what he wants, so whatever he has must be saved and hoarded (similar to the anal character in other classifications); (4) *marketing*—the person values himself only in terms of salability to others and is dependent upon personal acceptance by them; such a person becomes alienated and estranged from his actions and his own life forces, an automaton who is ruled by the institutions of industrial society; (5) *working*—the only productive type in this group, characterized by the ability to reason objectively, to love unselfishly, and to work productively. See *equilibration.*

**assisted reproductive technologies**   *ART* (q.v.).

**association**   Relationship. In psychoanalysis, association refers particularly to the relationship between the conscious and the unconscious. Associations may be free or induced. When a person without prompting is allowed to raise and to expand upon an idea or ideas, the process is known as *free association* (q.v.). Induced associations involve the giving of stimulus words to which the test-subject immediately replies with the next association that comes into his or her mind.

Jung used the term association method to mean the procedure; the tests were called association experiments.

**association, psychosis of**   *Induced psychotic disorder* (q.v.).

**association areas**   The largest part of the cerebral cortex; regions of the brain that link different parts of the brain, integrating the activity of the primary sensory areas of the cortex and linking them to motor areas of the cortex. Association areas provide the anatomical support for higher functions such as thought, perception, cognition, voluntary movement, memory, language, and emotional behavior. The primary, secondary, and tertiary sensory and motor areas, in contrast to the association areas, process aspects of a single sensory modality or motor function.

There are three major association areas: (1) the *parieto-temporal-occipital association cortex* integrates sensory functions with language; it plays a primary role in forming and controlling complex perceptions by combining information related to somatic sensation, hearing, and vision; see *heteromodal association cortex*; (2) the *prefrontal association cortex (PFC)* is involved in complex motor actions; it is responsible for maintaining the information needed for deciding on subsequent action; (3) the *limbic association cortex* is involved in motivation, emotion, and memory. See *limbic lobe; frontal lobe; occipital lobe; parietal lobe; temporal lobe.*

**association disturbances**   One of Bleuler's fundamental symptoms of the schizophrenias. The associations are the innumerable related threads that guide thinking, and in the schizophrenias they are interrupted and lose their contiguity. As a result, thinking becomes haphazard, seemingly purposeless, illogical, confused, incorrect, abrupt, and bizarre. Among the many possible association disturbances are clang associations, indirect associations, stereotypy in speech, dearth of ideas to the point of monoideism, *thought deprivation (blocking), naming* (echopraxia) or touching, pressure of thoughts, inappropriate application of cliches, *Klebedenken* (qq.v.), impoverishment of thought, replacement of thinking proper by a senseless compulsion to associate. See *semantic dissociation.*

**association experiment**   See *association.*

**association fibers**   See *commissure.*

**association of ideas**   The hypothesis that thinking is governed by two laws: (1) the law of contiguity—ideas or experiences that occur together frequently become associated in the mind; and (2) the law of resemblance—when two similar ideas or experiences occur, whatever has been associated with the first becomes associated with the second. If those laws alone are accepted as the basis of thinking, several features of thinking are left unexplained. The laws do not account for the concept of an individual, how to differentiate two persons or places with identical properties. Nor do they account for *compositionality*—a concept or meaning is composed of more

than separate contiguous or similar parts added together; the way they are combined is equally important. "A dog bites a man" and "a man bites a dog" are identical in the parts they contain; it is how they are combined, their composition, that determines the vast difference in their meanings.

**associationism**   The school of psychology that holds that mental development consists mainly of combinations and recombinations of basic, irreducible mental elements. See *connectionism; contextualism; reductionism.*

**associative learning**   Acquiring knowledge about the relation of one stimulus to another, as in classical conditioning, or about the relation of a stimulus to the subject's behavior, as in operant conditioning. *Habituation* and *sensitization* are forms of associative learning. In *nonassociative learning*, the subject is exposed to only one type of stimulus.

**associative mating**   Mating of those with like genes. See *selection.*

**associative thinking**   In group therapy, verbal catharsis that deals with immediate problems, rather than with traumatic events that occurred in childhood.

**associativity**   The property of long-term potentiation whereby weak stimulation of a synaptic input, which will not elicit an increase in synaptic strength, can lead to the onset of LTP if strong stimulation is simultaneously applied to an independent input to the same postsynaptic cell.

**assortative mating**   The mating of individuals who resemble one another in some particular, such as intelligence or hair color. Since there is likely to be some genetic basis for any such quality, assortative mating implies the mating of genetically similar individuals; but the term *inbreeding* is used to refer to the mating of related people.

**assumptions, group**   See *basic assumptions group.*

**astasia**   The inability to stand, when there is no organic reason for the disability. See *astasia-abasia.*

**astasia-abasia**   A form of hysterical ataxia with bizarre incoordination and inability to stand or walk, even though all leg movements can be performed normally while sitting or lying down.

**astereognosis**   Loss of ability to perceive the shape and nature of an object and inability to identify it by superficial contact alone, in the absence of any demonstrable sensory defect; sometimes called *tactile agnosia* (q.v.), although in astereognosis there is a defect in the higher correlation of proprioceptive sensations as well. Some use astereognosis for minor defects in which the patient cannot recognize form, and tactile agnosia for more profound defects in which there is inability to identify objects. Astereognosis follows lesions of the *parietal lobe* (q.v.), especially in the posterior portions.

**asterixis**   A lapse of posture consisting of momentary loss of a fixed position of the hands or arms followed by a jerking recovery movement that restores the limb to its original position; also known as *flapping tremor*, it usually occurs in association with tremulousness in patients with some degree of central nervous system dysfunction secondary to metabolic disorders, such as liver disease and uremia. It has also been reported as a side effect of diphenylhydantoin.

**asthenia**   Want or loss of strength, debility, diminution of the vital forces.

**asthenia, neurocirculatory**   Described as *irritable heart* by Jacob DaCosta in 1871, hence known also as *DaCosta syndrome*; other terms that are approximately equivalent are *cardiac neurosis, DAH (disordered action of the heart), effort syndrome, hyperdynamic-adrenergic circulatory state, hyperkinetic heart syndrome, soldier's heart, vasoregulatory asthenia*. Neurocirculatory asthenia is characterized by palpitations, shortness of breath, labored breathing, subjective complaints of effort and discomfort, all following slight exertion. Other symptoms may include dizziness, tremulousness, sweating, and insomnia. See *anxiety neurosis; hyperventilation syndrome; panic attack*.

**asthenic personality (disorder)**   Characteristics are easy fatigability, low energy, lack of enthusiasm, diminished capacity for enjoyment, and oversensitivity to physical and emotional stress. See *neurasthenia*.

**asthenic type**   *Leptosomic type*, characterized by the general impression of a deficiency in volume combined with an average unlessened length, so that the subject appears taller than he really is (see *constitutional type*). The head of the asthenic rises like a bud upon a lean, long neck. In profile, the curve of the head is interrupted by sharp irregularities. In frontal outline, the face is of short egg form. The middle face is long in proportion to the rest, and the upper lip is short. The chest of the asthenic is long, narrow, and flat. The prominence given to the clavicle is accentuated by a stooping attitude. The cavity of the abdomen is poorly developed, while the limbs appear long and thin with lean muscles. The hips in the male are usually wider than the chest measurement, accentuating the waist. The skin tends to be pale, dry, and cold with scant subjacent fat.

As a psychological type, the asthenic is thought to be basically *schizothyme* (q.v.), thus constituting the bulk of the schizothymic group, although the athletic and dysplastic types also contribute to it. According to Kretschmer's theories, the asthenics may fall into any one of the three divisions accepted by him: namely, the *healthy* schizothymes (polite, sensitive types; world-hostile idealists; cold-hearted egoists); the *schizoids* (the predominantly hyperesthetic temperaments, including despotic or passionate types and unsteady loafers); and the *schizophrenics*.

The asthenic type corresponds fairly closely to the following types in other systems: the *habitus phthisicus* of Hippocrates, the *sensory, pneumatic, chlorotic, phthisic*, and *lymphatic* type with a disposition to tuberculosis of Rokitansky-Benecke, the *first combination* of De Giovanni, the *macroskelic* type of Viola, the *hypovegetative (dolichomorphic)* biotype of Pende, part of the *hypotonic* group of Tandler, the *asthenic habitus* of Bauer and Mills, the *narrow-chested* type of Brugsch, the *slender* biotype of Stockard, the *T type* of Jaensch, the *regressive* type of Lewis, the *ectomorphic* type of Sheldon, the *sthenoplastic* type of Bounak, and the *hyperontomorphic* type of Beau.

**asthenophobia**   Fear of weakness.

**asthenopia**   Weakness of vision or sight.

**asthma, bronchial**   Recurrent attacks of bronchiolar spasm, which traps air in the lungs and results in paralysis of the expiratory muscles, assumption of the inspiratory position, and use of the accessory muscles of respiration.

Asthma is the best known systemic allergy, consisting of immune system overreaction by antibodies or immunoglobulins, triggered by microscopic allergens. Genetic factors play an important role.

Because the disorder is a result of immune system and neurologic system interaction, emotional and psychological factors are often important in triggering or aggravating asthmatic attacks. Bronchial asthma was once considered one of the seven "classic" psycho-somatic disorders, and the asthmatic attack was interpreted as an anxiety equivalent related to threat of separation from the pro-tecting, encompassing mother and a cry for help. Maternal rejection was a recurrent motif in the history of such asthmatics, who were often of the obsessive-compulsive personality type with an anal-sadistic orientation.

**astraphobia, astrapophobia**   Fear of thunder and lightning.

**astroactin**   A protein that acts as a ligand for neuron–glia binding during neuronal migra-tion; under its direction, cells destined to form specific cortical layers migrate along radial glial fibers. See *axon growth; NCAM.*

**astrocytes**   Star-shaped *glia* (q.v.) that insulate neurons, provide nutrients, and form a sup-porting framework, especially during early embryonic development. They also recycle neurotransmitters. With oligodendrocytes, astrocytes form the group called *macroglia.* See *neuroglia.*

A key function of astrocytes is removal of neurotransmitters released by active neurons. They can also release neuroactive agents, termed *gliotransmitters,* such as glutamate, ATP, and serine. Because they are crucial in glutamate cycling, they are likely to be a factor in excitotoxic damage in the nervous system. They are central to the *neurovascular unit*—comprising neurons, astroglial cells, vascular endothelia, and their associated extracellular matrices—and thus are able to restrict and mediate neurovascular transmission. They modulate communication between neurons by modifying synaptic transmission through release of neurotransmitters and modulators.

The core feature of the *neuron doctrine* (q.v.) is polarized communication between neurons by action potentials. It is now known that neuronal communication is heavily influenced by nonneuronal cells. Glia do not fire action potentials, but they detect impulses in axons through membrane recep-tors that bind signaling molecules. This axon–glial communication results in intercellular communication at sites far removed from chemical synapses, and information is propa-gated through cells that are not neurons.

The astrocytes may provide a parallel system of information processing that interacts with neuronal communication but propagates over much slower time scales through a reticular

network of nonneuronal cells. There is grow-ing evidence of their involvement in the path-ogenesis of some nervous system disorders, including epilepsy, ALS, stroke, and hepatic encephalopathy.

**astrocytoma**   See *glioma; intracranial tumor.*

**astyphia**   Sexual *impotence* (q.v.).

**astysia**   Sexual *impotence* (q.v.).

**asyllabia**   A form of aphasia (agraphia or alexia); inability to combine individual letters (or sounds) into syllables. See *speech disorders.*

**asylum**   Originally, a place safe from violence or pillage. The ancients set apart certain places of refuge where criminals were protected, and the name later came to be applied specially to an institution that afforded a place of refuge or safety for the infirm or mentally ill.

**asymbolia**   *Asemia* (q.v.); inability to make or understand symbols or signs.

**asymbolia, pain**   A type of disordered recogni-tion of the body, as is seen in parietal lobe lesions, in which the patient, although able to perceive painful stimuli, "shows a mor-bid poverty of emotional reaction to them. In every case described the lesion has been found in the left hemisphere but the whole body shows the abnormal response to pain" (Mayer-Gross, W., et al. *Clinical Psychiatry,* 1960).

**asymbolia, visual**   See *visual aphasia.*

**asymmetry**   Lack of identity on both sides; in biology, unevenness or dissimilarity between the two sides of an organism (or organ). Asymmetry also refers to *organ placement* (e.g., the heart is normally on the left and the liver is on the right). In psychiatry, asym-metry is most commonly used in relation to laterality and in describing other differences between the two sides of the brain. See *cere-bral dominance; planum temporale.*

**asymmetry, brain**   Differences between the two sides of the brain and its parts, including dif-ferences in functional layout, architecture, and neurochemistry. One well-known anatomical brain asymmetry is reflected in the right fron-tal and left occipital *petalia*—impressions left on the inner surface of the skull by protrusions of one hemisphere relative to the other. In humans, the right frontal lobe often extends beyond the left anteriorly, and the left occip-ital lobe beyond the right posteriorly. Petulia are more prominent in right-handers.

The left hemisphere is normally domi-nant for language, logical processing, and mathematical reasoning. The left planum temporale, in the posterior portion of the superior temporal sulcus, is much larger (sometimes as much as ten times) than the right; it is the most prominent human brain asymmetry.

The right hemisphere is normally dominant for spatial recognition, shape recognition, emotion processing, and musical and artistic functions. The Sylvian fissure (separating the frontal and temporal lobes) is higher on the right than on the left.

Preferred hand use appears in the fetus, long before language ability is developed. Maturation of the right hemisphere precedes that of the right for the first 3 years of life; beginning at about 3 years of age with the development of language ability there is a shift to the left hemisphere. See *cerebral dominance*; *sex differences*.

**asymptomatic neurocognitive impairment (ANI)** See *HIV-associated neurocognitive disorders*.

**asymptotic** See *wish-fulfillment, asymptotic*.

**asyndesis** A language disorder in which there is juxtaposition of elements without adequate linkage between them. Images and meanings that are connected in the mind of the patient are superimposed on each other in a sentence without explanation as to what the connecting links are; to the listener, the language seems disjointed and disconnected. See *thinking-aside*.

**asynergia** Lack of coordination, as in *ataxia* and *decomposition of movement* (qq.v.).

**asynergia of Babinski, major** Incoordination in standing and walking as a result of involvement of the cerebellum.

**asynergia of Babinski, minor** As a consequence of involvement of the cerebellum, there results a decomposition of movements giving rise to a "breaking up" of simple acts; when the patient attempts to carry out such acts as kneeling on a chair, elevating the leg while in a supine position, or sitting up from a recumbent position, the movements are disjointed and awkward.

**asynodia** Failure of sexual partners to attain simultaneous orgasm; less commonly, sexual impotence.

**α-synuclein** *SNCA;* a presynaptic nerve terminal protein, the precursor protein for the non–β amyloid component of the amyloid plaques found in Alzheimer disease; its pattern of expression coincides with the distribution of *Lewy bodies* (q.v.) in several neurodegenerative disorders.

Allele-length variability in the dinucleotide repeat sequence (REPı) of the SNCA gene promotor (located on chromosome 4) is associated with an increased risk of severe, familial *Parkinson disease* (q.v.). The SNCA protein is the principal component of the Lewy bodies characteristic of Parkinson disease. It has been suggested that mutant α-synuclein overpowers the capacity of *UPS* (q.v.) to eliminate abnormal protein, thus leading to neurodegeneration. Through a similar mechanism, two other mutants associated with familial PD—UCHLı (on chromosome 4), which impairs deubiquitination, and parkin (on chromosome 6), which impairs ubiquitination—decrease the ability of UPS to clear abnormal proteins.

Normally, α-synuclein is also degraded by autophagy, but pathogenic α-synuclein mutants act as uptake blockers on the autophagy pathway, inhibiting both their own degradation and that of other substrates.

**ataque de nervios** A culture-bound or culture-specific syndrome, often classified as a dissociative trance disorder, reported in Puerto Rico and among Hispanics from other parts of the Caribbean. The ataque consists of a short-lived paroxysm of dissociative, anxiety, somatoform, impulsive, and depressive symptoms, typically precipitated by sudden stress. Dissociative symptoms include trancelike states, narrowing of awareness, perceptual distortions, depersonalization, loss of consciousness, and partial or total amnesia for the episode.

**ataraxia** Absence of anxiety or confusion; imperturbability; untroubled calmness; inner harmony. See *psychotropics*.

**atavism** Mental or physical traits that are dormant for one or more generations and then reappear. The *collective unconscious* of Jung may be regarded as atavistic, particularly when its components are expressed overtly in the daily life of the person (as in schizophrenia).

**ataxia** Absence or lack of order; incoordination. In this general sense it may refer to the absence of order of any bodily function or system, physical or mental. It is most commonly used in the field of neurology to designate a loss of power of muscular coordination or delay in initiating responses with the affected limb. Ataxia may be due to brain or spinal cord pathology; it is a common manifestation of cerebellar dysfunction. Ataxia is a neurological dysfunction of motor coordination that can affect gaze, speech, gait, and balance. The etiology of ataxia encompasses toxicities, metabolic dysfunction, autoimmunity, paraneoplasms, and genetic factors. *Huntington disease* (q.v.) is the best-known ataxia; related to it are the *spinocerebellar ataxias, Wilson disease*, and *neuroacanthocytosis* (qq.v.) The first autosomal dominant gene for a hereditary ataxia (spinocerebellar ataxia, *SCA1*) was discovered in the 1990s. Since then, more than 25 loci for autosomal dominant spinocerebellar ataxias have been identified, as have about 10 loci for autosomal recessive phenotypes. See *polyglutamine disorders*.

Autonomic or vasomotor ataxia refers to imbalance of the sympathetic and parasympathetic nervous systems.

Stansky considered *intrapsychic ataxia*, a lack of coordination between thoughts and feelings, a cardinal symptom of schizophrenia.

**ataxia, hysterical**   See *astasia-abasia*.

**ataxia, locomotor**   See *tabes*.

**ataxia-telangiectasia (AT)**   *Louis-Bar syndrome*; the second most common cause of progressive cerebellar ataxia in childhood after *Friedreich ataxia* (q.v.); it is an autosomal recessive disease due to *ATM* (AT mutated) gene. Characteristics are progressive cerebellar ataxia (and also involvement of substantia nigra), oculocutaneous telangiectasia, immune defects (often manifested in severe infections, such as recurrent pneumonia), predisposition to lymphoreticular malignancies, progeric changes, gonadal abnormalities, and other endocrine disorders. Hypersensitivity of AT cells to ionizing radiation is diagnostic, placing it in a group of human diseases known as *genomic instability syndromes* (q.v.), which result from defective responses to specific DNA lesions. AT protein coordinates cellular responses to double strand breaks in DNA. The breaks activate the protein to turn on the repair network. ATM protein is unable to do this. Progressive neurodegeneration in AT is probably due to cumulative damage during development.

**ataxic gait**   *Tabetic gait*, due to loss of proprioceptive sense in the extremities as a result of posterior column disease. The patient walks on a wide base, slapping his feet, and typically watching his legs and feet so he will know where they are. See *tabes*.

**ataxic paraplegia**   Unsteadiness of station and gait in association with paraplegia.

**ataxophemia**   Impaired coordination of words; incoherence.

**atelesis**   Absence of integration or successful completion; used to refer to three major dysjunctions in schizophrenia: dysjunction of inner world and environment (autism), dysjunction of ego and the contents of consciousness (*splitting* or *ego anachoresis*), and dysjunction of experience contents and the elementary forms of mental perception (*destruction of categories*).

**ateliosis**   *Dwarfism* (q.v.); incomplete development; the term may refer to psychic infantilism or puerilism, to mental retardation, or to physical dwarfism (microsomia).

**atenolol**   A *beta blocker* (q.v.).

**atephobia**   Fear of ruin, and especially the fear of ruin if one does not curb one's reckless impulses.

**athetosis**   Irregular, writhing, slow, objectively purposeless movement with some apparent pattern, occurring mainly in the toes and fingers, in the form of extension and flexion and spreading of the digits.

Athetosis results from a lesion in the extrapyramidal pathways, usually the corpus striatum, or from other lesions that interrupt the circuit of the suppressor reaction between cortical areas 4s and 4.

**athletic type**   Robust, strong, vigorous, sthenic, possessing a well-developed muscular system with resultant physical activity and prowess. Kretschmer's athletic type is characterized by a strong development of the locomotor apparatus, so that the bones and muscles stand out in plastic relief. The head shares in the overdevelopment of the skeleton, as is usually demonstrated by prognathous jaws and marked occipital protuberance. The frontal facial outline is steep egg-shaped. The neck is strong and the shoulders are large. The trunk tapers down from the broad shoulder girdle, so that the trunk outline from the front appears inverted trapezoid. The limbs are relatively long, the hands and feet are large, and the fingers are often blunt, thick, and acromegaloid in character. The skin is thick, of good turgor, moderately tinted, and medium as to sweat secretion.

As a psychological type, the athletics were assumed by Kretschmer to be basically *schizothymic*, like the asthenics and the majority of the dysplastics. According to his theories, they constitute a considerable proportion of the total group of schizothymes, although a decidedly smaller one than do the asthenics, and they may also fall into any one of his three divisions of the schizothymes group, that is, the healthy schizothymes, the schizoids, and the schizophrenics (see *asthenic type*).

The athletic type thus described corresponds approximately to the following types in other systems: the *muscular* type of Rostan, the *second (plethoric) combination* of De Giovanni, the *normosplanchnic* type of Viola, the *hypertonic* type of Tandler, the *sthenic* type of Mills, the *medium* biotype of Davenport, the *normal* type of Aschner, the *mesoskelic* type of Pende, part of the *hypercompensatory* type of Lewis, and the *mesomorphic* type of Sheldon.

**athymia** 1. Apathy, emotional indifference, or unresponsiveness. 2. Unconsciousness. 3. Mental retardation. 4. Melancholia. 5. Absence of the thymus gland.

**ATM family** A group of proteins that participate in cell cycle progression by linking signals from growth factor receptors and internal checkpoints to the cell cycle machinery. The ATM proteins are members of the *kinase* superfamily (q.v.) and include the gene product of the *ataxia telangiectasia mutated* (ATM)-related family of proteins and the catalytic subunit of DNA-activated protein kinase *RAFT1* (also called *FRAP* or *mTOR*) and of the homolog yeast genes *TOR1, TOR2,* and *TEL1.*

RAFT1 mediates the potent immunosuppressant effects of *rapamycin,* and it is an important regulator of dendritic mRNA translation.

**atomistic psychology** Any psychology based on the doctrine that perceptions, thoughts, and all mental processes are built up through the combination of simple elements or atoms. According to the doctrine of atomism, the physical universe (or, as is sometimes taught, the whole universe, both physical and mental) is composed of simple, indivisible, and minute particles or atoms. Many thinkers have endeavored to interpret atomism from a psychical point of view, treating the atoms either as *mind stuff* or as composed of sense elements. Mind stuff, a term first used by

W. K. Clifford, is the elemental material held to be the basis of reality and to consist internally of the constituent substance of mind and to appear externally in the form of matter. "Psychoanalysis is an *atomistic psychology* which attempts to derive complex entities from the action of a synthetic principle (association, conditioning, integration) on or about a basic unit. A conative principle is used as an atomic unit to reconstruct the molecules of experience" (Kardiner, A. & Spiegel, H. *War Stress and Neurotic Illness,* 1947).

**atonic** Relating to or characterized by lack of tone or vital energy. It may refer to the whole body, to a particular system of the body, or to single organs, especially to contractile organs.

**ATP** Adenosine triphosphate, a purine that is an intracellular energy source and also a neurotransmitter involved in intercellular signaling between a wide variety of cells. In addition to its rapid actions in intercellular signaling, it also acts as a growth and trophic factor by regulating the two most important second messengers, cytoplasmic calcium and cAMP. Purinergic receptors have been identified in all major classes of glia, including Schwann cells in the peripheral nervous system and oligodendrocytes, astrocytes, and microglia in CNS. See *OXPHOS.*

**atrabiliary, atrabilious** *Obs.* Depressed or melancholic.

**Atreus complex** See *Medea complex.*

**atrophic dementia** *Obs.* Abiotrophic atrophic dementia; presenile brain disease, such as *Pick disease* (q.v.).

**atrophic lobar sclerosis** See *Little disease.*

**atrophy, progressive muscular** See *amyotrophic lateral sclerosis.*

**atropine** An anticholinergic drug. See *cholinergic.*

**atropine coma therapy (ACT)** The use of atropine sulfate to induce coma in the treatment of psychoses, first reported by Forrer in 1950. Greatest benefit has been reported in tense, anxious, and agitated psychotics. See *central anticholinergic syndrome.*

**atropine syndrome** *Central anticholinergic syndrome* (q.v.).

**attachment** Bond, link, and in particular the affective tie between infant and caregiver. The mother is often the primary attachment figure, but the child can bond with many other responsive persons, including other children. See *μ-receptor*.

John Bowlby's *attachment theory* postulates a universal need to form close affectional bonds; disruption of those bonds heightens vulnerability to depression or despair. The attachment behaviors of the infant (e.g., proximity seeking, smiling, clinging) are reciprocated by adult attachment behaviors (e.g., touching, holding, soothing). The experience of security is the goal of the attachment system, an open biosocial homeostatic regulatory system. The infant's signals of moment-to-moment changes in his or her state are understood and responded to by the observer, thus achieving regulation. In states of uncontrollable arousal, the infant will seek physical proximity to the caregiver in the hope of soothing and the recovery of homeostasis. The infant's past experiences with the caregiver are aggregated into representation systems that Bowlby termed *internal working models*. See *bonding*.

Attachment strategies are the nonconscious, implicit, behaviorally based representations of how to relate to others that are developed in infancy before the explicit memory system associated with consciously recalled images or symbols is available. A secure attachment style results in an integrated sense of self, a stable self-concept, and a capacity to reflect on and modulate one's own affects. Insecure forms of attachment involve some degree of compromise in caregiving effectiveness, resulting in suboptimal or disorganized attachment patterns.

Disorganized attachment results from failure of the caregiver to protect the child from overwhelming distress and, in particular, failure to provide reassurance and protection under conditions in which the caregiver may have contributed, inadvertently or intentionally, to the child's distress.

Disorganized and controlling forms of attachment behavior expose the infant to excessive unmodulated stress. Disorganized attachment behavior springs from contradictory models of the self that generate incompatible behavioral and mental tendencies. For example, the parent or caregiver may engage in frightened or frightening interactions with the infant, who then faces the paradox of the parent who is the source of protection is at the same time a source of threat. A perceived environmental threat leads a securely attached infant to approach the parent for protection; but if the parent communicates apprehension, hostility, or helplessness, the child may think that he or she is the cause of the parent's distress and be afraid to approach the parent.

Family environmental factors—including inconsistent parenting or disciplining, maternal psychologic unavailability, parental withdrawal, conflicting affective cues or role-confused responses to the infant, negative-intrusive or hostile responses, and failure to respond to clear affective signals from the infant—are the one set of factors that have been most consistently related to dissociative phenomena and other internalized forms of conflict in later life. Maternal *psychologic unavailability* (q.v.) and disorganized attachment in the first 2 years of life predict *dissociation* (q.v.), independent of concurrent abuse. Maternal hostile or intrusive behaviors, on the other hand, are only weak predictors. The hidden traumas of caregiver unavailability and interactive dysregulation are believed to contribute to the early hyper- or hyporegulation of stress response mediated through the limbic hypothalamic-pituitary-adrenocortical axis.

Disorganized attachment lies at the core of *borderline personality disorder* (q.v.); it is the developmental precursor to the dissociated self-with-other schemas (sometimes called *splitting*) found in BPD. It has been suggested that *dissociative identity disorder* (q.v.) is a variant of attachment disorder, and that disorganization of attachment may be more central to the development of dissociation than the trauma itself.

**attachment disorder of infancy** Reactive attachment disorder of infancy and early childhood, characterized by marked disturbance in social relatedness that begins before the age of 5 years; also sometimes *failure to thrive*. The care of such children has been grossly deficient, either because of persistent disregard for the child's basic emotional needs (for comfort, stimulation, affection, etc.) or physical needs (food, housing, protection from physical abuse or sexual assault, etc.) or because of repeated changing of the primary caregiver so that stable attachments are not made.

DSM-IV distinguishes two subtypes of reactive attachment disorder in infancy or early childhood: (1) inhibited—with failure to initiate developmentally appropriate social interactions, hypervigilance, frozen watchfulness and (2) disinhibited or diffuse—lack of selectivity in social attachment, such as overfamiliarity with relative strangers. See *μ-receptor*.

**attempted suicide** Uncompleted suicide, survival following an apparently suicidal act. Some writers prefer the terms *deliberate self-poisoning, deliberate self-injury, deliberate self-harm (DSH)*, or *parasuicide* to indicate that the behavior was not accidental while making no assumption about the presence of a desire for death. See *deliberate self-harm syndrome*.

**attempters** People who try to commit suicide but do not kill themselves. Between 10% and 20% of attempters go on to become completers—they do kill themselves. Although there is some overlap between the two groups, *suicide completers* and *attempters* are distinct populations. Conservative estimates place the ratio of attempters to completers at 8:1. An average of 3 men commit suicide for every 1 woman. The ratio is reversed for suicide attempts. Similarly, although suicide rates are highest in those over 50, suicide attempts are much more likely to occur in the young. The peak period for attempts is between 20 and 24 years.

**attention** Conscious and willful focusing of mental energy on one object or one component of a complex experience and at the same time excluding other emotional or thought content; the act of heeding or taking notice or concentrating. Attention depends on consciousness and is thus a part of what is meant by the more general term *sensorium* (q.v.). *Attention span* (also known as *perceptual span*) is the number of briefly presented objects that can be recalled immediately; it is used as a test of immediate *memory* (q.v.).

There are at least three types of attention: alerting, orienting, and executive. They are control systems that work closely together. Alerting attention, also termed sustained attention and vigilance, refers to the ability to increase and maintain response readiness in preparation for an impending stimulus. Phasic alertness, which is task specific, is a foundation on which other attentional functions rest. (Intrinsic alertness is a general cognitive control of arousal.) Parietal and frontal sites are involved in alerting, as is the noradrenaline system.

*Orienting attention* is the ability to select specific information from among multiple sensory stimuli; it is also called scanning or selection. Different brain areas are involved in the specific subroutines of the orienting process: pulvinar, superior colliculus, superior parietal lobe, temporoparietal junction, superior temporal lobe, and frontal eye fields.

*Executive attention* is also known as supervisory, selective, conflict resolution, and focused attention. Its role is the monitoring and resolution of conflict between computations in different neural areas. Such computations involve planning or decision making, error detecting, new or not well-learned responses, conditions judged to be difficult or dangerous, regulation of thoughts and feelings, and the overcoming of habitual actions. Included is *metacognition*, the monitoring and control of one's own cognition, emotion-regulation, self-regulation, effortful control, and inhibitory control. Cognitive conflict tasks activate the dorsal ACC (anterior cingulate cortex) and deactivate the rostral ACC; affect-related tasks have the opposite pattern. The ACC and lateral PFC are involved in executive attention; they are target areas of the mesocortical dopamine system.

The *Israeli High-Risk Study* (David Rosenthal) suggested that (1) poor attentional skills may be a strong predictor of the later development of psychiatric disorder in a high-risk population and (2) poor attention is linked to, or is a manifestation of, a core deficit in schizophrenia.

**attention, deterioration of** Bleuler lists this as one of the fundamental symptoms of the schizophrenias, where often there is seen an impairment in the ability to heed, observe, and concentrate on external reality. This fundamental symptom appears to be related to deterioration of affectivity (another fundamental symptom) and the patient's loss of interest in his or her surroundings. The impairment of attention is inconstant and shifting, for attention may appear normal when it is directed to something the patient wants to do. Inability to concentrate is seen also in other psychiatric disorders, but in this latter case it is almost always secondary, i.e., a result of emotional pressure, whereas in the schizophrenias it appears to be primary.

**attention and information processing (AIP)** The basic neural steps that prepare the subject for response to a stimulus. The brain is constructed to receive and respond to significant stimuli, and information received through the sensory channels is sorted into relevant categories and distributed to various parts of the brain, which analyze and process the information.

Attention involves extensive areas of the brain (i.e., there is no single "attention center"), but it appears to be more dependent on the reticular formation (concerned with alertness and vigilance) and the right hemisphere than on other areas. Once the stimulus is received, inputs are sent to the cerebellum, reticular formation, and thalamus. Stimuli that eventually become conscious go to special neurons of the thalamus and then to the cortex. Each kind of sensation goes to a primary sensory area of the cortex, next to the secondary sensory area, then to the association areas (which elaborate sensory information and join the various kinds of input to make a meaningful whole), and finally to the motor areas.

A lesion on one side of the brain may produce an attentional defect ("neglect") of the other side. A woman may apply makeup to only one side of her face, for example, or a man may shave only one side of his face. See *sensory neglect*.

**attention deficit hyperactivity disorder** *ADHD*; attention deficit disorder (ADD); attention deficit disorder with hyperactivity (ADDH); hyperkinetic disorder; symptoms include inattention, excessive motor activity, and impulsivity. Hyperactivity is manifested in restlessness and poorly organized excess activity that is haphazard, inconsistent, and lacking in clear goal orientation. The child fidgets, is always "on the go" or "running like a motor," and has difficulty sitting still. He frequently disrupts others at play and at work.

Other symptoms include specific learning deficits such as dyslexia; perceptual-motor deficits; defective coordination; lack of response to discipline and antisocial behavior, especially in adolescence; interpersonal relationships marred by obstinacy, stubbornness, negativism, bullying; emotional lability, low frustration tolerance; and temper outbursts. In addition, neurologic examination of such children often uncovers "equivocal" abnormalities, or soft signs, such as transient strabismus, mixed and confused laterality,

speech defects, or borderline EEG record. See *handicap, emotional*. In both children and adults, ADHD is associated with cognitive deficits, especially a disturbance of executive functions such as cognitive flexibility, initiation, interference control, planning and organization, response inhibition, self-monitoring, and working memory. Functional neuroimaging studies suggest abnormality of *frontal-striatal-thalamic-cortical (FSTC) circuitry* (q.v.) in ADHD during the performance of executive function tasks. Reduced activation in the cingulate cortex appears to be related to deficits in attention reallocation after committing errors. See *adult ADHD*.

One of the most consistent findings in ADHD is reduced performance on tasks of *motor response inhibition*, the voluntary act of stopping an ongoing response. The deficit is seen in both children and adults with ADHD and is stable over time. Motor inhibition activates the medial frontal and dorsolateral prefrontal cortex. Deficit in motor response inhibition is familial, and it may be a marker of genetic vulnerability to ADHD.

The syndrome appears early in life (in infancy or by the age of 7 years), is more common in boys (perhaps by as much as 10 times the incidence in girls), and affects 3%–7% of school-age children and 4%–5% of adults. There is a family pattern, manifested in an increased frequency of the disorder in siblings and in the childhood history of parents (especially fathers). Heritability (meaning that if one identical twin has it, the other will have it too) ranges from 65% to 90%, comparable to schizophrenia and bipolar disorder. Many genes are probably involved in the production of the disorder; there are suggestions that genes on chromosomes 5, 6, 16, and 17 harbor ADHD genes. Each gene confers a very low added risk—roughly 1%–3%—of developing ADHD.

Comorbidity is high (in 50%–75%) and includes major depression, bipolar disorder, anxiety disorders, personality disorders, oppositional and antisocial behavior, learning disabilities, alcohol and other substance abuse, self-medication with excessive doses of nicotine or caffeine, bulimia nervosa, and in some adults breathing-related sleep disorders.

*Attention deficit disorder without hyperactivity* is similar, but instead of hyperactivity and impulsivity there are apathy, daydreaming, and insufficient motivation in pursuing goal-directed activities such as schoolwork, household tasks, or employment.

It is recognized that the syndromes are heterogeneous and almost certainly encompass several distinct subgroups. The syndromes described have been given different names, including brain damage behavior syndrome, central nervous system deviation, *minimal brain dysfunction (MBD)*, postencephalitic behavior disorder, *choreatiform syndrome*, hyperactive child syndrome (HACS), Strauss syndrome, and infantile hyperkinetic syndrome. Because of the heterogeneity of the group to which any of the foregoing labels apply, some workers advocate the abolishment of all of them and call for more intensive efforts to describe discrete subgroups and identify their etiologic mechanisms.

Psychostimulants such as amphetamines or methylphenidate are generally effective in reducing hyperactivity and disruptive behavior, and some reports indicate that such drugs also improve academic performance. At the present time, between 1% and 2% of North American children receive psychostimulants as treatment for hyperactivity. Monoamine oxidase inhibitors have also been used successfully with such children; the mechanism of action appears not to be the same as that mediating their antidepressant effects.

**attention junkie**  A person who is pathologically dependent on applause, acclaim, approval, or other signs of acceptance by others; often applied to the hysteroid dysphoric and narcissistic personality disorder (NPD). See *hysteroid dysphoria*.

**attentional blink**  The result of interference with attention to visual stimuli. When the subject is required to identify two stimuli that are presented briefly in close succession, the first stimulus interferes with the ability to identify with the second stimulus for a period of about 500 milliseconds.

**attentional dysfunction**  Defective selective or sustained attention, one of the most consistently reported abnormalities in adult schizophrenics.

Reaction time measures selective attention; continuous performance tests measure sustained attention. It has been suggested that impaired ability to focus attention interferes with the acquisition of cognitive and social competence skills, and that the appearance of such dysfunction in children may identify specific subgroups who may be at increased risk of schizophrenia.

**attention-getting**  Any means of gaining attention and recognition when the ego is starved for them, as observed most often in a child who feels unloved. At first the child will attempt to do whatever he or she feels the parents like and will gain their attention. If this is not successful, the child may develop temper tantrums or other behavior disorders, preferring a display of displeasure or even a harsh disciplinary measure to no attention at all.

**attitude**  Readiness to act or react in a certain direction. See *analytic psychology*.

**attitude passionelles**  See *hysteria*.

**attitude therapy**  Originally, a process of treating children by working with the disturbed attitudes of their parents. Nowadays, a type of reeducative psychotherapy that focuses on the current attitudes of the patient, their distortions, their origins, and their present purpose. In this type of therapy, the patient is helped to adopt attitudes that make for harmonious relationships as substitutes for his or her maladaptive attitudes.

**attitude tic**  Tonic rigidity of the head or a limb, such as torticollis.

**attitudinal pathosis**  Thorne's term for a type of personality disorder, seen frequently in compensation and postaccident cases, in which the patient's attitude and self-righteous belief that because he was injured he cannot work or deserves special consideration forms a central core in all his thinking about the effects of his injury. Kamman distinguishes this reaction from *traumatic neurosis* (which term he would reserve for latent psychoneurosis precipitated by accident) and from *compensation neurosis* (where, although it is usually unconscious, the basic motive is the desire for cash compensation), mainly because of the conscious volitional element in attitudinal pathosis. This disorder is presumed to fall somewhere between psychopathic personality and traumatic neurosis. See *compensation neurosis*.

**attitudinal type**  One or the other of two types of introvert and extravert attitudes toward the world and oneself, in the Jungian system of psychology. "The introvert turns in upon himself, is absorbed in his inner world, while the extravert turns outward to the world, and is much more concerned with what goes on there than with his own private experiences. Both of these types he [Jung] subdivides into thinking, feeling, intuition, and sensation types. That is, there may be a thinking introvert, a thinking extravert, a feeling introvert or extravert and so on" (Thompson, C. *Psychoanalysis: Evolution and Development*, 1950). Introversion and extraversion are *attitudinal types*; thinking, feeling, intuition, and sensation are *functional types*. Jung believes that—probably by constitutional determination—every person is a combination of one or the other attitudinal type plus one functional type of the four. "Whereas the functional type describes the way in which the empirical material is specifically grasped and formed, the attitudinal type introversion-extraversion characterizes the general psychological orientation, i.e., the direction of that general psychological energy which Jung conceives the libido to be.... The functional type to which he belongs would be in itself an index to a man's psychological character. It alone, however, would not suffice. In addition, his general psychological attitude, i.e., his way of reacting to what meets him from without or within, must be determined. Jung distinguishes two such attitudes: extraversion and introversion. They represent orientations that essentially condition all psychic process—the reaction habitus, namely, through which one's way of behaving, of subjectively experiencing, and even of compensating through the unconscious is given" (Jacobi, J. *The Psychology of C. G. Jung*, 1942).

**attonity** Stupor with complete or almost complete immobility. Bleuler believed that the condition occurs most frequently in the catatonic form of schizophrenia, though it is also observed in states of depression; it is then known as melancholia attonita. Other authorities consider that the latter designation refers also to the catatonic type of schizophrenia.

**attributable risk** The absolute difference in rates of a disorder between those exposed and those not exposed. See *risk factor*.

**attribution** Assignment of credit or responsibility. An *attribution error* is incorrect assignment of etiological significance, as in overestimating the influence of psychological factors (*dispositional attribution*) or environmental factors (*situational attribution*) in attempting to explain behavior.

**attribution of beliefs** Inferring what another is thinking, believing, or intending to do, typically on the basis of cues from the other's motion or facial expression. Attributions of beliefs, specifically false beliefs, emerge at about 4 years of age and may be unique to humans. Like mentalizing or *theory of mind (q.v.)*, of which it is a part, attribution is associated with a neural network that includes medial frontal cortex (MFC), posterior cingulate cortex, superior temporal sulcus, temporal poles, and the temporoparietal junction. MFC appears to play the major role in such attributions; the more superior part of the region is involved in actions, the inferior part with feelings and outcomes.

**attribution theory** See *cognitive strategies*.

**atypical antipsychotic** A *psychopharmacologic agent* (q.v.) that is an efficacious antipsychotic without producing extrapyramidal symptoms (EPS). Because some of the so-called atypical drugs are, at least sometimes, associated with EPS, the current preferred term is *second generation antipsychotic*. The drugs so classified show less dopamine blockade compared with greater serotonin blockade in comparison with first generation drugs, but it is by no means certain that such a difference by itself accounts for the novel features of these medications. The first atypical introduced was clozapine; it was soon followed by risperidone, olanzapine, quetiapine, ziprasidone, aripiprazole, and amisulpiride. They have antimanic, and perhaps also antidepressant and prophylactic properties in bipolar disorder.

**atypical childhood psychosis** A pervasive development disorder, with onset between 30 months and 12 years of age, consisting of grossly impaired emotional relationships, labile or flattened or inappropriate affect, catastrophic reactions to ordinary stress, resistance to change with ritualistic and repetitive behavior, motility disturbances, self-mutilation, etc. Other terms that have been applied to this disorder are atypical development, symbiotic psychosis, and childhood schizophrenia. See *autism, early infantile; developmental disorders, pervasive*.

**atypical depression** Depression characterized by mood reactivity, anxiety, and reverse vegetative signs (hyperphagia rather than appetite loss, hypersomnia rather than early awakening), leaden paralysis, and hypersensitiviy to rejection. *Partial atypical syndrome* refers to patients with mood reactivity and only one of the other features; *full atypical syndrome* designates patients with mood reactivity and two or more of the associated features.

Atypical depressions may be preferentially responsive to monoamine oxidase inhibitors or selective serotonin reuptake inhibitors, and resistant to tricyclic antidepressants.

**atypical development**  A term used by some (notably Rank, Putnam, and Kaplan) as a diagnostic label for those children whom others would classify as having childhood schizophrenia or early infantile autism. See *atypical childhood psychosis.*

**atypical paranoid disorder**  See *paranoia.*

**atypical psychoses**  Syndromes that do not fulfill the accepted criteria for schizophrenic, delusional, or mood disorders. The term is nonspecific, although some writers have attempted to apply it to particular syndromes in a more specific way. See *reactive psychosis; remitting atypical psychosis.*

The more frequent use of the term as a nonspecific, "wastebasket" category includes syndromes that occur only at a particular time (e.g., postpartum psychosis) or within a particular cultural setting (e.g., koro, lata, piblokto); syndromes with unusual features, such as a persistent auditory hallucination; and syndromes about which the available information is not sufficient to establish a diagnosis.

**audible thought**  A type of auditory hallucination in which the voice is projected into the patient himself, as though he could hear his own thoughts. Such hallucinations with almost no sensory components are commonly designated as *inner voices.* Baillarger referred to them as *psychic hallucinations.* These are *hallucinations of conception* rather than of perception. Patients may use the term "soundless voices" to refer to essentially the same phenomenon. See *first-rank symptoms; thought hearing.*

**audile**  Ear-minded; i.e., understanding better by hearing than by seeing.

**audiogenic seizure**  Convulsion or fit induced by exposure to intense sounds of high frequency.

**audit**  Evaluation; *review* (q.v.). Medical audit is also known as *medical care evaluation (MCE)*; when the care under review has been provided by nonphysicians, the process is termed *patient care audit.*

Medical care evaluation studies are retrospective assessments of the quality of care or the nature of its utilization; they include investigation of suspected problems, analysis of the problems identified, and a plan for corrective action.

*Claims review* is also a retrospective assessment of the appropriateness of a claim for payment for a service rendered; it includes a determination that the claimant is eligible for reimbursement for the services provided, that charges are consistent with customary fees or published institutional rates, and that the service provided was necessary.

**audition**  Hearing. The left hemisphere usually takes precedence over the right in processing speech sounds and performing sophisticated language function; the right hemisphere is primary in processing tonal stimuli and music. See *auditory nerve*

**audition, thought**  A form of auditory hallucination in which everything the patient thinks or speaks is repeated by the voices; also known as *thought echoing* or *echo des pensées* (qq.v.).

**auditory aphasia**  *Word-deafness*; a subcortical aphasia in which the patient distinguishes words from other sounds but does not understand them, so that his own language sounds to him like a foreign tongue. Repetition is impaired.

**auditory aurae**  A form of epilepsy described as sensory seizures in which buzzing noises may occur suddenly, last a short period of time, and then disappear without the patient's having a grand mal attack. This would indicate a focus in the temporal lobe. In grand mal attacks, the patient occasionally may have an auditory aura just prior to the grand mal seizures, as a warning that a convulsive seizure is about to occur.

**auditory cortex, primary**  The part of the temporal cortex devoted to the analysis of sounds; it also retains specific memory traces about the behavioral significance of selected sounds. Like the primary visual cortex and the primary *somatosensory cortex* (q.v.), it has a systematic organization that reflects that of its sensory epithelium, the cochlea—a tonotopic map. The extent of the representational area may be a "memory code" for the level of behavioral significance of sound: the greater the importance, the larger the area tuned to that sound.

**auditory feedback**  See *feedback.*

**auditory hallucination**    See *haptic hallucination*.

**auditory hyperacuity**    See *Asperger syndrome*.

**auditory nerve**    Also, *acoustic nerve*; the eighth cranial nerve. It is a sensory nerve with two separate portions, the *cochlear* or auditory nerve (hearing) and the *vestibular* nerve (orientation in space). The cochlea is a coiled fluid-filled tube that fits into the temporal bone at the base of the skull. Sound pressure fluctuations are transmitted to the cochlea in several steps: by vibrations of each eardrum, by conduction through three small middle ear bones, and production of pressure waves within the cochlea to displace the basilar membrane. Vibrations of the eardrum or tympanum are relayed via the middle ear bones—the malleus, incus, and stapes—and initiate pressure waves in the cochlear fluids. The pressure waves set in motion the basilar membrane, on which the organ of Corti and their cells ride. The organ of Corti is an assembly of supporting cells and of inner and outer hair cells supported by a flexible basilar membrane. Signals from each inner hair cell are related to the brain via afferent fibers of cranial nerve VIII.

The cochlea contains two classes of hair cell, inner and outer. The electrical signals of inner hair cells relay information about the acoustic environment—speech, music, or other sounds in the outside world. The outer hair cells provide *otoacoustic emissions* (*OAEs*) that amplify acoustic energy in the cochlea and contribute to cochlear frequency selectivity. They convert sound-induced motion of the cochlear partition into changes in membrane potential that immediately modulate neurotransmitter release at synapses on the auditory afferent. From the cochlear nuclei, second-order neurons proceed through the trapezoid body and lateral lemnisci to the medial geniculate bodies. From here, auditory radiations are projected to the auditory cortex. First-order neurons of the vestibular nerve pass from the receptor cells in the vestibular ganglion (*Scarpa ganglion*) to the vestibular nuclei, and thence to the cerebellum.

Symptoms of cochlear nerve involvement include tinnitus, deafness, and, in the case of supranuclear disorders, auditory aphasia or word-deafness. Symptoms of vestibular nerve involvement include vertigo and nystagmus.

**auditory peripheral hallucination**    An auditory illusion (mainly of voices) experienced as a result of auditory sensory stimulation, as the pouring of water, rumpling of paper, or a person's walking.

**auditory processing**    The capacity for processing language that is heard (i.e., through the auditory channel). Component skills include selective attention, auditory attention, discrimination of speech vs. background noise, discrimination of individual speech sounds, memory for auditory information, sequencing of auditory information, and cognitive information processing.

**auditory span**    The number of digits (or letters, or words) that can be repeated after one hearing; determination of auditory span is a common test of immediate memory.

**Auffassung**    In Kraepelin's terminology, passive registration of information, as contrasted with *Aufmerksamkeit*, which denotes active, voluntary attention. Although Auffassung may be disturbed in the acute and terminal phases of schizophrenia (dementia praecox, in his termiology), it is Aufmerksamkeit that is a characteristic and consistent feature of schizophrenia.

**Aufgabe**    See *set*.

**Aufmerksamkeit**    See *Auffassung*.

**augmentation**    In treatment with drugs, one form of *coactive strategy* (q.v.) in which one or more drugs are added to the current drug in order to enhance the specific pharmacodynamic and therapeutic effects of the current drug, presumably through some specific pharmacodynamic mechanism.

**aulophobia**    Fear of seeing, handling, or playing a flute or similar wind instrument.

**aura**    A premonitory symptom that warns of some approaching physical or mental disorder. It disappears or loses its force after it has performed its function of warning.

In the grand mal type of epilepsy, an aura precedes loss of consciousness in about 60% of cases (the others are known as the "thunderclap" variety). The aura localizes the epileptogenic focus in the brain and thus appears in many forms, depending upon the specific location of the lesion: (1) *psychic aurae*—complex mental states such as feeling of unreality, or feeling of familiarity and déjà vu and déjà fait, disembodied feeling, intense but inexplicable fear; (2) *sensory aurae*—olfactory and gustatory hallucinations, visual hallucinations with complex scenes or simple flashes of light or balls of fire, auditory hallucinations of words, phrases, or merely crude sounds, and various paresthesiae; (3) *visceral aurae*—vertigo, epigastric discomfort; (4) *motor aurae*—as in cursive epilepsy.

**aura cursoria** Aimless running that occurs immediately before a seizure. See *aura*.

**auroraphobia** Fear of northern lights.

**autagonistophilia** A *paraphilia* (q.v.) in which sexual arousal and orgasm are contingent upon displaying oneself in a live show, i.e., being observed performing on stage or on camera. The observer's condition (if the stage or camera performance by the partner is a necessity for sexual arousal) is *scoptophilia* (scopophilia), not *voyeurism* (qq.v.).

**autarchic fiction** The infant's feeling of omnipotence in the stage of primary narcissism. For a time after birth, the infant is in the undifferentiated phase of consciousness; he is ignorant of any sources of pleasure other than himself and there is, at this stage of objectivation, no differentiation of the mother, or other objects, from himself. The breast is thought of as a part of his own body, and his slightest gestures are followed by satisfaction of his instinctive nutritional needs. This gives rise to the autarchic fiction of false omnipotence. See *narcissism, primary*.

The infantile ego only unwillingly orients itself to objects, which at this stage are seen only as ego substance that satisfies instinctual demands. Thus there is only ego and non-ego. Soon, however, reality makes increasing demands. Perceptions and memory system are differentiated, and the ego defends itself against stimulation by shutting off the perceptive system, by mastery through "fascination" (empathy), or by mastery through swallowing and introjection. The infant develops the attitude that objects exist only for the ego's satisfaction, and the purified pleasure ego perceives anything unpleasant as non-ego. The ego believes itself to be omnipotent, but this is disproved by experience and frustration. The ego then comes to believe that the parents are omnipotent and partakes of their omnipotence by introjection.

**autarchy** Supreme, autocratic power, absolute sovereignty; used in psychiatry in reference to the early infantile period, when no demands are made on the child and, insofar as possible, his instinctual demands are satisfied immediately. During this period the child is indeed absolute ruler—the slightest cry brings

instinctual gratification, there is no need to deny himself pleasure, and there need be no deferral of pleasure.

**autassasinophilia** Stage-managing one's own murder, reported as an extreme form of *masochism* (q.v.).

**autemesia** Idiopathic vomiting, usually psychogenic in origin.

**authoritarianism** See *irrational authority*.

**authoritative imperative** The pressing directives emanating from the superego that subconsciously direct behavior; the commanding voice of parental or social rule in the subconscious mind. According to Stekel, a compulsion is always a substitute for an imperative. The current (adult) imperative is always a resonance of infantile imperatives. "One may say that neurotics run after their infantile imperatives. The imperative apparently leads to an action which, however, in reality consists only of an inhibition" (Stekel, W. *Compulsion and Doubt*, 1949).

**authority complex** A group of emotionally invested, mostly unconscious ideas centering around the concept of authority. A person will react to authority just as he did originally, although he will not be aware of this fact. Unconsciously overdetermined reactions to authority either in the direction of rebellion against it or in submission to it are common in neurotic patients.

**autism** 1. *Autistic disorder* (q.v.).

2. Phantasy-thinking; a form of thinking almost entirely of a subjective character; if objective material enters, it is given subjective meaning and emphasis. Autism generally implies that the material is derived from the subject himself and is often unconscious, appearing in the nature of daydreams, phantasies, delusions, hallucinations, etc. Autism, *dereism*, and *introversion* are closely allied to one another (qq.v.). Some authorities speak of the autistic temperament, meaning by it the introverted, retiring type that shrinks from all contact with life.

Autism, when it is a pervasive and generalized dereistic life-approach, is one of the fundamental symptoms of the schizophrenias (Bleuler). In pathological autism, the effort is to maintain an insulated, closed system in order to eliminate the unknown and the unpredictable. In the autistic life-approach, the "Me" predominates, often to the exclusion of the "Not-Me," external reality gradually loses more and more of its significance, and the patient is attuned to and guided only by the inner workings of his being. He is unable to turn his energies onto objects outside himself. He exaggerates the importance of inner physical sensations as well as his own ideas and emotions. He becomes involved in pseudophilosophical speculations and has no time for mixing with his peers. He feels different from others, complains that he has never realized his potentialities, and is concerned with establishing an identity for himself.

**autism, early infantile** *Autistic disorder* (q.v.); a pervasive developmental disorder first described by Kanner as early infantile autism in terms of (1) primary symptoms, including (a) withdrawal and (b) anxious, obsessive desire to maintain the status quo; and (2) secondary symptoms, including (a) exceptional object relationships, (b) intelligent, pensive facies despite low intelligence and, often, auditory impairment, (c) language disturbances, (d) monotonously repetitive motor behavior, and (e) fear of moving objects and loud noise.

**autism spectrum disorder** ASD; in ICD-10 the term includes, in addition to *autistic disorder*, atypical autism, *Asperger disorder*, *Rett disorder*, overreactive disorder, *childhood disintegrative disorder*, and pervasive developmental disorder, which are believed to be biologically related to autism (qq.v.). It is characterized by pervasive abnormalities in socioemotional communication and stereotypical and obsessional behaviors.

High-functioning autism and Asperger disorder are commonly grouped together, but recent research suggests that they may have different neurobiological underpinnings. Further, in about 50% of boys with fragile X syndrome, the expanded repeats are associated with ASD symptoms. See *developmental disorder, pervasive.*

The serotonergic (5-HT) system in nonautistic humans modulates social behavior, the amygdala response to facial emotion, and repetitive behaviors; accordingly, it is believed that the 5-HT system may be implicated in the etiology of autistic spectrum disorder. See *5-HTTLPR.*

**autisme pauvre** Literally, impoverished autism; term for the schizophrenic's withdrawal and detachment from reality that is not a deliberate retreat into phantasy life but is instead a product of will and affect disturbances which cut him off from meaningful contact with his environment.

**autismus infantum** Early infantile autism. See *autism, early infantile.*

**autistic** Mental activity that is more or less subjective and removed from reality. See *autism.*

Infancy research has demonstrated that the infant engages actively with the environment and, at least for short periods, regulates incoming stimulation even during the first months of life. Such data cast doubt on the classical theory of a stimulus barrier and a normal autistic phase, if that is defined as disinterest in or failure to register and respond to external stimuli. It seems more likely that the infant's social nature is intrinsically determined and begins to unfold from the earliest days of life.

**autistic disorder** *Autism*; a pervasive developmental disorder first described by Kanner (1943) as *early infantile autism*, manifested in primary symptoms (which included withdrawal and an anxious, obsessive desire to maintain the status quo) and secondary symptoms (exceptional object relationships; intelligent, pensive facies despite low intelligence and, often, auditory impairment; language disturbances; monotonously repetitive motor behavior; and fear of moving objects and loud noise). The disorder is four times more common in males than in females.

Symptoms appear early in life (by the age of 3 years), with delays in social develoment, communication, and play. Characteristic are self-absorption, inaccessibility, aloneness, and inability to relate. The child seems to lack awareness of the existence or feelings of others. The most specific deficit apparent by 1 year of age is a tendency to look at others less than do other children, and to orient less to people who call the child by name. Objects take preference over people, and failure to adhere to the social conventions appropriate to the child's age is marked. When approached by others, for example, body stance is stiff and rigid, he does not smile and seems to be looking past the people talking to him. He may invite playmates home after school, but after they arrive he shuts himself alone in a room without explanation. In autistics, here is a disproportionate impairment in a specific aspect of social cognition—the ability to mentalize, to attribute mental status to others. See *theory of mind*.

Language disturbances are frequent, with pronominal reversals, an inability to accept synonyms, and sometimes echolalia. The child speaks in a monotone, or speaks with abnormal volume, pitch, stress, or rhythm of speech. Words are used idiosyncratically and stereotyped speech mannerisms intrude repeatedly, even though they are irrelevant to the topic of conversation. Facts are understood, but they are not well integrated into concepts. The child seems barren of developmentally appropriate imaginative activity. Approximately 60% of autistic children are mentally retarded, but a few autistics demonstrate *splinter skills*, i.e., they are gifted in particular areas, such as calculations, drawing, or music. See *Asperger disorder*; *idiot savant*.

Motor reactions and play activities are markedly abnormal. The autistic child manifests a predilection for rhythmical movements—rocking, jumping, whirling, head-banging—which may be so frequently and insistently repeated that they may cause physical injury. Motor skills, such as kicking a ball or tying shoes, may be acquired only with difficulty. The child is obsessed with details but does not integrate the particulars; he is preoccupied with parts of objects or unusual objects. He may spend his entire play period spinning the wheels of a tricycle rather than riding it; he may stare for hours at the spinning of the drier in the laundromat. Patterns of interest are restricted, solitary play activities are preferred, and if the child's repetitive play is interrupted the result may be a rage reaction. Behavioral disturbances, including severe tantrums, externally directed aggression, and self-injury are frequent. See *orderliness, organic*.

The autistic's obsessiveness with details and failure to integrate the particulars suggest a lack of synchrony between the inferior frontal cortex and the more detail-oriented visual areas in the back of the brain. Individual brain regions, particularly prefrontal cortex, may have hyperefficient internal communications but defective interaction with distant brain regions, such as those in other hemispheres. The longer fiber tracts that connect to *mirror neurons* (q.v.) are poorly organized; the *fusiform face area* (q.v.) is not activated when autistics look at people.

Incidence estimates of autistic disorder vary; currently it is believed that the prevalence rate is 1/500 for the full syndrome, and 1/166 for autism spectrum disorder. A genetic cause of the disorder is suggested by the following findings:

(1) significant incidence of autism in identical twins and in the siblings of autistic children. Siblings born after one autistic child are 215 times more likely to become autistic than siblings of nonautistics; the likelihood is twice as high if the first autistic child is female (probability 14.5% as compared with the overall probability of 7%). If there are already two autistic sibs in a family, the likelihood of the next child being autistic rises to 35%; (2) high male to female ratio; (3) association with other genetic and neurologic conditions, such as congenital rubella, phenylketonuria, trisomy 21, and Schilder disease.

Autistic disorder is a heritable neurodevelopmental disorder characterized biologically by enlargement of the head and brain and abnormalities of serotonin neurotransmission. It may be several genetic diseases with different genes that may be specific to different manifestations of autism, e.g., whether it appears in boys or girls, whether it develops early or late. The s (short) *5-HTTLPR* (q.v.) allele of the serotonin transporter gene is associated with the larger structural brain volumes in autistic children; the brain volume differences in autistic disorder appear to be most robust before the age of 4 years and to diminish with age.

There is evidence for genetic linkage on chromosomes 7q, 9 (associated with language acquisition), 11 (characteristic of families with only males affected), 4 (associated with females affected), 10 (especially in so-called regression autism, when the child acquires normal language by age 3 but language then regresses), and chromosome 3 (associated with early-onset autistic disorder). Other chromosome regions that may be involved include 2q, 15q11–13, 16p, and X. Elevated fetal testosterone may also be related to autistic disorder. See *Angelman* syndrome; *EMB theory*.

**autistic fantasy**  Excessive daydreaming as a substitute for human relationships or more direct and effective action in dealing with conflicts or stressors.

**autistic objects**  Normal early experience includes (1) autistic objects—feelings of a hard, angular impression on the skin, experienced as if the skin were shelllike, and associated with a diffuse sense of danger (in the paranoid-schizoid mode represented by phantasies of the skin surface as a protective armor); and (2) *autistic shapes*—a feeling of softness that will later be associated with ideas of security, safety, relaxation, warmth, and affection. See *autistic-contiguous position.*

**autistic-presymbiotic** Early disturbances (during the infant's first 6 months) in mother-infant bonding produce two types of pathology: (1) bonding failure, leading to psychoses of the autistic-presymbiotic type (*nuclear schizophrenia*), or (2) affectional psychopaths. See *antisocial personality.*

**autistic psychopathy** See *Asperger syndrome.*

**autistic psychosis** See *symbiotic infantile psychosis.*

**autistic-contiguous position** The most primitive psychological organization, a sensory-dominated and presymbolic area of experience whose meaning is generated by the organization of sensory impressions, particularly at the skin surface. The autistic-contiguous position antedates the paranoid-schizoid and depressive positions described by Melanie Klein. See *dialectic; depressive position; paranoid-schizoid position.*

Associated with the autistic-contiguous position is a unique form of anxiety: the fear that one's sensory surface might be dissolved, with a feeling of falling or leaking into endless, shapeless space. Breakdown of the autistic-contiguous organization leads to implementation of rigid, autistic defenses. See *autistic objects, depleted depression.*

**autoaggression** See *deliberate self-harm syndrome.*

**autocastration** A rare form of *self-mutilation* (q.v.), consisting usually of cutting the scrotum and testes from the external genitalia; even more rare is total ablation of the genitalia (i.e., penis as well as testicles). When it occurs, autocastration is almost always indicative of a schizophrenic process.

In early psychoanalytic writings, reference was sometimes made to *anticipatory autocastration*—a symbolic demasculinization or self-punishment that wards off actual castration or punishment by the father (or the superego, the gods, etc.). Feminine behavior in boys was often interpreted in this way; by acting like a girl, the boy placates the threatening father and avoids real *castration* (q.v.).

**autocatharsis** Self-expression, especially as a form of therapy wherein the patient is encouraged to write down his experiences, thoughts, and feelings in order to rid himself of disturbing emotions.

**autocentric** Self-centered.

**autochiria** *Obs.* Suicide.

**autochthonous delusion** Primary delusion, i.e., one that arises as an immediate experience, out of the blue, with no external or objective cause or explanation, but nonetheless with a strong feeling of conviction. Autochthonous delusions are characteristic of the schizophrenias; unlike delusions seen in other psychiatric disorders, they are not a disturbance of perception in which the subject tries to rationalize changes that he perceives in himself or in the outside world. Neither are they disturbances of apperception or intellect, for the subject can understand what specific objects in external reality are. Rather, autochthonous delusions are disturbances of symbolic meaning: because the legs of a chair are twisted, the world is twisted.

**autochthonous idea** A psychic disturbance of a delusional character in the sphere of judgment, characterized by the existence of a persistent idea, which the patient believes is put into his mind by an influence foreign to him. The idea seems to exist by itself, beyond the control of the patient, who, most of the time, attributes the existence of such ideas to some malevolent cause. See *autochthonous delusion.*

**autochthony** The state of originating in an organ itself, independent of any essential influences outside of the organ in question. See *autochthonous delusion.*

**autocoid** A substance released by a cell that acts on receptors of the cell itself. The typical role of an autocoid is to regulate transmitter release; the membrane receptor that is acted upon is an autoreceptor.

**autodysosmophobia** An obsessive fear or delusion that the person himself has a vile or repugnant odor; often combined with *automysophobia* (q.v.).

**autoecholalia** *Verbigeration* (q.v.).

**autoechopraxia** A form of stereotypy in which the patient, usually schizophrenic, constantly repeats an action that he or she had formerly experienced. Kraepelin says that "the patients stand or kneel for hours, days, or still longer, on the same spot, lie in the most uncomfortable positions in bed, fold their hands spasmodically, even till pressure-sores appear, take up the position of fencing" (*Dementia Praecox*, 1919).

**autoerotic asphyxiation**   See *hypoxyphilia*

**autoeroticism, autoerotism**   Havelock Ellis invented the term "autoerotism" to mean "the phenomena of spontaneous sexual emotion generated in the absence of an external stimulus proceeding, directly or indirectly, from another person" (*Studies in the Psychology of Sex*, 1919).

Common usage has made autoerotism synonymous with masturbation. The latter, however, is a special subdivision of autoerotism. The term onanism has likewise been diverted to mean masturbation or autoerotism, though, as Ellis says, "Onan's device was not auto-erotic, but was an early example of withdrawal before emission, or coitus interruptus" (ibid.).

In classical psychoanalysis, *autoeroticism* is also a phase in the development of object relationships (see *ontogeny, psychic*). The drives are present from the beginning of life and at first are amorphous energy potentials in the undifferentiated psyche. Since there are no object relationships at birth, these energies are, perforce, directed to the infant himself. This is the period of autoeroticism, when no distinction is made between the self and the non-self, when little if any heed is paid to the external environment.

Autoerotism is followed by the narcissistic stage out of which objects develop. Freud appears to have held concurrently three contradictory views on the nature of the earliest relationship to the environment; in one view autoerotism was considered primary, in another, narcissism, and in still another, the most primitive relationship was considered to be primary object love. See *narcissism, primary*.

According to Melanie Klein ("*The Origin of the Transference*"), autoerotism and narcissism are present from birth as part of the infant's first relation to objects (primarily the mother). This conceptualization contradicts Freud's view of autoerotic and narcissistic stages that preclude any kind of object relation.

**autofellatio**   Putting one's own penis into one's mouth. "A considerable portion of the population does record attempts at self-fellation, at least in early adolescence. Only two or three males in a thousand are able to achieve the objective, but there are three or four histories of males who had depended upon self-fellation as a masturbatory technique for some appreciable period of time—in the case of one thirty-year-old-male, for most of his life" (Kinsey, A. C. et al. *Sexual Behavior in the Human Male*, 1948).

**autofetishism**   Hirschfeld's term for the state of loving a material object (e.g., article of clothing) of one's own possession. The object acts as a sexual excitant.

**autoflagellation**   Hirschfeld's term for the act of whipping oneself as a sexual excitant.

**autogenic training**   A technique used to elicit the *relaxation response* (q.v.), consisting of six exercises: (1) focus on feelings of heaviness in the limbs; (2) cultivate a sense of warmth in the limbs; (3) concentrate on heart rate, (4) breathing, (5) warmth of the upper abdomen, and (6) coolness in the forehead. Autogenic training is often used in conjunction with reciprocal inhibition psychotherapy and other forms of *behavior therapy* (q.v.).

**autogeny, autogenic**   See *endogenous; endogeny*.

**autognosis**   Knowledge of oneself.

**autohypnosis**   *Self-hypnosis.* Autohypnotic phenomena are reported frequently in persons with *dissociative identity disorder* (q.v.): spontaneous trances (often described as spacing or tuning out), *enthrallment* (total engrossment in a single activity, such as reading a book or watching a film), spontaneous age regression (reliving periods from the past, with age-appropriate vocabulary and mental content), negative hallucinations (percepts and stimuli are not consciously registered), the ability to ignore or block out pain, out-of-body experiences or depersonalization.

**autohypnotic amnesia**   *Repression* (q.v.), as opposed to normal forgetting.

**autoimmunity**   An immunologic aberration in which antibody or sensitized lymphocyte reacts with the organism's own tissue. It is commonly believed that autoantibody attacks tissue and thereby causes autoimmune diseases (AID)—among which are lupus erythematosus, rheumatoid arthritis, mysasthenia gravis, scleroderma, and perhaps ulcerative colitis and some types of rheumatic heart disease. An alternative hypothesis is equally tenable—that autoimmunity may be due to genetically determined immunologic deficiencies that render the organism unable to respond immunologically to antigens (e.g., bacterium, virus, myoplasm, or other microorganism) that a normal immune system would readily eliminate. Autoantibodies may be a secondary mechanism that eliminates the tissue killed or damaged by the antigen or that protects the attacked organ from further damage. See *immune hypothesis.*

Human leukocyte antigens (HLAs) are the distinguishing markers of tissue types. There are more than 80 marker substances and hence thousands of possible combinations that are crucial to the regulation of the body's natural immune defense system. The gene complex of HLA is located on the short arm of chromosome 6. In many autoimmune diseases (including juvenile diabetes, myasthenia gravis, rheumatoid arthritis, systemic lupus, and perhaps narcolepsy) particular HLA types are found much more frequently than in the general population. The strongest association between an HLA substance and human disease was reported in 1971 by Paul Terasaki: HLA-B27, which is found in fewer than 6% of Americans, is present in more than 90% of persons who develop ankylosing spondylitis. HLA profiles are associated with disease susceptibility to a greater extent than any other known *genetic marker* (q.v.) in humans.

**autoinfection, mental** *Obs.* Kornfeld's term (1897) for a psychotic state in which the person believes himself wrong and brings every misfortune and unpleasant event into relation with his delusion.

**autoinhibitor** A type of *neuromodulator* (q.v.).

**autointoxication** Toxicity secondary to absorption of the waste products of metabolism or of the products of intestinal decomposition.

**autokinesis** Self-movement; frequently used in a specific way to designate the phenomenon of seeing and tracing the "movement" of a stationary pinpoint of light in a dark room. Persons with high autokinetic perception are said to demonstrate greater ego autonomy and more independent, nonconforming attitudes.

**autokinetic phenomenon** Perception of varying degrees of apparent movement by a stationary light; when exposed to a pinpoint of light at a distance of 12 feet in a totally dark room for 10 minutes, some subjects experience no apparent movement while others report varying amounts of movement.

**autologous transplant** A tissue transplant in which a patient's own progenitor cells are moved, expanded in culture, and then transplanted back into the disease-affected region.

**autology** Study of the self; self-analysis.

**automatic drawing** The execution of drawings without a person's conscious volition, but often after being directed to do so in a hypnotic trance. Automatic drawing is used in hypnoanalysis, much as dreams are used in psychoanalysis. Automatic drawing can be done in a hypnotic trance (hypnotic drawing), or after awakening if the person has previously, during the state of hypnosis, been instructed to do so.

**automatic memory** *Procedural memory* (q.v.).

**automatic obedience** *Command automatism;* following the orders of another blindly, without critical or automatic judgment. It may be induced through hypnosis and it appears spontaneously in the catatonic form of schizophrenia. "The patients carry out any commands whatsoever, even if it is against their will, as for example putting out their tongue when they know a pin will be stuck into it" (Bleuler, E. *Textbook of Psychiatry,* 1930). See *automatism; echopraxia.*

**automatic seizures** A type of *psychomotor epilepsy* (q.v.).

**automatic writing** Writing without conscious volition, while in a hypnotic trance. See *automatic drawing.*

**automatism** A condition in which activity is carried out without conscious knowledge on the part of the subject. Automatic actions and speech are seen in clear form in the catatonic form of schizophrenia in which incessant repetition may prevail without the patient's awareness. Automatisms are common also in other clinical states, particularly in those associated with a *fugue* (q.v.) and in epilepsy. See *automatic obedience.*

**automatism, postictal** See *epilepsy.*

**automatism, primary ictal** A type of psychomotor epilepsy. See *epilepsy.*

**automatization** The process whereby an action becomes routine and automatic, without conscious effort or direction.

**automaton conformity** The course of blindly adopting the pattern of culture of one's environment and bowing submissively to its dictates: the person accepts the way to live, to feel, and to think as implicitly or explicitly recommended by the group. The effects of culture on personality were greatly emphasized by Fromm. Man has today become aware of himself as a separate entity. The growing realization of his separateness gives him a sense of isolation and a longing to return to the earlier feeling of solidarity with others, so he uses certain irrational methods of relating back to the group. These are termed mechanisms of escape and include sadomasochism, destructiveness, and automaton conformity.

**automonosexualism**   *Rare. Narcissism* (q.v.).

**automysophobia**   Unreasonable fear that one's body is dirty or emits a repugnant odor.

**autonepiophilia**   Paraphilic infantilism; a *paraphilia* (q.v.) in which sexual arousal and orgasm are dependent on the subject acting as or being treated as an infant. The subject may need to wear diapers, for example, in order to become sexually aroused.

**autonoetic consciousness**   Awareness of the self. See *chronesthesia.*

**autonomasia**   A type of amnestic or nominal *aphasia* (q.v.), characterized by an inability to recall names or substantives.

**autonomic affective apparatus**   Kempf recognized two major divisions of body systems, the autonomic apparatus and its projicient apparatus. The sensory streams from the autonomic apparatus constitute the affective cravings or feelings, and the sensory streams flowing from the projicient apparatus constitute the kinesthetic stream (*Psychopathology,* 1921).

**autonomic arousal disorder**   Characteristics are autonomically mediated symptoms (other than pain) that are not part of another psychiatric disorder or general medical condition; sometimes classified as a somatoform disorder. Symptoms are persistent or recurrent, and they may appear in any of the following organ systems: cardiovascular (e.g., palpitations), respiratory (e.g., hyperventilation), gastrointestinal (e.g., aerophagia), genitourinary (e.g., dysuria), and skin (e.g., flushing). Many of these conditions were termed *psychosomatic* (q.v.) in older terminologies.

**autonomic epilepsy**   *Diencephalic epilepsy;* sympathetic epilepsy; parasympathetic epilepsy; a sudden, diffuse discharge of the autonomic nervous system in otherwise normal persons. In some, symptoms are primarily of sympathetic discharge; in others, symptoms are primarily of parasympathetic discharge. Usually, however, symptoms are mixed.

Penfield in 1929 described predominantly sympathetic seizures consisting of fever, flushing, tearing, sweating, salivation, hiccupping, and shivering, which he termed *diencephalic autonomic epilepsy.* In this case a ball valve tumor of the third ventricle had resulted in compression of adjacent hypothalamic nuclei. Cushing in 1932 reported on parasympathetic outbursts occurring in response to intraventricular injections of pituitrin and pilocarpine. Symptoms included profuse sweating, flushing, fall in blood pressure, lowering of temperature and basal metabolic rate, and increased peristalsis in the stomach and intestines. See *epilepsy.*

**autonomic failure**   See *PAF.*

**autonomic nervous system**   ANS; vegetative nervous system; a series of cerebrospinal nuclei and nerves with widely distributed ganglia and plexuses that subserve the vegetative functions of the body. In its peripheral ramifications the system is characterized by a series of synaptic junctions situated outside the central nervous system. There are two primary divisions: (1) the *parasympathetic,* or craniosacral, and (2) the *sympathetic,* orthosympathetic or thoracicolumbar. This subdivision is based upon the point of outflow from the central nervous system, the distribution of peripheral ganglia, the general antagonism in physiologic effects on visceral tissues most of which receive innervation from both divisions, and the response to pharmacologic agents. Each peripheral division of the autonomic nervous system is characterized by a two-neuron chain and consists of two histologic elements, the preganglionic neuron which terminates in a peripheral ganglion, whence the postganglionic neuron of the second order carries impulses to their destinations on the viscera. No impulse goes directly to an organ of termination.

The autonomic nervous system is under control of higher centers, the most important of which is the hypothalamus. The hypothalamus is the chief subcortical center for the regulation and integration of sympathetic and parasympathetic activities. The anterior and medial nuclei of the hypothalamus are chiefly concerned with parasympathetic functions, while the lateral and posterior hypothalamic nuclei are chiefly concerned with sympathetic regulation.

**autonomous ego functions**   Basic psychological capacities that form the basis for the development of the *ego* (q.v.), such as attention, arousal, social relatedness (typically manifested in the infant as pleasure or smiling when held), and motivation.

**autonomous speech** *Glossolalia* (q.v.).

**autonomous superego** The normal superego, which demands that the ego behave in a "good" way, in contrast to a *heteronomous superego* (q.v.), which demands that the ego behave in accordance with what is expected at the moment.

**autonomy** The quality or state of being self-governing. The living organism does not represent merely an inactive element but is, to a large extent, a self-governing entity. The biological process therefore is not entirely a result of external forces, but is in part governed by specific biological forces that are endogenous. See *respect for autonomy.*

**autonomy, sense of** Erickson's phrase for that aspect of the ego that allows it to maintain its identity and to continue its integrative work even during the regressive pull of the middle game transference. Like the similar *cohesive self* (Kohut) and *object constancy* (Kernberg), the sense of autonomy is a measure of ego strength.

**autonomy vs. doubt** One of Erikson's eight stages of man. See *ontogeny, psychic.*

**autopathy** Disease or disorder without apparent cause.

**autophagy** 1. Self-eating; biting or eating one's own flesh.

2. In times of stress or starvation, the process whereby cells digest their own cytoplasm and portions of their membrane to provide nutrients.

**autophilia** Self-love; narcissism.

**autophobia** Fear of being alone; fear of one's self.

**autoplasty** The process of adapting by changing one's self, rather than by altering the external environment. Autoplastic adaptation may be normal and healthy (the patient's change in the course of psychoanalytic treatment, for example, which results from an autoplastic identification with the analyst), or it may be neurotic (as in symptom formation). See *alloplasty.*

**autopsy, psychological** Retrospective study of a completed suicide that aims to reconstruct the events or circumstances immediately surrounding the death and to identify some of the factors that might have contributed to the suicide. Data are obtained from any informants who might reasonably be expected to have some knowledge of the subject's social, psychological, or medical status prior to the suicide, e.g., family members, work associates, teachers and classmates, counselors, physicians, and hospital personnel.

**autopsychic delusion** A delusional concept referring to one's own personality; a delusion related to the outside world is an *allopsychic delusion*; when it has to do with one's own body, it is called a *somatopsychic delusion.* This classification was suggested by Wernicke.

**autopsychic orientation** Appreciation of oneself, of one's own personality, one's psychic self. When a person is aware that changes take place in his personality, he or she is said to possess intact autopsychic orientation.

**autoreceptor** A receptor that controls the synthesis and release of neurotransmitters within the neuron on which it is located; sometimes called the presynaptic receptor to distinquish it from the postsynaptic receptor that is part of the feedback loop mechanism that mediates neurotransmitters originating from the antecedent neuron. Autoreceptor is the preferred term, however, because such receptors are located on the cell body and dendrites as well as in the presynaptic position on the nerve terminal. See *neuromodulator.*

**autoregulation** See *autoreceptor; neuromodulator.*

**autosadism** *Masochism* (q.v.).

**autoscopic hallucination** The experience of seeing one's body appear for a moment or two, usually in front of the subject.

**autoscopy** *Autoscopic psychosis*; seeing one's "self" or "double," usually as the face and bust that imitate the movement and facial expressions of the original, as if being a reflection in a mirror (and thus called a *phantom*). The double typically appears misty, hazy, or semitransparent, and associated auditory, kinesthetic, and emotional perceptions are frequent. The hallucinatory experience rarely lasts longer than a few seconds. The most common emotional reactions are sadness and bewilderment. Two forms of autoscopy are recognized: (1) symptomatic autoscopy, on an organic basis (such as irritative lesions in the temporoparietal lobes); and (2) idiopathic autoscopy, presumably a wishfulfilling mechanism.

**autosomal recessive** See *recessiveness.*

**autosome** A nonsex chromosome; there are 22 homologous pairs of autosomes in humans. Two sex chromosomes form the 23rd pair.

**autosuggestion** According to Charcot, an internally generated idea that has arisen by independent dissociation from the ego. Like a *suggestion*, it operates unconsciously and, because it is dissociated from the complex of the ego's stable associations, with impunity.

**autosymbolism** Hallucinations that represent, in symbolic form, what is thought or felt at a given instant. Autosymbolism is a phenomenon of the hypnagogic state, when neither full sleep nor full waking is predominant. It consists, essentially, of translation of thoughts into pictures.

**autotelik** Pertaining to behavior and traits that express the central aims of the person, such as self-preservation.

**autotomia** In zoology, severance of a part of the body. According to Ferenczi, "A similar tendency for freeing oneself from a part of the body which causes pain is demonstrated in the normal 'scratch-reflex,' where the desire to scratch away the stimulated part is clearly indicated, in the tendencies to self-mutilation in catatonia and in the like tendencies symbolically represented in the automatic actions of many tic patients" (*Further Contributions to the Theory and Technique of Psycho-Analysis*, 1926).

**autotopagnosia** *Somatotopagnosia*; inability to identify or orient the body or the relation of its individual parts, i.e., a defect in appreciation of the body scheme. This type of agnosia occurs in lesions of the thalamoparietal pathways of the cortex in the region of the angular gyrus.

**auxiliary ego** In psychodrama, a person who identifies consciously with all the subject's expressions and purposes, thus strengthening the subject's ego. The auxiliary ego, acting in the subject's behalf, is a genuine prolongation or extension of the subject's ego. "An auxiliary ego operating upon the instinctive level is a function known as an "alter-ego." Illustrations of an alter-ego are the mother to her child, the lover, or the friend....In the case of an interpersonal difficulty, the consulting psychiatrist becomes an auxiliary ego of two or more persons involved" (Moreno, J. L. *Sociometry 1*, 1937).

**avalanche conduction** Spread of nerve impulse to many more neurons so that an effect disproportionate to the initial stimulus is produced. See *law of avalanche*.

**AVED** Ataxia with isolated vitamin E deficiency; an autosomal recessive neurodegenerative disorder with symptoms similar to those of *Friedreich ataxia* (q.v.) but without cardiomyopathy or impaired glucose metabolism. Retinopathy and retinitis pigmentosa are reported in about a third of patients. It is more prevalent in North African and other Mediterranean populations. Incorporation of α-tocopherol (vitamin E) into very-low-density lipoproteins through the α-tocopherol transfer protein (TTPα) is impaired. As a consequence, concentrations of vitamin E in plasma are usually less than 10% of normal values. AVED is caused by mutations in the *TTPA* gene that encodes TTPα. Vitamin E is a powerful lipid-soluble antioxidant that effectively scavenges peroxyl radicals in cell membranes. Vitamin E deficiency can severely damage neuronal membranes through lipid peroxidation and cause neuronal degeneration by chronic *oxidative stress* (q.v.).

**Avellis syndrome** (George Avellis, German laryngologist, 1864–1916) A bulbar syndrome due to involvement of the vagus nerve and the bulbar portion of the spinal accessory nerve. Symptoms are homolateral paralysis of the soft palate, pharynx, and larynx and contralateral dissociate hemianesthesia, with loss of sensations of pain and temperature but not of touch and pressure.

**average expectable environment** See *affectomotor storms; facilitating environment.*

**aversion reaction** A response of avoidance or turning away from disturbing or frightening stimuli.

**aversion therapy** *Deterrent therapy*; negative conditioning; in particular, *chemical aversive conditioning* of alcoholism and alcohol abuse in which the ingestion of alcohol is paired with an aversive stimulus (such as vomiting, electrical shock, or thoughts of undesirable consequences) so that the ingestion of alcohol in itself comes to evoke aversive thoughts or responses. Techniques include the use of chemical agents such as emetine to produce vomiting (chemical aversion therapy) and electroshock (electrical aversion therapy). See *behavior theory; CAC; relapse prevention.*

**aversive control** One of the *decelerative* (q.v.) forms of behavior therapy. It involves presentation of a noxious stimulus (such as an electric shock applied to the forearm, exposure to substances with a noxious smell or taste, such as Tabasco sauce, or spraying the face with a water mist) immediately following the undesired (usually aggressive) behavior. Any behavior that allows the subject to avoid the stimulus is thereby reinforced. See *reinforcement*.

Forms of aversive control include *escape learning* (a subject learns to get away from a place or situation that is uncomfortable or painful) and *avoidance learning* (the subject's anticipatory response prevents the aversive event from happening in the first place).

Aversive techniques, especially in the case of aggressive children, have raised many ethical concerns and are used much less frequently nowadays than they were in the 1960s.

**aviator's neurasthenia** "A chronic functional nervous and psychic disorder occurring in aviators and characterized by gastric distress, nervous irritabilities, minor psychic disorders, fatigue of the higher voluntary mental centers, insomnia, and increased motor activity." The condition is also known as *aeroneurosis* (q.v.), *staleness*, and *flying sickness* (Sladen, F. J. *Psychiatry and the War*, 1943).

**aviophobia**    Fear of flying.

**avoidance**    A defense mechanism, akin to *denial* (q.v.), consisting of refusal to encounter situations, objects, or activities because they represent unconscious sexual or aggressive impulses and/or punishments for those impulses. Avoidance is a major defense in *phobia* and *anxiety hysteria* (qq.v.).

**avoidance learning**    See *aversive control*.

**avoidant**    *Abient*; negatively oriented or moving away from; an avoidant drive or behavior or response is a situation that results in behavior drawing away from the stimulus. Withdrawal behavior and defense reactions are types of avoidant behavior.

**avoidant disorder**    Social *phobia* (q.v.). See *anxiety disorders of childhood*.

**avoidant personality (disorder)**    Characteristics are hypersensitivity to real or imagined rejection, needing uncritical acceptance before venturing into relationships, avoidance of close personal attachments, and low self-esteem. In DSM-IV, avoidant personality is in Cluster C (with dependent and obsessive-compulsive personalities).

**avoided relationship**    See *group tension, common*.

**avoiders**    See *anxiety typology*.

**AVT**    Arginine vasotocin; a nonapeptide found in the pineal gland that may be involved in the regulation of sleep.

**avulsion of brachial plexus**    See *pain syndromes*.

**awareness**    The state of being informed, alert, conscious, knowledgeable, or responsive. Awareness depends on level of *arousal* (q.v.) and comprises multimodal sensory and cognitive functions. No specific assessment criteria for awareness have been established. Different states of awareness range from full wakefulness, alertness, and responsivity to *coma* (q.v.), where there is no response or only a reflexive response to all stimuli.

Other degrees of awareness include the following:

*Drowsiness*—ability to be stimulated to full arousal by sound, light, or other nonnoxious stimuli

*Lethargy*—responsiveness to nonnoxious stimuli but inability to be brought to full arousal

*Stupor* (q.v.)—noxious stimuli necessary to raise level of arousal

*Coma* (q.v.)—no response or only reflexive response to all stimuli

Level of awareness is usually measured by assessing the subject's orientation to person, place, time, and social context; determining whether the patient can follow simple commands and complex commands; and by testing the subject's ability to localize tactile and noxious stimuli. See *attention*; *vegetative state*.

**awareness training**    See *self-monitoring*.

**Awl, William M.**    (1799–1876) American psychiatrist; one of the "original thirteen" founders of the Association of Medical Superintendents of America (the forerunner of The American Psychiatric Association).

**axial hyperkinesia**    Thrusting pelvic movements such as sometimes occur in tardive dyskinesia and other extrapyramidal disorders, in barbiturate and other drug intoxications, and as conversion symptoms.

**Axis IV, V**    See *DSM-III-R, DSM-IV*.

**axon**    The main conducting unit of the *neuron* (q.v.); it arises from a specialized region of the cell body called the *axon hillock*. The axon hillock and initial segment of the axon are about as long as the diameter of the cell body; they act as a trigger zone that integrates and tallies incoming signals. The membrane of the trigger zone is rich in voltage-gated $Na^+$ channels, which, when sufficiently activated, initiate an action potential that is propagated down the axon.

The axon itself is characteristically long, of uniform caliber, ensheathed by neuroglial or neurilemma cells, and specifically differentiated to conduct nerve impulses away from the dendritic zone. It also brings substances needed by the cell back to the cell body; some nerve cell poisons and some viruses (such as rabies) are transported by such reverse or retrograde flow.

The terminal portion of the axon is a bulbous outpouching, the bouton; this area is also referred to as the axon telodendria because most nerves have several different terminal branches whose membrane or cytoplasm is specifically differentiated for synaptic transmission or neurosecretory activities. Because of those specializations, the bouton is able to attach itself to the dendritic zone of a selected adjacent neuron and stimulate it to produce an electrical response. See *synapse*.

Neurotransmitters may be synthesized in the cell body of the neuron or in the axon; most are stored in synaptic vesicles or granules in the terminal portion of the axon, ready for release on demand. (See *exocytosis*.) Also within the terminal axon are the enzymes involved in the synthesis and degradation of neurotransmitters, and *mitochondria* (q.v.), which generate cellular energy from the metabolism of glucose.

**axon growth** Neuronal connections form during embryonic development when each differentiating neuron sends out an axon, tipped at its leading edge by the *growth cone*, which migrates through the embryonic environment to its synaptic targets, laying down the extending axon in its wake. The cells follow a supportive roadway formed by the radial glial fibers under the direction of the protein *astroactin*, which acts as a ligand for neuron–glia binding during neuronal migration. Axons reach their appropriate target regions in a highly stereotyped and directed manner. Their pathfinding is directed by the coordinated action of multiple guidance clues. One guidance factor involves "sticky" regions on cells known as *cell adhesion molecules* (*CAMs*). There are also cell-substrate adhesion processes, in which neuroblasts attach to and travel along noncellular lattices, scaffoldings, and membranes of proteins, sugars, and other molecules, formed in the extracellular environment.

Axon growth depends upon at least two types of cellular behaviors: simple linear growth along "monorails," punctuated by more complex decision-making behaviors at intermediate targets (choice points), as axons switch from one highway to another. Axons respond to the coordinated actions of four types of guidance cues: *attraction* and *repulsion* cues, which can be either short-range or long-range.

The guidance of axons over individual segments of their trajectories appears to involve the simultaneous operation of several, and in some cases possibly all four, of these guidance forces. Thus, an individual axon might be "pushed" from behind by a chemorepellent, "pulled" from afar by a chemoattractant, and "hemmed in" by attractive and repulsive cues.

In the developing brain, the radial glia lead to a layer of cells near the outer surface, the *preplate*. The migrating neurons arrange themselves between the preplate and the *subplate*, like the filling in a sandwich. Subsequent generations of young neurons continue to stream in from below, passing through the layers of neurons already in place and arranging themselves in overlying layers, until there are six in all.

**axon guidance** The means by which neurons are helped to find their way during neuronal migration until they reach their final destination. The first cells to migrate tend to stay close to their site of origin; cells that migrate later must therefore bypass all those that migrated earlier. How they find their way to their final, appropriate destination depends upon several factors, including cellular adhesion, repulsion by inhibitory factors on the surfaces of other cells (such as oligodendrocytes), *guidepost cells* that present themselves as intermediate targets along the path to the neuron's final destination, and trophic factors supplied by the target zones or cells.

**axonal spheroid** Focal swelling of an axon, usually in CNS, to many times its usual diameter. Spheroids are often filled with disorganized cytoskeleton and organelles; they are almost universal in CNS neurodegenerative disease (including Alzheimer disease, CJD, HIV dementia, multiple sclerosis, and Parkinson disease) and in traumatic brain injury. Axonal spheroids may arise as terminal end bulbs after axons degenerate, but they and smaller varicosities may also begin on unbroken axons. Often they appear as tandemly repeated swellings on axons, particularly at the nodes of Ranvier. This suggests that spheroids interfere with axonal transport from the cell body, leading to *Wallerian degeneration* (q.v.) of the distal axon, which leaves the proximal stump with a large end bulb.

**ayahuasca** A "magic plant" used in South America and, in particular, the western part of the Amazon basin, in religious rituals. The bark of the plant contains the alkaloid harmine, a hallucinogen, related to tryptamine.

**aypnia** Insomnia, sleeplessness.

**Ayruvedic medicine** See *complementary therapy.*

**AZT** *Zidovudine* (q.v.), formerly called azidothymidine, an antiviral drug used in the treatment of persons with *AIDS* (q.v.).

# B

**B type** See *eidetic imagery*.

**B₁** *Thiamine* (q.v.).

**B₆** *Pyridoxine* (q.v.).

**B₁₂** The vitamin cyanocobalamin, a precursor of the coenzymes methylcobalamin and 5-deoxy-adenosylcobalamin, which are needed for cell growth and replication and for the maintenance of myelin in the nervous system. See *posterolateral sclerosis*.

**baab-ji** See *miryachit*.

**babbling** A form of speech preceding articulate speech, characterized by sound combinations devoid of meaning. See *language acquisition*.

**Babcock sentence(s)** Any of the statements suggested by Babcock (1930) to test a subject's ability to learn new information and reproduce it immediately. One that is frequently used is: One thing a nation must have to become rich and great is a large secure supply of wood.

**Babinski reflex** Described by Babinski in 1898 and 1903, as extension of the toes instead of flexion when stimulating the sole of the foot. Great toe extension may also be elicited by other tests—see *Chaddock reflex, Gordon refkex, Oppenheim reflex*.

**Babinski syndrome** See *hemiasomatognosia*.

**Babinski-Nageotte syndrome** (Joseph François Felix Babinski, Paris physician 1857–1932, and Jean Nageotte, Paris histologist, 1866–1948) A bulbar syndrome produced by scattered lesions of the glossopharyngeal, vagus, spinal accessory (bulbar portion), and trigeminal nerves. Symptoms are homolateral paralysis of the tongue, pharynx, and larynx; homolateral loss of taste in posterior tongue; homolateral Horner syndrome; homolateral loss of pain and temperature sense in the face; homolateral asynergia and ataxia with a tendency to fall to the side of the lesion; contralateral hemiplegia, and contralateral dissociate hemianesthesia with loss of pain and temperature sense but preservation of touch and pressure.

**baby blues** Sadness, mood swings, and anxiety that appear in as many as 70% of mothers following delivery; the symptoms usually resolve within a week without medication or other specific intervention. In contrast is postpartum depression, consisting of major affective symptoms that appear within a few weeks following delivery. See *postpartum psychosis*.

**baby talk** A form of speech characterized by defective articulation of certain consonants; it is rapidly outgrown unless adults in the environment contribute to its maintenance by using it themselves in conversing with the child. In severe behavior disorders and schizophrenia, the patient may revert to this type of speech.

**BAC** Blood alcohol concentration. See *BAL*.

**BACE1** β secretase, one of the enzymes that cleaves amyloid precursor protein (APP). Amyloid-β peptide (Aβ) is a product of the sequential cleavage of APP by β- and γ-secretases.

**background object** See *dream screen*.

**backlash** A type of *feedback* (q.v.), referring to the effect of its own overt responses upon the organism.

**backup saccades** See *saccades*.

**backward masking test** A measure of the time it takes for a stimulus to be moved from the stage of stimulus reception to short-term memory. The subject is presented with a visual stimulus, such as the letter T, to determine his or her threshold of perception. Then the stimulus is presented and is followed almost immediately by a mask, such as a pattern of X's. The pattern of X's obscures the target stimulus (T, in this case) if the interval between T and X remains short. In normal subjects, the backward mask ceases to obscure the target stimulus after about 200 ms. In most studies schizophrenia patients demonstrate an excessive vulnerability to the mask, which begins to lose its effectiveness after only about 500 ms. See *iconic storage*.

**backwardness** Educational retardation due to extrinsic causes.

**bacteriophage** See *recombinant DNA*.

**bad object** In Kleinian usage, persecuting part objects (such as the breast or the penis), whole objects (such as mother or father), or representations or images of either part or whole objects that arise from the sadistic aggression of the infant's death instinct. The infant's oral sadism, arising from the death instinct and from the frustrating breast, produces hate; projection of that hate is experienced as the bad breast hating the infant. In the paranoid-schizoid position there occurs a *splitting* of self and object representations into all good and all bad, which remain separated until the depressive position, when internal bad objects are no longer projected. Instead, they are retained as forerunners of the primitive superego, which attacks the ego with guilt feelings. Good internal objects protect against the death instinct and later also protect against the attacks of the primitive superego. See *good object*.

Still later, the split "good" and "bad" self and object representations are integrated and neutralized into a total self and a total object.

Fairbairn calls the split internalized bad object the *rejecting object*. See *libidinal ego; paranoid-schizoid position*.

**bad self**   The tendency on the part of both analyst and patient to project on each other their guilty images of their instinct-ridden selves. Behind the shield of unconscious countertransference, an analyst may make the patient a whipping boy for his own unconscious image of his infantile instinctual self.

On his side, the patient tends to project his own instinctual urges onto the analyst and to castigate the analyst for them. See *identification; paranoid-schizoid position; projective identification*.

**bad trip**   An adverse effect of hallucinogen use, consisting of hallucinosis with marked anxiety or depression, ideas of reference, delusional ideas, fear of insanity, impaired judgment, and perceptual changes, such as depersonalization, derealization, hallucinations, and synesthesias. The trip ends usually in less than 2 hours.

**β-adrenergic hyperdynamic circulatory state**   Panic disorder or generalized anxiety disorder in which cardiac symptoms occupy the forefront of complaints: chest pain, palpitations, breathlessness, a feeling of oppression, dizziness, sweating, fatigue, headache, tremor, and nervousness. As described, it is approximately equivalent to cardiac anxiety state, cardiac neurosis, da Costa syndrome, or effort syndrome. Diagnostic criteria include induction of symptoms by administration of isoproterenol (a pure beta-adrenergic stimulant), com-

plaints of cardiac awareness and tachycardia at rest, circulatory hyperkinesis, and benefit from propranolol. The *panic attack* (q.v.) has many features related to β-adrenergic function, such as tachycardia, tremulousness, and sweating.

**bag lady**   See *street people*.

**bah tschi**   See *miryachit*.

**Bailey, Percival**   (1892–1973) Neurologist, neurosurgeon, neuropsychiatrist; best known for *Classification of the Tumors of the Glioma Group* and for his books on cytoarchitecture of primate and human brains.

**Baillarger, Jules**   (1809–1890) French psychiatrist; investigated manic-depressive insanity as *folie à double forme* (1853–1854) and *cretinism* (1873).

**BAL**   1. Blood alcohol level; the concentration of alcohol in the blood, expressed in various ways: in percent (grams of alcohol per 100 ml of blood); in mg % (mg/100 ml or mg/dl); and as *promille* (grams/liter). The BAL that is considered presumptive evidence of alcohol intoxication in most of the United States is 0.1% (100 mg% or 1.0 promille). Because alcohol diffuses uniformly to all tissues, the BAL or *BAC* (blood alcohol concentration) reflects the concentration of alcohol in the brain.

The typical behaviors associated with different BALs, and the approximate number of drinks per hour it would take a 160–180-lb drinker to achieve various levels, are as follows:

| BAL (%) | DRINKS/ HOUR | BEHAVIOR |
|---|---|---|
| .01–.05 | 1–2 | Lowered alertness and restraint, a "good" feeling, some impairment of judgment |
| .06–.10 | 4–5 | Decreased awareness and reaction time; impaired depth perception, distance acuity, peripheral vision, and glare recovery |
| .11–.20 | | Marked depression in motor functioning, clearly intoxicated, sometimes outbursts of anger, joy, weeping, shouting |
| .21–.25 | 6–10 | Severe motor disturbances, staggering, blurred vision; within this range, both social and addictive drinkers show impairments |
| .30 | | Semistupor |
| .35 | | Surgical anesthesia; some will die at this level |
| .40 | 21 (a quart of whiskey) | Coma |
| .50 | | Cessation of breathing and heartbeat may occur |

**HOURS REQUIRED FOR ELIMINATION OF ALCOHOL**

| NO. OF DRINKS | WEIGHT OF DRINKER (IN LB) | | | | |
|---|---|---|---|---|---|
| | 120 | 140 | 160 | 180 | 200 |
| 1 | 2.6 | 2.2 | 1.9 | 1.7 | 1.5 |
| 2 | 5.2 | 4.5 | 3.9 | 3.5 | 3.2 |
| 3 | 7.8 | 6.7 | 5.8 | 5.2 | 4.6 |
| 4 | 10.4 | 9.0 | 7.8 | 6.9 | 6.1 |
| 5 | 13.0 | 11.1 | 9.8 | 8.7 | 7.8 |
| 6 | 15.6 | 13.5 | 11.7 | 10.4 | 9.3 |

The *elimination rate* of alcohol from the body is correlated with the number of drinks ingested and the weight of the drinker (a drink is defined as 1 ½ oz of 86-proof liquor, 5 oz of 12% wine, or 12 oz of 4.5% beer).

2. British anti-Lewisite, a chelating agent used as an antidote for poisoning by ingestion of heavy metals, such as antimony, arsenic, bismuth, chromium, gold, lead, mercury, and nickel.

**balanced group** In group therapy, the result of mixing patients in accordance with clinical and personal criteria in order to prevent intensification of a specific problem or set of problems.

**balanced placebo design** A research technique that allows for the effect of the subject's belief about what treatment he has received, by giving the experimental drug to one group of subjects who believe they have been given a placebo and giving a placebo to a second group who believe they have received the experimental drug.

**balbuties** *Stammering* or *stuttering* (qq.v.). Some authorities differentiate among *balbuties praecox* (starting before the age of 3 years), *balbuties vulgaris* (onset between the ages of 3 and 7), and *balbuties tarda* (onset after the age of 7).

**Balint syndrome** (Rezsoe Balint, Hungarian physician, 1874–1929) Apraxia of gaze (the subject cannot shift gaze on command), optic ataxia (clumsiness of movements performed under visual guidance), constriction of the field of visual attention (tunnel vision), and visual simultanagnosia (inability to recognize the whole picture even though its elements are recognized). The syndrome is caused by bilateral parieto-occipital lesions in the convexity of the hemispheres.

**Ballet sign** (Gilbert Ballet, French neurologist, 1853–1916) *Ophthalmoplegia externa*; loss of movements of eye and pupil with preservation of autonomic responses, often associated with exophthalmic goiter and other forms of hyperthyroidism.

**ballism, ballismus** Sudden, rapid, violent, large-amplitude flinging and flailing movements. It may appear as part of levodopa-induced dyskinesia; it is often associated with damage to the subthalamic nucleus. See *LID*.

**ballistophobia** Fear of missiles.

**balmy** Lay term for crazy in the United States. Based on the mispronunciation of *barmy*, derived from Barming (Kent County, England), the site of a large psychiatric hospital.

**balneology** *Obs.* Study of waters used in baths.

**Baló disease** (Jozsef Matthias Baló, Hungarian neurologist, b. 1895–c.1979) Concentric demyelination. See *diffuse sclerosis*.

**Bamberger disease** (Eugen Bamberger, Austrian physician, 1858–1921) A neuromuscular disorder consisting of clonic spasms of the leg muscles that produce jumping motions.

**β-amyloid disorders** Also, *beta-amyloid disorders*, *β-amyloid related diseases*; a group of inherited and sporadic disorders characterized by abnormal deposits of *amyloid* (q.v.) within the tissues. In the heritable forms, a mutated parent protein or proteolytic fragment of a mutated parent protein precipitates to form amyloid fibrils. The position of the mutation may determine clinical manifesations. Within the group are the following:

1. Some types of familial *Alzheimer disease* (q.v.).

2. Hereditary cerebral hemorrhage with amyloidosis, Dutch type (HCHWA-D); see *amyloid angiopathy, cerebral*.

3. Hereditary cerebral hemorrhage with amyloidosis, Icelandic type, involving castatin C.

4. Familial amyloidosis, Finnish type, involving gelsolin.

5. Familial amyloidotic polyneuropathy; see *amyloidotic polyneuropathy, familial*.

6. The spongiform transmissible encephalopathies (also known as infectious amyloidoses, prion diseases), which are associated with various mutations in the coding region of the PRNP (PrP) gene on the short arm of human chromosome 20.

Three inherited forms of spongiform encephalopathy are known: Gerstmann-

Straussler-Scheinker syndrome (GSS), characterized by chronic cerebellar ataxia and dementia in association with multicentric amyloid plaques; CJD or *Creutzfeldt-Jakob disease* (q.v.); and *fatal familial insomnia (FFI)*, characterized by untreatable insomnia, dysautonomia, and atrophy of thalamic nuclei. See *prion; virus infections.*

**β-amyloid peptide** *A*β; also *beta-amyloid peptide*; its accumulation is a primary event in the pathogenesis of *Alzheimer disease* (q.v.). β-amyloid peptide is generated proteolytically from a large precursor molecule, APP, by the sequential action of two proteases, β-secretase and γ-secretase. A third protease, α-protease, competes with β-secretase for the APP and can preclude production of Aβ by cleaving the peptide in two. See *amyloid hypothesis; APP.*

**BANC** *Blink-alpha neurocircuit*; a hypothesized neural pathway that includes the pontine tegmentum, cerebellum, substantia nigra, midbrain tectum lateral geniculate bodies, and occipital cortex. The rate of eye-blinking during visual fixation is reportedly elevated in a high percentage of patients with schizophrenia.

**bangungut** A culture-specific syndrome reported among male Filipino and Laotian youths; death from cardiac arrhythmia initiated by frightening dreams; also called *Oriental nightmare-death syndrome.*

**baquet** See *Mesmer.*

**bar reflex** A pathological postural reaction consisting of involuntary following by one leg when the other leg of the recumbent patient is moved laterally or vertically. The bar phenomenon is seen mainly in cases with lesions of the prefrontal areas (especially in cases of brain tumor).

**baragnosis** Absence of ability to recognize weight of objects, generally tested by placing objects in the hand; indicative of parietal lobe lesion.

**barbaralalia** Speech disorder evident when the subject speaks a second or foreign language.

**barbed wire disease** Vischer's term for any reactive mental disturbance of prisoners, who are often held in barbed wire camps. Also called barbed wire psychosis. Characteristically, the prisoners show irritability and loss of memory for prewar occurrences. See *prison psychosis.*

**barbed wire psychosis** A psychosis reported in prisoners of war, characterized by irritability and loss of memory for prewar occurrences.

**barber's chair syndrome** A form of *agoraphobia* (q.v.) in which the subject feels trapped and unable to escape when confined in a barber's chair (or a dentist's or beautician's). Similar feelings occur in transportation phobias, such as fear of flying or riding in a bus or automobile.

**barbiturates** A group of central nervous system depressants that are chemical derivatives of barbituric acid (malonyl-urea); among them are phenobarbital, Amytal, pentobarbital, Seconal, Evipal, and Pentothal. There are many similarly acting sedative and hypnotic drugs that produce the same kinds of complications, abuse, and dependency as seen with the barbiturates; among them are alcohol, "minor" tranquilizers (e.g., meprobamate, the benzodiazepines), and hypnotics (e.g., chloral hydrate, ethchlorvynol, glutethimide, methaqualone, methyprylon, paraldehyde). See *dependence, drug; psychoactive substance dependence.*

Symptoms of intoxication (i.e., indicators of abuse or dependence) include lability of mood, disinhibition of sexual and aggressive impulses, irritability, garrulity, slurred speech, poor coordination, unsteady gait, impaired attention or memory, impaired judgment, failure to meet responsibilities, and other signs of impaired social, occupational, or academic functioning.

Withdrawal symptoms follow cessation or reduction of use in persons dependent on the substance(s): nausea, vomiting, malaise, weakness, autonomic hyperactivity (sweating, rapid pulse, elevated blood pressure), insomnia, orthostatic hypotension, coarse tremor of hands, tongue, or eyelids, and grand mal seizures (in 75% of those with barbiturate dependence who withdraw abruptly).

A withdrawal delirium occurs in some (in as many as 60% of abrupt barbiturate withdrawals), manifested by autonomic hyperactivity, disturbance of attention, and inability to sustain goal-directed thinking or behavior, impaired memory and orientation, altered sleeping/waking pattern and level of psychomotor activity, and perceptual disturbances manifested as simple misinterpretation, illusions, or hallucinations.

Prolonged heavy use of this group of substances may be associated with an amnestic syndrome, characterized by impairment of short-term memory (leading to failure to store memory, inability to retrieve memories and, sometimes, confabulation), but retention of immediate memory. More extensive impairment is seen with barbiturate *dementia* (q.v.).

**barebacking**  Also, going bareback, skin-to-skin, and raw sex; having anal sex without condoms.

**baresthesia**  Pressure sense.

**barognosis**  The sense of weight differences, usually by lifting objects in the hand.

**barophobia**  Fear of (the pull of) gravity or of falling; fear of being overweight.

**Barr bodies**  Sex chromatin; a densely staining chromatin patch on the inner surface of the nuclear membrane, first described by Barr and Bertram in 1949. It was originally believed that the sex chromatin consisted of parts of both the X chromosomes that the female possesses, but currently most workers subscribe to the "Lyon hypothesis"—early in the embryonic development of the female one X chromosome in each cell is inactivated and becomes the sex chromatin. The number of Barr bodies is always less than the number of X chromosomes possessed.

**barrier**  Boundary; limit; obstruction; separation. In psychiatry, the word is generally used in four contexts: (1) the neurophysiologic, to refer to the functional obstruction of the free flow of constituents of the blood into the brain (see *blood–brain barrier*); (2) the interpersonal, to refer to an absent or defective ability to form adequate relationships with people—the *schizophrenic barrier* is thus considered a type of autistic behavior based on an ego defect, although the phrase is on occasion used to refer to lack of relatedness between different parts of the schizophrenic's personality; (3) in projective testing where *barrier response* is used to indicate a response that emphasizes the periphery of a percept and highlights the boundary (e.g., "turtle with shell," "man in armor"). Responses that emphasize weakness and permeability (e.g., "a gaping wound," "a torn rug") are called *penetration responses*. Schizophrenic patients tend to have fewer barrier responses and more penetration responses than neurotic or "normal"

subjects; and (4) ethical—in relation to transference and countertransference issues (e.g., undue familiarity, using information gained from the patient for the therapist's personal gain, soliciting contributions from a patient).

**Bartley v. Kremens**  See *consumerism*.

**Bartschi-Rochaix syndrome**  See *cervical migraine*.

**baryglossia**  *Obs.* Thick, heavy speech, usually implying a disorder of the tongue.

**barylalia**  An indistinct and thick speech, observed principally in patients with an organic lesion, often in the central nervous system (Broca area).

**baryphonia**  A heavy quality of voice; generally deep and hoarse.

**basal ganglia**  Masses of gray matter lying deep within each cerebral hemisphere, consisting of five large, interconnected subcortical nuclei: the caudate nucleus and *putamen* (together called the *corpus striatum, striatum,* or *neostriatum*), globus pallidus (or pallidum, *pleostriatum*), subthalamic nucleus, and substantia nigra. Some investigators have included the *claustrum*; the amygdala, and the ventral striatum (or limbic striatum), which comprises the nucleus accumbens, the olfactory tubercle, and the nucleus of the stria terminalis. See *striatum*. The *lenticular* (or *lentiform*) *nucleus* refers to the outer putamen and the medial globus pallidus; it nestles within the head and body of the C-shaped caudate, lateral to the thalamus. The caudate roughly parallels the shape of the lateral ventricle; near its tail lies the amygdala, which is now considered to be part of the *limbic lobe* (q.v.).

Each of the three input structures of the basal ganglia (putamen, ventral striatum, and caudate nucleus) projects to both output structures (medial globus pallidus and substantia nigra pars reticularis). The striatum receives three cortical inputs (corticostriate projections): (1) sensory motor cortices, (2) association cortices, and (3) limbic cortex.

Most thinking about the basal ganglia divides these structures into two parallel systems:

1. The dorsal striatal-dorsal pallidal system (including caudate nucleus, *putamen*, globus pallidus). The dorsal system is linked tightly to sensorimotor function and is the main target of the nigrostriatal system. These

cortical areas are thought to be involved in the motor planning that occurs before motor acts. Importantly, the dorsal striatum is not strictly a "motor" structure. A large part of the caudate nucleus and parts of the anterior putamen receive inputs primarily from the association cortex. Striosomes provide local links, especially in the caudate nucleus and anterior putamen, for limbic as well as motor processing.

2. The ventral striatal-ventral pallidal system (nucleus accumbens or limbic striatum and related structures, ventral pallidum). The ventral system is the main target of the limbic midbrain dopamine system and is tightly linked to core structures in the limbic system, including the hippocampal formation and the amygdaloid complex. The ventral striatal-ventral pallidal system is critical to behaviors based on reward and reinforcement. The ventral system may be a key executive system by which the hippocampus engages the motor system.

Structurally and functionally the basal ganglia are part of the *fronto-striato-pallido-thal-amo-frontal loop* (*FSPTFL*), which goes from the posterior portions of the orbitofrontal cortex through the ventral striatum (ventromedial caudate and accumbens nuclei), ventromedial pallidum, certain medial thalamic nuclei, and back to the orbitofrontal cortex. The basal ganglia are associated intimately with brain structures thought to be involved in cognitive processing. Outflow from the basal ganglia is preferentially directed toward the frontal lobes, and the basal ganglia receive their most massive inputs from forebrain regions. The basal ganglia are involved in goal-directed behavior, in learning related to motor and cognitive action plans, and in action planning itself or its neuromodulation.

Lesions of the basal ganglia produce various types of involuntary movements, such as *athetosis, ballism, chorea, dystonia*, and *tremor* (qq.v.).

Dopamine is synthesized in the striatum and substantia nigra; *Parkinson disease* (q.v.) is caused by degeneration of the nigrostriatal system. *Huntington disease* (q.v.) is caused by degeneration of intrastriatal cholinergic neurons and of the GABA-ergic system, which projects from the striatum to the globus pallidus and substantia nigra. *Hemiballism* (q.v.) is caused by damage to one subthalamic

nucleus. *Tardive dyskinesia* (q.v.) is produced when alteration of dopaminergic receptors by long-term treatment with phenothiazines or butyrophenones causes hypersensitivity to dopamine and its agonists.

Basal ganglia dysfunction is also associated with Gilles de la Tourette syndrome. It has also been implicated in the production of *obsessive-compulsive disorder* (q.v.), in which the subject is unable to suppress responses to irrelevant stimuli. The FSPTFL has also been hypothesized to be involved in the neuropathology of schizophrenia.

**basal nucleus of Meynert**   See *substantia innominata*.

**Basedow disease**   Hyperthyroidism or overactivity of the thyroid gland. Karl A. von Basedow, German physician (1799–1854), described exophthalmic goiter in 1840, characterized by enlargement of the thyroid gland, protrusion of the eyeballs, rapid heart action, fine muscular tremors, and so-called general nervousness. It is as commonly called Graves disease and less frequently Begbie, Marsh, Parry, Parsons, or Flajani disease. See *thyrotoxicosis*.

**basic anxiety**   Horney's term for a feeling of loneliness and helplessness toward a potentially hostile world. This concept is more comprehensive than Freud's "real" anxiety (*The Neurotic Personality of Our Time*, 1937).

**basic assumptions group**   In group therapy, a small group of 7 to 12 members in which the leader refuses to participate in group decision making or structuring. The name emphasizes the major regressive processes that characterize such a group.

The first is a *dependency assumption*: the leader, who is perceived as omnipotent, fails to live up to that demand; the group first denies and then devalues the leader; finally the group seeks a substitute.

The second is the *fight-flight assumption*: the leader is expected to protect the group from infighting by helping it deny intragroup hostility and project aggression onto external enemies.

The third operates under a *pairing assumption*: a focal couple in the group symbolizes the group's hope that the couple will reproduce itself and thereby preserve the group's threatened identity.

**basic conflict**   Horney's term for the intrapsychic struggle between opposing neurotic trends, such as self-effacing vs. expansive solutions, or proud self vs. despised self. See *conflict, central.*

**basic emotions** Happiness, fear, anger, disgust, sadness; contrasted with *moral emotions* (q.v.).

**basic fault** See *fault, basic.*

**basic mistakes** In Adlerian psychology, incidents, concepts, and attitudes of early childhood that have determined or contributed to a person's lifestyle, which must be corrected if the patient is to be helped. See *constancy.*

**basic rule** The fundamental precept governing the activity of the patient in psychoanalytic therapy: to think aloud, and by means of *free association* (q.v.) to overcome censorship and resistance to unconscious content.

**basic trust** In normal development, the infant's sufficient sense of security and comfort in his relationship with the parent(s) to allow him to cede his *grandiose self* ("I am perfect and you admire me") to the *idealized parental image* ("You are perfect and I am part of you"). This is the first step in recognizing the parent(s) as different from the self, and early basic trust is thus the basis for the ability to sense and test reality. See *cohesive self; grandiose self; relatedness.*

**BASIC-ID** An acronym devised to refer to what A. Lazarus, the originator of *multimodal therapy*, considers the core elements in human life and conduct: behaviors, affective processes, sensations, images, cognitions, interpersonal relationships, and drugs (for mnemonic reasons, the biologic is represented by drugs).

Multimodal therapy, also known as *multimodal behavior therapy*, is a form of brief psychotherapy that utilizes many techniques drawn from different sources without necessarily accepting the theory or system underlying each technique. In multimodal therapy, a *modality profile* is constructed for the patient that consists of a chart listing both problems and proposed treatments for each of the elements in the BASIC-ID. This enables the therapist to devise the best method or combination of treatment approaches for each patient and avoids the difficulties inherent in trying to fit every patient into the same form of therapy.

**basiphobia** Fear of walking, usually related to fear of collapse and death, rather than to fear of objects encountered while walking.

**basistasiphobia** *Stasibasiphobia* (q.v.).

**BASK** Behavior–affect–sensation–knowledge, the different dimensions of functioning and awareness that normally are connected with and consistent with one another. The BASK model of *dissociation* (q.v.) emphasizes the incongruity or dissonance that is often found either within one personality or between several alters in dissociative identity disorder.

**basket cells** See *neocortical neurons.*

**basophile adenoma** Tumor of the anterior lobe of the pituitary gland, characterized by a pluriglandular symptom complex (*Cushing syndrome*). The symptoms are adiposity of the body and face but sparing the limbs, amenorrhea and hypertrichosis in women, acrocyanosis with cutis marmorata, hypertension, purple striae distensae, at times polycythemia and peculiar softening of bones, and frequently hyperglycemia. See *intracranial tumor.*

Young adults are more commonly affected and duration of life is about 5 years following appearance of symptoms. Psychoses develop in approximately 25% of cases; they are commonly of the manic, melancholic, or anxious-agitated variety. In another 35% of cases, there are marked personality changes, usually in the direction of apathy.

**basophobia** *Basiphobia* (q.v.).

**basostasophobia** *Stasibasiphobia* (q.v.).

**Bastian law** (Henry C. Bastian, English neurologist, 1837–1915) In severe crush or complete interruption of the spinal cord, there results a total and permanent loss of reflexes with flaccid paralysis; death ensues within a few days or weeks.

**bath, continuous** Formerly used in the management of excited and delirious patients, a tub with continuous inflow and outflow of water at a constant temperature of approximately 98°F. The patient lies in a canvas suspended in the tub, with his or her body immersed in water.

**bathmophobia** Fear of stairs, escalators, or crossing a threshold.

**bathophobia** Fear of depths or heights, as in the fear of losing control of oneself while in a high place or a fear of falling from a height and thus being killed.

**bathroom phobia** A fear of the toilet or bathroom, seen often in children and persons with obsessive-compulsive disorder. The phobia is frequently expressed as a fear of falling into the toilet, of being attacked by some monster coming from it, or as a fear of being infected.

As a rule, such phobias represent a condensation of ideas of dirt (representing anal-erotic temptations) with ideas of castration.

**bathyesthesia**   Deep sensibility of the part of the body beneath the surface.

**batophobia**   Fear of (being on or passing) high objects or buildings.

**batrachophobia**   Fear of frogs.

**battarismus**   *Stammering; stuttering* (qq.v.); hesitating speech.

**battered child syndrome**   Term coined by pediatrician C. H. Kempe in the 1960s denoting physical injuries to children secondary to intentional acts of omission or to repeated, volitional, excessive beatings, by a parent or caretaker. Other than the obvious immediate dangers to the child's life and adequate physical growth, it is possible that such cruelty and abuse may constitute a long-term hazard in that it predisposes to a psychic development along the lines of delinquency and violence. See *psychopathic personality*; *dissociative disorders*.

The parents of abused or battered children show as wide a variation in character and personality makeup as do people in general; a small percentage of them can be classified as borderline psychotic, while only a few are overtly psychotic. Many, however, have poor self-esteem and a lack of self-confidence, difficulty in extracting pleasure from daily living, social isolation, a past history of abuse within their own families, and a lack of empathy with their child's needs. Such factors are often expressed in problem drinking, repeated job loss, unwanted and early pregnancies, unrealistic expectations of their children, and an inability to maintain children on various behavior and school schedules, (Coltoff, P. & Luks, A. *Preventing Child Maltreatment: Begin with the Parent*, 1978).

The first forensic book on sexual assaults on children was published in 1857 by Ambroise Tardieu. Sexual abuse of children—including incest, rape, and sexual relations between adults and children—appears to be rooted in defective family functioning. To describe it only in terms of violence by an adult against an innocent victim is an oversimplification. Incest, for example, involves at least three people— the incestuous pair and the nonparticipating parent—and each of them plays an essential role in sustaining the situation (Rosenfeld,

A. A. *Journal of the American Medical Association 240*, 1978). See *victim*.

**battering**   Repeated physical or sexual assaults (*spousal abuse*) by an intimate partner within a context of coercive control. The primary intent and function of battering is the intimidation and control of another, and to that service batterers use threats, taunts, and ridicule. Such psychological abuse may be an important precursor to subsequent physical aggression in battering couples. See *domestic violence*.

**battle fatigue**   See *shell shock*.

**Battle sign**   (William Henry Battle, London surgeon, 1855–1936) Postauricular and subconjunctival ecchymosis in cases of fracture of the base of the skull. See *raccoon eyes sign*.

**battology**   Continual reiteration of the same words or phrases in speech or writing.

**Bayle disease**   Antoine Bayle, French physician (1799–1858), first described it in 1822. *Obs. General paresis (q.v.)*; dementia paralytica.

**β-CCE**   β-carboline-3-carboxylic acid ethyl ester, a high-affinity benzodiazepine-receptor ligand that blocks the anticonvulsant, anxiolytic, and sedative-hypnotic actions of benzodiazepines.

**Bcl2**   B-cell leukemia/lymphoma 2; a protein that promotes the survival of neurons by stabilizing mitochondrial membranes and decreasing oxidative stress. See *apoptosis*.

**bdelygmia**   A Hippocratic term for morbid loathing of food. See *anorexia nervosa*.

**BDI**   *Beck Depression Inventory* (q.v.).

**BDNF**   Brain-derived neurotrophic factor. A frequent polymorphism, at nucleotide 196, is an amino acid substitution of valine to methionine, resulting in val66met. Persons with one or two met alleles (instead of the more common val allele) have measurably lower ability to perform tasks of learning and memory. Although the met allele variant of BDNF does not affect risk for schizophrenia, it may contribute to the cognitive impairments found in subjects with schizophrenia. See *neurotrophic factors*.

**BEAM**   Brain electrical activity mapping, an imaging technique that provides a topographic display of scalp-recorded signals from the EEG electrodes. It is sometimes called *spectral photography*. See *neurometrics; NMR*.

**Beard, George Miller**   (1840–1883) American psychiatrist; introduced the term *neurasthenia* in a paper, "Neurasthenia or Nervous

Exhaustion," *Boston Medical and Surgical Journal LXXX*, 1869.

**Beard disease** An old term for *neurasthenia* (q.v.).

**beating** Flagellation. Beating phantasies accompanying masturbation were discussed as a form of perversion by Freud. In the girl, beating phantasies typically go through three stages of development; first the father is beating a sibling, next he beats the girl herself, and finally he beats the other children againbut these are boys and need not be siblings. In the boy, beating phantasies develop in two stages: in the first, the father is beating the boy, and in the second it is the mother who is beating him. In both sexes, the phantasies originate from an incestuous attachment to the father; the boy evades the threat of homosexuality by transforming the beating father into the beating mother, while the girl transforms herself in phantasy into a man and derives masochistic pleasure from what appears on the surface to be a sadistic phantasy.

**beaxolol** A *beta blocker* (q.v.).

**Bechtereff-Mendel reflex** (V. M. Bechtereff, Russian neurologist, 1857–1927, and Kurt Mendel, German physician, 1874–1946) The cuboidodigital or dorsocuboidal reflex; striking the outer part of the dorsum of the foot normally produces a dorsal flexion of the toes; in abnormal conditions, such as pyramidal tract disease, there is plantar flexion.

**Beck Depression Inventory (BDI)** A scale of 21 items designed to provide a quantitative assessment of depressive disorders. The subject is asked to rate each statement on a scale from zero to three to indicate the severity of depression.

**Bedlam** The Priory of St. Mary of Bethlehem, founded in London in 1247, turned into a mental hospital in 1402 and incorporated in 1547 as the Hospital of St. Mary of Bethlehem. The proper name of this first English mental hospital became a common appellation for "lunatic asylum" in general and, still later, synonymous with states of frenzy, excitement, wild tumult, and pandemonium.

**beer goggles effect** The optical aids or other cues that make members of the opposite sex appear more attractive after the observer has a few drinks.

**Beers, Clifford W.** (American layman, 1876–1943) In 1909 founded National Committee for Mental Hygiene (now called National Association for Mental Health); wrote *A Mind That Found Itself*.

**Beevor sign** (Charles Edward Beevor, British neurologist, 1854–1908) Upward excursion of the umbilicus, observed when the lower half of the abdominal muscles are paralyzed.

**beggar, emotional** The type of person who is always "holding his mental palm out to people, yet always expecting it to be slapped down." The emotional beggar has been unable to detach himself from his parents (usually the parent of the opposite sex). He always looks for more, no matter how close to the parent he has managed to attach himself. "His general reaction to people is a suckling one" (Hinsie, L. E. *Understandable Psychiatry*, 1948).

**behavior** The manner in which anything acts or operates. A hungry man seeks food; the seeking constitutes behavior. Food gets into his stomach; the stomach acts and reacts, that is, it exhibits physiology or pathology.

Behavior is a complex interaction among (1) the genes, (2) brain anatomy, (3) the biochemical state of the brain, (4) the ways by which a person was reared and taught, (5) the way the person has been treated by society, and (6) the stimuli impinging on the person. Brain modules assume their identity by a combination of what kind of tissue they start with, where they are in the brain, and what patterns of triggering input they get during critical periods in development.

**behavior, chaotic** Extreme disorderliness in organizing one's humdrum affairs, with respect to the time to be made available for different needs, the necessary money for various expenditures, or the disposition of personal effects.

**behavior, collective** The behavior that results when every individual in a group, an assemblage, or a public is moved to think and act under the influence of a mood or state of mind, in which each shares and to which each contributes.

Elementary forms of collective behavior can be seen in the street crowd, the acting crowd, the expressive crowd, the mob, the gang, the panic, the riot, the stampede, and the mutiny; intermediate forms in mass behavior, the public, public opinion, the party, and crusades; and more highly organized forms in propaganda, advertising, religious movements, nationalistic movements, fashion, reform, and revolution.

**behavior contract**  A negotiated agreement that details in writing the conditions under which a person will do something for another person; often useful in promoting an exchange of positive reinforcement among family members. See *contract therapy*.

**behavior control**  See *forced treatment*.

**behavior disorders**  A group of psychiatric disorders in children and adolescents that are not secondary to somatic diseases or defects or to convulsive disorders and that are not part of a well-defined psychosis or psychoneurosis (see *conduct disorders*). In DSM-IV they are classified with the disruptive behavior and attention-deficit disorders.

The primary behavior disorders are considered to be reactions to an unfavorable environment; they appear as problems of personality development, as persisting undesirable traits or unfavorable habits (the so-called habit disorders, including nail-biting, thumb-sucking, enuresis, and temper tantrums), as delinquency or conduct disorders (truancy, fighting and quarreling, disobedience, untruthfulness, stealing, forgery, setting fires, destruction of property, use of alcohol, use of drugs, cruelty, sex offenses, vagrancy, etc.), as certain neurotic traits (such as tics and habit spasms, sleepwalking, overactivity, and fears), and as problems of school and general educational or vocational difficulties. In the past, children with such disorders were referred to as "problem children." See *oppositional disorder*.

**behavior disturbance, interictal**  See *temporal lobe syndromes*.

**behavior genetics**  *Behavioral genetics* (q.v.).

**behavior language**  *Body language* (q.v.); in children, use of actions to communicate before the child has learned to speak. Crying, fretting, anxiety, quiescence, satiety, smiling, and self-activity are the words of a language the infant uses before acquiring the capacity to produce articulate sounds. See *organ jargon*.

**behavior modeling**  See *modeling, behavior*.

**behavior modification**  See *behavior therapy*.

**behavior reversal**  A behavior technique in which more desirable responses to interpersonal conflict situations are practiced under the therapist's supervision.

**behavior theory**  A theory of the genesis of neurotic behavior, based on learning theory; among its leading exponents are Eysenck, Jones, and Wolpe. The theory postulates that neurotic symptoms are learned patterns of behavior that are unadaptive. If neurotic symptoms are learned, then they should be amenable to "unlearning," and behavior therapy is directed to the inhibition and/or extinction of the learned neurotic responses.

Particular forms of *behavior therapy* (q.v.) include assertiveness training, aversive therapy, biofeedback, conditioning, contract therapy, delay therapy, flooding, implosion, modeling, reciprocal inhibition and desensitization, shaping, system substitution, and systematic desensitization. See *BASIC-ID; behaviorism*.

**behavior therapy**  Also refers to *behaviour therapy; behavior modification; cognitive behavior therapy (CBT)*: application of the methods and findings of experimental psychology to the alteration of maladaptive behavior. The origins of behavior therapy are mainly to be found in two reports: (1) *Psychotherapy by Reciprocal Inhibition* (1958), in which Joseph Wolpe describes his work on experimental neurosis, leading to the technique of systematic desensitization; and (2) *Science and Human Behavior* (1953), in which B. F. Skinner describes how the effects on learning of the consequences of behavior could be applied therapeutically. See *behavior theory*.

Behavior therapy assumes that a person's behavior is a way of adapting to the environment and not necessarily a reflection of some kind of underlying psychopathology. In consequence, the first step is *behavior analysis*—assessing what symptoms affect functioning and what stimulates (precedes) or maintains (reinforces) them—rather than any attempt to fit the symptoms into a particular diagnostic category. Concrete goals are set, and specific behaviors (*target behaviors*) are selected for change. Therapy is typically brief, directive, structured, and focused on the here and now. The treatment plan is tailored to the subject's specific needs, and the treatment itself is monitored closely so that it can be modified as needed until the goals of therapy can be achieved.

Many different techniques have been developed within the framework of behavior theory, including assertiveness and social skills training, exposure methods, and self-control procedures such as *biofeedback, cognitive behavior therapy*, and *contingency management* (qq.v.). *Assertiveness* and *social skills training* help the patient to express positive or negative emotions clearly. *Behavioral rehearsal* (one or more practice sessions in expressing appropriate reactions to situations that are difficult for the patient), *modeling* (q.v.), and *information feedback* (in which patient and therapist act out troublesome situations and the therapist comments on the patient's behavior) are specific techniques that may be used. See *social skills training*.

**behavioral addictions**  Pathologically repetitive or compulsive activities that resemble drug addiction because of their characteristics, such as strong cravings or urges to indulge in the activity, continued engagement in self-destructive behavior despite adverse consequences, inability of affected persons to control their abnormal activity, and a conscious feeling of being unable to stop.

Pathological gambling is the disorder that most resembles drug addictions. Some studies suggest that drugs and gambling stimulate some of the same biochemical pathways. Compulsive overeating and bulimia (but not anorexia, where behavior is rigidly controlled and there is no high) also simulate addiction. Sex addicts obsess about whatever their favorite practice is, never get enough, feel out of control, and experience serious disruption of their lives. Compulsive shoppers often report that their shopping binges are precipitated by feelings of depression and anxiety, and the shopping can generate a temporary druglike high before the shopper crashes into depression, guilt, anxiety, and fatigue. Compulsive shoppers often end up with huge debts and their houses stuffed with unused merchandise.

Having one addiction lowers the threshold for developing another. Men are overwhelmingly represented among sex addicts and outnumber women by about 2 to 1 in gambling and substance abuse; women are prone to the "mall disorders"—eating, shopping, and kleptomania. FMRI studies indicate that the highs and lows of winning money, abusing drugs, or anticipating a gastronomical treat involve similar activation of the mesolimbic dopamine system.

**behavioral analysis**  A way of examining patterned behavior at the micro level based on operant theory and social learning models of transactions. The basic assumption is that the most important determinants of behavior are in the external environment, and that analysis of events that vary together with behavior makes it possible to predict future behavior. Focus is on the presence and effects of reinforcers and punishers.

**behavioral ecology**  *Socioecology;* the ethological approach to the study of behavior and, in particular, how the anatomy and physiology of particular brain structures relate to species-typical social behaviors such as which features of an organism's sensory world are relevant to its natural responses, and why. Behavioral ecology studies the interactions between the organism and its environment that determine the actions of the organism that contribute to its survival and reproduction; included are such behaviors as habitat selection, social grouping, competition for mates, dominance and territoriality claims, food seeking, and antipredator activity.

As social beings, primates must be able to evaluate the consequences of their own behavior, to predict the probable behavior of other individuals, and to weigh the balance of advantages and losses even as all the factors in the equation are in constant flux—and all this in a context that is constantly in flux. (See *choice*.) Such social skills require complex cognition: an ability to represent long, linear dominance hierarchies, to remember who is doing what to whom, and to manipulate this information to one's own advantage. Many social skills depend on visual and auditory cues and the sensory neocortical areas, particularly in the temporal lobe, that are involved in the processing of such information. See *face cells*.

**behavioral family therapy**  *BFT*, a systematic approach to single-family interventions, developed primarily for use in the treatment of alcohol and substance use disorders. Typically, it consists of at least 18 sessions, which include connecting with the family, assessment, psychoeducation, communication skills training, and problem-solving training.

**behavioral genetics**  The branch of genetics that is concerned with genetic determinants of behavior and behavioral disorders. To date, all behavioral disorders investigated have shown evidence of genetic influence.

Among the most heritable disorders is autism, although until the 1970s it was generally thought to be environmental in origin. Other disorders with substantial genetic influence include Alzheimer disease, schizophrenia, major mood (affect) disorder, and reading disability. Disorders with weaker evidence of genetic influence include antisocial personality, eating disorders, specific language disorder, panic disorder, and Gilles de la Tourette syndrome. See *heritability; personality.*

**behavioral medicine** "An interdisciplinary field concerned with the development and integration of behaoral and biomedical science, knowledge and techniques relevant to health and illness and the application of this knowledge and these techniques to prevention, diagnosis, treatment and rehabilitation" (Schwartz, G. E. & Weiss, S. M., *Journal of Behavioral Medicine 1*, 1978).

In the 1970s behavioral medicine began to be differentiated from *psychosomatic medicine* (q.v.) and to be defined as including (1) psychophysiological intervention through biofeedback, (2) direct psychological intervention in medical problems to provide alternative, or adjunctive approaches to traditional pharmacologic or surgical treatment, and (3) primary prevention.

**behavioral model** See *learning theory, social.*

**behavioral neurochemistry** Study of the relations between chemical substances in the brain and behavior—including neuroregulatory substances, genetic control of transmitter agents, different roles of compounds in different areas of the brain, pharmacogenetics, biochemical effects of receptor excitation, interactions between different agents within the brain, actions of drugs on enzymatic and metabolic processes within the brain, and the relation of all such biochemical events to psychological events and behavior.

**behavioral neurology** *Behavioral neuroscience; brain sciences;* the branch of neurology that links normal and abnormal behaviors to functioning of specific areas or regional systems of the brain, such as the finding that stopping and starting motor tasks is a frontal lobe function and that perseveration or motor inertia is therefore suggestive of frontal lobe disturbance. One of its basic goals is elucidation of the neural mechanisms underlying cognitive processing. The basic science of behavioral neurology is *neuropsychology* (q.v.). See *neuropsychiatry.*

**behavioral reaction** See *personality disorders.*

**behavioral rebound** See *amphetamines.*

**behavioral rehearsal** See *behavior therapy.*

**behavioral sciences** A multidisciplinary pursuit of knowledge that seeks to understand the roots of behavior in individuals, groups, and cultures, and in all conditions, normal, exceptional, and pathological. The behavioral sciences include the natural sciences, the social sciences, and the humanities; of particular relevance to psychiatry are the subjects studied by *behavioral genetics, behavioral neurochemistry, behavioral neurology, neuropsychiatry,* and *neuropsychology* (qq.v.).

**behaviorism** A term coined by J. B. Watson in 1913 to indicate that all habits may be explained in terms of conditioned glandular and motor reaction. "Behaviorism holds that the subject matter of human psychology is the *behavior or activities of the human being.* Behaviorism claims that 'consciousness' is neither a definable nor a usable concept; that it is merely another word for the 'soul' of more ancient times" (*Behaviorism*, 1924).

Classical behaviorism asserted that the proper subject for psychology was not the operation of the mind but rather the examination of objective, observable behavior. Behavior was to be understood in terms of the stimulus-response formula; the organism thus is essentially passive and can only react to stimulation. The leading psychologists of the next generation were trained in Watson's orbit—Clark Hull, B. F. Skinner, Kenneth Spence, and E. L. Thorndike. Modern behaviorism, as exemplified by Skinner's *operant behaviorism,* eschews a mechanistic view of human nature. The core theme of operant behaviorism is that activities of the organism bring consequences that shape and influence further action. It is the environment that produces the consequences, so it is the environment that shapes, influences, and determines a person's behavior. Behavior that elicits positive consequences (rewards) will tend to be repeated—*positive reinforcement* in Skinner's terminology. Negative consequences (punishment, in the form of either aversive stimulation or withdrawal of a positive stimulus) will tend to be avoided, and behavior that removes aversive stimulation will tend to be repeated (*negative reinforcement*).

*Behavioral engineering* refers to systematic control of the environmental conditions that shape the behavior of people (Skinner, B. F. *Walden Two,* 1948; *Science and Human*

*Behavior*, 1953; *Beyond Freedom and Dignity*, 1971). See *conditionalism; operant conditioning*.

In 1960, *Plans and the Structure of Behavior* (by George Miller, Karl Pribram, and Eugene Galanter) called for a replacement of standard behaviorism and its reflex arc. It proffered a *cognitive or cybernetic* approach to behavior in terms of actions, feedback loops, and readjustments of action in the light of feedback. The reflex arc was to be replaced by the *TOTE* unit (for "Test–Operate–Test–Exit"). The computer made it legitimate in theory to describe humans in terms of plans, images, goals, and other mentalistic conceptions. Current emphasis on cognitive psychology has overshadowed behaviorist theory, which is now largely of historical interest.

**behaviorist tradition**   See *cognitive neural science*.

**Behçet syndrome**   A syndrome that may be allergic in nature consisting of recurrent iritis, aphthous lesions of the mouth, and ulcerations of the genitalia, all of which run a benign course. Some cases show neuropsychiatric complications in addition, and these indicate a much more serious prognosis; they include episodic or progressive brain stem syndromes, meningoencephalitic syndrome, and organic confusional syndrome.

R. N. De Jong (*Neurologia 9*, 1964) suggested that Behçet syndrome is one of a group of related symptom complexes (rather than disease entities) and that multiple and diverse etiologies, such as virus or allergy, may be involved. The other syndromes included in the grouping are as follows:

1. *Harada syndrome*—uveitis, retinochoroidal detachment, cataract, and meningoencephalitis

2. *Vogt-Koyanagi syndrome*—bilateral uveitis, vitiligo, alopecia, poliosis, dysacousia, often accompanied by meningoencephalitis

3. *Fuch syndrome*—headache, fever, cyanosis, swelling of the face, ulceration of the mucous membranes, and conjunctivitis

4. *Klauder syndrome*—fever, vesicular eruption of hands and feet, and eruption of the mucous membranes and orifices

5. *Stevens-Johnson syndrome*—fever, severe and generalized maculopapular or vesicular or erythema multiforme-like eruptions of the orificial mucosa

6. *Reiter syndrome*—arthritis, nonspecific urethritis, and conjunctivitis

**Behr syndrome**   (Carl Behr, German physician, 1874–1943) A familial disorder that begins in infancy and manifests by temporal nerve and optic atrophy, ataxia, loss of coordination, and mental retardation.

**Bekhterev, Vladimir**   (1857–1927) Russian neurologist and psychiatrist; professor and director of the clinic for mental and nervous illnesses at St. Petersburg Military Medical Academy. Independently of Pavlov, he developed a theory of conditioned reflexes and assumed the existence of two psychological systems—the subjective, whose basic method of study is introspection, and the objective, whose basic method is the conditioned reflex. He described Bekhterev nucleus (the superior nucleus of the vestibular nerve), Bekhterev nystagmus (due to destruction of the labyrinth), and Bekhterev disease (chronic polyarthritis progressing to immobility of a number of joints).

**bel-2**   An oncogene that prevents lymphocytes from undergoing *apoptosis* (q.v.) in leukemia. It may play some role in preventing neuronal death, suggesting that it might be of value in neurodegenerative disorders such as Parkinson disease and Alzheimer disease.

**belief type**   According to Ferenczi, there are two fundamental types of personality from the standpoint of belief. There are those who have a tendency to "blind beliefs"; they accept statements without any question. The tendency derives from the time the child is disillusioned about his own omnipotence and dependence upon others, originally upon his parents, later upon anyone in authority. There is the second type, constituting "blind disbelief"; it is a phase of disillusionment in the power of the parents or other superior people.

**Bell, Luther V.**   (1806–1862) American psychiatrist; one of the "original thirteen" founders of the Association of Medical Superintendents of America (the forerunner of The American Psychiatric Association); *Bell mania* (q.v.).

**Bell, Sir Charles**   (1774–1842)   Born in Edinburgh, the son of a Scottish Episcopalian clergyman; moved to London 1806. He demonstrated the separate functions of the anterior (motor) and posterior (sensation) roots of the spinal nerves—the Bell-Magendie law.

**Bell disease**   Collapse delirium, delirious mania; the most severe of the manic type of manic-depressive psychosis. See *Bell mania; manic-depressive psychosis*.

**Bell mania**   Luther V. Bell (*American Journal of Insanity 6*, 1849) described 10 patients who died suddenly and whose autopsies failed to reveal an adequate explanation (nowadays termed *negative death autopsy*); the term Bell's mania was used to describe this entity, although later it was more commonly called *lethal catatonia, exhaustion death*, or *deadly catatonia*. The clinical picture consists of severe agitation, mutism, high fever, dehydration, delusions, hallucinations, and rapid death.

**Bell palsy**   See *facial nerve*.

**belladonna**   *Atropa belladonna; deadly nightshade; henbane*; an anticholinergic hallucinogen containing the alkaloids atropine, hyoscyamine, and scopolamine. Anticholinergic hallucinogens produce not only hallucinations but also clouding of consciousness and loss of memory for the period of intoxication.

As dosage is increased, symptoms of atropine poisoning become more obvious: dilatation of the pupils, weakness, clumsiness, mental confusion, speech disturbances, visual and auditory distortions, and hallucinations. With still higher doses, there are thought blocking, disorganization of thought and performance, feelings of unreality and alienation, loss of contact with reality, and difficulty in distinguishing between external reality and internal thoughts and feelings. Finally, coma may develop and the subject may die.

**belladonna alkaloids**   Anticholinergic and parasympatholytic drugs. See *cholinergic*.

**belle indifférence**   (F. "beautiful indifference") See *hysteria*.

**belonephobia**   Fear of needles.

**belongingness**   A feeling of being a part of or being accepted by another person or group. A lack of this feeling is often a complaint of schizophrenic patients. See *autism*.

**Benda, Clemens E.**   (1899–1975) German-born neuropathologist and psychiatrist who came to the United States in 1936; mental retardation, especially *Down syndrome* (q.v.).

**Bender, Lauretta**   (1897–1987) American neuropsychiatrist; Visual Motor Gestalt test; child psychiatry, especially schizophrenia and brain damage.

**Bender Visual-Motor Gestalt test**   A projective technique consisting of nine geometrical figures that are copied by the subject; devised by Lauretta Bender and first described by her in 1938. Its chief applications are to determine retardation, loss of function, and organic brain defects in children and adults, and in the study of personality deviations that show regressive phenomena. It is of limited usefulness in the study of psychoneuroses and psychosomatic disorders.

**bends, the**   See *caisson disease*.

**Benedikt syndrome**   (Moritz Benedikt, Austrian physician, 1835–1920) The symptoms following a lesion of the red nucleus in the midbrain which involves the oculomotor fibers passing through the midbrain: homolateral oculomotor paralysis and contralateral hyperkinesis.

**beneficence**   Goodness, kindness, or the performance of such acts toward others. In medical ethics, beneficence generally refers to preventing harm from befalling others (*nonmalfeasance*) and, in addition, acting to promote the well-being of others.

**beng**   See *cannabis*.

**benign**   In medicine, referring to a disorder with good prognosis, as opposed to *malignant*. It does not refer to the intensity of the clinical syndrome. A benign psychosis may be extremely intense, as the benign stupor state, from which the patient generally recovers or experiences appreciable amelioration.

**benign thunderclap headache**   A severe headache of very sudden onset resembling headaches of subarachnoid hemorrhage. See *headache*.

**Benommenheit**   Literally, a benumbing; Bleuler's term for one of the acute syndromes of the schizophrenias in which there is a slowing of all psychic processes but no dejection of mood or self-deprecatory ideas. Patients with Benommenheit are unable to deal with any relatively complicated or unusual situation; they make mistakes and show marked apraxia and impaired comprehension. Compare *Ganser syndrome*.

**Benton Visual Retention Test**   A test of visual memory, visual perception, and visuoconstructional ability consisting of three sets of 10 designs that are copied and then drawn from memory or selected from a multiple-choice presentation.

**Benzedrine dependency**   Symptoms include an inability to abstain from the drug, need for increasing dosage (high tolerance is developed, e.g., 1500 mg may be the usual daily dose), insomnia, restlessness, irritability, gross errors in judgment, loss of impulse control (especially aggressive impulses), ideas of reference and delusions of persecution, and hallucinosis with auditory and visual hallucinations. The hallucinosis usually clears within 4 or 5 weeks; males are much more prone to develop such symptoms than females. See *amphetamines*.

**benzodiazepine abuse** Two patterns are distinguished: use confined to benzodiazepines over long periods of time, and use in the context of multiple drug or alcohol abuse.

Many abusers ingest several hundred milligrams of diazepam a day, and some ingest as much as 1000 to 1500 mg. Some patients in methadone-maintenance programs ingest diazepam shortly before or immediately after taking their daily methadone to accentuate its mild sedative-euphoric effect. Alprazolam has a similar abuse pattern among opiate addicts.

Persistent abuse of benzodiazepines (and other sedatives) typically produces neuropsychological deficits similar to those occurring in alcoholics: impairment in memory, verbal and nonverbal learning, and in speed and coordination. Sedative-type dependence in general requires a slow withdrawal schedule, and benzodiazepines with a long half-life (such as diazepam) need a longer withdrawal period that those with a short half-life.

**benzodiazepine receptors** The neuronal binding sites for benzodiazepines; they are concentrated in the hippocampal formation, prefrontal cortex, amygdala, hypothalamus, and thalamus. Functionally and structurally, the benzodiazepine receptors are coupled to the GABA receptor and, with an associated chloride channel, they form a supramolecular receptor complex. They potentiate GABA by increasing the rate of opening of the chloride channel; the amount of time the channel is open is thus increased and more chloride ion enters the neuron, rendering it less excitable. This is the mechanism of the anxiolytic effect of benzodiazepines. Nonbenzodiazepine sedative hypnotics, in contrast, act directly on the chloride channel and not on the benzodazepine receptor.

There are at least two form of benzodiazepine receptor: $BZ_1$ and $BZ_2$. The latter appears to be more relevant to the anxiolytic effects of benzodiazepines, and most benzodiazepine receptors in the limbic system are of this variety.

**benzodiazepines** A family of *antianxiety agents* (q.v.), characterized chemically by the fusion of a benzene ring and a seven-atom diazepine ring. They act as sedatives at low dosage, as anxiolytics at moderate dosage, and as hypnotics at high dosage. They have a higher therapeutic index and lower abuse potential than the other *sedatives-hypnotics* (q.v.), with the possible exception of buspirone.

Currently, the benzodiazepines are used in the treatment of general anxiety, panic disorder, phobias, and bipolar disorder. They are also used as anesthetic adjuvants, muscle relaxants, and anticonvulsants (especially alprazolam and clonazepam).

The primary effect of benzodiazepines is to augment the action of *GABA* (gamma-aminobutyric acid), the major inhibitory neurotransmitter in the central nervous system. Benzodiazepines increase the frequency of GABA-mediated openings of chloride channels. The resultant increase in chloride permeability increases the negative potential across the neuronal membrane (*hyperpolarization*), making it less excitable. See *receptor complex, supramolecular*.

The first benzodiazepine, chlordiazepoxide, was introduced in 1960. Of the many benzodiazepines now available, diazepam, lorazepam, alprazolam, and triazolam have the most rapid onset of action. Alprazolam is approximately 10 times as potent as diazepam; triazolam may be as much as 100 times as potent as diazepam.

The most common unwanted effect of benzodiazepine treatment is sedation, which may appear as a hangover on the day following bedtime ingestion. *Rebound insomnia*, a worsening of sleep below baseline level on the nights following discontinuation of the drug, is particularly likely with short-acting benzodiazepines such as triazolam. Dependence and withdrawal symptoms are most likely to develop when a benzodiazepine has been used over a long period of time and is abruptly withdrawn. Withdrawal symptoms include malaise, insomnia, tachycardia, dizziness, faintness, confusion, excessive sweating, depression, and irritability. Delirium, convulsions, and paranoid psychosis may also occur.

**benztropine** A cholinesterase-like antiparkinsonian agent. See *cholinergic*.

**BEP** *Brief and emergency psychotherapy* (q.v.).

**berdache** A variant of *gynemimesis* (q.v.) reported in many native North American tribes, from Alaska to the Yucatan. The berdache typically shows gender cross-coding in prepubertal years (e.g., interests more typical of girls than of boys, feminine body movement); he may experience a spiritual revelation during a trance state while an adolescent, and thereafter he dresses and works as a woman. He is accepted by the community and may legitimately be sought after as a wife.

**bereavement**  Loss, most often used to refer to the loss of a loved one through death. The feelings of anguish and desolation and accompanying symptoms and signs constitute a psychiatric syndrome of depression (at least by DSM-III standards) even though the affective state is a normal reaction to loss. In the older literature, the distinction was often drawn between normal *mourning* and the pathological states of *melancholia* and *depression* (qq.v.).

Three stages of bereavement have been described: (1) a feeling of numbness and unreality, which lasts from a few hours to several days; (2) dejection and sadness, typically with insomnia and loss of appetite; about a third of bereaved people feel they did not do enough for the dead person, and about a fifth blame some other person(s) for their loss; (3) a stage of acceptance, with gradual abatement of stage 2 symptoms.

Even though bereavement is normal, studies have shown that bereaved subjects are immunosuppressed and may be vulnerable to physical illness. Older widowers have increased mortality during the first 6 months of bereavement, due mainly to cancer, cardiovascular disease, accidents, suicide, and cirrhosis of the liver. The particular illnesses associated with the increased mortality suggest that lifestyle factors, such as increased use of tobacco and alcohol, may be the responsible agents.

**bereavement, conjugal**  See *conjugal bereavement*.

**Bergen fraction**  A plasma factor claimed by some to be characteristic of schizophrenia; its effect, when injected into trained rats, is to impede their rope-climbing performance. The name comes from J. R. Bergen and his colleagues at the Worcester Foundation. Bergen suggested (1968) that the *Frohman factor* (q.v.) is identical to Bergen fraction, and that both are an alpha-2 globulin.

**Berger rhythm, Berger wave**  See *electroencephalogram*.

**beriberi**  *Thiamine deficiency* syndrome (q.v.), most often appearing in cultures where polished white rice is the dietary staple, in alcoholics, and in people with long-continued food fads. Symptoms include anorexia, irritability, and weight loss, with later involvement of the cardiovascular system (wet beriberi) or the nervous system (dry beriberi). Polyneuropathy (*burning feet syndrome*) and *Wernicke encephalopathy* are the most common manifestations of nervous system involvement (qq.v.).

**Berkson bias**  See *life-course epidemiology*.

**Berne, Eric**  (1910–1970) Canadian-born psychoanalyst, in United States after 1936; transactional analysis, group treatment.

**Bernheim, Hippolyte-Marie**  (1840–1919) French psychotherapist; hypnotism and suggestibility.

**Bessman-Baldwin syndrome**  See *imidazole syndrome*.

**best interests doctrine**  See *custody*.

**bestiality**  Any type of human behavior that resembles that of beasts; more specifically, sexual congress between humans and animals. See *sodomy*.

**beta alcoholism**  Although no physical or psychological dependence is demonstrable, drinking in this type of alcoholism leads to physical complications, such as in the gut, liver, pancreas, heart, vascular system, kidney, lungs, striate muscle, brain, mechanisms of resistance and defense (manifested in proneness to infections and high incidence of certain types of malignancy), and complications of other coexisting illnesses. This type of alcoholism is sometimes called somatopathic drinking. See *alcoholism*.

**beta arc**  See *alpha arc*.

**beta blocker**  A synthetic agent that blocks beta-adrenergic receptors, with consequent antihypertensive, antiarrhythmic, antimigraine, and antitremor effects. In psychiatry, such drugs have been used in schizophrenia and in some organic conditions (including adults with autism) for their antiaggressive effect, for anxiety-related tremors, and in anxiety disorders and panic states, particularly when somatic manifestations are prominent. They have also been used, with varying results, in the treatment of neuroleptic-induced akathisia. See *antianxiety agents*.

**beta elements**  See *alpha-function*.

**beta error**  Also known as Type II error—failure to find a statistically significant difference when an actual difference exists.

**beta rhythm or wave**   See *electroencephalogram.*

**beta test**   A set of mental tests used in the U.S. Army in 1917–18, designed for illiterates. Instructions are given in signs and the material is pictorial in character, in contrast to alpha tests, which are carried out verbally.

**beta-adrenergic state**   See β-*adrenergic hyperdynamic circulatory state.*

**beta-amyloid disorders**   Also, β-*amyloid disorders* (q.v.).

**beta-amyloid peptide**   Also, β-*amyloid peptide* (q.v.).

**beta-endorphin**   See *enkephalins.*

**beta-lipotropin**   See *enkephalins.*

**betel chewing**   A practice of some Asians and Pacific Islanders: the areca palm tree nut is wrapped in the betel tree leaf and flavored with burnt lime, and then chewed. When mixed with saliva, the mixture releases arecoline, an anticholinergic and CNS stimulant similar to *nicotine* (q.v.). The practice can produce dependence and other health problems, such as cancer of the mouth.

**betrayal traumas**   Events, and patterns of events, that involve failure or desertion by a parent or partner in a moment of need, such as emotional or sexual abuse by a parent, or marital rape. Terrifying events (such as gruesome accidents or wanton brutality) produce arousal and anxiety, while betrayal traumas tend to produce *dissociation* (q.v.) and gaps in memory and awareness. When betrayal traumas are also terrorizing and life-threatening, they are most likely to harm basic systems of cognition, emotion, behavior, *attachment* (q.v.), and other symptoms of complex PTSD. See *post-traumatic stress disorder.*

**Bettelheim, Bruno**   (1904–1990) Vienna-born psychologist, psychoanalyst; emigrated to United States in 1939; Director of Sonia Shankman Orthogenic School at University of Chicago until he retired in 1973; treatment of autistic children; *Love Is Not Enough* (1950), *A Good Enough Parent* (1987). Many have disputed his claims, concerning both his academic and experiential credentials and his treatment results.

**Betz cell**   (Vladimir Aleksandrovich Betz, Russian anatomist, 1834–1895) See *frontal lobe.*

**bewildered**   A term often used to describe the lost, dazed, perplexed, puzzled patient who appears to be confused but shows a sort of numb apathy about his confusion. Bewilderment is often associated with con-

scious ambivalence, with dereistic or autistic thinking, with preoccupation, and with vacuity or sterility of thinking. See *Benommenheit.*

**BFPP**   Bilateral frontoparietal *polymicrogyria* (q.v.).

**BFT**   *Behavioral family therapy* (q.v.).

**β-glucuronidase deficiency**   A *mucopolysaccharidosis* (q.v.) characterized by excessive dermatan sulfate in the urine, hepatosplenomegaly, dysostosis multiplex, white cell inclusions, and mental retardation. See *klotho.*

**bhang**   Also, beng, churus; an infusion made from cannabis. See *marijuana.*

**BHMCO**   Behavioral health managed care organization.

**Bianchi, Leonardo**   (1848–1927) Italian psychiatrist and neurologist.

**Bianchi syndrome**   Hemiplegia, hemianesthesia, agraphia, apraxia, and alexia, due to a lesion of the left parietal lobe.

**bias**   In statistics, any factor that distorts the representativeness of results.

**biased apperception**   Seeing things only as one wants to see them, considered by Adler a prerequisite for social participation since, without it, social movements would be stifled by indecisiveness. The person who cannot make a move unless he or she is certain to be right, for example, cannot usually move very much.

**biastophilia**   *Raptophilia*; paraphilic *rape* (q.v.).

**biblioclast**   One who destroys or mutilates books.

**biblioklept**   One who steals books.

**bibliokleptomania**   Compulsion to steal books.

**bibliomania**   Intense desire to collect and possess books, especially rare and curious ones.

**bibliophobia**   Fear of or aversion to books.

**bibliotherapy**   Use of reading as an adjunct to psychotherapy. Books may be recommended to patients for various reasons: (1) to help the patient understand better his or her own psychological and physiological reactions to frustration; (2) to remedy insufficient or erroneous knowledge; (3) to facilitate communication between patient and therapist by helping the patient understand the terminology of therapy; (4) to stimulate the patient to discuss and verbalize certain problems by helping to remove the fear, shame, or guilt related to those problems; (5) to stimulate the patient to think constructively between interviews; (6) to reinforce accepted social and cultural patterns and thereby inhibit certain infantile patterns of behavior; (7) to stimulate the patient's imagination and give him or her vicarious satisfactions which reality cannot afford without danger; (8) to enlarge the patient's sphere of interest; and (9) as an adjunct to a program of vocational rehabilitation. The reading matter recommended must, of course, be selected individually for the specific patient, depending on the goals of therapy, the intellectual capacities of the patient, and his or her stage of achievement in therapy.

**biceps reflex**   A deep reflex; patient's forearm is placed halfway between flexion and extension and slightly pronated; examiner's finger is on the tendon, and a blow on this digit results in flexion of the patient's forearm. This reflex depends upon the musculocutaneous nerve for its afferents and efferents; its center is $C_{5-6}$.

**Bichat, Law of**   (Marie Francois Xavier Bichat, French anatomist, 1771–1802) According to Bichat there are two great body systems, the vegetative and the animal. The former provides for assimilation and augmentation of mass, while the latter provides for the transformation of energy, "that is, for the relations with the environment." The two systems "are in inverse ratio of the development in ontogenetic evolution—the greater the development of the vegetative system, the less developed is the system of relation" (Pende, N. *Constitutional Inadequacies*, 1928).

**Biedl-Moon-Laurence syndrome**   See *Laurence-Moon-Biedl syndrome*.

**Bielschowsky disease**   (Max Bielschowsky, German neuropathologist, 1869–1940) See *Tay-Sachs disease*.

**bilingualism**   *Polyglossia*: a person's ability to communicate in two or more languages. It has generally been found that educating a child in one language interferes with his or her ability to pass examinations in a second, and the interference is greater the more "minor" the one language and the more elaborate the second. Initially interpreted as evidence that bilingualism interfered with or lessened intellectual capability, the data are now seen as supporting the view that particular skills acquired through one language may not be wholly available for transfer to a second, especially if the two languages are quite different.

Even people who have been fluent speakers of a second language since childhood need extra brain power to speak their nonnative tongue. The site of that extra power seems to be the putamen, which has not previously been linked to language learning but was thought to be involved mainly in the production of rote movements.

**bilis**   *Colera* (q.v.).

**bill of rights**   For psychiatric patients (and inpatients in particular), a listing of the civil rights that merit particular attention and protection, including the right to treatment (including the right not to be confined in a mental institution if only custodial care and not active treatment is provided), the right to refuse treatment, the right to have the least amount of and the least invasive treatment (this includes the least restrictive environment and related concepts), the right not to be subjected to unusual or cruel or hazardous treatments without express and informed consent, the right of due-process protection (for children as well as adults), the right to legal counsel, the right to a humane environment with adequate staffing, etc. See *consumerism*.

The term has been applied to legislation that seeks to eliminate the discrimination against mental patients by insurance companies and managed care organizations.

**bimodality**   The potentiality of functioning in two ways, most often used to refer to cerebral dominance or lateralization. See *cerebral dominance*.

**binary concept**   Kraepelin's early hypothesis that bipolar illness (manic-depressive insanity) and schizophrenia (dementia praecox) are distinct entities. An alternative concept is that psychosis occurs along a continuum of defect states, extending from unipolar depression (the least severe) through bipolar disorder and schizoaffective psychosis to schizophrenia (the most severe).

**binding**   1. Temporal synchronization of different neuronal assemblies, which correspond to stored neural representations, or codes.

2. Receptor binding. See *synapse*.

**Binet-Simon tests**   (Alfred Binet, French psychologist, 1857–1911, and Theodore Simon, French physician, 1873–1961) Tests of intellectual capacity, which is expressed as the intelligence quotient (IQ), introduced in France in 1905 as a result of studies made to determine whether children could be educated as the new laws required. The Stanford revision of the tests for use with American children was made in 1916, although they had already been introduced into the United States by Goddard in 1910.

**binge buying, binge spending** *Oniomania (q.v.).*

**binge drinking** Spree drinking; drinking in bouts; in Jellinek's typology, *epsilon alcoholism* (q.v.). See *alcohol use, unhealthy.*

**binge eating disorder** *BED*; voracious eating during a discrete time period (i.e., for a matter of minutes or up to 2 hours), during which the subject feels unable to stop eating or to control what or how much will be eaten. The binge-eater can easily recognize the binges as being abnormal and very different from other eating behavior. Eating is more rapid, it begins even though the person does not feel hungry, it continues despite satiation and feeling uncomfortably full, it replaces regular eating hours, and it is often done in secret because the subject is embarrassed by his eating behavior and does not want others to know he cannot control it.

Binge eating is characteristic of *bulimia nervosa*, where it is commonly coupled with *purging* (qq.v.). See *night-eating syndrome.* BED symptoms at some point in their lives were reported by 3.5% of women, 2% of men; bulimia by 1.5% of women, 0.5% of men; anorexia by 0.9% of women, 0.3% of men. The number of years symptoms were present was 8.3 years in bulimia, 8.1 years in BED, and 1.7 years in anorexia. Criteria for at least one other DSM-IV disorder (mood disorders, anxiety disorders, impulse control disorders, and substance use disorders) were met by 94.5% of patients with bulimia, 78.9% of those with BED, and 56.2% of those with anorexia (National Comorbidity Survey Replication, 2001–2003).

**Binger, Carl A. L.** (1890–1976) American psychoanalyst; psychosomatic medicine.

**Bing-Neel syndrome** See *macroglobulinemia, Waldenstrom's.*

**Bini, Lucio** (1908–1964) Italian psychiatrist. Co-discoverer (with Ugo Cerletti) of electric convulsive therapy, first demonstrated in Rome on March 28, 1938. The idea of inducing convulsions electrically rather than pharmacologically was Cerletti's, but the elaboration of the technique and bitemporal placement of the electrodes was Bini's.

**Binswanger, Ludwig** Existential analysis; case of Ellen West (1944; girl with fear of becoming fat; Binswanger's treatment applied principles of existential analysis to clinical psychi-

atry and psychopathology; the patient was diagnosed as schizophrenic although today her condition would probably be labeled bulimia nervosa).

**Binswanger, Otto** (1852–1929) Swiss-born psychiatrist, professor of psychiatry and director of mental hospital in Jena 1882–1919. Co-workers in Jena included Oskar Vogt (1870–1959), Korbinian Brodmann (1868–1918), and Hans Berger (1873–1941). Binswanger described encephalitis subcorticalis chronica progressiva in 1894; it came to be called *Binswanger disease.* His *Epilepsy* (1899) became a standard text.

**Binswanger disease** Subcortical encephalopathy. Early clinical features are episodes of mild upper motor signs (drift, reflex asymmetry, incoordination), gait disorders (small-step gait, marche à petit pas, magnetic gait, apraxic-ataxic gait, or Parkinson gait), imbalance, urinary frequency and incontinence, and extrapyramidal signs (hypokinesia and rigidity) as well as depression and mood changes.

**bioavailability** The degree to which a drug administered is distributed throughout the body and thus available for action at the desired receptor sites. See *absorption.*

**biobehavioral shift** A relatively sudden advance in development that occurs at around 2 or 3 months of age. It is characterized by a change in the infant's EEG patterns; more clearly social and instrumental usage of smiling, babbling, and similar behaviors; and increased tolerance for stimulation.

**biochemical marker** See *biomarker.*

**biodynamics** J. H. Masserman's system of psychoanalytic psychiatry (*The Practice of Dynamic Psychiatry*, 1955). The four principles of biodynamics—motivation, milieu, adaptation, and conflict—are stated as follows: (1) all organisms are actuated by their physiologic needs; (2) every organism reacts to its own interpretations of its milieu in terms of its individual needs, special capacities, and unique experiences; (3) whenever an organism's goal-directed activities are frustrated by external obstacles, the organism either changes its techniques to reach that same goal or changes its goal; (4) when two or more urgent motivations conflict so that the adaptive patterns attendant to each are mutually exclusive, the organism experiences anxiety and its somatic and muscular behavior becomes either ambivalent, poorly adaptive, and ineffectively substitutive (neurotic), or progressively more disorganized, regressive, and bizarrely symbolic (psychotic).

**bioethics**   See *ethics, biomedical*.

**biofeedback**   "An instrumental procedure that senses, records, and provides the subject with information about those physiological functions in relation to which there is usually no awareness or voluntary control" (Moldofsky, H. in *Psychiatry Update III*, ed. L. Grinspoon, 1984). Even though they are not conscious, such autonomic nervous system functions are subject to learning (visceral learning, physiologic self-regulation, learned automatic control). In theory, a subject can learn to control his internal organs and vital functions; it might therefore be possible for a patient with essential hypertension to learn how to reduce his blood pressure. Vital functions, such as blood pressure, are not maintained at a constant level, hence their fluctuations can be treated as responses and reinforced appropriately. The use of biofeedback and operant reinforcement (see *operant conditioning*) has been successful in regulating a number of bodily processes in laboratory experiments; attempts to transfer the learned visceral responses to real-life situations, however, have often failed. See *behavior therapy*.

Some of the classic studies in biofeedback include Miller's at the Rockefeller Institute in 1968, Kamiya's at the University of California in 1969 on alpha EEG rhythm, Shapiro et al. (hypertension, 1970), Weiss and Engel (arrhythmias, 1971), Sterman (seizure disorders, 1973), Menninger and Sargent (migraine, 1973), and Budzynski and coworkers (tension headache, 1973).

**biofidelity**   The quality of being lifelike in appearance or responses; often refers to dummies used in safety investigations of motor vehicles or in demonstrations of cardiopulmonary resuscitation.

**biogenetic mental law**   "In his embryonic life man passes through the anatomical forms of primordial times. The same law is valid for the mental development of mankind. Accordingly, the child develops out of an originally unconscious and animal-like condition to consciousness; first to a primitive, and then slowly to a civilized consciousness" (Jung, C.G. *Contributions to Analytical Psychology*, 1928). See *polymorphous perverse*.

**biogenetics**   See *genetics*.

**biogenic amines**   See *amine; neurotransmitter*.

**biographic sketch**   Used in the field of objective psychobiology (Adolf Meyer) to refer to the life history of the patient as the latter records it. To facilitate the recording Meyer devised what he called *The Life Chart*, consisting of topical guides for the person who is writing his biographic sketch. The life chart typically consists of three columns—one for life events, one for physical illness, one for mental illness—enabling the evaluator to highlight the time relations between episodes of physical and mental illness and potentially stressful events in the subject's life.

**biography in depth**   The use of established psychoanalytic knowledge to contribute to the understanding of the personality of the subject being studied. See *pathography*.

**biohazard**   Potential danger from biological sources, as opposed to chemical or mechanical dangers. The alleged dangers of recombinant DNA research, for example, are biohazards of molecular biological research.

**bioinformatics**   Computational genomics; computerized processing of biological information and development of the instruments that will make it possible. Bioinformatics includes writing computer programs to "annotate" the genome, identifying and analyzing all its genes.

**biolinguistics**   The study of the biological underpinnings of language such as the factors that enhance or retard language development and the neurophysiology of language disorders. See *linguistics; neurolinguistics*.

**biological clock**   See *clock, biological*.

**biological marker**   *Biomarker* (q.v.).

**biomarker**   *Biological marker*, a characteristic that can be measured and evaluated objectively as an indicator of normal or pathogenic biological processes, susceptibility or vulnerability to disease, exposure to toxins, or responses to a therapeutic intervention (such as pharmacologic agents or dietary changes). The following description of types of biomarkers emphasizes the way they are used in the early detection of neurodegenerative disorders.

*Clinical biomarkers*: As an example, in mild cognitive impairment (MCI), the clinical features of isolated impairment in recent memory, relative preservation of cognitive functions in other domains, and normal performance of activities of daily living define a group with a 12%–15% risk of developing Alzheimer disease within a year, compared to a risk of 1%–2% in age-matched normal subjects. A potential marker of early Parkinson disease is loss of olfaction, which is associated with dopamine dysfunction before motor symptoms appear. A potential marker of vulnerability to the development of attention deficit hyperactivity disorder (ADHD) is motor response inhibition deficit.

*Biolochemical markers*: Many serum and cerebrospinal fluid tests have been developed for early detection of neurodegenerative disorders, but their specificity and sensitivity have been limited.

*Genetic markers* (q.v.).

*Neuroimaging markers*: *PET* and *SPECT* (qq.v.) measure in vivo neurochemistry. Different ligands have been used to target dopaminergic activity and microglial activation, for example, and radiopharmaceuticals that bind to β-amyloid have been developed. *MR spectroscopy* (q.v.) has been used to measure psychoactive drugs in the brain as well as brain GABA levels. *MRI* (q.v.), fMRI, dMRI, and DTI have also been used to study the occurrence and progression of brain lesions, the cortical areas involved in a given cognitive process, and nerve fiber tracking and connectivity within the central nervous system.

**biomedical ethics**    See *ethics, biomedical.*

**biometrics**    Quantification of psychopathological differences between subjects, specifically by assessing each subject across multiple dimensions. In psychiatry those dimensions include sensation, perception, cognition, learning, psychophysiological reactions, and personality traits and characteristics. Cognitive psychological measures employ tasks that tap particular functions; used in conjunction with brain imaging, these measures identify the brain regions involved in such functions. Any abnormality in functioning that is found to be characteristic of a particular psychiatric disorder would then point to a specific brain region as being related to the development of that disorder.

**biometry**    The measurement of life; specifically, calculation of the probable duration of life and study of all the factors, endogenous and exogenous, that enter into the determination of the duration of life.

**bion**    The energy vesicles through which the orgone (life energy) manifests itself, according to Wilhelm Reich's theory. See *orgone.*

**bionics**    The study of biological functions and mechanisms from the point of view of applying them to electronic devices, such as computers.

**bionomics**    *Ecology* (q.v.); bionomic factors are those external, environmental factors that limit the development of an organism.

**biophilia**    Instinct of self-preservation.

**biopsychosocial model**    A perspective or conceptualization of disease emphasizing that all diseases have biological, psychological, and social components. George Engel is usually credited with introducing the concept, derived from his work in psychosomatic medicine.

**biosphere**    The realm or sphere of life in which the total biological process takes place. The biosphere includes both the individual and his or her environment not as interacting parts of constituents that have an independent existence, but as aspects of a single reality that can be mentally separated only by abstraction. The limits of life extend as far as the organism is able to exert an influence on the events outside of it. (Biosphere corresponds to the German term *Lebenskreis*.)

**biostatistics**    Vital statistics; the numerical representation of conditions associated with life.

**biosynthetic cargo**    See *Golgi apparatus.*

**biotaxis**    See *network; taxis.*

**biothanatos**    *Obs.* Suicide.

**biotype**    All individuals who equal each other *genotypically*, whether or not their *phenotypical* appearance may show any obvious resemblance. The phenotypical features of two individuals belonging to the same biotype may be dissimilar to a considerable extent, since every hereditary predisposition has a certain amount of variability of manifestation.

**biotypology**    The systematic study or doctrine of biotypes. Although the genetic concept of biotype applies to individuals equaling each other *genotypically*, it has been taken in the field of constitutional studies, especially by the Italian school, to indicate the phenotypical constellation of all characteristics making up the "somatic-psychic individuality" of a human being, including the morphological, physiological, and psychological aspects of the given type.

**biperiden**   An anticholinergic drug. See *cholinergic*.

**bipolar cells**   BPCs; see *neocortical neurons*.

**bipolar disorder (BPD)**   Affective (mood) disorder characterized by episodes of both mania and depression; manic-depressive disorder, mixed type.

Dunner and others differentiate between *bipolar I*—affective illness that has included mania of severe enough degree to require hospitalization—and *bipolar II*—affective illness with a history of hospitalization for depression and a history of hypomania, but the manic element has not been severe enough to require hospitalization. In some classifications, *cyclothymic disorder* is included within the bipolar II category, which is viewed as an intermediate phenomenological type that lies between unipolar II depression and bipolar I. Bipolar II disorder denotes the presence of hypomanic episodes, or milder manic episodes that do not cause impairment in functioning. Bipolar II patients are more likely to have a history of other mental disorders; they display more chronic symptoms that are predictive of poorer treatment response.

In DSM-IV, bipolar disorders are divided into Bipolar I, with the following subtypes: single episode; most recent episode hypomanic; most recent episode manic; most recent episode mixed; most recent episode unspecified; and Bipolar II, involving at least one major depressive episode and at least one hypomanic, but not manic, episode.

A course subtype, with rapid cycling, describes bipolar disorder with four or more full mood episodes in a 12-month period.

Substance abuse comorbidity is high: 60% in bipolar I disorder and 50% in bipolar II. The most commonly used substances are alcohol (33%), marijuana (16%), stimulants (9%), and cocaine (9%). Bipolar disorders increase the risk for suicide and are associated with poorer response to treatment and greater functional impairment.

Youths with bipolar disorder (*pediatric BPD*) are more severely ill and have a higher genetic loading than adult-onset cases. Typical symptoms are high levels of irritability and agitation (rather than euphoric mood), explosive and even violent outbursts, hyperarousal, grandiosity, oppositionalism, and disinhibited behaviors.

The lifetime risk of bipolar disorder in the general population is in the range of 1%–2%. The concordance rate for bipolar illness in dizygotic twins is approximately 15%, in monozygotic twins approximately 65%. Several valid linkages of both BPD and schizophrenia have been demonstrated to genomic regions; 8p22 and 10p14, 18p11, 13q32, and 22q11 are all susceptibility loci for both. See *affect(ive) disorder; cyclothymia; mania; manic-depressive psychosis; unipolar depression*.

**bipolar double bind**   See *double bind*.

**bipolar self**   In Kohut's terminology (self psychology), internalized psychic structures ranging from self-assertive ambitions derived from the *grandiose self* (q.v.) at one pole, to values and ideals derived from internalization of the idealized parent imago at the other. It replaces the id, ego, and superego of Freudian psychology. See *idealization*.

**bipolarity**   *Ambivalence* (q.v.).

**bipotentiality, sexual**   See *ambitypic*.

**Birnbaum, Karl**   (1878–1950) German psychiatrist; forensic psychiatry.

**birth, anal**   In psychoanalytic theory, sexual fantasies or dreams directly connected with anal erotism such as a wish to be reborn through the anus.

**birth, multiple**   In biology and vital statistics the term applies to all instances in which women produce more than one child at the same birth. The tendency to multiple births seems to run in certain families, although it has not yet been proved that it is based on a specific hereditary factor.

*Twins* (q.v.) come about once in every 90 births in most of the American and European countries. The proportion of fraternal to identical twins is approximately 3:1.

*Triplets* occur once in about 8000 births. They also may be identical or "unmatched" multiples, that is, developed either from one egg or from three separate eggs. The third possibility is that only two members of a set of triplets are identical, developed from one egg, and the third is a fraternal, developed from a different egg.

*Quadruplets* are reported by Scheinfeld to occur once in about 700,000 births, with only a few sets surviving. Here the following combinations are possible: (1) all four identicals; (2) three identicals and one fraternal; (3) two identicals and two fraternal; and (4) most rarely, all four fraternals.

The birth of five humans at one time is believed to have occurred spontaneously not more than 60 times in the last 500 years. In most cases, however, these *quintuplets* perished soon after birth.

With the increasing use of *fertility-inducing drugs* since the 1960s, there has been an increase in multiple births. The drugs used are those that stimulate the pituitary to produce gonadotropins or, if the pituitary produces none, gonadotropins themselves are used in an attempt to stimulate the ovary directly. It has been estimated that multiple births occur in about 20% of women treated with such drugs.

**birth control**   Regulation of the number or spacing of offspring, either by measures designed to prevent conception or by termination of pregnancy once conception has taken place. Two factors have significantly altered the complexion of birth control in recent years. One is the development in the 1960s of intrauterine contraceptive devices and of the contraceptive pill. The other is the 1972 decision of the United States Supreme Court that invalidated restrictive abortion laws. Those two developments made both contraception and termination of pregnancy easier and safer to achieve, with relative certainty, and removed from the realm of criminal behavior. The last aspect is of particular relevance to psychiatry because before the 1972 decision the major legal rationale for abortion was danger to the prospective mother's mental health, a danger that society expected the psychiatrist to foretell.

**birth injury**   Any damage to the fetus-neonate as a result of the birth process; often used in a more limited way to refer to brain damage due to the birth process (including that due to instrument delivery). See *brain damage.*

**birth trauma**   The act of being born is believed to mark a radical upheaval from both the psychical and physical points of view. Rank believed that some people are always attempting to reconstruct the conditions of intrauterine existence. Freud, however, suggested that Rank overestimated the importance of birth upon the psyche of the infant. "We certainly may not presuppose that the fetus has any kind of knowledge that it is in danger of annihilation"; the fetus can only sense "a wholesale disturbance in the economy of its narcistic libido" (*The Basic Writings of Sigmund Freud,* 1938).

Ferenczi agreed; what Rank called birth phantasies Ferenczi termed coital phantasies.

**bisexuality**   Presence of the qualities of both sexes in the same person. The term is synonymous with hermaphroditism, although the latter term appears to have gained almost exclusive reference to the organic manifestations of the condition. The term intersex, introduced by Goldschmidt, is used "to designate hermaphrodites as individuals who started out either male or female from a genetic standpoint but who after a certain period completed their sexual development in the opposite direction. In the intersex there is first a female phase and later a male phase, or vice versa, and in the second phase a typical mixture of both sexes exists" (Young, H. H. *Genital Abnormalities, Hermaphroditism and Related Adrenal Diseases,* 1937). See *ambisexual.*

In the classical sense a bisexual or hermaphroditic person is one "who has the gonads and external genitalia of both sexes and is capable of living as either a man or a woman." (ibid.).

At the present time there is a tendency to use the term in a more limited fashion, to describe persons who, for a significant time after the period of adolescence, consciously feel, think and alternately react psychically, erotically, or orgastically to members both of the same and of the opposite sex. See *androgyneity; gender identity; gender role.*

In 60% of human societies, bisexuality is both common and socially accepted. Some small island communities in Melanesia, for example, accept as normal that all adolescent males will at some point engage in homosexual anal intercourse. But even in those societies exclusive homosexuality over an entire lifetime is rare.

In societies in which all men show homosexual behavior, 30% to 50% of women do. Only 50% of bisexual women have had their first lesbian experience by the age of 25, only 77% by the age of 30; some do not have their first lesbian experience until they are in their 40s. Only 4% of bisexual women have more than 10 homosexual partners in a lifetime, compared with 22% of bisexual men. Fewer than 1% of women in any society are exclusively homosexual throughout their lives (Baker, R. *Sperm Wars,* New York: Basic Books, 1996).

**bit**   See *information theory.*

**biting mania**  A form of epidemic or mass hysteria reported in 15th-century Germany: a nun began to bite her associates compulsively, and the impulse spread throughout convents in Germany, Holland, and other parts of Europe.

**biting stage**  A subdivision of the oral phase of libido development. Abraham divided this phase into two parts. One is the sucking stage and the other, in consequence of the appearance of teeth, is the biting stage. Based on the nature of the fixation, the oral character will be (1) submissive or receptive, if the fixation takes place in the sucking stage, or (2) aggressive, if in the biting stage. See *oral character.*

**bitufted cells**  BTCs; see *neocortical neurons.*

**bivalence**  See *ambivalence.*

**bizarre hyperactive seizures**  See *frontal lobe seizures.*

**bizarreness**  Striking incongruity or eccentricity; discordant, disharmonious, contradictory behavior such as is seen frequently in schizophrenic patients.

**BLA**  The basolateral nucleus of the *amygdala* (q.v.).

**blackout**  1. Loss of consciousness, usually secondary to brain anemia or oxygen deprivation. When the loss of consciousness is only partial, gray-out is the term applied; this is seen frequently in pilots when they rapidly change altitude, as in a dive.

2. A period of memory loss for events and behavior during periods of intoxication (usually with alcohol), even though the subject's actions and state of consciousness during that period were not grossly abnormal as observed by others. Typically, the blackout follows moderate drinking, and the drinker converses reasonably and carries out elaborate activities without obvious signs of intoxication, but the next day the drinker has no memory of what he or she said or did. Such blackouts (sometimes called *dim-outs* to differentiate them from the acute syncopal episodes described in definition 1) are probably due to a failure of memory consolidation and, to a lesser extent, retrieval. The sharpness of the rise and fall of the blood alcohol level appears to have some role in the production of blackouts, but its mechanism of action is not well understood. Blackouts are indicative of beginning, but still reversible, brain damage (*intermediate brain syndrome due to alcohol*). They precede by months or years two major hallmarks of alcohol addiction: loss of control and prolonged drinking bouts. See *alcoholism.*

**bladder, automatic**  The filling and spontaneous evacuation of the urinary bladder occurring in cases of transsection of the spinal cord.

**"blame" psychology**  The tendency of persons with serious inhibitions in social competitive relationships to find expression for these inhibitions in hatred and persecution of some blameless scapegoat. It also permits the individual to harbor a secret grandiose conception of himself. See *projection.*

**blank hallucination**  A general term that includes the *Isakower phenomenon*, the *dream screen* of Lewin, and the *abstract perceptions* of Deutsch and Murphy; it refers to certain uncanny experiences of sensations of equilibrium and space, such as unclear rotating objects, rhythmically approaching and receding objects, sensations of crescendo and decrescendo, typically localized in the mouth, skin, and hands and at the same time in the space immediately surrounding the body. Most often such feelings occur in stress situations, when falling asleep, and in dreams. They are believed to be defensive repetitions of responses to early oral deprivation and to reflect the infant's subjective experience of being overwhelmed by excitation in the early traumatic situation. Their appearance in an analytic session suggests that primal scene material is approaching.

**blanket group**  See *structured group.*

**blast concussion**  See *postconcussion neurosis.*

**blastophthoria**  Degenerative effect on germ cells of poisons such as alcohol and lead. See *fetal alcohol syndrome.*

**blathering**  See *chatterbox syndrome.*

**blepharospasm**  Spasmoid closing of the orbicular muscle; a winking tic; *blinking* (q.v.). Blepharospasm is a focal dystonia characterized by chronic intermittent or persistent involuntary closure of the eyelids; typically, it is the first symptom of *tardive dystonia* (q.v.). Blepharospasm can be accompanied by oromandibular dystonia (*Meige syndrome*). Most commonly, blepharospasm starts with increased frequency of blinking to a variety of stimuli, such as bright light and stress, and progresses to chronic involuntary bilateral spasm involving both eyes. Eye closure can be so severe as to make vision, and therefore walking and driving, difficult. Injection of botulinum toxin into the muscles of the eyelids is the treatment of choice.

**Bleuler, Eugen** (1857–1939) Swiss psychiatrist; schizophrenia.

In 1911, Bleuler suggested the term schizophrenia to replace dementia praecox. His monumental treatise, *Dementia Praecox or the Group of Schizophrenias*, differentiated between the fundamental and the accessory symptoms of schizophrenia.

**blind, double** See *double blind*.

**blind hatred** A state of self-righteous rage described in narcissistic personality (disorder) and characterized by exaggerated grandiosity (a defense against a damaged self-concept) and assignment of others to a subhuman status. Blind hatred may appear as an explosive reaction of vengeful hostility and physical or verbal violence to some kind of insult. See *chaotic state*; *rage*.

**blindism** Mannerisms and habitual movements seen in blind patients, and particularly in children, such as repeated rubbing of the eyes, shaking and rolling the body, poking at the eyes, shaking the hands when excited and, if there is some vision, fanning the fingers in front of the eyes. Usually the blindism is given up as the child grows older.

**blindness, circumferential** See *field defect*.

**blindness, cortical psychic** Usually due to bilateral occipital lobe lesions producing a loss of topographical orientation, optic memory image, and spatial orientation.

**blindness, mind** Psychic blindness; objects and space dimensions are seen by the eye, but the patient has an erroneous idea of the size of objects and the three dimensions of space. Sometimes he sees objects as flat, or as small (see *micropsia*). Uncertainty over object relationships may be a basic element in the development of such symptoms.

**blindsight** A form of *implicit perception* demonstrated by patients who have sustained damage to the primary visual cortex (V1), most commonly a result of head trauma, cerebrovascular accident, or tumor. The damage produces a contralesional visual field defect. Patients report no awareness of a stimulus in their damaged field, but when forced to choose a property of the stimulus (e.g., is it red or green, is it moving or immobile) they perform better than chance.

**blink-alpha neurocircuit** *BANC* (q.v.).

**blinking** The act of shutting and opening the eyes quickly. Blinking is a reflexive response to irritation by a foreign body, but everyday blinking is not a reflex. It is initiated by signals from the brain, most likely the basal ganglia. Blinking rate is an index of general attention; it increases at times of distress or distraction and decreases during extended periods of high concentration. It may also increase with anxiety or embarrassment. Blinking is sometimes a *tic* (q.v.), and involuntary, repetitious blinking is the first symptom of tardive dyskinesia. See *blepharospasm*.

**BLM** Bucco-lingual-masticatory syndrome, the most common form of *tardive dyskinesia* (q.v.).

**block, partial genetic** See *chromosome; genetotrophic disease*.

**block design test** A performance test in which the subject tries to match standard designs using colored blocks; used as a measure of intelligence and as an indicator of deterioration in brain damage and in the schizophrenias. The test largely reflects visuospatial construction skills.

**blocking** *Thought deprivation*'; sudden cessation in the train of thought or in the midst of a sentence. The patient is unable to explain the reason for the sudden stoppage, which may occur in the absence of intellectual defect or sensorial disorder. "Often thinking stops in the middle of a thought; or in the attempt to pass to another idea, it may suddenly cease altogether, at least as far as it is a conscious process (blocking). Instead of continuing the thought, new ideas crop up which neither the patient nor the observer can bring into any connection with the previous stream of thought." (Bleuler, E. *Dementia Praecox or the Group of Schizophrenias*, 1950). It is usually experienced by the patient as unpleasant. Bleuler considered a positive response by a patient to the question of whether he had ever experienced thought-deprivation pathognomonic of schizophrenic association disorder. See *obstruction*.

In experimental psychology, blocking consists of temporary complete cessation of work during a period of continuous practice. Blockings of this sort are more frequent in schizophrenics than in others.

**blocking, counterimpulse in** The opposite of the impulse that is blocked. Kraepelin particularly stressed that counterdrives may cause blocking. Bleuler points out that "the denial of any impulse is so very often associated with a counter-impulse that, in stressing the counterimpulse, we only emphasize a different aspect of the same process, but we do not gain a new perspective" (*Dementia Praecox or the Group of Schizophrenias*, 1950).

**blood injury phobia** A common simple phobia consisting of exaggerated fear of the sight, experience, or even discussion of blood, operations, injuries, or minor pain. Typically, exposure to the stimulus produces vasovagal syncope (fainting). A common manifestation of blood injury phobia is *belonephobia* (fear of needles).

**blood–brain barrier** *BBB*; a selective barrier between the blood and brain interstitial fluid formed by the endothelial cells that line cerebral microvessels. The BBB supplies the brain with essential nutrients and mediates efflux of waste products; it regulates ionic and fluid movements between blood and brain to provide an optimal medium for neuronal function; it protects the brain from fluctuations in ionic composition (e.g., following a meal or exercise) which would disturb synaptic and axonal signaling. Tight junctions between adjacent endothelial cells force most molecular traffic to take a transcellular route across the BBB.

The blood–brain barrier is impaired in many disorders: stroke, trauma, infections (encephalitis, meningitis, HIV, sepsis), multiple sclerosis, neurodegenerative disorders (Alzheimer and Parkinson diseases), brain tumors, and epilepsy.

**BLS** Blessed Rating Scales comprising BLS-C (concentration scale), BLS-D (dementia), BLS-I (information), and BLS-M (memory). In addition to cognition, the BLS evaluate functional capacity, personality, and habits.

**BMPs** Bone morphogenetic proteins, members of the transforming growth factor-β (TGF-β) superfamily of growth and differentiation factors. One member of the BMP family, BMP-9, appears to be synthesized in the vicinity of developing cholinergic neurons and induces the expression of the cholinergic gene locus in these cells. Its action as a cholinergic differentiation factor suggests its potential use in the treatment of diseases affecting cholinergic neurons.

**BNCT** *Boron neutron capture therapy*; used in the treatment of glioblastoma multiforme, a rare brain cancer that is usually fatal within 6 months. The patient is injected with a boron compound that concentrates in tumor cells; then the tumor site is irradiated with neutrons that react with the boron atoms and self-destruct, thereby releasing radiation that kills the cancerous cells.

**boarding-out system** A system under which psychotic patients receive care as boarders in private homes. See *domicile; Gheel Colony*.

**bodig** The Guam islanders' name for Parkinson-dementia-amyotrophic lateral sclerosis; they also called it *lytico*, and it was not until recently that it was recognized that they are the same, and that the condition is unique to Guam.

**body buffer zone** The degree of physical proximity to a second person that is experienced as uncomfortable by the subject. For most persons, the body buffer zone to the rear is significantly larger than frontal distances. Several studies have also indicated that a positive correlation exists between size of body buffer zone and degree of aggressivity.

**body build, index of** A standard devised by Eysenck in his studies on the relationship between somatotype and psychosis. The IB consists of a measurement of stature and transverse chest diameter:

$$IB = \frac{stature \times 100}{transverse\ chest\ diameter \times 6}$$

**body dysmorphic disorder** *Dysmorphophobia*; one of the *somatoform disorders* (qq.v.). Dysmorphophobia consists of an obsessive preoccupation, sometimes of delusional degree, with an imagined defect in appearance, most commonly of the skin, hair, or nose. The majority of patients try to hide the perceived defect (e.g., with a wig, beard, or unusual clothing). Insight is lacking, and no amount of reassurance or even surgical measures to repair the imagined deformity decrease the patient's distress. The risk for suicide is high, especially when corrective surgery fails.

**body ego** That part of the perceiving portion of the ego around which all concepts of one's own ego are grouped. The body ego consists of the psychic representations of one's body and self—the memories and ideas connected with the body along with their cathexes. At first the various parts of the body, and eventually the body as a whole, occupy a particularly important place in the psyche throughout life. See *schema*.

The ego perceives not only external stimuli but also inner, mental processes (ideas, wishes, thoughts, strivings, sensations, and fantasies). External stimuli are intercepted by the sense organs and led to the central nervous system. Here they leave traces in the form of memories and ideas whose nature depends upon the particular sense organ that has received the stimulus (sight, hearing, touch). These precipitates in the psyche of external experiences, together with the internal processes, such as thinking, imagination, feelings, emotions, and visceral sensations, form the psychic body scheme or image. The nucleus around which all concepts of one's own ego are grouped is the body ego, whose main function is perception (Nunberg, H. *Principles of Psychoanalysis*, 1955).

Federn used the term "bodily ego-feeling" to refer to the body ego. See *body image; phantom limb.*

**body image**   The concept that each person has of his or her own body as an object in space, independently and apart from all other objects. The body is always in space and experiences are not possible without this conception of our body, or body image, since we live as human beings with a body. See *body ego; schema.*

The body image or *body identity* is the conceptualization of the body's structure and functions that grows out of the awareness of the self and one's body in intended action. Schizophrenic children are often deficient in the ability to localize, discriminate, or give pattern and meaning to body perceptions. "Thus, they lack body images that are integrated, stable in time, and clear in form. One child walked about all day feeling her body. Another observed the motions of her hand in fascination and addressed it as a baby" (Goldfarb, W. *International Psychiatry Clinics 1*, 1964). See *phantom limb.*

L. C. Kolb (*Schizophrenia, An Integrated Approach*, ed. A. Auerback, 1959) distinguishes between *body percept* (or *body schema*) and the *body concept*. The body percept is the postural image one has of one's body as it functions outside of central consciousness; it is organized over the years, mainly on the basis of incoming kinesthetic and tactile perceptions. The body concept, or conceptual image, includes the perceptions, thoughts, and feelings which the ego has in reference to viewing its own body.

**body language**   The expression of feelings or thoughts by means of bodily movements. See

*amygdala; physiognomonic communication; primitive psychosomatic language.*

**body of Luys**   (Jules Bernard Luys, French physician, 1828–1898) See *subthalamus.*

**body protest**   A term coined by Esther L. Richards to indicate that physical dysfunctions may serve as outlets for worries, disappointments, frustrations, etc. See *fixation hysteria.*

**body recognition**   See *face recognition.*

**body scheme**   See *body ego.*

**body-centered therapy**   A group of therapies whose common goal is the altering of self-image or personality through work with the physical body, either exclusively or as a major component of the therapy. Among the major ones are *bioenergetics, Rolfing (structural integration), Feldenkrais method (functional integration), body-centered psychotherapy* (a major form of which is called *Hakomi method*), *psychomotor therapy* (developed by Albert Pesso), *Lomi work* (developed by Robert Hall, Ellisa Hall, Catherine Flaxman, and Richard Heckler), and *Alexander technique* (developed by F. Mathius Alexander).

The various body-centered therapies work with the body in different ways: (1) slow, precise movements, as in the Feldenkrais method, t'ai chi, and Alexander technique; (2) expressive movements and stressful postures, used to access emotionally charged material, as in bioenergetics and dance therapy; (3) the manipulation of body tissue, as in Rolfing; (4) the body as an expression of character, as in bioenergetics, body-centered psychotherapy, and psychomotor therapy; (5) general conditioning and toning of the body to enhance health, feelings of well-being, and the development of the skills of self-defense and personal control, as in yoga and the Asian martial arts.

Bioenergetics is an offshoot of Reichian therapy developed by Alexander Lowen and John Perrakos.

In Rolfing, the intention is to create changes in the subject's self-image and personal feelings through integration of the myofascial system (the system that binds and gives shape to the muscles of the body) and the integration of the whole body to the field of gravity.

The Feldenkrais method uses heightened attention to the fine details of slow, gentle movement, whether the practitioner manipulates the subject's limbs or the subject makes the movements guided by a leader. The object is to enhance the subject's body image and thereby improve movement functions (Feldenkrais, M. *Awareness Through Movement*, 1972).

Body-centered psychotherapy is the most directly psychological method. In both the Hakomi method, developed by Ron Kurtz, and the psychomotor therapy of Pesso, the therapist combines discussion, action, and awareness as a way of gaining access to important emotional material.

**body-packer syndrome**  Drug overdose as a result of the ingestion of multiple small packages of contraband drugs (most commonly cocaine) in order to transport them. Rupture of the package or leaking from semipermeable wrappings (such as condoms) results in acute drug intoxication and, often, death.

**bogeyman**  A spirit or goblin who will punish the child for misbehavior; often interpreted psychoanalytically as externalized pre-superego, i.e., a projection onto persons in the external world of the internalized parental prohibitions that are the forerunners of the *superego* (q.v.).

**Bogorad syndrome**  *Crocodile tears syndrome*; profuse tearing during eating or drinking, due to a seventh nerve lesion and subsequent misdirection of regenerating nerve fibers. Nerves that formerly supplied the salivary gland are diverted to the lacrimal glands. Affected subjects usually also show some degree of residual facial paralysis.

**BOLD**  Blood oxygenation level-dependent. See *fMRI*; *imaging, brain*.

BOLD is a measure of brain activity, most of which is spontaneous neuronal activity. Identifying patterns of coherent BOLD activity is one approach to the analysis of functional connectivity within the brain. It has been found that the coherent spontaneous activity observed in the brain during its resting state contributes to intertrial variability in human behavior. Variations in structured, coherent spontaneous activity in the brain have been reported for several pathological states, including Alzheimer disease, ADHD, autistic disorder, blindness, depression, epilepsy, schizophrenia, and spatial neglect following stroke.

**bombesin**  A gastric peptide that may be the hormonal signal of gastric satiety; in humans,

it produces a potent inhibition of normal feeding.

**bonbon sign**  One form of the buccal-lingual-masticatory syndrome, consisting of pressing the tongue against the cheek. See *tardive dyskinesia*.

**bondage**  A form of overt sexual masochism in which erotic pleasure depends on the subject's being humiliated, endangered, and enslaved; bondage appears to be more frequent in men and more often than not with a homosexual orientation. Bondage may account for as many as 50 deaths annually in the United States, typically through a combination of suicidal wishes and accident.

**bonding**  Mutual dependency; in particular, the early mother–infant symbiosis, a tension-easing relationship that begins in utero and attains its peak intensity between the first and sixth postnatal months (in many ways equivalent to Mahler's *symbiotic phase*). The prime objective of bonding is preservation of the life of the infant, who is in a state of psychophysiologic lability with rapidly shifting internal states—*affectomotor storms* (q.v.). The mother–infant bond is the prototype of all subsequent object relationships. A primal failure to bond leads to overtly self-serving narcissism, expressed in affectionless psychopathy and psychopathic personalities.

**bone-pointing**  Death produced by a magic spell cast by a witch doctor into the victim's spirit. Pointing the bone is to some extent analogous to those patients with malignant disease whose realization of impending death is so terrible a blow that they die before the disease appears to have advanced enough to cause death.

**Bonhoeffer, Karl**  (1868–1949) Berlin psychiatrist; symptomatic (organic) psychoses, acute exogenous reactions. *Bonhoeffer sign* is the loss of normal muscle tone in chorea.

**Bonnet syndrome**  See *Charles Bonnet syndrome*.

**Bonnier syndrome**  (Pierre Bonnier, French physician, 1861–1918) Symptoms resulting from a lesion involving the acoustic, glossopharyngeal, and vagus nerves: paroxysmal vertigo (Ménière disease), contralateral hemiplegia, aphonia, dysphagia, and loss of gag reflex.

**border zone**  See *transcortical aphasia*.

**borderline personality (disorder)**  *BPD*; characteristics are instability in multiple areas of functioning (behavior, mood, self-image, interpersonal relationships); impulsive behavior that is potentially self-destructive; shifting, inappropriate, or uncontrolled emotions; feelings of emptiness and boredom, cannot tolerate being alone, suicidal threats, self-mutilation, identity disturbance with uncertainty about self-image, long-term goals, values. See *borderline psychosis*.

The symptom domains of BPD may be grouped into the following:

1. *Cognitive-perceptual*: including cognitive distortions (episodes of numbing, depersonalization, derealization, schizotypal cognition, lapses in judgment, brief stress psychosis) and identity problems (uncertainty about self-image, values, goals, or sexual orientation; anhedonia and other dysphoric affects, long-term feelings of emptiness, labile self-concept, pessimism, boredom). BPD subjects misperceive the world, their relationships, and their own role in cause and effect. Psychosocial adversity gives rise to traumatic memories that impair functioning, such as flashbacks and ruminative recall of traumatic events. Repetitive trauma influences the development of personality structure and processes, resulting in failure to develop an integrated self-system with well-defined interpersonal boundaries, and difficulty in establishing intimacy and attachment. BPDs process information about themselves and their world in maladaptive ways. Trauma gives rise to powerful expectations about the interpersonal environment and the expected actions of others.

2. *Affective dysregulation*: affective lability (affective instability and overreactivity, generalized hypersensitivity, labile anger, irritability); pervasive instability and ambivalence, resulting in fluctuating attitudes, erratic or uncontrolled emotions, and a general capriciousness and undependability. Their mood shifts quickly to resentfulness, anger, anxiety, dejection, or depression. Their despair is genuine but is also a means of expressing hostility, a covert instrumentality to frustrate and retaliate. Their obstructiveness, pessimism, and immaturity bring them misery and inflict pain on others.

3. *Impulsive-behavioral dyscontrol*: core symptoms are insensitivity and short latency to acting on urges, leading to impulsive self-harm and self-damaging behaviors such as spending sprees, sexual indiscretions and promiscuity, gambling, inappropriate or uncontrolled anger, temper outbursts, physical fights, self-mutilation, and recurrent parasuicide or suicide threats or gestures. Suicide attempts are reported in as many as 73% of borderline patients admitted to hospital, with an average of 3.4 lifetime attempts per patient. With a completed suicide rate of 4% to 10%, BPD is one of the most lethal of psychiatric disorders. Other inappropriate behavior includes alcohol and drug abuse, anorexia, and bulimia. BPD patients often create tensions with their therapists by not leaving when the session is over throwing objects, canceling appointments without notice, not paying the bill, behaving seductively or quitting therapy prematurely. Because they are impulsive, unpredictable, and often explosive, others are commonly uncomfortable in their presence so that they elicit rejection rather than support.

4. *Interpersonal psychopathology*: avoiding responsibility, BPD subjects place added burdens on others. Unstable, intense interpersonal relationships alternate between overidealization and devaluation. Insecure attachment is manifested by separation protest, proximity seeking, feared losses and frantic attempts to avoid real or imagined abandonment, and inability to tolerate solitude. BPD subjects are impatient and irritable unless things go their way. They may be pervasively aggressive in interpersonal relationships, including a violent attack on their own body or that of another. This inadequacy in their capacity to represent aggression-related attachment ideationallly puts them at risk of violent acts in the context of intimate interpersonal relationships.

Approximately 2% of the population meets criteria for BPD as thus described. It is more often diagnosed in women and is more widespread among first-degree relatives of those with the disorder. BPD falls within DSM-IV's cluster B of personality disorders, along with antisocial and narcissistic types.

BPD has been viewed as an *attachment* disorder (q.v.); it overlaps, but is distinct from, *DESNOS* (q.v.), which is considered a disorder of self-regulation. Disorganized attachment lies at the core of BPD and is characterized by unintegrated schemas of self-with-other involving an attachment figure. Severe chronic traumatization in childhood leads to complex PTSD or *PTPD* (q.v.); less severe traumatization is associated with BPD. See *trauma*.

In *cognitive therapy* (q.v.), the symptoms of the BPD patient are viewed as maladaptive schemata. The typical ones are as follows: (1) abandonment and loss (which may express themselves as feelings that the patient will always be alone and unsupported by others); (2) unlovability; (3) excessive dependence; (4) subjugation (the belief that one must accede to the desire of others or else face abandonment); (5) mistrust; (6) inadequate self-discipline (impulsivity and an inability to control oneself); (7) fear of losing emotional control; (8) guilt, the conviction of being a "bad" person; and (9) emotional deprivations, the feeling that one's needs can never be met. See *transference-focused psychotherapy*.

**borderline psychosis** An inexact term, often used to describe a patient who is potentially psychotic (usually schizophrenic) but has not, as yet, broken with reality. See *ambulatory schizophrenia; pseudoneurotic schizophrenia*. "To this group belong queer psychopaths, abortive paranoids, the many 'apathic' individuals whom one may call hebephrenoid personalities, all the types who, as adults, retain or regain a large part of their primitive narcissism because they are able to answer narcissistic hurts with simple denials and with protective increase in their narcissism; they tend to react to frustrations with the loss of object relationships, although this loss frequently is only partial and temporary" (Fenichel, O. *The Psychoanalytic Theory of Neurosis*, 1945).

The term "borderline" was originally used to describe patients who were not overtly psychotic (and thus by definition too ill to be placed on the couch) and yet did not respond well to classical psychoanalytic treatment. The term was extended to include several groups of patients who had been described and labeled by various clinicians: as-if personality (Deutsch), ambulatory schizophrenia (Zilboorg), preschizophrenic disorder (Rapaport, Gill, Schafer), pseudoneurotic schizophrenia (Hoch, Polatin), latent schizophrenia (Federn), latent psychosis (Bychowski), and borderline schizophrenia (Kety, Rosenthal). R. Grinker, B. Werble, and R. Drye (*The Borderline Syndrome*, 1968) applied the term to patients they did not consider schizophrenic or preschizophrenic; since then the concept

of borderline personality disorder that is distinct from the psychoses and also from other *personality disorders* (q.v.) has gained wide acceptance. Some authors hypothesize that borderline personality disorder may be more closely related to affective disorders than to schizophrenic disorders. See *borderline personality*.

**boredom** A feeling of unpleasantness due to a need for more activity, or a lack of meaningful stimuli, or an inability to become stimulated. The last form is generally considered pathological and may be expressed as a need to maintain the status quo and as a stubborn clinging to stimuli that are without interest or meaning to the subject. Pathological boredom usually represents a defense against libidinal or aggressive strivings.

In the analyst, an important type of *countertransference* (q.v.). Patients who resist by not communicating their feelings often induce feelings of nonrelatedness and boredom, and sometimes drowsiness, in the analyst. Boredom is also characteristic of one type of therapist *burnout* (q.v.); masochistic defenses are expressed in feelings of discouragement, loss of interest in psychoanalytic therapy, anger over victimization by patients, self-pity because the analyst is unloved and unappreciated. Kleinians interpret therapist boredom as the result of negative projective identification—the patient is projecting so as to interfere with the therapist's mental processes. "I am bored and not understanding the patient's material because the patient is arousing anxiety or hostility in me."

**boron neutron capture therapy** *BNCT* (q.v.).

**bottom-up** See *top-down*.

**bouffées délirantes** In the French nomenclature, acute delusional psychoses with a favorable outcome and no evidence of a strong genetic link to schizophrenia. They are reported as culture-specific syndromes in West Africa and Haiti, where typical symptoms are sudden outbursts of psychomotor excitement and aggression, with visual and auditory hallucinations or paranoid ideation. See *psychosis, reactive*.

**boundary** 1. The limits that mark off the self from the object; those limits are blurred at primitive developmental levels. Phantasies or fears of merger, for example, suggest a lack of stability in the differentiation between self and other.

2. Boundary has also been used to refer to situations that confront one with the impermanence of life, the uncertainty of the world, or the knowledge of one's impending death. See *out-of-the-body experience*.

3. The invisible line that separates the participants in a relationship and allows each to maintain a separate identity and to fulfill the obligations and responsibilities that are implicitly or explicitly understood as being part of his or her role. Boundary refers to the limits imposed, explicity or implicitly, on a professional relationship as distinct from a nonprofessional relationship. The limits may be formulated as rules or guidelines; their purpose is to maintain the therapeutic efficacy of the relationship and to protect patients from any harm to which their status as patients might render them peculiarly vulnerable.

*Boundary violations* refer to stepping over that invisible line that separates the professional from the client or the physician from the patient, using the power imbalance between therapist and patient to exploit the patient. In psychotherapy, boundary violations by the therapist reflect *countertransference* problems and a breaking of the rule of *abstinence* (q.v.), no matter what rationalizations may be elaborated in an attempt to excuse them. Boundary variables include therapist neutrality, confidentiality, informed consent, fee policy, and time or length or location of sessions. Obtaining informed consent for procedures and treatments, for example, serves the dual purpose of empowering the patient and protecting the therapist. The exploitative therapist does not wish to empower the patient, and hence does not request consent before starting therapy. The psychiatrist must eschew current or future personal relationships with patients, and avoid taking on as a patient anyone with whom there has been a prior personal relationship.

Once therapy begins, a firm boundary must be maintained between the therapist's personal and professional lives. Transference and countertransference issues can shape even the briefest of relationships, and transference never entirely disappears. It is obviously impossible for the therapist to have no transference-based reactions to a patient, but part of the professional contract with any patient is that the therapist will not act on such reactions. The therapeutic setting must

guarantee safety from any kind of exploitation so patients can experience and explore their transference reactions. See *countertransference; transference*.

Most boundary violations follow a similar pattern over time, beginning with subtle manifestations that may seem to be no more than exaggerated and flattering courtesy, followed by informality and demonstrations of friendliness (e.g., giving of gifts by the therapist, meetings outside regular sessions, unusual payment arrangements), progressing to therapist self-disclosure, and then to a dating relationship facilitated by the rescheduling of sessions to the end of the day. In the final phase, touching, hand-holding, hugging, and sometimes overtly sexual contact occur.

**boundary disorders** Schizoaffective disorder, schizophreniform disorder, and schizotypal personality disorder, the three main disorders within the schizophrenia spectrum that do not fulfill the DSM-IV criteria for any of the schizophrenic disorders.

**boundary extension** A type of memory distortion in which observers report having seen not only information that was physically present in a scene, but also information that they have extrapolated from sources outside the scene's boundaries. See *object recognition*.

**bouquet de malades** The distinctive odor said to be characteristic of psychiatric patients.

**Bourneville disease** (Désiré-Magloire Bourneville, Paris neurologist, 1840–1909) *Tuberous sclerosis* (q.v.).

**bouton, presynaptic** A knob-like outpouching at the terminal portion of the axon that contains the synaptic vesicles (which store neurotransmitters) and voltage-gated $Ca^{2+}$ channels. With each action potential, the channels open to permit an influx of calcium ions, which trigger *exocytosis* (q.v.). See *axon; neuron; neurotransmitter; synapse*.

**bouts of ritual making** See *ritual-making*.

**Bovarism** (From the title character in the novel *Madame Bovary*, by Gustave Flaubert) Confusion of daydreaming with the facts of the perceptual world; failure to differentiate between phantasy and reality.

**bovina fames** *Obs.* (L. "oxlike hunger") *Bulimia* (q.v.).

**bovine spongiform encephalopathy** BSE; mad cow disease; one of the transmissible spongiform encephalopathies (q.v.). It begins in the cow with signs of anxiety, restless, and aggressive behavior. With progression, the animal becomes unable to rise from a lying position, posterior ataxia develops, and body weight is lost despite normal appetite. Death usually occurs between 2 weeks and 6 months after onset of symptoms.

BSE was first diagnosed in 1986, in the U.K. Most cases have been found in cattle between 2 and 8 years of age. The source of BSE is believed to be scrapie-contaminated sheep products contained in cattle feed. It is generally believed that new-variant CJD (v-CJD) in humans is due to the transmission of BSE in contaminated beef.

Humans have always been exposed to Creutzfeldt-Jakob disease (q.v.), but because its spread requires either the direct ingestion or injection of infected tissues it has remained a sporadic disease. Polymorphism at residue 129 of human PrP (where either methionine or valine can be encoded) determines the ability of human PrP to form type 4 PrP$^{Sc}$ and to generate the neuropathological phenotype of vCJD. All those affected in the UK vCJD epidemic were 129MM homozygotes, and most were less than 30 years old.

**Bowlby, E(dward) John M(ostyn)** (1907–1990) English psychiatrist and psychoanalyst who introduced the term "maternal deprivation" and emphasized early mother–child interactions. He demonstrated that early attachment was not because of Freudian "orality" but rather an innate survival strategy catalyzed by the sustained and loving maternal touch. He helped to rectify the overemphasis of classical Freudian analysis on childhood phantasy and its neglect of real trauma. His renowned trilogy, Attachment and Loss, was begun in 1963 and completed in 1979.

**boxer's dementia** Dementia pugilistica; boxer's traumatic encephalopathy; chronic cerebral disorder seen in boxers, especially those who have sustained many blows to the head. A similar disorder is seen in high divers such as those in Acapulco, each of whom may dive two or three times a day from a high cliff. The dementia is slowly progressive, with pathologic changes similar to those seen in postencephalitic parkinsonism. Frequent symptoms are tremor, dysarthria, slowed movement, unsteady gait, intellectual impairment, lack of drive, irritability, and sometimes pathological jealousy. See brain injury; punch-drunk.

**BPRS** Brief Psychiatric Rating Scale (q.v.).

**BPSD** Behavioral and psychological symptoms of dementia, differentiated from the cognitive and functional domains of dementia. Physical aggression and paranoid (or other) delusions are the key symptoms in terms of severity, frequency, and impact. Other symptoms are agitation, wandering, misidentifications, hallucinations, sleep disturbances, affective disturbances, anxiety, and phobias. BPSD are similar in all forms of dementia, but some of the symptoms are particularly prominent in certain types. The symptoms in vascular dementia are similar to those in Alzheimer disease. In frontotemporal dementia (Pick disease), prominent features are personality changes, indifference, and disinhibition. (See frontal lobe dysfunctions). In Lewy body dementia, prominent features are auditory hallucinations, delusions, and sleep disturbances. In all, course of BPSD and response to both psychological and pharmacological treatments are independent of the underlying dementia as reflected in cognition.

**brachial plexus avulsion** See *pain syndromes*.

**brachium conjunctivum** See *cerebellum*.

**brachuna** Acrai; nymphomania or satyriasis.

**brachy-** Combining form meaning (abnormally) short.

**brachycephaly, brachycephalism** A skull with shortened anteroposterior diameter. See *cephalic index*.

**brachylineal** Brachymorphic.

**brachymorphic** Relating to or characterized by brachymorphy; a constitutional type that is shorter and broader than the normal, corresponding roughly to the *pyknic type* of Kretschmer (q.v.) or the megalosplanchnic type of Viola.

**brachyskelic** Characterized by an excessive shortness of the legs. See *pyknic type*.

**brachytypical** Synonymous with *brevilineal* and *brachymorphic* (qq.v.).

**Bradley, Charles** (1902–1979) American pediatrician and child psychiatrist. While Medical Director of the Emma Pendleton Bradley Home in East Providence, R.I. (founded by his great-uncle and named for the latter's neurologically impaired daughter), Charles Bradley was the first to note the benefit of psychostimulants in the treatment of attention deficit hyperactivity disorder. In 1948 he founded the Department of Child Psychiatry at the University of Oregon Medical School.

**brady-** Combining form meaning slow, from Gr. *bradys*.

**bradyarthria** Slowness of speech, due to some disorder in the central or peripheral apparatus connected with speech. See *bradylogia*, the implication of which is psychological (emotional) origin.

**bradyglossia** Slowness of speech because of impaired mobility of the tongue, which may be due to local tongue or mouth pathology or to more distant neural lesions (e.g., hypoglossal nerve, cerebellum, cerebrum).

**bradykinesia, bradykinesis** Slowness of movement and difficulty in initiating movement. It is characteristic of Parkinson disease and other neurological disorders involving the striatum; it is also seen in depression as part of psychomotor retardation. It is elicited by asking the patient to tap a finger or the heel.

**bradylalia** Abnormal slowness of speech; bradyarthria. It may, like bradylexia, be occasioned by organic or psychological pathology or both. It is common in depressed states.

**bradylexia** Abnormal slowness in reading; it may be associated with mental retardation or other brain dysfunction, or it may be one manifestation of psychomotor retardation in depressive states.

**bradylogia** Slowness of speech; bradyarthria. Some use the terms interchangeably; others use bradyarthria to refer to organically determined slowness of speech and bradylogia for slowness determined by psychological factors.

**bradyphasia** Slowness of speech.

**bradyphrasia** Slowness of thought.

**bradyphrenia** Sluggish mentality. It is used by some as the equivalent of mental retardation, by others as the equivalent of psychomotor retardation. Bradyphrenia may be symptomatic of any acquired disorder that interrupts the functioning of intelligence. Slowness in thinking is often associated with states of intense emotion, as in severe anxieties and depressions; in the latter there may be a marked paucity or such a profusion of ideas as to lead to great difficulty in concentrated thinking.

Bradyphrenia, like intellectual retardation, may be initial, that is, slowness in starting, or consistent, that is, slowness in continuing. Bradyphrenia is focal when there is retardation in the presence only of disagreeable or painful ideas; it is diffuse when it is vague and unvarying irrespective of the topic in mind.

**bradypragia** Slowness of action, with the implication that the cause is organic (as generalized slowing in myxedema or other deficiency states). Some use the term also for psychomotor retardation of psychologic origin, which most would term *bradyphrenia* (q.v.)

**braid-cutting** A perversion (paraphilia), relatively rare nowadays, consisting of the cutting of the hair from the victim; it is a form of sadism combined with a fetishistic preference for hair.

Psychoanalytically, braid-cutting is interpreted as expressing the idea, "I am the castrator, not the castrated one," and often also the complementary idea, "I am only a pseudocastrator, not a real castrator." The knowledge that the hair will grow back is an important part of the reassurance that the subject gains from the act in that it proves to him that castration need not be final.

**braidism** The theory of hypnosis named after James Braid, English surgeon (1795–1861), who in 1843 published *Neurypnology, or, the Rationale of Nervous Sleep*, considered in relation with animal magnetism.

**brain** The part of the nervous system within the skull, the major organ of mental activity; it includes the cerebrum, midbrain, cerebellum, pons, and medulla.

At birth, the human brain weighs approximately 350 grams; by 1 month of age its weight increases to 420 grams; by the age of 1 year it is half the adult weight of 1400–1600 grams (1600 g = 3 lb). See *neuron*. The brain contains about 100 billion neurons, each of which may have over 1000 synapses (some cortical neurons may approach 20 to 200 times that many). It is not size alone that distinguishes the human brain, but the size in relation to weight. The brain is roughly three times the mass of a monkey or ape of our size. It grows 340% in size after birth, compared to 70% growth of the rhesus brain, due to vastly expanded temporal, parietal, and especially prefrontal areas.

The resting human brain represents only 2% of total body mass but consumes 20% of the body's energy, most of which supports ongoing neuronal signaling. The component that consumes most of the brain's energy is spontaneous neural activity. See *BOLD; fMRI*.

**brain control** Affecting behavior by physical manipulation of the brain; includes electrical or chemical stimulation of discrete areas of the brain, electroconvulsive treatment and psychosurgery (which is also known as functional neurosurgery, sedative neurosurgery, psychiatric surgery, etc.). As distinguished from neurosurgery, *psychosurgery* (q.v.) refers to the selective destruction of areas of the brain for the primary purpose of altering thoughts, emotional reactions, personality characteristics, or social response patterns (Valenstein, E. S. *Brain Control*, 1973).

**brain damage**  Intracranial birth injury or its results; among the most important causes are excessive or otherwise abnormal compression due to abnormal presentations, contracted pelvis, or instrumentation; excessive longitudinal stress producing tears of the dura and rupture of venous sinuses; certain methods of resuscitation, which predispose to sinus rupture; prematurity, which predisposes to intracranial hemorrhage. See *organic syndrome*.

**brain death**  Permanent, irreversible cessation of the functions of the organism as a whole, including control of respiration and circulation, neuroendocrine and homeostatic regulation, and consciousness. Because many areas of the supratentorial brain (e.g., neocortex, thalamus, basal ganglia) cannot accurately be tested for clinical function in a comatose patient, most bedside tests for brain death directly measure the function of the brain stem alone.

In 1995, the American Academy of Neurology published guidelines for determining brain death in adults:

1.  Demonstration of coma (patient never shows eye opening, even on noxious stimulation; no facial expression; mute)

2.  Evidence for the cause of coma

3.  Absence of confounding factors, including hypothermia, drugs, and electrolyte and endocrine disturbances

4.  Absence of brain stem reflexes

5.  Absence of motor responses (at most, residual spinal activity may generate slow body movements, such as finger jerks, undulating toes flexion, pronation-extension reflex)

6.  Apnea (patient requires controlled artificial ventilation)

7.  A repeat evaluation after a further 6 hours is advised, but the time period is arbitrary

8.  Confirmatory laboratory tests are required only when specific components of the clinical test cannot reliably be evaluated. EEG shows absence of electrocortical activity; cerebral angiography and transcranial Doppler sonography document the absence of cerebral blood flow; radionucleotide cerebral imaging such as PET shows the *hollow skull sign*, confirming the absence of neuronal function in the whole brain (*functional decapitation*).

In a patient who is mechanically ventilated, validated neurological tests are used to assure irretrievable absence of brain (brain stem) function; in nonventilated patients, irretrievable absence of heartbeat and of breathing are evaluated. Brain death can be diagnosed with an extremely high rate of probability within hours to days of the original insult. (Laureys S. *Nature Reviews Neuroscience 6*: 899–909, 2005). See *brain injury; vegetative state*.

**brain development**  See *cerebral cortex, development of*.

**brain disorder**  In DSM-I, any psychiatric syndrome caused by or related to impairment of brain tissue function; also known as *organic psychosis, organic reaction type, organic brain syndrome (OBS)*, and in DSM-IV as *Delirium, dementia, and amnestic and other cognitive disorders*. See *organic syndrome*.

**brain fag**  Brain fatigue from too much thinking demanded of students; reported as a culture-specific syndrome in West Africa. Symptoms may include difficulties in concentration and memory, vague pains in the head and neck, and blurred vision.

**brain imaging**  See *imaging, brain*.

**brain injury**  Head injury; damage to the brain, most frequently caused by trauma, stroke, or brain tumor. See *cerebrovascular accident; cerebral compression; CIDS; concussion; intracranial tumor*.

*Traumatic brain injury (TBI)* is the leading cause of acquired cognitive disability and the leading cause of long-term disability in children and young adults. In the United States, TBI has an incidence of 1.5–2.0 million people per year with an overall prevalence of 2.5–6.5 million people with permanent impairment. Motor vehicle accidents account for approximately 45% of cases, falls for 20%, assaults for 12%, sports for 10%, firearms for 6%. Neurologic deficits persist in 5%–10% of those who survive; post-traumatic seizures develop in 5% of those who have had closed head injuries and in half of those with compound skull fractures and laceration of the brain. Preexisting psychopathology is frequently intensified by the injury, and other psychiatric conditions may occur as a result of psychological responses to the trauma or of cognitive deficits produced by the injury. The greater the duration of post-traumatic amnesia (PTA), the greater the likelihood of persisting cognitive deficits. Almost all subjects with a history of brain injury are hypersensitive to medications and other drugs.

Brain trauma may be fatal, or it may result in various levels of brain damage. The results of brain injury include *brain death*, persistent vegetative state (*PVS*), and minimally conscious state (*MCS*). Both patients who are brain dead and patients in the PVS (persistent vegetative state) are "hopelessly damaged and permanently unconscious." But in contrast to brain dead patients, those in PVS recover cyclical alteration of arousal patterns. This does not herald the recovery of consciousness, but it does show the existence of residual brain stem function. The recently described minimally conscious state is further distinguished from PVS by the presence of reliable but inconsistent awareness of oneself or the environment. Activation after deep-brain stimulation or other forms of neuromodulation might be useful in MCS patients with widely preserved networks to sustain recovery if properly assisted. See *CIDS*.

Sequelae may appear immediately or develop as long as 2 years following the injury. They include the following:

1. Mood changes, especially depression. The risk of suicide is significantly increased among brain-injured persons.

2. Personality changes, such as exacerbation of preexisting traits, or the appearance of completely different characteristics, including the development of specific syndromes (perhaps reflecting the area of injury). See *boxer's dementia; convexity syndrome; orbitomedial syndrome.*

3. Aggressiveness, agitation, and violence—variously termed disinhibition syndrome, episodic dyscontrol, intermittent explosive disorder, and organic aggressive syndrome.

**brain plasticity** The brain's ability to change its structure and function during maturation, learning, environmental challenges, or pathology. Changes in the adult brain involve many levels of organization, ranging from molecules to systems, with changes in neural elements occurring concomitantly with changes in supportive tissue elements such as glia and blood vessels.

**brain reward circuit** It includes the mesocorti-colimbic dopaminergic network, spanning the prefrontal cortex (PFC), amygdala, and mesencephalon, and also the thalamus and cerebellum, which are associated with the processing of salient stimuli. Within PFC, orbitofrontal cortex and anterior cingulate cortex mediate the sustained activation of goal-directed behavior (including drug-seeking). See *reward*.

**brain reward system** See *reward system*.

**brain scan** See *encephalography; imaging, brain; radioisotopic; tomography*.

**brain sciences** See *behavioral neurology*.

**brain stem** Includes the *medulla, pons* and *cerebellum, midbrain,* and *thalamus* (qq.v.); it contains the sensory and motor nuclei of the different cranial nerves and the more diffusely organized nuclei that make up the reticular formation, which mediates aspects of arousal. The neural systems of the brain stem integrate visual and vestibular information with somatosensory inputs, and brain stem nuclei control eye and head movements. Surrounding the narrow ventricle of the midbrain is the *periaqueductal gray*, which is crucial for fight/flight behavior and associated autonomic events.

Transection of the brain stem above the level of the vestibular nuclei and below the red nucleus produces *decerebrate rigidity*, with a posture of exaggerated standing and an increase in extensor tone.

**brain syndrome associated with systemic infection** Organic reaction complicating disorders such as pneumonia, typhoid fever, rheumatic fever, scarlet fever, malaria, influenza, smallpox, and typhus; also known as infective-exhaustive psychosis, acute toxic encephalopathy, acute toxic encephalitis, and acute serous encephalitis. The chief types of reaction, which occur mainly in children, are delirious, epileptiform, stuporous or comatose, hallucinatory, and confusional. The most common form is the toxic delirium.

**brain tissue transplants** See *Parkinson disease*.

**brain trauma** See *brain damage; cerebral compression; CIDS; concussion; contusion, brain; organic syndrome.*

**brain tumor**  See *intracranial tumor.*

**brain wave**  See *electroencephalogram; neurometrics.*

**brain-damage behavior syndrome**  See *attention deficit hyperactivity disorder; organic syndrome.*

**brain-derived neurotrophic factor**  BDNF. See *neurotrophic factors.*

**brainstorm**  An inspirational thought or new perception of the world, often accompanying bursts of electrical activity within the limbic system. Such limbic seizural activity may be precipitated by psychologic stress and also by toxins and any metabolic imbalance.

Brainstorm has also been used to refer to any sudden disturbance in brain functioning and, more recently, to any sudden insight or new idea. The latter meaning is retained in the popular use of brainstorm as a verb, meaning to meet with others to exchange ideas in an atmosphere free of the ordinary constraints of logic and orthodoxy, in the hope that such freedom of associations will encourage new insights or creative solutions to problems.

**brainwashing**  *Menticide* (q.v.).

**Brawner decision**  See *criminal responsibility.*

**breakdown, nervous**  A popular, inexact term for the appearance of neurotic or psychotic symptoms of enough severity to impair significantly the person's ability to cope with the demands of his or her current life. The term implies a relatively sudden onset of disability and/or a readily discernible fall from a previously maintained level of performance or adaptation.

**break-off**  A phenomenon that occurs in aviators when flying alone, at high altitudes, and when relatively unconcerned about flying details; the phenomenon consists of a feeling of physical separation from the earth. It is more frequent in emotionally unstable flyers and can itself precipitate an acute phobic reaction that may develop into a general fear of flying.

**breakthrough**  In psychoanalytic therapy, sudden resumption of progress after a period of doldrums, resistance, or inactivity. See *working-through.*

**breakthrough pain**  *BTP;* a transitory exacerbation or flare-up of pain of moderate or severe intensity that occurs in patients with *chronic intractable pain.* See *pain syndromes.*

**breast complex**  Psychoanalytic term for substitution of the possessed penis for the mother's breast that has been denied or withheld from the boy. The breast complex may be expressed in the phantasy of vagina dentata (a vagina with teeth), where the vagina represents the mouth that originally wanted to tear off the mother's breast. The complex may also be expressed in breast envy, which in turn may be expressed in that type of overt homosexuality in which the penis of the subject and/or his partner unconsciously represents the breast.

**breathing-related sleep disorder**  *Hypersomnia* or *insomnia* (qq.v.) due to sleep apnea, central alveolar hypoventilation syndrome, or some other breathing disorder. See *sleep disorders.*

The most common cause of sleep apnea (*sleep-induced respiratory impairment*) is obstruction or occlusion of the airway by atonic or excessive tissue—*obstructive apnea.* Another type of apnea is due to defective brain stem regulation of breathing; see *apnea, central.* The number and length of the apneic periods determine the extent of cardiovascular involvement and change in oxygen saturation. Apnea is associated with bradycardia and behavioral and electroencephalographic arousal; it often terminates with a loud snore, body jerks, sleep talking, or tachycardia. In addition to disturbing sleep, apnea also produces chronic fatigue and sleepiness during the day. Sleep apnea is associated with hypertension, right heart failure, secondary polycythemia, nocturnal cardiac arrhythmias, and possibly sudden, unexplained nocturnal death. Treatment may include nasal continuous positive airway pressure, surgical resection of portions of the soft palate, or tracheostomy. Obesity associated with hypersomnia is sometimes termed the *pickwickian syndrome* (q.v.).

**breeder hypothesis**  The theory that schizophrenia is caused by the social conditions under which many schizophrenics live: poverty, isolation, being single or an unskilled worker, living in the center of cities, etc. In opposition to the breeder hypothesis is the *drift hypothesis:* it is the schizophrenic illness that propels the patient into such conditions as social isolation and poverty.

**Breuer, Joseph**  (1841–1925) Viennese neurologist; published (1895), with Freud, *Studien uber Hysterie.*

**bribe**  In psychoanalysis, a compromise. The symptoms of a neurosis are regarded as symbolic representations of repressed impulses. At first the ego rejects the symptoms; later it becomes reconciled with them, since they afford a certain protection to the security of the ego. The symptoms are accepted by the ego in the nature of a bribe, but the acceptance carries certain favorable elements. For instance, there is the so-called secondary gain from suffering. The repressed impulse is released in the guise of symptoms; the patient does not recognize the released impulse in its new manner of expression. Moreover, in order to placate the superego, or inner conscience, the ego bribes it by suffering.

**Brickner, Richard** (1896–1959) American neurologist; multiple sclerosis, physiology of the frontal lobes.

**bridging** Bridges are social behaviors that connect groups. A person who travels from one location to another to engage in drug use or sexual behavior is bridging the geography or space between the locations. Travel can link urban areas of high HIV seroprevalence to rural areas of low seroprevalence. Male sex workers (*MSWs*, who trade sex for money) often bridge sexual and drug-use networks in different cities.

**brief and emergency psychotherapy (BEP)** A form of short-term, intensive psychotherapy developed by L. Bellak as an extension of his experience with the emergency psychotherapy of depression and with crisis intervention in a walk-in clinic. Based on dynamic psychotherapy and particularly on ego psychology, intensive brief and emergency psychotherapy is systematic, focused, and highly conceptualized. It is usually limited to five sessions.

**Brief Psychiatric Rating Scale** *BPRS;* a 16-item scale with nine general-symptom items, five positive-symptom (of schizophrenia) items, and two negative-symptom (of schizophrenia) items. Each item is scored on a seven-point severity scale (the higher the number, the more severe the symptom), resulting in a range of possible scores from 16 to 112. The average patient with schizophrenia entering a clinical trial typically scores 33.

**brief psychotherapy** *Brief dynamic psychotherapy; short-term therapy; time-limited psychotherapy;* any form of psychodynamic psychotherapy designed to produce therapeutic change within a short period of time (usually 20 sessions or less, sometimes up to a year with a frequency of one or two sessions per week). Brief dynamic psychotherapy is based on psychoanalytic principles; behavior therapy

and cognitive therapy are also time-limited, but they do not rely on change in personality dynamics. See *behavior therapy; cognitive therapy; psychodynamic psychotherapy; psychotherapy.*

Most forms of brief psychotherapy are highly specific in the selection criteria applied to potential patients, since it is considered crucial to exclude patients whom experience has shown to be unresponsive. Most do not encourage the development of a regressive transference, and although transference issues that emerge during treatment are dealt with, there is equal emphasis on disturbances in current relationships. The early termination that is characteristic of such approaches means that specific attention must be given to conflicts over loss and separation. Short-term therapy is typically circumscribed, focused (see *focal conflict*), and action oriented, concerned with immediate crises and with ways of dealing with the social unit or matrix of which the patient is a part. "Basic principles which are generally adhered to include early formulation of the problem, focusing, bypassing areas of resistance, and accepting, indeed sometimes strengthening defenses rather than challenging them" (Barten, H. H. *Brief Therapies*, 1971). The success of short-term therapy appears to be related to the following variables: easy accessibility to permit speedy restoration of equilibrium; modifying therapy techniques in accordance with the shifting needs of the patient and trials of different modalities should the patient fail to improve; and maximal utilization of ancillary persons and agencies (*community supportive network*).

J. Burke, H. White, and L. Havens divide the principal types of short-term dynamic psychotherapy into (1) *interpretive*—which stresses insight produced by the therapist's interpretations; (2) *corrective*—where the therapist is more active, directive, and manipulative; and (3) *existential*—where pressure is exerted by limiting time and through an increase in the therapist's empathy.

Among the many different forms of brief dynamic therapy are the following:

1. STAPP (Peter Sifneos)—see *short-term anxiety-provoking psychotherapy.*

2. TLP (James Mann)—see *time-limited psychotherapy.*

3. Broad-focused short-term dynamic psychotherapy (Habib Davanloo)—selection

criteria are broader than most brief psychotherapies, and patients with long-standing severe characterological deficits are accepted. Emphasis is on the patient's way of defending against real feelings by means of repetitive confrontation.

4. Malan-Tavistock-British School— evolved from the work of Michael Balint (focal psychotherapy) and David Malan at the Tavistock Clinic in London. Malan emphasizes two configurations: (1) the patient's aim, the perceived threat that makes its expression dangerous, and defensive efforts to ward off anxiety and (2) a repetitive pattern of relationships demonstrated with the therapist (transference relationship), current interpersonal relationships, past and present relationships with parent figures or siblings. Of major importance is the parent-transference linking interpretation, which analyzes the connection between the way the patient relates to the therapist and the way of relating to parental figures in the past.

5. ITP (Klerman and Weissman)—see *interpersonal psychotherapy.*

**brief psychotic disorder**   DSM-IV term for what was previously called brief reactive psychosis.

**brief reactive psychosis**   *Brief psychotic disorder* (DSM-IV); any reaction to major stress that is of psychotic proportions, with impaired reality testing and emotional turmoil, and a return to the premorbid level of functioning within 1 month. See *schizophreniform disorder.*

**brief stimulus therapy (BST)**   A type of electroconvulsive therapy in which the current is modified so that the average electrical energy needed to produce a seizure is much less than with the usual method. It is claimed that BST gives as satisfactory clinical results as classical ECT, with the added advantage of reducing or even eliminating confusion. A disadvantage of BST is that patients are more fearful than with the classical method; this can be overcome by using pretreatment barbiturates.

**Briggs law**   A law of Massachusetts named after L. Vernon Briggs (1921); the law provides that a person indicted by the grand jury who has previously been convicted of a felony, or who is known to have been indicted for any other offense more than once, will be examined by a psychiatrist-expert appointed by the State Department of Mental Health. The examiner is not asked to determine whether the accused can distinguish between right and wrong or whether the accused acted because of an irresistible impulse; instead, the psychiatrist is asked whether the accused suffers from a mental illness severe enough to affect his or her responsibility and to require treatment in a mental hospital. See *criminal responsibility.*

**Brigham, Amariah**   (1798–1849) American physician and alienist; founded *American Journal of Insanity* (1844), now the *American Journal of Psychiatry;* "moral treatment."

**bright child**   A child of superior ability; some writers make the following distinction: (1) bright child—a child of average intellectual endowment with an ability to perceive, grasp, and absorb communicated knowledge more quickly than his or her peers; (2) superior child—one with an extraordinary capability in some special field; (3) gifted child—one with a specific talent, usually overdeveloped in relation to other abilities, which may be at a bright, average, or dull level; (4) prodigy—a rare type of superior child who from the earliest stage of life shows an unusual and practically untrained capability in one or more fields.

**bright light therapy**   *Phototherapy* (q.v.).

**Brill, A. A.**   (1874–1948) First American psychoanalyst; translated Freud's works into English.

**Briquet, Paul**   (1796–1881) French psychiatrist; author of a monumental treatise on hysteria (1859), which is consequently termed Briquet syndrome.

**Briquet syndrome**   *Hysteria; somatization disorder* (qq.v.); P. Briquet was the first to describe hysteria systematically, in 1859. Some use the eponym to refer specifically to the polysymptomatic form of hysteria with many visits to different physicians, excessive medications, excessive hospitalizations, and excessive surgery. Criteria for the diagnosis of Briquet syndrome include (1) vague or dramatic medical history beginning before the age of 35 years; (2) a history of multiple symptoms (usually not less than 20) severe enough to interfere significantly with the patient's life or to require medication or a visit to a physician; and (3) a lack of any medical explanation for the symptoms.

**Brissaud syndrome**   (Edouard Brissaud, French physician, 1852–1909) Infantilism due to thyroid dysfunction; *cretinism* (q.v.).

**British school** Also, *object relations school*; associated particularly with Melanie Klein, W. R. D. Fairbairn, Michael Balint, Wilfred Bion, and D. W. Winnicott. They transformed psychoanalysis from a drive-reduction theory into a theory based on the developmental primacy of internalized and external object relations. See *affectomotor storms; bad object; conflict paradigm.*

**broad thumb-hallux syndrome** See *Rubenstein-Taybi syndrome.*

**broad-focused psychotherapy** See *brief psychotherapy.*

**Broca, Paul** (1824–1880) French surgeon and neuroanatomist; the first to localize the faculty of language to a restricted brain area; named the limbic system and deduced its functional importance on the basis of its persistence as an anatomic unit throughout evolution.

**Broca area** Traditionally, one of the speech areas of the brain. It lies in the frontal lobe above the lateral fissure, immediately anterior to the region of the cortex which, when stimulated, leads to movements of the muscles involved in speech. *Broca aphasia* is sometimes equated with "expressive" difficulties, although it is clear that the deficits are not limited to expressive language since the comprehension of distinctions in meaning conveyed by syntax can also be impaired. Broca area is the region which contains the learned programs for control of the musculature of speech. After destruction of this region, speech is slow and hesitant and also agrammatic, i.e., preposition, conjunctions, and auxiliary verbs are often omitted. These findings suggest that the Broca area has a major role in the production of grammatically correct language.

**Broca motor aphasia** *Anterior aphasia; agrammatism; expressive aphasia*; comprehension of both speech and writing is intact but expression is impaired (a nonfluent aphasia). Expression both in speech and writing is severely affected; utterances may be reduced to mere grunts; repetition is always impaired. In milder cases, consonants are slurred and sentences lack the functor words that hold normal speech together (articles, auxiliary verbs, tenses); the result is agrammatism (also called telegram or telegraphic speech). Speech is slow, effortful, and poorly articulated. The patient has difficulty in finding words but nonetheless makes sense because only speech

production is disturbed. Sometimes the patient is totally mute. Some, however, can still swear fluently and they can often sing. Some patients have a full understanding of spoken and written language and are painfully aware of their deficits. Many of those affected, however, have difficulty as well in understanding the parts of language that signal grammatical structures; these are left out in their own speech.

Since there is difficulty in both the production and the understanding of language, the deficit would appear to be in the processing of phonological or syntactic structure. Damage is in the left posterior inferior region of the left frontal lobe (Broca area), usually extending to the third frontal gyrus (Brodmann areas 44 and 45). Because the Broca area is located near the motor cortex and the underlying internal capsule, a right hemiparesis and homonymous hemianopsia (loss of vision) are almost always present.

**Broca speech area** (Paul Broca, Parisian anthropologist and surgeon, 1824–1880) The motor speech area; areas 44 and 45 of Brodmann; the inferior end of the motor area in the third left frontal convolution. See *Broca area; Broca motor aphasia; preadaptation.*

**Brodmann, Korbinian** (German neurologist, 1868–1919) In 1909 he demonstrated the characteristic cytoarchitecture of the cortex, which is arranged in six layers (numbered from the most external, layer 1, to the deepest, layer 6, which is adjacent to the white matter below the cortex). On the basis of cell size and density and which layers are present, he subdivided the cortex into 50 structural areas ("Brodmann areas"), most of which have specific functions. His functional classification of cortical areas continues to be the one most widely used.

**broken windows theory** Physical disorder theory; the theory that certain characteristics of the physical environment increase the likelihood that one will experience personal stress events. Physical disorder in the environment, such as deteriorating housing or vandalism, is a psychological stressor that increases adverse health outcomes. Complementing this theory is the *stress reduction hypothesis*, that living amidst physical disorder may increase the use and abuse of alcohol and drugs as maladaptive coping behavior or self-medication. See *social disorganization theory.*

**bromidism** Bromide intoxication that may be manifested in several ways: (1) simple intoxication, with mental dulling, memory disturbances, enfeeblement, tremor (especially of the hands, face, and tongue), ataxia, incoordination, acneform dermatitis, fetid breath, and coated tongue; (2) delirium, with disorientation in all spheres; (3) hallucinosis, with marked fear reactions; in contrast to delirium tremens, bromide hallucinosis lasts weeks rather than days; (4) schizophreniform psychosis; or (5) pseudoepilepsy.

**bromidrosiphobia** Fear that one's body odor is offensive.

**bromidrosis** Perspiration with foul odor.

**bromocriptine** A dopaminergic antiparkinsonian drug.

**brontophobia** Fear of thunder; astraphobia. It is related in part to the dread of allegedly demonical phenomena of nature, akin to personalization of such phenomena by primitive humans; it may also be related to fear of real persons, and especially of the father or father figure.

**brooding** Anxious or moody pondering, usually about very abstract matters; also termed intellectualization or *Grübelsucht* (q.v.). Brooding is seen frequently in obsessive-compulsive neurotics as a *thinking compulsion*, a need to worry very much about apparently insignificant things.

**brooding mania** Morbid impulse to meditate long and anxiously; obsessive doubting. See *folie du doute*.

**brooding spells** One of Rado's subdivisions of obsessive attacks is called *spells of doubting and brooding*: a swinging back and forth between the same pros and the same cons without reaching a decision. Since this may invade any mental activity, the patient soon finds he can trust no belief, no memory, not even his own observations, and as a result he must check and recheck his every move, to make sure that it has been right. See *obsessive-compulsive disorder*.

**Brown-Séquard syndrome** (Charles Brown-Séquard, French neurologist, 1817–1894) Hemisection of the spinal cord (as in cord tumor, syringomyelia, stab wound, etc.) producing homolateral lower motor neuron paralysis in the segment of the lesion, homolateral upper motor neuron paralysis below the lesion, homolateral anesthesia in the segment of the lesion, homolateral hyperesthesia below the lesion, homolateral loss of proprioception, vibratory and two-point discrimination below the lesion, contralateral hyperesthesia in the segment of the lesion, and contralateral loss of pain and temperature below the lesion.

**Brudzinski sign** (J. Brudzinski, Polish physician, 1874–1917) Flexion of the lower limbs produced by passive flexion of the head on the chest; indicative of meningitis.

**Brueghel syndrome** See *Meige syndrome*.

**brujeria** See *rootwork*.

**Brunet tests** A developmental scale designed for use with infants as young as 1 month.

**Bruns sign** (Ludwig Bruns, German neurologist, 1858–1916) Headache, vertigo, and vomiting associated with sudden movements of the head, occurring in cases of tumor of the fourth ventricle.

**brute pride** *Real pride*, i.e., pride based on self-assertive rage. See *domesticated pride*.

**bruxism** Gnashing or grinding of the teeth that occurs typically at night, during sleep. It is said to be especially common in alcoholics and to indicate repressed aggressivity or hostility.

**bruxomania** Grinding, pounding, or setting of the teeth apart from the normal activity of mastication. There results a loosening of the teeth and a bleeding of the gums.

**BSEP** Brain stem-evoked potential. See *neurometrics*.

**BSR** Brain-stimulation reward. See *reward*.

**BST** *Brief stimulus therapy* (q.v.).

**buccal onanism** *Fellatio* (q.v.).

**buccal-lingual-masticatory syndrome** See *tardive dyskinesia*.

**buccolingual dyspraxia** The subject cannot puff out his or her cheeks, whistle, or blow out a match; it is frequent in *aphasia* (q.v.). See *apraxia*.

**buffer memory** See *short-term memory*.

**buffoonery psyiosis** *Faxenpsychosis*; a form of hyperkinetic catatonia (catatonic excitement) in which the patient constantly makes disconnected caricatured grimaces and gestures. This psychosis probably represents a flight into disease as an escape from reality. "One has the impression that these patients want to play the buffoon, though they do this in a most awkward and inept fashion. They contrive any number of stupidities and sillinesses, such as beating their own knees, interchanging pillows for blankets when they go to bed, pouring water out on the floor instead of into a cup, lifting doors off their hinges. The patients will do all this while they are seemingly well oriented. As a rule they speak very little or not at all and what they have to say is, in the main, completely illogical cursing or other nonsense. Undoubtedly the "faxen-psychosis' has an origin similar to that of the Ganserian twilight state. It usually involves individuals who for some unconscious reason pretend to be mentally deranged" (Bleuler, E. *Dementia Praecox or the Group of Schizophrenias,* 1950). See *factitious disorders; Ganser syndrome.*

**bufotenin** Dimethylserotonin. An analogue of serotonin that, unlike serotonin itself, is psychotomimetic and produces effects similar to those seen following lysergic acid or mescaline administration. It has been suggested that conversion of serotonin into bufotenin rather than breakdown by monoamine oxidase into 5-hydroxyindole acetic acid may be of significance in the etiology of endogenous psychoses.

**bug, cocaine** *Formication*; one of the more common unpleasant tactual paresthesiae that may appear during withdrawal of cocaine in a cocaine addict. The patient typically interprets the sensation as an itching, biting, crawling, or sticking due to an insect. See *Magnan sign.*

**bug phobia** Fear of small animals such as insects, spiders, and flies. Although animal phobias are usually distorted representations of the passionate, sexual, aggressive, "animal-like" father, fears of small animals may be a direct projection of one's own drives. Creatures of this sort commonly represent genitals, feces, or little children (brothers and sisters).

**bugger** Colloquial for a homosexual who practices anal intercourse, from *bougre,* a French word for heretics, and particularly for certain types of Bulgarian origin; later it came to refer to a person who practiced sodomy, or to a homosexual male. In modern French, the word has no sexual implication. See *sodomy.*

**Buhler tests** A developmental scale designed for use with infants from birth up to school age.

**bulbar** Referring to the bulb. See *medulla oblongata.*

**bulbocapnine** One of the drugs used relatively early in the many experiments of H. H. DeJong in experimental production of catatonia.

**bulbotegmental reticular formation** See *reticular formation.*

**bulesis** The motivational or volitional apparatus; the will. See *abulia.*

**bulimarexia** See *restricters.*

**bulimia** Insatiable hunger with voracious eating; also known as cynorexia, eclimia, lycorexia; frequently used as an equivalent of *bulimia nervosa* (q.v.), but sometimes it is used to refer to the bulimic subtype of *anorexia nervosa* (q.v.). See *restricters.*

**bulimia nervosa** Fames canina; phagedena; phagomania; polyphagia; one of the *eating disorders* (q.v.), characterized by uncontrolled *binge-eating* episodes and *purging* (qq.v.) or other compensatory behavior to prevent weight gain. It occurs in persons of normal weight (where problems of self-induced vomiting or laxative abuse are the rule) as well as in people who are overweight. (If bulimia occurs during an episode of anorexia, the diagnosis is anorexia nervosa, bulimic type.)

Binges may occur many times a day or two or three times a week; they last from several minutes to several hours and end, not because of satiation, but because of nausea, severe abdominal pain, somnolence, or self-induced vomiting. The food is usually consumed in isolation, often late in the day upon returning home from work or school. Typically the food is high in carbohydrates and of a texture that is easily swallowed. After a binge, the bulimic is likely to feel guilty, depressed, and disgusted with himself or herself. The binge is followed by compensatory self-induced vomiting, laxative abuse, or pathologically extreme exercise. Chronic concern about body weight and shape is common. See *gorger-vomiter.*

Alcoholism and other substance abuse, suicidal gestures and attempts, stealing, self-mutilation, and sexual disorders (ranging from promiscuity to a total lack of interest or desire in sex) are often associated with bulimia nervosa.

Bulimia nervosa appears to be a relatively common disorder among females; males account for no more than 5% of those who come to clinical attention. Onset is usually in the teens. In several surveys of female college students, between 30% and 45% admitted to binge eating, but probably not more than 10% would fulfill the criteria for bulimia nervosa. The long-term course of the disorder is highly variable.

Bulimia may be associated with a number of physical consequences of both overeating and purging, including fluid and electrolyte abnormalities, decalcification leading particularly to problems of dentition, gastric dilatation, and even spontaneous rupture of the stomach.

**bullying** A complex and abusive behavior that involves a pattern of repeated aggression with a deliberate intent to harm or disturb a victim despite apparent victim distress, and a real or perceived imbalance of power allowing the more powerful child (or group of children) to attack a physically or psychologically vulnerable victim.

Bullying is a sign of potential psychiatric illness in both the bully and the victim. Bullies have a significant incidence of physical and emotional abuse in their past and a higher incidence of adjustment and conduct disorders. Bullies are likely to have long-lasting psychiatric consequences from their bullying behavior. Victims often develop anxiety and depressive disorders as a result of traumatization. Bullying is not always limited to physical abuse; it is often combined with psychological bullying.

**bullying, relational** Socially manipulative behavior intended to hurt others, such as spreading rumors about them, dropping them as a friend, or ostracizing them from the "in" group. Such bullying interferes with the victims' social enjoyment at school and makes them feel less safe there. It encourages some boys, particularly, to bring a weapon to school. Relational bullying can also affect the victim's life outside as manifested by generalized social anxiety, loneliness, and depression.

**Bumke, Oswald** (1877–1950) German psychiatrist and neurologist.

**buprenorphine** A derivative of thebaine, it is a partial μ-opioid agonist and a weak κ-opioid antagonist. Buprenorphine has been used in combination with naloxone for opiate addiction and cocaine dependence. In clinically used doses, the effects of buprenorphine are similar to full μ-opioid agonists such as morphine or methadone. At higher doses buprenorphine acts like an opioid antagonist. This ceiling effect decreases the risk of overdose and limits its abuse liability. Its slow dissociation from the opioid receptors allows flexible dosing ranging from several times a day to three times per week.

**bupropion** Among antidepressant medications, sustained-release (SR) bupropion has been the most commonly used medication for pharmacotherapy of smoking cessation. It blocks reuptake of norepinephrine and dopamine, and these effects may attenuate tobacco withdrawal symptoms. Bupropion also blocks nicotine receptors, which may attenuate the rewarding effects of smoking.

**burning feet syndrome** Sensory neuropathy with foot paresthesias: the feet feel as if they are on fire. The syndrome occurs with different vitamin deficiencies such as *beriberi* and *pyridoxine* deficiency (qq.v.).

**burnout** A syndrome of physical, emotional, or attitudinal exhaustion characterized by impaired work performance, fatigue, insomnia, depression, increased susceptibility to physical illness, reliance on alcohol or other drugs of abuse for temporary relief with a tendency to escalation into physiologic dependency, and in many cases suicide. The syndrome is generally considered to be a stress reaction to unrelenting performance and emotional demands stemming from one's occupation; others consider it a depression, and still others label it a life-management difficulty.

Different manifestations of burnout in therapists have been described: one characterized by masochistic defenses and typically expressed in *boredom* (q.v.); another characterized by narcissistic defenses. See *narcissistic countertransference*.

**Burton, Robert** (1577–1640) Oxford Dean of Divinity; he wrote about his own childhood experiences, recognizing the role of anger in the genesis of depression, in *Anatomy of Melancholy* (1621).

**buspirone** A partial agonist at the $5\text{-HT}_{1A}$ receptor; buspirone is an antianxiety agent that is not related pharmacologically to the barbiturates, benzodiazepines, or other sedative/hypnotic agents. Its mechanism of action is unknown. It does not demonstrate anticonvulsant or muscle relaxant effects, and it does not affect GABA binding. It has no significant affinity for benzodiazepine receptors, but it shows high affinity for serotonin receptors and moderate affinity for brain dopamine receptors. It does not exhibit cross-tolerance with benzodiazepines or other sedative/hypnotic drugs, and it appears to be less sedating than other *antianxiety drugs* (q.v.).

**Buss-Durkee Hostility Inventory** *BDHI*; the most widely used self-rated measure of aggression; it consists of 75 items on seven scales (Assault, Indirect Aggression, Irritability, Negativism, Resentment, Suspicion, and Verbal Aggression). A newer version, the *Buss-Perry Aggression Questionnaire*, includes only four scales (Physical Aggression, Verbal Aggression, Anger, and Hostility) and appears to be primarily a trait measure of aggression.

**Butler, John S.** (1803–1890) American psychiatrist; one of the "original thirteen" founders of Association of Medical Superintendents of America (forerunner of American Psychiatric Association).

**buying spree** Oniomania.

**BWAM** Brain wave activity measurement. See *neurometrics*.

**BWS** Battered wife syndrome. See *domestic violence; wife battering.*

**by-idea** *Metaphoric paralogia*; the secondary or manifest thought or concept onto which the primary or latent idea is displaced in dreams and thinking disorders. A by-association displaces the basic thought, leading to a *derailment* of thought or speech.

**BZRA** Benzodiazepine receptor antagonist; BZRAs are used to treat insomnia. They improve various parameters of subject sleep measures such as sleep latency and total sleep time. They are associated with a variety of side effects, including daytime drowsiness, physical dependence, impairment of motor abilities (resulting in falls and other accidents), anterograde amnesia and other cognitive impairments, and respiratory depression. Current research on insomnia treatment has focused on selective $GABA_A$ modulators such as gaboxadol, which differs from traditional GABA agonists by enhancing slow wave activity during NREM, promoting deep NREM sleep stages, and enhancing overall sleep efficiency.

# C

**CA** 1. Abbreviation for chronological age. 2. *Catecholamine* (q.v.). See *epinephrine*.

**CAA** *Cerebral amyloid angiopathy*; a Mendelian variant of small vessel disease, characterized by the deposition of amyloid in the walls of leptomeningeal and cerebral cortical blood vessels. Clinical manifestations include recurrent or multiple lobar hemorrhages, cognitive deterioration, and ischemic strokes. Rupture of structurally weakened arteries results in cerebral hemorrhage. Several autosomal dominantly inherited forms are due to mutations in the amyloid precursor protein. The $\varepsilon 4$ allele of APOE is associated with enhanced beta-amyloid deposition in the cerebral vasculature and earlier disease onset. Patients with CAA-related hemorrhage show an excess of the $\varepsilon 2$ allele, which may predispose to rupture of amyloid-laden vessels. See *VaD*.

**CAC** *Chemical aversive conditioning*; the use of sensitizing agents such as disulfiram in the treatment of alcoholism. See *aversion therapy*.

**cacergasia** *Obs.* Inadequate functioning of body or mind.

**cachectin** See *cachexia*.

**cachexia** A chronic catabolic state, associated with certain infections and malignancies, characterized by weight loss that continues despite consumption of an adequate diet. A factor or factors—termed *cachectin*—produced by endotoxin-stimulated macrophages, inhibits the activity of lipogenic (fat-producing) enzymes, and triglycerides are mobilized from adipose tissue with resultant weight loss. See *anorexia nervosa; hypophysial cachexia*.

**cachinnation** Canchasmus; inordinate laughter without apparent cause, observed most frequently in the hebephrenic form of schizophrenia.

**caco-** Combining form meaning bad, vitiated, distorted; from Gr. *kakos*, bad, evil.

**cacodaemonomania** A delusion that one is, or is about to be inhabited by or possessed of, a devil or some evil spirit.

**cacogenic** Giving rise to a deteriorated race or offspring; the opposite of *aristogenic* or *eugenic* (q.v.).

**cacogeusia** A bad taste; a frequent complaint in idiopathic epilepsy, in patients receiving tranquilizer therapy, and in somatic delusional states.

**cacolalia** *Coprolalia* (q.v.).

**cacophoria** See *euphoria*.

**cacosomnia** *Obs.* Sleeplessness.

**cacothymia** *Obs.* Any mental affection with depravation of the morals (Tuke, DH. *A Dictionary of Psychological Healing*, 1892).

**CADASIL** Cerebral autosomal dominant arteriopathy with subcortical infarcts and leukoencephalopathy; a Mendelian variant of small vessel disease due to mutations in *Notch3*. The ectodomain of the Notch3 receptor accumulates within blood vessels and produces a degeneration of vascular smooth muscle cells. The nonamyloid angiopathy involves small arteries and capillaries in the brain and in other organs. See *VaD*.

Recurrent transient ischemic attacks usually begin in mid-adulthood and may include stroke. By the age of 65, two-thirds of subjects are demented. Cognitive impairment includes deficits in episodic memory, attention, and executive and visuospatial functions. Small lacunar lesions and diffuse white matter abnormalities are particularly prominent within the temporopolar white matter.

**cadherins** See *adhesion, cellular*.

**cadiva insania** (L. "falling or epileptic insanity") *Obs.* Epilepsy.

**CAE** *Childhood absence epilepsy* (q.v.).

**caelotherapy** *Pastoral counseling* (q.v.).

**Caenis syndrome** A triad of genital self-mutilation, hysterical personality disorder, and eating disorder. (Neptune, god of the sea, raped Caenis and subsequently granted her wish that her genitalia be ablated so that she could never again be violated.)

**Caesar mania** *Obs.* "A feeling of being absolute master of life and death among savages" (Bleuler, E. *Textbook of Psychiatry*, 1930)

**cafard** Severe *depression; melancholia* (qq.v.). Cafard (or cathard) is also the name of a culture-bound syndrome described in Polynesia and similar to *amok* (q.v.).

**caffeine intoxication**   *Caffeinism*, due to the ingestion of substances containing caffeine: coffee, tea, cola drinks, hot chocolate, cocoa, cold remedies, and some analgesics. Caffeine is a weak psychostimulant and is used mainly to alleviate mild degrees of fatigue. Coffee contains 100–150 mg of caffeine per cup, tea about half as much, and cola about one-third as much. Intake of more than 250 mg of caffeine may produce symptoms of intoxication: restlessness, nervousness, excitement, insomnia, flushed face, diuresis, gastrointestinal disturbances, muscle twitching, rambling flow of thought and speech, tachycardia or cardiac arrhythmia, ringing in the ears, periods of inexhaustibility, and psychomotor agitation. Convulsions, respiratory failure, and death have been reported with doses above 10 g.

**caffeine use disorders**   These are classified within the substance-related disorders and include caffeine intoxication, caffeine anxiety disorder, and caffeine sleep disorder. Caffeine withdrawal is not recognized as a disorder in DSM-IV.

**Caffey syndrome**   *Shaken baby syndrome* (q.v.).

**CAG repeats**   See *trinucleotide repeat.*

**CAGE**   A four-question screening instrument for the detection of alcoholism devised by Ewing and Rouse; the letters of the acronym refer to the key word in each question—(1) Have you ever felt you should *Cut* down on your drinking? (2) Have people *Annoyed* you by criticizing your drinking? (3) Have you ever felt bad or *Guilty* about your drinking? (4) Have you ever used a drink as an *Eye*-opener (a drink first thing in the morning to steady your nerves or get rid of a hangover)?

**CAH**   Congenital adrenal hyperplasia; see *adrenogenital syndrome.*

**Cain complex**   Brother complex; rivalry, competition, aggression, or destructive impulses directed against a brother.

**cainophobia, cainotophobia**   Neophobia. See *kainotophobia.*

**Cairns stupor**   Akinetic or diencephalic stupor: stupor, rigidity, postural catatonia, absence of spontaneous movement and emotion. See *akinetic mutism.*

**caisson disease**   Diver's paralysis, the bends, tunnel disease; circulatory disturbance in the nervous system, observed when a person, subjected to high air pressure (e.g., in diving or working under compressed air in a caisson) returns too suddenly to normal atmosphere.

There is a question as to whether the sudden release of pressure causes air emboli in the brain and spinal cord or whether the blood vessels dilate, giving rise to congestion and stasis. Pathologically, the spinal cord shows softening and necrosis.

The symptoms are acute in onset with headache, pains in the epigastrium, limbs, and back, sufficient to double the patient up (the bends), dizziness, dyspnea, nausea, vomiting, coughing, and partial or complete paralysis, usually of both lower extremities. Cerebral symptoms may occur, such as aphasia, double vision, confusion, coma, and convulsions.

**Cajal, Santiago Ramòn y**   (1852–1934) Spanish physician, anatomist, and histologist. In 1891 he formulated the principle of *dynamic polarization* (q.v.) and made countless contributions to the neurosciences (e.g., neuronal plasticity, transplantation of nerve tissue, and nerve regeneration).

**calamitous relationship**   See *group tension, common.*

**calamity by appointment**   The physical and emotional disabilities that often follow successful removal of primary brain tumors; the disabilities may be more severe than those produced by the tumor.

**calcarine area**   See *occipital lobe.*

**calcium acetyl homotaurinate**   *Acamprosate* (q.v.).

**calcium channel**   $Ca^{2+}$ channel; an *ion channel* (q.v.) that regulates the rapid entry of $Ca^{2+}$ into the neuron; the influx can trigger various processes, including neurotransmitter release, modulation of synaptic transmission, generation and control of neuronal firing patterns, mechanisms of memory, excitotoxic cell death, and alterations of gene expression. To control calcium influx, neurons have many calcium-permeable ion channels, of different types.

Voltage-dependent calcium-sensitive channels are of two types: (1) high voltage-activated (HVA) calcium channels, which include the N-, L-, and P-types; many neurotransmitters inhibit HVA channels, diminishing transmitter release and thereby exerting a presynaptic inhibitory (autoinhibitory) effect; and (2) low voltage-activated (LVA) calcium channels are the T-type channels, which mediate repetitive bursting, pacemaking activity, and secretion by the neuron. Some calcium channels are receptor-activated rather than voltage-activated.

Organic calcium channel blockers prevent calcium influx by acting on drug-specific receptors that are linked to calcium channels. At least some anticonvulsants appear to act on LVA channels. See *glutamate; ion channel; ion pump; migration, neuronal; NMDA receptor; second messenger.*

**calcium channel blockade**   See *verapamil.*

**calcium-calmodulin-dependent protein** *CaMKII* (q.v.).

**callipedia**   *Obs.* The desire to give birth to a beautiful child.

**callomania**   *Obs.* Love of beauty and grace; the delusion that one is beautiful.

**callosal gyrus**   *Cingulate gyrus* (q.v.).

**callosal syndromes**   See *corpus callosum.*

**callosotomy**   A surgical procedure that severs only the *corpus callosum* (q.v.), either in part or in its entirety. Commissurotomy, the usual split-brain procedure, severs the corpus callosum and also the anterior commissure, and it may sever the posterior and hippocampal commissures as well.

**calmodulin**   *CaM*; it interacts with calcium channels to mediate calcium-dependent inactivation of the channels, and to transduce the signal from calcium entry through the channels into various intracellular signaling pathways. A single CaM molecule is both necessary and sufficient for calcium-dependent inactivation.

**calpains**   Cysteine proteases activated by calcium that cleave various substrates, including cytoskeletal proteins. One theory of memory proposes that calpain exposes receptors that are hidden deep within the cell's membrane, rendering them more sensitive to neurotransmitters; the resulting strengthening of existing synapses and freeing-up of new synapses account for short-term and long-term memory. See *apoptosis.*

**CAM**   1. Cell adhesion molecule. CAMs are proteins that form sticky regions on the surface of cells that link to similar molecules on other cells, thereby guiding the *neuroblast* (q.v.) to its proper destination. CAMs can serve as repellants as well as attractants; when they recognize molecules on certain cells they guide the neuron away from those cells rather than to them. In addition, some CAMs activate the receptor for fibroblast growth factor, initiating a series of internal cellular events that ultimately produce neurite outgrowth. 2. Complementary and alternative medicine. See *complementary medicine.*

**Camberwell Family Interview**   *CFI*; a semistructured interview used to assess *expressed emotions* (q.v.). Important elements are an ability to share a focus of attention with another person in conversation, the degree to which a speaker's communications are well defined and complete as opposed to amorphous or fragmented, and the coherence and comprehensibility of speech. The schizophrenic or a family member may make unknown or ambiguous references ("The two women came in and I didn't like her."). Reference failures may reflect the speaker's difficulties in the area of concept definition.

**camisole**   A canvas shirt with very long sleeves, used to restrain a violently psychotic person; popularly known as a straitjacket. The shirt is put on and securely laced, and then the patient's arms are folded and the ends of the sleeves are fastened behind the back.

**CAMKII**   *Calcium-calmodulin-dependent kinase II*, an enzyme that adds phosphate groups to other proteins. It is synthesized in the dendrites and plays a key role in synapse strengthening linked to learning and memory.

**camouflage, neurotic**   The endeavor to disguise neurotic symptoms. "The patient wishes to be obedient to the compulsions imposed by the neurosis, but at the same time he feels impelled to make his behavior conform to the requirements of his social milieu" (Reik, T. *American Imago* 2, 1941). See *obsessional rehearsal.*

**cAMP**   Cyclic adenosine monophosphate, an intracellular *second messenger* that can act either directly on a target protein or *ion channel* (qq.v.) or, more commonly, indirectly by activating a protein kinase, which phosphorylates a number of substrate proteins inside the cell. The cAMP pathway is believed to regulate long-term potentiation (LTP) by inhibiting protein phospatases; this opens a gate to allow the transmission of signals for LTP and thereby enhances synaptic responses to subsequent stimuli. The early phase of LTP requires the presence of the cAMP pathway in the postsynaptic cell, but by itself that pathway does not enhance synaptic response. The cAMP pathway itself can function as a gate and regulate signal flow through other pathways. See *long-term memory.*

Although cAMP may be the oldest of the second-messenger systems, it usually acts in combination with other second-messenger systems. Neurotrophin-dependent survival and growth of neurons requires an elevation in cAMP, but cAMP by itself does not promote growth or survival.

**campimeter** A chart upon which the visual field is plotted or projected. See *field defect.*

**camptocormia** Functional bent back; first described by Brodie in 1837, named camptocormia by Souques in 1915. It consists of persistent lumbar pain, anterior bending of the trunk of the body, and an anthropoid posture with head and trunk parallel with the ground and the arms swinging. Often there is a history of trauma, and almost always there is an accompanying *impotence* (q.v.). Most cases reported have been in soldiers; Kosbab reported the only known case in a woman, in 1961. See *Sandler triad.*

**canalization** Restriction of behavior patterns, and particularly the choice of one way of satisfying a drive in preference to all other possible ways. Janet used the term to refer to substitutive discharge of tension.

**cancellation test** Any test in which the subject is instructed to strike out one or more specified symbols that are distributed irregularly within the test material. The symbols may be particular letters, numbers, words, or geometrical figures.

**cancer phobia** A fear of being eaten away or eaten up by neoplastic cells. The fear of being eaten up, whatever rationalized form it takes, is common in neurotics and is based upon fears of retaliation for having sadistically introjected an object. The dangerous introject may have different meanings on different psychic levels; thus it may represent a child, a penis, the breast, milk, etc. In like manner, the fear may be expressed in various ways—as a phantasy of *impregnation*, as a delusion or fear of being *poisoned*, as a fear of *infection*, etc.

**canchasmus** *Obs. Cachinnation* (q.v.).

**candidate gene** A gene within a chromosome region that is associated with a disease; the protein product of the gene suggests that it could be the basis of the disease in question. Cloned genes that map in the region of a mutant for involvement in the phenotype associated with a mutation are tested for *linkage* (q.v.) to the disease. See *SNPs.*

**cannabinoids** See *cannabis.*

**cannabis** Any of the psychoactive substances (*cannabinoids*) contained in the Indian hemp plant (*Cannabis sativa*); the most important one is δ-9- tetrahydrocannabinol (THC), which has both depressant and hallucinogenic effects. The dried leaves and flowering tops of the plant are commonly termed *marijuana* (q.v.) or *ganga*; the resin of the plant is called *hashish*. *Bhang* is a drink (infusion) made from cannabis; it is also known as *beng* and *churus*. Cannabis has been used as a therapeutic agent for glaucoma and as an antinauseant in cancer chemotherapy.

**cannabis delusional disorder** A rare, self-limited syndrome consisting of persecutory delusions, anxiety, depersonalization, visual or auditory hallucinations, and sometimes amnesia for the episode. It typically remits within a day. Chronic psychosis attributable solely to cannabis use is even more rare; it has been reported (under the names *hemp insanity* and *cannabis psychosis*) mainly in India, Egypt, and Morocco, and more in the late 19th and early 20th centuries than currently.

**cannabis organic mental disorders** *Cannabis use disorders* (q.v.).

**cannabis psychosis** *Cannabis delusional disorder* (q.v.).

**cannabis use disorders** Psychiatric disorders associated with the use of cannabis (marijuana). They are classified within the substance-related disorders and include cannabis dependence, cannabis abuse, cannabis intoxication, cannabis delirium, cannabis psychotic disorder, cannabis mood disorder, cannabis anxiety disorder, cannabis sleep disorder, and cannabis sexual dysfunction. See *amotivational syndrome; marijuana.*

**cannibalistic fixation** The fixation of the libido and/or aggressive energy at the late oral or biting phase. This may lead to later cannibalistic impulses, such as the phantasy of biting and eating, swallowing, and incorporating a hated object.

**Cannon, Walter B.** (1871–1945) American physiologist, whose broad-ranging studies led ultimately to enunciation of the principles of homeostasis ("wisdom of the body"). His experiments in diagnostic roentgenography stimulated his interest in esophageal and gastrointestinal motility and subsequently to recognition of the role of the autonomic nervous system, humoral transmission, and "sympathin." From that point he turned to a study of shock and the role of the adrenal medulla and then to investigation of the central nervous system basis for emotion.

**Cannon hypothalamic theory of emotion** Cannon and Bard offered a more modern version of Head's thalamic theory: afferent impulses from peripheral receptors may evoke patterned efferent "emotional" responses directly through reflex pathways at the thalamic level and/or indirectly through arousal of "conditioned responses" at the cortical level, which in turn release diencephalically integrated patterns of emotional response from cortical inhibition. At the same time, upward discharges from the activated diencephalon reach the cortex, thus adding a patterned "quale" to the sensory experience and transforming the "object-simply-apprehended" to the "object-emotionally-felt."

**Capgras, Jean Marie Joseph** (1873–1950) French psychiatrist. See *Capgras syndrome.*

**Capgras syndrome** The delusional belief in the existence of identical doubles of significant others or of oneself or both, such as the delusion that one's spouse has been replaced by one or more imposters. See *misidentification, delusional.* The syndrome was first described in 1923 by J. Capgras and J. Reboul-Lachaux and is also known as *illusions of doubles, illusion des sosies,* or *illusions of false recognition.* It is to be distinguished from defects of memory, perception, or recognition, hallucination, illusion, and *prosopagnosia* (q.v.).

One variant is the autoscopic type in which the patient sees his or her "double" in nearby persons or objects; another is the hallucinatory autoscopic variant, a major theme in some of Edgar Allan Poe's stories (1839) and Dostoyevsky's novel *The Double* (1846). The syndrome of misidentification of persons may occur at any age, typically the result of a combination of psychopathologic and neuropathologic etiologies. Robin Maugham wrote of a visit to his uncle, W. Somerset Maugham, then 90 years of age. WS asked: "Do you know my nephew Robin? He's a very pleasant person." R replied: "But I am Robin." Later that morning, WS asked Robin: "Does my nephew look like you?"

The syndrome may develop following a change in significant interpersonal relationships, which leads to negative feelings so different and alien to the subject that he rejects the idea that they could be attributable to the previously loved person. They must, instead,

be due to an imposter or double. Such delusions occur as part of a paranoid schizophrenic picture, as well as in organic disorders and affective psychoses. The Capgras syndrome has also been reported following both localized and general organic brain disease, including frontal lobe trauma, subarachnoid bleeding, dementia, temporal lobe epilepsy, and increased intracranial pressure.

In the Capgras delusion, splitting provides a good object, the "real" one, to be admired and revered, and a bad object, the "impostor" or the "double," to be criticized and hated. The delusion is also described as a negative misidentification in that it denies the genuineness of a known person (though admitting a resemblance). In contrast, the *Frègoli phenomenon* (the *illusion de Frègoli,* the *illusion of a negative double*) is a positive misidentification, consisting of a belief that a persecutor has assumed the guise of various people whom the subject encounters in his or her daily life. (Frègoli was an actor famed for his ability to alter his appearance.) See *intermetamorphosis syndrome.*

**captation** *Obs.* Used by Descourtis to denote the first stage in hypnosis.

**captative attitude** The early ego's appraisal of the external world solely in terms of the self. See *narcissism.*

**captivation** Max Hirsch's term for the state of light hypnosis; Hirschlaff called the state one of *pseudohypnosis.*

**caput obstipum** *Obs.* See *torticollis.*

**carbamates** See *sedatives/hypnotics.*

**carbamazepine** An *anticonvulsant* drug (q.v.) that has also been used in the treatment of bipolar mood disorders.

**carbohydrate metabolism** The nervous system depends on glucose for most of its energy and uses other sugars only poorly, if at all. Yet there is little glucose storage in nervous tissue, so its functioning depends on how much glucose is circulating in the blood.

*Hyperglycemia* is abnormally high blood glucose. It is a prominent feature of untreated *diabetes mellitus,* characterized by an inability of cells to oxidize glucose. The resultant hyperglycemia leads to glycosuria (a spillover of excess blood glucose into the urine), polyuria, and ketosis (incomplete combustion of long-chain fatty acids). Unless hyperglycemia is severe enough to result in coma, few mental symptoms can be attributed to it. An acute organic syndrome with disturbed behavior may signal impending coma; accompanying physical signs include rapid pulse, low blood pressure, dehydration, and a smell of acetone on the breath.

*Hypoglycemia* is abnormally low blood glucose. It is a popular diagnosis but a rare condition, except for hyperinsulinism induced by therapeutic insulin. It also occurs in insulinoma (a pancreatic tumor), glycogen storage disease, alcoholism, and liver disease. Symptoms are due to sympathetic nervous system stimulation (weakness, palpitations, tachycardia, sweating, tremor, ataxic gait) and to inadequate cerebral supply of nutrient (slowed thinking, irritability, aggressiveness, anxiety and other mood changes, sometimes confusion). With progression, somnolence alternates with agitation and finally the patient lapses into coma. Persisting hypoglycemia or, more rarely, repeated minor hypoglycemic episodes may lead to personality changes, paranoid thinking, memory disturbances, and dementia.

Many inborn errors of carbohydrate metabolism have been identified, including lactose intolerance (deficiency of lactase in the intestinal mucosa results in malabsorption of ingested lactose); galactosemia (inability to utilize ingested galactose because of absence of two enzymes); and at least eight forms of glycogen storage disease, each due to the lack of a specific enzyme in glycogen catabolism, resulting in deposition of abnormal quantities of glycogen or its intermediates in various organs. See *galactosemia*.

**carbon dioxide inhalation therapy**  A form of somatic treatment introduced in 1945 by von Meduna (who also introduced Metrazol convulsive treatment for schizophrenia); rarely used nowadays. In $CO_2$ inhalation therapy, the patient breathes from a cylinder containing a mixture of 30% $CO_2$ and 70% $O_2$ to the point of unconsciousness. Treatments are given two or three times a week, sometimes to as many as 100 treatments. The method is of limited usefulness; those who find it of some value feel that it is best suited to traumatic hysteria with dissociation, to conversion symptoms of recent origin, and to anxiety hysteria.

**Card Sort**  See Wisconsin Card Sort(ing) test.

**card sorting**  See *sorting tests*.

**cardiac neurosis**  See asthenia, neurocirculatory.

**cardiazol**  Metrazol. See *Metrazol treatment*.

**cardiospasm**  See *achalasia*.

**care**  In medicine, provision of services to help a patient or client deal with his or her illness. Care includes therapeutic interventions directed toward ameliorating or curing illness or disability as well as a range of supervising, monitoring, and managing activities that will improve the quality of the recipient's quality of life. In mental health epidemiologic surveys, care is often divided into the following:

1. *Formal care*, which includes
   a. *general medical care* (general practitioner, family physician, company doctor, cardiologist, gynecologist or other physician; nurse; occupational therapist; or other health professional who is not a social worker or counselor); and
   b. *specialty care* (psychiatrist, psychologist, psychiatric social worker, etc.);
   c. *human services care* (social worker or counselor in a social or government agency, in a private office, or general health-care setting); and

2. *Informal care* (minister, priest, rabbi, self-help group, telephone hotline, spiritualist, herbalist, natural healer/therapist, folk healer, "santero", astrologer, "sobador", psychic, medium).

**care, alternate level of**  See *ALC*.

**carebaria**  Unpleasant head sensations, such as pressure or heaviness in the head.

**caregiver**  Any person involved in the identification or treatment or prevention of illness, and in the rehabilitation of patients. The *primary physician* (typically, the general practitioner in the community to whom the patient comes for help, no matter what the nature of the problem or illness) is often termed the front-line caregiver. Another type of caregiver is the indigenous worker—the person from the population being serviced who has had special training in diagnostic or treatment techniques and whose function is "to find out from the residents of the neighborhood how they saw their needs, and to explore with them the ways in which we [i.e., the professionals of the Community Mental Health Center] could or could not be helpful" (Peck, H. B., Roman, M. & Kaplan, S. R. *Psychiatric Research Report 21*, APA, April 1967). A third type of caregiver, the indigenous therapist, is a member of a community who uses sociologic circumstances peculiar to the predominant ethnic and culture groups of that community in an attempt to correct, ameliorate, or modify physical and/or mental disorders. A fourth type of caregiver is the family and sometimes also the patient's social support network. See *care; enabler.*

**CARE-HD**   Coenzyme $Q_{10}$ and remacemide evaluation in Huntington disease; a study of the ability of such therapy to delay disability in patients with early HD. The coenzyme is a substrate for mitochondrial electron transport, and remacemide is an NMDA glutamate antagonist. The rationale of the study is that mitochondrial energy defects and glutamate-mediated excitatory neurotransmission act as *propagating factors* (q.v.) in HD. A similar study of possible *neuroprotection* in Parkinson disease is *DATATOP* (qq.v.).

**carezza**   Also karezza; coitus prolongatus, *coitus reservatus* (q.v.).

**cargo selection**   See *Golgi apparatus.*

**carnosine**   A dipeptide, β-alanyl histidine, that is highly concentrated in olfactory areas of the brain. It is a derivative of histamine, but its function in brain is not known.

**carotodynia**   Pain in the malar (cheek) region, in the back of the neck, and about the eyes due to pressure on the common carotid artery.

**carpal tunnel syndrome**   Numbness, tingling, and other painfulparesthesias in the hands and fingers (especially the middle three), frequently worst at night. It is often misdiagnosed as somatization, but it is due to compression of the median nerve in the carpal tunnel (as in fracture or arthritis of the wrist) or to *pyridoxine* (vitamin $B_6$) deficiency (q.v.). The latter may occur as a side effect of treatment with monoamine oxidase inhibitors. The syndrome may also be a manifestation of repetitive strain disorder (repetitive stress injury).

**carphology**   *Crocidismus*; *trichologia*; *floccillation*; aimless picking or plucking at the clothes or bed coverings, a frequent symptom in the deliria and dementias.

**carrier**   See taint carrier; trait carrier.

**carrier screening**   See *genetic screening.*

**cART**   Combination antiretroviral therapy; also known as highly active ART, or *HAART* (q.v.).

**cascade**   A small but steep waterfall. The term is used in neuroscience to describe serial

activation along a neural pathway (in other registers, the "domino effect" is used in similar fashion). Induction of a protein at the beginning of the pathway stimulates another protein(s) farther down the path; that protein, in turn, stimulates other proteins still farther down the path, and so on until the final point or target is reached. See *caspase cascade; cytokines.*

**cascade model**   In information processing, a process in which later stages can begin before completion of earlier stages. This is in contrast to the *discrete model*, in which computations at any stage must be completed before the subsequent step can be taken.

**case ethics**   See *casuistry.*

**case management**   One of the models through which services are provided to patients; its focus is on early identification of potential high-cost cases (e.g., through hospital preadmission certification) and the development of alternative treatment plans. Once a high-cost case is identified, the patient case manager (PCM) or gatekeeper (q.v.) typically conducts a telephone assessment by conferring with the patient's attending physician, in order to define the problem, develop treatment objectives, target a discharge date, and coordinate follow-up outpatient care. See *managed care.*

The term encompasses a wide range of actual practices. In some settings, case managers function as primary therapists; in others, they are ombudsmen who negotiate with service providers on behalf of clients; in still others they are facilitators who work with the patient's physician, family, and insurance carrier to formulate cost-effective approaches to treatment in order to reduce costs and achieve optimal outcomes.

**case mix**   The relative frequency of different types of patients treated at a particular site. In prospective payment approaches, a hospital's case mix is determined by principal and secondary diagnoses, age, discharge status, operating room procedures, and significant or substantial comorbidities and complications.

**case-control study**   See *methodology.*

**casework, social**   One of the major divisions of *social work* (q.v.), along with social group work and community organization or social welfare planning. Its concern is with social relationships and its goals are release of individual capacities and the relief of environmental pressures.

**CASH** Comprehensive Assessment of Symptoms and History; a structured interview designed to record current symptoms and past history; it is more detailed than the *PSE* and *SADS* (qq.v.) and better able to detect negative symptoms of schizophrenia as well as symptoms of the schizophrenic spectrum of disorders (rather than only the symptoms of core schizophrenia). Other scales have been designed that focus specifically on schizophrenia and include not only current manifestations and past history but also the changes in symptoms over time. Among the latter are *SANS* and *SAPS* (qq.v.).

**caspase cascade** Cell death is the outcome of a genetically programmed intracellular cascade, which is centered on the activation of *caspases* (q.v.). A proapoptotic signal that the cells have been stressed or damaged or has received an order to die culminiates in the activation of an initiator caspase which, in turn, activates effector caspases (the executioners), which then make selected cuts in key proteins resulting in cellular disassembly. See *apoptosis*; *apoptotic pathway*.

**caspases** A family of cystein proteases that cleave proteins at specific aspartate residues and have a key role in inflammation and mammalian *apoptosis* (q.v.).

**castration** Surgical removal of the ovaries (ovariectomy, oophorectomy) or of the testes (orchidectomy). The result in females is loss of the ability to produce ova and elimination of estrus, and in males loss of the ability to produce sperm. Castration is now used only for medical reasons (e.g., control of prostatic and breast carcinomas). For eugenic purposes, sterilization by vasectomy or salpingectomy is preferred to castration, since it affects only reproductive capacity, whereas castration affects both reproductive capacity and secondary sex characteristics.

When performed or occurring after puberty, castration has in neither sex such drastic effects as are observed following surgical removal of the sex organs in early life, when the secondary sex characteristics of the organism have not yet developed. Castration before puberty results in *eunuchoidism* or eunuchism—the development of the secondary sexual characteristics of the opposite sex. Eunuchoid women are recognizable by male body proportions, deep voice, and hairiness of body and face, and eunuchoid men by large hips, narrow sloping shoulders, absence of beard and body hair, high-pitched voice, etc.

In psychoanalytic theory castration means loss of the penis, and the castration complex refers to the boy's fear of loss or injury to his penis, and the girl's concern that she lacks a penis. The castration complex is typically associated with the phallic stage of psychosexual development, and the manner in which the castration complex is handled determines in large part the fate of the *Oedipus complex* (q.v.). See *autocastration; penis envy; ontogeny, psychic.*

**castration anxiety** Fear of genital loss or injury. See *anxiety*. The castration complex has its origins in the pregenital stage of development. From the time of birth, the infant suffers various deprivations and losses. They are indelibly imprinted on the psyche and appear later in the form of character traits, depending on the way they were solved or resolved in the early years.

**castration complex, active** The ideas centered around the fear of losing the penis and the emotions linked with these ideas. The passive castration complex is the idea that the penis has already been lost and/or the wish to lose the penis.

**castrophilia** *Obs.* See *transvestitism.*

**castrophrenia** *Nooklopia* (q.v.).

**casuistry** The science of dealing with matters of conscience and questions of right and wrong in conduct. The term is often used in a derogatory sense to refer to the highly specific rules used by casuists and the certainty they express about the unacceptability of specific types of conduct. The casuist's approach to *case ethics* is to apply practical traditions (e.g., the Jewish halachah, the Catholic casus conscientiae, Protestant case morality, common law), based on experience with concrete modes of behavior, rather than to try to develop abstract and general principles.

**CAT** Choline acetyltransferase (q.v.).

**cat cry syndrome** A cytogenetic abnormality consisting of deletion of the distal portion of the short arm of chromosome number 5; manifestations include a high, piercing, catlike cry due to laryngomalacia (*cri-du-chat*); mental retardation, microcephaly, moonlike facies, hypertelorism, bilateral epicanthus, low-set ears, tiny external genitalia, laryngeal abnormalities, and abnormal palmar dermatoglyphs. The syndrome was first described in 1963 by L. Lejeune.

**CAT scan** Computed axial tomography scan (CT scan is preferred). See *imaging, brain; tomography.*

**catabolic** Pertaining to, or characterized by, *catabolism* (q.v.). In constitutional medicine, the term refers to the anabolic-catabolic balance. The catabolic biotype includes the microsplanchnic, dolichomorphic, and sympathicotonic type of other classifications.

**catabolism** In physiology and general medicine, *destructive metabolism* or a series of changes by which complex bodies are broken down into simpler forms.

**catabythismus** *Obs.* Suicide by drowning.

**cataclonia, cataclonus** Rhythmic convulsive movements, especially when psychically determined.

**catagelophobia** Fear of ridicule. See *agoraphobia.*

**catalepsy** Abnormal maintenance of postures or physical attitudes; also called *carus catalepsia, flexibilitas cerea* (*waxy flexibility*). Its possible manifestations include masklike facies, posturing, resistance to movement, decreased spontaneity, and negativism. Catalepsy is often associated with other motor abnormalities, such as echopraxia, echolalia, and command automatism.

*Rigid catalepsy* refers to taut and rigid "waxlike postures"; it is also called *congelatio, gelatio* (frozen postures), *lead pipe rigidity.* Cataleptic states are most frequently observed in catatonic schizophrenia, in epilepsy, and among patients with cerebellar lesions or lesions of the frontocerebellar pathway. At one time they were reported frequently as a manifestation of hysteria. See *catatonic schizophrenia.*

**catalepsy, artificial** Catalepsy occurring during induced hypnosis.

**catalepsy, epidemic** Cataleptic states appearing simultaneously in many persons, as a consequence of imitation or identification.

**catalexia** A type of reading disability characterized by a tendency to reread words and phrases.

**catalogia** Catalexia; cataphasia; logoclonia; verbigeration (qq.v.).

**catalysator, catalyzator** An external stimulus that serves to loosen inhibitions; a catalyzer.

**catalytic agent** In group psychotherapy, a patient who activates catharsis in other patients.

**catamite** *Rare.* A male (the term implies a young boy) who adopts a passive or receptive role in homosexual activity. See *active.*

**catamnesis** The medical history of a patient following a given illness, the so-called follow-up history; sometimes used to refer to the history of the patient and his or her illness following the initial examination.

**cataphasia** The repetition of words or phrases, seen in pronounced form in catatonic schizophrenia. See *stereotypy; verbigeration.*

**cataphora** A form of coma that may be interrupted by transitory states of partial consciousness; *coma somnolentium.*

**cataphrenia** *Pseudodementia* (q.v.).

**cataplexy** Temporary paralysis or immobilization; loss of antigravity muscle tone without loss of consciousness, often precipitated by emotional excitement. Cataplexy is usually associated with *narcolepsy* (q.v.). It is exacerbated by alpha-1 noradrenergic blockers and improved by amphetamine and related drugs and by antidepressants. It results from triggering, during a waking period, activity of the neurons that suppress muscle tone in REM sleep.

**cataplexy of awakening** See *sleep paralysis.*

**cataptosis** Galen's term for an epileptic or apoplectic seizure.

**catastrophe theory** The belief that the act of sexual intercourse is destructive to the penis.

**catastrophic behavior** A term introduced by Kurt Goldstein in 1939 to describe a type of behavior disorder that seemed more or less characteristic, of patients suffering from aphasia. This symptomatic behavior takes the form of an inability to carry on a simple course of action once it is interrupted. The patients "become agitated and fearful and more than usually inept when presented with once simple tasks that they can no longer do." Other symptoms of the catastrophic reaction include outbursts of anger, tearfulness, shouting, swearing, refusal, compensatory boasting, and sometimes aggressive behavior. The catastrophic reaction to brain injury is seen more frequently in patients with left hemisphere damage. In contrast, the *indifference reaction* (q.v.) is more frequent in right hemisphere damage.

**catastrophic reaction** Seen typically in patients who have suffered a stroke involving the left hemisphere: restlessness, irritability, anxiety, tearfulness, hyperemotionality, and uncooperativeness.

**catastrophic thinking**  In *obsessive-compulsive disorder* (q.v.), the feared element in obsessional thinking, the misfortune or disaster that the patient anticipates will befall him/her or loved ones should he not perform the compulsion called for by his obsessional thought.

**catathymia**  In psychoanalysis, the existence in the unconscious of a complex that is sufficiently charged with affects to produce effects in consciousness.

**catathymic amnesia**  Circumscribed loss of memory that is limited to a single experience. For example, a patient with clear memory for all other events had no memory for circumstances connected with her pregnancy.

**catathymic crisis**  Usually, an isolated, nonrepetitive act of violence that, though occurring suddenly, develops from a background of intolerable tension. See *impulse control disorders; explosive disorder*.

**catatonia**  A lowering of tension; in psychiatry it refers to a group of postural and movement abnormalities, such as catalepsy, stupor, hyperkinesiae, stereotypies, mannerisms, automatisms, and impulsivity. The most commonly observed clinical signs are immobility, staring, mutism, stupor, withdrawal, refusal to eat, posturing, rigidity, perseveration, echophenomen, automatic obedience, and hyperkinesiae. Modern descriptions of the clinical condition were first given in 1874 by Kahlbaum, who considered it a nosologic entity. Kraepelin, however, applied it to a subtype of schizophrenia, where it occurs in one of two general forms: catatonic stupor, associated with muscular rigidity or flexibility, and catatonic excitement, associated with overactivity, stereotypies, hyperkinesiae, and impulsivity. In fact, catatonia is more often associated with mania, melancholia, and psychotic depression than with schizophrenia. It is also seen in autism and in association with general medical conditions (such as metabolic disorders), drug intoxications (including the neuroleptic malignant syndrome and toxic serotonin syndrome), and neurological disorders (such as seizure disorders, encephalitis, and frontal circuitry disorders). The similarities between catatonia and parkinsonism suggest that aberrant signaling in the basal ganglia is central to both disorders.

M. A. Taylor and M. Fink (*American Journal of Psychiatry 160*, 2003) have proposed that catatonia be recognized as a distinct nosologic syndrome with three categories: nonmalignant catatonia (*Kahlbaum syndrome*), delirious catatonia (including delirious mania and excited catatonia), and malignant catatonia (characterized by acute onset of excitement, delirium, fever, autonomic instability, and catalepsy). Exposure to antipsychotic agents, both typical and atypical, usually worsens catatonia or induces the malignant form.

Antipsychotic drugs precipitate a malignant syndrome in patients with catatonia, so it is important to differentiate between *catatonic schizophrenia* (q.v.) and other forms of catatonia. About 80% of patients with catatonia will show symptomatic improvement after a challenge dose of lorazepam or amobarbital.

**catatonia, deadly**  See *Bell mania*.

**catatonia, depressive**  Synonymous with, but rarely used today for catatonic stupor. See *catatonic schizophrenia*.

**catatonia, lethal**  See *Bell mania*.

**catatonia, manic**  *Rare*. Catatonic excitement. See *catatonic schizophrenia*.

**catatonia mitis**  A mild and relatively short course of catatonia, with stupor and immobility as the principal symptoms. More extensive catatonic syndromes are termed *catatonia protracta*.

**catatonic schizophrenia**  One of the subgroups of schizophrenia (in the older literature, dementia praecox) that may appear as a chronic form or as an acute episode in the course of a schizophrenic pattern. As with any type of schizophrenia, the fundamental symptoms afford the basis for the diagnosis, although the subgrouping into the catatonic type is largely dependent upon certain secondary or accessory symptoms—catalepsy, stupor, hyperkinesiae, stereotypies, mannerisms, negativism, automatisms, and impulsivity.

Onset is acute in 41% of cases; in 31% of cases chronic paranoid symptoms precede the development of catatonic symptoms, and in the remaining cases the onset is subacute. In general, symptoms may be seen to fall into one of two categories: (1) catatonic stupor, including catalepsy, stupor, and negativism; and (2) catatonic excitement, including hyperkinesiae, stereotypies, mannerisms, automatisms, and impulsivity.

Catalepsy may appear as immobile or masklike facies, as posturing, resistance to movements, decreased spontaneity in movement, or less commonly, as *cerea flexibilitas* (waxy flexibility). The hyperkinesiae include arbitrary, automatic, pseudospontaneous movements, while the stereotypies include movements, actions, posturings, speech, writings, or drawings that are monotonously repetitive and that bear little obvious relationship to external reality.

*Schnauzkrampf* (q.v.) is a particular type of stereotypy. Mannerisms are not necessarily stereotyped, but they are nonetheless inappropriate, inadequately modifiable, and caricature-like. Negativism may appear in several forms: (1) external negativism, or negation of commands; (2) inner negativism, or oppositional thoughts (actually a type of intellectual ambivalence, but often misinterpreted as "obsessive thinking"); (3) active negativism, the active opposition of commands; (4) passive negativism, which often appears as stubbornness or uncooperativeness; (5)command-negativism, or doing exactly the opposite of what is ordered. Automatisms may also be expressed in various ways, such as echopraxia or echolalia (forms of command-automatism), or as fugues, self-injuries, or coprolalia. Impulsivity is commonly seen in catatonic schizophrenia and on occasion can lead to suicidal attempts or homicidal outbursts.

**catatonoid attitude**  Stereotyped behavior that substitutes for the emotional response that would be expected in a social situation. For example, the same vacant smile adorns the person's countenance when he hears his friend's story of a recent personal tragedy as when he is told an uproarious anecdote.

**catatony**  A rarely used Anglicized form of catatonia.

**catchment area**  See *community psychiatry*.

**catchup saccades**  See *saccades*.

**catecholamine**  *Adrenergic amine*; the group includes dopamine (DA), norepinephrine (NE, also known as noradrenaline), and epinephrine (adrenaline). The biosynthetic pathway for the catecholamines is as follows: tyrosine → dihydroxyphenylalanine → dopamine → norepinephrine → epinephrine.

Within the brain, the catecholamines function as neurotransmitters. About 1% of neurons use dopamine as a neurotransmitter; another 1% use norepinephrine. Because their postsynaptic effects are mediated by chemical reactions, they are slower in action than acetylcholine, whose rapid action is mediated by the opening of specific ionic channels in the neuroreceptor molecule. See *neurotransmitter; synapse.*

Epinephrine neurons, relatively few in number, are concentrated in the brain stem. Noradrenergic neurons occur in small groups throughout the brain stem; the largest concentration is in the locus coeruleus. Dopamine neurons are concentrated in the midbrain. They have been studied extensively because of the discovery that Parkinson disease and schizophrenia are alleviated by drugs that interact with dopamine neurons. See *adrenergic receptor; dopamine.*

**catecholamine hypothesis**  In relation to affective disorders, the hypothesis states that some or all depressions are associated with a relative deficiency of norepinephrine at functionally important adrenergic receptor sites in the brain and that elations (manias) are associated with an excess of such amines. It is no longer believed that depression is the result of a single monoamine deficiency. See *serotonin hypothesis.*

**categorical attitude**  *Abstract attitude* (q.v.).

**categorical imperative**  In psychoanalysis, the equivalent of *blanket demand*. The superego, for instance, is said to exercise its duties by the rigid "yes" or "no" rule, by the "all or none" law.

**categorical perception**  In language studies, discrimination of the acoustic events that distinguish phonetic units. A change of 10 ms in the time domain changes /b/ to /p/, and equivalently small differences in the frequency domain change /p/ to /k/. Each language uses a unique set of only about 40 distinct elements, phonemes, which change the meaning of a word (for example, from /bat/ to /pat/). Infants can discriminate these subtle differences from birth. See *language acquisition.*

**categorical system**  An all-or-none approach to the classification of disorders; on the basis of specified thresholds, a subject falls within the disease category or does not (e.g., subject must show 6 of 11 symptoms or signs to qualify for the diagnosis of X). Critics of the system point out that the thresholds are often arbitrary, that the use of all-or-nothing diagnostic categories obscures potentially important clinical information, and that there is extensive overlap or comorbidity among categories.

Categorical cutoffs ignore the impairment that occurs in below-threshold cases. In addition, they are not always appropriate in populations with different lifestyles than the countries in which they have been developed. In child psychiatry, categorical approaches fail to consider important sources of variance, such as developmental stage, gender, informant (teacher vs. parent vs. child), ethnicity, and comorbidity. See *dimensional system*; *nosology*.

**categorical thinking** See *physiognomonic thinking*.

**categorization** A decision about an object's kind, requiring generalization across members of a class of objects even though they have different shapes, colors, etc.

**categorization, symbolic** A type of abstract thinking that requires the subject to make a mental diagram of relationships in order to answer the question posed; it is used as a measure of dominant parietal lobe functioning. An example is: What is the relationship to you of your brother's mother? Of your brother's mother-in-law?

**categorizing** See *selective attention*.

**category mistake** To mix elements from different realms on the incorrect assumption that they are alike in kind. Ethics, for example, deals with values, biology with facts; if science be likened to a ship belonging to the material world, then ethics is a nonmaterial set of beliefs that should guide the ship's tiller.

**category test** Seven sets of stimulus figures (a total of 208 items) are shown to the subject; the first six sets are organized according to six principles, and the seventh set is a mixture of previously shown items. The subject presses a key to indicate the principle used in each item shown.

**catharsis** In psychiatry the term was first used by Freud to designate a type of psychotherapy. Psychiatric symptoms or symbols are looked upon as disguised representations of forgotten and repressed ideas or experiences. When the latter are brought back into the sphere of consciousness and lived out fully (in a therapeutic sense), the method is called catharsis. *Abreaction* and *catharsis* are often used synonymously.

**catharsis, activity** In psychotherapy, especially in activity group psychotherapy, the expression of unconscious preoccupations and conscious intent through *action* rather than through language.

**catharsis, community** Abreaction in a group, as in *psychodrama* (q.v.).

**catharsis, emotional** *Catharsis; abreaction* (qq.v.).

**cathect, cathecticize** To charge with, to infuse with psychic energy. See *cathexis*.

**catheterophilia** A *paraphilia* (q.v.) in which the necessary condition for sexual gratification is that a catheter or other foreign body (e.g., swizzle stick, garter snake) be inserted into the urethra.

**cathexis** Concentration of psychic energy on a given object; investment of the psychic energy of a drive in a conscious or unconscious mental representation such as a concept, idea, image, phantasy, or symbol. Included are the following types:

1. *Ego-cathexis*—when the psychic energy is attached to the conscious division of the ego. Hence, the expressions ego-libido and narcissism arise. Some use the term *self-libido* or *autolibido* in contradistinction to *object-libido*.

2. *Phantasy-cathexis*—when psychic energy is attached to wish-formations or phantasies or to their original sources in the unconscious. Both ego-cathexis and phantasy-cathexis are associated with primary narcissism.

3. *Object-cathexis*—psychic energy that is attached to some object outside the subject or to its representation in the mind of the subject. Object-cathexis is less stable or fixed than the other forms, because it is associated with manifestations of secondary narcissism, which, in turn, are less durable than those of the primary kind.

When there is an overcharge of psychic energy in an object, the term *hypercathexis* is used; when an undercharge, *hypocathexis*. Other words are often prefixed to the term cathexis: (1) to signify the quality of the charge—adjectives, as in affective-cathexis, libidinal-cathexis, erotic-cathexis, instinctual-cathexis; nouns, as in word-cathexis, thought-cathexis, thing-cathexis, or (2) to express the degree of cathexis, as in hyper-cathexis, hypocathexis, acathexis.

**cathisophobia** Fear of sitting.

**CATIE** Clinical Antipsychotic Trials of Intervention Effectiveness, a multicenter, multiphase, multidrug study of the most actively marketed antipsychotics. CATIE is a practical clinical trial, falling between naturalistic observational studies and methodologically rigorous RCTs (randomized control trials). The initial trials found few differences between first-generation antipsychotics and second-generation antipsychotics; the second-generation antipsychotics may show superiority in the most severely affected subgroup of patients with schizophrenia.

A total of 1493 patients entered phase 2 of the study, the results of which suggested a superiority of olanzapine in length of time to drug discontinuation. In the phase 2 "tolerability" study, clozapine showed a nearly three-fold increase in time until drug discontinuation compared with the three new antipsychotics (olanzapine, risperidone, and quetiapine). There was a significantly greater side effect burden with clozapine, however: weight gain, increased metabolic measures, sialorrhea, sedation, and agranulocytosis.

The CATIE results make it clear that to find the right drug for each patient often requires sequential trials of medications; patients vary greatly in their responsiveness to, and tolerability of, different antipsychotic drugs.

**cation channel** See *ion channel*.

**catochus** *Obs.* Catalepsy, especially that phase of ecstasy or trance in which the patient is conscious but cannot move or speak.

**cauda equina** The spinal roots projecting to and from the lumbar and sacral segments. During development, the vertebral column lengthens more than does the spinal cord within it, so that at birth the spinal cord ends at the level of the third lumbar vertebra (in adults, at the first lumbar vertebra). The space around the cauda equina is the *lumbar cistern*, from which cerebrospinal fluid is withdrawn by *lumbar puncture* without danger of damage to the spinal cord itself.

**caudate** A C-shaped mass of gray matter that arches posteriorly and then turns foward to end in the *amygdala* (q.v.). The caudate nucleus is part of the *basal ganglia* (q.v.). Huntington disease is characterized by atrophy of the caudate nucleus; OCD is associated with functional hyperactivity of the right caudate nucleus.

**causalgia** *Reflex sympathetic dystrophy* characterized by a sensation of burning pain in the distribution of a peripheral nerve, associated with glossy skin devoid of hair or wrinkles.

Other associated changes include swelling, redness, sweating, and curling of the nails. Causalgia is usually due to irritation of a nerve by injury; the median or sciatic nerves are most commonly involved. See *pain syndromes*.

**CAVD** A measure of intelligence, devised by Thorndike, consisting of a battery of four tests: completion, arithmetic, vocabulary, and direction-following.

**cavum septi pellucidi** A cavity separating the two layers of the septum pellucidum. In the fetus, the separation is normal, and ordinarily it shrinks before birth and disappears before adulthood. Brains of schizophrenic patients show an increase in prevalence of cavum retention, one of the several manifestations of structural abnormalities of the limbic region in schizophrenia.

**CB1** A cannabinoid receptor. See $\Delta^9$-*THC*.

**CBA** *Cost/benefit analysis* (q.v.).

**CBD** *Corticobasal degeneration* (q.v.).

**CBT** *Cognitive behavior therapy* (q.v.).

**CCC** Citrated calcium carbamide; like *disulfiram*, an alcohol-sensitizing (aversive) agent, used outside the United State in chemical aversive conditioning. Its use in this country was curtailed by its high rate of serious side effects, including cardiac toxicity, hepatitis, and risk for Malory Weiss syndrome. See *relapse prevention*.

**CCI** Calcium channel inhibitor (or blocker); the major ones in use in the United States are *diltiazem*, nifedipine, and verapamil. Although their primary use is as antihypertensive agents, they have also been used in psychiatry in the treatment of migraine, convulsive disorders, mood disorders (particularly mania), Gilles de la Tourette syndrome, tardive dyskinesia, and neuroleptic malignant syndrome (NMS), and as an antidote for hypertensive crises associated with monoamine oxidase inhibition. See *calcium channel; ion channel*.

**CCK** Cholecystokinin (q.v.).

**CD95L** *Fas* (q.v.).

**CDC** Centers for Disease Control, an agency of the U.S. Public Health Service; one of its publications is *MMWR*, the *Morbidity and Mortality Weekly Report*.

**CDD** *Childhood disintegrative disorder* (q.v.).

**CDR** Clinical Dementia Rating scale, a global staging scale consisting of six categories that are rated for impairment and then synthesized into a global rating that indicates degree of impairment. The scale evaluates memory, orientation, judgment and problem-solving, community affairs, home and hobbies, and personal care.

**CDRS** Clinical Dementia Rating Scale (of Hughes); assesses orientation; memory, problem solving, activities of daily living, and social interactions.

**CDT** Clock-drawing test; a cognitive screening test that is sensitive to changes in visual-analytic function, attention, and executive functions. It is predictive of cognitive decline in normal populations; and the CDT score reflects the severity of dementia. CDT performance is mediated by the left posterior temporal and the bilateral parietal regions. See *cognitive screening instruments.*

**%CDT** Carbohydrate-deficient *transferrin*, an indicator of heavy alcohol use (five or more drinks/day) during the 2 weeks preceding the time the blood is drawn for testing. Transferrin is a glycoprotein produced in liver cells; it transfers iron from the intestine to cells and organs that need iron to function. Heavy alcohol intake interferes with the manufacture of transferrin, which becomes deficient in carbohydrate sidechains. Under normal conditions, about 1% to 2% of transferrin is carbohydrate deficient; with heavy drinking, the deficiency can rise to 10%. Clinical studies have found that a %CDT of 2.6% is indicative of heavy drinking, and 50%–70% of heavy drinkers have a %CDT higher than 2.6%. A 30% decrease from baseline %CDT indicates that the subject has been abstinent (or has reduced alcohol intake substantially) since the time of testing; a 30% increase, on the other hand, suggests that the subject has increased alcohol intake substantially since the last test. The test may give a false positive result in about 5% of subjects who are not heavy drinkers.

**CEA** *Cost-effectiveness analysis* (q.v.).

**CED** Cell death abnormal; the genes that govern the specific steps in apoptosis. See *apoptotic pathway.*

**cell adhesion molecule** *CAM* (q.v.).

**cell assembly** See *equipotentiality.*

**cell death** Destruction of the cell, either appropriate or inappropriate. Appropriate cell death in most cases is programmed and takes the form of *apoptosis* (q.v.). Inappropriate cell death is unanticipated destruction of a cell that, under normal circumstances, was not programmed to die. Such destruction may take an apoptotic, necrotic (the most typical), or mixed form; see *necrosis, neuronal.*

**cellular enzymes** See *cytosolic proteins.*

**cene-, coene-** Combining form meaning common or general, from Gr. *koinos.*

**cenesthesia** The general sense of bodily existence (and especially the general feeling of well-being or malaise), presumably dependent on multiple stimuli coming from various parts of the body, including sensations of internal organ activity even though these are not necessarily on a conscious level. Such sensations are projected to the *insula* (q.v.), from which they are forwarded to the orbital frontal cortex.

**cenesthopathy** Any localized distortion of body awareness, such as the feeling that a hand has become like jelly; less commonly the term is used to refer to a feeling of general physical ill-being.

**cenophobia** See *kenophobia.*

**cenotrope, coenotrope** Instinct; behavior characteristic of all members of a group having the same biological and experiential background.

**censorship** In psychoanalytic theory, a nonspecific term referring to the critical and evaluative scrutiny to which any instinctual quality or drive impulse is subjected before it is allowed to pass into a higher level of mental organization. Both ego and superego have censorship functions and most typically, at least in the adult, these require some modification of the original drive.

**centering** Goldstein's term for perfect integration of the organism with its environment.

**centimorgan** cM; measure of genetic distance in which the probability of a recombination occurring is 1%; it corresponds roughly to a physical distance of a million bases. Some markers on genetic maps currently in use are as close as 3 centimorgans, while others may be 30 centimorgans or more apart. See *mapping, genetic.*

**central anticholinergic syndrome** *Atropine syndrome*; symptoms include hallucinations, anxiety, short-term memory loss, disorientation, and agitation; seen frequently in patients receiving combinations of psychotropic drugs because of the additive anticholinergic effects of tricyclic antidepressants, the weaker phenothiazines and antiparkinson agents. The syndrome often responds to simple reduction of anticholinergic drug, but in life-threatening situations (as in massive overdosage with tricyclic antidepressant) intramuscular physostigmine can be used as a specific antidote. See *atropine coma therapy.*

**central aphasia**    *Wernicke aphasia* (q.v.).

**central apnea**    See *apnea, central.*

**central conflict**    Horney's term for the intrapsychic struggle between the healthy, constructive forces of the real self and the neurotic, obstructive forces of the idealized self. In general, the central conflict involves the whole self (and not just part of the self, as is the case with basic conflict), is more severe than basic conflict, and is encountered during the course of psychoanalytic treatment.

**central dogma**    See *DNA.*

**central excitatory state**    See *summation.*

**central executive function**    See *short-term memory.*

**central integrative field factor**    The sum total of previous experience that forms the basis for *apperception* (q.v.) and incorporation of new experiences.

**central issue**    In Mann's terminology, the particular theme on which the work of brief psychotherapy will focus. It is different from the complaints voiced by the patient, since they are derived from the central issue. The central issue itself is typically an affective statement to the self of how a person feels now and has always felt about the self. It is formulated to include time, affects, and the image of the self. The last will be found to fall within one of the five categories of feeling about the self: glad, sad, mad, frightened, or guilty. See *time-limited psychotherapy.*

**central nervous system**    *CNS*; it consists of six bilaterally paired divisions—spinal cord; *medulla; pons* and *cerebellum; midbrain; diencephalon;* and *cerebral hemispheres* (qq.v.).

**central nervous system deviation**    See *attention deficit hyperactivity disorder.*

**central pain syndrome**    See *pain syndrome, central.*

**centralist psychology**    The subdivision of psychology that emphasizes the role of higher brain centers in determining behavior. In contrast to this is *peripheralist psychology* (including behaviorism), which attributes the major role in behavior to the receptor and effector organs.

**centration**    Piaget's term for prolonged involuntary attachment of a sensory modality to one part of a field, producing perceptual errors of exaggerations and distortions. Motor behavior based on perception (such as drawing tasks) is often secondarily affected and may thus be used to differentiate between the neurologically impaired, with perceptual distortions, and the emotionally disturbed, with thought disturbances.

**centrencephalic epilepsy**    Generalized (in contrast to focal) epilepsy,  in which extensive areas of both hemispheres are simultaneously activated by epileptic discharge from some midline center (probably the thalamus). See *centrencephalic system; epilepsy.*

**centrencephalic system**    Penfield's term for a hypothesized central structure of neurons in the brain stem responsible for the coherent unity of mental processes; in many respects, the centrencephalic system is similar to the *reticular formation* (q.v.).

**centrifugal**    Radiating or flying off from a center. See *centripetal.*

**centrioles**    See *cytoplasm; neuron.*

**centripetal**    Directed toward the center. In psychiatry the term implies a moving toward the psyche. It is said, for example, that psychoanalysis is a centripetal psychology because of its bias towards a minute and detailed analysis of the patient's associations.

The opposite of centripetal forces (of the mind) are *centrifugal* ones. Jung was the outstanding upholder of the centrifugal point of view, the principal representation of which is his *collective unconscious.*

**centrolobar sclerosis**    See *sclerosis, diffuse.*

**centromere**    The "waist" of a chromosome, a tapered area that separates the arms of the chromosome. In some chromosomes, such as C1, the arms are approximately equal in length; in others, such as C19, the arms at the top are shorter than the arms at the bottom.

**centrosome**    A small body near the cell nucleus, composed of two centrioles and associated pericentriolar material. It replicates before cell division and then, by way of protein cables that radiate from it, helps pull the duplicated chromosomes apart into the daughter cells. The centrosome helps to maintain appropriate microtubule organization and cell cycle progression. It is the focal point in generating the poles of mitotic spindles and the organizing center at other stages of the cell cycle. It is within the centrosome that accumulating proteins, which might otherwise clump together into insoluble inclusion bodies, are linked with ubiquitin molecules and marked for degradation by proteasomes. See *UPS*.

The Cdk2 enzyme, when activated by another enzyme, cyclin E, helps drive cells through the division cycle. The Cdk2–cyclin E (Cdk2-E) complex prods cells to begin making DNA and acts as a trigger to tell the dividing cell to copy its centrosome.

**CEOP** Chronic external ophthalmoplegia plus (typically, ptosis, and myopathy). See *mtDNA*.

**cephalalgia** *Headache*; sometimes a *somatoform disorder* (qq.v.).

**cephalea, epileptic** A type of visceral epilepsy, more common in children than adults, in which paroxysmal headache is the most prominent symptom.

**cephalic index** A measure of head size obtained by dividing the maximal breadth of the head by its maximal length and multiplying by 100. Medium heads (*mesocephaly*) have an index number from 76.0 to 80.9 cm. Long heads (*dolichocephaly*) have an index below 76.0 cm. Broad or short heads (*brachycephaly*) have an index of 81.0 cm or over.

**cephalogenesis** In embryological development, the stage that follows notogenesis and is associated with the origin of the primordia of the head. This stage is initiated by the appearance of the neural plate, the primordium of the nervous system, and the formation of the head fold that delimits the head end of the embryo from the extraembryonic blastoderm. The neural plate forms the floor of the neural groove, which is bounded along both borders by a neural fold developing subsequently into the neural tube, lined with neural ectoderm, from an overlying epidermal ectoderm. The cephalic portion of a neural tube produces three dilatations that later become forebrain, midbrain, and hindbrain, the primordia of the future cerebrum, cerebellum, and pons and medulla oblongata. The later steps in cephalogenesis lead to the formation of the face and the head as well as of the eyes and the ears.

**CERAD** Consortium to Establish a Registry for Alzheimer Disease; its assessment protocol contains a short battery of neuropsychological tests, of memory (word list memory, word list recall, and word list recognition), language (verbal fluency and naming), and intellectual status and constructional praxis (by the MMSE).

**ceraunophobia** *Keraunophobia* (q.v.).

**cerea flexibilitas** See *catalepsy*.

**cerebellar fit** Tonic or cerebellar fits were originally described by Hughlings Jackson in connection with tumors of the vermis. The patient suddenly loses consciousness, falls to the ground, and develops cyanosis; the pupils are immobile and dilated. There is no tongue biting or incontinence. The head is retracted, the back arched, the upper extremities extended and adducted with the forearm pronated, the wrist and hand are flexed and everted. The lower extremities are extended and the toes plantar flexed. There is no clonic phase; the phenomenon is one of decerebrate rigidity.

**cerebellar fossa** See fossa, posterior cranial.

**cerebellar gait** In diseases of the cerebellum, the patient walks unsteadily with a "drunken," wobbly gait. There is lack of association between the movements of the legs and body, so that in walking, the body either lags behind, or is abruptly brought forward, and there is a tendency to reel to one side.

**cerebellar outflow tremor** See *tremor*.

**cerebellar speech** In diseases of the cerebellum, the speech may be jerky, explosive, irregular, and scanning. This condition is also called *asynergic* or *ataxic speech*.

**cerebellum** The "little brain"; a large, oval structure with a laminated appearance that lies in the posterior fossa of the skull behind the pons and medulla. It is joined to the brain stem by three symmetrical tracts, the cerebellar peduncles, consisting of two inferior peduncles (the *restiform body*) and the superior peduncle (*brachium conjunctivum*). It appears grossly to be divided into two lateral lobes, the cerebellar hemispheres, and an unpaired median lobe, the vermis. Although the cerebellum constitutes only 10% of the total volume of the brain, it contains more than half its neurons (~50 billion). Each *Purkinje cell* (q.v.) receives input from approximately 200,000 axons (*parallel fibers*) from granule cells and integrates information from the pontine nuclei and inferior olive. *Climbing fibers* convey information from the inferior olive and each fiber forms multiple synapses with a single Purkinje cell.

Automatic information processing takes place in cerebellar circuits, leaving prefrontal circuits to solve new problems with non–routine informationprocessing.

The cerebellum consists of a thin outer mantle of gray matter (the cerebellar cortex), white matter, and three pairs of deep nuclei—*dentate* (which projects laterally out of the cerebellum), *fastigial* (from the medial roof), and *interposed* (including what are also called the *globose* and *emboliform*) nuclei.

Functionally, the cerebellum is divided into: (1) the *flocculonodular lobe* (or *vestibulocerebellum*), the most primitive part; its input is entirely vestibular and it governs eye movements and body equilibrium during stance and gait; lesions in this area cause disturbances of equilibrium, ataxia (e.g., swaying or staggering), plurosthotonus, titubation, skew deviation of the eyes, nystagmus, and vertigo; (2) the *spinocerebellum* (or *palaeocerebellum*), which extends through the central portion of the vermis and cerebellar hemispheres; it governs the execution of limb movement and regulates muscle tone; lesions in this area produce hypotonia, rebound, tremor, or dysarthria (e.g., scanning speech); (3) the *cerebrocerebellum* (or *neocerebellum*), the lateral part of each cerebellar hemisphere; its input is entirely pontine and its output is by way of the dentate nucleus to the thalamus and thence to the motor and premotor cortex; it is involved in the planning, initiation, timing, and accuracy of movements; it compares motor commands with ensuing motor action and compensates for errors and inaccuracies; lesions of the dentate nucleus result in delays in beginning and ending movement, action or intention tremor most marked at the ending of a movement (*terminal tremor*), dysmetria, *decomposition* of multijoint movement, dysdiadochokinesia, or deficits in timing and in ability to judge elapsed time. The anterior lobe of the cerebellum may be damaged by the cumulative effect of alcohol over many years. Since this area is concerned with leg and trunk stability, the typical alcoholic stumbles around and cannot sit straight in a chair.

During the 1990s evidence increasingly accumulated that the cerebellum is far more than a specialized control box for movement. Studies indicated that it participates in many brain functions, ranging from the analysis of sensory information, to telling time, to solving puzzles, and cognition. The cerebellum coordinates muscle tone, posture, and eye and hand movements, on the basis of sensory information that it receives from every part of the body. The information is then synthesized into body maps at the cerebellum's anterior and posterior ends. The cerebellum plays a large part in programming the details needed for automatic execution of skilled movements. In the decision to play a short piece on the piano, for instance, the initial plan for movement arises in the cortex. Impulses from the cortex go to the basal ganglia and lateral cerebellum, where some kind of program is written for the eye movements involved in reading the music and the contractions of the hand and arm muscles that will be involved in playing the piece. Those instructions are then passed to the motor cortex and transmitted to the muscles. The cerebellum further acts as a monitor of actual performance and corrects errors in the duration, timing, and coordination of the movements involved in the willed action. In addition to all the foregoing, the cerebellum is necessary for the learning of motor skills.

Learning occurs in both the cerebellar cortex and the deep cerebellar nuclei; memories can be stored at both sites; the component of learning that occurs in the cerebellar cortex is critical for regulating the timing of movements; learning that occurs in the cerebellar cortex can be transferred partially or completely to long-term memory in the deep cerebellar nucleus; there is evidence that the cerebellum sends signals to some brain areas involved in cognition but not movement.

Decreases in the size of the cerebellum have been found in patients with schizophrenia (using magnetic resonance or other brain imaging technology).

**cerebral amyloid angiopathy** *CAA* (q.v.).

**cerebral anemia** An inexact, descriptive term for reduced blood flow to the brain. The diminished blood supply may be in the brain as a whole (generalized cerebral anemia) or it may be limited to one or more specific areas of the brain (local cerebral anemia). Generalized cerebral anemia may be acute, as in cardiac failure or in psychological or physiological shock, or it may be chronic, as in pernicious anemia, leukemia, other blood dyscrasias, repeated blood loss, cerebral arteriosclerosis, or cachexia.

Symptoms of acute cerebral anemia include roaring in the ears, spots before the eyes, swaying, weakness, apathy, somnolence, unconsciousness, profuse sweating, and cold, pale skin. Symptoms of chronic cerebral anemia include headaches, feeling of pressure in the head, roaring in the ears, dizziness, insomnia, or drowsiness, and in many cases progression to an organic reaction with memory disturbances, delusions, and hallucinations.

Local cerebral anemia is seen in cerebral arteriosclerosis, intracranial tumor, vasospasm, hypertensive encephalopathy, etc. Symptoms include fleeting pareses, transient aphasias, temporary sensory disturbances, hemianopsia, and focal convulsive twitches. See *cerebral arteriosclerosis; vascular dementia.*

**cerebral aqueduct**  See *ventricle.*

**cerebral arteriosclerosis**  Degenerative changes in the arteries and arterioles of the brain ("hardening of the arteries"), the most common causes of which are (1) primary degeneration of the intima; (2) degeneration secondary to high blood pressure; (3) endarteritis (usually syphilitic); (4) thromboangiitis obliterans; (5) polyarteritis nodosa or periarteritis nodosa; and (6) temporal arteritis. The effect of progressive occlusion of cerebral blood vessels is an impairment of circulation in the regions they supply, with resultant impairment in function even before any vessel is completely blocked. See *cerebrovascular accident.*

Manifestations vary with the area(s) of the brain impaired and with the type of pathology. In a relatively small group of subjects, a clear-cut succession of strokes produces enough brain tissue damage to cause *dementia* (q.v.), referred to as arteriosclerotic dementia or arteriosclerotic psychosis, multi-infarct dementia, or vascular dementia. There are disturbances in memory, abstract thinking, judgment, impulse control, and personality. Onset is often insidious, and the course of deterioration is patchy and fluctuating, rather than steadily progressive as in dementia of the Alzheimer type.

Pathologically, the primary changes are in the elastic tissues, especially in the internal elastic membrane of the cerebral arterioles. Two major types of pathology are seen: (1) hyperplastic degeneration, which produces focal parenchymatous lesions and mainly neurologic symptoms (convulsions, aphasia, agnosia, apraxia, paralysis of the upper motor neuron type, senile tremor, chorea, athetosis, parkinsonism, and often signs of visual impairment); mental changes appear relatively late in the course of the disorder; (2) hypoplastic degeneration, which produces gross hemorrhagic softenings and mainly mental symptoms: signs of frontal lobe damage such as *witzelsucht* (q.v.), callousness, and euphoria; basal ganglia signs such as impulsiveness and whining; temporal lobe signs such as depression and visual hallucinations; and with parietal lobe involvement, hypochondriacal trends frequently appear. In addition, there are general intellectual dulling with memory defects, emotional lability, self-centeredness, hostility to all change, paranoid trends, loosely constructed delusions, confusion, and finally profound dementia.

**cerebral compression**  Any degree of head injury (concussion, brain contusion, or cerebral laceration) that is followed by intracranial hemorrhage. The latter may be subdural (which is twice as common) or extradural. Acute subdural hemorrhage is usually the result of severe cerebral laceration; extradural hemorrhage is usually due to laceration of the middle meningeal artery by fractured bone, and in this case the posterior branches of the artery are more frequently involved than the anterior.

**cerebral cortex development**  The cerebral cortex develops in a precisely ordered sequence:

1. 7th week (in utero)—postmitotic cells in the ventricle region move up to form the cortical plate

2. 10th–11th week—the cortical plate expands and afferent fibers that will ultimately make connections with the overlying cortex begin to appear in the intermediate zone beneath the cortical plate

3. 11th–13th week—the cortical plate becomes bilaminate, with an inner and an outer zone

4. 14th–15th weeks—cells move up into the intermediate zone, and the ventricular zone begins to disappear

5. 16th week through early postnatal stage—cells migrate from the intermediate zone into the cortical plate

In both the migration process and the differentiation of the neuronal precursors once they have reached their destination, the outer layers of the cortex are the last to form and mature. Layers V and VI (the deeper layers) show extensive neuronal maturation at 7 months in utero, while cells in layer II have not begun to differentiate. At birth, the neurons in layer III are close to maturity, while the pyramidal cells in layer II have just begun to differentiate.

**cerebral dominance** The tendency for certain functions of the brain to be concentrated on one side. In right-handed persons, for example, functions such as language tend to be concentrated in the left hemisphere—called left cerebral dominance or left hemispheric dominance. The dominant hemisphere is the one that is organized to express language and handle symbolic functions; it processes information in a sequential, logical, rational, analytic, linear fashion. The nondominant hemisphere processes information in a holistic, parallel, simultaneous fashion; it deals with relational perception, visuospatial information, and orientation. Cerebral or hemisphere dominance is also referred to as *lateralization* or *bimodality*. See *planum temporale*.

It was Roger Sperry and Michael Gazzaniga who found that each hemisphere carries an independent awareness of the self. Instead of saying that the left hemisphere is specialized for language, it may be more accurate to say it is specialized for symbolic-conceptual representation. The right hemisphere deals with nonsymbolic-direct-perceived representations, those large chunks of experience that do not employ language. But it is not totally true that the right hemisphere is completely devoid of language ability. It may be capable, after some practice, of decoding a word such as "horse." It will have difficulty, however, when presented with a more symbolic one such as "faith."

There is a relation between hemisphere dominance and handedness, but the two are not identical. Approximately 90% of humans are right-handed (*dextral*), and approximately 97% of these show left-hemisphere speech and language localization, whereas only 3% show right-hemisphere lateralization or bilateral language representation. These relationships shift to 70% and 30%, respectively, in the left-handed.

The left hemisphere is also dominant for sign language, even though lexicon and grammar are spatially organized in sign language and the right hemisphere is ordinarily dominant for spatial recognition.

There is evidence that the two sexes differ in their patterns of cerebral asymmetry and in the rate of maturation of cognitive functions in the two hemispheres. Girls, for instance, show right-hemisphere specialization for spatial processing later than do boys; this may indicate retention of greater plasticity of the brain for a longer period in girls. Such plasticity may be reflected clinically in a lower incidence in girls of developmental dyslexia, developmental aphasia, and autism, all of which are characterized by prominent language deficits. Further, patients with epilepsy, mental retardation, cerebral palsy, stuttering, and dylexia have a higher than normal incidence of left-handedness.

**cerebral embolism** See *cerebrovascular accident.*

**cerebral hemispheres** The two halves of the brain, each hemisphere consisting of cerebral cortex, the underlying white matter, three deep-lying nuclei (the *basal ganglia, hippocampus,* and *amygdala*), the *insula,* and the *limbic lobe* (qq.v.). See *dominance, cerebral; hemisphericity.*

Distinct hemispheres developed in early reptiles in the Triassic Era (245 million years ago). In the later mammals of the Jurassic Era (210 million years ago), the hemispheres swelled enormously and assumed all but the most basic automatic responses such as control of breathing and heartbeat.

**cerebral hemorrhage** See *cerebrovascular accident.*

**cerebral palsy** *Little disease* (William John Little, English surgeon, 1810–1894); *spastic diplegia; atrophic lobar sclerosis*; congenital diplegia; congenital spastic paralysis. A congenital disorder of unknown cause, consisting of bilateral symmetrical gliosis and atrophy of the nerve tracts, and in particular of the pyramidal tracts. Manifestations include weakness and spasticity of the limbs, ataxia, athetosis, seizures, and delayed growth and development. The thighs are adducted, the knees rub together, the legs cross in progression (*scissors gait*), and the child walks on its toes (pes equinovarus). Affected children may also show learning disabilities or some degree of mental retardation. Symptoms are predominantly spastic in 65% of cases, athetoid in 25%, and ataxic in 10%.

In the United States, about 5000 children are born each year with cerebral palsy. There are about 500,000 cases in the United States and about half of those suffer from severe forms of the disease. Incidence is 1.1 of every 1000 single pregnancies, 12 of every 1000 twin pregnancies, and about 108 of every 1000 twin pregnancies in infants whose twin died before birth. Incidence is higher than average among children with a low birth weight. Incidence is also higher than average among the Amish. See *glutaric aciduria.*

**cerebral peduncle**  See *midbrain.*

**cerebral thrombosis**  See *cerebrovascular accident.*

**cerebration**  Lewes used this term for "cerebral actions consecutive on a perception"; today it generally means any kind of conscious thinking.

**cerebrocerebellum**  Neocerebellum. See *cerebellum.*

**cerebromacular degeneration**  See *Tay-Sachs disease.*

**cerebrospinal fluid**  See *ventricle.*

**cerebrotonia**  A personality type, described by Sheldon, associated with the ectomorphic body build and characterized by restraint, inhibition, alertness, and a predominantly intellectual approach to reality.

**cerebrovascular accident**  *CVA; apoplexy;* thromboembolic *stroke;* gross or focal cerebral damage secondary to ischemia (which accounts for 85% of episodes) or hemorrhage into the brain (10% of episodes) or into the subarachnoid, subdural, or intraventricular spaces. Included within the ischemic group is the transient ischemic attack or *TIA* (q.v.).

Thromboembolic stroke is often a manifestation of cerebral arteriosclerosis and occurs chiefly in old age, although children with an acute infectious disease, young adults with cerebral syphilis, and young and middle-aged alcoholics may also develop *cerebral thrombosis.* Three-quarters of all strokes occur in people over the age of 75 years. CVA is the third leading cause of mortality and morbidity in the United States (behind heart disease and cancer); 35% of stroke victims die within 3 weeks, and at least half of the survivors will be disabled. See *cerebral arteriosclerosis.*

The patient who suffers a CVA may awaken in the morning completely paralyzed on one side of the body, monoplegic, or aphasic. Thromboembolic stroke may also occur during the daytime, especially when the patient is inactive.

Cerebral hemorrhage occurs most frequently as a result of arteriosclerosis or hypertension or as a complication of alcoholism. It also occurs in children and young adults with congenital abnormalities of the cerebral vasculature, such as aneurysms. Since hypertension of the essential type is so frequently familial, death from cerebral hemorrhage correspondingly runs in families.

The exciting causes are such acts as straining at stool, coughing, retching, coitus, violent emotion, or heavy eating, all of which elevate the blood pressure. Thus hemorrhage frequently occurs in the daytime during periods of activity. Unconsciousness occurs suddenly, and the patient topples over or falls to the ground. Coma may gradually deepen and the patient may die in a few hours. More common is a coma of several days' duration during which the patient may rouse a little and then lapse back into deep coma. Some patients gradually recover consciousness and survive the attack.

*Cerebral embolism* creates the same clinical picture as cerebral thrombosis, but emboli are usually multiple and the syndrome may be more bizarre. The commonest causes of emboli are (1) diseases of the heart—as with auricular fibrillation and coronary occlusion with mural thrombi, which may break off and become embolic to the brain; or as in bacterial endocarditis, with valvular vegetations, which may become dislodged and flow to the brain; and (2) pulmonary diseases, with septic emboli lodging in a cerebral vessel, damaging the wall of the vessel and producing one or more brain abscesses and sometimes meningitis. Cerebral embolism comes on suddenly, without warning, and severe general symptoms appear as in hemorrhages. There may be convulsions and coma. Death may occur in a few hours when the embolus has lodged in a vital area. The embolism may produce only softening, but most frequently hemorrhage also. It is the most frequent cause of sudden hemiplegia in childhood.

The clinical picture in patients who survive depends on the type of lesion, the specific region of the brain that has been damaged, and the brain structures connected to that region. Depression is the most frequent psychiatric disorder; it occurs in 30% to 50% of victims and is likely to be particularly severe when the lesion is in the left frontal lobe. See *aphasia; catastrophic behavior; frontal lobe; occipital lobe; parietal lobe; temporal lobe*.

**cerebrum**  The major portion of the brain; the *forebrain* (q.v.) or prosencephalon.

**ceremonial, compulsive**  See *compulsive ceremonial*.

**ceremonial, defensive**  A more or less elaborate pattern of actions unconsciously devised by a person as a defense against anxiety and compulsively executed by him or her whenever this anxiety threatens. In traumatic neuroses, for example, many patients have symptoms that are chiefly unconscious defense reactions against the original trauma.See *compulsive ceremonial*.

**Cerletti, Ugo**  (1877–1963) Italian neuropsychiatrist; in 1938, with L. Bini, introduced an electrical form of convulsive therapy.

**certification**  Designation of competence by a professional review body; those so certified by the American Board of Psychiatry and Neurology, Inc. (ABPN) are issued diplomas indicating that they have passed the required examinations and hence are termed diplomates.

In Utilization Review procedures, the *certification process* refers to *review* (q.v.) of the case record to determine whether health care is necessary, and if the type or level of care and the site in which it is rendered are appropriate.

Certification is also used to refer to the process of completing the necessary documents in *commitment* proceedings (q.v.).

**certification, admission**  See *review*.

**certify**  To formally declare a person insane.

**ceruloplasmin**  An alpha-globulin that contains almost all the copper in blood serum. Among other substrates, ceruloplasmin acts on serotonin and norepinephrine. One theory, no longer considered tenable, was that schizophrenia is due to a genetic defect or metabolic error that produces an abnormal ceruloplasmin, *taraxein*, which fails to neutralize noxious metabolites such as adrenoxine and adrenolutin.

**cervical migraine**  *Cervical vertigo syndrome; Bartschi-Rochaix syndrome*; headache, dizziness, stiffness of the neck, vertigo, and paresthesiae due to cerebral artery compression.

**CES**  Cranial electrotherapy stimulation, consisting of transcranial application of extremely low-dose electrical current to the brain (600 microamperes or less), from a wallet-sized device through electrodes attached to the ears. It has been used to treat chronically aggressive, treatment-resistant neuropsychiatric patients.

**c.e.s.**  Central excitatory state. See *summation*.

**CET**  1. Computed electroencephalographic topography, a surface imaging technique used in the assessment of brain function. The EEG or evoked potential is recorded by 16 to 32 sensors, and the amount of activity of each EEG frequency (alpha, delta, theta, etc.) is measured at each sensory position and expressed as a color on the brain map. See *imaging, brain; pixel*.

2. Cerebral electrotherapy; *electrosleep* (q.v.). Low-intensity pulses of direct current that some have claimed to be of value in the treatment of depression, anxiety, and insomnia.

3. *Cognitive enhancement therapy* (q.v.).

**CFF**  Critical flicker fusion. See critical flicker fusion test; flicker.

**CFI**  *Camberwell Family Interview* (q.v.).

**CFS**  *Chronic fatigue syndrome* (q.v.).

**CGG repeats**  See *trinucleotide repeat*.

**CGI**  Clinical Global Impression.

**cGMP**  Cyclic guanosine monophosphate, a *second messenger* that can act either directly on a target protein or *ion channel* (qq.v.) or, more commonly, indirectly by activating a kinase, which phosphorylates a specific protein inside the cell. *NO* (q.v.) stimulates synthesis of cGMP in neurons and glial cells of the cerebellum.

**CGRP**  Calcitonin gene-related peptide. See *neuropeptides*.

**Chaddock reflex**  (Charles Gilbert Chaddock, American neurologist, 1861–1936) Dorsal extension of the great toe, induced by stroking the skin over the external malleolus. This is one of several pathological reflexes that may be seen when the lower motor neuron is released from the normal suppressor effect of higher centers, as in pyramidal tract lesions.

**chaerophobia**  *Chairophobia; cherophobia*; fear or avoidance of rejoicing, gaiety; a fear of showing that one is happy or content.

**chaining**  Linking, connecting; *perseverative chaining* is one form of loosening of associations described in schizophrenic patients.

Example: Schizophrenic subjects are asked to describe one colored chip so that their audience can pick it out from among a group of colored chips. Schizophrenics reveal an impaired ability to generate appropriate cues under such circumstances; listeners (both normal subjects and other schizophrenics) were unable to select the correct chip on the basis of the cues provided. One defect apparent in the schizophrenic subjects' descriptions was the use of immediately preceding descriptors, rather than descriptors of the particular chip—a defect termed perseverative chaining.

**chains**   See *neuroethology*.

**chairophobia**   *Chaerophobia* (q.v.).

**Chakrabarty**   The defendant in *Diamond Commissioner of Patents and Trademarks v. Chakrabarty*. Ananda Chakrabarty was a molecular biologist who invented a genetically engineered bacterium capable of breaking down crude oil, and in 1960 the U.S. Supreme Court held that such a live, human-made microorganism is patentable subject matter.

**chalasis**   Inhibition of resting posture. Hines, in her studies on the maturation of excitability in the precentral gyrus, describes chalastic foci that cause inhibition of resting posture.

**chalastic fits, postdormital**   See *sleep paralysis*.

**challenge**   Originally, provoking an immune response in a previously sensitized subject by administering an antigen or allergen. Currently used in a more general sense, to refer to testing the function of a biological system by activating the system with a stimulus whose effect on a normal system is known and comparing the response obtained to the response that would be expected of the normal system. An example is administering thyrotropin-releasing hormone (TRH) and then measuring the amount of thyroid-stimulating hormone (TSH) released; subjects with depression typically show a blunted or diminished release of TSH in comparison with control subjects.

**challenged, physically**   See *disability*.

**chameleon effect**   The tendency of humans to imitate each other automatically when interacting socially. Imitative behavior is crucial for the development of social cognitive skills. The more people tend to imitate others, the more they tend to be empathic.

**chance action**   An action that is executed by mere chance and has no conscious aim or purpose, but nevertheless subserves the execution of an unconscious intention. Under this heading Freud distinguishes three separate categories: (1) habitual actions such as fingering one's hair; (2) actions that are usual under certain circumstances, such as doodling and coin-jingling; and (3) isolated chance actions. One example of the last variety might be the loss of a wedding ring on the honeymoon, indicating an unconscious wish to dissolve the marriage.

**chandelier neurons**   CHCs (chandelier cells); GABA-ergic interneurons that synapse exclusively with pyramidal cells. Chandelier neurons exert powerful regulatory (inhibitory) control over pyramidal cell output. Cognitive deficits in schizophrenia are due in part to GABA (inhibitory) interneuron abnormalities; the parvalbumin-expressing chandelier class of neurons is most clearly implicated. In schizophrenia there is relative insufficiency of resource allocation between competitive systems, sometimes discussed in terms of hypofrontality or frontotemporal dysconnectivity. See *hypofrontality hypothesis*; *neocortical neurons*.

**changing, compulsive**   A symptom found in some obsessive-compulsives; changing may involve anything, anywhere: personal habits, dress, work, social relations, opinions, etc. The changing is an effort to bring the world into accord with the patient's system. Through compulsive changing the patient avoids the reality that the world does not obey his or her compulsive system.

**channeling**   Also, trance channeling; mediumship. The person who provides channeling is variously termed a fortune-teller, guru, healer, *medium*, shaman, or witch doctor. He or she assembles an audience and then voluntarily goes into a trance in which he surrenders himself to the "guide" or "source" who will speak through him. See *folk medicine*.

**channels of communication**   See *communication*.

**chaotic families**   See *family types*.

**chaotic state**   A mixed state of anger compounded with shame and anxiety, described in narcissistic personality (disorder). At its height the subject experiences panic with fears of flying apart, loss of body integrity, and of a fragmenting identity. See *autistic objects*; *autistic-contiguous position*; *blind hatred*.

**chaperone, molecular**   See *molecular chaperone*.

**chaperone proteins**  A family of cellular proteins that mediate the correct folding of other polypeptides, and sometimes their assembly into oligomeric structures; they are not components of those final structures, however. They prevent misfolding and aggregation and in some cases appear to be able to unfold already misfolded proteins and help them attain the correct conformation. They assist polypeptides in folding by inhibiting alternative assembly pathways that would produce nonfunctional structures. See *protein conformational disorders*; *protein folding*.

Molecular chaperones have essential roles in many cellular processes, including protein folding, targeting, transport, degradation, and signal transduction. Of the families of molecular chaperones, the most prominent are HSPs (heat shock proteins), especially HSP100, HSP60, HSP70, and HSP90.

**chaperones, apoptotic**  They herd together inactive *caspases* (q.v.) to increase their local concentration and ease them into conformations that promote their action.

**Chapman conceptual breadth test**  The subject sorts sets of 30 cards into categories that vary in level of specificity.

**character**  In current usage, approximately equivalent to *personality* (q.v.); it consists of the totality of objectively observable behavior and subjectively reportable inner experience. It includes the characteristic (and to some extent predictable) behavior-response patterns that each person evolves, both consciously and unconsciously, as his or her style of life or way of being in adapting to his environment and in maintaining a stable, reciprocal relationship with the human and nonhuman environment.

Some authorities define character as learned attributes originating primarily in early life experience and personality as the combination of temperament and character. See *character defense*; *character structure*.

**character analysis**  Psychoanalytic treatment of a character disorder. See *character defense*.

**character defense**  *Personality* (q.v.), viewed as a grouping of defenses that have been developed by the subject as a routine way of coping with reality. In the early 1920s, many psychoanalysts had become pessimistic about the value of therapy. Reich (*Character Analysis*, 1949) pointed out that many chaotic analyses are the result of failure to recognize a latent negative transference.

A *negative transference* is commonly hidden behind the character traits of the person, which serve as a protective armor against stimuli from the outer world and against his or her own libidinous strivings. The character armor serves as a compact defense mechanism, and this *character resistance* or character defense must be overcome if the analysis is to proceed. The ego employs other mechanisms of defense, such as repression, regression, reaction-formation, isolation, undoing, introjection, turning against the self, reversal, and sublimation, but they correspond essentially to a single experience, whereas the character represents a specific way of being and is an expression of the total past.

Reich's classification included four main types, differentiated on the basis of the clinical picture: (1) *compulsive character*; (2) *hysterical character*; (3) *masochistic character*; and (4) *phallic-narcissistic character* (qq.v.).

Another classification is based on the libidinal level that is believed to have been a primary determinant of the character structure: (1) *oral aggressive character*; (2) *oral receptive character*; (3) *anal character*; (4) *phallic character*; (5) *urethral character*; and (6) the mature or *genital character* (qq.v.).

**character neurosis**  Used by most authorities to refer to *personality disorders* (q.v.). In psychoanalysis the expression has acquired a nosologic implication. A neurotic character, in terms of mental deviation, occupies a position between the healthy and the clear-cut neurotic personality. See *character defense*.

**character structure**  Personality; a relatively permanent constellation of habitual ways of reacting to the world, connoting only habitual attitudes developed as reactions to life situations; not to be confused with *temperament*. See *character; character defense*.

**charas, churus**  Hashish (in India). See *cannabis; marijuana*.

**Charcot, Jean-Martin**  (1825–93) French neurologist and psychiatrist; localizaωtion of function in cerebral disease; hysteria; hypnosis; the first modern physician to make a serious attempt to treat emotional disorders on an individual psychotherapeutic basis.

**Charcot-Marie-Tooth disease**  (*Jean-Martin Charcot*, q.v.; Pierre Marie, French physician, 1853-1940; Howard Henry Tooth, English physician, 1856–1926); *CMT*; *peroneal muscular atrophy; neural progressive muscular atrophy*; an inherited, slowly progressive, demyelinating peripheral neuropathy, transmitted usually as a Mendelian dominant (less frequently it is X-linked, rarely it is an autosomal recessive disorder), more often affecting males. The disease typically begins between the ages of 5 and 10 years, with wasting of the small muscles in the peripheral limbs secondary to degeneration of the peripheral nerves and spinal cord. Both sensory and motor axons are affected; the disease can originate from defects in myelin (type I) or axons (type II).

The muscular wasting results in a steppage gait, a "fat bottle" calf when the lower calf is wasted, and "inverted champagne bottle" limb when the lower third of the thigh is wasted. Children with the disease may walk on their toes. In adulthood, the disease produces abnormalities of gait, foot deformities, or loss of balance. Impaired dorsiflexion of the foot leads to a frequent complaint of tripping over objects on the floor and ankle sprains. Involvement of the hands leads to difficulty in manipulating small objects, in zipping, and in buttoning. The disease runs a slow course and may become arrested at any stage; it does not shorten life, and there are no associated intellectual changes. Tooth independently described the peroneal form (peroneal muscular atrophy).

CMT is the most common inherited peripheral neuropathy, with an estimated prevalence of one in 2500. In the majority of autosomal dominant CMT families, the disease locus demonstrates linkage to DNA markers on chromosome 17. The specific genetic defect consists of duplication of a small portion of chromosome 17: about 500,000 DNA bases (out of the total of approximately 130 million base pairs that form the normal chromosome) are duplicated in the middle of the upper arm of the chromosome. If the chromosome with the deletion is passed on to the next generation, the result may be a different, milder, disorder—*HNPP* (hereditary neuropathy with liability to pressure palsies).

**Charcot syndrome**  *Multiple sclerosis* (q.v.).

**charge of affect**  "That part of the instinct which has become detached from the idea, and finds proportionate expression, according to its quantity, in processes which become observable to perception as affects" (Freud, S. *Collected Papers*, 1924–1925) See *cathexis*.

**Charles Bonnet syndrome**  A rare condition consisting of isolated visual pseudohallucinations that are persistent or repetitive and often, but not always, associated with lesions of the visual system or other brain pathology. Most of the cases reported have been in the elderly. The syndrome was first described by the Swiss philosopher Charles Bonnet in 1769. K. Gold and P. Rabins (*Comprehensive Psychiatry 30*, 1989) have suggested the following criteria for diagnosis of the syndrome: (1) the visual halluincations are formed, complex, persistent or repetitive, and stereotyped; (2) the subject recognizes that the hallucinations are unreal; (3) there are no associated or concurrent primary or secondary delusions; and (4) there are no hallucinations in other modalities.

**charm**  Light hypnosis; *hypotaxis* (q.v.).

**chastity, conjugal**  The state of husband and wife living in celibacy.

**chatterbox syndrome**  Blathering; cocktail party syndrome; general mental retardation with the exception of language skills, which are unimpaired or even overdeveloped; seen in some hydrocephalic children. See *Williams-Beuren syndrome*.

**chattering mania**  *Obs.* Uncontrollable urge to talk gibberish; pressured speech.

**checkers**  Those persons suffering from *obsessive-compulsive disorder* (q.v.) whose major symptom is pathological doubting that requires incessant examining or verifying to be sure that there is no reason for concern. For example, the person so afflicted might have recurrent doubts about whether the gas has been turned off and feels compelled to return to the kitchen to check the controls on the stove. But as soon as he or she is out of the kitchen, the doubt returns and another check must be made.

**cheese effect**  Hypertensive crisis due to the interaction of monoamine oxidase inhibitors with tyramine, a potent vasopressor. Tyramine is formed when bacteria in food provide the enzyme that decarboxylates the amino acid tyrosine. Many foods contain tyrosine, but over 75% of the hypertensive reactions reported with MAOI use, and almost all the resultant deaths, have been associated with the ingestion of cheese. See *TSF*.

**cheimaphobia**  Fear of cold.

**cheiro-**  See *chiro-*.

**ChEIs**  Cholinesterase inhibitors. See *anticho-linesterases*.

**chelation**  The act of binding, fixing, or attaching chemically; specifically, formation of a bond between a metal ion and another molecule, as in the chelation of the iron ion by the porphyrin ring in heme. Chelating agents, such as British anti-Lewisite (see BAL) and/or versenate, are used in the treatment of heavy metal poisoning to form stable compounds with the toxic metal, which can then be eliminated safely from the body without exerting their toxic effects on tissues.

**chemical aversive conditioning**  *CAC* (q.v.). See *aversion therapy*.

**chemical dependency**  Generic term relating to psychological or physical dependence, or both, on an exogenous substance. See *dependence, drug*.

**chemical neuroanatomy**  See *neuroanatomy, chemical*.

**chemoaffinity hypothesis**  The specificity of neural connections depends on selective chemical affinities that exist between individual neurons; axons select particular pathways by recognizing specific molecular cues in their environment. See *axon guidance*.

**chemoattractant**  See *axon growth*.

**chemokines**  Proinflammatory cytokines with the ability to attract and activate leukocytes. Chemokines and their receptors are important in the regulation of a variety of normal functions in the brain, including those of neurodevelopment, intercellular communication, and neuronal survival.

Disturbances in chemokine levels can be induced by infectious agents. The increased risk for schizophrenia in adulthood associated with prenatal exposure to common viruses could be a consequence of cytokine disturbances induced by those viruses. CCR5 is the chemokine receptor; its gene often carries an allele characterized by deletion of a 32-bp segment. That allele has been associated with susceptibility to various immune-related and autoimmune diseases, and recently to schizophrenia of late onset.

**chemopallidectomy**  Injection of alcohol into the globus pallidus, used in the therapy of basal ganglia hyperkinetic disorders.

**chemopsychiatry**  The application and effect of chemical substances in psychiatry. See *psycho-tropics*.

**chemoreception**  Perception of smell and taste; see *interoception*; *sensation*.

**chemorepellent**  See *axon growth*.

**chemotaxis**  *Chemotropism* (q.v.).

**chemotropism**  *Chemotaxis*; oriented growth of axons, guided by gradients of diffusible chemicals released by the target cells with which the axons will make their final connections. See *axon guidance*.

**cheromania**  The manic form of bipolar manic-depressive) illness.

**cherophobia**  *Chaerophobia* (q.v.).

**Chiarugi, Vincenzo**  (1759–1820) Italian physician; in 1789 published his landmark hospital regulations (*Regolamento*) for care of the mentally ill: history for each patient, standards of hygiene, recreational and occupational therapies, minimal restraint, and respect for individual dignity. *Della Pazzi in Genere e in Specie* (On Insanity and Its Classification) 1793–4, described insanity as due to impairment of the physical structure of the brain. Chiarugi divided mental illnesses into melancholia, mania, and amentia.

**child, emotionally handicapped**  See *handicap, emotional*.

**child, gifted**  See *bright child*.

**child, pseudo-mature**  See *adultomorphization*.

**child abuse**  Maltreatment or neglect of a child by parent(s) or other caretakers; intentional exploitation or misuse of a child. It includes a number of subtypes, including the following:

1. *physical abuse*—infliction of injury on a child under 18 years of age by a parent or caretaker;

2. *sexual abuse*—often considered to be a subtype of physical abuse, usually involving genital contact ranging in severity from gentle fondling to forcible rape resulting in physical injury;

3. *neglect*—failure of the parent or caretaker to provide the child with adequate physical care and supervision; general neglect, systematic poisoning, and physical violence are sometimes euphemistically labeled *nonaccidental injury*;

4. *psychological abuse*—many children who are not physically abused are deliberately made to suffer painful psychological states, such as fear, rejection, and loneliness.

Physical and sexual abuse result in both immediate and long-term sequelae in the child victims, including impairment in social, psychological, and cognitive functioning.

Abused children may manifest one or more of the following symptom patterns:

1. "Traumatic" reaction with fearfulness, anxiety, and related symptoms: sleep disturbances, insomnia, nightmares, fear reactions extending to phobic avoidance of all males; hypervigilance, anxiety and fear in relating to adults, expecting punishment and criticism.

2. Paranoid reactions and inability to establish trusting relationships with adults; the child considers all potential love objects to be unpredictable.

3. Poor self-image, often assuming the abuse is a consequence of his or her own behavior; sometimes this is hidden behind compensatory fantasies of grandiosity and omnipotence. The *damaged goods syndrome* refers to the abused child's feeling of having been damaged or altered by the sexual encounter.

4. Depression, sometimes with suicidal behavior.

5. Poor school performance.

6. Use of primitive defenses, such as denial, projection, and splitting.

7. Post-traumatic stress disorder.

In 1994, more than 3 million children in the United States were reported to child protective service agencies. More than 1 million of these cases were substantiated as victims of maltreatment. Physical abuse was involved in 21%, sexual abuse in 11%, neglect in 49%, and other forms of maltreatment in 19%. Nearly 90% of deaths from child abuse or neglect involved children under 5 years of age. It is estimated that up to 10% of abused children die, and that at least 25% suffer serious neurological damage with impairment of intelligence. According to most experts, there are 15 to 20 actual cases of maltreatment for each one reported.

Between 25% and 30% of females, and 10%–16% of males (=40 million children in the United States) experienced some form of sexual abuse in childhood, ranging from sexual fondling to intercourse. The peak age of abuse for victims is 9–12 years. Most often, the abuser is a man who is known to the child. Nationally, adolescents are perpetrators in 20% of the reported cases of child sexual abuse.

**child analysis** Psychoanalytic treatment of children that requires major modifications of the classical analytic technique. More activity is required of the analyst, for one thing, and play therapy must often substitute for free associations as a way to elicit the significant psychodynamic factors. See *play therapy*.

**Child ego state** See ego state, adult; transactional analysis.

**child guidance** Preventive or prophylactic measures directed toward the goal of minimizing the chances of mental and emotional disorders developing in adult life. Child guidance strives to influence the child's developmental familial and social milieu mainly through education, support, insight, and understanding, directed toward both the child's immediate family (especially the mother) and such influential parent surrogates as the family physician or pediatrician, the school nurse, the teacher, and the minister.

**"child is being beaten"** See *beating*.

**child maltreatment** See *child abuse*.

**child molester** See *pedophilia*.

**child neglect** Disregard, indifference, or inattentiveness to the needs of a child by the person(s) responsible for the child; as a result, the child experiences avoidable suffering and/or is denied elements that are essential to the adequate development of his or her physical, intellectual, or emotional capacities. Child neglect is estimated to be three or four times as frequent as child abuse. See *battered child syndrome; child abuse*.

Indicators of neglect include (1) physical signs, such as malnutrition, fatigue, and poor hygiene; and (2) behavioral signs, such as poor school attendance, drug or alcohol use, repeated ingestion of harmful substances, exploitation and role reversal (in which the child becomes the parent's caretaker), and other behaviors that suggest inadequate or inappropriate parental supervision or failure to obtain requisite medical attention. See *attachment disorder of infancy.*

**child of an alcoholic** Adult child of an alcoholic (*ACA, ACOA*), a status that is sometimes conceptualized as a form of *codependency* (q.v.). ACOAs are often part of a mutual-help movement, operating on Twelve-Step group principles and sometimes under Al-Anon auspices.

**child prodigy** See *bright child*.

**child psychiatry** The branch of psychiatry dealing with disorders of children and adolescents, including the study of normal psychological, physical, and social development, parenting, education, and learning. Basic research in child development has focused on studies of object attachment, cognition, psycholinguistics, affective states, and bonding. Clinical research has extended the understanding of the pervasive developmental disorders, learning disorders, Tourette syndrome, eating disorders, classification and epidemiology of psychiatric disorders in childhood, affective disorders and suicide, and the rights of the child in the juvenile justice systems.

**child rapist**  See *pedophilia*.

**child-centered**  In educational psychology, a school whose primary concern is fulfilling the child's present needs rather than preparing him or her for adult life.

**child-guidance therapy**  The treatment of emotional problems of children by the simultaneous therapy of the child and its parents, especially the mother.

**childbirth, envy of**  According to some authorities the boy has an envy of the girl's ability to bear children, which in its intensity matches the girl's envy of the boy's penis. Fenichel does not believe this to be the case. He points out that both boys and girls may have a "passionate wish to give birth to babies, a wish that is doomed to frustration," since little girls can in no possible way bear children any better than can little boys (Fenichel, O. *The Psychoanalytic Theory of Neurosis*, 1945).

**childhood**  The period of life from birth to puberty. See *developmental levels*.

**childhood, land of**  Jung's expression to describe "that time in which the rational consciousness of the present was not yet separated from the "historical soul,' the collective unconscious, and thus not only into that land where the complexes of childhood have their origin but into a prehistorical one that was the cradle of us all (Jacobi, J. *The Psychology of C. G. Jung*, 1942).

**childhood absence epilepsy**  *CAE;* a familial disorder characterized by nonconvulsive seizures—sudden, brief impairments of consciousness accompanied by a generalized, synchronous, bilateral, 2.5–4 Hz spike and slow-wave discharge (SWD) in the EEG. During the seizure, the child usually does not respond to commands and may stare with open eyes; after the seizure, there may be no recollection of ictal events. The absences start between 3 and 8 years of age and generally occur many times each day (up to ~200 per day); they are not a result of visual or other sensory stimuli. About 70% of patients show spontaneous remission, often around adolescence.

**childhood disintegrative disorder (CDD)**  Also called *Heller disease, dementia infantilis*; a pervasive developmental disorder characterized by seemingly normal development for at least the first 2 years of life, with severe developmental regression and loss of acquired skills (such as language, social skills, motor skills, play behavior, and bladder and bowel control) before the age of 10 years. Mental retardation is usually severe. Behavior is often restrictive, repetitive, and stereotyped, and attempts to interrupt their preoccupations or routines are often met with strong resistance, tantrums, or outbursts of aggression.

**childhood memories**  See *hypnosis*.

**childhood psychosis**  See atypical childhood psychosis; developmental disorders, pervasive.

**childhood schizophrenia**  *Early onset schizophrenia (EOS)* is currently used to refer to onset of symptoms of *schizophrenia* (q.v.) before the age of 18 years, *very early onset schizophrenia (VEOS)* to onset before the age of 13 years. Most VEOS occurs in boys, who overall account for twice as many early onset cases as do girls. The two youngest reported patients manifested symptoms at 3 years and 5.7 years, indicating that the justifiable diagnosis of schizophrenia in children under the age of 6 is exceedingly rare.

As childhood schizophrenia is currently defined, the most frequently noted symptoms are auditory hallucinations (the presenting symptom in 80% in one study), flat or inappropriate effect, delusions (the presenting symptom in 63%), formal thought disorder, and visual hallucinations (the presenting symptom in 37%). Autistic children, by contrast, manifest none of these symptoms.

Children affected with schizophrenia also show cognitive, neuropsychological, and linguistic deficits and abnormalities of event-related potentials, skin conductance, and eye movements similar to those reported in adults with schizophrenia. Whether they also show signs of hypofrontality in PET studies remains an unsettled issue. (Asarnow, R. F. and Aranow, J. R. *Schizophrenia Bulletin 20*, 1994) See *communication deficits; discourse skills*. It is estimated that as many as 1% of all schizophrenic disorders manifest themselves in patients younger than 10 years of age, and 4% before age 15. Males predominate in childhood schizophrenia, but not in adolescent-onset cases. Prognosis is relatively poorer with early onset, particularly in children who are shy, introverted, withdrawn, and cognitively impaired in the premorbid period.

Until well into the 1960s there was no general consensus about the dividing lines between schizophrenia in childhood, infantile autism (Kanner), symbiotic infantile psychosis (Mahler), and many other pervasive developmental disorders, and the terminology as applied in the literature of that time is often incompatible with current usage of the same terms. One confounding factor is that the child often does not have the verbal and cognitive skills required to express symptoms in the same way that adult schizophrenics do. Another confounding factor was failure to differentiate between indicators of potential risk factors for the illness and symptoms of the disease itself. Thus, Bender could say: "We now define child schizophrenia as a maturational lag at the embryonic level in all areas which integrate biological and psychological behavior; an embryonic primitivity or plasticity characterizes the pattern of the behavior disturbance in all areas of personality functioning. It is determined before birth and hereditary factors appear to be important. It may be precipitated by a physiological crisis, which may be birth itself, especially a traumatic birth" (Caplan, G. *Emotional Problems of Early Childhood*, 1955). See *atypical childhood psychosis; autism, early infantile; developmental disorders, pervasive; symbiotic infantile psychosis*. In her descriptions of what she then called childhood schizophrenia, Bender emphasized the following symptoms:

1. Vasovegetative—undifferentiated homeostatic functions; unpredictable temperature responses in illness; flushing, sweating, color changes, cold extremities; disturbed rhythm of sleeping and fluctuation in and out of torporous states of consciousness; disturbances in eating, elimination, and respiration; growth discrepancies; soft visceral tone leading to many "psychosomatic disturbances";

2. Motility—undifferentiated reactions and hypersensitivity to external stimuli; lack of suppression of early reflex patterns (e.g., startle response); soft muscular tone, plasticity, awkwardness, infantile posture; insecurity

with new motor patterns; residual primitive reflex patterned activities; oral mannerisms; head-turning and whirling (whose persistence after the age of 6 years she considered almost pathognomonic);

3. Dependence on contact with others—motor compliance; wooden, mechanical voice;

4. Disturbances in the perceptual, thought, and language spheres, with incongruous early and late patterns; and

5. Deep concern with problems of identity, body image, body functions, and orientation in time and space.

**childhood sexual abuse** CSA. See *child abuse; pedophilia*.

**childhood trauma** See *trauma*.

**child-penis wish** In psychoanalytic psychology, the wish for a child with which, in her psychosexual development, the little girl replaces her wish for a penis. The little girl's first love object is the mother, since it was she who provided the first satisfactions of life, nourishment, warmth, etc. As the child develops, her strong attachment to her mother is replaced by an attachment to her father. This takes place in an atmosphere of hatred for the mother. Although there are many obvious sources for this hatred of the mother—the unavoidable necessity in the child's development of frustrating her insatiable desire for the breast; the birth of a sibling who deprives the little girl of the mother's exclusive attention; the frustration (with threat and disapproval from the mother) of the child's masturbatory activities, which the mother herself had unwittingly stimulated; the other necessary restrictions associated with education; and finally the strong ambivalence of the child's impulses toward her mother—Freud believed that in the girl's turning from her mother to her father the main and specific factor is her wish for a penis (Freud, S. *New Introductory Lectures on Psychoanalysis,* 1933) See *penis envy*.

Having given up her love for her mother, who, too, is found to be castrated and therefore cannot satisfy her daughter's desire for a penis or the sexual phantasies associated with her masturbation, the little girl turns her love toward her father. She has not, however, relinquished her wish for a penis, which, in effect, her mother has refused her, and which she now expects from her father. Also, her passive instinctual impulses have gainedthe upper hand, since a certain amount of activity was surrendered along with clitoral masturbation. A symbolic equation, child = penis, comes into effect, and the wish for a penis is replaced by the wish for a child. The girl's strongest wish now is for a child by her father and she enters into the *Oedipus complex* (q.v.).

Freud envisioned the little girl's resolution of the oedipal situation as "precisely analogous" to that of the little boy, but there were many differences that he never fully explained. The girl entered the oedipal phase because of her absence of masculinity, and ended the phase by symbolically recapturing masculinity in the form of a baby. That entailed a prolongation and incomplete resolution of the oedipal phase leading, according to Freud, to a weaker superego, less capacity to sublimate her drives, and more inner-directed drive energy (erotogenic masochism) than in the boy. At the present time, even psychoanalysts disavow Freud's androcentrism and his theories of "normal" female masochism and of an inherent moral and cultural weakness in the woman.

**children at risk**   See *risk*.

**chimera**   In Greek mythology, a fire-breathing monster with the head of a lion, the body of a goat, and the tail of a serpent. In genetics, the term is used to refer to a *transgenic* animal (q.v.).

**China white**   *MPTP* (q.v.).

**Chinese medicine**   See complementary therapy.

**Chinese menu approach**   Use of checklist(s) as a means of describing clinical phenomena or generating diagnoses on the basis of objective phenomena that can easily be identified or recognized. The technique is often viewed as sacrificing the intuitive aspect of clinical practice for the reproducible certainty of counting bits of information that may be irrelevant to the patient's condition.

**chionophobia**   Fear of snow.

**chipping**   Controlled use of opiates; it is believed that long-term chippers account for a large number of opiate users.

**chips**   A device that permits the investigator to scan rapidly all 23 chromosomes from one or more persons, and to determine their allelic variations. See *DNA*.

**chiro-**   Combining form meaning hand, from Gr. *cheir*.

**chirography**   Handwriting analysis.

**chiromania**   *Obs.* Masturbatic psychosis; compulsive masturbation.

**chi-square test**   A statistical test, developed originally by Karl Pearson, that measures the significance of differences occurring between groups. In a group of 500 cases of lobar pneumonia treated with penicillin, for example, the overall cure rate was 94%. But not all cases were treated with the same batch of penicillin: 100 cases were treated with batch A penicillin and 98% were cured; 100 cases treated with batch B and 89% were cured; 100 cases with batch C and 95% were cured; 100 cases with batch D and 92% were cured; and 100 cases with batch E and 96% were cured. In this imaginary example, the chi-square test could be applied to ascertain whether the different cure rates in different groups are due only to chance or whether, all other relevant factors being equal, the different results are due to different effectiveness of the individual batches of penicillin.

**chloride channel**   *See benzodiazepines; ion channel.*

**choc fortuit**   *Obs.* (F. "accidental shock") Binet's term (1887) to denote an accidental shock or psychic trauma, usually of a sexual character and influential in modifying subsequent adjustment of the person.

**choice**   Selection; the act of selecting or deciding; discrimination among options or rewards. Choice, decision, and decision-making are used interchangeably in social cognitive neuroscience.

Reliable prediction underlies decision-making. The choices available may be between a reward that will be given immediately and one that will be given later. In such cases, the value of each option is discounted according to the expected time until delivery. See *time discounting*. The choice may also be between alternatives, mutually exclusive options. Such a choice depends not only on what one hopes to gain, the *expected value*, but also by how one hopes to feel afterward. In making a choice, 24 areas in the brain are more active under conditions of ambiguity or uncertainty than under conditions of risk. Among these regions are the amygdala, OFC, and DMPFC. By contrast, the dorsal striatum is preferentially activated during the risky condition. As the dorsal striatum is implicated in reward prediction, the result indicates that ambiguity lowers the anticipated reward of decisions.

Missed opportunities due to wrong choice typically produce *regret*, a cognitively mediated emotion triggered by the capacity to reason counterfactually. See *counterfactual thinking; reward.*

**choice of neurosis**   See *compliance, somatic.*

**choked disk**   See *papilledema.*

**cholecystokinin**   *CCK;* an octapeptide neurotransmitter that may play a role in eating disorders, movement disorders, and schizophrenia. It is found in the neuritic plaques of Alzheimer disease. It coexists with GABA and dopamine. See *hypothalamic-pituitary-adrenal (HPA) axis; peptide, brain.*

**choleric type**   In constitutional medicine, one of the four classical temperamental and constitutional types of antiquity. Galen attributed the irritability of this type to the predominance of the yellow bile over the other three humors (or fluids) of the human organism. See pyknic type.

**choline acetyltransferase**   CAT; the enzyme that catalyzes the reactionof choline with acetylcoenzyme A to form acetylcholine (which is then destroyed by acetylcholinesterase). In the brains of subjects with *Alzheimer disease* (q.v.), CAT activity is reduced by 60%–90%; it is generally believed that this reflects a lower rate of acetylcholine production and, consequently, inadequate acetylcholine for neurotransmission. The assumption that the fundamental defect in Alzheimer disease is reduced central cholinergic activity is known as the cholinergic hypothesis.

**cholinergic**   Referring to neurons that are activated by or secrete *acetylcholine* (q.v.) and to endogenous agents (such as neurotransmitters) or drugs that stimulate the action of parasympathetic postganglionic nerves. In the latter sense, cholinergic is equivalent to *parasympathomimetic.* (For sympathomimetic agents, see *adrenergic.*)

The cholinergic system, which includes the medial septum, the diagonal band of Broca, and the nucleus basalis of Meynert (a small region of the globus pallidus), projects directly to the hippocampus, cingulate gyrus, and neocortex. Most of the neurons that project to the cortex originate in the Meynert nucleus; those neurons are markedly diminished in number in Alzheimer disease. The acetylcholine system is involved in the encoding of memory. See *cholinergic hypothesis.*

The cholinergic system is enhanced by (1) parasympathomimetics, such as acetylcholine, pilocarpine, lecithin, and choline and (2) anticholinesterases (q.v.).

The cholinergic system is blocked by (1) parasympatholytics, including anticholinergics and antimuscarinics, and spasmolytics; among these are the belladonna alkaloids, atropine, homatropine, and hyoscine (scopolamine), naturally occurring antimuscarinic agents; papaverine, and also the heterocyclic (tricyclic and tetracyclic) antidepressants and the phenothiazines and (2) cholinesterase, antiparkinsonian agents such as benztropine and trihexyphenidyl, and phencyclidine (PCP). Cholinergic antagonists may impair cognitive functions.

**cholinergic hypothesis**   The theory that *Alzheimer disease* (q.v.) is due to a deficiency of acetylcholine in the brain. Cholinergic innervation of the cerebral cortex arises from the nucleus basalis of Meynert in the basal forebrain, and in Alzheimer disease the basal nucleus shows a significant loss of the large cholinergic cell bodies. Furthermore, the activity of choline acetyltransferase (CAT, the enzyme that catalyzes the production of acetylcholine from choline and acetylcoenzyme A) is markedly reduced in the Alzheimer brain, supporting the idea that the basic defect is an inadequacy of acetylcholine for neurotransmission. See *choline acetyltransferase.*

**cholinergic systems**   Cholinergic interneurons are found in the dorsal striatum (caudate nucleus and putamen) and ventral striatum, including the nucleus accumbens, olfactory tubercle, and ventral pallidum. These striosome patches are relatively free of acetylcholinesterase activity, while acetylcholinesterase activity is more abundant in the extrastriosomal matrix. The neostriatum contains the encoding of all five muscarinic receptors.

**cholinesterase**   See *acetylcholine; elementary process.*

**chorea**   A movement disorder characterized by irregular, spasmodic, involuntary movements of the limbs or facial muscles. Choreic movements are jerky, irregular, and quasi-purposive. Unless otherwise modified, chorea usually means *Sydenham chorea* (q.v.), or St. Vitus dance.

**chorea nutans**   A hysterical symptom characterized by rhythmical nodding; also called chorea oscillatoria, though the latter term properly refers to rhythmical hysterical movements seen in any part of the body.

**chorea oscillatoria**   See *chorea nutans.*

**chorea saltatoria**   A form of chorea in which the patient involuntarily jumps rhythmically or irregularly.

**chorea-acanthocytosis**   See *neuroacanthocytosis.*

**choreatiform syndrome**   See attention deficit hyperactivity disorder.

**choreiform**   Resembling chorea, choreoid.

**choreoacanthocytosis**   A rare familial disorder of the basal ganglia with tics, choreiform movements, dysphagia, muscle atrophy, and dementia. Acanthocytes (*spur cells*) are present: a contracted red blood cell with spurlike projections.

**choreoathetosis**   Purposeless, quick, jerky movements that occur distally; or sinuous, writhing movements that occur proximally; or both.

**choreomania**   Dancing mania; epidemic chorea. During the 14th and 15th centuries such epidemics were prominent in western Germany, where they were known as *Tanzwut*; later they were called *chorea Germanorum* to distinguish the condition from *chorea Anglorum* (Sydenham chorea).

**choriomeningitis, acute lymphocytic**   A virus infection, spread by mice, involving the leptomeninges, the ependyma of the ventricles and the choroid plexuses, and ganglion cells of the brain. Children are most commonly affected, and complete recovery is the rule.

**chorion biopsy**   *Chorionic villus biopsy; CVS* (chorionic villus sampling); excision of chorionic (placental) tissue to obtain a sampling of fetal cells that are then examined for chromosome abnormalities. The technique is painless, and tissue is taken directly through the cervix rather than by means of a needle biopsy through the abdominal wall, as in amniocentesis. Chorion biopsy can provide a larger sample of fetal tissue than can be obtained by amniocentesis, and the test can be performed earlier. Further, it provides material for immediate examination in contrast to amniocentesis, where the sample of amniotic fluid must first be cultured before it can be analyzed for chromosomal irregularities. Some studies have suggested, however, that the technique may be associated with a higher incidence of spontaneous abortion (1% increase in risk) and of

missing or undeveloped fingers or toes in the fetus (0.03% risk vs. a normal risk of about 0.005%).

Coupled with DNA probes (q.v.), new techniques for analyzing human genetic material through recombinant DNA methods, chorion biopsy may make it possible to detect almost any of the genetic disorders for which a faulty gene is known to exist (among them cystic fibrosis, phenylketonuria, and galactosemia, three of the most important genetic disorders among white Americans; sickle cell anemia, various forms of thalassemia or Cooley anemia, hemophilia, and Duchenne muscular dystrophy)

**choroid plexus**   Site of production of CSF in the adult brain; it is formed by the invagination of ependymal cells into the ventricles, which becomes richly vascularized.

**ChR2**   See *opsin.*

**chrematistophilia**   A *paraphilia* (q.v.) in which the necessary condition is that the relationship with the partner be on a monetary basis: the partner must charge the "client" or otherwise force him to pay for sex, or must rob or blackmail him. The term is sometimes broadened to include sellers as well as clients, e.g. "compulsive" hustlers, prostitutes, and sexual blackmailers (so long as such activity is needed for their own sexual arousal and is not merely their way of making a living).

**chrematophobia**   Fear of money; rare in the United States, where chrematomania is the more common condition.

**chrematorrhea**   Spending spree.

**chromatin**   *Chromatin* is a tightly wound amalgam of DNA, *histones,* and other proteins. The 46 DNA molecules that make up the diploid human genome are very long and thin. All are tightly packed into a nucleus, looping by attachment to an underlying matrix. As condensed as it is, the packed tangle must allow transcription of individual genes and the replication of all chromosomes. One complete new genome must be sorted our for inheritance by each daughter cell. If gene expression is to occur, the chromatin tangle must be opened up to allow the cell's gene-reading apparatus to gain access to the genetic material. This is accomplished by transcription factors and coactivators which attach different chemical tags, such as acetyl or phosphyl or methyl groups, to certain histone proteins. When they are attached to histones, the different chemical groups make the DNA more accessible and the activity of specific genes is boosted. Chromatin is loosened, or tightened, as needed for cell function. See *DNA*.

**chromatin remodeling** See *epigenetic mechanisms.*

**chromatolysis** Changes in the cell body as a result of injury to the nerve: the cell body and the nucleus swell, the basophilic endoplasmic reticulum (*Nissl substance*) breaks apart and disperses to the periphery of the cell body, and often there is an increase in RNA and protein synthesis within the cell. If the cell body itself is destroyed, the neuron in the central nervous system will certainly die; in the peripheral nervous system, the neuron may be able to regenerate itself. Severance of the axon will sometimes cause cell death. In other cases, the neuron is able to regenerate an axon; if it contacts a new target cell it resumes at least some degree of functioning and the cell body usually returns to its former appearance. If it fails to make connections with other cells, however, the neuron will atrophy and die.

**chromatophobia** Fear of a color or of colors in general.

**chromesthesia** A form of synesthesia in which colors are seen in association with the other forms of sensation, and especially in association with sounds (colored hearing).

**chromidial neuroplasm** See *neuron.*

**chromidrosis** Colored perspiration.

**chromomere** Minute nodules in the chromosomes of a cell nucleus that form a chain of chromatic bodies, particularly in the early stages of mitosis, and are strung like beads on a fine thread. They show persistent differences in size and distribution and presumably have also different chemical compositions. There are sound reasons for believing that many chromomeric nodules are too small to be visible. See *chromosome.*

**chromophobia** Fear of color(s); chromatophobia.

**chromosomal, chromosomic, chromosomatic** The adjectives refer not only to the minute chromosome particles themselves into which the scattered chromatin of a cell nucleus separates at the beginning of cell division, but are also used to characterize that part of the mechanism of heredity that is based on the activities of the chromosomes.

**chromosomal mapping** Chromosomal mapping is done by correlating the disease trait with DNA sequence variations, which are identified by restriction fragment-length polymorphism (RFLP) analysis. Any difference in the physical properties of a given DNA fragment between individuals is called a *polymorphism.* If a polymorphism correlates (or cosegregates) with the phenotypic disease trait, it suggests that the gene(s) for that trait is (are) on the same DNA fragment.

A growing number of familial neuropsychiatric disorders have now been "mapped" to specific chromosomal loci using recombinant DNA technology. These include Gaucher disease, Huntington disease, Duchenne muscular dystrophy, myotonic dystrophy, von Recklinghausen neurofibromatosis, and the familial forms of Alzheimer disease, manic-depressive illness, and amyloidotic polyneuropathy.

**chromosome** A dark-staining, compacted length of *DNA* (q.v.) in the nucleus of the cell that contains the genes. Chromosomes are formed from portions of the long string of the three billion nucleotide bases that constitute DNA. In the human, there are 46 chromosomes of varying length and base composition, arranged as 22 pairs of autosomes and a pair of sex chromosomes, or heterosomes (XX in the female, XY in the male). Each of the 23 chromosomes has a characteristic length and sequence of bases and therefore carries unique genetic information.

The specificity of DNA depends entirely on the sequence of its bases. The complete set of DNA sequences carried on all the chromosomes is the genome. See *gene.*

The largest human chromosome consists of 250 million base pairs; the smallest contains about 48 million base pairs. The identical members of a pair of chromosomes are homologues. The full complement of 46 chromosomes is termed the diploid number. During *mitosis*, the two strands of the DNA double helix unwind, and each resulting strand serves as a template for the formation of a new strand. *Meiosis* is a similar process that occurs in sexual reproduction; each strand, with its haploid number of 23 chromosomes, is assigned to a gamete (egg or sperm); the haploid gamete of one partner (the female, for example) pairs with the haploid gamete from the male to form a new cell (the zygote) with 46 chromosomes (23 pairs). The zygote has the full diploid number of chromosomes, but in a new combination: in each pair of genes, one homologue has come from the mother, the other from the father.

In the interphase nucleus, individual chromosomes occupy discrete patches (*chromosome territories*), which are separated by channels (the *interchromosomal domain*). RNA transcripts are apparently formed at the surface of the territories and then deposited in interchromosomal domain channels for further processing and transport. Within individual chromosome territories the chromatin fiber is highly contorted, looping back and forth betweeen the nuclear interior and the periphery.

Why do chromosomes move? Knowledge of how chromosomes are organized and of how the metabolic activities within the nucleus are related to its different substructures is still rudimentary, but it seems likely that some movements are linked to DNA replication, consistent with the proposal that DNA replication occurs at a fixed number of sites within the nucleus, called *replication factories*. Chromosomes move to the factories to initiate their replication.

How do the neurons and chromosomes know where to go? Tips of the growing neuronal processes, *growth cones*, make the necessary navigational decisions guided in part by diffusible attractive factors. Guidance signals can be attractive or repulsive, diffusible or substrate bound. Attractive and repulsive guidance mechanisms are mechanistically related and switched from one to the other by cyclic nucleotide levels within the growth cone. In general, elevation of cyclic nucleotide levels promotes attraction, and lowering their levels results in repulsion.

It is estimated that over 15 million Americans suffer from one or more birth defects, 80% of which are due to genetic changes. Genetic factors are responsible for 50% of all miscarriages, for at least 40% of all infant deaths, and for 80% of mental retardation in the United States. As many as 30% of all pediatric and 10% of all adult hospital admissions in the United States and Canada stem directly from genetic disorders.

**FREQUENCY OF CHROMOSOMAL ABNORMALITIES IN LIVE BIRTHS, BY MOTHER'S AGE**

| MATERNAL AGE | RISK OF DOWN SYNDROME | TOTAL RISK OF CHROMOSOMAL ABNORMALITIES |
|---|---|---|
| 20 | 1/1,667 | 1/526 |
| 30 | 1/952 | 1/385 |
| 33 | 1/602 | 1/286 |
| 35 | 1/378 | 1/192 |
| 38 | 1/173 | 1/102 |
| 40 | 1/106 | 1/66 |
| 42 | 1/63 | 1/42 |
| 45 | 1/30 | 1/21 |

*SOURCE*: Reprinted with permission from the American College of Obstetricians and Gynecologists.

The most common of the lethal genetic diseases is cystic fibrosis, which affects 1 in every 1800 births in the United States. Duchenne muscular dystrophy, one of the most common sex-linked disorders, affects 1 of every 3000 males born in the United States. Huntington disease affects 1 in every 10,000 births. Phenylketonuria (PKU) affects 1 in every 12,000 births. Type A hemophilia affects 1 of every 10,000 males.

Among the 3500 or more diseases recognized as genetic disorders are albinism, alkaptonuria, cystinuria, pentosuria, galactosemia, anidiria, microphthalmus, arachnodactyly, adenosine deaminase deficiency, Lesch-Nyhan syndrome, chondrodystrophy, sickle cell disorder, color blindness, epiloia, Tay-Sachs disease, Wilson disease, retinoblastoma, and neurofibromatosis.

Many believe that certain forms of epilepsy, manic-depressive (bipolar) disorder, schizophrenia, Pick disease, Alzheimer disease, and some forms of alcoholism are largely of genetic origin. Hormonal abnormalities that are recognized as genetically determined are diabetes insipidus, diabetes mellitus, and one form of goitrous cretinism. Diseases known to be due to gross chromosome abnormalities are Down syndrome, Turner syndrome (with XO sex chromosomes instead of XX or XY),

Klinefelter syndrome (XXY), superfemale (XXX), and chronic granulocytic leukemia.

**chromotopsia** A condition, most often due to ingestion of certain drugs, in which all objects appear to be of the same color or hue.

**chronaxia, chronaxy** The shortest duration a current of a certain defined strength takes to flow through a nerve in order to produce a muscular contraction.

**chronesthesia** The sense or feeling of time, the ability to place oneself in time and to imagine the distant future and the distant past. It is a type of consciousness of the self—*autonoetic consciousness.*

**chronic alcoholism** An obsolete term for alcoholism. The contrasting term "acute alcoholism" is now rarely used; it means severe intoxication by alcohol.

**chronic brain syndrome** See *organic syndrome.*

**chronic dementia** *Obs.* Dementia praecox (schizophrenia).

**chronic fatigue syndrome** *CFS*; a syndrome of unknown origin consisting of debilitating fatigue of at least 6 months' duration and some degree of functional impairment, not caused by any other identifiable clinical condition. Associated symptoms include headaches, sleep disturbances, difficulties with concentration, and muscle pain. No single definition is universally accepted; some include within the definition postviral fatigue syndrome, *EBV syndrome* (q.v.), and *myalgic encephalitis (ME).* The latter refers to gross abnormal muscle fatigue after relatively mild activity, with pain and a variety of symptoms suggestive of disturbances of the central nervous system.

CFS is usually described as an illness that occurs mainly in young adults; but it has been reported in children and in the elderly. Duration ranges from months to decades. In most reports, women account for 70% or more of cases.

Theories of etiology abound and many different treatment approaches have been advocated. A review of the literature on randomized controlled trials and controlled trials by P. Whiting et al. (*Journal of the American Medical Association 286,* 2001) concluded that GET (graded exercise therapy) and CBT (cognitive behavior therapy) showed promising results; immunoglobulin and hydrocortisone showed some limited effects, but overall evidence for their usefulness was inconclusive. The studies included a total of 2801 participants. Many other interventions were included in the studies but none of them demonstrated significant beneficial effects.

Because many CSF patients have shown evidence of active viral infection and immunologic changes, some researchers have hypothesized that the condition is a manifestation of Epstein-Barr virus infection. But as many as 80% of asymptomatic, healthy controls show equally strong evidence of such infection.

**chronic mentally ill** A generic term for patients with severe mental illness (most often schizophrenic and organic disorders), who need continuing care for long periods and at varying levels of intensity in accordance with their changing needs and their responsiveness (or lack of it) to treatment measures. Their plight was highlighted by *deinstitutionalization* (q.v.), since it was recognized that for many patients what had happened was more appropriately termed *transinstitutionalization*—a shift out of the hospital and into other institutions such as jails, nursing homes, and other *domiciles* (q.v.). The *young adult chronic patient* is a subgroup of patients between 18 and 35 years of age with severe and persistent dysfunctions combined with alternating abuse and underutilization of mental health services. As generally reported, over half of the patients in this group are diagnosed schizophrenic; others are diagnosed severe personality disorder or neurosis, organic mental disorder, mental retardation, or specific learning disability.

**chronobiology** The study of biological rhythms. See *clock, biological; rhythms, biological.*

**chronophilia** A *paraphilia* (q.v.) in which sexual satisfaction depends on the age of the partner; most frequently, the partner must be of a pronouncedly different age than the subject (*chronophilic disparity*). The term includes ephebophilia (adolescents are the sexual object), gerontophilia (the partner must be older, of parental or grandparental age), nepiophilia (infants), and pedophilia (juveniles).

**chronophobia** A neurotic fear of time. This is the most common psychiatric disorder in prison inmates, and sooner or later almost all prisoners suffer chronophobia to some degree. The duration and immensity of time are often terrifying to the prisoner, and the passage of time throws him into a panic. The frequency of chronophobia in prisoners has led to the condition's being called *prison neurosis*.

Chronophobia appears suddenly, without warning, at the time the inmate comes to grips with his sentence. The introductory phase of imprisonment is ordinarily marked by hopes and plans for a new trial or the like, by uncertainty, and by a studied indifference or carefree attitude. After the novelty of prison has worn off and the real length of the sentence is felt, chronophobia sets in. The prisoner goes into a panic, usually while in his cell, and fears his enclosure and restraint, but this apparent claustrophobia arises from fear of time, as represented by the prison. After the first attack, more or less constant anxiety, restlessness, insomnia, dissatisfaction with life, numerous hypochondriacal complaints, and progressive inability to adjust himself to his surroundings appear. The intensity of the crisis usually passes within a few weeks or months, though mild relapses may occur. But the prisoner becomes essentially a phlegmatic, indifferent automaton who serves the rest of his sentence by the clock and lives wholly in the present, one day at a time.

**chronotaraxis**  Confusion for time, as for date, season of year, time of day, and overestimation or underestimation of duration of time; this symptom has been reported as occurring as a result of bilateral lesions of the dorsomedial and anterior thalamic nuclei.

**chronotherapy**  Treatment of *delayed sleep phase syndrome* (DSPS) (q.v.) based on a sleep-wake phase angle physiology. The complaint is that the subject cannot fall asleep at the desired time and has difficulty awakening in the morning. It is believed that such subjects are unable to phase advance; i.e., they cannot move their sleep times ahead to earlier, more conventional hours. Treatment consists of a phase delay of approximately 3 hours on each consecutive day. The schedule must be rigidly maintained, for if the subject is allowed a late night, the original complaints recur. See *circadian rhythm sleep disorder*.

**CHT**  The high-affinity choline uptake transporter. Dysregulation in the capacity of CHT to transport choline is associated with the decline in cholinergic transmission in Alzheimer disease. There is evidence that increases in the capacity of the CHT in the right prefrontal cortex are specifically associated with attentional performance.

Monaminergic neurotransmitter transporter polymorphisms have also been linked to cognitive disturbances, but the interactions between the regulation of monaminergic and cholinergic systems are not fully understood.

**chthonic**  Relating to the depths of the earth. Jung described psychic archetypes as the chthonic portion of the mind.

**Chubby Puffer syndrome**  Sleep apnea in an obese child with large tonsils and adenoids, which occlude the air passages during sleep. There is some evidence that sudden infant death syndrome may be due to sleep apnea.

**chunking**  1. A type of cognitive therapy useful for the insomnia of ruminative, intrusive thinkers; the patient is trained to connect randomly occurring thoughts into logical groups, which then become easier to control.

2. A method of facilitating storage of information. See *short-term memory*.

**churus**  See *cannabis*.

**cibophobia**  Fear of food; sitophobia.

**CIDI**  Composite International Diagnostic Interview (World Health Organization).

**CIDS**  CNS injury–induced immunodepression. CNS injury induces a disturbance of the normally well-balanced interplay between the immune system and the CNS, leading to secondary immunodeficiency and, in some cases, infection. Infection is a highly relevant complication in three major injury conditions of CNS—stroke, traumatic brain injury (TBI), and spinal cord injury (SCI). CNS injury activates the HPA axis, and sympathetic and parasympathetic nervous systems. Through the release of noradrenaline, glucocorticoids, and accetylcholine, a systemic anti-inflammatory response is mounted that negatively affects the function and composition of the innate and adaptive immune systems. As a consequence of the resulting immunodepression and breakdown of immunological barriers, infection develops. The risk of infection is further increased because such patients are hospitalized under intensive care conditions and the CNS lesion itself may lead to dysphagia, aspiration, bladder dysfunction, etc. Systemic infection increases morbidity and mortality and leads to worsening of outcome.

**cilia**  See *asymmetry*.

**ciliospinal reflex**  A superficial reflex; scratching or pinching of the skin on the side of the neck produces dilation of the pupil; strong light and accommodation must be avoided in this test.

**cinaedi**   Males who adopt the passive or receptive role in homosexual activity. See *active*.

**CIND**   Cognitive impairment, no dementia; at least twice as prevalent as dementia at ages over 65 and associated with more functional impairment and institutionalization than occurs in the healthy elderly. Nearly half of subjects with CIND progress to dementia over a 5-year period.

**Cinderella syndrome**   Simulation of neglect, or false accusation of neglect by a child, such as an adopted child's allegation (unfounded) that her stepmother made her do all the household chores and then left her unclothed in a snowdrift while the stepmother went off to the movies with her other children.

**cineseismography**   A photographic system for recording and measuring abnormal involuntary movements; its great advantage is that it obviates the need to attach any devices to the subject.

**cingulate cortex**   See *anterior cingulate cortex*.

**cingulate gyrus**   The arched, crescent-shaped convolution on the medial surface of the cerebral hemisphere that lies immediately above the corpus callosum. Also known as gyrus cinguli; callosal gyrus. Part of "Papez circuit." See *Papez's theory of emotion*.

The *anterior cingulate cortex (ACC)* (q.v.), on the medial surface of the frontal lobe; contributes to performance monitoring by detecting conditions under which errors are likely to occur. The region has rich anatomical connections with association, limbic, and motor cortices.

**cingulate signs**   Bilateral lesions of the cingulate gyri may cause apathy, akinesia, and mutism. See *anterior cingulate cortex*.

**cingulotomy**   Cingulumotomy; a type of *psychosurgery* (q.v.) in which small portions of the cingulum bundle are coagulated bilaterally; the procedure has been beneficial in treatment-resistant psychosis and in chronic alcoholism and drug addiction.

**CIP**   Caudal intraparietal area; see *intraparietal sulcus*.

**cipher method**   A method in secret writing. Freud referred to the cipher method of dream interpretation, in which every sign is translated into another sign of known meaning, according to an established key.

**circadian**   See *rhythms, biological*.

**circadian clock**   The timekeeper or pacemaker for circadian rhythms, which are fluctuations of biochemical, physiological, and behavioral phenomena that have a periodicity of approximately 24 hours in a constant environment. These genetically determined biological rhythms have evolved in response to the 24-hour astronomical cycle to which all organisms are exposed.

Circadian rhythms are genetically determined, and the free-running period is very similar among individuals of a single species. The free-running period of human rhythms changes with age, suggesting that humans differ from other animals in the precision of their timekeeping. The basis of circadian function is transcription of clock genes (such as *tim* and *per*) and synthesis of the proteins they encode. When the protein products are degraded, gene transcription begins again and the cycle is reestablished. The *suprachiasmatic nucleus (SCN)* of the hypothalamus is the principal circadian pacemaker in mammals. Circadian behavioral responses are driven by an internal clock and also reset (or entrained) by light. The 24-hour variation in sleep propensity is regulated by opposing homeostatic and circadian mechanisms. The homeostatic system governs the probability of falling asleep; the circadian system promotes wakefulness and, in humans, consolidates sleep into the characteristic 8-hour sleep bouts. Serotonin levels vary diurnally with the light/dark cycle: high levels in daylight, varying inversely with melatonin, which shows high levels in darkness.

*Zeitgebers* (time setters) shift the rhythms by advancing the phase of the clock at certain parts of the circadian cycle and by delaying the phase when impinging on other parts of the cycle. According to the *humoral phototransduction model*, the blood contains chronobiological photoreceptors that act in concert with melatonin or other antioxidants to shift the phase of the clock. See *clock, biological; SCN*.

**circadian desynchronosis**   *Circadian rhythm sleep disorder* (q.v.).

**circadian rhythm sleep disorder**   *Circadian desynchronosis; sleep-wake schedule disorder*; a *sleep disorder* (q.v.) consisting of sleep disruption as a result of a mismatch between the schedule imposed by environmental conditions and the subject's own sleep-wake pattern. The sleep disruption leads to excessive sleepiness or insomina. Various types have been described, such as *delayed sleep phase*, with persisting inability to fall asleep or awaken as early as desired; and the desynchronized type, when the subject is sleepy when he or she should be awake, awake when he should be sleeping, as a result of night-shift work or frequently changing shifts of work (shift work type), or due to recent or repeated travel across more than one time zone (*jet lag* type). The effects of long-term shift work on workers who do not adjust adequately to it have been termed the *shift maladaptation syndrome, irregular schedule disorder*, and *hypernychthemeral syndrome.*

**circuit, Papez**    See Papez's theory of emotion.

**circuit, reverberating**    Lorente de Nò's hypothesis to explain enduring reflex responses to a single stimulus; the hypothesis assumes that several internuncial neurons are intercalated between the sensory fibers and the anterior horn cells and that these several neurons discharge in sequence rather than simultaneously and thus produce an enduring *cerebral excitatory state* and enduring reflex discharge.

**circular dementia**    Kraepelin's term for a form of schizophrenia characterized by alternating phases of excitement and depression.

**circular psychosis**    See *mania; manic-depressive psychosis.*

**circulatory psychosis**    Confused mental state associated with cardiovascular failure.

**circumscription, monosymptomatic**    The condition of having only a single symptom. See *monoideism; monomania.*

**circumstantiality**    A disorder of associations seen in schizophrenics in which too many associated ideas come to consciousness because of too little selective suppression. Many things that are implicit in ordinary conversation are explicitly communicated and, typically, to an absurd and bizarre degree. One of Bleuler's patients, for example, wrote the following letter to his mother: "I am writing on paper. The pen I use for it is from a factory called Perry & Co., the factory is in England. I am assuming that. After the name Perry Co. the city of London is scratched in; but not the country. The city of London is in England. That I know from school."

Some patients who are aware of their circumstantiality will describe an accompanying subjective experience of feeling that the central idea has not been communicated until all of its facets have been considered in detail. This same sort of uncertainty and doubt about adequacy of communication may be seen in obsessional disorders where it usually appears as overmeticulousness, precision, or ostentatious honesty. See *Klebenbleiben.*

Circumstantiality also occurs in epileptic dementia. Preoccupation with peripheral details is also often a feature of the interictal behavior syndrome in patients with temporal lobe epilepsy (complex partial seizures). It may be expressed not only in speech but also in writing (hypergraphia), as in writing lengthy letters or diaries filled with minutiae.

**cis-acting element**    A regulatory genetic element located in the same DNA molecule as the gene being regulated.

**cistern, lumbar**    See *cauda equina.*

**cisternae**    See *Golgi apparatus*

**cistern(al) puncture**    A technique for gaining access to the subarachnoid space by means of introduction of a needle into the cisterna magna. Cistern puncture is performed when lumbar puncture is for some reason impossible; it is also used for the injection of air or opaque media for diagnostic purposes and for the introduction of therapeutic substances. It is contraindicated in cases of tumor or abscess in the posterior fossa, in cases of increased intracranial pressure, and when the cisterna magna is likely to be obliterated by inflammatory adhesions. See *suboccipital puncture.*

**cisvestitism**    Dressing in the clothes of one's own sex, but in clothes inappropriate to one's station of life, as when an adult dresses as a child or a child as an adult, or a civilian as an army officer. See *transvestitism.*

**CIT**    See *crisis intervention team model.*

**cittosis**    *Pica* (q.v.).

**CJD**    *Creutzfeldt-Jakob disease* (q.v.).

**CL- channel**    See *GABA.*

**C-L psychiatry**    Consultation-liaison psychiatry. See *consultant; consultation-liaison.*

**claim, neurotic**    Horney's term for the belief held by certain patients (whom Freud called "the exceptions") that they are in some way superior and that others should fulfill their wishes and needs.

**claims review**    See *audit; review.*

**CLAMS**    Clinical Linguistic and Auditory Milestone Scale, a screening test for defects in language development, developed by Arnold Caputo, Bruce Shapiro, and Frederick Palmer.

The test compares the child's language development with standardized receptive and expressive milestones for the age period between 1 week and 36 months.

**clang association**   An association based on similarity of sound, without regard for differences in meaning; most frequently observed in the manic phase of manic-depressive disorder and in the schizophrenias. See *homonym.*

**clarification**   See *interpretation.*

**clasp knife phenomenon**   Seen in spastic patients (such as those with lesions of the premotor area of the brain), it consists of the sudden disappearance of resistance to passive movement.

**class, social**   Rank, estate, station, or status within a society or group; a grouping of people based on similarity in income, education, vocation, etc.

While some sociologists define social class (or stratum) largely in economic terms, others stress similarity of lifestyle, attitudes, or prestige. A. B. Hollingshead and Fritz C. Redlich (*American Social Review 18*, 1953) studied the urbanized community of New Haven, Connecticut, in 1950 and 1951, in an attempt to define the relationship between social class and mental illness. They used the following categories:

   *Class I*—business and professional leaders, including a long-established core group of interrelated families and a smaller upwardly mobile group of new people.

   *Class II*—managers or less ranking professions; four of five in this category are upwardly mobile.

   *Class III*—salaried administrative and clerical workers; small business owners.

   *Class IV*—working class; semiskilled or skilled manual workers; education within this class usually ends with graduation from grammar school.

   *Class V*—semiskilled factory workers or unskilled laborers, who usually have not completed elementary school.

Hollingshead and Redlich found an inverse relationship between social class and mental illness; the significant division was between Class V and all the other classes. See *neuroses, class differences in.*

**classes of drugs**   See *psychopharmacological agents.*

**classical technique**   See *parameter.*

**classification**   See *DSM-III; DSM-IV; nosology.*

**claudication, cerebral intermittent**   A vasomotor phenomenon in which transient spasm and closure of the lumen of an artery occurs, temporarily depriving a part of the brain of its blood supply, producing transitory hemiplegia. This condition is usually observed in the course of *cerebral arteriosclerosis* (q.v.).

**claudication, mental**   Transitory spasm of the blood vessels of the brain. Some authors hold that mental claudication may be responsible for sudden fleeting episodes of mental confusion.

**claustrophilia**   A pathological desire to be confined and enclosed within a small space—the exact opposite of claustrophobia. Claustrophilia is a manifestation of a strong tendency to withdraw in a somatic way and is seen in many catatonic episodes. It has been suggested that certain criminals have adopted a psychopathic reaction pattern, thus inviting incarceration, which represents a protected withdrawal from unbearable environmental tension. In such cases claustrophilia is interpreted psychoanalytically as an escape from the world and a tendency to return to the womb. A disposition to claustrophilia is often seen in asthmatics, who symptomatically withdraw into their own respiratory cavities. Such patients show a predilection for introversion and isolation, often with a strong need for solitude and silence.

**claustrophobia**   Fear of being locked or shut in; fear of enclosed places, such as tunnels, elevators, theaters, classrooms, boats, or narrow streets. Like all phobias, this fear may represent a feared temptation (e.g. a fear of sexual excitement which in some patients is manifested in feelings of constriction and painful vegetative sensations, or a fear of phantasies of being in the mother's womb, or a fear that one might not escape his or her own excitement once it has reached a certain intensity), or it may represent punishment for yielding to temptation, or (as is most common) it may represent a combination of both the foregoing. See *agoraphobia.*

**claustrum**   See *basal ganglia.*

**clavus**   Severe head pain, sharply defined, and typically described as feeling like a nail is being driven into the head; usually regarded as a conversion symptom.

**clear twilight state**   See *epileptic equivalent.*

**cleft, synaptic**   See *neurotransmitter; synapse.*

**Clèrambault-Kandinsky complex**   (Gatian G. de Clèrambault, 1872-1934, French psychiatrist) *Erotomania* (q.v.).

**client** A purchaser of services or goods; in nonmedical settings used instead of patient to refer to the recipient of mental health care.

**client-centered psychotherapy** *Nondirective therapy*; developed by Carl Rogers and originally (1938-39) called *passive therapy* or *relationship therapy*. Client-centered psychotherapy eschews the medical model and instead employs a growth model: each person has inherent capacities for self-understanding and for constructively changing ways of being and behaving, and the goal of therapy is to release those capacities in order to facilitate healthy change and growth. That can best be done in a relationship with certain definable qualities: the therapist's genuineness or congruence (the therapist's openness about his or her own feeling state about the patient, whether positive or negative), unconditional positive regard and nonjudgmental acceptance of the client as he or she is, and accurate empathic understanding of the client. Individual psychotherapy is viewed as one example of all constructive interpersonal relationships, and its processes and philosophy have been used in group therapy, marital therapy, and in many settings that are quite separate from formal psychotherapy: the intensive group experience to facilitate personal growth, encounter groups, person-centered teacher-training programs (including programs for medical educators), community organization, and intercultural and international relationships. In all these settings, the emphasis is on the qualities of the relationship, and in recent years a particular focus has been on the power structure within those relationships and the effects of self-empowerment on the participants.

**climacophobia** Fear of stairs.

**climacteric** Pertaining to the involutional period, characterized in the woman by cessation of menses, less definitely characterized in men.

**climacteric melancholia** *Involutional psychosis* (q.v.).

**climacterium** A critical period of life; most commonly, in present-day usage, the involutional period when the endocrine and reproductive glands undergo a decrease in functional activity. In the male, the climacterium is generally considered to fall between the ages of 50 and 65 years; in the female, between 40 and 55 years. See *developmental levels; involutional psychosis.*

**climacterium, male** An ill-defined syndrome in males, in middle life, and thought of as analogous to the menopause in females. The major symptoms are usually nocturnal frequency, fatigue, indecision, flushes, decreased sexual desire, and decreased erective and intromissive potency. Various other symptoms may be present also. It is a moot question whether this syndrome constitutes a separate and distinct clinical entity, or whether it is a symptomatic manifestation of a psychoneurotic breakdown in middle life, revolving, in the main, around psychogenic impotence and anxiety. In a very small percentage of cases, a true organic, or gonadal, endocrine etiology, secondary to testicular atrophy and degeneration, has been diagnostically validated by means of androgen and gonadotrophic assays of the urine.

**climax** Peak; acme; often used synonymously with *orgasm* (q.v.).

**climbing fibers** See *cerebellum.*

**clinical genetics** See *genetic epidemiology.*

**clinical marker** See *biomarker.*

**clinical poverty syndrome** Slowness, underactivity, reduced emotional responsivity, and impaired ability to communicate (as manifested, for example, in a wooden expression, monotonous voice, lack of gesturing, poverty of speech content). The clinical poverty syndrome is a type of long-term impairment or disability that tends to persist in many schizophrenics even after acute symptoms have subsided.

**clinical psychologist** See *psychologist.*

**clinicoeconomics** Health care economics; the application of economic principles to analysis of the utilization of health care resources, including analysis of the relative costs and benefits of diagnostic procedures and clinical treatments.

**clioquinol** A Cu/Zn chelator that has been reported to inhibit and reverse the Cu/Zn-mediated aggregation of β-amyloid in post-mortem brain samples from patients with Alzheimer disease.

**clitoris** A part of the female external genitalia. It is about an inch and a half in length and is composed of two corpora cavernosa capped by a glans. In psychoanalytic theory, the first genital belief of the child is that everyone possesses a penis (phallic sexual monism). The little girl regards her clitoris as an undeveloped penis. Deutsch stressed that in the beginning of the phallic stage the clitoris possesses for the girl the same pleasure-giving capacities as the penis has for the boy. There is clitoral primacy just as there is phallic primacy.

**cloaca**  The common opening of the rectum and urethrum in the embryo. The anal membrane ruptures later, and the rectum acquires its own orifice. In psychoanalysis, emphasis is placed on the child's cloaca theory, that babies are expelled by way of the anal aperture.

**clock, aging**  See *aging, theories of*.

**clock, biological**  *Cerebral pacemaker; circadian clock*; a self-sustained oscillator with a period of about 24 hours which controls a temporal program of cellular metabolism to facilitate adaptation to daily environmental changes. It regulates the internal temporal order and timing of hormonal, physiologic, and behavioral rhythms. The intrinsic period of the human circadian pacemaker averages 24–25 hours and, contrary to earlier beliefs, does not shorten with age but, rather, throughout the life cycle remains stable and precise in measuring time. The neural mechanism involved is believed to be located in the *suprachiasmatic nucleus* (SCN) of the inferior hypothalamus. See *aging, theories of; rhythms, biological*.

Cyanobacteria are the simplest organisms that display circadiation rhythms; in them, the gene cluster of *kaiA, kaiB*, and *kaiC* (*kai* means cycle in Japanese) is essential for the circadian oscillation, which is based on negative feedback control of their expression. Similarly, in *Drosophila* and *Neurospora* the clock genes *Drosophila per* and *Neurospora frq* are repressed by their products PER and FRQ, respectively.

Jet lag and the effect of changes in work shift reflect physiological derangements of circadian organization, and it is hypothesized that the same neural mechanism is responsible for the periodicity of various neuropsychiatric disorders. Circadian rhythms appear to be regulated by at least two subsystems, one regulating the sleep-wake cycle and the second regulating body temperature, cortisol secretion, and REM sleep propensity. It has been hypothesized that changes in the relative relations of these two systems are involved in the production of depression.

**clock drawing**  A neuropsychological assessment instrument in which the subject is asked to draw a clock with the hands indicating a time specified by the examiner (e.g., "2:30" or "11:20"). It has been in use since the 1950s to assess neurocognitive functioning. Widely accepted as a quick, reliable, and nonthreatening test for dementia, the clock drawing test was believed to be valid across cultures and easy to administer in a wide range of settings. Some recent studies have cast doubt on its predictive accuracy for probable dementia, particularly in a multicultural population.

**clock-driven behavior**  Endogenous rhythmic behavior. See *clock, biological; rhythms, biological*.

**clomipramine**  The three-chloro analogue of imipramine, the most potent serotonergic uptake inhibitor of the tricyclic antidepressants. In the United States, it is used chiefly in the treatment of obsessive-compulsive disorder; in other countries, it has been used also as an *antidepressant* (q.v.).

**clonal deletion theory**  Now called *negative selection*; Burnet's theory that a cell-intrinsice suicide program leads to *apoptosis* (q.v.).

**clonazepam**  A benzodiazepine drug with *anticonvulsant* properties (q.v.). It has also been used in the treatment of bipolar mood disorders.

**clone**  A group of organisms that have originated from a single individual by asexual reproduction. Since all these organisms must be endowed with the same hereditary equipment, it may generally be assumed that differences in their phenotypical appearance are due to modifying conditions of their environment. See *modification*.

**clonic convulsion**  Convulsion characterized by alternate contraction and relaxation of muscular tissue.

**clonidine**  An imidazoline derivative used primarily as a hypertensive agent; an alpha-2 noradrenergic agonist that inhibits bulbar sympathetic cardioaccelerator and vasoconstrictor centers and decreases norepinephrine release from the brain. In psychiatry, it has been used in mood disorders, obsessive-compulsive disorder, and akathisia.

**cloning, molecular**  The series of procedures involved in inserting DNA from one organism to another; a gene is copied, and the copy is transferred to a vector, usually a virus. The vector then makes multiple copies to produce *recombinant DNA* (q.v.).

**cloning, positional**  Progressively narrowing a large region of a gene that contains a suspected gene mutation, using gene mapping techniques, in order to establish that the gene does, in fact, contribute to the disease in question or to susceptibility to the disease. Once its role in the disease has been established, the biological action of the disease gene and the way it contributes to the disease can be determined. Positional cloning refers to identification of a particular gene at the DNA level; it makes possible the identification of a gene in the complete absence of knowledge of how the gene works and what it produces. See *behavioral genetics.*

**clonus** A rhythmical series of contractions in response to the maintenance of tension in a muscle, often appearing in pyramidal lesions as a manifestation of exaggerated tendon reflexes.

**clonus, ankle** A clonic rhythmical tremor of the foot elicited by placing the leg in semiflexion, · holding the leg with one hand, grasping the foot with the other, and briskly dorsiflexing the foot one or more times. See *clonus.*

**clonus, patellar** Patellar clonus is elicited by extending the leg, grasping the patella (kneecap) between index finger and thumb, and briskly pushing the cap down one or more times. See *clonus.*

**closed group** A therapy group to which no new patients are added in the course of treatment or after treatment has proceeded for a time. See *open group.*

**closing-in** A symptom of constructive apraxia in which the patient tends to close in on the model when performing constructive tasks. For example, when attempting to copy from a model, the patient moves toward the model; or, in setting-up exercises, he will bring his hands ever closer to those of the demonstrator. The symptom, which becomes worse with an increase in the difficulty of the task, may be the result of a fear of empty space, but more likely it represents an attempt to perform better when there is a disturbance in the ability to make an abstract copy from a concrete model.

**closure** Conclusion, resolution, ending; the process of reaching a decision or ending a debate.

**closure, law of and life-course** A person's course of life is described by a general law of Gestalt dynamics, the law of closure. This means that every uncompleted whole tends to a kind of continuation that is in accordance with the inherent system of that given whole. In the early phase of life only a few initial lines of

the life patterns are apparent, and the continuation patterns may take many different directions. The more the pattern nears completion, the less variation in the pattern continuation is possible.

**clouded states** See *epileptic clouded states.*

**cloudiness** See *sensorium.*

**clouding of consciousness** *Obtundation*; reduced clarity of awareness of the environment with reduced capacity to shift, focus, and sustain attention to environmental stimuli or to engage in goal-directed thinking or behavior. The subject appears drowsy, slow to react, muddled in thinking, and sometimes misinterprets external events. Clouding is part of the general disturbance in arousal that is characteristic of *delirium* (q.v.).

**Clouston, Sir Thomas Smith** (1840-1915) British psychiatrist and neurologist.

**clownism** A popular term denoting clownish, grotesque attitudes assumed by certain psychiatric patients; seen especially in the so-called *Faxenpsychosis, buffoonery psychosis* and, to a lesser extent, in the *Ganser syndrome* (qq.v.).

**clozapine** A dibenzodiazepine antipsychotic agent that was found effective in some patients with treatment-resistant schizophrenia, diminishing psychotic symptoms and even negative symptoms; the first of the "atypical" neuroleptics. It is a dopamine receptor antagonist and appears to act more selectively than traditional neuroleptics on mesolimbic and mesocortical dopamine tracts, with less effect on nigrostriatal tracts. It does not cause tardive dyskinesia or tardive dystonia. It is more likely than other neuroleptics to produce agranulocytosis, however, and for that reason was withdrawn from the U.S. market.

**club drugs** Include cocaine, crystal methamphetamines (crystal), amyl nitrites (poppers), Ecstasy, gamma-hydroxybutyrate (GHB), ketamine (special K), and Viagra.

**clumsiness** Difficulty in performing skilled movements that a normal subject of the same age could perform with ease; the difficulty is not due to cognitive, intellectual, or gross sensory deficits. Clumsiness in children is sometimes called *developmental apraxia* and is often associated with speech or reading problems, as in *attention deficit hyperactivity disorder* (q.v.) or minimal brain dysfunction.

**clumsiness, arranged** An unconsciously prepared inaptitude through which the neurotic prevents himself from properly performing certain acts that he secretly fears. In a general sense, arranged clumsiness is an escape mechanism by means of which the performance of certain acts is avoided through the pretense of lack of skill.

**clumsy gait**   See *waddling gait.*

**cluster, personality**   An aggregation of personality disorders. DSM-III-R, for example, recognized:

> *Cluster A*—the odd, eccentric group; included are the schizotypal, schizoid, and paranoid personalities; at an interpersonal level, such types tend to withdraw.
>
> *Cluster B*—with dramatic presentation, impulsive acting out, and unpredictable behavior; included are the borderline (characteristically, with no impulse control), antisocial (no conscience), and narcissistic (no humility) personality disorders; in interpersonal relations, such types tend to exploit others.
>
> *Cluster C*—anxious and fearful; included are the avoidant, dependent, passive-aggressive, and obsessive-compulsive personality disorders; in interpersonal relations, such types tend to comply.

**cluster headache**   In ICHD-II, the category of cluster headache and other trigeminal autonomic cephalalgias includes cluster headache and paroxysmal hemicrania. Cluster headache has also been called *migrainous neuralgia* and is described as a syndrome characterized by paroxysms of severe pain, usually located in the frontotemporal region and eye, lasting for as long as 2 hours and occurring several times during a 24-hour period. Each bout of headaches tends to last a few weeks and then recur after a free interval of several months or even a year. Etiology is unknown; treatment is symptomatic, with oral ergotamine. Some writers use the term to refer to any atypical facial neuralgia that is not *migraine* (q.v.), including histamine cephalalgia, ciliary neuralgia, and sphenopalatine neuralgia (vidian neuralgia, Sluder syndrome).

**cluster trigeminal autonomic cephalalgias**   Include cluster headache and chronic paroxysmal hemicrania. See *cluster headache; headache.*

**cluttering**   Rapid, jerky speech with faulty phrasing patterns, as a result of which the child's language is at times unintelligible. Cluttering is a language and speech disorder within the group "specific developmental disorders"

in DSM-III-R. It is commonly associated with motor awkwardness and personality and behavior changes (e.g., behavior is erratic, disorganized, impulsive, untidy). Other language disorders such as delay in beginning to speak, reading disability, and spelling disability are common. Family history frequently reveals clutterers in the same family and the condition is often mistaken for stammering. Like stammering, it is more common in boys, but cluttering tends to persist throughout life and the cluttered speech is characteristic. It is hurried, even precipitate (tachylalia), and confused.

In DSM-IV, cluttering is not a separate entity; instead, it is treated as an associated feature of expressive and receptive language disorders. Probably the most famous clutterer was the Reverend W. A. Spooner, Warden of New College, Oxford, whose word confusions have come to be known as *spoonerisms*. Typical examples include "The two great English poets, Kelly and Sheets" (for "Shelley and Keats") and "The Lord is a shoving leopard" (for "loving shepherd").

Cluttering is also sometimes called *agitolalia.*

**Clytemnestra complex**   This refers to the wife who kills her husband so that she may possess one of his male relatives.

**cM**   Centimorgan. See *mapping, genetic.*

**CME**   Continuing medical education.

**CMHC**   Community Mental Health Center. See *community psychiatry.*

**CMMS**   Columbia Mental Maturity Scale, designed primarily for use with patients with cerebral palsy.

**CMP**   Competitive medical plan; chronic mental patient; see *chronic mentally ill.*

**CMT**   Chronic motor tics. See *tic.*

**CMV**   Cytomegalovirus. See *cytomegalic disease.*

**CNV**   Contingent negative variation; *readiness potential*; in testing event-related potentials, the negative voltage that builds slowly in the subject who is warned of the imminence of a target. The CNV is generally interpreted as an indicator of arousal or anticipation. It is reduced in amplitude in many schizophrenics and in other disorders as well, but in the latter it returns to normal when patients are in clinical remission while it remains abnormal in schizophrenics in remission. See *evoked potential.*

**CO**   Community organization, community organizer. See *social policy planning.*

**coactive strategy**  In pharmacotherapy, the simultaneous use of two or more drugs to achieve a positive response. Included are *combination*, in which each of the drugs used has a unique and different mode of action, the net effect of which is a greater response than would be achieved with any of the drugs used alone, and *augmentation*, in which one or more drugs are added to the current drug regimen in order to enhance the specific pharmacodynamic and therapeutic effects of the current drug. An example of a combination strategy is the conjoint use of a tricyclic antidepressant and a monoamine oxidase inhibitor; lithium augmentation is often used when patients do not respond adequately to an antidepressant drug alone.

**co-alcoholic**  Codependent on alcohol. See *codependency*.

**coat components**  See *Golgi apparatus*.

**cocaine**  An alkaloid obtained from the coca bush (Bolivia, Peru), used as a topical anesthetic in ear, nose, and throat surgery, and in dentistry and ophthalmology. It is a powerful psychostimulant that produces a sense of exhilaration and a decreased sense of fatigue and hunger. It has a high potential for abuse and dependence. See *dependence, drug*.

Cocaine activates positive reinforcement by blocking the reuptake of dopamine in the central nervous system. Of the various dopamine receptor subtypes identified, the $D_3$ receptor is the most likely to be involved in cocaine abuse: it has an unusually high affinity for dopamine and is localized within limbic dopaminergic areas.

In addition to abuse and dependence, the following mental disorders may be associated with cocaine use: intoxication, withdrawal, delirium, psychotic (delusional) disorder, mood disorder, anxiety disorder, sleep disorder, and sexual dysfunction.

Cocaine ("coke") may be taken orally, often with alcohol; with this route of administration, peak toxicity is reached about 1 hour after ingestion. It may be sniffed ("snorted") in powder form, producing effects in 1 to 3 minutes and lasting for 30 minutes. It may be smoked, as with *freebasing* and *crack* (qq.v.). Intravenous use is particularly frequent in combined opioid and cocaine users (the combination is called a *speedball*). Intravenous administration produces a *rush* (q.v.). If quickly and frequently repeated, it induces a *crash*: a rapid shift from exhilaration to dysphoria, apprehensiveness, ideas of reference, delusions of persecution, ringing in the ears, *snow lights* (q.v.), or other hallucinations.

Cocaine psychotic disorder may resemble a functional paranoid disorder, with hypervigilance, suspiciousness, and fixed delusional beliefs.

A similar condition may develop with chronic use of amphetamine, methylphenidate, and appetite suppressants.

**cocaine bug**  See *Magnan sign*.

**cocaine delirium**  An organic mental syndrome that develops within 24 hours of cocaine use; it may appear in both the naive experimenter and the chronic user. Symptoms consist of an admixture of anxiety, irritability, fear of impending death, and disorientation, often with accompanying hyperpyrexia or life-threatening hypertension.

**cocaine delusional disorder**  Persecutory delusions developing shortly after use of cocaine during a period of long-term use, usually with ideas of reference, aggressiveness and hostility, anxiety, and psychomotor agitation.

**cocaine intoxication**  Symptoms include tachycardia, pupillary dilation, elevated blood pressure, sweating or chills, nausea and vomiting, visual or tactile hallucinations, and maladaptive behavior such as fighting, grandiosity, hypervigilance, impaired judgment, and psychomotor agitation. Cocaine exerts a generalized sympathomimetic effect on the vascular system and may thus induce cardiac arrhythmias and severe hypertension, which may lead to cerebral hemorrhage. It may also induce myocardial infarction and status epilepticus.

**cocaine withdrawal**  Despite clearcut evidence of extreme dependence, chronic cocaine users report symptoms, generally mild, during withdrawal; temporary feelings of fatigue or a "letdown," depression, disturbed sleep, and increased dreaming.

**cocaine use disorders**  Classified within the substance-related disorders: cocaine dependence, cocaine abuse, cocaine intoxication, cocaine withdrawal, cocaine delirium, cocaine psychotic disorder, cocaine mood disorder, cocaine anxiety disorder, cocaine sleep disorder, and cocaine sexual dysfunction.

**cocainism**  Cocaine poisoning or cocaine dependency

**cocainomania**  Craving for cocaine.

**cochlear nerve**  See *auditory nerve.*

**Cockayne syndrome**  Mental retardation associated with dwarfism, wizened countenance, photosensitive skin, and cerebellar and ocular involvement ("salt and pepper"-like abnormalities of the retina).

**cocktail party syndrome**  See *chatterbox syndrome.*

**co-conscious, co-consciousness**  "Conscious states that we are not aware of, simply because [they are] not in the focus of attention but in the fringe of the content of consciousness. The term would also include pathologically split-off and independently acting co-conscious ideas or systems of ideas such as occur in hysteria, reaching their apogee in conscious personalities and in automatic writings" (Prince, M. *The Unconscious,* 1916).

In psychoanalysis the term preconscious is in general equivalent to co-conscious.

**code, labeled line**  A mechanism for identifying the modality of a stimulus that reflects receptor specificity; the receptor responds only to a particular stimulus energy under natural conditions (e.g., auditory, vestibular, gustatory, or visual), and even if excited artificially by direct electrical stimulation it will elicit the same sensation.

**code, professional**  An articulated statement of role morality as perceived and agreed on by the members of the profession itself. Such codes are often criticized as lacking adequacy and comprehensiveness because they emphasize a limited number of moral principles but ignore others. Specifically in medicine, at least in the past, they have tended to focus on the obligations of the professional but have managed at the same time to ignore patient autonomy. See *ethics.*

**codependency**  A pattern of self-defeating, learned behaviors that is hypothesized to develop within one or more members of a dysfunctional family (or other social unit), characterized by overattachment (*dependent bonding*) of the subject on another person, fear of rejection or abandonment by that person, a need to deny or suppress all feelings lest the person be displeased (leading to emotional paralysis and an inability to participate in loving relationships), and increasing inflexibility and rigidity of response in order to avoid the dangers of spontaneity or loss of control.

Codependency is a popularized term, but there is little evidence to support its existence as a bona fide psychiatric disorder. It was first applied to the families ("codependents") of alcoholics, whose manipulativeness and charismatic charm often entangle a large number of family members, coworkers, and social contacts within a web of unspoken rules and oppressive regulations whose end result is to prevent open expression of feelings and direct dealing with personal and interpersonal problems. Empirical studies support a stress and coping model as the significant factor in the behavior of a family with a chemically dependent member.

Although sometimes discussed in terms of distorted communication, codependency refers to all the effects that alcoholics (and/or gamblers, sex addicts, substance abusers, bulimics, anorexics, and similar "compulsive" behaviors) have on the people around them, including those persons' attempts to affect the alcoholic. See *communication deviance; enabler.*

**codification**  The act of systematizing or classifying; in communications theory, the phrasing of signals in such terms as to be understandable to others.

**coding region**  See *gene; gene functions.*

**codon**  The smallest unit of a *gene* (q.v.), consisting of three adjacent nucleotides, that is able to specify an amino acid residue in the synthesis of a polypeptide chain. See *DNA.*

**coefficient, correlation**  See *correlation.*

**coefficient, regression**  See *correlation.*

**coenaesthetic schizophrenia**  G. Huber's term (1957) for a chronic of bodily sensation and by associated vegetative, motor, and sensory symptoms. According to Huber, this form is steadily progressive and is organically determined by disturbances in the diencephalic and thalamic areas.

**coene-**  See *cene-.*

**coercion**  Any threat of sufficient force that no rational person would reasonably be expected to resist. Strong or forceful recommendations, particularly when given so as to overcome a patient's irrational fear about a procedure or plan for treatment, do not ordinarily consititute coercion. Threatening to commit a patient or hospitalize him involuntarily if he does not accept the proffered treatment, however, often falls within the definition of coercion in that it has removed the patient's freedom of choice. Because even under identical conditions, and given identical choices, not all would choose the same course of action, valid consent must include freedom of choice and lack of coercion to make one choice, provided that more than one course of action is available. Physicians tend to rank survival as the most important choice, no matter what the alternatives, whereas many patients consider pain or disability more significant in determining choice than the prospect of mere survival. See *informed consent*.

**coercive philosophy**  The attempt to force others by argument to believe things.

**coercive treatment**  See *forced treatment*.

**Coffin-Lowry syndrome**  See *histones*.

**cog wheel rigidity**  Also, cog wheeling; alternating periods of resistance and relaxation in response to repeated flexion and extension movements of a limb by the examiner; typical of Parkinson disease.

**cognition**  In a broad sense, *information processing* (q.v.); more commonly, however, it denotes a relatively high level of processing of specific information, including thinking, memory, perception, motivation, skilled movements, and language. The *hippocampus* (q.v.) contains the neural circuitry crucial for cognitive functions such as learning and memory.

Cognition refers to the perceptual and intellectual aspects of mental functioning, as differentiated from *conation* (q.v.) and the emotional aspects. Cognition refers to the use, handling, or manipulation of what is known or perceived and the ability to evaluate what is perceived in terms of what is already known. Cognition includes thinking and the mental processing of information; it refers to both the perception of reality and the manipulation of internal representations of reality; it is intimately related to the acquisition and use of language. Among specific functions that may be assessed in determining the intactness or adequacy of cognition are orientation; the ability to learn necessary skills, to solve problems, to think abstractly, to reason, and to make judgments; the ability to retain and recall events; mathematical ability (e.g., calculation) and other forms of symbol manipulation; control over primitive reactions and behavior; language use and comprehension; attention; perception; and praxis (e.g., writing, the ability to draw or copy). See *abstract attitude; cognitive science*.

*Dementia* (q.v.) refers to global loss of cognitive function with a duration of more than

3 months but with no clouding of consciousness. See *cognitive defects*.

**cognition, paranormal**  Obtaining knowledge by means outside of the normal process of perceiving or thinking, as in *extrasensory perception* (q.v.).

**cognition, primary**  The earliest way of viewing the world, when there is no clear distinction between self and non-self, inside and outside. Arieti relates the primary process to this level of cognitive organization and suggests that schizophrenia consists of regression to the level of primary cognition as a way of interpreting the world and the self-image in less frightening ways. See *object relations, narcissistic; object relations theory; primary psychic process; self-object*.

**cognitions**  In cognitive therapy, the thoughts or images in consciousness that appear almost automatically when one is confronted with a situation; what a person thinks in a situation and not what he or she thinks about a situation. Cognitions are differentiated from schemata, the silent assumptions or beliefs based on past experience that direct a person to attend to certain stimuli, to ignore others, and to value and perceive events in a certain way. Schemata thus account for cognitions, and analysis of a series of cognitions enables the therapist to infer the schema. See *cognitive therapy*.

**cognitions, depressive**  The characteristic thought content of patients with clinical *depression* (q.v.): ideas of present failure and inadequacy, hopelessness about the future, and ruminations about past misdeeds.

**cognitive**  In neuroscience, referring to mechanisms that can override or augment reflexive and habitual reactions in order to orchestrate behavior in accord with the subject's intentions; their function is to control lower-level sensory, memory and/or motor operations for a common purpose. The neural mechanisms for cognitive control extract the goal-relevant features of experiences for use in future circumstances. The prefrontal cortex (PFC), which has connections with virtually all sensory neocortical and motor systems and a wide range of subcortical structures, is centrally involved in this process. It provides the infrastructure for synthesizing the diverse range of information needed for complex behavior; with its widespread projections back to those systems, it is able to exert a top-down influence on a wide range of brain processes. See *conation*.

**cognitive ability**   Capacity for thinking, reasoning, or information processing. See *cognition*.

QTL studies have shown that the genetic contribution to cognitive ability is remarkably constant throughout life. In a sample of 240 pairs of octogenarian twins, the heritability (proportion of trait variance attributable to genetic agents) of general cognitive ability was 62%. Overall, data indicate that genetic agents account for 0.50 of the variance in general cognitive ability, shared environmental agents for 0.33, nonshared environmental agents for 0.17, and error of measurement for 0.10. Thus, genetic agents are indeed important in the determination of intellect and its closely related traits (such as working memory and spatial skills), but environmental and experiential agents are also critical. See *behavioral genetics*.

QTL studies have also shown that the gene for apolipoprotein-E is not only associated with late onset Alzheimer disease, but also with cognitive decline in an unselected sample of elderly subjects.

**cognitive abulia**   A lack of goal-directed activity on the basis of intellectual decline; seen in patients with *Alzheimer disease* (q.v.), who cannot carry a thought long enough to remember what to do next.

**cognitive anthropology**   *Ethnoscience* (q.v.).

**cognitive behavior therapy (CBT)**   Sometimes called cognitive restructuring; an active, structured, time-limited, and directive form of therapy, based on the belief that the way a person perceives and structures the world determines his or her feelings and behavior. Depression, for example, is an outgrowth of a tendency to view oneself in a negative way, and treatment is aimed at altering that cognitive schema by helping the patient gather evidence for and against his or her distorted self-view.

Cognitive therapy emphasizes how the patient came to think in certain ways about himself, the future, and the world. It was developed by Aaron T. Beck and is rooted in the work of Alfred Adler, George Kelly, and Karen Horney, with a number of its tactics derived from behavior modification. The cognitive view assumes that one assigns meaning and value to one's perceptions and experiences. Cognitive therapists work at the dual

levels of the symptom structure (manifest problems) and underlying *schema* (inferred structures). One's schemas are understood as directing rule-guided behavior. Cognitive schema are organized representations of prior experience that help a person to screen, encode, and categorize perceptions. They may be reactivated, however, by stimuli that are only remotely similar to the historically etiologic context and in relation to present-day reality are distorted, maladaptive, and exaggerated. The goal of therapy is to identify and correct the subject's distorted negative *cognitions*, to elucidate and challenge the underlying cognitive schemata, and to increase the patient's adaptive problem-solving repertoire. The subject's distortions are considered to be errors in information processing; in depression, the most common ones are *selective abstractions* (by taking a detail out of context, the person misses the significance of the total situation), *arbitrary inferences* (the person jumps to a conclusion despite contradictory or insubstantial evidence), *overgeneralizations* (a single incident is accepted as an invariable rule or consequence), and *magnifications* (specific details are given undue emphasis or significance). See *behavior therapy*; *dysfunctional attitudes*; *holistic healing*.

Although initially developed for depression and anxiety, CBT and its techniques have been adapted for personality disorders, eating disorders, schizophrenia and other psychotic illnesses, chronic pain, and substance abuse. Among the user-friendly cognitive and behavior change strategies: behavioral self-monitoring, activity scheduling, graded exposure, automatic thought recording, Socratic questioning, and cognitive restructuring.

CBT added to antipsychotic medication is now a first-line treatment for patients with schizophrenia in the United Kingdom; it has not been as widely used in the United States In schizophrenia, CBT focuses on delusions, hallucinations, and negative symptoms to reduce stress and disability. Psychosis is viewed on a continuum between normal and ill, as a reaction to stress. Psychotic symptoms can often be understood as a way for the patient to make sense of underlying cognitive dysfunction; the personal meaning of symptoms thus becomes an important consideration in therapy. To stop the hearing of voices from progressing to fixed beliefs, for example, CBT uses normalizing, socratic questioning, and inference chaining. To stop the progression of delusional beliefs to emotional and behavioral expression, CBT uses decatastrophizing, formulation, alternate strategies, and a focus on mastery.

Among the many variants of cognitive therapy are Ellis's rational-emotive therapy (see *rational psychotherapy*) and Meichenbaum's self-instructional training (SET). SET typically focuses on specific irrational beliefs the patient holds, making the patient aware of them and then helping the patient counter them by making appropriate comments while the patient is performing the behavior that has posed difficulties in the past.

**cognitive circuits**   One of the networks of the *frontal-striatal system* (q.v.). It includes (a) the dorsal cognitive, which are believed to play a role in complex cognitive processes such as working memory and the ability to establish and shift mental sets (see *executive function*) and (b) the ventral cognitive (also called the *lateral orbitofrontal circuit, socioemotional circuit,* or *contextual circuit*); projections from the orbitofrontal cortex are relayed to the caudate and thence to the dorsomedial nucleus of the thalamus; the ventral cognitive circuit is believed to play a role in response inhibition.

**cognitive conditioning**   A form of *conditioning* (q.v.) in which an aversive stimulus is paired with a thought, phantasy, or memory of the behavior to be modified or eliminated. In one method of treating smoking, alcoholism, and other addictive behaviors, the subject imagines vividly that he is smoking, drinking, etc., and while doing so administers an electric shock to himself. In time, the thought alone serves as a cognitive shock that discourages the behavior.

**cognitive control**   Self-regulation; the ability to inhibit inappropriate actions in favor of appropriate ones. Different brain regions contribute to cognitive control. Activation in the superior and inferior parietal lobes is related to sustained attention/vigilance, or set shifting, and effortful *attention* (q.v.). The basal ganglia and cerebellum are involved in learning about the frequency and timing of events (i.e., learning what to expect and when), and the posterior parietal region signals the prefrontal cortex when competing stimuli require top-down biasing of attention in favor of one

stimulus attribute or location over another. Each of these regions projects to and receives projections from PFC, thus providing a means for signaling prefrontal regions to help impose top-down control of behavior. Activation in the right inferior frontal gyrus likely reflects response inhibition, and activation in the cingulate gyrus likely reflects response conflict. In particular, the anterior rostral cingulate zone appears to be an "error-sensitive" region. See *anterior cingular cortex.*

**cognitive defects**   Cognitive dysfunctions; any of those signs and symptoms indicating impairment in the ability to recognize and understand reality; difficulties in perceiving, recognizing, judging, and reasoning are characteristic of organic mental disorders. When the degree of intellectual deterioration is such as to interfere with social or occupational functioning, the term *dementia* (q.v.) is often applied. The most common cognitive defects are impaired abstract thinking (as manifested in abnormally concrete interpretation of proverbs or inability to recognize the similarity between related objects), constructional difficulty (as in inability to reproduce geometrical designs), apraxia (inability to perform motor acts in the absence of paralysis or sensory disturbance), and impaired ability to name objects and similar aphasic disturbances. See *organic syndrome.*

Cognitive dysfunction is also a core feature of schizophrenia and is present in the majority of patients throughout the course of the illness. Although patients with schizophrenia score below healthy control subjects on all measures of cognitive functions, most affected are verbal learning, memory, psychomotor speed, and vigilance; least affected are attention span, perceptual discrimination, and basic linguistic abilities.

**cognitive disorders**   Included are *delirium, dementia,* and *amnestic disorders* (amnesia) (qq.v.). See *cognitive defects.*

**cognitive dissonance**   In information theory, *incongruity* (q.v.).

**cognitive dysmetria**   See *disconnection hypothesis.*

**cognitive enhancement therapy (CET)**   A multidimensional psychosocial treatment that targets the specific, discrete cognitive deficits of schizophrenia. Introduced by Gerard Hogarty (*Archives of General Psychiatry,* 2004), CET integrates computer-assisted training in neurocognition with social-cognitive group sessions. It is a recovery phase intervention for patients whose positive symptoms have been stabilized with antipsychotic medication. CET provides 1 hour a week (for 60 hours) of computer-assisted training in memory, attention, and problem solving, and 45 weekly sessions of 90 minutes of highly structured social-cognitive group therapy, focused on facial affect recognition, the ability to understand the "gist" of social interactions, social context appraisal, recognition of nonverbal cues, and *foresightfulness* (ability to foresee how others will feel or react to one's cues).

Other psychosocial treatments include the following:

1. *Cognitive Remediation Treatment* (CRT), consisting of exercises that are shaped to each patient's strengths and weaknesses. Task difficulty is gradually increased as performance improves, and treatment time focuses on individual areas of cognitive defect.

2. *Compensatory Treatment*, a manualized treatment with one-on-one coaching aimed at helping the patient to develop an individualized set of problem-solving strategies to improve attention, memory, and other cognitive functions.

3. *Social Skills Training* (q.v.).

**cognitive enhancers** Drugs that improve cognitive functioning in the organically impaired. See *nootropic*; *smart drugs*.

**cognitive ergonomics** The study of information exchange between humans and computers (or other machines).

**cognitive functioning** The way a person thinks and particularly how one's intrapsychic constructs prepare that person to assess and deal with external reality. See *cognitive style*.

**cognitive map** A neural representation of space. See *navigation*.

**cognitive mapping** Encoding in the brain of the relationships between a subject's location and environmental cues, an important part of spatial navigation. The hippocampus plays a major role in encoding such information.

**cognitive neural science** *Cognitive science*; *cognitive neuroscience*; a merger of cognitive psychology with neural science in an endeavor to understand the nature of mind and how it is related to the brain. With the abandonment of the *behaviorist tradition* (associated particularly with Hull, Spence, and Skinner), psychology no longer restricts its focus to the reflexive and observable aspects of behavior.

With the emergence of computers to model and test ideas about mind, *cognitive psychology* developed to explore language, perception, memory, motivation, and skilled movements in rigorous and stimulating experiments. Its recent merger with neural science has given rise to what is now called cognitive neural science. See *abstract attitude*.

The discipline employs an arsenal of methods, each of which provides information about a certain aspect of cognitive processes. Electrophysiological and functional imaging techniques (such as ERPs and MRI), together with adequate psychological procedures and behavioral measurements, can provide detailed spatiotemporal information about where and when a specific cognitive process is computed in the brain. This information can be linked to neuroanatomical data and, finally, neural network models of the processes in question can provide a framework for the development and testing of further hypotheses.

Cognitive science encompasses the disciplines of cognitive psychology, artificial intelligence, and large sections of philosophy and linguistics. Much of neuroscience, however, proceeds at a level of study where issues of representation and of the computer-as-model are not encountered. In consequence, one of the challenges to the field is how to join the cognitive aspects of language, perception, and problem solving to their neuroscientific and anthropologic roots.

**cognitive psychology** See *cognitive neural science; cognitive style; cognitive behavior therapy*.

**cognitive restructuring** See *behavior therapy; cognitive behavior therapy*.

**cognitive ritual** A mental activity used by an obsessive patient to reduce anxiety (in contrast to the obsession itself, which increases anxiety).

**cognitive science** *Cognitive neural science* (q.v.); an attempt to comprehend the structure of higher mental processes and the nature of knowledge typically using the electronic computer as model and blending contributions from various disciplines such as artificial intelligence, linguistics, psychology, anthropology, philosophy, and the neurosciences. Cognitive science was officially recognized around 1956. The psychologist George A. Miller fixes the date at 11 September 1956, at a Symposium on Information Theory at

MIT, where Allen Newell and Herbert Simon described the "Logical Theory Machine," the first complete proof of a theorem ever carried out on a computing machine; the young linguist Noam Chomsky outlined "Three Models of Language" demonstrating that language has all the formal precisions of mathematics; and Miller posited that the capacity of human short-term memory is limited to approximately seven entries.

To some extent cognitive science developed as a reaction against behaviorism and neurophysiology, both of which tried to explain complexly organized behaviors such as speaking as a consequence of environmental promptings. The currently dominant theory of human cognition is based on *symbolic computation* and emphasizes that organization stems from the organism itself, that central brain processes precede and determine the ways in which an organism carries out complex behavior. Patterns of generic relations, or schemata, are used to organize information, and cognitive skills are composed of rules that can be represented symbolically in the form, "If this, then that." See *connectionism; cognitive style*.

**cognitive screening instruments**   Tests used to detect impairments in thinking, reasoning, information processing, etc., that suggest the presence of dementia or other neuropsychiatric syndromes with cognitive defects. If positive, such tests indicate that more extensive neuropsychological examination is warranted. The tests, or batteries of tests, most frequently used by clinicians are the *MMSE,* CDT, Delayed Word Recall (Mini-Cog), Verbal Fluency, Similarity, and *Trail Making* (qq.v.).

**cognitive slippage**   P. E. Meehl's term for loosening of associations that he considered a core element in schizophrenia. (*American Psychologist 17*, 1962).

**cognitive strategies**   The mental plans used by a person to understand both self and environment. One approach to the question of how people perceive the causes of behavior is attribution theory, according to which (1) people tend to explain their own behavior in terms of situational events, and to perceive the behavior of others in terms of stable internal dispositions and personality traits, and (2) whatever reason is adduced to explain a given event influences subsequent feelings and behavior.

**cognitive style**   *Cognitive control;* the characteristic way in which a person organizes environmental stimuli, relates such information to other perceptions, ideas, and memories, and translates that information into a potential response. Cognitive psychology and in particular cognitive personality theory are concerned with how different cognitive styles develop in different people, and with how the different models of reality that people have affect their behavior. One of the major differences between Piaget's theories and Freudian theories of personality is the former's emphasis on formal thinking and cognitive maturation (rather than instinctual needs or affective states) as determinants of identity formation and the development of autonomy. See *cognitive behavior therapy*.

Information processing approaches view the person as a complex information processing system and use computer technology (such as artificial intelligence) to build models of human cognitive processes. Such cognitive science seeks to understand how symbols are recognized, how memories are retrieved, how learning develops, how problems are solved, etc. See *artificial intelligence*.

Specific cognitive peculiarities have been ascribed to the person with *narcissistic personality disorder*: (1) overt—impressively knowledgeable, decisive, opinionated, often strikingly articulate with a love of knowledge; (2) covert—knowledge often limited to trivia (*headline intelligence*), forgetful of details, impaired ability to learn new skills, language and speaking used for regulating self-esteem.

**cognits**   Neuronal assemblies or distributed functional networks of neurons that have specific cognitive functions. Processing of action words (e.g., kick, lift, throw) activates both language regions and motor cortical regions in parallel, indicating that semantic processing engages many cortical areas and is not confined to any single locus adjoining the Wernicke area.

**cohabitation**   See *coitus*.

**cohesion, social**   See *hedonism*.

**cohesive self**   *Core self;* the stable and adequately structured sense of one's identity, that one is the same person today as yesterday, even in the face of threats to self-esteem. See *self-object*.

According to Kohut, the self develops by means of a consolidation of three elements: the *grandiose-exhibitionistic self* (omnipotence, ambitious strivings for power and success), the *idealized parental image* (values and goals), and an intermediate area of skills and talents maintained by the tension between the other two. See *basic trust; grandiose self.* Optimal development, consisting of progressive consolidation of these elements into the cohesive self, requires sensitive, empathic, *good enough* parent figures (self-objects) whose *approbative mirroring* reflects the child's self-worth and thus encourages the development and maintenance of self-esteem and self-assertive ambitions. See *autonomy, sense of.*

Pathology results when the parent figures fail to empathize with the child's *exhibitionistic (mirroring) needs* and his or her *idealizing (merger) needs.* The pathology in narcissistic personality disorder is linked to an incompletely structured and unstable self whose cohesiveness is threatened by narcissistic injury; temporary breakup, enfeeblement, or disharmony of the self under such conditions reactivates needs for narcissistic sustenance.

**cohesive ties** See *discourse skills.*

**cohort** Those who belong to a group as defined by explicit criteria used by the investigator. A birth cohort, for example, comprises all those people born in a specific time period, such as all those born in the United States between 1976 and 1980.

**coin test** A test of tactile gnosis (recognition) in which the subject is required to estimate the size of coins touched; an underestimation of the size has been believed to be indicative of a lesion of the pyramidal system, but mass examination of normal subjects reveals that approximately 70% of those tested are unable to estimate coin size accurately, and that 90% underestimated the size.

**coitophobia** Fear of the sexual act.

**coitus, coition** Sexual intercourse per vaginam between male and female. In medicine, coitus, copulation, *cohabitation*, and sexual intercourse are used synonymously, though the words have a widely different meaning in their original context.

**coitus, external** *Perineal coitus.*

**coitus, incomplete** *Coitus interruptus* (q.v.).

**coitus a tergo** *Coitus more ferarum* (q.v.).

**coitus inter femora** *Obs.* Sexual relations by the insertion of the penis between the thighs of the partner.

**coitus interruptus** Cessation of sexual intercourse before emission; synonymous with *onanism.* (Popular usage, however, has equated onanism with masturbation.)

**coitus more ferarum** *Obs.* (L. "sexual intercourse in the manner of wild beasts") The carrying out of the act of heterosexual intercourse in the "natural" position of lower animals, that is, from the rear, and usually with the female on hands and knees. The penis is inserted into the vagina; when it is inserted into the rectum, the act is called anal intercourse. This latter practice is called *pederasty* (q.v.) when the partner is a boy, and *sodomy* (q.v.) when the sexual relation is with an animal through the vagina.

Coitus more ferarum is not sodomy, but is thought of as primitive. The axis of the vagina, in this position, is in direct correspondence with the axis of the penis in erection. This might indicate the primitive biological congruity of this position. Certain elements of tenderness, which are dominant in the so-called normal, or face-to-face, position, are, however, excuded in this approach.

**coitus oralis** *Obs. Fellatio* (q.v.).

**coitus per anum** Anal intercourse; termed *pederasty* (q.v.) when a boy is the receptive partner.

**coitus reservatus** *Carezza*; sexual intercourse in which the male partner delays or withholds his orgasm until the female partner has hers, or indefinitely as a means of birth control.

**colera** A culture-specific syndrome of Mayan (Guatemalan) Indians, consisting of violent outbursts, delusions, and hallucinations, often proceeding to an exhausted or stuporous state. Also called *bilis* or *muina.*

**collaboration** As used by Sullivan, a type of interpersonal relationship in which there is not only cooperation but also sensitivity to the needs of the other person.

**collapse delirium** Kraepelin's term for a condition, usually associated with high fever, characterized by marked disorientation, illusions, unsystematized delusions, and emotional variability; the condition is marked by physical collapse. This term is also sometimes used to refer to delirious mania (Bell mania).

**collateral** Any person related by blood to a series of siblings, but not descended from the same line of immediate ancestors. A first cousin is the most closely related instance of a collateral. The term also means "indirect" when applied to this line of descent of an individual or to the form of inheritance of a

Mendelian factor as characteristic of *recessiveness* (q.v.), that is, transmission of a trait to descendants of the siblings of a trait carrier.

**colleague-centered consultation**   See *consultant*.

**collecting, collection**   See *collecting mania; hoarding; soteria*.

**collecting mania**   The morbid impulse to collect, often related to anal erotism. See *coprophilia; hoarding; soteria*.

**collective attitude**   An *attitude* (q.v.) that is peculiar "not to one individual, but to many, at the same time, i.e., either to a society, a people, or to mankind in general" (Jung, C. G. *Psychological Types*, 1923).

**collective efficacy**   See *social disorganization theory*.

**collective insanity**   Ireland's term for psychosis of association. See *induced psychotic disorder*.

**collective psychosis**   Psychic defensive mechanisms utilized by an entire group in adapting to other cultures and societies. Freud's instinctual theories recognized two basic drives, sex and aggression. Freud felt that people's aggressive trends lead them and their culture to fatal conflicts. Human aggressiveness within a culture is diverted to people outside that culture's psychic mass. This diversion of hostile trends implies a process of projection of the superego's aggressive component, so that an individual's hostility can be ascribed to other groups. Flescher thinks that this paranoid projection is inherent in the formation of the mass and constitutes the collective psychosis.

**collective unconscious**   "All those psychic contents I term collective which are peculiar not to one individual, but to many, at the same time, i.e., either to a society, a people, or to mankind in general. The antithesis of collective is individual."

Jung refers to two divisions of the unconscious, the *personal* and the *collective*. The former "embraces all the acquisitions of the personal existence—hence the forgotten, the repressed, the subliminally perceived, thought and felt. But, in addition to these personal unconscious contents, there exist other contents which do not originate in personal acquisitions but in the inherited brain-structure. These are the mythological associations—those motives and images which can spring anew in every age and clime, without historical tradition or migration. I term these contents the collective unconscious." (Jung, C.G.

*Contributions to Analytical Psychology*, 1928). See *analytic psychology*.

**college, invisible**   A collection of individuals or of scientists with a feeling of allegiance to another and with frequent professional and social interactions. Although the term originated in the 17th century, it is now used to refer to a group of scientists who live in "disparate geographical locations, but who often attend the same conferences, who publish in the same journals, who invite each other to give presentations in their home institutions, and who share reprints of their research endeavors. It is through the political power of such 'colleges' that many of the changes in science are made" (Blashfield, R. K. *Schizophrenia Bulletin 8*, 1982).

**colloidal gold reaction**   See *Lange colloidal gold reaction*.

**coloboma**   A cleft or defect, especially of the eye; of significance in neuropsychiatry in that choroidoretinal coloboma is one of the elements of a familial syndrome that also includes dysplastic body build and mental retardation. The coloboma appears as a white patch of exposed sclera below the optic disk and causes a scotoma in that region.

**colocalization**   Joint tenancy; used particularly to refer to the fact that more than one neurotransmitter may be contained in and released by a specific neuron. Typically, an amine neurotransmitter provides a specific signal to the receptor site of the next neuron, and a neuropeptide cotransmitter serves a longer-term modulatory function on adjacent cells. Such combinations of transmitters make possible a wide range of neuronal response; they also make it extremely difficult to predict specific response since the possibilities are not limited to the simple action of approximately 30 neurotransmitters but instead may involve over 400 different combinations of transmitters. See *amine; amino acids; peptide, synapse*.

**color agnosis**   See *word blindness*.

**color hearing**   A form of *synesthesia*, characterized by a sensation of color when sounds are heard. See *sensation, secondary*.

**Columbia Mental Maturity Scale**   *CMMS* (q.v.).

**coma**   The deepest degree of stupor in which all consciousness is lost and there is no voluntary activity of any kind. Among the various conditions that may produce coma the most common are encephalitis, cerebral hemorrhage, cerebral thrombosis, cerebral embolism, subarachnoid hemorrhage, intracranial tumor, head injury, postepileptic coma, diabetic coma, hypoglycemic coma, hypertensive encephalopathy, uremic coma, acute alcoholism, intoxication with opiates or other sedatives, hypothalamic lesions, congestive attacks of general paralysis, hysterical trance, and catatonic stupor.

**coma scale** See *Glasgow Coma Scale.*

**coma somnolentium** (L. "coma of the somnolent") *Cataphora* (q.v.).

**coma vigil** *Agrypnocoma*; coma in which the eyes remain open. Coma vigil occurs in certain acute brain syndromes associated with systemic infection (the infective-exhaustive psychoses, also known as acute toxic encephalopathy, acute toxic encephalitis, or acute serous encephalitis). See *akinetic mutism.*

**combat exhaustion** Combat fatigue. See *shell shock.*

**combination** In genetics, the hereditary variations that represent the effect of *hybridization* and that occur in crossbred products originating from the union between two individuals with unlike hereditary equipment. Pearson used this term to refer to what he considers the earliest mechanism of learning: the unification of sensory impressions from the outside with perceptions arising from instinctual (internal) stimuli.

**combination strategy** See *coactive strategy.*

**combined degeneration of the spinal cord** See *posterolateral sclerosis.*

**cometophobia** Fear of comets.

**coming out** Acknowledging to oneself and to others that one is homosexual or prefers homosexuality to heterosexuality. Some writers believe that coming out is essential for optimal functioning as a whole person in someone with a homosexual orientation. In some instances, use of the term emphasizes the aspect of acknowledging or proclaiming one's sexual orientation to society in general; in others, the emphasis is on the value of acknowledging sexual orientation to oneself and to others of the same orientation.

**command automatism** *Automatic obedience* (q.v.)

**command negativism** See *negativism.*

**commensalism** See *symbiosis.*

**commissure** Transverse or commissural fibers; those portions of the white substance of the cerebral hemispheres made up of medullated nerve fibers connecting the two hemispheres. The commissural fibers are to be distinguished

from the two other types of myelinated nerve fibers found in the white matter: *projection fibers*, which connect the cerebral cortex with lower portions of the brain and spinal cord, and *association fibers*, which connect different portions of the same hemisphere. The *corpus callosum* (q.v.) is the largest commissure.

**commitment** Depriving a person of his liberty by putting him under the guardianship of another (whether mental hospital, prison, or other institution, or in the custody of a probation officer). In psychiatry, commitment is a process whereby one or more doctors explain to a court why a patient's mental problems necessitate forfeiture of his freedom. Such explanation is usually in the form of a certificate signed by the examining physician(s), and it is the process of completing this certificate that is properly labeled *certification.* In practice, however, the terms commitment and certification are interchangeable.

In recent years, *outpatient commitment* has been legalized in some jurisdictions. Clinicians advocate this form of coerced treatment in the community as a way to prevent clinical deterioration and hospitalization; civil libertarians denounce it as another way of depriving a person of his rights. In most states that allow outpatient commitment, the same criteria are used as with involuntary hospitalization: some version of mental illness plus current dangerousness. A few states have broader critieria, based on prevention of physical or psychiatric deterioration rather than dangerousness. Most outpatient commitment statutes do not permit physically forced medication.

**commitment, civil** Involuntary mental hospitalization of a person who is not charged with criminal conduct.

**commitment, criminal** Involuntary mental hospitalization of a person who is charged with violation of one or more criminal statutes.

**communicated insanity** See *folie á deux; induced psychotic disorder.*

**communication** The process of transmitting information from sender (*encoder*) to receiver (*decoder*). "The encoder is the originator of the message; the decoder is the recipient of the message; and the message is a response of an encoder which may be the stimulus for a decoder. Communication results when a response of an encoder is received as a stimulus for a decoder."

*Channels of communication* are differentiated according to the source and destination of the message. "The six major channels of human "face to face' communication, defined in terms of their source and destination, are: speech (*source*: vocal tract; *destination*: ear), kinesics (body movement; eye), odor (chemical processes; nose), touch (body surface; skin), observation (body surface; eye), and *proxemics* (body placement; eye)" (Kiesler, D. J. *The Process of Psychotherapy*, 1973).

The foregoing describes an informational approach to communication, emphasizing the content or meaning. Another approach is the interactional, which defines communication as a way of structuring and managing social occasions by behavioral means. Such an approach is concerned with how behavior is organized rather than with what it means.

The relational approach considers communication to be the overall system of relationships that are developed between people and by those people with their community and their habitat. An outgrowth of the relational approach is the double-bind model of psychopathology, which views schizophrenia as a distortion in the pattern of relationships between the subject and other persons rather than as a distortion in the behavior of the subject. See *double bind*.

**communication, disordered** *Distorted communication*; abnormal or deviant transmittal of messages. Examples include the following: (1) lack of clarity—about content (the message is difficult to interpret or decode), about receiver (to whom is the message being sent?), about form (is it a command, a question, an observation, or a hypotheses?); (2) lack of response—the answer given does not address the substance of the question posed, or it ignores the emotional accompaniment of the question, or a metaphorical answer is given to a concrete question; (3) inconsistency between verbal content and the feeling tone.

Family systems theory and family therapy practitioners have emphasized the *family pattern* (q.v.), which includes the interactional or communications style that the family develops. The more distorted that style, the more likely it is that some degree of psychopathology will be evident in one or more members of the family. Some workers, for instance, have found that schizophrenic families are characterized by a high incidence of

disordered communication. Among the patterns described are *amorphous communications*, which are vague, loose, and indefinite, and *fragmented communications*, which lack closure and are easily disrupted and poorly integrated.

By themselves, such observations cannot answer the question whether the deviant communication is a cause of the psychopathology or instead a reaction to it; at most they suggest that distorted intrafamilial communication may aggravate or perpetuate the psychopathology of individual family members. See *codependency; expressed emotions (EE)*.

**communication, nonverbal** Transmittal of information by means other than formal language. As with verbal communication, nonverbal messages may be factual, *indexical* (conveying information about the nature of the sender), or interactional. Erving Goffman (*The Presentation of Self in Everyday Life*, 1969) described four basic types of communicational relations: direct (the sender conveys a message through signals known to be understood by the receiver) and indirect (the message must be decoded by the receiver); symmetrical (sender and receiver send messages back and forth to each other) and asymmetrical (the sender and receiver roles are not reversible).

**communication deficits** Impaired ability to transmit meaningful messages to others, most commonly expressed as impaired linguistic skills. In children with schizophrenia, the chief communication deficits are based on loose associations, illogical thinking, and inadequate *discourse skills* (q.v.).

**communication deviance** Tendency toward a fragmented or amorphous conversational style, noted to be frequent in parents of schizophrenic offspring. Although first interpreted as a parental disturbance that predisposed to the development of schizophrenia, it is now recognized as a reaction of families to a schizophrenic member, a reaction that may secondarily aggravate the offspring's illness.

**communication disorders** Included are language disorder (expressive or mixed receptive-expressive), *phonological disorder*, and *stuttering* (qq.v.). See *developmental disorders, specific*.

**communication unit** The essential components of transmission of information from one person to another; these components are the *source* (the person sending the message), the *transmitter* (the motor apparatus through which the message will be expressed), and the *destination* (the person to whom the message is sent, who picks up the message through his or her receiver, or sensory apparatus). See *information theory*.

**communicative matching** Also referred to as *mutual cueing* (Mahler) or *goodness of fit* (Bergler) between child and mother (or other parent figure), and approximately equivalent to Kohut's concept of parental *mirroring* and Bion's concept of the *container-contained maternal function* (qq.v.). All these terms refer to the state, or its development, of interpersonal attachment that leads the mother to respond empathetically to her infant's needs and to remodel the infant's projections and send them back to him or her as additional scaffolding on which the child builds an identity separate from the mother's, an ability to test reality, an ability to self-regulate, an ability to think, and a sense of mastery and self-esteem. See *empathic failure; fit; grandiose self*.

**community, therapeutic** 1. A psychiatric or mental hospital that emphasizes the importance of socioenvironmental and interpersonal influences in the therapy, management, resocialization, and rehabilitation of the long-term patient. Self-control, dignity, and trust are employed rather than excessive imposed controls, restrictions, regimentation, and meaningless rituals. See *Herstedvester*.

The therapeutic community requires an organized social structure that becomes a therapeutic culture in which the living-learning-confrontation aspect engenders increasingly open communication between patients and staff and the opportunity for immediate feedback about patients' behavior and interactions.

2. A residential setting for the rehabilitation of drug abusers, consisting of a drug-free program combined with provocative encounter-group sessions with peers and drug counselors.

**community care** See *domicile; rehabilitation*.

**community divorce** See *divorce, stations of*.

**community feeling** The sense of relationship between the individual and the community. Adler states that out of community feelings "are developed tenderness, love of neighbour, friendship and love, the desire for power unfolding itself in a veiled manner and seeking secretly to push its way along the path of group consciousness" (Adler, A. *The Practice and Theory of Individual Psychology*, 1924).

**Community Mental Health Center** See *community psychiatry*.

**community organization** See *social policy planning*.

**community psychiatry** Public health psychiatry; the branch of psychiatry concerned with the provision and delivery of a coordinated program of mental health care to a specified population.

The core concept of the *Community Mental Health Center* is that it will function as the nucleus for mental health services of the community it serves—usually defined geographically and termed the *catchment area*. An essential element in the delivery of such services is *continuity of care*—often misinterpreted to mean that the patient has the same therapist throughout every phase of his treatment and rehabilitation program, although more properly it refers to the provision of an organizational structure that will guarantee that the patient receive whatever kind of care he needs at the time he needs it and will ensure a relatedness between past and present care in conformity with the therapeutic needs of the patient.

Many in the field believe that evaluation of psychosocial disorder should include not only analysis, but ultimately also manipulation of existing social structures and systems. Others term such direct social or community action social engineering and include it as a part of social psychiatry. Still others view this as an unwarranted and potentially dangerous assumption of political power that is beyond the realm of medicine.

**community reinforcement** A frequent addition to drug treatment programs that includes skills training, a job club, disulfiram therapy (for alcohol abusers), and relationship counseling. In many drug treatment programs, *contingency management* is also used: vouchers redeemable for goods and services are issued, contingent on the patient's providing drug-free urine specimens.

Limitations have been noted in contingency and reinforcement programs: (1) effects tend to weaken after the contingencies are terminated; (2) the cost of providing rewards and administering contingency management systems is high; and (3) many substance abusers do not respond to contingency management.

**comorbid insomnia** Previously termed secondary insomnia; insomnia that occurs in conjunction with a primary medical, psychiatric, or environmental condition.

**comorbidity** Occurrence or existence of more than one disease at the same time in the same subject. There is a high rate of comorbidity of alcoholism and depression; the presence of either predisposes the subject to the other, but the etiologic relationship of one to the other is unknown. See *depression, unipolar; dual diagnosis.*

There is evidence that patients with mood disorder and comorbidity with any other psychiatric disorder are at high risk for completed suicide. The comorbidity hypothesis of schizoaffective disorder postulates that it represents the chance association in one subject of all the factors responsible for two different disorders, schizophrenia and mood disorder.

Among some of the commonly cited comorbidities are the following:

Anorexia nervosa: 5%–85% have depressive symptoms.

Bulimia nervosa: 35%–75% have a mood disorder.

Fragile X syndrome: 73%–100% have attention deficit hyperactivity disorder (ADHD).

Learning disability: 10%–92% have ADHD.

Major depression: 40% have a personality disorder.

Obsessive-compulsive disorder (OCD): 35% or more have depression (reactive); 40% have other anxiety disorders (reactive); 24% have learning disabilities; 20% have minor motor tics; higher than expected incidence of Sydenham chorea, choreoathetosis, and Gilles de la Tourette disorder.

Panic disorder, agoraphobia: 65%–70% experience an episode of major depression at some point in their lives; mitral valve prolapse in 35%–50%.

Pervasive developmental disorders: most also have symptoms of ADHD.

Substance abuse: 20% have recurrent major depression; 10% have dysthmic disorder.

Tourette disorder: 40% have OCD (which may be an alternate manifestation of the Tourette "gene") and other anxiety disorders; 21%–54% have ADHD; higher than expected incidence of personality disorders and mood disorders.

**companion, imaginary** It has often been observed that a child will create an imaginary companion and will endow this product of phantasy with the qualities of reality. The imaginary companion will have a name, a definite appearance, and personality—even an imaginary family created for it, and so on.

Imaginary companions are created mostly by only children, or by children whose siblings are much older, or who for any reason are without real playmates. The imaginary companion fulfills the child's need for intimate companionship and friendship and serves an important function in his or her emotional life. The imaginary companion is freely taken into confidences from which parents are distinctly barred and becomes "someone to tell troubles to" and "to share secret pleasures with." In general, the imaginary companion is so created by the child that it has everything the child desires but lacks. The play *Harvey* presents an amusing and not dissimilar instance of this imagery; a huge white rabbit is created as an imaginary companion. Though it is an animal and the imaginary creation of an adult, its origin and function are much the same as those of the imaginary companions of children. See *hallucinatory game; transitional object.*

**companion, phobic** See *agoraphobia.*

**comparative psychiatry** *Cultural psychiatry*; that branch of psychiatry concerned with the definition of culture, interactions between the culture and the individual, culture-specific syndromes, the influence of the culture on the mental health of members or groups within the culture, and epidemiological or clinical observations of the differences between cultures in their definitions of health and illness and the cross-cultural variation in incidence or prevalence of syndromes and symptoms. When the focus is on different cultures, rather than differences within a single culture, the term *transcultural psychiatry* may be used. Comparative psychiatry has also been termed *social psychiatry, ethnopsychology,* and *clinical sociology.* See *community psychiatry.*

Sometimes, *cross-cultural psychiatry* is used as a more general term to include comparative psychiatry (as defined above), *psychological anthropology* (the use of psychodynamic and other psychological theory to interpret the relationships between the different elements of society and culture), and *medical anthropology* (the use of anthropological methods to analyze variation between cultures in their conceptualization of illness and care-taking roles, including the study of culture-bound syndromes and non-Western systems of healing). See *anthropology; ecology*.

**compartmentalization**   Isolation; keeping separate parts of one's personality that should be kept together; psychic fragmentation.

**compensation**   Counterbalancing an inequity, making restitution for a loss, correcting an inferiority or loss (in somatopathology, typically by hypertrophy of tissue or by increased functioning of the organ or system in question), providing a substitute for something that is unacceptable or unattainable. See *overcompensation*.

**compensation neurosis**   1. Kempf so classifies a neurosis in which there is "persistent striving to develop potent functions and win social esteem initiated by fear of impotence or loss of control of asocial cravings" (*Psychopathology*, 1921).

    2. *Desire neurosis; indemnity neurosis*; a form of traumatic neurosis induced by desire of monetary recompense. It is believed that some people after sustaining an injury may develop a neurosis in the hope of gaining financially (and otherwise) as a result of the injury. See *epinosic gain*. Compensation neurosis has been defined as "a state of mind, born out of fear, kept alive by avarice, stimulated by lawyers, and cured by verdict." The degree and duration of the neurosis are often inversely proportional to the extent of injury. See *insurance hebephrenia; attitudinal pathosis*.

**compensation schizophrenia**   N. D. C. Lewis's term for a type of schizophrenia characterized by overcompensation for feelings of inferiority. Delusions of grandeur form the core of the psychosis.

**compensation-ideal**   Adler's term for substitution of some superior image in dreams or phantasy for an inferior one, a reflection of the desire for power and mastery.

**competence, competency**   In the medical setting, decisional capacity or ability to exercise autonomy. See *respect for autonomy*.

    Competence is a *substantive legal standard* (q.v.) that is defined in different ways in different jurisdictions: in terms of ability to communicate a choice, ability to under-

stand relevant information, ability to manipulate information rationally, to reason about the risks and benefits of potential options, to appreciate the nature of one's situation, to express a choice, and to understand what the consequences of that choice might be. The concept of competence focuses on the process of making a decision and the ability to choose between alternative courses of action. Competence is often described in terms of capacities for particular tasks, such as *personal care capacity* (q.v.). See *emancipation*.

**Competence Assessment Tool**   See *MacCat-T*.

**competing responses**   A form of behavior therapy, used particularly to treat tics. The subject is taught isometric tension of muscles that oppose the muscle groups involved in tic behavior. The subject with a tic consisting of backward jerking of the head, for example, is taught to contract the anterior muscles of the neck and slowly bring the chin down toward or on the chest. Once the subject has learned the response, he or she is instructed to initiate it at the first moment of awareness of an oncoming bout of symptoms, and to continue it for a minute or more.

**competitive inhibition**   See *narcotic antagonist*.

**complacency principle**   W. B. Cannon formulated the thesis that "instincts" and "drives" are attempts on the part of the organism to maintain its optimal body economy (*homeostasis*). R. B. Raup called it the principle of complacency, thereby indicating that every organism is a physiological system that tends to preserve its stationary condition or to restore the stationary condition as soon as it is disturbed by any variation occurring within or outside the organism.

**complaint habit**   Kanner's term for *hypochondriasis* (q.v.) in children.

    At various times and in connection with a variety of situations children are known to complain of various aches and pains that clearly are emotionally rather than physically caused. For example, one child may complain of severe headache the morning of a day on which a feared test is to be given at school; another may complain of stomachache when some particularly disliked food is served, but these are *isolated*, not habitual, complaints.

    The complaint habit refers to a *habitual* way of reacting by means of complaints of bodily disorder, according to definite patterns. In some instances the pattern has been set by the child himself, out of certain material from his own experience. If a real stomachache or a real cough has kept the child from school, which he happens to dislike, and has brought all sorts of kindly attentions, comforts, and privileges not ordinarily forthcoming, it may be found thereafter that a great desire for all this as a relief from some stress or other will be heralded by a stomachache or cough which, though felt and complained about, is not real. More often the pattern is suggested to the child by observation of his environment. If he notices that mother or father seems always to be relieved of this or that chore by reason of the complaint of headache or backache, the child, too, will be found feeling and complaining of headache or backache when the performance of some hated task is expected (*Child Psychiatry*, 1948).

**complementarity**  A state of harmony or balance between the emotional needs of the interacting members of a group, or the degree to which such a balance has been achieved. N. W. Ackerman (*The Psychodynamics of Family Life*, 1958) describes a *minus form* of complementarity in family role relations that is limited to neutralization of the disintegrating effects of conflict and anxiety. The *plus form*, in addition to such neutralization, promotes further growth and creative development in the family unit and in the individual members of the unit.

**complementarity, reciprocal**  In sociology, the postulate that moral and social codes, rather than being arbitrary conventionalities that are antagonistic to emotional drives, are an intrinsic factor in human functioning and that homeostasis exists in relation to the social environment fully as much as it exists in relation to the internal milieu.

**complementary**  Mutually supplying each other's lack; used most often to refer to a type of relationship within a family, or between husband and wife. In a *complementary* relationship, behavior of one sort by one partner—such as dominance—is met by behavior of another sort, in this case submission, by the spouse. In a *symmetrical* relationship, both partners exchange the same kind of behavior—both are giving, or both are domineering, for example. In contemporary America, a husband often has to deal with a wife who demands a symmetrical relationship on the one hand, and insists that she be treated as an equal, but at the same time demands that her husband dominate her in a complementary relationship. Such an incompatibility of messages constitutes paradoxical communication, or what has been termed by Bateson, Jackson, and their co-workers, a *double bind* (q.v.).

**complementary medicine**  CM; complementary therapy; alternative medicine; *folk medicine*; *holistic healing* (qq.v.). Complementary medicine is preferred to the popular term, *alternative medicine*, because the therapies included are regarded as supplements to, rather than a replacement of, orthodox medicine. Other terms have included fringe medicine, and unconventional medicine, unorthodox medicine, natural medicine.

John E. Cooper (in Andrews, G and Henderson, S. *Unmet Need in Psychiatry*, Cambridge University Press, United Kingdom, 2000) subdivides currently available complementary therapies into:

A. Systems available before 1790 (when homeopathy was developed)

1. Traditional *Chinese medicine* (acupuncture, moxibustion, herbal remedies, hiatsu, and tai-chi-chuan). These are linked by the principles of life energy, *qi*, which has two component forces, *yin* and *yang*. Yin is associated with darknesss, rest, earth, inwardness, downwardness, femaleness, and water. Yang is associated with light, activity, energy, expansion, upwards, maleness, and fire. The human body is supposed to contain a large number of invisible channels or meridians, along which these two components of *qi* must flow for normal life and functioning; when they are in balance, all is well. By placing fine needles in special points along the meridians, *qi* can be stimulated to get the flow and balance back to norrmal. In *moxibustion* the same points are stimulated by burning a very small piece of dry vegetable fluff on them for a few seconds. The same points can also be stimulated by pressure, massage, or electricity.

2. *Ayurvedic medicine* (India). possibly older than the Chinese system, ayurvedic medicineis based upon a concept of a life force (*ojas*), which needs to be in balance. The five basic elements—fire, water, earth, air, and ether—are combined in the body in various and individually different proportions to produce three "humors" which influence health and temperament. The balance can be corrected by such things as certain foods, drinks,

sexual gratification, light, fresh air, and spiritual activity.

3. Western herbal medicine

B. Developed after 1790

1. Emphasis on the technique (useful for anything): hypnosis and relaxation, laying on of hands (spirit healing), naturopathy, crystal therapy, iridology, metamorphic technique, and reflexology (soles of feet). Iridology and reflexology both depend upon the idea that the whole body is represented in miniature on one small part of itself; for iridology it is the iris of the eyes, for reflexology the soles of the feet.

2. Emphasis on specific remedies for particular ailments: homeopathy, bach flower remedies, aromatherapy, and color therapy

3. Effect limited to one system or part of body: osteopathy, chiropractic, colonic lavage, Alexander technique (posture), and rolfing (painful massage to relieve tensions by relaxing and repositioning muscles)

4. Distant healing (most act by facilitating or balancing a 'life force' or vibrations): radiesthesia; radionics. A unique feature is that the physical presence of the person being healed is not required.

**complementation, gender**   Part of the process of gender identification in which the person recognizes the other sex as "other" and "not me," and recognizes the other sex as reciprocating but being different from one's own. See *gender identification*.

**completers**   See *attempters*.

**complex**   Complex of ideas; neurogram; a group of unconscious or repressed ideas interlinked into a whole, which besets the individual, impelling him or her to think, feel, and perhaps act after a habitual pattern. Jung, who introduced the term, described it as the grouping of psychic elements about emotionally toned contents. Jones described it as a group of emotionally invested ideas partially or entirely repressed. Morton Prince defined complex or neurogram as a set of ideas connected to specific experiences and linked with emotions, so that when one of the ideas belonging to an experience comes to mind the experience as a whole is recalled.

Fundamental psychic conflicts, usually derived from the stages of infantile sexuality, are the typical source of complexes. Thus one speaks of the Oedipus, Electra, and castration complexes.

**complex partial seizures**   *Temporal lobe epilepsy* (q.v.); psychomotor seizures. See *epilepsy*.

**complex readiness**   The tendency of unconscious feelings or impulses to find substitute expression in the behavior or routine of everyday life, as in lapses in speaking, reading, and writing.

**compliance**   Self-effacing submission or obedience to the overt or implied demands of others; often, oversubmissiveness is implied. It frequently occurs as part of the obsessive-compulsive character's defensive system. According to Laing, compulsive compliance is also characteristic of the schizoid or narcissistic personality, where it is used to hide the true self. See *false self*.

**compliance, motor**   A type of response noted in many schizophrenic children, in whom light palm contact is enough to make them turn or change position. Such children show marked dependence on contact with others—they melt into the lap of the examiner and show many disturbances in motility. See *childhood schizophrenia*.

**compliance, patient**   Adherence to a prescribed treatment regimen, used most commonly in reference to taking medications in the amount and frequency recommended. Lack of compliance is a major factor in apparent treatment failures and in relapse of chronic patients.

**compliance, somatic**   The degree to which the individual's organic structure coincides with his or her psychological mechanism in the symptomatic expression of pathological defenses. In conversion symptoms, for instance, the entire cathexis of the objectionable impulses is condensed onto a definite physical function. The ability of the affected function to adsorb this cathexis is its somatic compliance. The function may be chosen because the organ in question presents a *locus minoris resistentiae* (see *organ inferiority*), or because the erogeneity of the afflicted part corresponds to the unconscious phantasies seeking expression (as in the case of a person with oral fixations who, when symptoms are developed, will show primarily oral symptoms), or because of the situation in which the decisive repression occurred (the organ or function under highest tension at the decisive moment is likely to become the seat of disturbance), or because of the organ's ability to symbolize the unconscious drive in question (thus convex organs such as the hand, nose, and breasts may symbolize the penis and represent masculine wishes).

**compliance, strategic** In paradoxical therapy, change based on the patient's acceptance of or obedience to the therapist's directive. A well-known compliance-induction procedure is the *Devil's Pact*, in which the patient is induced to promise that he will carry out a plan before he is told what the plan is. See *paradoxical therapy*.

**component impulse** Partial impulse; any of the various pregenital or preadult manifestations of drive and particularly, in the case of the libidinal drive, those infantile activities and impulses that will later become subordinate to the adult genital organization. Among the component impulses are sucking, biting, touching, defecating, urinating, looking (voyeurism), exhibiting, sadism, and masochism—all of which, although they may be detectable in adulthood, will generally be expressed as forepleasure activities and will remain subservient to genital primacy. See *genitality*.

**componential analysis** *Ethnoscience* (q.v.).

**compositionality** See *association of ideas*.

**comprehension** Understanding, especially as opposed to mere apprehending or cognition. In examining the sensorium, mental grasp, and capacity of a patient, the examiner often presents him with a comprehension test, which commonly consists of having the patient read or listen to a narrative paragraph and then asking him questions to determine how much he grasped of the significance of the story.

**compression** *Condensation* (q.v.).

**compromise-distortion** In contradistinction to compromise-formation that occurs in normal and neurotic development, Freud used the term compromise-distortion to describe an analogous process in a psychosis. Owing to a compromise between the resistance of the ego and the strength of the idea under repression, the return of the repressed idea becomes distorted into a delusion or a hallucination. "A circumstance quite peculiar to paranoia...is that the repressed reproaches return as thoughts spoken aloud" (Freud, S. *Collected Papers*, 1924-25).

**compromise-formation** In psychoanalysis, a substitutive idea or act representing a repressed conflict. As a consequence of the ego's contacts

with reality, four typical danger situations arise, each derived from some stage of infantile sexuality: (1) danger of separation, i.e., loss of the love object; (2) danger of the loss of love; (3) danger of castration; and (4) danger of the loss of superego approval, i.e., guilt. See *anxiety*.

All psychogenic symptoms are compromises, for they arise on the basis of repressed material and thus serve to give release to the pressure or tension resident in the repressed complex.

**compulsion** A repetitive, stereotyped, and often trivial motor action, the need for whose performance insistently forces itself into consciousness even though the subject does not wish to perform the act. Failure to perform the act generates increasing anxiety; completion of the act gives at least temporary surcease of tension. Compulsions are ego-alien and therefore always resisted. See *obsession*.

The compulsion involves a volitional disability in that the subject acts intentionally but not voluntarily, and although he can perform the action he cannot refrain from performing it even though he has good reason to do so. The compulsion is an intentional but involuntary action. See *impulse control disorders; volition*.

**compulsive buying** Problematic buying behavior, also called compulsive shopping, spendaholism. There is doubt that such behavior warrants classification as disease, even though it can lead to serious adverse consequences, such as family conflict, divorce, bankruptcy, illegal activities such as writing bad checks and embezzlement, and even suicide attempts.

**compulsive ceremonial** A term used to describe the ritualistic behavior that is characteristic of obsessive-compulsive disorder. According to Freud, this ritualistic behavior demonstrates the use of two types of defense mechanisms in particular: "undoing" and "isolation." Through motor means, that is, by a gesture or act that is symbolic and is repeated countless times, the patient tries to undo an undesirable or traumatic experience. For example, a patient with a washing compulsion is undoing a previous dirtying action (either real or imaginary). The dirtying action is usually masturbation, which by anal regression (characteristic of the obsessive-compulsive) is conceived of as dirty. Through order, routine, and system the obsessive-compulsive tries to isolate his experiences and rid them of their emotional concomitants. In analysis he finds it extremely difficult to associate or to experience any emotional reactions no matter how exciting his ideas may be.

Compulsive ceremonials often center around the taboo of touching, such as routines concerning which objects should not be touched and which should, and, in the latter case, in which order the objects should be touched. Such rituals frequently concern routines to be followed in washing or bathing, but they may involve any ordinary daily activity such as crossing thresholds or handling doorknobs.

**compulsive character** *Anal character* (q.v.); *anankastic personality*; a type of *character* (q.v.) manifested in a pedantic concern for orderliness, a tendency to collect things, and thriftiness or avarice. Thinking is circumstantial and ruminative in type. This character armor is a defense against sadistic and aggressive impulses. See *character defense.*

**compulsive masturbation** An ill-defined term used with various meanings by different authors. Some use it synonymously with habitual masturbation or pathological masturbation, i.e., when masturbation is preferred to sexual intercourse or when masturbation is used, not occasionally to relieve sexual tension, but so frequently as to indicate a disturbed capacity for sexual satisfaction. Others apply the term to the constant impulse to masturbate that is seen in some children, who stimulate their genitals frequently, without regard to their environment, and usually without accompanying sexual erotic phantasies. More properly, the term is confined to repetitive masturbatory activity performed without adequate sexual feelings or without any accompanying sexual feelings.

Used in a more general sense as synonymous with habitual, pathological, or overfrequent masturbation or masturbatory *pseudosexuality*, the term compulsive masturbation implies a disturbance in the capacity for satisfaction. Such cases are often based on (1) conflicts over hostility and aggressiveness, especially in those who are afraid to manifest overt defiance; or (2) conflicts over the expectation of punishment, for which masturbation may represent a substitute; or (3) conflicts over "perverse" sexual impulses, where masturbation is felt to afford a higher

pleasure than can be achieved in reality; or (4) attempts to forestall threatened depression, which typically is related to unsatisfied yearnings for love and narcissistic supplies; or (5) use of masturbation to withdraw from reality in those who are neurotically inhibited, shy, and afraid of interpersonal relationships.

**compulsive personality (disorder)** Also known as anal personality, anankastic personality; in DSM-IV, in Cluster C of *personality disorders* (q.v.). Order, parsimony, and obstinacy are key traits; the compulsive person is overconcerned with conformity and adherence to standards. Such a person is rigid, overinhibited, overconscientious, overdutiful, indecisive, perfectionistic, and inordinately scrupulous. Yet the veil of smiling submissiveness and compliance often drops to reveal stubbornness, obstructionism, pettiness, irascibility, avarice, possessiveness, arrogance, and pretentiousness. See *anal character.*

**compulsive symptoms** Compulsions and the orderly and systematic behavior exhibited by the obsessive-compulsive in order to protect himself against anal-erotic instinctual demands. He protects himself against a rebellion of sensual and hostile demands (such as murder and incest), which through regression have become anal-erotic in nature. He accomplishes this by doing things in a compulsive systematic way, according to a prearranged plan or routine, to avoid the danger associated with spontaneity. The systematization is especially noticeable with respect to money and time.

The drives, however, "usually sabotage orderliness and clinging to a 'system.' They may reappear in the form of disorder or events that disturb the system" (Fenichel, O. *The Psychoanalytic Theory of Neurosis*, 1945). Furthermore, the obsessive-compulsive is never certain that he has provided enough rules to govern all possibilities, that he knows all the rules well enough, or that the unconscious drives have not actually permeated the systems themselves. The compulsive often pressures others to follow his systems in an effort to ensure their validity.

The systematization of the obsessive-compulsive leads him to make false generalizations. All ideas are classified into certain mutually exclusive categories. Thus the likelihood of an unforeseen new event (which would be interpreted as a dangerous temptation) is excluded. See *compulsion; obsession; obsessive-compulsive disorder.*

**compulsive-obsessive psychoneurosis** See *obsessive-compulsive disorder.*

**computation, symbolic** See *cognitive science.*

**computational theory** The theory of mental operations that treats beliefs and desires as *information*, incarnated as configurations of symbols. Intelligence is computation by reason of its processing of symbols: arrangements of matter that have both *representational* and *causal* properties, that is, they simultaneously carry information about something and take part in a chain of physical events. The brain acts like a computer with many elements that are active to a degree, corresponding to the *probability* that some statement is true or false, and in which the activity levels change smoothly to register new and roughly accurate probabilities.

A symbol is connected to its referent in the world by the sense organs; this is its causal role. The sensory image triggers a cascade of templates or similar circuits, providing an opportunity to which a symbol can be inscribed. The unique pattern of symbol manipulations triggered by the first symbol mirrors the unique pattern of relationships between the referent of the first symbol and the referents of the triggered symbols - the *inferential role. Together* the causal and inferential roles of a symbol determine what it represents. Causal and inferential roles tend to be in synchrony because natural selection designed both perceptual systems and inference modules to work accurately, most of the time, in this world. The human brain uses at least four major formats of representation. One format is the visual image, which is like a template in a two-dimensional, picturelike mosaic. Another is a phonological representation, a stretch of syllables that is played like a tape loop in mental operations, planning mouth movements and imagining what the syllables sound like. A third format is the grammatical representation: nouns and verbs, phrases and clauses, stems and roots, phonemes and syllables, all arranged into hierarchical trees. The fourth format is *mentalese* (q.v.) (Pinker, S. *How the Mind Works*, New York: Norton, 1997).

**computer electroencephalographic topography** See *imaging, brain.*

**computer-assisted cognitive therapy** First used in 1990, a computer program developed for the treatment of depression. It used written text to provide information on depression and a model that simulated dialogue between therapist and patient. Since then, programs have expanded to the use of multimedia formats to engage patients, teach the basic methods of standard cognitive therapy, and reinforce learning. Interactive self-help exercises build skills for using *cognitive behavior therapy* (q.v.).

**COMT** Catechol *O*-methyltransferase, a metabolic enzyme that is the principal regulatory factor determining the functional effects of synaptic dopamine in the frontal cortex. Two genetic forms of COMT occur in humans, one with the amino acid valine (Val) at position 108, the other with the amino acid methionine (Met) at 109. Because all people have two genes for each of their proteins, they carry three possible forms of COMT: Val-Val, Val-Met, or Met-Met. The val allele is associated with high enzymatic activity and consequently low extracellular dopamine levels, while the met allele is associated with significantly reduced enzyme activity and high extracellular dopamine levels. Frontal cortex-related neurocognitive dysfunction is more common with the Val-Val genotype, suggesting that more rapid dopamine metabolism in the cortex may be related to neuropsychologic deficits. The low activity met allele is characterized by greater task-dependent frontal efficiency (i.e., decreased magnitude and activation for a given level of task performance) and associated cognitive advantages (e.g., working memory enhancement). But it is also associated with abnormal affective behaviors, such as bipolar disorder and major depression.

The COMT gene, on chromosome 22q11, has been linked with schizophrenia, and also with 22qDS, the 22q11 deletion syndrome. See *velocardiofacial syndrome.*

**conarium** The point of contact of mind and body in Cartesian philosophy. The basic tenet of this philosophy is that the human mind is a thinking substance in intimate association with the body. The Cartesian conarium was renamed the id by Freud, who regarded it as the place in which the instincts are localized and from which they spread to diverse sections of the body and the mind.

**conation**   Striving, inclination, tendency to do actively or purposively. Many psychologists distinguish among three categories of mental functioning: the cognitive (perceptual or intellectual), the emotional, and the conative. Conation includes instincts, drives, wishes, and cravings.

**concatenated ideas**   Interconnected or interdependent ideas.

**concentration**   See *attention*.

**concentric demyelination**   Baló disease. See *diffuse sclerosis*.

**concentric method**   A concept of stratification of the personality employed by Laignel-Lavastine. Five concentric zones of personality are recognized: psychic, nervous, endocrine, visceral, and morbific. Personality difficulties and psychiatric symptoms result from abnormalities in any zone, or in any combination of zones.

**concept, body**   See *body image*.

**conception-hallucination**   See *hallucination of perception*.

**conceptive phase**   See *proceptive phase*.

**conceptual structure**   See *semantics*.

**concordance**   1. Agreement; in statistics, used primarily in twin studies to refer to the proportion of a representative sample of affected twins whose co-twins are or will be similarly affected. Concordance is the tendency for twins to have the same illness. To be contrasted with *frequency*, which refers only to incidence of illness among twins, without regard to incidence in their co-twins.

2. In literary and linguistic computing, a list of words that shows the frequency and locations for each item in a written text. If one wished to know how often Freud used the word "ego," a concordance of his writings would give the answer.

3. Compliance of a patient with the treatment regimen prescribed.

**concordance, probandwise**   The risk of illness in co-twins of proband twins.

**concrete attitude**   *Concretism*; a need for environmental immutability such that any sudden or unanticipated change in the environment may provoke an overreaction. Such concretism is found in dementia and other organic disorders and also in some patients with schizophrenia or borderline personality disorder. See *abstract attitude*.

**concrete operational stage**   One of the stages described by Piaget in the development of mature thinking; the sequence proposed by Piaget begins with the *sensorimotor stage* (q.v.), followed by the *preoperational*, the *concrete operational* and, finally, *fully (formal) operational* ideation (which includes the capacity for abstraction and categorization). See *propositional thinking*.

**concrete operations**   See *adolescence*.

**concrete thinking**   Also, *concretism*; preference for the literal (denotative) meaning; an under-inclusive bias. See *physiognomonic thinking*.

**concretism**   The antithesis of abstraction in thought and feeling; a concretely thought concept is one that has grown together or coalesced with other concepts. Such a concept is not abstract, not isolated, and independently thought, but always related to the sense-conveyed material of perception. See *concrete attitude*.

**concretization**   The act of making or being concrete and specific, as opposed to general and abstract. In psychiatry, the term generally connotes an overemphasis on specific detail and on the events of immediate experience especially in the subject's verbal productions, in which case the concretization is considered to be an association defect. See *association disturbances; reification; connotation*.

For example, a university student with an IQ of 134 gave the following concretistic responses to a word association test: "My father always "has a head and shoulders' " and "If I were queen I would "be seated and have a scepter.' "

**concretizing attitude**   A tendency to transform abstractions about their life into concrete representations, as shown by the schizophrenic patient who felt his wife was poisoning his life and developed the delusion that she was poisoning his food.

**concurrent review**   See *review*.

**concussion**   Widespread paralysis of brain function, due to a blow on the head, with a strong tendency to spontaneous recovery, and not necessarily associated with gross organic brain damage. Experimental evidence suggests that this functional disturbance is due to a direct physical injury to the neuron that is reversible, the rate of recovery being proportional to the severity of the injury. See *cerebral compression*.

**condensation**   *Compression*; the process whereby an idea is made to contain all the emotion associated with a group of ideas. The condensation of latent thoughts, memories, and phantasies in a dream operates like a magnet, gathering together out of the whole reservoir of past and present-day experiences all those pertinent to the magnet. See *dream*.

**conditional release**  An involuntary outpatient commitment order issued upon a patient's release from hospital. Such *outpatient commitment* (q.v.) may provide significant benefits, such as reducing the amount of inpatient care required, increasing patient compliance, and providing protective oversight for those considered dangerous to themselves or others. Its use is controversial, however, in that it gives little opportunity for voluntary engagement and depends more on the legal system than on the medical care system. Further, it may be contrary to legislative intent if legislation requires evidence of failure of voluntary treatment before legal measures are instituted.

**conditionalism**  Approximately equivalent to the Jungian concept of determinism and to the Skinnerian concept of *contingency*. Causality is relative rather than absolute, and effects are dependent upon (contingent upon, conditional upon) certain other things occurring. Turning a key in the ignition may be a necessary condition to start a motor, but it will not always start even when the key is turned. See *behavior therapy; behaviorism*.

**conditioned cueing**  In substance abuse and *addiction* (q.v.), the process whereby previously neutral stimuli that are paired to drug experiences develop both motivational and reinforcing significance (salience).

**conditioned place preference (CPP)**  A technique used to study the motivational properties of a drug in animals. The animal receives a specific drug in a suitable vehicle while the animal is in a unique environment that has a specific odor, color, or texture. On the next day, the animal receives the vehicle instead of the drug and is placed in another conditioning environment. After several such cycles, the animal is given the opportunity to spend time in either of the environments. CPP allows the testing of both the rewarding properties of a drug (the animal can show a preference for the drug-paired environment) and its aversive properties (the animal can actively avoid the drug-paired environment).

**conditioning**  A procedure in which an adequate stimulus (e.g., presentation of food, causing salivation in the experimental animal) is paired with an inadequate stimulus (e.g., ringing of a bell, which of itself has no effect on salivation) until the previously inadequate stimulus is by itself able to evoke the response. The original, adequate stimulus (food, in the above example) is termed the unconditional stimulus (US), and the response to the unconditional stimulus is termed the unconditional response (UR). The other stimulus (ringing of a bell in the above example) is termed the conditioned or conditional stimulus (CS), and the response to it once conditioning is established is termed the conditioned or *conditional response* (CR).

Because conditioning as thus defined was first described by I. P. Pavlov, it is often known as *Pavlovian conditioning*. It is also known as *classical conditioning* or *respondent conditioning*.

**conditioning, aversive**  See *aversion therapy*.

**conduct**  1. As a rule the word conduct refers to the action or behavior of the total individual rather than to parts of him or her (such as movement of an extremity as an isolated act).

2. Self-conscious and self-regulatory behavior as determined by the standards set for the person by his or her social environment.

**conduct disorder**  *Behavior disorders* (q.v.); a disruptive behavior disorder of childhood characterized by repetitive and persistent antisocial activities that violate the rights of others and are clearly beyond the usual pranks of childhood. Symptoms may include verbal or physical aggression directed against others (e.g., bullying, fighting, destruction of property, fire-setting, breaking and entering, cruelty to people or animals, use of a weapon that could cause serious physical harm); often repeated violation of age-appropriate social norms and rules (e.g., truancy or work absences, use of alcohol or other substances before the age of 13, staying out at night despite parental prohibitions); stealing, with or without confrontation of a victim (e.g., shoplifting, forgery, mugging, armed robbery); and "conning" others in order to gain personal advantages or avoid responsibilities.

The reported rates range from 4% to 9%, with a frequency four to five times higher in boys than in girls. Median age of onset in boys is 7 years, in girls 13 years. See *oppositional disorder*.

**conduction aphasia**  Symptomatically similar to *Wernicke aphasia* (q.v.) in that output is fluent, retention and naming are impaired, but comprehension is preserved, and there are phonemic substitutions (mispronunciations) rather than verbal paraphasias. Patients show great difficulty repeating sentences spoken to them and in reading aloud (although they can read silently with good comprehension). Speech is semantically abnormal, but the Wernicke area provides normal comprehension. Writing may be disturbed; spelling is poor, with omissions, reversals, and substitutions of letters. The lesion is in the arcuate fasciculus, which connects the Broca area and the Wernicke area.

**cones** See *photoreceptor*.

**confabulation** Production of erroneous statements made without a conscious effort to deceive, or statements or actions that involve unintentional but obvious distortions; determined amnesia; spontaneous narrative reports of events that never happened; false memory; replacing memory loss by phantasy or by reality that is not true for the occasion. The gaps in memory are filled by all sorts of *confabulations* or *fabrications* that are narrated in great detail and with perfect appearance of lucidity (thus sometimes termed opportune confabulation). See *amnesia; amnestic syndrome; reduplicative memory deception*.

Korsakoff distinguished *simple confabulation* (errors in the temporal ordering of real memories) and *fantastic confabulation* (bizarre, patently impossible statements unrelated to actual memories). Confabulations are also divided into *provoked confabulations*, triggered by questioning or strong suggestions (overt or implied) from others, and *spontaneous confabulations*, unrelated to any external trigger. Provoked confabulations can be induced in healthy subjects when they are pushed to retrieve details of an inaccurate or nonexistent memory. See *false memory*.

Spontaneous confabulations, on the other hand, occur in a setting of disorientation (which is always present in the early stages) and profound derangement of thought, due to failure to suppress evoked memories that do not pertain to ongoing reality. The patient seems to re-experience an earlier event as if it were real and occurring in the present. Memory traces that do not pertain to ongoing reality intrude and come to dominate current thought and behavior. The patient is convinced of the veracity of his or her narrative and may even act according to it. The story seems to be invented but always contains elements of true events.

Spontaneous confabulation is usually based on disturbance in the basal forebrain and posterior orbitofrontal cortex. It can also result from destruction of the dorsomedial thalamic nucleus, as in *Korsakoff psychosis* (q.v.). Korsakoff originally termed spontaneous confabulations *pseudoreminiscences*.

Confabulation is to be differentiated from *pseudologia fantastica* (q.v.), which occurs mainly in the "psychopathic" group and in other conditions in which acting-out is prominent. In pseudologia fantastica, the phantasy is believed only momentarily and will quickly be dropped if the patient is confronted with contradictory evidence. The confabulator, in contrast, will stick steadfastly to his or her story.

In describing the perceptual, thought, and language disturbances of schizophrenic children, W. Goldfarb terms *confabulations* those misconceptions that the child is seeing different people when he or she is really seeing the same person in different settings. See *object constancy*.

**confabulosis** A type of symptomatic psychosis characterized by systematized confabulations in a setting of relatively clear consciousness; other than confabulations, memory disturbances are mild, and orientation is relatively intact. Confabulosis typically occurs during the stage of recovery from an acute brain syndrome.

**confidence, diagnostic** See *sensitivity*.

**confidence level** A quantitative expression of the degree of reliability of an inference; a 5% level of confidence, for example, is a statement that the particular inference would be wrong 5% of the time. Thus the percentage specified is seen to be negatively related to the degree of confidence involved, and a small percentage denotes a high degree of confidence or a low degree of uncertainty.

**confidentiality** In the medical setting, one element of the right of the patient to privacy, i.e., to have privileged communication with the therapist. Disclosure of information gained within the therapeutic relationship without the permission of the patient is a breach of confidentiality. Such a breach may be allowed under limited and specific circumstances, e.g., to prevent harm to others that might result if confidentiality is not breached. Even in such instances, however, the probability that such harm will occur must be high, and the consequences of not breaching confidentiality must be of considerable magnitude. See *notification, anonymous*.

Issues of privacy are also important in discharge planning, particularly for elderly patients. Placement in a residence and the use of home health aides, for example, may significantly jeopardize the patient's liberty, autonomy, and privacy. In the United States, federal law is especially restrictive about disclosure of information concerning treatment for alcoholism or drug dependence.

**configural interpretation** Evaluation of a test on the basis of the pattern or profile of responses to the entire test, rather than depending on a single score as the measure of a variable. Often a battery of tests is administered, and even though they might all be measuring the same general area, they do so in a different way or with a different emphasis. The pattern of responses to all the tests provides a better assessment of the subject's strengths and weaknesses in the area than any one test could offer.

**configuration** 1. Gestalt. See *Gestalt psychology*.

2. In the card-sorting tests devised by David Reiss and his colleagues to measure the indigenous family culture, the amount of information on the cards that is used by the family members as they work at the task together. High-configuration families recognize subtle patterns and sort the cards accordingly. High configuration does not depend on intelligence or education but is rather a reflection of the family's optimism about its ability to solve a problem through diligent work (Reiss, D. *The Family's Construction of Reality*, 1981). See *family culture, indigenous*.

**conflict** Incompatibility; battle or struggle; opposition; nability to complete a response, either because it is blocked by some environmental condition (frustration) or because the response is incompatible with other response tendencies of the subject (intrapsychic conflict). See *frustration*.

**conflict detouring** See *scapegoating*.

**conflict of interest** See *informed consent*.

**conflict paradigm** In psychodynamics, the theory that pathology is caused by frustration of drives and the attempt to gratify them or to defend against their unwanted expression

(thus, also called the *drive-defense-conflict* model). Self psychology (e.g., Kohut) and object relations theory (e.g., Melanie Klein) emphasize relationships with objects, both external and internalized, from the very beginning of life, rather than instinctual discharge and the gratification of drives. The object relations theory of pathogenesis is a *deficit-relationship* model. See *mirroring deficits*.

**Conflict Tactics Scale** A self-administered 18-item scale to measure violence within relationships, assessing behaviors that a person might exhibit during an argument with a partner.

**confluence** 1. In individual psychology (Adler), the flowing together of several instincts into a single object. 2. In genetics, the combined influence of heredity and environment.

**confrontation** See *interpretation*.

**confrontation, reality** See *social therapy*.

**confusion** A state of disordered orientation; a disturbance of consciousness in the sense that awareness of time, place, or person is unclear. See *organic syndrome*.

Some clinicians differentiate between anamnestic and deliriant confusion. *Anamnestic confusion* consists of a disturbance of orientation and perception secondary to domestic dislocation, such as transfer of an older person to a nursing home. Such confusion can sometimes be prevented by informing, describing, or demonstrating in advance the changes the person is likely to encounter.

*Deliriant confusion* occurs mainly at night and may be accompanied by severe agitation. Usually it is due to inadequate cerebral oxygenation, as when an already embarrassed cardiovascular or cerebrovascular system is compromised by nocturnal vagotonia combined with hypnotic medication. Because those with deliriant confusion appear to have relatively normal mental functioning during the day and develop confusional episodes only at night, they are sometimes referred to as *sundowners*.

**confusion psychosis** See *cycloid psychosis*.

**confusional state, acute** 1. Disordered memory and orientation, characteristic of some types of *delirium* (q.v.). There is a short-term memory deficit; amnesia is both retrograde (impaired recall of memories formed prior to the onset of delirium) and anterograde (impaired ability to register new information following the onset of delirium). Disorientation typically involves both time and place; disorientation in person is rare.

2. *Reactive confusion*; an acute stress reaction, occurring typically in adolescents when they are placed in an unfamiliar environment, such as college, and are expected to manifest a degree of psychological maturity that they have not as yet achieved. The reaction is precipitated by some minor frustration and is characterized by rage, followed by the confusional state itself (inability to concentrate, estrangement, depersonalization, feelings of loneliness, sometimes impulsive suicidal attempts). Unless the subject is otherwise predisposed to the development of psychosis, the acute confusional state is self-limiting and the subject slowly reintegrates his or her ego defenses.

**confusional states**   According to Rosenfeld (a follower of Melanie Klein), extreme forms of narcissistic object relations that are defenses against primary envy, characterized by the simultaneous presence of opposite perceptions and emotions, where good and bad, external and internal cannot be split and differentiated. They appear most prominently in schizophrenia, hypochondriasis, severe psychosomatic illnesses, and addictions. See *ambivalence; envy, primary*.

**congelatio**   *Obs.* Rigid state of the body in catalepsy; same as *gelatio*. See *catalepsy.*

**congenital**   Existing or possessed since birth. In biology applied to an attribute, or anomaly, possessed and manifested by an individual since birth. See *hereditary; teratology.*

**congenital hypomyelination (CH)**   See *myelin disorders.*

**congophilic**   Having an affinity to Congo red dye, such as the amyloid deposits within the senile plaques of *Alzheimer disease* (q.v.).

**congruent**   Consistent, dependable; in harmony with or concordant with what would generally be considered proper, reasonable, or appropriate. Rogers emphasizes the need for the therapist to be congruent; that is, to be dependably real and to act in accordance with the feelings or attitudes he is in fact experiencing, rather than to adopt a stereotyped demeanor (e.g., of loving acceptance) that is rigidly maintained no matter what happens between him and his client. See *mood-congruent.*

**conjoint family therapy**   See *family therapy.*

**conjoint marital therapy**   See *matrix, therapeutic.*

**conjugal bereavement**   Loss of a spouse (typically through death), among the most potentially stressful of commonly occurring life events. It is associated with increased medical mortality, onset of panic attacks in susceptible subjects, and suppression of mitogen-induced lymphocytic stimulation (which may be related to the onset or course of physical illness following bereavement).

**conjugal paranoia**   Morbid jealousy of the marital partner that constitutes the sole or primary delusion of an underlying paranoia or paranoid schizophrenia. See *jealousy, morbid.*

**conjugal unit, isolated**   The expected and usual pattern of marriage in the United States, in which young men and women mingle freely, choose their own partners, and set up their own household separate from relatives. Such a unit is in marked contrast to the *extended family*, characteristic of most of the rest of the world, where a new family is received into a group that is economically, psychologically, and socially experienced in family living. The extended family includes parents, children, and persons united by kinship or marital ties; the *nuclear family* is limited to parents and their children.

**conjunctive**   Sullivan's term for that which promotes harmony among different and even contradictory factors and situations. See *motivation.*

**Conn syndrome**   *Aldosteronism* (q.v.).

**connection weight**   See *parallel distributed processing.*

**connectionism**   The *neural network* approach, which attempts to explain both observable behavior and its neurophysiological basis in terms of networks of simple, neuronlike processing units; an associationist theory of cognition which assumes that the mind is a large set of simple elementary units connected with one another in a network. Mental processes are interactions between units that are individually simple but have complex results in the overall patterns that occur in the network. Units excite and inhibit each other throughout the network simultaneously—in parallel operations rather than in a sequence. Knowledge consists of the connections between pairs of units that are distributed throughout the network rather than being stored in localized structures. Because of those characteristics, connectionism is sometimes referred to as *parallel distributed processing* (q.v.). See *cognitive science.*

Connectionism challenges the main assumptions of modern cognitive science and its belief that human cognition is based on symbolic computation, the idea that knowledge and mental processes involve structures of symbols and transformations of symbolic expressions. The theory assumes that patterns of generic relations, or *schemata*, are used to organize information in specific situations, and that cognitive skills are composed of rules that can be represented symbolically in the form, "if this, then that."

Association theorists, on the other hand, believe that complex cognition can be explained in terms of elementary structures and processes. They show how performance that seems to reflect knowledge of representations of rules or schemata can in fact occur because there are connections in a network.

**connectionism, cellular** The regional specialization view of brain functioning, the belief that regions of the brain are specialized for different functions (e.g., language, vision, and hearing) and that neurons are localized in functional groups (sometimes called parallel distributed systems). It is the connections between the many elements, not the contribution of any one of them, that makes it possible to process complex information. This view of brain functioning, currently the favored theory, is an outgrowth of the studies of J. Hughlings Jackson, Karl Wernicke, and Ramón y Cajal. See *aggregate field view; parallel distributed processing.*

**connectionist model** In the connectionist model of associative memory, words (or various word features) are represented as networks of interconnected nodes. Organized into local networks, nodes are activated in parallel in such a way that a word activates or primes a local network of related associates.

In the connectionist model of acquisition and expression of complex behavior, cerebral cortex function is considered at four levels of the cortical system—cell, module, tissue, and global—that integrate learning experiences to produce a coherent functioning system. The cellular level processes information and modifies neuronal behavior; the modular level enables computation and learning within a cortical column; the tissue level activates different inputs in parallel and integrates successive learning experiences; and the global level integrates functions from different cortical regions to produce behavior. Prefrontal cortex is believed to be crucial to the operation of the system.

**connexins** Proteins that form gap junctions.

**connexon** See *gap junction.*

**connotation** The significance of a word as it applies to a whole class rather than to a specific or concrete embodiment of the word. Thus the connotative meaning of the word chair would include all the qualities essential to any chair and would be most closely indicated by the phrase *chair in general as a physical entity.* This is to be distinguished from *denotation*, or denotative meaning, which (in this case) would refer to certain chairs or to a specific chair.

It has been noted that schizophrenics typically demonstrate a reduction in their connotation ability and are able to define words only as they apply to specific objects and not in their general sense as representative of a group or class. As a result, there is relative overemphasis on denotation and thinking comes to be pathologically concretized (see *concretization; holophrastic*). This would also appear to be an important factor in the schizophrenic's overliteralness and inability to use metaphor.

**Conolly, John** (c. 1794–1866) British psychiatrist; psychotherapy.

**consanguinity** In contradistTinction to affinity or the relation by marriage, consanguinity means relation by blood or descent from a common ancestor within the same family stock. See *kinship.*

**conscience** Those psychical organizations that stand in opposition to the expression of instinctual actions. Conscience relates to the moral and esthetic and ethical attitudes of the individual. According to psychoanalysis, when the parental attitudes, prohibitions, and commands take up their position in the unconscious to form the superego, it is the superego that is conscience. Later in development, when the child begins to emulate others outside the family circle and develops an ego-ideal, he acquires another conscience. There is, however, a continuity between the two. See *superego.*

The function of conscience is to warn the ego to avoid the pains of intense guilt feelings. "Conscience becomes pathological when it (a) functions in too rigid or too automatic a manner, so that realistic judgment about the actual outcome of intended actions is disturbed ("archaic superego') or (b) when the breakdown toward "panic' occurs and a greater or lesser sense of complete annihilation is experienced instead of a warning signal, which is the case in severe depressions." (Fenichel, O. *The Psychoanalytic Theory of Neurosis*, 1945).

**conscious** 1. As a noun, the conscious denotes a particular division of the psyche. In such use it is practically synonymous with *consciousness*. 2. It is used less frequently as an adjective descriptive of a function of consciousness or of the conscious realm as a perceptive faculty. As such, it is synonymous with aware, having knowledge of, present in the field (or realm) of consciousness.

**consciousness** *Sensorium* (q.v.); consciousness includes the following:

1. *Self-knowledge*—building an internal model of the world that contains the self, reflecting back on one's own mode of understanding.

2. *Access to information*—access-consciousness has four obvious features. First, we are aware, to varying degrees, of a rich field of sensation. Second, portions of this information can fall under the spotlight of attention, get rotated into and out of short-term memory, and feed deliberative cognition. Third, sensation and thoughts come with a emotional flavoring. Finally, an executive, the "I," appears to make choices and pull the levers of behavior. Exercising the will—forming and carrying out plans—is dependent on the frontal lobes, which act as a controller that selects a plan from a hubbub of competing agents. See *vigilance*.

Each of these features discards some information in the nervous system, defining the highways of access-consciousness. Information must be *routed* and made accessible to a computation when it is relevant, insofar as that can be predicted.

3. *Sentience*—subjective experience, phenomenal awareness, raw feelings, first-person present tense, "what it is like" to be or do something.

Different levels of consciousness are often differentiated clinically: alert wakefulness, lethargy, obtundation, stupor, and coma. The neural correlates of the level of consciousness

(e.g., awake, asleep, attentive, or drowsy) should be distinguished from the neural correlates of specific phenomenal content (such as a green apple versus an orange). This distinction reflects our everyday experience of the phenomenal distinction between being conscious (as opposed to being unconscious) and being conscious of X (as opposed to not being conscious of X). The level of consciousness can be thought of as an enabling factor (like neuronal arousal mediated by the ascending reticular activating system) that is required for awareness but does not directly reflect specific conscious experiences.

**consciousness, clouding of** See *sensorium*.

**consciousness, splitting of** When a set of experiences, a mental constellation, exists, as in hysteria, essentially alone in consciousness, without associations with other components of consciousness, it is said that there is a splitting of consciousness.

**consciousness raising** The process of increasing a subject's awareness of himself—including recognition not only of the subject's needs but also of how the subject relates to his environment and how the culture of which he is a part fosters attitudes and stereotypes about people and subgroups within the culture. Most commonly, consciousness raising is a group process that may use discussion groups (*rap sessions*) as its primary vehicle.

**consensual light reflex** When light enters the pupil of one eye only, causing the iris of the other eye to contract.

**consensual validation** See *parataxic distortion*.

**conservator** Protector; guardian; a person or institution designated to protect the interests of another. The conservatorship procedure is a way of protecting and preserving the property of persons with a serious debility (mental and/or physical), whose condition falls short of incompetency or, if actual incompetency exists, where there is a disinclination to declare the person incompetent because of the stigma attached thereto.

**consolidated memory** See *consolidation; long-term memory*.

**consolidation** The process by which labile new memories are stabilized into long-lasting memories; protein synthesis within neurons is a key molecular step of the process. Memory representations are transferred over time between brain areas, typically from hippocampus to neocortex. Neocortical areas provide dedicated processors for perceptual motor or cognitive information. The parahippocampal region mediates convergence of this information and extends the persistence of neocortical memory representations. The hippocampus encodes the sequences of places and events that compose episodic memories, and links them together through their common elements. The hippocampus functions as a temporary store for new information, but permanent storage depends on a broadly distributed cortical network.

Memory consolidation comprises two types, fast (molecular) and slow (reorganization of brain regions at a system level). The fast type consists of morphological changes required for the initial stabilization of memories in hippocampal circuits: synaptic activation leads to recruitment of second messenger systems, activation of transcription factors, and synthesis of new proteins. This cascade of events results in the growth of new synaptic connections and restructuring of existing synaptic connections. The changes take place in the first few hours that follow learning, and interference with any of the changes blocks memory formation. Similar treatments outside the period of consolidation do not disrupt memory.

System consolidation is a gradual and slower reorganization of the brain regions that support memory. Experience is initially encoded in parallel in hippocampal and cortical networks. Subsequent reactivation of the hippocampal network reinstates activity in different cortical networks. This coordinated *replay* across hippocampal-cortical networks leads to gradual strengthening of corticocortical connections, which eventually allows new memories to become independent of the hippocampus and to be gradually integrated with preexisting cortical memories.

Memories are labile not only after learning but also after reactivation or retrieval. The cascade of cellular events that lead to memory consolidation is recapitulated each time a memory is retrieved. Noradrenergic transmission is involved not only in initial consolidation, but in reconsolidation as well. Every retrieval operation triggers a reconsolidation process that allows new information to be integrated within the background of the past. Old memories are therefore modified and reinforced as a result of retrieval. Retrieval and

reconsolidation update and strengthen rather than weaken or wither a dynamic memory trace. Hippocampal BDNF (brain-derived neurotrophic factor) is required for the initial consolidation of long-term memory, but not for reconsolidation, which instead is dependent on the transcription factor Zif268. See *long-term memory; memory.*

**constancy**  Steadfastness or stability; Adler assumed a constancy of personality, i.e., that a person remains fundamentally the same once his personality has been well established in early childhood. Such constancy of personality constitutes the *lifestyle* of the person, the characteristic way in which he pursues his long-range goals. See *individual psychology.*

In object relations theory, constancy refers to an inner coherence underlying the changes and unpredictability of perceptions and sensations; the cognitive processes underlying rule extraction, cognitive integration, and elaboration and organization of the world perceived and the objects within it as enduring and stable, despite their moment-to-moment variations; stable and internal representations of self and others; ordering and analyzing symbolic representations; keeping the "word" and the "thing" clearly defined and appropriately separated. See *identity diffusion; object relations theory; separation-individuation.*

**constancy, object**  See *autonomy, sense of; evocative memory; object constancy.*

**constellation**  A group of allied thoughts, centering around a nuclear idea.

**constitution**  The relatively constant physiological composition and biological makeup of the human organism that determines the individual's reaction, successful or unsuccessful, to the stress of environment, including *diathesis* (q.v.), or vulnerability to disorder.

From Hippocrates to the present there have been systems of constitutional types and diseases, which changed in content and could be more finely subdivided when further knowledge was added. Up to the 19th century, all diseases not localized in the pathology of a single organ were constitutional. When the knowledge of pathogenesis advanced, the number of these so-called constitutional diseases was correspondingly reduced.

Concepts of heredity and constitution have become practically inseparable, although it is clear that the constitution is not to be identified with either the genotypical structure or the phenotypical makeup of a person. While the phenotype is the changeable picture of the manifest appearance of an organism and is always modified by its external life-situation, constitution represents a relatively constant state of the person and classifies this person according to his biological values. It is therefore best understood as an auxiliary concept of medical classification and general pathology.

Among the different constitutional types described in the literature are the following: hyperadrenal, hyperpituitary, hyperthymic, hyperthyroid, hypoadrenal, hypopituitary, hypothyroid, and post-traumatic (qq.v.) See character; constitutional type; habitus.

**constitutional** Pertaining to those elements in the biological and physiologic makeup of an organism that are inherent and relatively constant. The concept of constitution is based on the differentiation of three factors determining the final nature of the organism: the inherited elements that make up the genotype and are again transmissible, the peristatic conditions of the environment, and the dispositional response of the individual organism. See *constitution; hereditary.*

**constitutional psychology** The theory that personality and other specific psychological characteristics are associated with particular types of physical constitution.

**constitutional type** The constellations of traits, morphological, physiological, and psychological, that are assumed to be associated with tendencies to certain diseases, physical and mental. Often used in a wider sense to include types of body and mind, even where no relations to any particular tendency to disease is postulated. See *constitution.*

The first typological system was developed by Hippocrates, who described a tendency to apoplexy, the *habitus apoplecticus* (q.v.), in persons of thick-set, rounded appearance, and a tendency to pulmonary tuberculosis; the *habitus phthisicus* (q.v.), in persons of slender, angular appearance. This dichotomizing system was extended by Galen to four human types that were related to the four fluids or humors assumed to form the basis of the body. The *sanguine* type was thought to owe his enthusiasm to the "strength of the blood," the *melancholic* type was said to be sad because of the overproduction of the "black bile," the *choleric* type was irritable owing to

the predominance of the "yellow bile," and the *phlegmatic* type was sluggish because of the abundance of "phlegm."

Harvey's discovery of the circulation of the blood had the twofold effect of focusing attention on the blood as the important humor, and of emphasizing the role of the blood vessels. It was Haller who demonstrated the loose connection between the blood and the temperaments, and thereby paved the way for modern typologists to describe their types in terms of anatomical systems instead of humors.

The discovery of the internal secretions and their effect on the morphology of body and mind led to a classification of types on the basis of altered secretion of one of these glands. The prefixes *hyper-*, *hypo-*, and *dys-* were employed to indicate oversecretion, undersecretion, or qualitatively altered secretion. The main typological systems developed on the basis of these concepts were those of the modern French, Italian, German, and American typologists.

In psychiatry, the typological system of Kretschmer has been the most influential one (*pyknic, asthenic, athletic,* and *dysplastic* types on the physical side; and *cyclothymic* and *schizothymic* temperaments). In the modern *American* school, the most systematic and effective work has been done by Draper (*panels of personality*), Davenport (*fleshy, slender,* and *medium* biotypes), Stockard (*lateral* and *linear* types), Lewis (*regressive, hypercompensatory,* and *normally compensating* types), and Sheldon *ectomorphic, mesomorphic,* and *endomorphic* types).

Well-known *English* typologists are E. Miller, Spearman, and Cohen, and in the modern *Dutch* school Hymans and Wiersma.

**constitutive pathway** See *vesicles.*

**constraint of thought** The idea that one's thoughts are under the influence of others. The same idea of constraint applied to movements is called *constraint of movement.* It is to be noted that psychiatric usage differentiates between constraint and *constriction* (q.v.).

**constriction** When applied to thinking or movement, this term implies a reduction in range or variability. Constriction is associated with diminished spontaneity. Psychiatric usage differentiates between constriction and *constraint of thought* (q.v.).

**construct validity** See *validity.*

**constructional apraxia** Inability to manipulate objects in the environment. When asked to reproduce simple geometric patterns with matches, for example, the patient is unable to connect the separate parts correctly; the end result is disorder and chaos. *Dressing apraxia* (q.v.) is a type of constructional apraxia. The impairments in constructional apraxia are not related to intelligence, nor are they due to motor or sensory deficits. The patient with this kind of apraxia often recognizes his errors. See *apraxia; Gerstmann syndrome.*

**constructive** Synthetic, as opposed to reductive; used particularly to refer to elaboration of unconscious products such as dreams and phantasies.

**consultant** In traditional medicine and psychiatry, an advisor to the treating physician on matters of diagnosis, treatment, rehabilitation, etc. Ordinarily, the consultant is a specialist whose expert advice is sought by the attending physician or, sometimes, by the patient. The consultant may or may not meet directly with the patient, but ordinarily he does not take actual charge of a case; instead, he advises or counsels the attending physician, although his advice is *patient-oriented.*

Another type of consultation is *colleague-centered*; here the consultant-specialist meets with one or more colleagues to advise, counsel, or educate them in the area of his specialized knowledge. Questions about the management of specific patients may legitimately be raised during the course of colleague-centered consultation, but the primary focus of the consultant is not a single patient, but the other physician(s).

Still another type of consultation is *agency-centered*; here it is the entire organization or agency with whom the consultant meets and tries to help.

Consultation psychiatry may refer to any of the above types of consultation performed by a psychiatrist. Often, however, it is limited to the activity of the psychiatrist (diagnostic, therapeutic, teaching, research, etc.) in the nonpsychiatric parts of a general hospital; when used in this sense, it is synonymous with *consultation-liaison psychiatry* (C-L psychiatry) is concerned primarily with psychiatric and psychosocial problems associated with physical illness. Currently, the term C-L psychiatry has been replaced by *psychosomatic medicine* (q.v.)

**consultation-liaison** In the 1980s the favored term for what had previously been called consultation psychiatry and liaison psychiatry; it is the subspecialty of psychiatry that focuses on psychiatric morbidity among physically ill and somatizing patients, and on the provision of consultation and education for nonpsychiatric health workers in general hospitals or any other clinical setting. See *consultant; psychosomatic medicine.*

**consumerism** In medicine, the movement to guarantee high quality of care and protection of the rights of patients (see *advocacy*). In psychiatry, consumerism has focused on the civil rights of patients, and particularly on the *right to treatment*, enunciated by Dr. M. Birnbaum, who noted in 1960 that the due process of law does not allow the mentally ill person who has committed no crime to be deprived of his liberty by indefinitely institutionalizing him without medical treatment.

Judge D. Bazelon's decisions (1966) in *Rouse v. Cameron* and *Lake v. Cameron* emphasized that the least restrictive alternative is the desideratum, that less treatment, rather than more, is the acceptable objective.

In *Wyatt v. Stickney* (1971), the court concluded that treatment requires a humane environment and "adequate" staffing (as defined by standards of staff/patient ratios, floor space, individualized treatment plans, etc.). One of the standards stated that patients have the right not to be subjected to unusual or hazardous treatment procedures without their expressed and *informed consent*. This led ultimately to the establishment of a *bill of rights* (q.v.) for patients, limiting the incursions that can be made into patients' freedoms in the name of treatment (see *informed consent*). The *Willowbrook Consent* (1972) ruled that the mentally retarded also have a right to protection from harm, and their rights were spelled out in 23 steps, standards and procedures dealing with programming, staffing, and the environment.

In *O'Connor v. Donaldson* (1975), the court ruled that no nondangerous person can be custodially confined if he can survive safely in freedom. In *Bartley v. Kremens* (1976), the Pennsylvania court extended due-process protections and provision of legal counsel to children committed to mental facilities by their parents.

In a number of decisions subsequent to the foregoing, the right of patients not to be subjected to unusual or hazardous treatment has been extended to include the *right to refuse treatment*, concern for which has been heightened by a growing awareness of the potential misuse of psychotechnology as a means of social control. At issue also is what the courts consider to be unusual, invasive, intrusive, or high-risk treatments—judgments that seem to physicians to ignore very often the clinical and human realities with which they must deal. See *forced treatment; Rogers decision.*

**consumerist movement**   See *radical psychiatry.*

**contact-shunning personality**   See *mirroring deficits; narcissistic personality.*

**container**   Container-contained maternal function; in Bion's conceptualization of tension regulation, all those elements (in mother, analyst, etc.) that help the infant or analysand hold parts of the self intact and separate from the object. See alpha-function. In the concretely bounded and calm receptiveness provided by the analytic setting, the analyst is often seen, not as a real object, but as a container into which all the anxieties and other unwanted feelings and parts of the analysand are evacuated. The concept is similar to Kohut's concept of transmuting internalization (see self-object). See affectomotor storms; communicative matching; empathic failure; fit.

**contamination**   *Agglutination; neologism;* an error of speech characterized by amalgamating a part of one word with that of another. Bleuler gives as an example the neologism "gruesor," derived from gruesome and sorrowful.

**contempt**   See *manipulative personality.*

**content analysis**   Interpretation of a subject's production on the basis of what is said, rather than on the basis of how it is said. The interpretation of symbols in a patient's dream, for example, is content analysis.

**contentious**   Quarrelsome. Some patients, particularly those with a manic syndrome and those in the early stages of a paranoid reaction, feel that they and others are being treated unfairly; they see slights when none is present or intended, as a result of which they incessantly quarrel about discrimination.

**context frames**   See *object recognition.*

**context processing**   The ability to represent and actively maintain information required to select and execute task-appropriate behavior. It is a part of *working memory* and of *executive function* (qq.v.). Context processing has been associated with activity in the middle frontal gyrus (which includes Brodmann area 9). In schizophrenia, disorganization symptoms are more highly correlated with dysfunction in this region than are other symptoms.

**contextual circuit**   See *frontal-striatal system.*

**contextual cuing**   A form of implicit memory that results in improved performance in spatial configuration tests, such as a visual search task, when display patterns are repeated.

**contextualism**   The theory that the quality of experience is as significant as the events themselves in determining the memory of the experience. The older *associationism* theory held that memory and other mental structures were assemblies or clusters of linkages, and that simple addition of one subassembly to another produced behavior that was more complicated but not different in kind.

**contingency**   See *conditionalism.*

**contingency contracting**   See *contract therapy.*

**contingency management**   See *community reinforcement.*

**contingent observation**   A behavior therapy technique, used especially in aggressive young children: the child who shows signs of previolent behavior is removed to the perimeter of a group for a defined period.

**contingent restraint**   A behavior therapy technique used especially with severely aggressive patients; immediately upon appearance of the undesirable behavior the patient is immobilized with physical restraints.

**continuation maintenance therapy**   See *preventive therapy, long-term.*

**continued stay review**   See *review.*

**continuing vegetative state**   Persistent *vegetative state (q.v.).*

**continuity, social**   Maintenance of cultural forms in succeeding generations. The family, school, play group, and church are some of the major agencies involved.

**continuity of care**   See *community psychiatry.*

**continuous amnesia**   See *amnesia, psychogenic.*

**continuous epilepsy**   A form of *epilepsy* (q.v.) that includes the *polyclonia epileptoides continua* of Choroschko, the epilepsia corticalis continua of Kozhevnikoff, and the epilepsia partialis continua of Wilson, characterized by myoclonic attacks in single muscular groups; it is limited to one side of the body and consciousness is retained during the attacks.

**continuous group**   *Open group* (q.v.).

**continuous performance test**  *CPT*; a measure of *vigilance* (q.v.), to detect impaired pattern recognition and sustained concentration and alertness. Example: the subject is instructed to detect a particular letter, such as X, in a series of letters presented one at a time for brief periods, from 40 msec to 200 msec, and separated by brief intervals, from 100 msec to 1500 msec. A related test is the *span of apprehension* test: the subject is required to detect, for example, whether the letter T or the letter F is flashed on the screen. At times the target letters appear alone, and at other times they are embedded in two, four, nine, or more different letters. The test has several variations, including:

> *CPT-AX*—the subject presses a button only when the target letter follows another designated letter, e.g., press X only when it follows A.
>
> *CPT-double*—the subject presses a button each time two identical letters are presented consecutively.

Many workers have reported that the performance of schizophrenic patients on both the CPT and the span of apprehension test is inferior to that of nonschizophrenic controls. Both tests also tend to elicit poor performance in patients with coarse brain disease, especially in those with lesions of the dorsolateral prefrontal cortex.

**continuous sleep treatment**  A symptomatic method of treatment in which the patient is sedated with any of a variety of drugs; the aim of treatment is to provide 20 hours of sleep per day, for periods up to 3 weeks in more agitated patients. Klaesi, in 1922, introduced continuous sleep treatment with barbiturates. The method is seldom used today.

**contract, interactional**  See *contracting*.

**contract therapy**  Also known as *behavioral contracting* and *contingency contracting*; a form of behavior therapy in which a systematic way of scheduling the mutual exchange of reinforcements between the patient and his family or friends is established for the purpose of modifying reinforcement contingencies that maintain the undesirable behavior. During the initial interview the therapist may suggest to the patient and his family that if each of the family members learns to accommodate to the requests of the others, each might in turn be able to enjoy the fulfillment of more of his own desires and privileges. Then specific statements of privileges (reinforcements), responsibilities (responses), sanctions for contract violations, and bonuses for contract compliance are drawn up and negotiated. A type of microsocial engineering, behavioral contracting may not only change family conflict into positive interaction, but it may also train the family in a pattern of conflict resolution that can be used indefinitely (Stuart, R. B. *Journal of Behavior Therapy and Experimental Psychiatry 2*, 1971).

**contracting**  Agreeing that if no one person engages in certain behaviors, the other person will engage in certain other behaviors. In Sager's model, a contract is a set of assumptions and expectations of the self and partner with which each person approaches the relationship. They come from various aspects of childhood development, cultural norms, need and wishes of the family of origin, and internal dynamically based needs. From these individual contracts, couples join to form a system with its own dyadic rules, the *interactional contract*. See *contract therapy*.

**contraction, habit**  See *tic*.

**contraindication**  A reason for not doing something; more specifically, a feature or complication of a condition that countermands the use of a therapeutic agent that might otherwise be applied. Active pulmonary tuberculosis and aortic valvular insufficiency, for example, are ordinarily considered to be contraindications to the use of electroconvulsive therapy in depression.

**contrary sexual**  *Obs.* A homosexual; *homosexuality* (q.v.).

**contrasexual psyche**  Jacobi's term for the "repressed side" in Jung's theory of analytical psychology. Jung maintained that there is a male and a female side to everyone, the side that is not dominant being repressed; i.e., in the male the female side is repressed and vice versa. "The second stage of the individuation process [self-realization through Jungian analysis] is characterized by the meeting with the figure of the 'soul-image,' named by Jung the anima in the man, the animus in the woman. The archetypal figure of the soul-image is the image of the other sex that we carry in us, both as individuals and as representatives of a species. One experiences the elements of the opposite sex that are present in one's own psyche in the other person. One chooses another, one binds one's self to another, who represents the qualities of one's own soul" (Jacobi, J. *The Psychology of C. G. Jung*, 1942).

**contrasuggestibility** *Negativism* (q.v.).

**contrectation** Tumescence or swelling of the penis; erection.

**control** In clinical psychiatry, control is often used to refers to *self-control*, the conscious suppression or limitation of one's own impulses, wishes, tendencies, etc. It may also refer to the direction or regulation of other people, machines, etc.

In experimental psychiatry, control refers to regulation of all known variables in the experimental situation except the variable that is under investigation. This is an attempt to ensure that whatever effects are produced will be a function of the experimental variable and not due to extraneous factors. In assessing the value of a particular drug in the treatment of depression, for instance, a "control group" may be formed by patients matched in age, clinical condition, and treatment conditions to the "experimental group," the only difference being that the control group does not receive the drug while the experimental group does. In such an experiment, a *placebo* (q.v.) may be used in place of the drug under investigation to mimic more closely all the extraneous factors that may influence the response of the experimental group to the experimental drug.

**control, loss of** See *alcoholism*.

**control, social** The influence upon the behavior of a person exerted by other persons, particularly as members of a social group or of a society. The formal control of society over its members exemplified by law and by institutions derives its effectiveness in large part from their conformity to the folkways, the mores, and public opinion. See *Scull dilemma*.

**control analysis** Psychoanalytic treatment of a patient by a trainee in analysis whose therapeutic methods are under the close supervision of (i.e., are being "controlled" by) an experienced analyst.

**control training** Any treatment and rehabilitation program that aims to teach the alcohol abuser techniques of handling drinking problems. Such an approach is open to goals other than total abstinence and recognizes that some alcohol abusers can both reduce alcohol intake and reduce problems connected with drinking without maintaining total abstinence for the rest of their lives.

**controlled clinical trial** See *randomized clinical trial*.

**controlled drinking** Alcohol ingestion that is moderated to avoid intoxication or other harmful effects of drinking; applied particularly to subjects who have manifested signs of alcohol dependence in the past. *Controlled drug use* implies a noncompulsive type of substance use that minimizes untoward drug effects and does not interfere with functioning. There is controversy as to whether alcoholics can attain a status of controlled drinking. The disease concept of alcoholism implies that until a cure is found for the basic illness, the person with the disease is never cured and abstinence must be the goal of treatment. Nonetheless, clinical studies regularly report that some alcoholics have been able to return to social, controlled drinking without following a progressively deteriorating course.

**Controlled Oral Word Association Test** A measure of *verbal fluency*. The subject is asked to name as many words as possible beginning with C, F, and L in three separate 1-minute segments.

**contusion, brain** A diffuse disturbance of the brain, secondary to head trauma, with edema and multiple intracerebral hemorrhages, most commonly at the poles of the hemispheres. Typically, cerebrospinal fluid pressure is raised and this plays an important part in the production of symptoms (coma, stupor, drowsiness, or confusion). A late result of the edema of the brain may be localized, severe demyelination. Although a patient may recover rapidly and completely from cerebral contusion, persistent disabling symptoms are extremely common. The three cardinal late symptoms are headache, dizziness, and mental disturbances (typically, a mild dementia, with inability to concentrate, memory impairment, and anxiety). See *post-traumatic constitution*.

**convergence** See *accommodation*.

**convergence, neuronal** Integration of signals from many other cells by a single target or receptor cell; the opposite of neuronal divergence.

**conversion** Symbolic representation of psychical conflict in motor or sensory manifestations. By symbolization, repressed instinctual tendencies gain external expression; usually the symbolization also contains the defense set up against the instinctual impulses.

**conversion disorder** One of the *somatoform disorders* (q.v.); formerly called conversion hysteria. Traditionally, conversion disorder and dissociative disorder were subtypes of *hysteria* (q.v.). What was formerly called conversion hysteria was placed in the category of somatoform disorders because it met the general criteria of a condition with multiple physical symptoms that could not fully be explained on the basis of any known non-psychiatric medical condition. Many studies, however, continue to support the notion of conversion and dissociative symptoms occurring in the same person and being of similar pathogenesis, and some classifications (among them, ICD-10) continue to include conversion symptoms within the *dissociative disorders* (q.v.). DSM-IV uses conversion as a behavioral descriptor only; it disavows any implication of a specific unconscious defense mechanism in its use of the term (thereby rendering the term meaningless).

Conversion symptoms resemble those of a neurologic or other general medical disorder affecting sensation (e.g., blindness, double vision, deafness, anesthesia) or voluntary motor function (e.g., impaired coordination, paralysis, mutism, urinary retention, seizures). Individual symptoms typically start and stop abruptly, but about one-quarter of patients develop other conversion symptoms during the succeeding 1 to 6 years. Some also include *autonomic arousal disorder* (q.v.) within the conversion disorders.

**conversion hysteria**   See *hysteria.*

**conversion of emotion**   The psychosomatic process through which an unconscious emotional conflict concerning the function of one organ is displaced upon and expressed, vicariously, through the energizing of the functional disturbance of another organ. In this process symbolic representation of organ function plays a major role.

Blushing is an example of the displacement of the erotic functions of congestion, tumescence, and erection from their primary phallic (clitoral or penile) glans, or head, onto the head (caput) of the body as a whole. In this process the body, as a whole, functions symbolically and unconsciously as a phallus, and is utilized to express and carry out conflicts that relate primarily to the genital area, and not primarily to the organ involved (Weiss, E. & English, O. S. *Psychosomatic Medicine*, 1949).

**conversion seizures**   *Pseudoseizures*; psychogenic or non-epileptic seizures. See *conversion*

*disorder.* Most patients with conversion seizures have clear-cut dissociative symptoms in addition to their seizures. During an interview or therapy session, they often stare blankly and recurrently enter spontaneous trance states with subsequent amnesia. If the trance state is not interrupted promptly, it often evolves into conversion seizures during the interview. In *dissociative identity disorder*, an *alter* may create conversion seizures to express rage over childhood abuse, which the host personality has dissociated from awareness (qq.v.).

Conversion disorder is reported frequently in Turkey, where pseudoseizure is the most prevalent form. There is a large overlap with other *dissociative disorders* (q.v.), and a strong relationship to childhood trauma.

**conversion therapy**   *Reparative therapy* (q.v.).

**convexity syndrome**   Symptoms produced by a lesion of or near the lateral surface of the frontal lobe, most frequently negative symptoms such as apathy, indifference to the environment, loss of drive and ambition, or deterioration of social behavior often manifested as disheveled and dirty appearance. Motor inertia, catalepsy, and posturing are frequent. If the pathology is in the dominant hemisphere, there are also deficits in language and verbal thinking (which is impoverished, vague, and without detail), impaired verbal fluency, stereotyped speech with verbigerative and perseverative utterances, dyspraxia, and, sometimes, Broca or transcortical aphasia. The convexity syndrome is sometimes called the *pseudodepressive syndrome*. See *frontal lobe dysfunction.*

**convulsion**   An involuntary, violent muscular contraction; a fit. See *epilepsy.*

**cooperative psychotherapy**   See *multiple psychotherapy.*

**coordinated epilepsy**   A type of focal seizure in which the movements seem purposive and voluntary but are repeated aimlessly without accomplishing what appears to be their goal. See *epilepsy.*

**coordination**   In group and family therapy, the amount of agreement and cooperation between subjects who are asked to solve a problem or work at a task together. In family therapy, coordination reflects the family's conception of how it is treated by the outside world, high coordination indicating its feeling that the world treats it as a unitary group and what one member does reflects on the entire family. See *family culture, indigenous.*

**coordination disorder** A motor skills disorder (within the group, specific developmental disorders, and not secondary to known physical disorder such as cerebral palsy) consisting of clumsiness, delays in achieving motor milestones (crawling, sitting), poor performance in sports, poor handwriting, etc. See *developmental disorders, specific.*

**coparental divorce** See *divorce, stations of.*

**copharmacy** Combined or concurrent medication strategies, used particularly in managing chronic or treatment-resistant disorders where *monotherapy* (q.v.) gives only inadequate control of more severe episodes and is insufficient for the satisfactory control of chronic disorders.

**COPI** Coat complex I; see *Golgi apparatus.*

**coping** Adjusting; adapting; successfully meeting a challenge. Coping mechanisms are all the ways, both conscious and unconscious, that a person uses in adjusting to environmental demands without altering his goals or purposes.

**copro-** Combining form meaning feces, filth, from Gr. *kopros.*

**coprolagnia** Sexual pleasure from handling feces. See *anal eroticism.*

**coprolalia** Literally, fecal speech; *coprophrasia*; the involuntary utterance of vulgar or obscene words, seen in some schizophrenics who play with words as though they were feces. See *Gilles de la Tourette syndrome.*

**coprophagy** Ingestion of feces.

**coprophemia** Obscene speech; scatalogia; most commonly presenting as a type of *paraphilia* (q.v.) in which uttering obscene words or phrases is a necessary condition for sexual excitement in the subject.

**coprophilia** Love of feces or filth; a *paraphilia.* According to psychoanalysis, *anal erotism* (q.v.) possesses two chief aspects, the first concerned with the retention and expulsion of fecal material, and the second with pleasure in the product itself. During the stage of sphincter training the aim is twofold—to perform regularly and not to soil. The discipline associated with anal training is later carried over in the form of character traits, while a certain quantum of libido remains fixed in its original form. A third possibility exists, that interest in the product is later transferred to other objects that resemble or symbolize feces, even though there may be no conscious awareness of the resemblance.

Thus Ferenczi traces the development from feces through its various forms of symbolizations: mud pies, sand, pebbles, marbles, buttons, jewels, coins, currency, securities, etc. Hence ownership of valuables is traced chiefly, but not exclusively, to early anal interests; that is, it is a coprophilic interest. See *hoarding; soteria.*

Coprophilic interest may also be sublimated in such forms as painting, sculpting, or cooking. Some patients exhibit coprophilia more literally. Thus one patient hoarded his feces as earlier he had hoarded his money. Another "decorated" himself with feces. A third said she loved her feces "as if it were her child." A fourth could experience sexual potency only when thinking of feces.

**coprophobia** Fear of rectal excreta, sometimes seen in obsessive-compulsive disorder. More typically, the fear is expressed symbolically, as fear of dirt or of contamination (e.g., fear of an infectious disease, or fearing to touch anything lest the patient acquire some ailment). Coprophobia is generally a reaction-formation against unconscious coprophilic impulses, which are derivatives of the anal stage. See *anal eroticism.*

**coprophrasia** *Coprolalia* (q.v.).

**coprostasophobia** Fear of becoming constipated.

**copulatory phase** See *proceptive phase.*

**copying mania** *Amurakh; echopraxia* (qq.v.).

**CoQ** Ubiquinone. See *OXPHOS.*

**core gender identity** See *gender identity.*

**core self** *Cohesive self* (q.v.).

**corneal reflex** Bilateral blinking induced by touching the cornea with a wisp of cotton. The afferent nerve of the corneal reflex is N. V, its efferent is N. VII, and its center is in the pons.

**cornealpterygoideal reflex** Touching the cornea is followed by contraction of the external pterygoid, which produces deviation of the lower jaw of the opposite side.

**Cornell Word Form (CWF) test** A modification of the word-association technique devised to distinguish "normals" from subjects with neuropsychiatric and psychosomatic disorders in a way not apparent to the subject. The test is used primarily in industrial psychology. It consists of a list of stimulus words, each of which is followed by two response words. The subject is asked to encircle whichever of the two words seems to him to be the most related to the stimulus word; e.g., mother—mine, woman.

**countershock**　See *type A.*

**corpora quadrigemina**　Four raised eminences, arranged in pairs, on the dorsal surface (tectum) of the midbrain. The two superior colliculi and the two inferior colliculi make up the four corpora. The superior colliculi are optic reflex centers and receive fibers from the lateral geniculate body via the superior quadrigeminal brachium. The more prominent inferior colliculi are associated with the auditory system and are the termination of the lateral lemniscus. The inferior colliculi project to the medial geniculate body via the inferior quadrigeminal brachium.

**corpus callosum**　The largest connective structure in the brain, consisting of over 190 million axons that transfer information between the two cerebral hemispheres. The connections are primarily excitatory, integrating information between the two hemispheres. After crossing the midline, callosal axons grow into the contralateral hemisphere toward their designated target regions, usually homotopic to their region of origin, and then innervate the appropriate cortical layer.

There are three other telencephalic commissures (the anterior commissure, the hippocampal commissure, and the massa intermedia), and two midbrain interhemispheric pathways (the posterior and habenular commissures).

Most of our knowledge of callosal function comes from patients with *AgCC* (agenesis or hypogenesis of the corpus callosum) and "*split brain*" patients, who have undergone a commissurotomy, a surgical procedure that severs the corpus callosum as well as the anterior commissure. Research on the split brain had its origins with Roger Sperry in the early 1960s. He noted that although callosal *commissurotomy* produces a *disconnection syndrome*, with absence of callosal transfer of sensory information and a deficiency in bimanually coordinated motor activity, the procedure leaves motivation, consciousness, and voluntary action relatively intact. He proposed that the two sides of the brain are differently involved in rational, verbal thinking and in nonverbal imagery. According to the dynamic dual pathway model of language, syntax and semantics are lateralized to the left hemisphere and prosody to the right hemisphere. The corpus callosum is the main path for coordination of the lateralized information, particularly for coordinating syntactic and prosodic information. See *cerebral dominance.*

Although primary AgCC has a surprisingly limited impact on general cognitive ability, in more than half the reported cases performance IQ and verbal IQ are significantly different. Impairments are consistently noted in abstract reasoning, problem solving, generalization, category fluency (the ability to list multiple items that belong to a semantic category, for example, names of animals), phonological processing, rhyming, comprehension of syntax, linguistic pragmatics (impaired comprehension of idioms, proverbs, vocal prosody, and narrative humor), and expressive language (e.g., difficulties in the verbal expression of emotional experience or *alexithymia*). Specific traits associated with commissurotomy and primary AgCC include emotional immaturity, lack of introspection and self-awareness, impaired social competence, general deficits in social judgment and planning, and interpersonal conflict both at home and at work due to misinterpretation of social cues. Social situations require extremely rapid processing of very complex information that is typically handled within lateralized regions (that is, lexical and affective processes) and therefore may be particularly sensitive to corpus callosum abnormality. It has often been noted that the deficits in AgCC overlap with the diagnostic criteria for autism (Paul, L. K. et al. *Nature Reviews Neuroscience 8,* 2007).

In *callosal syndromes* (*disconnection syndromes, split-brain syndromes*), the patients act as if their two hemispheres were functioning independently. As an example, the shirt may be buttoned with one hand and immediately thereafter unbuttoned by the other hand (the *alien hand syndrome*).

Various callosal syndromes have been described, including: (1) anterior lesion—ideokinetic dyspraxia in the hand ipsilateral to the dominant hemisphere, and constructional dyspraxia in the hand contralateral to the dominant hemisphere; and (2) posterior (splenium) lesion—alexia of the field of vision opposite to that of the side of the lesion. Other symptoms include an inability to tie one's shoes with the eyes closed; difficulties in writing and reading; and astereognosis or graphanesthesia of the hand on the same side as the dominant hemisphere.

Mental changes are more frequently observed in cases of tumor of the corpus callosum than in any other part of the brain, including the frontal lobe. Apathy, drowsiness, and memory defect are the most common disturbances, but there may be depression, anxiety, and epileptiform convulsions.

**corpus striatum**   See *basal ganglia*.

**correctional psychiatry**   That branch of *forensic psychiatry* (q.v.) which deals with mental health care within the prison system. Among the problems faced by the mental health professionals who work in jails and prisons are ensuring the availability and quality of needed mental health care, management of the suicidal patient, prevention of suicide, special consideration for women and for the developmentally disabled, treatment of offenders with mental illness (including those in maximum security settings and in outpatient settings), homosexual victimization and assaults, violence, and malingering.

**corrective emotional experience**   1. One of the briefer and more direct techniques advocated by Alexander to expedite psychotherapy. In this technique, the therapist temporarily assumes some particular role to bring the patient more quickly to an awareness of transference relationships and to other personal insights and reorientations.

2. In a more general sense, providing an opportunity in the therapeutic setting to repeat an early unpleasant event and thus to reconsider it in more objective terms, and to learn how to deal more effectively with similar events should they recur.

**correlation**   Mutual relation; tendency to concomitant change in two variables. If the change, whether positive or negative, in one is accompanied by a like (i.e., in the same direction) change in the other variable, the correlation is positive with a maximal coefficient of +1. If an increase in one corresponds to a decrease in the other (or, vice versa, a decrease in one corresponds to an increase in the other), the correlation is negative, with a maximal coefficient of -1. If there is no change in the second variable, the correlation is 0.

The most commonly used measure of correlation is Pearson's coefficient of correlation, while the best method describing an individual in terms of the degree to which he possesses the factors that vary *independently* of one another is constituted by the analysis of a person according to "independent variables" as devised by Spearman, Cohen, and others (see *constitutional type*).

With factors that are related, the change that takes place in one factor for a unit change in the other can be computed; this statistic is known as the *regression coefficient*. Computation of this allows the value of one factor to be estimated when the value of the other factor is known. Even when the correlation is very high, however, the error of this estimate may be large.

Evidence of association is not necessarily evidence of causation, and the possible influence of other factors common to the ones for which correlation is discovered must always be recognized. "*Correlation does not imply direct causation* and must not under any circumstances be so interpreted without *additional experimental proof*." (Eysenck, H. J. *Handbook of Abnormal Psychology*, 1960).

Eysenck cites a study of the relationship between early weaning and the later appearance of oral aggressive character traits (see *character defense*). The finding that mothers who practiced early weaning had children who developed oral aggressive traits was interpreted as evidence that early weaning causes aggression. But "this argument clearly has no logical validity at all; there are many other alternative hypotheses which account equally well for the observed facts. One alternative...may be called the hereditary theory. Using the same facts as before we may argue that aggressive parents wean their children early, and that the children inherit the parents' aggressiveness....The second alternative theory can be called the reaction theory. According to this hypothesis, aggressive children behave aggressively to their mothers, reject the breast, etc. They therefore cause their mothers to wean them early....Many other possibilities could be envisaged, but these two will suffice to show that the known facts cannot be used to support the environmental theory in any unequivocal manner. Essentially, the facts offered are *correlational*." (ibid.).

**correlative**   Pertaining to the values of a reciprocal relation between biological phenomena as indicated by the method of *correlation* (q.v.).

**cortex, cerebral** The most anterior portion of the telencephalon; the cerebral cortex is made up of the two cerebral hemispheres, each of which is subdivided into the frontal lobe, parietal lobe, occipital lobe, temporal lobe, and insula. Strictly speaking, the rhinencephalon is not considered part of the cerebral cortex, although by implication the rhinencephalon is included where the term cerebral cortex (or cerebrum) is used. For a description of function, see under the various divisions of the cortex—e.g., *frontal lobe, temporal lobe, parietal lobe, isocortex.*

**cortex, olfactory** See *rhinencephalon.*

**cortex, visual** See *occipital lobe.*

**cortical spreading depression** See *migraine.*

**cortical word blindness** See *word blindness.*

**corticalization** *Encephalization* (q.v.).

**corticobasal degeneration** *CBD;* a late-onset neurological disorder manifested as one of two clinical syndromes: (1) rigidity and at least one of the following cortical signs—apraxia, corticosensory loss, or alien limb phenomenon; (2) asymmetric rigidity, dystonia, and focal reflex myoclonus. Like progressive *supranuclear palsy* and *frontotemporal dementia* (qq.v.), CBD is a tauopathy with tau-positive inclusions in both basal ganglia and cortical structures. Depression and apathy are frequent; some patients show irritability and agitation. Delusions, hallucination, disinhibition, and anxiety are less common.

**corticostriate projection** See *basal ganglia.*

**cortico-striato-spinal degeneration** Spastic pseudosclerosis; Creutzfeldt-Jakob disease (q.v.).

**corticotropin-releasing factor (CRF)** Also, corticotropin-releasing hormone (CRH); a 41-amino acid peptide chain released from the hypothalamus; CRF stimulates the release of ACTH and other POMC (pro-opiomelanocortin) products from the pituitary; ACTH in turn stimulates the synthesis and release of cortisol and other glucocorticoids from the adrenal cortex; cortisol, the primary adrenocortical hormone in humans, exerts feedback effects at each of the preceding levels. See *hypothalamic-pituitary-adrenal (HPA) axis; peptide, brain.*

One of the most consistently reported abnormalities in Alzheimer disease is reduction in CRF immunoreactivity in the neocortex and in CRF concentration in the frontal and temporal cortex and in the caudate nucleus.

Bipolar depressed patients have a blunted ACTH secretory response to CRF when compared to control subjects; no such difference in ACTH response is found in recovered patients (i.e., the abnormality is a marker of the depressed state rather than a trait marker of bipolar disease). The fact that there is blunted ACTH response to CRH, despite hypercortisolism, indicates that the defect in depression is at the hypothalamic level and not in the pituitary or adrenal glands.

**corticotropin-releasing hormone** *CRH.* See *hypothalamus.*

**cortisol** A glucocorticoid stress hormone that has a panoply of central and peripheral effects mediated by two intracellular specialized glucocorticoid receptor subtypes: the high-affinity type I receptor or mineralocorticoid receptor (MR), and the low-affinity type II receptor or glucocorticoid receptor (GR). Recent data suggest that direct antagonism of GRs may be a future therapeutic strategy.

**COS** Childhood onset schizophrenia. See *EOS.*

**cosmic identification** Belief that one is the universe; a failure, on the part of the patient (usually a schizophrenic), to differentiate between himself and the outside world.

**cost shifting** In health care delivery systems, charging one patient group (e.g., private patients) more in order to balance losses incurred from caring for other patients (e.g., patients in federal programs such as Medicare).

**costal stigma** See *Stiller sign.*

**cost/benefit analysis (CBA)** Comparison of the costs of a program or technology to resulting benefits, with both costs and benefits expressed by the same measure (usually monetary). Because it requires that outcomes be quantified in monetary terms, this approach is rarely used in evaluations of mental health care.

**cost-effectiveness analysis (CEA)** Comparison of the costs of a program or alternative programs to the resultant benefits or effectiveness expressed in different measures. Costs are usually expressed in money, while benefits are expressed in such measures as number of lives saved or disabilities avoided or other objectives deemed worthwhile.

**Cotard syndrome** (Jules Cotard, French neurologist, 1840–87)

*Délire de négation(s);* a nihilistic delusion consisting of an intense sensation of death and disintegration (e.g., the subject feels his head or body has been destroyed, his family has been exterminated, he is penniless, etc.). The delusion is not chronic and unremitting but instead recurs intermittently.

The syndrome may be a manifestation of mood disorder or schizophrenia, but it may also be associated with organic disorders such as Alzheimer disease, and particularly with dysfunction of the nondominant cerebral hemisphere. Cases have been reported in patients with right frontotemporal lesions, temporal lobe epilepsy (where it may be an exaggerated form of the unreality and depersonalization phenomena so often seen in such cases), and parietal disorders. The relative contributions of frontal lobe and limbic system are uncertain (in the cases reported by M. Drake in *Psychiatric Journal of the University of Ottawa 13*, 1987), but that the limbic system contributes significantly is suggested by the fact that the delusional symptoms appeared mainly in the postictal setting.

**cotherapy** See *multiple psychotherapy*.

**cotranslational** See *cytosolic proteins*.

**cotransmission** See *linkage*.

**cotransmitter** A seconary neurotransmitter released along with a primary transmitter (such as serotonin or glutamate), whose action it typically enhances. Cotransmitters are often peptides; they produce long-lasting actions that the primary transmitter, because there is no uptake or degradative mechanism for them in the synaptic cleft.

Cotransmitters may also have behavioral effects of their own, distinct from their enhancement of primary transmitter action. Peptides, for example, often modulate homeostasis, particularly thirst (angiotensin), feeding (neuropeptide Y, galanin), and pain (enkephalins).

**co-twin control** A method used in biogenetics in which one member of an identical twinship is trained, treated, etc., while the other is not.

**co-twin control method** Developed by Gesell and Thompson for use in medical genetics: observational twin data are obtained from a few selected one-egg pairs, whose aptitudes or adjustment under different life conditions are then compared.

**coulrophobia** Fear of clowns.

**counseling** *Guidance* (q.v.); a type of psychotherapy of the supportive or reeducative variety; often the term is applied to behavioral problems not strictly classifiable as mental illness, such as vocational or school or marriage problems. See *psychotherapy*.

**counteraffect** See *inversion of affect*.

**countercathexis** *Anticathexis* (q.v.).

**countercompulsion** A compulsion secondarily developed to fight the original compulsion, when the patient finds himself deprived of the means to continue the performance of the original compulsion. The patient supplants the original compulsion with the new one in order to continue his compulsive behavior, e.g., the compulsion to keep silent is in opposition to the compulsion to talk.

**counterconditioning** A term for the types of behavior therapy described by the South African medical practitioner Joseph Wolpe in *Psychotherapy by Reciprocal Inhibition* (1958): systematic *desensitization* (q.v.), assertion or *assertiveness training* (q.v.), sexual retraining, and avoidance conditioning.

**counterfactual thinking** The mechanism by which "what is" is compared with "what might have been." Orbitofrontal cortex, which is connected with DLPFC regions involved in reasoning and planning as well as with limbic areas (important for emotion) and other areas providing access to multiple sensory modalities, is active in *reward* evaluation and comparison (q.v.).

**counterformula** A new formula often resorted to by a compulsive patient under certain (insurmountable) circumstances and consisting of the *exact opposite* of his hitherto established *tenet*. A tenet characteristic might be: "If I do not perform this action my father will die." Very often, however, it is impossible to carry out the particular action. When such an impossibility is encountered, the patient goes through a series of compulsions and obsessions until he eventually finds a solution, by amending his formula in the following manner: "My father will die if I do perform this action." The final version is called the counterformula (Stekel, W. *Compulsion and Doubt*, 1949).

**counteridentification** A form of *countertransference* (q.v.) in which the analyst identifies with the analysand.

**counterinvestment** *Anticathexis* (q.v.).

**counterphobia** Preference for or seeking of the very situation that the phobic person is, or was, afraid of. Probably the basic component of the pleasure derived from the counterphobia is the gratification that the person takes in the fact that indulging in the particular pleasure is now possible without anxiety. The counterphobic attitude is similar to the mechanism (seen normally in childhood and frequently in cases of traumatic neurosis) of striving to master excess anxiety through repeated coping with danger. Such repetition makes possible the transformation of passivity into activity; and it may also indicate libidinization of the anxiety or a flight into health.

**countershock** Nonconvulsive electrical stimulation usually applied for a 1-minute period immediately after an electroconvulsive shock. Some claimed that countershock relieves postconvulsive amnesia or confusion; others found that countershock may even increase amnesia.

**countertransference** The total reaction of the therapist, both the transference reaction and the realistic reaction, to all aspects of the patient's transference and general personality; the effect on the analyst's understanding or technique of the therapist's own unconscious needs and conflicts. Countertransference reactions, sometimes called analytic stumbling, are manifestations of the therapist's reluctance to know or learn something about himself. They may impair the analyst's interpretive capacity and his ability to deal with resistances by distorting the therapist's perception of the patient's unconscious processes.

Especially in the older literature, countertransference was viewed as an impairment of the analytic process. Beginning with Ferenczi, there was a shift in emphasis from the analyst as a "flawed" instrument to recognition of the transference-countertransference interaction as a facilitator in understanding the patient's preverbal or pre-oedipal phantasies. Kleinian (object relations) analysts in particular use countertransference feelings to understand the patient's transference and object representations.

In analytic treatment, the patient reexperiences early events, including traumatic ones, in relation to the therapist. As the patient reports his or her inner life, phantasies, affects, and memories of the past history of the analyst are stimulated. Countertransferentially, the analyst may be seduced, made angry, or defend against the patient's object representations. Countertransference issues emerge when the patient externalizes his bad objects and projects them onto the analyst, who must then "process" the *projective identification* (q.v.) of the patient. The analyst learns to recognize that a feeling state has been induced in him by the patient and allows himself to identify with the patient's self and object representation, to experience them, think about them, and understand them. In this way, the patient can reinternalize a modified version of what was projected in the first place. *Concordant identifications* refer to the analyst's identifications with the patient's self-representations; *complementary identifications* are the analyst's identifications with the patient's object representations. See *transference*.

Ideally, the analyst's unconscious mechanisms will be sublimated successfully into the qualities necessary for the practice of psychoanalytic technique. If this has not occurred, however, there may appear various undesirable countertransference manifestations. These may be acute, temporary, and short-lived, and such manifestations are often based on identification with the patient or on reactions to the specific content of the patient's productions.

More serious, however, are frequently recurring, long-lasting, or even permanent manifestations of countertransference; these are usually based on deeply ingrained personality disturbances of the analyst. Among the most frequent are reactions of irrational "kindness" and "concern"; irrational hostility and retaliation; anxiety reactions; blindness to the patient's resistances; *boredom* (q.v.); and arrogance and grandiosity. See *narcissistic countertransference*.

E. Etan et al. (*American Journal of Psychiatry* 162: 890–898, 2005) described the structure of countertransference phenomena in eight factors and found that several were highly correlated with the type of patient pathology:

Factor 1—overwhelmed/disorganized, most frequently reported by therapists treating patients with borderline personality disorder, narcissistic personality disorder, or disorganized and unresolved attachment problems (Cluster B, the dramatic/erratic disorders)

Factor 2—helpless/inadequate; also associated with Cluster B disorders

Factor 3—positive, with feeling of a positive working alliance; Cluster B disorders showed a negative correlation with positive countertransference

Factor 4—overinvolved, a sense of the patient as special, problems in maintaining boundaries such as self-disclosure or ending sessions on time; associated with this factor was borderline personality disorder

Factor 5—sexualized, feelings of sexual tension or of sexual feelings toward patient; associated with this factor were the Cluster B disorders

Factor 6—disengaged, feeling distracted, annoyed, or bored in sessions; associated with narcissistic personality disorder

Factor 7—parental/protective, a wish to protect and nurture patient; associated with this factor were the Cluster C (anxious) disorders

Factor 8—criticized/mistreated, fee lings of being unappreciated, dismissed, or devalued; significantly associated with this factor were the Cluster A (odd, eccentric) disorders

**countervolition**   Counterwill, as is evidenced frequently in dreams in the form of being physically unable to perform some action (such as running away) or being unable to attain some goal by reason of the particular dream situation (e.g., the dreamer wishes to visit his sweetheart but is unable to find her house, even though he has been there many times before).

**counterwill, hysterical**   An impulse or a wish, unconsciously determined, that expresses the opposite of a conscious wish. "A child who is very ill at last falls asleep, and its mother tries her utmost to keep quiet and not to wake it; but just in consequence of this resolution (hysterical counterwill) she makes a clucking noise with her tongue." (Freud, S. *Collected Papers*, 1924–25).

**counting, compulsive**   Arithmomania.

**coupling**   1. The capacity of hereditary characters to remain associated in several generations, without regard to the Mendelian principle of independent assortment. See *linkage*.

2. In neurotransmission, the binding of the transmitter to its receptor that activates the *transducer* (q.v.). Direct coupling occurs when the recognition site of the *neurotransmitter receptor* (q.v.) is part of the protein complex that includes the ion channel. Indirect coupling occurs when the neurotransmitter receptor is not part of an ion channel but is instead linked to enzymes. (Some authorities use coupling to refer only to what is described here as indirect coupling.) See *synapse*.

Rapidity of action is the leading characteristic of direct coupling.

In the central nervous system, such coupling occurs with the excitatory amino acids (such as glutamate and aspartate, which result in an opening of the $Na^+$ channel, depolarization, and increase in cell excitability) and the inhibitory amino acids (such as GABA and glycine, which result in an opening of the $Cl^-$ channel, hyperpolarization, and decrease in cell excitability).

Indirect coupling gives effects that are characteristically slow and long-lasting, hence it is sometimes described as neuromodulatory. Examples are the slow inhibition following opening of the $K^+$ channel by the opioid peptides, serotonin, and somatostatin.

**coupling receptor**   See neurotransmitter receptor.

**courtship phase**   See *proceptive phase*.

**cousin marriage**   See *intermarriage*.

**couvade**   A custom, found in some primitive tribes, consisting of the father taking to his bed during or shortly after the birth of his child, as though he himself had given birth to the child.

**cover-memory**   *Screen memory* (q.v.).

**CPP**   *Conditioned place preference* (q.v.)

**CPR**   Cardiopulmonary resuscitation.

**CPT**   *Continuous performance test* (q.v.).

**CR**   1. Conditional response. See *conditioning*. 2. Critical ratio; a measure of the significance or stability of a statistic, obtained by comparing the statistic to its standard error.

**crack**   Alkaloidal *cocaine* (free base) in a form suitable for smoking.

This almost pure form of cocaine is made by preparing an aqueous solution of cocaine HCl and adding ammonia (with or without baking soda) to alkalinize the solution and precipitate alkaloidal cocaine. It is usually sold as pure beige crystals (*rocks*). Crack melts at 98°C and vaporizes at higher temperatures, making it suitable for smoking in a "base pipe." Its name derives from the crackling noise it makes when heated. The rock can also be crushed, mixed with tobacco, and smoked in a cigarette.

Unlike *freebasing* (q.v.), crack smoking does not require preliminary mixing of the substance with a solvent to clear it of contaminants. The "high" it gives is more intense and more rapidly reached than that attained by snorting (inhaling) or injecting other forms of cocaine. Effects appear 4 to 6 seconds after inhalation and last 5 to 7 minutes; snorting, in contrast, produces effects in 1 to 3 minutes and they last 20 to 30 minutes. The intense, short high produced by crack is followed by a period of deep depression, so the user is compelled to continue use of the drug in order to regain the exhilaration, euphoria, and feelings of power and superiority it bestows.

Overdosage is frequent with crack. Cocaine is a central nervous system stimulant that increases heart rate and blood pressure. It may cause hyperpyrexia, seizures, angina pectoris, myocardial infarction, and ventricular arrhythmia. Many of the deaths caused by cocaine are believed to be due to seizures leading to anoxia. Other possible side effects include extreme anxiety, tactile hallucinations, loss of consciousness, and paranoid psychosis.

**crack house** Base house; the place where sales of *crack* (q.v.) are made and where users gather to indulge in smoking binges that may last for hours or days.

**Craik-O'Brien-Cornsweet illusion** See *filling in.*

**cranial neuralgia** See *neuralgia; pain.*

**craniofacial defects** Malformations of the brain and face, ordinarily developmental in origin and situated along the midline. Such defects include *anencephaly; craniosynostosis; encephalocele;* and *holoprosencephaly* (qq.v.).

**craniopharyngioma** See *intracranial tumor.*

**craniosynostosis** Early closure of one or more of the cranial sutures. The brain is forced to grow in directions where the bone is not resisting, leading often to multiple neurological defects. The most frequent form is *oxycephaly* (q.v.) due to closure of the coronal and lambdoid sutures. Closure of the coronal suture produces *acrocephaly;* closure of the sagittal suture produces *scaphocephaly.* There are more than 100 syndromes associated with craniosynostosis, including Apert, Crouzon, Pfeiffer, and Saethre-Chotzen syndromes. Familial cases of craniosynostosis are associated with mutations in FGF receptor genes *FGER1, -2, -3,* in *TWIST,* and in *MSX2.*

**cratomania** *Obs.* The monomania of power, preeminence, and superiority (Tuke, D. H.

A Dictionary of Psychological Healing, 1892).

**cravers** See *narcissistic personality.*

**craving** Intense desire for a certain object or experience, typically associated with the expectation of pleasure or relief from negative feelings. Craving refers to the strong desire and urge to drink (in the case of the alcoholic), to inject or ingest the drug of abuse, or to indulge in the compulsive behavior to which one is addicted (gambling, gorging, etc.).

**creative arts therapies** See *dance therapy.*

**creative imagination** *Creative work;* the process in which dormant, unrelated contents of the unconscious become associated with the organized labor of consciousness and accomplish something new.

**creative self** See individual psychology.

**creativity** Presentation of a new conception; investing something with a new character; producing a workable approach to an unsolved problem or a previously unrecognized opportunity. Typically, the new idea occurs suddenly, "in a flash," and the details are filled in later. It has been suggested that creativity evolves in four phases: preparation, incubation, illumination, and verification. Needed first is a base of knowledge or fund of information from which to draw; then an incubation period during which information is sorted, compared, or rearranged; the illumination phase is the "Eureka, I have it" stage; in the final stage the creator reorganizes and refines his concept until he can present a polished final product. Studies suggest that much of the thinking of the incubation phase takes place in the right hemisphere; the preparation and verification phases seem to be of left hemisphere origin. *Alexithymia* (q.v.) is sometimes described as the opposite of creativity.

**CREB** Cyclic AMP-response element binding protein, a transcription factor that plays an important role in long-term memory, and in tolerance to and dependence on cocaine and amphetamine and perhaps other drugs. CREB can respond to both the cyclic AMP and the $Ca^{2+}$ pathways. Cocaine or amphetamine leads to dopamine stimulation of D-1 receptors on neurons in nucleus accumbens and dorsal striatum, leading to CREB phosphorylation and activation of prodynorphin gene expression. The resulting dynorphin peptides are transported to striatal neurons, from which they inhibit release of dopamine, thus decreasing the responsiveness of dopamine systems. D-1 receptor mediated increases in dynorphin can thus be construed as a homeostatic adaptation to excessive dopamine stimulation of target neurons in nucleus accumbens and dorsal striatum that feed back to dampen further dopamine release

**credulity**    *Suggestibility* (q.v.). Bernheim and the Nancy School disagreed with the physiologic explanation of hypnotic phenomena proposed by Charcot and his followers. Instead, Bernheim believed that such phenomena were based on the psychologic power of suggestion, consisting of the transmittal of an idea from one person to another. Acceptance of the idea was no more than an exaggeration of a universal trait, credulity.

**cremasteric reflex**    A superficial reflex; stroking the inner and upper side of the thigh causes contraction of the cremaster and elevation of the testicle on the same side. The afferents of this reflex depend upon the femoral nerve, the efferents on the genitofemoral nerve; the center is $L_1$.

**cremnophobia**    Fear of precipices.

**cresomania**    The delusion that one is rich.

**crest cells, neural**    See *neural plate*.

**cretinism**    Hypothyroidism in infancy. Mental and physical signs usually appear at about the sixth month of life: apathy, lethargy, protrusion of the tongue, skin changes, thickening of features, prominence of abdomen, breathing difficulties (the "leathery" cry), defective speech, difficulty in posture and gait, generalized underdevelopment, and intellectual impairment (a form of deprivative amentia).

**Creutzfeldt, Hans Gerhard**    (1885–1964) German psychiatrist; *Creutzfeld-Jakob disease* (q.v.).

**Creutzfeldt-Jakob disease (CJD)**    Also, *spastic pseudosclerosis*; *cortico-striato-spinal degeneration; Heidenheim disease*; a rare, progressive, fatal, degenerative disease of the central nervous system, generally classified as an infectious disorder due to an unconventional slow virus or *prion* (q.v.).

Symptoms begin typically in the mid-50s, with speech disturbance, memory loss, confusion, progressive motor symptoms, and sometimes psychosis. CJD may begin with specific agnosias (e.g., symptoms began in a choreographer with inability to pirouette to the right while standing on his left leg although

he could perform the action while standing on his right leg). Later there are widespread neurologic disturbances such as gross ataxia, dysarthria, growing spasticity of the limbs, grotesque extrapyramidal movements, and myoclonus. Once it becomes clinically manifest, the dementia develops rapidly; characteristic are inertia, failure of attention, markedly defective registration and retention of recent experiences, and a tendency to confabulation. EEG shows paroxysmal bursts of high-voltage waves. Speech becomes an incoherent jumble, sphincter control is lost, and death ensues in 11 months on the average (range, 4–24 months), in a state of extreme emaciation.

The pathology consists of a spongiform encephalopathy (sometimes called *glional neurodystrophy*) with neuronal destruction, vacuolization in the cytoplasm of the remaining nerve cells, pronounced fibrous astrogliosis, and plaquelike formation. The pituitary stalk is always involved, and the pathologic process is seen also in the cerebral cortex, basal ganglia, cerebellum, and the anterior horn cells.

One case of CJD occurs per million population. It is usually sporadic although there is a strong inheritance pattern in 10% of cases (which may reflect a genetic susceptibility to infection rather than direct inheritance of the disease). In the United States, CJD accounts for about 250 deaths each year; it is found in one of every 3000 autopsied bodies. It is more frequent in males (two or three to one). A focus of CJD among Libyan Jews as compared with European Jews in Israel has been reported: 31.3 per million vs. the expected 0.4–1.9, a 16- to 78-fold increase). The high incidence is believed to be related to higher exposure to infected neural tissue among Libyan Jews. High rates have also been reported in central Slovakia and adjacent Hungary.

Four $PrP^{Sc}$ types have been observed in CJD: types 1 to 3 in classical (sporadic or iatrogenic) CJD and type 4 in vCJD (variant CJD). Polymorphism at residue 129 of human PrP (where either methionine or valine can be encoded) powerfully affects genetic susceptibility to human prion diseases. Humans have always been exposed to CJD, but because its spread requires either the direct ingestion or injection of infected tissues, CJD has remained a sporadic disease. Historically, the greatest risk has come from cannibalism. A polymorphism at position 129 of PrP provides some protection against kuru. In contrast, 129MM homozygotes are particularly susceptible to prion infection. In the U.K. vCJD epidemic, all the affected subjects were 129MM homozygotes, and most were less than 30 years old. (Carrell, R. W. *Science* *306*: 1692–1693, 2004)

CJD has been transmitted successfully from man to chimpanzees, monkeys, domestic cats, and guinea pigs. Probable human-to-human transmission has been reported in a recipient of a corneal graft, through root-canal dentistry, in craniotomy patients, in patients undergoing electroencephalography when the silver electrodes had been used previously in patients later found to have CJD, and in neurosurgeons and other physicians exposed to brain tissue during surgery or postmortem examinations. The incubation period is often given as approximately 2 years but is highly variable, with a probable range of 1½ to 50 years. See *beta-amyloid disorders; bovine spongiform encephalopathy; prion; virus infections.*

**CRF**   *Corticotropin-releasing factor* (q.v.).

**CRH**   Corticotropin-releasing hormone. See *hypothalamus.*

**cri-du-chat**   See *cat cry syndrome.*

**crime à deux**   *Folie à deux* (q.v.) in which one or more crimes are committed as part of the psych    otic behavioral pattern. The term was introduced by Moreau de Tours in 1893.

**crime and mental disorder**   There is no invariable relationship between crime and mental disorder, although criminals as a group have a greater incidence of psychiatric abnormalities than noncriminals. Many studies have shown that some degree of mental retardation is found in unexpectedly high frequency in prison inmates (20% to 25%, as opposed to the expected 1% to 3%); although such findings may indicate that the retardate is defective in his ability to control aggressive or other antisocial impulses, it may equally indicate that the retardate is less adept in escaping detection, more likely because of his suggestibility to be influenced by others to act against society, or is poorly equipped to defend himself once he is brought to trial.

Other disorders with a higher than expected incidence of crime are schizophrenia, epilepsy and other organic brain disorders, alcoholism (especially states of acute and pathological intoxication), drug use and abuse, amnesic episodes, and fugue states. The greatest

proportion of habitual offenders, however, rather than belonging to any of these categories, fall instead into the group labeled antisocial or psychopathic personality. Many of these have had an arrested emotional development, have learned a style of delinquent life in unfavorable psychosocial settings, have had no proper models for constructive identification, and have had to resort to models from disapproved subcultures (in Erikson's terminology, *malignant identity diffusion*), or have been reared in a society that aroused expectations in them but then denied them opportunity to fulfill those expectations

One of the major interests of the psychiatrist in crime and mental disorder, and in the criminally insane, revolves about the question of responsibility of the accused for the criminal action he is alleged to have committed. See *criminal responsibility.*

**criminal from sense of guilt**   A person with an unconscious need for punishment stemming from repressed oedipal wishes; the unconscious need propels him into commission of a crime for which punishment is certain.

**criminal hygiene**   The branch of mental hygiene of which the object is the "study and investigation related to the causes, prevention and treatment of the social-medico-psychological illness known for centuries as crime."

In taking into consideration the complexity of this problem in modern society, the science aiming at the study of crime has necessarily to deal with many aspects of the offender: heredity, environment, home, social, economical, and political factors, legal aspects, emotional and physical development, psychiatric investigation, etc. (Seliger, R. V. et al. *Contemporary Criminal Hygiene*, 1946)

**criminal intent**   "Criminal intent is a knowing disregard of criminal law (bearing in mind that ignorance of a law is no defense as knowledge of the law itself is presumed). Any person manifesting this disregard is an outlaw, that is to say, he is a criminal in the eyes of the law. Intent is often wrongly confused with motive; motive is merely that which impels" (Singer, H. D., & Krohn, W. O. *Insanity and Law*, 1924).

**criminal responsibility**   The culpability of a person, as determined   by due process of law, for any of his actions that are defined as criminal. Determination of such responsibility is a legal function, not a psychiatric one, although a psychiatrist may be called upon to present evidence to the court in order to aid the judge or jury in reaching a decision as to responsibility. Determination of responsibility varies with the laws of the state in which the accused is being tried, but in general all states base their laws on five famous judicial decisions or legal recommendations concerning criminal responsibility:

1. The *M'Naghten* (or McNaughton) *rule*, also known as the *right and wrong test* or the *knowledge test*—In 1843, Daniel M'Naghten shot and killed Drummond, private secretary to Sir Robert Peel. He had mistaken Drummond for the latter. For some years, M'Naghten had suffered from delusions of persecution and had finally woven Sir Robert Peel into his delusional system. He was determined to right his imaginary wrongs by killing Peel. When he was brought to trial, the court recognized that the killing was an outcome of his delusions of persecution; he was declared of unsound mind and committed to an institution for the criminally insane. Following this trial, the Judges of England enunciated two rules to determine the responsibility of an accused who pleads insanity as a defense: (a) to establish such a defense the accused, at the time the act was committed, must be shown to have been laboring under such defect of reason as not to know the nature and quality of the act he was doing, or (b) if he did know it, he did not know that what he was doing was wrong.

2. The *irresistible impulse test*, recommended as an addition to the M'Naghten rule in 1922—"A person charged criminally with an offense is irresponsible for his act when the act is committed under an impulse which the prisoner was by mental disease in substance deprived of any power to resist."

3. The *Durham decision*—a 1954 ruling by the United States Court of Appeals that "an accused is not criminally responsible if his unlawful act was the product of mental disease or mental defect." Prior to this decision, psychiatric testimony relating to the mental status of the accused was confined to a determination of whether the accused could distinguish right and wrong, or acted under an irresistible impulse at the time of the offense. Under the Durham test, however, the psychiatrist may give any relevant testimony concerning the mental illness issue.

4. *American Law Institue (ALI) test*—absolves the defendant of criminal responsibility if, because of a mental disease or defect, the defendant lacks substantial capacity to appreciate the criminality (wrongfulness) of his or her conduct or lacks the capacity to conform his or her conduct to the requirements of law.

5. *Brawner decision*—a 1972 ruling by the United States Court of Appeals for the District of Columbia that adopted the *American Law Institute Formulation* that "a person is not responsible for criminal conduct if at the time of such conduct as a result of mental disease or defect he lacks substantial capacity either to appreciate the wrongfulness of his conduct or to conform his conduct to the requirement of law."

Traditionally, the defense of nonculpability has been limited to very young children and the mentally disturbed. Controversy revolves about the question of defining "mentally disturbed." So long as the accused was clearly psychotic and obviously unable to understand what he was doing, it seemed only logical to absolve him of responsibility for his actions.

But studies of persons found not guilty by reason of insanity (NGRI) reveals that between 10% and 30% of such acquittees are diagnosed as having personality disorders, not as psychotic. In consequence, there is concern that the defense may be abused, particularly in the case of persons charged with violent crime. That concern has been reflected in recent tightening of the standards and procedures used to determine an accused person's culpability, both to prevent the misuse of the NGRI defense in the first place and also to protect the public against premature release of potentially dangerous people.

In 1984, a proposal to eliminate the volitional aspect of the Model Penal Code was adopted, and the new federal insanity test requires that "…at the time of the commission of the acts constituting the offense, the defendant, as the result of a severe mental disease or defect, was unable to appreciate the nature and quality of the wrongfulness of his acts."

**criminalism, compulsive** Frequent repetition of criminal acts in a compulsive manner. Like most symptoms of the obsessive-compulsive, such antisocial acts are closely related to feelings of hostility and aggression, often against the father. Because these acts are symptomatic, they afford only temporary relief and are therefore repeated.

**criminally insane** See *crime and mental disorder*.

**criminosis** Antisocial behavior; criminality. The word is patterned after neurosis and psychosis in form, but differs in that it does not specifically connote mental illness. It suggests instead that criminals be classified on the basis of the behavior they demonstrate unless they show clearcut evidence of mental disorder.

**crises, urban** See *social policy planning*.

**crisis hospitalization** Extended observation: the usual observation period in a hospital's emergency room is limited to less than 24 hours, but in EOUs (emergency observation units) this period can be extended to as many as 72 hours. Such units are often referred to as 72-hour beds.

**crisis intervention model** A model of illness that focuses on transitional-developmental and accidental-situational demands for novel adaptational responses. Because minimal intervention at such times tends to achieve maximal and optimal effects, such a model is more readily applicable to population groups than is the *medical model*. Typically, such intervention consists of brief psychotherapy to aid a person or group in coping with developmental crises (adolescence, parenthood, retirement, etc.) or accidental crises (bereavement, disaster, etc.). See *community psychiatry; medical model*.

**crisis intervention team model** *CIT*; a partnership between law enforcement, the mental health system, and consumers of mental health services and their families that strives to meet the needs of patients with mental illness in crisis situations. Police officers volunteer for the program, and after training about mental illness, the mental health system, and de-escalation of crisis, they become the first responders in the community. Essential to the success of the model is ongoing collaboration between the partners.

**crispation** Slight spasmodic or convulsive muscle contraction; *dysphoria nervosa*. The subject feels as if something were creeping or tingling within.

**criterion-referenced** See *test*.

**criterion validity** See *validity*.

**critical flicker fusion test** *CFF*; the subject is presented with sections of different colors on a rotating wheel and indicates at what point the colors fuse together without flickering. See *flicker*.

**critical period** During development, an irreversible decision point when the nerve cell becomes committed to one or another pathway of differentiation. There are similar critical periods in the development of behavior, both in the acquisition of sexual identity and in the development of social and perceptual (including language) competence. During critical periods the infant must interact with a normal environment if development is to proceed properly. See *psychophysics*.

Many neurolinguists believe that there is a critical period for *language acquisition* (q.v.), a time when the brain is prepared to construct a mental *grammar*, extending from about the age of 2 years (the onset of the two-word stage) to 12 years (qq.v.). The hypothesis remains controversial, and it has proved to be extremely difficult to test.

**critical point** The event, occurrence, or situation in which the patient's problem comes to a head and he mobilizes his resources for dealing with the problem. Slavson, who suggested the term, believes that in nearly all therapy an ultimum point is reached in the specific intrapsychic or environmental situation that is the culminating point of therapy. See *nuclear problem*.

**critical ratio** See *CR*.

**critical stimulus duration** *CSD*. See *mask*.

**criticizing faculty** See *superego*.

**crocidismus** *Carphology* (q.v.).

**Crocodile Man** A person whose murderous assaults were likened by his defense lawyers to attacks by a crocodile and attributed to a limbic system disorder that released impulses over which the subject had no control. See *episodic dyscontrol; explosive disorder*.

**crocodile tears** See *Bogorad syndrome*.

**cross impulse** An impulse that crosses the path of another impulse and thereby checks the further development of the latter. See *side impulse*.

**cross-association, telepathic** The phenomenon that occurs when a thought or phantasy in one mind suddenly intersects a thought or phantasy articulated by another. It is assumed that such factors as coincidence, intuition, suggestion, or sympathetic identification of the one individual with the other are not at play.

**cross-coding** In relation to gender, giving signals that are disharmonious as to one's sexuality; *gender transposition*. See *gender coding*.

**cross-cultural** Referring to the comparative study of phenomena as they appear in different societies, nations, and cultures. Cultural or cross-cultural psychiatry is concerned with mental illness in relation to the cultural setting in which it occurs. What is regarded in one culture as clearly pathological may be regarded as normal or even desirable in another. See *comparative psychiatry; culture-specific syndromes*.

**cross-cultural method** Comparison of different cultures or societies to determine the effect of a particular variable on behavior.

**cross-dependence** The ability of one drug to suppress the manifestations of physical dependence produced by another and to maintain the physically dependent state. See *cross-tolerance*.

**cross-dressing** *Eonism*; dressing in the clothes of the opposite sex. It may occur as *fetishistic transvestism* (garments of the other sex, typically underclothes or lingerie, are necessary for sexual arousal and orgasm), *nonfetishistic transvestism* (sporadic or episodic dressing in clothing of the opposite sex, but not because it is necessary for sexual arousal), *gynemimesis* or *andromimesis* (qq.v.), or as a part of *transsexualism* (q.v.). See *transvestitism*.

**cross-fostering** A strategy for investigating genetic factors in the development of any disorder in which offspring of normal biological parents are reared by adopting parents who manifest the trait or disorder under investigation. Most commonly, the cross-fostered subjects are compared with two other groups—one group consisting of offspring of parents with the disorder reared by normal adopting parents (*index adoptees*), the other consisting of offspring of normal parents reared by normal adopting parents (*control adoptees*).

**cross-gender disorder** See *gender identity disorder; transsexualism*.

**crossing over** The genetic mechanism by which a chromosomal linkage group is broken up, so that some of the linked genes are able to separate and to enter different gametes and new *recombinations*. The new linkage groups are again as permanent as those that preceded them. If there is only little crossing over between two genes, the linkage is said to be *strong* or *close*. If there is much crossing over taking place, it is said that the linkage is *weak* or *loose*. See *crossover; linkage; linkage analysis*.

**cross-linkage theory** See *aging, theories of*.

**cross-modal binding** Linking together information from different sensory modalities, such as sight and sound, that comes from the same stimulus. Although the world is experienced as a unified whole, sensory systems do not deliver it in that way to the brain. Signals from different sensory modalities are initially registered in separate brain areas, and cross-modal binding produces a unified experience of the world.

**crossover** 1. *Recombination* (q.v.). Crossover is an exception to Mendel's law of independent assortment. The term was first used in the context of linkage effects on the segregation of genes for different characters by Morgan and Cattell (1912). See *linkage; linkage analysis*.

2. A *crossover pattern* has been described in tests of readiness to respond: the normal subject takes advantage of the predictability of when a stimulus will be presented and responds more quickly to a stimulus beginning after a predictable interval than to a stimulus that begins after an unpredictable interval. In process schizophrenic patients, however (and also in patients with temporal lobe lesions and in some aged persons), as the length of intervals between stimuli increases, responses to a stimulus after a predictable interval become slower than responses to a stimulus after an unpredictable interval.

3. In drug studies, referring to an experiment in which two groups are matched, then the drug being assessed is administered to one of the groups but not the other; later (at the crossover) the drug is given to the other group and discontinued in the first group. In crossover studies, each subject serves as his own control.

**cross-sectional research** Examination of one or more variables under study at one point in time or among different age groups; for example, the number of new cases of schizophrenia occurring within different age groups in the United States in the year 2001. Each age group is compared with the other age groups in that year. This is in contrast to *longitudinal research*, which compares a subject or a group of subjects with itself at different times; for example, at age 20 and then again at age, 30, 40, 50, etc.

**cross-tolerance** *Reciprocal neuroadaption*; tolerance manifested to one drug that has not been previously administered or ingested, as a result of having already developed tolerance to another drug because of long-term administration of that other drug. One drug has the capacity both to prevent the withdrawal manifestations that would otherwise emerge upon discontinuation or removal of another, and to maintain a similar type of neuroadaptive state. Cross-tolerance may be manifested as a difficulty in inducing anesthesia for surgical procedures: a person who has developed tolerance to alcohol is also tolerant to volatile anesthetics or barbiturates, which in consequence do not produce the desired or anticipated level of anesthesia when administered in their usual amounts. See *cross-dependence; tolerance.*

**Crow type I schizophrenia** T. J. Crow (*British Medical Journal 280*, 1980) hypothesized that schizophrenia is a composite of two syndromes: type I, characterized by reversible delusions, hallucinations, and thought disorder with good response to neuroleptic treatment and possibly due to increased numbers of striatal and limbic dopamine receptors; and type II, characterized by frequently unremitting negative symptoms (flat affect, social withdrawal, poverty of thought content), poor response to neuroleptics, and a presumptive etiology of cell loss and structural brain damage, possibly due to a virus. See *negative symptoms.*

**crowding** See *spacing.*

**crowding, thought** Bleuler's term for enforced thinking. "In superficial contradistinction to obstruction, schizophrenics often feel a "crowding of thoughts'; they are forced to think." Bleuler adds that it is to be distinguished from obsessive thinking in that "in the former the obsession lies in the subject-matter, while in the latter it is in the process." (Bleuler, E. *Textbook of Psychiatry*, 1930).

**cryogenic** Relating to refrigeration, and especially to methods of producing very low temperatures. In neuropsychiatry, used particularly to describe methods of producing brain lesions; the technique is generally reported to produce less severe blood loss

and lower mortality than other types of surgery.

**cryptesthesia** A general term for clairvoyance, clairaudience, and other types of paranormal cognition in which the sensory stimulus is unknown. See *paranormal; extrasensory perception.*

**cryptogenic epilepsy** *Epilepsy* (q.v.) without known etiology.

**cryptogenic symbolism** Silberer's term for any form of pictorial representation or image formed in mental functioning. In other words, all functions of the mind, save the ideational, are represented by cryptogenic symbolism.

**cryptomnesia** A forgotten experience is recalled, but it appears to be completely new.

**cryptophasia** *Glossolalia* (q.v.).

**cryptophoric symbolism** See *metaphoric symbolism.*

**crystal gazing** A technique used in hypnoanalysis consisting of having the hypnotized subject observe a glass ball or a mirror and then produce associations. The subject is instructed to look at the glass and told that he will see in it things that he will describe to the analyst afterward.

**crystallized** Referring to the state that develops in some chronic users of phencyclidine (PCP): poor attention, dulling of thinking and reactions, loss of recent memory, decreased impulse control, lethargy, and depression.

**crystallized intelligence** The intelligence that is derived from what a person knows. See *fluid intelligence; intelligence.*

**crystallophobia** Fear of glass.

**CS** Conditional stimulus. See *conditioning.*

**Cs** *Conscious* (q.v.).

**CSA** Childhood sexual abuse. See *child abuse; pedophilia.*

**CSD** 1. Critical stimulus duration. See *mask.*

2. Cortical spreading depression; see *migraine.*

3. Chronic subjective dizziness; see *dizziness, chronic subjective.*

**CSR** Continued stay review. See *review.*

**CT** 1. Conduction time; see *nerve conduction; synapse.*

2. Computerized tomography; a structural imaging technique; uses ionizing radiation, a highly collimated X-ray beam that passes through the patient's head and then is recorded by CT detectors. Dense bone attenuates more of the X-ray beam than less dense tissue; the density of soft tissues lies between that of bone and air. Dense structures (like bone and

acute blood) appear brighter or whiter on CT tissues than less dense tissue (like CSF or fat). CT is relatively less expensive, quicker, and more available than MRI. CT is more sensitive than MRI in detecting acute hemorrhage and calcification and is superior in the depiction of bony architecture. A relative disadvantage is that, practically, CT imaging is limited to the axial or transverse plane. See *PET*.

**CT scan** Computed tomography scan; also, CAT scan (computed axial tomography scan). CT, developed in the 1960s, was the first method that allowed visualization and measurement of the brain in living subjects. See *imaging, brain; MRI; tomography*.

**CTS** *Carpal tunnel syndrome* (q.v.).

**cuboidodigital reflex** See *Bechtereff-Mendel reflex*.

**cue, minimal** The smallest quantum or most elemental aspect of a stimulus presentation that will elicit a response or a major portion of the total response. The responder is typically unaware of the significance or even the presence of the stimulus, and his response in many respects is similar to the conditional response in clinical or operant *conditioning* (q.v.). The mechanisms involved, at least at times, are also analogous to those operative in the production of temporal *summation* (q.v.) through subliminal excitation.

**cued memory** See *evocative memory*.

**cueing, mutual** See empathic failure; fit.

**Cullen, William (1710-1790)** A Scottish physician who emphasized the endogenous nature of mental disorders and their relationship to irritability of the nervous system; Dr. Benjamin Rush was among his students.

**cult** A group of people or a movement with a distinctive doctrine or set of strongly held beliefs whose dogma and ritual are typically contrary to the established one(s) within the community. In what has been termed a totalist cult, the characteristic dedication to the dogma and the leadership of the movement may lead to the use of unethically manipulative techniques of persuasion and control in order to fulfill the goals of the leaders and recruit new members. See *exit therapy*.

**cultural competence** Providing patients a context that is congruent with their cultural values and beliefs; application of knowledge, skills, experience, and personal attributes to respond respectively and effectively to people of all cultures, races, ethnic backgrounds, and religions in a manner that recognizes and

values the cultural differences and similarities and the worth of individuals, families, and communities and protects and preserves the dignity of each. Cultural competence is a continuing process of seeking cultural sensitivity, valuing diversity, and knowing about cultural mores and traditions of the populations being served. See *comparative psychiatry*.

Cultural considerations are increasingly important in the psychological and neuropsychiatric examination of patients, particularly as immigration has increased. Both the legal system and the medical system are part of the larger sociocultural system, and both are significantly influenced by the cultural backgrounds of the persons involved. Cultural competence involves understanding of the beliefs, assumptions, and expectations of both patient and therapist. The patient enters the clinical system with preconceived beliefs about the cause of illness and the best way to manage it. Clinicians, too, have cultural characteristics that reflect the professional training they have received in addition to their own family, social, economic, and ethnic backgrounds. The interaction between patient and clinician to a significant degree depends upon how much the patient feels comfortable in revealing to the therapist, and how much the therapist can be accepting, empathetic, and supportive of the patient.

Unless the patient is in a hospital or residential care facility, most of the clinician's decisions about treatment are implemented in the patient's space and under the patient's direction. The clinician must understand what the patient faces, when implementing a treatment strategy, in the beliefs, values, and conventions that were inherent in his or her rearing and which are shared by those who people his or her current environment.

The Outline for Cultural Formulation (OCF) developed by the DSM-IV Task Force is divided into five subsections: the cultural identity of the individual, the cultural explanation of the individual's illness, cultural factors related to the individual's psychosocial environment and levels of functioning, cultural elements of the relationship between the individual and the clinician, and overall cultural assessment for diagnosis and care.

**cultural process** The process by which the folkways, mores, and social values are transmitted from generation to generation and are modified in adjustment to social change.

**cultural psychiatry** *Comparative psychiatry* (q.v.).

**culture** The totality of the individual artifacts, behavior, beliefs, art, law, morals, customs, and any other capabilities and habits acquired by man as a member of society; what remains of man's past working on his present to shape his future. The distinction is made between material culture, including tools, shelter, goods, technology; and nonmaterial culture, including shared patterns of belief, feeling, and adaptation, which serves as a guide of conduct in the definition of reality, as well as values, customs, institutions, and social organization. Culture is usually assumed to depend largely on learning by one person from others in his society, but inherited elements of brain structure and function also contribute. See *collective unconscious*.

Some authorities, believing that species other than the human might have culture, prefer to define culture as socially transmitted adjustable behavior.

**culture shock** A type of *interface shock*. See *network*.

**culture-bound** Culture-specific; characteristic of or confined to a particular ethnic or cultural population. See *culture-specific syndromes*.

**culture-specific syndromes** Behavior disorders that appear to be limited to certain societies or cultural groups; by those groups they may or may not be considered illnesses or afflictions, but they typically have no clear-cut counterpart in Western nosology. Among such syndromes are *amok* (Malaya), *ainu*, *amurakh*, Arctic hysteria, *ataque de nervios* (Puerto Rico, Latin America), *bangungut*, bebainan, benzi mazurazura, berserk, bilis or *colera*, *bouffée delirantes*, *brain fag*, cathard (Polynesia), copying mania, *delahara*, *dhat*, *echul*, *falling out*, fighting sickness, frenzied anxiety state (Kenya), *ghost sickness*, *gi-gong*, *grisi siknis*, guria, *hwa-byung*, *Hsieh-Ping*, *imu* (Japan), jumpers (jumping Frenchmen of Maine and Canada), *juramentado*, *kimilue*, *koro*, kupenga, kwechitsiko, *lata*, *mal de ojo*, mal de pelea (Puerto Rico), menerik, mirachat or *miryachit* (Siberia), muina, olonism, Oriental nightmare-death syndrome, phil pob, piblokto or *piblokot* (polar Eskimos), pseudoamok syndrome, pseudonite syndrome (Sahara), *Puerto Rican syndrome*, *sangue dormido*, *shin-byung*, *susto*, *taijin-kyofusho*, Tropenkoller, Vimbuza,

voodoo death, Whitman syndrome (United States), wihtigo psychosis, wild man behavior (New Guinea), *windigo psychosis* (qq.v.). See *dissociation; possession trance*.

Among Xhosa children and adolescents in South Africa, ukuphaphazela ("fright") appears to be predominantly a cultural variation of sleep terror disorder, and school anxiety (brain fag syndrome) appears to be a cultural variant of conversion disorder. Amafufunyane ("possession by evil spirits") is correlated with possession trance disorder. Ukuphambana ("madness caused by evil spirits") and ukuthwasa (calling by ancestral shades to become a healer) are less discrete categories that may have developed indigenously to give meaning to more biologically based and more psychosocially influenced abnormal behavior, respectively.

**culturgen** An observable feature of a culture. Culturgens are processed by *epigenetic rules*, genetically determined procedures that direct the formation of the mind. The epigenetic rules of the mind bias the subject to choose certain culturgens in preference to others. The totality of all such choices in a population creates that group's culture and social organization. Genetic variation takes place in the epigenetic rules, and this variation accounts for at least some part of the variation in behavioral choices seen in a population. Individuals whose choices increase their inclusive genetic fitness are able to pass more of their genes along to future generations. As a result, the population as a whole has shifted toward certain epigenetic rules and the types of behavior favored by those rules. It is the epigenetic rules that are inherited because the genotype actually codes for the construction of the wiring pattern of the mind, which in turn encodes these rules. See *meme*.

**cunnilingus** Apposition of the mouth to the vulva or to any part of the external female genitals, usually clitoris.

**cunnus** Pudenda; vulva; female external genitalia.

**curanderismo** *Folk medicine* (q.v.) among Spanish-speaking people and, in particular, among Mexican-Americans. The folk healers themselves are curanderos (males) and curanderas (females). The curanderos are believed to have derived their calling as well as their rituals from divine inspiration. Their techniques typically involve herbal infusions, dramatic healing rituals, and prayer directed against a variety of physical and psychological symptoms such as *embrujo* (witchcraft), *empacho* (intestinal distress), *mal ojo* (evil eye), *mal puesto* (hexing), and *susto* (soul loss). Curanderismo is not viewed as competitive with or antithetical to medical treatment, which may be sought and followed concurrently. See *complementary medicine.*

**curdling**   *Rare.* Masselon's term for emotional dementia, referring to the fixation of affects upon infantile or early childhood experiences.

**cure, transference**   See *flight into health.*

**curiosity, infantile**   Curiosity concerning matters of a directly sexual nature, indulged in by most children at one time or another. Some children exhibit a kind of foolish, witless behavior, in order to delude their elders into regarding them as being "too young to understand" or even into altogether disregarding their presence. The purpose of the artifice is that by these means children can view and overhear various private things that they are not supposed to. See *pseudoimbecility.*

**Currens formula**   The ruling that a person is not responsible for a crime if he or she lacked "adequate capacity to conform his conduct to the requirements of the law." See *criminal responsibility.*

**curse, Ondine**   See *apnea, central.*

**curse, psychotic**   Profane speech in a mentally ill person, as in Gilles de la Tourette syndrome or as a complication of neuroleptic treatment of the syndrome.

**Cushing syndrome**   (Harvey William Cushing, American surgeon and neurologist, 1869–1939) Hyperadrenocorticism. See *basophile adenoma.*

**custodial care**   Any of a continuum of services in which protection  and monitoring of the patient, or protection of others from the patient's aggressive potential, are of paramount importance. Custodial care may include active medical intervention, but most often it is needed for chronically ill patients whose level of functioning is unlikely to change appreciably for the better, even though they may require continuing drug treatment and milieu therapy to prevent or retard further deterioration.

**custody**   Safekeeping, guardianship, protectorship, or the state of being guarded or protected. See *custodial care.* Most typically, the term is applied to children in the sense of which parent retains the control of and responsibility for the child in cases of divorce. Historically, custody has meant both ownership and protectorship. Until the middle of the 19th century, the father was usually awarded custody of the child in the same way that he had absolute control over all family property. With the Victorian era came the *tender years presumption*, that the young child needed the ministrations of a gentle mother more than the firmness and discipline that a father could provide. Children of prelatency years were generally awarded to their mothers, but it was not unheard of that as they grew older they would be shifted to the father's care. The approach in favor during most of the 20th century emphasizes the rights of children and would assign custody on the basis of what is in the best interest of the child—the *best interests doctrine.*

*Joint custody* refers to the sharing of custody by both parents, such as joint *legal* custody (the parents share decision making in all or specified areas, while the child resides with one parent), joint *physical* custody (the child spends a specified amount of time with each parent), or variousother arrangements.

**Cutter, Nehemiah**   (1787–1859) American psychiatrist; one of the "original thirteen" founders of Association of Medical Superintendents of America (forerunner of American Psychiatric Association).

**cutting**   See self-mutilation.

**CVA**   *Cerebrovascular accident* (q.v.).

**CVAH**   Congenital virilizing adrenal hyperplasia; see *adrenogenital syndrome.*

**CVS**   Chorionic villus sampling; see *chorion biopsy.*

**CWF**   *Cornell Word Form test* (q.v.).

**cyanocobalamin**   $B_{12}$ (q.v.).

**cybernetics**   The study of messages and communication in humans, social groups, machines, etc., especially in reference to regulation and control mechanisms such as *feedback* (q.v.). The term was devised by Norbert Weiner (1948) to include the entire field of control and communication theory; he envisioned its creation as a linkage of developments in understanding the human nervous system, the electronic computer, and the operation of other machines. See *information theory.*

**cyberphobia**   Unreasonable fear of direction or authority; fear of control, especially mind control (see *brain control; menticide*); fear of computers, computer technology, or the possibility that computer intelligence will supplant human intelligence.

**cyberstalking**   See *stalking.*

**cycad seed**   Used by the Chamorros in producing flour, it contains a neurotoxin, β-N-methylamino-L-alanine, which has been proposed to be the agent responsible for the high frequency of the Parkinsonism-amyotrophy-dementia complex of Guam - *Guam ALS-PDC (q.v.).*

**cycasin**   See *Guam ALS-PDC.*

**Cyclazocine**   See *methadone.*

**cycle, life**   See *developmental levels.*

**cycle, manic-depressive**   See *manic-depressive psychosis.*

**cycle length**   In recurrent disorders, such as major depressive disorder or bipolar disorder (manic-depressive psychosis), the period between the onset of one episode and the onset of the next, including the period of the first episode.

**cyclic addiction**   A syndrome originally described by Wulff that occurs most commonly in women and consists of periods of depression, feelings of ugliness, and overeating or over-drinking alternating with periods of normal or elated mood, feelings of beauty, and ascetic behavior. By psychoanalytical definition these patients show a pre-oedipal mother conflict with unconscious hatred of the mother and of feminity. Their urge to eat is an attempt to incorporate something to counteract feminity —milk, penis, child or narcissistic supplies which soothe anxieties. See *hysteroid dysphoria.*

**cyclic antidepressant**   A generic term that includes tricyclics (e.g., imipramine), tetra-cyclics (e.g., maprotiline), and similar antidepressant agents; heterocyclic has also been used as a generic term for the same agents. See *antidepressant.*

**cyclical depression**   Recurrent episodes of depression that may  or may not alternate with periods of exaltation.

**cycloid**   The type of personality characterized by alternating states of increased psychic and motor activity, usually with feelings of well-being, and of diminution of the same factors. The personality is said to alternate from the one to the other. Cycloid commonly describes the normal or usual personality of many who subsequently develop manic-depressive psychosis, although the development of the psychosis is not a necessary result of such a personality.

Cycloid and cyclothymia are regarded by many as synonymous, although the latter term generally refers to personality problems that are more than cycloid and less than manic-depressive reactions. See *affective disorders.*

**cycloid psychosis**   As used by Karl Kleist, *cycloid marginal psychosis* referred to an episode of atypical psychosis that did not fit clearly into either the schizophrenic or the manic-depressive category. See *remitting atypical psychosis.*

Leonhard and Perris used *cycloid psychosis* to denote atypical psychosis with delusions or hallucinations or both, with bipolar manifestations, and with good outcome (i.e., no chronic or residual defect state). Other symptoms, in order of frequency, are perplexity (the most frequent), motility disturbances, pananxiety, and ecstasy. Leonhard distinguished three forms, depending on which symptoms are predominant:

1. *Motility psychosis*—hyperkinetic or akinetic
   a. The hyperkinetic form may resemble manic or catatonic excitement, with many abrupt gestures and expressive movements that seem to be the result of autonomous mechanisms and not responses to environmental stimuli or depressions of the patient's mood.
   b. The akinetic form is like a catatonic stupor.
2. *Confusion psychosis*: thought disorder prominent, ranging from excitement and pressured thought at one pole to underactivity and poverty of speech at the other.
3. *Anxiety elation psychosis* (anxiety-blissfulness psychosis): periodic states of overwhelming anxiety and paranoid ideas of reference in the anxiety phase. The elation phase manifests itself most frequently in ecstatic blissfulness, expansive behavior, and grandiose ideas concerned with the mission of making others happy and of saving the world.

As described, cycloid psychoses are more frequent in females than in males, and affected patients are younger at the time of first admission than unipolars. Rates of both schizophrenia and affective illness in subjects' relatives are intermediate between the rates found in schizophrenics' and affectives' families. Although recurrences are frequent, they tend to be short-lived. See *reactive psychosis*.

**cyclophrenia**   *Rare. Manic-depressive psychosis* (q.v.); thymergasia.

**cycloplegic**   See *mydriasis*.

**cyclotaxia**   Seldom-used term for genetic or familial risk for increased depressive symptoms, aggression, and mania; applied to children who do not display the full syndrome (i.e., are "*subsyndromal*") of bipolar disorder. Many such children show clusters of symptoms of other disorders and as a result do not fit clearly into any single disorder described in the diagnostic manual.

**cyclothymia, -themia**   Mild fluctuations of the manic-depressive type that almost have the stamp of normal mood shifts come under the heading of cyclothymia. There need not be fluctuations from psychomotor overactivity to underactivity. Some cases give a history only of periodic excitements, while others have one of periodic depressions. See *affective disorders*.

The depressive phase may be clouded by the predominance of physical complaints, to which the term neurasthenia has been applied. Cyclothymia is classified as one of the bipolar disorders and is described as recurrent periods of abnormally elevated or expansive mood and of abnormally dejected mood or loss of interest or pleasure; the abnormal mood shifts must have continued for a minimum of 2 years, but they are not of such quality or severity as to meet the criteria for manic episode or major depressive episode.

**cyclothymic personality (disorder)**   Affective personality (disorder)—recurring variations of mood, ranging from elated "highs" (with ambition, energy, warmth, enthusiasm, optimism) to dejected "lows" (with pessimism, worrying, low energy, feelings of uselessness and futility). See *affective disorders; cycloid; cyclothymia*.

**cyclothymosis**   A term suggested by Southard for manic-depressive disorder.

**cynanthropy**   *Obs.* A symptom in which the patient believes himself to be a dog; it is sometimes seen in the hebephrenic form of schizophrenia.

**cynophobia**   Fear of a dog, or of rabies, sometimes called pseudohydrophobia; usually hysterical in character, the fear is sometimes precipitated by the bite of a dog.

**cynorexia**   Dog's appetite; *bulimia* (q.v.).

**CYP**   *Cytochrome P450 isoenzyme system* (q.v.).

**cypri(do)phobia**   Fear of sexual intercourse and, in particular, of venereal disease as a consequence of sexual activity.

**cyproterone acetate**   An antiandrogen, the European equivalent of *medroxyprogesterone* (q.v.); its trade name is Androcur.

**cystathianineuria**   A metabolic defect associated with mental retardation.

**cytheromania**   *Nymphomania* (q.v.).

**cytoarchitecture**   Cell structure; used primarily in neurohistology. See *Brodmann; isocortex*.

**cytochrome c**   See *OXPHOS*.

**cytocrome P450 isoenzyme system**   *CYP*; a group of gastrointestinal and hepatic isoenzymes responsible for the phase I oxidative metabolism of many drugs. More than 30 isoenzymes are known; they are subdivided into families and subfamilies. Many drugs inhibit isoforms different from the ones responsible for their own metabolism, thereby leading to potentially dangerous interactions with other medications. The major isoforms involved in the metabolism of psychotropic drugs are the 2D6, 3A3/4, 1A2, and 2C19 isoenzymes.

A drug metabolized by a given pathway is termed a *substrate*. It is often used to predict what the clinical effect will be of combining drugs, because many are substates for the same enzyme, active metabolites of drug may be metabolized by different isoenzymes than the parent drug, and genetic differences can influence the capacity of the liver to metabolize many substrates. See *drug metabolism*.

**cytogenetics**   Study of the structure and arrangement of chromosomes and genes within the nucleus and of the effects of quantitative chromosomal irregularities, typically by use of the light microscope.

**cytokines**   Small, secreted proteins that are produced by immune cells. They respond to viruses, bacteria, and other antigens, they effect cross-talk between immune cells and neurons, and they affect mood and behavior. They regulate growth and development, and they mediate inflammatory response. Cytokines act as intercellular mediators by binding to specific membrane receptors, which then signal through second messengers—often tyrosine kinases—to alter the target cell's behavior. Inflammatory cytokines include macrophage chemoattractant protein 1 (MCP1) and transforming growth factor β1 (TGFβ1). Interferons are antiviral, immunomodulatory, antiproliferative cytokines.

The group of structurally related cytokines consisting of interleukin-6 (IL-6), IL-11, IL-27, leukemia inhibitory factor (LIF), ciliary neurotrophic factor (CNTF), cardiotrophin 1 (CT-1), neuropoietin and cardiotrophin-like cytokine (CLC; also known as novel neurotrophin 1, NNT1), and B cell stimulating factor 3 (BSF3) has been given various names, including the *IL-6 family* (the first of the group to be recognized), the *gp130 family* (because all members signal through the gp 130 receptor), and the *neuropoietic* family (for its effect on hematopoietic and nervous systems).

Activation of the *maternal immune system* by respiratory infection can affect fetal brain development and the behavior of adult offspring. Respiratory infection and elevated cytokine levels in pregnant women, for example, significantly raise the risk of schizophrenia in the offspring. Elevated cytokine levels during pregnancy are also associated with other deficits in the offspring such as disturbed social interaction and autism, and prepulse inhibition of the acoustic startle response (a measure of sensorimotor gating). Whether these cytokines serve as direct effectors of injury or as neuroprotectants to repair damage has still to be determined. See *chemokines*.

**cytomegalic disease** Congenital cytomegalic inclusion body disease is a viral disorder (CMV) that may infect the fetus and produce mental retardation; inclusion bodies are demonstrable in the cells of cerebrospinal fluid, tissues, and urine. About 1 of every 200 live births is infected with the virus, and it has been estimated that at least 10% of those infected at birth will become mentally retarded.

Cytomegalovirus *retinitis* is one of the opportunistic infections to which subjects with *AIDS* (q.v.) are susceptible. It often occurs in conjunction with CMV *neuropathy*, a severe, multifocal neuropathy predominating in the cauda equina area, usually associated with CSF pleocytosis with polymorphonuclear reaction. CMV colitis and CMV pneumonitis are also frequently reported in subjects with CMV neuropathy.

**cytoplasm** The outer protoplasmic substance of a cell, exclusive of the nucleus and the cell wall. The matrix or ground substance contains numerous enzymes, most of the soluble precursors of the cellular pool, and various differentiated structures (organelles), including *centriole*, around which spindle microtubules are organized; *centromere*, with which spindle fibers become associated during mitosis and meiosis; *Golgi apparatus*, concerned with the elaboration or storage of various substances within the cell; *lysosomes*, containing hydrolytic enzymes that act on substances taken up by the cell; mitochondria, whose major function is phosphorylation; and *ribosomes*, containing proteins and several kinds of ribosomal RNA that are of central importance in genetic translation. The cytoplasm provides the substrate for gene action and regulates the expression of genetic information through chromosomal inheritance. In addition it contains the elements (e.g., mitochondria and other inclusion particles) responsible for extrachromosomal inheritance, which consequently is termed cytoplasmic inheritance. See *chromosome; gene.*

**cytoskeleton** The framework of the cell consisting of protein fibrillar elements that include *microfilaments* and *microtubules*. Microtubule-associated proteins (*MAPs*) promote the assembly and stability of the microtubules; they include MAP-1, MAP-2, and *tau* (q.v.). *Neurofilaments* are the most numerous of the fibrillar elements in axons; they are typically bundled together in *neurofibrils*. In Alzheimer disease and other degenerative brain disorders the neurofibrils are altered in some way and produce a characteristic lesion, the neurofibrillary tangle or *NFT* (q.v.). See *cytosol.*

**cytosol** The cytoskeletal (fibrillar) elements and soluble proteins (enzymes) within a nerve cell, transported down the axon by slow axoplasmic flow. The numerous enzymes the various metabolic reactions of the cell. The proteins of the *cytoskeleton* (q.v.) mediate the movement of organelles from one region of the cell to another and they anchor membrane constituents (e.g., receptors) to their proper locations on the cell's surface. The chief constituents of the cytoskeleton are fibrillar elements of three types: *microfilaments* (the thinnest), *microtubules* (the thickest), and *neurofilaments*.

**cytosolic proteins** These include (1) the *fibrillar elements* that make up the cytoskeleton (neurofilaments, tubulins, and actins), and (2) the numerous *enzymes* that catalyze the various metabolic reactions of the cell. Modifications that are important can be classified as *cotranslational*, occurring while the polypeptide chain is being synthesized, or *posttranslational*, occurring after the chain is completed.

# D

**D₁ receptor**  See *dopamine*.

**DA**  Dopamine.

**Da Costa syndrome**  Effort syndrome; neurocirculatory asthenia; soldier's heart. See *asthenia, neurocirculatory*.

**dacrygelosis**  *Obs.* Condition characterized by spells of alternate weeping and laughing; seen most frequently in hebephrenic schizophrenia.

**daemonic character**  The person who is his own worst enemy and throughout his life (unconsciously) brings ill fortune upon himself. See *accident proneness*; *masochism*.

**daemonophobia**  A morbid fear of ghosts, spirits, devils, etc.

**DAF**  Delayed auditory *feedback* (q.v.).

**DAG**  *Diacylglycerol* (q.v.).

**DAH**  Disordered action of the heart; the syndrome is known as neurocirculatory asthenia or effort syndrome.

**Dale's principle**  Dale's law; based on the work of Sir Henry Dale in the early 1930s, the principle states that a neuron releases a single transmitter from all its terminals. The original version has undergone considerable revision. It is now known that more than one *neurotransmitter* (q.v.) can be released from a single neuron; most often, the combination involves a biogenic amine or amino acid neurotransmitter with a neuropeptide as cotransmitter. The cotransmitter exerts a long-term modulatory effect on adjacent cells. Although approximately 30 neurotransmitters were known by 1987, the fact that they work in combination indicates that any satisfactory description of neurotransmission must make allowance for the 435 combinations of these transmitters that might occur.

**Daltonism**  Red-green color blindness.

**DALY**  Disability adjusted life year, expressed as *YLD* (year of life lived with disability) + *YLL* (year of life lost because of premature death); a statistic used to measure the economic burden associated with the mortality and morbidity of illness. When years lost through disability and disease are combined, mental disorders account for 9.1% of the worldwide burden of disease; in established market economies they account for 22.4% of the total burden of disease. The burdens attributed to the various mental disorders are as follows: unipolar depression, 6.7%; alcohol, 4.7%; dementia, 2.9%; PTSD, OCD, and panic disorder, 2.4%; schizophrenia, 2.3%; bipolar disorder, 1.7%; and drug abuse, 1.5%. (Andrews, G. and Henderson, S. *Unmet Need in Psychiatry—Problems, Resources, Responses,* Cambridge: Cambridge University Press, 2000).

**damaged goods syndrome**  One form of *battered child syndrome* (q.v.).

**Damocles syndrome**  Described in long-term survivors of cancer: increased concern about illness and death and a feeling of fragility about life and health, related to their physical vulnerabilities. The resulting loss of self-confidence adversely affects interpersonal relationships and the ability to compete in school or at work.

**dance, St. Vitus**  See *Sydenham chorea*.

**dance therapy**  *Dance movement therapy;* the use of movement as a process to promote the patient's growth, development, functioning, and ability to cope with and gain satisfaction from life. Body movement reflects inner emotional states, and changes in the way of moving can lead to changes in the patient's feelings and attitudes about himself, others, and the nonhuman environment. The dance therapist encourages the patient to express dynamic and symbolic material and to recognize and share his inner, emotional life within the interpersonal context of the treatment session.

The dance itself first developed as a formal performing art with emphasis on technique and following the forms and structure (choreography) imposed by others. The modern dance movement began in the early 1900s, emphasizing natural movements, spontaneity, and creativity rather than the rigid and impersonal forms of the formal art. Concurrently, other creative arts (drama, music, art, poetry, etc.) were explored as vehicles for self-expression, providing a means to bring the patient in touch with his inner emotional state at the same time that they reflected his personality, capabilities, and specific conflicts. Dance and the other *creative arts therapies* are also useful in making initial contact and establishing rapport with the patient, and in promoting socialization. *Psychodramatic movement therapy*, associated with the name of Fran Levy, incorporates *psychodrama* (q.v.) into dance therapy as a creative action-oriented approach to group and individual psychotherapy.

**dancing mania** *Choreomania* (q.v.).

**Dandy-Walker syndrome** Congenital atresia of the foramen of Magendie.

**danger situation** See *anxiety*.

**dangerousness** The state of being a peril or hazard. In the United States, almost all states now include dangerousness as one of the major criteria for involuntary commitment. Most laws define danger in terms of physical harm to other persons or to self (e.g., self-mutilation, suicide). Some include *passive dangerousness*—inability to provide for one's basic needs, leading to harm of self through neglect. Still another criterion has been proposed: the person is likely to suffer substantial physical or mental deterioration if not treated. See *police power*.

**DAP** *Draw-a-person* test (q.v.).

**dart and dome** The spike and wave type of electroencephalographic tracing seen in *petit mal epilepsy* (q.v.).

**Darwin, Charles Robert** (1809–1882) British naturalist; his demonstration of breeding experiments as a means of settling problems of ancestry anticipated modern *genetics*; in *On the Origin of Species by Means of Natural Selection or the Preservation of Favored Races in the Struggle for Life* (1859), he enunciated his theory of *evolution* (q.v.).

**Darwinism, Darwinianism** Both terms relate to the branch of biology that deals with, or is in favor of, the doctrine of Charles Darwin postulating the evolution of all forms of living organisms from a few forms of primitive life (see *evolution*).

**Dasein** "A being who is here"; a term used in *existentialism* (q.v.) to refer to the distinctive character of human existence, the capacity to become aware of one's own being at any particular point in time and in space and thereby to accept responsibility for what one is to become in the immediate future.

**DAT** 1. Dementia of the Alzheimer type. See *Alzheimer disease*.

2. Dopamine transporter; a Na$^+$/Cl$^-$ dependent transporter that is found on dopamine neurons. Both amphetamine and cocaine increase extracellular dopamine by interfering with DAT's ability to clear dopamine from the intercellular space. Cocaine and other chemically related drugs are nonselective, competitive inhibitors of monoamine transporters. Amphetamine-like drugs, on the other hand, are substrates for monoamine transporters and lead to redistribution of vesicular monoamines into the cytoplasm, and a reversal in the direction of neurotransmitter transport. Dopamine is associated with feelings of pleasure and reward. DAT densities are affected in several brain disorders, including Parkinson disease, Wilson disease, Lesch-Nyhan disease, Tourette syndrome, major depression, and ADHD.

**data base** See problem-oriented record.

**DATATOP** Deprenyl and tocopherol antioxidative therapy of parkinsonism; a study of the ability of such therapy to delay disability or extend life in patients with early Parkinson disease. A similar study of possible *neuroprotection* in Huntington disease is *CARE-HD* (qq.v).

**date rape** Enforcing nonconsensual sexual intercourse on a date. Like other victims of *rape* (q.v.), the victim feels guilty and responsible for what happened, and particularly since it is the perpetrator's word against the victim's she may come to doubt the adequacy of her objections to the sexual activity that ultimately occurred.

Sexual violence, as manifested in rape and date rape, is often the result of the interaction of seven variables in the perpetrator: sexual arousal in response to aggression, dominance as a sexual motive for sexual acts, hostility toward women, attitudes accepting of violence against women, psychoticism, the nature of the person's prior sexual experience, and opportunity for sexual activity.

**date rape drug** Usually, a sedative-hypnotic given surreptitiously to an otherwise unwilling partner to facilitate intercourse. One frequently used *party drug* is GHB (q.v.). Another date rape drug is flunitrazepam, a benzodiazapine sold in the United States as a street drug called roach, *roofies*, or roSHAY. While media publicity about such drugs is framed to warn women that men may slip flunitrazepam into their drinks, another potential result of media articles is to instruct unscrupulous men in its use.

**Dauerschlaf** Prolonged sleep treatment with drugs (usually barbiturates), used mainly in status epilepticus, acute psychotic episodes, and drug addiction.

**day center** An outpatient or aftercare unit, ordinarily with a nonmedical staff, designed to provide company for the lonely, occupation for the handicapped, and meals for people unable to shop or cook for themselves.

**day hospital** A type of treatment for mentally ill patients consisting of a psychiatric hospital program (including individual and group psychotherapy, somatic treatment, nursing care, social case work, psychological evaluation, occupational and recreational therapy) in which the patient participates during the day but, at night, returns to home, family, and community. The first day hospital was set up by Dr. Ewen Cameron at the Allan Memorial Institute, Montreal, in 1946. In 1954, the first *night hospital* (with patients partaking of hospital care at night but returning to their homes and occupations during the day) was established at the Montreal General Hospital. Both the day hospital and the night hospital are types of *partial hospitalization*, another form of which is the weekend hospital. See *domicile*.

**daydream** Reverie; an ongoing series of brief associated thoughts or images, triggered by internal or external stimuli, and typically related to current life concerns or unaddressed challenges. Daydreams serve an appeasing function, in that they give partial release to strong, unconscious affects. Daydream is often used interchangeably with *phantasy* (q.v.), but phantasy is more elaborate and continuous, composed more of pure imagination than memory, and directed at self-amusement, distraction, or escape.

**daymare** Anxiety attack; panic attack. See *panic; panic disorder.*

**DBS** *Deep brain stimulation* (q.v.).

**DBT** *Dialectical behavior therapy* (q.v.).

**DC** *Dichorionic* (q.v.).

**DD** Depersonalization disorder. See *depersonalization; dissociative disorders.*

**DDIS** *Dissociative Disorders Interview Schedule* (q.v.).

**de Clérambault syndrome** *Erotomania* (q.v.).

**de Lange syndrome** *Amsterdam retardation*; a type of mental retardation with associated and highly variable minor physical manifestations, including low stature, mild microcephaly, low forehead, heavy confluent eyebrows, depressed bridge of the nose, flaring nostrils, small mandible, low-placed ears, micromelia and/or phocomelia, limitation of extension at the elbow joints, clinodactyly of the little fingers, low-placed thumb, webbing of the second and third toe, and hypertrichosis. Cause is unknown; the syndrome was first described by Cornelia de Lange in 1933 and is sometimes known as the Amsterdam type of retardation because it was described in subjects in that area.

Some authorities differentiate two types: (1) the Brachman-de Lange type, or Amsterdam dwarf disease, with retarded bone maturation, short arms and fingers, and prominent features; and (2) the Bruck-de Lange type, with broad neck and shoulders, muscular hypertrophy, and a wrestler like appearance.

**deadly nightshade poisoning** *Strychnomania;* belladonna intoxication. Deadly nightshade is a plant of the genus Solanum. Poisoning may follow ingestion of the black berries of the plant. The mouth and tongue become dry and vision is impaired; any or all of the following symptoms may then appear: visual hallucinations, mutism, restlessness, unresponsiveness, widely dilated pupils, disorientation and confusion, with increasing agitation. The patient then falls into a deep sleep and awakes asymptomatic but with amnesia for the agitated period. During the disturbed period, a misdiagnosis of acute schizophrenic reaction is commonly made.

**deadly quartet** See *metabolic syndrome.*

**deafferentation** See *pain syndromes.*

**deafferented state** See *akinetic mutism.*

**deafferentiation** Elimination or loss of afferent stimuli. Sleep was once believed to be a temporary shutting down of mental and biological activity due to deafferentiation.

**deafness, prelingual** Hearing impairment that develops before speech is learned. Prelingual deafness interferes markedly with speech and language development.

**deafness, word** *Auditory aphasia* (q.v.).

**de-analize** To shift an instinct from the anal region to another object or form of expression. For example, interests in feces may later be expressed as interests in mud, still later in money, securities, etc.

**death**   Cessation of life, physical and mental; total and permanent cessation of the functions or vital actions of an organism. For some psychiatric patients the term "death" does not imply cessation of life; instead, it is regarded simply as a preliminary step to rebirth. In others, death may represent punishment for carrying out a forbidden impulse, such as incest. Or it may represent reunion with the oedipal love object. Another symbolic meaning of death occurs in depressive states, in which suicide unconsciously represents the means by which the death of another is accomplished.

With the development of technology that permits life support of patients for long periods of time after they might otherwise have died, many new questions about death have arisen. There is continuing controversy in both medicine and law concerning the definition of death, whether death is to be defined in terms of cessation of brain activity or cessation of measurable cardiac function, whether artificial or technologic mimicry of certain "essential" functions can be equated with life, etc. In some states in the United States, death has been defined in statutes in an attempt to provide a societal determination of the answer to the ethical questions surrounding the controversy.

**death, autopsy negative**   See *Bell mania.*

**death, neuronal**   See *pruning.*

**death anxiety**   A form of depression in which fear of death, poverty, etc., is the most prominent complaint.

**death domain**   A protein–protein interaction domain consisting of a sequence of 80 amino acids that is found in *Fas, TNF,* and RIP (qq.v.). The death domain is necessary if the receptor is to trigger the cell-death pathway. MORT1/FADD, TRADD, and RIP all use their own death domains to link up with other death domain–containing proteins.

**death drive**   According to Melanie Klein, primary envy is the emotional representative of the death drive and the most painful feeling the baby has to face. Massive projective identifications based on envy are a type of narcissistic object relations, attempts to spoil or destroy the breast or the creativity of mother and father. See *death instinct; object relations theory.*

**death instinct**   Freud (1933) specifically characterizes the death instinct as primary masochism and points out that it seems to be necessary to destroy some other thing or person in order not to destroy ourselves, so as to guard against our primary impulse to self-destruction. The ambiguity of Freud's concept appears in the shifting emphasis on different aspects of it. In *The Ego and the Id* (1923), he declared that sadism is the representative of the death instinct. Finally, in *An Outline of Psychoanalysis* (1940), he described the death instinct as a destructive, aggressive, sadistic assault on the organism that may be diverted outward or stored in the superego. The silent pull toward the inorganic state is deemphasized.

In *Beyond the Pleasure Principle* 1920), Freud first recognized the death instinct as an independent drive. He came to believe that not all mental processes were subject to the pleasure-pain (pleasure-unpleasure) principle and that there was a phylogenetically older principle, the repetition-compulsion principle. The latter operates to restore a previous condition of pleasure and harmony, whenever noxious stimuli cannot adequately be handled by the pleasure-pain principle. Since the repetition-compulsion tends to restore the status quo, Freud reasoned that it must ultimately tend to return the organism to the earliest state of all, namely that of inanimate existence; thus, the manifestations of the repetition-compulsion principle were called the death instinct, and it was presumed that deflection of the death instinct onto objects in the external world constituted the *aggressive instinct.* The aggressive or death instinct aims at destroying the outside world, which is the source of disturbing stimuli; but disturbing stimuli may also come from within by means of an increase in (sexual) libido. As the sexual instincts develop, this increase in libido is accompanied by a transformation of narcissistic libido into object libido. The primal masochism, directed originally against the narcissistic libido, is now projected onto the objects of the libido in the outside world as *sadism.*

The death instinct operates in the oral phase, which thus is often termed the cannibalistic stage; for gratification of hunger also destroys the object. In the anal phase, the destructive instinct appears as soiling, retention, and other means of defiant rejection of the disturbing external world. In the phallic phase, phantasies of piercing, penetration, or dissolution of the object betray the operation of the destructive instinct. Genital sadism appears in the form of hatred, which normally is restricted by love and persists only as the activity involved in taking possession of the love object. In the genital phase, there is fusion of the destructive instinct with the sexual instinct, and the destructive instincts, if not completely paralyzed by the sexual instincts, are at least restrained by them. In certain psychiatric conditions, however, there is a greater or lesser defusion of the instincts; this is seen particularly in depressive psychoses and in certain forms of schizophrenia.

Freud's hypotheses about the death instinct have by no means achieved universal acceptance in psychoanalytic circles, and many feel that although destructiveness may accompany any response pattern, it is not an instinct or drive in itself but is rather a maladaptive or misdirected expression of the single instinct to live. The only aim of instinct is to reduce the physiological stimulus or disequilibrium and to maintain optimal tension, i.e., life.

**death phobia**  Unrealistic or excessive morbid fear of dying, most  commonly an outgrowth of the idea of death as a punishment for death wishes against other persons, or of the idea of death as the ultimate in relaxation consequent upon orgastic relief of one's own excitement, or of the idea of death as a reunion with a dead person.

**death rate**  The ratio of the number of persons dying within a specified period, usually a year, to the number who were in the original group. In institutional statistics, the death rate is usually calculated as the ratio of deaths to the average number under treatment during the period. The number of admissions and the total number under care have been used incorrectly as the base for the death rate.

**death trance**  A state of apparent death; so-called suspended animation as may be seen in hysteria and catatonic schizophrenia.

**debility**  Asthenia.

**debriefing**  A type of psychoeducation, usually for a large group, following a disaster. It provides the opportunity for ventilation of feelings within a supporting group, normalizing responses, and education about the participants' responses to the event. Results have generally been better if the debriefing is given by someone who already had a connection with the group, such as a fellow survivor or a relative of a participant.

**decadence**  The retrogression of a person or society that results from social rather than from physical or biological change. See *degeneration*.

**decapitation, fear of**  One manifestation of castration anxiety.

**decarceration**  See *Scull dilemma*.

**deceitfulness**  See *dysfunctional attitudes*.

**decelerative**  In behavior therapy, techniques designed to reduce target behavior(s) by producing neutral (i.e., nonrewarding) or negative consequences when the undesired behavior is shown.

**decentering**  The ability to limit one's own self-centered (narcissistic) view of what is going on about him or her.

**deception**  Simulation; *malingering* (q.v.).

**decerebrate rigidity**  A syndrome of exaggerated posture in continuous spasm of muscles produced by transection of the brain at a prepontine level. The extensor muscles are particularly affected and exhibit lengthening and shortening (clasp-knife) reactions. See *brain stem*.

**decidentia**  *Obs.* Epilepsy.

**decision**  Selection of an option, making a choice, solving a question. See *choice; counterfactual thinking; neuroeconomics; orbitofrontal cortex; regret; reward*.

**decision support system**  See *information system, executive*.

**decision tree**  See *algorithm, clinical*.

**decisions, legal**  See *consumerism*.

**declarative memory**  *Explicit memory; propositional memory, reference memory*; a form of *long-term memory* (q.v.) that is explicit and conscious, consisting of information based on specific facts or data. It is the ability to encode and recall facts, events, and arbitrary associations. Declarative memory is a group of memory functions requiring conscious retrieval of specific facts and events, which can be brought to mind verbally as a proposition or nonverbally as an image. Brain regions important to declarative memory include the medial temporal lobe (MTL), including hippocampus, parahippocampus, and amygdala; medial diencephalon; basal forebrain; prefrontal cortex, subcortical nuclei, and cerebral white matter pathways. The amygdala, in the dorsomedial portion of the temporal lobe, is vital to emotional and autonomic behavior and is interconnected with regions involved in memory consolidation; damage to the amygdala itself does not impair the ability to learn new information if it is emotionally neutral. Learning a conditioned fear response, however, is highly dependent on the amygdala.

In the diencephalon, the structures most often implicated in amnesia are the dorsomedial nucleus of the thalamus, the mammillary bodies of the hypothalamus, and the mammillothalamic tract connecting them. Basal forebrain structures, rich in acetylcholine, play a role in modulating memory processes that occur in other brain systems. Disruption of prefrontal systems is associated with source memory deficits and temporal ordering, the ability to recall the spatial and temporal contexts within which information was originally acquired.

The ability to search and retrieve information from long-term memory is a function of subcortical nuclei and white matter systems. Damage results in slowed information processing, inefficient learning, and poor recall.

Declarative memory is subdivided as follows:

1. *Episodic memory*—personal memory of specific time-and-place events (less commonly, episodic memory is used interchangeably with working-memory)

2. *Semantic* or *reference memory*—facts, general information, knowledge of concepts and rules.

The other major form of long-term memory is *procedural memory* (q.v.). See *memory; MTL*.

**decompensation** Recurrence or exacerbation of an illness, and in particular schizophrenia, because the mechanisms that had served to correct it are no longer adequate to maintain an acceptable or desirable level of functioning.

**decompose** To divide oneself or another into separate and distinct personalities.

**decomposition** Division of a person into separate components, or, more correctly, personalities.

**decomposition of movement** *Asynergia*; described by Babinski, it is characterized by irregularity in the successive flexion or extension at the various joints, instead of steady, well-timed movements. See *cerebellum; disorganization*.

**decriminalization** The act or process of removing acts or deeds from the category of criminal behavior. Decriminalization programs are those that remove certain types of juvenile offenders from the juvenile justice system and handle them instead under a child welfare or other noncourt system. The term has also been applied to the 20th-century tendency to label as sickness many behaviors that in earlier times were considered criminal or immoral.

When applied to substance use, decriminalization often refers to redefining use as less serious a crime than before and, consequently, as less severely punished (e.g., substituting a warning or fine for a previously mandated arrest or imprisonment). The term is also used to refer to redefining drug use as legal, and not a crime of any degree; this is more correctly termed *legalization*.

**decursus morbi** Clinical course of an illness, used particularly to describe the different paths, trajectories, and outcomes demonstrated by different patients with the same illness.

**dedifferentiation** Loss of higher levels of organization and function; regression; usually applied to the simultaneous acceleration and retardation of development found in schizophrenic children and approximately equivalent to what Bergmann and Escalona termed *fragmentation of the ego*, to Erikson's *interference with psychoembryological schedule of ego functions*, to what Eckstein and Wallerstein termed *fluctuating ego states*, and to Rank's *atypical development*.

**DEEG** Depth EEG; see *ECoG*.

**deemed status** Certification that a facility or unit has satisfied appropriate standards in consequence of which it can be delegated to perform self-regulation and monitoring that would ordinarily be the responsibility of an external regulatory agency.

**deep brain stimulation (DBS)** Initially developed as a treatment for Parkinson disease, used also to control seizure activity in epilepsy. One technique used is *SANTE* (Stimulation of the Anterior Nucleus of the Thalamus for Epilepsy): electrode(s) implanted into the brain, a pacemaker-like generator implanted elsewhere (often in the chest) and a connecting cable between them which is tunneled under the skin through the neck. A similar, but closed-loop, device is *RNS* (responsive neurostimulator system): electrodes are implanted at the sites in the brain of seizure onset; they monitor the EEG and respond to abnormal activity by delivering an electrical impulse to abort seizures and prevent them from spreading.

DBS has also been used to alleviate symptoms of disorders resistant to other treatments, such as chronic pain, tremor, and dystonia. More recently, it has been used in combination with optical neuromodulation and neuroimaging methods such as *magneto-encephalography* (q.v.) to identify the specific cells involved and the timing of their reactions to electrical stimulation. See *opsin*.

**deep reflex** Any one of the tendon and periosteal reflexes, which include the ankle jerk, jaw jerk, knee jerk, and the Bechtereff-Mendel biceps, pectoral, radial, suprapatellar, tibio-adductor, triceps, and ulnar reflexes.

**deerotize** To remove libidinal cathexis from the psychic representation of an object.

**defaulter** Also *drug defaulter*; the patient who does not follow the recommended dosages of prescribed drugs.

**defect** See *disease*.

**defect, ego** Unstable or poorly organized *ego* (q.v.).

**defect psychosis** *Obs.* Mental retardation; feeblemindedness.

**defective, mental** One who is subnormal intellectually; feebleminded. See *retardation, mental*.

**defemination** See *eviration*.

**defense (defence)** A mental attribute or *mechanism* or dynamism that serves to protect the person against danger arising from his impulses or affects. See *anxiety; defense mechanisms*.

The ego arises in response to the frustrations and demands of reality on the organism; it learns to follow the reality principle. But the id follows the pleasure principle only, so that often there are conflicts between the two. This is the essential neurotic conflict. The superego may take either side, and if the world and external reality appear to the ego to be sources of temptation, the conflict may appear to be between the world and the ego. The mechanisms of defense are developed as a means of controlling or holding in check the impulses or affects that might occasion such conflicts.

The various motives for the development of defense mechanisms are (1) anxiety, arising when the ego believes the instinct is dangerous; (2) guilt, with anxiety of the ego

toward the superego and fear of annihilation or decrease of narcissistic supplies; (3) disgust, when the ego must reject the impulse or it will have to be vomited out; and (4) shame, a fear of being looked at and despised if the impulse is not rejected.

When successful, the ego defenses are called *sublimations*. The instinctual drives find an adequate discharge in these sublimations. When unsuccessful, however, defenses are considered pathogenic. The opposed pregenital impulses do not find discharge but continue to gain strength because their physiological bases remain active. A breakthrough may occur, resulting in neurotic symptoms that express simultaneously both a repressed drive and the defense against it.

Various defense mechanisms have been described. Anna Freud (The Ego and the Mechanisms of Defence, 1948) lists the following: regression, repression, reaction-formation, isolation, undoing, projection, introjection, turning against the self, reversal, and sublimation or displacement of instinctual aims (qq.v.). O. Fenichel (The Psychoanalytic Theory of Neurosis, 1945) includes regression, repression, reaction-formation, isolation, undoing, projection, introjection, sublimation, displacement, denial, postponement of affects, affect equivalents, and change in the quality of affects.

Evidently both Anna Freud and Fenichel use introjection and identification interchangeably, although technically introjection is the mechanism by which *identification* (q.v.) is accomplished. Some of the names seem not so much to describe different defenses as to suggest different ways of viewing the same mechanism. Both dissociation and repression, for example, refer to ways of avoiding the unpleasant, the threatening, or the dangerous. In repression, unpleasant content is removed from awareness, while in dissociation, danger is avoided by shifting from one state of consciousness to another. See *character defense*.

**defense interpretation** Ego and superego interpretation; in psychoanalytic therapy, an interpretation that brings to consciousness the kind and sources of defensive resistances used by the patient.

**defense mechanisms** In DSM-IV, *coping styles*; automatic psychological processes that protect the subject against anxiety and from awareness of external dangers or stressors.

A *defensive functioning scale* is proposed that recognizes the following levels of adaptation:

1. High adaptive level, characterized by optimal balance between conflicting motives. Typical mechanisms at this level include anticipation (which promotes the consideration of realistic, alternative responses); affiliation (seeking support from others); altruism; *humor*; self-assertion; self-observation; *sublimation*; *suppression* (qq.v.).

2. Mental inhibitions or *compromise formation* level; typical mechanisms include *displacement*; *dissociation*; intellectualization (overuse of abstract thinking or generalizations to minimize disturbing feelings); *isolation* of affect; *reaction formation*; *repression*; *undoing* (qq.v.).

3. Minor image-distorting level; typical mechanisms include *devaluation*; *idealization*; *omnipotence* (qq.v.).

4. Disavowal level; typical mechanisms include *denial*; *projection*; *rationalization* (qq.v.).

5. Major image-distorting level; typical mechanisms include *autistic fantasy*; *projective identification*; *splitting* of self-image or image of others (qq.v.).

6. Action/withdrawal level; typical mechanisms include *acting out* (q.v.); apathetic withdrawal; help-rejecting complaining; passive aggression (see *passive-aggressive personality*).

7. Defensive dysregulation level; typical mechanisms include delusional *projection*; psychotic *denial*; psychotic *distortion* (qq.v.).

**defense psychosis** *Obs.* A general term used by Freud to emphasize the defensive value of a psychosis.

**defiance-based strategy** See *paradoxical therapy*.

**defiant rage** In Rado's terminology, the angry resistance or opposition to demands and orders, as in the child whose temper tantrum more or less obviously expresses the idea "I won't." Defiant rage is a typical reaction, at least in the American culture, to bowel training; opposed to this reaction is guilty fear and fearful obedience, which arise in response to the mother's punishments, threats, and demands for expiation. The resulting conflict between the opposing tensions of defiant rage and guilty fear is of particular significance in the genesis of obsessive behavior. See *obsessive attack*.

**deficiency, mental** Mental retardation; intellectual inadequacy, feeblemindedness, hypo-

phrenia, oligophrenia, oligergasia. In the 1952 nomenclature (DSM-I), the term denoted intellectual defect existing since birth, without demonstrated organic brain disease or known prenatal cause. As thus used, the term was equivalent to an older term, familial or idiopathic mental deficiency. Mental retardation is the term preferred currently. See *retardation, mental*.

**deficit model** An explanation that relates disorder to a lack of some element that would be expected to be present. The *alexithymic deficit model* of psychosomatic symptoms, for example, posits that the symptoms result from the direct shunting of arousal into the endocrine and autonomic nervous system, due to absent or diminished psychological processes that would be mobilized in the average person.

In linguistics, the deficit hypothesis is the view that because of the relative barrenness of their backgrounds, some children have not acquired a broad enough range of grammar and vocabulary to allow them to express the complex ideas that will be needed for success in school. The opposing view (the *difference hypothesis*) holds that the nonstandard varieties of speech can express ideas of any complexity, and that the child from a working-class or ethnic minority background might not have the opportunity or motivation to use language in demanding or challenging contexts.

**deficit symptoms** In schizophrenia, *negative symptoms*; included are affective flattening or blunting; alogia, thought blocking, or poverty of speech; apathy, avolition, loss of intentionality, and passivity; and anhedonia or asociality. Increases in negative symptoms are associated with more severe degrees of deterioration.

**deficit type schizophrenia** A form of schizophrenia in which negative or deficit symptoms are prominent, enduring, and not caused by medication, depression, or lack of environmental stimuli. Characteristic symptoms include loss of fluency and spontaneity of verbal expression (alogia, poverty of speech), blunted affect, impaired ability to initiate or persist in various tasks (volition), impaired ability to experience pleasure (anhedonia) or to form emotional attachments to others, and impaired ability to focus attention on some specific activity or task in a sustained manner.

See *latent schizophrenia; schizophrenia, models of; schizophrenia, residual.*

**deficit-relationship**   See *conflict paradigm.*

**definitive**   Conclusive; serving to define or separate from others of a class or group. In diagnosis and classification of psychiatric disorders, for example, definitive symptoms are those necessary to distinguish between related disorders.

**defloration scruple**   *Rare.* Hirschfield's term for a compulsion neurosis in young men about to marry; it implies a dread of being the first one to "injure" a woman and carries with it also the fear of castration on the part of the male.

**defusion**   In psychoanalysis, the separation or detachment of the instincts, so that they operate independently. Normally, the energy of the aggressive or death instinct is fused with the sexual. With regression, however, the unification and organization of part-instincts crumble; the destructive instincts are freed and often work directly against the sexual instincts. This is the process of defusion, which in severe form will lead to such prepotency of the destructive instincts that negation of life is the result.

**degeneration**   *Deterioration* (q.v.); reduction to a lower type of personal and social conduct as defined by existing moral and organic laws to which the person is expected to conform. Often the term is used in a pejorative sense to imply a sexual offense.

**degeneration psychosis**   A group of atypical affective psychoses that show, in addition to the more typical manic-depressive symptoms, periodic hallucinosis, stupor, excitement, and paranoid phases. The term *degeneration* refers to the genetic loading found in families in which such variants occur. See *phasophrenias; reactive psychosis.*

**degenerative psychosis**   *Obs.* Any psychosis with regressive tendencies or manifestations; by some, used in a more specific way to refer to organic psychoses with irreversible dementia.

**dégénérés superieurs**   *Obs.* (F. "high-class degenerates") Magnan's term for sexual deviates whose perversions inspire achievement in some special field of endeavor—social, artistic, ethical, etc. An example is the sadistic pedophile who built and maintained a home for disadvantaged children.

**degenitalization**   *Desexualization* (q.v.).

**deglissando**   See *glissando.*

**dehumanization**   Subjecting a person to an environment lacking in personal warmth and respect (e.g., privacy, courtesy). Many reformers of the 1960s emphasized the dehumanizing elements of mental hospitalization. See *deinstitutionalization.*

Imprisonment and warfare are characteristically dehumanizing. Compassion, reason, and love are among the first casualties of war, and the oppressor and the oppressed are equally likely to commit barbaric acts. *Humiliation* (q.v.) is often a part of dehumanization. See *violence.*

**deinstitutionalization**   Discharge from hospital to community, particularly of those chronically mentally ill patients who would otherwise be kept in hospital for long periods of time. Full rehabilitation of the so-called chronic patient requires more than placement in appropriate residential settings, however. Also needed are *mainstreaming*, helping the deinstitutionalized patient to function as a member of the community, and *normalization*, all those interventions whose aim is to eliminate or minimize behavior that would identify the patient as being abnormal in the eyes of his fellows. See *domicile.*

**déjà entendu**   (F. "already heard, perceived") The feeling, not demonstrable in fact, because it never was associated with reality, that one had at some prior time heard or perceived what one is hearing in the present.

**déjà eprouvé**   (F. "already experienced, tested, tried out") The feeling that an act or experience in which the subject has never in fact engaged, has already been carried out by him.

**déjà fait**   (F. "already done") P. Marie's term for a type of paramnesia in which the patient believes that what is happening to him now has happened to him before. Thus one hebephrenic believed he had experienced exactly 1 year before, everything that was happening to him at the time. See *reduplicative memory deception.*

**déjà pensé**   (F. "already thought") The feeling that what one is thinking has been thought about some time in the past. "The déjà vu and déjà pensé phenomena that are a part of many psychomotor attacks...suggest that many of them are associated with disorders localized to the temporal lobes" (DeJong, R. N. *American Journal of Psychiatry CVII,* 1951).

**déjà raconté** (F. "already told, recounted") A forgotten experience, particularly one from the distant past, is recalled, and the person feels as if he had known all the time that the experience had been told to him. The term is also applied to the conviction of the patient in psychoanalysis that he has already related an episode to the analyst, when in fact he has not.

**déjà voulu** (F. "already desired") P. Marie's term for a type of paramnesia in which the patient believes that his present desires are exactly the same as the desires he had some time before. See *déjà fait; déjà vu.*

**déjà vu** (F. "already seen") Feeling of familiarity. Upon perceiving something that he has never seen before, a person has the distinct feeling that he had had the experience some time in the past. Freud suggested that déjà vu feelings correspond to the memory of an unconscious phantasy; the experience probably represents a combination of ego defenses in a situation that both symbolizes and stimulates the revival of an anxiety-provoking memory or phantasy. The ego defenses include wish-fulfillment (in the form of "Don't worry; you have been in the same situation before and came out all right") and regressive reanimation of omnipotent feelings (in the form of predicting the future).

**dejection** Melancholy. The word dejection refers to the mood-tone change that is part of a clinical depression and is approximately equivalent to the word depression as used by the layman. In psychiatry, *depression* (q.v.) has a more specific meaning (referring to a syndrome) and should not be used when only a lowered mood tone is meant (a symptom).

**Déjérine, Jules-Joseph** (1849-1917) Swiss-born French neurologist; described various medullary syndromes, paralyses, muscular dystrophies, and neuropathies. He also described word blindness in 2 papers published in 1891 and 1892. The first patient suffered from word blindness (alexia) with writing impairment (agraphia); the second suffered from pure word blindness, without agraphia.

**Déjérine-Sottas syndrome** (**DSS**) *Hereditary hypertrohic insterstitial neuropathy*; a myelin disorder. Compared with *Charcot-Marie-Tooth disease* (q.v.), it involves a more extreme loss of muscle control and appears earlier, usually in the first two years of life, delaying milestones of development such as walking. It

leads to complete crippling. Patients may die of related disorders such as failure of the diaphragm muscles to maintain breathing during pneumonia.

**DeJong, H. Holland** (1895-1956) Dutch psychiatrist, in later years in the United States; production of symptoms of mental illness in animals (especially catatonia).

**delahara** A culture-specific syndrome in Philippine women similar to *amok* (q.v.).

**Delay, Jean** (1907–1987) French psychiatrist; introduced electroencephalography into France; originated modern psychopharmacotherapy when in 1952, with Pierre Deniker and other colleagues, he reported on the effect of chlorpromazine on psychotic symptoms; introduced the term "neuroleptic."

**delay therapy** *Response prevention*; a behavioral management technique used with obsessive-compulsive subjects in which the usual ritualistic response is prevented or postponed.

**delayed auditory feedback** See *feedback.*

**delayed awakening** See *sleep paralysis.*

**delayed sleep phase syndrome** See *circadian rhythm sleep disorder; chronotherapy.*

**delayed stress syndrome** *Post-traumatic stress disorder* (q.v.).

**deletion** Omission; in genetics, a chromosomal abnormality in which part of a chromosome breaks off during cell replication and gives rise to a smaller than normal chromosome. The *cat cry syndrome* (q.v.) is associated with deletion of chromosome 5.

**deliberate self-harm syndrome** Conscious and willful inflicting of painful, destructive, or injurious acts on one's own body without intent to kill. Typically, the subject feels mounting tension and an impelling impulse to act, followed by a feeling of relief after the injury has been inflicted on the self. The most frequent self-destructive behavior is wrist cutting; other reported acts include abrasion, amputation (e.g., tongue or ear), biting, burning, enucleation of the eye, genital mutilation including castration, removal of the tongue, head banging, ingestion of medication and other objects, jumping from heights, hair pulling, and insertion of foreign bodies into the urethra.

The syndrome most commonly begins in late adolescence and continues for many years. It probably occurs most often in borderline or schizophrenic patients, in order to

(1) relieve feelings of depersonalization; (2) lessen inner tension; (3) solve genital conflicts; (4) reassure the subject that he or she is alive by seeing his own blood; (5) deny inability to control the body by planning its destruction. Also called *autoaggression, focal suicide, parasuicide, self-attack, symbolic wounding*. See *self-mutilation; attempted suicide*.

**delibidinization**   Technically, the act of removing libido from an object. In practice, this term is used to refer to an interpersonal relationship that is predicated on spiritual, objective, or nonemotional grounds. In certain Jewish forms of culture, for example, the father's authority rests primarily on his status as an exponent of the religious and scholarly tradition, rather than on the status of comforter, nurse, or donor of material or emotional comforts. Insofar as is possible his personality is delibidinized.

**delictive acts**   Offenses against the law.

**Delilah syndrome**   Promiscuity in a woman for whom seduction of the partner is equated with rendering him weak or helpless, something she would like to have achieved with her dominating and exploitative father.

**delinquency**   Behavior by a juvenile that is in violation of the criminal law; behavior that if occurring in an adult would be considered a crime. No uniformly acceptable definition of either delinquency or crime is possible by reason of the fact that the line between what is normal and what is criminal, deviant, immoral, or improper varies from state to state, from country to country, from culture to culture, and from one time to another. Further, the age at which an offense is defined as crime rather than delinquency is by no means fixed; under certain conditions, certain times, in certain regions, it may be as low as 14 years or as high as 21 years. In the case of juvenile offenders, moreover, there has been a tendency to broaden the definition of delinquency to include violations of regulations that would not ordinarily be considered crimes, such as truancy and running away from home.

By reason of the shifting and uncertain definition of what constitutes delinquency, it has been difficult to gather reliable data on its incidence, and it has proved impossible to pinpoint a specific, single cause for delinquent behavior. In any one juvenile offender, it may well be that a genetic, biological, psychological, or social factor has been of paramount significance in producing the behavior that is identified as delinquency. Yet even in the individual youth such behavior is much more likely to be the result of many factors, and it is their simultaneous action at a particular period of the offender's life that has been crucial in the evolution of that behavior.

All in all, it is generally agreed that delinquents or juvenile offenders resemble their nondelinquent peers psychologically and psychodynamically more than they differ from them. The number who suffer from a clear-cut psychiatric disorder or from mental retardation is small, notwithstanding the many popular misconceptions to the contrary.

**delinquent, defective**   *Obs.* A juvenile offender who is mentally retarded; used more often in a legal than in a medical or clinical context, to give recognition to the special needs of the mental retardate who happens to enter into the criminal justice system.

**délire**   (F. "delirium") A nebulous term, which sometimes refers to *delirium*, at other times to *delusion* or to *compulsion* (qq.v.). In general, the term could best be described as referring to a complex or system of ideas that forms a prominent part of the patient's mental condition.

**délire à quatre**   (F. "quadruple insanity") A psychiatric constellation, usually consisting of systematized delusions of persecution, involving four people. The delusions are found first in one person, and then are taken over, as in a contagious disease, by a second, third, and fourth person. See *induced psychotic disorder*.

**délire chronique**   In the French nomenclature, paranoid states without deterioration of personality. They are subdivided into *focused*, with a single delusional theme, and *unfocused*, in which several areas of mental activity are affected. See *paranoia completa*.

**délire crapuleux**   (F. "dissolute delirium") Delirium tremens.

**délire de négation**   Nihilistic delusion. See *Cotard syndrome*; *negation, delusion of*; *nihilism*.

**délire d'emblée**   (F. "delirium at one blow") A delusion that is fully formed and developed at the time of its first appearance, equivalent to the autochthonous or primordial delusion of other systems. See *autochthonous delusion*.

**délire d'énormité**   (F. "mania of vastness") Delusion of grandeur; *megalomania* (q.v.).

**délire ecmnesique**   (F. "ecmnesic delirium") See *ecmnesia*. Pitres's term for preoccupation with events that transpired years before. He describes the condition in conjunction with hysteria, pointing out that the patient in this state lives almost entirely in the past.

**délire en partie double**   (F. "double-entry delirium") Induced "insanity"; folie à deux. See *induced psychotic disorder.*

**délire terminal**   See *hysteria.*

**deliria oneirica**   *Obs.* "These deliria are constituted of scenes from dreams, changing, varied, and uninterrupted, the subject being as if he were in a somnambulic dream. These occur generally at night, but sometimes they continue after waking. On recovery the patient has no recollection of his delirium" (Bianchi, L. *A Text-Book of Psychiatry*, 1906).

**delirium**   A cognitive disorder with relatively global impairment, consisting of deficits of attention, arousal, consciousness, memory, orientation, perception, and speech or language. Also frequent are changes in the sleep-wakefulness cycle and abnormal psychomotor activity. These clinical features are accompanied by diffuse EEG abnormality, which may reflect reduced synthesis of various neurotransmitters in the brain, particularly acetylcholine.

Onset is typically rapid (in a matter of hours or days), and course is rapidly fluctuating. Ordinarily the condition is reversible. Usually, delirium is a hypoactive disorder and difficult to distinguish from dementia. The description of hyperactive delirium in terms of excitement and agitation stems from the florid clinical stereotype manifested chiefly in younger patients.

The most common causes are medications, drugs (delirium may occur as part of intoxication by or withdrawal from psychoactive substances such as alcohol and the amphetamines), infections, avitaminoses, endocrinopathies, and metabolic disturbances; but delirium can occur in the course of any brain disorder. Specific groups have been found to be at particularly high risk for the development of delirium: the elderly, children, post cardiotomy patients, burn patients, patients with preexisting brain damage, and patients with drug addiction. See *clouding of consciousness; confusional state, acute.*

Delirium includes a diversity of neuropsychiatric states, other names for which include acute brain syndrome with psychosis, acute confusional state, acute reversible psychosis, *dysergastic reaction*, exogenous psychosis, infective-exhaustive psychosis, metabolic encephalopathy, oneiric state, reversible cognitive dysfunction, toxic encephalopathy. Greek and Roman writers used phrenitis to refer to delirium and recognized it as one of the three main types of mental disorder (the other two being mania and melancholia).

Delirium at one time was used in a general way to indicate insanity, psychopathy, and almost any psychopathologic manifestation; now obsolete, such usage explains the appellations persecutory delirium (paranoia), touching delirium (compulsive touching), etc.

**delirium, emotional**   Morel's term for the mental state in which the patient unqualifiedly accepts a false idea.

**delirium, initial**   *Obs.* A delirious reaction of toxic-infectious origin in which delirium appears before the fever is at its height. The term *fever delirium* is similarly used to indicate a delirious reaction occurring at the height of the fever, while *collapse delirium* is sometimes used for delirium following high fever.

**delirium, metamorphosis**   *Obs.* The state in which the patient believes that his or her body is transformed into that of a beast.

**delirium, micromaniacal**   The delusion that one is a little child or a dwarf with shrunken limbs.

**delirium, subacute**   "A syndrome in which incoherence of thought, speech and movement appear together with perplexity, in a setting of clouding of consciousness, fluctuating in degree. The state may follow a typical delirium or appear independently. It may persist over a considerable period, weeks or months, outlasting the signs of the underlying physical illness, but always ending in recovery" (Mayer-Gross, W. et al. *Clinical Psychiatry*, 1960).

**delirium ambitiosum**   (L. "conceited delirium") *Obs. Megalomania* (q.v.).

**delirium è potu**   (L. "delirium from drinking") Delirium tremens; used by some to refer to pathological intoxication. See *alcoholic intoxication.*

**delirium ebriosorum**   (L. "delirium of drunkards") Delirium tremens.

**delirium ferox**   (L. "wild, savage, fierce") A psychiatric state characterized by violence.

**delirium grave** Collapse delirium. Also used by some to refer to delirious mania (*Bell mania*).

**delirium mite** (L. "mild, calm, gentle") A mental state characterized by low, delirious muttering. See *muttering delirium*.

**delirium mussitans** *Muttering delirium* (q.v.).

**delirium of interpretation** Sérieux and Capgras suggest that there are but two forms of paranoia. One is the *delirium of interpretation*, characterized by delusions of persecution; the other is the *delirium of revindication*, which has to do with a delusional organization based upon the urgency to gain justice for alleged offenses perpetrated against the patient. *Delirium* in this sense signifies a delusional, not a delirious state.

**delirium palingnosticum** The delusion that what one is experiencing in the present is a repetition of past experiences. See *déjà fait; déjà vu.*

**delirium sine delirio** Delirium tremens without hallucinations; alcohol withdrawal state that has not progressed to the full picture of delirium tremens.

**delirium tremens** Alcohol withdrawal delirium; delirium with onset during withdrawal from alcohol, often precipitated by intercurrent infection or injury.

The syndrome begins suddenly with fever, rapid pulse, leukocytosis, profuse perspiration, headache, anorexia, nausea, weakness, and dehydration. Along with the tremor, ataxia and hyperreflexia are seen, and all these appear to be due to an encephalosis involving mainly the fronto-ponto-cerebellar pathways. Increased cerebrospinal fluid pressure and increased globulin in the cerebrospinal fluid are usual, and in about 50% of cases a mild transitory albuminuria is seen. Epileptiform convulsions may also occur; these *rum fits*, as they are sometimes called, are probably due to pyridoxine (vitamin $B_6$) deficiency.

The delirium itself begins within a few days after onset of the disorder. Persecutory delusions are common and are usually in reference to a gang of the same sex or some obvious castration fear. These delusions may lead to suicide or homicide. Illusions are frequent and are easily suggested. Visual hallucinations are the most common of the hallucinatory elements, and these are typically of animals, such as snakes or rats, which symbolize mainly sexual fears (pink

elephants, incidentally, are most uncommon). Haptic hallucinations, of animals crawling over the skin, are also seen, but many of these are probably illusions based on paresthesiae. Auditory hallucinations, when they occur, are usually of a derogatory or homosexual nature. In the midst of the delirium, disorientation is marked; there is loss of attention and impairment of memory, most marked for recent memory. There is an incontinence of emotions—panic, anxiety, and terror most commonly, although some few show euphoria or indifference to their hallucinations and illusions. Misidentification is common, and patients are highly suggestible and can easily be made to confabulate.

The delirium usually lasts 3 to 6 days; the patient usually has amnesia for the delirium and frequently returns to his pattern of heavy drinking and thus there is often an early repetition of the syndrome. Auditory hallucinations usually indicate that the course will be prolonged. In uncomplicated cases, death is rare (3% to 4%). If there is not full recovery, there is usually progression into a Korsakoff syndrome (in about 15% of cases).

The pathological picture consists of nuclear destruction of the nerve cells, with all degrees of granular degeneration and disintegration of the nuclei. In most patients, the cortex is mainly affected, but in those tending clinically to progress into a *Korsakoff psychosis* (q.v.), the brain stem is affected to a greater degree.

Terms formerly used for delirium tremens include enomania, oinomania, the *horrors*, and *Saunders-Sutton syndrome.*

**delta alcoholism** The usual type of alcoholism seen in France and wine-drinking countries, characterized by increased tolerance, adaptive cell metabolism, and withdrawal symptoms, but rather than typical loss of control the delta alcoholic is unable to go on the "water wagon" for even 1 or 2 days without withdrawal symptoms. This type of alcoholism is also known as inveterate drinking.

Some would include herein the French category *alcoolisation*, the regular (usually daily) consumption of relatively large amounts of alcohol that results in a general undermining of health and a shortened life span, but no specific complications and no physical or psychological dependence. See *alcoholism.*

**delta EEG activity** See *sleep.*

**delta rhythm or wave**   See *electroencephalogram.*

**delta sleep**   See *sleep.*

**delta TSH**   The maximal TSH (thyroid-stimulating hormone) response to exogenous doses of TRH (thyrotropin-releasing hormone). The delta TSH is blunted in approximately 25% of patients with depression, and failure of the response to normalize with clinical recovery may be predictive of relapse.

**delusion**   A false belief that is firmly maintained even though it is contradicted by social reality. While it is true that some superstitions and religious beliefs are held despite the lack of confirmatory evidence, such culturally engendered concepts are not considered delusions. What is characteristic of the delusion is that it is *not* shared by others; rather, it is an idiosyncratic and individual misconception or misinterpretation.

Further, it is a thinking disorder of enough import to interfere with the subject's functioning, since in the area of his delusion he no longer shares a consensually validated reality with other people.

Like hallucinations, delusions are condensations of perceptions, thoughts, and memories and can be interpreted much the same as hallucinations and dreams. Delusions are misjudgments of reality based on projection. The sequence of events in the form of delusions is often seen to be as follows: the patient's relationship to objects is an archaic, ambivalent one; he attempts to incorporate the object, which then becomes a part of his own ego; the object is then reprojected into the external world and becomes the persecutor. Persecutory delusions thus represent projections of the patient's bad conscience; since the superego (conscience) is usually an introjected object of the same sex, the struggle against the superego represents also a struggle against the patient's homosexuality. The imagined persecutors, however, not only threaten and punish the patient; often also they are perceived as tempters who lead the patient into sin or weaken his potency. "This can be explained by the fact that...the hallucinations and delusions of reference represent not only the superego but also, at the same time, the (ambivalent) loved object; the sexual wish for this object is perceived as a destructive sexual influence that emanates from him" (Fenichel, O. *The Psychoanalytic Theory of Neurosis,* 1945). See *paranoia.*

## CLASSIFICATION OF DELUSIONS

Nonexistence: nihilism; nihilistic delusion; délire de négation

  of being dead: necromimesis

  of not having a body: Cotard's syndrome; acenesthesia

  of memory or orientation being lost: negativistic amnesia

  if one stops, so will the world: ergasiophobia

  denial of existing body change, illness, defect: anosognosia

Involving one's body: somatopsychic delusion

  of being beautiful: callomania

  of being physically deformed: dysmorphomania; dysmorphophobia; dismemberment complex

  part(s) of one's body are larger: macromania; macrosomatognosia; délire dénormité

  part(s) of one's body are smaller: micromania; micromaniacal delirium; microsomatognosia

  that one's penis is small or has shrunken or retreated into one's abdomen: koro; small-penis complex

  of having been changed into a woman: eviration

  that one's sex has changed: metamorphosis sexualis paranoia

  that one has a double: heutoscopy

  of infestation: dermatozoic delusion; Ekbom's syndrome; parasitophobia

  of animals crawling under the skin: formication

  of having a vile or repugnant odor: automysophobia; autodysosmophobia

  that one has changed into an animal (or, less common, that one can change others into an animal): delirium of metamorphosis; metamorphosis delusion; melancholia zoanthropia; zoanthropy

  into a cat: galeanthropy

  into a wolf: lycanthropy; lycomania; insania lupina; melancholia canina

  into a horse: hippanthropy

  into a dog: cynanthropy; melancholia canina

Involving self or personality: autopsychic delusion

  of loss of memory: negativistic amnesia

  déjà fait: delirium palingnosticum

  of having become another person: appersonation; appersonification

  with a religious content: hieromania

  of guilt, sinning, having committed some unpardonable sin: enosimania

  of grandiose ability (special mission or purpose): delusion of omnipotence; megalomania; ambitious mania; Caesar mania; delirium grandiosum; folie (or délire) ambitieuse; Napoleon complex; cosmic identification; délire dénormité; delirium ambitiosum; expansive delusion

  when delusion is clearly contradicted by reality: delusion of orientation; double orientation

  of grandiose identity:

  of being God: theomania

  of being the universe: cosmic identification

  of being of divine or celestial origin: uranomania

  of being of distinguished or royal parentage: Mignon delusion; family romance

  of being of superior intelligence: sophomania

  of being loved by another: aidoimania; delusional loving; erotomania; Clérambault complex; phantom lover syndrome

Involving the outside world: allopsychic delusion

  of having an imaginary companion: Doppelganger

*continued*

### CLASSIFICATION OF DELUSIONS CONTINUED

of one's spouse or sexual partner having been unfaithful: conjugal paranoia; delusion of infidelity; Othello syndrome; virginity scruple

of persecution, harrassment, libel, slander, undue influence, external control: delirium of interpretation; delusional perception; self-referential delusion; misomania; sensitiver Beziehungswahn; Wahnstimmung

of being watched: delusion of observation

that being wronged warrants legal redress: litigious mania; delirium of revindication; reformist delusion

that one's mind is controlled by an outside agency: Clérambault-Kandinsky complex

that one's thoughts are influenced by others: constraint of thought

of possession by evil spirit, of being poisoned by the devil: cacodaemonomania

that one is to be subjected to homosexual attack: Kempf disease; homosexual panic

of being influenced by an imposter: delusion of false recognition

that a known person has been replaced by an imposter: Capgras syndrome; illusion of doubles; illusions of false recognition

that a persecutor has adopted the form of a known person: Frégoli phenomenon; illusion of a negative double; intermetamorphosis syndrome

**delusion, partial**  A delusion about which the subject has doubts, seen frequently in subjects who are recovering from an acute delusional state in which the false idea was firmly held.

**delusion, secondary**  A delusion that is based upon a primary one. "When the patient is convinced that the physician wants to murder him and after taking medicine he feels indisposed, then it is a conclusion, based on logical probability, that the physician has prescribed poison (secondary delusion)" (Bleuler, E. *Dementia praecox; or the Group of Schizophrenias*, 1911).

**delusion of grandeur**  In the *PSE* glossary (see *Present State Examination*), these delusions are divided into *delusions of grandiose ability* (the subject believes he has been chosen by destiny or some higher power for a special mission or purpose) and *delusions of grandiose identity* (the subject believes he is rich, titled, famous, or related to royalty or prominent people). See *megalomania*.

**delusion of guilt**  The conviction that one is responsible for adverse conditions, usually combined with the feeling of a need to expiate or atone for the suffering that others have had to endure because of one's actions. Delusions of guilt are prominent in severe depressions.

**delusion of influence**  The conviction that one is being controlled by outside forces beyond one's control.

**delusion of observation**  Delusion of reference; delusion of being watched. See *reference, ideas of*.

**delusion of poverty**  The conviction that one is penniless, without resources. Delusions of poverty may be seen in any depression, but they appear to be particularly frequent in the delusional states of old age (late paraphrenia).

**delusion of reference**  *Self-referential delusion*; the conviction that whatever happens in the world has an intended meaning for the subject: if there happens to be a group of people standing on the street corner, the person is convinced they are talking about him; the houselights dim in an electrical storm, but the person is convinced it was intended for him, either to annoy him or send him a message, etc. The delusion of reference is typically a part of a paranoid persecutory system and the patient misinterprets anything that happens in reality as a sign that his imagined persecutors are about to succeed in harming him. See *reference, ideas of*.

**delusional disorders**  Paranoid disorders. See *paranoia*.

**delusional loving**  *Erotomania* (q.v.).

**delusional mood**  *Wahnstimmung* (q.v.).

**demand**  See *feeding, self-demand*.

**demand language**  See *language disability*.

**demand reduction**  Educational, treatment, and rehabilitation efforts directed at reducing the desire for something (most commonly, psychoactive drugs).

**dement**  A person with an absence or reduction of intellectual faculties in consequence of known organic brain disease. Earlier writers used the term for deteriorated schizophrenics. Thus, the paranoid dements of Kraepelin are those with unstable and unorganized delusions, apparent marked reduction in intellectual capacities, and a break in psychic unity.

**dementia**  A cognitive disorder with amnesia, aphasia, apraxia, agnosia, and defects in executive functioning. The major forms of dementia are dementia caused by Alzheimer disease; vascular dementia; dementia due to head trauma, to Pick disease, to Creutzfeldt-Jakob disease, to Huntington disease, and to Parkinson disease; and substance-induced persisting dementia (as with alcohol, inhalants, and the sedative-hypnotic-anxiolytic family of drugs).

The most common mix of pathologies in the brains of persons with dementia is the combination of Alzheimer disease and cerebral infarcts.

Characteristic is a dysmnesic syndrome progressing to full dementia, with deterioration of previously acquired intellectual abilities of sufficient severity to interfere with social or occupational functioning and to impair the patient's capacity to meet the ordinary demands of living. Intellectual disintegration is manifested in impairment of memory, abstract thinking, or judgment, and defects in counting, calculation, and general knowledge (any or all of which are often termed *cognitive deficits*). In addition, disintegration of feeling and striving as well as personality change or impaired impulse control typically appear at some point in the development of the disorder. See *organic mental disorders*.

In past years, dementia had various meanings. It was once synonymous with madness, insanity, and lunacy; in the early part of the 17th century it was synonymous with delirium. Nowadays it tends to be imited to primary memory loss on an organic basis, and in the usage of at least some it connotes irreversibility. *Deterioration* also refers to loss of intellectual faculties, but without intimating a specific cause and without stressing the permanency of the change. *Regression*, on the other hand, emphasizes reversibility, and with Freud the term came to refer primarily to emotional disturbances rather than to loss of intellectual ability. See *schizophrenic dementia; organic syndrome*.

**dementia, acute** *Obs.* Anergic stupor, such as seen in catatonic stupor and hysterical trance states; in the past it was considered a distinct nosological entity.

**dementia, primary** Endogenous dementia, such as senile and presenile dementias of the Alzheimer type.

**dementia, relative** See *higher dementia*.

**dementia, simple depressive** *Stuporous dementia*, one of Kraepelin's subdivisions of schizophrenia. The syndrome is characterized by depression, resembling that seen in the depressive phase of manic-depressive disorder; the projection mechanism appears to a greater or lesser degree. The condition often leads toward periodicity, but not with the same sharpness that marks clear-cut depressive states.

**dementia, simple senile** See *Alzheimer disease*.

**dementia apoplectica** Apoplectic attacks, associated with *cerebra arteriosclerosis* (q.v.), may be due to hemorrhage or to softening of brain tissue. Usually there are prodromes of variable duration; they may appear as headache, dizziness, fainting attacks, together with ideational and emotional changes. Depending upon the nature and severity of the arteriosclerotic process, the apoplectic ("stroke") condition may be followed by diffuse cerebral atrophy, giving rise to the organic type of dementia. Clinically the last condition is known as apoplectic dementia. See *cerebrovascular accident*.

**dementia dialytica** An aluminum-induced encephalopathy, with progressive mental deterioration, paranoid ideas, and psychotic behaviors occurring in patients undergoing dialysis; accompanying neurological signs include dysarthria, dysnomia, dyspraxia, and seizures. All the foregoing are aggravated during and immediately following dialysis, and within 6 months of onset of the syndrome most patients have died.

**dementia infantilis** *childhood disintegrative disorder* (q.v.).

**dementia paralytica** (L. "paralytic dementia") See *general paresis*.

**dementia paranoides gravis** "Those paranoid morbid states, which begin with simple delusions, but which as time goes on terminate in severe so-called deterioration, a *peculiar disintegration of the psychic life*" (Kraepelin, E. *Psychiatrie*, 1893).

The *milder* type of paranoid schizophrenia, hallucinatory feeblemindedness, Kraepelin called *dementia paranoides mitis*, when the patient has hallucinations and "the substance of the personality seems to be less seriously damaged." Today the term is used only occasionally and even then not in the diagnostic sense assigned to it by Kraepelin.

**dementia paratonita progressiva** A. Bernstein's term for catatonic schizophrenia, which he also sometimes called *paratonia progressiva*.

**dementia praecocissima** According to DeSanctis, this condition, occurring in young children, sometimes as early as the fourth year, is characterized by a more or less abrupt appearance of catatonia. Stereotypy, fixed postures, negativism, angry outbursts, echolalia, and emotional blunting are particularly noticeable. Marked intellectual deterioration is present.

Kanner believed that dementia praecocissima includes a variety of pathological conditions. "Some of the cases are indistinguishable from childhood schizophrenia (Bromberg), others represent rapidly progressing brain diseases (Lutz; Schilder).

"Rapid disorganization after a fairly normal start is encountered in small children on rare occasions and offers baffling problems of diagnosis. Some cases prove to belong to the group of Heller's disease (*dementia infantilis*), some few are cases of Tay-Sachs disease with or without the characteristic eye ground findings, others are instances of even more unusual cerebral disease processes" (Kanner, L. *Child Psychiatry*, 1948). See *developmental disorders, pervasive*.

**dementia praecox** A term coined by Morel in 1857 to describe those psychoses ("vesania") with a poor prognosis, i.e., those ending in deterioration (dementia) and incurability. Praecox refers to the fact that the onset of the disorders occurs early in life—typically in adolescence. In the years following the introduction of this term, various symptom complexes were described that later were included in the group, dementia praecox.

Thus Kahlbaum described catatonia, Hecker described hebephrenia, Pick and Sommer described simple deterioration, and Zieber described paranoia. In 1896, Kraepelin made the important differentiation between manic-depressive psychosis and dementia praecox, and he included the aforementioned entities as subgroups of dementia praecox. He, too, emphasized the poor prognosis in dementia praecox and believed that those cases that could be cured permanently or arrested for very long periods were really instances of manic-depressive psychosis.

In 1911, Bleuler introduced the term *schizophrenia*, which in present-day psychiatry has largely replaced the term dementia praecox. Bleuler rejected the latter term because, in his experience, dementia was not a constant end product of the disorder (or group of disorders), and because at least 40% of cases did not manifest gross disturbances until after their 25th year.

Some contemporary authorities, and particularly European psychiatrists, continue to use the term dementia praecox in a fairly restricted sense to refer to "nuclear" or "process" schizophrenia, i.e., unquestionable cases with a high tendency to deterioration and little tendency to remission or recovery. See *schizophrenia*.

**dementia praesenilis** See *senium praecox*.

**dementia pugilistica** *Boxer's dementia* (q.v.).

**demography** The statistical study of populations, including births, marriages, mortality, health, geographic distribution, and population shifts.

**demonolatry** Worship of a demon or devil.

**demonomania** Morbid dread of demons; *entheomania*. Freud noted that the original pleasurable affect associated with an act, such as masturbation, may first be repressed, then transformed into anxiety, which contains features of punishment in it and brings dread of an evil spirit as the next stage.

**demophobia** Morbid fear of crowds; ochlophobia. See *agoraphobia*.

**demorphinization** The process of gradual or rapid withdrawal of morphine in the treatment of addicts.

**Demosthenes complex** The neurotic need to achieve mastery over inferiority feelings through words and language in the process of speaking. See *overcompensation*.

**demyelination** Destruction of the myelin sheaths of nerve fibers. There is a large group of demyelinating diseases of the nervous system, characterized by foci of demyelination. These foci are usually in the white matter and vary in size, shape, distribution, and in the acuteness of the pathological process. Classification of these disorders is unsatisfactory; their etiology is unknown, their differential pathology is indistinct, and clinical forms are often transitional, presenting features common to more than one of the specific diseases recognized. The four major forms, divided on the basis of clinico-pathologic manifestations, are acute *disseminated encephalomyelitis* (following acute infections); disseminated myelitis with optic neuritis (*Devic disease*); *multiple sclerosis* (disseminated sclerosis); and *diffuse sclerosis* (Schilder disease, Baló disease, etc.) (qq.v.).

**demyelination, concentric** Baló disease. See *diffuse sclerosis*.

**denarcissism** The state of being unselfish, altruistic.

**dendrite** The principal signal reception and processing site on the neuron. The dendrites of each pyramidal neuron are highly branched and contain thousands of synapses made by axons from almost as many neurons. They are thin (~ 1 μm in diameter), and many are decorated with thousands of fine, twiglike projections, the dendritic *spines,* where synaptic signals impinging on the dendrite are first processed. The dendrite contains highly specialized receptors that recognize and bind the neurotransmitter released by *exocytosis* from the terminal *axon* of an adjacent *neuron* (qq.v.). The nerve impulse thereby generated is conducted to the axon of its own neuron. See *synapse.*

Dendrites are a major source of peptides released in the brain. Some of them act at presynaptic terminals and modulate transmitter release retrogradely. Others act on the cell of origin as well as on neighboring cells to exert autoregulatory effects.

Much of the processing machinery is contained in the *postsynaptic density (PSD),* a highly organized biochemical apparatus attached to the cytosolic surface of the postsynaptic dendritic membrane. PSD contains neurotransmitter receptors and associated scaffolding proteins and enzymes; it organizes signal transduction pathways at the postsynaptic membrane. Each neuronal type has a specialized and highly regulated set of dendritic, voltage-gated, ion channels, which change during development and can be modulated by neurotransmitters. Dendrites perform the neuron's computation, receiving and adding up the signals coming in from other neurons through the synapses. Dendrites respond to signals by strengthening or weakening their synapses; their morphology, synapses, and ionic channels undergo constant activity-dependent modulation.

**dendrophilia, dendrophily**   Love of trees, which may be phallic symbols.

**deneutralization**   Resexualization or reaggressivization, as a result of which energy that had previously been neutralized and thereby made available to the ego in noninstinctual form for its secondary-process work reappears as overtly sexual or aggressive. Thus, what had been an aid to the ego in solving its problems has become, again, a problem that the ego must solve. See *neutralization.*

**denial**   Refusal to admit the reality of, disavowal of the truth of, refusal to acknowledge the presence or existence of. Known also as *negation,* denial is a primitive *defense* (q.v.), that centers on splitting. Because denial must ignore data presenting themselves to the perceptory system and garnered by the memory apparatus, such a defense can operate only in the undeveloped, infantile psyche, or in persons whose ego is weak or disturbed (as in the psychoses), and even so, denial succeeds best against single internal perceptions of a painful nature. Denial and negation are also used, more loosely, to refer to any form of *resistance* (q.v.).

The person with narcissistic personality disorder denies his dependency by identifying himself with his idealized self-images. He typically disavows or negates disappointing experiences or "slides around the meaning of events in order to place the self in a better light," leading to a shaky subjective experience of ideas. In antisocial personality disorder of the passive parasitic type, the subject denies aggression and transforms it into ruthless exploitation.

**deniers**   See *anxiety typology.*

**denotation**   See *connotation.*

**dentate gyrus**   Gray matter composed of three layers situated above the hippocampal gyrus in the medial frontal lobe. The molecular layer is continuous with the *hippocampus* (q.v.) in the hippocampal fissure. The granular layer consists of tightly packed spherical neurons, the granule cells, the axons of which pass through the polymorphic layer and terminate on the dendrites of pyramidal cells in the hippocampus. The *perforant path,* the key interconnection between hippocampus and neocortex, terminates in the dentate gyrus.

**dentate nuclei**   See *cerebellum.*

**dentatorubral-pallidoluysianatrophy**   *DRPLA*(q.v.). See *trinucleotide repeat.*

**deolepsy**   Delusion of being possessed by a god.

**deontology**   A theory of ethics that holds that what is morally right is independent of the ends for judging the means and that it is incorrect to define morality in terms of ends and means. Like utilitarian theories of ethics, deontologic theories may be monistic (holding that there is a single rule or principle from which all others may be derived) or pluralistic (holding that there is more than one basic and irreducible principle), and they may focus on acts or on rules that encompass classes of acts. See *utilitarianism; utilitarianism, act.*

**deorality**  A state in which instinctual activity, formerly connected with the oral region, is expressed through some other agency. The pleasure of suckling at the breast may in later life assume the form of a pleasure in being morally dependent upon a maternal person.

**deoxyribonucleic acid**  *DNA*. See *chromosome*.

**depatterning**  D. E. Cameron used this term almost synonymously with regressive ECT. He used intensive ECT and prolonged sleep with chlorpromazine and barbiturates to treat chronic paranoids.

**dependence, drug**  *Substance dependence; chemical dependence*; a biopsychosocial syndrome associated with the use of a psychoactive drug (or class of drugs) and characterized by behavioral and other responses that always include giving use of that drug a sharply higher priority over other behaviors that once had significantly greater value. The user experiences an intense desire to take the drug on a continuous or periodic basis in order to experience its psychic effects, and sometimes to avoid the discomfort of its absence. Although often used interchangeably, addiction and drug dependence are not the same. Addiction refers to a behavioral disorder manifested in craving for and repetitive dosing with a drug; dependence is a physiological effect of a drug and typically develops in an addicted person as a complication of repetitive dosing with the drug. Repeated drug exposures often produce tolerance to the drug, but they can also produce sensitization or reverse tolerance. See *addiction*.

Drug dependence consists of a cluster of cognitive, behavioral, and physiologic phenomena, not all of which are necessarily present in each instance, or to the same degree. DSM-III had used the broad concept developed by Griffith Edwards and Milton Gross, which included social, behavioral, and biological components. DSM-IV requires that three or more of the following be present: indications of tolerance (e.g., need for increased amounts of the substance to achieve intoxication or the desired effect) or withdrawal (e.g., taking the substance to relieve or avoid withdrawal symptoms); the substance is often taken in large amounts or over a longer period than intended; *salience* of drug-seeking behavior relative to other important priorities, e.g., use of the substance consumes an inordinate amount of the user's time in activities necessary to obtain it, use it, or recover from its effects, or important social, occupational, or recreational activities are replaced or reduced by use of the substance; persistent desire (*craving*) or unsuccessful attempts to reduce or control use; and continuation of drinking despite awareness that use of the substance is likely to have caused or exacerbated a persistent or recurrent physical or psychological problem.

Common to many addicted persons who develop drug dependence is an inability to inactivate the dopaminergic fibers in the mesolimbic system which project to the nucleus accumbens in the limbic forebrain. The development of tolerance and addiction to morphine is thought to involve antiopioid systems that include some types of glutamate receptor.

The substantial numbers of persons who are addicted to and develop dependence on both alcohol and other drugs suggest that there is a generalized vulnerability to substance dependence. Some authorities disagree, however, believing that there is a specificity of the genes contributing to that vulnerability. In adolescents and young adults, the triad of alcohol, marijuana, and cocaine abuse is frequent. See *heritability*.

**dependence, oral**  The unconscious wish for maternal protection, to be encompassed by the mother, to regain the peace, protection, and security of her sheltering arms. This stems from the original intense and forgotten gratifications of the infantile nursing period, when the infant's prehensile mouth anchored it to the mother's nipple and breast. To the child, to be fed means to be loved, i.e., to be protected, ergo, to be secure.

**dependence, physical**  A state of physiologic adaptation (neuroadaptation) to regular intake of a psychoactive substance, manifested in development of tolerance and emergence of a withdrawal or abstinence syndrome when administration of the drug is suspended or the drug is displaced from its site of action. The *withdrawal syndrome* (q.v.) may be relieved in whole or in part by readministration of the drug. The psychological and physical symptoms and signs of the withdrawal syndrome are characteristic for each drug type and for the specific biological system, or species. See *neuroadaptation*.

**dependence, psychological** Habituation; a condition in which repetitive use of a psychoactive substance produces a subjective sense of need for that drug, either to produce pleasure or to avoid negative effects associated with abstinence from the drug. The sense of need is sometimes referred to as an intense craving for, or a compulsion to take, the drug(s).

**dependence potential** The risk that the user of a psychoactive substance will develop psychological or physical dependence on it. The dependence potential can often be assessed in animal experiments in a preclinical phase of drug testing.

**dependence-producing drug** A drug that is capable of producing a state of psychic or physical dependence in the user. The characteristics of the state of drug dependence, once developed, vary with the type of drug involved. The drug may be used medically or nonmedically without necessarily producing such a state.

**dependency** State of being reliant on others. Dependency reflects needs for mothering, love, affection, shelter, protection, security, food, warmth, etc. In Horney's terminology, morbid dependency is a form of self-effacement manifested in a compulsive need to surrender to and unite with a stronger person.

**dependency, alcohol** See *alcoholism*.

**dependency, drug** See *dependence, drug*.

**dependency assumption** See *basic assumptions group*.

**dependent bonding** See *codependency*.

**dependent personality (disorder)** Characteristically, the dependent personality type places responsibility for his own life onto others, subordinates his own needs to theirs, has persisting low self-esteem, and cannot tolerate being alone.

**depersonalization** A nonspecific syndrome in which the subject feels that he has lost his personal identity, that he is different or strange or unreal. Derealization, the feeling that the environment is also strange or unreal, is usually part of the syndrome. Other frequent symptoms are mood changes (e.g., dejection, apathy, bewilderment, or a feeling of emotional emptiness or numbing); difficulty in organizing, collecting, and arranging thoughts; and cephalic paresthesiae (e.g., numbness of head or a feeling that the brain has been deadened). Depersonalization has been reported in depression, hysterical and dissociative states, schizoid personality, schizophrenia, toxic psychoses, temporal lobe epilepsy, and in states of fatigue. It most commonly occurs in the third and fourth decades and is more common in women. It may last for 1 or 2 years before disappearing spontaneously; it rarely responds to treatment of any sort. See *dissociative disorders*.

M. Roth (*Proceedings, Royal Society of Medicine 52,* 1959) has described a more specific syndrome, the *phobic anxiety-depersonalization neurosis* (sometimes also called pseudo-schizophrenic neurosis). In this neurosis, phobic anxiety is combined with depersonalization; the patient often complains of giddiness, swaying feelings, and fears of collapse or loss of self-control in public. Roth suggests that the neurosis may be at least in part related to some disorder of the temporal lobes, the limbic system, or the cerebral mechanisms regulating awareness. PET studies of brain metabolism do not suppport the primacy of temporal lobe phenomena in depersonalization; they suggest instead that more extensive associational brain networks, including the visual, somatosensory, and auditory processing pathways, are involved in addition to areas responsible for an integrated body schema.

It has also been suggested that depersonalization is a variant of endogenous depression and good response to treatment with imipramine has been reported. G. Langfeldt (*Proceedings, Royal Society of Medicine 53,* 1960) used the terms depersonalization and derealization to describe syndromes characterized by experiences of a particular type of disturbance of volition and the self that are found usually only in schizophrenia. Unlike similar phenomena in neurotic states, those in the schizophrenic are always experienced as originating outside the self, and the patient has no insight into his own condition.

When a person cannot feel his or her bodily senses, emotions are also difficult to recognize as such, and the person with depersonalization often complains of being emotionally numb. A rape victim, for example, described how she felt during the attack: "I didn't feel there, it was as though I was floating on the ceiling and watching everything happen. When I think about it now, I just feel numb." Depersonalization can be viewed as an unconscious control mechanism to quell or suppress (and repress) overwhelming affects like terror, horror, and helplessness. See *dissociative disorders*.

**depersonification** Being acknowledged as somebody else. In the depersonifying mother-child relationship, the narcissist's mother does not acknowledge the child as a person in his own right but instead casts the child as a representative of the parent's world. She sends the message that the child must become an adult or a quasi-parent—*adultomorphizatio n* (q.v.), with a *pseudomature* child the result.

The borderline's mother sends the message that any effort by the child to separate or *desymbiotize* will result in withdrawal of nurturance. Growth and development mean disaster; success means failure.

One form of depersonification is seen in the *parentified* child, where the child is cast in the role of the parent. See *role reversal*.

**depleted depression** According to Kohut, the reaction of an unhealthy self to disruption of a self-object relationship or a narcissistic insult; the self experiences the deepest anxiety one can experience, not fear of physical annihilation but fear of loss of humanness or psychological death (hence also called *disintegration anxiety*). See *autistic-contiguous position*.

**depolarization** Decrease in the resting membrane potential, which has an excitatory effect on the neuron in that it increases the cell's ability to generate an action potential. See *action potential; resting membrane potential*.

**depolarization block** A possible mechanism of action of neuroleptics, consisting of slowly developing changes in presynaptic dopamine terminals leading ultimately to a decrease in the firing rate of dopamine neurons. Feedback activation of presynaptic neurons—characterized by increased activity of tyrosine hydroxylase, increased dopamine turnover, and increased electrophysiological activity—occurs within hours of receptor blockade. It persists for days or weeks but is gradually replaced by reduction to (or below) baseline, with diminished tyrosine hydroxylase activity and dopamine turnover and the development of depolarization block in increasing numbers of neurons.

**Depo-Provera** Trade name for medroxyprogesterone acetate, an *antiandrogen* (q.v.).

**depopulation** Reducing the residents or population of an area, facility, etc.; in psychiatry, used particularly to refer to the shifting of patients from one system (e.g., psychiatric hospitalization) to another (e.g., the criminal justice system). See *chronic mentally ill*.

**depot neuroleptic** A long-acting form of antipsychotic drug that is administered parenterally, usually by intramuscular or subcutaneous injection, as maintenance therapy. Esterification of fluphenazine, for example, markedly extends the drug's duration of effect, and a single injection of fluphenazine decanoate may be effective in controlling symptoms for 2 or more weeks. Because the depot form of the drug is released slowly, over so long a period, each dose administered is typically much larger than that required when the drug is given by mouth 1 or more times a day. In consequence, such maintenance therapy is sometimes termed *megadose* treatment (q.v.).

**depressant, brain** Central nervous system (CNS) depressant, including alcohol, the barbiturates, methaqualone, chloral hydrate, GHB (gamma-hydroxybutyrate), and an enormous variety of other synthetic sedatives and hypnotics. These substances have in common the ability to cause a degree of drowsiness and sedation or pleasant relaxation, but they may also produce "disinhibition" and loss of learned behavioral control as a result of their depressant effect on higher centers of the brain, a property that accounts for the seemingly "stimulant" effects of alcohol. All such drugs have the potential to induce cross-tolerance and changes in the nervous system that lead to withdrawal syndromes, which can be life-threatening. "Minor tranquilizers" of the *benzodiazepine* (q.v.) type, such as diazepam and chlordiazepoxide, are probably best placed in the general depressant group, although they also have some distinctive features: the benzodiazepines have less potential to induce serious withdrawal states (possibly because they are much longer acting) and are generally far safer drugs in clinical practice than the barbiturates. See *sedatives/hypnotics*.

**depressio apathetica** *Obs.* See *anxietas praesenilis*.

**depression** A clinical syndrome consisting of a lowering of mood tone (feelings of painful dejection or an irritable mood), loss of interest or pleasure in comparison with the subject's premorbid state, psychomotor retardation or agitation, and difficulty in thinking or concentration. Complaints of fatigue or loss of energy and of feelings of worthlessness or guilt are common. The depressed patient often has recurrent thoughts of death, and a significant number of depressed patients attempt suicide or make plans to do so. Biological symptoms of depression include sleep disturbance (insomnia or hypersomnia), diurnal variation of mood, loss of appetite, loss of weight, constipation, loss of libido, and, in women, amenorrhea.

As used by the layman, depression typically refers only to the lowering of mood tone (dejection, sadness, gloominess, despair, etc.) See *affective disorders; depression mechanisms; depression, psychotic; involutional psychosis; manic-depressive psychosis; melancholia; psychoneurotic depression.*

**depression, atypical**　A depression characterized by mood reactivity, anxiety, and reverse vegetative signs (hyperphagia rather than appetite loss, hypersomnia rather than early awakening), leaden paralysis, and hypersensitivity to rejection. *Partial atypical syndrome* refers to patients with mood reactivity and only one of the other features; *full atypical syndrome* designates patients with mood reactivity and two or more of the associated features.

Atypical depressions may be preferentially responsive to monoamine oxidase inhibitors and resistant to tricyclic antidepressants.

**depression, classification of**　For the DSM-IV classification, see *depressive disorders.*

An older scheme after Kraepelin classified manias and depressions (or melancholias) under the general heading Affective Psychosis, as follows: (A) Manic-Depressive Psychosis: (1) Manic (a) hypomania; (b) acute mania; (c) delirious mania (Bell mania); (d) chronic mania; (2) Depressive (a) simple depression; (b) acute depression; (c) depressive stupor; (3) Periodical psychoses; (a) recurrent mania; (b) recurrent melancholia; (c) alternating insanity; (4) Mixed states; (a) maniacal stupor; (b) agitated depression; (c) unproductive mania; (d) depressive mania; (e) depression with flight of ideas; (f) akinetic mania; (g) perplexity state; (B) Involutional Melancholia: (1) depressed type (agitated depression); (2) paranoid type depression, primary. See *unipolar depression.*

**depression, psychotic**　Melancholia; in the 1968 revision of psychiatric nomenclature

(DSM-II) psychotic depressive reaction refers to those severely depressed patients with gross misinterpretation of reality (including delusions and hallucinations) who do not have a history of previous depressions or of marked mood swings, but whose symptoms are reactive (i.e., attributable to some identifiable experience) and of psychotic degree.

In DSM-III, a major depressive episode is more specifically identified as "with psychotic features" when there is gross impairment in reality testing, as manifested by hallucinations, delusions, mutism, or stupor.

**depression, recurrent**　A mood disorder characterized by more than one episode of depression. A patient who has had only one episode has a 50% chance of another; with two episodes, the risk increased to 50% to 90%; with three or more episodes, it rises above 90%.

**depression, secondary**　See *unipolar depression.*

**depression mechanisms**　Over the years, many theories of the mechanism of depression have been proposed. Most of them reflected the latest findings in studies of the pathophysiology of depression, and while some of them have been discarded—at least in part—they nonetheless highlight phenomena that occur in depression and which must, therefore, be explained by any theory of depression. Among the proposed mechanisms are the following:

1. Monoamine hypothesis (biogenic amine hypothesis): depression reflects an imbalance in noradrenaline or serotonin. This theory does not explain why the effects of antidepressants occur only after several weeks of treatment. It may be that changes in brain gene expression that are elicited only after chronic treatment might explain the delay of effects.

2. Neuropeptides: dysfunctions in growth hormone, in the thyroid axis, in opioid receptors, and in substance P have all been posited as central to depression.

3. Circadian regulation: abnormalities in the circadian regulation of sleep, temperature, and activity cycles.

4. Infectious agents, in particular, viruses.

5. Neuroimmune mediators: among the mechanisms of disease (such as necrosis, degeneration, and neoplasia), inflammation can best explain the highly variable waxing

and waning course of depression. *Cytokines* (q.v.) influence various CNS functions that are dysregulated in major depression— sleep, food intake, cognition, temperature, and neuroendocrine regulation.

6. Genetics: major depression is a familial disorder in which first-degree relatives carry a threefold increase in risk. Major depression has an estimated heritability of 31%–42%, which is much lower than the 70% heritability estimated for schizophrenia and bipolar disorder. No genetic linkage or association with depression has yet been confirmed. At present there are no linkage or association genetic findings that have been adequately confirmed and accepted.

**depression spectrum**  A type of major depression characterized by families in which males are alcoholic and females are depressed.

**depressive anxiety**  The specific anxiety observed in a person afflicted with depression. "The anxiety lest the good objects and, with them, the ego should be destroyed, or that they are in a state of disintegration, is interwoven with continuous and desperate efforts to save the good objects both internalized and external" (Klein, M. *Contributions to Psycho-analysis 1921–45*, 1948).

**depressive crash**  Abrupt onset of severe depression, usually in response to frustration or disappointment, as in acute depressive reaction of the hysteroid dysphoric to abandonment or rejection.

**depressive dementia**  Kraepelin's designation for a special subdivision of schizophrenia. The syndrome resembles that of simple depressive dementia, save that all symptoms are more intense and the course of the illness is protracted. Rarely used in the United States.

**depressive disorders**  A group of mood disorders, including major depressive disorder (major depression; manic-depressive disorder, depressed type) and dysthymic disorder.

The majority of depressed patients treated with SSRIs and selective SNRIs do not attain remission, perhaps because of their lack of effect on dopamine neurons. It has been suggested that there is a *dopamine dysfunction subtype* of depression, characterized by a poor response to antidepressants that act primarily on serotonergic or norepinephrine neurons.

#### PREVALENCE OF MOOD DISORDERS

| | PREVALENCE (IN %) | |
|---|---|---|
| DISORDER | LIFETIME | CURRENT |
| Major depressive episode | | |
| Any episode | 6 | 2.2 |
| Unipolar only | 5 | 1.8 |
| Bipolar | 1 | 0.4 |
| Dysthymia* | 3 | 1.6 |
| Any mood disorder | 8 | 5.1 |
| Subsyndromal depression | 7 | ? |

* Twenty-five percent of these have had double depression within the past six months; 50% have a lifetime diagnosis of double depression.

[*Source*: Reprinted with permission from Regier et al., *Archives of General Psychiatry 45*: 977, copyright American Medical Association, 1988.]

**depressive episode, major**  Major depression; *unipolar depression* (q.v.). Symptoms are those of *depression* (q.v.); in addition, DSM-IV describes "cross-sectional" symptom features that may occur in major depressive episodes that are part of bipolar disorder as well as those that occur in major depressive disorder. They are as follows:

1. Melancholic features—lack of pleasure in activities or lack of reactivity to usually pleasurable stimuli, depression regularly worse in the morning, early morning awakening, marked psychomotor retardation or agitation, anorexia or weight loss, excessive or inappropriate guilt; the quality of the depression is felt to be distinctly different from the sadness or grief that is part of bereavement.

2. Atypical features—mood reactivity, reverse vegetative symptoms, sensitivity to rejection.

3. Catatonic features—such as immobility (catalepsy, waxy flexibility) or stupor; extreme agitation; negativism; peculiarities of movement such as posturing, stereotypies, mannerisms, grimaces; echolalia or echopraxia.

**depressive neurosis**  See *psychoneurotic depression*.

**depressive personality (disorder)**  Characteristics of the person with depressive personality disorder: (1)quiet, passive, unassertive; (2) gloomy, pessimistic, cannot have fun; (3) self-critical, self-reproaching, self-derogatory; (4) skeptical, hypercritical, complaining; (5) conscientious, self-disciplining; (6) brooding, given to worrying;

(7) preoccupied with inadequacy, failure, and negative events. Depressive personality has similarities to but is distinct from dysthmic disorder. It lacks the persistent depressed mood and vegetative symptoms seen in dysthmic disorder and is expressed instead in personality traits or dispositions, often of a cognitive nature.

**depressive position**  A concept introduced by Melanie Klein (1935) to refer to the most mature form of psychological organization; it follows the paranoid-schizoid position and reaches a peak during the second half of the first year of life. (See *paranoid-schizoid position; separation-individuation*.) It is distinguished by a shift from part-object to whole-object relationships: mother and father are perceived as subjects and not merely as objects. Thoughts and feelings are experienced as personal creations, for which the child feels responsible. Together, these developments make it possible for the child to experience *guilt*, the pain that one feels in response to real or imagined harm that one has done to someone about whom one cares. This generates a new form of anxiety, that the child's anger has driven away or harmed the person(s) he or she loves (*abandonment depression*). Working through the depressive position results in the capacity to mourn; the child mourns separation from the mother, but that separation is necessary if he or she is to develop as an independent person and become capable of genuine intimacy. At the same time, primitive defenses such as splitting, idealization, omnipotence, and denial gradually decrease in intensity and the reality principle begins to replace the pleasure principle. Object permanency develops, and the child is then able to enter into the oedipal stage.

Failure to work through the depressive position (and, in consequence, the incapacity to mourn), is the result of persisting abandonment depression, a typical result of inadequate *communicative matching* or *fit* (qq.v.) between mother and child.

Contrary to Freud's view, Klein and her followers believe that object relationships exist from the very beginning of life and that the first dramatic psychic experience is the loss of unity with the mother at the time of birth. In arguing that working through of the depressive position is the central problem in development, Klein replaced the Oedipus complex with preoedipal trauma as the fundamental factor disposing to psychopathology.

**depressive spectrum disorder**  *DSD* (q.v.).

**depressive stupor**  See *stupor, benign*.

**deprivation**  Failure to meet adequately the needs or wants of another; denial or withdrawal of the physical or emotional supplies needed by another. Maternal deprivation refers to failure of the mother or caregiver to supply the child with appropriate emotional support and positive experience in interpersonal relationships. See *battered child syndrome; child neglect; maltreatment*.

**deprivation, thought**  *Blocking* (q.v.).

**deprivational dwarfism**  See *psychosocial dwarfism*.

**deprivative amentia**  Mental retardation (amentia) due to the lack of some constituent of the complete development of the brain. Among the several deprivative factors, three are well recognized. First, involvement of the endocrine glands, particularly the thyroid, associated with cretinism; second, malnutrition (nutritional amentia); third, lack of sensory stimuli (amentia due to sense deprivation, isolation amentia).

**deprogramming**  All those measures used to counteract the effects of brainwashing; reindoctrination of a subject in the values, customs, beliefs, or philosophy that he has rejected and deserted in favor of a different ideology. The underlying assumption is that the new ideology has been adopted under pressure or undue influence, but such an assumption raises many ethical questions as to the person's right to decide for himself, the limits of paternalism, etc. See *brain control; menticide; sensory deprivation*.

**depth psychology**  The psychology relating to the realm of the unconscious, in contradistinction to the psychology of the conscious part of the mind. In psychoanalysis (Freud), depth psychology may be represented by the id and superego; in analytical psychology (Jung), by the collective unconscious.

**DER**  Disulfiram ethanol reaction. See *Antabuse*.

**derailment**  Abnormal deviation or disorganization of psychic processes.

**derailment of volition**  A type of *parabulia*, most commonly seen in schizophrenic disorders, in which tangential, insignificant, and irrelevant impulses replace consistency of aim and purpose. Dependability and deliberation give way to whimsy, and goal-oriented behavior disintegrates into a disorganized flurry of contradictory wishes, ill-sustained passions, and short-lived causes.

**derealization**   The feeling of changed reality; the feeling that one's surroundings have changed, that the world is unreal. If severe enough, this feeling of changed reality may be expressed as a feeling of imminent or actual catastrophe. See *depersonalization; dereism; dissociative identity disorder.*

**dereism**   Mental activity that deviates from the laws of logic and experience and fails to take the facts of reality into consideration. In many schizophrenic states, psychic activity is largely expressed without respect to the realities of life. When a patient firmly believes that, as the Redeemer, he cures all illnesses by a simple gesture, his or her thinking is said to be out of harmony with facts, that is, dereistic. "The separation of associations from experience naturally facilitates dereistic thinking in its highest degree, which is actually based on the very fact that natural connections are ignored" (Bleuler, E. *Textbook of Psychiatry*, 1930). See *autism; depersonalization.*

**dereliction of duty**   See *negligence.*

**derivative**   See *substitute formation.*

**dermatitis artefacta**   Self-induced skin lesions, a *factitious disorder* (q.v.).

**dermatome**   The skin area supplied by the dorsal root of a single nerve segment.

**dermatophobia**   Fear of skin (-lesion).

**dermatosiophobia**   Fear of (acquiring a) skin disease.

**dermatozoic**   Of or pertaining to the sensation of animals in the skin. Dermatozoic delusions, also called *formication* (q.v.), are seen in toxic psychosis and in some (usually female) patients with depression.

**DES**   *Dissociative Experiences Scale* (q.v.).

**desaggressivization**   Neutralization of the aggressive drive (just as desexualization is neutralization of the sexual drive), so that the energy that would ordinarily be discharged is made available to the ego for carrying out its various tasks and wishes according to the secondary process.

**descriptive**   Concerned with the observable and the objective, rather than with the internal forces that may affect or determine overt behavior. Thus, *descriptive psychiatry* typically refers to any system of psychiatry that is based primarily on the study of symptoms and phenomena; often contrasted with *dynamic psychiatry*, which is primarily concerned with internal, unconscious drives or energies that are presumed to determine behavior.

**descriptive ethics**   See *ethics; ethics, descriptive.*

**descriptive validity**   See *validity.*

**desensitization**   1. Time-dependent accentuation of a receptor's responsiveness or refractoriness to a stimulus (agonist). *Homologous* desensitization is limited to a specific agonist; for example, the loss of adenylate cyclase responsivity is only to the catecholamine agonist, and responsivity to other neurotransmitters or hormones remains intact. *Heterologous* desensitization refers to a general decline of responsivity, which extends to other stimulating agents that would ordinarily activate adenylate cyclase. Desensitization is a refractory state induced in a ligand-gated ion channel by exposure to a high concentration of the ligand. A refractory state that occurs in voltage-gated channels after activation is termed *inactivation.*

2. Also *systematic desensitization*; a variant of reciprocal inhibition psychotherapy of particular value with some phobic patients. The procedure entails three maneuvers: (1) the subject is trained in relaxation; (2) during those training sessions an anxiety hierarchy is constructed, consisting of a list of stimulus situations that provoke anxiety grouped according to themes and then ranked from most to least anxiety-provoking; (3) when the subject is as relaxed as he can be, he is asked to imagine a scene that includes the least anxiety-provoking situation. The scene is presented again and again until the subject can tolerate it without anxiety. The therapist then proceeds to the next rung on the ladder until even the most anxiety-provoking situation can be tolerated in phantasy. Almost always, as it turns out, what the subject can imagine without anxiety he can experience in reality without anxiety. See *behavior theory; behavior therapy.*

**deséquilibrés**   (F. "unbalanced persons") Magnan's term for those affected by what was then known as inherited neurasthenia.

**desexualization**   *Degenitalization*;   neutralization of the sexual drive so that the energy that would ordinarily be expended in immediate id discharge (the primary process) is held up and made available to the ego for its various tasks and wishes according to the secondary process.

**designer drug** Any version of a regulated drug whose chemical structure has been modified so that it falls outside the restrictions placed on the regulated drug it imitates. Current law requires that the exact chemical structure and name of an individual compound be specified before it can be controlled. Addition of a single fluoride or carbon molecule to a regulated drug, for example, will change a drug enough so that the modification is no longer a controlled substance, even though it may be even more potent than the original regulated compound. It is estimated that the amphetamine series of drugs has between 2000 and 3000 variations, many of which are more hazardous than the amphetamines that are already regulated.

**desire** A wish, a longing for, a craving, an inclination. With the development of fuller knowledge of the unconscious, the term desire was applied to many impulses or tendencies of that part of the psyche. In the unconscious are impulses, the antitheses of conscious desires or wishes, that press for overt expression. They are regarded as biological urges or "wishes" or "desires," in contradistinction to personal wishes.

**desire neurosis** *Compensation neurosis* (q.v.).

**DESNOS** Disorder of extreme stress not otherwise specified; used to indicate *complex PTSD* by those who describe a secondary adaptation to the core symptoms of post-traumatic stress disorder as a personality disorder, *post-traumatic personality disorder* (q.v.).

**desocialization** The process of withdrawing or turning away from interpersonal contacts and relationships, such as seen commonly in schizophrenics, who tend to replace social behavior and language habits with personal, highly individual behavior.

**despair** Erikson describes *integrity vs. despair* as one of the eight stages of man. See *ontogeny, psychic*.

**despeciation** The presence in a person of a number of extreme variants of physical characteristics, such as a scaphoid shoulder blade, a supernumerary breast, a deformed earlobe, an anomalous distribution of hair. The variants, when alone, have little pathogenic value

or meaning, but the accumulation of them in a single individual is regarded as a sign of biological inferiority or despeciation (Apert). J. Bauer uses the term *degeneration* to refer to such marked deviations from the type of the species.

**destiny, neurosis of** *Moral masochism; fate neurosis* (qq.v.). This type of neurotic ailment afflicts the person who unconsciously arranges all of his life's experiences so that he is in the position of suffering continual reverses, while he consciously holds that destiny or fate brings them. His friends will always remark on his bad luck and continual ill-fortune. Moreover, he invariably tends to blame his fate for his continual reverses, being unaware that he is responsible for them himself. See *failure through success; masochism; masochistic personality*.

As the "all-consuming task of his life" this neurotic has in the first place the "mastery of guilt-feelings," which he hopes to accomplish through his own suffering, and thus ingratiate himself with an implacable superego. Second, the patient turns all of his life's activities into situations where he can experience this suffering. In Fenichel's words, he uses his environment solely as "an arena in which to stage his internal conflicts." All real-life actions "are repetitions of childhood situations or attempts to end infantile conflicts rather than rational undertakings."

**destrudo** E. Weiss coined this term to denote the energy associated with the death or destructive instinct (*Imago*, 1935). It is the opposite of *libido*, the energy of the instinct Eros. See *Thanatos*.

**desymbiotize** See *depersonification*.

**desynchronization** See *alpha blocking*.

**desynchronosis** Temporal disorientation, or feeling out of place or displaced in time relationships. See *circadian rhythm sleep disorder*.

**detached affect** An idea that is unbearable to the ego whose associated affect is separated from it and persists in the psychical sphere. Its affect attaches itself to other ideas, which are not in themselves unbearable.

**detachment** Separation; divorce from emotional involvement. See *detached affect; somnolent detachment*.

**detention** *Commitment* (q.v.); involuntary hospitalization.

**deterioration** Worsening of the clinical condition; progressively increasing impairment in functioning. See *regression; dementia*.

Intellectual deterioration generally refers to diminution or impairment of the ability to remember, together with disorders attendant upon memory losses. Intellectual deterioration is characteristic of patients with destructive processes in the cerebral cortex.

In schizophrenia, deterioration tends to occur early in the disease and is concentrated in the 5 years after symptomatic onset.

**deterioration, emotional** Occurs mainly in patients suffering from schizophrenia: the patient becomes careless and indifferent about the surroundings and people around him or her and shows no adequate emotional reaction to environmental stimuli.

**deterioration index or quotient** An index of the degree of intellectual impairment, based on comparison of scores on those tests of the Wechsler-Bellevue that show little or no decline, with scores on those tests that generally show a steep age decline. The tests that do not decline are often termed "Hold" tests: information, vocabulary, picture completion, and object assembly; those that do decline are often termed "Don't Hold" tests: digit span, arithmetic, block design, digit symbol. The deterioration index, or DI, is computed as follows:

$$DI = \frac{Hold - Don't\ Hold}{Hold}$$

**deterioration reaction type** When regression, accompanied as a rule by delusions and hallucinations, is a principal characteristic of a psychiatric syndrome, as it is in schizophrenia, Adolph Meyer classified the syndrome as a deterioration or deteriorated reaction type.

**deterioration scale** See *GDS*.

**determinant, dream** The real or principal motive or reason responsible for the production of the dream, since it is true that even if "dreams are always abundantly overdetermined, one determinant is invariable in the dreams of neurotics." This invariable factor is called the "dominant determinant" and is in direct connection with the dreamer's most important conflict. To discover the dominant determinant is no easy task: most of the time it is not revealed through association and may be discovered only by the use of the interpreter's intuition (Stekel, W. *The Interpretation of Dreams*, 1943).

**determinative idea** The goal or end result toward which thoughts progress. One of the schizophrenic's disturbances of associations is an inability to keep to the determinative idea or to focus his attention on a central goal. See *association disturbances*.

**determiner** A cause or determinant; in genetics, a *gene* (q.v.).

**determining quality** A term used by Freud in describing hysteria. He states: "Tracing an hysterical symptom back to a traumatic scene in question fulfills two conditions—if it possesses the required *determining quality* and if we can credit it with the necessary *traumatic power*" (*Collected Papers*, 1924–25). For example, a hysterical symptom of vomiting was attributed to the shock of a railway accident. This derivation of the symptom lacks determining quality, although it may be said to possess traumatic power. However, on further analysis this accident woke the memory of another event that had happened previously, during which the patient saw a decomposing corpse, a sight that aroused in her horror and disgust. This connection now supplies the determining quality for the hysterical symptom of vomiting. The antecedent experience justifiably gave rise to a high degree of disgust.

**determining tendency** See *set*.

**determinism** "The concept...that our actions can change nothing in the events of life which were firmly established through causal connection, and that man is not free to dispose of his own will and to choose between good and evil in his actions" (Bleuler, E. *Textbook of Psychiatry*, 1930). See *environmentalism*; *free will*.

**determinism, biological** A structure of social explanation that uses basic concepts in anatomy, evolutionary theory, genetics, and neurobiology; it posits that biology is destiny, and that the differences among individuals and between sexes, ethnic groups, and races in status, wealth, and power are based on innate biological differences in temperament and ability. According to Stephen Jay Gould, the major conceptual error of the theory was the determinist's conversion of the abstract idea of intelligence into a thing, a single entity, located in the brain. Once viewed as a unit, methods were developed to measure it and reduce it to a single number for each person through the statistical method. The error is not in the arithmetic but in the supposition that, having gone through the mathematics, one has produced a real object.

In the older mental retardation literature, biosocial determinism referred to the extent to which hereditary or other biologic factors determined the degree of disability.

**determinism, biosocial**  *Obs.* In mental retardation, recognition that the degree of disability is due neither to biologic nor social factors alone, but to their combination.

**determinism, linguistic**  See *Sapir-Whorf hypothesis.*

**deterrent therapy**  See *aversion therapy.*

**detouring, conflict**  See *scapegoating.*

**detoxification**  The process of withdrawing a person from an addictive substance in a safe and effective manner.

**detumescence**  Subsidence of erection and genital engorgement. See *contrectation; tumescence.*

**deuteropathy**  A secondary disease, disorder, or symptom.

**Deutsch, Helen Rosenbach**  (1884–1982) Polish-born psychoanalyst, first woman to be analyzed by Freud, founded Vienna Psychoanalytic Institute; emigrated to United States in 1935; *The Psychology of Women* (1944); *"as-if" personality* (q.v.).

**devaluation**  A defense mechanism consisting of attribution of exaggerated negative qualities to self or others when faced with emotional conflicts or stressors. See *envy.*

Devaluation of others is one of the best discriminators of narcissistic personality disorder (the others being sense of superiority, high achievements in school or at work, sense of uniqueness, and hostile or suspicious reactions to other people's envy). See *narcissistic personality.*

**developmental**  Referring to the process of maturation and the changes that occur in an organism or structure over time. The term has been used in two ways: (1) in a temporal sense, to indicate that the time during which a pathogenic process actively damages the nervous system is limited to fetal or perinatal life; disorders of neural development in this sense are, by definition, early and nonprogressive; and (2) to refer to the elaborate neurobiological mechanisms controlling the process of development; in this second, and currently more frequent, usage, the abnormal processes can continue to act postnatally and thus are progressive. Developmental studies attempt to describe the changes that do occur and to determine the causes of developmental differences. See *developmental psychobiology; ontogeny, psychic.*

Developmental disorders are usually first evident in infancy or childhood; included are mental retardation, pervasive developmental disorders, and specific developmental disorders.

**developmental articulation disorder**  A type of *language retardation*, believed to be due to lag in cerebral maturation (in which heredity may be a significant factor), consisting of deviant production of speech sounds, such as distortion, substitution, or omission of one or more sounds (e.g., g, r, s, or th).

**developmental disorders**  Manifestations of the child's struggle for mastery at various stages of development; such manifestations are not disorders per se. Included are such symptoms as nonhunger crying in the baby, stranger anxiety at 6 to 12 months of age, separation anxiety at 18 to 30 months, negativism and tantrums around 2 years of age, and crankiness or transitory fears in children from 3 to 5 years old.

Others use the term in a different sense, to refer to infantilism or slow rate of development, or to a group of childhood conditions, including autism, mental retardation, epilepsy, childhood spasticity, speech problems, and some disorders of speech and hearing.

**developmental disorders, pervasive**  A group of childhood disturbances characterized by severe distortions in the timing, rate, and sequence of the psychological functions basic to the development of language, communications, and social skills in general. The category includes *autistic disorder, Rett disorder,* childhood disintegrative disorder, and *Asperger syndrome* (qq.v.).

In DSM-IV, pervasive developmental disorders have been placed in Axis I (they were previously in Axis II).

**developmental disorders, specific**  A group of childhood disturbances characterized by a lag, delay, or deviance in the development of a specific function, such as reading, speaking, or arithmetic ability, and not explicable in terms of mental age or inadequate schooling. These disorders frequently coexist with other disorders (e.g., conduct disorders, attention deficit disorders). Included within the group are (1) language and speech disorders (articulation disorder, stuttering, cluttering, expressive language disorder, receptive language disorder); (2) academic skills disorder (reading disorder, expressive writing disorder, arithmetic disorder); and (3) motor skills disorder (*coordination disorder*).

Except for the pervasive developmental disorders, the term "developmental" has been eliminated from DSM-IV: what were formerly termed academic skills disorders are called learning disorder, and developmental recessive language disorder is termed mixed receptive-expressive language disorder.

**developmental dysphasia** Specific language impairment (SLI), characterized by defects in expressive language and articulation (*expressive dysphasia*) and also, in the more severe forms, by defects in the comprehension of language (*receptive dysphasia*). Some studies suggest that it is a genetically produced impairment in the ability to construct a mental grammar that does not impair other cognitive abilities.

**developmental failures** Rinsley (1989) described three possible types of developmental failure: (1) failure of both separation and individuation, associated with psychosis or borderline personality disorder; (2) failure of separation but not of individuation, associated with narcissistic personality disorder; and (3) failure of individuation but not of separation (a theoretical possibility only, in that no such case has ever been described).

**developmental hyperactivity** See *learning disability, specific.*

**developmental levels** Divisions of the life cycle in terms of chronological age; the following levels are generally recognized: (1) neonatal period, from birth to 1 month; (2) infancy, from birth to 1 year; (3) early (preschool) childhood, from 1 to 6 years; (4) midchildhood, 6 to 10 years; (5) late childhood or preadolescence, 10 to 12 years; (6) *adolescence* (q.v.), 12 to 21 years; (7) adulthood or maturity, beginning at 21 years and ending with old age according to some, but with others ending at (8) the involutional period or climacterium, 40 to 55 years for women, 50 to 65 years for men; (9) old age or the senium, beginning at 65 or 70 years. See *ontogeny, psychic.*

**developmental lines** Often used as approximately equivalent to stages or phases of development, although the phrase *lines of*

*development* (q.v.) was used by Anna Freud in a very specific way. See *developmental phases.*

**developmental linguistics** Also, developmental psycholinguistics; the study of *language acquisition* (q.v.).

**developmental neuropsychiatry** The specialized area of child and adolescent psychiatry that emphasizes the brain mechanisms involved in developmental disorders such as mental retardation syndromes and learning disabilities, which render the child vulnerable to neuropsychiatric disorders.

**developmental phases** The different stages through which the organism passes during its life span, often described separately for different organ systems or functions. Each stage usually shows characteristic impulses and features, and it presents its own challenges that must be met if development is to proceed normally. Psychosexual development, for example, was described by Freud in terms of libidinal phases: oral phase, anal phase, phallic phase, latency, and genitality. Object relationships were described in terms of autoerotic, narcissistic, homoerotic, heteroerotic, and alloerotic stages. Erikson described lifelong personality development in terms of the oral sensory stage (where the dominant issue is trust vs. mistrust), muscular-anal stage (autonomy vs. shame and doubt), locomotor-genital stage (initiative vs. guilt), latency (industry vs. inferiority), puberty and adolescence (ego identity vs. role confusion), young adulthood (intimacy vs. isolation), adulthood (generativity vs. stagnation), and stage of maturity (ego integrity vs. despair). Gesell described landmarks of normal behavioral development in the child from birth to 6 years in terms of motor and sensory behavior, adaptive behavior, and personal and social behavior. Piaget described cognitive development in terms of sensorimotor phase, preoperational phase, concrete (operational) phase, and formal (abstract) phase. See *fixation.*

Emotional disorders arise when environmental pressures interfere with the maturational timetable, or when one or more *lines of development* (q.v.) come into conflict with environmental demands.

**developmental psychobiology** The study of the relationship between emotional experiences in childhood and later pathology, of the biological determinants of behavior and its psychological components, of the effects of the external environment on the development of the central nervous system. Developmental psychology is a broad field that includes

(1) ethology and comparative psychology, with emphasis on how behavioral traits enable the organism to meet environmental demands and how they are maintained in the face of natural selection; (2) toxicology and teratology, with emphasis on the particular susceptibility of immature organisms to environmental events; and (3) the neurosciences, with emphasis on how the nervous system develops and its relationship to reproduction, communication, learning, memory, sleep, etc.

Animal studies have shown that early separation from the mother disrupts neurochemical and neuroendocrine growth processes, sleep-wake organization, emotional behavior, and immune reactivity. Psychosocial dwarfism appears to be a similar phenomenon in humans, and when the stressful situation is removed, the growth retardation, bizarre eating behavior, and growth and adrenocorticotrophic hormone abnormalities of such children disappear. See *psychosocial dwarfism; failure to thrive.*

**developmental psychology**    Study of the processes of maturation of the intellectual, emotional, attitudinal, and social aspects of the organism with particular emphasis, in the human, on the childhood and adolescent years. Jean Piaget's theories (called *genetic epistemology*) recognized the importance of cognitive learning processes and concept formation in the young child, and he described the regular stages of intellectual development. In the period of *sensorimotor intelligence* (the first 2 years of life), the child learns to use senses and muscles to deal with external events, and he begins to symbolize, i.e., to represent things by word or gesture. In the period of *representative intelligence* (2 to 7 or 8 years), words and other symbols are used to represent the outer world and inner feelings. He begins to understand relationships—spatial, temporal, and mathematical (grouping, sizes, qualities, etc.). Although Piaget emphasized the internal processes of development, he also noted their dependence on an environment conducive to learning the necessary skills.

**developmentalism**    The genetic, longitudinal view of human behavior.

The term is used to describe Gesell's emphasis on maturation as a biological process in a cultural setting. Each level of development of children's behavior is determined and standardized on the basis of long-term studies; there is little concern with interpretation of the inner life of the child.

**developmentally disabled abuse**    Children and adults with developmental disabilities are at approximately 1½ times greater risk than the nondisabled for being physically and sexually abused. Up to 90% of instances involve sexual offenses. Prior to their 18th birthday, 39%–68% of girls and 16%–30% of boys with developmental disabilities are sexually abused, most frequently by family members, paid caregivers, and others with disabilities.

The developmentally disabled are also vulnerable to *institutional abuse*—physical, sexual, emotional, or neglectful behavior and abuse in a managed institutional setting.

**deviant, deviate**    Any person differing markedly from what is accepted as the norm, the average, or the usual. Probably the most common use of the term is in relation to the sexual form. See *sexual deviation; deviant, sexual.* See *pedophilia.*

**deviation, average**    See *mean deviation.*

**deviation, conjugate**    See *oculomotor nerve.*

**deviation, ego**    See *ego deviant children.*

**deviation-amplifying feedback**    *DAF*; positive feedback; a process whereby the output of a system is fed back into the system with the effect of increasing or decreasing the output of the system. The vicious circle—and its opposite, the virtuous circle—are examples of deviation-amplifying feedback. DAF is a mechanism wherein a small and relatively insignificant variation leads to consequences of major proportions. It may be the mechanism at work in brief therapy, where small therapeutic interventions can foster behavioral alterations of appreciable magnitude.

**Devic disease**    Neuromyelitis optica; ophthalmoneuromyelitis; disseminated myelitis with optic neuritis. An acute demyelinating disease that is sometimes self-limited but which in 50% of cases is relapsing, progressive, and fatal. It consists of massive foci of demyelination in the optic nerves and chiasma and spinal cord, which may undergo softening and cavitation. Etiology is unknown and there is no definitive treatment.

**Devil's Pact**    See *compliance, strategic.*

**dexamethasone**  See *DST*.

**dextrality-sinistrality**  See *cerebral dominance; laterality*.

**dextrophobia**  Fear of objects to the right.

**ΔosB**  A transcriptional regulator that modulates the synthesis of certain AMPA glutamate receptor subunits and cell-signaling enzymes. An up-regulation of posttranslationally modified forms of this regulator occurs in the nucleus accumbens and dorsal striatum in response to dopamine stimulation and to addictive drugs such as cocaine; when overexpression is prolonged, the rewarding effects of cocaine are increased. See *addiction*.

**DFP**  Diisopropylphosphorofluoridate; an organophosphate which, in rats, reduces the number of both the muscarinic and the nicotinic receptors in the hippocampus, striatum, and parts of the cortex. The result is a learning deficit that persists for as long as 3 weeks after DFP is administered. The finding is of interest because of the claim of many that the *gulf war syndrome* (q.v.), and the cognitive deficits of which many affected subjects complain, are due to exposure to organophosphates. See *psychotomimetic*.

**DHA**  Docosahexaenoic acid; see *omega-3 fatty acids*.

**dhat**  Also, *jiryan*; a culture-specific syndrome reported in India, consisting of anxiety, feelings of exhaustion, and somatic concerns related o seminal emission. Similar syndromes are seen in other countries and bear different names: *sukra prameha* (Sri Lanka), *shen-k'uei* (Taiwan), *shenkui* (China).

**DI**  *Deterioration index* (q.v.).

**diabetes mellitus**  See *carbohydrate metabolism*.

**diabetic exophthalmic dysostosis**  *Xanthomatosis* (q.v.).

**diaboleptics**  Maudsley's term for those who claim to have supernatural communications.

**diacylglycerol**  *DAG; DG*; an intracellular second messenger. One of the three second messenger systems is diacylglycerol-inositol (the others are cAMP and arachidonic acid). Diacylglycerol and *inositol* are produced within the cell by receptor-activated phospholipase C. DAG, in turn, activates protein kinase C, while inositol acts on the endoplasmic reticulum to release calcium from endogenous stores. See *neuromessenger*.

**diagnosis**  Four statistics document the accuracy of diagnostic procedures: *sensitivity*,

*specificity* (qq.v.), positive predictive power, and negative predictive power. See *nosology*.

**diagnosis, negative**  Diagnosis by means of exclusion; "wastebasket" diagnosis.

**diagnostic confidence**  See *sensitivity*.

**dialectic**  Reasoning by an exchange of ideas and opinions; the Socratic techniques of logical discussion with the aim of exposing false ideas and uncovering truth. According to Thomas Ogden, experience is the dialectical interplay of three modes or processes through which perception is attributed meaning in a particular way: the depressive, the paranoid-schizoid, and the autistic-contiguous.

Psychopathology appears when the dialectic collapses in the direction of one or another of the three modes. See *autistic-contiguous position; depressive position; paranoid-schizoid position*.

**dialectical behavior therapy (DBT)**  A type of *cognitive behavior therapy* (q.v.), originally developed (by Marcia Linehan) to treat suicidal and other dangerous, severe, or destabilizing behaviors in patients with borderline personality disorder (BPD). A focus on stabilizing patients and achieving behavioral control is balanced with acceptance, compassion, and validation of the patient. DBT's biosocial theory posits a pervasive deficit in the ability to regulate emotions in BPD, a deficit that is maintained by transactions between the subject's emotional vulnerability and the environment's pervasive pattern of invalidation of the vulnerable subject. *Invalidation* describes indiscriminate rejection of the communication of private experiences, punishment of emotional display but intermittent reinforcement of emotional escalation, and the consistent message that emotional problems are easier to solve than they really are.

DBT combines basic behavioral procedures of skills training, exposure-based procedures, cognitive restructuring, contingency management, and problem solving with validation, mindfulness practices, reciprocity, and attention to the patient-therapist relationship. Therapy begins with *radical acceptance*: patients accept who they are, not what they want to be; they come to recognize their self–harming behaviors and suicide attempts as dysfunctional responses to profound stress; they have two choices, to change or to stay miserable. Patients pledge to stay alive and not attempt suicide no matter what their mood. The patient and therapist collaborate in drawing up a prioritized list of specific behavioral targets for change.

The next step is *distress tolerance*. Patients learn to notice when their emotions begin to stir, allow their feelings to build up, and then let the emotional storm pass, without doing anything. Such self-observation is called *mindfulness*, not a means of avoidance but an exercise in feeling and enduring emotional pain, and learning that emotion need not rule behavior. *Chain analysis* is a moment-to-moment reconstruction of the interactions and sensations preceding destructive behavior, used to understand behaviors targeted for change and to break the chain of events that produced them.

Once they have committed themselves to change and have demonstrated their ability to endure some degree of distress, patients learn the many specific social and behavioral skills that can combat depression, anxiety, and other negative emotions. The therapist helps the patient to establish behavioral control and to master skills, to address issues of self-respect and individual goals, and to identify behaviors that interfere with therapy or with quality of life. Progress in changing targeted behaviors is monitored daily by the patient, whose diary card is reviewed with the therapist.

DBT customarily consists of one session per week with the therapist, a weekly 2¼-hour skills training group, and as-needed telephone calls to the therapist if the patient is about to perform a self-destructive act. Part of the original contract setting is that such calls are not permitted when the self-destructive act has already been performed. Individual therapists and group skills trainers meet in a weekly consultation team meeting.

**dialogue, therapeutic**   See *therapeutic alliance*.

**diamine**   Any substance that contains two amine groups. See *amine; epinephrine; ergotropic; serotonin*.

**Diana complex**   The wish of a female to be a male. See *transsexualism*.

**diaphragma sellae**   See *meninges*.

**diaschisis**   Impaired information processing not only at the site of a brain lesion but also in downstream pathways connected to the lesion site.

**diathesis**   Constitutional disposition, or predisposition, to some anomalous or morbid condition "which no longer belongs within the confines of the normal variability, but already begins to represent a potential disease condition." These various *diathetic* conditions are distinguished by the fact that diathetic individuals respond with abnormal or truly pathological reactions to physiological stimuli, such as foods, or other ordinary conditions of life, such as sunlight, that are borne by the majority of individuals without injury (Pende, N. *Constitutional Inadequacies*, 1928) See *constitution; disposition; personality; temperament*.

**diathesis stress model**   The hypothesis that schizophrenia and *schizotypal personality disorder* (SPD) are schizotypes that share the same genetic liability (diathesis) for schizophrenia. Interactions with the environment determine which of these schizotypes later decompensate to schizophrenia.

**DIB**   Diagnostic Interview for Borderlines (see *borderline personality; borderline psychosis*). A semistructured interview that includes a systematic review of social adaptation, impulse/action patterns, affects, psychotic episodes and experiences, and interpersonal relationships described by John Gunderson, Jonathan Kolb, and Virginia Austin (*American Journal of Psychiatry 138*, 1981).

**dichorionic**   *DC*; describing twins who have developed separate placentas and chorions. Approximately one-third of monozygotic twins and all dizygotic twins are dichorionic. See *monochorionic*.

**dichotic listening test**   Two different strings of numbers are presented simultaneously through dual-track headphones, one to each ear, and the subject is asked to recall all the numbers presented.

**dichotomous thinking**   A cognitive distortion, typical of *borderline personality disorder* (q.v.), in which the experiences of everyday life are assessed as either all good or all bad. Persons with BPD habitually overreact to minor shortcomings on the part of a relative or significant other. They idealize in a manner just as unrealistic as the hatred engendered by a negative experience. Extreme reactions give rise to extreme emotions and, often, to extreme behaviors (especially impulsive and destructive acts).

**DID**   *Dissociative identity disorder* (q.v.).

**didactic**   Fitted or intended to teach; used often to refer to formal teaching lessons, such as lectures, in contrast to discussion groups or seminars. Didactic psychoanalysis is also known as training or tuitional analysis. See *training analysis.*

**didactic group psychotherapy** A strictly tutorial practice in which outlines, texts, and visual aids are used for teaching patients in special subjects.

**diecious** Two-housed; applied to species whose members are sexually distinct (as in the human, where individuals are identified as male or female). In general, this implies that what males do is masculine, what females do is feminine, and what both do (or can do) is sex-shared, bisexual, or *ambisexual* (q.v.).

**dielectric barrier** See *ion channel.*

**diencephalic anterograde amnesia** Impaired learning of new declarative information following pathology in the medial thalamic or hypothalamic regions.

**diencephalic epilepsy** *Autonomic epilepsy* (q.v.).

**diencephalic stupor** *Cairns stupor* (q.v.).

**diencephalic syndrome** Abnormalities of endocrine, autonomic, and mental functions due to disruption of neural pathways between the pituitary and *hypothalamus* (q.v.).

**diencephalon** Between-brain; forebrain; it consists of the *thalamus* and *hypothalamus* (qq.v.), which lie between the cerebral hemispheres and the midbrain.

**diencephalosis** A term used to refer to any of the many possible disturbances or functional alterations of the diencephalon or its interconnections. The following symptom groups are included: (1) lack of restraint and inhibition, (2) paradoxical coexistence of opposed functional disturbances, (3) alterations of biological rhythms, (4) various endocrine dysfunctions, (5) abnormalities of growth and development, (6) certain forms of psychopathy, (7) vascular lability, (8) dysthermia, (9) electroencephalograph abnormalities, and (10) cranioradiographic abnormalities (Pende, N. *Medicina 6,* 1957).

**dietary chaos syndrome** See *restricters.*

**dietary restriction** A decrease in the amount of food consumed over time (caloric restriction) or a decrease in the frequency of meals (intermittent fasting).

**difference hypothesis** See *deficit model.*

**differential fertility** See *fertility, differential.*

**differential reinforcement schedules** See *accelerative.*

**differential therapeutics** The matching of therapies available with the patient's or family's needs; tailoring therapy to the patient or group to be treated; the process of choosing the therapy to be recommended.

**differentiation subphase** See *separation-individuation.*

**difficult child** See *temperament.*

**diffuse sclerosis** "A group of progressive diseases usually occurring early in life and characterized pathologically by widespread demyelination of the white matter of the cerebral hemispheres, and clinically in typical cases by visual failure, mental deterioration, and spastic paralysis. Both sporadic and familial cases are encountered. The aetiology of these disorders is unknown and there is no general agreement as to their classification. At present their resemblances to one another appear to outweigh their differences and they are therefore included under a common title" (Brain, W. R. *Diseases of the Nervous System,* 1951). The various entities that Brain includes are *encephalitis periaxialis diffusa (Schilder disease), centrolobar sclerosis, encephaloleukopathia scleroticans, progressive degenerative subcortical encephalopathy, leukodystrophy,* leukoencephalopathia, myeloclastica primitiva, *encephalomyelomalacia chronica diffusa, concentric demyelination (Baló disease),* Krabbe disease, *Scholz disease,* and *Pelizaeus-Merzbacher disease.* It has been suggested that some of this group are caused by specific biochemical defects affecting different stages in the metabolism of myelin.

The demyelination typically begins symmetrically in both occipital lobes and spreads forward. Onset is usually before the age of 14; males are more frequently affected than females. Symptoms may begin acutely or insidiously and include headache, giddiness, visual impairment progressing to blindness; diplopia, nystagmus; spastic diplegia, aphasia and/or spastic dysarthria, epileptiform attacks, and progressive dementia. Survival period is rarely longer than 3 years after the onset of symptoms. There is no known treatment.

**diffusion tensor imaging** A variation of *MRI* (q.v.).

**DiGeorge syndrome** See *velocardiofacial syndrome.*

**digestive epilepsy** The commonest form of *visceral epilepsy* (q.v.).

**digit span**   The examiner reads a series of numbers, and the subject is asked to repeat them. The number of digits remembered is the digit span. It partly reflects visual short-term working memory, as do arithmetic tasks. See *short-term memory*.

**digit symbol substitution task**   A timed test in which the subject is shown a row of nine boxes, each with a letter and a corresponding symbol; he or she is then presented with numbers and is asked to write the corresponding symbol under each number. The test largely reflects visuo-motor functioning.

**dihybrid**   A hybrid individual differing in two hereditary characters, or hereditary traits based on two pairs of genes. See *hybrid*.

**diisopropyl fluorophosphate**   See *psychotomimetic*.

**dikephobia**   Fear of justice.

**dilapidation**   *Deterioration; dementia* (qq.v.).

**diltiazem**   A calcium-channel blocker. See *CCI*.

**dimensional system**   In *nosology* (q.v.), the conceptualization of diseases as developing on a continuum, in contrast to the *categorical system* (q.v.), in which dichotomous variables (present and absent) define each component of the syndrome or disease. A dimensional diagnosis has three or more ordinal values, which can range from a 3-point scale (at a minimum) to a continuum. In the classification of personality disorders, for example, the dimensional system views personality traits as continuously distributed in populations and personality pathology as extreme variants of these traits. Any dimensional diagnosis can be made categorical by setting a cut-off point.

Compared with the categorical approach, the dimensional approach gives greater power to detect treatment effects, less attenuation and greater precision in estimates of effect sizes, and better ability to detect signals; it incorporates a greater amount of potentially relevant information, has better predictive and discriminating power, is more stable over time and less affected by minor shifts in psychopathology, and has higher levels of reliability. Dissatisfaction with the categorical approach, exemplified by *DSM-III* and *DSM-IV*, has led to the conceptualization of diseases occurring on a *spectrum* (qq.v.)

In the anxiety and mood disorders, genetic data are more compatible with a dimensional than a categorical approach. Epidemiologic data also suggest that depression is best conceptualized as a continuously distributed syndrome rather than as a discrete diagnostic entity. A dimensional approach is needed to prepare for the future inclusion of genetic, neurobiologic, and biochemical elements to psychiatric diagnosis. Identifying disease-related *endophenotypes* is one step in this direction; another proposed step is *prototype matching* (qq.v.).

Dimensional approaches are not free of drawbacks, however. Dimensional self-report scales, for instance, have significant limitations such as difficulties in determining duration and persistence, and their almost exclusive focus on current state. Key questions in adopting dimensional approaches in childhood disorders are how to take into account the developmental pathways and the mechanisms involved in symptom progression, the age-related variations in scales and measurements, the neuroscience findings, and the integration of information obtained from multiple informants.

**diminished capacity**   Diminished responsibility, partial insanity, partial responsibility. See *insanity defense; criminal responsibility*.

**diminutive visual hallucination**   *Lilliputian hallucination* (q.v.).

**dimorphic**   *Ambitypic* (q.v.).

**dim-out**   *Blackout* (q.v.).

**DIMS**   Disorders of initiating and maintaining sleep; the insomnias. See *sleep disorders*.

**dinomania**   Dancing mania; *choreomania* (q.v.).

**Diogenes syndrome**   *Hoarding; squalor syndrome* (qq.v.).

**dionism**   Heterosexuality. See *uranism*.

**diplegia**   Bilateral paralysis of corresponding parts of the body.

**diplegia, congenital spastic**   *Cerebral palsy* (q.v.).

**diploid**   The original stage in the maturation of a reproductive cell, in which the number of chromosomes is full, that is, not yet halved by the reduction division following the first or equation division. See *chromosome; meiosis*.

**diploid mode**   The normal number of chromosomes—in humans, 46.

**diplopia**   Double vision; due to paralysis of the ocular muscles, which causes the image of an object to fall upon noncorresponding portions of the two retinae. See *oculomotor nerve*.

**diplopia, monocular**　A condition in which two images are seen with one eye. The existence of true monocular diplopia is questioned and when present is regarded as a sign of hysteria.

**dippoldism**　Flogging of (school) children. The German schoolteacher Dippold was tried and convicted of manslaughter for flogging a child to death. Thereafter the act of *flagellation* (q.v.) came to be known as dippoldism.

**dipsomania**　Enomania; *oinomania*; *posiomania*; a type of *alcoholism* (q.v.) characterized mentally by a variety of responses peculiar to the drinker. Some become shy and retiring; others quite boisterous and pugnacious; still others exhibit paranoid reactions. The alcoholic bout and its results last as a rule for several days, rarely for several weeks. Dipsomania is usually regarded as a symptom of some more fundamental disorder, such as psychopathic personality, epilepsy, or schizophrenia. Bleuler includes dipsomania among the acute syndromes in the schizophrenias.

**direct analysis**　A form of psychoanalytically oriented psychotherapy, advocated by John Rosen for treatment of schizophrenics, in which the therapist enters into the patient's delusional system and confronts him with interpretations of the meaning of his symptoms and behavior. Because such interpretations are based on the therapist's guesses about the patient's unconscious, the method is often referred to as wild analysis.

**directed thinking**　See *intellect.*

**directive**　In psychiatry, and particularly in the areas of psychotherapy and counseling, directive refers to an active and often authoritarian approach in which the therapist gives advice, suggests or demands that the patient follow certain courses of action, etc.

**dirty urine**　See *urine, dirty.*

**DIS**　Diagnostic Interview Schedule; see *NIMH-DIS.*

**disability**　A limitation of function secondary to a disorder of a specific organ or body system. *Handicap* refers to the obstacles encountered by the person in pursuing his goals because of his disability, often described in terms of the degree of economic, emotional, social, or physical dependence resulting from the disability. A handicap reflects the interaction between the disability, on the one hand, and both the disabled person and his architectural, attitudinal, social, and legal environment on the other. In current socialese jargon, *physically challenged* is used to refer to the disabled or handicapped person.

To be noted is that in practice its meaning is defined by the policy that covers the disability. Social Security offers disability benefits through Social Security Disability Insurance and Supplemental Security Income. The Contract with America Advancement Act of 1996 abolished substance use disorders as a cause of disabling impairment. Addictive disorders in the presence of other psychiatric or medical disorders may qualify, but only if the patient would remain disabled if he stopped using alcohol or drugs. The Americans with Disabilities Act (ADA) of 1990 offers protection from discrimination in the workplace against those who suffer disabilities. ADA applies to those suffering from addictive disorders, but in limited and specific ways. The law distinguishes between alcohol and illegal drugs, and protects those addicted to each differently. Recent case law has reduced the ADA protections afforded to addicted persons.

**disabled (dab)**　See *scrambler mice.*

**disadvantaged**　Lacking assets; a social psychiatry vogue term of the 1970s denoting persons or groups who are economically poor and/or members of minority groups. Disadvantages typically include deprivations in housing, education, work opportunity, and medical (and particularly prenatal) care and are associated with family disruption, faulty identity formation or malignant identity diffusion, and excessively high rates of juvenile offenses and of admissions to state mental hospitals.

**disappointment**　See *regret.*

**disaster**　Sudden and unexpected loss, reversal, injury; catastrophe or *trauma* (q.v.). Three stages of early reaction are recognized: (1) initial shock and disorganization because of immobilizing and overpowering anxiety; (2) dependency and suggestibility with passive and almost blind acceptance of direction from others; (3) reorganization and recovery, with a return of control and independence often accompanied by apprehensiveness and repetitive descriptions of the incident and the rescue efforts. See *post-traumatic stress disorder; traumatic neurosis.*

**disavowal**　Repudiation; *denial* (q.v.). See *defense mechanisms.*

**DISC1** Gene *disrupted in schizophrenia-1*, a candidate schizophrenia gene. One missense mutation produces a depression-like phenotype; another mutation alters prepulse and latent inhibition, which model information-processing deficits in schizophrenia. Both mutations reduce binding of the gene to phosphodiesterase-4B (PDE4B), suggesting that it is altered DISC1-PDE4B binding that underlies the behavioral phenotypes.

**discharge** 1. An unloading, release, dismissal. In neurophysiology, synonymous with *firing*, the delivery of excitation from one neuron to the next. In mental hospital statistics, the dropping of a patient from the rolls because of termination of services (patients transferred to other facilities and patients who die are not usually counted as discharges).

2. Seminal emission, ejaculation.

3. Release or seepage of purulent material from a wound.

**discharge of affect** An energetic reaction to an affective experience that includes the whole range of voluntary and involuntary reflexes, by which, according to experience, the emotions—from weeping to a clear act of revenge—are habitually worked off.

**discharge rate** The ratio of the number discharged within a given period (usually a year) to the total number in the original group. In institutional statistics this rate is usually approximated by relating the number discharged in a given period to the number who were admitted during the same period. See *readmission*.

Example: If there are 620 admissions to a mental hospital during the calendar year, and if there are 527 discharges from that hospital during the same year, the discharge rate is 85%.

**dischronation, dyschronation** *Chronotaraxis* (q.v.).

**disconnection hypothesis** In schizophrenia, abnormal connectivity between neurons leads to disintegration of the neuronal dynamics underlying response and perception, expressed as an inability to form new stimulus-response links (impaired emotional learning) or stimulus-stimulus links (impaired perceptual learning). In terms of cognition, this could be expressed as *cognitive dysmetria* and, at lower levels, a disruption of perceptual learning and inference (i.e., perceptual dysmetria). Abnormal perceptual learning is manifested as inhibitory deficits on electrophysiological measurements such as P50 inhibition (reflecting dysfunction in the septohippocampal cholinergic system involved in sensory gating), as deficits in context processing because of failure to use contextual cues to inhibit their responses, and as errors in predictive coding because of loss of synchronization between GABA-ergic interneurons and pyramidal cells (schizophrenic patients show a selective decrease in the axon terminal density of GABA-ergic chandelier neurons, which synapse exclusively with pyramidal cells).

Schizophrenia is a miscoordination of distributed neural networks that would normally function in an integrated and time-linked manner. Andreasen et al. coined the term *cognitive dysmetria* to emphasize the temporal dimension of neural disconnection in schizophrenia, hypothesizing an underlying lack of connectivity in cortical-cerebellar-thalamal-cortical circuitry (Andreasen, N. C., Paradiso, S. and O'Leary, D. S., *Schizophrenia Bulletin 24*: 203–218, 1998)

**disconnection syndromes** Speech disorders due to destruction of the *corpus callosum* (q.v.) which prevents the cerebral hemispheres from communicating with each other.

**discontinuous analysis** Interrupted or staggered analysis, especially a reduction in the frequency of sessions as part of gradual and planned termination of psychoanalytic treatment.

**discourse skills** In communicating with another, linguistic devices that make it easier for the listener to understand what the speaker is trying to say. Both adults and children with schizophrenia often fail to provide the listener with enough links to previous utterances (*cohesive ties*) or enough references to people or events mentioned earlier (*referential cohesion*) to make it easy, or even possible, for the listener to understand what or whom is being talked about. Schizophrenics tend also to stray from the subject being discussed into comments about the immediate surroundings (*exophora*). In addition, children with schizophrenia often use fewer than normal connecting signs (conjunctions) between contiguous clauses, less repetition of words or word roots (*lexical cohesion*), and frequent omissions of previous clauses (*ellipsis*) that the listener needs in order to make sense of what is being said.

**discrete model** See *cascade model*.

**discriminanda** See *intelligence*.

**disease** A state that places a person at risk of adverse consequences, including physical or psychological impairment, activity restrictions, or role limitations. Treatment is directed toward preventing or ameliorating such adverse consequences. To some extent, the definition of disease is dependent upon the culture in which it occurs, because an adverse consequence in one culture may not be viewed as such in another. Further, the presence of a genetic variation that is of minimal or no risk to the person carrying it is not sufficient to constitute a disease.

Many words have been used to refer to conditions whose definitions to date have been generally unsatisfactory; among them are *abnormality, affliction, condition, defect, deviation, disability, disfigurement, disorder, disturbance, dysfunction, impediment, illness, injury, lesion, reaction, variant,* and *wound*.

"Illness and disease are closely related, but diseases are more robust ontologically than illnesses. They are regarded as entities having characteristic signs and symptoms with known or discoverable underlying 'mechanisms' and, ultimately, known or discoverable etiologies." C. Culver and B. Gert (*Philosophy in Medicine*, 1982) suggest instead the term *malady* to designate any condition in which there is something wrong with the person. "A person has a malady if and only if he has a condition, other than his rational beliefs and desires, such that he is suffering, or at increased risk of suffering, an evil (death, pain, disability, loss of freedom or opportunity, or loss of pleasure) in the absense of a distinct sustaining cause." See *abnormality*.

In medical anthropology, disease refers to whatever biological reality underlies the disorder in question; illness refers to the social construction of the disease (e.g., the explanatory model that is favored by the culture).

**disease concept** In relation to alcohol dependence in particular, less commonly to other forms of chemical dependence as well, recognition that such substance use is the manifestation of a chronic, progressive, and potentially fatal biogenetic and psychosocial disease characterized by tolerance and physical dependence manifested by a loss of control, as well as diverse personality changes and social consequences. The disease concept views addiction as a pathological process in and of itself; it emphasizes sobriety as a goal, since there is no known cure for the disease itself. This contrasts with the psychological viewpoint, which admits of the possibility of learning to use alcohol or other drugs responsibly despite a previous period of addiction to those drugs. See *alcoholism*.

**disease narcissism** Ferenczi's term for overevaluation (hypercathexis) of parts of the self that are not involved in a disease process. An example is the soldier whose lower jaw had been almost entirely blown away by a shell, leaving his face grossly deformed. However, he paid little attention to his injury, and was instead concerned with his diet and the appearance of his fingernails, demanding that the nurse manicure him daily.

**disengagement** Detachment; breaking free from involvement or commitment. See *aging, theories of*.

**disengagement theory** The hypothesis that the older person most likely to achieve satisfaction and contentment is the one who can accept the inevitability of reduced social and personal interactions with advancing age. See *aging, theories of*.

**dishabituation** 1. In neurophysiology, re-establishment of responses to a repeated stimulus that the organism has come to ignore; overriding *habituation* (q.v.) by a sensitizing stimulus. A person living beside an airport is likely to become habituated to (i.e., to ignore) the sound of airplanes flying overhead. Should a plane burst into flames and crash into his building, it is likely that for some time after he would be acutely aware of (i.e., sensitized to) the noise of each plane in the air above him. See *sensitization*.

2. According to A. K. Nyman of Lund University, a phenomenon characteristic of borderline ("nonregressive") schizophrenia consisting of hypersensitivity, overreactions to, and intense, unpleasant feelings aroused by involuntary scratching, sounds, gestures, etc. See *habituation*.

**disharmony, affective** Lack of conformity of the emotional reaction and the ideational content; characteristic of schizophrenic disorders.

**disinhibited syndrome** A frontal lobe syndrome, associated with pathology in the orbitofrontal system; see *orbitomedial syndrome*.

**disinhibition**   Removal of an inhibition. The inhibitory function of the cerebral cortex can be reduced by various agents—for instance, alcohol. If such a cortical function is impaired or reduced in its activity, the inhibitory influences of the cortex are diminished or removed and then a disinhibition takes place, indicating that without the high cortical control, lower vegetative or emotional functions are manifested. At all levels of the nervous system, a balance is maintained between excitatory and inhibitory influences. With increasing complexity of the nervous system there is a tendency for hierarchical integration, with higher centers normally exerting an inhibitory influence over lower centers. When those higher centers are removed, whether by organic lesions (e.g., neoplasms and cerebrovascular accidents) or by drug effects (e.g., depressant effects of alcohol and barbiturates), they can no longer inhibit or suppress the lower centers. The result is disinhibition—a surge of *release phenomena* reflecting excitation at the lower level. The cortex, and in particular portions of the frontal lobe, ordinarily inhibits the limbic system, including the hypothalamus. Interruption of the connections between the cortex and the limbic system may produce disinhibition of emotional expression (with pathological laughing or crying), sham rage, or episodic dyscontrol with outbursts of agitated, aggressive behavior.

**disinhibition syndrome**   *Explosive disorder* (q.v.).

**disintegrated type**   In the system of constitutional types described by E. R. and W. Jaensch, a psychological state associated with the T type (tetanic) of *eidetic imagery* (q.v.).

**disintegration**   Disorganization of psychic processes. See *integration; disruption*.

**disintegration anxiety**   See *depleted depression*.

**disintegrative disorder**   A pervasive developmental disorder characterized by loss of language, social, play, or motor skills, or of bowel or bladder control after what appears to be normal development for at least the first 2 years of life. The child manifests impaired social interaction and communication and restricted patterns of behavior and interest, similar to that seen in *autistic disorder* (q.v.).

**disintegrative psychoses**   In ICD-9 (see *International Classification of Diseases*), disorders in which normal development for the first few years is followed over a period of a few months by loss of social skills and speech and severely disordered emotions, behavior, and relationships. Most such psychoses are organic in origin.

**disjunctive**   See *activation*.

**disjunctive suppressant**   *Nonreciprocal suppressant* (q.v.).

**dislocation of memory**   Holland's term for complete but temporary forgetfulness or amnesia.

**dismemberment fear**   The fear that one is losing part of one's body, expressed most often by patients with involutional psychoses or schizophrenia. In some cases, different parts of the body are projected onto the outside world and return in the form of persecutors. Such a mechanism is clearly illustrated in the example of the depressive menopausal woman who feared she was going to cut off all her fingers every time she held a knife in her hand. She later developed a persecution complex in which five different enemies were following her (Schilder, P. *Psycho-therapy*, 1938).

**disorder**   See *disease*.

**disordered behavior, classification of**   See *adaptational psychodynamics*.

**disorders of impulse control**   See *impulse control disorders*.

**disorganization**   Loss or reduction in the usual or expected degree of organization, structure, or systematization, or evenness of performance. Disorganization may be indicative of structural damage to any organ whose ability to function is thereby compromised. Disorganization of movement, a type of dyssynergia that is also known as *decomposition of movement*, indicates cerebellar dysfunction and is characterized by a jerky, broken, "by the numbers" quality of movements that are ordinarily performed smoothly and easily. Mental or *personal disorganization* usually refers to a significant inability of the person to organize and maintain his living in a reasonably orderly, predictable, and integrated fashion. Such disorganization is seen particularly in organic mental disorders, schizophrenia, and acute manic episodes, although the term is sometimes applied loosely to any person who does not meet the standards of the observer's desire for organization and orderliness.

**disorientation**   Impairment in the understanding of temporal, spatial, or personal relationships. See *organic syndrome*.

**disparagement, mania for** Janet's term for "one who feels himself to be a weakling and has a terrible dread of effort, has a different idea of competition. His aim is to triumph, not by raising himself, but by lowering his rival. Thus it is that the psychasthenic secures a partial and thrifty success by preventing others from acting....In many instances, an additional factor is his dread of others' success." (*Psychological Healing*, 1925).

**disparity, chronophilic** See *chronophilia*.

**displaced child syndrome** A form of separation phenomenon, often precipitated in a child by the birth of a sibling. Symptoms include a mixture of irritability, discouragement, jealousy of siblings, and feelings of rejection by other children.

**displacement** 1. Transference of the emotions (affective cathexis) from the original ideas to which they are attached—to other ideas. Schizophrenic patients exhibit displacement of affects to a remarkable degree. What are seemingly the most inconsequential thoughts may be heavily emotionalized. One schizophrenic patient would go into a state of uncontrollable rage over his shoestrings, another became ecstatic over the word "there." The displacement of affects presupposes also the displacement of ideas.

2. Shifting of id impulses from one pathway to another. When, for instance, aggression cannot express itself through direct motor discharge, as in fisticuffs, it may take the pathway of verbalization. Displacement manifests itself also with regard to organic zones. The instincts shift, for example, from the oral to the anal, to the genital zones, or to any other erotogenic zone. In conversion hysteria a psychic complex may be displaced upon any potentially acceptable organ structure. Or all the issues connected with genitality may be displaced to the oral zone. Displacement "from below upward" is a common phenomenon.

Dreams afford notable examples of displacement, where an important latent thought may be represented as an insignificant detail in the manifest content. Similarly, the affective accompaniment may be very strong with the least important dream thought, but feeble with the most important thought. Displacement may also be achieved by reversal; e.g., representing the inside as the outside, the bottom as the top, etc. See *dream*.

**displacement transferences** See *transference*.

**disposing mind and memory** *Obs.* "A sound mind, capable of making a will; remembering the property to be disposed of and the persons who are the natural objects of bounty, and comprehending the manner in which the property is to be distributed" (Singer, H. D. and Krohn, W. C. *Insanity and Law*, 1924).

**disposition** 1. Susceptibility to a disease, vulnerability. 2. *Temperament* (q.v.); relatively consistent qualities of mood or behavior characteristic of a person that allow a degree of predictability of his reactions to particular situations. 3. Prevailing humor or mood.

**disposition, constitutional depressive** *Dysthmic disorder* (q.v.).

**disposition, constitutional manic** The type of personality that has more or less a "manic" tinge throughout life. "The manic temperament of such people disposes to over-hasty acts and to a thoughtless manner of living in general, when it is not restrained by a particularly sound understanding and a particularly good morality. For that reason we find here on the one hand snobbish, inconsiderate, quarrelsome and cranky ne'er-do-wells, who have no staying powers in their transactions, but on the other hand "sunny dispositions,' and people endowed with great ability, amounting sometimes to genius, and not rarely gifted with artistic ability who possess a tireless energy." (Bleuler, E. *Textbook of Psychiatry*, 1930). Bleuler says these people have the *manic mood*. The term constitutional mania is used by some as an equivalent to "endogenous mania," or mania without clear-cut precipitating factors.

**disposition system** See *systematized complex*.

**dispositional attribution** See *attribution*.

**disruption** Sudden loss of organization; although disruption is often used synonymously with *disintegration* (q.v.), the latter term more properly is reserved for slow or gradual loss of organization.

**disruptive behavior and attention-deficit disorders** Included are attention deficit hyperactivity disorder, conduct disorder, and oppositional defiant disorder.

**disseminated encephalomyelitis, acute** Acute perivascular myelinoclasis; an acute demyelinating disease occurring in the course of infection with the causal virus of one of the exanthemata (e.g., measles, mumps, smallpox, chickenpox, vaccination, antirabic inoculation).

**disseminated sclerosis**   *Multiple sclerosis (q.v.).*

**dissimilation**   See *assimilation.*

**dissimulation**   The act of pretending or feigning; *denial* (q.v.).

**dissociate**   To split off some part or component of mental activity, which component then acts as an independent unit of mental life. See *dissociation.*

**dissociate-dysmnesic substitution reaction**   Adolf Meyer's term for conversion hysteria, which emphasizes the fundamental role of memory dissociation in the development of symptoms. See *hysteria.*

**dissociation**   1. Separation of psychologic experiences and events that are normally related, leading to a distortion of experience and of the meaning of personal and interpersonal events; exclusion from consciousness and inaccessibility of voluntary recall of mental events of varying degrees of complexity, including mental and somatic aspects. Dissociative experiences occur normally in everyday life, in the form of absorption in and total attention to particular activities (with an associated imperviousness to distracting events), daydreaming, night dreaming, and *phantasy* (q.v.). Dissociation may also be imposed through hypnosis. *Normative* or nonpathological dissociation is used (1) for mental processing, as in anticipating, rehearsing, creating, planning, and considering how to do things differently; (2) for escape or disengagement from a negative experience; and (3) to reinforce worthy activities—for example, giving full attention to an activity may enhance performance and mood and reduce boredom or stress. See *positive dissociative experiences.*

Dissociation is the experience of having a mind in which there can be two or more independent streams of consciousness flowing concurrently, allowing some thoughts, sensations, and behaviors to occur simultaneously or outside awareness, as in altered states of consciousness (*ASC*). Most non-Western cultures describe culturally patterned dissociative symptoms—major discontinuities of consciousness, memory, identity, and behavior, such as nonpossession trance states and *kinetically induced dissociation* (rhythmic music and dance, commonly a part of religious observances). Such indigenous

ASC phenomena are usually considered normal and appear to be socially sanctioned expressions of disowned and unremembered aggression and sexuality. See *culture-specific syndromes.*

2. Dissociation is sometimes equated with schizophrenic *splitting* (q.v.), in which ideas are separated from their consonant affects. An example is the patient who laughed heartily while describing his delusion that he had been cut into a million pieces. For other abnormal forms of dissociation, see *dissociative disorders.*

**dissociative disorders**   A group of disorders characterized by alterations in the normally integrated functions of identity, memory, or consciousness. The disturbance may be sudden or gradual in onset, and transient or chronic in duration. In older classifications, the dissociative disorders were called hysterical neurosis, dissociative type, or conversion hysteria with predominantly mental symptoms.

In the dissociative disorders, the disorder is not the fact that dissociation is present, nor that it was deployed as a defense in the face of trauma, but that severe dissociation and its ramifications continue in the absence of immediate trauma. Such continuing or recurring dissociation has been subdivided into the following:

1. *Primary dissociation*—the intrusion into consciousness of fragmented memories of trauma, usually in sensory rather than verbal form, such as intense waves of feelings or flashbacks. Such intrusions are cued by reminders of past traumatic events and are associated with psychophysiologic arousal. Primary dissociation is characteristic of *posttraumatic stress disorder* (q.v.). Neuroimaging studies of primary dissociation have found lower than normal activation of the anterior cingulate cortex (involved in regulation of emotional, cognitive, and autonomic responses) and of medial prefrontal cortex (consistent with hyperarousal in reaction to the misperception of the intrusion as a current threat, rather than as a memory of past trauma).

2. *Secondary dissociation,* sometimes called *peritraumatic dissociation*—abnormalities of the sense of self and somatosensory awareness, such as the feeling that the mind has left the body and is observing the traumatic act

from afar. Secondary dissociation is characteristic of *depersonalization* disorder (q.v.). It is not associated with intense fear or arousal; instead, there is a general dampening of feeling and behavior ("freezing") and often a feeling of helplessness.

3. *Tertiary dissociation*—ego states or complex identity states that may represent different components of one or more traumatic experiences or the varying conflicts, deficits, and coping strategies involved in trying to live in a difficult world.

Dissociative disorders are among the most common comorbid disorders in borderline personality disorder, conversion disorder, eating disorders, gender identity disorder, and substance use disorders (qq.v.).

In DSM-IV, the dissociative disorders include dissociative *amnesia*, dissociative *fugue*, *dissociative identity disorder* (multiple personality disorder), *depersonalization* disorder, *trance disorder*, and *Ganser syndrome* (qq.v.). See *hysteria*.

Many authorities believe that dissociation is a normal defense mechanism that may evolve over time into a maladaptive or pathological process. In this view, dissociative phenomena exist on a continuum and become maladaptive only when they exceed certain limits in intensity and frequency, or occur in inappropriate contexts.

**Dissociative Disorders Interview Schedule**  *DDIS*; a 131-item structured interview devised by Ross. It inquires about consciously perceived and endorsed symptoms of several mental disorders, and its false positive rate for dissociative identity disorder is said to be less than 1% in clinical populations.

**Dissociative Experiences Scale**  *DES*; devised by Bernstein and Putnam as a screening instrument for dissociative disorders, including dissociative identity disorder.

**dissociative fugue**  See *fugue*.

**dissociative identity disorder**  *DID*; formerly known as *multiple personality disorder* (*MPD*); one of the *dissociative disorders* (q.v.), characterized by the presence of two or more relatively distinct and separate subpersonalities in a single person, as in Dr. Jeckyll and Mr. Hyde, or in Morton Prince's case of Miss Beauchamp, or in Cleckley and Thigpen's case of Chris Sizemore (Eve).

Although previously considered rare, MPD has been reported in increasing numbers since the late 1970s. Greater awareness of the disorder has permitted identification of a relatively specific historical antecedent with which it appears to be associated: child abuse, most commonly neglect or physical and sexual child abuse. Each alternate personality appears to deal with a related set of affects, such as rage in response to abuse or sexual affects and conflicts stemming from sexual abuse.

How many of the growing number of MPD cases atre responses to suggestions from the therapist, and how many of those cases are truly a result of child abuse, are matters of intense controversy. See *false memory.*

There appears to be a relationship between MPD and temporal lobe epilepsy. Perhaps as many as 33% of patients with temporal lobe epilepsy experience dissociative episodes, and some such patients develop DID. It has been hypothesized that the dissociation is a product of intensely dystonic affects characteristic of the interictal period in temporal lobe epilepsy.

In multiple personality, the original personality is termed the primary personality, and the dissociated or split-off personality is termed the secondary personality, or the *alter.* The alter personalities (there are rarely less than three) may be of the opposite sex, of different races and ages, and from a family different from the family of origin. The most common subordinate personality is childlike.

There is generally amnesia during each personality state for the existence of the others and for the events that took place when another personality was dominant. Sometimes, however, personalities are aware of (co-conscious with) all or some of the others to varying degrees and may experience the others as friends, companions, or adversaries. DID usually has its onset by the age of 8 years, although it may not be diagnosed until adulthood. Women account for 75% to 95% of reported cases.

There are two major clusters of dissociative symptoms in DID: switching from one personality to another with concomitant amnesia (i.e., full dissociation from consciousness), and partially dissociated intrusions by alter personalities into executive functioning and sense of self. In its description of DID, DSM-IV includes the switching and amnesia cluster, but not the cluster of partially dissociated intrusions.

The following dissociative symptoms of DID are listed (approximately) in the order of frequency with which they are reported:

1. Amnesia is the most frequently reported symptom; it may be manifested in various ways, including *fugue, microamnesia* (qq.v.), time loss, being told of disremembered actions, finding unfamiliar objects among one's possessions, finding objects are unexpectedly missing, encountering people the patient does not recognize who introduce themselves as familiar with or friends of the patient, finding evidence of recent actions that the patient does not remember, being told of disremembered actions, amnesia for childhood, amnesia for personal identity, temporary loss of well-practiced knowledge or skills.

2. *Conversion* (q.v.) and other somatoform symptoms are the second most commonly reported group of symptoms; DSM-IV classifies them as somatoform rather than dissociative disorders.

3. The third most common dissociative symptom is hearing voices, usually "in the head" but sometimes reframed as "like the voice of conscience"; DSM-IV includes only command hallucinations in this category.

4. *Depersonalization* (q.v.); this is not included in DSM-IV's list of dissociative symptoms.

5. *Trance* states (q.v.)—periods of nonresponsiveness during which the patient manifests a blank stare; not included in DSM-IV.

6. *Self-alteration* (q.v.), feeling as if one's body, thoughts, or urges belong to someone else.

7. *Derealization*, feeling that the world has changed or is unreal.

8. Subjective awareness of the presence of other personalities.

9. Identity confusion, not knowing one's name.

10. Flashbacks, similar to those seen in PTSD, which is extensively comorbid with DID.

11. Psychotic-like symptoms: auditory hallucinations may appear as hearing the voices of alters, or hearing the auditory part of flashbacks; visual hallucinations may appear as seeing alter personalities either mentally or externally, or as the visual component of flashbacks. Both forms of hallucination may also be genuinely psychotic.

12. Schneiderian *first-rank symptoms* (q.v.), such as "made" actions, "made" feelings, "made" impulses, voices arguing or commenting, thought withdrawal, and thought insertion (Dell, P. F. *Psychiatric Clinics of North America 29*: 1–26, 2006)

It has been suggested that DID is a variant of *attachment* disorders (q.v.). Disorganization of attachment may be more central to the development of dissociation than the trauma itself.

Neuroimaging studies have reported that DID is associated with volume reductions in both amygdala and hippocampus, but with relatively greater reduction in the amygdala. (Vermetten, E. et al., *American Journal of Psychiatry 163*: 630–636, 2006)

**distortion**   The process of disguising, hiding, or otherwise modifying unconscious mental elements so that they are allowed to enter consciousness, whose censoring mechanisms would not allow them access to consciousness in undisguised form.

There are many ways in which distortion may be effected, e.g., dropping out (repression) of associative links between conscious content and unconscious impulse, displacement of activity onto a substitute object, replacement of objectionable impulse with another one that is associatively connected.

**distortion by transference**   Misperceptions of the analyst or analytic situation based on *transference* (q.v.). The accusation that the analyst is bored or uninterested may be an expression of the childhood wish for more love and attention from mother rather than an accurate appraisal of the analyst's current attitude toward the patient.

**distractibility**   See *mania.*

**distributed processing**   Apportionment of different elements of a system or function to different sites. In the central nervous system, for instance, different components of a single behavior (e.g., the perceptual and motor elements of language) are localized in different regions of the brain; interconnections between those different parts makes the final behavior possible. See *connectionism.*

Attention, for instance, is a distributed process involving extensive areas of the brain. Each of the areas contributes, and although some parts (especially, the right hemisphere) are more important than others, there is no "attention center." Similarly, object knowledge is stored in a distributed system. Information about specific features is probably stored close to the cortical regions mediating perception of those features. Memory functions are organized around fundamentally different information storage systems.

**distributive analysis** In objective *psychobiology* (q.v.), the analysis of information gained about the patient "is distributed by the physician along the various lines which are indicated by the patient's complaints and symptoms, by the problems which the physician himself can recognize, by the patient's imaginations concerning the present and the past as well as by actual situations, attitude to the future and outstanding features of his personality" (Diethelm, O. *Treatment in Psychiatry*, 1936).

**disulfiram** See *Antabuse*.

**diurnal** Occurring each day, or in the daytime, as opposed to occurring at night (nocturnal).

**DIVA** Digital intravenous angiography, a method of visualizing the major blood vessels supplying the brain.

**divagation** Rambling thought and speech.

**divergence, neuronal** Transmission of a signal from one neuron to many target cells; the opposite of neuronal convergence.

**diversional therapy** In occupational therapy, tasks given primarily for the amusement and distraction of the patient.

**divorce, emotional** A type of marital relationship in which the partners live in separate worlds; contrasted with *mutuality*, which refers to normal interaction between the partners and a give-and-take relationship. Emotional divorce appears to be much more frequent in parents of schizophrenics than in other parents. See *family therapy*.

**divorce, stations of** As described by Bohannan (1973), the various issues that confront a divorcing couple: (1) *emotional divorce*—the loss of face and involvement preceding separation (see *family therapy*); (2) *legal divorce*—one person leaves the house and legal proceedings are initiated; (3) *economic divorce*—reduction in income for each of the couple, property settlement, and other economic entanglements; (4) *coparental divorce*—negotiating the transition to remaining parents while no longer being spouses; (5) *community divorce*—reorganization of friendship networks; (6) *psychic divorce*—reestablishing autonomy as a single person.

**divorce therapy** A subspecialty of marriage and family therapy consisting of counseling and support for partners who are in the process of terminating their formal, contractual relationship. Major forms are (1) individual treatment for a divorcing person; (2) family counseling with focus on parenting and separation, or counseling each parent separately with the children concerning establishment of separate households; (3) divorce groups, consisting of task- or information-oriented sessions with same-sex persons at various stages in the separating process; and (4) divorce mediation, consisting of helping the couple deal with practical issues such as property settlement and visitation rights; this proffers a therapy model as an alternative to the more usual legal adversary model. See *marital therapy*.

**Dix, Dorothea Lynde** (1802–87) American reformer in the care of psychiatric patients.

**dizygotic** *DZ*; Pertaining to a twin pair produced by two eggs; preferable to the synonymous fraternal, nonidentical.

**dizziness, chronic subjective (CSD)** A feeling of swaying, often set off by motion cues such as being in crowds of people, around flashing light stimuli, or in heavy traffic. About 1% of the United States population has CSD. Of those studied, 60% had primary or secondary anxiety disorders; about 37% had some CNS disorder, including migraine, postconcussional syndrome or traumatic brain injury, or dysautonomias (Staab, J. et al. *Archives General Psychiatry*, February 2007).

**D-KEFS** Delis-Kaplan Executive Function System, a battery of 9 tests assessing executive function. The tests are trail making, verbal fluency, design fluency, color-word interference, sorting, twenty questions, word context, Tower test, and proverbs test.

**DLB** Dementia with Lewy bodies; see *Lewy body dementia*.

**DLPFC** Dorsolateral *prefrontal cortex* (q.v.); DLPFC has reciprocal connections with brain regions that are associated with motor control (basal ganglia, premotor cortex, supplementary motor area), performance monitoring (cingulate cortex), and higher-order sensory processing (association areas, parietal cortex). DLPFC supports regulation of behavior and control of response to environmental stimuli. It is the nonemotional PFC; the *orbital prefrontal cortex* (q.v.) is the emotional PFC.

Impairment of reflective, mechanistic behavior is most evident following DLPFC damage. See *prefrontal cortex*.

When subjects suppress a memory, DLPFC is active. At the same time, activity in hippocampus is decreased. It is possible that people with PTSD are deficient in their ability to recruit this network. Just as DLPFC may dampen activity in hippocampus to manage memory, it may dampen activity in amygdala when people try to put a positive spin on a bad situation. Some studies have found heightened amygdala activity and decreased prefrontal cortex activity in depressed subjects, perhaps indicating that they are less able to tap into the neural networks for reappraisal.

**DMA**   A phenylethylamine *hallucinogen* (q.v.).

**DMPEA**   See *pink spot*.

**dMRI**   Diffusion MRI produces MRI-based quantitative maps of microscopic, natural displacements of water molecules that occur in brain tissues as part of the physical diffusion process. When water movement is impeded by obstacles such as brain tissue (including cell membranes, fibers, and macromolecules), those obstacles can be measured by the amount of diffusion distance reduction. dMRI produces images of brain activation from signals that are directly associated with neuronal activation, rather than through changes in blood flow. For example, the water diffusion coefficient decreases by 30%–50% in brain tissue within several minutes of occlusion of the middle cerebral artery. dMRI has become the imaging modality of choice for the management of stroke patients because of its ability to assess lesion severity and extension at a stage when tissue is still salvageable. See *fMRI*; *MRI*.

In *DTI* (diffusion tissue imaging), diffusion is described by an array of nine coefficients that fully characterize how diffusion in space varies according to direction. The most advanced application of DTI is fiber tracking in the brain. Whereas fMRI provides information about the cortical areas involved in a given cognitive process, connectivity studies provide information on the structural/dynamic wiring that determines how those areas are networked. DTI is increasingly being used to identify subtle connectivity anomalies in various dysfunctions, such as brain tumors, dyslexia, multiple sclerosis, and schizophrenia.

**DMT**   Dimethyltryptamine. See *hallucinogen*.

**DNA**   *Deoxyribonucleic acid;* a nucleic acid that contains deoxyribose in its sugar component. It is found in the nuclei and mitochondria as a long chain of deoxyribose molecules, linked to which are the purine bases adenine (A), thymine (T), guanine (G), and cytosine (C). DNA is the information archive of the cell, but proteins do all the work of the cell and ultimately dictate all biological processes and cellular fates. In mitochondria, DNA is single-stranded; in chromosomes, it is double-stranded: two antiparallel strands wind around a spool, the *nucleosome*. The nucleosome is composed of protein molecules, the histones. Each nucleosome carries a double turn of DNA. Nucleosomes are stacked together in groups of six or eight in a spiral braid, which makes a fiber, *chromatin*. Chromatin makes up the fine structures of chromosomes, 23 pairs of which are packed into the cell nucleus. See *chromatin; chromosome; histones; nucleosome*.

DNA serves two functions: (1) reproduction—self-duplication for transfer to new cells or new offspring and (2) synthesis of proteins. In both cases, the double strands of DNA separate. In sexual reproduction, each strand is assigned to a gamete and pairs with a similar strand from the mate's gamete to provide a new cell with a full set of chromosomes.

In protein synthesis, the strand acts as a template for RNA which, in turn, acts as a template for the synthesis of proteins. This role of DNA is described in the *central dogma*: whenever the cell needs to manufacture a new protein, it must retrieve a copy of the protein's specifications from the coiled stacks of its DNA library; DNA is duplicated within the cell nucleus and transcribed into *RNA* (q.v.) in the cytoplasm, where it is translated into the synthesis of protein(s). See *transcription*.

The winding DNA has been compared to a spiral staircase (the *double helix* model of Watson and Crick), the sides of which consist of monotonously repeating deoxyribose sugar molecules joined by phosphate bonds. The millions of rungs of the ladder are formed by two weakly bonded purine nucleotides that face each other within the helix and contain the genetic code. The code consists of only four bases that are always paired with the same partner within the helix: adenine with thymine (A : T), and guanine with cytosine (G : C).

Triplets of bases (*codons*) constitute genetic "words" specifying particular amino acids. Although these four chemical "letters" make up the whole alphabet, the long chain of them in the DNA molecule constitutes a tape of coded instructions with almost infinite variations. Each human cell contains a full 6 feet (2 meters) of DNA, which occurs as a long string of approximately 3 billion pairs of nucleotide bases. The genes constitute about 1 percent of the nucleotide bases; most of the genome does not encode proteins or regulatory information and, in consequence, is often labeled *junk DNA*. See *noncoding DNA*.

The sequence of hundreds or several thousands of subunits in a gene gives the living cell orders for manufacture of a particular protein. It is estimated that the human *gene* system or *genome* (qq.v.) is composed of about 30,000 genes. DNA's four nucleotide letters can occur in 64 different combinations of three: ATA, ATC, and so on. Because these 64 triplets need code only for the insertion of 20 amino acids, different combinations sometimes code for the same thing. Both TTA and TTG, for example, code for the amino acid leucine. In addition to 61 DNA trios, or codons, for amino acids, there are three codons for a "stop" command, telling the ribosome to stop adding amino acids to a protein. When the cellular machinery transcribes DNA into RNA, the letters change, but the stop signals remain in place.

In other words, DNA contains the genetic blueprint of the organism in chemical language. It is a reservoir of information needed to maintain cellular integrity as well as to respond to environmental challenges. The information is expressed in a series of steps regulated partly by information contained within the DNA itself and partly by environmental signals. Regulation of gene expression by environmental signals is basic to homeostasis and adaptation, including learning and memory.

**DNA probe**  See *probe*.

**DNA variation**  Difference in the nucleotide code. Humans share at least 99.9% of the nucelotide code in their genome; diversity of human beings at the genetic level is encoded by less than 0.1% variation in DNA. The most common form of DNA variation in humans is the *SNP* (q.v.).

**D-O psychiatrist**  Directive-organic psychiatrist; Hollingshead and Redlich so designated that group of psychiatrists whose orientation is biological and whose psychotherapeutic approach is directive and authoritarian.

**dodge, insanity**  Fictitious defense of insanity designed to evade punishment for a criminal act. See *criminal responsibility*.

**DOES**  Disorders of excessive somnolence. See *sleep disorders*.

**Dole-Nyswander program**  See *methadone*.

**dolichocephaly**  See *cephalic index*.

**dolichomorphic**  Relating to long, thin stature. Dolichomorphic is equivalent to *microsplanchnic* of Viola and corresponds closely to Kretschmer's *asthenic type* (qq.v.).

**doll's eye maneuvers**  *Oculocephalic maneuvers* (to elicit the oculocephalic reflexes); testing a subject's extraocular movements by moving the head and noting how the eye changes position in relation to the orbit. Absence of such movements is indicative of brain stem disease; in supranuclear disease, however, the eyes fail to move on volition but can be deviated by the oculocephalic reflex.

**domatophobia**  Fear of being confined in a house.

**domestic violence**  *Family violence*; included are child and spouse homicide, spouse abuse, wife battering, child abuse, child sexual abuse, severe child neglect, adolescent abuse, sibling abuse, parental abuse, and abuse of the elderly. The family is the most frequent single locus for all violence, including homicide. Violence is estimated to occur in at least 50% of American families.

Some use the term in a more limited way, to refer only to *spousal abuse*: violent acts between adults who are involved in an intimate relationship. The acts range from shoving to aggressive acts of beating (assault, battery), false imprisonment, and homicide. Acts of physical aggression between domestic partners occur in approximately 1 in 6 American homes. Three of 4 women who are killed in the United States are murdered by domestic partners, and 75% of spousal assaults occur at the time of separation or divorce. See *battered child syndrome; child abuse; infidelity; victim; wife battering*.

**domesticated pride**  Rado's term for the pride and overevaluation of self seen in the obsessive patient, whose pride is based on guilty fear and its resultant humiliation, which have been repressed. Such a patient has no awareness of the guilty fear that is the foundation on which his pride rests; this is in contradistinction to the individual with real pride in his self-assertive rage. Domesticated pride is also known as *moral pride.*

**domicile**  Dwelling; residence. *Domiciliary care* is a generic term referring to a spectrum of housing or residential settings ranging from a highly structured, intensively supervised facility to a loosely organized living arrangement that provides patients maximal independence and minimal supervision. Successful *deinstitutionalization* of long-term, chronic mental patients depends upon a combination of continuing medical supervision and regulation of psychopharmacological treatment with the organization technology to ensure ready access to whatever level of psychiatric care their changing needs may require.

Included within the spectrum of settings are (1) *chronic care hospitals*, which provide a high level of continuous nursing care and/or rehabilitation as well as immediately available medical attention; (2) *skilled nursing facilities* or *therapeutic residential centers*, which provide 24-hour nursing care or supervision in a community-based facility; (3) *health-related facilities*, most often operated in association with a skilled nursing facility, to provide institutional care less extensive than available in a skilled nursing facility or chronic care hospital; (4) *intermediate care facilities* or *community treatment houses*, which provide 24-hour nursing care or supervision on a temporary basis, typically in a converted residence or similar homelike setting; (5) *halfway houses*, nonmedical facilities that promote socialization and provide patients with a place to stay until a suitable residence is available; (6) *residential facilities, residential care homes*, or *board and care homes*, which provide room and board and limited personal assistance in a group or family setting within the community; (7) *social rehabilitation facilities*, which provide 24-hour services in a group setting to persons who need temporary assistance, guidance, or counseling; (8) *satellite housing*, apartments or single-family houses that do not provide live-in staff but do offer some professional supervision and access to assistance in emergencies. Variants of satellite housing are landlord-supervised apartments and *Fairweather lodges*. The latter are operated by patients themselves, with only occasional visits by professionals (Fairweather, G. et al. *Community Life for the Mentally Ill*, 1969). Other experimental settings include *Soteria House*, a residence for first-admission, unmarried schizophrenic patients between 15 and 30 years of age; the setting is usually drug-free (including antipsychotic agents) and the staff is nonprofessional. The *Missouri Foster Community Program* is patterned after the Gheel Colony in Belgium and provides full integration of former patients into the community.

**dominance**  1. *Cerebral dominance* (q.v.).

2. High ranking on the socioeconomic scale. See *SES.*

3. The genetic mechanism by which one member of an allelic pair of hereditary factors is endowed with the capacity of expressing itself so strongly that it prevails in the hybrids over the contrasting factor and determines the visible appearance of a hybridized individual either completely or, at least, predominantly. The phenotype of any hybrid inheriting a *completely dominant* character from one of the parents exhibits no manifestations of the suppressed, or *recessive*, factor and is thus enabled to appear as a pure-bred organism in spite of its heterozygosity (see *recessiveness*).

The terms dominance and recessiveness are relative rather than precise and exact, and different authorities use the terms in different ways. Some, for example, define a dominant gene as one that causes expression of the disease when present in one parent, and a recessive gene as one that causes expression only when present in both. Genes that always cause the disease are termed fully *penetrant*, while those that cause it only irregularly are termed partially penetrant.

X-linked dominant diseases are rare. Autosomal dominant diseases are more frequent, and either father or mother can transmit the gene to offspring of either sex. The phenotype appears in every generation, and each child has a 50/50 chance of developing the disorder. Huntington disease is transmitted as an autosomal dominant; it is due to a single mutation on the short arm of chromosome 4.

**dominance, cerebral**  See *cerebral dominance*

**dominance test**  See *Wada dominance test.*

**dominant**  1. A phenotype caused by one allele is said to be dominant with respect to a phenotype caused by a second allele if an individual carrying both alleles shows the former and not the latter phenotype.

2. Referring to *cerebral dominance.*

**dominant determinant**  See *determinant, dream.*

**dominant mentality**  See *group tension, common.*

**Don Juan**  (The Chronicle of Seville relates that Don Juan Tenorio killed Comendador Ulloa at night and carried off his daughter. The father was buried in the family chapel and his statue was erected there. The statue and chapel were destroyed by fire. To end the profligate's debauchery the Franciscan monks lured and killed him and spread the rumor that Don Juan had insulted the Comendador on his tomb and that the new statue had dragged the Don to hell.)

In psychiatry the term Don Juan refers to a type of male *hypersexuality* (q.v.). Sexual activities are aimed toward contradicting inferiority feelings by proof of erotic successes. The Don Juan type is little interested in his woman partner of the moment; for having proved that he can excite her sexually, he must then allay his doubts about his ability to excite other women and so moves on to another conquest. The condition depends on intense narcissistic needs and fears of loss of love, with a pregenital and sadistic coloring of the total sexuality. The Don Juan type of erotomania is frequently a defense against unconscious homosexual impulses.

**Don Juan of achievement**  Fenichel's term for a type of narcissistic personality disorder (although not so-named at the time), characterized by omnipotent behavior, undue independence, leadership qualities, lack of tenderness, infidelity, desire to be a great or renowned person, and being always in a hurry.

**donatism**  Donato (professional name of the Belgian "magnetizer" Alfred d'Hont, 1845–1900) demonstrated the role of imitation in hypnosis; the term donatism was given to that form of hypnosis in which imitation forms an important part.

**doorknob phobia**  A phobia in which the situation to be avoided (because it produces anxiety) is the touching of a doorknob. On first examination the anxiety seems to be related to touching an object believed to be dirty, as a doorknob must be. Thus the patient is protected against anal-erotic wishes to be dirty or to soil, for in magical thinking the characteristics of an object are communicated by touching it. As Fenichel points out, however, occasionally what appears to be only a protection against anal-erotic wishes may in reality be a protection against other impulses altered by regression, so that they seem to be anal-erotic impulses. He explains that the goal of all impulses involves touching an object, whether it be another person or one's own body. In this way, for example, the patient can achieve security against a wish to masturbate.

"Not infrequently a wish to masturbate that has been warded off has been altered by regression, so that the phobia appears to be a protection against anal-erotic wishes to be dirty or to soil" (*The Psychoanalytic Theory of Neurosis,* 1945).

**dopamine**  A *catecholamine* (q.v.) that is believed to be involved in the development of schizophrenia and in other neuropsychiatric disorders, including drug dependence. Dopamine appears to have an important general role in the neuromodulation of exploratory and appetitive behaviors, including alcohol-seeking behavior. Low doses of ethanol have an excitatory effect on dopaminergic neurons in the *ventral tegmental area* (*VTA*), suggesting the possibility that ethanol provides a pharmacological reward that facilitates alcohol-seeking behavior for its euphorigenic effects. See *addiction; alcoholism.*

Dopamine neurons occur in the midbrain, in at least four tracts:

1. *Nigrostriatal,* which accounts for approximately 70% of the total brain content of dopamine. The nigrostriatal tract is part of the extrapyramidal motor system; its cell bodies are in the substantia nigra and it projects to the basal ganglia (chiefly the caudate nucleus and putamen). The hypokinesia of Parkinson disease is due to degeneration of nigrostriatal dopamine neurons; it is usually alleviated by administration of levodopa. It is probable that the nigrostriatal tract is also involved in the motor (catatonic) symptoms of schizophrenia and in the parkinsonian side effects of neuroleptics.

2. *Tuberoinfundibular,* which originates in the hypothalamus and projects to the

pituitary; neuroleptic drugs elevate prolactin levels by blockading dopamine receptors in the anterior pituitary.

3. *Mesolimbic*, which originates in the ventral tegmental area and projects to the limbic system, including the nucleus accumbens and amygdala. The mesolimbic system is important in the reinforcement of eating, sexual behaviors, and perhaps in addictive "drive states" which are similarly stereotypic, repetitive, and relentless in their nature.

4. *Mesocortical*, which originates in the ventral tegmental area and projects to the cortex of the frontal and temporal lobes. Drugs that act selectively on the limbic and cortical dopamine systems are also antipsychotic, suggesting that disturbance of these pathways may be involved in the development of schizophrenia. See *dopamine hypothesis*.

The clinical potency of the older neuroleptic drugs is highly correlated with their affinity for dopamine receptors (and is not related to their ability to compete for other receptors, such as alpha-adrenergic, serotonergic, histaminergic, opiate, or muscarinic cholinergic receptors). Dopamine exerts its effect through interaction with at least two types of dopamine receptor: $D_1$, linked to stimulation of cyclic adenosine monophosphate (cAMP), and $D_2$, associated with an inhibition of the adenylate cyclase activity that stimulates cAMP. Both these receptors are concentrated in the basal ganglia, which is involved in the control of movement; it is likely that they are largely responsible for the extrapyramidal side effects of neuroleptic therapy. Schizophrenia, however, is expressed primarily in cognitive and emotional symptoms, not in movement disturbances.

Drug effects on dopaminergic neurotransmission include (1) inhibition—the amino acid analogues alpha-methyltyrosine and alpha-methyldopa (Aldomet), by competitive inhibition; reserpine, by inhibiting vesicular storage of dopamine; the older neuroleptic drugs, by blocking dopamine receptors; and (2) augmentation—the precursor amino acid Levodopa, by enhancing dopamine receptors; bromocriptine, by direct agonist effect at dopamine receptors; cocaine, methylphenidate, and amphetamine, by inhibiting the uptake and inactivation of dopamine; monoamine oxidase inhibitors, by interfering with enzymatic degradation of dopamine.

**dopamine hypothesis of addiction** Increased dopamine transmission in the nucleus accumbens and the basal ganglia underlies the reinforcing responses to drugs of abuse. The dopamine increases are not directly related to reward (pleasure) per se, but to the prediction of reward and to salience (reflecting motivation, drive); dopamine increase motivates procurement of more drug regardless of whether the effects are pleasurable. See *addiction*

Dopamine is crucial for the rewarding effects of the psychomotor stimulants. It is important, but probably not crucial, for the rewarding effects of the opiates, nicotine, cannabis, and ethanol. The dopamine transporter hypothesis of cocaine addiction assumes that cocaine addiction results from the binding of cocaine to the dopamine transporter (DAT) and to the resultant inhibition of dopamine reuptake. But dopamine is rewarding even in DAT-deleted mutant mice, suggesting that noradrenaline and serotonin transporters (NET and SERT) are involved. Dopamine uptake in the medial prefrontal cortex, a cocaine reward site, is mediated primarily by NET. Cocaine is no longer rewarding in mice with both DAT and SERT knocked out. See *reward*.

**dopamine hypothesis of reinforcement** Dopamine is crucial to positive reinforcement. Most normally rewarding stimuli are ineffective as reinforcers in dopamine-compromised animals.

**dopamine hypothesis of reward** See *reward*.

**dopamine hypothesis of schizophrenia** The theory that schizophrenic disorders are related to or caused by some abnormality in the metabolism of dopamine in the brain; specifically, that relative overactivity of mesolimbic, mesocortical, or nigrostrial dopaminergic neurons (or supersensitivity of dopamine receptors) may be present in at least some schizophrenics. The increase may be responsible for specific symptoms, such as delusions or hallucinations, or for specific mechanisms, such as attentional impairment. See *epinephrine*.

Hyperdopaminergic transmission is unlikely to be the primary or sole event in either the etiology or pathogenesis of schizophrenia. Research on schizophrenia focused on the dopamine system for almost 20 years and produced little of substantial value. Revisions of the dopamine hypothesis posit diminished dopaminergic activity in the prefrontal cortex underlying negative symptoms and reciprocal dopaminergic hyperactivity in the mesolimbic pathways to be responsible for psychotic symptoms. It seems very clear now that, whatever the abnormality underpinning schizophrenia, it does not reside solely within the dopamine system. See *schizophrenia, models of*.

It is currently believed that schizophrenia is more likely due to an imbalance between multiple neurotransmitter systems, including serotonin and glutamate as well as dopamine. A low concentration of $5\text{-HT}_2$ receptors in the frontal cortex, for example, or a dysplasia of glutamate afferents to the frontal cortex, may be a critical abnormality that establishes the substrate necessary for sensitivity to dopaminergic manipulations.

**dopamine stabilizer**  A partial agonist or partial mixed-action antagonist to dopamine. In low dopaminergic states, such a compound increases dopamine release; but in states of high dopaminergic tone, such a compound acts as antagonist.

**dopamine transporter**  *DAT* (q.v.).

**dopaminergic systems**  These include dopaminergic neurons in the substantia nigra pars compacta and the retrorubral area. The first system, the *mesostriatal pathway*, projects to the entire neostriatum, whereas the VTA, also called the *mesolimbic pathway*, terminates in the ventral striatum.

Tardive dyskinesia (a Parkinson-like syndrome) demonstrates a severe loss of catecholaminergic neurons in the substantia nigra pars compacta. Conversely, in schizophrenia, it is thought that the mesolimbic dopaminergic system is overactive and that the mesocortical dopaminergic system has reduced activity.

The observation that cells of the dopaminergic systems fire in relation to rewarding stimuli and reward conditioned stimuli, taken with the presence of $D_1$ and $D_2$ receptors on cholinergic interneurons, has suggested that dopamine plays a key role in the documented plasticity of response of tonically active neurons (*TANs*) during reward-based learning. See *addiction*.

**doping**  Use of substances to improve an athlete's performance.

Among those most commonly used are steroids, psychostimulants, opioids, antihistamines, beta blockers, and blood transfusions. Screen testing for one or more of such substances is now routine in national and international sports competitions.

**Doppelganger phenomenon**  A reduplicative paramnesia consisting of the delusion that a double of a person or place exists elsewhere. One patient, for example, after brain injury came to believe that he had been relocated and was in a hospital in a different city. The phenomenon suggests nondominant parietal lobe pathology and is related to other disturbances of recognition. See *Capgras syndrome; nonrecognition; parietal lobe; prosopagnosia; sensory neglect*.

**Dora**  The subject of a case history written by Freud in 1901 and published in 1905 as "Fragment of an Analysis of a Case of Hysteria." Freud's writings include four other extensive case histories: Little Hans (see *Hans*), the *Rat-Man, Schreber*, and the *Wolf-Man* (qq.v.). The case of Dora was used to illustrate how Freud interpreted dreams and how symptoms could be understood in terms of the repressed parts of mental life.

Dora had been referred to Freud by her father when she was 19. She was subject to fits of depression, irritability, suicidal ideas, and vengeful outbursts. During the 11-week treatment period, it became evident that Dora felt she had been handed over to Herr K, her middle-aged admirer, in return for his toleration of the sexual relationship between her father and Herr K's wife. Beginning at the time Dora was 14, Herr K had made sexual overtures to her. She was both excited and disgusted by his advances and rejected them. Thereafter, she developed a feeling of pressure in the upper part of her body, and fits of coughing accompanied by aphonia or mutism, which sometimes persisted for weeks.

Dora's attacks of coughing and aphonia/mutism were believed by Freud to coincide with Herr K's absences, suggesting that speech had no value for her since her loved one was not there to hear it. The pressure in the upper body Freud interpreted as a displacement from below of feelings of genital engorgement. Dora broke away from treatment before the meaning of all her symptoms was understood.

**doraphobia**  Fear of the skin of animals.

**Dorian love**  Male *homosexuality, pederasty* (qq.v).

**doromania**  Compulsive gift giving.

**dorsal pathway**   See *visual stream.*

**dorsocuboidal reflex**   See *Bechtereff-Mendel reflex.*

**dorsolateral PFC**   *DLPFC* (q.v.).

**dorsolateral prefrontal cortex**   *DLPFC* (q.v.).

**dorsomedial nucleus**   MD; a nuclear group of the *thalamus* (q.v.) containing at least three different neuronal types: medial or magnocellular, lateral (parvocellular or fascicular), and posterior or multiform. It is subdivided into three distinct segments, each of which projects to a specific prefrontal cortical region. A lateral segment projects to the superior frontal convexity, which is part of the dorsolateral prefrontal cortex (DLPFC). Input is from the same prefrontal regions, from the entorhinal cortex (the major cortical input to the hippocampus), and from the amygdala and inferior temporal gyrus via the inferior thalamic peduncle.

**dose dependence, therapeutic**   Development of physical and psychological dependence on a prescribed drug even though the patient has never exceeded the prescribed dose. Seen most frequently with sedative-hypnotic drugs after long-term use, therapeutic dose dependence is related to rebound of REM sleep and deterioration of sleep patterns that occur when the drug is withdrawn.

**dosing, targeted**   See *targeted-dose strategy.*

**dotage**   Senile dementia. See *Alzheimer disease.*

**double bind**   This term is approximately equivalent to dilemma and is used particularly to refer to a type of interaction once believed to be characteristic of families containing schizophrenic members. The parent of a schizophrenic, for example, is perceived by the patient as emitting signals of an incongruent nature. The parent encourages the patient to express a courageous opinion, but when that opinion is expressed disparages it as unloving, disloyal, or disobedient. As a result of repeated entrapment in the double bind, which can be neither ignored nor attacked directly by commenting on the incongruity, the schizophrenic learns to strip all his communications of material that might be maltreated in this way.

A. Ferreira (*Archives of General Psychiatry,* 1960) terms the double bind a "unipolar message" that is not confined to schizophrenia. What is particularly frequent in schizophrenia is that the contradictory messages emanate from a single (unipolar) source, usually the mother. In delinquent behavior, on the other hand, the source of the messages is split (bipolar), with message A emanating from the father and message B (a comment about message A with the effect of opposing or destroying it) emanating from the mother, or vice versa. Ferreira calls this the "split double bind."

**double bind, therapeutic**   See *paradoxical therapy.*

**double blind**   Referring to a research method, used primarily in drug investigations, in which neither subject-patient nor rater-evaluator knows whether the drug being studied or a placebo is being administered. Use of the double-blind method, advantageous as it may be from a research point of view, raises certain ethical questions when the subjects of the study are humans. The physician who permits his patient to be a subject, for example, has to some degree abrogated responsibility for the care of the patient by relinquishing control over selection of the particular treatment modality. For another thing, conventional treatment is being withheld from those subjects who are in the experimental group, while those in the control group are not given the opportunity to receive what may turn out to be a therapeutic breakthrough in the treatment of their condition. Double-blind experiments, in other words, put the experimenter into a double bind, the only solution to which would appear to revolve about obtaining fully *informed consent* (q.v.) from the subjects of the experiment.

**double bouquet cells**   DBCs; see *neocortical neurons.*

**double depression**   A condition in which a major depressive episode occurs in a subject with preexisting chronic minor depression (dysthymic disorder) of at least 2 years' duration.

**double helix**   See *DNA.*

**double orientation**   Bleuler's term for the schizophrenic's ability to maintain some adequacy in day-to-day functioning and at the same time to believe sincerely in the most contradictory and phantastic delusions, such as the patient who works conscientiously as an elevator operator and at the same time feels that he is the president of the United States. Also known as *delusion of orientation.*

**double personality**   See *dissociative identity disorder.*

**double simultaneous tactile sensation** The ability of the subject to perceive that he has been touched in two places at the same time. This is usually acquired by the age of 6 years and is considered an index of biological sentiency, level of organization, and discrimination of environmental changes. It is often late in developing or otherwise defective in childhood schizophrenics and in children with attention deficit disorder; it is also often impaired in patients with diffuse brain damage (e.g., cerebral arteriosclerosis). The *face-hand test* (q.v.) is designed to measure such impairment.

**double superego** The double conscience sometimes seen in *psychic dualism*. The two consciences, or superegos, are usually antagonistic and regard each other vigilantly and belligerently. One conscience is usually considered masculine, the other feminine because it often demands subservience, total goodness, and conscientiousness.

**double thinking** An infrequently used term with unclear definition; some authorities use the term synonymously with *thought-hearing*. See *first-rank symptoms*.

**double-agentry** See *informed consent*.

**doubles, illusion of** See *Capgras syndrome*.

**doubt** See *ontogeny, psychic*.

**doubt, obsessive** An uncertainty that persistently forces itself on the mind of the person and cannot be banished or reasoned away. Obsessive brooding and doubt may represent sexualization of thought, and their unconscious content is the same as in other symptoms of the obsessive-compulsive: bisexuality, ambivalence (love vs. hate), and id impulses vs. superego demands. See *obsession*.

**doubting mania** Obsessive doubting in which the patient finds it necessary to say "no" to everything. The patient raises objections to whatever comes into his mind from within or without. See *folie du doute*.

**doubting spells** See *brooding spells*.

**Down syndrome** (John Langdon Down, English physician, 1828–96) Congenital acromicria; Langdon Down disease; autosomal trisomy; trisomy 21; mongolian idiocy (obsolete). An autosomal anomaly that produces mental retardation; the syndrome was first described by Down in 1866. The general frequency of the disorder is approximately 1 in every 600 to 650 births. Three chromosomal types are recognized:

1. Trisomy 21, which accounts for 95% of cases, is due to *nondisjunction* during meiosis (i.e., before fertilization); the 21st pair of chromosomes fails to separate, resulting in a germ cell with 24 rather than 23 chromosomes. When such a germ cell unites with a normal germ cell during fertilization, the resulting organism contains 47 rather than the normal complement of 46 chromosomes. Incidence is related to maternal age. The estimated risk for women under 35 years of age is less than 0.2%; for women 35 to 40 years of age, 0.9%; for women 40 to 45 years of age, 1.4%; and for women over 45, 2.5%.

2. *Translocation* type due to fusion of two chromosomes; typically, extra genetic material does not remain in position 21 as an extra chromosome but instead attaches itself to chromosome 15 (thus called 15/21 translocation). The number of chromosomes is normal (46), but the chromosome receiving the excess of genetic material is abnormally elongated. The translocation form can occur at any maternal age and is heritable. Having once appeared, it has a 20% to 30% likelihood of recurring in subsequent pregnancies with the same parents.

3. *Mosaicism*, the least frequent type, is due to nondisjunction of chromosome 21 after fertilization, resulting in a mixture of normal and trisomic cell lines.

Pathologically, the brain is small, and there are widespread defects in the cortical cell layers and in the number of ganglion cells. Whole gyri may be faulty in development. The process apparently is stationary, for regressive changes are not seen. There are many signs characteristic of trisomy 21, but not all are seen in each case. In one reported series, the signs appeared with the following frequencies; slanting of the palpebral fissures (88%), hyperextensible joints (88%), flabby hands (84%), brachycephalic skull with flat occiput (82%), ear anomalies or small lobules (80%), diastasis recti (76%), high-arched palate (74%), irregular alignment of teeth (68%), flat nipples (56%), epicanthus (50%), speckling of the iris (30%), heart murmurs (28%), double-zoned iris (22%), and pathologically open fontanels (16%) (Levinson, A., Freidman, A. and Stamps, F. *Pediatrics 16*, 1955).

Mentally, the subject is usually docile and tractable and may give an appearance of higher mental capacity than is really present because of imitativeness. The majority have a mental age of 4 to 7 years, although there are variations from moronity to pronounced idiocy. A few are hyperactive and sometimes destructive.

**downlow**  Used originally to refer to "straight" men who have sex with men. The man "on the downlow" identifies himself as heterosexual, and even though he may have frequent male sex partners he denies that he is either bisexual or gay. Men on the downlow typically use targeted and discreet strategies to seek male partners, such as going to sex clubs or seeking partners on the Internet. Substance use is almost always present and often plays a role in partner-seeking strategies. Black and Latino MSMs may be more reluctant than whites to label themselves as gay (Miller, M. Serner, M. and Wager, M. *Journal of Urban Health 822 (Suppl 1):* i26–i34, 2005).

The use of the term has been expanded to refer to any kind of sexual activity by a male or a female with a person other than the spouse; this use emphasizes the need for secrecy rather than the sex of the object choice. A magazine advertisement for a restaurant asked: "Dining on the Down Low? Eat here while keeping your affair of the heart a secret."

**down-regulation**  *Tachyphylaxis*; progressive desensitization (i.e., reduced sensitivity, decreased reaction); usually used to refer to the effects of neurohormones and pharmacological agents on brain cell receptors. The therapeutic effects of antidepressants, for example, may be achieved by down-regulation of central β-adrenergic receptors due to increased concentration of norepinephrine at the synapse. See *up-regulation.*

**doxogenic**  Induced by one's own ideas, opinion, or belief about what should happen.

**dram shop laws**  Legislation that regulates the selling or serving of alcohol (from dram, meaning a small drink or draft of spirits), including attachment of legal liability to anyone who serves alcoholic beverages.

**dramatic moments**  See *stalking.*

**dramatism**  Flamboyant or histrionic behavior.

**dramatization**  The part of the manifest dream that appears as an action or situation; representation in the manifest dream of an action or situation evolved from the latent thoughts by the dream mechanisms. It is the subjective

attempt within the psyche to project anxiety and control stimuli. The mechanisms may attempt to draw a unity from the conflicting forces of many years, balancing and neutralizing affects. Different persons may represent conflicting parts of the psyche. If a balance is not achieved, the dream may leave a disagreeable affect or anxiety. See *dream.*

**dramatogenic**  J. L. Moreno's term to denote people "especially sensitive for collective experiences and able to dramatize them easily...Just as there are some people who are photogenic, there are some individuals who are dramatogenic..." (*Sociometry VI,* 1947).

**drapetomania**  Uncontrollable impulse to wander; dromomania. See *simple senile deterioration.*

**Dravet syndrome**  A rare, intractable epilepsy syndrome in which prolonged generalized tonic, clonic, or tonic-clonic seizures occur between 2 and 9 months of age followed by myoclonic, tonic-clonic, absence, and partial seizures in the second year of life. The syndrome is associated with delayed psychomotor and speech development, and ataxia.

**drauci**  Males who adopt the passive role in homosexual activity. See *active.*

**draw-a-person test**  *DAP*; a method of personality analysis based upon the interpretation of drawings of the human figure. Although figure drawings had been used by many workers in the field, it was Karen Machover who in 1949 outlined a system of interpretation that was correlated with clinical diagnostic categories.

**DRD2**  D$_2$ dopamine receptor gene.

**dread**  Anxiety related to a specific danger situation. Freud stated that in proper usage the term anxiety should be reserved for the original reaction of helplessness in a traumatic situation where no specific danger situation is expected. The term dread should be used for the anxiety that relates to a specific danger, i.e., "when it has found an object." (Freud, S. *The Problem of Anxiety,* 1936; *Group Psychology and the Analysis of the Ego,* 1922).

**dread, nameless**  According to Bion, the infant's terror of the unknown, related to the mother's inability to use *reverie* or the *alpha-function* (qq.v.) to contain the infant's anxiety and other unwanted feelings.

**dream**  A psychic phenomenon occurring during *sleep* (q.v.) in which thoughts, images, emotions, etc., present themselves to the dreamer, usually with a definite sense of reality. Dreams safeguard sleep; they foster solution in phantasy of needs and conflicts too dangerous for solution in reality; they provide an outlet for the discharge of instinctual tension; they allow a working through of destructive and traumatic experiences that defy the coping capacities of the waking state.

According to psychoanalytic theory, the recollected dream emerges as the "manifest dream content," which tends to be constructed out of events in the recent past. The "latent dream content" is uncovered by analysis of the manifest content, usually by means of free association. The day's residues (events of the waking day) establish contact with repressed, unconscious impulse(s), which attempt to find fulfillment in the material of the latent thoughts. The unrecognizability, strangeness, and absurdity of the manifest dream are partly the result of translation of thought into archaic modes of expression and partly the result of the restrictive and disapproving dream censorship of events in the dream.

The processes that transform the latent into the manifest content are called the *dream work*. They include *condensation, displacement, dramatization, secondary elaboration,* and *symbolization* (qq.v.).

Dream research has cast doubt on some of the teleological explanations that have traditionally been used in psychological theories. Dreaming does not appear to be a unique response to a specific psychological experiential factor; instead, it serves to maintain or reestablish homeostasis on a neurophysiologic-biological level as well as on a psychological one. It is not an unconscious wish that determines dreaming; rather, neurophysiologic changes in the sleep-wakefulness apparatus provide opportunities for representation of unconscious wishes, which "ride along on" the waves of neurophysiologic disequilibrium, as it were, but which can hardly be credited with primary responsibility for dream production itself. Furthermore, it seems unlikely that repression is a major factor in producing amnesia for dreams, the majority of which are followed by a period of deep sleep that inhibits or prevents memory consolidation.

**dream, artificial** Any dream that is apparently induced by sensory stimulation. Freud cites from Maury, who, when his neck was lightly pinched during sleep, dreamed that a blister was being applied.

**dream, color in** The color in a dream may have significant meaning, including any or all of the following: to camouflage or to identify specific portions or excretions of the body; representation of a specific affect system; synaesthetic representation of other sensory systems; to serve as a screen for traumatic experiences. Dreaming in color may also reflect some kind of neurophysiologic disturbance, for such dreams have been reported frequently in patients with epilepsy, migraine, and drug intoxication.

**dream, counterwish** According to Freud, certain dreams seem not to be associated with a wish; in fact they seem to convey a counterwish. An impotent patient dreamed he had syphilis. He said that if he had syphilis it would signalize potency to him.

**dream anxiety disorder** *Nightmare* (q.v.).

**dream censorship** Dreams are highly disguised representations of unconscious impulses that are under the constant rule of censoring influences. "The stricter the domination of the censorship, the more thorough becomes the disguise, and, often enough, the more ingenious the means employed to put the reader off the track of the actual meaning" (Freud, S. *Interpretation of Dreams*, 1933).

**dream content** The material of which the dream is composed. Dreams have a latent dream content, made up of dream thoughts and manifest dream content, usually presented in a highly symbolic form.

**dream ego** Jung's term for "a mere fragment of the conscious ego" that is active during the dream stage. "In a dream, consciousness is neither fully awake nor fully extinguished; there is still a small remnant of consciousness.... It is rather a limited ego, sometimes peculiarly transformed or distorted.... Hence it happens that we find ourselves in situations like those in real life, but rarely exercise thought or reason about them" (*Contributions to Analytical Psychology*, 1928).

**dream function** According to Freud, "the dream is the (disguised) fulfillment of a (suppressed, repressed) wish" (*The Interpretation of Dreams*, 1933)

Jung holds that the general function of dreams is to reflect "certain fundamental tendencies of the personality, either those whose meaning extends over the whole life, or those that are momentarily of most importance. The dream gives an objective statement of these tendencies, a statement which does not trouble itself about conscious wishes and convictions" (*Contributions to Analytical Psychology*, 1928).

**dream induction** The production of a dream through hypnotic stimulation. Such dreams may be "artificially stimulated on command during hypnosis or they may be posthypnotically suggested, to appear later during spontaneous sleep." Both the induction and the interpretation of this type of dream play an important part in the technique of hypnoanalysis (Wolberg, L. R *Hypnoanalysis*, 1945).

**dream pain** Hypnalgia; pain occurring during the dream state.

**dream stimulus** The exciting cause of a dream. It may be an internal or external sensory stimulus, an internal (organic) physical stimulus, or a stimulus from the psyche itself.

**dream within a dream** "The inclusion of a certain content in 'a dream within a dream' is therefore equivalent to the wish that what has been characterized as a dream had never occurred" (Freud, S. *The Interpretation of Dreams*, 1933). The attitude that the dreamer assumes toward it constitutes a repudiation of it.

**dreamy state** A state of arrested consciousness, akin to epileptiform seizures, but unaccompanied by convulsions. The patient suddenly passes off into a dream world, often with olfactory, auditory, or visual hallucinations, and usually recovers within a few minutes. Such states are most commonly associated with temporal lobe lesions. See *temporal lobe dysfunction*.

**dreher mutation** An autosomal recessive mutation in the mouse; because it affects cell proliferation and neuronal migration, it is used for the experimental study of those processes.

**dressing apraxia** The patient is unable to don his clothes properly, putting his jacket on upside down, for example. Dressing apraxia is a form of *constructional apraxia* (q.v.); it is seen most commonly in parietal lobe lesions, such as occur in Pick disease. See *apraxia*.

**DRG** Diagnosis-related group, a type of case mix for prospective reimbursement purposes based on the diagnosis of patients treated.

**DRI** Differential reinforcement of incompatible behavior. See *accelerative*.

**drift hypothesis** See *breeder hypothesis*.

**drinking behaviors** The conditions under which alcohol is ingested (e.g., how much, what type, how often, under what circumstances) and the effects (health, familial, social, occupational, etc.) associated with particular patterns of ingestion.

Under *alcoholism* (q.v.), DSM-II differentiated *episodic excessive drinking* (episodes of intoxication, with clear-cut alteration in behavior or impairment of coordination or speech, occurring at least four times a year), *habitual excessive drinking* (more than 12 episodes of intoxication a year), and alcohol addiction.

**drive** A motivational state, urge, or impulse based upon bodily needs that arouses and directs voluntary action in order to achieve satiation. In classical psychoanalytic psychology, two drives are distinguished, the sexual or erotic and the aggressive or destructive. See *instinct*.

**drive reduction theory** See *reductionism*.

**drive psychology** A drive-conflict-defense theory of human behavior, such as Freud's psychoanalytic psychology. See *conflict paradigm*.

**drive-defense-conflict** See *conflict paradigm*.

**drivel** Drooling or, by extension, uncontrollable flow of foolish or silly speech. Drooling of saliva is frequent in parkinsonism, including the form induced by neuroleptic drugs.

**driveling** Fluent jargon-filled speech, a characteristic of Wernicke receptive aphasia. See *jargon aphasia; Wernicke aphasia*.

**driveling dementia** *Rare*. Kraepelin's term for "the general decay of mental efficiency" observed in the terminal states of certain syndromes of schizophrenia.

**drivenness, organic** Kahn and Cohen's term for the overactivity of the brain-damaged subject, which is attributed to defective brain stem organization. See *organic syndrome*.

**driving, psychic** Continuously repeated playback of psychodynamically significant material that has been recorded on a device such as a tape recorder. If the psychic driving is in response to the patient's own verbal cues, it is termed "autopsychic"; if it is in response to cues verbalized by others but based on the patient's known psychodynamics, it is termed "heteropsychic." The values of psychic driving are said to include penetration of defenses, elicitation of hitherto inaccessible material, and the setting up of a dynamic implant. See *implant, dynamic.*

**DRL** Differential reinforcement of low rate behavior. See *accelerative.*

**DRO** Differential reinforcement of other behavior. See *accelerative.*

**dromolepsy** A short spurt of running occurring just prior to and generally ending in an epileptic attack. By many it is believed to be the beginning of the attack. It is known also as *procursive epilepsy.*

**dromomania** An abnormal impulse to travel; used by Hirschfeld to denote the desire to escape from a disagreeable sexual situation. It is also known as *vagabond neurosis.*

**dromophobia** Fear of (running across) a street.

**drop attack** A fleeting loss of muscle tone that causes the subject to fall without any loss of consciousness; it may be caused by transient ischemia within the vertebrobasilar system.

**dropout** A student who leaves school before completing a grade or before graduation; a patient who withdraws from and terminates treatment. In the latter case, the term generally implies that the therapist has not concurred in the patient's decision to terminate.

**Drosophila per** See *biological clock.*

**DRPLA** Dentatorubropallidoluysian atrophy, a *polyglutamine disorder* (q.v.) that is common in Japan. It has the same molecular defect as *Haw River syndrome* (HRS), a disorder reported in an African-American family from North Carolina. DRPLA is related to a polyglutamine expansion in atrophin-1; the primary targets of neuropathology are the cerebellum (dentate nucleus), red nucleus, globus pallidus (external segment), and the subthalamic nucleus.

**drug** Any chemical entity or mixture of entities, other than those required for the maintenance of normal health, the administration of which alters biological function and possibly structure. Drugs may be used for the diagnosis, prophylaxis, treatment, or alleviation of disease (and are then called medications, therapeutic agents, remedies, etc.), or for nontherapeutic purposes (designated nonmedical use, substance abuse, unsanctioned use, or self-administered).

**drug abuse, drug misuse** Misuse is generally preferred to abuse as being less judgmental, but the terms are virtually synonymous. A drug is generally considered to be misused if its use is (1) unlawful or unsanctioned by a society or a group within that society, (2) hazardous in that it is likely to produce dysfunction or harm in the user, (3) dysfunctional, in that it impairs psychological or social functioning, or (4) harmful, in that it has caused tissue damage or mental illness in the user; or (5) if the drug is a licit pharmaceutical substance used other than for acceptable medical purposes, or (6) if the drug is used in excess or contrary to medical directions, or (7) if the drug is inappropriately prescribed.

For a minority of writers, drug misuse is used only in the sense of (7), while drug abuse is applied to all the other patterns described. See *dependence, drug.*

In 2006, pain relievers headed the list of drugs tried by new users, followed by marijuana, tranquilizers, cocaine, ecstasy, stimulants, inhalants, sedatives, LSD, heroin, and PCP (National Survey on Drug Use and Health, Substance Abuse and Mental Health Services Administration)

**drug addict** A person who is physically dependent on one or more psychoactive substances, whose long-term use has produced tolerance, who has lost control over his intake, and who would manifest withdrawal phenomena if discontinuance were to occur.

**drug addiction** A chronic disorder characterized by the compulsive use of a substance, resulting in physical, psychological, or social harm to the user and continued use despite that harm. See *addiction.*

**drug defaulter** See *defaulter.*

**drug free** Not currently using any psychoactive substance.

**drug holiday** Temporary discontinuation (or, less commonly, lowering of dosage) of a drug in order to reduce or avoid development of tolerance to the drug or to prevent the development of serious side effects that are more likely to occur with prolonged administration of the drug. The length of drug holiday varies—it may be for a weekend, for a week, or for a month. Once the holiday is over, the drug is usually reinstated, either immediately or in rapidly increasing amounts, to its previous level.

**drug interactions** See *interactions, drug.*

**drug intoxication** Disruptions in physiological functioning, mood states, or cognitive processes due to excessive consumption of a drug.

**drug metabolism** It characteristically occurs in two phases. Phase I involves modification of the drug by introduction of a functional group (such as a hydroxyl moiety), in most cases by the *cytochrome P450 isoenzyme system* (q.v.). Phase II reactions involve conjugation of metabolites produced in Phase I. Most antipsychotics, as well as TCAs and SSRIs, are metabolized by the CYP 2D6 enzyme. CYP 2D6 polymorphisms are known to result in differential drug metabolism and individually specific dosing schedules. For example, rapid metabolism genotypes can result in very low drug levels of some SSRIs and hence poor drug response, whereas slow metabolism genotypes produce unexpectedly high drug levels often associated with adverse drug reactions.

**drug misuse** Any use of a drug that varies from a socially or medically accepted use; *drug abuse* (q.v.).

**drug problem, drug-related problem** Use of a drug that is causing or threatening to cause significant impairment of the user's mental or physical health or social adjustment. At times, the drug may be only contributing to such impairment, rather than being the sole causal agent-for example, use of hallucinogens may contribute to the precipitation of onset in schizophrenia. Within the public health context, a drug problem may be deemed to exist in relation to a particular drug if the health authorities judge that it is causing significant harm to a significant percentage of the population, or threatening to do so.

A drug problem may result from the use of a dependence-producing drug or one without this property (e.g., LSD), or from the use of a potentially dependence-producing drug before the individual has progressed to dependence (e.g., accidental overdose at an early stage of heroin use). Conversely, dependence may occur without any obvious immediate drug problem (e.g., dependence on caffeine). In practice, many people who misuse drugs will both develop dependence and incur accumulating drug-related problems, but conceptually "dependence" and "drug problem" are distinct. See *dependence, drug*.

**drugs, classes of** See *psychotropic*.

**drug-trafficking** The selling and portage of drugs; its psychiatric significance is its unquestionable relation to violence and homicide.

**drunken gait** Staggering gait, seen not only in acute alcoholic intoxication but also in other drug intoxications, polyneuritis, multiple sclerosis, general paresis, and brain tumors.

**DSA** *Digital subtraction angiography*; an imaging technique in which fluoroscopic images of blood vessels are converted into digital information. Before contrast material is introduced, a radiographic image is taken of the area in which the blood vessels under investigation are located. Images made after contrast material is injected are compared with the before image, and anything common to both is "subtracted" from the image. What remains is an image of the vessel through which the contrast material flows. See *imaging, brain*.

**DSD** 1. *Depressive spectrum disorder*, a subtype of unipolar primary depressive illness characterized by alcoholism or antisocial disorder, or both, in first-degree relatives of the depressed subject. 2. *Depression sine depression*, or *masked depression*, when the affect disorder is hidden or disguised by symptoms suggesting other disorders, such as psychosomatic illnesses or conversion hysteria.

**D-serine** A D-amino acid which is synthesized from L-serine in astrocytes; it is released by glutamate and binds to the glycine site of the NMDA receptors. It thus regulates glutmatergic neurotransmission and is considered a neurotransmitter. The brain enzyme that makes D-serine, *serine racemase*, was cloned in 1999.

**DSH** Deliberate self-harm. See *attempted suicide*.

**DSIP** Delta sleep-inducing peptide; may be involved in the regulation of sleep.

**DSM-I** *Diagnostic and Statistical Manual of Mental Disorders*, 1st edition (1952); the official nomenclature of the American Psychiatric Association. It included, for the first time, experience that did not derive solely from mental hospital data, such as World War II military experience and data from clinics and private practice. In labeling most of the categories "reactions" it moved away from the concepts of constitutional and assumed organic factors, stressing instead the psychosocial and adaptational aspects and the transitory nature of many of the functional disorders.

**DSM-II** *Diagnostic and Statistical Manual of Mental Disorders*, 2nd edition; the 1968 revision of the nomenclature of mental disorders, prepared by the Committee on Nomenclature and Statistics of the American Psychiatric Association. See *nomenclature, 1968 revision.*

**DSM-III** *Diagnostic and Statistical Manual of Mental Disorders,* 3rd edition (1980), prepared by the Task Force on Nomenclature and Statistics of the American Psychiatric Association. The aim of this classificatory system was to provide clear descriptions of diagnostic categories while avoiding insofar as possible bias in favor of any particular theory of etiology. The manual suggests criteria that would warrant inclusion in each of the categories; most of the proposed criteria are based on clinical judgment and have yet to be validated in terms of other correlates, such as prognosis and response to particular forms of treatment. Although in a general way modeled after *ICD-9-CM* (International Classification of Diseases, 9th edition, 1978, clinical modification for use in the United States), DSM-III is not compatible with it in every instance because it is of greater detail or reflective of more recent evidence than was included in ICD-9-CM. Further, DSM-III employed a *multiaxial classification* that coded data on each of the axes, on the assumption that attention to more than one clinically relevant parameter of a disorder will provide greater specificity and objectivity and a firmer basis for identifying subtypes.

**DSM-III-R** Revision of DSM-III, 1987. Most of the changes from DSM-III (q.v.) have been indicated in appropriate entries, and the aim and format of the revision remain essentially as described for DSM-III itself. The five axes of DSM-III-R are as follows:

Axis I—Clinical Syndromes and V Codes (conditions not attributable to a mental disorder that are a focus of attention or treatment)

Axis II—Developmental Disorders and Personality Disorders, which generally begin in childhood or adolescence and persist without remissions or exacerbations into adult life

Axis III—Physical Disorders and Conditions

Axis IV—Severity of Psychosocial Stressors

Axis V—Global Assessment of Functioning on a nine-point scale

**DSM-IV** The 1994 revision of the *Diagnostic and Statistical Manual of Mental Disorders.* Its major

differences from DSM-III-R are (1) reconceptualization of *organic mental disorders* (q.v.); (2) more extensive description of the longitudinal course of mood disorders; (3) replacement of Axis IV with a psychosocial and environmental checklist to provide more specific description of the influence of these factors on illness; (4) placement of developmental disorders (autism and learning disorders) in Axis I, as a result of which Axis II contains only personality disorders and mental retardation; (5) placement of premenstrual dysphoric disorder (formerly called LLPDD) under depressive disorders; (6) incorporation of childhood avoidant disorder and overanxious disorder into social phobia and generalized anxiety disorder; (7) inclusion of new diagnoses, such as bipolar II disorder, acute stress disorder, feeding disorder of infancy or early childhood, catatonic disorder due to a general medical condition, narcolepsy, breathing-related sleep disorder, and three additional forms of pervasive developmental disorders— Rett disorder, childhood disintegrative disorder, and Asperger disorder; (8) description in the appendix of postpsychotic depression of schizophrenia; (9) addition to the appendix of three axes for further study—a defense functioning scale (defense mechanisms); a Global Assessment of Relational Functioning (GARF) Scale with a focus on families and couples rather than only on the individual; and a Social and Occupational Functioning Assessment Scales (SOFAS), a rating of individual functioning (a modification of what formerly was Axis V); (10) a glossary of culture-specific syndromes; (11) expansion and reconceptualization of the V-codes (other conditions that may be a focus of clinical attention); and (11) removal of self-defeating personality disorder from the appendix because of a paucity of evidence regarding its existence as a discrete entity.

DSM-IV-TR is the text revision of DSM-IV, published in 2000.

**DSPS** *Delayed sleep phase syndrome;* a circadian rhythm disorder in which sleep onset is delayed by several hours. The subject does not sleep until past the normal sleep onset time and, in consequence, is not able to get up until well into the next day. The condition usually begins in adolescence; in many instances, it is familial. Treatment is bright light (10,000 lux for 30 minutes) administered in the early-morning hours.

**DSS**  *Déjérine-Sottas syndrome* (q.v.).

**DST**  *Dexamethasone suppression test*; a measure of the degree to which cortisol suppression is overcome. Dexamethasone, a glucocorticoid, ordinarily suppresses or inhibits the hypothalamic-pituitary system, as manifested in a lowered cortisol (ACTH) level for up to 48 hours. Some patients with a clinical depression overcome the usual inhibiting effect of cortisol; in such *nonsuppressors*, the cortisol level quickly returns to pretest levels. Nonsuppression is a positive DST, and it may reflect a relative lack of norepinephrine or a relative excess of serotonin in the central nervous system. Maintenance of DST nonsuppression may be a marker for early relapse in depressed patients. See *hypothalamic-pituitary-adrenal axis*.

The test shows highest sensitivity in very severe, especially psychotic, mood disorders; it is less sensitive and less consistent in other mood disorders. Its clinical utility therefore is limited—a positive test is no guarantee of significant response to antidepressant treatment, and a negative response is certainly no reason for withholding treatment.

**Δ⁹-THC**  The active ingredient of cannabinoids, whose effects on central nervous system include deficits in memory and cognition, catalepsy, tremor, and decreased body temperature. CNS effects are believed to be due mainly to CB1, one of the most abundant neuromodulatory receptors in the brain and expressed at high levels in hippocampus, cortex, cerebellum, and basal ganglia. A second G protein-coupled cannabinoid receptor, CB2, is found mainly in immune tissues, and there may be a third cannabinoid receptor, CB3. Cannabinoid receptor antagonists can block the nicotine-induced release of presynaptic dopamine in the nucleus accumbens, and they may prove useful in smoking cessation.

**DTI**  Diffusion tissue imaging; see *dMRI*.

**dual diagnosis**  An inexact term because of the way it is used by different workers. Currently, for many psychiatrists, it denotes coexisting substance use disorder and psychiatric disorder, although originally it meant "functional" psychosis or neurosis superimposed on mental retardation (see *pfropfschizophrenia*). Particularly in the field of addiction medicine and addiction psychiatry, it refers to multi-drug abuse; in other usages, it

indicates *comorbidity* (q.v.) of any two disorders. See *MICA*.

In nicotine, alcohol, and illicit drug use, comorbidity rates of major depression range from 32% to 54%; of post-traumatic stress disorder, from 22% to 43%. ADHD and schizophrenia are also frequently associated with substance use disorders. Persons with co-occurring substance use disorders and severe mental illness are highly prone to relapse to substance abuse.

**dual personality**  See *dissociative identity disorder*.

**dual stream model**  See *speech processing*.

**dual task coordination**  See *DLPFC*.

**dual track narcissism**  In Kohut's terminology (1971), the grandiose self ("I am perfect") and the idealized parental image ("You are perfect and I am part of you"). See *basic trust; cohesive self*.

**dual transference therapy**  Treatment of the same patient by two therapists, sometimes advantageous when the patient needs both support and confrontation with reality issues but is unable to accept both from the same therapist. It is theorized that providing two therapists enables a fragile ego to differentiate more clearly between good and bad mother images as a step toward ultimate fusion and integration of those images.

**dual unity**  See *symbiotic stage*.

**dualism, psychic**  Coexistence of double consciousness or of two fairly distinctly formed superego streams (double conscience) as in *multiple personality*, where one personality may alternate with a second with complete amnesia of the active personality for the behavior of the inactive one, or where the two personalities live side by side, one or the other being predominant periodically but still influenced by the inactive one. But such co-conscious mentation may also be a normal phenomenon, as when one writes a letter and at the same time listens to the radio. Usually, however, when the co-conscious thinking is pathological, each of the co-conscious organizations strives to drive the ego in a different direction. Psychic dualism is perhaps responsible for critical self-observation, the ability of one conscious stream to observe the remainder of the personality. See *alternating personality; dissociative identity disorder*.

**dual-trace hypothesis**  The theory that short- and long-term memory (and perhaps other memory stages) are sequentially linked; others have more recently proposed that instead they are based on independent processes acting in parallel.

**due process**   See *rule of law.*

**dullard**   See *moron.*

**dulling**   Obnubilation, clouding of consciousness, hampered ability to concentrate or think; productive of intellectual or affective depression.

**dumbness, word**   See *Broca motor aphasia.*

**dummy**   1. *Placebo* (q.v.). 2. The silent player (as in bridge). See *Lacan, Jacques.*

**Dunham, H. Warren**   (1906–85) Sociologist; epidemiology of mental disorders; *Mental Disorders in Urban Areas* (with Robert E. L. Farris, 1939), *Community and Schizophrenia* (1965).

**duplicative reaction**   A perceptual disturbance described most commonly in schizophrenic children; because he does not conceptualize objects as continuing and unitary when they are out of direct sensory contact, the schizophrenic child is "seeing the same person in different settings or at different times thinks he is seeing more than one person" (Goldfarb, W. *International Psychiatry Clinics 1*, 1964). See *object constancy.*

**dura mater**   See *meninges.*

**durable power of attorney**   See *advance directive.*

**Durham decision, Durham test**   See *criminal responsibility.*

**duty to protect**   See *Tarasoff decision.*

**duty to warn**   See *Tarasoff decision.*

**dwarfism**   Extreme deficiency in stature; *microsomia;* usually divided into the following three special forms:

1. Dwarfs with regular physical proportions and normal psychic development, going under such names as *nanosomia primordialis, heredo-familial essential microsomia,* and *pygmeism.*

2. Dwarfs with a serious hypogenesis of the skeleton except for a very large skull, falling under the heading of Paltauf's *nanism.*

3. Dwarfs with a combination of infantilism and premature senility, known as Gilford's *progeria* or the *senile nanism* of Variot and Pirronneau.

4. In addition to these specific forms, there is a heterogeneous group of *infantilistic* dwarfisms, or nanisms, of endocrine origin. See *growth hormone.*

**DWI**   1. Diffusion-weighted imaging. In boxer's dementia (punch-drunkenness, the

effects of repetitive blows to head), routine brain imaging with CT and MR typically fail to reveal abnormalities until after the onset of clinical abnormalities. L. Zhang et al. (*American Journal of Neuroradiology,* January, 2003) report that microscopic brain damage from TBI can be detected with DWI before it can be seen on clinical images. DWI is sensitive to water molecule motion and thus can reveal microscopic changes in brain tissue; by measuring diffusion, researchers can detect changes in the microstructure of brain.

2. Driving while intoxicated.

**dwindles**   *Failure to thrive* (q.v.) in the older person, sometimes manifested as the *tea and toast syndrome* (q.v.).

**dyad**   In social psychiatry, a two-person relationship.

**dying, stages of**   E. Kubler-Ross (*On Death and Dying,* 1969) posits five: (1) denial; (2) anger ("Why me?"); (3) bargaining; (4) depression; and (5) acceptance and increasing detachment.

**Dyke Davidoff syndrome**   Hemiatrophy of the brain, manifested by mental retardation, seizures, facial asymmetry, and contralateral hemiplegia (Gorlin, R. J. et al. *Modern Medicine 38,* 1970).

**dynamic**   Relating to the operation of mental forces or energy.

**dynamic apraxia**   Impaired ability to perform continuous movements, suggestive of pathology of the premotor cortex. See *apraxia.*

**dynamic mutations**   See *anticipation.*

**dynamic polarization**   *Neuron doctrine;* a principle formulated by Cajal in 1891. Dendrites and cell bodies are the perceptive regions of the neuron (a term introduced that same year by Waldeyer); they conduct the neural signal toward the axon, which in turn transmits it toward other nerve cells. The principle became the cornerstone of neurobiology and was the foundation for the development of the synapse concept.

**dynamic psychiatry**   See *descriptive.*

**dynamics**   Used interchangeably with *dynamism(s)* (q.v.). See *psychodynamics.*

**dynamism**   The action of psychic structures and the forces behind the action; "a specific force operating in a specific manner or direction" (Healy et al. *The Structure and Meaning of Psychoanalysis,* 1930) While the authors cited prefer dynamism to mechanism, the latter is more commonly used. See *defense; mechanism.*

**dynamopsychism**    G. Geley's theory of libido or energy. The unconscious is the seat of both lower and higher functions, but the latter are purposely kept in abeyance during normal life in order to maintain the sense of limitation and deficiency necessary for ambition and progress. Thus a person forgets, because too much knowledge would remove the spurring to further efforts. But with impending death, the sense of limitation and deficiency is no longer necessary, so that the higher faculties are allowed to appear. The mind then becomes clearer and sharper, and certain manifestations such as clairvoyance and telepathy may occur (*From the Unconscious to the Conscious*, 1921).

**dynorphins**    One of the three major families of endogenous opioid peptides, the other two being *endorphins* and *enkephalins* (qq.v.). The opioid peptides appear to be part of a signaling system that relates to pain perception, mood regulation, and learning. The precursor of the dynorphins is *prodynorphin*, located chiefly in the hypothalamus, basal ganglia, and brain stem. See *peptide, brain; peptides, opioid.*

**dysapocatastasis**    *Obs.* Restless discontent.

**dysarthria**    Difficulty in articulation; partial impairment of articulatory speech.

**dysautonomia, familial**    *Riley-Day syndrome*; an autosomal recessive disorder of the autonomic nervous system manifested in the first year of life, usually in Ashkenazi Jews, with such symptoms as excessive sweating and salivation, defective lacrimation and temperature control, blotchy skin, hypertension with postural hypotension, and emotional lability. The child is prone to recurrent physical crises and also shows difficulty in organizing complex behavior and in adapting to change, reminiscent of the behavior of some childhood schizophrenics. Some workers have reported decreased serum dopamine beta-hydroxylase in dysautonomic patients.

**dysbasia**    Difficult or distorted walking.

**dysbulia, dysboulia**    Disturbance in the will or in the volitional aspects of the personality. See *will disturbances.*

**dyscalculia**    See *acalculia.*

**dyschezia**    Inadequate evacuation of the stool from the rectum, commonly found in children who suffer from constipation.

**dyscontrol, emergency**    See *adaptational psychodynamics.*

**dyscopia**    Inability to cope with day-to-day problems, often followed by withdrawal into depression. Dyscopia occurs frequently in the aged as a mixture of lack of resilience and lack of inner strengths and knowledge to manage the difficulties encountered because of failing strength, multiple medical disorders, and feelings of powerlessness, abandonment, and rejection.

**dysdiadochokinesia**    Impaired ability to perform rapid alternating movements, to sustain a regular rhythm, or to sustain an even amount of force; suggestive of cerebellar disease.

**dyseneia**    Defective articulation secondary to deafness.

**dysequilibrium syndrome**    Seen in patients undergoing hemodialysis, when a shift in osmotic gradient between brain and blood causes cerebral edema: headache, nausea, and in a small percentage of patients delirium or stupor, which may be accompanied by convulsions.

**dysergasia**    Adolf Meyer's term for those psychiatric syndromes that are presumably associated with disordered physiology of the brain. The dysergasias are generally known as toxic psychoses, one of the chief symptoms of which is *delirium* (q.v.).

**dysesthesia**    Distortion of the sense of touch.

**dysexecutive syndromes**    Malfunctioning within the various distributed networks that support *executive function* (q.v.) can be manifested in various ways:

> *Abulic-akinetic syndrome:* medial prefrontal cortex (anterior cingulate) dysfunction, with hypo/akinesis, impaired initiation, impaired persistence, decreased responsivity to environmental cues, blunted affect, apathetic/abulic comportment, depressive syndromes
> *Disinhibition syndrome:* orbitofrontal cortex dysfunction with inhibitory failure, perseveration
> *Dysexecutive syndrome:* dorsolateral prefrontal cortex dysfunction with loss of set (task goal), reduced response repertoire, reduced generativity, decreased response flexibility, impaired error monitoring, inefficient learning, poor free recall/ top-down retrieval (recognition is better maintained)

*Environmental dependency:* release of parietal exploratory behavior because of absence of frontal inhibition; stimulus-bound, defects in utilization behavior

*Frontal-striatal:* defects in cognitive flexibility, reward, punishment

*Frontal white matter:* slowed processing speed

**dysfluency** Impaired ability to control the smooth flow of speech production, as in *cluttering, stuttering*, and *aphasia* (qq.v.).

**dysfunctional attitudes** Maladaptive beliefs; extreme and relatively rigid beliefs that guide thinking, emotional reactions, and behavior. Patients with dysfunctional attitudes are more chronically ill, less treatment responsive, or more prone to relapse. Such attitudes are the focus of many treatment approaches, such as *cognitive behavior therapy* (q.v.).

Dysfunctional attitudes are prominent in various personality disorders. Frequently reported maladaptive beliefs include *entitlement* ("I am superior to others and deserve special privileges"); *deceitfulness* ("I can avoid punishment or maintain control if I am dishonest about some of my actions")*;* and *sexual provocativeness* ("The best way to become accepted—or to control others—is by stimulating them sexually"). See *entitlement.*

**dysgenesis** 1. Faulty development and infertility in general. 2. More specifically, a condition in which hybrids are sterile among themselves, but fertile with members of either parent stock.

**dysgenic** A genetic term describing various biological conditions that have a detrimental effect on the hereditary qualities of a stock or tend to counteract improvement of a species through influences bearing on reproduction. In a more general sense, the term denotes any factor that is in contrast with eugenic principles by tending to impair the qualities of future generations. See *eugenics.*

**dysgeusia** Impairment or perversion of the sense of taste.

**dysglucosis** Any disturbance in the blood sugar level, and particularly those disturbances in which the central nervous system (cortex, diencephalon, hypothalamus, or hypophysis) plays some role.

**dysgnosia** *Obs.* Intellectual impairment or anomaly.

**dysgraphia** *Dysorthography;* defective ability to write. As seen clinically, dysgraphia is often dissociated in that the patient is unable to write spontaneously but is able to copy from printed material to script or vice versa. Dissociated dysgraphia is an almost constant finding in patients with primary reading retardation and in the *Gerstmann syndrome* (q.v.). See *legasthenia; reading disabilities.*

**dysidentity** A term suggested by Rabinovitch to refer to what he considers the characteristic and basic problem of childhood schizophrenia: the child's inability to experience a clear-cut self-percept and to appreciate identities, their boundaries and limits. See *body image.*

**dyskinesia** Distortion of voluntary movements; involuntary muscular activity, such as a tic, spasm, or myoclonus. It includes both chorea (hyperkinetic, purposeless, dancelike movements) and dystonia (sustained, abnormal muscle contractions). See *LID.*

**dyslexia** *Pure word blindness;* alexia; reading disorder; usually grouped within the learning disorders or academic skills disorders when it occurs as a developmental disability. Some writers use dyslexia specifically to indicate a developmental disability, and alexia to indicate acquired word blindness as a result of lesions in the left occipital cortex and splenium, the posterior portion of the corpus callosum that connects the visual cortex of one hemisphere with the other.

Dyslexia is manifested by an inability to read effortlessly or with understanding, a severe disability that reveals itself initially in difficulty in learning to read, and subsequently by erratic spelling and deficits which affect written as opposed to spoken language. Dyslexic children are particularly impaired in phonemic processing—the ability to associate letters with the sounds they represent. Usually, however, they can understand other signs or symbols of communication, such as traffic signs. Learning to read alphabetic languages such as English depends on developing an awareness that printed characters (*graphemes*) correspond to phonemes, the smallest meaningful unit of sound that can change the meaning of a word. Proficiency in decoding words into their phonemic segments (*phonemic awareness*) is considered by many to be the core deficit in dyslexia. One can predict which children will have a struggle with reading on the basis of their ability to manipulate phonemes within spoken words (for example, knowing that saying 'plane' without the /n/ sound is 'play'). Although dyslexia was originally described as a defect in visual processing, it is now recognized that it is better conceptualized as a cluster of language-related conditions in which reading problems reflect impairment in the representation and manipulation of phonemes (the individual units of sound that are combined in speech to make words). The different conditions may have distinct etiologies. At least two types have been described:

1. A form of language disorder, with a history of delayed receptive and expressive oral language acquisition; sometimes persists to some degree. Although most of those affected overcome their speech difficulties, they may continue to manifest poor auditory discrimination (in the absence of any hearing loss) and find it hard to blend phonemes to form words or to recognize whole word letter patterns (orthography) without need for phonological mediation. Such children have been found to score as many as 20 points lower on verbal as compared with non-verbal intelligence tests. See *specific language impairment*.

Alexia may be combined with agraphia (writing impairment); affected subjects cannot read or write or connect visual symbols, such as letters, with the sounds they represent. The condition has sometimes been associated with lesions of the angular or supramarginal gyrus (in the parieto-temporal-occipital association cortex).

2. Problems of visual perception and memory; perception of simple material is usually adequate, but the deficiency appears when the child is asked to differentiate parts of complex figures. Affected subjects have problems with perception of shapes of words. Letters may seem to weave on the page, transposing themselves or dancing off the edge. Reversals of letters (b for d) and words (saw for was) are frequent; they are sometimes based on a lack of firm unilateral cerebral dominance. See *word blindness*.

Dyslexia has classically been considered a cognitive disorder. It is not due to intellectual inadequacy as such and is not open to explanation in terms of a lack of sociocultural opportunity or inadequate teaching techniques. Secondary (reactive) emotional problems are frequently identified, but the condition is not thought to be an outcome of a primary emotional resistance to learning. It is possibly a specific maturational delay which will, in many instances, show positive responses to remedial help, especially if this is provided at a relatively early stage. Several genes are believed to be linked to dyslexia; one of them, DYX3, has been mapped to chromosome 2.

No specific dyslexia risk gene has yet been identified by gene mapping or genome-wide scanning, although different studies have reported four potential susceptibility loci—on chromosomes 2, 3, 6, and 18. Other studies employing *phenotypic dissection* (q.v.)—measuring the different components that contribute to the dyslexic syndrome—have found that measures of phonological, orthographic, and rapid-naming skills are significantly heritable, and that those components are overlapping rather than independent. *DCDC2*, a gene on chromosome 6, and *ROBO1*, a gene on chromosome 3, have been linked to *reading disability* (q.v.). Different genes may increase dyslexia susceptibility in different populations.

For some, at least, a core feature appears to be a temporal processing deficit, expressed as difficulty in identifying or sequencing short-duration sensory inputs. Affected subjects have trouble distinguishing syllables such as "ba" and "da" that begin with consonant sounds that last only tens of milliseconds. Because they cannot hear the distinct parts of spoken words, they have difficulty associating those spoken words with the letters that represent those sounds. They have similar "fast element" recognition problems in other sensory modalities, including vision (rapid automized naming) and touch. If touched in rapid succession on two different fingers, they cannot identify the fingers. Their capacity for segmentation of successive sensory stimuli can often be sharpened, however, by remedial training in which stimuli are presented in slower forms ("stretched").

*Fast ForWord* is an information strategy that combines acoustically modified speech with explicit phonological, language, and reading intervention in a series of neuroplasticity-based training exercises disguised as computer games. Neuroplasticity-based intervention aimed at improving RAP thresholds and sharpening acoustic/phonetic processing has an impact not only on oral language, but also on reading decoding and comprehension skills. It does so by "re-mapping" brain areas that are important for these functions. In addition to significantly improved reading in the trained dyslexic group, fMRI results showed "normalization" (increased activity) in the left-hemisphere temporoparietal language region, which is normally active during phonological processing but is not active in children and adults with dyslexia.

About half of subjects with dyslexia also have achromatopsia (color blindness—they see objects not as colors but as shades of gray) or color agnosia (they can match colors but cannot name them).

**dyslexia, literal**  The inability to distinguish individual letters within a word which itself can be read; often a letter surrounded by numbers can be read more easily than if surrounded by other letters.

**dyslogia**  Incoherence of speech.

**dyslysimelia**  Localized muscle contractions, which may be painful, occurring in both lower limbs during relaxation or sleep. The term is commonly shortened to *dyslysis*.

**dyslysis**  *Dyslysimelia* (q.v.).

**dysmegalopsia**  Illusory change in the size or shape of an object that is perceived visually; sometimes called the *Alice in Wonderland effect*. When the object is perceived as smaller than it actually is, the illusion is termed *micropsia*; if the object appears to be enlarged, it is termed *macropsia*.

**dysmentia**  Pseudoretardation; impaired performance on psychological tests secondary to psychological factors.

**dysmetabolic syndrome**  See *metabolic syndrome*.

**dysmetria**  Improper measuring of distances required for muscular acts.

**dysmimia**  Inappropriate mimicry.

**dysmnesia**  Impaired memory. See *memory; organic syndrome*. The term is sometimes used, either by itself or in the form of "the dysmnesic syndrome," to refer to reversible Korsakoff-like syndromes that may be seen after a delirium, especially in the middle-aged and older. The patient has amnesia for the acute delirious episode but in addition has difficulty in retaining recent events and a faulty orientation. Generally the syndrome clears rapidly within a few days, but occasionally it may abate only slowly, over a period of weeks or months.

**dysmorphic delusion**  *Dysmorphic somatoform disorder; dysmorphophobia* (qq.v.); a fixed, false belief that some part of one's body is defective—nose, eye, ear, etc. See *monosymptomatic hypochondriacal psychosis*.

**dysmorphic somatoform disorder**  Preoccupation, but not of delusional degree, with some imagined defect in one's physical appearance. See *dysmorphophobia*.

**dysmorphomania**  *Dysmorphophobia* (q.v.).

**dysmorphophobia**  The conviction that some physical defect is noticeable to others when appearances are in reality normal. Described by Morselli in 1886. Dysmorphophobia by proxy was reported by R. Laugharne in 1997: the patient was preoccupied not with her own appearance but with how her potential offspring might look.

Dysmorphophobia may be manifested as an obsessive fear or, more commonly, a delusional conviction of being physically deformed or otherwise abnormal; sometimes the term is used loosely to refer to any hypochondriacal complaint of delusional intensity. When the patient presents with a single complaint, the condition is sometimes called *monosymptomatic hypochondriacal psychosis* (q.v.) and is generally found to lie somewhere along the paranoia/paraphrenia/paranoid schizophrenia axis. In general, the more exposed to full view is the area of supposed deformity, the worse is the prognosis.

**dysnisophrenia**  Psychopathy; *psychopathic personality* (q.v.); a general term for the heterogeneous psychopathic disorders.

**dysnomia**  *Anomic aphasia* (q.v.).

**dysorexia**  Impaired or perverted appetite. See *eating disorders*.

**dysorthography**  *Dysgraphia* (q.v.).

**dysostosis, diabetic exophthalmic**  *Xanthomatosis* (q.v.).

**dysostosis multiplex**  See *mucopolysaccharidosis*.

**dyspareunia**  A sexual pain disorder characterized by persistent genital pain before, during, or after intercourse. It is much more frequently described in females, but it can occur in males.

**dysperception**  Any impairment or abnormality of *perception* (q.v.).

**dysperception, metabolic**  A term suggested by Bella Kowalson (1967) as a substitute for dementia praecox or schizophrenia to emphasize the wide variety of perceptual changes that have been observed in schizophrenic patients and the probable metabolic basis for such changes.

**dysphagia** Difficulty in eating; it may be organically or psychically determined, but the term generally implies an organic etiology.

**dysphagia globosa** *Globus hystericus* (q.v.).

**dysphasia** A general term for any disorder of the symbolic function of speech, that is, the comprehension and expression of meanings through words. The most common dysphasia seen clinically is *aphasia* (q.v.). Other abnormalities that frequently accompany the language disturbances are as follows: ideokinetic dyspraxia of the ipsilateral hand (patients are physically able to do things, but not on command; they have no trouble brushing their teeth in the morning, but when asked to demonstrate it they cannot do it); buccolingual dyspraxia (cannot puff out cheeks, whistle, or blow out a match); dysgraphia of the ipsilateral (and sometimes the contralateral) hand; weakness or paralysis of the contralateral hand; weakness or paralysis of the contralateral extremity. See *developmental disorders, specific; dysphasia, developmental.*

The most common cause of aphasia is head trauma, which produces 200,000 cases in the United States each year. The next most frequent cause is stroke, which gives 100,000 cases of aphasia each year.

**dysphasia, developmental** *Specific language impairment (SLI)*; some studies suggest that it is a genetically produced impairment in the ability to construct a mental grammar that does not impair other cognitive abilities.

**dysphemia** *Stuttering* (q.v.); stammering.

**dysphonia** Disturbance in vocalization; like *dysarthria* (q.v.), a disorder of the mechanical process of speech.

**dysphoria** Dejection; disaffection; dysthymia; unhappiness; dissatisfaction with life or self, often manifested as underestimation of self on any or every level.

**dysphoria nervosa** *Crispation* (q.v.); fidgets.

**dysphoric disorder, late luteal phase** *LLPDD* (q.v.); premenstrual dysphoric disorder.

**dysphoric disorder, premenstrual** *LLPDD* (q.v.).

**dysphoric separation anxiety** See *abandonment depression; separation anxiety; separation-individuation.*

**dysphrasia** Impaired speaking due to intellectual defects.

**dysphrasia, imitative** *Echolalia* (q.v.); echophrasia.

**dysplasia** Abnormal tissue development. The term came into prominence in psychiatry particularly through the studies of Kretschmer on body configuration. According to him, there are three basic types of physique among psychiatric patients: the asthenic, athletic, and pyknic. The fourth, called the dysplastic, is a heterogeneous group, "varying much among themselves, of which any one group contains only a few members." Among the types described under this heading are elongated eunuchoids, those with polyglandular syndromes, infantilism, and hypoplasia.

**dysplastic type** In Kretschmer's system of constitutional types, a form of physique that varies markedly from the average form of one of the main types called *asthenic, pyknic,* and *athletic* (qq.v.). Most dysplastic subjects fall either into the category of elongated *eunuchoidism* with tower skull and, in the female, with masculinism, or into the groups of polyglandular *fat abnormalities* and *infantilism*; their psychological makeup was held by Kretschmer to be basically *schizothymic* (q.v.).

The anomalies of the dysplastic type are comparable to the *sterile, atrophic* constitutions described by Carus and to Bauer's *status degenerativus.*

**dyspraxia** Partial impairment of the ability to perform skilled movement, with no associated defect in the motor apparatus; characteristic of nondominant parietal lobe disorders.

**dysprosodia** Inability to express mood properly, even though it is experienced normally (unlike subjects with emotional blunting). To the listener, dysprosodic speech sounds foreign. Dysprosodia is suggestive of nondominant frontal lobe disturbance. See *aprosodia.*

**dysregulation** Lack of ability to control impulsive behavior related to strong positive and negative affects, a lack of ability to comfort oneself when strong affects give intense physiologic outcomes, problems in turning attention toward other aspects, and difficulties in organizing and coordinating activities to achieve one's goals. One frequent manifestation of emotional dysregulation is *lability* of the affect (q.v.).

**dysrhaphic** Dysontogenetic; referring to disturbances of development and particularly to developmental disorders of the central nervous system, such as the *Arnold-Chiari malformation* (q.v.).

**dysrhythmia, dart and dome**   See *pyknolepsy*.

**dysrhythmia, major**   See *hypsarrhythmia*.

**dysrhythmia, paroxysmal cerebral**   *Epilepsy* (q.v.).

**dyssocial**   Outside the norms of the group in relation to values, ideals, ethics, etc.; in psychiatry, it usually implies that the pathology is not wholly endogenous and may be the result of having been reared in or having lived in a subgroup whose social code differed from that of the general society. Kernberg defines dyssocial reaction as normal or neurotic adjustment to an abnormal social environment or subgroup with antisocial behaviors. See *antisocial personality; sociopathic personality disturbance*.

**dyssomnias**   Sleep disorders including primary *insomnia*, primary *hypersomnia, narcolepsy, breathing-related sleep disorder, circadian rhythm sleep disorder*, and nocturnal *myoclonus* (qq.v.).

**dyssymbiosis**   A pathological type of symbiosis between mother and child in which the child uses psychotic defenses to control the degree of closeness to the mother. He must maintain a symbiotic relationship since the separation from the mother is experienced as annihilation; but he must also maintain control over the relationship, which, if it becomes too close will result in engulfment by the mother. See *symbiotic infantile psychosis*.

**dyssymbole**   A state of mind characterized by the inability to formulate conceptual thoughts upon personal topics or to discriminate the gradations of personal emotions in language intelligible to others. Dyssymbole is certainly apparent in some schizophrenics, but many physicians believe that it is present in all schizophrenics. Whether dyssymbole represents a defect in the patient's semantic power or is indicative of a more basic emotional deficiency is not known.

**dyssynergia**   Failure to work in unison or harmony, such as is seen in the motor and gait disturbances that follow cerebellar lesions. See *disorganization*.

**dyssynergia cerebellaris myoclonica**   See *Hunt syndrome*.

**dysthymia**   1. In DSM-III-R one of the *depressive disorders*, consisting of a chronic (over 2 years) pattern of "down" or "low" days outnumbering symptom-free days; in addition to dejected mood, the most frequent symptoms are altered eating and sleeping habits (loss of appetite or overeating, insomnia or hypersomnia), lowered energy and self-esteem, difficulty in concentrating, and ideas of suicide or wishing to be dead. In time, major depressive episodes may be superimposed on the chronic condition (*double depression*). The DSM-III-R definition is similar to a usage that had approached obsolescence, applying dysthymia to depression of less intense degree than that found in manic-depressive psychosis and associated in addition with neurasthenic and hypochondriacal symptoms.

2. Eysenck's term for the group of symptoms found in patients with a high degree of neuroticism and a high degree of introversion.

**dysthymic disorder**   Depressive neurosis; neurotic depression; one of the *depressive disorders* (q.v.) characterized by lowered mood tone and a variety of other symptoms, some of which are almost always present, reflecting the chronic nature of the disorder. Among the other symptoms are poor concentration, indecisiveness; loss of enjoyment of sex, praise, rewards, or other ordinarily pleasurable conditions; unrelenting feelings of tiredness, ineffectiveness, inadequacy, inability to cope, or being slowed down; less active or talkative than usual; poor appetite or overeating; insomnia or hypersomnia; irritability or poorly controlled anger; brooding, self-pity, feelings of hopelessness; recurrent thoughts of death or suicide. See *psychoneurotic depression*.

**dystonia**   Abnormal muscle tone, including both excessive or exaggerated tone, as in muscle spasm, and deficient or absent tone; persisting posture of a body part, which can result in grotesque movements and distorted positions of the body. Dystonia is characterized by involuntary movements and abnormal and often painful postures. While it may be psychogenic, it is more often a side effect of pharmacotherapy, such as tardive dyskinesia. Abnormal increases in sensory cortical representations—such as the high decibel levels of "rock" music—can also lead to dystonia. See *tardive dyskinesia*.

**dystonia, acute**   A neurologic side effect of neuroleptic drugs (and other drugs that block dopamine $D_2$ receptors) characterized by intermittent or sustained uncoordinated spasmodic movements of the head, neck, and limbs. The movements take many forms, including torticollis, retrocollis, opisthotonus, oculogyric crises, macroglossia, grimacing, dysarthria, dysphasia, and stridorous respiration. It generally begins during the first or second day of treatment and is most likely to occur in young males.

**dystonic** Relating to abnormal (muscular) tension. The psyche or personality is said to be dystonic when it is not in harmony either with itself or with its environment.

**dystrophia adiposogenitalis** *Frohlich syndrome* (q.v.).

**dystrophy, argyrophilic** See *Alzheimer disease.*

**dystrophy, reflex sympathetic** See *pain syndromes.*

**dystropy** A term used by Adolf Meyer, meaning abnormality of behavior.

**dystychia** See *euphoria.*

**DZ** *Dizygotic* (q.v.).

# E

**EAA** Excitatory amino acid (neurotransmitter), including aspartate and *glutamate* (q.v.). At least three different subtypes of EAA receptors are known: (1) the *NMDA receptor* (q.v.), which is activated by NMDA and also by ibotenate, glutamate, and aspartate; (2) the *kainate* receptor, which is activated by kainate and also by glutamate and quisqualate; and (3) the *AMPA* receptor, which is activated by AMPA and also by glutamate and quisqualate. See *excitotoxicity.*

**EAAT2** Excitatory amino acid transporter-2, the promotor of a gene for the major glutamate transporter in CNS. See *glutamate.*

**EAATs** Excitatory amino-acid transporters, a family of membrane proteins essential to *glutamate* uptake (q.v.). EAAT1 and EAAT2 are predominantly glial and are found in the hippocampus. EAAT3 is expressed in neurons of the hippocampus and elsewhere in the brain. EAAT4 and EAAT5 are also neuronal; the former is found in Pukinje cells in the cerebellum, the latter in the retina.

**EAP** *Employee assistance program* (q.v.).

**ear pulling** Pulling of the ears is believed by Kanner to be a substitute for thumb-sucking; in psychoanalysis it is believed to be a masturbatory equivalent.

**Earle, Pliny** (1809–1892) American psychiatrist; hospital administration; in 1877 published statistical study entitled *The Curability of Insanity.*

**early infantile autism** See *autistic disorder.*

**early warning signs** *EWS*; see *prodromal symptoms.*

**easy child** See *temperament.*

**eaten, fear of being** Whether conscious or unconscious, the fear of being eaten originates early in the development of the infant's ego during the oral stage. During this stage the infant develops the normal aim of pleasure or satisfaction through eating and, in a more general sense, through the incorporation of objects. Frustrations of this erotic aim of eating or incorporating and fears of such frustration are of frequent occurrence. These anxieties take the form of a fear of being eaten, because of infantile animistic thinking, which assumes that what the infant feels and does will also take place in the world around it. Fear of being eaten may have another function—it may serve as a cover for castration anxiety, disguised by being distorted through regression into the older fear of being eaten.

**eaten, phantasy of being** The phantasy of being eaten or incorporated frequently occurs as part of a certain type of relationship to a love object. In this relationship the patient's only aim is "to become part of a more powerful personality" whom the subject overestimates to an enormous degree, though having at the same time no interest in or idea about the partner's real personality. Those who have this sort of aim, attitude, and phantasy (sometimes described as merger-hungry) are characterized by an overwhelming feeling of inadequacy and inordinate need for self-esteem. As a result they can never give love but have an extreme need to feel loved.

**eating disorders** *Limosis*; dysorexia; heterorexia; currently, the category includes *anorexia nervosa, binge eating, bulimia nervosa,* and in some classifications *pica* and *rumination* (qq.v.). Changes in eating habits occur as symptoms in many conditions, including bereavement, substance abuse, and mood disorders. See *night eating syndrome; obesity.*

**eating without saturation** See *night-eating syndrome.*

**EBA** Extrastriate body area, perhaps a specialized area for recognition of the human body and body parts. See *face recognition.*

**EBL** Emotional body language. See *amygdala.*

**EBM** *Evidence-based medicine* (q.v.).

**EBV** Epstein-Barr virus syndrome, also known as *chronic mononucleosis, myalgic encephalomyelitis,* and *postviral syndrome.* See *chronic fatigue syndrome.*

**EC** *Entorhinal cortex* (q.v.).

**ECA** The NIMH *epidemiologic catchment area* study of incidence and prevalence of mental disorders in the United States. See *prevalence.*

**ECB** Executive Control Battery, designed to elicit manifestations of executive dyscontrol, such as perseveration, echopraxia, field-dependent behavior, inertia, and stereotypies.

The subtests are as follows: (1) Graphical Sequence Test, (2) Competing Programs Test, (3) Manual Postures Test, and (4) Motor Sequences Test.

**eccentric paranoia**  See *amorous paranoia*.

**Eccles, John C.**  (1903–1997) Australian neuroscientist; studied at Oxford under Sir Charles Sherrington; shared the 1963 Nobel Prize with Alan Hodgkin and Andrew Huxley for his work on excitatory and inhibitory synapses; dominated the field of neuroscience for decades. *The Physiology of Nerve Cells*; *The Physiology of Synapses*.

**ecdemomania, ecdemonomania**  Morbid impulse to travel or wander about. See *Alzheimer disease*.

**ecdysiasm**  A tendency to disrobe in order to provoke useless erotic stimulation in the opposite sex. See *exhibitionism*.

**écho des pensées**  (F. "echo of thoughts") The imagined sound reproduction of the patient's thoughts; audible thoughts (see *first-rank symptoms*). A special form of auditory hallucinations in which the acoustic verbal images of the thought itself are projected outside in such a way that whatever the subject thinks, he hears repeated in speech. See *Gedankenlautwerden*.

**echo phenomena**  Kraepelin's term for *echolalia* and *echopraxia* (qq.v.).

**echo principle**  Imitative patterning, such as is seen in children who exhibit certain behavior or behaviorisms similar to those seen in their parents but not necessarily indicative of inheritance. For example, a child learns to speak English or French not because of specific genetic predisposition, but because English or French is spoken in his or her home.

**echo sign**  *Rare*. A speech disorder observed in epileptic patients characterized by the repetition of a word in some part of a sentence; *logoclonia* (q.v.).

**echo speech**  *Echolalia* (q.v.).

**echoencephalography**  A technique of neurodiagnosis in which ultrasound is transmitted to the brain and its echo is recorded on an oscilloscope. A shift in echo may indicate the presence of a space-occupying mass.

**echoing, thought**  *Écho des pensées* (q.v.).

**echokinesis**  *Echopraxia* (q.v.).

**echolalia**  Pathological repetition by imitation of the speech of another, seen in some patients with the catatonic form of schizophrenia and

also in Alzheimer disease and other cerebral degenerative disorders.

**echomatism**  *Echopraxia* (q.v.).

**echomimia**  *Echopraxia* (q.v.).

**echopalilalia**  Senseless repetition (re-echoing) of words spoken by another person.

**echopathy**  Pathological repetition through imitation of the actions or speech of another. It occurs most frequently in the catatonic phase of schizophrenia, when the patient assumes the postures, gestures, and speech of another in "mirror" form. See *echopraxia*; *echolalia*.

**echophrasia**  *Echolalia* (q.v.).

**echo-planar MRI**  *EPI*; an improved form of conventional *MRI* (q.v.) that approaches real time in its recording of radio signals from the brain. Use of rapidly oscillating magnetic field gradients and high-speed software allow it to collect several hundred lines of data at a time, rather than the one line collected by conventional MRI.

**echopraxia**  Repetition, by imitation, of the movements of another; the action is not a willed or voluntary one, and it has a semi-automatic, compulsive, and uncontrollable quality. A catatonic patient acted as the "mirror image" of his physician, assuming every posture and gesture of the physician while he was in the room with him. Various forms of echopraxia have been labeled: *copying mania; echokinesis; echomatism; echomimia*.

"Contrasting with negativism is the so-called automatic obedience, showing itself in echopraxia (repetition of actions seen), echolalia (repetition of words heard), and flexibilitas cerea (the maintenance of imposed postures)" (Henderson, D. K. & Gillespie, R. D. *A Text-Book of Psychiatry*, 1936). See *amurakh*.

**echul**  A culture-specific syndrome described in Native Americans in southern California consisting of sexual anxiety and convulsions related to severe stress, such as death of a child or spouse.

**eclactisma**  A synonym for epilepsy, in part descriptive of the movements of the lower limbs during the grand mal seizure.

**eclampsic amentia**  *Obs*. Formerly applied to cases of mental retardation associated with epileptiform convulsions in early infancy.

**eclecticism**  In psychiatry, the selection of compatible features from diverse (and, often, superficially incompatible) systems of metapsychology in an attempt to combine whatever is valid in any theory or doctrine into an integrated, harmonious whole.

**eclimia** *Bulimia* (q.v.).

**eclipse, cerebral** Short-lived loss of consciousness, or loss of perception and motor power, in chronic cerebral circulatory insufficiency. Such episodes are not syncopal, nor do they give evidence of cardiac arrest, lowered blood pressure, or the neurovegetative manifestations characteristic of carotid sinus syncope.

**eclipse, mental** Janet's term for the "stealing" of ideas from patients, particularly from patients with schizophrenia, who claim that whenever they have an idea, someone takes it away. See *first rank symptoms*.

**ECM** 1. External chemical messenger; *pheromone* (q.v.). 2. Extracellular matrix. See *metalloproteinases*.

**ecmnesia** *Rare.* Anterograde amnesia. See *délire ecmnesique; retrograde amnesia.*

**ecnoea** *Obs.* Mental disorder or disease.

**ecnoia** A type of fear reaction seen in children consisting of prolongation of what began as a normally motivated sudden fright; for days or weeks the child is startled by everything and sheds tears at the slightest provocation. During this period, sleep, appetite, and excretory functions may be affected.

**ECoG** Electrocorticogram; an *electroencephalogram* (q.v.) obtained by placing electrodes directly on the brain cortex rather than on the scalp. In a depth EEG (*DEEG*), intracerebral electrodes are inserted into deeper cortical or subcortical tissues. Both DEEG and ECoG show increased amplitude of electrical activity as compared with the usual scalp EEG.

**ecological systems model** This model views disease and disorder not only as a deviance of the person, but also as a reflection of deviance or disequilibrium in that series of social and biological systems with which the person articulates. See *medical model; community psychiatry.*

**ecology** Study of the mutual relationships between living things and their environment. One of its basic principles is that no form of life can continue to multiply indefinitely without eventually coming to terms with the limitations imposed by its environment. Ecology includes such studies as the differential incidence of mental disorder in various populations and the distribution of crime and delinquency within a specified geographical area. The psychiatric ecologist (or social psychiatrist) is particularly interested in why one person falls ill while his neighbor (or sibling, parent, etc.) maintains good health. "The responses to stress vary from case to case between the widest extremes. The reasons for the variation lie in *genetical and constitutional differences* between individuals as well as in *developmental and psychological ones.* Genetical data are among the few solid facts we have, and hypotheses about the role of social factors in mental disease which take account of them are bound to be more fruitful than those which ignore them" (Mayer-Gross, W. *Clinical Psychiatry,* 1960). Ecology is also known as *bionomics*; psychiatric ecology is often called *social psychiatry.* See *behavioral ecology; community psychiatry; comparative psychiatry.*

The ecological model provides a network approach to psychosocial disorder that may try to manipulate the expectations that impose specific roles on subsystems, and this is the model that involves itself most directly in social engineering and community action. In such a model, the primary role of the psychiatrist is as a change agent in social action and community organization, who uses his or her knowledge of group process to mediate and reconcile opposing forces that produce social disequilibrium and to stimulate new approaches through interpersonal transactions. See *social policy planning.*

**ecomania** *Obs.* Morbid attitude toward the members of one's family. Also *oik(i)omania.*

**economic divorce** See *divorce, stations of.*

**economics** A social science that studies the production, distribution, and consumption of goods and services and, in particular, how individuals and societies seek to meet their needs and wants when available resources are in short supply. Typical methods of evaluation include *cost-benefit analysis* and *cost-effectiveness analysis* (qq.v.).

Technological advances in medicine have resulted in increased costs, not only because they often require more expensive procedures or more expensive drugs, but also because they increase the size of the population that might benefit from the new treatment. Most new drugs and procedures improve efficacy only marginally over already available interventions, and the cost of their development might be more effective if allocated to improving the performance of the health care system in delivering existing treatments. An important principle of economic evaluation is to take a broad, societal perspective on health cost and benefits, and this requires more than comparison of one drug or procedure to another. Economic evaluation must also give attention to the relevant findings of other fields, such as behavioral science, epidemiology, political science, psychology, social marketing, etc. (Suh, G.-H. *International Pscyhogeriatrics* *19*: 993–1002, 2007). See *FFS; managed care; translational research*.

**Economo disease**  (Konstantin von Economo, Austrian neuropathologist, 1876–1931) See *encephalitis, epidemic*.

**ecophobia**  See *oikophobia*.

**ecosystem**  The balance attained within a society, population, or group between competing and mixed components, variation in any one of which requires commensurate change in all other components.

**écouteur**  One who obtains gratification through listening to sexual accounts; eavesdropper; the auditory counterpart of a *voyeur* (q.v.).

**écouteurism**  Sexual pleasure obtained from sounds or listening to the sexual or toilet activities of others. See *voyeurism*.

**ecphoria**  Evocation of an *engram* (q.v.) by a memory or by an experience similar to the one stored in the engram.

**ecstasy**  1. Trance states in which religious ideation or similar ideas of dedication and complete surrender occupy almost the entire field of consciousness; it was also known as *contemplatio, ébriécation celeste, phrenoplexia*, and *status raptus*.

2. Street name for MDMA. See *hallucinogen*.

**ECT**  *Electric convulsion therapy*; *ECS* (electroconvulsive shock); a form of somatic treatment for certain psychiatric conditions in which electrical current is applied to the brain through two electrodes placed on the skull. ECT was developed in the 1930s, when it was believed that epilepsy (convulsive disorder) and schizophrenia were mutually exclusive. Additional studies and experience with the treatment revealed that there was, in fact, no "natural" antgonism between the two disorders, and that convulsive treatment was of major benefit in depression rather than schizophrenia. It is true, however, that the therapeutic results of ECT are dependent on convulsive activity in the brain, and not on the production of peripherally manifested convulsions.

Although ECT has been in use for over 80 years, its mechanism of action and how its most significant adverse effect, memory loss, is caused are unknown. There is experimental evidence for the involvement of many factors: supersensitivity of receptor-mediated responses in the hippocampus or down-regulation of those receptors; neuropeptides; the anticonvulsant effects of ECT; and electrophysiologic changes in the prefrontal cortex.

As developed in Rome by Cerletti and Bini, ECT employed bilateral placement of the two electrodes on the temporal areas of the skull. Current was applied through a specially constructed machine, whose main features are a stop for time regulation to fractions of a second and a voltameter for regulation of the voltage applied. The desired generalized convulsion is ordinarily obtained with voltage varying between 70 and 130 volts applied for 0.1 to 0.5 seconds—a strength lower than the densities used in the direct stimulation of neural tissue in sensory prosthesis studies or with the diathermy needle, and far less than those of the cardiac defibrillator.

The technique of administration has been modified since ECT was first used. Many clinicians now premedicate the patient with atropine to reduce bronchial secretions and to inhibit the vagal discharge that accompanies convulsion; they use a rapid-acting barbiturate of short duration at the lowest dose that will induce general anesthesia; and they use a muscle relaxant (such as succinylcholine) to prevent fractures. Oxygen 100% is administered by mask for a short period immediately following administration of the muscle relaxant and anesthetic, and again throughout the period of apnea following the convulsion.

ECT is a remarkably safe procedure, whether administered with or without a general anesthetic. The question of whether ECT can ever produce persisting electroencephalographic changes when administered in the usual way remains moot. The most controversial area is that of persisting memory defects, but most studies have failed to demonstrate impairment that persists more than a month or two after the last treatment. No studies have demonstrated impairment in the capacity to acquire new memories.

Bilateral electrode placement continues to be the most commonly employed method in all countries, but there are many advocates of unilateral ECT who claim that such a modification reduces posttreatment confusion and is as effective as bilateral placement.

The major indication for ECT is clinical depression, for which results with ECT therapy remain superior to improvement rates with antidepressant drugs. ECT is also indicated in manic patients when response to neuroleptics or lithium is inadequate. The main indication for ECT in acute schizophrenic episodes is lack of response to neuroleptics and persistence of symptoms to a degree that necessitates continued hospitalization. It is probably of limited value in chronic schizophrenia.

The major drawback of ECT is the high relapse rate; it has not yet been determined if that rate is higher or lower than the relapse rate with antidepressant drugs. Probably the only absolute contraindication to ECT is increased intracranial pressure. It is worthy of note that the risk of death in severe depression is high enough to outweigh any side effects that ECT may produce.

**ectoderm**   See *embryonic disc.*

**ectodomain shedding**   See *metalloproteinases.*

**ectomorphic**   In Sheldon's system, a constitutional type characterized by predominance of its third component (linearity); that is, the physical structures developed from the *ectodermal* layer of the embryo. Persons of this type are contrasted with the *endomorphic* and *mesomorphic* types and correspond roughly to Kretschmer's *asthenic* type.

**ectopic gray matter**   Islands of neurons that failed to complete their migration to the cortex during development; they have been reported in about 5% of males with schizophrenia and are presumed to reflect abnormal brain development.

**ectopic release**   Spillover of neurotransmitter from the extrasynaptic region, rather than direct release from the active zone of the presynaptic terminal. In ectopic release, the neurotransmitter may diffuse extensively along the cell membrane and activate receptors in extrasynaptic regions or at neighboring synapses. At some cholinergic synapses, for example, ectopic release can activate the predominantly extrasynaptic $\alpha 7$ nicotinic receptor subtype.

**ectype**   Outstanding or unusual type; types of physical or mental constitution that vary considerably from the average. From the physical point of view, two ectypes are recognized, the megalosplanchnic (brevilineal, brachymorphic) and the microsplanchnic (longineal, dolichomorphic). There are two corresponding personality ectypes, the introverted and the extraverted.

**edema, angioneurotic**   *Quincke disease; angioedema*; giant urticaria; a chronic condition consisting of recurrent episodes of localized, painless swellings of the subcutaneous tissue or submucosa of various parts of the body. The disease may be fatal if the edema involves the glottis and larynx. It appears as a rare hereditary form due to a lack of inhibitor of complement ($C_1$ esterase inhibitor deficiency), and as a sporadic form which is often an allergic or anaphylactic reaction to infectious, toxic, or autotoxic processes. Despite its name, angioneurotic edema is not considered to be primarily of psychological origin, although emotional upsets may sometimes trigger the reaction in the sporadic form.

**edipism**   (From Oedipus, who tore out his own eyes) *Rare.* Self-inflicted injury to the eyes.

**editing, transcript**   See *transcription.*

**EDR**   Electrodermal response. See *psychogalvanic reflex.*

**EDS**   Excessive daytime sleepiness, characteristic of *narcolepsy* (q.v.).

**education, compensatory**   Any program designed to enrich intellectual and social skills in disadvantaged children as early in their lives as possible; probably the best known example of such early intervention is the *Head Start* Program, begun in 1965 by Julius B. Richmond, M.D. Despite early reports that cast doubt upon the value of the program, most long-term studies have found that the program did in fact increase the social competence of disadvantaged children and raised their IQ scores.

**education, progressive**   A movement within the field of education, founded by John Dewey, that emphasizes the needs of the individual and the individual's capacity for self-expression and self-direction.

**educational psychology**   The branch of psychology concerned with the derivation of psychological principles and methods that can be applied directly to problems of education.

**educational-socialization model**  A model of illness that views a   population as a social system containing people who have certain roles. This is a sociologic approach that asks how well are people fulfilling their roles, and whose focus is often on newcomers to the group (children, immigrants, etc.) and on refitting to appropriate roles those who have deviated (rehabilitation and tertiary prevention of residual defects). See *medical model; community psychiatry.*

**education**  Sullivan's term for central processes, i.e., whatever lies between receptor functions and effector functions.

**EE**  *Expressed emotions* (q.v.).

**EEG**  *Electroencephalogram* (q.v.).

**EEG activation**  Any of the various procedures used to elicit or enhance abnormal EEG activity, such as sleep deprivation, stimulation with a flashing strobe light (photic stimulation), or hyperventilation. See *electroencephalogram.*

**EFAs**  Essential fatty acids; see *omega-3 fatty acids.*

**effectiveness**  See *efficacy.*

**effectiveness research**  In contrast to *efficacy research* (q.v.), it emphasizes external validity or generalizability by conducting studies under conditions that include usual patients, routine practice settings, and routine clinical providers.

**effector protein**  *Transducer* (q.v.).

**effeminated man**  Passive male, often implying that the male is homosexual.

**efferent**  See *afferent; reflex.*

**efficacy**  The ability to produce the desired effect(s). In psychopharmacology, referring to a drug that produces the intended effect under ideal conditions; efficacy is usually determined by comparing drug-treated patients with a randomized, double-blind, placebo-controlled, parallel group. *Effectiveness* refers to the drug's ability to produce the intended effect under usual practice conditions; the term further implies that the effect is maintained over time.

**efficacy expectancy**  See *social learning theory.*

**efficacy research**  Typically, it emphasizes internal validity by controlling for as many variables as possible in order to focus on a single research variable or question. Efficacy studies are a critical first step in establishing

the likelihood that an intervention will result in the desired outcome, in comparison with a placebo or a well-defined alternative under highly controlled conditions. See *effectiveness research; evidence-based medicine.*

**effort syndrome**  A type of anxiety neurosis or anxiety reaction, approximately equivalent to soldier's heart, neurocirculatory asthenia, or, in current terminology, hyperventilation syndrome. See *hyperventilation syndrome; asthenia, neurocirculatory.*

**egersis**  *Obs.* Intense wakefulness.

**ego**  In psychoanalytic psychology, that part of the psychic apparatus that is the mediator between the person and reality. Its prime function is the perception of reality and adaptation to it. The ego is the executive organ of the reality principle and is ruled by the *secondary process.* The various tasks (functions) of the ego include perception, including self-perception and self-awareness; motor control (action); adaptation to reality; use of the reality principle and the mechanism of anxiety to ensure safety and self-preservation; replacement of the primary process of the id by the secondary process; memory; affects; thinking; and a general synthetic function manifested in assimilation of external and internal elements, in reconciling conflicting ideas, in uniting contrasts, and in activating mental creativity. Unlike the id, the ego has an organization (i.e., it is not chaotic), it can generate coordinated action, and it is ruled by the secondary rather than the primary process. Its functions develop gradually, dependent upon physical maturation (and particularly, the genetically determined growth of the central nervous system) and upon experiential factors. See *libidinal ego; object relations theory.*

From the standpoint of analytical psychology (Jung), the ego is "a complex of representations which constitutes the centrum of my field of consciousness and appears to possess a very high degree of continuity and identity." The ego "is not identical with the totality of my psyche, being merely a complex among other complexes. Hence, I discriminate between the ego and the Self, since the ego is only the subject of my consciousness, while the Self is the subject of my totality: hence it also includes the unconscious psyche. In this sense the Self would be an (ideal) factor which embraces and includes the ego. In unconscious phantasy the Self often appears as a super-ordinated or ideal personality" (Jung, C. G. *Psychological Types*, 1923).

**ego, central** Fairbairn's term for the conscious self that deals with reality, approximately equivalent to Freud's ego. The central ego idealizes the parents and forms the ideal object; the combination of central ego with ideal object strives to maintain good relationships with the parents in order to adapt.

**ego, collective** The ego is not only a product of the individual, but it also reflects the group and its concepts. See *collective unconscious*.

**ego, effective** The ego that has learned how to adapt itself to the environment and deal with it *effectively*, as differentiated from the infantile ego—helpless at birth and therefore *ineffective* in this respect.

**ego alteration, reactive** A type of anticathexis—that is, expenditure of energy in maintaining the repression of libidinal or aggressive impulses—in which the ego is altered by a reaction formation against the particular libidinal impulses. Freud gives the example of the compulsion neurosis in which an exaggeration of the normal character traits of pity, conscientiousness, and cleanliness is found. These character traits are the antithesis of the anal-sadistic impulses repressed by the compulsion neurosis (*The Problem of Anxiety*, 1936).

**ego analysis** In psychoanalytic treatment, the uncovering and interpreting of the ego's (and superego's) defenses against impulses. Libido analysis and ego analysis go hand in hand in treatment: libido analysis, for example, discovers what it is that has been repressed, while ego analysis discovers why the infantile ego found it necessary to repress the impulse in the first place. See *object relations theory*.

**ego anxiety** The threat of internal dangers to the ego in contrast to fear, which refers to the threat of external dangers to the ego. See *anxiety*.

**ego boundary** A concept introduced by Federn to refer to "the peripheral sense organ of the ego." The ego boundary discriminates what is real from what is unreal. Because the boundary is flexible and dynamic, it will vary in accordance with different ego states. There are two main ego boundaries, the inner and the outer. The inner ego boundary is the boundary toward the repressed

unconscious. This is strengthened by countercathexes (anticathexes) and thus is able to prevent the entrance of repressed material. Its flexibility is demonstrable in hypnagogic states and in normal falling asleep, where the ego and its boundaries lose cathexis and unegotized material enters. The external or outer ego boundary is the boundary toward stimuli of the external world. The external ego boundary includes the sense organs but it is more than mere summation of these, for the sense of reality of an object comes not alone by stimulation of a sense organ but further requires that the non-ego material impinge upon a well-cathected external ego boundary. If the boundary loses cathexis, these perceptions, no matter how vivid, will have a strange, unfamiliar, or even unreal quality. See *derealization*.

**ego cathexis** See *cathexis*.

**ego center** P. Schilder's term for the nucleus, or inner part of the ego, surrounded by a peripheral part of the ego in the same manner that the nucleus of a cell is enclosed by the protoplasm. According to Schilder, some sensations are particularly close to this hypothesized nucleus, and specifically pain, sexual excitement, and an`xiety seem to be in the very center of the personality. Thus, the importance of surgical operations varies in accordance with the part of the body operated upon: operations on genitals, breasts, or eyes threaten the body parts that are nearer than others to the center of the ego (*Psychotherapy*, 1938).

**ego defect** Any abnormality of ego functioning. See *ego*.

**ego deviant children** Beres's diagnostic label for those children whom others would classify as having childhood schizophrenia or early infantile autism. See *autistic disorder; childhood schizophrenia*.

**ego distortion** An inexact, general term that is approximately equivalent to "ego impoverishment," "ego deviation," or "ego immaturity." Some writers, however, use "ego distortion" in a more specific sense to refer to an inability to use the usual ego functions of defense in adapting to painful reality. Thus, S. Nacht (*International Journal of Psycho-Analysis 39*, 1958) differentiates between (1) the classical disturbances of ego function, which stem primarily from memory falsifications of past experiences that are distorted by unconscious phantasies of the patient, and (2) ego distortion, where the ego is injured by objectively harmful events that occurred in reality rather than in phantasy.

**ego drive**  Impulse toward self-preservation, ego maximation, and group conformance, the development of which is deeply rooted in biological constitution and markedly influenced by the social nature of man's existence. Also called *ego instinct.*

**ego erotism**  Narcissism. See *ego libido.*

**ego fragmentation**  See *dedifferentiation.*

**ego functions**  Included are reality testing, judgment, sense of reality, regulation and control of drives, object relations, thought processes, adaptive regression in the service of the ego, defensive functions, stimulus barrier, autonomous functions, synthetic functions, and mastery-competence. See *ego.*

**ego identity**  That sense of identity which "provides the ability to experience one's self as something that has continuity and sameness, and to act accordingly" (Erikson, E. *Childhood and Society,* 1950). The term refers particularly to the degree to which the boundaries of the physical and the mental self are clearly delineated; those whose ego identity is confused are believed by many to be especially vulnerable to schizophrenia.

"Identity is the unconscious directional pattern or sensing apparatus whereby the individual orients himself to others and to his environment. In part it consists of identifications and representations of relationships with primary love-objects.... Ultimately it must represent a temporally persistent, coordinate system whereby the self is located. Identification, by contrast, should probably be used to describe the process whereby external objects and the exchanges with them are partially or totally represented in the psychic apparatus, and subsequently subjectified or equated or correlated with the representations of the self" (Suslick, A. *Archives of General Psychiatry 8,* 1963).

**ego instinct**  Defined by Jones as all the nonsexual instincts. See *ego drive.*

**ego libido**  Narcissistic libido; an ambiguous term reflecting Freud's view (later abandoned) that all libido is stored in the ego during the earliest stage of development—the stage of primary narcissism. See *narcissism, primary.*

**ego maximation**  Ego drives to maintain feelings of personal adequacy in competitive situations. See *self-maximation.*

**ego motor control**  The control exerted by the ego over one's motor activities. The human infant learns to substitute "actions for mere discharge reactions" by acquiring a tolerance for the tension that arises from stimuli and results in immediate reaction. According to Fenichel, learning to walk, to control the sphincter, and to speak "are the main steps in the development of the mastery of physical motor functions." See *ego.*

**ego neurosis**  See *traumatic neurosis.*

**ego psychology**  A general trend in psychoanalytic theory that emphasizes ego functions and object relations early in life, rather than id instincts. In *The Ego and the Id* (1923), Freud held that all libido is stored in the id and whatever is drawn into the ego as narcissism must therefore be secondary. In later writings, although inconsistently, he referred to object love as the most primitive type of relationship to the environment.

Anna Freud shifted the emphasis of psychoanalytic theory from the id's drives to the ego's attempts to control the drives through elaborate defense mechanisms. She, and the ego psychology that followed her shift in emphasis, focused on the defenses and their expression in the form of psychopathology when they were unable to contain the drives.

In 1952 Heinz Hartmann, generally considered the leader of the "United States school" of ego psychology, introduced the notion of object constancy—the constancy that a child achieves when the relationship to its love object remains stable. This requires object permanence, in which a mental representation of the object persists in the object's absence, a cognitive achievement of the first year of life. Object constancy probably develops during the end of the second year and is a precursor of the capacity to love another person in a stable fashion, regardless of the state of one's needs.

Hartmann emphasized adaptation to the external world and primary object relations, thereby bringing psychoanalytic theory closer to a two-person, relationship theory. Nonetheless, when object relations appear and how they develop, remain highly controversial topics. Some maintain that autoerotism is primary and that the infant makes no distinction between self and nonself at the first stage of development. Others believe that narcissism is the primary state, in which the infant perceives others only as an extension of the self. Still others, following Melanie Klein's lead, insist that the infant is object-related from the very beginning, although her theory views instinctual drives (and the death instinct in particular) as the basis for object relationships. See *object relations theory*. Kohut, and some of Klein's followers (e.g., Fairbairn, Winnicot), also believed that object relations are present from the very beginning but emphasized the nature of the relationship with the caretaker rather than instincts as the determinant of development.

**ego resistance** Much of the resistance to be overcome in analysis is produced by the ego, "which clings tenaciously to its anti-cathexis." The ego "finds it difficult to turn its attention to perceptions and ideas the avoidance of which it had until then made a rule, or to acknowledge as belonging to it impulses which constitute the most complete antithesis to those familiar to it as its own." This resistance of the ego is known more specifically as *repression resistance*. It appears as *transference resistance* (q.v.): the repression constantly exerted by the ego is in this case related specifically to the person of the analyst and thus appears in the analysis in different and more definite ways than simple repression resistance.

Another category of ego resistance is related to the gain of the illness. Symptoms in warding off dangerous instinctual impulses both relieve anxiety and serve as a means of gratifying these instinctual impulses. The ego opposes the renunciation of both the gratification and relief that are "based upon the inclusion of the symptom in the ego."

In analytic treatment there are also resistances that derive from sources other than ego. These are (1) the "'resistance of the unconscious' or of the id, which derives from the 'repetition-compulsion,'" and (2) the "resistance of the super-ego," which derives from "the sense of guilt or need of punishment" (Freud, S. *The Problem of Anxiety*, 1936).

**ego retrenchment** The act of diminishing or removing the need for a given function of the ego. Thus, inhibitions may make it unnecessary for the ego to form symptoms in order to appease an unconscious impulse.

**ego split** A psychoanalytic term designating the phenomenon in which the ego may develop several divergent yet coexisting attitudes toward the same thing. This situation exists (1) in the normal personality; (2) in neuroses; and (3) in psychoses.

In the normal person, "The ego can take itself as object, observe itself, criticize itself." In particular, Freud describes that faculty of the ego that serves and criticizes the ego, which he names *superego*. This is one example of a split in the ego, and the self-observation and self-criticism demonstrate the existence of two attitudes toward whatever is being done by the person at the time. See *splitting*.

In neuroses, two contrary and independent attitudes are always present as regards some particular behavior, for the ego's defensive efforts to ward off danger are never completely successful and the weaker attitude that is repressed nevertheless leads to "psychological complications," such as the neurotic symptoms.

In psychotic episodes, patients may describe how, even during acute hallucinatory and delusional states, one part of their mind was watching in an objective way the remainder of the patient and his feelings, behavior, and thoughts. This is particularly clear in those catatonic patients who, after the attack has ended, can report coherently on all their behavior and upon all that was going on about them during a catatonic episode in which they appeared to be completely out of contact.

**ego stability** Health, strength, maturity, or normality of the ego. The usual differentiating criteria of the more normal ego, in contrast to the neurotic one, are the following: (1) less severe primitive or infantile hostility (id); (2) less severe self-punitive archaic conscience drive (superego); (3) fewer magical defensive systems; (4) less infantile omnipotent (wishful) thinking; and (5) enhanced object reality functioning.

**ego state, adult** In *transactional analysis* (q.v.), the analyzing, deciding, computerlike aspects of the ego which emphasize the objective and the rational. The child ego state creates the wanting part of the person, but the adult ego state decides whether the want can be fulfilled, and how that fulfillment can be achieved.

**ego states** Dissociated partial identities that fall short of having full *alter* (q.v.) formation or are separated incompletely from the usual state of consciousness. An organized system of behavior and experience whose elements are bound together by some common principle; unlike alters, the boundaries of ego states are relatively permeable. In DSM-IV, they are labelled DDNOS, dissociative disorder not otherwise specified. See *dissociation*.

**ego strength** The degree to which the ego's functions are maintained, even in the face of wide variations in the supply of instinctual energy to the ego; the effectiveness with which the ego discharges its various functions, such as developing anxiety tolerance, impulse control, and sublimation. A strong ego will not only mediate between id, superego, and reality, and integrate these various functions, but further it will do so with enough flexibility so that energy will remain for creativity and other needs. This is in contrast to the rigid personality in which ego functions are maintained, but only at the cost of impoverishment of the personality. See *ego*.

**ego stress** Broadly speaking, anything requiring adaptation maneuvers on the part of the ego, although usually the term implies that the strain is such as to require unusual defensive reactions. The stress itself may arise from the external world (the demands of reality), or from within (the pressure of the id for discharge and gratification of drives or superego demands). As stress increases so will defenses until distortion may result or even alteration of the ego. Responses may vary from normal emergency reactions (phantasy, reaction-formation, etc.), to exaggerations of normal function (somatization), to partial withdrawal (depersonalization, dissociation), to transitory ego rupture (panic, oneiric episodes), to retreat with phantasies (psychoses), to complete disintegration (suicide).

**ego subject** When the ego is the object of its own instincts (ego instincts), the ego is called the ego subject. "Originally, at the very beginning of mental life, the ego's instincts are directed to itself and it is to some extent capable of deriving satisfaction from them on itself. This condition is known as narcissism and this potentiality for satisfaction is termed autoerotic. The outside world is at this time, generally speaking, not cathected with any interest and is indifferent for purposes of satisfaction. At this period, therefore, the ego-subject coincides with what is pleasurable and the outside world with what is indifferent (or

even painful as being a source of stimulation)" (Freud, S. *Collected Papers*, 1924–25).

**ego suffering** Guilt feelings or any of their substitute expressions such as attempts at atonement, punishment, or remorse. See *guilt*. While present in many psychiatric syndromes, including the character disorders, ego suffering is most evident in depressive states.

**ego weakness** Ego defect; ego deficit; it includes deficiencies in *anxiety tolerance*, *impulse control*, and *sublimation*. See *ego; ego strength*.

**ego-alien** *Ego-dystonic* (q.v.).

**egocentrism** 1. A lack of full differentiation between self and object. According to Piaget, each developmental move to a higher level of cognitive organization has characteristic forms of egocentrism. In the earliest sensorimotor period, egocentrism is manifested in a literal inability to differentiate between self and object and, correspondingly, in lack of object permanence. In the preoperational subperiod, attempts to engage in symbolic thinking are at first limited by a failure to differentiate between the symbol and its referent. In the period of concrete operations, probability is not appreciated and there is inadequate differentiation between mental constructions of the self and facts. At adolescence, hypothetic-deductive reasoning is initially limited by the unrealistic belief that others are as preoccupied with the adolescent as he himself is. See *hypothetical-deductive thinking*.

2. Term proposed by Healy, Bronner, and Bowers (*The Structure and Meaning of Psychoanalysis*, 1930) as clearer and less confusing than *egoism* (q.v.).

**ego-dystonic** Anything that is unacceptable to the ego. Stimuli from any source that are rejected by the ego or that are prevented from reaching the ego for its consideration are called ego-dystonic. Its opposite is *egosyntonic* (q.v.).

**ego-dystonic homosexuality** A seldom-used term, listed for a short time in the official American Psychiatric Association nomenclature but deleted in 1987 because there was no evidence of its scientific validity. The term was applied to a sustained pattern of overt homosexual arousal in a person who explicitly complains that such responses are unwanted and a source of distress. Further, such a person desires to acquire or increase heterosexual responsivity so that heterosexual relations can be intitiated or maintained. If there are persons who fit such a description they must be few, since a 5-year literature search (1981–1986) uncovered only 13 references to the term. Any such case would be classified as sexual disorder not otherwise specified.

**ego-ideal**   That part of the ego devoted to the development of parental substitutes (parental imagos) and in which the parental imagos are laid down. "Identifications take place with these later editions of the parents as well, and regularly provide important contributions to the formation of character; but these only affect the ego, they have no influence on the super-ego, which has been determined by the earliest parental imagos" (Freud, S. *New Introductory Lectures on Psycho-Analysis*, 1933). See *father-ideal*.

The ego-ideal may change from time to time as newer identifications are made. When the person's own narcissism is threatened, it is usually withdrawn from the ego-ideal of later development and regresses to what is called the narcissistic ego-ideal, namely, the mental image of perfection that the child constructs of himself. See *ego; superego*.

**egoism**   Selfishness; the condition of evaluating things in terms of oneself and of one's personal interests. When the self-centeredness is heavily laden with a sense of self-importance, it is called *egotism*.

**egoity**   Egohood; personality; individuality.

**egology**   A term devised by S. Rado to mean study of the ego, the "I."

**egomania**   Exaggerated self-centeredness.

**egomorphism**   Attribution of one's own needs, desires, motives, etc., to someone else; the tendency to build a system of thought and interpret the reactions of others in terms of one's own ego needs—*projection* (q.v.). It has been suggested that the interpretations a psychiatrist makes to a patient are based on the egomorphism of the physician. This is one factor that has led psychoanalytic training institutes to require their students to undergo psychoanalysis. See *training analysis*.

**egopathy**   Hostile behavior due to a psychopathically exaggerated sense of self-importance. Egopathic patients are characterized by a strong egocentric trend that compels them to deprecate others in their constant aggressive and unconceding attitude.

**ego-syntonic**   Referring to the acceptability of ideas or impulses to the ego, which receives the impulses as consonant and compatible with its principles. Its opposite is *ego-dystonic* (q.v.).

**egotheism**   Self-deification.

**egotism**   See *egoism*.

**egotistic suicide**   See *anomie*.

**egotropy**   Adolf Meyer's term for egocentricity or *narcissism* (q.v.).

**egregorsis**   Egersis; intense wakefulness.

**EHR**   Electronic health-record system.

**EIA**   *ELISA* (q.v.).

**EID**   Emotional intensity disorder; *borderline personality disorder* (q.v.). See *STEPPS*.

**eidetic**   Pertaining to or characterized by clear visualization (even by a voluntary act) of objects previously seen. Eidetic images (also known as primary memory images) are clearer and richer in detail than the usual memory images and are also more intense and of better quality. Except that the subject recognizes the eidetic image as a memory experience, the phenomenon is analogous to a hallucination. Visual eidetic imagery is more common than auditory. Such imagery is rare in adults. See *eidetic imagery*.

**eidetic imagery**   Generally, a psychological phenomenon intermediate between the ordinary visual memory image and the afterimage. E. R. Jaensch observed that eidetic imagery occurs in 60% of children under 12, but that it persists after adolescence only in two constitutional types, the *Basedow* type and the *tetany* type, or, as they are usually called, the B type and the T type.

The eidetic image differs from the ordinary memory image by the following details: (1) it possesses a pseudo-perceptual quality; (2) it is superior in clearness and richness of detail, and this clearness is less dependent upon the organization of its content; (3) it is more accurate (mimetic) in its reproduction of detail; (4) it is more brilliant in coloration; and (5) it requires more rigid fixation of the eye for its arousal. It differs from the afterimage by the following characteristics: (1) it may be aroused by a more complicated and detailed object; (2) it is superior in clearness and continues longer in the visual field; (3) it is subject to voluntary recall, even after the lapse of considerable time, as well as to voluntary control; (4) it requires a shorter length of exposure and less rigid fixation for its arousal; and (5) it is more dependent upon factors of interest.

The B type is nearer to the memory image and has been observed only in persons with Basedow disease or the tendency to it. The T type, in which the imagery approaches the afterimage, has been found in subjects whose blood calcium and potassium show either definite evidence of tetany or changes in the direction of it.

**eidetic personification**   In Sullivan's terminology, any holdover or representation of previous experiences that influences current behavior.

**eidetic type**   Constitutional type characterized by a particular kind of *eidetic imagery* (q.v.) and by associated differences in other psychological qualities as well as in certain physiological, biochemical, and clinical features. There are two eidetic types, the *integrated* and the *disintegrated*.

**Eigengrau**   *Phosphene* (q.v.).

**eight stages of man**   See *ontogeny, psychic*.

**Einfuehlung**   *Empathy* (q.v.).

**Einheitpsychose**   Unitary psychosis, a concept held by Griesinger (and others) that all psychiatric symptoms are manifestations of a single psychosis and that it is impossible to separate them or classify them into specific entities.

**eisoptrophobia**   Fear of mirrors.

**ejaculatio deficiens**   *Obs.* Absence or diminution of ejaculation; ejaculatory impotence. See *impotence*.

**ejaculatio praecox**   The ejaculation of semen and seminal fluid during the act of preparation for sexual intercourse, i.e., before there is penetration; classified as an orgasm disorder within the group of *sexual dysfunctions* (q.v.).

Psychoanalysis views ejaculatio praecox (premature ejaculation) as usually based on a feminine orientation or a sadistic desire to soil the woman or intense urethral eroticism. Typically, such patients have marked masturbatory guilt. The sexual partner is identified with the mother, and the patient aims to have his genitals touched by the woman and then to ejaculate as though he were passing urine. This is in part determined by infantile narcissism, in that the penis and urinary activities are thought to exercise an irresistible charm over the woman. The praecox patient can only receive love, and his exhibitionism is a hostile attitude of contempt for the woman. In ejaculatio praecox there is a defiant relapse into the infantile uncontrolled emptying

of the bladder; in this way, the person takes revenge on every woman for the disappointments in love he suffered as a child at the hands of his mother.

**ejaculatio retardata**   Unduly delayed ejaculation during sexual intercourse; a type of *sexual dysfunction* (q.v.) that is often based on narcissistic and sadomasochistic object relations.

**ejaculation**   Sudden expulsion of semen from the penis. How often a man ejaculates (by any means, including masturbation, intercourse, and nocturnal emission) reflects his rate of sperm production. From early puberty to the age of about 30 years, on average, a healthy male produces around 300 million sperm a day and ejaculates three to four times a week. By the age of 50 years, the numbers are about 175 million sperm a day and two ejaculations a week; by the age of 75 to 90 years, about 20 million a day and less than once a month.

When he masturbates, a man expels about 5 million *sperm* (q.v.) for every hour since he last ejaculated. Most sperm are killers when they are young and blockers when they are old. Masturbation between acts of intercourse usually results in an ejaculate with fewer sperm, but they are younger, more active, and mixed with fewer older sperm than would be the case had there been no masturbation (Baker, R. *Sperm Wars*). New York: Basic Books, 1996).

**ejaculatory impotence**   See *impotence*.

**Ekbom syndrome**   1. Restless legs syndrome, consisting of irregular, intermittent paresthesiae of the legs and a need to move the legs for relief. When it occurs spontaneously it is often associated with low serum iron. Akathisia as a side effect of neuroleptic administration is similar and may also be associated with iron deficiency. Even though not anemic, such patients have low serum iron and percentage saturation, and high total iron-binding capacity. Further, the lower the serum iron, the more severe the akathisia.

2. Dermatozoic delusions. See *dermatozoic; Morgellons disease; parasitophobia; restless legs syndrome*.

**elaboration, secondary**   One of the four mechanisms of dream-making, which are (1) condensation, (2) displacement, (3) dramatization, and (4) secondary elaboration. The psychic material from which the dream is derived is transformed by these four mechanisms into the picture of the dream as it appears to the dreamer.

**élan vital** Bergson's term for the creative life-force or life-impulse, the basis of evolutionary progress.

**elation** An affect consisting of feelings of euphoria, triumph, intense self-satisfaction, optimism, etc.; an elated, though unstable, mood is characteristic of *mania* (q.v.).

**elbow jerk** See *triceps reflex.*

**elective mutism** See *mutism, elective.*

**Electra complex** *Obs.* The female Oedipus complex. Electra, the daughter of Agamemnon, induced her brother Orestes to wreak vengeance on their mother, Clytemnestra, and her new husband, Agamemnon's brother, for having together murdered Agamemnon. The dark broodings over the fate of her beloved hero-father possessed the wedlock-scorning Electra till death.

**electroconvulsive therapy** *ECT* (q.v.).

**electrocorticogram** *ECoG* (q.v.).

**electrodermal response** See *psychogalvanic reflex.*

**electroencephalogram (EEG)** The graphic record of the electrical activity of the brain, usually obtained by means of electrodes attached to the scalp. The regular, spontaneous oscillations of the electrical potential of the brain are amplified and recorded on an oscillograph. Characteristic changes in type, frequency, and potential of the brain waves occur in various intracranial lesions.

The *alpha rhythm* (q.v.), also known as the Berger wave, is the most common wave form of the adult cortex. It is found mainly in the parietooccipital area when the subject is at rest and consists of smooth, regular oscillations at a frequency of 8–13 Hz. It is usually diminished ("blocked") by sensory stimulation and mental activity.

*Beta* activity (14–30 Hz) is associated with alertness. The *delta rhythm* (1–3 Hz) is an abnormal rhythm often found when the subject is in light sleep. The *theta rhythm* (4–7 Hz) occurs most frequently in the temporal region. Other rhythms are the *fast* (80–200 Hz) and the *ultrafast* (200–600 Hz).

Various techniques are used to accentuate abnormal waves or to bring out latent abnormalities, among them overventilation, natural or drug-induced sleep, *photic driving* (rhythmic optic stimulation with a stroboscope), chemical stimulation (especially with

Metrazol, and often combined with photic driving), and hydration induced by Pitressin, alcohol, hypoglycemia, or oxygen lack. Such *activated* EEGs, however, often give false positives and are therefore even more difficult to interpret than the standard record. See *neurometrics.*

**electroencephalograph** The apparatus used in making a graphic record of the electrical activity of the brain.

**electroencephalography** The process of recording the electrical activity of the brain; the recording itself is the electroencephalogram (EEG). Electrodes are applied to the scalp (or directly to the brain), and eight or more matched channels simultaneously record the amplified brain potentials on graph paper as it passes beneath galvanometer pens. Usually the EEG is recorded under conditions of nonattentive wakefulness, overbreathing, and natural sleep. Deviations from normal or usual brain wave patterns (*dysrhythmias*) may be correlated with underlying disease such as epilepsy, cerebrovascular abnormalities, neoplasm, and infection. See *evoked potential; tomography.*

**electronarcosis** Electric narcosis; "subconvulsive" electroshock therapy consisting of an initial tonic phase similar to that of conventional ECT and a clonic phase whose development is limited or prevented by continued electrical stimulation (usually for a period of 7 minutes). Most clinical reports indicate that electronarcosis is less effective and produces more undesirable side effects than conventional ECT. See *electroconvulsive therapy.*

**electronic media** See *media.*

**electro-oculograph (EOG)** See *polysomnogram.*

**electrophobia** Fear of electricity.

**electrophysiological battery** See *Quantitative Electrophysiological Battery.*

**electroplexy** *Electroconvulsive therapy* (q.v.).

**electrosleep** Electrical transcranial stimulation (ETS) developed in Russia in the 1940s and reported to be effective in the treatment of chronic anxiety, depression, and insomnia. A relaxed state is induced by means of transcranial application of a low-intensity electric current.

**electrostimulation** Electric shock, usually of painful intensity, used as a technique of negative conditioning in *aversion therapy* (q.v.).

**elemental anxiety** See *panic, primordial.*

**elementary process** D. Nachmansohn's theory of neural excitation and transmission:

excitation of the neural membrane results in a dissociation of bound acetylcholine into an active form (the ester); free acetylcholine acts on a protein receptor and thereby increases the permeability of nerve membrane to ions. Thus, bioelectric potential is generated and acts as a stimulus to adjoining nerve segments or to the synapse, resulting in propagation and transmission of the impulse. Meanwhile, the free ester of acetylcholine undergoes hydrolysis by the enzyme cholinesterase, and the protein receptor returns to its resting condition. The barrier to ionic movement is thus reestablished. See *action potential.*

**elfin-face syndrome** *Williams-Beuren syndrome* (q.v.).

**Elgin checklist** A list of behavioral activities that occur frequently in a psychotic population but rarely in a normal one.

**elimination disorders** Functional *enuresis* and functional *encopresis* (qq.v.).

**elimination rate (of alcohol)** See *BAL.*

**ELISA** *EIA*; enzyme-linked immunosorbant assay, used to screen blood for HIV antibodies. See *AIDS.*

**ellipsis** Omission of one or more words or ideas, leaving the whole to be understood or completed by the reader or listener. Ellipsis is frequent in dreams, symptom formation, and other types of primary process thinking. Much of the effort in psychoanalytic treatment is directed toward uncovering the omitted ideas as a way of understanding the symptoms. See *discourse skills; primary process.*

**Ellis, Henry Havelock** (1859–1939) British sexologist.

**elongation, transcript** See *transcription.*

**elopement** In psychiatry, escape; absenting oneself from a mental hospital without permission.

**ELSI Program** The Program on the Ethic, Legal, and Social Implications of human genome research, established as a branch of the National Center for Human Genome Research at the National Institutes of Health (United States). The program addresses the ethical questions raised by genetic testing, such as the following.

A woman learned through genetic testing that she carries a gene for schizophrenia. Who will counsel her? If she consults a physician about the advisability of childbearing, will her insurance carrier or her employer find out? Could she be dismissed from her position because of the risk she carries? Or does she enjoy protection from job discrimination under the Americans with Disabilities Act? If she becomes pregnant, is it possible to determine if the fetus has inherited the gene? What preventive strategies can be devised if she does have children?

**emanative** Indirect but often powerful effects of psychopharmacologic agents on self-concept and social interactions.

**emancipated** Free, independent. In legal language, emancipation is the legal process by which minors are released from the custody, control, and authority of their parents. An *emancipated minor* is a person below the age of majority who exercises general control over his or her life and as a result is able to claim the legal rights of an adult.

**emancipation** 1. Legal aknowledgement by the state of a person's capability by the granting of autonomous rights; the legal process by which minors are released from the custody, control, and authority of their parents. Typically, emancipation is considered in terms of the *competence* of the minor involved.

2. In psychoanalysis, detachment of instinctual qualities with particular reference to the Oedipus complex as it reappears at puberty. Oedipal strivings are dormant during the latency period, but at puberty they are reanimated and to them is added a current of sensuality. The child is obliged to relive the earlier complex, following which in normal instinctual growth he frees himself from the libidinal attachment to the parents and from dependence upon parental authority. The emancipation leads to heterosexual object-choice.

**emancipation disorder** A disorder of late adolescence or early adulthood characterized by symptomatic suggestions of a conflict over independence in situations where the subject has moved to what he considers a position of desirable freedom from parental control. The symptomatic suggestions include indecisiveness, paradoxical overdependence on the advice of the parents he wants to break away from, excessive dependence on peers, homesickness that contradicts the desire to be free, etc.

**emasculation** Castration; physical eviration; eunuchism.

**EMB theory** *Extreme male brain theory* of autism (q.v.).

**embarrassment psychosis** *Sensitiver Beziehungswahn* (q.v.).

**embitterment, chronic** One of the "states of mind" characteristic of narcissistic personality disorder consisting of an internal dialogue in which other people or "the fates" are unfairly abusing the self. Two forms have been described: blustery-outgoing, and sullen-withdrawing (Horowitz, W. *Psychiatric Clinics of North America*, 1989). The dialogue has also been referred to as *self-talk*. See *narcissistic personality*.

**emboliform nuclei** See *cerebellum*.

**embolism, cerebral** Brain obstruction; emboli (i.e., plugs or stoppers, usually detached clots) arising from the pulmonary circulation, from thrombosis of the arteries of the neck and head, or from vegetations on the heart valves, may interfere with cerebral circulation, causing cerebral softening and neurological or psychotic symptoms. Stupor or coma may be present with focal signs of hemiplegia or paralysis. Irritability and anger, dulling of general intelligence, and memory defects may occasionally be observed. See *cerebrovascular accident; multi-infarct dementia*.

**embololalia, embolalia** A type of speech disorder, frequently associated with stuttering, in which the patient interpolates short sounds or words that are out of place in the structure of the sentence.

**embolophrasia** *Obs.* "A melancholic subject in my clinique became quite oppressive, because he interlarded his speech with 'really, now.' 'Really now, you cannot understand, really now, how much I suffer, really now....' This dysphrasic disorder goes under the name of *embolophrasia*" (Bianchi, L. *A Textbook of Psychiatry*, 1906).

**embrujo** See *curanderismo*.

**embryogenesis** The shaping of an embryo, which depends not only on specific patterns of gene expression, but also on the physical forces acting on the epithelial sheet, including the tugging, bending, folding, and sculpting of tissues.

**embryonic disc** At about 3 weeks after fertilization, the embryonic disk is evident, with three layers of cells which are the basis for three main groups of tissues in the body. The future *ectoderm* differentiates into the ectoderm proper and the *neural plate*, which thickens and dips to form the *neural groove*. It grows deeper, curves around to close at the top thereby forming the *neural tube*. While the neural tube is forming, two strips of cells are pinched from the edges of the neural folds. Known as *neural crest cells*, they will form part of the ANS (autonomic nervous system).

**emergence** *Epigenesis* (q.v.); the theory that mind or consciousness arises from living matter that has reached a certain state of complexity; the term emergence is used to indicate that such an end result is not predictable from a consideration or knowledge of its constituent parts. Emergence is antireductionistic and emphasizes that although the different parts are essential, the final whole that is constructed from them is qualitatively much more than a mere summation of the individual components. See *general systems theory*.

**emergency** An unforeseen set of circumstances in which a catastrophic outcome is thought to be imminent unless immediate action is taken.

**emergency emotions** *Fight-flight responses* (q.v.). See *adaptational psychodynamics*.

**emetophobia** Morbid dread of vomiting. See *anorexia nervosa*.

**emic** Referring to socially unique, intracultural phenomena, such as amok, koro, and lata. See *culture-specific syndromes; etic*.

**emission tomography** A category of neuroimaging that includes *PET* and *SPECT* (qq.v.).

**emotion** Feeling; mood; *affect* (q.v.). In current usage, emotion and affect are used interchangeably, although some use *emotion* to refer primarily to the consciously perceived feelings and their objective manifestations, and *affect* to include also the drive energies that are presumed to generate both conscious and unconscious feelings.

Developmental psychobiology views emotions as behavioral adaptations that have occurred during evolutionary development as attempts to achieve control over survival-related problems, such as predators, food, reproduction, and communication. They are genetically programmed responses that have been maintained because they have increased the chances of the organism's survival. Emotions consist of complex psychological and physiological states that, among other things, reflect the organism's *value*—the organism's ability to sense whether events in its environment are desirable. *Feelings* are mental representations of physiological changes that characterize and are consequent upon processing emotion-eliciting objects or states. Feeling states do more than to add subjective coloring to an experience; they also influence such functions as decision making and interpersonal interactions. There is accumulating evidence that emotion and feeling are mediated by distinct neuronal systems.

The amygdala, a critical structure in emotional perception, contributes to perceptual value judgments, such as making trustworthy decisions in relation to the facial appearance of others. The ventromedial prefrontal cortex provides access to feeling states associated with past decisions as the organism contemplates a decision of similar nature in the present. Better predictive judgments are mediated by means of enhanced awareness of bodily states of arousal. Damage to the ventromedial prefrontal cortex may have no consequence for intellectual function, but it leads to patients making personally disadvantageous decisions. See *moral emotions*.

For Adler, emotions do not determine goals and hence are never the cause of undesirable or antisocial behavior; rather, goals are set in accord with cognitive processes (even though the subject may not be consciously aware of these). Emotions are generated secondarily to suit those goals, and to permit and support what the subject intends to do. "People are not emotionally disturbed; they are deficient in their social movement, in their goals, in their form of social integration, because they have wrong concepts about themselves" (Dreikurs, R. in *Contemporary Psychotherapies*, ed. M. Stein, 1961).

"The usual way of thinking about the emotional experiences and their facial or other bodily manifestations is that the emotional experience is excited by the perception of some object, and that the emotional feeling then expresses itself in the bodily manifestations in question" (*Encyclopaedia Britannica*, 14th ed.). See *Cannon hypothalamic theory of emotion; ergotropic; Papez's theory of emotion*.

The James-Lange Theory of Emotions states that the so-called expressions or bodily changes are the direct results of the perception of the exciting object, and that the emotion is just the feeling of these bodily changes as they occur.

**emotion, Papez's theory**  See *Papez's theory of emotion*.

**emotional aggression**  Belligerent and contemptuous behavior toward the partner, characteristic of men involved in *domestic violence* (q.v.), rather than less verbally hostile forms of aggression or disagreement (e.g., criticism, disagreement, or defensiveness). See *aggression; battering; domestic violence*.

**emotional body language**  See *amygdala*.

**emotional deprivation**  Inadequate or inappropriate interpersonal and environmental relationships, especially in the early years of development; isolation of an infant from its mother to the degree that identification with the maternal figure is not made, with the result that personality development is impaired. The validity of the general proposition regarding the adverse effects of emotional deprivation has been established by two sets of observations—studies of children who were reared in institutional settings and whose difficulties reflected early distortions in personality development; and studies of infants' reactions to separation from their mothers. See *anaclitic depression; developmental disorders; object relations theory; empathic failure; victim*.

**emotional divorce**  See *divorce, stations of; family therapy*.

**emotional intensity disorder**  EID; *borderline personality disorder* (q.v.). See *STEPPS*.

**emotional memory**  Representation of a positive or negative affect associated with specific stimuli, typically reflected in autonomic nervous system activation, attraction, or avoidance rather than in conscious recollection.

**emotional release therapies**  See *experiential therapy*.

**emotionality, pathological**  A variety of emotional responses characterizing one type of *psychopathic personality* (q.v.), which are usually held under control in the presence of superior strength or police force. The most common pathological emotion is pugnacity. A person afflicted with this type of malady is uncivil and bullying, and scorns the rights of others. Pathological emotionality is also shown by inordinate bragging, by the person's acting the part of a beggar in order to gain money or favors, or by his or her enacting sadness for purposes of attention. In all these instances there is a certain slyness or cunning.

**emotionally handicapped**  See *handicap, emotional*.

**emotionally unstable personality**  A *personality trait disturbance* (q.v.) characterized by excitabiliity, ineffectiveness, and poor judgment when under even minor stress; poorly controlled hostility, guilt, and anxiety; formerly called psychopathic personality with emotional instability. Some workers consider *EUCD* (emotionally unstable character disorder) to be a mood dysregulation and have reported successful results with long-term lithium treatment. Arthur Rifkin et al. (*Archives of General Psychiatry 27*, 1972) define EUCD as a disorder with chronic maladaptive behavior patterns characterized by short mood swings, both depressive and hypomanic. In their experience, most patients are adolescent girls, with difficulties in accepting reasonable authority and in being appropriately self-reliant. They are often overactive, abuse drugs, avoid schoolwork, malinger, and may be sexually promiscuous.

**emotions, Cannon-Bard theory**   See *Cannon hypothalamic theory of emotion.*

**empacho**   See *curanderismo.*

**empathema**   *Obs.* Ungovernable passion.

**empathic**   In Burrow's phylobiology the organism's primary feeling-motivation and response. Contrasted with affects or projective feeling. See *empathy.*

**empathic failure**   Inability to understand another's subjective experience, most often used to refer to parental or maternal failure to respond appropriately to the child's emotional needs. Empathic failure is allied to defective *mirroring* (Kohut), *mutual cueing* (Mahler), *communicative matching*, or interpersonal attunement in the mother–child relationship; to inadequacy of the *container-contained maternal function* (Bion); to lack of parent–child goodness of *fit* (q.v.); and to inability to react selectively to the child's grandiose-exhibitionistic (mirroring) and idealizing (merger) needs. See *empathy.*

Self psychology avers that repeated empathic failures by the parents, coupled with the child's responses to them, are the basis of almost all psychopathology. Mahler observed that failure of the mother to support empathically her child's contrasting strivings for autonomy and fusion may lead to a collapse of the child's omnipotence. Modell notes that the mother's empathic failure at the time when the child is developing a sense of self propels him into a precocious and vulnerable sense of autonomy. Similarly, Masterson and Rinsley described a type of empathic

failure characteristic of mothers of borderlines: the mother depersonifies her child by giving him the message that any attempt to separate or individuate will provoke a withdrawal of maternal nurturance. This produces a lifelong *failure script*, and any movement toward succeeding provokes severe separation anxiety (*abandonment depression*, q.v.). In the narcissistic personality, depersonification by the mother demands that the child achieve, but only in relation to her. The result is *adultomorphization* (q.v.) or a pseudomature child, who needs approbative mirroring to an excessive degree in order to maintain his fragile sense of inner cohesiveness (D. B. Rinsley, *Developmental Pathogenesis and Treatment of Borderline and Narcissistic Personalities*, 1989).

**empathize**   To diagnose; to recognize and identify the feelings, emotions, passions, sufferings, torments through observing their symptoms is to *realize intellectually, to understand* them, in a remote way to identify oneself with the patient, without ever having personally experienced those feelings.

On the other hand, to place oneself in the position of the patient, to get into his skin, so to speak, to be able to duplicate, live through, *experience* those feelings in a vicarious way, is closely to identify oneself with another, to *share his feelings with him*, to sympathize, from the Greek *syn*, together with *pathos*, suffering, passion. See *sympathy.*

**empathy**   *Vicarious introspection* (Kohut); *Einfuehlung* (Freud); *intersubjective resonance*; a form of cognition that enables one to comprehend another person's subjective experiences from his own unique perspective, understanding not only the feelings that motivate his actions but also the conflicts and compromise formations that constitute the totality of his self-experience. See *theory of mind.*

Empathy is not compassion, but affect attunement is the first step in the empathic process of understanding and accepting the subjective validity of the other person's point of view. Freud's writings contain only two sentences on empathy, both in *Group Psychology and the Analysis of the Ego* (1921), and one of them is a footnote. He suggested that identification, by way of imitation, leads to empathy, "the mechanism which enables us to take up any attitude at all towards another's mental life" and "plays the largest part in our understanding of what is inherently foreign to our ego in other people."

In psychotherapy, empathy is, in addition, a mode of inquiry that allows the therapist to understand the patient's reported experiences. As Thomas Ogden (*The Primitive Edge of Experience*, 1989) points out, it is the analyst's own emotionally colored perceptions that lead to an understanding of the patient. Since most of these are unconscious, the analyst must learn to make use of his or her own shifting unconscious state in order to understand the patient's subjective experiences. The patient is not confronted with what would be considered defensive behavior or resistance from the traditional psychodynamic perspective; instead, the therapist remains in tune with the patient's subjective experience, which is accepted as legitimate and adaptive.

Lack of empathy is described as a characteristic trait of narcissistic personality in DSM-III-R. Despite its frequency in such patients, clinical studies have not found it to be a good discriminant, since it occurs also in many other types of psychopathology. Parents who are unable to empathize adequately with their children set the scene for various types of psychopathology in those children. See *empathic failure*.

**empirical** Depending or based on experience and observation rather than on hypothesis, intuition, or theory. An empirical problem is one that can be solved by the collection and analysis of appropriate data through the use of relevant statistical techniques.

**empirical self** See *self*.

**empiricism** A school of philosophic thought that claims that the only source of knowledge is observable fact or objective experience. Watson's behaviorism is a form of empirical psychology. See *rationalism*.

**employee assistance program** *EAP*; an occupational-industrial program originally designed to detect possible alcoholism on the basis of the subject's work performance and to refer the subject for appropriate consultation and treatment. The program was designed to keep the worker on the job; objective performance criteria were set as a way of promoting compliance with treatment aims and of ensuring that dismissal from the job or other sanctions would not be based on moralistic judgments about alcoholism. The counselor or therapist in the program was often a recovering alcoholic, and a mutual-help "twelve-step" approach (similar to that used in AA) was typical.

From its initial focus on alcohol-related problems, the EAP concept expanded to include other drugs, and then to include other problems in living that might affect job performance adversely—psychiatric illness, family crises, legal entanglements, career and retirement planning, etc. With the broadening of focus there came a need for additional professionals with competence in areas other than alcoholism and substance abuse, and with that arose the need for better-defined levels of professional competencies in those who were dealing with the troubled employee through the EAP mechanism. In consequence, EAPs nowadays are likely to be staffed by persons trained as traditional mental health workers (e.g., clinical psychologists, psychiatric social workers, certified counselors), and the number of staff whose only training is the experience of having themselves experienced alcoholism or other chemical dependency is diminishing.

**empowerment** See *recovery model*.

**empresiomania** *Obs.* Pyromania (q.v.).

**emprosthotonos** A forward bending of the body. It is the opposite of opisthotonos. See *arc de cercle; camptocormia*.

**empty speech** Speech without meaning, as in *Wernicke aphasia* (q.v.).

**emptying reflex** See *gastrocolic reflex*.

**EMR** Educable mentally retarded.

**EMS** *Eosinophilia-myalgia syndrome* (q.v.).

**emulation** Conscious, willful copying or imitating of another. Emulation is to be differentiated from *identification* (q.v.), which is an unconscious process.

**enabler** 1. A mental health paraprofessional, indigenous to the community, who assists the mental patient in adjusting to life within his community. The enabler may take a patient into his home, or may help the patient to manage his own apartment and routine of living. See *caregiver*.

2. Any person, organization, or institution whose actions or policies have the effect of facilitating the continuation of substance abuse or dependence (including alcoholism).

**enantiodromia** "'A running counter to.' In the philosophy of Heraclitus the concept was used to designate the play of opposites in the course of events, namely, the view which maintains that everything that exists goes over into its opposite." Jung quotes from Zeller (*History of Greek Philosophy*): "From the living comes death, and from the dead, life; from the young, old age; and from the old, youth; from waking, sleep; and from sleep, waking; the stream of creation and decay never stands still" (Jung, C. G. *Contributions to Analytical Psychology*, 1928).

**enantiomer**  Mirror-image forms of the chiral amino acids, known as *d* (dextro) and *l* (levo). Most frequently, they occur in the l form (e.g., levodopa). In similar fashion, the double helix of DNA could twist to the left or right, but it almost always takes the right turn. The two different forms of chiral chemicals often interact in different ways when administered to organisms: one form of ibuprofen is three times stronger than the other, and one thalidomide enantiomer controls morning sickness of pregnancy while the other interferes with fetal growth. Most chemical syntheses produce equal amounts of both enantiomers; it would clearly be advantageous to be able to control the amount of each enantiomer that is produced, and preliminary studies indicate that application of a magnetic field will produce an almost pure single enantiomer.

**enantiopathic**  Tending to induce an opposite passion.

**encapsulation**  Enclosure in a capsule or sheath; the process of walling off from surrounding areas, as in encapsulation of a brain abscess. Used in clinical psychiatry to refer particularly to the ability of some schizophrenic patients to keep their delusional life almost completely separated from their routine life in the real, external world. See *double orientation*.

**encephalitis**  Any inflammatory process involving the brain. Etiologic agents include the following:

1. Bacterial—syphilis, other spirochetal; tuberculosis, other mycobacteria; meningococcal.

2. Viral—poliomyelitis; cytomegalovirus; encephalitis lethargica; smallpox; chickenpox (varicella); herpesviral; measles; rubella (German measles); rabies; lymphocytic choriomeningitis; mumps; enteroviral (Coxsackie virus, echovirus); AIDS.

3. Slow virus—Creutzfeldt-Jacob disease; subacute sclerosing panencephalitis; progressive multifocal leukoencephalopathy; kuru.

4. Mosquito-borne viral encephalitis—Japanese encephalitis; Western equine encephalitis; Eastern equine encephalitis; St. Louis encephalitis; Australian encephalitis; California encephalitis.

5. Tick-borne viral encephalitis—Far Eastern encephalitis (Russian spring-summer encephalitis); louping ill.

6. Rickettsial and other arthropod-borne diseases—Rocky Mountain spotted fever; louse-borne typhus; mite-borne scrub typhus; malaria; trypanosomiasis.

7. Toxoplasmosis.

8. Mycoses—coccidioidomycosis; cryptococcosis.

9. Trichinosis, other helminthiases.

10. Encephalitis of chorea, encephalopathy of rheumatic fever.

11. Other.

**encephalitis, epidemic**  Encephalitis lethargica; von Economo encephalitis; popularly known as sleeping sickness. First described by von Economo in Vienna in 1917; by 1918 the epidemic had reached Germany and Great Britain, and by 1920 the whole world. There was another peak incidence in 1924, but if the virus that is presumed to have been the etiologic agent now exists at all, it is not known to have produced an epidemic since 1927.

The major reason for continued interest in this type of encephalitis is the discovery that it tended to persist in diverse chronic forms for many years after initial infection. Among the chronic stage syndromes are the following:

1. Parkinsonism, with rigidity of posture and movement, and subsequent appearance of tremor (in idiopathic Parkinson disease, the sequence of symptoms is the reverse);

2. Sleep disturbances, including lethargy, insomnia, narcolepsy, or inversion of the sleep pattern;

3. Disturbances of vision, including misty vision, slight inequality of pupils, some impairment of accommodation, weakness of conjugate conversion, or oculogyral spasm;

4. Involuntary movements, such as torsion spasms, tremors, and tics, many of which were commonly misinterpreted as being primarily of psychologic origin;

5. Disturbances of respiratory rate and rhythm;

6. Rarely, metabolic and endocrine disorders, probably due to hypothalamic

involvement; among these are obesity, polyuria and polydipsia, and hyperthyroidism;

7. Mental disturbances, particularly depression and, in children, behavior disorders of a restless and aggressive kind. See *attention deficit hyperactivity disorder.*

**encephalitis, purulent**   Brain abscess.

**encephalitis, traumatic**   A term suggested by Osnato and Giliberti (1927) to replace postconcussion neurosis, because of actual cerebral injury in cases of concussion. In current usage, the term traumatic encephalopathy has superseded both older terms. See *traumatic encephalopathy.*

**encephalitis periaxialis diffusa**   Schilder disease. See *diffuse sclerosis.*

**encephalization**   *Corticalization*; in higher mammals the cerebral cortex has taken over more and more the task of controlling and exerting a regulative function on bodily processes and on emotions. In the human being this process of encephalization has reached its highest degree. In humans, the cerebral cortex governs not the somatic system alone, but all systems involved in emotional expression, psychological tensions, fears, and phobias. The lower animals are regulated by the hypothalamus and other centers. In the human, the lower centers cooperate in directing the behavior but are themselves increasingly dominated by the cortex.

**encephalocele**   A neural tube defect caused by a gap in the skull, which results in herniation of the meninges and brain tissue through the cleft in the skull. It can occur in the occipital, parietal, or frontonasal regions.

**encephalogram**   An X-ray of the skull following replacement of cerebrospinal fluid by air by means of lumbar puncture.

**encephalography, radioisotopic**   See *MRI.*

**encephaloleukopathia scleroticans**   See *diffuse sclerosis.*

**encephalomalacia**   Softening of the brain.

**encephalomyelomalacia chronica diffusa**   See *diffuse sclerosis.*

**encephalopathy**   Disease of the brain.

**encephalopsychosis**   Southard's term for psychosis associated with cerebral lesions.

**encephalopyosis**   Brain abscess.

**encephalosis**   A degenerative brain process produced by infectious disease. Clinically, it is characterized by headache, irritability, apathy, stupor, and convulsions. Pathologically, there occur petechial hemorrhages, anemic infarcts,

endarteritis of small vessels, degeneration of ganglion cells, and brain hydration.

**encephalotrigeminal angiomatosis**   See *Sturge-Weber syndrome.*

**ENCODE Project (ENCyclopedia Of DNA Elements)**   A consortium of research centers with the goal of identifying all functional elements in the human genome sequence. Such a complete catalog would include protein-coding genes, non-protein-coding genes, transcriptional regulatory elements, and sequences that mediate chromosome structure and dynamics.

The pilot phase began in September 2003 with the funding of eight projects that involve the application of existing technologies to the large-scale identification of a variety of functional elements in the ENCODE targets, specifically genes, promoters, enhancers, repressors/silencers, exons, origins of replication, sites of replication termination, transcription factor binding sites, methylation sites, deoxyribonuclease I (Dnase I) hypersensitive sites, chromatin modifications, and multispecies conserved sequences of yet unknown function. Other groups have since joined the ENCODE Consortium. These include groups focused on comparative sequencing, on coordination of databases for sequence-related and other types of ENCODE data, and on studies of specific sequence elements.

**encoding**   In communications, the process of translating data (i.e., a message) into signals (a code) that can be carried by a communication channel.

In studies of memory, encoding refers to the processes that heighten or favor retrieval. It is a function of long-term potentiation (*LTP*, q.v.). Encoding may be shallow (such as no more than reading the word to be remembered) or deep (thinking of the meanings of the word and of its emotional significance), simple or elaborate. The deeper the level of encoding, and the more elaborate the encoding, the greater the success of retrieval. The *encoding specificity principle* states that the retrieval cue and the memory trace must have something in common if retrieval is to occur; that is, the retrieval cue must to some extent reinstate the original conditions of encoding. See *communication.*

**encoding, neural**   See *stimulus transduction; transducers.*

**encopresis, functional** An elimination disorder consisting of involuntary defecation not due to organic defect or illness, occurring in a child who is 4 years of age or older. The term is also applied to voluntary but inappropriate passage of stool, such as defecating into the clothes or on the floor. Encopresis may be associated with constipation, which, if severe enough, can lead to overflow incontinence.

**encounter group** *T-group* (q.v.).

**end plate, motor** That part of a nerve fiber making functional contact with the muscle spindle of an effector organ.

**end pleasure** In psychoanalysis, the culmination of the sexual act in the mature, genital stage of psychosexual development. The term emphasizes the subservience of pregenital satisfactions to adult genitality.

**endocannabinoids** *Cannabinoids* (q.v.) in the brain and other tissues. Endocannabinoids are unconventional neurotransmitters, traveling from a postsynaptic to a presynaptic neuron—the opposite direction to typical neurotransmitters. Several cannabinoid receptors have been identified; CB1 is one of the most abundant neuromodulatory receptors in the brain. It is expressed in high levels in hippocampus, cortex, cerebellum, and basal ganglia. In hippocampus, a major function of endocannabinoids is to regulate GABA release; in the cerebellum, endocannabinoids affect both GABA synapses and glutamatergic synapses.

**endocytosis** Inward budding of vesicles from the plasma membrane, as in envelopment of a neurotransmitter. Envelopment of a neurotransmitter within a synaptic vesicle of the terminal *axon* (q.v.), to be released on demand when the neuron is stimulated. See *exocytosis*.

**endogamy** Restriction of marriage to members of one's own social, religious, or cultural group.

**endogenous, endogenic, endogenetic** In psychiatry, referring to conditions that are based primarily on special hereditary-constitutional factors, thus originating predominantly *within* the organism itself and affecting the nervous system *directly*.

Schizophrenic and manic-depressive psychoses are the most characteristic types of endogenous disorders, while the so-called *symptomatic* psychoses that arise—as a secondary symptom of organic diseases in part of the body other than the nervous system—

from causes *outside* the nervous system, even though *within* the body, are classified as exogenous.

When used with depression, endogenous (or autogenic, autonomous, endogenic, or endomorphogenic) denotes a biological, somatic, or nonreactive condition (termed *melancholia* in DSM-III). See *exogeny*.

**endomorphic** Sheldon's term for the body type characterized by a predominance of its first component (circularity), that is, the physical structures developed from the *endodermal* layer of the embryo. Persons of this type are contrasted with the *mesomorphic* and *ectomorphic* (qq.v.) types and correspond roughly to Kretschmer's *pyknic type* (q.v.).

**endomusia** Silent recall of a melody; often appears as a type of obsessive thought.

**endonuclease** See *recombinant DNA*.

**endopeptidase** Proteinase. See *peptidases; protease*.

**endophenotype** A heritable quantitative trait that predicts the liability to or risk for disease with a heritable neurophysiological, biochemical, endocrinological, neuroanatomical, or neuropsychological constituent of the genetic disorder that is a more immediate result of the genetic defect than the clinical syndrome.

**endoplasmic reticulum** See *Golgi apparatus*.

**endopsychic** Characterizing something as being within the mind or psyche; those mental mechanisms that occur completely within the mind; thus, *psychic suicide* is determined by the same processes that determine physical suicide, but in the case of the former the processes work endopsychically. Endopsychic structure refers to the structure of the psyche itself: the conscious, the preconscious, and the unconscious, the ego, the superego, and the id are all parts of the endopsychic structure.

**endoreactive** Endogenous; not related to external events. An unfortunate term in that the internal events to which the patient is supposedly reacting are usually unknown to him or her, in which case use of "reactive" would seem to be inappropriate.

**endorphins** One of the three major families of endogenous opioids, the other two being the *dynorphins* and the *enkephalins* (qq.v.). Beta-endorphin is a 31-amino-acid peptide, *beta-lipotropin*, found in the pituitary. The precursor of beta-lipotropin is *pro-opiomelanocortin (POMC)*, which also gives rise to ACTH.

POMC is found in the arcuate nucleus of the hypothalamus and sends axons to many limbic and brain stem regions. In addition to modulating pain perception, the endorphins may be involved in modulating mood and response to stressful stimuli. See *peptide, brain; opioid peptides.*

**enduring**  A duration of stressful events of 6 months or more; acute stressors are those that last less than 6 months.

**enelicomorphism**  *Adultomorphism* (q.v.).

**enema addiction**  The frequent and habitual taking of enemas to gratify deep, hidden, unconscious character needs, but usually rationalized "for health." See *anal eroticism.*

**energizer**  See *psychostimulants; psychotropics.*

**energy homeostasis**  See *hypothalamus.*

**energy lack**  Fatigue, a nonspecific symptom; among psychiatric disorders, it is most frequent in alcohol or substance abuse, bereavement, depression, schizophrenia, and sleep disorders.

**enforced treatment**  See *forced treatment.*

**enfrenzy**  *Rare.* To madden, enrage; to goad into agitation or violence.

**engineering**  Manipulation of knowledge for practical uses. Genetic engineering refers to alteration of genetic information for practical uses.

**engrafted schizophrenia**  See *Pfropfschizophrenia.*

**engram**  In neurology, a neuronal pattern of an acquired skilled act; the neural representation of learning or memory; the collection of neural changes that have occurred in processing information and storing it in memory; sometimes called *memory trace.* The term has been used somewhat loosely in psychiatry to refer to the persisting psychical traces (usually in the form of an unconscious or latent memory) of any experience.

**engrossment**  The involvement of the father with his newborn; the developing bond between them is characterized by perception of the newborn as attractive or even perfect, a desire to touch and hold the baby, elation following the birth of the child, and an increased sense of self-esteem and worth within the family.

**enhancer element**  See *gene functions.*

**enhancers**  See *noncoding DNA.*

**enissophobia**  Fear of reproach.

**enkephalins**  Also, encephalins; one of the three major families of endogenous opioids, the other two being the *dynorphins* and the *endorphins* (qq.v.). The precursor of the enkephalins is *proenkephalin*, which contains several pentapeptides with opioid activity and is distributed widely in the brain from the highest cortical to the lowest spinal levels. See *peptide, brain; opioid peptides.*

**enlightenment effect**  The result of knowing a theory, as when a theory's predictions come true because the people to whom the theory applies have learned about the theory. That particular enlightenment effect is termed *self-fulfilling prophecy.*

**enmeshment**  A form of faulty family functioning consisting of overinvolvement of family members in one another's lives.

**enomania**  *Dipsomania* (q.v.).

**eNOS**  Endothelial isoenzymes of NOS. See *NO.*

**enosimania**  *Obs.* Obsessional belief that one has committed an unpardonable sin.

**enosiophobia**  *Obs.* Unwarranted fear of having committed an unpardonable sin.

**ensemble**  In neurophysiology, a *network* (q.v.) of neurons.

**enshrinement**  See *mummification.*

**entatic**  Invigorating, aphrodisiac.

**enteroptosis**  Ptotic habitus.

**entheomania**  *Obs. Demonomania.*

**enthrallment**  See *autohypnosis.*

**entitlement**  1. The rights granted to a person or group by law or regulation.

2. A characteristic disturbance of the self-concept in narcissistic *personality disorder* (q.v.) consisting of an expectation or feeling that one is due special favors without having to assume reciprocal responsibilities. Such a person expects always to get the best and to be first; he feels he has the right to extract both sadistic and exhibitionistic gratification from the other (whom he dehumanizes). Entitlement is related to another criterion for narcissistic disturbance, interpersonal exploitativeness, which is often the means by which the feelings of entitlement are gratified. See *dysfunctional attitudes.*

**entomophobia**  Fear of insects.

**entorhinal cortex**  *EC;* the main route by which the neocortex communicates with hippocampus. The EC is an anterior extension of the parahippocampal gyrus, a relay station between prefrontal cortex and hippocampus and a component of the novelty detection circuit comprising PFC, hippocampus, para-hippocampus, and cingulate. The entorhinal cortex is a multilevel buffer, holding "real sensory" information while hippocampus compares it with internal representations to detect "familiarity" versus "novelty." The entorhinal cortex is involved in processing episodic, autobiographical, and recognition memory and in associative learning. Grid cells in the medial EC form part of a spatial coordinate system for navigation; other cells encode information about head direction. See *place cells*.

**entrainment**  See *rhythms, biological*.

**entrance events**  See *life event*.

**entropy**  A measure of the unavailable energy in a thermodynamic system; a measure of the unavailable information in an information system, usually "in terms of the number of a priori equiprobable states compatible with the macroscopic description of the state—that is, it corresponds to the amount of microscopic information missing in the macroscopic description" (Goldstine, H. H. *Science 133*, 1961).

The term is used more loosely in psychoanalytic theory to refer to the affective cathexis unavailable for displacement in a psychodynamic system. Freud pointed out that as one grows older there is a "striking diminution" in the movements of "mental cathexes." Some people lose mental plasticity prematurely, whereas others retain it far beyond the usual age limit. "So that in considering the conversion of psychical energy no less than of physical, we must make use of the concept of an *entropy*, which opposes the undoing of what has already occurred." (Freud, S. *Collected Papers*, 1924–25)

**enuresis**  Involuntary passage of urine after the age by which full control of urinary excretion (bladder control) should have been attained (an elimination disorder). It may be organic in origin (e.g., neurologic or urologic disorders), or it may be functional.

Functional enuresis may be nocturnal (bedwetting), diurnal, or both. Enuresis occurs independently of normal REM dream periods and is no longer considered a dream-related disorder. It is considered primary if it is not preceded by a period of at least 1 year during which bladder control has been maintained; by definition, then, primary functional enuresis has its onset by the age of 5. Secondary

functional enuresis, which appears after bladder control has been established, usually has its onset between the ages of 5 and 8. Enuresis is about twice as common in males as in females and tends to abate with time and finally disappear. By the age of 8 years, only about 1 of every 100 males is enuretic, while the condition is almost nonexistent by that time in females.

Despite its name, that even "functional" enuresis may often be on an organic basis is suggested by the findings that approximately 75% of enuretics have a first-degree relative with a history of the disorder, and that concordance for enuresis is significantly higher in monozygotic than in dizygotic twins.

According to psychoanalysis, enuresis may represent nocturnal masturbation (Jones), exhibitionistic impulses (Abraham), or penis envy. Freud and Ferenczi noted a relationship between bedwetting and fire-setting and considered enuresis as a urethral-erotic trait. Subsequent studies have failed to confirm the relationship they reported.

**environment**  Milieu; everything surrounding a person; the aggregate of external elements that stimulate and influence an organism, including physical, biological, social, and cultural factors.

In quantitative genetics, environmental refers to all nonheritable factors, including nontransmissible DNA somatic mutations, unstable DNA sequences, and imprinting.

**environment, neutral**  A physical and social environment that imposes no specific or rigid limitations or demands upon the patient. "Psychological determinants for what appear to be the same maladjustments may be quite different, and because of that, they require different situations. Since a therapy group supplies a neutral environment, each member can take from it whatever his needs may be. The aggressive child finds relief from his anxiety…while the shy and withdrawn one overcomes his fears" (Slavson, S. R. *An Introduction to Group Therapy*, 1943).

**environmentalism**  The view that attributes all that we are to nurture (typified by the "schizophrenogenic mother" concept). After the 1950s, it gave way to *determinism* (genes determine behavior), and, most recently, to *probabilism* (a view that considers both nature and nurture, positing that genes determine the likelihood of behaviors).

**envy**  A desire to possess what belongs to another, usually with resentment of the other's advantage or endowment. Inordinate envy, both conscious and unconscious, is one of the pathological features of object relations in the narcissistic personality (but not a highly discriminating feature). Devaluation of others is often a defense against envy. The phantasied ideal self compensates for feelings of frustration, rage, and envy, while the unacceptable image of the self is dissociated and projected onto others. Primary envy is a manifestation of the *death drive* (q.v.), according to Melanie Klein. See *identification; primary envy.*

**enzygotic**  Of the same egg; usually the term refers to identical (homozygotic) twins.

**enzyme**  A cell protein that catalyzes a substance within the cell, the enzyme's *substrate,* without itself being altered or destroyed. Typically, the enzyme is specific for the substrate upon which it acts. See *chromosome.*

**enzyme induction**  Increase in liver enzyme activity caused by a drug, resulting in more rapid metabolism and elimination (and, consequently, lower blood levels) of the drug than would otherwise be expected.

**EOG**  Electro-oculograph. See *polysomnogram; sleep.*

**eonism**  *Cross-dressing* (q.v.). Named after the Chevalier d'Eon (1728–1810), a transvestite who was a French diplomat to the court of Catherine the Great and was subsequently exiled to England.

**EOS**  Early-onset schizophrenia, usually defined as onset before the age of 18 years. *VEOS,* very early onset schizophrenia, begins before the age of 13 years; this is termed *COS* (childhood onset schizophrenia) by some writers. The earliest reported cases had onset at 3 and 5.7 years. EOS and VEOS occur twice as frequently in boys as in girls, usually with an insidious onset. See *schizophrenia.*

**eosinophilia-myalgia syndrome**  *EMS*; an eosinophil count greater than 1000 cells/mm³ and generalized myalgias in the absence of infection or neoplasm. The syndrome has occurred in patients taking L-*tryptophan* and may be fatal (in 15 of 1321 cases in one survey). Frequently accompanying the eosinophilia and myalgia are muscle weakness, mouth ulcers, abdominal pain, dyspnea, and various rashes or alopecia. The condition is believed to be due to a contaminant or alteration in a subset of tryptophan manufactured by a single company, rather than to tryptophan itself.

**eosophobia**  Fear of dawn.

**EP**  Evoked potential. See *neurometrics.*

**EPA**  Eicosapentaenoic acid; see *omega-3 fatty acids.*

**ependymal cells**  *Glia* (q.v.) that line the ventricles and the spinal canal. They are covered with fingerlike microvilli and allow certain molecules from the brain to pass into the CSF. See *neuroglia.*

**ependymoma**  See *glioma; intracranial tumor.*

**ephebiatrics**  The branch of medicine that treats the development and pathology of adolescence; the specialty of diseases of adolescents.

**ephebophilia**  A *paraphilia* (q.v.) in which sexual arousal and orgasm are dependent upon the partner being an adolescent. See *pedophilia.*

**ephedra**  A plant extract also known as *ma huang.* Its active component is *ephedrine,* a mixed sympathomimetic agent that enhances the release of norepinephrine from sympathetic neurons and stimulates alpha- and beta-adrenergic receptors. At lower doses, it improves mood and heightens alertness; at higher doses, it causes anxiety, restlessness, and insomnia. Prolonged use leads to neurotoxicity with depletion of brain monoamines and may induce psychosis, severe depression, mania or agitation, hallucinations, sleep disturbance, and suicidal ideation.

**ephemeral mania**  See *mania transitoria.*

**ephialtes**  *Obs.* Nightmare.

**EPI**  1. *Echo-planar MRI* (q.v.).
 2. Eysenck Personality Inventory.
 3. Extrapyramidal involvement, referring to drug-induced symptoms (the more usual term for this is EPS).

**epicritic sensibility**  The ability to appreciate light touch and its localization; point discrimination; discrimination of moderate variations; distinguished from protopathic.

**epidemic chorea**  The convulsive dances of the Middle Ages that spread among the population like an epidemic. See *choreomania.*

**epidemiology**  The study of health and illness in human populations, and in particular the variations in the distribution of specific disorders in populations and the factors that influence that distribution. *Descriptive epidemiology* examines the patterns of occurrence of diseases and other health-related outcomes in populations according to sociodemographic characteristics, such as age, gender, race, social class, geographic area, and time. *Analytic epidemiology* examines the relationships between *risk factors*, or antecedent exposures, and health outcomes. Epidemiologic studies not only identify independent risk or protective factors but also quantify the strength of their relative contribution to the risk of disorder.

The findings of such studies are usually expressed in terms of (1) *incidence*: the number of new cases that appear during a specified time period, such as the number of first admissions to mental hospitals during 1 year; and (2) *prevalence*: the number of cases of any mental disorder that exist currently within the population. *Point prevalence* is the number of cases that exist at a specific point in time, such as the number of schizophrenics in a population on January 1, 1990; *period prevalence* is the number of cases that exist within a defined period of time, such as a month or a year; *lifetime prevalence* is the number of persons who have had a mental disorder in their lifetimes.

Knowledge of the magnitude of a disorder (i.e., its prevalence and the incidence rates) and the patterns of risk for the occurrence of a disorder may suggest ways in which that disorder can be prevented.

**epigastric aura** See *aura*.

**epigastric reflex** See *abdominal reflex*.

**epigenesis** Those genetically determined processes that give direction and stability to the organism in its development of species-specific end states. In the case of the nervous system, epigenetic processes ultimately determine the integrative power of the brain. See *emergence*.

Epigenesis also refers to any process or factors added to or interacting with the heritable genotype (i.e., to the process of gene-environment interaction during development). Epigenic rules are the neurobiological constraints imposed, for example, on cognitive processing of information, resulting in a channeling of mental development in specific directions.

**epigenetic** Four definitions of epigenetic are currently in use in the literature:

1. Referring to transmission and perpetuation of information through meiosis or mitosis that is not based on the sequence of DNA, but on changes in the regulation of gene expression or changes in the function of gene products. The changes in phenotypic gene expression persist across at least one generation. The genotype does not change, and the epigenetic manifestation is transmitted independently of the DNA sequence itself. This can occur at the level of cell division. One type of epigenetic regulation, for example, is caused by adjustments in the shape of chromatin, composed of bundles of DNA and certain fundamental proteins. By changing shape and becoming either more or less compact, chromatin can alter which genes are expressed.

2. Meiotically and mitotically heritable changes in gene expression that are not coded in the DNA sequence itself; the altered patterns of gene expression can occur through several mechanisms, based on DNA, RNA, or proteins; an example is imprinting, in which the expression status of a gene depends upon the parent from whom it is derived; one copy of a gene is transcribed normally, while the homologous copy is silenced for many cell generations;

3. The mechanisms for stable maintenance of gene expression that involve physically marking DNA or its associated proteins; this allows genotypically identical cells (such as all cells in an individual human) to be phenotypically distinct (e.g., a neuron is phenotypically distinct from a liver cell). By this definition, the regulation of chromatin structure is equivalent to epigenetics.

4. Epigenetic also describes phenomena that are a result rather than a cause of illness, such as the manifestations of gene–environment interaction during development. Such phenomena are characteristic of the illness and may even be used as diagnostic indicators.

**epigenetic mechanisms** *Chromatin remodeling*; enzymatic modification of chromatin structures that can up- or down-regulate gene expression in a manner that is transmissible to daughter cells. There is increasing evidence of an association of such mechanisms with regulation of complex behavior, including abnormalities in several psychiatric disorders, including depression, drug addiction, schizophrenia, Angelman syndrome, fragile X syndrome, Prader-Willi syndrome, Rett disorder, and Rubinstein-Taybi syndrome.

The fundamental unit of chromatin is the *nucleosome* (q.v.). Chromatin is activated by histone acetylation, which allows transcription of individual genes. Chromatin remodeling permits small groups of nucleosomes to become more, or less, activated so that access of the transcriptional machinery to specific promoter regions is enhanced, or inhibited, respectively. The best known remodeling mechanism in brain is the post-translational modification of histones—by acetylation, ADP-ribosylation, methylation, phosphorylation, or ubiquitylation. Such remodeling is associated with activation or repression of genes by synaptic activity. *Rett disorder* (q.v.), for example, is an epigenetic disorder because it is caused by mutations in the gene that encodes the transcriptional repressor MeCP2. Deficiency of MeCP2 results in global reduction in cortical synaptic excitation and a shift towards inhibition of synapses in cortical neurons.

Another example is schizophrenia. There is evidence that hypermethylation down-regulates genes, such as *reelin*, in GABAergic neurons; this disrupts synchronization in neural networks and leads to impaired higher brain function in schizophrenia.

**epigenetic principle** Each stage of development is dominated by one or more characteristic crises that must be resolved if development is to proceed along regular lines; if such adaptational demands are not met, all subsequent phases will reflect that failure in some type of maladjustment (physical, emotional, cognitive, or social). See *ontogeny, psychic.*

**epigenetic regulation** See *gene functions.*

**epigenetics** The study of heritable modifications of DNA or its associated proteins that are not due to changes in the DNA sequence. See *epigenetic.*

Epigenetic changes occur during gestation, neonatal development, puberty, and old age. The epigenome is most vulnerable to environmentally induced alterations during embryogenesis, when DNA synthesis is rapid and DNA methylation patterning and chomatin structure required for normal development are established. See *epigenetic mechanisms.*

**epigenomes** Catalogs of nongenetic controls of gene function. See *junk DNA.*

**epilempsis** Hippocratic term for epilepsy.

**epilepsia corticalis continua** See *continuous epilepsy.*

**epilepsia cursiva** *Obs.* A symptom of epilepsy with apparently aimless running about. See *procursive epilepsy.*

**epilepsia partialis continua** (L. "partial continuous epilepsy") Kozhevnikoff originally described this rare motor variant of epilepsy:

"It differs from the general myoclonic type in that the twitching is limited to one segment of the body, nearly always a peripheral part such as the wrist and fingers, is practically continuous between the paroxysmal fits, and on the whole partakes of the form less of movements than of irregular, individual muscular contractions" (Wilson, S. A. K. *Modern Problems in Neurology*, 1929). See *continuous epilepsy; virus infections.*

**epilepsy** A paroxysmal, transitory disturbance of brain function that develops suddenly, ceases spontaneously, and exhibits a conspicuous tendency to recurrence; a state of neuronal hyperexcitability characterized by massive hypersynchronous discharges from large numbers of neurons in the brain. Epilepsy is fundamentally a circuit phenomenon, and seizures are possible only because the brain is organized in a series of interconnected neuronal networks. The initially localized hyperexcitability spreads into surrounding neuronal networks, where it might be either counterbalanced by inhibitory mechanisms or, after involving more and more neurons, cause a clinically visible seizure. A different mechanism is seen in absence seizures, where abnormal synchronization of the thalamocortical network, rather than an excessive recruitment of neurons, causes the seizures. The typical epileptic attack, or fit, or *convulsion*, consists of the sudden onset of loss of consciousness, with or without tonic spasm and clonic contractions of the muscles. There are many forms of epilepsy, which vary depending upon the site of origin, the extent of the area involved, and the nature of the etiological factors; at the present time the term also includes transient episodes of sensory or psychic disturbances. Epilepsy, in short, is not a disease but a symptom, consisting of recurrent episodes of changes in the state of consciousness, with or without accompanying motor or sensory phenomena. Epilepsy has also been called *paroxysmal cerebral dysrhythmia.*

Among the many older terms for epilepsy are caduca passio, cadiva insania, caducus morbus, cataptosis, decidentia, eclactisma, epilempsis, St. Valentine's disease, St. John's evil, faunorum ludibria, grande nevrose,

Herculeus morbus, hieronosus, hylephobias, insania cadiva, lues divina, magnus morbus, malum caducum, morbus astralis, and morbus sacer.

The average frequency or expectancy of epilepsy in the general population is 1 in 200; but persons with one epileptic parent have a higher expectancy (1 in 35), and those with both parents epileptic have a much higher expectancy (1 in 10). For each person who develops seizures during his or her lifetime, it is said that there are 20 more with a predisposition to the affliction. There is no difference in incidence between the sexes, although epilepsy tends to begin earlier in the female.

It is customary to divide epilepsy into two major groups on the basis of etiology: (1) *genuine* or *idiopathic* or *cryptogenic* epilepsy, in which there is no known local, general, or psychological cause. Idiopathic seizures are assumed to be mainly genetic in origin. Many of the genes implicated in idiopathic epilepsies code for ion channels, but for most idiopathic epilepsies the genes involved remain unknown. (2) *symptomatic* epilepsy, in which an organic basis is demonstrable. Approximately 25% of all epileptics fall clearly within the symptomatic group. But as the horizons of neurology widen to include more recent pathological, physiological, and biochemical advances, it can be anticipated that specific etiologic agents will be demonstrable in an increasing number of cases. Epilepsy is an uncontrolled discharge of cortical or subcortical neurons, a physiochemical disturbance that could be produced by any number of agents. See *grand mal epilepsy.*

Within the *symptomatic* group of epilepsies are those due to (1) local causes—intracranial infection, brain trauma, congenital abnormalities, degenerative diseases such as Pick disease, various circulatory disturbances of the brain, etc.; (2) general causes—exogenous poisons, anoxemia, endocrine disorders, metabolic disorders (uremia, hypoglycemia, alkalosis, eclampsia, and hypertension of pregnancy), etc.; and (3) psychogenic causes.

In regard to the psychogenic group, there is little evidence that epileptic seizures, as distinct from hysterical fits, are ever purely psychogenic, but it is well recognized that the individual attack may be precipitated by fear, excitement, or other strong emotions. See *epileptic dementia; epileptoid personality; temporal lobe epilepsy.*

The *idiopathic epilepsies* have no known local, general, or psychological cause; this is a large and heterogeneous group that suffers from a predisposition to convulsions, the nature of which is not yet understood. This predisposition in some cases seems to be largely hereditary in origin, but not all workers would subscribe to the view that idiopathic epilepsy is essentially a hereditary disorder. What is inherited is not epilepsy itself, but rather a predisposition to the development of convulsions under certain conditions, i.e., the physical basis of a cortical dysrhythmia. And only a small proportion of those with this cortical dysrhythmia become epileptic.

The onset of epilepsy is often difficult to determine, for minor attacks may not be recognized, and major attacks (25%) may be only nocturnal, especially in children. The first seizure occurs before the age of 20 in 75% of cases.

Epilepsy is divided into types on the basis of etiology, as discussed above; it may also be subdivided on the basis of physical manifestations. The International League Against Epilepsy subdivides epileptic syndromes into the following:

I. Idiopathic epilepsy syndromes, focal or generalized
  A. Benign neonatal convulsion
  B. Benign focal epilepsy of childhood
  C. Childhood absence epilepsy
  D. Juvenile myoclonic epilepsy
II. Cryptogenic or symptomatic epilepsy, focal or generalized
  A. West syndrome (infantile spasms)
  B. Lennox-Gastaut syndrome
  C. Epilepsia partialis continua
  D. Temporal lobe epilepsy
  E. Frontal lobe epilepsy
  F. Post-traumatic epilepsy
III. Other epilepsy syndromes of uncertain or mixed classification
  A. Neonatal seizures
  B. Febrile seizures
  C. Reflex epilepsy
  D. Adult nonconvulsive status epilepticus

**epileptic character** See *epileptoid personality; interictal behavior syndrome; temporal lobe epilepsy.*

**epileptic clouded states** Psychotic reactions occurring in epileptics. At times, either preceding or following a convulsive attack, the epileptic may manifest a dazed reaction with deep confusion or excitement, anxiety, and bewilderment. Associated with this, there may be violent outbreaks, hallucinations, fears, or ecstatic moods with religious exaltation.

**epileptic cry** Sometimes called *initial cry*; a peculiar, discordant cry or yell occasionally uttered at the beginning of an epileptic fit, just before respiration is arrested. It is due to the expulsion of air through the glottis, which is narrowed at the time of the tonic spasm.

**epileptic dementia** Progressive mental and intellectual deterioration that occurs in a small number of epileptics—probably not more than 5%, and there are many famous epileptics, such as Helmholtz, Flaubert, and Dostoyevsky, who showed no such dementia. It seems more likely to occur when the attacks have begun early in life. Both the dementia and the convulsions are probably expressions of some undetected physiological abnormality, although some believe that the dementia is a result of neuronal degeneration secondary to vascular disturbances during the convulsive episode.

In a small group of epileptics, more complicated clinical psychiatric syndromes are seen, with mainly depressive or schizophrenic symptoms. These patients show that epilepsy and schizophrenia are not mutually exclusive, even though a belief to the contrary provided a rationale for electroconvulsive treatment. See *epileptoid personality; temporal lobe epilepsy.*

**epileptic equivalent** For some, any attack in an epileptic that is neither a grand mal nor a petit mal episode. Others use the term to indicate psychomotor epilepsy. See *temporal lobe epilepsy.*

**epileptic personality** *Epileptoid personality* (q.v.).

**epileptic psychopathic constitution** See *epileptoid personality.*

**epileptic psychoses** See *epileptic dementia.*

**epileptoid personality** Also, *epileptic personality*; both terms are used in different ways by different writers. Sometimes the terms imply a true epileptic character; at other times they refer to reactions to the chronic invalidism of epilepsy. In either case, the term is applicable to fewer than 20% of epileptics, and *epileptoid*

(or *explosive*) is therefore preferred to *epileptic* personality.

The characteristics highlighted in most descriptions of epileptoid personality are rigidity, egocentricity, selfishness, religiosity, seclusiveness, explosive outbursts of emotion, and extreme rage reactions when frustrated. Children especially become frenzied when refused their wishes. Enuresis is also common. Probably the most frequently described abnormality is morose egotism. Only one feature supports the belief in a specific epileptod constitution; viz., phantasies of death and rebith, which are more common here than in any other illness. See *epileptic dementia; explosive disorder; temporal lobe epilepsy.*

**epiloia** See *tuberous sclerosis.*

**epinephrine** The active hormone of the medullary portion of the adrenal glands, $C_9H_{13}NO_3$, often referred to by its proprietary name, Adrenalin. Epinephrine is a potent vasopressor drug; it increases blood pressure, stimulates heart muscle, accelerates heart rate, and increases cardiac output.

There is evidence that epinephrine and other catecholamines are involved in the pathophysiology of mood disorders. See *catecholamine hypothesis; dopamine hypothesis.*

The Two-Disease Theory of Depression includes (1) the *norepinephrine* (NE) (or catecholamine) hypothesis: depression in one subgroup of depressives is caused by low brain norepinephrine, and mania by high brain epinephrine; (2) the *serotonin* hypothesis: depression in another subgroup is due to low brain serotonin, mania by high brain serotonin. Research has not yet proved that there is a NE defect in depressed patients, but there is much evidence to suggest that many antidepressants may exert their effect through NE.

The Cholinergic Hypothesis: Although the cholinergic system has not been as extensively studied at this point, there is good evidence that it may play a role in mood disorders. Drugs that stimulate acetylcholinergic activity can induce depression in control subjects, exacerbate depression in depressed patients, and decrease symptoms in manic episodes.

**epinosic gain** Secondary advantages accruing from an illness, such as gratification of dependency yearnings or attention seeking. "In the traumatic neuroses, *secondary gains* play an even more important role than in the psychoneuroses; there are certain uses the patient can make of his illness which have nothing to do with the origin of neurosis but which may attain the utmost practical importance.... Obtaining financial compensation or fighting for one creates a poor atmosphere for psychotherapy, the more so if the compensation brings not only rational advantages but has acquired the unconscious meaning of love and protecting security as well" (Fenichel, O. *The Psychoanalytic Theory of Neurosis*, 1945). See *bribe*; *compensation neurosis*.

**epiphenomenalism**  The belief that the mental world is without causal efficacy, that thoughts, feelings, and impulses occur within our subjective experience but do nothing. Such an assertion ignores the direct effects that the brain can be demonstrated to have on mental functioning. Subjective, first-person mental phenomena have causal efficacy in the world and carry critical causal information about human behavior.

**epiphenomenon**  An event that occurs with, is associated with, or is superimposed on another event, but which is not considered to be caused by that other event. See *correlation*.

**episodic amnesia**  Loss of memory for a specific happening without anterograde or retrograde extension, considered to be on the basis of repression and not primarily organic in nature.

**episodic disorders**  Impulse disorders. See *episodic dyscontrol*.

**episodic dyscontrol**  A syndrome first described by Bach y Rita et al. (1971) consisting of violent outbursts with loss of control over aggressive behavior upon minimal provocation, often related to alcohol ingestion or occurring in a setting of alcoholism, and frequently with a history of hyperkinesis and truancy in childhood. Aurae and postictal states are seen in some cases, and aggressive use of automobiles is a frequent manifestation. Functional abnormalities of amygdalar or other limbic regions are suspected in such cases but often cannot be demonstrated. Psychotherapy and treatment with tranquilizers have generally been ineffective; many patients, however, respond well to diphenylhydantoin or other anticonvulsants.

In DSM-IV, episodic dyscontrol is considered a disorder of impulse control. In contrast to aggressive sociopathy, with which it can be confused, episodic dyscontrol is often associated with amnesia for the aggressive outburst;

dyscontrol patients typically feel tension before the event and relief afterwards, and no matter how ego-syntonic the event is at the time, most patients later feel great remorse and guilt.

**episodic memory**  Brodmann area 10 is involved in episodic memory encoding and retrieval and, compared with normals, is hyperactive during performance of a working memory task in subjects with schizophrenia, while area 9 is hypoactive. Such a reversal suggests that in schizophrenia less efficient strategies, such as episodic memory, are used in maintaining information. See *declarative memory*.

Episodic memory is also important to the ability to imagine nonexistent events and to simulate future happenings. A core brain system is involved that includes prefrontal and medial temporal lobe regions, as well as posterior regions, such as the precuneus and the retrosplenial cortex. *Theory of mind* (q.v.) uses the same core brain system (Schachter, D. L. et al. *Nature Reviews Neuroscience 8*: 637–661, 2007).

**episodic paroxysmal anxiety**  *Panic disorder* (q.v.).

**episodic representation**  Neural firing patterns that encode the sequence of events composing a unique, personal experience.

**epistasis**  A type of gene–gene interaction, when two alleles at different loci interact in a nonadditive fashion on a phenotype. In one form of epistasis, the phenotypical expression of one hereditary factor masks, or prevents, the manifestation of another factor that concerns the same organ, although it is not allelic to the factor with the greater expressivity. The factor exercising the masking effect is called *epistatic*, while the hidden factor is said to be *hypostatic*.

The result of *epistasis* is similar to that produced by a *dominant* character. However, there is a significant difference between the phenomena of dominance and epistasis. While a dominant and a recessive factor are always alleles of each other, an epistatic and a hypostatic factor are merely related to the same trait or organ, but they are not the two members of an allelic pair. See *dominance*.

**epistemic**  Relating to the need to know, considered by many to be one of the basic motives of human behavior.

**epistemophilia**  The love of knowledge or the impulse to inquire into things; said by psychoanalysts to receive its earliest important stimulation during the phallic phase, although preliminary preparation is gained through interests in other and earlier erotogenic zones, particularly the oral and the anal. The many subsequent manifestations of the impulse to learn are regarded as sublimations of the several varieties of infantile sexuality.

**epithalamus**   A zone of brain tissue above the thalamus composed of (1) *habenular ganglion* or *trigone*, a depressed triangular area anterior to the superior colliculus; (2) *pineal body*, which lies between the superior colliculi; (3) *posterior commissure*, some of whose fibers connect the two superior colliculi.

**epitope**   An immunological determinant of an antigen; antigenic determinant; any site on an antigen to which an antibody can bind. The chemical structure of the binding site determines the specificity of the antibody that enters into the antigen-antibody combination.

Epitope is also used to refer to a member of the same family (e.g., bacteria, toxins, antigens) that exerts a muted or less intense effect in comparison with the prototype.

**EPO**   *Erythropoietin* (q.v.).

**epoch**   *Stage* (q.v.).

**epochal amnesia**   "In the epochal type of amnesia a person, perhaps after a shock, suddenly loses all memory for lost epochs; it may be for days and even for years of his preceding life. In the case of Mr. Hanna, studied by Boris Sidis, the amnesia was for his whole previous life, so that the subject was like a new-born child" (Prince, M. *The Unconscious*, 1916).

**epochal multiple personality disorder**   *Sequential multiple personality disorder*; a type of dissociative identity disorder (DID) in which switches into alter personalities are rare, but when one alter does take over it is for a long time, during which all other alters remain dormant. Because of the length of the periods, and the apparent shock of other alters when they do return, Kluft has termed this the *Rip Van Winkle* form of DID.

**EPS**   Extrapyramidal symptoms, including acute dystonic reactions, akathisia, parkinsonism, tardive dyskinesia, and tardive dystonia. EPS are the most common side-effects of neuroleptic agents.

**EPSDT**   Early and periodic screening, diagnosis, and treatment. Often an essential element in

any *prospective* study of disorder, but increasingly subject to stringent limitations because of ethical issues involved. Subjects must be told what is being done to and for them as part of *informed consent* (q.v.); but such action may become a self-fulfilling prophecy, as labeling theory would predict.

**epsilon alcoholism**   A pattern of paroxysmal drinking bouts, during which the alcoholic drinks for days or weeks on end until he collapses; following recovery from one episode, he may stay dry for weeks or months until the next bout. Epsilon alcoholism is also known as *dipsomania*, or *paroxysmal* or *periodic drinking*. See *alcoholism*.

**equilibration**   Maintenance or restoration of constancy and stability; *homeostasis* (q.v.). Piaget described intelligence in terms of equilibration—adapting to and compensating for an ever-widening range of internal and external changes. This involves *assimilation*, the integration or incorporation of external elements into the structure of the developing intelligence, and *accommodation*, adapting to new data or new conditions that remain external to the subject and do not become a part of the subject's structure. See *concrete operational stage*; *developmental psychology*; *propositional thinking*.

**equine encephalomyelitis**   A virus infection of the central nervous system transmitted by mosquitoes from bird and wood-tic reservoirs. Two immunologically distinct types are recognized: (1) western, with lower mortality (c. 10% and more complete recovery, usually within 1 or 2 weeks) and (2) eastern, with higher mortality (c. 65%) and severe sequelae in those who do recover (e.g., mental defect, epilepsy, spastic palsies).

**equinophobia**   Fear of or aversion to horses.

**equipotentiality**   The theory, most commonly attributed to Lashley, that while each area of the brain performs a given function, all areas of the brain have equal potential to perform every task for which the brain is ultimately responsible and that mental functions cannot be localized to a specific brain region. Lashley's work suggested that it was the amount of brain mass destroyed, rather than the specific area, that determined the extent of deficit, and that physical damage to the brain results in nonspecific behavioral impairment. Equipotentiality is the direct opposite of the *localization* theory: individual behaviors are strictly associated to a specific neurologic substrate, and injury to particular areas of the brain produces specific behavioral sequelae. Behavioral patterns are built up gradually over long periods of time through the connection of particular sets of cells, *cell assemblies.* With time, more complex behaviors come to be formed out of sets of cell assemblies, called *phase sequences,* which inevitably involve some equipotentiality.

It was Donald Hebb, a study of Karl Lashley, who suggested that learning and memory involve changes in neuronal circuits and that every psychological function is due to activities in a *cell assembly,* in which nerve cells are connected in specific circuits or neural networks. See *connectionist model; network; parallel processing.*

**Equus-Laingian view**   Romanticization or eroticization of madness, ranging from a tendency to overvalue the positive aspects of bipolar illness while minimizing the negative, painful ones to a conviction that all psychopharmacologic interventions in such illnesses are oppressive, intrusive, and contraindicated. The term was suggested by K. R. Jamison and F. K. Goodwin (*Psychiatry Update II,* ed. L. Grinspoon, 1983).

**ER**   Endoplasmic reticulum; see *Golgi apparatus.*

**era**   *Stage* (q.v.).

**erbfest**   *Inheritable* (q.v.).

**Erdheim's tumor**   Craniopharyngioma.   See *intracranial tumor.*

**erectile disorder, male**   *Impotence* (q.v.); the male counterpart of female sexual arousal disorder, consisting of inability to attain or maintain an adequate erection until completion of the sexual activity.

**erective impotence**   See *impotence.*

**eremiophobia, eremophobia**   Fear of a lonely place or solitude.

**eremophilia**   *Obs.* Morbid desire to be alone.

**erethism**   *Obs.* Pathologic irritability, sensitivity, excitability, or overactivity; often used to denote sexual erethism, which may be manifested as erotomania, nymphomania, satyriasis, etc.

**erethizophrenia**   Exaggerated cortical excitability.

**erethizophrenic**   Pertaining to or suffering from erethizophrenia. J. R. Hunt's term, equivalent to *cycloid.*

**ereuthophobia**   *Erythrophobia* (q.v.).

**erg**   A general term for a unit of work, functioning, or activity.

**ergasia**   Adolf Meyer's term for the total of functions and reactions of an individual, in contradistinction to the functions of individual organs or parts of the human organism. It embraces the concept known as the *personality as a whole* and refers to those responses of a person that represent the results of the activity of many of his or her parts.

**ergasiatry**   Adolf Meyer's term for psychiatry.

**ergasiology**   Adolf Meyer's term for psychology.

**ergasionomania**   *Obs.* Compulsion to work, to keep busy.

**ergasiophobia**   Fear of functioning or acting, generally associated with an underlying dread that if movement takes place something disastrous will happen; related to the magical feeling that what happens to oneself also happens to the environment. A patient may believe that if he or she stops functioning or moving, the world will do the same.

**ergasthenia**   *Obs.* Fatigue or debility due to overwork or excessive functioning.

**ergodialeipsis**   Action that ceases before it is completely carried out. It occurs most commonly in schizophrenia and appears to be a type of *blocking* (q.v.).

**ergomania**   Compulsion to work, "workaholism."

**ergonomics**   The science and engineering of human factors involved in adapting to work conditions or to the general environment.

**ergoreception**   Afferent activity relating tissue energy and metabolic needs.

**ergotherapy**   *Occupational therapy; praxitherapeutics* (qq.v.).

**ergotism**   Chronic poisoning with ergot alkaloids, one of the most powerful of which is isoergine (lysergic acid amide). In the 17th and 18th centuries, ergotism was a common condition in Europe and the United States, resulting from eating contaminated rye bread. As seen at that time, ergotism was of two types: (1) gangrenous—dry gangrene of the extremities, the affected portions of which finally fall away; and (2) convulsive—with paresthesiae of skin and extremities, vertigo, tinnitus, headaches, vomiting, diarrhea, painful muscular contractions, epileptiform convulsions, and hallucinations.

**ergotropic**   Having the quality of turning to, predisposing toward, or preparing for action. Hess and others applied this term to that portion of the diencephalic subcortical system that integrates sympathetic with somatomotor activities and prepares the body for positive action. The other division of this system is called the trophotropic; the latter integrates parasympathetic with somatomotor activities and promotes protective and recuperative behavior patterns.

Much of the work of experimental psychiatry since the mid-20th century has been devoted to attempts to define more specifically the neurophysiological bases of emotion in the belief that this will open the way to a better understanding of emotional disorders. Hess's proposal that the reactions of the organism to environmental change are effected by a subcortical system coordinating visceral, somatic, and psychic functions is an example of one way in which the general problem has been attacked.

The significance of Hess's hypothesis depends upon recognition of the brain as a communication system, whose functional integrity is maintained by neural excitation and transmission, which in turn depend upon metabolic production of energy and its transformation into neural activity. If disordered or abnormal behavior is considered to be due, possibly, to some fault in this communication system, either because of defective transmission of the impulse or because of abnormal response of the nerve cells involved, the problem becomes one essentially of production or destruction of metabolites and the enzyme systems involved.

Emotions and emotional behavior depend upon the functional integrity of a subcortical coordinating system, which in turn depends on the balance and interaction of two opposing functional systems—the ergotropic, whose neurohumor may be *norepinephrine* (q.v.), or dopamine and the trophotropic, whose neurohumor may be *serotonin* (q.v.).

**Erichsen disease**  Railway spine; less commonly, railway brain; post-traumatic stress disorder with physical symptoms relating to the spine.

**Erikson, Erik H.**  (1902–1994) German-born psychoanalyst of Danish parentage; friend and disciple of Freud and analyzed by Anna Freud; emigrated to United States in 1933. Many orthodox Freudians considered him a heretic for the theory he developed that the ego and the sense of identity are shaped over the entire life span and not only in infancy

(he coined the term "identity crisis"); eight stages of man—humans operate in and are molded by a social matrix that includes political, economic, and social systems (see *ontogeny, psychic*); psychobiography (of Mohandas K. Gandhi, 1969, and Martin Luther, 1958); *Childhood and Society* (1950); *Identity and the Life Cycle* (1959); *Youth: Change and Challenge* (1963); *Insight and Responsibility* (1964); *The Life Cycle Completed* (1982); *Vital Involvement in Old Age* (1986).

**Erickson, Milton H.**  (1901–1980) American psychiatrist; hypnotherapy, brief strategic psychotherapy; founder of American Society of Clinical Hypnosis; *Experiencing Hypnosis: Therapeutic Approaches to Altered States* (with Ernest Rossi), *Hypnotherapy: An Exploratory Casebook* (with Ernest Rossi), *Time Distortion in Hypnosis* (with Leslie Cooper).

**ERISA**  The federal (U.S.) Employee Retirement Income Security Act of 1974, which regulates health benefits and insulates health plans from the legal consequences of restricting care. It does not require employers to offer any health benefits, nor does it dictate what benefits must be offered. Under most circumstances, it preempts state law concerning health benefits and claims for damages against health plans.

**Erklaren**  Jasper's term for the type of etiologic statement about a psychiatric condition that is based on an objectively verifiable conclusion, such as "This paranoid syndrome is due to amphetamine intoxication." Jaspers contrasted Erklaren, "explanation," with Verstehen, an "understanding" of the dynamics based on an intuitive grasp of the connection between the psychiatric manifestations and the subject's life, such as "This paranoid syndrome is based on the patient's doubts about his masculinity after being rejected by his love object."

**erogeneity**  The state or quality of being erogenous. See *anality; orality.*

**erogenous zone**  An organ or organ system that is invested with libidinal energy. Of the many erogenous zones, three are particularly important in psychoanalytic psychology: the oral, the anal, and the genital. See *anal eroticism; genitality; ontogeny, psychic; orality.*

**Eros**  (Gr. *Erōs*, the god of love) The life instinct or drive. See *death instinct; instinct.*

**erotic countertransference**  *Sexualized countertransference* (q.v.).

**erotic epilepsy**    A type of epileptiform focal seizure in which the patient experiences spells of intense erotic sensation; first reported by T. C. Erickson (*Archives of Neurology & Psychiatry 53*, 1945) in a 43-year-old housewife, in whom a small vascular tumor was later disclosed on the medial surface of the cerebral hemisphere, impinging upon the motor and sensory representation of the genitalia. See *epilepsy*.

**eroticism**    See *erotism*.

**eroticize**    To charge with libidinal or erotic energy. Any part of an object or person may be invested with the erotic instinct, that is, eroticized (libidinized).

**erotism (eroticism)**    A condition characterized by the instinctual quality called "love" or Eros. Thus, one speaks of erotism relating to body zones, such as anal, oral, and genital erotism; or to psychic structures, such as ego-erotism (narcissism); or to objects outside the body or mind, such as alloerotism.

**erotism, ego**    See *narcissism; ego libido*.

**erotization**    *Libidinization*; the act of erotizing or state of being erotized. During infancy the body becomes erotized, notably those parts of the body called erotogenic zones. All forms of activity subsequent to the stage of infantile sexuality may and usually do undergo erotization. Character traits, ideas, actions of all sorts, hobbies, recreations, etc. are erotized.

**erotized anxiety**    A paradoxical reaction to anxiety in which, instead of flight from the source of anxiety, the tendency is to head directly toward the source and enjoy it.

**erotized repetitive hangings**    Also, *eroticized repetitive hangings*; accidental death by hanging, which is initiated in order to produce neck constriction and cerebral hypoxia as a way of heightening sexual excitation. H. Resnik (*American Journal of Psychotherapy 26*, 1972) presents evidence of at least 50 such deaths each year in the United States. The subjects, usually teenagers or young adults, are nude or partially clothed; nearby sexually exciting materials or literature suggests that the hanging has been part of a masturbatory act.

**erotocrat**    A person of powerful sexuality.

**erotodromomania**    *Obs.* Hirschfeld's term to denote the impulse to travel as an escape from some painful sexual situation.

**erotogenesis**    The springing or origination of libidinal or erotic impulses. In *Three Contributions to the Theory of Sex*, Freud suggested that the sexual instincts in humans are complex and result from impulses coming from several sources, among them the oral, anal, and phallic zones.

**erotogenetic**    *Erotogenic* (q.v.).

**erotogenic**    Relating to or having its origin in the libidinal or erotic instinct; commonly applied to libidinal impulses that are expressed through special body areas or erotogenic zones (genitals, mouth, anus, urethra).

**erotogenic masochism**    *Primary masochism*; one of the three types of masochism described by Freud—"the lust of pain." It is the form commonly implied by the term *masochism* (q.v.), when masochism is a requisite condition for sexual gratification. The self-destructive tendencies arising from the death instinct are to a large extent disposed of early in life by displacement onto objects in the outer world; this is the origin of mastery, the will to power, and true sadism. The part which is not so disposed of remains as the original erotogenic masochism, elements of which can be traced through all the developmental stages of the libido: oral (fear of being devoured), anal (desire to be beaten by the father), phallic (castration phantasies), and genital (in situations characteristic of womanhood, the passive or receptive part in coitus and the act of giving birth).

**erotographomania**    Compulsion to write love letters. The letters are generally written anonymously.

**erotolalia**    Sexually obscene speech, especially in reference to the use of such speech during sexual intercourse as a means of enhancing gratification. This term emphasizes the sexual content of speech in contrast to the obscene or socially taboo speech of coprolalia, which term is more properly limited to verbal expression of excretory processes.

**erotomania**    *Aidoiomania; delusional loving; de Clérambault-Kandinsky complex*; a syndrome that occurs almost exclusively in females, consisting of the delusional belief that a man, usually older and of higher social status, is deeply in love with the patient; described in 1922 by G. G. de Clérambault. Some authors regard the syndrome as a denial of unconscious homosexual impulses; most, however, interpret it as a grandiose phantasy constructed as a defense against a narcissistic injury that has made the patient feel unloved or unlovable.

Mary V. Seeman (*Archives of General Psychiatry 35*, 1978) distinguishes two types of delusional loving: (1) phantom lover syndrome, a fixed and unshakable conviction that one is loved, usually by an "ordinary" person; the syndrome is found most often in poorly integrated, schizophrenic women and survives repeated confrontations with reality; (2) erotomania proper or *de Clérambault syndrome*, which occurs in healthier, sexually active, aggressive women who develop intense but short-lived delusions about a man whom they admire for his wealth, power, or position. As time brings more denials of the reality of their beliefs, such women give up the man in question and move on to another with whom they repeat the cycle.

Sometimes erotomania is used as an equivalent of *hypersexuality* (q.v.).

**erotopathy**   Any abnormality of the sexual impulse; *paraphilia* (q.v.).

**erotophobia**   Aversion to sex, including avoidance or denial of sexual feelings; sexual aversion disorder. See *sexual dysfunctions*.

**erotophonophilia**   A type of *paraphilia* (q.v.), in which sexual arousal and orgasm are dependent upon sacrificial killing of the partner; lust murder. See *sadism*; *rape*.

**ERP**   1. Event-related potential; *evoked potential* (q.v.).

2. Exposure and Response Prevention; see *exposure methods*.

**error**   Errors of memory are distinguished from forgetting and false recollections through one feature only, namely, that the error (false recollection) is not recognized as such but finds credence. According to Freud, back of every error is a repression. More accurately stated: the error conceals a falsehood, a disfigurement which is ultimately based on repressed material (*The Basic Writings of Sigmund Freud*, 1938).

**error attribution**   See *attribution*.

**errorless learning**   A training approach designed to compensate for impairments in neurocognition that impede or restrict skill acquisition; it has been used extensively with the developmentally disabled and other neurologically impaired patients to teach new skills and curb maladaptive behavior. More recently it has been used in patients with schizophrenia. Based on the theory that learning occurring in the absence of errors is stronger and more durable, it has four components: (1) the task to be learned is broken down into component parts; (2) training begins with simple tasks that have a high likelihood of success; (3) training proceeds through hierarchically ordered exercises in which the tasks are gradually made more difficult; proficiency at each level is reached by using multiple instructional aids (e.g., prompts, visual cues, guided instruction); and (4) performance within each component is overlearned through repetitive, successful practice and a rich schedule of positive reinforcement.

**erstarrende    Rückbildungspsychose**   Stiffening involutional psychosis. See *paraphrenia*.

**erythema multiforme**   See *Stevens-Johnson syndrome*.

**erythrism**   In medicine and anthropology, a condition characterized by the presence of red hair in certain regions of the body, notably in the beard and pubic zone, where it contrasts with the color of the remainder of the body hair. In constitutional medicine it is considered a stigma of the *asthenic, microsplanchnic* physique and its tendency to tuberculosis. See *asthenic type*.

**erythroblastosis fetalis**   See *icterus gravis neonatorum*.

**erythroedema polyneuropathy**   *Acrodynia* (q.v.).

**erythrophobia**   Fear of red. The fear is most commonly associated with blood, although, as with other fears, anything identified with the original fear may act as a substitute for it. For example, the fear of blood may be expressed as the fear of red, of anything that is red; the fear may then spread to all colors; the fear of colors may then give way to that of certain localities in which colors are prominent. Fears amass with great facility; moreover, as fears grow they tend to appear less associated with the original one, until finally the fear seems thoroughly illogical and unrelated to any previous experiences.

The conscious fear is often symbolic of an unconscious and antithetic impulse. Thus, the fear of blood may be related unconsciously to a wish for it. The wish may be a sadistic expression connected with the castration phantasy or one of its many subsequent symbolic expressions.

Erythrophobia is often manifested as a fear of blushing, possibly related to genitalization of the face or head and exhibitonistic impulses: the red face is feared as if it were the exposed penis.

**erythropoietin**   *EPO*, the hematopoietic growth factor; a glycoprotein that is a member of the type I cytokine superfamily. It maintains optimal tissue oxygenation by regulating the number of erythrocytes, and it mediates injury-related tissue protection. It is a neuroprotective factor in hypoxic-ischemic, traumatic, excitotoxic, and inflammatory injuries, where it inhibits apoptosis in tissue adjacent to the lesion. It also modulates nitric oxide synthesis and neurotransmitter release, and it antagonizes leakiness of the blood–brain barrier that is induced by vascular endothelial growth factor or inflammation. See *ischemic tolerance.*

**ES**   Embryonic *stem cell* (q.v.)

**E-S theory**   Empathizing-systemizing theory. See *sex differences.*

**escape drinking**   See *alcoholism.*

**escape learning**   See *aversive control.*

**escapism**   In psychoanalytic treatment, a form of *resistance* (q.v.) consisting of a wish to escape from painful reality to the security of childhood. It may manifest itself as an accentuation of symptoms.

**ESL**   1. "English is their second language," used particularly to refer to children whose parents' native tongue is a language other than English, in consequence of which the children are reared speaking the other language even though when they go to school they will be expected to be familiar with English.

2. "English as a second language," a specialized field of education.

**ESN**   Educationally subnormal.

**esophageal neurosis**   Psychogenic disturbances of the swallowing functions of the esophagus, usually manifested by choking on food, inability to get it down, or the sensation of a foreign body in the upper region of the esophagus (*globus hystericus*). The major unconscious emotional basis for the symptom is the rejection of, or defense against, the process of "incorporation," which represents a guilty oral aggressive (castrative) wish.

**esophageal reflux**   See *achalasia.*

**esophoria**   See *heterophoria.*

**ESP**   *Extrasensory perception* (q.v.).

**espiritismo**   A form of *folk healing* (q.v.) culturally specific to Puerto Ricans, based on the belief that the world is inhabited by spirits that require one or more incarnations in human bodies before they can finally accomplish their mission of union with God. Some spirits (*causas*) have trouble reaching that goal and intrude on people during their dreams or enter their bodies, causing physical and psychiatric illness. The affected person consults an *espiritista* (medium or spiritualist) either in a private session (*consulta*) or at regularly held meetings (*reuniones*). Several seances may be needed to convince the spirit of its wrongdoing and to get it back on track. Herbal medicines, prayers, and consultation with physicians may all be advised by the *espiritista*. See *complementary medicine; folk medicine.*

**Esquirol, Jean Etienne Dominique**   (1772–1840) French physician who specialized in treatment of the mentally ill. He was Pinel's favorite pupil. In 1817 at the Salpétrière, he inaugurated the first official course on mental disease; his textbook, *Des Maladies Mentales*, was published in 1837.

**essential fatty acids (EFAs)**   *Phospholipids*, the major form of lipid in all cell membranes. The two major *omega-3 fatty acids* (q.v.) are DHA (docosahexaenoic acid) and EPA (eicosapentaenoic acid).

**essential tremor**   See *tremor.*

**EST**   Electroshock therapy. See *ECT.*

**est**   Erhard Seminar Training, a consciousness-expanding technique developed by Werner Erhard; usually given as a 60-hour seminar that takes place on two consecutive weekends. Est is an eclectic integration of Eastern and Western philosophies, of various psychological theories and practices, and of motivation techniques from the business world; in the 1970s it was one of the most popular of the human-potential movements.

**EST sequences**   Expressed sequence tagged sequences; short sequences of DNA from known genes, used to identify unknown genes. The DNA sequence in which the unknown gene is located is compared with a collection of sequences from known genes.

**esthesia**   Sensibility; capacity for sensation. Used frequently as a combining form.

**esthesiogenesis**   The production of a reaction in a sensory zone.

**estrangement, inner**   Federn's term to refer to the feeling that external objects, even though well perceived, have a strange, unfamiliar or unreal quality. He considered estrangement to be characteristic, nosologically and clinically, of the depressive psychoses (while depersonalization is characteristic of the schizophrenias). Federn ascribed estrangement to a failure of cathexis of the external ego boundary, one of whose functions is to identify non-ego (external objects) as real and familiar. This failure is due to a primary disturbance in the bodily ego feeling, which is derived from the narcissistic libido (the sexual energy investing the ego).

**état lacunaire** Arteriosclerotic brain degeneration, consisting of diffuse vascular atrophy of the corpus striatum (much more rarely the thalamus) due to widespread enlargement of perivascular spaces.

**état marbré** Status marmoratus. See *torsion dystonia.*

**ETD** *Eye tracking dysfunction* (q.v.). See *pursuit eye movements; SPEM.*

**eternity, fear of** By this term Fenichel designates one in the group of fears of "surroundings that imply the loss of the usual means of orientation," such as fear of cessation of customary routine, fear of death, fear of uniform noises, etc. The patient who has such fears is particularly afraid of a loss of control over infantile sexual and aggressive impulses, and then projects onto the outside world his own fears of losing control. A concept such as eternity, in which the normal assessment of time loses its significance, is seen as a great threat to him, for it means a loss of the forces protecting him against his own unconscious unmastered sexual and aggressive impulses (*The Psychoanalytic Theory of Neurosis*, 1945).

**ethanol** Ethyl *alcohol* (q.v.).

**etheromania** Ether drinking; ether was drunk as an inebriant in many parts of the world in the early 13th century, and in some European peasant communities it rivaled alcohol in popularity. This form of inebriety is now rare.

**ethical imperative** The inexorable disciplinary power of moral principles exerted upon one's mental life and behavior. It represents "the wish of the moral self, the endeavor of the nobler side of man leading the ego to higher and better things in life." One may also speak in terms of "the upward aspiration of man," which in fact constitutes the admonitions of the moral consciousness in the life of an individual (Stekel, W. *The Interpretation of Dreams*, 1943).

**ethical principles** See *ethics, biomedical.*

**ethical self** See *superego.*

**ethics** That branch of philosophy concerned with the moral life and consisting of consideration of one's ordinary actions, judgments, and justifications as a means of discovering what one ought to do and of determining what actions are morally good, acceptable, or right, and what actions are unacceptable or wrong. Ethics is more than morality, which refers to any system of beliefs and values against which behavior is judged. Ethics comes into being when morality itself is problematic, and when conflicts arise between opposing moral systems or sets of values (Pellegrino, E. *Bulletin, New York Academy of Medicine* 54, 1978).

Codes of professional ethics, despite their names, more often address themselves to matters of professional etiquette than to questions of morals. They typically enjoin the physician to do what he or she deems best for the patient and ignore the possibility of conflict between the value systems of the patient and the physician.

Some writers differentiate between *general normative ethics*, or ethical theories, and *applied normative ethics*, the attempt to apply the principles to specific problems that call for concrete decisions. Normative ethics is concerned with what ought to be. *Nonnormative ethics*, on the other hand, is concerned with what attitudes and codes do operate in fact. The study of how moral codes differ from one society to another, termed *descriptive ethics*, is one nonnormative approach. Another is *metaethics*, which is concerned with the logic of moral reasoning and the meanings of the fundamental concepts of ethics, such as rights, obligations, and responsibilities.

**ethics, applied** The use of ethical theory in the solution of practical, moral, and social problems, such as capital punishment, cognitive enhancement, genetic research, racism, and warfare. The premise of such applications of ethics is that moral problems are the cause rather than merely a significant aspect of the social conditions under study. Applied moral philosophy strives for greater clarity, avoidance of logical fallacies, consideration and understanding of the appropriate moral concepts, and critical examination of the arguments propounded in attempting to find solutions to moral problems.

**ethics, biomedical** *Bioethics*; a form of applied ethics, consisting of the application of general ethical theories and principles to the problems actually encountered in medical practice, delivery of health care, medical and biological research, and public policy determinations affecting health and illness.

Because it is applied ethics, biomedical ethics cannot be confined to a systematic analysis of moral principles but must instead be continuously subject to scrutiny and revision in terms of the applicability of provisional principles to actual cases. Medical practice is particularly concerned with the following *ethical principles*: beneficence, autonomy, dignity, integrity, justice, nonmalfeasance, and vulnerability. See *beneficence; respect for autonomy; utilitarian principle; utilitarianism; vulnerability principle.*

**ethics, community**   Focus on an ethic of community obligation in which individual interests must be submerged. Professional and ethical codes are forms of community ethics.

**ethics, descriptive**   A history of different ethical theories or concepts, usually including illustrations of different aspects of ethics from which students or readers are expected to select those views that are applicable to the conditions or dilemmas that confront them.

**ethics, situation**   A monistic form of act utilitarianism ethical theory that holds that there is one fundamental or basic principle, and that what one must do is determine the meaning of that principle in the situation at hand. The right or morally correct action is whatever will, all in all, cause the most good or prevent the most evil. To a situation ethicist, rules are summarizations of the wisdom of the past rather than determinants of a specific course or action that one must take. See *utilitarianism, negative.*

**ethnology**   The branch of anthropology that deals with the division of humankind into races or cultures and studies the origin, history, customs, and institutions of those various racial or cultural groups. Although "race" and "ethnicity" are often used interchangeably, *race* is more properly used to refer to shared physical characteristics of a group, while ethnicity refers to identification with a presumed shared heritage.

**ethnopsychology**   See *comparative psychiatry.*

**ethnoscience**   Also known as *componential analysis, ethnosemantics,* and *cognitive anthropology,* ethnoscience comprises the organized study of the thought systems of people in other cultures and sometimes in our own. Ethnoscientists search for the ways in which knowledge of a culture's rules is reflected in the behavior of natives, and especially in their speech. An ethnoscientific description attempts to write a set of rules for a culture so complete that an outsider could use them to behave appropriately in that culture.

**ethnosemantics**   Cognitive anthropology; systematic collection of data concerning the naming, classifying, and concept-forming abilities of people living in remote cultures and then describing in formal terms the nature of their linguistic and cognitive practices.

**ethology**   1. The study of group behavior as it is reflected in the mores and customs of a human group.

2. More commonly, the study of the behavior of animals in their natural habitat. Some of the key concepts of ethology are *instinct* (q.v.), imprinting, and social releaser. See *releaser, social.*

**ethopropazide**   An anticholinergic drug. See *cholinergic.*

**ethosuximide**   An *anticonvulsant* drug (q.v.).

**ethyl alcohol**   Ethanol; see *alcohol.*

**ethylamine**   See *neurotransmitter.*

**etic**   Referring to phenomena that, if not universal, at least are not culturally bound. See *emic.*

**etiology**   The division of medical science relating to the cause of disease. The cause of general paresis is the germ of syphilis; not all patients with syphilis develop general paresis. Etiologic studies also involve investigations into the nature and response of the tissues of the host as well as of the response of the total personality to the results of the disease.

**ETS**   Electrical transcranial stimulation; *electrosleep* (q.v.).

**eu-**   Combining form meaning good, well, advantageous.

**EUCD**   Emotionally unstable character disorder. See *personality trait disturbance.*

**eudemonia, affective**   Flight into mental illness as an escape from frustrating or frightening reality. The *Ganser syndrome*, certain cases of *hypochondriasis*, and *Faxenpsychosis* (qq.v.) are instances of affective eudemonia. This term emphasizes secondary gains, which are particularly prominent in these cases.

**euergasia**   Adolf Meyer's term for wholesome or normal mental functioning; orthergasia.

**eugenic**   Used in its original sense, the ideology or methods of preventive medicine in *applying* genetic principles to human health conditions as postulated by eugenics.

**eugenics**   This term was coined by Francis Galton in 1883 to denote the systematically organized efforts of preventive medicine to improve average human qualities through the observation of *heredity*. Galton's introduction of the word "study" into his final definition—"the study of agencies under social control that may improve or impair the racial qualities of future generations, either physically or mentally"—makes it clear that he was thinking of such studies as would be the foundation of plans. Eugenics is thus complementary to *euthenics*, which aims at the betterment of the human race by studying the *environmental* conditions of human beings and differs from *genetics*, which is the branch of natural science that studies the origin, transmission, and manifestation of hereditary characters.

Eugenic measures are (1) *positive*, to encourage reproduction by persons biologically most highly qualified (*aristogenic*), or (2) *negative*, for the reduction or stoppage of parenthood among those least qualified physically and mentally (*cacogenic*).

Society has long tried to control heritable disorders. In 1757 Sweden passed a law forbidding epileptics to marry on eugenic grounds. During the early 1900s, many laws calling for sterilization of the mentally retarded were passed in various states in this country. More recently, other nations have used the same argument of eliminating alleles that produce undesirable phenotypes in what have been viewed by others as genocidal efforts. Such misuses of medical knowledge have highlighted the dangers of uncontrolled application of genetic principles as well as the ethical issues involved.

Many heritable disorders can be detected prenatally, and most people would not fault a program of voluntary detection (by means of amniocentesis, for example) followed by voluntary abortion of genetically defective fetuses. Such programs, however, have not been notably successful.

In the case of severe illnesses, for which there exists no cure or effective treatment and whose victims must be supported by public funds, the question inevitably arises as to the advisability of mandating a program for prenatal detection and then of mandating abortion of those fetuses found to be defective. There are many objections to such a program concerning who will decide what disorders are severe enough to warrant such action, who has the right over the body of the fetus and the body of the woman who carries it, what is an acceptable quality of life, and what the rights to procreational privacy are.

**eugeroic** Producing good arousal; used to describe drugs with stimulant properties, such as modafinil.

**Euler-Chelpin, Ulf Svante von** (1905–1983) Swedish physician and physiologist; discovered noradrenaline in 1946 and confirmed that it is stored within the nerve fibers; shared Nobel prize in 1970 with Julius Axelrod and Bernard Katz for work on the chemistry of nerve transmission; research on prostaglandins, hypertension, and arteriosclerosis.

**eumorphic** Well-formed; according to the classification of constitutional types by the Italian school, this term means "built along normal lines."

**eunuch** A male *castrated before puberty* and subsequently developing the secondary sexual characteristics of a female. See *castration*.

**eunuchoid** In constitutional medicine, the physical appearance of a male whose secondary sexual characteristics resemble those of a female. See *hypogenital type*.

**euphoria** Abnormal sense of well-being. See *mania*.

Various terms have been suggested for varying degrees of feelings of happiness and unhappiness: euphoria, a feeling of physical well-being, relaxation, and happiness; *eutychia*, a state of general satisfaction; hypertychia, an excited elation with acceleration of physical and mental activity; ecstasy, a state of exaltation, exhilaration, or trance; *cacophoria*, a generalized feeling of unhappiness; apathy, a lack of interest and feeling; and *dystychia* or anhedonia, a loss of the ability to enjoy. See *depression; dysphoria; dysthymia*.

**euphoria, indifferent** Elation and cheerfulness that lack emotional depth. Bleuler applies this term to apparent euphoria in the schizophrenic, where seemingly marked euphoria is often expressed in the same sentence, side by side with marked depression or indifferent expressions. Indifferent euphoria is an instance of the lack of homogeneity of mood and of the dissociation between mood and verbal expression, which are almost pathognomonic of schizophrenia.

**euphoriants** See *psycholeptica*.

**euphoric apathy**   An expression used by Jung to refer to happy indifference, analogous to the "belle indifference" of the hysterical subject.

**eupraxia**   Normal ability to perform coordinated movements.

**eurhythmia**   In constitutional medicine, harmonious body relationships.

**eurotophobia**   Fear of female genitals.

**euryplastic**   A constitutional type described by Bounak, corresponding to the *pyknic* type in Kretschmer's system and the *megalosplanchnic hypervegetative* constitution of Pende.

**eusthenic**   In comparison with the *oligosthenic* and *phthinoid* divisions of the *asthenic* type in Kretschmer's system of constitutional types, this denotes the asthenic variety, which is relatively the most vigorous and the closest to the *athletic*.

**eustress**   Any kind of stress with a beneficial effect on the subject, such as stress that promotes learning.

**eutelegenesis**   In genetics, synonymous with *artificial insemination*, denoting the technical process of artificially impregnating a female with the sperm of a male without any contact between the two.

**euthanasia**   Applies mainly to the measures by which physicians alleviate, or seek to remove, the distress attending the approach of death in the course of a chronic disease. According to this concept, the removal of pain is regarded as essential for an "easy death."

In a more specific sense, the term implies not only an easy, painless death, but also the means of terminating life by legally putting to death every sufferer from an incurable disease who prefers this kind of death to being tormented for a lengthy period before an eventual, painful death. This particular procedure is commonly known as "mercy killing" and is legal in some countries. In the United States it has been advocated by small groups of physicians subscribing to the belief that, with adequate safeguards, euthanasia should be legalized "to allow incurable sufferers to choose immediate death rather than await it in agony." These advocates of euthanasia hold that most of the legal and religious arguments against mercy killing are founded on emotion rather than on reason.

Within the province of eugenics, it is the method of infanticide—that is, the destruction of infants with marked congenital defects—that has at certain times been prac-

ticed as a form of euthanasia that seemed advisable for the particular purposes of race betterment. It was in Plato's *Republic* and in ancient Sparta—whose population was essentially military and had become accustomed to looking at marriage chiefly as a means of supplying new soldiers—that infanticide was urged for the first time and actually practiced, upon the decision of the ephors, when a child was unlikely to become a vigorous citizen (soldier). Numerous tribes and nations, at one time or another, have sought to destroy their unfit, in order to prevent them from becoming a burden to themselves and to society.

**euthenics**   In contrast to *eugenics*, which aims at improving the biological qualities of future human generations with the aid of data gained from the observation of heredity, euthenics relates to the study of environmental conditions tending to improve the human race. See *peristasis*.

**euthymia**   Joyfulness or mental tranquility; bienaise.

**eutonia sclerotica**   A feeling of intense physical well-being experienced by some patients with multiple sclerosis, even when the disease itself is far advanced. See *multiple sclerosis*.

**eutychia**   See *euphoria*.

**evaluated time**   A description of phases or periods of life with an assessment by the subject of the feeling tone aroused by them. According to D. Chiriboga (*Journal of Gerontology 33*, 1978), 60% of subjects aged 16 to 67 years rate the teens and twenties as the best time of life, and another 18% rate the thirties as best. No one chose the later years as best.

**evaluation**   Measurement of worth or value; assessment of the degree of success in achieving a predetermined objective. Evaluation requires that concrete objectives or achievement tasks be set, that the measures and indices for assessing success be specified, that degrees of success be defined in terms of output expected within stated periods of time, and that the information obtained be fed back into the system so that the program can be altered as indicated. Evaluation aims to determine the effectiveness, efficiency, and scope of the system under investigation, to define its strengths and weaknesses and thereby to provide a basis for informed decision-making.

**evaluation, false**   A. Adler's term for under-evaluation of other persons or objects and overevaluation of personal achievement or aims.

**evasion**   See *paralogia*.

**event-related potential**   *ERP*; a succession of waves corresponding to the sequential processing of information by the subject. The sensory *evoked potential* (q.v.) is dependent upon the stimulus alone (e.g., auditory or visual), whereas the event-related potential is dependent also on the context in which the stimulus appears (e.g., whether it is expected or is a surprise). Some elements of the ERP are determined by the physical stimulus and the state of the afferent pathways ("exogenous" processes); others reflect the prior experience, expectation, or semantic processes of the subject ("endogenous" processes). At least in some brain regions, these different processes appear to involve different neurons.

Exogenous processes are mediated by stable cells, which respond to physical features of the stimuli independent of their meaning. Endogenous processes are mediated by *plastic cells*, whose firing patterns are correlated with subsequent behavioral responses and not with the physical features of the stimulus.

The *brain-stem-evoked potential* (*BSEP*; sometimes referred to as the *far-field evoked potential*) is a special type of exogenous ERP. The auditory BSEP is a sensitive measure of lateral lemniscus functioning, and the somatosensory BSEP is equally sensitive to the functional status of the medial lemniscus. See *neurometrics*.

$P_{300}$ (q.v.) is a late-appearing component of the ERP. Its amplitude increases with unpredictable, unlikely, or highly significant stimuli and thereby constitutes an index of mental activity. Both adult schizophrenics and children at risk for schizophrenia show a reduction in late positive amplitude in comparison with control subjects.

**eversion theory**   See *aging, theories of*.

**evidence-based medicine**   *EBM*; medical practice that is based on information produced from well-designed empirical experiments in which outcomes are carefully measured for a well-defined treatment compared with a placebo treatment, no treatment, or an alternative treatment. Such information is adapted and applied to meet the specific circumstances and clinical needs of the patient, whose specific values and preferences are incorporated in a process of shared decision making.

**evidence-based   psychiatry**   Decision-making based upon data regarding the likely impact of different treatments on specific outcomes for specific populations; distinguished from tradition-based methods of using expert opinion (the BOGSAT method—a bunch of guys sitting around a table).

**evil, St. John's**   *Obs.* Epilepsy.

**eviration**   Emasculation; feminization; sometimes used also to indicate a delusion in a male that he has become a woman.

**evocative memory**   *Cued memory; object permanency*; the ability to summon up a consistent inner image or representation of another person: "I can remember what you look like when you are not here with me." It is the cognitive-perceptual (mnemonic) aspect of *object constancy* (q.v.), whose other part is an affective component: "I can remember what you look like when you are not here with me, and it makes me feel good."

*Object constancy* begins to develop by 18 months of age and is essentially complete by 30–36 months, reflecting the child's ability to differentiate between self-representations and object-representations. Evocative memory is essential to a sense of selfhood, to a child's ability to profit from the tension-easing and creative outlets that play provides, and for the productive use of phantasy, which is the basis for effective foreplanning. See *separation-individuation*.

**evoked potential**   A specific electroencephalographic response to sensory stimulation, such as a light flash, a musical tone, a click, or a photograph. Included are the *sensory evoked potential* and the *event-related potential* (qq.v.). Because attention disturbances are frequent in some schizophrenic disorders, average evoked potential (AEP) techniques have been widely used to investigate perceptual dysfunction in such patients. See *neurometrics; P50 sensory gating*.

**evolutility**   The capability of an organism to exhibit change in growth and other aspects of the physical structure as a result of nutrition.

**evolution**   Development; unfolding. In biology, the process by which living things have acquired their present form. The theory of evolution proposed by the British naturalist Charles Darwin (and independently but almost simultaneously by A. R. Wallace), that the more complex forms of life are descended from more primitive forms, provided much of the basis of modern biology. In *On the Origin of Species by Means of Natural Selection or the Preservation of Favored Races in the Struggle for Life*, published in 1859, Darwin argued that progress was a result of natural selection, exercised through competition. Although Darwin implied that acquired characteristics, if helpful to survival of a species, would be transmitted by inheritance to succeeding generations, modern genetics has recognized that mutations, and not acquired characteristics, are transmitted genetically and are subject to the same processes of natural selection as are all other inherited traits. See *mutation*.

By extension, Darwin's theory was interpreted by some to mean that the key to social progress was control of the unfit and not of their environment, which they would only recreate in any event. Such control, perhaps through sterilization or other ways of limiting reproduction, would provide the answers to crime, poverty, mental illness, etc. Many laws mandating sterilization of mental retardates, epileptics, and others believed to be carriers of defective or undesirable genes were an outgrowth of such interpretations, which are generally disavowed nowadays because of their ethical implications. See *psychopolitics*.

**evolutionary developmental psychology** *Evolutionary psychology* (q.v.) is a Darwinian approach to human behavior which views the ontogeny of the human mind as a process of the genes being expressed over time. Evolutionary developmental psychology postulates an inherited gene–environment system in which genes unfold, the environment selectively activates or inhibits certain genes, and the genes themselves choose a conducive environment. Genes determine individuals who seek environments conducive to their phenotypic expression; succeeding generations inherit the gene–environment system that is thereby created. Within such a system are domain-specific modules that have evolved in the species, such as cognition, language, and mathematics. Also included are evolved psychological structures that have been optimized for age-appropriate learning in a co-evolved milieu. Family relationships—between parent and child, with siblings and kin—are also products of evolution.

Not all offspring have an equal chance of *reproductive success* (q.v.); according to *parental investment theory*, this inequality is mirrored in a differential investment of resources (giving more to offspring with a greater chance of further propagation). One manifestation of this inequality is the greater likelihood of parental abuse of children with congenital defects.

Fitness for successful competition for resources is believed to be the basis for social behavior, as well as attachment, dominance, and aggression. Evolutionary psychologists attempt to identify the selection pressures that have shaped human psychology and relate them to specific cognitive mechanisms that operate in humans. Evolution has been largely a process of genes adapting to changing environments, but the mechanisms that evolved during the early hunter-gatherer phase of human natural history do not necessarily mesh well with modern environments (Bjorklund, D. F. and Pellegrini, A. D. *The Origins of Human Nature: Evolutionary Developmental Psychology*, Washington, D.C.: American Psychological Association, 2002).

**evolutionary psychology** Named by the anthropologist John Tooby and the psychologist Leda Cosmides, evolutionary psychology combines cognitive psychology with evolutionary biology. The former explains the mechanics of thought and emotion in terms of information and computation; the latter explains the adaptive design of living things in terms of selection among replicators.

**EWS** Early warning signs; see *prodromal symptoms*.

**exaltation** *Obs.* Mania.

**examination anxiety** Freudian term for the anxiety attendant on examinations intensified by experiences of the past, usually unconscious, that had to do with "the punishments we suffered as children for misdeeds we had committed."

**exanthropia** *Obs.* What was called the third stage of melancholia, namely, dislike for society.

**exaptation** Adaptation of an old organ to a new function (Darwin's "pre-adaptation") or the adaptation on a non-organ (bits of bone or tissue) to an organ with a function. Occasionally a machine designed for a complicated improbable task can be pressed into service to do something simpler.

**exceptions type**   "The exceptions" type was first described by Freud; such persons, because of early frustrations, arrogate unto themselves the right to demand lifelong reimbursement from fate. This behavior is intensified if they are required to contradict a deep inner doubt as to their right to compensation. See *entitlement*.

**excessive daytime sleepiness**   Difficulty in staying awake that occurs daily for at least 3 weeks, or for recurrent periods of shorter duration. See *sleep disorders*.

**excitatory amino acid**   *EAA* (q.v.).

**excitatory state, central**   See *summation*.

**excitatory synapse**   A *synapse* (q.v.) that results in the flow of positive ions into the neuron, with the result that the intraneuronal compartment is less negatively charged and better able to develop an *action current* (q.v.).

**excited melancholia**   *Motor melancholia*; agitated depression. See *involutional psychosis*.

**excitement, catatonic**   See *catatonic schizophrenia*.

**excitement, constitutional**   *Obs.* Kraepelin's term for manic temperament.

**exciting object**   See *bad object*.

**excitotoxicity**   Excessive stimulation of excitatory amino acid receptors, especially NMDA, which triggers a cascade of cell death. (See *EAA*.) It has been hypothesized that some neurodegenerative diseases and CNS damage secondary to hypoxia-ischemia or trauma are due to the release of excessive amounts of EAAs, which then act as endogenous excitotoxins. In Huntington disease, for example, an accumulation of levodopa (because of defective conversion of levodopa to dopamine) could be neurotoxic; but in addition, the lack of dopamine needed to regulate striatal excitatory neurons could result in release of an excess of glutamate (the major EAA) onto cells already overstimulated by levodopa. The toxin MPTP (1-methyl-4-phenyl-1,2,3,6-tetrahydropyridine) can mimic the destruction of nigrostriatal dopaminergic neurons seen in Parkinson disease. MK-801, an EAA receptor blocker, can protect the rat against dopamine neuron damage that follows direct injection with MPTP. In Alzheimer disease, it is possible that *beta amyloid* has an excitotoxic effect on neurons and makes them more susceptible to damage by EAA receptor agonists. See *amyloid; glutamate*.

**exclusion criteria**   See *SADS*.

**executioner proteins**   See *apoptosis*.

**executive function**   *Executive performance*; a broad range of cognitive processes that coordinate or conjoin discrete, lower-level functions, including sensory, motor, cognitive, memory, and affective domains that contribute to decision making and enable the performance of complex, often novel high-level tasks. Executive skills include anticipation, goal selection, planning and organization, ability to establish goals, initiation of action, self-monitoring and inhibition of inappropriate action, use of feedback, ability to maintain or shift a mental set, interference control, response inhibition, flexibility in response to changing contingencies, and working memory. Executive dysfunction affects other cognitive areas, such as visuospatial abilities, set-shifting, the ability to encode and retrieve new memories, and the *organizational approach* (q.v.). See *context processing*.

Many executive functions previously assumed to be exclusively prefrontal are in fact subserved by distributed neural networks that include the anterior cingulate cortex, basal ganglia, possibly the dorsomedial thalamic nucleus and cerebellum, and the ventral mesencephalon. Inhibitory control is a multi-domain executive function critical for flexible interaction with changing task demands. It is thus incorrect to use the terms executive control and frontal lobe functions interchangeably.

Disturbances in executive function can be manifested in various ways. See *dysexecutive syndromes*.

**executive information system**   See *information system, executive*.

**executive organ**   The organ that is used for the execution of responses to stimuli. "In the infant the technique of mastery has two chief executive organs, the hand and the mouth, the eye being the leading auxiliary organ." (Kardiner, A. and Spiegel, H. X. *War Stress and Neurotic Illness*, 1947). When hunger is the stimulus, response to it is executed by way of the mouth; when the stimulus is the desire to grasp at an object, response to it is executed by means of the hand.

**executive system**   Generally included as part of *cognition* (q.v.), it is a process or set of processes whose primary purpose is to facilitate adaptation to novel situations, involving planning, initiation of action, and inhibition of inappropriate action. See *executive functions*; *information system, executive*.

**exhaustion death**   See *Bell mania*.

**exhaustion psychosis**   See *infective-exhaustive psychosis*.

**exhaustion stage**   See *general adaptation syndrome*.

**exhaustive psychosis**   *Collapse delirium* (q.v.). Binswanger subdivides exhaustive psychosis into *exhaustion stupor; exhaustive amentia;* and *delirium acutum exhaustivum*.

**exhibitionism**   A *paraphilia*, within the group of *sexual disorders* (qq.v.), consisting of repeated exposure of the genitals to strangers; the exposure itself gives sexual excitement and no further contact is sought with the victim. See *flasher*.

Paraphilic exhibitionism is much more common in males, but it is believed to occur in females also. Its prevalence in the female is unknown, however, since female exhibitionists are almost never reported to the police. Paraphilic exhibition of the penis is termed *peodeiktophilia*.

Exhibitionism is also used to describe non-paraphilic behavior that is not specifically sexual but reflects a need for constant attention and admiration. Exhibitionism of this type is a key trait of the narcissistic personality and is closely related to the grandiosity observed in that personality. In object relations psychology, the *exhibitionistic self* is equivalent to the *grandiose self* (q.v.). See *narcissistic personality*.

**exhibitionistic self**   See *grandiose self*.

**exhilaration**   See *manipulative personality*; *narcissistic personality*.

**existential anguish**   See *ontological insecurity*.

**existential neurosis**   Chronic meaninglessness, apathy, and aimlessness, which typically arise within a person who sees himself as nothing more than an embodiment of biological needs and a player of social roles. See *existentialism*.

**existentialism**   A system of philosophy particularly associated with Jean-Paul Sartre, Martin Heidegger, Karl Jaspers, and Søren Kierkegaard. Existential philosophy is essentially of European origin and is a reaction to the realization that technology and a belief in pure rationalism, logical positivism, or similar philosophies have only alienated man from society and from himself. Existentialism rejects the Hellenic view of man as a man of detached, logical reason and instead emphasizes the Hebraic view of man as a man of faith and a concrete, individual doer. See *humanistic psychology*.

Philosophy in the Western world before the time of Kierkegaard tacitly accepted Parmenides's belief that if a thing cannot be thought, it cannot be real. Yet existence cannot be thought—it can only be lived; thus, reason must ignore existence completely or reduce it to nothingness. For Kierkegaard, existence was not a matter of speculation but a reality in which the individual is personally and passionately involved; the decisive encounter with the Self is in the Either/Or of choice. For Heidegger, existence is a Being spread over a field or region that is the world of its care and concern. This field of being is called *Dasein* (q.v.). In the everyday world, none of us is a private Self confronting a world of external objects; we are simply one among many—"the One," a fallen state in that we have not yet become a Self and recognized our mortal, feeble, impotent nature. Sartre and his followers, representing a small part of existential philosophy, emphasize the despair of a world from which God has departed, and their themes include "Alienation and estrangement; a sense of the basic fragility and contingency of human life; the impotence of reason confronted with the depths of existence; the threat of Nothingness, and the solitary and unsheltered condition of the individual before this threat" (Barrett, W. *Irrational Man*, 1958).

In psychiatry, existentialism forms the philosophic background for "existential analysis," which in the main is represented by Europeans trained originally as psychoanalysts (e.g., Ludwig Binswanger). The existential group does not consider itself divorced from the body of orthodox psychoanalytic theory and method, but it looks to existentialism rather as a more extensive and practicable approach to the patient and his or her world. Existential analysis is considered to have appeared in reaction to existing inadequacies in the various schools of thought in psychopathology. See *logotherapy*.

*Existential analysis* places more emphasis on conscious experience than does classical psychoanalysis and is more confrontational than person-centered counseling. It assumes that a person's decisions about life give meaning to life, and the therapist is active in asking difficult questions to high-light the subject's decision-making process. Decisions can be seen as choosing the unknown future or the familiar past (the status quo). Choosing the future is anxiety-provoking but nonetheless desirable, for by giving meaning to life it promotes continued growth. To tolerate the anxiety associated with choosing the future, it is necessary to develop *hardiness*, an attitude of commitment, confidence in the ability to control, and a perception of the new as challenging rather than threatening.

Choosing the past, on the other hand, brings guilt and the feeling of missed opportunity. It narrows perspectives, obstructs learning, enforces conformity, and ultimately leads to boredom, stagnation, meaninglessness, and despair.

**EXIT** Executive interview (of Royall); assesses executive functions.

**exit events** See *life event*.

**exit therapy** Mobilization of whatever ties to the outside world remain in order to guide a person out of a cult with which he or she has become entangled.

**exocytosis** Extrusion of a neurotransmitter from its synaptic vesicle. Triggered by the calcium ion entering the presynaptic terminal bouton through voltage-gated $Ca^{2+}$ channels, the vesicle fuses with the membrane of the bouton and the neurotransmitter is released into the synaptic cleft. See *axon; vesicles*.

**exogenous, exogenetic, exogenic** Descriptive of physical or mental disorders caused predominantly by factors acting either from outside the body or from another part of the body (outside the system). See *endogenous*.

**exogeny, exogenism, exogenesis** In medicine, originally the pathogenetic process of only those morbid conditions caused by factors acting from outside the body; in psychiatry, it includes disorders caused by influences of pathological processes outside the nervous system.

**exon** A region of a *gene* (q.v.) that will be translated into an amino acid sequence that will, in turn, direct the synthesis of a protein; about 1% of the genome is spanned by exons. Exons are arranged in discontinuous segments interspersed with *introns*, sequences that do not code for an amino acid sequence but may contain regulatory information. Introns, in addition, are critical to alternative splicing,

which makes it possible for one gene to make several different proteins.

*DNA* (q.v.) is first transcribed into RNA; then the introns are spliced out; the remaining exons are joined together into a more functional sequence of RNA; and units of the new sequence attach appropriate amino acids into a growing protein chain. Protein synthesis takes place on the ribosomes within the cytoplasm. See *chromosome; transcription*.

**exophora** Diversions from the central track or issue; in conversation, strayings into tangential subjects. See *discourse skills*.

**exophoria** See *heterophoria*.

**exophthalmic dysostosis** *Xanthomatosis* (q.v.).

**exophthalmic goiter** *Thyrotoxicosis* (q.v.).

**exorcist syndrome** A type of homophobia expressed in attacking homosexual(s) physically or psychologically, or both. An example is the gay-basher who arranges to be propositioned by a gay man, has sex with him, and then beats him or even kills him; such behavior is frequently interpreted as the basher's way of ridding himself of (i.e., exorcising) his guilt of his own bisexuality or latent homosexuality. The physiological attack is seen in attempts of "...the self-righteous in high places of homophobic power, influence, and authority..." to discriminate against gays, lesbians, and any whose lifestyle they consider appropriate and what they consider to deviate from what they would impose on all of society as the only acceptable norm. John Money, who suggested the term, considers both forms to be manifestations of malignant bisexuality (*Gay, Straight, and In-Between: The Sexology of Erotic Orientation*. New York: Oxford, 1988).

**exotic psychoses** *Obs. Culture-specific syndromes* (q.v.).

**expansiveness** Lack of restraint in feelings and actions and especially overvaluation of one's own work. Sometimes used to refer to megalomaniacal trends; thus, delusions of grandeur and omnipotence are called expansive delusions. Horney uses the term to refer to a type of neurotic solution of inner conflicts based on identification with the idealized self and expressed in the form of narcissism, perfectionism, arrogance, and vindictiveness, or as other qualities consistent with mastery. See *megalomania*.

**expectable environment** See *affectomotor storms; facilitating environment*.

**expectant analysis**   See *focused analysis.*

**expectation, anxious**   Apprehensiveness, particularly in situations that involve something novel, unexpected, unexplained, or uncanny.

**expectation neurosis**   *Obs.* Anxiety that develops over the anticipated performance of an act; performance anxiety. Such anxiety is often a symptom of *agoraphobia* (q.v.). See *performance anxiety.*

**expected value**   See *choice.*

**expediter**   In social psychiatry, a person (or mechanism) who routes a patient through the network of social subsystems with which he or she articulates and effects linkages between those systems, as part of the total treatment and rehabilitation plan. See *ecology; community psychiatry; enabler.*

**experiential therapy**   A group of treatments that use controlled emotional experiences and training in recognizing and gaining better control over one's feelings and body as a way to achieve inner growth and self-actualization. See *alternative psychologies.*

*Emotional release therapies*, often short-term and intense, emphasize an understanding of the messages being transmitted from the body as a way to recognize inner tensions and restore physiological balance. Within this group are encounter group therapy, Gestalt therapy, and *primal scream therapy*. Some therapies (among them *bioenergetic psychotherapy*, and rolfing or Structural Integration) use body contact as the most direct way to recognize tensions. See *Gestalt therapy; rolfing; T-group.*

*Emotional control therapies* emphasize gaining greater control over the body through specific training. Included are *transcendental meditation* (*TM*) and *yoga psychology* (qq.v.). Religious and inspirational therapies include *faith healing* (q.v.) and Christian Science.

Cognitive emotional therapies include rational-emotive therapy (RET) and Glasser's reality therapy. See *cognitive behavior therapy; rational psychotherapy.*

**experimental conflict**   An artificial situation created through hypnotic suggestion in order to demonstrate to the patient his inner attitude toward the real conflict; an *experimental neurosis* (q.v.) induced by the hypnotist to bring the subject to awareness of his motivations.

**experimental neurosis**   *Artificial neurosis*; disorganized behavior that appears in the experimental subject in response to inability to master the experimental situation. Such behavior was noted by Pavlov in his dogs, when the animals were unable to discriminate between sounds of similar pitch or test objects of similar shape. Experimental neuroses have been induced in other animals as well—chimpanzees, cats, goats, pigs, etc.

Neurotic symptoms are based on involuntary emergency discharges that supplant the usual control mechanisms. The latter are insufficient because more excitation than can be mastered is presented, or (as in experimental neurosis) innocuous stimuli operate as traumatic precipitants in releasing an accumulation of unmastered tensions.

**experimental psychology**   The study of behavior by empirical methods, with an emphasis on sensation and elucidation of the ways in which a stimulus leads to a subjective experience. The founders of experimental psychology are generally considered to be Gustave Fechner, Herman Helmholtz, Ernst Weber, and Wilhelm Wundt. Experimental psychology was an outgrowth of positivism, which also engendered behaviorist psychology and its emphasis on the properties of the stimulus and the objectively observable responses it elicits. See *behavior therapy.*

**experimenter effects**   The often unrecognized, or unacknowledged, influence of the bias of the experimenter upon the results obtained in an experiment. Common examples are subtly suggesting the choice the subject should make, accepting (and reporting) only evidence that supports the experimenter's hypothesis, or telling the subject in advance what the outcome of the experiment is expected to be. See *suggestion.*

**expiation**   Atoning for, or making satisfaction for, a misdeed. According to Rado, obsessive attacks are derived from the temper (rage) tantrums of childhood, but in the obsessive patient the discharge of rage is slow and incomplete since it is always opposed by guilty fear. The latter, in turn, must be followed by expiatory behavior, just as in the child the mother's punishment and threats led to fearful obedience.

Such expiatory behavior would be considered by some as an expression of moral masochism. See *masochism.*

**explanatory delusion**   Bleuler's term for delusions that give reasons for the false belief. A patient who believes that men are persecuting him explains the delusion by "showing" that they open his mail, that they publish photographs of him, that they assemble to discuss methods of injuring him.

**explication**   Explaining, interpreting, or exploring the meaning of; trying to make sense of a situation. Explicatory coping strategies include causal explanation, rationalization, wit and mirth, confabulating, dreaming, hallucinating, and depersonalization.

**explicit memory**   *Declarative* or *propositional memory*, such as autobiographical memory. See *long-term memory*.

**explicit role**   See *role*.

**exploitative behavior**   In an uncertain environment, choosing familiar options with known rewards. *Exploratory behavior*, in contrast, is choosing unfamiliar options with riskier, but potentially more advantageous, outcomes. Decision making typically entails switching between exploitative and exploratory behavior. Exploitative decision making is associated with activation of the striatum and ventromedial prefrontal region; activation of the frontal pole of PFC is characteristic of exploratory decisions.

**exploitative character**   Fromm's term for the character pattern described by Abraham as *oral aggressive* (see *character defense*). Instead of viewing character structure as the result of libido sublimation or reaction formation, the cultural school of psychoanalysis sees the character types as basic attitudes in the process of socialization and coping with each particular life situation. Accordingly, Fromm believes that such a person develops in a frustrating atmosphere and hence comes to feel that one can have only what one takes and that the only source of security lies in exploiting others. When threatened with danger, the exploitative character tries to manipulate the situation by flattery, cajoling, aggression, or any other means.

**exploitativeness**   Making use of others for one's own gain, with the implication that the other's needs or desires are ruthlessly ignored or dismissed; often expressed as greediness, appropriation of others' ideas or property, and *entitlement* (q.v.). Exploitativeness is characteristic of both the narcissistic personality and the antisocial personality.

**exploiting type**   See *assimilation*.

**exploratory behavior**   See *exploitative behavior*.

**explosion readiness**   Readiness to explode, or burst forth violently. See *explosive disorder*.

**explosive diathesis**   A clinical subdivision of the traumatic psychoses.

**explosive disorder**   Intermittent explosive disorder is one of the *impulse control disorders* (q.v.) consisting of serious aggressive outbursts (e.g., assault or destruction of property) that are grossly out of proportion to any identifiable stressors. Between episodes, the subject may show impulsive or aggressive behavior, but it does not have the explosive nature characteristic of the disorder. *Catathymic crisis* is used by some writers for a single episode that is not repeated.

There may be associated nonspecific EEG abnormalities suggestive of subcortical or limbic system involvement, soft neurologic signs, a history of hyperactivity, or accident proneness. The condition is sometimes referred to as *epileptoid personality*, particularly when the subject presents evidence of an aura or postictal changes in the sensorium.

**explosive personality disorder**   Also, *epileptoid personality* (q.v.); characterized by intense irritability, particularly after the ingestion of alcohol; the irritability sometimes leads to acts of violence that appear unmotivated, that is, automatic. See *episodic dyscontrol; traumatic neurosis; traumatic psychosis*.

**exposure in vivo**   See *behavior therapy*.

**exposure methods**   Techniques used in *behavior therapy* (q.v.); their aim is to extinguish anxiety and other symptoms by repeated, controlled exposure of the patient to the feared situation. At one level, modeling may be used to allay the patient's anxiety by having him or her observe the desired reaction being performed by someone else. At another level, systematic *desensitization* (q.v.) may be used to reduce anxiety by gradual increments in the fear level of trial situations. At still another level, exposure may be rapid and fear-inducing as in flooding or *implosion* (q.v.). *In vivo exposure*, exposure to the real situation, appears to be the most effective approach in the treatment of obsessional behavior. See *imaginal exposure*.

**exposure, self-directed**   In treatment of phobia, the homework tasks required of the patient outside therapy sessions: entering into and remaining in phobic situations hitherto avoided. Some workers enhance instructions to the patient with manuals describing the rationale for self-directed exposure (also called *programmed practice*).

**expressed emotions (EE)**   In studies of schizophrenics and their families, high relapse rate was found to be related to frequency and quality of EE, defined as criticism, hostility, and overinvolvement expressed by the family toward the patient. Relapse was particularly high (79%) in high-EE-high-contact families (i.e., families in which patients spent 35 hours a week or more with their families) as compared with a relapse rate of 29% in high-EE-low-contact families (Brown, G. W. et al. *British Journal of Psychiatry 121*, 1972).

A similar association between high EE and relapse has been found in depression, bipolar illness, and obesity, suggesting that high EE may be a situation-specific coping response to the poor social functioning of the ill family member. On the other hand, the finding that family intervention programs that change EE attitudes in families result in lower relapse rates is consistent with a theory of causal relationship between the two. See *communication, disordered.*

**expressible**  Penetrant. See *dominance.*

**expressive aphasia**  *Broca motor aphasia* (q.v.).

**expressive dysphasia**  See *developmental dysphasia.*

**expressive therapy**  A method of treatment in which the therapist's dominant aim is to help the patient to bring out, talk about, act out, or emotionally express all ideas and feelings so that both the patient and the therapist come to know the dynamic emotional roots of the patient's symptoms and illness. Through encouragement and by bringing about a reversal of the *covering up* (or normal) defensive mechanism, expressive therapy endeavors to *uncover* the roots of mental emotional illness. As epitomized in psychoanalysis, the main purpose of expressive therapy is, through a reversal of the repressive defensive mechanisms, to shift the material from the unconscious realm into the realm of conscious thought.

On the other hand, *suppressive therapy* tends to cover up, to keep down, and to strengthen the repressive, defensive forces of the personality. As such, suppressive therapy tries to build up the forces of concealment of the self toward hidden portions of itself, while expressive therapy brings about painful but valuable self-revelation. Suppressive therapy tends to maintain and continue the individual's comfortable and peaceful illusion of himself, while expressive therapy becomes painfully disillusioning and thus aims in the direction of self-realization and reality.

**expressive variety**  The number of different things that can be said (or expressed) by combining words (or other symbols) in different ways. The expressive variety of *language* (q.v.) is so great that it would be impossible to store each whole sentence as a separate entity. As an example, "The patient related two phantasies." Also possible are "The patient related four phantasies" and "The patient related ten phantasies." In theory, there could be as many sentences in this series alone as there are numbers; in fact, the number is infinite, since any sentence stating the highest nameable integer (call it N) could be followed by the sentence, "The patient related (N + 1) phantasies," and so on. The example sentence contained 5 words; most sentences, of course, are much longer; in scientific journals and texts, they typically range from 27 to 54 words. Assuming that all of the sentences in the world are 20 words in length and that they come from 10 different categories of ideas, one would have, even at such a low estimate, a total of $10^{20}$ sentences—1 hundred million trillion.

If language were merely a learning process of childhood, and if a child were able to learn one different sentence every 5 seconds, the process would require a learning period of about 1 hundred trillion years in order to achieve only a modest language capacity. The expressive variety of language is achieved not because of learning but because of a body of innate knowledge that endows the child with the ability to construct a mental *grammar* (q.v.) for any of the languages of the world (therefore it is sometimes referred to as Universal Grammar).

Rather than storing whole sentences, the brain stores words and their meanings (this is the part of language that is largely learned), plus patterns into which words can be placed (the rules of language or the mental grammar); e.g., "The patient referred to N phantasies," "An X is not a Y." This provides maximal variety at minimal storage cost. Further, it allows the language user to recognize as well as to create novel examples of any pattern, regardless of whether they have been heard or used before.

**expressivity**  The extent to which a given phenotype is manifested in an individual. See *chromosome; dominance.*

**extended stay review**  Concurrent review of a continuous hospital stay that equals or exceeds the period defined in that hospital's utilization review plan.

**exteriorization** The act of objectivizing one's interests and affects.

**external chemical message** ECM; *pheromone* (q.v.)

**externalization** In discussing the Thematic Apperception Test, Bellak (in Abt, L. E. & Bellak, L. *Projective Psychology*, 1950) defines externalization as "those apperceptive processes which function on a preconscious level and can therefore readily be made conscious." The writer thereby differentiates between, on the one hand, projection as an unconscious defense mechanism that leads to extreme and pathological distortion of reality, and, on the other, the apperceptive distortions that make up the subject's responses in "projective" tests.

R. D. Chessick (*Archives of General Psychiatry 27*, 1972) defines externalization as a dual process, consisting first of projecting and second of manipulating, perceiving, and selectively reporting on external reality so that it will conform to and thus validate the subject's projections.

Horney used the term to refer to the experiencing of any intrapsychic process as occurring between oneself and others. In active externalization, the feelings toward oneself are experienced as feelings toward others; in passive externalization, feelings toward others are experienced as being directed by others toward oneself. (In Horney's system, projection is the shifting of responsibility or blame for one's own undesirable qualities onto others.) See *projection*.

**externalizing behaviors** See *internalizing behaviors*.

**externalizing/internalizing** A classification used by T. M. Achenbach (*Psychological Monographs 80*, 1966) to classify children on the basis of the psychiatric symptoms that manifest at the time of referral. Externalizing symptoms include acting-out and antisocial behavior and a turning against others; internalizing symptoms include excessive inhibition, anxiety, somatization, and depression. Some studies suggest that externalizers are likely to be more disturbed in adulthood (as measured by global mental health ratings) and have a higher incidence of schizophrenia than internalizers. See *internalization*.

**exteroception** Perception of touch, which is represented in the parietal somatosensory cortices. Sherrington included sensation of pain and temperature within touch, but unlike touch and other bodily feelings, pain and temperature are inherently associated with emotion. See *interoception; sensation*.

**extinction** In neurophysiology, disappearance of excitability to a previously adequate stimulus. Immediately after application of a stimulus to a nerve, there occurs a progressive depression of excitability of that nerve; at the point at which the nerve or focus becomes completely inexcitable, extinction is said to have occurred. In studies on memory, extinction refers to eradication of previously reinforced but no longer useful memories.

In subjects with unilateral brain damage, the ability to detect brief single visual stimuli on either side but an inability to detect a contralesional stimulus that is presented concurrently with an ipsilesional stimulus. Extinction for visual and tactile stimuli is found in occipitoparietal lesions; it is a defect of visual and tactile attention (and hence is also termed inattention). The subject is able to perceive stimulation in the affected sensory area when this is the only area stimulated; but if stimulated in some other area of the visual or tactile field he cannot recognize the stimulus object in the affected area.

In operant conditioning, extinction refers to the weakening and ultimate disappearance of the conditioned response when it is not reinforced or rewarded. See *amygdala*.

**extinction, order of** In genetic family studies, the statistical estimate of families dying out in a certain generation because of lack of reproduction.

**extra-axial** See *intra-axial*.

**extracampine** Outside the (usually visual) field of perception.

**extracampine hallucination** "Hallucinations which are localized outside of the sensory field in question. In the nature of the thing one deals mostly with visions, the patient sees with perfect sensory distinctness the devil behind his head, but it may also concern the sense of touch; thus the patient feels how streams of water come out from a definite point of his hand" (Bleuler, E. *Textbook of Psychiatry*, 1930).

**extractive disorders** See *adaptational psychodynamics*.

**extrapunitive** See *intropunitive*.

**extrapyramidal system** The name given to the motor system that was believed to control movement in parallel with but independent of the corticospinal (pyramidal) motor system; the *basal ganglia* (q.v.) were its major components.

The term is currently in disfavor because many other parts of the brain participate in voluntary movement; the basal ganglia and corticospinal system are interconnected rather than independent of each other; and the basal ganglia are involved in cognitive and affective functions in addition to motor functions. The term survives mainly as "extrapyramidal symptoms" (EPS), referring to symptoms of basal ganglia dysfunction that occur frequently as side effects of treatment with neuroleptics.

**extrasensory perception (ESP)** Paranormal cognition; acquisition of knowledge without using any of the known senses. Included are the following: (1) *telepathy*, the transfer of information from one mind to another; (2) *clairvoyance*, obtaining knowledge of objective events or conditions not known at the time by anyone else (such as telling what a specific page of a closed book contains); (3) *precognition*, knowing of an event before it has in fact occurred; and (4) *psychokinesis*, the ability to manipulate matter at a distance through willpower alone and without the use of any known physical means. (For another use of this term, see *psychokinesia*.)

**extrastriate body area** *EBA*; a region in the right lateral occipitotemporal cortex that appears to be organized for processing the visual appearance of the human body and body parts. See *face recognition*.

**extraversion** Disposition to turn one's interests upon or find pleasure in external things. Jung speaks of active extraversion, when the libido is "deliberately willed," and passive extraversion, "when the object compels it, i.e., attracts the interest of the subject of its own accord, even against the latter's intention" (*Psychological Types*, 1923).

The act or process of extraverting is *exteriorization*. Currently, extraversion most commonly denotes an "outgoing" personality type—gregarious, sociable, impulsive, uninhibited, optimistic, carefree, etc. There is some evidence that extraversion may be associated with low cortical arousal (and introversion with high cortical arousal). Arousal level is in large part determined by the reticular activating system. See *reticular formation*.

**extraverted type** When "the state of extraversion becomes habitual," Jung speaks of the person as possessing the extraverted type of personality. When introversion is habitual, the personality is of the introverted type. "Thus in both *general attitude* groups (the *extravert* and *introvert*) individuals with regard to *function* (i.e., reaction to a stimulus or event) may be either (1) *rational* (a) thinking, (b) feeling, or (2) *irrational* (c) intuitive, or (d) sensational" (Jung, C. G. *Psychological Types*, 1923). See *general attitude type*.

**extreme male brain theory** The *EMB theory* of autism proposes that individuals on the autistic spectrum are characterized by impairments in empathizing alongside intact or even superior systematizing. Characteristic behaviors seen in *autistic disorder* (q.v.), such as insistence on sameness, repetitive behavior, obsessions with lawful systems (e.g., train timetables), islets of ability (e.g., calendrical calculation), precocious understanding of machines, and superior attention to the detection of change, all involve a strong interest in rule-based prediction and therefore can be read as signs of hypersystematizing. See *sex differences*.

**extroversion, extrovert** Incorrect, but frequent spellings of extraversion, extravert.

**eye movement, rapid** See *sleep; REM sleep*.

**eye tracking** See *pursuit eye movements; SPEM*.

**eye tracking dysfunction** ETD. See *pursuit eye movements; SPEM*.

**eyelash sign** In unconsciousness due to functional disease, such as hysteria, stroking the eyelashes will make the lids move, but no such response occurs in organic brain lesions, such as apoplexy, fracture of the skull, or other severe head trauma.

**eye-roll sign** An index of susceptibility to hypnosis developed by psychiatrist Spiegel; the subject is directed to roll his eyes upward as far as possible and at the same time to lower his eyelids slowly. The amount of white space showing under the corneas is scored from zero (no space or "eye-roll") to five. Low scores are not hypnotizable; they tend also to be critical, controlling personality types who favor thinking over feeling. The readily hypnotizable high scorers tend to be uncritical and gullible people who are "feelers" rather than "thinkers."

**eyes, dancing** A characteristic feature of myoclonic encephalopathy of infants, whose other typical symptoms are somatic myoclonic ataxia and irritability.

# F

**FAB** Frontal Assessment Battery; a fast, short test to assess frontal lobe dysfunction. It comprises six subtests: conceptualization, verbal fluency, motor series, conflicting instruction, go–no go, and prehension behavior.

**fabrication** See *confabulation; Korsakoff psychosis*.

**Fabry disease** An inborn error of glycosphingolipid metabolism, transmitted by an X-linked gene, characterized by the systemic accumulation of glycolipids and by deficiency of the enzyme ceramide trihexosidase. (Other inborn errors of lysosomal storage and glycosphingolipid metabolism are metachromatic leukodystrophy, Gaucher disease, and Tay-Sachs disease.)

**face cells** Found primarily in the inferior temporal cortex (IT) and superior temporal sulcus (STS), face cells are neurons that respond at least twice as vigorously to faces or components of faces (such as eyes or mouths) as they do to other complex visual stimuli. The IT cortex is more important for processing facial identity, whereas STS is more involved in processing facial expressions (including eye gaze direction) and other "biological motion" inputs. See *behavioral ecology; fusiform face area*.

The evidence supports the idea that there are separate routes for face detection and face identification, with face detection being supported by a subcortical route. Studies have implicated the superior colliculus, pulvinar, and amygdala as the main structures on this fast pathway.

The adult subcortical face-processing route functions in newborns and is responsible for the patterns of face-related stimulus preference that are seen at that age. The subcortical route not only detects the presence of faces and orients the newborn towards them, but it might also activate relevant cortical regions, such as the lateral occipital, fusiform, and orbitofrontal cortices. Early enhancement of activity in selected cortical areas might assist in the recruitment of these specific cortical areas for face processing and social cognition.

**face recognition** The ability to identify individual faces despite their similarities; the perception that a face being seen is a face that has been seen previously. An allied ability is to deduce how another person is feeling from his or her facial expression. The two functions appear to be carried out by different visual pathways in the brain, which use different elements of the visual information contained by the image of a face. Face recognition is mediated by a well-demarcated, distributed hierarchical neural system, the core of which consists of bilateral occipitotemporal regions in the extrastriate visual cortex, most notably the right fusiform gyrus, the inferior occipital gyri, and the anterior temporal cortex. See *fusiform face area; object recognition*. The fusiform face area (FFA) is selectively activated by images of faces, and images of fearful faces also activate the amygdala. The amygdala, unlike FFA, is activated by fearful faces even if those faces are not consciously perceived or attended.

There is evidence that a region in the right lateral occipitotemporal cortex—the *extrastriate body area (EBA)*—is a specialized system for processing the visual appearance of the human body and body parts (*body recognition*). The EBA is anatomically distinct from the retinotopic cortex, fusiform face area, and the parahippocampal place area. See *social cognitive neuroscience*.

Reduced facial recognition memory and decreased extraversion have been correlated with schizotypal personality traits and schizophrenia, and smaller right posterior fusiform gyrus volumes have been reported in patients with schizophrenia.

**face validity** See *validity*.

**face-hand test** *Fink-Green-Bender test*; a test of diffuse cerebral dysfunction. The subject, whose eyes are closed, is touched simultaneously on the cheek and the dorsum of the hand; retesting is done with the eyes open. Ten trials are given: eight face-hand (divided between four contralateral and four ipsilateral), and two interspersed combinations of face-face and hand-hand stimulation. Results are considered positive if the subject fails consistently to identify both stimuli within

10 trials. By the age of 7, normal children respond with a negative test. Positive results are seen not only in cases of cerebral dysfunction in children and adults, but also in schizophrenic children. See *double simultaneous tactile sensation.*

**facial nerve** The seventh cranial nerve. It is primarily a motor nerve that originates in the posterior pons and supplies the stapedius muscle of the middle ear and the superficial musculature of the face and scalp. Parasympathetic fibers supply the glands and mucous membranes of the pharynx, palate, and nasal cavity. The facial nerve also has some sensory fibers that carry taste from the anterior tongue. Lesions of the facial nerve may be peripheral (*Bell palsy* or *prosoplegia*), nuclear, or supranuclear.

In peripheral facial paralysis, the following signs will be seen on the affected side: drooping mouth, inability to whistle or wink or wrinkle forehead, tearing of eye, loss of deep facial sensation, food collecting between cheek and gum, and paralysis of the flaccid (lower motor neuron) type.

In the nuclear type of facial palsy, the above signs are also seen and, in addition, contralateral hemiplegia due to pyramidal involvement. In the supranuclear type of facial palsy, the paralysis is of the spastic (upper motor neuron) type, the frontalis muscle is spared because of its bilateral cortical innervation, and reflexes and emotional responses are retained. Supranuclear facial paralysis is often associated with homolateral hemiplegia or monoplegia.

**facies, ironed-out** The facial expression of patients with general paresis. The loss of tone of the muscles of expression gives the face the appearance of having been "ironed-out" or flattened.

**facies, mongolian** A disfavored term for the facial appearance of a patient with *Down syndrome* (q.v.); characteristic features are slanted palpebral fissures, small ear lobules, irregular alignment of teeth, and large tongue or lips.

**facilitating environment** Winnicott's term for the maternally provided empathy and appropriateness of response to the infant's cues about his or her needs. This is closely related to the *average expectable environment* (Hartmann), the functioning of the *good enough mother* (Winnicott), *mutual cueing* (Mahler), parental *mirroring* (Kernberg), and the *container-contained maternal function*

(Bion). See *communicative matching; empathic failure; fit.*

**facilitation** In neurophysiology, shortening of the central reflex time (the synaptic delay, i.e., that portion of the total latent period of a reflex that is due to passage of impulse through internuncial neurons) either by giving a second stimulus soon after the first, or by increasing the strength of the stimulus. Facilitation is to be differentiated from *summation* (q.v.). See *reinforcement.*

The above definition refers to local facilitation. It is known that facilitation (or suppression) from a distance may also occur, especially in motor areas of the cortex. The existence of bands of facilitation and suppression in the cortex has been established by Dusser de Barenne et al.

In genetics, facilitation refers to that form of interaction between hereditary and environmental factors in which a genetic tendency to a particular malformation or abnormality becomes manifest only under conditions of gestational stress.

**FACS** 1. *Facial Action Coding System*, a method of describing any facial expression objectively in terms of the basic muscle units that produce it and of the measurement of each unit's timing, intensity, and extent of bilateral symmetry.

2. Fellow of the American College of Surgeons.

**factitial** Factitious; artificial. A factitial disease, such as hypoglycemia factitia, is any symptom, syndrome, injury, or illness that is self-inflicted. See *Munchhausen syndrome.*

**factitious disorders** A group of disorders whose physical or psychologic symptoms are produced by the subject and are under voluntary control; *pathomimicry*. In contrast to *malingering* (q.v.), there is no apparent goal other than to assume the role of patient.

Factitious disorder many be manifested as (1) a factitious history only, (2) feigned illness, or (3) creation of actual pathophysiology. Differentiation from malingering depends on the intentionality of deceit in factitious disorder, in contrast to the unconscious deception of somatoform disorder. Women are 20 to 40 times more frequently affected than men, and they often work in medically related occupations. Their symptoms and signs typically consist of the following:

1. Factitious fever, either simulated by manipulation of a thermometer or stimulated

by self-infection (e.g., injecting saliva, urine, or other contaminated substances intravenously or subcutaneously);

2. Simulated illnesses, such as dermatitis artefacta (self-induced skin lesions); factitious bleeding disorder produced by surreptitious ingestion of dicumarol or coumadin; factitious hypoglycemia, typically induced by injecting insulin or ingesting oral hypoglycemic agents;

3. Chronic wounds— usually exacerbating preexisting lesions;

4. Self-medication, which the patient hides from his or her physician.

Factitious disorder with psychological symptoms formerly included the *Ganser syndrome* (q.v.), which is now classified as a dissociative disorder. Chronic factitious disorder with physical symptoms (*Munchhausen syndrome*, q.v.) is also known as *hospital addiction syndrome*, and patients are called *hospital hoboes*. Physical symptoms, presented so convincingly that multiple hospitalizations are the rule, may include acute abdominal and neurologic complaints, hemorrhage, skin rashes and abscesses, or involvement of any organ system.

*Factitious disorder by proxy* (a controversial diagnostic entity) refers to a person who produces symptoms in another, such as a mother who produces symptoms in her child so that she can indirectly assume a sick role. In such a situation, it is the mother who receives the diagnosis of factitious disorder by proxy. Should it happen that the child, for any reason, colludes with the mother in producing the symptoms, the child would be diagnosed as having factitious disorder, the mother as having factitious disorder by proxy.

**factor** In genetics, practically identical with *gene.*

**factorial** Pertaining to a genetic factor or a combination of factors.

**factorial design** A method of research in which two or more variables are manipulated deliberately to allow study of the interaction between them as well as the main effect of each variable.

**facultative** Having the power to live or operate under other conditions; that is, nonobligatory. In psychiatry, most commonly applied to homosexuality *faute de mieux* (q.v.), and to other cases in which homosexuality is symptomatic of specific neurotic conflicts. See *homosexuality, male.*

**FADD** Fas-associated death domain protein; an adaptor protein whose death domain interacts with the *death domains* of the receptors for *Fas* to activate the cell's apoptotic machinery (qq.v.)

**Fahr disease** Idiopathic nonarteriosclerotic symmetrical calcification of cerebral vessels, especially in the basal ganglia, first described in 1930 by T. Fahr, a German neurologist (1877–1945). It is a rare, slowly progressive, hereditary disorder characterized by the following:

1. Movement disorders, including Parkinson-like syndromes, choreoathetosis, cerebellar ataxia, and paralysis; and

2. Neuropsychiatric manifestations, including progressive dementia, schizophreniform psychosis, and depression. Some authorities distinguish two subtypes: one with onset around 30 years of age and with psychosis as the initial manifestation, and the other with onset around 50 years of age and with dementia as the initial manifestation.

**failure script** See *abandonment depression; empathic failure.*

**failure through success** A term used by Freud to describe the self-injuring conduct of those who, on the verge of achieving a long-desired aim, renounce it, obtaining gratification through its renunciation. Examples are "the clinical assistant who for so long desired to become professor and renounced the position on his predecessor's sudden death," or "the girl who withdrew from the beloved man at the sudden death of his wife, her rival." It is a moral veto, which occurs only when it is preceded by a period of phantasy that anticipates the misfortune or the death of the rival (Reik, T. *Masochism in Modern Man*, 1941). See *destiny, neurosis of; masochism; obedience, deferred.*

**failure to thrive** Also nonorganic failure to thrive (*NFTT*) and *attachment disorder of infancy* (q.v.); a nonorganic disorder of the first 2 years of life characterized by marked deceleration of weight gain and growth and slowed acquisition of developmental milestones. Several subtypes have been described: Type I, in which the caregiver both undernourishes and understimulates the infant; Type II, in which the caregiver provides adequate stimulation but, because of misinformation or lack of resources, fails to provide adequate nutrition; and Type III, in which the mother reacts with anger or depression to the infant's struggle for autonomy, which is then typically expressed in behavioral disturbance based on food refusal but not in any developmental abnormalities.

At least in Types I and II, such distortions in early life experience bespeak a poor prognosis in the long run; persisting defects in physical or intellectual development and behavior problems are the rule rather than the exception. See *psychosocial dwarfism*.

**failure to warn**   See *warn, duty to*.

**Fairbairn, Ronald**   (1889–1964) Scottish psychoanalyst; object relations theory; *Psychoanalytical Studies of the Personality* (1952).

**Fairweather lodges**   See *domicile*.

**faith cure**   Improvement (less frequently, cure) as a result of faith or confidence of the patient in the therapist and/or the therapeutic method, probably a response to supportive psychotherapy, and to prestige suggestion and persuasion.

**faith healing**   A form of *folk medicine* (q.v.) found in many fundamentalist Christian denominations in the United States, with an emphasis on personal testimonials of successful healing, coming forth in a group meeting with the complaint(s) and being prayed over by the healer and the elders of the church. See *complementary medicine*.

**fallacia**   *Obs.* An illusion or hallucination.

**fallectomy**   See *salpingectomy*.

**fallen fontanel syndrome**   *Susto* (q.v.).

**falling out**   A culture-specific syndrome, reported among black Americans and black Caribbeans, consisting of sudden collapse and inability to move, see, or speak. See *culture-specific syndromes*.

**Falret, Jean-Pierre**   (1794–1870) French psychiatrist; in 1854, Falret and Baillarger independently described recurring attacks of mania and melancholia in the same patient.

**Falret, Jules Ph. J.**   (1824–1902) French psychiatrist; in 1879 described "folie circulaire" and "mixed states," which he considered to be transitory stages between attacks of mania and depression.

**false alarm rate**   See *vigilance*.

**false confession**   A statement, usually made under pressure, that one has committed a crime of which he or she is not guilty. *Innocence Projects* use DNA analysis from crime scenes to exonerate innocent persons. Approximately 25% of such cases have involved false confessions

arising from inappropriate police interrogations. Persons with mental impairment appear to be disproportionately represented within that group. Mentally ill defendants, particularly defendants with psychotic disorders, are significantly less likely to understand their interrogation rights than defendants who are not mentally ill. Disorganization of thought, deficits in executive functioning and attention, and impaired decision making, for instance, could contribute to self-incrimination.

Some police interrogations employ psychological manipulation to obtain "confessions." *Minimization techniques*—such as feigning sympathy, offering a moral justification for the crime, or shifting blame—are used to placate accused suspects and lead them into a false sense of security. *Maximization techniques*—such as presenting false evidence—attempt to browbeat the suspect into confessing. Persons with mental illness may be more susceptible to both.

**false consensus**   Believing that others would do what the person chooses to do as an individual, often expressed as conformity to the perceived reaction of one's peers. *Torture* can sometimes be understood as, at least partly, a crime of socialized obedience. Subordinates not only do what they are ordered to do, but what they think their superiors would order them to do.

**false ego**   See *Lacan, Jacques*.

**false memory**   *Pseudomemory*; a memory of a past event, usually of a traumatic experience, that is not supported by fact. In the 1990s, the concept of a false memory syndrome was developed in an attempt to explain the marked increase in the number of cases of multiple personality disorder and of allegations by adults of having been traumatized and sexually abused during childhood years. Some authorities suggested that at least some instances of multiple personality and some allegations of childhood sexual assault were based on suggestions or interpretations of the therapist, or that they represented retrieval of childhood phantasies rather than memories of actual experiences. *False memory syndrome* described a condition in which a person's identity and interpersonal relationships revolve about a memory that, although unfounded, is strongly believed and maintained despite evidence that challenges the memory. Other authorities dismiss the concept of false memory syndrome as being without scientific foundation, calling it a "rhetorical pejorative."

Memory is malleable. Witnesses of a scene may pick up information from sources other than the scene itself; they combine bits of memory from different experiences; leading questions or other forms of misinformation contaminate their memories; witnesses talk to one another at the scene and cross-contaminate each other's memories. Studies have shown that imagination can affect autobiographical information; imagination can lead people to remember their past in ways that conform to their wishes about the past and to deny the events that actually occurred. Multiple identities can be "created" and elicited easily from many normal people. People can come to construct memories of abuse, for instance, even if they have not personally experienced it.

**false recognition, illusions of** See *Capgras syndrome.*

**False Self** Winnicott's term for an external, compliant aspect of a person, contrasted with the True Self, an internal, authentic, and uncompliant aspect. Organized reactions to maternal failure, such as nonempathy or not relating to the child as he or she really is, form the False Self. The analytic setting provides an opportunity for the patient to find a place to resume suspended True Self activity. See *impingement.*

Laing stressed the false self of the schizoid (narcissistic) patient, the compulsively compliant appearance that is presented to the world devoid of hatred or other "negative" feelings. According to Laing, the schizoid splits into a secret true self and a body associated with the false self. He also splits himself from the world and tries to do everything by himself, oscillating between merger with the object and isolation (rather than oscillating between genuine relatedness and separation, as the normal person does). The false self system arises as a defense against *ontological insecurity* (q.v.) in a person whose true self in childhood was not adequately confirmed or mirrored.

**falsehood, unconscious** A false or untrue statement made by a person without intention or without his being aware of its false nature.

**falsification, memory** See *confabulation; Korsakoff psychosis.*

**falsification, retrospective** The addition of false details and meanings to a true memory; especially common in paranoid schizophrenia,

where past experiences may be related to conform with the delusional system.

**falx cerebelli, cerebri** See *meninges.*

**fames canina** *Obs.* Bulimia.

**familial** A normal or morbid trait tending, or observed, "to run in families." As the hereditary origin of such a trait is not proved by the mere observation of its occurrence in several members of the same family, the use of the expression "familial" is to be interpreted in the sense that in the particular case of a disease or another trait the genetic basis either is not to be stressed or is as yet unknown. See *heredity.*

**familial alcoholism** Pattern of alcoholism occurring in more than one generation within a family, due to either genetic or environmental factors.

**familial hemiplegic migraine** *FHM;* characterized by obligatory motor aura symptoms that consist of unilateral motor weakness or paralysis, and usually visual, sensory, or aphasic symptoms as well. The aura is usually unilateral. Some FHM patients have atypical severe attacks with impairment of consciousness (coma) or prolonged hemiplegia that last several days. About 20% of FHM families show progressive cerebellar ataxia or permanent nystagmus. See *migraine.*

FHM is genetically heterogeneous. Different missense mutations in *CACNA1A* (on chromosome 19), the gene coding for the pore-forming $\alpha_1$-subunit of $Ca_v2.1$ (the voltage-gated $Ca^{2+}$ channel), are associated with type 1 FHM (FHM1). Missense mutations in *ATP1A2* (on chromosome 1q23), the gene encoding the $\alpha_2$-subunit of the $Na^+/K^+$ ATPase, have been reported in two familes (FHM2).

**familianism** A sociological and psychological term emphasizing the tendency to maintain strong intrafamilial bonds, ties, and demands, culturally transmitted and inherited, and making for intensely compact family life and solidarity.

**familiarity** One aspect of recognition of previously encountered information: the more frequently an event has been observed the more likely it is to be recognized on the basis of familiarity alone Repetition affects the integration of information rather than its retrieval; it establishes familiarity independent of the context of the information or its relationship to other mental contents. See *memory.*

**famille névropathique (F. "neuropathic family")**  A group of degenerative diseases in which Charcot included hysteria, since heredity, he felt, was the unique originating cause.

**family, artificial**  Used in research especially in schizophrenia; introduced by N. E. Waxler (*Family Process 13*, 1974), who created artificial families composed of parents of normal or schizophrenic children paired with normal and then schizophrenic offspring from other families. She found that the schizophrenic child gave only minimal disruption to normal parents; that schizophrenic parents have little effect on normal children; but that schizophrenic children showed significant improvement in cognitive performance after working on a task together with normal parents.

**family, extended**  See *conjugal unit, isolated*.

**family, nuclear**  Traditionally defined as a married couple with children under the age of 18 years in the home. The number of such households has been declining in the United States and many European countries since the 1960s. The number of people living with nonrelatives (e.g., unmarried female-male couples, homosexual couples, friends sharing an apartment) has been increasing.

**family based association**  A method used in genetic studies that compares the frequencies of the mutant allele in patients who have the disorder with its frequencies in their unaffected siblings. See *behavioral genetics*.

**family care**  The boarding out of chronic patients (usually schizophrenics, tractable mental retardates, or senile cases) with relatives or, more commonly, with unrelated guardians. The patient is absorbed not only into the guardian's home but into the life of the local community as well. Perhaps the best known organized system of family care is the *Gheel Colony* (q.v.) in Antwerp, Belgium.

**family counseling**  See *genetic counseling*.

**family culture, indigenous**  The structure of a family such as its belief about itself, its conceptions about its relation to the social world in which it lives, its hierarchy of power and influences, and the openness of its boundaries to outsiders. Various objective measures of different aspects of such structures have been developed, among them *coordination* and *configuration* (qq.v.).

**family evaluation**  "One or more family interviews conducted to assess the structure and process of family interactions, to determine how the family influences and is influenced by the behavior and symptoms of its individual members, and to gather the data necessary to decide whether family treatment is possible and indicated" (Grunebaum, H. & Glick, I.D. in *Psychiatry Update II*, ed. L. Grinspoon, 1983).

**family group intake**  See *intake, family group*.

**family identity**  A family's experience of itself as a group, including its distance from or closeness to the outside world, its traditions and feelings of continuity with the past, and its feelings of internal cohesion.

**family intervention**  Family therapy; the term is most frequently used to refer to treatment that involves the family members of alcohol and drug addicts and is designed to benefit the target patient as well as the family constellation.

**family pattern**  The style of living within a family, and particularly the quality of the relationship between parents and child. Among the different family patterns described are *symbiotic* unions, where parent and child form an inseparable bond; *family sacrifice*, where the child is rejected and excluded from the family; *open*, when the family has friends, entertains, and is active in the community; and *closed*, when the family shuns contact with the outside. Some workers have found that families of schizophrenics are often symbiotic unions or are closed, and that more demonstrate family sacrifice than do families of nonschizophrenics.

**family romance**  See *romance, family*.

**family social work**  "Family social work is a field of organized practice having to do with human relationships. Its main purpose is to help individuals deal effectively with difficulties experienced in relating themselves to others in their families and in their communities. This practice is based on a growing body of knowledge about human beings as functioning members of society and it employs the technique and art termed social case work" (*Social Work Year Book*, 1939).

**family studies**  1. In family therapy, the formal, quantitative investigations of family process and clinical descriptions of family life and family therapy.

2. In genetics and epidemiology, case-controlled investigations of illness in the relatives of patients or in normal controls.

**family systems interview** A diagnostic-therapeutic interview conducted over one or two sessions very early in the treatment process as a way of understanding the contexts in which the symptomatic behavior is distinctively present or absent, and as an opportunity to observe the reactions of the family as various subjects are discussed.

**family therapy** A professionally organized attempt to ameliorate disturbances in the marital or family unit, primarily through nonpharmacologic means with an emphasis on relationships and behavior patterns rather than on individual pathology. The goal is more satisfying ways of living for the entire family and not just for one family member.

Nathan Ackerman's seminal paper, "The Family as a Social and Emotional Unit," appeared in 1937 in the *Bulletin of the Kansas Mental Hygiene Society*. In 1959 Don D. Jackson introduced the phrase *conjoint family therapy* to describe the situation in which the whole family works with the same therapist in the same room at the same time. In the same year, Jackson founded the Mental Research Institute, whose staff included Dick Fish, Jay Haley, Jules Riskin, Virginia Satir, Paul Wazlawick, and John Weakland.

In family therapy, the focus is on the way relationships are structured within the family rather than on intrapsychic events within an identified patient, on the context within which events occur rather than on a search for specific causes of particular diseases. Family therapy often follows a biopsychosocial systems model (often referred to as *family systems therapy*) rather than a biomedical linear model. It is process-oriented rather than outcome-oriented and looks for patterns of interaction and the function that the symptom or "problem" fulfills within the family system.

The family is viewed as a rule-governed, change-resistant transactional system sustained by the conformity of the family members to the operational objectives of the system. The dysfunctional family, for instance, often fails to support children in their movement away from the family and hampers their individuation and social maturation. Family therapy attempts to improve the social functioning of the whole family so that no generation will inhibit the individuation and separation of an adjacent generation.

Family psychotherapy is based on the hypothesis that the patient's psychosis is a symptom manifestation of a problem involving all members of the family (Bowen, M., in *Schizophrenia—An Integrated Approach*, ed. A. Auerbach, 1959). Bowen and his coworkers find that the father, the mother, and the patient (the *interdependent triad*) are the primary members involved. These investigators have further noted that in all their schizophrenic families there is a striking emotional distance between the parents (*emotional divorce*) that is maintained by a combination of controlled positiveness and physical distance. In such families, both parents are immature and true family teamwork is never possible. Instead, one parent will seize authority and make decisions for himself and his spouse, forcing the latter into a submissive, helpless role. This pattern has been termed *overadequate-inadequate reciprocity*.

**family therapy, strategic** Brief family therapy that emphasizes the role symptoms play in maintaining a dysfunctional or pathological family system. Highly structured team interviews and paradoxical task assignment are frequently used. Strategic family therapy is associated with the "Palo Alto School" (Haley, Wazlawick, influenced by Bateson and Erickson and by Selvini-Palazzoli and her coworkers in Milan). See *paradoxical therapy*.

**family therapy, structural** Developed by Minuchin, originally for use with economically disadvantaged families with multiple problems, it focuses on the structuring of interaction patterns (e.g., disengagement, enmeshment, rigidity, triangulation) that have been dysfunctional when used in the nuclear family's efforts toward conflict resolution. Existing structures are challenged, subsystem boundaries are clarified, the family system is organized hierarchically, and more functional interaction patterns are developed, starting in the therapy sessions themselves. Structural family therapy has been applied beyond the multiproblem family and is said to be of particular value in families with psychosomatic illnesses.

**family therapy, systematic** A form of communication therapy in which the family system is redefined in various ways as working for its own best interests in its apparent dysfunction. As an example, the dysfunction is recognized as a way to avoid change that would be even more threatening to the family than the dysfunction is. Characteristic of systematic family therapy is a radical neutrality of therapeutic attitude. It is associated with Selvini-Palazzoli, Boscolo, Cecchin, and Prata.

**family types**  Alanen of Helsinki University (Finland) reports that two general types of families can be distinguished in the group of schizophrenics: chaotic and rigid. Intrusive parent–child relationships are found in both, but in rigid families possessive and restrictive parental attitudes predominate, whereas in chaotic families the parents are unable to separate themselves psychologically from their children, often hold unusually fanatical or deviant norms, and are excessively inconsistent.

**family violence**  See *domestic violence.*

**fanaticism**  Excessive, unreasonable zeal on any subject, such as religion; fanaticism, like litigiousness, is extremely frequent in paranoids, whose zealotry in the espousing of causes may approach the delusional.

**fantastic confabulation**  See *confabulation.*

**fantasy**  See *phantasy.*

**fantasying, active**  A psychotherapeutic procedure in which the patient is asked to relate his spontaneous imagery. An analysis of these fantasied images enables the physician to find out the roots of the patient's conflicts. If it becomes possible to show the patient these unconscious connections, he is in a position to recognize the source of his conflicts and is able to bring the conflict within the sphere of conscious insight and control (Baynes, H. G. *Mythology of the Soul,* 1940).

**FAP**  Fixed action pattern. See *instinct.*

**FAS**  *Fetal alcohol syndrome* (q.v.).

**Fas**  Also known as *Apo1, CD95L;* fas and *TNF* are important extracellular actvators in the mammalian immune system. The cognate receptors for these cytokines contain cytoplasmic *death domains* (q.v.) that activate the cell's apoptotic machinery through interaction with the death domains of the adaptor proteins *FADD* (Fas-associated death domain; also called *MORT1*) and *TRADD.*

**fasciculus cuneatus**  *Tract of Burdach,* located in the posterior white column of the spinal cord between the fasciculus gracilis and the posterior gray column. The fasciculus cuneatus carries proprioception and vibratory sensation fibers from the upper limbs. These fibers terminate in the nucleus cuneatus at the

medulla, whence arise internal arcuate fibers, some of which proceed to the homolateral restiform body and most of which cross to form the medial lemniscus of the opposite side.

**fasciculus gracilis**  *Tract of Goll,* located in the posterior white column of the spinal cord next to the posterior (dorsal) median septum. The fasciculus gracilis carries proprioception and vibratory sensation fibers mainly from the lower limbs. These fibers terminate in the nucleus gracilis at the medulla, whence arise internal arcuate fibers, some of which proceed to the homolateral restiform body and most of which cross to form the medial lemniscus of the opposite side.

**fascinating gaze**  In hypnosis, fixation of the eyes of the hypnotist on the subject.

**fascination**  When a desire for mastery of some factor in the environment cannot be gratified, a partial mastery of it is sometimes achieved by means of identification with it. This reaction is called fascination. For example, if an infant is seen paying rapt attention to a rattle which the mother waves before it, a phase preliminary to mastery can be assumed. But if mastery is not possible because the rattle is beyond reach, or perhaps because the knack of reaching has not yet been learned, there still remains the rapt attention, which becomes greatly intensified. The infant, so to say, loses itself in the sight and sound of the rattle and thus becomes one with it, and through identification, a partial mastery is achieved by way of fascination.

**fascinum**  (L. "witchcraft") An ancient belief that certain people possess "the evil eye," because of which they are capable of fascinating and injuring others by looking at them.

**FASPS**  Familial advanced sleep-phase syndrome, due to a mutation of the gene *hPer2,* on chromosome 2. The mutation speeds up the circadian clock of affected subjects, who are "early birds", rising as early as 4 a.m.

**FAST**  See *GDS.*

**fastigial nuclei**  See *cerebellum.*

**fat depletion syndrome**  See *lipodystrophy.*

**fatal familial insomnia**  *FFI*; an inherited form of spongiform encephalopathy characterized by untreatable insomnia, dysautonomia, and severe atrophy of thalamic nuclei. See β-*amyloid disorders.* Like CJD or *Creutzfeldt-Jakob disease* (q.v.), FFI is associated with a double point mutation in the PRNP gene. In both disorders, a mutation at codon 178 results in the substitution of asparagine for aspartic acid. There is a second mutation at codon 129, which codes for either methionine (in 62% of Caucasian populations) or valine (in 38%). Homozygosity for either one predisposes to infectious forms of spongiform encephalopathies, such as kuru and CJD, or affects the age of onset of inherited Gerstmann-Straussler-Scheinker syndrome. When the codon 178 mutation is combined with the presence of methionine at position 129, the result is FFI; when the codon 178 mutation is combined with the presence of valine at position 129, the result is CJD.

**fate neurosis**  Failure in one's career as a result of unconscious need for punishment; a type of moral masochism. See *destiny, neurosis of; masochism.*

**father, vaginal**  A motherly, unaggressive, feminine kind of husband or father, who typically has significant conflicts revolving about unconscious identification with his own mother.

**father fixation**  Inordinate attachment to the father. See *fixation; Oedipus complex.*

**father substitute**  See *mother surrogate; surrogate.*

**father-ideal**  A psychoanalytic term for the father component of the ego-ideal. Jones writes: "If we inquire into the matter and origin of the ego-ideal, we discover that it is compounded of two constituents, derived from the Father and the Self respectively—the original (primal) narcissism of the infant becomes in the course of development distributed in four directions, the actual proportion in each of these varying enormously with different individuals. *One* portion remains in an unaltered state attached to the real ego; that is probably the one concerned in the genesis of hypochondria. A *second* portion is deflected from any direct sexual goal and becomes attached to the ideal of the parent, leading to adoration, devotion, and general overestimation. It is important to bear in mind that to begin with this process is much more a matter of narcissistic identification than of any form of object-love. A *third* is transferred on to an ideal ego, and is one of the constituents of the 'ego-ideal.' The *fourth* is gradually transformed into object-love. Now the second and third of these commonly fuse during the latency period of childhood or even earlier. The form assumed by the resulting ego-ideal is largely derived from the ideas and mental attitudes of the father, the bond being effected through the second portion of the narcissistic libido mentioned above—that attached to what may be called the *father-ideal*. On the other hand, the energy that gives the ego-ideal its significance is wholly derived ultimately from narcissistic libido. There are three routes for this: (1) directly from the original narcissism of the primary ego (third portion mentioned above); (2) via the attachment to the *father-ideal* (second portion); (3) via the regression of narcissistic identification with the father that often takes place after a disappointment at the lack of gratification of object-love (fourth portion) " (Jones, E. J. *Papers on Psycho-Analysis*, 1949). See *ego-ideal; superego.*

**father-imago**  See *image.*

**fatigue state**  See *hypoglycemia.*

**fatigue syndrome**  See *chronic fatigue syndrome.*

**fatty acids**  See *omega-3 fatty acids.*

**fatuity**  Feeblemindedness; sometimes used synonymously with dementia of any kind.

**fault, basic**  Balint's term for impairment of narcissism based on inadequate mother-infant bonding and expressed as a feeling that one is defective or damaged. See *partialism, persistent.*

**faulty action**  *Symptomatic act* (q.v.).

**faunorum ludibria**  *Obs.* Sometimes meaning nightmare, and at other times referring to epilepsy.

**faute de mieux**  (F. "for want of anything better") In psychiatry, this term is ordinarily used to refer to so-called accidental homosexuality, in which a person chooses a same-sexed person as a sexual object when no other-sexed person is available.

**Faxenpsychosis**  *Buffoonery psychosis* (q.v.).

**FE65**  A cytoplasmic scaffold protein. See *Alzheimer disease.*

**fear**  A reaction to real or threatened danger, with many of the same psychological and physiological elements that characterize *anxiety* and *stress* (qq.v.).

When the senses pick up a threat—a loud noise, a scary sight—the information takes two different routes through the brain:

1. An immediate fear response—the brain automatically activates the amygdala, the fear center and emotional core of the brain, which tags information with emotional significance. The amygdala triggers the fear response, consisting of (a) activation of the hypothalamus

and pituitary, causing the adrenal glands to release high levels of the stress hormone cortisol; (b) activation of the sympathetic nervous system, increasing activity in the heart (blood pressure and pulse rise), lungs (hyperventilation), sweat glands, and nerve endings (whose tingling produces goosebumps); (c) adrenaline shoots to the muscles preparing the body for fight or flight, and the senses become hyperattentive to potential new threats; and (d) digestion shuts down to conserve energy (sometimes with vomiting, involuntary defecation or urination).

2. The thalamus processes sensory information (sights, sounds, smells, touch); it breaks down incoming visual cues by size, shape, and color, and auditory cues by volume and dissonance, and then signals the appropriate parts of cortex. Olfactory and tactile stimuli, however, go directly to the amygdala, as a result of which smells often evoke stronger memories or feelings than do sights or sounds. The cortex analyzes the raw sights and sounds, enabling the brain to become conscious of what it is seeing or hearing. The hippocampus stores the new information coming in from the senses, along with the emotional baggage attached to the data during their trip through the amygdala. If the alert is warranted, the cortex signals the amygdala to maintain the alert; if it is not necessary, prefrontal cortex (PFC) acts as a brake and shuts down the emergency response.

Should it happen that too much cortisol is released, or its high level is too long maintained as part of the immediate fear response, cells in the hippocampus are short-circuited. The subject has difficulty in organizing the memory of the stressful experience; memories of it lose their context and become fragmented.

**fear, guilty**   Rado's term for the fear that dire consequences are in store for one because of a misdeed (or forbidden impulse). Guilty fear is thus a derivative of the dread of conscience. It is a prominent feature of the obsessive syndrome, where it opposes the patient's defiant rage and leads, ultimately, to repression of the latter. See *obsessive attack*.

**fear, impulse**   A fear that arises within the subject, more or less directly from an instinctual source. It is contrasted with real fear, which is associated with some real object in the environment. The fear of being in a dark place is a real or a "reality" fear. The fear of imminent collapse and death, while in excellent health, is an impulse fear.

**fear learning**   Fear learning involves the lateral and basolateral parts of the amygdala, where the association between incoming fearful and neutral stimuli leads to potentiation of synaptic transmission. These parts project to the central amygdala (CeA), whose efferents to the hypothalamus and brain stem trigger the autonomic expression of fear. CeA expresses numerous neuropeptides and neuropeptide receptors, including high levels of receptors for vasopressin and oxytocin. Vasopressin enhances aggressiveness, anxiety, and stress levels and the consolidation of fear memory. Oxytocin decreases anxiety and stress and facilitates social encounters, maternal care, and the extinction of conditioned avoidance behavior. Vasopressin and oxytocin modulate activity in CeM (medial part of CeA) neurons in opposite ways through the activation of distinct elements of an inhibitory network.

**fear of**

    **air:** aerophobia

    **animals:** zoophobia

    **anything new:** kaino(to)phobia; neophobia

    **bacilli:** bacillophobia

    **bad men:** pavor sceleris; sclerophobia

    **barren space:** cenophobia; kenophobia

    **bearing a monster:** teratophobia

    **bees:** apiphobia; melissophobia

    **being afraid:** phobophobia

    **being alone:** autophobia; eremiophobia; monophobia

    **being beaten:** mastigophobia

    **being buried alive:** taphephobia

    **being dirty:** automysophobia

    **being enclosed:** clithrophobia

    **being laughed at:** catagelophobia

    **being locked in:** claustrophobia; clithrophobia

    **being looked at:** scopophobia

    **being overweight:** barophobia

    **being tied up:** merinthophobia

    **being touched:** (h)aphephobia; haptephobia

    **birds:** ornithophobia

    **blood:** hematophobia; hemophobia

    **blushing:** ereuthophobia; erythrophobia, sekimen-kyofu

**books:** bibliophobia
**brain disease:** meningitophobia
**burglars:** scelerophobia
**cancer:** carcinomatophobia
**cats:** ailurophobia; geleophobia; gatophobia
**change:** kainophobia; kainotophobia; neophobia
**childbirth:** maieusiophobia
**choking:** anginophobia; pnigophobia
**clowns:** coulrophobia
**cold:** cheimaphobia; psychropophobia
**color(s):** chromatophobia; chromophobia
**comets:** cometophobia
**confinement:** claustrophobia
**contamination:** coprophobia; molysmophobia; mysophobia; scatophobia
**corpses:** necrophobia
**(crossing a) bridge or river:** gephyrophobia
**(crossing a) street:** dromophobia
**(crossing a) threshold**: bathmophobia
**crowds:** demophobia; ochlophobia
**cumbersome pseudoscientific terms:** hellenologophobia
**dampness:** hygrophobia
**darkness:** achluophobia; nyctophobia; scotophobia
**dawn:** eosophobia
**daylight:** phengophobia
**death:** necrophobia; thanatophobia
**definite disease:** monopathophobia
**deformity:** dysmorphophobia, shubokyofu
**demons:** demonia; demonomania; entheomania
**depths:** bathophobia
**devils:** demonophobia; satanophobia
**dirt:** mysophobia; rhypophobia; rupophobia
**disease:** nosophobia; pathophobia
**dizziness, vertigo:** illyngophobia
**dogs:** cynophobia
**dolls:** pediophobia
**dust:** amathophobia
**eating:** cibophobia; phagophobia; sitophobia
**electricity:** electrophobia
**emptiness:** kenophobia
**enclosed spaces:** claustrophobia
**entering a body of water**: equaphobia
**escalators:** bathmophobia
**everything:** pamphobia (*Obs.*); panphobia; panophobia; pantophobia
**examination:** examination phobia

**excrement:** coprophobia; scatophobia
**eyes:** ommatophobia
**failure:** kakorrhaphiophobia
**falling:** barophobia
**fatigue:** kopophobia
**fearing:** phobophobia
**feathers:** pteronophobia
**feces:** coprophobia
**female genitals:** eurotophobia
**fever:** febriophobia; fibriphobia; pyrexiophobia
**filth:** mysophobia; rhypophobia; rupophobia
**filth (personal):** automysophobia
**fire:** pyrophobia
**fish:** ichthyophobia
**flash of lightning:** selaphobia
**flogging:** mastigophobia
**floods:** antlophobia
**flutes:** aulophobia
**flying:** aerophobia; aviophobia
**fog:** homichlophobia
**food:** cibophobia; phagophobia; sit(i)ophobia
**foreigners**: xenophobia
**forests:** hylophobia
**frogs:** batrachophobia
**functioning:** ergasiophobia
**germs:** spermophobia
**ghosts:** phasmophobia
**girls:** parthenophobia
**glass:** crystallophobia; hyelophobia
**God:** theophobia
**gravity:** barophobia
**hair:** trichopathophobia; trichophobia
**heat:** thermophobia
**heaven:** siderophobia; uranophobia
**heights:** acrophobia; bathophobia; hyposophobia
**hell:** hadephobia; stygiophobia
**heredity:** patroiophobia
**high buildings or objects**: batophobia
**horses:** equinophobia
**houses:** domatophobia; oikophobia
**human beings**: anthropophobia
**humiliation:** catagelophobia
**ideas:** ideophobia
**impending death:** meditatio mortis; thanatophobia
**infinity:** apeirophobia
**injury:** traumatophobia
**innovation:** neophobia
**insanity:** lyssophobia; maniaphobia
**insects:** acarophobia; entomophobia

**jealousy:** zelophobia
**justice:** dikephobia
**knives:** aichmophobia
**large objects:** megalophobia
**left:** levophobia; sinistrophobia
**lice:** ptheirophobia
**light:** photophobia
**lightning:** astraphobia; astrapophobia; keraunophobia
**loneliness:** erem(i)ophobia; monophobia
**machinery:** mechanophobia
**many things:** polyphobia
**marriage:** gamophobia
**materialism:** hylephobia
**medicine(s):** pharmacophobia
**men:** androphobia
**mental illness:** phrenophobia
**metals:** metallophobia
**meteors:** meteorophobia
**mice:** musophobia
**mind:** psychophobia
**mirrors:** eisoptrophobia; spectrophobia
**missiles:** ballistophobia
**moisture:** hygrophobia
**money:** chrematophobia
**motion:** kinesophobia
**myths:** mythophobia
**naked body:** gymnophobia
**naming, being named:** onomatophobia
**needles:** belonephobia
**neglecting duty:** paralipophobia
**Negro(es):** negrophobia
**night:** noctiphobia; nyctophobia
**noise or loud talking:** phonophobia
**northern lights:** auroraphobia
**novelty:** kainophobia; kainotophobia; neophobia
**odor (personal):** autodysosmophobia; automysophobia; bromidrosiphobia; jikoshu-kyofu, olfactory reference syndrome
**odor(s):** olfactophobia; osmophobia; osphresiophobia
**open space(s):** agoraphobia; agyiophobia
**pain:** algophobia; odynophobia
**parasites:** parasitophobia
**people:** anthropophobia; phobanthropy
**physical love:** erotophobia
**places:** topophobia
**pleasure:** hedonophobia
**points:** aichmophobia
**poison:** iophobia; toxi(co)phobia
**poverty:** peniaphobia
**precipices:** cremnophobia

**public places:** agoraphobia
**punishment:** poinephobia
**rabbits:** lagophobia
**rabies:** cynophobia
**railroads or trains:** siderodromophobia
**rain, rainstorms:** ombrophobia
**rats:** rodentophobia; lagophobia (less correctly)
**rectal excreta:** coprophobia
**rectum:** proctophobia
**red:** erythrophobia
**reproach:** enissophobia
**responsibility:** hypengyophobia
**ridicule:** catagelophobia
**right:** dextrophobia
**rivers:** potamophobia
**robbers:** harpaxophobia
**(the) rod:** rhabdophobia
**ruin:** atephobia
**sacred things:** hierophobia
**scabies:** scabiophobia
**school:** scholionophobia
**(receiving a) scratch:** amychophobia
**(the) sea:** nautophobia; thalassophobia
**self:** autophobia
**semen**: spermatophobia
**sex:** genophobia
**sexual intercourse:** coitophobia; cypri(do)phobia
**sharp objects**: belonophobia
**shock:** hormephobia
**ships (drowning):** nautomania; nautophobia
**sin:** hamartophobia
**sinning:** enosiophobia; peccatiphobia; scrupulosity
**sitting:** cathisophobia; thaasophobia
**sitting down:** kathisophobia
**skin disease:** dermatosiophobia
**skin lesion:** dermatophobia
**skin (of animals):** doraphobia
**sleep:** hypnophobia
**small objects or animals:** microbiophobia; microphobia
**smothering:** pnigerophobia
**snakes:** ophidiophobia
**snow:** chionophobia
**solitude:** erem(i)ophobia; monophobia
**sounds:** acousticophobia; phonophobia
**sourness:** acerophobia
**speaking:** lal(i)ophobia
**speaking aloud:** phonophobia
**speed:** tachophobia
**spiders:** arachn(e)ophobia

**stairs:** bathmophobia; climacophobia

**standing up:** stasiphobia

**standing up and walking:** stasibasiphobia

**stars:** siderophobia

**stealing:** kleptophobia

**stillness:** eremiophobia

**stories:** mythophobia

**strangers:** xenophobia

**streets:** agoraphobia; agyiophobia

**string:** linonophobia

**success:** polycratism

**sunlight:** heliophobia

**symbolism:** symbolophobia

**syphilis:** syphilophobia

**talking:** lal(i)ophobia

**tapeworms:** taeniophobia

**taste:** geumaphobia

**teeth:** odontophobia

**thinking:** phronemophobia

**thirteen:** triskaidekaphobia

**thunder:** astra(po)phobia; brontophobia; keraunophobia; tonitrophobia

**time:** chronophobia

**travel:** hodophobia

**trembling:** tremophobia

**trichinosis:** trichinophobia

**tuberculosis:** phthisiophobia; tuberculophobia

**vaccination:** vaccinophobia

**vehicles:** amaxophobia

**venereal disease:** cypridophobia; cypriphobia

**voids:** kenophobia

**vomiting:** emetophobia

**walking:** basiphobia

**water:** aquaphobia; hydrophobia; nautophobia

**weakness:** asthenophobia

**wind:** anemophobia

**women:** gynophobia; horror feminae

**words:** logophobia

**work:** ergasiophobia; ponophobia

**writing:** graphophobia

**fear, real** See *fear, impulse; anxiety.*

**feature-detector system** A sensitivity, presumably inborn, to particular types of stimulation; sometimes called *pre-wiring.* The human infant, for example, is particularly tuned to respond to features of human behavior, and even at 2 months of age, long before he can talk or understand speech, he shows a special sensitivity to human speech sounds.

**febrile psychosis** *Obs.* Infective-exhaustive psychosis.

**febriphobia** Pyrexeophobia; fear of fever.

**feces-child-penis concept** According to psychoanalysis, many factors connected with the anal stage have significant bearing upon the Oedipus and castration complexes. As Freud says: "The handing over of feces for the sake of (out of love for) someone else becomes a prototype of castration; it is the first occasion upon which an individual gives up a piece of his own body (it is such that feces are invariably treated by children) in order to gain the favor of some person whom he loves. So that a person's love for his own penis, which is in other respects narcissistic, is not without an element of anal-erotism." The same reasoning applies to the concept of child and the breast, and the symbolic equation breast-feces-penis-child is at the root of many pregnancy phantasies (Freud, S. *Collected Papers*, 1924–25)

**Fechner, Gustav Theodor** (1801–1887) German physicist, psychologist, philosopher.

**fee for service** *FFS* (q.v.)

**feeblemindedness** Mental deficiency; oligophrenia; hypophrenia. See *retardation, mental.*

**feeblemindedness, affective** Ferenczi's term for pseudodementia, diminution in intellectual capacities secondary to anxiety, depression, or other emotional states.

**feeblemindedness, epileptic** Sometimes during the course of epilepsy there is a steady decline of intelligence that may result in a greater or lesser degree of dementia. See *epileptic dementia.*

**feeblemindedness, hallucinatory** See *dementia paranoides gravis.*

**feedback** In psychiatry, information given to patients about the nature and effects of their behavior, in the form of direct comments, videotape replays, role playing, etc. Also, communication to the sender of the effect his original message had on those to whom it was relayed. Feedback may alter or reinforce the original idea; it is a function that is basic to correction and self-correction. See *cybernetics.*

Feedback is positive when it increases the level or probability of future behavior ("the more you eat the more you want" phenomenon), negative when it decreases the level of future behavior (e.g., food intake, which decreases the likelihood of eating in the near future).

Auditory feedback is the hearing of one's own speech. When this is delayed (as by transmitting the subject's voice to him through special headphones after a temporal delay of 200 to 300 milliseconds), the normal person shows dramatic changes in speech. He begins to stutter, vocal intensity increases, words become slurred, pitch is distorted, speech slows, and various emotional disturbances and other psychophysiological changes occur. In contrast, *delayed auditory feedback (DAF)* often has no adverse effect on the speech of schizophrenic children, a finding that has been interpreted to mean that the schizophrenic child excludes hearing as a basis for continued monitoring of his speech.

**feedback, alpha**   See *alpha wave training.*

**feedback, information**   See *behavior therapy.*

**feeding, self-demand**   In infant feeding, the modern concept that the infant is a reacting human being and should be fed whenever he is hungry. Everything else being equal, the child will cry when hungry and at the time he should be fed. This is opposed to the Spartan attitude that requires that the infant be fed every 4 hours, regardless of his physiological needs, and that, even when hungry, he should be made to wait until the scheduled feeding time. During the first 2 or 3 weeks of life, hunger stimuli make themselves apparent at rather irregular intervals, but thereafter the normal infant settles gradually into a time schedule of his own.

**feeding disorder of infancy or early childhood**   Failure to gain weight, regardless of whether food intake is adequate, in the absence of any demonstrable gastrointestinal disorder or other general medical condition.

**feeding problem**   A common type of behavior disorder in which the child will not eat at all, or only under certain conditions, or shows any number of untoward and unusual reactions if and when he or she does eat.

**feeling**   Sensation; *affect* (q.v.); emotion; empathic reaction. Contrasted with *cognition* and *conation* (qq.v.). See *emotion.*

**feeling, undirected**   See *feeling-apperception.*

**feeling type**   The second of Jung's four functional types of personality. With the first (*thinking*) type it constitutes the *rational* class of *functional* types.

**feeling-apperception**   "The nature of feeling-valuation may be compared with intellectual apperception as an *apperception of value.* An

*active* and a *passive* feeling-apperception can be distinguished.... Active feeling is a *directed* function, an act of will, as for instance, loving as opposed to being in love. This latter state would be *undirected,* passive feeling, as, indeed, the ordinary colloquial term suggests, since it describes the former as activity and the latter as a condition. Undirected feeling is *feeling-intuition*" (Jung, C. *Psychological Types,* 1923).

**feeling-into**   A literal translation of the German *Einfuhlung*; empathy (q.v.).

**feelings analysis**   See *transactional analysis.*

**feigned bereavement**   A false tale of death of a loved one presented by the subject as a major factor in development of the grief of which he or she complains. It is probably a variant of the *Munchhausen syndrome (q.v.).*

**Feldenkrais method**   *Functional integration.* See *body-centered therapy.*

**fellatio**   Oral stimulation of the penis.

**fellatrice**   A female who performs fellatio.

**felt needs**   See *need.*

**female orgasmic disorder**   Inhibited female orgasm; anorgasmia. See *sexual dysfunctions.*

**femaleness**   See *feminine.*

**feminine**   Referring to a set of sex-specific social role behaviors, unrelated to procreative or nurturant biological function, that identify the person as being a girl or woman. Contrast with *femaleness,* which refers to anatomic and physiologic features relating to the female's procreative and nurturant functions. See *gender identity.*

**feminine masochism**   One of the three types of *masochism* (q.v.) described by Freud as an expression of what he considered to be the characteristic passivity and receptivity of feminine nature.

**feminine traits in male**   According to Adler, the following are feminine traits that the male neurotic perceives in himself either consciously or unconsciously: passive attitude, obedience, softness, cowardice, memory of defeat, ignorance, lack of capacity, and tenderness. The person attempts to overcome these characteristics by developing hatred, defiance, cruelty, and egoism.

**femininity**   In contrast to the concept of *femaleness,* which is primarily related to the proper sex chromosome structure of XX individuals, femininity refers to a female's possession of the typical and well-developed secondary sex characteristics of a woman. See *sex determination.*

**feminism** 1. The social system or viewpoint that assigns equality to the sexes, an orientation espoused by the feminist movement. 2. Based on the assumption that the word is formed in the same way as *racism* and *sexism* (qq.v.), feminism is used by some in a directly opposite way to refer to the social system that assigns to women the status of inferior, undesirable, etc.

In most cultures, gender is the primary element of social classification and social relationships, but since the 1960s it has become increasingly evident that both cultural and scientific conceptions of masculinity and femininity are grossly inadequate.

While social classifications reduce complexity and provide simple models for self-definition, sex stereotyping can lead to conflicts for both sexes and particularly for females. Current emphasis is on integrative conceptualizations that focus on the ways in which the sexes are alike more than they are different, and on dualistic conceptualizations that recognize the important differences between the sexes but emphasize the feminine as a valid alternative to the masculine.

**feminization** See *ambitypic*.

**fentanyl** A synthetic analgesic used for the rapid control of pain. A *designer drug* (q.v.) analogue of fentanyl, called China white, is marketed as a solution and sold for street use as a powder. It can also be taken by rubbing on the buccal mucosa and gargled, and by sniffing or smoking. It is 50 to 100 times more potent than morphine and can cause overdosage symptoms even in amounts that are difficult or impossible to detect in urine. Overdosage can be treated with naloxone. See *MPTP*.

**Féré phenomenon** See *psychogalvanic reflex*.

**Ferenczi, Sandor** (1873–1933) Hungarian psychoanalyst; "active" analysis.

**Ferri, Enrico** (1856–1929) Italian forensic psychiatrist.

**fertility, differential** A degree of reproductiveness that differs from that of the normal population; used in genetics to refer to the effect on fertility of subjects with a hereditary disorder. Their effective fertility may be lowered by biological, psychological, or sociological factors; the degree of lowering is a measure of the selective disadvantage associated with the disorder in question.

**fertility, net** The number of children of carriers of a hereditary trait who reach the age group that corresponds to the manifestation period of the trait in question.

**festination gait** Involuntary inclination to hurry one's gait, typical of *Parkinson disease* (q.v.). See *propulsion gait*.

**fetal abuse** A mother's abuse or neglect of her unborn child. See *battered child syndrome*. Fetal abuse appears in several forms: the mother will not seek prenatal care, refuses treatment designed to benefit the fetus, continues behaviors that are known to pose a risk to the fetus, etc. Fetal abuse presents more medico-ethical problems than does child abuse, for several reasons. The law has not yet answered the question of whether a fetus is a person; if the mother is competent, she has the right to accept or refuse any kind of treatment; the mother has a right to her own body integrity; a person cannot generally be forced to undergo an invasive procedure in order to save another's life; and more often than not the treatments being urged on the patient (e.g., blood transfusions, caesarean section) carry their own risks to the health and life of the mother.

**fetal alcohol syndrome** *FAS*; an alcohol-related birth defect (ARBD) consisting of a pattern of retarded physical and mental growth, with associated cranial, facial, limb, and cardiovascular anomalies, that is found in 30% to 50% of the offspring of severely alcoholic mothers. The most frequently reported abnormalities are prenatal or postnatal growth deficiency, microcephaly, developmental delay or mental retardation; short palpebral fissures, a short upturned nose with sunken nasal bridge and a thin upper lip; abnormal palmar creases, and septal or other cardiac defects.

Damage to the fetus by maternal alcoholism is one of the most common recognizable causes of mental retardation. Affected children generally do not "catch up" in their growth patterns, even when given a nutritionally adequate diet. The basis for the syndrome is believed to be a direct toxic effect of alcohol or one of its intermediate breakdown products on the fetal brain.

Many other abnormalities have been ascribed to the effects of alcohol on the fetus, but it remains controversial as to how many of them are due to alcohol alone and as to the level of maternal alcohol consumption that will produce them. There is no established safe dose of alcohol during pregnancy, nor does there appear to be a safe time to drink.

**fetal hydantoin syndrome**  See *gestational epilepsy.*

**fetal screening**  See *genetic screening.*

**fetal trimethadone syndrome**  See *gestational epilepsy.*

**fetalism**  Penrose's term for the signs of *mongolism (Down syndrome)*, many of which appear to be remnants of fetal existence.

**fetish**  A fetish is a material object of any kind (idol, charm, talisman) that embodies mysterious and awesome qualities and from which supernatural aid may be expected.

In psychiatry, the love object of the person who suffers from the *paraphilia* (q.v.) called fetishism—usually a part of the body or some object belonging to or associated with the love object, such as female undergarments. The fetish replaces and substitutes for the love object, and although sexual activity with the love object may occur, gratification is possible only if the fetish is present or at least fantasied during such activity. Typical also is the ability of the fetishist to obtain gratification from the fetish alone, in the absence of the love object. The most common fetishes—shoes, long hair, earrings, undergarments, feet—are penis symbols or serve to avoid complete nudity of the female, and fetishism is thus considered to be a means of denying castration fears. Such denial of the woman's lack of a penis by the adult male presupposes a degree of splitting in the person's ego that ordinarily is found only in cases with a defective or severely limited ego.

Fetishism, almost exclusively a male disorder, tends to be chronic. *Kleptomania* (q.v.), an almost exclusively female disorder, is an impulse disorder rather than a paraphilia, but in some women compulsive stealing may be sexually exciting.

Fetish and fetishism are also used to refer to current rules and conventions that are misapplied or unduly revered.

**fetishism, adherent**  Hirschfeld's term for the form of fetishism in which clothing is donned by the fetishist. See *fetishism, coherent.*

**fetishism, beast**  A paraphilia in which "touching furs or animal skins produces peculiar and lustful emotions (analogous to hair-, braid-, velvet-, and silk-fetishism)." (Krafft-Ebing, R. v. *Psychopathia Sexualis*, 1908).

**fetishism, coherent**  Hirschfeld's term for "the attraction which is exercised, for many people far more than is normal, by stuffs, and objects which are not donned or thrown over the body as clothing, but are brought into immediate contact with the body surface;" *Sexual Pathology* (1939).

**fetishism, foot**  See *retifism.*

**fetishistic transvestism**  Also called transvestic fetishism. See *cross-dressing; transvestitism.*

**fetotoxin**  A compound that, when taken during pregnancy, can produce acute toxic damages to the fetus. Most psychopharmacologic agents are neither teratogenic nor fetotoxic (exceptions are lithium, the anticonvulsants carbamazepine and divalproex, and perhaps MAOIs). Used late in pregnancy, however, many agents can lead to a series of short-term toxic effects in the newborn, such as the transient jitteriness, suckling problems, hyperexcitability, cardiac arrhythmias, urinary retention, and intestinal motility disorders that have been associated with use of antidepressant drugs. See *teratogen.*

**Feuchtersleben, Ernst von**  (1806–1849) German psychiatrist; author of *Lehrbuch der aerztlichen Seelenkunde.*

**FFA**  *Fusiform face area* (q.v.).

**FFI**  *Fatal familial insomnia* (q.v.).

**FFS**  *Fee for service*; a reimbursement system for health care in which the provider of care (hospital, physician, or other approved provider) is paid a set fee for the particular service provided. The system was introduced in the 1960s and 1970s as a way to expand access to health care. The result was that increased supply created increased demand, and critics of the system asserted that unnecessary health care was being provided at the expense of other social services.

In the 1990s, *managed competition* was introduced to control the rise in health care costs. It utilized two mechanisms: (1) managed care (q.v.) and (2) competition between health care systems and plans for patients on the basis of cost and quality. Although such measures reduced the provision of care and slowed the escalation of costs, it soon became clear that more than ineffective or unnecessary care was being eliminated. Increased patient co-payments, for example, reduce the use of all health care services, not just unnecessary ones.

Another management tool has been introduced as a way to improve access and at the same time improve quality of care—*pay for performance* (P4P), which establishes incentives for providers to deliver care that third parties deem appropriate to achieve both highest quality standards and best outcomes. Critics claim that P4P is no more than another form of FFS, that clinical decisions will still be made by third parties, that the practice guidelines used to set standards for high-quality care ignore individual patient needs and preferences, that the programs do not address the problems of misuse or overuse of services, that tracking process and outcomes involves extremely high administrative costs, and that guidelines may ultimately be driven by forces with an inherent bias to deliver more expensive care (e.g., pharmaceutical companies, developers of new technologies).

**FGA** First-generation (conventional) antipsychotic.

**FHM** *Familial hemiplegic migraine* (q.v.).

**FHRDC** Family History Research Diagnostic Criteria; an instrument designed to obtain screening information through the family history method. The criteria have good reliability and high sensitivity and specificity for core schizophrenia but are considered weaker for the evaluation of milder spectrum disorders.

**Fiamberti hypothesis** (A. M. Fiamberti, 20th-century Italian psychiatrist) The theory that schizophrenia is due to a deficiency of acetylcholine, perhaps secondary to toxic-infectious influences.

**fibrillar elements** See *cytosolic proteins*.

**fibrillation** Slow, vermicular twitchings of individual muscle fibers or bundles, occurring anywhere in the body, without producing movements of muscles or joints; the condition is mainly indicative of slow degeneration of anterior horn cells (nuclear masses of motor cells).

**fibriophobia** Ungrounded fear of developing a fever.

**fibromyalgia** *FM*; characterized by (1) a host of regional somatic and visceral pain syndromes, such as irritable bowel syndrome, temporomandibular disorder, tension headache, idiopathic low back pain; and (2) augmented central processing of pain, with *tender points*, including both hyperalgesia (increased painfulness to normally painful stimuli) and allodynia (pain in response to normally nonpainful stimuli) throughout the body. There is increasing evidence that baseline differences in the function of the ANS, the hypothalamic-pituitary-adrenal axes, and pain processing systems in large part represent diatheses that predispose individuals to subsequently develop chronic regional or widespread pain.

Some authorities consider fibromyalgia to be a variant of *chronic fatigue syndrome* (q.v.).

**fibronectin** An extracellular matrix glycoprotein secreted by fibroblasts; in neural adhesion it interacts with integrins. See *adhesion, cellular; neurotrophins*.

**fiction, autarchic** The false belief of the child in its own omnipotence. At the beginning of extrauterine life the infant is ignorant of any sources of pleasure other than those within itself: the infant even thinks of the breast as a part of its body. Ferenczi called this the period of unconditional omnipotence. The infant tries to cling to this feeling of omnipotence and only unwillingly orients itself to objects. This is the basis for the frequency of masturbation in children when they are weaned: they turn to themselves for pleasure rather than recognize their dependency upon the environment.

**fiction, directive** A term used by Adler to describe the phantasy or idea of superiority that a person originally conceives as a subjective compensation for a feeling of inferiority. The person uses the phantasy or idea and reacts to as if it were an absolute truth.

**fictional finalism** See *individual psychology*.

**fictive kin** Genetically unrelated people who are called kin and claim the emotions ordinarily directed at kin; the most familiar example is the spouse. Marriages make in-laws into natural allies, and that is one reason why in all cultures marriages are alliances between clans, not just between spouses.

**fidgetiness** Fidgety state. Increased motor activity, more frequently used in reference to children than to adults. Winnicott distinguishes three causes of fidgetiness: anxiety, tics, and chorea.

**fidgets** Vague uneasiness, usually accompanied by restless movements. Fidgets or creeps were colloquial terms for the disease or morbid symptom called *dysphoria* (q.v.).

**fiduciary relation** In law, the trust between patient and physician, including the expectation of confidentiality and undivided loyalty on the part of the physician.

**field defect** The field of vision is the limit of peripheral vision, the area within which an object can be seen while the eye remains fixed on some one point. The normal visual field has a definite contour, any change in which from the normal constitutes a field defect.

The various visual field defects (with their common causes) are (1) *circumferential blindness* or *tubular vision* (hysteria, optic or retrobulbar neuritis), consisting of a concentric contraction of the visual fields;

(2) *total blindness* in one eye (complete lesion of optic nerve on same side); (3) *hemianopia* or hemianopsia, loss of one-half of the visual field, which may be (a) homonymous, i.e., loss of vision in the temporal half-field on the same side as the lesion and loss of vision in the nasal half-field of the other eye (lesions posterior to optic radiation); or (b) heteronymous with loss of vision in the same half-field (usually the temporal) of both eyes (chiasmal lesion); or (c) unilateral hemianopia with loss of vision in the nasal or temporal half-field of one eye (perichiasmal lesion); (4) *quadrantic hemianopia* or *quadrantanopia* (partial involvement of optic radiation), with loss of vision in one quadrant of the visual field, usually homonymous. See *occipital lobe*.

**field dependence**    An expression of the degree of reliance on the environment to provide a definition of the self. The field-dependent person uses the visual context to establish spatial orientation, whereas the field-independent person relies more on postural and gravitational cues. Females in general are more field dependent than males, and field dependence tends to decrease with age in both sexes.

**fields of Forel**    See *subthalamus*.

**fight-flight assumption**    See *basic assumptions group*.

**fight-flight responses**    *Emergency emotions*; adaptive physiological changes that occur in an organism confronted with an emergency. On the basis of his work with animals, Cannon hypothesized that stressors activated catabolic functions (mediated by the sympathetic or adrenergic ystem) and inhibited anabolic functions (mediated by the parasympathetic or cholinergic system). In consequence, the animal was prepared to fight the attacker or to flee.

**figure**    In psychoanalytic psychology particularly, this term, in combination with other nouns denoting familial or close interpersonal relationships (e.g., father figure, mother figure, authority figure), is approximately equivalent to substitute, replacement, representative, or surrogate.

**figure, helpful**    In the child's world of phantasy, a male or female fairy creature with so much love, understanding, and sympathy that the child could turn to it for help in any need.

**figure-ground**    See *ground*.

**filicide**    Parental *infanticide* (q.v.); murder of one's child. If the child is less than 24 hours old, the term neonaticide is used. See *Medea complex*. Child murder includes the following: (1) altruistic homicide to relieve suffering, sometimes associated with suicide; (2) acutely psychotic killer; (3) killing an unwanted child; (4) child maltreatment (fatally battered child); and (5) spouse revenge.

**filling in**    A perceptual phenomenon in which a visual attribute (e.g., color, brightness, texture, motion) is perceived in a region of the visual field even though such an attribute exists only in the surround. The phenomenon is observed in various situations: (1) when some region of the visual field is deprived of visual input, such as a blind spot or scotoma; this is the reason the patient often does not realize that such a defect exists, for no odd region has been perceived in the visual field.; (2) when steady fixation is maintained; the contrast of an object in the peripheral visual field gradually decreases and finally the object becomes invisible, and the area it occupied is filled in the visual features of the surround (the *Troxler effect*); (3) illusions, such as the regions between two vertical lines appearing to be darker than the regions outside the lines (the *Craik-O'Brien-Cornsweet illusion*), or vertical achromatic gratings separated by a horizontal dark band are perceived as if an illusory grating crosses the gap to connect the upper and lower gratings.

**filopodia**    See *growth cone*.

**filtering**    See *selective attention*.

**final tendency**    The ultimate goal or aim of the neurosis. Adler was the first to point out "the presence of a final tendency in the structure of every neurosis." In this respect he was guided by both Janet's theory of the *idée fixe* and Wernicke's concept of *overcharged idea* (q.v.).

**finger agnosia**    See *agnosia*.

**finger gnosis**    See *parietal lobe*.

**finger painting**    Direct manipulation of the paint with the fingers and hands to achieve a graphic effect. Finger painting is used as a projective technique, the assumption being that finger painting is a form of expressive behavior, the analysis of which reveals significant characteristics of the subject. Finger painting was developed by Ruth F. Shaw (1934) as an educational technique, and it has also been used as a part of psychotherapy and play therapy, and by occupational therapists in rehabilitation of spastic patients, the deaf, and the blind.

**finger tapping test** The subject taps with alternate index fingers on a device that records the number of taps for 10-second periods.

**fingers, insane** Inflammation at the end of a finger or toe (called a *whitlow*) seen in residents of psychiatric hospitals, usually a reflection of poor hygiene and a low level of care.

**Fink-Green-Bender test** *Face-hand test* (q.v.).

**firesetting** See *pyromania*.

**firewater myth** The popular but discredited belief that Native American Indians are constitutionally unable to handle alcohol. As a group, Native Americans have the highest alcohol-related death rates of all ethnic groups in the United States; some studies suggest that they are less sensitive than normal to the physiologic and subjective effects of alcohol.

**firing** *Discharge* (q.v.).

**first admission** A person admitted for the first time to an institution of a given class (e.g., mental hospital or institution for the retarded).

**first attack** An illness occurring for the first time, regardless of whether it results in hospitalization, is a first attack.

**first half deprivation** See *sleep deprivation*.

**first messenger** See *neurotransmitter receptor*.

**first pain** Sharp, pricking pain, associated with rapidly conducting δ fibers.

**first-line treatments** In treatment guidelines or other recommendations by expert consensus, those treatments that are considered appropriate as initial treatment for a given situation; a *treatment of choice* is one that carries an especially strong first-line recommendation. *Second-line treatments* are those considered reasonable choices for patients who cannot tolerate or do not respond to first-line treatments. *Third-line treatments* are those used only when referred alternatives have not been effective.

**first-order relatives** *First-degree relatives,* who share 50% of a person's genes—siblings, parents, and children. *Second-order relatives* share 25% of a person's genes—aunts, uncles, nieces, nephrews, grandchildren. *Third-degree relatives* share only 12.5% of a person's genes.

**first-pass effect** In pharmacokinetics, binding of a drug and metabolism by the liver before it reaches the systemic circulation for distribution throughout the body.

**first-rank symptoms** A group of symptoms described by Kurt Schneider, and used by him and his followers as a basis for making a diagnosis of *schizophrenia* (q.v.). It is now recognized that the symptoms can also occur in other disorders, such as *dissociative identity disorder* (q.v.). The first-rank symptoms include the following:

A. Hallucinations
   1. *Audible thoughts*
   2. Hearing voices arguing
   3. Hearing voices commenting on the subject's behavior

B. Changes in thought process
   4. *Thought insertion*—the experience that the subject's thoughts belong to others who have intruded their thoughts upon the subject
   5. *Thought withdrawal* or thought interruption by some outside person or force (castrophrenia; *mental eclipse*; nooklopia)
   6. Thought broadcasting—the subject's private thoughts are known to others

C. Delusional perceptions
   7. Attributing highly personal meaning to perception(s) without any comprehensible justification

D. Somatic passivity
   8. Body sensations that the subject attributes to outside forces, such as X-rays or hypnosis

E. Other external impositions
   9. "Forced" or *"made" impulses*—the subject is being forced to do things that he does not want to do
   10. Made volition—the subject is being forced to want things he does not really want
   11. Made feelings—the subject is being made to feel emotions or sensations (often sexual) that are not his own

Schneider worked in Munich in the 1930s and during the period of 1945–1955 occupied Kraepelin's chair in Heidelberg. Even though he accepted the wider post-Kraepelinian concept of schizophrenia that had begun with Bleuler, he and his followers held to a more narrow delineation than was upheld by most American psychiatrists.

In the International Pilot Study of Schizo-phrenia (IPSS, 1973), 57% of the patients diag-nosed schizophrenic by the nine participating countries demonstrated first-rank symptoms. Although long thought to be pathognomonic of schizophrenia, first-rank symptoms have also been recognized in patients with bipolar disorder and in *dissociative identity disorder* (q.v.).

**fit** 1. Consonance or *complementarity* (q.v.) in a dyadic relationship, most often applied to the mother–child relationship. Being totally helpless and dependent, the infant needs an empathic, loving, soothing, competent, powerful yet benevolent caretaker to protect him and ensure his survival. Goodness of fit is one measure of the mother's ability to respond appropriately to the cues her infant gives her about his needs. Mahler referred to such interactions as *communicative matching* or *mutual cuing*. Related concepts include the *good breast* (Klein), the *container-contained* function (Bion), *mirroring* (Kohut). See *empathic failure*. 2. Convulsion; epileptic attack.

**fitness** The ability of an organism to survive and reproduce in a given environment; phe-notypic fitness. The Darwinian concept of natural *selection* (q.v.) refers to the rewarding of organisms of higher phenotypic fitness. *Genetic fitness* refers to the organism's genetic contribution to the next generation, not to the organism's phenotypic characteristics. Inclusive fitness, a sociobiological concept, is the fitness of the individual plus the individu-al's influence on the fitness of nondescendant relatives; it is one element of kin selection, enhancing the survival and reproduction of those to whom the organism is related, even if that involves actions that decrease the organ-ism's own fitness.

**fits of horrific temptation** See *temptation, horrific*.

**fixate** In psychoanalysis, to retain excessive amounts of libidinal or aggressive energy in one or more of the infantile structures to which they were originally attached. See *ontogeny, psychic*.

**fixation** In psychoanalysis, persistence of the libidinal or aggressive cathexis of an object of infancy or childhood into later life. Fixation generally implies pathology and this con-notes that the amount of energy retained at the infantile level is greater than is normal.

In the normal person, even though earlier levels persist along with higher levels of psy-chic development, most psychic energy is concentrated in the higher levels. When the energy retained at lower levels exceeds the normal amount, the term "fixation" is appli-cable. Fixation is indicative of a weak spot in psychic structure that may predispose to neu-rosis. See *inertia, psychic; ontogeny, psychic*.

Closely related to fixation is *regression* (q.v.), for when the latter occurs it is typically to an object or mode of gratification on which the person was fixated that he or she regresses.

In social work, fixation is "a form of aber-rancy of affection in which there is exagger-ated devotion to someone, usually, in the parental role, as mother fixation." (Hamilton, G. *A Medical Social Terminology*, 1930).

**fixation hysteria** Conversion hysteria in which the area or function affected is one that is, or had previously been, the site of some organic disorder. An example is conversion paraly-sis of an arm broken earlier in an accident. Closely allied to fixation hysteria is *pathohys-teria*, wherein a chronic disease process is itself productive of hysterical symptoms. A more general term for the latter phenomenon is *pathoneurosis*. See *immobilization paralysis*.

**fixation point** In psychoanalytic psychology, the different neuroses and psychoses are con-sidered to be reflections of a fixation of psy-chic energy at given foci or fixation points—schizophrenia, for example, at the autoerotic stage; melancholia at the oral sadistic phase; hysteria at the early genital level; obsessional neurosis at the anal stage.

**fixed idea** See *idée fixe*.

**fixed pupil** A pupil that does not react to light, to accommodation, or to convergence.

**fixed-interval (FI) schedule** See *reinforcement schedule*.

**fixed-ratio (FR) schedule** See *reinforcement schedule*.

**flagellantism** Erotic stimulation from whip-ping or being whipped.

**flagellation** The act of whipping as a sexual excitant. See *dippoldism; masochism; sadism*.

**flagellomania** *Flagellantism* (q.v.).

**flapping tremor** *Asterixis* (q.v.). Rapid burst of flexion and extension in the wrist and meta-carpophalangeal joints similar to the flapping of a bird's wings; such a *tremor* (q.v.) is indic-ative of hepatic failure.

**flash** See *amphetamines*.

**flash suppression**  The perceptual suppression of a monocular stimulus on flashing a different stimulus to the opposite eye, while keeping the original stimulus on the other eye.

**flashback**  1. *Posthallucinogen perception disorder; hallucinogen persisting perception disorder*; recurrence of one or more of the perceptual symptoms (e.g., hallucinations, misperceptions, illusions) that were part of the subject's reaction to a hallucinogen in the past. The flashback lasts from seconds to hours and is sometimes precipitated by fatigue, alcohol intake, or marijuana intoxication, although often there is no identifiable precipitant. Flashbacks are believed to occur in 25% or more of hallucinogen users. Because they occur without warning and during a drug-free period, the symptoms are markedly distressing and are often interpreted as an indication of losing control or "going out of my mind." 2. Flashback is also characteristic of *dissociative identity disorder, post-traumatic stress disorder*, and other dissociative disorders where it appears as re-experiencing in the here and now a traumatic event of the then and there; an intrusive memory or sensory recollection of a past experience.

**flashbulb memory**  Personal moments that stand out especially vividly, and which seem to be remembered accurately rather than being distorted with each recall; they are apparently "burned" into the subject's brain because the original experience was so powerful. Something similar is seen in victims of post-traumatic stress disorder. See *memory*.

**flasher**  Exhibitionist; so called because of the way in which the genitals are exposed—many exhibitionists clothe themselves solely with a topcoat, and when they chance upon their victim open the coat quickly to display their genitalia. See *exhibitionism*.

**flattening**  In psychiatry, a disturbance of affectivity. Flattening of affect (or "flat affect") is rarely seen outside the schizophrenic group, although affect block, which is seen also in obsessive-compulsive patients, may be difficult to differentiate from flattening. Flattening of the affect consists of a general impoverishment of emotional reactivity or failure to react appropriately to affect-tinged stimuli. The affect-flattened patient is often described as emotionally bleak or dull, colorless, unresponsive, cold, removed, apart, uninvolved, or unconvincing. The patient himself may complain that reality seems far away, that nothing has meaning for him, or that his emotional responses seem forced, false, and unreal.

**flavism**  The presence of yellow hair in certain regions of the body in contrast with the stronger, darker hair on other parts of the body. In constitutional medicine, like *erythrism*, it is considered a stigma of the *asthenic, microsplanchnic* physique and its tendency to tuberculosis.

**flavor**  See *gustation*.

**fletcherism**  (Horace Fletcher, 1849–1919, American dietitian) The belief that each bite of food must be masticated thoroughly before it is swallowed, and that liquids should be ingested only in small sips; often includes an injunction as to the specific number of times each mouthful should be chewed.

**flexibility, waxy**  See *catalepsy*.

**flexion reflex (of the leg)**  A deep reflex; patient's leg is semiflexed at the knee; the examiner's finger grasps the tendons of the semimembranosus and semitendinosus muscles; this finger is tapped, resulting in contraction of these muscles and flexion of the leg.

**flicker**  Flutter; rapid change in frequency of stimulation (usually auditory or visual) producing corresponding change in the visual or auditory perception. In the case of vision, for example, a flickering light will be perceived as such until brightness of the light or frequency of the flicker is increased to a certain point (*critical flicker frequency*); at this point, the stimulus will be perceived as a single, continuing stimulus (fusion). See *critical flicker fusion test*.

**flight**  Fleeing or running away, to escape danger. See *fugue*.

**flight into disease**  "By means of *flight into the disease* one achieves definite aims through the disease; by an attack of rage one achieves a yielding; by a fainting spell, a new hat; and by the more protracted disease one gets a pleasant sojourn in a sanatorium. By means of all these one can at the same time compel consideration, secure care and tenderness, obtain power over others who have to adjust themselves to the disease, extort an allowance, evade tasks from the simple household duties up to the terrors of the trenches" (Bleuler, E. *Textbook of Psychiatry*, 1930). See *epinosic gain*.

**flight into health**  *Transference cure* or *improvement*; a relinquishing of symptoms that occurs not because the patient has resolved his or her neurosis, but rather as a defense against further probing by the analyst into painful, unconscious material.

**flight of ideas**  A near-continuous flow of speech that is not disjointed or bizarre, but that jumps rapidly from one topic to another, each topic being more or less obviously related to the preceding or to adventitious environmental stimuli. Flight of ideas is characteristic of acute manic states: in bipolar disorder and in acute manic syndrome of schizophrenia. N. Cameron termed flight of ideas "topical flight": "The manic in his talk keeps to social trails of communication, even though he may change his direction on them at every moment; the schizophrenic does not keep to social paths, but makes his own trail as he goes" (*The Psychology of Behavior Disorders*, 1947).

**floccillation**  *Carphology* (q.v.); aimless picking or plucking.

**flocculonodular lobe**  See *cerebellum*.

**flogger**  One who whips; flagellator.

**flooding**  *Implosion* (q.v.).

**flow chart**  See *algorithm, clinical*.

**flow states**  Also called optimal experiences; see *positive dissociative experiences*.

**flowback**  The collection of material that flows out of the vagina some time after intercourse. The main part of it is the seminal fluid from the man, almost all of which is ejected from the vagina. To this the woman adds a quantity of mucus from her cervix. See *sperm*.

**fluctuating ego states**  See *dedifferentiation*.

**fluency**  Easy flow of speech. Fluency disturbances, seen frequently in schizophrenic subjects, include unnecessary or excessive pauses, hesitations, false starts, repetitions of sounds, syllables, words, and phrases, as well as shifts in the speed of flow of speech.

**fluent aphasia**  *Wernicke aphasia* (q.v.).

**fluid intelligence**  Also known as *g*; the ability to learn and to organize an effective task plan by activating appropriate goals or action requirements. See *crystallized intelligence*; *intelligence*.

**fluidity**  Mobility; in Kurt Lewin's theory of personality, fluidity refers to the permeability of boundaries between the different regions or subsystems of the person. Lewin uses the term accessibility for the permeability of the personality boundaries to external stimulation.

**flush reaction, alcohol**  See *alcohol flush reaction*.

**flutter**  A sensory submodality; flutter is felt when touching an object that vibrates at frequencies between –5 and –50 Hz. Flutter is primarily mediated by rapidly adapting cutaneous mechanoreceptors.

**fMRI**  Functional magnetic resonance imaging; the imaging technique most frequently employed in evaluation of neuropsychiatric patients. By coupling changes in local cerebral blood flow with neural activation, fMRI allows noninvasive evaluation and localization of motor, sensory, and cognitive deficits or symptoms. With blood oxygen level–dependent (BOLD) contrast, neural activation is followed by an increased number of red blood cells carrying oxyhemoglobin flow. fMRI allows the study of brain activity without the use of either ionizing radiation or the injection of radiopharmaceuticals needed in SPECT and PET. The temporal and spatial resolution of fMRI are better than those of PET or SPECT. Limiting head motion is esssential for obtaining high-quality images. Like other MR techniques, patient claustrophobia may be an issue. Typically, baseline images are acquired with the patient at rest. Then the patient performs a specific task and another set of images is acquired.

**FMR-1 gene**  See *fragile X syndrome; trinucleotide repeat*.

**FMRP**  Fragile X mental retardation protein, whose gene is mutated in *fragile X syndrome* (q.v.). FMRP is needed for protein synthesis near synapses in response to stimulation; if it is lacking or mutated, synaptic stimulation fails to increase protein synthesis.

**focal clonic seizures**  See *frontal lobe seizures*.

**focal conflict**  A specific emotional problem that is identified as the major issue to be confronted in brief dynamic psychotherapy. Typically, it is the conflict between a feeling or desire and the person's enduring value system that has led to frustration and the development of various defenses and compromises. See *brief psychotherapy*.

**focal dystonia**  *Dystonia* (q.v.) confined to a specific set of muscles, as in writer's cramp, seamstress's cramp, or musician's cramp.

**focal suicide**  See *deliberate self-harm syndrome*.

**focused analysis**  *Selective analysis* (q.v.); directed analysis; a modification of the orthodox psychoanalytic technique (which is termed by Glover *expectant analysis* because the analyst waits and follows the spontaneous unfolding of the patient's psyche with leisurely, free-floating, analytical attention). In the focused or selective analysis, interpretations are purposively geared to a particular aspect of the patient's pathology—particular defenses, particular shades of transference, particular types of conflict, and particular stages of instinctual needs that seem to be of paramount importance.

**focused delirium**   See *délire chronique*.

**focusing disturbance**   A disturbance of adaptability that may occur in patients with organic brain disease: some tasks can be performed when approached one way, but not if they are approached in any other way.

**folding**   Bending or flexing; *protein folding* is the process by which a protein acquires its native tridimensional structure. Each protein normally has a unique and stable folded structure, but in *protein conformational disorders* (q.v.) the polypeptide chain adopts an alternative structure, which is associated with the pathogenesis of the disease.

**folic acid**   A vitamin essential for carrying various one-carbon groups in metabolism. Folic acid deficiency occurs with inadequate dietary intake (as in alcoholism, poverty, food faddism), malabsorption diseases, and use of medications that inhibit it or interfere with its absorption. Megaloblastic anemia is the most common result of folic acid deficiency; peripheral neuropathy may also occur, but not as commonly as in vitamin $B_{12}$ deficiency. The most frequent psychiatric abnormality in folate-deficient subjects is mood disorder.

**folie (F. "insanity")**   The French distinguished *mental alienation* and insanity (*folie*), considering the former in a generic sense, while they used folie to denote a psychiatric condition acquired by a person who had previously been in good mental health.

**folie à deux**   (F. "double insanity") Folie à deux has been known by a number of names: *induced psychotic disorder* (q.v.), shared paranoid disorder (DSM-III), *communicated insanity*, double insanity (Tuke), *folie simultanée* (Régis), *folie imposée* (Lasègue and Falret), *folie induite* (Lehmann). It was first described by William Harvey in 1651 in a pair of sisters. Usually, one partner is dominant (the inducer) and has a psychotic illness (most often, schizophrenia). The delusions and hallucinations become shared by the passive partner (recipient), who may or may not have a coincidental schizophrenic or delusional disorder. Cognitive impairment, poverty, and shared traumatic life experiences may be vulnerability factors, but

the outstanding risk factors are isolation and pathological intimacy. Ninety percent of cases occur within family settings, most commonly between sister and sister, next most commonly between mother and child. The shared delusions are generally persecutory or hypochondriacal in nature. Continued close proximity prolongs the process, as does living in poverty (Boughton, D. P. and Popkin, M. K. Mummification and folie a deux. *Comprehensive Psychiatry 30*: 26–30, 1989).

In *folie simultanèe*, both persons have a psychotic illness occurring simultaneously. In *folie imposèe*, the dominant partner has a psychotic illness and the recipient is not psychotic. In *folie communiquèe*, both have psychoses but become ill in sequence. In *folie induite*, a psychotic person, usually hospitalized, adopts the delusions of a fellow-patient in addition to his own.

**folie à double forme**   *Obs.* (F. "insanity in double form") Manic-depressive psychosis.

**folie à quatre**   (F. "quadruple insanity") The appearance of the same delusions in four members of a family. Bleuler cites the following case: "At one time we had in Burgholzli four siblings (two brothers and two sisters) who all had the same persecutory and religious delusions. It turned out that one sister, the most intelligent of the four, was the first to become ill; she imposed her delusions on the others. She deteriorated severely and later developed catatonic symptoms. The second sister could eventually be released, but had to be readmitted later. The two brothers managed to maintain themselves outside the hospital. There was no doubt that the two sisters were really schizophrenic; and we had excellent reasons for believing that the two brothers were also schizophrenic, not only because they never recovered completely afterwards, but also because of their peculiar modes of life already before the acute attack." (*Dementia Praecox or the Group of Schizophrenias*, 1950). Bleuler considered this a form of induced schizophrenia. See *induced psychotic disorder*.

**folie à trois**   (F. "triple insanity") The appearance of the same delusions in three members of a family. See *folie à deux; induced psychotic disorder*.

**folie circulaire**   (F. "cyclic insanity") Falret's term for manic-depressive psychosis, circular or alternating type.

**folie communiquée** (F. "infectious insanity") *Folie à deux* (q.v.).

**folie d'action** (F. "madness of movement, action") Brierre de Boismont's term for moral and emotional insanity.

**folie démonomaniaque** (F. "demonomaniacal insanity") *Demonomania* (q.v.).

**folie des grandeurs** (F. "insanity of greatness") *Megalomania* (q.v.).

**folie des persécutions** (F. "insanity of persecutions") Paranoid psychosis.

**folie du doute** (F. "insanity of doubt") *Doubting mania*, today usually subsumed under the heading of anxiety neurosis or obsessive-compulsive disorder. "The fear of responsibility expresses itself in the compulsion to examine repeatedly whether a match thrown away no longer burns, whether the doors of closets are locked, whether letters are sealed, or whether a mistake was made in calculating (doubting mania, *folie du doute*)." (Bleuler, E. *Textbook of Psychiatry*, 1930). Falret introduced the expression as a nosological entity, calling it *la maladie du doute*. At an earlier date Esquirol termed the same condition *monomanie raisonnante*; Baillarger referred to it as *monomanie avec conscience*; at other times it was known as *alienation partielle*; Oscar Berger named the condition *Grübelsücht*.

**folie du pourquoi** (F. "craze of 'why'") Question-asking insanity; Fragesucht; a manifestation of obsessive-compulsive disorder.

**folie gémellaire** (F. "twin-insanity") Psychoses in twins occurring simultaneously.

**folie hypocondriaque** (F. "hypochondriacal insanity") Neurasthenia.

**folie imitative** (F. "imitative insanity") *Folie à deux* (q.v.).

**folie imposée** (F. "imposed insanity") See *folie à deux; induced psychotic disorder.*

**folie induite** (F. "induced insanity") See *folie à deux.*

**folie instantanée** (F. "momentary insanity") Mania transitoria (q.v.).

**folie morale** (F. "moral insanity") See *moral insanity.*

**folie morale, acquired** Kraepelin's term for antisocial behavior that masks an underlying schizophrenic disorder, which breaks through in the form of acute psychotic states with delusions, auditory hallucinations, and agitation or stupor.

**folie pénitentiare** (F. "penitentiary insanity") Prison psychosis. See *Ganser syndrome.*

**folie raisonnante** (F. "reasoning insanity") *Folie du doute* (q.v.).

**folie simulée** (F. "feigned insanity") Feigned psychosis.

**folie simultanée** (F. "simultaneous insanity") See *folie à deux.*

**folie vaniteuse** (F. "conceited insanity") *Megalomania* (q.v.).

**folk medicine** *Folk healing;* the interrelated beliefs, behaviors, treatment techniques, and medicines that have evolved indigenously within specific cultural settings to cope with illness and injury. Folk medicine includes unorthodox forms of medical care, such as the *voodoo* of the Haitians, *santeria* of the Cubans, *espiritismo* of the Puerto Ricans, *curanderismo* of Spanish-speaking people, folk healing, charismatic faith healers, and rootworkers. See *complementary medicine.*

**folk soul** A group mind, the presence of which is deduced from the way each member displays properties and modes of reaction not present when he or she remains outside the group. The folk soul is considered a sort of transcendental supermind that possesses more good than the individual minds that contribute to it. The following terms are approximately equivalent to folk soul: *group mind* (McDougall); *general will* (Rousseau); *collective consciousness* (Renan); *social consciousness* (Espinas, Durkheim, Wundt); and *group consciousness* (Heard). Many do not accept the concept of group mind and instead would explain collective reactions like communism and anarchism as racial neurosis (see *collective psychosis*). Freud explains group psychology on the basis of individual identification of one member with another, secondary to the sharing of a common emotional situation.

**folklore** Folk wisdom or folk learning; suggested by Thoms in 1846. Folklore is the sum-total of relics (which have survived, through tradition, from earlier primitive-culture stages) of cultural monuments in word and art: historical accounts, legends and myths, adages and sayings, beliefs, customs, magic practices, folk remedies, household prescripts, fairy tales, fables, and songs (words, music, dances).

**folkways** Group habits or customs; the whole system of behavior patterns characteristic of a group; the accepted or expected ways of performing the nearly infinite number of minor rituals of normal social living.

**Folling test**    See *phenylketonuria*.

**follow-back**    See *follow-through*.

**follow-through**    A type of follow-up technique in research in which the investigator examines the subjects (both experimental and control) in childhood and then reevaluates them at intervals until they reach the age at which he measures the outcomes in which he is interested.

Particularly when they are used to monitor the development of children or others at risk, such follow-up studies have disadvantages, such as the period of time required, changing concepts of nosology over time, development of different diagnostic or treatment techniques over time, and the ethical questions of how the researcher can maintain a role of uninvolved, objective observer if a treatable condition is detected or if a new treatment is developed that will alter the natural course of the condition under study. See *risk; vulnerability factor*.

*Follow-back* approaches the problem from the other end of the temporal spectrum. The experimental group is formed by persons diagnosed as suffering currently from the disease under study. Their development is then traced retrospectively—by the examination of birth records, school performance, and medical history, for example—in an attempt to identify the significant factors in the development of the disorder. This method also has drawbacks, including the unavailability of some of the records considered crucial in at least some of the subjects.

**follow-up**    Pursuing or repeating an earlier action, including assessment of the effects of an earlier action. To the clinician, the term generally means aftercare and monitoring of the patient's response to initial and subsequent interventions. To the researcher, the term is likely to mean periodic evaluation or *follow-through* (q.v.).

**folly**    The clinical syndrome known in the early part of the 19th century as *folly* was roughly the equivalent of what is today known as schizophrenia; Guislain (early 19th century) used the terms folly and paraphrenia interchangeably.

**fomes ventriculi**    (L. "foreign body as "contagium-carrier of the stomach' ") Hypochondriasis.

**foot fetishism**    *Retifism* (q.v.).

**foot-drop gait**    See *steppage gait*.

**foramen, foramina**    See *ventricle*.

**forced alimentation**    *Forced feeding*; feeding in opposition to the will of the person being fed, as is frequently done in the treatment of patients with anorexia nervosa, persons who try to commit suicide through starvation, and prisoners on hunger strike. All such cases raise ethical questions about the rights of the person involved to refuse treatment and about the authority of the treater to override that person's autonomy.

**forced groping**    Forced grasping. See *frontal lobe dysfunction*.

**forced impulses**    See *first-rank symptoms*.

**forced phantasy**    A technique devised by Ferenczi, based upon his finding that there is a type of person who "both in analysis and life is particularly poor in phantasies, if not actually without them, on whom the most impressive experiences leave no apparent trace." He advocated forcing affect into the memories, as by asking the patient to fabricate or guess about the memories, or even by telling him what he should have felt and phantasied.

Ferenczi believed that phantasies should be forced only at the end of a psychoanalysis. Moreover, he believed that there are mainly three topics that lend themselves to forced phantasies: (1) positive and negative phantasies of transference, (2) phantasies relating to infancy, and (3) onanistic phantasies (*Further Contributions to the Theory and Technique of Psycho-Analysis*, 1926). See *guided affective imagery*.

**forced treatment**    Coercive or enforced treatment; imposition of a treatment procedure or therapeutic regimen on a patient against his or her will. In the United States, Standard 9 of the Wyatt v. Stickney decision (1972) states that patients have a right not to be subjected to unusual or *hazardous treatment* procedures without their expressed and informed consent, after consultation with counsel or an interested party of the patient's choice. Specified as high risk or as less commonly used treatments were lobotomy, electroconvulsive therapy, and aversive reinforcement conditioning—treatments considered by the courts to be invasive or intrusive. Since then, the concept has been broadened to the right to refuse treatment as part of the growing concern over the potentiality of misuse of psychotechnology to achieve behavior control or social control. See *consumerism*.

**forebrain**  Prosencephalon, from which develop the telencephalon (which forms the cerebral cortex, striate bodies, rhinencephalon, lateral ventricles, and the anterior portion of the third ventricle) and the *diencephalon* (q.v.). The diencephalon is the conduit for ascending sensory information, whereas the telencephalon is the highest-order processor of neural function.

**foreconscious**  *Preconscious (q.v.).*

**Forel, fields of**  (Auguste Forel, Swiss psychiatrist, 1848–1931) See *subthalamus.*

**forensic**  Relating to public policy, especially that formulated in judicial decisions. Forensic psychiatry (legal psychiatry) refers to the application of psychiatry in the courts of law. See *advocacy; consumerism; forced treatment; forensic psychiatry.*

**forensic proof**  The standard that testimony must meet in order to be probative. Proof of *guilt* beyond a reasonable doubt, for instance, requires a mass of evidence, each element of which must exclude every plausible inference except guilt. Many physicians and biomedical scientists feel that the law demands more certainty and concreteness than any probabilistic science can provide. Almost all states, however, require a "reasonable" degree of medical certainty rather than absolute certainty and thus allow medical testimony that reflects the current degree of knowledge within the field.

**forensic psychiatry**  The application of psychiatry to law and to the goals or ends of the legal system. Forensic psychiatry developed largely in relation to lawyers' efforts to save their clients from a death sentence. It first involved citing "facts" about insanity, intent, competence, etc., and then spread to include other areas, such as decisions about whether a psychiatrist is negligent in his or her treatment of patients, and about whether persons are compensable for mental suffering they have endured.

Other psychiatric-legal issues i nclude child custody, child abuse, domestic violence, testamentary capacity. See *crime and mental disorder; criminal responsibility.* A broader area is the portion of *health law* (q.v.) that pertains to psychiatry. See *correctional psychiatry.*

**forepleasure**  Physical and psychical antecedents to final genital action and end pleasure. During the phase of infancy, libido is invested in many erotogenic zones—mouth, anus, skin, muscles, eyes, nose, etc. During the pregenital stage, stimulation of these zones constitutes an end pleasure, but with the advent of genital primacy the pregenital zones are subordinated to the genital; hence, they later become a forepleasure.

**foreseeability**  In relation to protecting the potential victim(s) of a patient's violence, three variables are important: (1) whether there is a threat to a named victim; (2) whether the patient has a history of violence, and (3) whether the patient has a credible motive. When two or three of these conditions are present, courts almost always find that violence is foreseeable and that the duty to protect exists.

**foresight**  See *frontal lobe.*

**foresightfulness**  Foresightedness; provision for the future based on past experience and insight into the effect one's own actions are likely to have on the actions of others. In *cognitive enhancement therapy* (q.v.), the ability to predict how others will react to the social cues one presents to them. See *empathy; theory of mind.*

**forgetfulness, organic**  Memory disturbances based on organic disorders. See *amnesia.*

**forgetting**  Inability to remember, a reflection of a failure of communication between the nerve cell assemblies crucial to *memory* (q.v.). In general, three causes can be distinguished:

1.  Storage loss—because of decay of the neuronal connections that represented the information, or because of displacement from storage by new information.

2.  Retrieval failure—retrieval is greatly affected by the presence or absence of relevant cues, and also by the internal cues provided by mood. Hypnosis can sometimes alter the mood state and thus facilitate retrieval, but the belief that there is no true forgetting, and that hypnosis can recover "seemingly" forgotten memories, is without substance. The "memories" produced under hypnosis have proved to be highly unreliable.

3.  Encoding deficiency—insufficient information was stored in the first place and provides no basis for differentiating between wanted and unwanted information.

**formal operations**  See *hypothetical-deductive thinking; propositional thinking.*

**formants**  The resonant frequencies that, like notes in a musical chord, make up each vowel sound (such as the "e" in "see"). Formant frequency patterns convey the sounds of language and are used to estimate SVT length. See *vocal tract normalization*.

**format, treatment**   The specifics of how treatment will be delivered: duration, intensity, focus, identification of subsystems involved (e.g, individual, marital, or family), relationship to concurrent therapies or position in a sequence of planned interventions, who is included in therapy, where it takes place, etc.

**formes frustes**   (F. "defaced, worn, blurred forms") Indefinite or less significant or atypical symptoms or types of a disease.

**formication**   *Magnan sign; cocaine bug*; a tactile hallucination found in some cocaine abusers consisting of the feeling that ants or other small insects are moving in or under the skin; first described by Magnan and Saury in 1889. It is relatively rare and when it does appear it is usually in association with intravenous use of the drug.

**formicophilia**   A subtype of *zoophilia* (q.v.) in which sexual arousal and orgasm are dependent upon the sensations produced by small bugs or other creatures crawling or nibbling at the skin, most frequently in the genital or anal areas or around the nipples. See *paraphilia*.

**fornication**   Sexual intercourse on the part of an unmarried person.

**fornix**   An arched white fiber tract lying beneath the corpus callosum, extending from the hippocampus and terminating in the mammillary body. See *Papez's theory of emotion*.

**fossa, posterior cranial**   *Cerebellar fossa*; the hindmost and largest depression of the base of the cranium, containing the cerebellum, pons, medulla oblongata, and the fourth ventricle. The roof of the posterior cranial fossa is the *tentorium cerebelli*, which is formed by dura mater overlying the cerebellum; that roof supports the occipital lobe of the cerebral cortex. *Infratentorial* refers to what lies below the tentorium, that is, the contents of the posterior cranial fossa; *supratentorial* refers to what lies above.

**Foster Kennedy syndrome**   (Foster Kennedy, New York neurologist, 1884–1955) See *olfactory nerve*.

**Fothergill neuralgia**   (Samuel Fothergill, English physician, 19th century) See *tic douloureux*.

**fouetteuse**   A female flogger or flagellator.

**founder population**   A group of people descended from a limited number of common ancestors, who have not intermarried much with outside groups because of various factors such as geography, language, religion, etc. Because of their homogeneity, founder populations are ideal for the study of genetics and inheritance.

**Fournier tests**   (Jean Alfred Fournier, French dermatologist, 1832–1914) Used to verify the presence of equilibratory ataxia in walking: the patient is commanded to rise quickly from a sitting position; he is asked to rise and walk, then stop quickly on command; he is requested to walk and turn about quickly on sharp command.

**fourth ventricle**   See *ventricle*.

**Foville syndrome**   (Achille L. Foville, French neurologist, 1799–1878) A form of *hemiplegia alternans* (q.v.) with contralateral hemiplegia and homolateral paralysis of the abducens and facial nerves.

**FOXP2**   One of a family of proteins that are key regulators of gene expression during embryogenesis. The protein is encoded by a gene on chromosome 7. Disruption of FOXP2 results in severe speech disorder characterized by difficulty in controlling the fine mouth movements required for speech, coupled with deficits in many aspects of language processing and grammatical skill.

**FPDD**   Familial pure depressive disease (in Winokur's terminology).

**fractional analysis**   A brief therapy method introduced by Alexander: psychotherapy is suspended for calculated intervals while the patient works through insights already attained and prepares to gain more.

**Fragesucht**   Compulsion to ask irrelevant questions even though not particularly interested in the answers.

**fragging**   The use of explosives (typically, the fragmentation grenade, hence the name for the action) in an assault on a superior officer; said to have been more frequent in the Vietnam war than in previous wars. The hypothesized relationship between fragging and disinhibition of aggressive impulses by a variety of drugs has not been firmly established.

**fragile X ataxia syndrome**   See *FXTAS*.

**fragile X syndrome**   The most common form of inherited mental retardation, with the highest incidence of all X-linked diseases, caused by an abnormality of the X chromosome. Clinical manifestations in males include moderate to severe mental retardation, large head, long face, large ears, and large testicles (macroorchidism). Estimated incidence is one in 1,250 males and 1 in 2,500 females.

Females who inherit the defect are often not affected, because females have a second copy of the X chromosome that usually compensates for the abnormal form. All males who inherit the fragile X are affected, although between 20% and 50% of them are asymptomatic. Asymptomatic male carriers pass the gene to their daughters, who are also asymptomatic, but in the third generation the syndrome typically appears in females as well as males.

Many males and some females with the defective gene are severely retarded. Others are of normal intelligence but have a learning disability, such as inability to learn arithmetic or other tasks involving the use of abstract symbols, or behavior problems with short attention span and hyperactivity. In some reports, over 75% of subjects with fragile X syndrome also have ADHD. Contrary to earlier claims, there is little evidence for an association between fragile X and autism. See *attention deficit hyperactivity disorder; developmental disorders, specific.*

In the fragile X syndrome, the tip of the long arm of the abnormal X chromosome is connected to the rest of the chromosome by only a slender thread and is easily broken, hence the term fragile X. Fragile X sites of affected subjects are much larger than the corresponding sites in normal subjects and in asymptomatic carriers.

The gene responsible for the syndrome, *FMR-1*, was identified in 1991; in the same year a DNA test for it was developed that allows prenatal diagnosis of the defect. Soon thereafter, the specific mutation responsible for the syndrome was identified within *FMR-1*, a highly polymorphic CGG (cytosine-guanine-guanine) repeat. This *triplet repeat* is amplified in successive generations as reflected in increasing disease severity or earlier onset in successive generations (the *Sherman paradox*). See *anticipation.*

Sufferers have more than 200 CGG repeats in the 5′ untranslated region of the fragile X mental retardation 1 gene (*FMR-1*), compared with 60 or fewer in normals. The expanded disease alleles derive from phenotypically normal individuals who carry an intermediate number of unstable repeats, which in

the case of fragile X ranges from 60 to 200. Some of these *premutation carriers* have been found to develop a new form of progressive neurodegeneration by Pen Jin et al. (*Neuron* 39: 739–747, 2003), who found that human premutation repeats alone can lead to neurodegeneration, and that the effect depends on the abundance and length of the repeat. See *FXTAS.*

**fragmentation** Breaking apart; in psychodynamics, it usually refers to a dissolution of the ego into psychotic states (sometimes called *micropsychotic* episodes) and a loss of the sense of self that represent a regressive response to stress or the influence of psychoactive substances. Manifestations may include panic states, fears of flying apart, dread of immediate death or annihilation, loss of bodily integrity, and diffusion of body identity.

**fragmentation of thinking** A disturbance in association, frequent in schizophrenia, in which even such basic concepts as "father" and "mother" become vague and obscure and the thinking processes become so confused that they cannot result in a complete idea or action, but merely in vague movements. Bleuler called this a primary symptom of schizophrenia and believed it to be due to associations no longer following the logical pathways indicated by past experience. Instead, associations easily take new and seemingly illogical pathways, and thinking becomes bizarre. Thus, two ideas, fortuitously encountered, are combined into one thought. Associations lack the concept of purpose. When the symptom is of mild degree, it may be noticed only that the patient gives generalized rather than precise answers. Thus, one patient, asked to give the location of London, said "Europe" rather than "England" (*Dementia Praecox or the Group of Schizophrenias*, 1950).

**fragmented communications** See *communication, disordered.*

**frame** The concepts of frames and scripts are predicated on the belief that few situations we encounter are really new. Technically, frames describe static situations, while scripts characterize a dynamic set of actions appropriate to a given set of circumstances. See *script.*

**Frankenstein factor** *Antitechnology bias*; specifically, the fear that advances in macromolecular chemistry, immunology, etc., will make possible the creation of a monster or threat that can easily escape the control of its originator.

**Frankl, Viktor** (1905–1997) Austrian psychiatrist who developed *logotherapy* (q.v.), considered the "third school" of Viennese psychotherapy after the "first school" of Freud and the "second school" of Adler. *Man's Search for Meaning* (1946), *Man's Search for Ultimate Meaning* (1997).

**FRAP** See *ATM family.*

**free association** The trends of thought or chains of ideas that spontaneously arise when restraint and censorship upon logical thinking are removed and the subject orally reports everything that passes through his mind. This fundamental technique of psychoanalysis assumes that the analysand will bring forward basic psychic material and thus make it available to analytical interpretation.

Many questions have arisen in regard to the validity of free association as a method of gaining access to the unconscious. Freud's descriptions of his technique make it clear that the associations recorded were by no means free and spontaneous, but instead were often suggested to the patient and subtly forced on him. In the case of *Little Hans* (q.v.), whose father played the role of analyst under Freud's direction, Freud indicated that Hans often had to be told what his father believed his next thought should be. "His attention had to be turned in the direction that his father was expecting something to come" (Wolpe, J. and Rachman, S., in Rachman, S. *Critical Essays on Psychoanalysis*, 1963).

**free radical** Radical ion; a chemical entity that has an unpaired electron and also an electrical charge. In biological systems, most free radicals are based on oxygen; an important example is the superoxide ion, symbolized $O_2^-$. The "leakage" of high-energy electrons from the mitochondrial electron transfer chain causes the formation of the reactive oxygen species (ROS), $O_2^-$, and hydrogen peroxide. In the presence of reduced cellular iron, hydrogen peroxide generates the highly toxic hydroxyl radical OH–. Free radicals are highly reactive and potentially toxic, attacking cellular membranes, proteins, and nucleic acids. Many organ systems possess mechanisms to deactivate free radicals: deactivating enzymes such as superoxide dismutase (SOD), or scavengers such as vitamin C and vitamin E, which capture the extra electron of the radical and become radicals themselves but are less toxic. All such deactivators or detoxicants are often called *antioxidants*. The brain is highly vulnerable to free radical effects because it is highly oxygenated yet relatively poor in antioxidants.

Free radicals are produced during the metabolism of dopamine, and it has been suggested that Parkinson disease is related to free radical damage in the substantia nigra. They have also been implicated in schizophrenic "burnout." The dopamine-blocking effect of neuroleptics increases the amount and rate of dopamine turnover in the brain; this could result in the increased production of free radicals that, through lipid peroxidation, could damage membranes and cells in or near brain areas high in catecholamine content. In the same way, tardive dyskinesia could result from increased free radical formation. Glutamate toxicity may be based on the production of free radicals; when glutamate binds to the NMDA receptor, a channel opens to permit an excessive inflow of calcium ions, which activate calcium-dependent proteases that produce free radicals. See *aging, theories of.*

**free will** The concept that people are free to dispose of their own will; that they can choose between alternatives in such manner that the choice is entirely uninfluenced by factors not consciously controlled by them. The opposite of free will is *determinism* (q.v.).

**freebasing** Increasing the potency of *cocaine* by extracting pure cocaine alkaloid, the free base, and then inhaling the heated vapors through a cigarette or water pipe. Extraction is simple and requires only baking soda and a source of heat, but many cocaine abusers extract the alkaloid by mixing it with ether and acetone. This is dangerous because the mixture is explosive and highly flammable. See *crack.*

**freedom to choose** See *coercion.*

**Freeman, Walter J.** (1895–1972) American psychiatrist and neurologist; psychosurgery.

**free-running** See *rhythms, biological.*

**freezing** Periods of bradykinesia and immobility, particularly when walking in narrow spaces, seen often in Parkinson disease. See *trauma.*

**Fregoli phenomenon** See *misidentification, delusional; parietal lobe; sensory neglect.*

**frenetic** See *phrenetic.*

**frenzy** *Obs.* Extreme excitement and mental agitation; sometimes considered synonymous with mania.

**frequency bands** The different spontaneous oscillations of the electrical potential of the brain. Oscillations are a prominent feature of neuronal activity, and the *synchronization* (q.v.) of oscillations reflects the temporally precise interaction of neural activities and is a likely mechanism for neural communication. The oscillations have been classified into different frequency bands: delta, 1–3 Hz; theta, 4–7 Hz; alpha, 8–13 Hz; beta, 14–30 Hz; gamma, 30–80z; fast, 80–200 Hz; ultra fast, 200–600 Hz. See *electroencephalogram*.

**frequency, flicker (fusion)** See *flicker*.

**FRET** Fluorescence resonance energy transfer, the process by which an excited fluorophore (the donor) transfers energy to another molecule (the acceptor) when the emissions spectrum of the donor overlaps the absorption spectrum of the acceptor. The distance over which energy transfer is 50% efficient, the Förster distance, is typically 20–60 A, making FRET useful as a spectroscopic ruler for distance measurements in proteins. It is used, for instance, to measure intracellular aggregation of polyglutamine proteins, which are implicated in diseases such as Huntington disease. See *VSDI*.

**Freud, Anna** (1895–1982) Vienna-born lay analyst, daughter of Sigmund Freud; *The Ego and the Mechanisms of Defence* (1936); play therapy; psychoanalysis of children and adolescents.

**Freud, Sigmund** (1856–1939) Austrian neurologist and psychoanalyst; founder of psychoanalysis; concepts of the libido, regression, repression, transference, sublimation, id, ego, superego, Oedipus complex, etc.; psychopathology of dreams; evaluation of infantile experiences.

**Freud syndrome** Repression. Janet called it "…an interesting symptom; it explains certain remarkable phenomena, such as monstrous and sacrilegious longings. It will continue to form a part of mental pathology under the name of 'Freud's syndrome' " (*Psychological Healing*, 1925).

**Freudian slip** See *symptomatic act*.

**friction** In social work, "conflicts arising out of unlike temperaments or emotional needs which, instead of resolving themselves in a constructive manner, continue on a level of chafing and irritation. *Family Friction*—a generalized tension or irritation in any combination of family life, excepting when otherwise distinguished; *Marital Friction*—the spouse being the patient; *Parental Friction*—between the parents of a minor child, the child being the patient; *Parent–Child Friction*—between parent and child, either being the patient" (Hamilton, G. *A Medical Social Terminology*, 1930).

**Friedmann complex** (Max Friedmann, German neurologist, 1858–1925) See *narcolepsy; posttraumatic constitution*.

**Friedreich ataxia** *FRDA*; an autosomal recessive degenerative disease, the most common hereditary ataxia with an estimated prevalence of 1 in 50,000 to 1 in 100,000. It affects males more frequently. It is characterized by progressive gait and limb ataxia, sensory neuropathy, nystagmus, intention tremor, weakness of the legs, kyphoscoliosis, dysarthria, and, because of early degeneration of the pyramidal tracts, development of pes cavus (clubfoot deformity). (When accompanied by peroneal atrophy, the condition is termed *Roussy-Lévy syndrome*.) Onset is between 5 and 15 years of age. The disorder is slowly progressive and most patients are confined to a wheelchair by their late 20s and dead by the age of 30. There is little evidence that FRDA causes either mental retardation or dementia.

Pathologically, there is degeneration of the posterior columns and spinocerebellar tracts of the spinal cord, mainly in its lower portion, and of the pyramidal tracts. FRDA is a *trinucleotide repeat* disorder, but an unusual one in that it is transmitted as an autosomal recessive with little evidence for genetic *anticipation*, and onset in middle age or later is uncommon (qq.v.). The mutant gene is X25, in the critical region for the FRDA locus on chromosome 9. The gene encodes the protein frataxin. In normal chromosomes, 10 to 20 copies of the GAA repeat occur, whereas nearly 95% of FRDA chromosomes contain between 200 and 900 repeats. The GAA-repeat expansion inhibits transcription of *FRDA*, whereas point mutations adversely affect protein expression, function, or stability. Frataxin is a mitochondrial protein; there are at least five hypotheses about its function: iron transport, iron storage, antioxidant activity, stimulation of oxidative phorylation, and biosynthesis of iron-sulfur (Fe-S) centers (ISCs). There is evidence that frataxin acts as a storage protein for intramitochondrial iron, keeping it in a nontoxic, bioavailable form;

but it is more likely that a recently identified mitochondrial ferritin performs this function. All in all, data suggest that mitochondrial iron accumulation might be a distal consequence of an earlier, proximal effect of frataxin deficiency. The neurodegeneration associated with FRDA may well be the result of a multistep cycle that includes Fe-S deficiency, which leads to iron accumulation, resulting in oxidative stress, which leads to Fe-S deficiency.

**friendly** In computer language, relatively easy to use by those not versed in computer science. It takes a great many circuits (VLSIC, very large scale integrated circuits) to make a system easy to learn and friendly to use, and the person–machine interface may remain a barrier to effective use of the computer that is not friendly.

**fright** A reaction to an unexpected danger. According to Freud, "Fright is the name of the condition to which one is reduced if one encounters a danger without being prepared for it; it lays stress on the element of surprise." This element of surprise distinguishes fright from both fear and apprehension. "Apprehension denotes a certain condition of expecting a danger and preparation for it, even though it be an unknown one; fear requires a definite object, of which one is afraid" (*Beyond the Pleasure Principle*, 1922).

Surprise appears to be an essential element in the traumatic neurosis as well. Apprehension does not produce a traumatic neurosis; rather, it prepares the organism for oncoming excitation. In fright, the organism is unprepared, so that it is overwhelmed by the excitation.

**frigidity, sexual** Female sexual arousal disorder, consisting of lack of sexual desire, or lack of pleasure or sexual excitement in response to adequate stimulation, typically leading to avoidance of genital contact with a sexual partner; analogous to sexual impotence in the male.

*Total frigidity* includes complete anesthesia; absence of sexual interest; vaginismus, with or without dyspareunia—and women so afflicted will generally tolerate intercourse only if forced.

More common than total frigidity is some type of *relative frigidity*, among the more frequent of which are the following: (1) *vaginal hypoesthesia*, with sensitivity limited to the clitoral area; (2) sudden abrupt cessation of excitement before orgasm, even though there has been pleasure during intercourse, during both clitoral stimulation and vaginal friction; some women of this group, in their search for satisfaction, appear insatiable in their sexual demands and may go from one partner to another hoping that each new experience will bring orgasm; (3) orgasm achieved, but only under certain conditions—such as concurrent beating or rape phantasies—or only with certain men; (4) whatever the degree of satisfaction obtained during intercourse, the sexual act is followed by anxiety, tension, insomnia, guilt feelings and depression, or physical complaints.

**Frohlich syndrome** (Alfred Frohlich, Viennese neurologist, 1871–1953) Frohlich syndrome or *dystrophia adiposogenitalis* described in 1901 is caused by a chromophobe adenoma that destroys the anterior lobe of the pituitary gland occurring mainly during the pre- or postadolescent period. It is characterized by eunuchoidal obesity, alteration of the secondary sex characters, metabolic disturbances, and change in body growth—gigantism, hypoplastic genitals, polyuria, polydipsia, and increased sugar tolerance.

**Frohman Factor** A protein factor found in the serum of schizophrenics isolated by C. E. Frohman and colleagues. The factor alters the anaerobic metabolism of chicken red blood cells. It has been suggested that the Frohman Factor is the same as the *Bergen fraction* (q.v.).

**Froin syndrome** (George Froin, Viennese physician, b. 1874) High protein content of the cerebrospinal fluid (0.5% or more) associated with xanthochromia, massive coagulation, and pleocytosis. Froin syndrome is seen mainly in chronic meningitis, especially syphilitic, in obstruction of the spinal subarachnoid space by cord tumor or epidural abscess, and in cases of polyneuritis and Landry paralysis.

**Froment sign** In patients with essential tremor, passive movements of a limb elicit a rhythmical resistance while voluntary action occurs in another body part. The sign may also be found in patients with Parkinson disease, but it is not the same as cog wheel rigidity.

**Fromm-Reichmann, Frieda** (1890–1957) German-born psychoanalyst; director of psychotherapy, Chestnut Lodge Sanitarium; Washington School of Psychiatry and Psychoanalysis; psychotherapy of schizophrenia.

**frontal lobe**  The portion of the cerebral hemisphere in front of the central sulcus and above the lateral fissure. The principal areas of the frontal lobe, as designated by Brodmann, are as follows: area 4 (*precentral gyrus*; principal motor area); immediately in front of 4 is area 6 (*premotor area*; a part of the extrapyramidal tract circuit); in front of this, area 8 (which is concerned with the eye movements and pupillary changes); and in front of this, at the frontal poles and continuing along the inferior surface of the frontal lobe, areas 9, 10, 11, and 12 (which are frontal association areas). See *prefrontal cortex*.

According to Luria, the frontal lobes have four functions: (1) generating plans for action; (2) programming the components, or subroutines, of actions; (3) monitoring ongoing activity with reference both to the goal and to environmental shifts (*self-analysis*); and (4) correcting the course of activity already in progress.

Functions include motor behavior (such as initiation of and persistence in fine motor tasks and rapid sequential movements, as in typing); expressive language; global orientation; right spatial recognition; the ability to concentrate on or attend to a task in a sustained manner (which also depends on the reticular system of the brain stem); abstract problem solving and abstracting ability; judgment; the capacity to form social judgments and read social situations and to form emotional attachments to others; the ability to control motor actions intentionally, based on thinking or reasoning; the ability to think serially and sequentially, and to plan for the future by anticipating or predicting what will happen based on previous experience. The frontal lobe is concerned not with the intellectual functions of analysis, synthesis, and selectivity but with the adjustment of the personality as a whole to future contingencies in the light of past experience. The prefrontal regions in humans are therefore concerned with *foresight*, imagination, and the apperception of the self, and these psychological functions are invested with emotion by way of the association fibers which link the hippocampus and the cingulate gyrus with the prefrontal region on the one hand and with the thalamus and hypothalamus on the other. (See *prefrontal cortex*.) The frontal lobes appear to be responsible for controlling and shaping emotions, which are largely the products of

the limbic system. Together, these two brain areas exert their influence on the hypothalamus, which controls the endocrine system and the autonomic nervous system.

In the human, the prefrontal cortex is the signal largest region of the brain; it accounts for more than 25% of the total cortex, almost twice the size of that of the chimpanzee. See *hypofrontality hypothesis*.

**frontal lobe absence**  See *frontal lobe seizures*.

**frontal lobe dementia**  *Frontotemporal dementia* (q.v.). Prominent features include personality change, apathy, indifference, disinhibition, loss of insight, distractibility, and symptoms of manic-depressive psychosis. Those symptoms are often divided into three clusters: ritualistic-stereotypic, antisocial-impulsive, and apathetic-ahygienic.

**frontal lobe dysfunction**  When the frontal lobes are damaged or destroyed, the ability to synthesize signals from the environment, assign top priorities, or make balanced decisions is impaired. The control made possible by the frontal-limbic connections is weakened, and behavior becomes erratic and unpredictable. Life may also become an endless round of oftentimes purposeless activity, or just the reverse, the patient is immobilized by *aspontaneity*.

Manifestations of frontal lobe dysfunction include the following:

1. Impaired short-term memory store, impaired concentration; sometimes right spatial neglect. See *sensory neglect*.
2. Language and comprehension disturbances:
   a. loss of verbal fluency (as in Broca aphasia or transcortical aphasia)
   b. difficulty suppressing irrelevant associations (*intrusions*), verbigeration
   c. inability to anticipate or predict consequences of action, to foresee what is likely to happen on the basis of past experience
   d. inability to formulate an approach to complex problems that extend over time
   e. dissociation of speech from action (e.g., a patient told to squeeze a ball when he sees a light turned on says, "I must squeeze the ball"; but when he sees the light he fails to carry out the action)

f. impaired abstraction, with difficulty understanding metaphors, similes, and parables (the inability to assume the *abstract attitude* described by Goldstein)

g. *aprosodia* (indicates nondominant frontal lobe disease), which includes:

*motor aprosodia*—the ability to comprehend emotions but inability to express them; speech is monotonous, with difficulty in repeating sentences with prosodic affective variation, but with excellent comprehension of the affective components of speech and gesturing. Often there is inappropriate emotional expression or a lack of affective accompaniments to speech, giving a bland, colorloss quality to the subject's communications (often misinterpreted as blunted affect).

*sensory aprosodia*—inability to understand affect expressed by others, a type of fluent aphasia associated with a posterior lesion in the nondominant temporal lobe.

h. destruction of the frontal association areas (9, 10, 11, and 12) may produce facetiousness (*witzelsucht*), blunting, with a fatuous, shallow mood incongruous to the situation; changes in moral and social behavior, loss of interest, intellectual deterioration, and distractibility.

3. Motor abnormalities: motor impersistence, inertia, impaired rapid sequential movements, catatonic behavior, and stimulus-bound behavior (e.g., echopraxia, gegenhalten), loss of learned complex behavior, stooped and shuffling gait. Cells of the precentral gyrus (*Betz cells*) control voluntary movements of skeletal muscle on the opposite side of the body via the pyramidal tracts; irritative lesions in this area may give convulsive seizures (Jacksonian epilepsy). Destructive lesions in area 4 produce flaccid paralysis; spasticity will occur if area 6 and intermediate cortex are also involved. *Forced grasping* is often seen following destructive lesions of area 6.

4. Specific syndromes associated with frontal lobe dysfunction are the *convexity syndrome* and the *orbitomedial syndrome* (qq.v.), most commonly caused by head trauma associated with motor vehicle accidents.

**frontal lobe seizures** Several forms of frontal lobe seizures have been described. Most are brief (sometimes less than 1 minute), occur in clusters, are frequently associated with sleep, often show no postictal confusion, and are not associated with a specific aura. Frontal seizures of all types tend to be associated with convulsive and nonconvulsive status epilepticus (*NCSE*); the latter may last for hours or even days. See *epilepsy*.

B. C. Jobst and P. D. Williamson (*Psychiatric Clinics of North America 28*: 635–651, 2005) propose the following classification:

*Hypermotor seizures*: also, *complex partial seizures of frontal lobe origin*; *bizarre hyperactive seizures*. These consist of sudden and sometimes explosive automatisms of highly complex behavior, such as jumping out of bed, running around the room, yelling, screaming, shouting obscenities, barking, and pelvic thrusting or aggressive sexual behavior (but no accompanying sexual sensations). During the automatism, the patient is often awake but unable to control motor behavior. They usually end as suddenly as they begin. They have been associated mainly with seizure onset in orbitofrontal cortex and anterior medial frontal regions, including the cinguate gyrus.

*Focal clonic seizures*, consisting of clonic movements of the face or unilateral extremities which increase in severity and spread to other areas. See *Jacksonian epilepsy*. If the seizures do not subside, they are termed *epilepsy partialis continua*.

*Tonic SMA (supplementary motor area) seizures*, with sudden tonic posturing of one or more extremities and, usually, head and eye deviation contralateral to the seizure origin. They may be preceded by an aura of unilateral or bilateral sensory symptoms, such as pulling, pulsing, numbness, or tingling. They may occur in clusters of as many as 100 per night.

*Frontal lobe absence*: staring or absence spells, trancelike states or immobility and unresponsiveness. Absences may last minutes, hours, or days, and many terminate in a generalized convulsion. EEG shows a frontally predominant irregular spike-wave pattern, *spike-wave stupor*. Onset is in the frontal polar or medial frontal region.

*Autosomal dominant nocturnal frontal lobe epilepsy (ADNFLE)*: seizures are brief, frequent, nocturnal, of the bizarre hyperactive or asymmetrical tonic type. Onset is in the teens, with a dominant family history of frontal lobe seizures. ADNFLE is associated with missense mutations of the gene for the neuronal nicotinic acetylcholine receptor $\alpha_4$ subunit (*CHRNA4*) on chromosomes 20q13.2 and 15q24 or the beta-2 subunit on chromosome I (*CHRNB2*).

*Rasmussen encephalitis* (q.v.).

**frontal-striatal system**  Networks of cortical and basal ganglia pathways that are organized into segregated, *parallel circuits*. Projections from different regions of the cortex to separate components of the striatum (the caudate nucleus and putamen) are relayed to the *thalamus* (q.v.) and thence back to the cortex (almost exclusively the frontal cortex). There are at least five circuits that fall within two functional groups:

1. *Motor circuits*, involved in higher level motor skills such as initiating, maintaining, and sequencing complex movements:
    a. Sensorimotor
    b. Oculomotor
2. *Cognitive circuits*, which are involved particularly in the *executive function* (q.v.):
    a. Dorsal cognitive, with projections from the lateral prefrontal cortex to the caudate and thence to the *dorsomedial nucleus* (q.v.) of the thalamus; the dorsal cognitive circuit is believed to play a role in complex cognitive processes, including working memory and the ability to establish and shift mental sets.
    b. Ventral cognitive (also called the *lateral orbitofrontal circuit*, the *socioemotional circuit*, or the *contextual circuit*); projections from the orbitofrontal cortex are relayed to the caudate and thence to the dorsomedial nucleus of the thalamus; the ventral cognitive circuit is believed to play a role in response inhibition.

    c. *Affective-motivational circuit*; projections from the paralimbic cortex (posteromedial orbitofrontal and anterior cingulate) to the *nucleus accumbens* of the striate and thence to the dorsomedial nucleus of the thalamus; this circuit plays a role in emotional or reward-based information processing.

**frontal-striatal-thalamic-cortical (FSTC) circuitry**  Five parallel and partially segregated reciprocal loops that interconnect neurons in prefrontal cortex and subcortical structures, including striatum (caudate nucleus, putamen) and thalamus, and other basal ganglia such as globus pallidus and subthalamic nucleus. These circuits subserve complex cognitive abilities such as planning and execution of multistep tasks in the context of ongoing distractions and new information.

1. The dorsolateral prefrontal subcircuit appears to subserve working memory, novel problem solving, self-monitoring, planning, cognitive flexibility, and the use of organizational strategies during the encoding of information.
2. The orbitofrontal subcircuit is involved in response inhibition and regulation of emotions.
3. The anterior cingulate gyrus circuit mediates goal-directed behaviors and the voluntary allocation of attention, monitors conflict between response choices, and controls emotion.
4. The oculomotor subcircuit, projecting from the frontal eye fields, is involved in the voluntary control of eye movement.
5. The motor subcircuit is important in programming and control of movement.

**frontal-subcortical circuits**  Parallel segregated circuits linking the frontal lobe with subcortical structures (striatum, globus pallidus/substantia nigra, thalamus). Behaviorally relevant circuits include the *DLPFC*, the *frontostriatal-thalamic circuit*, the *orbitofrontal cortex*, and the *medial frontal cortex* (qq.v.).

**frontostriatal-thalamic circuit**  One of the *frontal-subcortical circuits* (q.v.), seemingly involved in comparing current state with expected state, and leading to pathological doubt in obsessive-compulsive disorder.

**frontotemporal dementia**  *FTD; frontal lobe dementia; Pick disease*; circumscribed cortical atrophy, lobar sclerosis; dementia due to focal degeneration of the frontal or anterior temporal lobes. Neuropsychiatric symptoms occur early in the course of the disease and begin with profound personality and behavioral changes and a progressive change in language, rather than with the memory defects characteristic of Alzheimer disease. Impairment of attention and executive functions are the first cognitive signs of FTD.

Like *Alzheimer disease* (q.v.), FTD occurs more in women than in men, and average age of onset is 55 years. The Pick body is characteristic—an inclusion body of abnormal, straight filaments that have some poorly understood relationship with the paired helical filaments characteristic of Alzheimer disease.

The personality changes are typically expressed in three clusters: ritualistic/sterotypic; antisocial/impulsive; and apathetic/ahygienic. Prominent features include disinhibition, loss of insight, apathy, disorganization, aspontaneity, indifference, lack of personal hygiene, mental rigidity, inflexibility, hyperorality, and speech reduction. The paradoxic combination of the apathetic patient, who is emotionally and attentionally disengaged, with disinhibited, socially inappropriate, compulsive, perseverative, or impulsive behaviors is characteristic. Echolalia and mutism may be prominent, and some patients manifest gluttony and sweet food preferences. Apathy appears without the characteristic sadness, crying, and expressions of worthlessness and suicidal ideation seen in depression. Obsessive, compulsive, stereotypical, and repetitive behaviors are related to striatal pathology. The often described jocularity (witzelsucht) and childishness (moria) occur fairly infrequently. Patients may be particularly sensitive to the extrapyramidal side effects of neuroleptics.

The language changes include two type of progressive aphasia: progressive nonfluent aphasia (*PNFA*) and progressive fluent aphasia. In PNFA, speech is halting and distorted with frequent phonological substitutions and grammatical errors. Pathology is prominent in the perisylvian language areas, particularly the insular and Broca areas. In progressive fluent aphasia (also called *semantic dementia*) speech is fluent but becomes progressively devoid of content words. Anterior temporal lobe atrophy is prominent, typically greater on the left side.

FTD is more common in men. Approximately 40% of cases show an autosomal dominant pattern. FTD is genetically heterogeneous; mutations in the *tau* gene on chromosome 17, and in the *presenilin* 1 gene have been demonstrated in some families, and there is also linkage to chromosome 3 and chromosome 9. Abnormalities of tau and ubiquitin metabolism affect primarily frontal and temporal structures.

The frontotemporal dementias constitute up to 10% of all dementias and are particularly prevalent among those with onset before age 65. See *FTDP; Pick complex; primary progressive aphasia; VaD.*

**frontotemporal lobar degeneration** *FTLD*; includes three syndromes: (1) semantic dementia (SD) features a progressive fluent aphasia and visual agnosia; (2) primary progressive nonfluent aphasia (PNFA); and (3) *frontotemporal dementia* (q.v.) with prominent behavioral changes.

In SD, speech remains fluent and well articulated but becomes progressively devoid of content words; the language and other nonverbal cognitive deficits reflect a breakdown in semantic memory. Consistently there is atrophy of the anterior temporal lobe (typically left > right). Most patients have ubiquitin-positive tau-negative inclusions.

In PNFA speech is faltering and distorted with frequent phonological substitutions and grammatical errors, but the semantic aspects of language remain intact. Most patients have tau-positive pathology, either classic Pick body positive FTD, corticobasal degeneration, or Alzheimer disease. The main locus of pathology is in the perisylvian language areas, particularly the insular and Broca area.

**frottage** Sexual perversion in which orgasm is induced by rubbing against the clothing of the sexual object as occurs when the subject is pressed close to others in a throng or crowded public transportation. A person so afflicted is a *frotteur* (q.v.).

**frotteur** (F. "one who rubs") One who gains sexual excitement through the sense of touch by rubbing against somebody. The term usually implies that the act of touching or being touched is not directly or overtly genital, or at least that there is some measure of disguise. For example, some subjects are sexually stimulated when they are pressed closely by others as often happens when they are in a crowd.

Some authorities use the term to mean direct genital or sexual activity so long as it does not include union of the genital organs.

**frotteurism**   *Frottage* (q.v.). The DSM definition of this paraphilia emphasizes that the frotteur's sexual object is nonconsenting.

**frozen watchfulness**   An alert but inhibited appearance observed in many children who have suffered abuse, as part of the reactive attachment disorder they develop.

**frq gene**   See *rhythms, biological.*

**frustration**   Denial of gratification by reality, sometimes spoken of as external frustration to distinguish it from the thwarting of impulses by forces in the unconscious or also in consciousness.

Internal frustration means the checking of instinctual impulses by forces in the unconscious, chiefly by the superego.

**frustration tolerance**   The ability to withstand tension arising from a buildup in instinctual demand that is not immediately relieved or gratified. Development of tension or frustration tolerance is essential for achieving active mastery by the ego; low frustration tolerance and/or the need for immediate instinctual gratification are indicative of severe ego weakness.

**FSPTFL**   The fronto-striato-pallido-thalamo-frontal loop, believed to be the critical circuitry in the pathogenesis of *obsessive-compulsive disorder* (q.v.); it runs from posterior portions of the orbitofrontal cortex, through the ventral or ventromedial caudate and accumbens nuclei, then through the ventromedial pallidum and some medial thalamic nuclei, and finally back to the orbitofrontal cortex. See *basal ganglia.*

**FSTC circuits**   See *frontal-striatal-thalamic-cortical (FSTC) circuitry.*

**FTA-ABS**   The fluorescent treponemal antibody absorption test for syphilis; the test is extremely sensitive and highly specific, with less than a 1% incidence of false-positive reactions.

**FTD**   *Frontotemporal dementia* (q.v.).

**FTDP**   Inherited frontotemporal dementia and Parkinsonism; FTDP-17 is linked to chromosome 17, with mutations in the tau coding regions. It is characterized by behavioral, cognitive, and motor disturbances, and by frontotemporal atrophy associated with gliosis and the formation of intraneuronal tau-containing deposits. See *frontotemporal dementia.*

**FTLD**   *Frontotemporal lobar degeneration* (q.v.).

**Fuch syndrome**   See *Behçet syndrome.*

**fugue**   *Dissociative fugue*; the subject suddenly leaves home or work and begins to wander or goes on a journey that has no apparent relation to what he or she had been doing, with amnesia for the past. During the fugue there is confusion about personal identity or, particularly in fugues of longer duration, assumption of a new identity. The fugue is usually brief—hours to days—with spontaneous and rapid recovery. Recurrences are rare. Fugues appear often to be precipitated by a desire to escape an intolerable situation. See *dissociation; hysteria.*

Fugues may occur in temporal lobe epilepsy, alcohol and other drug intoxication, or as a part of dissociative identity disorder or catatonic excitement.

**Fulton, John Farquhar**   (1899–1960) American physician; neurophysiology (especially hypothalamus, cerebellum, autonomic nervous system); history of science and medicine.

**function complex**   In analytic psychology, a mechanism through which a function operates. No matter what *function type* (q.v.) predominates, daily living requires many ad hoc adjustments. One such is the function complex called the *persona* (q.v.), a mask or outer appearance that is adopted as a temporary expedient to fit in with the environment. The persona and other function complexes may be used by any of the function types.

**function engram**   For Jung, an inherited, archaic residue. "The symbol is always derived from archaic residues, or imprints engraven in the very stem of the race, about whose age and origin one can speculate much, although nothing definite can be determined. It would certainly be quite wrong to look to personal sources for the source of the symbol, as for instance repressed sexuality. At best such a repression could only furnish the libidosum which activates the archaic imprint. The imprint (engram) corresponds with a functional inheritance whose existence is not contingent upon ordinary sexual repression, but proceeds from instinct differentiation in general" (*Psychological Types*, 1923).

**function pleasure**   Enjoyment of functioning or doing or exercising one's own capacities. Function pleasure is obtained when an act can be accomplished without anxiety; such pleasure is the basis for subsequent repetitions of situations that originally induced excitation and anxiety, as is seen frequently in children who enjoy endless repetitions of the same game or of the same story, which has to be retold in exactly the same words.

**function type**   The generic name for Jung's various types: feeling, thinking, intuitive, and sensation. "These types, which are based upon the root-functions and which one can term the thinking, the feeling, the intuitive, and the sensational types, may be divided into two classes according to the quality of the respective basic function: viz., the *rational* and the *irrational*. The thinking and feeling types belong to the former. The intuitive and sensational to the latter" (*Psychological Types*, 1923).

The characters of introversion and extraversion are ways of regarding reality rather than methods of adaptation to reality; hence, they are called attitude types. Any one of the four functional types may occur in either of the two *general attitude* groups—the *extravert* or the *introvert*; i.e., there are: (1) thinking, (2) feeling, (3) intuitive, (4) sensational extraverts, and introverts, or eight varieties of psychological type in all. See *analytic psychology*.

**functional**   Relating to performance or execution; in psychiatry, refers to disorders that are without known organic basis, thus often (incorrectly) equated with "psychogenic" or emotional. A functional disturbance is one in which the performance or operation of an organ or organ system is abnormal, but not as a result of known changes in structure. Although psychogenic disorders are functional, in that their symptoms are not based upon any detectable alterations in the structure of the brain or psyche, it is not true that all functional disorders of the psyche are of emotional origin—no more so than functional heart murmurs are based on emotional conflict.

A drug-induced, temporary disturbance in synaptic transmission, for example, may produce many alterations in thinking, affect, and behavior. Since such a disturbance does not depend upon structural changes in the brain, it is properly termed "functional"; yet it can hardly be considered to be of psychogenic origin. See *organic*.

**functional assessment stages**   See *GDS*.

**functional budgeting**   In this system of resource allocation and control, the budget is not constructed according to line items (*inputs*), but instead according to functions or activities carried out by the departments or components of an organization (*outputs*). Resources are then assigned for the accomplishment of the organization's objectives. Thus, the budget focus is where it should be, on the programs of the organization designed to achieve its goals. Functional budgeting is an essential element of *strategic planning* (q.v.).

**functional decapitation**   See *brain death*.

**functional genomics**   See *genome*.

**function-way, archaic**   In analytical psychology, thinking, acting, and feeling characteristic of the primitive type of mind. While discussing *regression* Jung says: "…Since man has spent relatively only a few thousand years in a cultivated state, as opposed to many hundred thousand years in a state of savagery, the archaic function-ways are correspondingly extraordinarily vigorous and easily reanimated. Hence, when certain functions become disintegrated through deprivation of libido, their archaic foundations begin to operate in the unconscious" (*Psychological Types*, 1923).

**functor words**   See *aphasia*.

**fundamental symptom**   Bleuler differentiates between fundamental and accessory symptoms of the schizophrenias. The fundamental, primary, or principal symptoms are those that are pathognomonic of *schizophrenia* (q.v.). The accessory symptoms, by contrast, while they may overshadow the fundamental symptoms in their intensity, are not the essential or basic elements because they occur also in other diseases, particularly in the organic brain syndromes. The fundamental symptoms include autism; disturbances in the associations, in the affect, in the person, in the will, in attention, in activity and behavior; ambivalence (of affect, intellect, or will); and schizophrenic dementia.

**Funkenstein test**   (Daniel Hertz Funkenstein, American psychiatrist, b. 1910) See *Adrenalin-Mecholyl test*.

**funnel plots**   See *publication bias*.

**fureur génitale**   *Obs.* Bruisson's term for nymphomania and satyriasis.

**furiosi**   (L. "those full of madness, raging, fury") A subdivision of the insane recorded in the old Roman laws. Those who were violent and maniacal were called *furiosi*; those exhibiting dementia or feeblemindedness were termed *mente capti*.

**"furlough" psychosis** An episode of the acute schizophrenic type secondary to the sudden emotional readjustments required by a military furlough or leave. Dynamically, the outbreak of the psychotic behavior seems to be related to the sudden release of the soldier from military authority, on which he has become dependent. Symptoms appear suddenly a few days after the apparently well-adjusted person has returned home. Affect becomes inappropriate, delusional trends and ideas of reference are prominent, and suicidal tendencies are frequent. In the ensuing week or two, severe confusion with blocking of thought processes becomes marked. Gradual improvement occurs within 2 months, irrespective of any particular form of therapy. The patient cannot return to duty, because flattening of affect and unpredictable behavior usually remain (*American Journal of Psychiatry 102*, 1945–1946). See *schizophreniform disorder*.

**fusiform face area** *FFA*; the lateral fusiform gyrus in the occipitotemporal region in the extrastriate visual cortex. FFA is specifically activated in response to faces. The superior temporal sulcus is activated during visual gaze tasks and is involved in processing the changeable aspects of the face. FFA, on the other hand, is more strongly activated during identity tasks and processes nonchangeable aspects of the face. It was long believed that face processing takes place separately from that of other objects in a face-specific processing module. But the fusiform area can also show similar activations in response to birds, cars, or other objects in people who have experience with these stimuli. See *face cells*; *face recognition*.

The fusiform gyrus processes the structural, static properties of faces, which are reliable indicators of personal identity. Regions more anterior and dorsal in the temporal lobe (such as the superior temporal gyrus and sulcus) are involved in processing information about the changeable configurations of faces, such as facial expressions and eye and mouth movements. The superior temporal cortex processes information about biological motion, the basis of social attribution. Specific movement cues appear to generate attributions of animacy, intentionality, and agency. (*Animacy* is the subjective impression that a stimulus is alive; agency refers to the subjective impression of a willful, goal-directed action.)

Both patients with schizophrenia and persons with schizotypal personality show reduced facial recognition memory. In schizophrenia, reduction in both extraversion (a heritable personality trait often used as a measure of sociality) and facial memory is correlated with a smaller than normal volume of the right posterior fusiform gyrus.

**fusion** 1. In psychoanalysis, the union of the instincts. Normally during the early infantile months the two primal instincts, life and death, operate separately. Later they fuse to a greater or lesser extent. In psychiatric conditions there is often some defusion of the instincts.

For example, when the ego is threatened by an external danger associated with a genital impulse, the latter is repressed and regression to the anal-sadistic level follows. Several possibilities then occur regarding the redistribution of libido. "A part regresses and fuses with the hate instincts to constitute sadism" (Jones, E. *Papers on Psycho-Analysis*, 1938). See *instinct*.

2. In the literature on dissociative identity disorder, fusion refers to the moment during successful treatment when the alters have ceded their separateness and the patient has attained a single personality. See *integration*.

3. See *flicker*.

**futility, medical** The situation in which a therapy that is hoped to benefit a patient's medical condition will predictably not do so on the basis of the best available evidence. See *brain death*; *vegetative state*.

**future shock** A term coined by Alvin Toffler (1970) to refer to the psychological syndrome occurring when the subject is continuously overwhelmed by frequent, sudden, and abrupt changes in the environment.

**FXTAS** *Fragile X-associated tremor/ataxia syndrome*, found in some older male carriers of the fragile X premutation expansion. The subjects, in their 50's and older, develop progressive gait instability and intention tremor, often with progressive cognitive and behavioral difficulties such as reclusive or irritable behavior, memory loss, deficits of executive function, and dementia.

Premutation expansions (50–200 CGG repeats) of the fragile X mental retardation 1 (*FMR1*) gene are frequent in the general population, occurring in approximately 1 of every 259 females and in 1 of every 813 males.

# G

*g* In psychometrics, general intelligence in the sense of reasoning and ability to solve novel problems; it is consistently linked to the integrity and function of the lateral PFC, which supports the executive control of action and attention. Gf is fluid intelligence, "on the spot" reasoning and novel problem-solving ability, related to analytical intelligence; it is strongly related to working memory. Gc is crystallized intelligence, overlearned skills and static knowledge, such as vocabulary.

Psychometric *g* is highly heritable, and the heritability of intelligence increases with age—as we grow older, our phenotype reflects our genotype more closely. A strictly environmental theory would predict the opposite.

**g factor** The hypothesized causal entity underlying the phenotype of general intelligence as measured by IQ scores, defined operationally as what diverse tests of cognitive ability have in common. Charles Spearman (1904) introduced the term as a neutral signifier of general cognitive ability that avoided the many connotations of "intelligence."

**G protein** Guanosine triphosphate-binding protein; also called *N protein* (nucleotide-binding regulatory protein). The ubiquitously distributed G proteins link an array of receptors at the cell surface, including many neuroreceptors (among them the α- and β-adrenergic, dopamine, muscarinic acetylcholine, opioid, rhodopsin, serotonin, substance K, and THC receptors), to a variety of intracellular effectors that lie along or near the inner cell membrane. The effector is an enzyme that converts an inactive molecule within the cell to an active one, the second messenger. This activated molecule initiates various intracellular responses, such as inhibiting or promoting adenylyl cyclase activity, phosphodiesterase, and phospholipase C or other second messengers. G proteins couple with many neurotransmitters; in consequence, they receive and direct large amounts of information arriving from diverse sources within the brain. See *glutamate.*

G proteins consist of three protein subunits (α, β, and γ) and function as on-off switches for cellular signaling. In the off position, guanosine diphosphate (*GDP*) is tightly bound to the α subunit. When the membrane receptor is activated, it interacts with the G protein, which goes into the on position. Guanosine triphosphate (*GTP*) replaces GDP, and the protein dissociates into two complexes, the α subunit and the βγ subunit, both of which can activate effectors.

In addition to coupling with a number of metabotropic receptors (G protein–coupled receptors), G proteins sometimes gate ion channels directly. (Some receptors also gate ion channels directly, without linkage to G proteins. Among them are the nicotinic acetylcholine and the AMPA, GABA, glycine, and NMDA classes of glutamate receptors.) See *ion channel; neurotransmitter receptor; second messenger.*

Alterations in the structure of G proteins (such as by genetic or somatic mutations) may increase or decrease their activity and lead to serious pathophysiologic consequences, including *pseudohypoparathyroidism* (Albright hereditary osteodystrophy), hypersecretion of growth hormone and acromegaly, McCune-Albright syndrome (hyperfunction of one or more endocrine glands), and testotoxicosis (precocious puberty secondary to hypersecretion of testosterone by Leydig cells). Abnormalities in the function or expression of G protein signaling pathways have been reported in patients with schizophrenia.

**G spot** *Grafenberg spot* (after Ernest Grafenberg, 1881–1957); an area on the anterior wall of the vagina described in popular literature as a highly erogenous area that is palpable at least in some women during sexual arousal. It is a zone of glandular tissue surrounding the urethra (hence termed the paraurethral glands) and may be responsible for the release of fluid through the urethra at the time of orgasm. It is analogous to the male prostate.

**GABA** Gamma-aminobutyric acid; an amino acid *neurotransmitter* (q.v.). GABA and *glycine* are the major inhibitory transmitters in the CNS (glutamate is the major excitatory transmitter). Inhibitory synaptic action is mediated by receptor channels selective for chloride, i.e., inhibitory transmitters open Cl– channels. The concentration of Cl– is high on the outside of the cell and low inside. The influx of Cl– adds to the negative charge inside the cell, while efflux of K+ removes positive charge. Thus, opening either Cl– or K+ channels leads to a positive or outward current and a net hyperpolarization.

Benzodiazepines and barbiturates act as GABA agonists and increase inhibitory tone; they bind to GABA receptors and enhance the Cl– flux through these channels in response to GABA. See *benzodiazepine*; *ion channel*; *receptor complex, supramolecular*.

**GABAergic systems** Most neurons in the striatum are GABAergic. Also particularly rich in GABA are the globus pallus and substania nigra partidis reticulata (SNpr). Inhibition of GABA-containing neurons in the external globus pallidus releases (disinhibits) subthalamic neurons from their tonic inhibition by the external globus pallidus; the result is choreiform movements such as those in Huntington disease. Similarly, striatal activation may lead to nigral inhibition and consequenctly to thalamic activation because of disinhibition of the latter.

GABA transmission regulates synaptic integration, the probability and timing of action potential generation, and plasticity in principal neurons. Interneurons that use GABA as their transmitter do far more than just inhibiting other neurons; they also generate and maintain network oscillations, which orchestrate the activation of neural assemblies.

**GABA-receptor** See ion channel; receptor complex, supramolecular.

**Gabob** The hydroxyl derivative of GABA (gamma-aminobutyric acid).

**GAD** Generalized anxiety disorder (q.v.).

**GAF** *Global assessment of functioning*; a scale that rates psychological, social, and occupational adjustment or performance on a 10-point range from 100 (no symptoms and superior functioning in a broad range of activities) to 10 (persisting or imminent danger of severely hurting self or others, or persisting inability to maintain personal hygiene).

**gagging** See *gustation*.

**GAI** Guided affective imagery (q.v.).

**gain of function effect** In genetics, a mutation that either enables the affected protein to be active in a new way that is different from its

usual action, or increases a preexisting function of the affected enzyme. In *amyotropic lateral sclerosis* (q.v.), about 10% of cases are associated with a dominant *SOD1* mutation with a gain of function effect.

**galactosemia** An autosomal recessive disorder (in which the patient is homozygous for the gene) consisting of an absence of the enzyme galactose-1-phosphate uridyl transferase, which is essential for the conversion of galactose-1-phosphate to glucose-1-phosphate. Galactose-1-phosphate accumulates in erythrocytes, liver and kidney tissue, brain, and lens, with resultant impairment of tissue metabolism. Mental retardation may in large part be prevented by early administration of a galactose-free diet.

**galanin** A neuropeptide; its functions include regulation of appetite and hormone secretion.

**galeanthropy** The delusion that one is a cat.

**galeophobia** Fear of cats; also *ailurophobia*, *gatophobia*.

**Galgenhumor** *Gallows humor* (q.v.).

**galli** Devotees of the ancient goddess Astarte (13th–15th centuries B.C.), who emasculated themselves and thereafter dressed as women. Astarte came to be known as Atargatis, the "Syrian goddess," in the Hellenistic world (3rd century B.C.–3rd century A.D.).

**gallows humor** *Galgenhumor*; humorous and comical behavior in the face of disaster or death. Gallows humor is seen most frequently in the organic psychoses, and particularly in delirium tremens.

**Galt, John Minson II** (1819–1862) American psychiatrist; forensic psychiatry, psychiatric records research.

**Galton, Sir Francis** (1822–1911) Mathematician; invented the correlation coefficient, the weather map, and the systematic use of psychological questionnaires. After the publication of *On the Origin of Species* by his cousin, Charles Darwin, Galton became interested in the measurement of individual differences and the influences of heredity on mental and physical development. He gave particular attention to the tendency for exceptional talents to run in families.

**galvanic skin response** *GSR*. See *psychogalvanic reflex*.

**gambling** Game playing for money, which may be normal (social gambling) or pathological. Pathological gambling is an *impulse* *control disorder* (q.v.), which has some or all of the following characteristics that serve to differentiate it from social gambling: (1) progressive, with a continuous or periodic loss of control over gambling; (2) preoccupation with gambling and with obtaining the money it requires; (3) getting a "high" from gambling, a euphoric state often referred to by the gambler when he or she indicates that it is action that is sought, and not merely money; (4) tolerance—the gambler places larger and larger bets or needs to take bigger and bigger risks; (5) withdrawal symptoms—the gambler becomes restless or irritable when attempting to control or stop, with the result that most such attempts are unsuccessful; (6) losing is intolerable, and when it happens the gambler tries to "get even" and win everything back at once, abandoning earlier careful strategies for risky, injudicious moves ("chasing" one's losses); (7) jeopardizes his career or interpersonal relationships by gambling away all his savings, missing work, losing jobs, allowing gambling to take precedence over every other aspect of life, repeated lying about the extent of gambling, and failure to fulfill his many promises to reform; (8) reliance on others to bail him out of his desperate financial situation; (9) a stage of frenzy or desperation in which anything will be done to finance gambling ("crossing the line")—loan sharks, forgery, fraud, theft, embezzlement, etc.; (10) a need to continue gambling despite his conviction that he will lose (and his increasingly sloppy play guarantees defeat). In the later stages, depression (sometimes with suicide attempts), stress-related physical illnesses, or the phantasy of starting life over with a new identity may develop. Some authorities classify pathological gambling as one of the OCD spectrum disorders.

Pathological gambling is twice as frequent in men as in women. Women gamblers typically begin later in life, and more for escape than for the ""action" or excitement of the game. They tend to become addicted more quickly (3 or 5 years as compared with 20 to 30 years in men).

The most frequent course of the syndrome is a single episode lasting a year. Of those who have been diagnosed as pathologic gamblers, 62% report one episode in their lifetime,11% report two episodes, and only 27% report three or more episodes.

**games**  See transactional analysis.

**gamete**  A specialized sexual cell that unites with another germ cell to form a zygote. Among animals, male gametes are *spermatozoa* and female gametes are *eggs* or *ova*. Gametes are always haploid and genetically pure, because they contain only one member of a given factor pair. Since the formation of a gamete involves a reduction of 50% in the amount of genetic material carried, each gamete has only half of the factorial equipment of an ordinary body cell and never shows the hybrid character of the individual producing it. See *chromosome*.

**gamma alcoholism**  The usual type of alcoholism seen in the United States, Canada, and other Anglo-Saxon and hard-liquor-drinking countries, characterized by increased *tolerance* (q.v.), cellular adaption to the repeated ingestion of the depressant substance, precipitation of a *withdrawal* or *abstinence* syndrome ("shakes," compulsive craving, convulsions, hallucinations, delirium; see *delirium tremens*) when alcohol intake is halted, and loss of control as defined above. This type of alcoholism is also known as *essential, addictive, regressive, malignant,* or *idiopathic.* See *alcoholism.*

**gamma rhythm**  The work mode of the brain, consisting of oscillations in the fast range (30–90 Hz). Gamma oscillations are triggered when the reticular formation puts the brain into a state of arousal. They bind visual processes across the two sides of the brain so that the more than two dozen areas in each hemisphere that are involved in seeing can be brought together as one experience. Gamma oscillations have been proposed to represent reference signals for temporal encoding, sensory binding of features into a coherent percept, and storage and recall of information. Gamma rhythm also operates in processing hearing, smelling, and the sensation of touching. See *alpha rhythm, electroencephalogram.*

**gamma synchrony**  See *synchronization.*

**gammacism**  Common speech defect (the "baby talk") of young children who replace the velars (g,k) with corresponding dentals (d,t).

**gamma-glutamyl transferase**  *GGTP* (q.v.).

**gamma-hydroxybutyric acid**  *GHB* (q.v.).

**gamo-**  Combining form meaning marriage, (sexual) union, from Gr. *gamos.*

**gamonomania**  Desire to marry.

**gamophobia**  Fear of marriage.

**gang** An intimate social group characterized by a high degree of close personal contact among its members, who share common values or standards of behavior. Largely an urban phenomenon, the gang is a subculture whose interests and attitudes are typically different from, and sometimes even in direct conflict with, those of the larger society. The usual gang comprises male youths. A gang of adult men is often organized around criminal activity; delinquents are more often members of gangs than are nondelinquents, but not all youth gangs are overtly antisocial by any means.

**ganga, ganja** The second grade of *marijuana* (q.v.), with a higher quality and quantity of resin than found in bhang, the first grade. See *cannabis*.

**ganglia, basal** See *basal ganglia*.

**gangliosides** Glycolipids that contain sialic acid; they are found in almost all cells but are especially abundant in CNS and may have an important role in regulating neuronal excitability. The main ganglioside in human plasma is GM3. An autosomal recessive form of epilepsy has been described which begins in the first year of life, involves mainly generalized tonic clonic (grand mal) seizures not associated with any focal abnormalities on EEG or MRI, and produces a marked decline in motor and verbal development as well as severe visual impairments. The affected child had a single region of homozygosity on chromosome 2, with a nonsense mutation (C694T) in the gene *SIAT9I*. The mutation abolishes the activity of GM3 synthase, which normally triggers the first step in the production of CNS gangliosides by transferring a sialic acid residue to lactosylceramide to form GM3. GM3 and its derivatives were completely absent in the affected members of the family (Simpson, M.A. et al. *Nature Genetics 36*: 1225–1229, 2004).

**gangliosidosis, G$_{M1}$** An autosomal recessive disorder due to deficiency of the lysosomal enzyme beta-galactosidase (which maps to chromosome 3p1). Generalized gangliosidosis, the infantile type, has early onset of mental retardation, seizures, facial and skeletal dysmorphisms, and hepatosplenomegaly. Death usually occurs by 2 years of age.

**gangliosidosis, G$_{M2}$** Autosomal recessive lipid storage disorders caused by either (1) mutations in the alpha chain, resulting in *Tay-Sachs disease*; or (2) mutations in the beta chain, resulting in *Sanhoff disease* (qq.v.).

**Ganser syndrome** (Sigbert J. M. Ganser, German psychiatrist, 1853–1931) *Nonsense syndrome; syndrome of approximate answers; syndrome of deviously relevant answers*; in 1897 Ganser described a syndrome of a twilight state (or clouding of consciousness), memory disturbances, *vorbeireden* ("talking at cross purposes"), sudden appearance and disappearance of symptoms, and the presence of hysterical stigmata. Since the original description, other signs and symptoms have been viewed as characteristic: approximated answers, somatic conversions, auditory pseudo-hallucinations, disorientation, perceptual disturbances, fugue, and conversion symptoms.

The syndrome is often observed among prisoners who, it is held, hope to be treated leniently by the court because of their malady. The subject seldom does anything correctly. When shown a watch reading 3:30, he may say it reads 5:00; when shown a glove, he says it is a hand; he designates a quarter as a dollar bill and a key as a lock. In addition, behavior may be bizarre, with episodes of excitement or stupor, as though the subject were acting out an artificial psychosis (neuromimesis).

There is controversy as to whether the syndrome is predominantly dissociative, as DSM-IV considers it, or a transient psychosis. It is often viewed as an attempt to deal with a "no-way-out" situation by "going crazy" in persons who are predisposed by reason of organic or functional impairment (e.g., schizophrenic spectrum personality disorder). Many who develop the syndrome show signs of organicity, and it has been noted that vorbeireden is strikingly similar to regressive metonymy, the first symptom of asensory or jargon aphasia.

**Ganymede** In medieval Europe, gay. In Greek mythology, Ganymede was a youth raped by Zeus, and some scholars trace the derivation of the Latin word *catamitus* (used by first-century Romans to refer to a male prostitute who took the "passive" role in homosexual activity) to Ganymede.

**gap junction** The space between the two neurons of an electrical synapse; a cellular specialization that bridges the cytoplasm of adjacent cells, providing the main structural element of electrical synapses. Gap junctions are formed by a family of proteins, the connexins. Each of the neurons, presynaptic and postsynaptic, contains a cyclindrical hemicylinder or *connexon*. The two *hemichannels* connect within the gap junction to form a communicating channel that allows the electrical stimulus to pass from the presynaptic to the postsynaptic neuron. The gap junction corresponds to what is termed the synaptic cleft in chemical synapses.

The normal extracellular space is about 25 nanometers across (one six-hundredth the width of a hair), but the cleft between the presynaptic and postsynaptic cells at an electrical synapse is approximately 3.5 nanometers. The gap between chemical synapses is only slightly wider, 20–40 nanometers, but the nerve signal cannot leap it electrically; instead, chemical neurotransmitters seep across the gap to receptors on the postsynaptic membrane. See *neurotransmitter*.

**Gardner-Diamond syndrome** *Painful bruising syndrome*, or *autoerythrocyte sensitization*, first described by F. H. Gardner and L. K. Diamond (*Blood 10*, 1955). Tingling, burning, or stinging sensations often develop in the areas that will be involved in the painful swelling and erythema that later evolve into ecchymoses. The lesions may occur alone or in clusters, they vary in size from several centimeters to encompass the whole limb, and typically they arise close to a recent trauma (including surgery). A period of emotional distress preceding the development of the syndrome is so common that it is sometimes referred to as *psychogenic purpura*. Unpredictable remissions and disabling recurrences are the rule, and no fully effective therapy is known. Immunopathogenic mechanisms appear to be of etiologic significance. The syndrome has been observed much more frequently in women than in men.

**gargalesthesia** Sensation of tickling.

**gargoylism** See *mucopolysaccharidosis*.

**garment addiction** Transvestophilia; *transvestitism* (q.v.).

**GAS** 1. Global Assessment Scale; a structured interview designed not only to detect the presence of symptoms but also to measure their change over time.

2. *General adaptation syndrome* (q.v.).

**gastrocolic reflex** *Emptying reflex* (q.v.); contraction of the colon following stretching of the muscle wall of the stomach (as by filling of the stomach).

**gastropaths, false** Dèjèrine and Gauckler so designated those who express food phobias.

**gatekeeper** In community psychiatry, an extramural, nonprofessional person whose role in the community (e.g., bartender, policeman, playground worker) is such as to allow him to observe segments of the population for signs of stress, disharmony, disaffection, and discord. He may receive specialized training from the Community Health Center (at orientation sessions) so that he can function as a liaison worker between the Center and the community.

Gatekeeper is sometimes synonymous with patient case manager (PCM) and primary care physician (PCP), whose function is to channel a patient's access to medical services in nonemergency situations. In HMOs, PPOs, and other systems of *managed care* (q.v.), the gatekeeper may be a physician (typically, from family practice, internal medicine, pediatrics, obstetrics-gynecology, or osteopathy). Nonphysicians may also be gatekeepers: nurses, nurse practitioners, physician assistants, social workers, or psychologists. See *case management*.

**gatekeeper variables** See *recidivism*.

**gateway drugs** Those substances of abuse—alcohol and marijuana—that provide the major portals of entry into abuse of other drugs. They are considered particularly dangerous because they are believed by so many to be relatively harmless.

**gating** Screening out irrelevant stimuli; inhibiting, suppressing. The gating theory of schizophrenia proposes that schizophrenics are characterized by a deficit in inhibiting (gating) irrelevant sensory input; in comparison with normal persons, they respond more to irrelevant features of situations or tasks and less to the central or significant issues. See *ion channel*; *spinal gating, $P_{50}$ sensory gating*.

In normal subjects, a prepulse low-level stimulus blunts the startle response (as measured by the eye blink reflex); in schizophrenics it does not, and there is evidence that the deficit is linked to dopamine overactivity.

Sensory-gating deficits are also found in acutely psychotic manic patients, suggesting that the psychotic state per se involves catecholamine systems. The difference between the two types of patients is that the deficit persists after remission in schizophrenics but disappears with remission of a manic episode. Further, sensory-gating deficits have been reported in schizophrenics' relatives even though they do not give evidence of any disorder that would warrant the diagnosis of schizophrenia.

**gatophobia** Fear of cats; also *ailurophobia, galeophobia.*

**Gaucher disease** (Philippe Gaucher, French physician, 1854–1918) An autosomal recessive *glycolipid storage disease* (q.v.) consisting of deficiency of the enzyme β-glucosidase glucocerebrosidase (the gene for which is located on chromosome 1); glucocerebroside accumulates because it is not adequately broken down to ceramide and glucose. The result is a lipid histiocytosis, with depositions of keratin in the reticuloendothelial cells of liver and spleen and in ganglion cells of the cerebral cortex, basal ganglia, and cerebellum.

Onset is usually between the ages of 6 and 12 months, typically in Jewish females. Symptoms include listlessness, apathy, head retraction, hypertonicity, bulbar signs, and sometimes mental retardation. Associated typical findings are hepatosplenomegaly, pancytopenias, and bone lesions. Diagnosis is by measuring the activity of leukocyte acid β-glucosidase, which is greatly decreased. Clinical manifestations widely, probably because different mutations of the β-glucosidase locus produce very mild forms of the disease. See *lysosomal storage disorder.*

In the United States, 2000–3000 cases are diagnosed each year. Three different mutations of the gene have been identified that together account for 97% of all cases among Ashkenazi Jews. As a result, carriers can be identified (heretofore, identification depended upon the appearance of the disease within the family).

Currently, only the type 1 form of *Gaucher disease*, which is characterized by glucocerebrosidase deficiency in the absence of neuropathology, has been successfully treated by enzyme replacement therapy. The neuropathologic forms of the disease (types 2 and 3) are refractory to therapy.

**Gault decision** A 1967 decision by the U.S. Supreme Court mandating fair and accurate fact-finding procedures for juveniles when serious punishment could be inflicted should they be found guilty. The rights thereby guaranteed the juvenile include the right to notification of the specific charges, the right to counsel, the right against self-incrimination,

and the right to confront and cross-examine the accusers. The decision stemmed from the case of an Arizona adolescent, Gerald Gault, who had been accused of making an indecent telephone call. Under the law of that state he could have been committed to a state industrial school for 6 years.

**gay** A person whose erotic contacts are limited to another person of his or her own gender. Many whose romantic attachments are to members of their own gender object to the term "homosexual" to describe themselves because it seems to refer solely to sexuality, whereas their orientation means far more to them than sexual behavior. Further, homosexual was coined (in the late 19th century) in the context of pathology. Gay, in contrast, antedates homosexual by at least several centuries, it is more precise in that it describes persons who are conscious of their orientation, and it is applicable to both men and women. The current tendency, however, is to use gay for men and "lesbian" for women.

**gay-basher** See exorcist syndrome; homophobia.

**Gayet-Wernicke encephalopathy** *Wernicke encephalopathy* (q.v.).

**GBMI** Guilty but mentally ill. See *offenders, mentally disordered.*

**Gc** Crystallized intelligence; see *g.*

**GCSE** Generalized convulsive *status epilepticus* (q.v.).

**GDNF** Glial cell line–derived neurotropic factor; see *ibogaine.* The GDNF-related family includes GDNF, neurturin, persephin, and artemin (also known as neublastin or enovin).

**GDP** Guanosine diphosphate. See *G protein.*

**GDS** *Global Deterioration Scale,* a description of levels of cognitive performance for use in assessing the extent of mental deterioration in the elderly person. In addition to a general description of changes, the scale includes objective changes in behavior that are expressed as *functional assessment stages (FAST).*

In the GDS staging system, stage 1 indicates that the patient has no subjective or clinically evident impairment; at stage 2, there is subjective deficit only; at stage 3, subtle cognitive deficits are manifested which may interfere with executive tasks (this stage is sometimes called MCI (mild cognitive impairment); at stage 4, deficits are clearly manifest and typically interfere with instrumental activities. In uncomplicated Alzheimer disease, the stages proceed in ordinal fashion, and any deviation from that pattern suggests that something other than Alzheimer disease is a complicating factor or is the primary cause of the subject's cognitive impairment.

Many studies have confirmed the prognostic significance of the system. After 4 years, dementia had developed in no stage 1 subjects, in 15% of stage 2, and in almost 70% of stage 3.

**Gedankenlautwerden**  Auditory hallucination consisting of hearing voices that speak the subject's thoughts as he or she is thinking them. If the thoughts are repeated immediately after the subject thinks them, the phenomenon is termed *ècho de la pensèe*.

**Gegenhalten**  See *paratonia*.

**gelasmus**  Spasmodic laughter, observed in hysteria and the schizophrenias, and in some organic (especially bulbar) diseases of the brain.

**gelastic epilepsy**  A form of *epilepsy* (q.v.) in which laughter is a part of the seizure pattern, usually due to a lesion in the left temporal region.

**gelatio**  *Obs.* Rigid state of the body in *catalepsy* (q.v.), as though it were frozen.

**Gélineau syndrome**  (Jean Baptiste Edouard Gèlineau, French neurologist, 1828–1906) Idiopathic *narcolepsy* (q.v.).

**Genain quadruplets**  David Rosenthal conducted (1964) the now-classical studies of the Genain quadruplets (identical, monozygous schizophrenic women, discordant for the severity of their psychosis; i.e., varying forms and severity of psychopathology), which demonstrated that some aspect of the disorder is genetically transmitted.

**gender coding**  The signals that a person gives as to his or her sexuality, including both gender identity and gender role. Gender coding reflects sex differences that are specific to reproduction (e.g., impregnation, gestation) as well as those that are due to hormonal differences (e.g., growing a beard, developing breasts), behavioral characteristics that may largely be dependent on hormonal influences on the brain (e.g. competitive aggressiveness, nurturance of the young), and socially sanctioned or imposed roles (e.g., occupational differences, styles of clothing and grooming).

In one person, all levels of coding may be congruent with each other; in another person, there may be different degrees of incongruity or disharmony between them (*cross-coding*).

**gender complementation**  That part of gender identification in which the person recognizes the other sex as "other" and "not me." See *gender coding*.

**gender dysphoria**  Dissatisfaction with one's genital anatomy, which is experienced as incongruous with or contradictory to one's gender identity or gender role. See *cross-dressing; transvestitism*.

**gender identification**  The process of recognizing the qualities and attributes that are considered to be part of one's sex; this includes identifying and separating one's self from those elements considered to be characteristic of the other sex (gender complementation). See *gender coding*.

**gender identity**  The inner conviction that one is male, female, ambivalent, or neutral. Gender role is the outward appearance or image that one gives, through behavior and manner, that indicates he or she is to be classed as male or female. Both gender identity and gender role are established in accordance with the sex of assignment and rearing; they are clearly evident by 18 months of age and for the most part irreversible after 30 months of age, hence often called *core gender identity*. (This dating is in contrast to the classical theory that assigns differentiation between the sexes to the much later oedipal period.) Ordinarily, both gender identity and gender role are the same, although transvestitism or cross-dressing is a notable exception. Gender role and gender identity are to be distinguished from sexual identity, which is biologically determined. See *gender coding; gender identification*.

**gender identity disorder**  *Cross-gender identification*; dissatisfaction with one's assigned sex and identification with the opposite sex. The person feels that he or she has the typical feelings and reactions of the opposite sex, may feel that he or she has been born with the wrong sex, and may feel it necessary to change (by hormone treatment or sex-reassignment surgery, for example) the primary and secondary sex characteristics in order to simulate the opposite sex (*transsexualism*).

**gender recognition**  See *face recognition*.

**gender role** The behavior and appearance that one presents in terms of what the culture considers to be "masculine" or "feminine." That the gender role and sexual identity are not wholly determined by genetic constitution is demonstrated by pseudohermaphrodites who were reared contrary to their chromosomal sex; in all such cases, the gender role and orientation are congruent with the assigned sex and rearing, rather than with the biological sex. See *gender coding; gender identity.*

**gene** That which is responsible for the manifestation of traits, whatever its chemical nature. Most definitions in current use limit and specify the chemical to be DNA; the gene is then viewed as a fragment of *DNA* located along the *chromosome* (q.v.). It is a locus of cotranscribed exons, which are blueprints for the assembly and regulation of proteins, the body's building blocks. Each gene constitutes a tape of instructions, written in the four-letter hereditary code of base pairs (the *codon*). The gene is a mixture of exons and introns; the *exon* codes for the sequence of amino acids that will be assembled to create a *protein* (q.v.). *Introns* are intervening sequences that often contain regulatory information.

A codon is the gene's code word for an amino acid and consists of a triplet of bases. In an exon, a sequence of CCA followed by CAG, for instance, tells the cell that in making a particular protein, the amino acid proline will be followed by the amino acid glutamine.

The cell "reads" the orders issued by its DNA by building a "copying machine"—mRNA (messenger RNA), a nucleic acid similar to DNA except that the base uracil (U) replaces DNA's thymine. For each base in the DNA, RNA lays down a complementary base: base C whenever base G occurs in DNA, and base A whenever base T occurs. It edits out meaningless parts and then moves out of the cell nucleus into the ribosomes, protein producers that are scattered throughout the cell. Here a second form of RNA—transfer RNA or tRNA—calls in a batch of amino acids, and the ribosomes link them together in the order dictated by the original codon to form the protein. See *transcription.*

If there is an alteration in even the smallest part of the chain of amino acids, the entire protein may not function properly or it may not function at all. Defects in working proteins, caused by mutations in their parent genes, are responsible for much of the burden of human disease. To transform a single fertilized egg cell into an adult human body and then keep that body alive and healthy, each of the 22,000 genes must adjust its activity to precise degrees and at precise times and locations. It is estimated that 10% of the genes in the human genome are involved in the production of diseases; 25% of the genes are believed to contribute to functions of the brain and nervous system. See *gene functions.*

Genes occur as functionals sections of the 23 pairs of chromosomes contained in the nucleus of every body cell. Chromosomes are randomly broken up in each generation by crossing-over; the gene is a portion of chromosome which has survived enough generations to act as a unit of natural selection. Genes are not distributed equally along the chromosomes but are often found in clusters. Some chromosomal regions are gene rich and others relatively gene poor. Within intergenic regions there is a great deal of DNA with unique sequences of unknown function, and also long stretches of tandemly repeated sequences, known as *satellite DNA.* Although every cell possesses a full copy of the *genome* (q.v.), it is believed that each type of cell uses only its own special subset of genes, the remainder being turned off permanently.

Genome researchers estimate that there are 22,000 genes in the human, and about 3.2 billion base pairs in the genome. Because there is no punctuation in the tape of instructions to indicate where each gene stops or starts, identification of individual genes has been difficult and has required development of elaborate technology.

The 22,000 genes in the human genome code for about 400,000 proteins. To understand their role in disease, it is necessary to find out how multiple genes and proteins interact, how they are turned on and off, how they are instructed to increase or decrease their activity, how that affects the proteins for which they code, and how the multiple genes and proteins interact with the environment.

The complex organization of the genome and the multitude of regulatory and modifying elements acting on genes and their protein products make gene boundaries ambiguous, so it is difficult to establish an adequate structural and functional definition of a gene.

Gene duplication is one mechanism for the emergence of new proteins. Modifications in gene regulation can place a protein in a different location with different functions, as can gene sharing. When genes are duplicated, modified, or shared, the changed concentration of the genes may generate new molecular functions. Proteins can specialize for a new function while retaining their ancestral roles. See *genetic disorder; inheritance.*

**gene expression**   At the molecular level, transformation of genes (or operons) into functional proteins and enzymes that direct and catalyze cellular metabolism and differentiation. Most genes are not constantly active; each gene is ordinarily dormant and in order to be expressed it must be turned on by a signal box positioned just before the part of the gene that contains the codon for a particular protein.

In learning, and other persistent changes in mental functions, alterations of gene expression induce changes in patterns of neuronal connections by altering the strength of synaptic connections and through structural changes that alter anatomical connections between neurons. See *transcription.*

Transfer RNA (tRNA) plays a central role in gene expression. It makes possible the accurate synthesis of cellular proteins, in conjunction with the ribosome, by mediating the orderly addition of amino acids to growing polypeptide chains in response to genetic instructions encoded in messenger RNA.

**gene functions**   The gene has two functions: (a) the *template function* provides each gene, in each cell of the body (including the gametes), the ability to replicate reliably and to provide succeeding generations with (i.e., to transmit) copies of each gene; the template can be altered only by mutations and not by social experience of any sort (it is transmissible but not regulated); (b) the *transcriptional function,* the ability of the gene to direct the manufacture of specific proteins in any given cell and thereby to determine the structure, function, and other biological characteristics (the phenotype) of the cell in which they are expressed. In any given cell type, only a fraction of genes (ca. 10%–20%) are expressed or transcribed; the others are suppressed.

In addition, there are two regions in a gene: (a) the *coding region* encodes mRNA which in turn encodes a specific protein;

(b) the *regulatory region*, usually upstream of the coding region, comprises two DNA elements: the *promotor element*, where the enzyme DNA polymerase begins to read and transcribe the DNA coding regions into mRNA, and the *enhancer element*, which recognizes protein signals that determine in which cells, and when, the coding region will be transcribed by the polymerase. Thus, a small number of proteins (*transcriptional regulators*), by binding to different segments of the enhancer element, determine how often RNA polymerase binds to the promotor element and transcribes the gene. Internal and external stimuli (such as different steps in the development of the brain, hormones, stress, learning, and social interaction) alter the binding of the transcriptional regulators to the enhancer element. In this way, different combinations of transcriptional regulators are recruited. This aspect of gene regulation is often termed *epigenetic regulation.*

All bodily functions, including all functions of the brain, are susceptible to social influences, which are biologically incorporated in altered expression of specific genes in specific nerve cells of specific regions of the brain. Because social influences are not incorporated in the sperm and egg, they are regulated but not genetically transmitted; instead, they are transmitted culturally (by learning).

**gene sequencing**   Determining the specific order of the hundreds or thousands of DNA nucleotides (base pairs) in a gene that provide instructions for manufacture of a particular protein. Once the specific order has been determined, it can be used to detect abnormalities, such as the large number of triplicate repeats in Huntington disease.

Comparison of gene sequences shows that strikingly similar proteins are encoded in the genomes of organisms as distantly related as yeast and mammals. Nucleated cells evolved more than 1.5 billion years ago, and the great majority of the proteins of the time have been perpetuated in myriad descendant cells. The function of one member of a gene family can often be deduced from that of its known relatives. Once a gene has been identified, annotators can often guess what it does by comparing its sequence of DNA letters with that of genes whose function is already known. Because of the unity of evolution, the sequence of every human gene is recognizably similar to the equivalent gene in other organisms.

**gene transfer** Introduction of genetic material from one organism into the cells of another (the host). Gene transfer is an essential part of gene therapy for various disorders, and it is also used as a means of studying brain function.

**genealogy** Although in a sense identical with the actual pedigree of an individual or with the demonstration of such a pedigree in the form of a genealogical family tree, the term applies to the scientific study, or the proper historical account, of the biological descent of persons, or a group of persons, from a certain number of ancestors. Such studies aim to provide a complete list of ancestors for as many generations as possible and to clarify the relationship of a person with the families of a given population group, rather than to investigate either the biological qualities of these families or the variations of certain hereditary family traits in successive generations.

**gene-environment interactions** $G \times E$; the effects on the neural substrate of a disorder of environmental pathogens and a candidate gene(s) for the disorder; the convergence of environmental and genotypic effects within the same neural substrate. Reliable findings of gene–environment interactions provide clear evidence for a neural pathways connecting gene, environmental pathogen, and disorder. The gene–environment interactional approach assumes that environmental pathogens cause disorder and that the effect of genes is to influence susceptibility to these pathogens. Such an approach moves beyond the often fruitless search for single genetic polymorphisms and recognizes that genes showing no connection to disorders in genome-wide scans may nonetheless be connected to a disorder through unrecognized gene–environment interactions.

A *candidate gene* (q.v.) can provide information about where—in body, cell, and molecule—the environmental pathogen's effect on disorder occurs. The concordance of MZ twins for even highly heritable disorders, however, is less than perfect, pointing to the existence of nongenetic contributing causes, such as maternal stress during pregnancy, maternal substance abuse during pregnancy, low birth weight, birth complications, lack of normal parental care during infancy, childhood

physical maltreatment or sexual abuse, childhood neglect, premature parental loss, exposure to family conflict and violence, stressful life events involving loss or threat, substance abuse, toxic exposures, and head injury.

All environmental *risk factors* for psychopathology are characterized by *response heterogeneity*, which is associated with pre-existing individual differences in temperament, personality, cognition, and autonomic physiology—all known to be under genetic influence. One example is maltreated children. Those whose genotype confers low levels of MAO-A expression more often develop conduct disorder, antisocial personality, and adult violent crime than children with a high activity MAO-A genotype. See *COMT*; *serotonin transporter gene*.

**gene/protein approach** See *linkage analysis*.

**general adaptation syndrome** The various changes in the body in response to or as defense against stress. Selye distinguishes three stages in this syndrome: the *alarm reaction*, in which adaptation is not yet acquired; the *stage of resistance*, in which adaptation is optimal; and the *stage of exhaustion*, in which the acquired adaptation is lost again. The hypophysis–adrenal interrelationships, which largely determine the various elements of the syndrome, are as follows: the stress agent, or stressor, acts not only upon the cells of the *target organ* but also acts upon the anterior pituitary and stimulates the latter to produce ACTH; in certain circumstances it may also induce a release of somatotropic hormone (STH). ACTH, in turn, induces the adrenal cortex to produce *glucocorticoids* (such as cortisone). The latter exert primarily an inhibitory effect upon the various target organs—catabolism, diminution of granuloma formation and of allergic responses, etc. STH, on the other hand, by stimulating connective tissue, enhances defensive reactions in the target organs—anabolism, augmentation of granuloma formation and of allergic responses, etc. This action occurs by means of direct sensitization of the connective tissue elements to *mineralocorticoids* (such as desoxycorticosterone) and also by stimulating the adrenal cortex to produce mineralocorticoids. This latter corticotrophic effect, however, depends upon the simultaneous availability of ACTH. Thus, the target organ response to stressors depends largely upon the balance between STH and the mineralocorticoids on the one hand, and ACTH and glucocorticoids on the other.

**general attitude type**   Jung's expression for the total mental cast or psychic makeup that statically determines a person's general attitude independently of or in advance of the external stimulus. This conception aggregates all human beings into two groups of extraverts and introverts. See *extraverted type; introversion.*

With regard to the person's dynamic reaction to a life stimulus, Jung classifies all humankind into *functional types* (q.v.) and also into two classes: (1) *rational* and (2) *irrational.*

**general medical care**   See *care.*

**general   medical   conditions**   Nonpsychiatric (organic) disorders, used in DSM-IV to refer to any nonpsychiatric condition that gives rise to a psychiatric disorder. The term represents an attempt to avoid the obsolete   organic-nonorganic   dichotomy. (Substance-induced disorders remain a separate category.) In addition to the group of cognitive disorders (including dementias, delirias, and amnestic disorders), the major presentations are catatonic disorder and personality change due to a general medical disorder. Such personality change, called organic personality disorder in DSM-III-R, is manifested in any of the following subtypes: labile, disinhibited, aggressive, apathetic, and paranoid.

**general paresis**   *General paralysis of the insane (GPI), dementia paralytica, Bayle disease*; the most malignant form of (tertiary) neurosyphilis consisting of direct invasion of the parenchyma of the brain producing a combination of both mental and neurologic symptoms. General paresis was first described by Haslan in 1798, and again by Bayle in 1822, and by Esquirol in 1826. The term general paralysis of the insane was first used by Delaye in 1824, and the relationship of the disorder to syphilis was first suggested in 1857 by Esmarch and Jessen. Identification of the spirochete as the cause, rather than merely a predisposing factor, was made possible in 1911, when Noguchi demonstrated their presence in the brains of paretic subjects.

Pathology includes shrinking and atrophy of brain substance and a thickening of the dura mater. Lymphocytes, plasma cells, and giant cells infiltrate the meninges and the brain itself, where the ganglion cells show severe large areas of softening.

Mental symptoms may appear in various forms: as (1) simple dementia, the most common type, with deterioration of intellect, affect, and social behavior; (2) paranoid form, with persecutory delusions; (3) expansive or manic form, with delusions of grandiosity; or (4) depressive form, often with absurd nihilistic delusions. No matter what the form, intellectual functions show increasing impairment, with loss of more and more memory, confabulation, disorientation (especially in the area of time), carelessness in personal appearance and hygiene, irritability and restlessness, alcoholic excesses, and sexual aberrations.

Neurologic symptoms and signs that may appear are (1) epileptiform attacks, which occur in 50% of cases; (2) Argyll Robertson pupil; (3) tremor, most on voluntary movement, that tends to affect the perioral musculature and also the muscles of the hands and fingers so that writing becomes tremulous, and words and letters are often left out or transposed; (4) vacant, masklike facies, giving patient a wrinkle-free, youthful appearance; (5) impaired oculomotor activity; (6) optic atrophy; (7) impaired motor function, including ataxia, poor coordination, unsteady gait, weakness; (8) slurred speech (dysarthria); and (9) hyperactive reflexes (but hyporeflexia if tabes dorsalis coexists); (10) loss of bladder and bowel control. There are few or no sensory changes, unless tabes coexists.

**general systems theory**   "A set of related definitions, assumptions, and propositions which deal with reality as an integrated hierarchy of organizations of matter and energy. General systems behavior theory is concerned with a special subset of all systems, the living ones" (Miller, J. G. *Behavioral Science 10*, 1965). General systems behavior theory is an attempt to develop an embracing general theory of human behavior the behavior of man by identifying the organized, interacting components that make up the system; by defining the controls that keep those subsystems or fields stable and in equilibrium; and by establishing the roles, relationships, inputs, outputs, and routes of flow within the hierarchy of subsystems that make up the whole. General systems theory thus provides a holistic approach to the study of human behavior and attempts to integrate the different conceptions of how each subsystem operates from a wide variety of disciplines and specialties in a search for the general truth inherent in all. See *emergence*.

**generalization**   Applying to a whole group or class of conclusions, ideas, judgments, etc., based upon experience with a limited number of the class. While generalization is an essential element of conceptualization in the processes of normal thought, it attains particular significance in psychiatry in that one of the many thought disorders in schizophrenia is the tendency to overgeneralize and to treat the concrete as though it were abstract.

**generalized absence syndrome**   A nonconvulsive seizure that typically occurs in childhood, characterized by a sudden, brief impairment of consciousness, cessation of ongoing activity without loss of postural tone, and 3 Hz rhythmic cortical discharges of generalized onset. Usual duration is 5–10 seconds; several episodes can occur daily.

**generalized amnesia**   See *amnesia, psychogenic*.

**generalized anxiety disorder**   *GAD*; anxiety neurosis; *overanxious disorder* (in a child or adolescent). Characteristics are unrealistic or excessive worrying and apprehensive expectation about life circumstances, need for reassurance, symptoms of autonomic hyperactivity and hyperarousal (e.g., trembling, palpitations, sweating, exaggerated startle response), and resulting difficulty in attention and concentration so that social and occupational functioning suffers. The worrying is intrusive and pervasive and cannot be controlled. Characteristically, the person with GAD perceives even neutral stimuli as threatening: "Yes, my teacher said my report was good, but she said I might have referred to additional sources than the ones I cited."

GAD typically develops during the period of the late teens to the late 20s; it is a chronic condition that persists for a decade or longer. Incidence is estimated as between 3% and 4% per year. It is more common among women, the unmarried, racial-ethnic minority members, and persons of low socioeconomic status. Comorbidity is frequent; as many as 60% also have major depressive disorder, 40% have dysthymia, 37% have alcoholism, and 34% suffer from social phobia.

In DSM-IV, *overanxious disorder* of children was eliminated as a diagnosis and incorporated under GAD. Worries in children range

from usual events, such as being on time for school, to disasters, such as hurricanes, floods, or earthquakes. The average age of onset of childhood GAD is 8.8 years.

Over the years, diagnostic criteria for GAD have shifted away from physical symptoms to psychic symptoms, although more than 50% of patients with GAD in primary care present with somatic symptoms only. DSM-IV, for example, lists as physical symptoms only restlessness or feeling "on edge," easy fatiguability, difficulty in concentrating or mind "going blank," irritability, muscle tension, and sleep disturbance.

It is estimated that the genetic contribution to GAD (i.e., heritability) is approximately 30%; more than half the variance is accounted for by extrafamilial factors, not by a shared environment.

**generation**   The act of producing offspring, or the biological process by which reproduction is accomplished, or a group of offspring produced. In the last sense the term may mean that the given offspring are (1) of the same genealogical rank, as a stage in the succession of natural descent; (2) a series of siblings within one family as the offspring of the same parents; (3) a particular group of persons within the general population, living at the same time; or (4) people of the same period.

As a statistical concept, the term refers to the average duration of life in a species or group.

**generativity**   The general impulse for procreation in the human race. "Generativity is primarily the interest in establishing and guiding the next generation or whatever in a given case may become the absorbing object of a parental kind of responsibility" (Erikson, E. *Childhood and Society*, 1950). *Generativity vs. self-absorption* is the seventh of Erikson's eight stages of man. See *ontogeny, psychic*.

**generator potential**   See *transducer potential*.

**generic**   *Biol.* Pertaining to a genus, as compared with specific.

**genes, modifying**   All those genes that have some influence on the effect of any particular gene; for all practical purposes, the modifying genes are all the genes other than the one under specific study, for even genes that produce a single large effect are subject to modification and qualification by the entire remainder of the genetic constitution.

**genetic, genetical**  Whereas *genetical* is used exclusively in the sense of pertaining to the province of genetics, the term *genetic* has two meanings: (1) it is synonymous with *genetical*; (2) produced or predetermined by a gene or a combination of genes—practically identical to *hereditary*; and (3) referring to development or genesis, not necessarily related to hereditary mechanisms.

**genetic block**  See genetotrophic disease.

**genetic counseling**  *Family counseling; genetic guidance*; the process of helping people understand and adapt to the medical, psychological, and familial implications of genetic contributions to disease. The process includes interpretation of family and medical histories to assess the chance of disease occurrence or recurrence; education about inheritance, testing, management, prevention, resources, and research; and counseling to promote informed choices and adaptation to the risk or condition. Providing accurate information on recurrence risks is important, but equally important is determining that those being counseled are well enough to receive the information and to participate actively in discussions about it.

Genetic counseling can offer parents and siblings the opportunity to express their feelings of guilt and blame and to restructure those feelings on the basis of a better understanding. It can also promote health-enhancing behaviors, recognition of any signs of relapse, and development of coping strategies and behaviors to deal with the illness and with the stigmatization family members may be subjected to. Family members may be blamed for causing their loved one's illness, they may have their own mental health questioned, or they may be rejected by friends. Stigmatization leads to increased withdrawal, isolation, and sense of burden; to exacerbation of medical conditions; to decreased social network size, emotional support, and quality of life; and to decreased likelihood of seeking or accepting treatment.

**genetic directive**  Determination of form, structure, behavior, function, etc. by genes or heredity, basically a description of the *genotype* as opposed to the *phenotype* (qq.v.).

**genetic disorder**  Disease or defect due to a misreading of the genetic code. See *chromosome; gene*.

Wrong nucleotides may be added, others may be deleted, still others may be substituted or rearranged. Any of these possibilities will alter or erase a polypeptide or enzyme that is essential for one step in a metabolic pathway; consequently, a biochemical block develops at the expected site of action. The absence of the usual end product of the metabolic pathway may produce disease, and/or the accumulation of intermediate products (that would ordinarily have been broken down and removed) may produce disease.

An example of the former kind is succinylcholine sensitivity, due to absence of the enzyme pseudocholinesterase. Phenylketonuria and galactosemia, on the other hand, are examples of the second kind of mutation, where accumulation of an intermediate metabolic substance (or a derivative) is responsible for development of characteristic symptoms.

Since the entire process of transmitting the instructions carried within

DNA to amino acids is a mechanical one, once a mutation has occurred it will be copied faithfully forever after. Traditionally, genetic disorders have been divided into mendelian and multifactorial traits. See *gene–environmental interactions; inheritance; mendelian laws*.

**genetic diversity**  Variation in the coding sequence of genes in one population as compared with another. *Gene sequencing* (q.v.) has made it possible to draw phylogenetic trees relating organisms on the basis of similarities in their genes rather than shared physical characteristics. The current world population of 6 billion people descends from a few tens of thousands of progenitors who inhabited Africa some 150,000 to 200,000 years ago. Such small populations can maintain only a limited degree of genetic diversity—typically, only a few common variants in the coding sequences of each gene in their genome. Moreover, the few thousand generations of subsequent exponential expansion have been too few on an evolutionary time scale to alter the spectrum of common variation substantially. As a result, the modern human population has much less intraspecies genetic variation than, for example, chimpanzees—raising the prospect that it will be possible to catalog all the common variants (alleles) of all human genes.

**genetic drift**  A change in succeeding generations of the frequency of certain genes, due to chance rather than to selection.

**genetic epidemiology**  *Clinical genetics*; study of the patterns of incidence, prevalence, and covariance of a disease and disorders related to it in families. The goal of genetic epidemiology is to infer models of genetic transmission of the disease being studied and to differentiate genetic from nongenetic causes. See *genetics.*

**genetic epistemology**  Piaget's theory of cognitive or intellectual development, described as occurring in stages; each stage is a prerequisite for the one that follows it. See *concrete operational stage; developmental psychology; equilibration; scheme; propositional thinking.*

**genetic fitness**  See *fitness; phenotypic fitness.*

**genetic guidance**  See *genetic counseling.*

**genetic heterogeneity**  Descriptive of a trait or disease that can be caused by mutations at any one of several loci. Genetic heterogeneity is one source of major errors in linkage studies, in that the disorder being investigated may show linkage to one locus in one family and to another locus in a different family.

**genetic isolation**  Prevention of different populations of a species from mating; it is one of the primary mechanisms for the creation of a new species. If two groups never mate, their genes are likely to diverge.

**genetic loading**  See *diathesis-stress model.*

**genetic mapping**  See *mapping.*

**genetic marker**  An inherited trait that occurs in association with another disease often enough to support the assumption that the second disease is at least in part genetically determined and that its gene occupies a chromosomal location close to the gene for the inherited trait. See *autoimmunity; restriction enzyme.*

Gene markers are DNA sequences of known chromosomal location that show many variants in the general population. The inheritance patterns of different markers are compared with the inheritance pattern of the disease itself. If a particular variant is consistently inherited with the disease, then the disease gene must be located near the marker. The DNA marker is the combination of varying-sized fragments resulting from a restriction enzyme's cutting of DNA. In order to be traced in pedigree studies, the marker must occur in various forms (alleles)

that are inherited in a simple mendelian pattern; that permits identification of the parent and grandparent from whom the subject has inherited the marker. See *linkage analysis; PCR.*

Genetic studies try to find the chromosomal location of the genes that confer vulnerability. There are three complicating factors that make the search difficult: (1) behavioral traits are polygenic in nature and more than one gene is involved in determining different aspects of the trait; (2) no matter how many genes are involved (they are known collectively as quantitative trait loci), at least some of them are likely to display incomplete penetrance; and (3) the probability of phenocopies (a disorder of a nongenetic type that clinically is identical to genetically influenced variants).

To overcome these obstacles, geneticists study informative pedigrees to determine if any sort of marker is transmitted through families in parallel with transmission of the disease. RFLPs are often used. They are specific patterns of electrophoretically displayed fragments that are produced by digesting the chromosomal DNA with certain enzymes. Certain patterns may be transmitted with the disease, and this suggests where within these fragments a genetic variant might be found.

Two kinds of probes are used: (1) random probes that bind at different sites and thus scan the entire genome; and (2) candidate genes that seem likely to be linked to the known physiology of the disease are used as a probe to examine the electrophoretic pattern of chromosome fragments.

DNA markers have been used to map several major human genetic diseases whose underlying physiological mechanisms were unknown, a strategy termed *reverse genetics.* Examples are Huntington disease, Wilson disease, cystic fibrosis, neurofibromatosis, and a form of familial Alzheimer disease.

Various strategies are used to study diseases suspected of being at least partly genetic in origin:

1. *Twin studies* endeavor to hold the family environment constant and compare the degree to which illness occurs in genetically identical monozygotic twins versus dizygotic twins. In *schizophrenia,* the risk for illness in MZ twins of patients is at least 3-fold greater than the risk in DZ twins of patients, and a

40- to 60-fold greater risk in MZ twins than in the general population; in *bipolar* affective disorder, there is concordance for illness in 79% of MZ twins, in 19% of DZ twins; in *alcoholism*, 26% in MZ twins, 12% in DZ twins; in *panic* disorder, 31% in MZ twins, 0% in DZ twins.

2. *Adoption studies* and *cross-fostering sudies* attempt to separate the contribution of genes and environmental factors shared among subjects reared in the same home. Despite limitations, in the aggregate these studies have yielded evidence for a genetic role in a number of mental illnesses. These are crucial first steps, but the evidence gathered does not directly implicate a specific gene. To do that, the researcher uses sophisticated statistical techniques to decide whether a specific gene or chromosomal fragment is involved:

3. *Segregation analysis* compares the observed frequency of an illness in a pedigree with a pattern that would occur if a hypothesized mode of inheritance (e.g., one of the monogenic patterns or polygenic transmission) were true. The main limitation of the method is that findings may be compromised by etiologic heterogeneity, which would invalidate pooled family data or population data and would thus be relatively insensitive to single-gene effects.

4. *Linkage analysis.* To overcome these obstacles, a more sensitive assay technique called *linkage disequilibrium* is used. Instead of looking for a simple association, say, between depression and a genetic marker, it statistically compares the prevalence of the marker in depressives to its prevalence in the population at large. Used in the right circumstances, linkage disequilibrium can detect even tiny genetic contributions. It may be more sensitive in detecting monogenic inheritance than polygenic inheritance, however.

5. Linkage analysis examines the familial patterns of illness in one or more families to discover whether an illness is cosegregating (i.e., being inherited together with) a genetic marker whose location on one of the chromosomes is known.

**genetic redundancy**    See *aging, theories of.*

**genetic screening**    Systematic search for persons in a population who possess certain genotypes that (1) are associated with existing disease or predispose to future disease (because of genetically determined susceptibilities to environmental agents, for example), (2) may lead to

disease in their descendants, or (3) produce other variations of interest but not known to be associated with disease.

It is conventional to screen (1) blood of newborns (*newborn screening*) for the hyperphenylalaninemias, the tyrosinemias, the amino acidopathies, the galactosemias, and aberrations of thyroid hormone biosynthesis and (2) urine of newborns for disorders of amino acid or monosaccharide metabolism and transport.

*Fetal screening* permits detection of genetic disease in the fetus and thus permits selective termination of pregnancy. With the use of recombinant DNA, restriction enzymes, and oligonucleotide probes, it has become possible to detect many more diseases than previously and the methods pose fewer dangers to the fetus than earlier methods.

*Carrier screening* aims to identify persons heterozygous for a gene for a serious recessive disease, and it is now common to screen young adults in relevant high-risk ethnic communities to initiate genetic counseling for indications of Tay-Sachs, beta thalassemia, and sickle cell heterozygosity. Screening to identify persons with variant phenotypes, such as alpha-1 antitrypsin deficiency, has become a form of epidemiologic research to discover the natural history of the variant.

**genetic testing**    For many diseases the benefits of genetic testing are uncertain and the potential risks great—e.g., insurance and employment discrimination. See *ELSI Program.*

**genetic vulnerability**    Inherited predisposition to developing an illness, either because of a heavy loading of those factors that contribute to the development of the illness or because of inadequate resistance or defenses against the illness. The concept implies that the vulnerability is an actual or measurable variation in structure or function, that it is continuous and chronic, and that the affected person carries the constitutional susceptibility even during periods of health. This is in contrast to the stress concept of psychiatric illness, which implies that in the well state a person is equivalent to a normal control and it is only when stress appears that he deviates from the normal. See *risk; risk factor.*

**genetics**    Study of heredity and inheritance, of the transmission of traits from one individual to another, either through simple cell division or the more elaborate sexual processes; study of how genes are transmitted from generation to generation.

**genetics, pathophysiological** Search for and study of the biological variables (including vulnerabilities and markers) that are related to the gene(s) presumed to be the cause of the disease in question. Schizophrenia, for example, is generally believed to have a significant genetic component, but whether only a single gene is involved is unknown. Pathophysiological genetics searches for any type of neurochemical or psychophysiological abnormality that may be a link between the responsible gene(s) and the full clinical picture of unquestionable schizophrenic disorder. The search includes studies of family members to determine if, and how frequently, they also manifest the same physiological abnormality even though they do not develop a schizophrenic disorder. Uncovering such *endophenotypes* (who bear some of the inherited physiological abnormalities or vulnerabilities or markers, but are not schizophrenic) is one step toward determining if schizophrenia is a heterogeneous group of subtypes and what the range of subtypes is.

**genetophobia** Stigmatization of and fear of the effect of a genetic disorder on the subject discovered to have an abnormal gene or chromosome. Often the significance of a discovered defect is impossible to predict, but the mere fact that it is discovered may influence those who know about it to treat the subject in such a way that the diagnosis becomes a self-fulfilling prophecy.

**genetotrophic disease** A disease "in which the genetic pattern of the afflicted individual calls for an augmented supply of a particular nutrient (or nutrients) for which there develops, as a result, a nutritional deficiency" (Williams, R. J. et al. in *Management of Addictions*, ed.

E. Podolsky, 1955). "On the basis of our studies with rats it seems likely that the basic etiologic factor in human alcoholism is genetotrophic, and that the sociological and psychological factors so generally considered as fundamental factors are only precipitating factors for the development of the clinical syndrome" (ibid.). The factor described is believed to depend on one or more partial genetic blocks: "Briefly described, such a block involves a heritable trait that is characterized not by a complete inability to carry out a specific enzymatic transformation, but

by a diminished potentiality for producing the biochemical change. This in turn leads to an augmented requirement for some specific nutritional factor or factors" (ibid.).

**genial** *Biol.* Pertaining to or having the particular genetic quality or the individual manifestations of a *genus*.

**geniculate bodies** The medial and lateral geniculate bodies are part of the posterior nuclei of the thalamus. The medial geniculate body receives auditory fibers from the cochlear nuclei (via the lateral lemniscus) and from the inferior colliculus. It sends fibers to the temporal cortex (Heschl gyrus) via the auditory radiation, which ascends through the internal capsule. The lateral geniculate body receives most of the fibers of the optic tract; it sends fibers to the visual cortex (around the calcarine fissure) via the optic or geniculocalcarine radiation, which ascends through the internal capsule.

**geniculate neuralgia** See *neuralgia*; *pain*.

**genital character** The mature type of *character* (q.v.), no longer dominated by the pleasure principle. The subject shows features characteristic of the preceding stages, but in a combination conducive to the greatest effectiveness. The mature character is able to care for and contribute to the welfare of another. During the pregenital stages, the management of instinctual energies was largely of an autoerotic and narcissistic character; now, since the object of the genital impulses is outside the person himself, the instincts strive toward alloerotic (homosexual and heterosexual) expression. See *character defense*.

**genital love** The type of object love characteristic of the genital or adult stage; adult, mature, nonambivalent object love.

**genital primacy** In psychoanalytic psychology, genitality is divided into two principal substages. The first is the phallic phase. The second is reached only at puberty; it is the stage of late genital, or complete genital primacy. See *ontogeny, psychic*.

**genital retraction syndrome** *Koro* (q.v.).

**genitality** A general term referring to the genital components of sexuality, and sometimes used to refer to adult sexuality; but genitality is evident before genital primacy is complete, as in childhood and adolescent genital masturbation. "In time, the genitals begin to function as a special discharge apparatus, which concentrates all excitation upon itself and discharges it all no matter in which erogenous zone it originated. It is called genital primacy when this function of the genitals has become dominant over the extragenital erogenous zones, and all sexual excitations become finally genitally oriented and climatically discharged" (Fenichel, O. *The Psychoanalytic Theory of Neurosis*, 1945).

**genitalize**  To displace genital libido, as onto a nonsexual (but predisposed) organ in hysteria, where libido is discharged, but inadequately and incompletely.

**genital-psychical development**  A psychoanalytic term that stresses the importance of psychosexual, developmental, emotional maturation as a true basis for genito-sexual potency—in contrast to mechanical, anatomical, physiological, and orgastic criteria that give rise to pseudopotency and the masking of impotence. Genito-sexual potency is characterized by the ability to love in the adult sense and by a free, full, and satisfactory orgasm as well. Genito-sexual pseudopotency is manifested in a masturbatory preoccupation with personal, orgastic, and tactile sensation. Even though orgasm in the pseudopotent may be deceptively satisfactory, it is frequently entirely dependent upon thinly disguised perversion stimuli and perversion auspices. Genito-sexual pseudopotency is associated with self-love and self-satisfaction; in contrast, the genito-sexual potency of the psychosexually mature is strongly marked by love of and consideration for the partner. See *impotence; sexual disorders.*

**genius**  A generic, nonspecific term used loosely to denote an individual child or adult of markedly superior intellectual, emotional, volitional, affective, or creative abilities.

**genocopy**  A genetic imitator, such as all those genetic disorders that can present a clinical picture of schizophrenia.

**genogram**  Graphic representation of the history and the relationship structure of the family, emphasizing the connection between events and patterns; the genealogy of a family; family tree. In family therapy, the genogram is a means of identifying intergenerational continuities and the ways in which the past determined both the expressed and the unexpressed expectation that family members have of one another.

**genome**  The archive containing the sets of instructions for each type of cell; a generic representation of the full gene set of an organism (in the human, estimated to be 22,000 genes). It gives directions to generate a 10- to 50-trillion-celled organism from a single egg, and the life instructions that guide the cells from birth to adolescence, maturity, and death. Each tape of the archive contains a long sentence, spelled out in evolution's four-letter programming code. See *chromosome; DNA; gene; genomics.*

**genomic imprinting**  The phenomenon in which maternal and paternal genomes contribute differentially to the developing embryos of their offspring, as in *Angelman syndrome* and *Prader-Willi syndrome* (qq.v.). In both, mental retardation is the foremost symptom, and both are disorders of chromosome 15. Yet the associated symptoms are almost the exact opposite in the two disorders: hyperactivity in Angelman syndrome, and bradykinesis and obesity in Prader-Willi syndrome. In Angelman syndrome, the deletions are in the chromosome 15 inherited from the mother; in Prader-Willi syndrome, the deletions are in the paternally derived chromosome.

**genomic instability syndromes**  A group of diseases due to defective repair responses to DNA lesions. *Ataxia telangiectasia* (q.v.) is due to mutation of the AT protein, which normally coordinates responses to double strand breaks in DNA. Defects in the response to single strand breaks lead to *AOA1* and *SCAN* (qq.v.).

**genomics**  A term coined in 1986 by Thomas Roderick for the systematic study of complete genomes, i.e., mapping, sequencing, and analyzing genomes. Currently, emphasis is moving to genome function, and genome analysis is now divided into structural genomics and functional genomics. *Structural genomics* represents an early phase of genome analysis—the construction of high-resolution genetic, physical, and transcript maps of an organism. The ultimate physical map of an organism is its complete DNA sequence. *Functional genomics* refers to the development of methods to assess gene function by making use of the information and reagents provided by structural genomics.

The *Human Genome Project (HGP)* was organized in 1990 with the goal of constructing a complete genetic map of the human genome. The genome comprises three billion bases of DNA; the vast majority of it—perhaps 95%, so-called *noncoding DNA* (q.v.) —does not encode proteins or regulatory information. The HGP directed its attention first to relatively small genomes of important experimental organisms—bacteria, yeast, flies, and worms—were attacked first, to serve as pilot projects designed to refine the tools for automated sequencing and computational analysis of genomic information. In 1995, the first complete bacterial genome was produced—the 1.8 Mb *Haemophilus influenzae*. In 1998, the genome of the first multicellular organism—the 97 Mb DNA sequence of the roundworm *Caenorhabditis elegans* was published. It confirmed that the number of distinct genes required to template a complex organism such as the fruit fly (which has some 13,000 genes) was not much greater than the ca. 6000 carried in the genome of the single-celled baker's yeast.

The Human Genome Project was completed in 2003, and in 2004 the International Human Gene Sequencing Consortium published a description of the finished human gene sequence. The analysis suggested that humans have 20,000–25,000 genes, down from estimates a decade earlier of more than 100,000 genes. In 2007, the genome of DNA discoverer James Watson was sequenced, the first time an individual's genomic map had been completed.

**genophobia**   Fear of sex.

**genotropism**   Szondi's hypothesis that latent recessive genes determine instinctive or spontaneous choice reactions. This is manifested in one way by attraction of libido between persons possessing similar gene stock. The *Szondi test* (q.v.) was constructed to demonstrate this hypothesis experimentally, and it was Szondi's belief that the test subject chooses a particular picture because his or her corresponding need system is in a state of tension.

**genotype**   The totality of replicators contained in an organism's physicochemical genetic makeup; strain; selected line. Heredity refers to the transmission of genotypes from the parents to their children. See *replicator*.

The term genotype was coined by the Danish botanist Johannsen in connection with his pure-line theory, in order to distinguish the factorial structure of an organism from its manifested *phenotype* (q.v.). According to this theory, all individuals descended from a common ancestor by asexual reproduction have an identical genotype and will continue to breed true, regardless of environmental differences, forming lines genetically pure for all their characters. Although originally the term meant the sum of all inherited predispositional characters of an individual, it has become customary to use it now in the sense of a particular *predisposition* (q.v.) underlying an individual disease.

**genu**   Knee; used to describe any structure that is bent like a knee, such as the genu of the internal capsule (the angle formed by the union of its two limbs) or the genu of the corpus callosum (the ventral curve at the anterior end of its body).

**genus**   In biology, this term signifies a group of related species and classifies the group as ranking above a species and next below a subfamily.

**geology, medical**   Study of the influence of rocks, minerals, and other elements of the earth on health and disease. One specific application is in epidemiology, where the geographic distribution of trace elements (e.g., selenium) in soil and food is compared with rates of mental illness in those areas.

**geophagia, geophagy**   Dirt eating; a form of *pica* (q.v.).

**gephyrophobia**   Fear of crossing a bridge or river.

**GERD**   Gastroesophageal reflux disease; *achalasia* (q.v.).

**geriatric psychiatry**   *Psychogeriatrics*; the branch of psychiatry that deals with disorders of old age; it aims to maintain old persons independently in the community as long as possible and to provide long-term care when needed. Its future hinges on research into Alzheimer disease and other dementias of late life, which, if prevented, would allow 90% of the people over 75 years of age to be free of physical and mental disability instead of the 50% to 75% who now are free of such disorder.

**geriatrics**   The science of curing or healing disorders and ailments of old age. See *geriatric psychiatry*.

**geriopsychosis**   A term suggested by Southard for psychoses of the senescent period; senile psychoses.

**germinally affected**   Equivalent to the German term, *keimkrank,* describing an organism (1) as being heterozygous for some recessive character and thus carrying the predisposition for the trait in its genotype without manifesting it phenotypically; or (2) as a homozygote for any kind of hereditary character with inhibited manifestation.

**gerocomy** The belief, or practice, that an older man absorbs virtue and youth from younger women.

**gerontalism** Impersonating or adopting the characteristics of an older person; it is sometimes reported as a *paraphilia* (q.v.) when sexual arousal and orgasm are dependent upon playing such a role and being treated as an older person by the sexual partner. Paraphilic gerontalism is at the opposite end of the age scale from paraphilic *juvenilism* (q.v.).

**gerontology** The study of old age.

**gerontophilia** A *paraphilia* (q.v.) in which sexual arousal and orgasm depend upon the partner being older (e.g., parent- or grandparent-aged); such a paraphilia is also described in terms of a chronophilic or age disparity (along with pedophilia, ephebophilia, etc.).

**gerontophobia** See *ageism*.

**gerophilia** Same as *gerontophilia*.

**Gerstmann syndrome** (Josef Gerstmann, American neurologist, 1888–1969) A symptom complex described by Gerstmann in 1940 consisting of finger agnosia, right-left disorientation, acalculia, and agraphia. There may be various additional features, such as constructive apraxia, amnestic reduction of word finding, disturbed ability to read, impaired color perception, absence of optokinetic nystagmus, and disturbance of equilibrium. The agraphia often takes the form of dissociated *dysgraphia*. Presence of the Gerstmann syndrome implies definite parietal lobe pathology, usually in the neighborhood of the angular gyrus. See *parietal lobe dysfunction*.

Most present-day neurologists question the usefulness of the concept, in that the deficits forming the syndrome are no more closely linked than are a score of other combinations of behavioral deficits.

**Gesell, Arnold L.** (1881–1961) Founder and director (for 37 years)of Yale Clinic of Child Development.

**Gesell developmental test** A series of 27 age-level recorded observations and reactions to standardized situations from birth through the first 5 years of life. At each age level an inventory of activities is divided into four categories of behavior: (1) Motor; (2) Adaptive; (3) Language; and (4) Personal-Social. Each of these categories of behavior is evaluated by observing the infant or child in a number of standardized situations.

**Gestalt psychology** A school of psychology that is concerned primarily with perceptual processes. Its development is associated particularly with Max Wertheimer, Wolfgang Koehler, and Kurt Koffka. An outgrowth of opposition to traditional association psychology, it maintains that aspects of perception reflect the brain's innate capacity to order simple sensations.

"Gestalt psychology holds that the whole or total quality of the image is perceived. This is in contrast to association psychology, which states that stimuli are perceived as parts and built into images. According to gestalt psychology, the organization of the stimuli into the image is based upon laws of perception which include proximity, similarity, direction, and inclusiveness of parts of the stimuli. The perceptual experience is a gestalt or *configuration* or pattern in which the whole is more than the sum of its parts. Organized units or structuralized configurations are the primary form of biological reactions. In the sensory field, these gestalten correspond to the configuration of the stimulating world.

"The organism has a 'gestalt function' which is defined as thatfunction of the integrative organism whereby it responds to a given constellation of stimuli as a whole, the response being a constellation or pattern or gestalt which differs from the original stimulus pattern by the process of the integrative mechanism of the individual who experiences the perception. The whole setting of the stimulus and the whole integrative state of the organism determine the pattern or response.

"There is a tendency not only to perceive gestalten but to complete gestalten and to reorganize them according to principles biologically determined by the sensory motor pattern of action which may be expected to vary in different maturation or growth levels and in pathological states organically or functionally determined" (Bender, L. *Child Psychiatric Techniques,* 1952).

**Gestalt therapy** A holistic form of psychotherapy that emphasizes heightened emotionality, understanding the autonomic and musculoskeletal messages transmitted by the body, and helping the subject get in touch with the primitive wisdom of the body. The person acts out a variety of roles in life and during therapy learns to recognize what is symbolized by those patterns of activity and to take responsibility for conflicts within himself and attitudes toward others that contribute to his problems.

During the treatment session, the therapist considers not only what the patient says but how he is saying it—his voice inflection, posture, gestures, breathing patterns, etc. Change is viewed as a subintellectual process and the here-and-now is all important. Gestalt therapy employs role-playing and other techniques to promote the subject's growth process and to develop his full potential.

Developed by Fritz Perls, Gestalt therapy is used in both individual and group therapy. It draws from many sources, including psychoanalysis, Jung's ego psychology, Reich's character armoring, existentialism, phenomenology, and behavior theory.

**gestational epilepsy** Seizures that appear only during pregnancy. The incidence of gestational epilepsy is relatively low, but it highlights the problems of management of the pregnant epileptic. Anticonvulsants appear to increase by two or three times the risk of congenital malformations in the fetus (especially cleft palate, cleft lip, and septal or other cardiac defects). *Fetal hydantoin syndrome* includes craniofacial abnormalities, limb defects, growth abnormalities, and mental retardation. *Fetal trimethadione syndrome* includes epicanthal folds, low-set ears, V-shaped eyebrows, ocular defects, short stature, developmental delays, and speech disturbances. See *epilepsy.*

**gesticulation, involuntary** A parakinesis, suggestive of a posterior or posteromedial frontal lobe lesion on the contralateral side; often observed in conjunction with a grasp reflex.

**gestural-postural language** A method or form of communication between persons by means of gestures and/or postures without resorting to the use of words. It is one form of communication by means of nonverbal language.

**geumaphobia** Fear of taste.

**Gf** Fluid intelligence; see *g.*

**GGTP** Gamma-glutamyl transpeptidase; also *GGT (gamma-glutamyl transferase)*; an enzyme that transports amino acids into cells. Most of the GGTP found in blood comes from the liver, and it has been used as a state marker for heavy drinking (and, thus, a monitor of abstinence in the recovering alcoholic). GGTP is a relatively sensitive marker of heavy alcohol consumption: between 70% and 80% of alcoholics who have recently been drinking heavily show elevated blood levels of GGTP, and between 70% and 80% of people with high levels of GGTP are found to be very heavy drinkers. Levels of GGTP are also elevated in severe cardiac or pulmonary disease, Crohn disease and ulcerative colitis, thyroiditis, and marked obesity, and in persons using benzodiazepines or phenytoin. Normal blood level of GGTP is 30 units per liter; heavy drinking increases the value, and when drinking ceases the blood level begins to decrease within 2 weeks.

**GH** *Growth hormone* (q.v.), which is synthesized and stored in somatotropes in the lateral wings of the anterior pituitary. GH is regulated by two hypothalamic peptides, GHRH (*GH releasing hormone*) and SS (*somatostatin*). GHRH stimulates GH output, and somatostatin inhibits it. The GH gene is on chromosome 17. See hypothalamic-pituitary-adrenal axis.

**GHB** *Gamma-hydroxybutyric acid;* it is produced endogenously by the metabolism of gamma-aminobutyric acid (GABA). It increases dopamine levels in the brain and acts on the endogenous opioid system.

It acts synergistically with alcohol to produce CNS and respiratory depression. An oral dose of 10 mg/kg can produce amnesia and hypotonia, of 30 mg/kg somnolence within 15 minutes, and in amounts over 50 mg/kg it may abruptly induce coma, with depressed respiration and sometimes seizure like activity.

GHB has been used experimentally for the treatment of narcolepsy. It has been reported (mainly by Italian workers) to be effective in treating alcohol withdrawal and in preventing alcohol relapse. See *relapse prevention.* GHB is sold in health food stores and promoted (illegally in the United States) for sleep, weight control, and euphoric and anabolic effects.

**Gheel Colony** A boarding-out type of domiciliary care in Gheel,(now called Geel), Belgium, that has existed since the 13th century for the treatment of a large number of psychotic patients who reside in private homes in the community. See *domicile; family care.*

**ghost sickness** A culture-specific syndrome reported in American Indian tribes, consisting of multiple somatic symptoms and hallucinations associated with thoughts of death or of people who have died.

**ghrelin** A peptide expressed in the stomach, the *arcuate nucleus* (q.v.) of the hypothalamus, and elsewhere. Ghrelin is a natural appetite stimulant that alters synaptic inputs to POMC (propriomelanocortin) and NPY (neuropeptide Y) neurons in a direction opposite to that of *leptin* (q.v.).

**GHRH** GH releasing hormone. See GH.

**gibberish** Unintelligible and incoherent language seen in some patients with schizophrenia, who may regress to a stage in which language is founded on the principles of primitive mentality. The language of the patient is gibberish to those who cannot understand it, in much the same sense that dreams are gibberish, or that any mode of communication foreign to one is gibberish. See *jargon aphasia.*

**gifted** As used in child psychiatry, describing a child whose intelligence is in the upper 2% of the total population of his age. Often, however, the term is used more loosely to refer to a child who shows outstanding ability in any single area. See *bright child.*

**gigantism** A constitutional anomaly characterized by a stature greatly above the average (any height above 205 cm in white population groups) and by a corresponding excess of body mass. It is due either to a heredito-constitutional hyperplasia of the entire endocrine system or to a particular form of hyperfunction in the anterior lobe of the hypophysis during the period of growth of the person affected. This condition of hyperpituitarism may be primary or it may be secondary to genital hypofunction. Only in rare cases, glands other than the pituitary may be primarily implicated, for instance, the adrenal cortex or the pineal gland.

Among the various forms of gigantism are Berlinger's *gigantosomiaprimordialis*, Pellizzi's *precocious macrogenitosomia*, and *eunuchoid small gigantism*. The last consists of excessive growth, especially of the lower extremities, which takes place just before puberty and is associated with a hypogenesis of the secondary sexual characteristics. It is often found in the phthisic or dolichomorphic types of constitution and may correct itself in later years, unless it is complicated by active pulmonary tuberculosis. The syndrome has also been reported as a residuum of rheumatic encephalitis.

**gigantism, eurythmic** *Gigantosomia primordialis* (q.v.).

**gigantosomia primordialis** Berlinger's term for the extremely raresyndrome of *gigantism* with normal sex development.

**Gilles de la Tourette syndrome** *GTD; Tourette disorder* (q.v.).

**Gjessing syndrome** Recurrent episodes of catatonic stupor or excitement occurring in schizophrenics and associated with phasic variations in the nitrogen metabolism; first described by R. Gjessing in 1938. The syndrome is related to inadequate metabolism of dietary protein, leading to periods of nitrogen retention that are concurrent with hyper- or hypokinetic episodes. Dietary regulation is sometimes enough to control such patients; in others, thyroid administration increases nitrogen output with corresponding improvement in mental state. See *periodic catatonia.*

**glabella tap test** Tapping the glabella (the most prominent point on the forehead between the two superciliary arches) with the index finger causes the orbicularis oculi muscles to contract so that both eyes blink. Normally, blinking stops after 5 to 10 taps; persistence of blinking beyond that is a positive sign (sometimes called *Myerson sign*) and suggestive of Parkinson disease. In patients with very loose skin, pinching a fold of skin on the patient's temple lateral to the external canthus may provide a better glabellar surface for tapping.

**glabellar sign** Inability to inhibit blinking in response to tapping of the forehead, suggestive of Parkinson disease.

**glabrous** Hairless; having a surface without projections. Glabrous skin is highly sensitive and discriminating, especially at the tips of the fingers. The two principle types of mechanoreceptors in the superficial glabrous skin are the rapidly adapting *Meissner corpuscle* and the slowly adapting *Merkel receptor.* There are two other types of mechanoreceptor in the subcutaneous tissue beneath both glabrous and hairy skin: the rapidly adapting *Pacinian corpuscle* and the slowly adapting *Ruffini corpuscle.*

**Glasgow Coma Scale** A measure of the degree of impairment of wakefulness, consciousness, and alertness, based on functioning in three areas: E (eye open, rated from not open to open spontaneously), M (motor response, rated from no response to obeys commands), and V (verbal response, rated from no response to oriented).

**GLBT** Gay, lesbian, bisexual, transsexual.

**glia** (Gr. "glue") *Neuroglia*; a web of supporting tissue in the central nervous system. The glia act as a scaffold that guides developing neuroblasts and axon growth cones to their proper destinations. The glia include *microglia*, of mesodermal origin, phagocytic scavengers mobilized by disease, injury, or death; *ependymal cells;* and *macroglia* (of ectodermal origin), which include *oligodendrocytes* (or oligodendroglia), *Schwann cells*, and *astrocytes*.

Neurons account for only a minority of cells in the brain; glia constitute approximately 85% of brain cells. Although classically described in terms of their supporting function, glia are now recognized to play a role in both neurogenesis and gliogenesis in adult life. Neuroepithelial cells in the early neural tube develop into radial glia, which are transformed into astrocytes at birth. In some areas of the brain, those astrocytes continue to produce not only glia but also neurons.

The microglia are not true glial cells but, rather, are macrophages, a group of white blood cells. They are debris scavengers located between neurons and along the blood vessels in CNS.

Ependymal cells lines the ventricles and the spinal canal. They are covered with fingerlike microvilli through which certain molecules pass from the brain into the cerebrospinal fluid.

Oligodendrocytes within the central nervous system and Schwann cells in the peripheral nervous system provide the myelin sheath that surrounds axons. The myelin sheath provides insulation that accelerates the velocity of conduction of action potentials down axons. The star-shaped astrocytes perform several functions: they are phagocytic scavengers that remove debris caused by cell injury: they take up neurotransmitters released into the synaptic cleft, they guide the migration of neurons during development: they participate in the formation of the blood–brain barrier and provide a vascular regulatory mechanism so that blood flow and oxygen consumption keep pace with neural activity.

Astrocytes recycle the neurotransmitter glutamate. Once released at a synapse, glutamate excites neurons until it is removed. Astrocytes handle about 90% of this glutamate clearance, but if overactivated or injured they may release glutamate instead of removing it. See *excitotoxicity.*

Glia may also have a key role in CNS disorders such as neuropathic pain, epilepsy, multiple sclerosis and neurodegenerative diseases such as AD, and they may be involved in the pathogenesis of schizophrenia and depression.

**glial guide cell** See *axon guidance; NCAM.*

**glial neurotrophic factors** See *GDNF.*

**Glick effect** Positive correlation between dropping out of school and subsequent marital instability ("marriage drop-out"); not observed in all studies.

**glioblastoma** See glioma; intracranial tumor.

**gliogenesis** See *glia.*

**glioma** The generic name for one of the commonest types of brain tumor. The gliomata (gliomas) account for approximately 50% of all intracranial tumors. They arise from glial cells and are composed predominantly of astrocytes or their embryonal precursors (medulloblasts, spongioblasts, astroblasts). By common usage, nearly all tumors of neuroepithelial origin are included in this term. In general, prognosis is unfavorable because gliomata tend to grow deep into the neural tissue; the more adult cell types (astrocytoma, oligodendroglioma, *ependymoma*) grow more slowly and are relatively benign, while the more immature cell types (*medulloblastoma*, spongioblastoma, or glioblastoma) tend to grow more rapidly, are more invasive, and are more malignant. See *intracranial tumor.*

**gliotransmitters** See *astrocytes.*

**glissando** Sliding up and down the musical scale; in neurology, glissando/deglissando refers to a gait disturbance: the subject walks with a shuffling gait, but as he moves from one point to another he accelerates to a near run and then gradually slows down to a stop. Such a gait is seen in Parkinson disease and also in the frontal lobe *convexity syndrome* (q.v.).

**global aphasia** The most severe aphasic syndrome, a combination of motor aphasia and a comprehension defect. Global aphasia is a nonfluent aphasia in which all language functions are lost; the patient cannot read, write, repeat, or name objects. Some patients can say spontaneously such overlearned words as goodbye and no. The lesions are in both the Broca and Wernicke areas and the arcuate fasciculus, the region of the left hemisphere that receives its blood supply from the middle cerebral artery. Usually there is an accompanying right hemiparesis, right hemisensory defect, and almost always a right homonymous hemianopsia.

**Global Assessment of Functioning**  *GAF* (q.v.).

**Global Deterioration Scale**  *GDS* (q.v.).

**globalist view**  In Chomsky's globalist view of *linguistic competence*, the capacity to acquire human language is due to a unique, genetically programmed part of the brain. Studies of the anatomical localization of language and of language development in children have long suggested that a large part of the process is innate. See *language; language acquisition*.

**globose nuclei**  See *cerebellum*.

**globus hystericus**  The sensation of a ball or globe that arises in the stomach area and progresses upward, being finally felt in the throat where it produces the feeling of strangulation.

Although the term suggests that the symptom is usually psychogenic in origin, the complaint is also frequent in patients with diaphragmatic hernia and esophageal reflux. In psychogenic cases, globus hystericus and other esophageal neuroses are often based on unconscious rejection of incorporation secondary to sexual or aggressive impulses (such as castration wishes). Disgust plays an important role and is probably a combination of temptation and rejection along with an ambivalent attitude toward incorporation. See *anorexia nervosa; eating disorders; esophageal neurosis*.

**globus pallidus**  One of the five nuclei of the basal ganglia (q.v.); the nucleus basalis of Meynert lies within the globus pallidus. The globus pallidus participates in both reward circuitry and movement; bilateral pallidal lesions are associated with anhedonia, depression, loss of drug craving, and extrapyramidal signs. See *cholinergic; striatofugal projections*.

**glorified self**  *Idealized self* (q.v.).

**glosso-**  Combining form meaning tongue, language, from Gr. *glōssa*.

**glossodynia**  An itching, burning sensation in the tongue and buccal mucous membranes.

**glossolalia**  *Autonomous speech; cryptophasia; idioglossia; polyglotneophasia; psittacism*; neologisms that simulate coherent speech. Despite the fact that they are expressed as unintelligible conglomerations of sounds, or written as series of unintelligible letters, such neologisms mimic normal speech by maintaining the distinctions of words, sentences, and even paragraphs. Glossolalia is most often seen in ecstatic and somnambulistic states, and, somewhat less commonly, in schizophrenia. If completely devoid of content, glossolalia is termed psittacistic, although some writers use glossolalia and psittacism interchangeably.

**glossopharyngeal nerve**  The ninth cranial nerve; it is motor to the stylopharyngeus muscle and sensory to the pharynx, soft palate, posterior tongue, and to the carotid body (for reflex control of respiration, blood pressure, and heart rate). The glossopharyngeal nerve also supplies taste buds in the posterior third of the tongue. Symptoms associated with lesions of this nerve include loss of gag reflex, loss of taste in posterior tongue, and deviation of uvula to the unaffected side.

**glossospasm**  Rapid protrusion and retraction of the tongue; the spasm generally lasts for several minutes.

**glossosynthesis**  *Neologism* (q.v.).

**GLS**  Glycolipid storage disease (q.v.).

**glucagon**  A hyperglycemic-glycogenolytic factor excreted by thealpha cells of the pancreas in response to hypoglycemia or stimulationby growth hormone of the anterior pituitary. Glucagon hydrochloride isa pharmacological preparation used to treat hypoglycemia (including thehypoglycemia of insulin coma therapy); it acts by mobilizing glycogen from the liver.

**glucocorticoids**  Steroid hormones secreted by the zona fasciculata of the adrenal cortex that bind to two subtypes of intracellular receptors: mineralocorticoid receptors and glucocorticoid receptors. Patients with glucocorticoid excess, either endogenous (Cushing syndrome) or exogenous (corticosteroid treatment), have a marked elevation in appetite and accumulate abdominal fat. Patients with glucocorticoid deficiency (Addison disease) have reduced appetite and weight loss. Reduced glucocorticoids have a potent effect to alter the ability of arcuate nucleus-derived peptides to increase or decrease food intake. See *general adaptation syndrome*.

**glucogenosis** *Von Gierke disease*; mental retardation due to a deficiency of glycogen-metabolizing enzymes, so that glycogen is deposited in the brain and other organs. See *carbohydrate metabolism*.

**glucoprivation** Decrease in level of circulating glucose, once believedto be the physiologic reason for hunger. See *carbohydrate metabolism*.

**Glueck, Eleanor Touroff** (1898–1972) Criminologist; with her husband, Sheldon Glueck, developed social prediction tables for early identification of delinquents.

**Glueck, Sheldon** (1896–1980) Lawyer, criminologist; juvenile delinquency; with his wife, Eleanor Glueck, developed controversial prediction tables based on 40 decisive factors in forecasting the appearance and level of criminal behavior.

**glue-sniffing** Inhalation, through the mouth or nose or both, of the aliphatic and aromatic hydrocarbons in glue (such as the glue used in making model airplanes). Glue-sniffing is one of the *psychoactive substance use disorders* (q.v.), and it is often practiced by very young children (9 to 12 years of age). Most inhalant abusers use other psychoactive substances as well. See *inhalant intoxication*.

**Glut1 transporter** Glucose transporter 1; a secondary active membrane transporter that clears the transmitter from the synaptic cleft after exocytoxic release. A mutation in the transporter gene causes Glut1 deficiency syndrome, symptoms of which include infantile seizures and developmental delay. Similarly, mutations in human glucose-6-phosphate transporter (G6PT) cause glycogen storage disease type 1b. See *transporter proteins*.

**glutamate** An excitatory amino acid (*EAA*), the brain's main excitatory neurotransmitter. It strengthens synaptic connections and consolidates new pathways throughout the brain. Virtually all brain cells have receptors that allow them to respond to glutamate, and over half the brain's 100 billion neurons generate the *neurotransmitter* (q.v.). In contrast, the brain has only about 10,000 dopamine-generating neurons. Glutamate does not simply excite neurons but through *mGlu receptors* (q.v.) can fine-tune neuronal signaling, slowing or accelerating transmission in specific brain circuits. The promotor of a gene for the

major glutamate transporter in CNS has been identified—excitatory amino acid transporter 2 (*EAAT2*). See *EATTs*.

Glutamate is toxic in excess. Excess glutamate with neuronal death is seen in many neurological disorders, including stroke, temporal lobe epilepsy, AD, ALS, HD, HIV-associated dementia, and growth of malignant gliomas. Glutamate may contribute to the loss of control that is characteristic of addiction, and glutamate dysregulation is believed to be a significant factor in the development of schizophrenia. See *glutamatergic model*; *neurotoxicity*.

Glutamate activates two types of receptors: ionotropic, which gate ion channels, and metabotropic, which are coupled to G proteins that affect intracellular metabolic processes.

The ionotropic receptors are named after the glutamate analogues that activate them: kainate, *AMPA*, and NMDA. The effects of all three are mediated by the opening of cation channels permeable to $Na^+$, thereby polarizing or "exciting" the neuron. AMPA and kainate receptors play the primary role in mediating fast excitatory postsynaptic potentials responsible for excitatory neurotransmission. The *NMDAR* (q.v.) is different; its channel is blocked by $Mg^{2+}$. Activation by kainate or AMPA receptor removes the block so that glutamate can open the NMDA channel, which is permeable not only to $Na^+$ but also to $Ca^{2+}$, an intracellular signaling ion (Goff, D. C. & Coyle, J. T. *American Journal of Psychiatry 158*, 2001). See *neurotransmitter receptor*.

*NMDA* (q.v.), the N-methyl-D-aspartate receptor, is a glutamate-gated ion channel that allows influx of calcium into the neuron. Calcium is required for neuronal plasticity, but in excessive amounts it causes cell death. *Phencyclidine* (PCP), a noncompetitive glutamate antagonist, acts by binding to the calcium channel associated with NMDA, preventing entry of calcium into the neuron.

Normally, glutamate is tightly bound in nerve endings or stored in astrocytes. Under conditions of oxygen deprivation, the membranes of the astrocytes fail, permitting large amounts of glutamate to spill out into the brain. The excess glutamate acts as an excitotoxin and overstimulates neurons with glutamate receptors; as a result, calcium floods the neurons and triggers a cascade of cell death. Drugs that block glutamate receptors (e.g., MK-801), if used early enough, might arrest cell death in cases of cerebrovascular accident, head trauma, and some cerebral degenerative diseases. See *excitotoxicity; Guam ALS-PDC.*

**glutamatergic** Referring to neurons that are activated by or secrete *glutamate* (q.v.), and to endogenous agents (such as neurotransmitters) or drugs that stimulate such neurons.

**glutamatergic model** *Glutamate hypothesis;* the theory that dysregulation of brain glutamatergic neurotransmission is a significant factor in the pathophysiology of schizophrenia. The model does not negate the *dopamine hypothesis* (q.v.); reciprocal relationships between forebrain dopaminergic and glutamatergic systems are well recognized, and dysregulation of one system would be expected to alter neurotransmission in the other. See *glutamate.*

The glutamate hypothesis of schizophrenia is based largely on the psychotomimetic effects of phencyclidine (PCP, "angel dust"), a noncompetitive antagonist of the N-methyl-D-aspartic acid (NMDA) subtype of glutamate receptors, which produces a schizophreniform psychosis that can consist of both negative and positive symptoms of schizophrenia.

**glutamine synthetase** An enzyme essential to brain nitrogen metabolism; it synthesizes glutamine from glutamate, ammonia, and ATP (adenosine triphosphate). It seems also to be an antioxidant. See *free radical.*

**glutaric aciduria** A genetic disorder of protein metabolism characterized by a buildup of highly toxic glutaric acid, which attacks muscle, liver, and brain tissue. Affected children are usually healthy for the first 6 months of life, but the disorder erupts under the stress of infection. Some children become comatose and die within 48 hours; those who survive the initial episode show progressive muscular atrophy and paralysis. Preliminary studies suggest that treatment of children at high genetic risk with a protein-restricted diet supplemented by riboflavin may prevent development of the disorder.

Glutaric aciduria is the leading cause of *cerebral palsy* among the Amish in Lancaster County, Pennsylvania. They number about 15,000 and are descendants of 200 Swiss immigrants who began to settle there in 1720.

It has been estimated that as many as 1 in every 7 Amish living today in the county is a carrier of the defective gene; 1 Amish child in 200 thus is likely to be stricken with glutaric aciduria. (If both parents are asymptomatic carriers, each child has a 25% chance of developing the disorder.) Among the Amish, glutaric aciduria is 10 times more common than diabetes and 100 times more common than childhood leukemia.

**gluteal reflex** A superficial reflex; stroking the buttocks causes contraction of the glutei.

**glycine** An amino acid *neurotransmitter;* glycine and *GABA* are the major inhibitory transmitters in the CNS (qq.v.). Glutamine stimulates binding of noncompetitive NMDA antagonists, such as PCP and MK-801. See *NMDAR.*

**glycolipid storage disease** *GLS;* accumulation of intermediate products of glycolipid catabolism because of a deficiency in the acid hydrolase enzymes that normally break them down. The most common one is Gaucher disease (types 1, 2, and 3), in which glucocerebroside is not adequately hydrolyzed to ceramide and glucose because of a deficiency of β-glucosidase glucocerebrosidase. Other glycolipid storage diseases are Tay-Sachs disease ($GM_2$ ganglioside accumulates), Fabry disease (ceramide trihexoside accumulates), Niemann-Pick disease, (sphingomyelin accumulates), Sanhoff disease, $G_{M1}$ gangliosidosis, fucosidosis, Krabbe disease, and metachromatic leukodystrophy. These result from the inheritance of defects of the genes encoding the catabolic enzymes required for the complete breakdown of glycolipids within lysosomes. See *Gaucher disease; lysosomal storage disorders; Niemann-Pick disease; Tay-Sachs disease.*

**glycosylation site** A position on a newly made protein where sugar molecules are added to mark the protein for transport to the cell membrane.

**gnostic** A term applied by the Dutch school of neurologists (Brouwer and Kappers) to designate the deep and epicritic sensations in contradistinction to the protopathic sensations that are considered as vital or paleosensations.

**GnRH** Gonadotropin-releasing hormone; a decapeptide that acts to release luteinizing hormone (LH) and follicle-stimulating hormone (FSH) from the pituitary; it has direct central stimulatory effects on sexual behavior, attention, and alertness. Norepinephrine stimulates its release, while gonadal steroids inhibit its release. See *hypothalamus*.

**God complex** E. Jones's (1915) term for what today would be termed narcissistic personality disorder, characterized by inflated self-confidence, phantasies of omnipotence, desires to display one's own person, intense need to be pleased and admired, sometimes a masking of grandiosity with caricatured modesty and social aloofness or pretended contempt for money, articulateness and love of language that often coexists with subtle learning defects and inattention. See *grandiose self*.

**going on being** See *impingement*.

**goiter** Enlargement of the thyroid gland. See *thyroiditis; thyrotoxicosis*.

**gold curve** See Lange colloidal gold reaction.

**Goldstein, Kurt** (1878–1965) German psychiatrist and neurologist; aphasia; gestalt psychology; self-actualization.

**Golgi, Camillo** (1843–1926) Italian psychiatrist and neuroanatomist who developed a histologic method for visualization of nerve fibers and neurons and described the morphology of glial cells. He also described the "Golgi internal reticular apparatus", an interlacing network of subcellular intracytoplasmic structures now known to have important cytometabolic functions. In 1906 he shared the Nobel Prize for Medicine or Physiology with Ramòn y Cajal. See *Golgi apparatus; reticulum*.

**Golgi apparatus** Also, Golgi complex; a polarized stack of compartments (*cisternae*) that is a key sorting system directing *biosynthetic cargo* from the *endoplasmic reticulum* (*ER*) to various destinations. The ER contains pre-Golgi intermediates that select protein that is properly folded. They return their sorting and targeting components to the ER for use in subsequent sorting of other cargo: newly synthesized proteins and lipids targeted to various extracellular and intracellular sites as well as proteins that are continually recycled between compartments as part of the transport machinery involved in *cargo selection*, vesicle formation, and targeting and fusion of vesicles. (A *vesicle* is any membrane-enclosed structure into which cargo is segregated.)

Golgi-processing enzymes lead to formation of the *trans-Golgi network* (*TGN*), where cargo is directed to the proper downstream compartment. Selection of cargo initiates vesicle formation, and sorting determinants on the cargo as well as cytosolic *coat components* direct cargo to the developing vesicle. Coat and targeting components form sorting machines that move cargo from one destination to the next. Vesicle coats recruit cargo; other components, *targeting determinants*, direct the vesicle to its destination. They identify the vesicle and its targets, and they mediate the docking and fusion of vesicles. Coat recruitment, cargo selection, and vesicle fusion are coordinated by *guanosine phosphatases*.

Although the traditional view has been that vesicles coated with *coat complex I* (*COPI*) direct *anterograde transport* of biosynthetic cargo, recent evidence indicates that it directs *retrograde transport* instead. Recycling by means of retrograde trafficking from the cell surface enables cells to balance and regulate outward membrane flow appropriately.

**Golgi neuron** A large neuron, found in the cerebellum.

**Goll, column of** (Friedrich Goll, Swiss anatomist, 1829–1904)Fasciculus gracilis (q.v.).

**gonad** A germ-gland; sexual gland.

**gonadocentric** Relating to the genitals as focal points. At puberty the sex urge becomes fully gonadocentric, with masturbation at the threshold and fringe of object love.

**good and evil test** See *criminal responsibility*.

**good breast** See *affectomotor storms; fit*.

**good enough mother** See *affectomotor storms; cohesive self; facilitating environment*.

**good object** In Kleinian usage, gratifying, loving, and protective whole or part objects or their representations that arise from splitting of self and object representations into all good and all bad during the paranoid-schizoid position. The gratifying breast is experienced as the good breast loving the infant. Good internal objects are regularly idealized, leading to fantasies of unlimited gratification by the objects. Internalization of the sense of being loved protects against the death instinct and its various manifestations. Good experiences diminish persecutory fears and primary envy and lead instead to gratitude and generosity. Projection of good inner objects onto new objects forms the basis of trust. Idealization of the object also limits aggression against it and attenuates the guilt associated with such aggression. See *bad object; primary envy; paranoid-schizoid position.*

**Goodenough test**   A test of a child's intellectual level of development based upon the subject's drawing of a human figure. The test was introduced in 1926 by Florence Goodenough, who standardized children's drawings to produce a test of intelligence.

**goodness of fit**   See communicative matching.

**Gordon Holmes rebound phenomenon**   (Gordon Holmes, British physician, 1876–1965) A test for ataxia, specifically illustrating the loss of cerebellar "check" on coordinated movement; if an attempt is made to extend the flexed forearm against resistance and suddenly let go, the hand or fist flies unchecked against the mouth or shoulder.

**Gordon reflex**   (Alfred Gordon, American neurologist, 1874–1953) Dorsal extension of the great toe, induced by compression of the calf muscle.

**gorger-vomiter**   A person with a form of *bulimia* (q.v.) in which the eating binges end in spontaneous or self-induced vomiting, followed by guilt and shame over loss of control, and depression. The depression is often severe, with suicidal ideas, starvation, and self-mutilation.

**governess psychosis**   "For decades, the idea has been preserved that governesses were especially prone to develop schizophrenia...a 'governess-psychosis'; and it has even been maintained that governesses suffer a particularly severe (and unpleasant) form of the disease" (Bleuler, E. *Dementia Praecox or the Group of Schizophrenias,* 1950). Statistics do not, in fact, indicate that incidence of schizophrenia is higher in governesses than in other vocations.

**Gowers sign**   A characteristic symptom of Duchenne muscular dystrophy: because of increasing muscle degeneration, the child must climb up his own trunk with his arms in order to rise from the supine position.

**Gowers tetanoid chorea**   (Sir William R. Gowers, English neurologist, 1845–1915) See *hepatolenticular degeneration.*

**gp120**   The envelope protein of the AIDS virus, a small portion of which attaches the virus to cellular receptors and thereby infects the cell. By antagonizing the normal functions of VIP receptors on neurons and glial cells, the virus or the infected macrophages cause neurons in the cortex to degenerate, producing a variety of debilitating dementias, rapidly progressing to death. See *AIDS dementia complex; vasoactive intestinal peptide* (VIP).

**gp 130 family**   See *cytokines.*

**GPCR**   G protein–coupled receptor, a cell surface protein that activates a *G protein* (q.v.). GPCRs constitute the most commonly used signal-transduction system and are key controllers of a number of physiological processes, including neurotransmission, cellular metabolism, cellular differentiation and growth, and inflammatory and immune responses.

**GPI**   General paralysis of the insane. See *general paresis.*

**G-protein**   See *G protein.*

**Graefe disease**   (Albrecht von Graefe, German ophthalmologist,1828–70)  See oculomotor nerve.

**Grafenberg spot**   See *G spot.*

**Graftschizophrenia**   *Pfropfschizophrenia* (q.v.).

**grammar**   The rules determining the allowable ways in which words can be combined to form sentences (*syntax*), as well as the manner in which those sentences are to be understood (*semantics*) and pronounced (phonetics) (qq.v.). It seems highly probable that concepts are stored in a mental lexicon of words and the concepts they stand for (a *mental dictionary*) and a set of rules that combines the words to convey relationships among concepts (a *mental grammar*).

A grammar is an example of a *discrete combinatorial system*: it samples and combines a finite number of discrete elements (words) so as to create larger structures (sentences) whose properties are distinct from those of their elements. For instance, "Analyst consults broker" is different from the meaning of any of the three words, and it is also different from the meaning of the same words presented in reverse order.Another noteworthy discrete combinatorial system in the natural world is the genetic code in DNA. The grammar is also *generative*; i.e., knowledge of general rules allows the user to generate new instances of those rules.

The linguist Noam Chomsky was the first to postulate the existence ofa Universal Grammar (UG), consisting of the basic design features of language, with a common plan of syntactic, morphological, and phonological rules that apply to all human languages. See *sign language*. The differences among languages result from a small set of individual options (like the items on a computer menu or checklist); choosing one or more of them does not change the basic operating system. Hundreds of universal patterns have been found in languages from all over the world. The largest number involve implications, "if…then". For example: if a language has X, it will also have Y; if the basic word order is subject-object-verb (SOV), it will have question words at the end of the sentence; if the basic word order is SVO (as in English), question words such as why and where will be placed at the beginning; if a language has a word for purple, it will have a word for red. See *expressive variety*.

**gramophone symptom** Mayer-Gross's term for a symptom seen often in *Pick disease* (q.v.): the patient repeats "with correct expression and diction an elaborate anecdote, seeming himself to be highly amused by it, and could not be stopped until he had told the whole story. After a short interval he would repeat his anecdote as something quite new" (*Clinical Psychiatry*, 1960).

**grand mal epilepsy** *Epilepsy* (q.v.) characterized by generalized tonic-clonic seizures; the convulsion or fit consists of a tonic spasm of all the limbs, rarely lasting longer than 30 seconds. This is followed by the clonic phase—a series of sharp, short, interrupted jerks that result from a series of interruptions of the tonic phase. Following cessation of these spasms, the patient may pass into a heavy sleep lasting for hours; some patients, in this *postictal phase*, evidence postepileptic automatism in which they wander, completely amnesic and disoriented, from the scene of attack (this may last for hours or days). Other patients become psychotic, maniacal, or even homicidal.

**grande attaque hysterique** See *hysteria*.

**grandiose self** Also, *grandiose-exhibitionistic self*; the effort of the child to be perfect and thereby, given *good enough* parents, to gain their affirmation of the child's self-worth and value. A pathological grandiose self may develop in the face of parental empathic failures.

Characteristics of the pathological grandiose self include exaggerated self-regard with unrealistic ideas about one's superiority, uniqueness, invulnerability, and limitlessness; a wish to display and exhibit the self; phantasies of outstanding success, power, and self-aggrandizement; insatiable craving for attention, approval, admiration, and love; overambitiousness, with unrealistically high goals and schemes; intolerance of imperfection; feelings of entitlement, expectation of special favors; a negative, hostile, devaluating attitude toward others; overweening, arrogant, pretentious, self-centered, boastful, and haughty in interpersonal relationships.

In normal self-object development, the child's early interactions are in the form of *self-object* relationships (q.v.), in which the other is experienced as an extension of the self. In the earliest form of grandiosity, the child had believed himself to be omnipotent (the autarchic fiction of false omnipotence: "I am wonderful and you admire me"); then he begins to recognize that his needs are being met by an all-powerful and perfect other (usually, the mother—"You are wonderful and I am part of you"). As self-object needs are met, there is increasing differentiation between self and object, and increasing awareness that the other is autonomous.

In her empathic responsiveness to her child, the mother reflects back to him the worth and value of what he has done or said, and such *mirroring* responses allow him to develop self-esteem and self-assertive ambitions. His grandiose-exhibitionisitic self is the attempt to elicit continuing approbation, by being perfect. Not all his actions will, of course, endear him to the mother. Even so, if she is generally responsive, affirming, approving, and consistent, the child can tolerate the inevitable failures of his own behavior (he learns from his mistakes and develops internal control and self-regulation) as well as the expectable lapses in her responsiveness. See *basic trust*.

It is in children of parents who are repeatedly inadequate in responding to their children (empathic failures) that psychopathology is seen. See *empathic failure; narcissistic personality*.

**grandiosity** See delusion of grandeur; megalomania.

**grandma's rule** *Premack principle* (q.v).

**Grantham lobotomy** Lobotomy performed by means ofelectrocoagulation of the ventromedial quadrant of the prefrontal lobe.

**granular atrophy** Vascular cortical atrophy.

**grapevine**  Rumor spread through underground channels; informal communication channels by which information is disseminated among persons and groups belonging to formal organizations.

**graphanesthesia**  A disturbance of graphesthesia (a function of the dominant parietal lobe), consisting of the inability to recognize letters that are traced one at a time on the palm of the hand while the subject's eyes are closed.

**graphemes**  Printed characters that correspond to *phonemes* (q.v.), the smallest meaningful unit of sound that can change the meaning of a word. See *dyslexia; language acquisition.*

**graphesthesis**  See *parietal lobe.*

**graphic function**  See *parietal lobe*

**grapho-**  Combining form meaning to write, from Gr. *graphein.*

**graphology**  The study of handwriting, especially in the sense of deducing some of the personality traits of the writer from a handwriting sample.

**graphomania**  Pressured writing or a compulsive need to write, often without regard to the worth of what is being written.

**graphophobia**  Fear of writing; a common form is severe anxiety or tremulousness if forced to sign one's name while being observed.

**graphorrhea**  Inordinate, uncontrolled, senseless writing, whose purpose seems to be to fill pages rather than to record or transmit a message.

**grasp reflex**  *Forced grasping; forced groping; instinctive grasp reaction. See frontal lobe dysfunction.*

**grasping and groping reflexes**  These reflexes are elicited when the palms and the fingers are stroked, causing a closure of the hand on the stimulating object. Normally this occurs in infants below 1 year of age, otherwise it is indicative of *frontal lobe* lesions (q.v.).

**gratification**  Satisfaction; in psychiatry, satisfaction of a person's needs or desires.

**Graves disease**  *Thyrotoxicosis* (q.v.).

**gray-out**  A relatively mild or partial loss of consciousness due to anemia of the brain or anoxemia such as occurs in high-altitude flying. A more complete or total loss of consciousness is a *blackout* (q.v.).

**Great Mother**  See *archetype.*

**greed**  See primary envy; oral sadism.

**Greenacre, Phyllis**  (1894–1989) U.S. psychoanalyst; *Trauma, Growth and Personality* (1952).

**Greenfield disease**  Infantile metachromatic leukodystrophy. See *diffuse sclerosis.*

**gregariousness**  See *herd instinct.*

**grey literature**  Information produced at all levels of government, academics, business, and industry in electronic and print formats not controlled by commercial publishing. Because of the growth of Internet technology, grey literature has become a mainstream source of information.

**GRF**  Growth hormone–releasing factor; see *growth hormone.*

**grief**  Sorrow or pain secondary to bereavement; sadness or remorse; normal mourning, as contrasted with *depression* (q.v.). See *melancholia.*

**Grieg disease**  *Hypertelorism* (q.v.).

**Griesinger, Wilhelm**  (1817–1868) German psychiatrist; *Mental Pathology and Therapeutics* (1845); described mental disorders as brain diseases, combined psychiatric and neurological clinics into a single department.

**grim**  See apoptosis.

**grimace**  A distorted facial expression or facial tic, often a result of organic neurologic disorder; in psychiatric syndromes, grimacing is most frequently seen in the catatonic group of the schizophrenias.

**Griselda complex**  (Griselda, or Griselidis, a paragon of purity, virtue, and endless patience, widely celebrated in medieval romances) Putnam's term for a father's complex in regard to his daughter. He unconsciously resents giving up his daughter to another man. Contemplation of the marriage of his daughter—the future mother—reactivates the older oedipal yearning for his own mother. The father's reluctance to give up his daughter to another man is often thinly disguised under the pretext of altruistic solicitude for the daughter's welfare.

**grisi siknis**  A culture-specific syndrome, reported among the Miskito of Nicaragua, consisting of headache, anxiety, unprovoked anger toward people in the immediate environment, aimless running, and falling down. See *culture-specific syndromes.*

**GRM3**  The metabotropic glutamate receptor 3, a regulator of glutamate neurotransmission. Single nucleotide polymorphisms in the GRM3 gene are associated with an increased risk of schizophrenia, reduced verbal fluency, and reduced levels of *N-acetylaspartate* in the DLPFC. *N*-acetylaspartate is an amino acid believed to be an index of neuronal function.

**grooming disorders** A group of disorders that, behaviorally, appear to be pathological exaggerations of actions that are a normal part of grooming in humans or animals. Included are obsessive-compulsive disorder (especially when fears of contamination lead to excessive handwashing or rituals related to excretory activities), trichotillomania (hair-pulling), compulsive face-picking, onychophagia (fingernail and toenail biting), and *rhinotillexomania* (nose-picking).

**groove, neural** See *neural plate.*

**ground** Background; the scenery, area, etc., on which the figures or objects in a picture appear to be superimposed. The *figure* is generally the part attended to, although the relationship of figure to ground may be reversed. Defective differentiation of figure and ground is common in the patient with organic brain disease, who as a result is almost always experiencing the uncertainty and instability that a normal person experiences only when confronted with ambiguous figures.

**group** Groups have been variously classified as (1) *primary,* characterized by intimate face-to-face associations, and *secondary*, where the members, typically without presence, are formally and impersonally associated; (2) *in-groups*, of which the person is a member and *out-groups*, to which he does not belong and with which his group is often in conflict; (3) *homogeneous* and *heterogeneous*; (4) *conflict* groups, e.g., nationalities, parties, labor unions, and gangs; and (5) *accommodation* groups, e.g., classes, castes, vocations, denominations.

**group analysis** Psychoanalytic group psychotherapy; resolution of individual conflict in a social network, where the symptom is reactivated and is translatable into communicative processes. Malcolm Pines (Tavistock Clinic), a pioneer in the application of psychoanalytic principles to the setting of group therapy, follows the proposition of Foulkes, one of the leading exponents of group therapy in England. The essence of the person is social, and neurosis and psychological disturbances generally arise in disordered social relationships that develop from the unconscious forces of love and hate. The highly individualistic neurotic position is essentially group disruptive. The individual's inner world is actualized in the group setting. As each group member represents a deviation from the norm of the community to which all belong, together the group members are the norm from which each deviates. See *group psychotherapy.*

**group feeling** *Herd instinct* (q.v.).

**group marriage** A family structure in which three or more adults (including at least one male and one female) live together, share labor and money and the bearing and rearing of children, and have sexual access to each other.

**group psychotherapy** *Group therapy*; a method of treating emotional disturbances, social maladjustments, and psychotic states in which two or more patients participate simultaneously in the presence of one psychotherapist or more.

The techniques in group psychotherapy vary to a great extent in accordance with the different schools of psychiatric thought and the preferences of individual psychiatrists and other psychotherapists. Slavson (*An Introduction to Group Therapy*, 1943) separates group psychotherapy under three major categories: activity, analytic, and directive.

1. *Activity group therapy*, which he originated, is suitable for children in latency. Children selected by criteria he had described are given the opportunity to act out their aggressions or withdrawal in the presence of a neutral, permissive, and understanding adult. The patients draw upon one another for support. The accessibility of the patients to each other and to the environment, and their interaction, generate certain inhibitive controls that improve the superego formation and strengthen the ego of each participant. Slavson believed that this type of therapy is predominantly ego therapy and is an experience in which character changes occur. He therefore recommended selecting patients on the basis of these two factors. No interpretation is given to the children and a minimal restraint of their behavior is exercised by the therapist and, at that, only when the group cannot bring itself under control.

2. *Analytic group psychotherapy* is a technique in which interpretation is given to the patients, activity and verbalization are encouraged and interpreted, and insight is evoked. In this technique the therapist is more active than he is in activity group psychotherapy, where he is predominantly a passive agent.

Slavson divided analytic group psychotherapy into three subdivisions: play group psychotherapy; activity-interview group psychotherapy; and interview psychotherapy. *Play group psychotherapy* is suitable for young children in the prelatency period, where the catharsis occurs through play with specially selected materials through which the children in the group can act out their preoccupations, phantasies, and anxieties. *Activity-interview group psychotherapy* has been designed by him for children in latency who suffer from severe psychoneuroses, who are given the opportunity to act out against each other and against their environment as in activity group psychotherapy, but interpretation of the latent meaning of the behavior is given by the children to each other and by the therapist. Spontaneous and planned discussions are held with individual children or with a number of the children in the group or the group as a whole. These are intended to stimulate understanding by the children of the meaning of their behavior and to evoke insight into the unconscious motivations and phantasies. *Interview group psychotherapy* is intended for adolescents and adults who are selected by definite criteria and are grouped together so that the patients would have a therapeutic effect upon one another. The basic criterion suggested by Slavson is syndrome (not symptom or diagnosis) homogeneity.

Other group psychotherapists do not use this criterion but group the patients without any special considerations, provided the patients can accept and gain from a group experience. In analytic group psychotherapy the procedure is the same as in individual psychotherapy. Since the patients are adolescents and adults, the catharsis occurs through verbalization and free association. The psychotherapist here, as in individual treatment, interprets, explores, and helps patients to uncover their repressed, guilt-producing, and anxiety-evoking feelings, attitudes, values, and behavior.

3. *Directive group treatment*, under which Slavson included such activities as didactic or therapeutically educational group work, particularly with psychotics, group guidance, group counseling, therapeutic recreation, and many other group efforts to help patients, particularly psychotic patients, adjust to their environment.

H. G. Whittington (*Clinical Practice in Community Mental Health Centers*, 1972) divides group therapies in relation to *control* and *expectation*. Control refers to the demands made of the patient, the limits imposed on him, and the structuring of the therapy situation. Expectation refers to the assumption that because of the group experience the patient can improve insofar as his feelings, thoughts, or behavior is concerned.

1. Group therapies with a relatively high level of control and expectation include the following. *In-hospital community meeting*, which is both psychotherapy and sociotherapy; it promotes a sense of shared plight among the participants. *In-hospital small group*, with a lower level of control and higher expectation; often focuses on insight derived from interaction with other patients and staff, on plans for posthospital adjustment. *Child activity group*, with high control and high expectation; helps the child to learn to trust an adult, to resolve conflict by discussion and compromise and to learn culturally valued skills. *Psychodrama*, with moderately high control and very high expectation; expects the patient to reexperience feelings and events and thereby to learn about himself and develop better ways of dealing with himself and others. *Adolescent group therapy*, with high expectation and high control. *Prevocational group*, prepares the patient to look for a job, effectively handle the interview situation, and then function adequately at work.

2. In the high-control/low-expectation group are the following. *Anaclitic group therapy*, to dampen the intensity of dependency strivings. *Addict and alcoholic groups. Social hour*, a large group after-care session that combines patient government, resocialization, remotivation, and recreation therapy as a way to encourage interpersonal relationships and minimize regression. *Boarding home group counseling.*

3. In the low-control/high-expectation group are the following. *Postemployment group*, for the patient moving from the prevocational group into active employment. *Marital group therapy. Expressive group therapy. T-group, sensitivity*, and *encounter groups*, typically to increase the quality of "humanness" in essentially normal people. *Family therapy.*

4. The *drop-in lounge* is a type of low-expectation/low-control situation; the patient consults with the staff member on duty if he experiences some adaptational failure, mixes with others who happen to be in the lounge at the time, etc.

**Group Relations Conferences, A. K. Rice** Offshoots in the United States of the conferences sponsored by the Tavistock Clinic in Leicester, England. Based on Rice's systems theory of organizations, the conferences provide a means of learning group, organizational, administrative, and leadership functions. They last a few days to 2 weeks and include *study groups* (small group meetings, organized around specific events), large group meetings, *intergroup exercises* (in which the entire group is brought together and is organized into ad hoc task forces to react with other groups, management, staff, etc.), lectures on group theory, and *application groups*, which provide participants the opportunity to discuss how to apply what they have learned to their home organizations.

**group selection** Lorenz's idea that an individual within a group would be willing to suffer a personal loss in fitness if that loss was more than compensated for by an increase in overall group fitness. It is generally acknowledged that group selection is a rare phenomenon.

**group superego** S. R. Slavson differentiated between the group superego and the infantile superego (*An Introduction to Group Therapy*, 1943). The group superego is an outcome of the adaptations to and experiences with various groups of people beyond the relationship with parents.

**group tension, common** In psychoanalytically oriented treatment of a group, the predisposition at any point of individual members to participate in a certain group theme. The theme may be a dominant *required relationship*, a defense against *avoided relationship*, which, because of his phantasies, the subject fears will be another disastrous or *calamitous relationship*. Common group tension, Ezriel's term, is approximately equivalent to the *dominant group mentality* of Bion (Ezriel, H. *Journal of Mental Science 96*, 1950).

**growth cone** A specialized structure along the terminal shaft and at the tip of an axon, by means of which the axon lengthens and extends. Connected with this extension are *filopodia*, finger-like projections from the growth cone that continually extend and retract during the period of axon growth. See axon growth; chromosome.

**growth factors** Promoters of cell division; in contrast to trophic factors, they are not essential for the survival of neurons.

**growth hormone (GH)** A polypeptide of 91 amino acids, produced by the somatotrophs in the anterior pituitary. Its secretion is controlled by two hypothalamic hypophysiotrophic substances: growth hormone-releasing factor (*GRF*), which stimulates its secretion, and somatostatin, which inhibits it. Growth hormone promotes and regulates somatic and particularly skeletal growth, and it influences carbohydrate, fat, and protein metabolism.

Deficiency of growth hormone results in *pituitary dwarfism* (*hypophysial dwarfism, nanism*); both familial and sporadic forms occur. It may be associated with insufficiency of other pituitary tropic hormones, with consequent failure of gonadal development and severely diminished thyroid and adrenocortical function. Excess growth hormone produces *gigantism, acromegaly* (qq.v.), and glucose intolerance.

In Alzheimer disease of early onset, and also in endogenous depression, the GH response to GRF is increased; it is decreased in schizophrenia, chronic alcoholism, and mental retardation. GH secretion is also stimulated by insulin. Approximately half of depressed patients have a blunted response on the insulin tolerance test (ITT), as have children and some schizophrenics. See *hypothalamic-pituitary-adrenal* (HPA) axis; peptide, brain.

**Grübelsucht** Brooding over trifles; seen most commonly in obsessive-compulsive disorder and in depressive psychoses.

**Gruhle, Hans W (1880-1958)** German psychiatrist and psychologist; phenomenology (especially schizophrenia and delusions) and social psychiatry.

**grumbling mania** "The patients, indeed, display exalted self-consciousness, are pretentious and high-flown, but by no means of cheerful mood; they rather appear dissatisfied, insufferable, perhaps even a little anxious. They have something to find fault with in everything, feel themselves on every occasion badly treated, get wretched food, cannot hold out in the dreadful surroundings, cannot sleep in the miserable beds, cannot have social intercourse with the other patients" (Kraepelin, E. *Manic-Depressive Insanity and Paranoia*, 1921).

**Grundsymptoma**  Basic or fundamental symptoms. Bleuler used this term to refer to the fundamental symptoms of *schizophrenia* (q.v.)

**GSR**  Galvanic skin response. See *psychogalvanic reflex.*

**GSW**  Gunshot wound(s).

**GTP**  Guanosine triphosphate. Various GTP-binding proteins in the terminal of the neuron are involved in synaptic vesicle replenishment and in the docking of synaptic vesicles that occurs before neurotransmitter is released.

The enzyme GTP cyclohydrolase 1 catalyzes the conversion of GTP to dihydroneopterin triphosphate, and thus it is a rate-limiting enzyme in the biosynthesis of tetrahydrobiopterin ($BH_4$), a cofactor for phenylalanine hydroxylase as well as for tyrosine hydroxylase, tryptophan hydroxylase, the O-alkylglycerolipid cleavage enzyme, and nitric oxide synthases. $BH_4$ plays a role in the control of phenylalanine catabolism and of neural and immune functions. See *G protein; neuromessenger; neurotransmitter receptor.*

**GTS**  Gilles de la Tourette syndrome. See *Tourette disorder.*

**Guam ALS-PDC**  Amyotrophic lateral sclerosis-parkinsonism dementia complex, found among Guam natives, the Chamorros; *Guaminina-ALS.* It sometimes destroys the motor neurons of its victims, producing a syndrome indistinguishable from ALS; at other times it produces a parkinsonian syndrome. See *amyotrophic lateral sclerosis.*

When first reported, in the 1940s, Guam ALS-PDC occurred at a rate 50 times that of the rate of occurrence of ALS in industrialized countries. It was hoped it might provide a model for neurodegenerative disease in general. In the intervening four decades, however, its incidence has declined dramatically and is now almost the same as in western countries. The ALS syndrome in particular is dying out, and more dementia cases without parkinsonism are being seen (a phenomenon sometimes called *Mariana dementia*, after the island chain that includes Guam).

Earlier research had identified the *excitotoxin* (q.v.) amino acid β-N methylamine l-alanine (BMAA) in the seeds of Guam's *cycad* trees, and it was proposed that BMAA might act as a slow toxin that damages nerve cells over the years. But various investigators were unable to reproduce those findings; still others noted that humans would need to consume about 100 kg of processed cycad flour per day in order to reach toxic levels. Further, BMAA is metabolized rapidly and transported poorly into the brain, casting doubt on its ability to produce any kind of neurologic damage.

Excitotoxicity may still be involved in the pathophysiology of the syndrome, however, or a combination of excitotoxins and neurotoxic metals in the environment. The emphasis currently is on the excitotoxin *glutamate*, or on another cycad toxin, *cycasin.* Cycasin's metabolite methylazoxymethanol (MAM), although not an excitotoxin, damages DNA. And a few researchers still believe aluminum, a known neurotoxin, may be implicated—but how aluminum enters the brain remains a mystery.

**Guamanina ALS**  See amyotrophic lateral sclerosis.

**guanosine phosphatases**  See *Golgi apparatus.*

**guidance**  A form of supportive psychotherapy in which the patient is counseled and instructed in ways to set and achieve specific goals and in ways to recognize and avoid areas of conflict and anxiety-provoking situations. Educational guidance refers particularly to helping the patient find the school or courses best suited to him on the basis of his intelligence, aptitudes, preferences, and available opportunities. Vocational guidance refers particularly to helping the patient find a job that is realistically suited to his capacities. Guidance is a relatively superficial type of psychotherapy and makes little attempt to deal with the unconscious motivants of behavior. It is based upon an authoritarian relationship in which the patient often overvalues the therapist and in which he must suppress any doubts or hostility against the therapist.

**guided affective imagery (GAI)**  A waking dream technique in psychotherapy, used particularly in brief therapy and group therapy. See *forced phantasy.*

**guidepost cells**  See *axon guidance.*

**guiding fictions** Adler's term for the principles by which one understands, categorizes, and evaluates his or her experiences.

**Guillain-Barrè syndrome** (Georges Guillain, French neurologist, 1876–1961, and Jean Alexander Barrè, French neurologist, 1880–1967) Acute infective *polyneuritis*; acute toxic polyneuritis; rheumatic polyneuritis; polyradiculoneuritis. An acute, diffuse disease of the nervous system, probably due to a virus, consisting of chromatolysis of the anterior horn cells and the posterior roots and of myelin degeneration of the peripheral nerves. Most cases occur in males between the ages of 20 and 50 years. Initial symptoms are headache, vomiting, fever, and pain in the back and legs. These are followed by sudden paralysis of the limbs, in all segments, and of the facial muscles. There is pain, numbness, and tingling in the limbs.

Cerebrospinal fluid protein is markedly elevated, but there are few or no cells. In sporadic cases the prognosis is good, but in some epidemics the mortality (usually from respiratory paralysis) is high. No specific treatment is known.

**guilt, guilt feelings** Realization that one has done wrong by violating some ethical, moral, or religious principle. Associated with such realization typically are lowered self-esteem and a feeling that one should expiate or make retribution for the wrong that has been done. See *forensic proof; shame.*

In psychoanalytic writings, the term usually refers to neurotic or pathological guilt feelings that do not appear justified by the reasons adduced for the guilt. Such guilt indicates a conflict between ego and *superego* (q.v.); the latter acts as an internal authority that stands between ego and id, compelling the person to renounce certain pleasures, and imposing punishment (loss of self-esteem, guilt feelings, etc.) for violations of its orders. The superego's prohibitions are often directed against impulses (and especially hostile and destructive ones) of which the subject is not consciously aware; but because they have incurred the superego's wrath, the end result is guilt. Guilt is a pain that one bears in response to real or imagined harm that one has done another person about whom one cares. It can only occur when others are experienced as subjects and not simply as objects. Thus, it appears as a new form of anxiety in

the *depressive position* (q.v.), the fear that one's anger has driven away the person one loves.

Guilt feelings are thus seen to be topically defined anxiety, the anxiety of ego toward superego. What is feared by the ego is that something terrible will happen within the personality (food, affection, love, or narcissistic supplies will be cut off) and that there will be a loss of certain pleasurable feelings, such as well-being and security. In its most severe form, the loss of self-esteem characteristic of guilt feelings becomes a feeling of complete annihilation, such as is seen in depression.

In Adlerian psychodynamics, guilt feelings are the demonstration of good intentions that one does not have (or is unable to effect or exercise). They occur when past transgressions are blamed for a present unwillingness to behave as one feels he should. Erikson describes initiative vs. guilt as one of the eight stages of man. See *ontogeny, psychic.*

**Guislain, Joseph** (1797–1860) Belgian physician; introduced work therapy in his institution for the mentally ill in Ghent.

**Gulf War syndrome** Multiple symptoms, ranging from subtle problems such as muscle aches and fatigue to gross indications of cognitive deficits and confusion, that many veterans from the 1991 Persian Gulf War have experienced. Cause is uncertain; the U.S. government has officially attributed the symptoms to stress, but many of the veterans and some researchers believe they are a manifestation of exposure to organophosphates (one of the ingredients of many chemical weapons and insecticides). See *DFP.*

**gull wing pattern** An MMPI profile said to be characteristic of pseudoneurotic schizophrenia.

**gumma, intracranial** A rare form of cerebral syphilis. The predominating pathological process is the gumma or syphiloma. This is an irregular or round granulomatous nodular growth, varying in size from that of a pinhead to a walnut; it is generally multiple. Occasionally, when single and of large size, it may produce symptoms of intracranial pressure with or without focal signs. The mental symptoms include the acute organic type of reaction, and consist of delirium, with a memory defect for recent events, and emotional lability. When there is evidence of increased intracranial pressure, a dull, stuporous state is common, with loss of sphincter control. The blood and spinal fluid findings may be similar to those observed in cerebral syphilis, and response to antisyphilitic treatment is fairly successful.

**Gunn synkinetic syndrome** See *synkinesia*.

**Gunther-Waldenstrom syndrome** *Porphyria, acute intermittent* (q.v.).

**gustation** A distributed neural process by which information conveyed to the brain through specialized taste, orosensory, and gastrointestinal fibers is integrated, so that the organism can engage in appropriate feeding behaviors. There are five *primary tastes*: salt, sweet, bitter, umami (a savory taste), and sour (acidic). The Japanese word *umami* is used to refer to the savory taste of food as produced, for example, by monosodium glutamate. Umami taste is found in vegetables, fish, meats, and cheese.

Nonprimary tastes, such as astringent, fatty, tartness, water, metallic, starchy, cooling, tingling, and pungent, result from the co-activation of taste and specialized somatosensosry neurons located in the oral cavity. These specialized neurons surround taste buds and include different classes of mechano- and chemo-receptors that transmit information on the food's texture, weight, and temperature to the brain, mainly via the trigeminal system.

In the oral chemosensory epithelia, *taste buds* contain 50–100 taste receptor cells (TRCs), which are distributed throughout the tongue, palate, epiglottis, and esophagus. TRCs are innervated on the palate by the chorda tympani, and on the anterior tongue by the greater superior petrosal nerve. These branches of the facial nerve transmit information about the identity and quantity of the chemical nature of the tastants. On the epiglottis, esophagus, and posterior tongue, TRCs are innervated by the lingual branch of the glossopharyngeal nerve and the superior laryngeal branch of the vagus nerve. These nerves are responsive to tastants but participate primarily in the brain stem–based arch reflexes that mediate *swallowing* (ingestion) and *gagging* (rejection). TRCs also contain receptors for many circulating hormones and neuropeptides, including aldosterone, antidiuretic hormone, leptin, neuropeptide Y, and cholecystokinin. Multiple nonsapid (i.e., not related to taste, flavor, or palatability) sensory and neurohormonal factors can affect how gustatory information is processed through multiple neural pathways.

The nucleus tractus solitarius (NTS) of the medulla receives information from taste-responsive cranial nerves, somatosensory inputs from the trigeminal system, and visceral (vagal) inputs that convey information about the physiological status of the gastrointestinal system. The NTS controls the production of *orosensory behaviors,* such as swallowing, licking, chewing, and mastication. The NTS taste information is forwarded to the taste thalamic nucleus, the venoposterior medial nucleus, and from there is projected to the primary taste cortex in the anterior insula cortex. Gustatory cortical neurons respond not only to taste inputs but also to olfactory inputs and to somatosensory inputs (e.g., mouth and jaw movements, temperature). Flavor perception depends on the convergence and integration of gustatory and olfactory information in the insula. The secondary taste cortex, the direct target of the gustatory cortex, is the orbitofrontal cortex (OFC). It is there that taste responses are modulated according to physiological state, as in the changing reward value of a food eaten to satiety (Simon, S. A. et al. *Nature Reviews Neuroscience 7*: 890–901, 2006).

**gustatism** See sensation, secondary.

**gustatory hallucination** See *haptic hallucination.*

**gustatory seizure** A form of epilepsy in which the sensation of a definite and usually peculiar taste is a part of the seizure pattern. The seizures are often also associated with sensations of peculiar odors. See uncinate fit.

**Guthrie test** See *phenylketonuria.*

**gymnophobia** Fear of a naked body.

**gynander, gynandromorph** An individual of a bisexual species, exhibiting a "sexual mosaic" of male and female characters as a result of the development of both types of sex tissue in the same organism.

Most specimens are *lateral* or *bilateral* gynandromorphs, male on one side of the midline of the body, and female on the other, with a sharp demarcation between the two kinds of tissue. In some instances, the distribution is in a ratio of about 1:3, or the head may be female and the rest of the body male.

It is assumed that on the male side there appear the sex-linked characters received from either the mother or the father; while the characters of the female parts show the presence in these parts of both the maternal and paternal X chromosomes, as though one of the X chromosomes had been eliminated from the male parts, leaving them XO, while the female parts are XX. "Such a gynander appears to have begun development as an XX female and at some early cell division to have lost one of the X chromosomes from part of the tissues" (Sinnott, E. W. and Dunn, L. D. *Principles of Genetics*, 1939).

**gynecomania**  Insatiable desire for women; *satyriasis* (q.v.).

**gynecomastia**  Enlargement of the male breast, in a minority of cases accompanied by galactorrhea. Gynecomastia may occur as a manifestation of some underlying abnormality, such as hepatic cirrhosis, thyrotoxicosis, or the Klinefelter syndrome; it may also be a side effect of drugs, including psychopharmacological agents. Adolescent gynecomastia occurs in some boys at the time of puberty; in most cases it is mild in degree and self-correcting. In a few, breast development is so marked as to require corrective mastectomy; it is presumed that such cases reflect atypical utilization of the estrogen produced by the testis or relative insensitivity to testosterone, which normally counteracts such estrogen effects.

**gynemimesis**  *Lady with a penis syndrome*; the full-time miming of a female by a person who has a penis. It may include hormonal feminization but stops short of genital, sex-reassignment surgery. Gynemimesis appears to be much more widespread than its counterpart in the female, *andromimesis* (q.v.), and it has

been reported in many different cultures. See *acault; berdache; hijra; mahu; xanith.*

**gynemimetophilia**  A *paraphilia* (q.v.), in which sexual arousal and orgasm depend upon the partner being a female impersonator.

**gynephilia**  Sexual love of a woman by a man (male gynephilia) or by another woman (female gynephilia).

**gynephobia**  Fear of women.

**gyno-**  Combining form meaning woman, female, from Gr. *gyne.*

**gynomonoecism**  A genetic female's capacity for developing spermatozoa in the ovary, at certain times. See *hermaphroditism.*

**gynophobia**  Morbid fear of women.

**gyrectomy**  One of the several surgical operations on the brain performed as a therapeutic measure in certain cases of mental illness. In the gyrectomy procedure, bilateral symmetrical removals of frontal cortex are carried out along fissure lines in order to preserve the normally functioning gyri. See *topectomy.*

**gyrencephalic**  Referring to the convoluted shape of the human cerebral cortex, with grooves or fissures (sulci) separating the gyri.

**gyrus**  See *sulcus.*

**gyrus, angular**  The posterior portion of the lower parietal region; the left angular gyrus is associated with speech function.

**gyrus, postcentral**  See *parietal lobe.*

**gyrus, precentral**  See *frontal lobe.*

**gyrus cinguli**  *Cingulate gyrus* (q.v.).

# H

**HAART** Highly Active AntiRetroviral Therapy; also known as *cART* (combination antiretroviral therapy). Available since 1996, HAART uses multiple (three or more) antiretroviral drugs, typically from at least two classes, to suppress human immunodeficiency virus (HIV) replication. Multiple classes are required because new mutations—including those that confer resistance to single drugs or classes—arise at prodigious rates and are "archived" in the form of proviral DNA. See *microglia*. Additionally, by reducing plasma viral replication to undetectable levels, HAART curbs CD4$^+$ T lymphocyte destruction, a major pathogenic feature of HIV disease. This partially restores immune function and impedes disease progression, but it does not eliminate the virus. The person infected with HIV must take medications for life (Ellis, R. et al. *Nature Reviews Neuroscience* 8: 33–44, 2007). See *pill fatigue*; *risk-taking behavior*; *STIs*.

**habeas corpus** (L. "you must have the body") In forensic psychiatry, a writ or order for a person being held in a hospital or other institution to appear before the court, so that a determination of the appropriateness or necessity for the confinement can be made.

**habenular ganglion** See *epithalamus*.

**habilitation** Producing or improving fitness through training, applied particularly to congenital disorders and disorders of early infancy.

**habit, accident** See *accident proneness*.

**habit, hysterical** Kretschmer distinguished two kinds of hysteria, *reflex hysteria* and *hysterical habit*. The latter is a hysterical reaction that begins as a conscious, voluntary process and gradually becomes automatic by repetition. See *reflex hysteria*.

**habit deterioration** The abandonment of integrated and socialized behavior in favor of disintegrated and personal behavior; regression; a failure of the habits appropriate to the patient's social standing.

**habit disorder** Also stereotypy/habit disorder; repetitive, nonfunctional behavior (such as hand waving, body rocking, head banging, nail biting, picking at face) that is injurious to the child or interferes markedly with normal activities. See *behavior disorders*.

**habit memory** One type of *procedural memory* (q.v.).

**habit reversal** A form of behavior therapy, probably most frequently used in the treatment of tics, stereotypies, and obsessive-compulsive disorder. It combines awareness training, contingency management, *relaxation training*, *competing responses*, and *self-monitoring* (qq.v.). See *behavior therapy*.

**habit training** Acquisition (by the young child) of specific behavior patterns mainly related to the functions of eating, elimination, sleep, and dress. To the behaviorist, training is in the nature of conditioning. To the psychoanalyst, habit and habit training have a different meaning: "A particular habit is for the child a defence against a particular unconscious fantasy or wish. His clinging to habit may be one of his main defences against the anxiety connected with aggressive impulses and fantasies in general" (Isaacs, S. in *On the Bringing Up of Children*, ed. J. Rickman, 1936).

**habit-forming** As a description of a drug, incidence of psychological craving or dependency in its users. The likelihood of psychologic craving is generally independent of proneness to physiological craving or addiction (q.v.).

**habituation** Cessation of a response upon repeated presentations of a stimulus; decrease or suppression of response to a repeated, nonnoxious stimulus; learned suppression of response to a repeated stimulus; repetition of a stimulus without reinforcement leading to a gradual loss of reflex behavior. Habituation is the simplest form of associative learning, in which response to a repeated, nonnoxious stimulus decreases or is suppressed. In this sense, habituation is *tolerance* (q.v.). It is characteristic of many drugs and is a significant factor in substance abuse, because increasing dosage of the substance is required in order to obtain the effect(s) produced by the initial dosage. See *addiction; dependence, psychological; sensitization*.

Habituation is the ability to disregard repetitive stimuli that are neither rewarding nor harmful, ceasing to respond to stimuli that prove to have no predictive value. Habituation allows the organism to disregard irrelevant stimuli. Habituation has both a short-term form lasting minutes and a long-term form lasting days and weeks. Habituation can be overridden (*dishabituation*) by a sensitizing stimulus.

Habituation leads to *homosynaptic depression*, a decrease in synaptic strength secondary to activity in the stimulated pathway. In habituation, repeated stimulation of the sensory neuron results in less calcium entering the presynaptic nerve terminal; as a result, less neurotransmitter is released and there is a decrease in the strength of the glutamate-mediated synaptic connections between sensory and motor neurons. Habituation is related to gating and is a way for the organism to "damp down" or decrease its responsivity to repeated stimuli. Schizophrenics have impaired startle habituation, an inability to decrease responding to more intense and stressful stimuli.

**habitus** In general medicine, constitutional disposition or tendency to some specific disease, in the sense of *habitus phthisicus* and *habitusa-poplecticus* as described by Hippocrates. Later the term was extended to include the type of physique associated with such tendencies by different typological schools of constitutional medicine and to the general characteristic appearance of the human body.

**habitus apoplecticus** (L. "apoplectic constitution") A thick-set, rounded physique, corresponding to Kretschmer's *pyknic type* and its equivalent in other systems.

**habitus phthisicus** (L. "consumptive constitution") Hippocrates's term for the tendency of certain persons to *pulmonary tuberculosis*. He ascribed a slender, flat-chested physique to such persons, and the term is used in a derived sense to indicate the type of physique corresponding approximately to Kretschmer's *asthenic type* and its equivalents in other systems.

**HACS** Hyperactive child syndrome. See *attention deficit hyperactivity disorder.*

**HAD** HIV-associated dementia. See *AIDS dementia complex.*

**hadephobia** Fear of hell.

**Haeckel biogenetic law** (Ernst Heinrich Haeckel, German naturalist, 1834–1919)

According to this formula, "The child is on a lower developmental level of mankind than the adult." In the child all the criminal drives of humanity are latent. Compulsive acts are viewed as protective measures against the evil of one's self. A neurosis arises when the instinctual criminal drives are too powerfully developed. (Stekel, W. *Compulsion and Doubt*, 1949). See *biogenetic mental law; polymorphous perverse.*

**haem(at)o-** See *hem(at)o-.*

**Hahnemann, Samuel** (1755–1843) German physician; disillusioned with medical practice, he formulated a new system of medicine and therapeutics that he named "homeopathy." He had an enlightened approach to the treatment of the mentally ill, and a holistic approach to public health.

**hair pulling** *Trichotillomania*; a *disorder of impulse control* (qq.v.); it is sometimes included within the obsessive-compulsive spectrum disorders. Patients with trichotillomania usually pull hair from the scalp, but eyelashes, eyebrows, legs, armpits, and pubic regions are also targets. Trichotillomania is more common in girls and begins in early childhood or adolescence. Of the early-onset cases, one-third develop it before the age of 10, and 14% before the age of 7. This form is usually benign and self-limited. Pulling and eating dolls' hair can be a first symptom. Later onset forms are likely to be chronic.

Of those affected, only 30% engage in *trichophagia*, and only about 1% will eat their hair to the extent requiring surgical removal. *Trichobezoar* formation (q.v.), while rare, is the most serious complication.

**Hakim disease** See *normal-pressure hydrocephalus.*

**half-life** T½; in pharmacology, the time necessary for the concentration of a drug in the blood to decrease by half after absorption and distribution are complete; the amount of time required for half the amount of drug administered to be excreted; it is typically measured in hours. A drug's half-life is a function of drug binding to tissue other than plasma or blood constituents and the clearance of the free or unbound drug. Half-life is used rather than time to complete excretion because the second half of excretion is very slow.

**half-show** A modification of the puppet show technique in psychotherapy of children in which the patient sees only that part of the puppet show that presents or states a problem in dramatic fashion. When the conflict is at its height, the show is stopped with the promise that it will be continued later. Then the subject or group is asked what should happen. The solutions suggested are colored by the child's own problems, and the child will try to unravel the conflict in terms of his or her own constitution, background, emotional involvement, and general level of maturity.

**halfway children** R. Geist's term for chronically ill children and adolescents who are neither well nor so sick as to require continuous, intensive inpatient care. Instead, their course is characterized by repeated in-and-out hospital stays and dependence on a complex system of hospital care, pharmacological treatments, surgical procedures, and artificial devices (*American Journal of Orthopsychiatry 49*, 1979).

**halfway house** A specialized residence for mental patients who are not sick enough to require full hospitalization, but not well enough to function completely within the community without some degree of professional supervision, protection, and support. See *domicile; family care.*

**Hall, G(ranville) Stanley** (1844–1924) American psychologist and sexologist.

**Hallervorden-Spatz disease** (Julius Hallervorden, German neurologist, 1882–1965; Hugo Spatz, German neuropathologist, 1888–1969) Now known as NBIA (neurodegeneration with brain iron accumulation); it is due to mutations in the gene that codes for pantothenate kinase 2, which is necessary for coenzyme-A biosynthesis and is targeted to mitochondria. NBIA is a rare, hereditary progressive pigmentary degeneration of the globus pallidus and substantia nigra, transmitted as an autosomal recessive. Onset is usually before adolescence, with rigidity, dystonia, choreoathetosis, spasticity, hyperreflexia, speech difficulties, and a gradually progressive dementia. Life span after onset of the disorder is shortest (1 to 2 years) in those with earliest onset; children with onset at 10 years or after may live as long as 20 years from the time of onset.

**Halloween effect** Hyperactivity and other behavioral and cognitive dysfunctions in response to ingestion of sugar, such as the candy given to children in the "trick-or-treat"

ritual of Halloween. Although many claims of such reactions have been made, all attempts to replicate them have failed. What few changes in activity have been found in response to sucrose and fructose challenges have, in fact, tended to be in the direction of decreased, rather than increased, activity. See *attention deficit hyperactivity disorder.*

**hallucinate** To have a sense perception for which there is no external reality (i.e., sensory stimulus). See *hallucination.*

**hallucination** *Fallacia* (*Obs.*). Perception of an external object when no such object is present; a type of imagery characterized by externalization and a continued belief that the experience is a perception of something outside the self rather than an internal thought or image. A paranoid patient, sitting alone in a quiet room, complains that his persecutors, who are miles away, speak directly to him in derogatory terms; moreover, he believes implicitly that he feels electrical stimuli over the entire body, the stimuli coming, he alleges, from a machine operated by his persecutors. The auditory and tactile stimuli have no source in the environment; rather they are sensations arising within the patient himself. A hallucination is a *sense perception* independent of any external stimulus. The *false beliefs* regarding persecutors are *delusions*; a delusion is a belief that is obviously contrary to demonstrable fact.

When the same paranoid patient, sitting alone in an otherwise quiet room, upon hearing the crackling of the floorboards, is firmly convinced that the crackling sounds like those of a telegraph ticker are messages from the persecutors to him (the patient), he misinterprets actual stimuli from the environment. An *illusion* is a false impression from a real stimulus. But the interpretation he makes of these stimuli is a *delusion*. See *illusion; delusion.*

**hallucination, autoscopic** The experience of seeing one's body appear for a moment or two, usually in front of the subject.

**hallucination, elementary** "As elementary hallucinations in the optic field we designate such unformed visions as lighting, sparks, and cloudlike partial darkening of the visual field, and in the acoustic field, the simple noises such as murmurs, knocks, and shooting" (Bleuler, E. *Textbook of Psychiatry*, 1930).

**hallucination, negative** Not a hallucination at all, but the condition in which the subject fails to see an object while apparently looking at it. The phenomenon can be induced through hypnosis.

**hallucination, psychic**  See *hallucination of perception.*

**hallucination of conception**  See *hallucination of perception.*

**hallucination of perception**  An auditory hallucination in which the patient hears the sound or noise as coming from outside himself, in contrast to *hallucination of conception* (or, in Baillarger's terminology, psychic hallucination), in which inner voices are heard.

**hallucinatory epilepsy**  A type of focal *epilepsy* (q.v.) in which complex hallucinations are the main part of the attack. The hallucinations are short-lived, paroxysmal, and irresistible in quality; they tend to be identical in each attack.

**hallucinatory game**  In children, the same factors that are responsible for illusions may produce reactions A. Stern called hallucinatory games (*Psychologies der fruhen Kindheit*, 1928). Such hallucinations differ from real hallucinations in their being actively created by the child instead of being felt as something foreign and externally induced. The child is fully aware of the unreality of these self-created objects and can easily banish them when tiring of them. A very young child's play store is largely a hallucinatory game: the business of the "store" is playfully transacted through pantomime and the use of hallucinated merchandiseand money. See *companion, imaginary.*

**hallucinogen**  *Psychedelic, psychotogenic, psychotomimetic* (drug); a chemical agent that induces alterations in perception, thinking, and feeling that resemble those of the functional psychoses without producing the gross cognitive impairments characteristic of organic mental disorders.

Two groups of hallucinogens are often distinguished: (1) indolealkylamines—LSD (lysergic acid diethylamide), DMT (dimethyltryptamine), psilocin, psilocybin; (2) phenylethylamines—mescaline, DMA, MDA (3,4-methylenedioxyamphetamine), and MDMA (ecstasy; 3,4-methylenedioxymethamphetamine). The dissociative anesthetics, such as *phencyclidine* (q.v.) and *ketamine*, are also hallucinogenic.

Most hallucinogens are taken orally; DMT is sniffed or smoked. Use is typically episodic rather than chronic, although dependence is recognized in addition to abuse, intoxication, and delirium. Effects are noted within 20 to 30 minutes after the drug is taken: pupillary dilatation, blood pressure elevation, tachycardia, tremor, hyperreflexia, and the psychedelic phase consisting of euphoria or mixed mood changes, visual illusions and altered perceptions, a blurring of boundaries between self and non-self, and often a feeling of unity with the cosmos. After 4 or 5 hours, that phase is replaced with ideas of reference, increased awareness of the inner self, and a sense of magical control.

Adverse effects include the following: (1) the *bad trip* (q.v.); (2) delusional disorder (hallucinogen psychotic disorder)—follows a bad trip; the perceptual changes abate but the subject becomes convinced that his perceptual distortions correspond with reality; the delusional state may last only a day or two, or it may persist and is then indistinguishable from a spontaneously occurring psychotic disorder, such as schizophrenia; (3) mood disorder—anxiety, depression, or mania occurring shortly after hallucinogen use and persisting for more than 24 hours; typically the subject feels that he can never be normal again and expresses concern that he has damaged his brain by taking the drug; (4) *flashback* (q.v.), also called hallucinogen persisting perception disorder.

**hallucinogen intoxication**  Symptoms include the following: marked anxiety or depression, ideas of reference, fears of losing one's mind, paranoid ideation, and impaired judgment; perceptual changes occurring in a state of full wakefulness, such as subjective intensification of perceptions, depersonalization, derealization, illusions, hallucinations, and synesthesia; and physical signs, such as pupillary dilation, tachycardia, sweating, palpitations, blurring of vision, tremors, and incoordination. See *hallucinogen.*

**hallucinogen use disorders**  These are classified within the substance-related disorders and include hallucinogen dependence, hallucinogen abuse, hallucinogen intoxication, hallucinogen persisting perception disorder (posthallucinogen perception disorder), hallucinogen delirium, hallucinogen psychotic disorder, hallucinogen mood disorder, and hallucinogen anxiety disorder.

**hallucinosis**  Persistent or recurrent appearance of hallucinations, usually in a clear intellectual field, without confusion or intellectual impairment; most commonly due to intoxication with alcohol or drugs, or following traumata such as surgical procedures and childbirth. Usually there is a slow return to normal within a period of weeks; if symptoms persist, the condition is generally considered to be a schizophrenic reaction. The most common form of acute hallucinosis is alcoholic hallucinosis. See *alcoholic hallucinosis; flashback; organic mental disorders.*

In DSM-IV, hallucinosis is classified on the basis of whether reality testing about the hallucinatory experiences is intact. In alcoholic hallucinosis, for example, if reality testing is impaired, the hallucinosis is termed substance-induced psychotic disorder with hallucinations; if reality testing is intact, it is termed substance-induced intoxication (or withdrawal) with perceptual disturbance.

**Halstead-Reitan Battery** A neuropsychological test for subjects 15 years of age and older. Among its 13 subtests are Tactual Performance (which assesses tactile recognition, motor speed, and the ability to form a visual "map"); Category test (which measures new learning and mental efficiency); Speech Sounds Perception (measures auditory-verbal perception); Rhythm test (measures attention, concentration, nonverbal auditory discrimination); and Finger Tapping (which compares motor speed for both sides of the body). The scores on the test yield an Impairment Index and a general indication of the level of brain dysfunction. It may take as long as 2 days to administer the battery. See *Luria-Nebraska Neuropsychological Battery; neuropsychological tests.*

**hamartophobia** Fear of error or sin. Commonly misspelled harmatophobia.

**Hamilton scale** The Hamilton Rating Scale for Depression consists of 24 items reflecting the subject's responses in a clinical interview to questions about feelings of guilt, suicide, sleep habits, etc. Each item is rated 0 to 4 or 0 to 2, with a maximum total range of 0 to 76.

**HAND** *HIV-associated neurocognitive disorders* (q.v.).

**Hand-Christian-Schüller syndrome** *Xanthomatosis* (q.v.).

**handgun violence** In 1976 there were 28,000 deaths (including homicides, suicides, and other fatalities) from firearms. In 1993, the number had risen to 40,230. Firearm injuries kill 40,000 and harm another 240,000 each year in the United States. More than a fourth of those who die are 15–24 years old. In 1991, firearm-related injuries were the eighth leading cause of death and the fourth leading cause of years of potential life lost before 65 years of age in the United States. Firearm homicide in males 15–19 years more than tripled in the 10 years between 1984 and 1993. More teenagers die from firearm injuries than all natural causes combined. The rates of nonfatal firearm-related GSWs were highest among males (68.7/100,000 population), persons 25–34 years (119.5), and African Americans (149.4). An average of 52,000 U.S. residents die each year with traumatic brains injuries (TBI). Firearms surpassed motor vehicles as the largest single cause of deaths associated with TBI in 1990. See *GSW; weapons.*

**handedness** See *cerebral dominance.*

**handicap** See *disability.*

**handicap, emotional** In educational psychology, a learning disability or behavioral disturbance of enough severity to render the affected child unable to function in the regular classroom. The emotionally handicapped child is of average or superior intellect, demonstrates no gross neurological disorder, but nonetheless is unable to learn or maintain satisfactory interpersonal relationships with peers and teachers. In addition, the child may overreact to what appears to the observer to be minimal stress, or he may develop any number of somatic or psychic symptoms in relation to ordinary school pressures, or he may show generalized unhappiness and disenchantment with living. See *attention deficit hyperactivity disorder.*

**handicap, mental** Mental retardation; see *retardation, mental.*

**hand-to-mouth reaction** Observed in young infants, bringing to the mouth and sucking all objects within reach. These may be parts of the infant's body (hand, foot) or any outside object. According to Gesell, this reaction disappears at about 12 months of age.

**hangover** The aftereffect ("*morning after*") syndrome following ingestion of alcohol or other sedatives, such as barbiturates. Symptoms include a bad taste, nausea, vomiting, polypnoea, pallor, irritability, sweating, and conjunctival injection. The syndrome may be a direct result of ethanol intoxication or due to effects of acetaldehyde, an intermediate metabolite that develops in the course of alcohol oxidation, or a result of toxic congeners contained in most forms of commercially available alcohol that extend and amplify the effects of alcohol itself.

**Hans** See *Little Hans.*

**HAP1** Huntingtin-associated protein 1. See *Huntington disease.*

**haploid** See *meiosis.*

**haploinsufficiency** Loss of one copy (one allele) of a gene is sufficient to give rise to disease. Haploinsufficiency implies that no dominant-negative effect of the mutated gene product has to be invoked.

**haplology** Omission of syllables in words because of speed in speech; seen often in mania and in schizophrenic syndromes in which there is pressure of speech.

**haplotype** Haploid genotype; all the known nucleotide sequences at a polymorphic site and closely linked genes that are inherited together. A haplotype is a long stretch of DNA at a given location on a chromosome, with a distinctive pattern of *SNPs* (q.v.). A sequence of 50,000 bases might contain 50 SNPs, which could come in as many as $2^{50}$ variations; but the same sequence might contain only 5 haplotypes (*patterns* of SNPs) that account for 80% or more of the population. Haplotyping thus promises to reduce significantly the amount of DNA that must be scanned in identifying associations between DNA and complex diseases. See *polymorphism.*

**Happy Puppet syndrome** A form of mental retardation characterized by protruding jaw and tongue, flat occiput, ataxic gait, epilepsy, a smiling but otherwise expressionless face, paroxysms of laughter, hypotonia, absent speech, abnormal EEG, and a variety of other congenital malformations. Etiology is unknown, although it is presumed to be of genetic origin.

**haptephobia** Fear of being touched.

**haptic deafferentation, selective** Total loss of the sense of touch and propriocception from the body, due to sensory neuropathy.

**haptic hallucination** Hallucination associated with the sensation of touch. A paranoid patient complained that his persecutors, operating an electrical apparatus hidden in the walls of the building, induced very disagreeable sensations over his body through the machine. Alleged persecutors reach the patient's body through many avenues, among which are the sensory zones. In clear-cut cases of schizophrenia the persecutors aspire to tempt the patient to engage in homosexual practices. Indeed, they constantly stimulate him sexually through the several sense areas. "He operates a machine that masturbates me" is a common expression among paranoid schizophrenic patients. The persecutors are said also to surround the patient with "bad sexual odors" (*olfactory hallucination*); they put "scum" (seminal fluid) in his food (*gustatory* or *taste hallucination*); they call him a sexual pervert with men (*auditory hallucination*); they grimace at him, meaning he is homosexual (*visual hallucination*).

**haptophonia** The hearing of noises or voices in response to tactile or haptic stimulation. One patient, for example, complained of hearing voices coming from his forearm, where there was the scar of an old injury.

**Harada syndrome** See *Behçet syndrome.*

**harassment, sexual** Unwelcome sexual advances, requests for sexual favors, and unwelcome verbal or physical conduct of a sexual nature within the work setting. In tangible or *quid pro quo* harassment, jobs, positions, promotions, or benefits are contingent upon the victim granting sexual favors to the co-worker or supervisor who holds controls or decides upon job benefits. Probably much more frequent (and much more difficult to prove) is abusive or *hostile environment* harassment, which involves unwanted or unwelcome action of a sexual nature that would make any reasonable person feel uncomfortable in such a work environment. The behavior may include unwelcome sexually oriented joking or teasing; unwelcome display of sexual depictions or objects; unwelcome propositioning or touching; or repeated sexual flirtation or suggestive gestures. The conduct must be more than merely offensive, but most court cases have not required that it cause a "tangible psychological injury."

Harassment outside the workplace is often, but not always, of a sexual nature, and takes many forms. In conjunction with the increasing reach of the Internet, which makes it easy to access personal data about other people online (especially via social networking and dating sites), *cyberstalking* has become a major form of harassment. See *stalking.*

**hardiness**   See *existentialism*.

**Hardy mutation**   (John Hardy, molecular geneticist, reported with A. Goate and coworkers, 1991) An APP (amyloid precursor protein) mutation, on chromosome 21, associated with early-onset familial Alzheimer disease. The mutation is a single nucleotide change, consisting of substitution of isoleucine for valine at codon 717. (At least two other substitutions at this position will also produce Alzheimer disease: substitution of either phenylalanine or glycine for the native valine.) The Hardy mutation is so rare that it cannot be the cause of all early-onset Alzheimer disease, which is itself so rare that its prevalence has not yet been quantified. Nonetheless, the Hardy mutation shows that aberrations in APP are sufficient, if not necessary, for the development of Alzheimer disease.

**Harlow, Harry**   (1905–1981) U.S. psychologist; pioneer in the study of social attachment. His major contributions were in the areas of learning, motivation, affection, and the role of early experience in the formation of parent–infant, filial, and pair (male–female) bonds in rhesus monkeys. He was noted for his use of "wire mothers" and "monkey therapists."

**harm principle**   The bioethical principle that interference with a person's freedom or autonomy is justified only when there is a reasonable likelihood that the person will cause harm to others. Clinically, this is translated into the dangerousness requirement for civil commitment or involuntary treatment.

**harm reduction**   *Harm minimization*; strategies to prevent or limit the adverse consequences of any activity (most commonly, psychoactive drug use), without necessarily affecting the activity itself. An example is needle and syringe exchange to counteract needle-sharing by drug users.

**harmatophobia**   A frequent misspelling of *hamartophobia* (q.v.).

**harmful drinking**   A pattern of alcohol use that is causing physical or mental damage to the drinker; it also may be producing social consequences. Harmful drinking is contrasted with *hazardous drinking*, which refers to potential damage that may occur if drinking continues. See *risk-taking behavior*.

**harmful use**   *Alcohol abuse*, one form of *alcohol use, unhealthy* (qq.v.).

**harmine**   See *psychotomimetic*.

**harpaxophobia**   Fear of robbers.

**Harris syndrome**   Hypoglycemic syndrome. See *hypoglycemia*.

**Hartmann, Heinz**   (1894–1970) Viennese-born U.S. psychoanalyst; *Ego Psychology and the Problem of Adaptation* (1939).

**Hartnup disease**   A pellagralike disorder caused by a genetic abnormality of tryptophan metabolism: instead of conversion into nicotinamide, tryptophan is converted into indican. A variety of mental symptoms may result, including anxiety, feelings of depersonalization, depression, delusions, hallucinations, delirium, confusion, irritability, apathy, emotional lability, and in many cases mental retardation. See *niacin deficiency*.

**hashish**   The resin of the Indian hemp plant. See *cannabis; marijuana*.

**hate**   See *aggression*.

**hate propaganda**   See *propaganda*.

**haut mal**   Major epileptic attack; grand mal seizure.

**Havisham syndrome**   *Hoarding; squalor syndrome* (qq.v.).

**Haw River syndrome**   See *DRPLA; trinucleotide repeat*.

**Hawthorne effect**   Named after the Hawthorne plant of Western Electric, where a study of industrial productivity (1927–1929) failed to allow for the effect of the investigators' presence and attention on productivity of the workers being observed. A similar effect has been noted in some studies of pharmacological agents in nursing home populations. The observed increases in subjects' interest, activity, socialization, and mood tone—originally attributed to the drug under study—were found to be a response to the increased attention given the subjects when they were visited daily by investigators and questioned about their feelings and their symptoms.

**hazard, moral**   In insurance terminology, a demand for services that is created by their being offered in the first place or determined to a significant degree by the relatively low cost of the insurance premium as compared with the cost to the beneficiary of the service provided by the policy. The term moral is applied because, at least to some degree, the benefit is used even though the service is not essential or would not have been sought had not the policy provided it as a benefit.

**hazardous behavior**   *Risk-taking behavior* (q.v.).

**hazardous drinking**   See *harmful drinking.*

**hazardous treatment**   See *forced treatment.*

**HBMIs**   Hybrid brain–machine interfaces; a technological development that allows continuous interactions between living brain tissue and artificial electronic or mechanical devices. Examples are electrical signals to stimulate brain tissue in order to alleviate pain, to control motor disorders such as Parkinson disease, to reduce epileptic activity, or to restore sensory functions (as does the cochlear implant).

**HBS**   *Homicidal Behaviors Survey* (q.v.).

**HCA**   Heterocyclic antidepressant drug.

**HCR-20**   Historical Clinical Risk Management 20, a rating scale of 20 items that have been found to be predictive of violence. The items include not only history but also current clinical presentation and environmental risk factors.

History factors: previous violence, age at time of first violence, poor social relationships, work problems, substance use, mental illness, psychopathy, early maladjustment, personality disorder, and failure of supervision by a correctional facility or mental health agency.

Clinical factors: lack of insight, negative attitude, active symptoms of mental illness, impulsivity, lack of response to treatment.

Risk factors: risk-management plans not feasible, exposure to conditions the might trigger violence, lack of support, noncompliance with remediation efforts, current stress.

**HD**   *Huntington disease* (q.v.).

**head direction cells**   See *place cells.*

**Head Start**   See *education, compensatory.*

**head trauma**   See *cerebral compressionl; concussion; contusion, brain; traumatic neurosis.*

**headache**   Cephalalgia; pain in the head, such as in the temples, over the eyes, or at the top or base of the skull. In *ICHD-II* (q.v.), headaches are divided into the following categories:

A. Primary Headaches
   1. Migraine: (a) without aura; (b) with aura; (c) chronic migraine
   2. Tension-type headache (TTH): (a) infrequent episodic; (b) frequent episodic; (c) chronic
   3. Cluster headache and other trigeminal autonomic cephalalgias: (a) cluster headache; (b) paroxysmal hemicrania; (c) short-lasting unilateral neuralgiform headache attacks with conjunctival injection and tearing (*SUNCT*)
   4. Other primary headaches: (a) hypnic headache; (b) primary thunderclap headache; (c) hemicrania continua; d) new daily-persistent headache (NDPH)

B. Secondary Headaches
   1. Headache attributed to head and/or neck trauma: (a) acute post-traumatic headache; (b) chronic post-traumatic headache; (c) acute headache attributed to whiplash injury; (d) chronic headache attributed to whiplash injury
   2. Headache attributed to cranial or cervical vascular disorder: (a) subarachnoid hemorrhage; (b) giant cell arteritis
   3. Headache attributed to nonvascular intracranial disorder: (a) idiopathic intracranial hypertension (IIH); (b) postdural puncture; (c) intracranial neoplasm; (d) postictal
   4. Headache attributed to a substance or its withdrawal: (a) medication overuse (MOH)
   5. Headache attributed to infection: (a) bacterial meningitis; (b) chronic postbacterial meningitis headache
   6. Headache attributed to disorder of homeostasis (systemic disorders, such as hypertension, hypoxia, hypercarbia, and hormonal and fluid disturbances)
   7. Headache or facial pain attributed to disorder of cranium, neck, eyes, ears, nose, sinuses, teeth, mouth, or other facial or cranial structures: (a) cervicogenic headache
   8. Headache attributed to psychiatric disorder: (a) somatization disorder; (b) psychotic disorder
   9. Cranial neuralgias and central causes of facial pain: (a) trigeminal neuralgia
   10. Other headache, cranial neuralgia, central or primary facial pain: (a) headache not elsewhere classified; (b) headache unspecified

In ICDH-II, all headache disorders present in a patient are separately diagnosed, allowing for more than one diagnosis. See *cluster headache; familial hemiplegic migraine; migraine; subarachnoid hemorrhage; tension-type headache.*

Headache is extremely common, occurring in as much as 80% to 90% of the population over their lifetimes. It may be the primary complaint of more than half the patients presenting themselves to an emergency room; of these, about 40% are related to infection and about 25% are tension headaches or migraine. Headaches suggestive of some type of intracranial lesion typically have one or more of the following characteristics: aggravated by changes in position, such as head movement, coughing, or straining; sudden onset of excruciating pain; awaken the subject from sleep; accompanied by vomiting.

**head-banging**  One of the many typical physical exertions commonly observed during a temper tantrum in small children. The child works up to a pitch of excitement and by almost every conceivable physical or muscular movement literally throws himself or herself all over the place. See *stereotypic movement disorder*.

**heading perception**  The moment-to-moment sense of where one is going. Humans sense their heading by tracking the image focus; the cortical neurons that respond selectively to image expansion are clustered in the MST (medial superior temporal) area of the brain. Those cells also detect the position of the expansion focus and correct for the displacement of that focus each time the eyes move. MST encodes both instantaneous heading direction and the path to that heading. Adjacent cortical areas project to hippocampal place cells that build a cognitive map of the environment. See *place cells*.

**head-knocking**  A habit developed by some infants that consists of bumping the head against the crib sides or other objects.

**headline intelligence**  A cognitive peculiarity seen in borderline and narcissistic personalities consisting of superficial knowledge about trivia but inability to study anything in depth; catchwords and phrases are combined into a veneer of opinionated familiarity with almost any topic. See *borderline personality; cognitive style; narcissistic personality*.

**head-rolling**  Rhythmical, semicircular movements of the head exhibited by some children before going to sleep. When sufficiently constant, this movement may be considered similar to tics. In some instances, the rolling of the head may be attributed to restraint of movement in the crib and, in other instances, to absence of play material (monotony). In other cases it may reflect the passivity of the fetus during intrauterine life. In these cases the rolling of the head is a hyperactive function that serves as a balance for the intrauterine inactivity. See *jactatio capitis nocturna*.

**health, mental**  See *mental health*.

**health care proxy**  See *advance directive*.

**health law**  The body of rules governing the provision of medical care, including not only the legislation formally enacted but also the regulations that have been devised to implement what is perceived as the intent of the legislation. Health law includes *forensic medicine* and *medical jurisprudence*. Forensic psychiatry is well recognized as a special area of psychiatry, but there is no widely used term (such as "psychiatry law") that corresponds with health law, and most writers use "law and psychiatry" or "legal regulation of psychiatry" to refer to laws and regulations that define the practice of psychiatry and govern the quadrangle of psychiatric care, i.e., the relationships between psychiatrists, their patients, third-party payers, and fourth-party monitors of health care. Specific issues with which law and psychiatry deal include the civil rights of patients, informed consent, competence to consent to treatment, involuntary treatment, commitment, confidentiality, judicial decisions that prohibit or limit certain treatments, advertising, employment contracts, double-agentry (and other matters related to "entreprenurial medicine" and the increasing corporatization of medicine), advertising, insurance practices that discriminate against psychiatric patients, billing practices, the psychiatrist's responsibility for the actions of patients, relationships with other nonmedical mental health professionals and paraprofessionals, and the definition of mental illness by courts or laws or insurance policies. See *consumerism; forced treatment; forensic psychiatry*.

**health maintenance organization**  *HMO* (q.v.).

**health policy**  The many roles of governmental and nongovernmental organizations in the prevention and treatment of illness, including planning for the directions that will be taken in promoting health and eliminating disease. See health law; *public policy*.

**health-related facilities**  See *domicile*.

**hearing alpha**  See *alpha rhythm*.

**Hebb, Donald O.**  (1904–1985)  Canadian neuropsychologist, best known for his neurophysiological postulate on learning, which appeared in his book *The Organization of Behavior* (1949). He proposed a distinction between STM (short-term memory), based on temporary electrical activation, and LTM (long-term memory), based on neuronal growth. Modern neuropsychology is based on Hebb's work with Wilder Penfield. Computer models of the brain are based on his ideas of the synapse and cell assembly. The physiological bases of learning and memory are based on Hebb's ideas of multiple memory systems, and long-term potentiation is the experimental analysis of Hebbian synaptic plasticity. His *Essay on Mind* (1980) is a summary of his ideas on the biological basis of mind and a sequel to *The Organization of Behavior*.

**Hebbian synapse** The characteristics of the synapse as described by Donald Hebb in 1949: homosynaptic plasticity, associativity, and input specificity. The strength of the connection between two neurons is increased when the firing of the postsynaptic neuron is closely associated in time with the firing of a presynaptic neuron. The synaptic strengthening that follows the coincidental firing of the two neurons is input specific; i.e., other synapses on either neuron remain unchanged. Since Hebb, heterosynaptic plasticity has also been recognized: a synapse can be strengthened by the firing of a modulatory interneuron, without the requirement that either presynaptic or postsynaptic neuron be active. See *synapse; synaptic plasticity*.

**hebephilia** *Ephebophilia* (q.v.).

**hebephrenia** A symptom complex now considered a chronic form of schizophrenia. In 1871 Hecker described hebephrenia and the heboid, and in 1896 Kraepelin included hebephrenia in the group dementia praecox. See *hebephrenic schizophrenia*.

**hebephrenia, depressive** Some patients with the hebephrenic form of schizophrenia run, for some time, a course that resembles the periodic changes observed in manic-depressive psychosis. When the constituents of a depression appear in hebephrenia, the state is known as depressive hebephrenia. When there is similarity to a manic phase, it is known as *manic hebephrenia*. See *schizoaffective disorder; schizophrenia, forms of*.

**hebephrenic schizophrenia** A chronic form of schizophrenia characterized by marked disorders in thinking, incoherence, severe emotional disturbance, wild excitement alternating with tearfulness and depression, vivid hallucinations, and absurd, bizarre delusions that are prolific, fleeting, and frequently concerned with ideas of omnipotence, sex change, cosmic identity, and rebirth (the so-called *phylogenetic symptoms*). The hebephrenic forms tend to have an early onset, usually before the age of 20. Bleuler classified as hebephrenic all those schizophrenias with an acute onset that were not characterized by catatonic symptoms (e.g., the manic, melancholic, amented, and twilight states) and also all those chronic forms where the accessory symptoms are not dominant. Others have depended upon the presence of the silly, inappropriate "teenager" symptoms to establish the diagnosis.

Hebephrenic schizophrenia in almost all reported series has been associated with a poor prognosis; i.e., with a relatively rapid deterioration and schizophrenic dementia. It is this form that contributes most heavily to the group termed nuclear or process schizophrenia by other workers.

**hebetude** Emotional dullness or lack of interest. It is most often observed in schizophrenia in which the pronounced withdrawal of interest from the environment and even from the patient himself causes the patient to appear thoroughly listless, unemotional, uninterested, and apathetic. See *affectivity disturbances; apathy*.

"In the severer forms of schizophrenia the *'affective dementia'* is the most striking symptom. In the sanatoria there are patients sitting around who for decades show no affect no matter what happens to them or to those about them. They are indifferent to maltreatment; left to themselves they lie in wet and frozen beds, do not bother about hunger and thirst. They have to be taken care of in all respects. Toward their own delusions they are often strikingly indifferent" (Bleuler, E. *Textbook of Psychiatry*, 1930).

An older meaning of hebetude included listlessness or apathy from any cause, physical or mental. It is still sometimes used in this sense.

**Hecker, Ewald** (1843–1909) German psychiatrist; known from his studies in hebephrenia (a term he coined.)

**hedoni-**  Combining form meaning, delight, enjoyment, pleasure, from Gr. *hedonē*.

**hedonic impact**  See *reward*; *salience*.

**hedonic level**  See *adaptational psychodynamics*.

**hedonism**  **1.** A philosophic doctrine in which pleasure or happiness is presented as the supreme good. In psychiatry, it refers to the seeking of certain goals because they afford some type of gratification. Hedonism, then, is in opposition to the doctrine that goals may be sought as ends in themselves, irrespective of the pleasure or gratification they give the person. See *hormism*.

 **3.** A form of *social cohesion* based on reward, in contrast to *agonic social cohesion*, which is based on avoidance of punishment.

**hedonistic utilitarianism**  See *utilitarianism, hedonistic*.

**hedonophobia**  Fear of pleasure.

**heel-to-knee test**  A test of ataxia; the patient in a recumbent position, with the eyes open or closed, is requested to raise the foot high, touch the knee with the opposite heel, and move the heel along the shin.

**Heidenhain syndrome**  Subacute presenile spongiform encephalopathy with occipital predilection and cortical blindness.

**Heidenheim disease**  *Creutzfeldt-Jakob disease* (q.v.).

**Heinroth, Johann Christian**  (1773–1843) Leipzig physician who was the first to propose that psychiatry be acknowledged as a discrete medical discipline; beginning in 1811 he occupied the first chair in psychiatry at Leipzig.

**heir of the Oedipus complex**  See *superego*.

**heliophobia**  Fear of sunlight.

**hellenomania**  Impulse or tendency to use complicated, cumbersome terms, frequently Greek or Latin, instead of readily understandable English words. The impulse is rampant in the field of psychiatric writing, as witness the list of (generally undesirable) terms under *fear of*.

 Interestingly enough, hellenomania is itself a pseudoerudite misnomer since literally it means a pathological love of Greeks or their country. The correct term for what is defined above is hellenologomania. In like fashion, hellenophobia is a fear of Greeks (a subtype of xenophobia), while hellenologophobia would denote a fear or avoidance of Greek terms.

**Heller disease**  *Childhood disintegrative disorder* (q.v.).

**helmet, neurasthenic**  A feeling of pressure over the entire cranium in certain cases of neurasthenia, as if from a tight-pressing helmet. See *lead-cap headache*.

**helper, magic**  Fromm's term describing a particular form of interpersonal relationship. Man has today become aware of himself as a separate entity. The growing realization of his separateness gives him a sense of isolation and a longing to return to the earlier feeling of solidarity with others. So he uses certain irrational methods of relating back to the group, and these are termed mechanisms of escape. One method is to seek to lean on another for support. The other person represents a power or authority who can be used for that purpose. Sometimes the individual expects the other person to solve all his problems for him and endows the person with almost magical omnipotence. This other person is then termed the magic helper. It is obvious that the person so endowed with magical power must himself be affected by it and to a degree be dependent on it. The power he has illustrates a form of *irrational authority* (q.v.), which is based not on competence but on a neurotic need for power.

**helping relationship**  A type of relationship, as defined by Carl Rogers, in which one of the participants intends that there should come about, in one or both parties, more appreciation, expression, or functional use of latent inner responses. Examples include mother and child, and teacher and student, as well as therapist and patient.

**helplessness, psychic**  The state that occasions the first expression of anxiety in early infancy. The prototype of anxiety, according to Freud, is the experience of birth; all later anxiety states are reproductions of this earliest experience with danger. Anxiety as experienced in later life is also a response to a danger situation.

**hematidrosis**  Bloody perspiration.

**hem(at)o-**  Combining form meaning blood, from Gr. *haima*, -atos.

**hematoencephalic barrier**  See *blood–brain barrier*.

**hematophobia**  See *hemophobia*.

**hemeralopia**  Day blindness; vision is poor by day, in bright light, and good in dim light; the opposite of *nyctalopia*. See *optic nerve*.

**hemeraphonia** Voicelessness during daytime, usually a symptom of hysteria.

**hemi-** Combining form meaning half, from Gr. *hēmi-*.

**hemiakinesia** See *sensory neglect*.

**hemianopic, hemianopsia** See *field defect*.

**hemianopsia, heteronymous** Bitemporal or binasal loss of vision.

**hemianopsia, homonymous** Loss of vision in the similarly situated (both right or both left) halves of one's eyes, i.e., in the nasal half of one eye and in the temporal half of the other. See *field defect*.

**hemiasomatognosia, hemisomatagnosia** *Hemisomatognosis* (q.v.).

**hemiatrophy, facial** *Parry-Romberg syndrome*; a trophic disorder, perhaps due to disturbance of the sympathetic nervous system, in which there is progressive wasting of some or all of the tissues of one side of the face, which as a result looks old and wrinkled. The disorder usually begins during the second decade; it causes no disability.

**hemiballism** Violent, uncontrollable shaking, twisting, and rolling movements involving one side of the body, occurring as a result of hemorrhage into the subthalamic body.

**hemichannels** See *gap junction*.

**hemichorea** Chorea affecting one side of the body only.

**hemichorea, preparalytic** Unilateral choreic movements preceding an attack of hemiplegia.

**hemicrania** In ICHD-II, paroxysmal hemicrania is included under *cluster headache* (q. v.).

**hemidepersonalization** *Hemisomatognosis* (q.v.).

**hemiopia** Hemianopia. See *field defect*.

**hemiparesis** Slight paralysis or weakness of only one side of the body.

**hemiplegia** A symptom complex rather than a disease, characterized by paralysis of one side of the body.

**hemiplegia, nocturnal** See *sleep paralysis*.

**hemiplegia alternans** Crossed paralysis; paralysis of one or more cranial nerves and paralysis of the arm and leg of the opposite side. Hypoglossal hemiplegia alternans involves the twelfth cranial nerve; *Weber syndrome* involves the oculomotor (third cranial) nerve. See *Foville syndrome*.

**hemiplegia cruciata** (Mod. L. "crossed hemiplegia") Paralysis of an upper extremity and of the lower extremity on one side and of the lower extremity on the other.

**hemiplegic gait** In patients with hemiplegia, the lower extremity is held stiffly and circumducted in walking, and the patient leans to the affected side.

**hemisomatognosis** *Hemidepersonalization; Babinski syndrome*; a disorder of body image in which the subject feels that one limb is missing, usually the left arm or leg. It often occurs in combination with hemiparesis and unilateral spatial agnosia. See *body image*.

Also, defective or absent awareness of one side of the body, as in the subject's denial of hemiplegia (*Babinski syndrome*) or blindness (*Anton syndrome*); some use hemiasomatognosia to differentiate this type of *sensory neglect* (q.v.) from the hemidepersonalization described above.

**hemispatial neglect** See *spatial neglect*.

**hemispheres, cerebral** See *cerebral hemispheres*.

**hemisphericity** *Cerebral dominance* (q.v.), or the hypothesis that some types of emotion or affective behavior are mediated through one hemisphere of the brain rather than the other. Some studies, for example, have found dysfunction of the right, nondominant hemisphere to be associated with affective disorders; others have found hysterical repression to be consistent with right hemisphericity and obsessive-compulsive traits to be consistent with left hemisphericity.

**hemo-** *Hem(at)o-* (q.v.).

**hemoclastic crisis** Reversal of the normal white blood cell and blood pressure response to the ingestion of protein. In the normal, ingestion of protein results in leukocytosis and rise of blood pressure. In contrast, hemoclastic patients show a fall in blood pressure, leukopenia, altered differential white blood count, and a reduction in the refractive index of the blood. Hemoclastic crisis is said to be particularly frequent in schizophrenia, depression, and anxiety states, and to be correlated with a poorer prognosis than in patients with a normal response.

**hemophobia, hematophobia** Fear of blood.

**hemorrhage, cerebral** See *cerebrovascular accident*.

**hemothymia** Passion for blood; impulse to murder.

**hemp insanity** See *cannabis delusional disorder*.

**hepatolenticular degeneration** *Tetanoid chorea of Gowers*; Westphal pseudosclerosis; progressive lenticular degeneration; *Wilson disease*. It is caused by mutations of the gene

*ATP7B* on chromosome 13q14.3. An autosomal recessive hereditary disorder of copper metabolism characterized by degeneration of the corpus striatum (especially the putamen) and cirrhosis of the liver, with decreased serum ceruloplasm and increased urinary excretion of copper and amino acids. The disease begins early in life (10 to 25 years of age) and is progressive. The initial symptom is usually tremor, which is increased by voluntary movement. This is followed by rigidity (similar to that seen in parkinsonism) dysarthria, dysphagia, and a vacant, expressionless appearance or a vacuous smile. Involuntary laughing and crying may occur and also some degree of intellectual deterioration.

In a certain number of cases, a zone of golden-brown granular pigmentation (the *Kayser-Fleischer ring*) can be seen in the cornea; some would distinguish these patients from those with Wilson disease and term the syndrome *Westphal-Strumpell pseudosclerosis*. Untreated cases are invariably fatal, half of them within 6 years from onset of symptoms. Treatment with penicillamine or BAL (British anti-lewisite, dimercaprol) to remove copper from the body may afford temporary amelioration. Psychotropic medication may be helpful but should be used cautiously because of hepatic abnormalities.

**hephephilia**  *Stuff eroticism*; a *paraphilia* (q.v.) in which sexual gratification depends upon contact with soft, smooth fabrics, such as silk or velvet.

**Heracles complex**  A father's hatred of his children. See *Medea complex*.

**herbalist**  Witch doctor.

**Hercules syndrome**  See *adrenogenital syndrome*.

**herd instinct**  *Group feeling*; group formation; the desire to be with others and to take part in social activities; *gregariousness*. From the psychoanalytic point of view this is not an instinct; rather, social and group phenomena are explained as results of identification, the origin of which is to be found in the jealousy and hostility of childhood. It is said that the first child is jealous of his successors and desires to get rid of them. If the jealousy is maintained, however, he will lose the admiration and love of his parents. He is eventually compelled to unite (to identify himself) with his brothers and sisters.

When identification takes place, it is followed by reaction formation, that is, sympathy with the rival replaces hostility. The identification with the leader is of the same order as the earlier identification with the father. The leader is a new ego-ideal.

**hereditary (hereditarial)**  Referring both to the mendelian mechanism by which physical or mental attributes are transmitted from one generation to another and to the inherited attributes to which an organism is predisposed by the presence of a certain gene or combination of genes.

"We usually call what is programmed in the chromosomes hereditary or genetic. The sum of what is biologically given (whether determined by genetics or intrauterine environment) is referred to as constitutional.... The unfolding of biologically given factors and their manifestation at critical periods in the life history are referred to as maturation, a somatically programmed schedule. The opposite of maturation is *involution*" (Redlich, F. C. & Freedman, D. X. *The Theory and Practice of Psychiatry*, 1966).

**heredity**  The process of inheritance as a biological phenomenon; the forces responsible for the resemblance between an individual and his ancestors, insofar as this resemblance is due to the operation of predisposing gene units rather than to the similarity of environmental influences.

The morphological equivalent of heredity is the mendelian mechanism based on the integrity of the chromosomes and their community from one cell generation to the next, while the science dealing with the study of heredity is usually called *genetics*. See *Mendelism*.

**heredo-familial essential microsomia**  See *dwarfism*.

**heritability**  In genetics, the proportion of trait/phenotypic variance in a population that is attributable to genetic agents. The highest heritability so far reported for any behavior dimension is cognitive ability, for which genetic factors increase in importance—to a high of as much as 80% later in life. Heritability in the range of 40% to 50% has been found for *personality* (q.v.), vocational interests, general intelligence, scholastic performance, spatial reasoning, and verbal reasoning. Heritability for memory is lower, as is speed of processing cognitive information. Studies also suggest significant heritability for information processing, EEG evoked potentials, cerebral glucose metabolism, self-esteem, social attitudes, and sexual orientation (Plomin, R. et al. *Science 264*, 1994).

The heritability of lifespan accounts for <35% of its variance. Two studies of human twins attribute most (> 65%) of the variance to nonshared (individually unique) environmental factors. In contrast to the findings on life-spans, strong genetic effects are found in late-onset cognitive declines.

**heritable** *Inheritable* (q.v.).

**hermaphrodism** *Hermaphroditism* (q.v.).

**hermaphrodism, psychical** Adler's term for the constant striving of the person to free himself from feelings of weakness, inferiority, and futility to attain self-confidence, superiority, and self-gratification. It is the conflict between the masculine and feminine components.

**hermaphroditism** *Intersexuality*; combination of the genital attributes of both sexes, with consequent ambiguity as to whether a person is male or female according to one or more of the usual criteria for sex; viz. (1) chromosomal (usually 46, XX for females, 46,XY for males; (2) H-Y antigen (typically recognized on 46,XY cells, but not on 46,XX cells); (3) gonadal (prevalently ovarian for females, testicular for males); (4) prenatal hormones, with either a feminizing or a masculinizing effect on the developing genitalia (and on certain portions of the brain); (5) morphologic sex of the internal and external genitalia (i.e., for females, uterus and oviducts; for males, testes, scrotum, and penis); (6) pubertal hormonal sex (i.e., feminization and the development of breasts and menses, or masculinization, with the enlargement of the penis, erectile capability, and beard growth); (7) the sex of assignment and type of rearing, which has a profound effect, in combination with all the foregoing, on the establishment of gender identity. See *androgen insensitivity syndrome; gender coding; gender identity.*

**hermaphroditism, androgen-induced** The effects of an excess of masculinizing hormone from the mother transmitted through the placenta to the gonadally female (46,XX) fetus. The excess hormone is usually due to a maternal or placental tumor.

**hermeneutics** The principles or methods of interpreting the meaning of the Bible, or the study of those principles; sometimes applied to the study of psychotherapy, in which case hermeneutic theory denotes the study of the rules or methods governing interpretation of the patient's productions (associations, dreams, etc.) during analytic treatment.

**hero syndrome** See *pyromania.*

**hero worship** According to Freud, a product of the need of the great majority of people "for authority which they can admire, to which they can submit, and which dominates and sometimes even ill-treats them." The need for such an authority is the longing of each person for the ideal or perfect father (*Moses and Monotheism*, 1939).

**hero-birth, primordial image of** The source of the pregnancy dream in the unconscious; the hero to be born represents the dreamer's individuality. See *primordial image.*

**heroin** See *opioid; opium.*

**herpes simplex encephalitis** After primary infection, the herpes simplex virus is retained throughout life in sensory ganglia and causes occasional recurrences that are not usually serious. Rarely, and in persons whose immune system is compromised, the virus may spread beyond the dorsal root ganglia either centripetally into the central nervous system or by causing a viremia and then *encephalitis* (q.v.).

**Herrick, Charles Judson** (1868–1960) American neurologist; comparative neurology; *The Evolution of Human Behavior.*

**Herstedvester** A town in Denmark known for the rehabilitation program in use in its Institution for Criminal Psychopaths. The program was a combination of group and individual treatment that provided a therapeutic community for the inmates. See *therapeutic community.*

**Hertwig-Magendie phenomenon** (Oscar Hertwig, German physiologist, 1849–1922, and François Magendie, French physiologist, 1783–1855) See *skew deviation.*

**hertz** (from German physicist Heinrich Hertz, 1857–1894, the discoverer of radio waves) Hz; a unit for measuring frequency; 1 Hz = one cycle per second.

**Herxheimer reaction** See *Jarisch-Herxheimer reaction.*

**Heschl gyrus** Brodmann area 41, on the upper surface of the temporal lobe in the posterior part of the superior temporal gyrus, under (and completely hidden by) the frontal operculum. It is the primary auditory association cortex, receiving stimuli from the cochlea through the medial geniculate body (a nucleus of the thalamus). Heschl gyrus appears to be responsible for tone recognition, intensity coding, and spatial localization of sound. More complex properties of sound, such as frequency-modulated tones and meaningful vocalizations, are also partially coded here. See *planum temporale*.

**hetaeral phantasy**   Phantasy in women of being, and in men of possessing, a courtesan or female paramour.

**hetero-**   Combining form meaning other, different, from Gr. *heteros*, the other, one of two.

**heterocentric**   Directed away from oneself; opposed to autocentric.

**heterochomatin**   Heterochromatin contains relatively few genes and can suppress the transcriptional activity of active genes that are translocated adjacent to it. It is thought to contain large protein complexes that propagate laterally along the chromatin fiber and silence genes with which they come into contact. The best known heterochromatin protein is *HP1* (heterochromatin protein 1), whose role is to interact with multiple nuclear proteins to assemble macromolecular complexes in chromatin. HP1 that is targeted to reporter genes inactivates transcription. The *Polycomb protein* is also involved in gene silencing; it binds exclusively to sites in euchromatin. *Ikaros* is a transcriptional regulator, inactivating genes by moving them from permissive loci in the nucleoplasm to a zone of transcriptional suppression near centromeric heterochromatin.

**heteroclite**   A person who deviates from the common rule, as opposed to *homoclite*, a person who follows the common rule and is ordinary, normal, healthy, etc.

**heterocyclic**   See *antidepressant*.

**heteroeroticism**   Attachment (cathexis) of libidinal energy to objects outside of oneself, and specifically to objects of the opposite sex. If one uses the term libido synonymously with Eros, then heteroerotism is heterolibido or object-libido.

Heteroeroticism is a phase in the development of object relationships (see *ontogeny, psychic*); its achievement constitutes the chief task of adolescence. At puberty, libidinal strivings that have been dormant during the period of latency (q.v.) reappear because of biological intensification of sexuality. In childhood, the person had come to recognize his sexual impulses as dangerous; at puberty, he returns to just that point in his sexual development where he had abandoned it earlier, and the fears and guilt connected with the Oedipus complex reappear. But overt sexuality now has a physiologically mature genital discharge apparatus, and finally, at about 16 or 17, the adolescent desexualizes his relationship with all but one (or more) unrelated persons of the opposite sex and the stage of heterosexuality is reached.

**heterogamous**   Relating to the structural and functional differences between the male and female gametes, as they appear in most animals and plants. See *syngamy*.

**heterogeneity, heterogeny**   Dissimilarity in the genotypical structure of individuals originating through sexual reproduction. See *homogeneity*.

**heterohypnosis**   Hypnosis induced by another, as opposed to autohypnosis.

**heterolalia**   Substitution of meaningless or inappropriate words for those meant or intended; malapropism.

**heteromodal association cortex (HMAC)**   A dispersed association system in the cerebral cortex related to secondary and higher-order associative functions that are involved in processing more than one type of information, such as the areas involved in perceiving the stimulus of a verbal question, understanding its content and appreciating the emotional "tone" in which it was delivered, planning an appropriate response, and generating that response. The HMAC areas are the dorsolateral prefrontal cortex, the inferior parietal cortex (supramarginal, angular, and inferior parietal gyri), and the superior temporal gyrus (*planum temporale*, q.v.). See *association areas*; *frontal lobe*; *limbic lobe*; *occipital lobe*; *parietal lobe*; *temporal lobe*.

The heteromodal association cortex has recently been proposed to play a key role in schizophrenia, in which there is a disturbance of normal symmetry, accounted for by a relative increase in the size of the right planum temporale. Normal asymmetry of the PT is lost in schizophrenia and this effect is apparently specific to this area of heteromodal association cortex, since the primary auditory cortex is not affected.

**heteronomous superego**   A special type of superego which demands that the ego behave according to what is expected at the moment. A person with such a superego is irresolute and weak, for his behavior at any moment is controlled by the desire to secure the approval of those about him; he is in constant fear of being criticized or punished—i.e., he has "social anxiety." This is in contrast to the normal autonomous superego, which demands only that the ego behave in a "good" way, according to a certain set of standards or ideals. The heteronomous superego is often an outcome of inconsistent handling of a child; he is made uncertain about the difference between good and bad and responds only to what he perceives as the demand of the moment.

**heteronymous hemianopia** See *field defect*.

**heterophasia** *Heterolalia* (q.v.).

**heterophemy** The saying of one thing when another is meant.

**heterophonia** *Heterolalia* (q.v.).

**heterophoria** Deviation of one eye because of muscular imbalance. Inward deviation is known as *esophoria*; outward deviation is *exophoria*; downward deviation is *hypophoria*; upward deviation is *hyperphoria*.

**heteroplasmy** Co-existence of both wild-type (normal) and mutant genes and their products. See *mitochondrial disorders*.

**heteroreceptor** A receptor that modulates the synthesis or release of neurotransmitters other than its own ligand. See *neuromessenger*.

**heterorexia** Alibert's term for morbid appetite; dysorexia. See *eating disorders*.

**heterosexuality** Sexuality (in all its manifestations, normal and deviant) directed to the opposite sex. See *genital character; genitality*.

"There is no conceivable way of quantifying the homosexual vs. heterosexual....If, for instance, Alexander the Great had sexual relations with hundreds of women and only two men, but one of the men (Bagoas) was unquestionably the erotic center of his life, the statistics would give us a highly misleading picture....At best these categories group together according to one arbitrarily chosen aspect of sexual actions—the genders of the parties involved—varieties of sexual behavior which may be more dissimilar than similar" (Boswell, J. *Christianity, Social Tolerance, and Homosexuality*, 1980).

**heterosis** The favorable influence of crossing on growth and other developmental properties of animals and plants, as exercised by an increase in heterozygocity in contrast to the decrease in vigor following inbreeding. It is best evidenced in the generation immediately following the cross, by greater size, larger parts, increased longevity, and higher resistance to disease. Hybrid vigor disappears rapidly under inbreeding. The mule is commonly cited as a hybrid animal whose vigor, hardiness, and resistance to disease are due to heterosis.

**heterosome** The sex chromosome, as distinguished from all other chromosomes (autosomes). See *chromosome; sex determination*.

**heterosuggestibility** The state of influencing another; the opposite of auto- or self-suggestibility.

**heterotopia** Congenital displacement of gray matter of the spinal cord into the white substance.

**heterotropia** *Strabismus* (q.v.); squint.

**heterozygousness** *Obs. Heterozygosity*; relates to the genetic condition of an organism whose two genes of a given factor pair are *different*. Only dominant characters can appear in the state of heterozygousness, while the heterozygotic condition of a recessive trait affects the organism merely "germinally." A heterozygotic individual transmits the trait to the offspring but is not able to manifest the trait in his own phenotype. See *heterosis; inbreeding*.

*Double heterozygousness* refers to the individual who has both dominant and recessive alleles for two linked genes. See *linkage*.

**heutoscopy** The false belief or delusion that one has a double.

**hexafluorodiethyl ether** A convulsant agent used in psychiatric treatment in the same capacity as ECT. The trade name is Indoklon.

**hexing** See *rootwork*.

**HGP** *Human Gene Project*. See *genomics*.

**HGPS** Hutchinson-Gilford progeria syndrome; see *progeria*.

**HHHO** See *Prader-Labhart-Willi syndrome*.

**HI** *Hyperglycemic index* (q.v.).

**HIAA** Hydroxyindoleacetic acid. See *indole; serotonin*.

**hibernation** Prolonged sleep therapy, especially when accompanied by a lowering of the body temperature. High dosages of chlorpromazine, for instance, were used to keep patients in a continuous semisomnolent state with a lowered body temperature; such treatment was called hibernation therapy.

**hiccup, hiccough**　A spasmodic myoclonous of the diaphragm producing a sudden inhalation of air that is interrupted by a spasmodic closure of the glottis, thus producing a sound that may simulate an ordinary cry or an unpleasant crow; also known as *singultus*.

**hid**　See *apoptosis*.

**hidden figures test**　The subject identifies a simple figure embedded in a more complex one by marking its outline.

**hidden self**　See *dissociative identity disorder*.

**hieromania**　*Obs.* Religious insanity.

**hierophobia**　Fear of sacred or religious things.

**HIF**　Higher intellectual function.

**high**　The pleasurable state induced by substance intoxication, as with alcohol or *marijuana* (q.v.).

**high utilizer**　See *adverse selection*.

**higher dementia**　Van Guden's term for inability to apply knowledge or make use of one's intelligence; also known as *parlor dementia* (Hoch) and *relative dementia* (Bleuler).

**high-risk behavior**　*Risk-taking behavior* (q.v.).

**high-volume hospital**　See *volume sensitive*.

**hijra**　A variant of *gynemimesis* (q.v.) reported in India. The hijras are a community of male-to-female transsexuals who undergo eunuchizing surgery and live as women. They are part caste, part cult, and have their own deity, the goddess Bahuchara Mata.

**hillock, axon**　See *axon*.

**hindbrain**　*Rhombencephalon*, from which develop the *metencephalon* (cerebellum, pons, part of the fourth ventricle) and the *myelencephalon* (medulla oblongata and part of the fourth ventricle).

**hindsight bias**　The tendency to impute causation to an action when a bad outcome is known. Such a bias tends to overestimate the number of deaths caused by adverse events. An extreme example of hindsight bias would be to conclude that beds are dangerous because most people die in bed.

**Hinkemann**　Term generally used in Germany for a castrated male. Hinkemann, the principal character of a play by the same name, written by Toller, lost his genitals as a result of injury sustained in World War I.

**hippanthropy**　The delusion that one is a horse.

**Hippel-Lindau disease**　See *von Hippel-Lindau disease*.

**hippocampus**　A phylogenetically ancient brain structure, the hippocampus lies deep within the cerebral hemisphere, in the *medial temporal lobe*, extending the length of the floor of the temporal horn of the lateral ventricles. It is an integral part of the limbic system and a main component of the neuroregulatory limb of the HPA. The hippocampal formation includes the hippocampus proper (Ammon's horn), subiculum, fimbria, *dentate gyrus*, and entorhinal cortex. The hippocampus receives input from the entorhinal cortex by way of the *perforant path*; it sends output to the subiculum, which has reciprocal connections with many areas of the brain, including the isocortex. The fibers of the hippocampus-fornix that innervate the hypothalamus originate in the subiculum.

The hippocampus, and in particular the posterior hippocampal formation, is a critical component of the medial temporal lobe (MTL) memory system. The hippocampus aids in converting short-term memories to long-term memories and in integrating multiple sensory inputs into one coherent memory. Memories are stored for long-term retrieval outside the MTL, in the neocortex. The hippocampus can serve as an index for information stored elsewhere in the brain. Its neurons are woven into autoassociative networks which have strong input and output circuitry with the rest of the brain and are specialized for holding contextual information. Hippocampal neuronal networks link the sequences of events and places that complete episodic memories; they also link continuing experience to stored episodic representation. See *cognitive functions*; *memory*; *MTL*.

Glucocorticoid homeostasis is critical to normal hippocampal function. Increased cortisol release caused by stress damages the hippocampus, and decreased hippocampal volume, such as reported in some patients with schizophrenia, increases vulnerability to stress. The hippocampus and amygdala link neocortical association areas with the hypothalamus, septum, midbrain, and medulla; disturbances in these linkages lead to a dissociation between neocortical-cognitive activities and hypothalamic-emotional reactions to those activities.

Clinicopathologic material from amnesic patients has generally identified where damage must occur to produce *amnesia* (q.v.): the medial temporal region, with emphasis on the hippocampus; and the midline diencephalic region, with emphasis on the mediodorsal thalamic nucleus and the mammillary nuclei. A hippocampal lesion interrupts exchange between the hippocampus and memory storage sites and thus interferes with the storage and consolidation of declarative memory. The most common cause of hippocampal lesions is inadequacy of oxygen supply secondary to difficult birth and delivery.

Patients with hippocampal damage demonstrate severe anterograde amnesia, with marked deficits in recent memory. They cannot remember where they had dinner last night or what they talked about. They cannot create new memories (declarative memory), but they can learn new skills (procedural memory) and they are able to perform mental arithmetic.

**Hippocrates** (460–377 B.C.) Greek physician, considered the father of medicine; his careful observation and description of various diseases separated medicine from philosophy and placed it on a scientific basis. The *Hippocratic oath* continues to represent the ideals of ethical professional conduct. Hippocrates and his followers developed a rudimentary classification of mental disorders; see *phrenitis*. Hippocrates and his followers also identified four temperaments: choleric (hostile, irritable, angry); sanguine (hopeful, warm, optimistic); melancholic (depressed, pessimistic); and phlegmatic (indifferent, unresponsive, apathetic). Each temperament (q.v.) was attributed to a particular balance between the different body humors (fluids: blood, phlegm, black bile, yellow bile).

**hippus** A condition in which the pupil alternately contracts and dilates on stimulation with light.

**Hirschfeld, Magnus** (1868–1935) German sexologist.

**histamine** Histamine is a neuromodulator, localized in the tuberomammillary nucleus of the hypothalamus. It appears to be involved in arousal, attentiveness, and in processes involving the *NMDAR* (q.v.), such as induction of long-term potentiation. See *neurotransmitter*.

**histaminergic system** See *tuberomammillary nucleus*.

**histiocytosis, lipid** See *Gaucher disease; Niemann-Pick disease*.

**histocompatibility complex** See *immune hypothesis of schizophrenia*.

**histones** A group of proteins that are crucial to many gene and DNA activities. They associate with DNA to form nucleosomes and thereby make it possible for large amounts of DNA to be packaged within the nucelus. They alter the accessibility of gene sequences to components of transcription and replication machinery by way of different modifications such as *acetylation* (addition of acetyl groups to amino acids in the amino terminus of the histone), *phosphorylation*, ubiquitination, and methylation. How one and the same event (phosphorylation of serine in H3) can lead to chromatin unfolding and gene action in one setting, and to condensation of chromatin and tight bundling of DNA in another setting, remains a mystery.

Since 1991, evidence has mounted suggesting that *MAP* (mitogen-activated protein) kinases activate genes by phosphorylating histone. Patients with *Coffin-Lowry syndrome*, a hereditary type of mental retardation that is often accompanied by facial and other deformities, have mutations in the Rsk-2 protein, one of the kinases in the MAP kinase pathway. H3, one of the five major histone proteins, is linked to the expression of genes involved in growth stimulation

**histrionic personality (disorder)** *Hysterical personality*; includes any or all of the following: vain, egocentric, attention-seeking, dramatic description of past symptoms and illnesses with a multiplicity of vaguely described complaints and overtalkativeness during the psychiatric interview; suggestibility; soft, coquettish, graceful, and sexually provocative, although frigid and anxious when close to attaining a sexual goal; easily disappointed, excitable, emotionally labile, and often unaware of inner feelings; dependently demanding in interpersonal situations; history of excessive operations and hospitalizations.

Such a manipulative adaptational pattern occurs in those with a tendency toward rigid repression of dysphoric emotion and a denial of threatening stimuli; hence, it has also been termed *repressive personality*. Conflicts in such patients are often centered around genital incest strivings or oral disappointments. See *character defense*.

**hit rate** See *vigilance*.

**HIV, HIV-1** Human immunodeficiency virus, AIDS virus; formerly called HTLV-III or LAV. See *AIDS*.

**HIV lymphoma** A central nervous system neoplasm to which HIV-infected persons are susceptible. Lesions tend to be single rather than multiple, with proliferation of atypical lymphocytes in a perivascular distribution. Early aggressive radiation therapy may increase the length and quality of life; without such treatment, mean survival is approximately 2 months. See *AIDS; AIDS dementia complex.*

**HIV meningitis** An acute aseptic meningitis that occurs soon after HIV infection. Symptoms include headache, fever, retro-orbital pain, meningismus, photophobia, cranial neuropathies, and sometimes transient encephalopathy. The symptoms typically resolve within 1 to 4 weeks. See *AIDS; AIDS dementia complex.*

*Cryptococcal meningitis* is a more serious form of meningitis that occurs in HIV-infected persons as a result of heightened susceptibility to opportunistic infection. Intravenous drug users and blacks are at much higher risk than other AIDS patients for cryptococcal meningitis. It is caused by infection with the common soil fungus *Cryptococcus neoformans*. Symptoms include headache, stiff neck, fever, and photophobia.

**HIV myelopathy** Vacuolar myelopathy in the spinal cord due to HIV infection and usually associated with *AIDS dementia complex* (q.v.). Manifestations include slowly progressive spastic paraphresis, sensory ataxia, sphincter disturbances, and impaired distal sensation without a clear-cut sensory level. HIV myelopathy may occur in as many as 20% of patients with AIDS.

**HIV neuropathy** The most common forms of neuropathy secondary to HIV infection are (1) Demyelinating peripheral nerve disease, which presents either as an acute demyelinating motor neuropathy similar to *Guillain-Barré syndrome* (q.v.) or as a more chronic syndrome with predominantly motor weakness. Symptoms and signs include hyporeflexia, weakness, vibratory loss, and electrophysiological abnormalities, such as slowed nerve conduction velocity. Most of those affected recover spontaneously. (2) Predominantly sensory neuropathy (PSN), which occurs in about 20% of patients with AIDS and in fewer patients with ARC. Symptoms and signs include acral paresthesias and dysesthesias, primarily affecting the balls of the feet and the toes; depressed ankle jerks; elevated vibratory threshold; nerve biopsy abnormalities, such as axonal loss and mild inflammation.

**HIV-associated dementia (HAD)** See *AIDS dementia complex.*

**HIV-associated neurocognitive disorders (HAND)** The results of neurodegeneration and synaptodendritic injury in HIV-infected subjects. Before *cART* (q.v.), severe and disabling dementia (HIV-associated dementia, HAD) affected ~20% of patients with advanced HIV disease. See *AIDS dementia complex*. In both the pre-cART and post-cART eras, up to 50% of patients experienced HAND. With the introduction of cART, there has been a tendency to improvement of overall cognitive performance in HIV, but the improvements are unevenly distributed. Some patients experience remarkable restoration of neurological status, whereas others benefit only partially and remain mildly or severely impaired.

*Asymptomatic neurocognitive impairment* (*ANI*) refers to mild neurocognitive deficits, established by neuropsychological testing, but not severe enough to interfere with everyday functioning. *Mild neurocognitive disorder* (*MND*), also known as *minor cognitive motor disorder* (*MCMD*), refers to cognitive deficits that interfere to a modest degree with everyday functioning. Persons with MND can typically continue to work, but in a less efficient manner. *HAD* describes individuals with multiple moderate to severe cognitive impairments that markedly disturb everyday functioning, and almost always render the person incapable of living independently. Most HIV-infected persons who suffer from neurocognitive disorders have ANI or MND.

HIV-associated neuropsychological deficits reflect widespread synaptodendritic injury, particularly in *FSTC circuits* (q.v.) and other parts of the brain that govern executive functions.

Memory disturbances tend to be in components of learning new information such as maintaining information in working memory and encoding, rather than accelerated forgetting. *Prospective memory* (q.v.) might also be affected.

**HMO** *Health maintenance organization*; an organized health care delivery system combining health care services with a prepaid fixed group rate. The HMO contracts to provide its enrolled members with comprehensive health care services for a fixed period (usually 1 year), in return for fixed premiums (usually payable monthly).

**HNPP** Hereditary neuropathy with liability to pressure palsies; familial recurrent polyneuropathy; tomaculous neuropathy; an autosomal dominant, demyelinating peripheral neuropathy. Like *Charcot-Marie-Tooth disease* (q.v.), HNPP has been mapped to chromosome 17.

HNPP is manifested in periodic episodes of numbness, muscular weakness, atrophy, and sometimes palsies that follow relatively minor compression or trauma to the peripheral nerves. Carpal tunnel syndrome and other entrapment neuropathies are also frequent.

**hoarding** The practice of collecting any number of objects, generally of limited size and of no practical use. Hoarding is seen most commonly in deteriorated schizophrenics, obsessive-compulsive disorder, and in organic cerebral disorders. Hoarding is one of the behavioral manifestations on which an opinion of *incompetency* (q.v.) may be based.

When hoarding leads to neglect of one's home or environment, it is sometimes referred to as the *Diogenes syndrome*. See *collecting mania*.

Hoarding has been reported as a relatively infrequent ritual in subjects with *obsessive-compulsive disorder* (q.v.). Huge quantities of useless and unneeded material are collected, and the patient spends hours in listing, cataloguing, organizing, and sorting the material, which may be so voluminous as to require rental or purchase of storage space. Any attempt by the subject or family members to discard even a part of the "collection" precipitates anxiety (and usually, also, a family argument). See *coprophilia; soteria*.

**hoarding type** See *assimilation*.

**Hoch, August** (1868–1919) American psychiatrist; described shut-in personality.

**Hoch, Paul Henry** (1902–1964) Hungarian-born neuropsychiatrist, emigrated to United States in 1942; somatic treatment, mental hospital administration, community psychiatry.

**Hoche, Alfred** (1865–1945) German psychiatrist; Hoche's tract, or fasciculus septomarginalis: the myelinated descending axons in the lumbar dorsal column near the posterior

septum; in the sacral cord they form a superficial, median triangular zone, the fasciculus triangularis.

**hodophobia** Fear of travel.

**Hoffer, Willi** (1897–1967) Austrian psychoanalyst; fled to London with S. Freud in 1938.

**Hoffmann (or Tromner) sign** (Johann Hoffmann, German neurologist, 1857–1919) In hemiplegia, due to organic brain disease, snapping of the index or ring finger produces flexion of the thumb.

**holding environment** A term introduced by Winnicott to refer to all nurturing aspects of the child's milieu, including actual physical holding and the mother's preoccupation with the infant. See *holding-soothing introject*.

Psychotherapy provides a holding environment by giving the patient protection and freedom to examine his or her internal self and to move back and forth between phantasy and reality. The use of medication can be part of a needed holding environment, particularly in the initial management phase when the disturbed or regressed patient is unable to tolerate an approach that is confined to dealing interpretively with transference and resistance.

**holding-soothing introject** The complex mnemonic-eidetic-affective endopsychic structure that underlies the growing child's object constancy and promotes a feeling of being soothingly held. Holding-soothing introjects reflect positive experiences with nurturant caretakers (good objects). See *container*.

In early infancy, two types of relatedness to the mother coexist: the relationship to the mother as *holding environment*, and the relationship to the mother as object. The former aspect of relatedness far outweighs the latter until *object constancy* develops, at about 18 months of age. Object constancy, the ability to perceive objects as having an existence of their own and also to summon the memory of the mother as a comforting, tension-easing other, depends in large part on evocative memory. See *borderline personality; empathic failure; object relations theory*.

**holergasia** A psychiatric disorder of such a nature as to involve the *whole* person. For example, schizophrenia and manic-depressive psychosis ordinarily are associated with a disorganization of the entire personality, and the syndromes are therefore known as holergastic reactions.

**holiday syndrome** Sadness, anxiety, or other emotional pain—reflected in increased rates of suicide, hospital admissions, and deaths in automobile accidents—occurring during the period between Thanksgiving and New Year's Day. The syndrome appears to be an expression of unmet dependency needs triggered by the reminiscing and loving aspects of the holiday season.

**holism** *Gestalt totality*; the thesis that the study of parts cannot explain the whole, because the whole is something different from the simple summation of its parts. The application of the holistic principle to the study of human beings has far-reaching implications. There are several sciences relating to the person, but no science of the person in its totality. From a holistic point of view, the human being is more than a mere aggregation of physiological, psychological, and social functions: the person as a whole has attributes that cannot be explained by the attributes of its constituent parts.

Adler particularly emphasized the need for the holistic approach in the understanding of personality; recognizing that the whole person cannot be understood by an analysis or dissection of his parts, he emphasized that he could be understood in terms of the goals he sets for himself and toward which he moves.

**holistic healing** A system of health care based upon the theory that health is the result of the body, mind, and spirit in harmony and that stress—whether from physical agents or social or psychological pressures—is the enemy of good health. Because a person's reaction to stress depends upon his perception of the world, which in turn is determined by his belief system, healing efforts must be directed toward eliminating the patient's self-limiting thoughts, distorted ideas, negative self-images, and other programmed attitudes that have disturbed the balance and harmony requisite for normal functioning. Self-direction, self-regulation, and self-actualization are important elements in achieving the inner balance essential for health. See *cognitive behavior therapy; complementary medicine.*

**holistic psychology** *Humanistic psychology* (q.v.).

**hollow skull sign** See *brain death.*

**Holmgren test** (Alarik Fritniof Holmgren, Swedish physiologist, 1831–97) A test for color blindness, which requires the subject to match skeins of different-colored yarn with standard skeins.

**holograph** A document in the handwriting of the purported author. Paulina Kernberg uses the term *holographic man* to refer to the patient who creates, in the diagnostic interviews, a vague, nebulous image of himself that is disconnected from present reality and actual past; the image changes from moment to moment as the analyst explores different aspects of the history. As a result, the diagnostician has a sense of unreality about the interaction, feeling unable to center on any concrete issue.

**holophrastic** Expressing a complex of ideas in a single word, as in some primitive languages that require a completely new word for any slight change in the total situation. Schizophrenics, who typically demonstrate a reduction in their connotation ability and a relative overemphasis on denotation, can be described as manifesting holophrastic association defects. See *connotation.*

**holoprosencephaly** Failure of the forebrain (prosencephalon) to differentiate into two cerebral hemispheres and diencephalon. It includes a wide range of phenotypes of varying severity. The brain is not subdivided into hemispheres and the olfactory bulbs are missing. Depending upon severity of the malformation, facial features may include short or absent nose, cleft upper lip, or a single eye located in the center (*cyclopia*). Holoprosencephaly may be due to genetic factors or to teratogens such as alcohol or retinoic acid.

**homatropine** An anticholinergic drug. See *cholinergic.*

**Homburger, August** (1873–1930) German psychiatrist; psychopathology of children.

**home, loveless** From the standpoint of mental hygiene, homes in which an inharmonious atmosphere prevails as the result of constant discord among the members of the family, and where the children are made buffers between quarreling parents who have "fallen out of love." This is the type of surrounding that breeds delinquency. In these loveless homes the children are constantly exposed to traumatic experiences that have a definite influence in the development of neuroses and other mental disturbances. Such loveless homes have a much greater deleterious effect upon the children's mental development than have broken homes, which seem to play a rather secondary role in this respect (Seliger, R.V. et al. *Contemporary Criminal Hygiene*, 1946).

**homebound**  Unable to leave one's residence. It appears as a symptom related to any of several psychiatric disorders: in depression, when the subject feels too exhausted to get out of bed; in schizophrenia, as part of a general withdrawal from reality and interpersonal contacts; in agoraphobia and panic disorder, to avoid triggering a panic attack; in delusional disorder, to avoid imagined persecutors. See *agoraphobia*.

**homeopathic principle**  See *isopathic principle*.

**homeostasis**  The status quo; the tendency of an organism to maintain a constancy and stability of its internal environment; the result of the various autonomic mechanisms that adjust and adapt the body as a whole to changes in the external or internal environment. Homeostasis is Cannon's term for a steady, balanced, internal constitution ("wisdom of the body"). Claude Bernard called it milieu interieur; Raup called it the principle of complacency. In general, rapid adjustments are made by the autonomic nervous system, while slower adjustments occur through chemical and hormonal influences. See *complacencey principle*.

**homeostatic equilibrium**  See *aim of instinct*.

**homeostatic index**  Any measure of the capacity to resist alteration of the status quo; the higher the homeostatic index, the more rapidly will an organism recover from any disturbing situation and return to normal balance.

**homeostenosis**  Inflexibility or narrowed range of homeostatic ranges available to an organism, characteristic of the aged and one of the factors that predisposes them to multiple disorders and to prolongation of any disorder they develop as compared with younger people.

**Homer proteins**  Scaffolding proteins that exist in complexes with metabotropic glutamate receptors (mGluRs). The gene encoding Homer proteins may play a key role in cocaine addiction. In mice, lack of *Homer2* mimics many aspects of the sensitization seen with withdrawal from repeated cocaine administration.

**homesickness**  An acute separation syndrome appearing in dependent persons when for any reasons they are removed from their usual sources of dependency gratification. See *separation anxiety*.

**homichlophobia**  Fear of fog.

**Homicidal Behaviors Survey**  *HBS*; a self-rating instrument consisting of 12 questions designed to help in assessing the presence of current or past violent/homicidal behaviors.

**homicidal mania**  *Obs. Homicidomania*. Any kind of mental disease where there is an attempt or desire on the part of a patient to kill.

**homicide**  The killing of one person by another. Legally, homicide is often divided into *murder* (premeditated homicide, killing with malice aforethought), *manslaughter*, and *infanticide*. Clinically, homicide is traditionally subdivided into a "normal" or nonpsychiatric group, and an "abnormal" group in which there is an associated psychiatric disorder.

Infanticide and murder-suicide (the person kills another and then kills himself or herself) are almost always in the abnormal group. Males are six to nine times as likely as females to kill. Homicide by women usually falls into the abnormal group, and *infanticide* (q.v.) is the most frequent form in women. Younger women tend to kill their children; older women, their spouses.

Normal homicide is twice as frequent as abnormal homicide; it is most often committed by young males, and victims are most likely to be family members or close acquaintances. Abnormal homicide tends to be committed by older people, and victims are usually family members. Probably the most frequently associated psychiatric disorder is depression; schizophrenia, especially of the paranoid type, alcoholism, and personality disorders have also been reported. See *victim*.

*Sexual homicide* refers to killing associated with a sexual offense.Sometimes it is a result of panic triggered by events surrounding the sexual offense. In other cases it is a *lust murder*—a form of *sadism* (q.v.), typically committed by a shy, introspective, inadequate man with an enduring pattern of sexual arousal to bizarre phantasies involving killing and cruelty. In contrast to other types of homicide, of which almost 60% are committed with firearms and only 2% by strangulation, strangulation is the method preferred by sexual killers.

**homicidophilia**  *Erotophonophilia* (q.v.).

**homilopathy**  Kraepelin's term for disease due to mental induction, including persecution mania of the deaf.

**homilophobia**  Fear of sermons; also, fear that in a group of people the others in the group might find something wrong with one's appearance, attire, or demeanor. See *agoraphobia*.

**homo-**  Combining form meaning one and the same, common, from Gr. *homos*; opposed to hetero-.

**homoclite**  See *heteroclite*.

**homocystinuria**  An inborn error of metabolism, transmitted as an autosomal recessive, associated with mental retardation and characterized by excretion of moderate amounts of the essential amino acid methionine and of an abnormal amino acid, l-homocystine, in the urine. The syndrome was first reported in 1962.

Clinical features include skeletal abnormalities similar to Marfan syndrome (pigeon breast or chicken breast), joint enlargement, fine and fair hair, and ectopia lentia. It may be associated with thromboembolic episodes.

**homoerotic**  Relating to or manifesting the erotic or libidinal instinct toward one of the same sex.

**homoerotism, homeroticism**  A general term for the objectivation of erotic or libidinal interests upon a member of the same sex. The impulse is subject to all the modifications of erotic impulses. It may be directly expressed (homogenitality); it may be sublimated (homoerotism or *homosexuality*, q.v.); it may be severely repressed; if so, the impulses may be subjected to reaction-formation, that is, they may appear as aversions against the homerotism; or they may be transferred into reality in symbolic form (delusions, hallucinations, etc.).

*Homoeroticism* is a phase in the development of object relationships (see *ontogeny, psychic*), and the term is generally applied to that period following the oedipal phase and lasting until adolescence, when libidinal energies are repressed and aggressive energies are redirected into elaborating a more effective web of defenses, including the superego, and into increasing mastery in the social sphere, in socially condoned and desirable competitiveness, conquest, and domination. See *latency*.

**homogamy**  In contrast to *panmixia*, this genetic term applies to the inbreeding conditions in isolated population groups composed of organisms with the same hereditary characteristics.

**homogeneity, homogeny**  Identical genotypical structure of two or more organisms of common descent, as found in the case of pure lines or in monozygotic twins.

**homogenic love**  Homosexuality. See *gay*.

**homogenitality**  Interest in the genitals of one's own sex. See *homosexuality*.

**homologous**  Referring to gene units that belong to the same pairs of *homologues*. See *allele*.

Homologous indicates similarity on the basis of shared ancestry, whereas analogous indicates similarity that is not genetically determined but has occurred by chance or through other mechanisms. The Schnauzkrampf of the catatonic is analogous to the snout of a pig, not homologous.

**homologue**  Evolutionary counterpart.

**homology**  In comparative biology, similarity based on common descent. See *allometry; analogy*.

**homonym**  A word that has same sound as another, even though the two words differ in meaning and often in spelling as well; *agnomenatio, homophone*, and *paranomasia* are approximate equivalents. Examples are here and hear, there and their. Ordinarily the listener is able to grasp the intended meaning of what is said because of the context in which it occurs.

In various conditions that interfere with attention and concentration, including manic states and organic confusional states, the subject fails to grasp the intended meaning, however, and any misinterpretation of the environment may be based on the more familiar meaning of the homonym. Thus the delirious child may believe that the Lord's prayer includes the phrase "Harold be thy name" rather than "hallowed be thy name." See *clang association*.

**homonymous hemianopsia**  See *field defect*.

**homonymous quadrantic field defect**  See *field defect*.

**homophile**  A lover of one's own kind; a gay person; specifically, a homosexual, and a term used especially by organizations that purport or attempt to represent homosexuals as a group. See *homosexuality*.

**homophily**  The theory that people seek out those similar to themselves; in the case of children, the theory receives support from the observation that exposure to deviant peers leads to increases in antisocial behavior, especially among those children who are psychologically susceptible to peer pressure.

**homophobia** Negative attitudes to homo-sexuals and homosexuality, reflecting both conscious and unconscious fears and reactions. Homophobia includes not only irrational and persistent fear of homosexuality (often manifested in extreme rage reactions to homosexuals—*gay-bashing*), but also the self-hatred experienced by gay men and women because of their homosexuality. Religious and other cultural taboos against homosexuality are a part of early learning and are reinforced by experience. They may be used unconsciously in denying one's own impulses, and successful denial, reaction formation, and other defenses are often rewarded by the environment. This in turn tends to perpetuate and intensify the defense so that the prejudice and discrimination against persons perceived to be of a homosexual orientation become increasingly entrenched or even ineradicable. As with sexism and racism, homophobia is frequently expressed in humor based on negative stereotypes (e.g., the effeminate male hairdresser or ballet dancer, the masculine female athlete or executive). The homophobic attitudes of gay people themselves may perpetuate such negative stereotypes.

**homophone** See *homonym*.

**homoplasmy** Presence of either wild-type (normal) or mutant genes and their products, but not the coexistence of both types (which is termed heteroplasmy). See *mitochondrial disorders*.

**homosexual** Relating to or directed toward one of the same sex.

**homosexual panic** An acute, severe episode of anxiety related to the fear (or the delusional conviction) that the subject is about to be attacked sexually by another person of the same sex, or that he is thought to be a homosexual by fellow workers, etc. First described by Kempf in 1920 and hence sometimes known as *Kempf disease*; symptoms include agitation, ideas or delusions of reference, conscious guilt over homosexual activity, hallucinations, ideas and threats of suicide, depression, and often perplexity. The panic state is typically precipitated by loss or separation from a member of the same sex to whom the subject is emotionally attached, or by fatigue, illness, fears of impotence, failures in sex performance, homesickness, etc. It may appear as the first acute episode in schizophrenic disorders, and it is more frequent in males than in females.

Sometimes, instead of overt sexual material, the anxiety is related to fears of undue malignant influence, physical violence, or impending death. Such an episode is termed *acute aggression panic*.

**homosexuality** Sexual orientation characterized by erotic attraction to others of the same sex; "contrary sexual"; feelings of love, emotional attachment, or sexual attraction to persons of one's own gender and/or sexual behavior with a person of the same sex. Homosexuality usually appears first in childhood and develops in adolescence and throughout adulthood.

Data on the frequency of homosexuality vary considerably and are marred by problems of definition as well as by the social stigma that prevents many subjects from identifying themselves in research samples. Hirschfeld (1920) estimated its incidence at 2% to 3%, Havelock Ellis (1936) at 2% to 5%, and Kinsey (1948) found that 4% of the white male population, 2% to 6% of unmarried women, and less than 1% of married women are exlusively homosexual. Including the predominantly homosexual, the bisexual, and the occasional homosexual obviously would add substantially to those figures, but it would seem that the commonly accepted figure of 10% of the general population is high, except perhaps in some cities. In the 1990s, the National Health and Social Life Survey in the United States, and similar British and French surveys, found that 2.8% of the males and 1.4% of the females identify themselves as homosexual, 4.9% and 4.1% report having had a same-gender partner since age 18, and 4.4% and 5.6% report that same-gender sex is "very appealing." Other data indicate that the incidence of male-male sexual activity since age 18 is 16.4% in the 12 largest cities surveyed; residents of those cities would correctly perceive that more than 5% of the male population is gay.

Cross-cultural studies have found homosexuality in all world regions, in all types of economies, settlement patterns, family and household types, and economic exchange systems.

Homosexuality is considered a nonpathological variant of human sexuality. DSM-III-R did not include the category *ego-dystonic homosexuality*, which was used in DSM-III to denote a sustained pattern of overt sexual arousal in a person who complained explicitly that such responses were unwanted and a source of distress. Further, the person so diagnosed wanted to acquire or increase heterosexual responsivity so that heterosexual relations could be initiated or maintained. In clinical practice, the term was almost never used, and it was therefore deleted from the 1987 revision.

Although most homosexuals engage in sexual activity, genital sexual behavior is by no means an absolute predictor or sign of sexual orientation.

Sexual behavior is not always congruent with sexual desire, patterns of sexual behavior fluctuate during a person's life, and behavior may be inhibited by intrapsychic conflict, societal pressures, or both. Heterosexuality and homosexuality are not dichotomous. For both heterosexual and homosexual persons, early sexual behavior (in childhood or adolescence) may be congruent or incongruent with the direction of adult sexual expression.

Some authors differentiate between overt homosexuality (physical sexual contact) and latent homosexuality (unrecognized or unconscious attraction, or recognized ideas and impulses not openly expressed). A less frequent subdivision is into *homogenitality* (genital sexuality), homosexuality (preference, phantasies, impulses without genital activity with another of the same sex), and *homoeroticism* ("well-sublimated" attraction or preference expressed in other than specifically genital or sexual activities).

Sexual brain organization is dependent on sex hormone and neurotransmitter levels occurring during critical developmental periods of the brain. Attempts to locate a "gay gene" or to correlate sexual preference with variations in brain anatomy (e.g., in various nuclei of the anterior hypothalamus and adjacent limbic area) or hormone levels (e.g., prenatal androgen excess or deficiency) have not been convincing, however. Both male and female homosexuality show a moderate degree of heritability. Higher concordance rates for homosexuality in monozygotic than in dizygotic twins, coupled with increased rates in biological siblings, suggest heritability, but the extent to which heritable factors underlie homosexuality remains an open question.

In general, the term "inversion" is equivalent to homosexuality. When "sex-role inversion" is used, however, it must be differentiatedfrom homosexuality. Homosexuality refers to sexual desires or activitybetween members of the same sex; sex-role inversion refers to adoption of the sex role and introjection of the psychologic identity of the opposite sex. The two may coexist, but more frequently one or the other is present alone. See *bisexuality*.

**homosexuality, female** A female's sexual orientation characterized by erotic attraction for, or behavior with, one or more other females, including emotional attachments, phantasies, desires, impulses, and sexual or genital contact. Female homosexuality is often referred to as lesbian or sapphic, after the isle of Lesbos, home of the classic Greek poet Sappho, who wrote of her erotic attachments to women. Since the 1960s, homosexual females have often preferred to be identified as lesbian, considering it less judgmental that "homosexual." The most common sexual activities in lesbian sex are stroking and massaging of the clitoris, stroking and massage of the breasts, licking and sucking of nipples, oral sex, and the pressing and rubbing together of the genitals (least common). The orgasm "success rate" is about twice as great if a women is stimulated by another woman, rather than by a man (Baker, R. *Sperm Wars*. New York: Basic Books, 1996). See *homosexuality*.

**homosexuality, latent** Sometimes used interchangeably with unconscious *homosexuality* (q.v.).

**homosexuality, male** A male's sexual orientation characterized by erotic attraction for, or behavior with, one or more other males; a male whose sexual phantasies are exclusively or nearly exclusively of others of the same sex. There may be men who are homosexual but unaware of their sexual orientation because of repression or denial of their phantasies. There are also some homosexual men who are conscious of their phantasies and sexual arousal patterns but cannot acknowledge their homosexuality because of social pressures or intrapsychic conflict.

*Homosexuality* (q.v.) has been reported in all cultures studied, and most men are capable of homosexual behavior. Incidental homosexuality, the choice of another man as sexual object when no women are available (*faute de mieux*), may occur in same-sex schools, the military, and prisons, even though homosexuality may not be the primary sexual orientation of the participants.

Since the late 1960s, homosexual males have often preferred to be identified as *gay* (q.v.), considering it less pejorative and judgmental than "homosexual."

Freud hypothesized at one time or another that fear of castration, intense oedipal attachment to the mother, narcissism, narcissistic object choice, and sibling rivalry with overcompensatory love for the rival were significant etiologic factors in male homosexuality. None of these hypotheses, however, proved to be of much value in the therapy of gay men. There is increasing suggestive evidence that male homosexuality, like heterosexuality, has a genetic or constitutional basis. F. J. Kallmann (*Heredity in Health and Mental Disorder*, 1953) long ago presented evidence of a genetic basis of homosexuality based on twin studies. Although these studies were flawed by methodological error, more recent reports support his conclusion and find (1) a significantly greater concordance of homosexual behavior in monozygotic than in dizygotic twins and (2) a significantly higher percentage of homosexual or bisexual brothers of gay men than of heterosexual men.

The view that homosexual object choice is determined by conflict evolving from faulty parenting (such as a close binding mother or a distant father) is not supported by recent observation, nor do psychological tests support the view that homosexuals are more disturbed psychologically than heterosexuals.

A clinical approach based on the theory that homosexuals must change their sexual orientation in order to live healthy and productive lives has proved to be harmful to the psychological well-being of homosexual men. Current approaches to gay men with concerns about sexual orientation are directed to internalized *homophobia* (q.v.), supporting a positive view of the self, and exploring other issues that affect self-esteem (Cabaj, R. P. *Journal of Homosexuality 15*, 1987; Isay, R. A. in *Contemporary Perspectives on Psychotherapy with Lesbians and Gay Men*, ed. T. Stein & C. J. Cohen, 1986).

In the United States and Europe, about 6% of men experience homosexual contact during their lifetimes, most often during adolescence. Over 80% of men who will ever show homosexual behavior have done so by the time they are 15 years of age, 98% by the time they are 20. For two-thirds of these men, the contact is genital, often involving anal intercourse. The majority of men who have sex with men (MSM) are bisexual; 80% also have sex with women (Baker, R. *Sperm Wars*. New York: Basic Books, 1996). See *bisexuality.*

**homosexuality, masked**   Unconscious homosexual impulses. For example, a married man, complaining that his wife was frigid, insisted on having solely anal intercourse with her, since this was much more gratifying to him than genital relations. The unique pleasure found exclusively in anal contact represented his masked homosexuality.

**homosociality**   A term coined by J. C. Fluegel to denote social relationship between members of the same sex.

**homosynaptic depression**   See *habituation.*

**homosynaptic plasticity**   A form of *synaptic plasticity* (q.v.).

**homozygocity**   *Homozygousness* (q.v.).

**homozygote**   A zygotic organism produced by the union of two similar gametes and therefore possessing two like genes of a given factor pair.

In the case of *recessive* mendelian inheritance, a hereditary character can be manifested only by those offspring who have inherited its predisposing factor from both parents and thus are homozygous for the character in question.

**homozygousness**   *Obs. Homozygosity; homozygocity*; the "germinally pure" condition of a person who inherits the same gene factor from each parent, so that in his organism the two genes of the given pair are *alike.*

Homozygousness of a dominant anomaly is very rare, as it can be assumed only when both parents of a diseased person are also patients. In the case of a recessive anomaly that can only appear in the phenotype of a homozygote, all trait carriers must be homozygotes. Consequently, the occurrence of such a recessive anomaly is not possible, unless both parents are either homozygotes or heterozygotes for the anomaly in question. See *recessiveness.*

Certain deleterious effects of inbreeding are now assumed to be due chiefly to the attainment of homozygousness rather than merely to the process of inbreeding itself. The frequent mating of persons closely related in descent must automatically result in a reduction of *heterozygosity* unless new mutations occur in these inbred lines. If the mutation rate is high, this may defer or prevent the attainment of homozygousness. See *heterosis; inbreeding.*

**Hoover sign** (Charles F. Hoover, American physician, 1865–1927)

Observed in organic hemiplegia and used for differentiating organic from hysteric hemiplegia; if the patient, lying on his back, attempts to raise the paretic leg, he unconsciously presses down forcibly the heel of the healthy leg; this accentuation does not occur in hysteria.

**Hopkins symptom checklist** *SCL-90-R* (q.v.).

**horizontal transmission** See *transmission, vertical.*

**horme** *Libido* (q.v.).

**hormephobia** Fear of shock.

**hormesis** A process in which exposure of a cell or organism to a sublethal level of stress increases the resistance of that cell or organism to a subsequent higher and otherwise lethal level of the same or different stress.

**hormism** Used by the school of psychology that holds that goals are sought for their own sake because of some intrinsic value, regardless of any pleasure attendant upon their attainment. McDougall believed that in humans and animals there are certain tendencies or urges that account for all forms of behavior, including abstract mental processes. Each tendency leads to a definite end or purpose. Hormism is thus opposed to hedonism, which states that goals are sought only because they give pleasure or gratification to the person. See *hedonism.*

**hormone** A chemical messenger produced by a tissue or organ that regulates or modulates the activity of another tissue or organ. See *neurohormone.*

**Horner syndrome** (Johann Friedrich Horner, Swiss ophthalmologist, 1831–1886) Caused by paralysis of the cervical sympathetic nerve, this condition has the following signs and symptoms: (1) miosis, (2) enophthalmos, (3) pseudoptosis, (4) occasionally ipsilateral vasodilatation and anhydrosis on the side of the face and neck.

**Horney, Karen** (1885–1952) Psychoanalyst and founder of the Association for the Advancement of Psychoanalysis (the Horney school of holistic psychology); female psychology, actual self, self-realization, basic anxiety;

*The Neurotic Personality of Our Time* (1937), *New Ways in Psychoanalysis* (1939). Horney was born in Germany and was a neurologist before she became associated with the Berlin Psychoanalytical Institute under the influence of Karl Abraham. She ultimately broke with Freud over his androcentric conception of female psychology; he viewed penis envy, for example, as a recognition of biological fact, while she viewed it as a screen for other early losses or developmental failures. She came to the United States in 1932 and was first with the Chicago Institute for Psychoanalysis, and then with the New York Psychoanalytic Institute until she formed her own Association.

**horror feminae** *Obs.* "The essential feature of this strange manifestation of the sexual life is the want of sexual sensibility for the opposite sex, even to the extent of horror, while sexual inclination and impulse toward the same sex are present" (Krafft-Ebing, R. v. *Psychopathia Sexualis,* 1908).

**horrors** *Delirium tremens* (q.v.).

**Horton syndrome** (Bayard T. Horton, contemporary American physician) See *histamine.*

**hospice** A program of care for the dying, a place where such care is provided, or both. The hospice movement has developed in recognition of the fact that there comes a point in medical care when cure is no longer a real possibility and attention must be directed toward comforting patients and families.

**hospital, day or night** See *day hospital.*

**hospital hoboes** See *Munchhausen syndrome.*

**hospitalism** See *anaclitic depression.*

**hospitalitis** A humorous term coined to emphasize the complete hospital conditioning (or dependency on the hospital) of a patient who is usually an utterly helpless or incompetent person before his admission to the hospital. It may be difficult for him to leave the hospital, and each attempt to prepare the patient for discharge results in an aggravation of symptoms. Also called *sanatorium disease.*

**host mother** See *surrogate mother.*

**host personality** Also, presenting or primary personality; in dissociative identity disorder, the alter that is in executive control most of the time.

**hostel** Lodging place, such as an inn; in psychiatry the term includes short-stay hostels, such as *halfway houses* and other rehabilitation units, and long-stay hostels, for patients who are unlikely to improve further but who do not require the intensive level of care provided in a hospital or nursing home.

**hostile aggression**   See *aggression*.

**hostile environment harassment**   See *harassment, sexual*.

**housebound**   Unable to leave one's residence. It appears as a symptom related to any of several psychiatric disorders: in depression, when the subject feels too exhausted to get out of bed; in schizophrenia, as part of a general withdrawal from reality and interpersonal contacts; in *agoraphobia* and *panic disorder* (qq.v.), to avoid triggering a panic attack; in delusional disorder, to avoid imagined persecutors.

**House-Tree-Person (HTP) test**   A type of projective test in which the subject is asked to draw a house, a tree, and a person.

**housewife's neurosis**   Also called *housewife's psychosis*; an obsessive-compulsive disorder characterized by constant preoccupation with cleaning house. Though justified by the patient, who explains that these exaggerated domestic activities are necessary in view of the danger inherent in the lack of hygiene in the place where she lives, in reality they disguise obsessive ideas concealed by the patient. According to Stekel, the inner "compulsions are covered up for many years until the decrease of the patient's working capacity, or the danger of complete isolation force the patient to confess her illness to other people" (*Compulsion and Doubt*, 1949). This is often the personality type of the woman who later develops an involutional psychosis.

More recently, the term *housewife's disease* or *housewife's syndrome* has been applied to a state of acute or chronic dissatisfaction and frustration that appears in some women as a type of mental stagnation secondary to marriage, motherhood, and separation from the stimulation of employment and free movement among people. Typical symptoms are loss of libido and fatigability at age 24–30, backache at age 30–35, and general somatic overconcern at age 40–55.

**housing instability**   Includes living in a shelter or runaway facility, having been asked to leave home, self-identifying as currently "homeless," or describing other related experiences, such as sleeping on the streets, in a park, on a subway train, or in an abandoned building.

**hovering tremor**   An early sign of Parkinson disease that often precedes the full-blown condition by several years, consisting of a fine tremor of the hand and fingers with 3 to 6 beats/sec that appears when the subject is asked to salute without resting his hand against his temple.

**HP1**   See *heterochromatin*.

**HPA axis**   *Hypothalamic-pituitary-adrenal axis* (q.v.).

**HPT**   *Hypothalamic-pituitary-thyroid axis*. See *hypothalamic-pituitary-adrenal axis*.

**HRB**   *Halstead-Reitan Battery* (q.v.).

**HRQoL**   Health-related quality of life.

**HSCL**   The Hopkins Symptom Checklist, a self-report inventory consisting of 58 items that are representative of the symptom patterns common in outpatients, including somatization, obsessive-compulsive, interpersonal sensitivity, anxiety, and depressive symptoms.

**HSCS**   High Sensitivity Cognitive Screen; an interview-based test that examines various cognitive domains, including memory, language, attention and concentration, visual and motor skills, spatial perception, and self-regulation and executive functioning. See *cognitive screening instruments*.

**Hsieh-Ping**   A culture-specific trancelike state, seen in Taiwan, characterized by tremor, disorientation, delirium, and ancestor identification, and often accompanied by visual or auditory hallucinations. The seizure may last from 30 minutes to several hours.

**HTLV-III**   Human T-cell leukemia virus, type III. See *AIDS; HIV*.

**HTP**   *House-Tree-Person test* (q.v.).

**5-HTP**   5-hydroxytryptophan, a *serotonin* precursor (q.v).

**Htt**   *Huntingtin*, the protein encoded by the gene that is mutated in *Huntington disease* (q.v.).

**5-HTTLPR**   A biallelic polymorphism located in the promoter region of the *SLC6A4* serotonin transporter gene, with short *(s)* and long *(l)* alleles that differ in size by 44 nucleotides. The l form provides for greater transcription and function of the serotonin transporter, resulting in less synaptic serotonin. SSRIs are believed to exert their effects through inhibition of the serotonin transporter, thereby increasing synaptic serotonin.

Individuals carrying the *s* allele are slightly more likely to display abnormal levels of anxiety, acquire conditioned fear responses, to develop bipolar disorder, and to manifest suicidal behavior compared with those homozygous for the *l* allele. Abnormal fear conditioning, a phenomenon dependent on the amygdala, is associated with 5-HTT function, suggesting that this structure mediates the effects of 5-HT on emotional behavior. The increased anxiety and fear associated with the *s* allele may reflect hyperresponsiveness of the amygdala to relevant environmental stimuli. The *s* allele is associated with numerous childhood psychiatric disorders and traits such as childhood-onset depression, aggression, ADHD in males, and with phenotypic traits directly relevant to autism, such as neuroticism, childhood shyness, and symptom severity and amygdala excitability in social phobia.

Gene polymorphism of the serotonin metabolizing enzyme, *tryptophan hydroxylase*, has also been linked to suicidal behaviors.

**Hu syndrome** *Paraneoplastic encephalomyelopathy/sensory neuropathy syndrome*; a set of neurological degenerative symptoms that occur as single or multifocal disorders. Neurological dysfunction is most often localized to dorsal root ganglia (in ca. 60% of patients) but may also appear in the cerebellum, brain stem, or limbic, motor, or autonomic nervous systems. There is a possibility that Hu proteins participate in splicing regulation in neurons in addition to their suggested role in the early development of postmitotic neurons.

**Hübner, Arthur** (1878–1949) German forensic psychiatrist.

**huffing** Deliberate inhalation of organic solvents to achieve a euphoric sensation or high. Like glue-sniffing, the procedure is habituating and is typically repeated at 5- to 15-minute intervals for hours. Also like glue-sniffing, the habit may produce severe damage to the nervous system, most commonly in the form of peripheral neuropathy.

**Human Genome Project** *HGP*; the aims are to sequence the genomes of the human and selected model organisms, identify all the genes, and develop the technologies requires to accomplish these objectives. See *genomics*.

**human potential** See *humanistic psychology*.

**human relations group** *T-group* (q.v.).

**human services care** See *care*.

**human surrogate** Euphemism for corpse or for a portion of a dead body.

**humanistic psychology** *Holistic psychology*; an orientation that rejects both the quantitative reductionism of behaviorism and the psychoanalytic emphasis on unconscious forces in favor of a view of man as uniquely creative and controlled by his own values and choices. Through experiential means, each person can develop his greatest potential, or *self-actualization*. Humanistic psychology is related to the *human potential* movement and its encounter groups, growth centers, sensitivity training, etc. See *mental health*.

Humanistic psychology is related to and draws from group dynamics, *existentialism* (q.v.), the person-centered approach in counseling (with its emphasis on expressing the self and also taking responsibility for one's actions), Jung's individuation as a process of achieving selfhood, and Asian philosophies with emphasis on meditation, body awareness, and peak experiences.

**humiliation** Feeling of being disgraced, shamed, debased, or ignominiously dishonored; it may represent a frustration of narcissistic aspirations and disapproval or punishment by the superego. Such feelings are frequent concomitants to the dejection of clinically depressed patients (loss of self-esteem). Provocation of others into actions that appear to warrant feelings of humiliation is seen often in *masochism* (q.v.). See *shame*.

Humiliation is also an act of debasing another. It is used by aggressors and oppressors to control their victims or subjects, by evoking feelings of inferiority, guilt, and absolute worthlessness. The traumatized victims feel sadness and despair on the one hand, and anger and revenge on the other.

**humor** Sometimes used as a defense against stress or conflict; it consists of emphasizing the amusing or ironic aspects of the conflict.

**humoral phototransduction hypothesis** The theory that light of sufficient intensity, falling on a vascular surface, sets in motion a process by which neuroactive gases transported in and regulated by blood-borne photoreceptors (for example, hemoglobin in erythrocytes) act in concert with melatonin or other antioxiants to shift the phase of the *circadian clock* (q.v.).

Timed bright light exposure is an effective treatment for sleep and circadian rhythm disorders, including jet lag, shift work sleep disturbance, age-related insomnia, and advance- and delayed-sleep phase syndromes. The largest shifts in rhythm, both advances and delays, occur at times during which people are usually asleep. If extraocular light exposure were effective, it would be possible to design more practicable treatment measures. But attempts to show that the human circadian response to light can be mediated through an extraocular route (such as the popliteal region) have not, in general, been effective.

**hunger, nervous** Urge to eat (orally incorporate) as a method of allaying anxiety or tension and of gratifying frustrated pleasure cravings. Obesity is frequently the secondary symptomatic result of such chronic and intense nervous hunger. Nervous hunger is an expression of intense dependence and stems back to the oral incorporative stage of infantile development.

Food addiction and cigarette addiction are closely related phenomena. Thumb-sucking, which is closely related to the use of pacifiers in infancy, with the thumb replacing the pacifier, is an early infantile prototype of nervous hunger. See *eating disorders.*

**hunger center** See *hypothalamus.*

**hunger strike, neurotic** Adler thus denotes the fear of eating, occurring mainly in females at about age of 17. There follows usually a rapid decrease in weight. The goal, to be inferred from the whole attitude of the patient, is the rejection of the female role. See *anorexia nervosa.*

**Hunt syndrome** Dyssynergia cerebellaris myoclonica, a syndrome characterized by myoclonic crises, cerebellar ataxia and dysarthria, and, usually, epileptic seizures.

**Hunter syndrome** A *mucopolysaccharidosis* (q.v.) characterized by a sex-linked (rather than autosomal) deficiency of sulfoiduronide sulfatase enzyme, with excessive dermatan sulfate and heparan sulfate in the urine. There is no clouding of the cornea, but in the more severe form death occurs usually by the age of 15 years; in the mild form, patients survive to the 30s or even 50s.

**huntingtin** A gene ubiquitously expressed both in and outside CNS, with its highest concentrations in CNS neurons and the testes. A mutation of the gene consisting of an expanded CAG tract of more that 35 repeats is translated into a corresponding polyglutamine stretch (polyQ) that make spiny neurons in the striatum particularly vulnerable to death; the result of the mutation is *Huntington disease* (q.v.).

*Huntingtin* is essential for establishing and maintaining neuronal identity, especially in cortex and striatum, and it protects against ischemic injury and excitotoxicity, to which cells are made more susceptible by the mutant protein. Normal (wild-type) *huntingtin*, but not the mutant, stimulates production of cortical BDNF (brain-derived neurotrophic factor); the mutated gene may affect the ability of BDNF to reach its striatal targets. All in all, it seems possible that the mutant gene is not solely responsible for the symptoms of Huntington disease; loss of the normal gene may reduce the ability of neurons to survive the toxic effects of the mutant proteins.

**Huntington, George** (1850–1916) American neurologist; hereditary chorea was first described by C. Waters in 1841 and again by Huntington, whose name it was given, in 1872. At that time he noted that he, his father, and his grandfather (all physicians) had observed the disorder in several generations of their patients.

**Huntington chorea** (G. Huntington, U.S. neurologist, 1850–1916) Chronic progressive chorea; adult chorea; currently known as *Huntington disease* (q.v.).

**Huntington disease (HD)** *Huntington chorea,* a rare, autosomal dominant, *polyglutamine disorder* (q.v.), characterized by tremor, chorea, rigidity, bradykinesia, dementia, and progression to death within 15 to 20 years of onset. Each child of an affected parent has a 50% chance of inheriting the disease. Incidence is approximately 6 cases per 100,000 persons in the western hemisphere, and it seems to occur more frequently among whites. It is known to affect about 30,000 persons in the United States.; 150,000 more are at risk. It is particularly rare in Japan and among North American and African blacks. Penetrance, the percentage possessing the gene who actually display the disease, is 100%.

HD is due to the mutation of the IT15 gene and a *triplicate repeat* (q.v.) on the short arm of chromosome 4. The gene encodes the protein, *Huntingtin (Htt).* The pathogenic proteins produced by the mutation aggregate into cytotoxic inclusions in neurons and in neuronal processes. The repeated nucleotide bases are cytosine-adenine-guanine (CAG); normally, the number of repetitions is around 20, whereas HD patients typically show at least 37 repetitions. There is an inverse correlation between the age of onset of HD and the number of repetitions; patients with more than 60 repetitions invariably present with juvenile-onset HD.

Htt is subject to ubiquitination, which normally targets proteins for degradation; in HD, there is reduced ability of Htt to be ubiquitinated and degraded. See *ubiquitin*. Htt is also subject to SUMOylation—covalent attachment of SUMO-1 to lysine residues—and there is evidence that SUMOylation can increase Htt accumulation, decrease aggregate formation (possibly increasing the amount of toxic oligomers), potentially mask a cytoplasmic retention signal, and promote nuclear repression of transcription. *Palmitoylation*, a post-translational protein modification, regulates Htt's normal function, and without palmitoylation the protein becomes cytotoxic.

Although it may appear at any age, average age at time of onset is 35–42 years, with choreic symptoms. *Juvenile HD* has onset of symptoms before the age of 20. When onset is in the 20s, striate rigidity is the most prominent manifestation; in late-onset patients (older than 50), intention tremor is often the most prominent.

Major signs and symptoms may be grouped into the following:

1. *Motor*—involuntary choreic movements (present in 90%); dysarthria (slowed, irregular, staccato speech broken by long silences); dysphagia (which may be expressed as asphyxia, aspiration, or choking); and ideomotor apraxia (apraxia of palpebral movements makes it impossible to open or close the lids). Gait is uncoordinated and interrupted by choreic movements, and postural instability leads to frequent falls.

2. *Other neurologic signs*—urinary or fecal incontinence is common; autonomic dysfunction occurs occasionally, as do convulsions.

3. *Cognitive*—all HD patients eventually develop dementia, characterized by decline of frontal subcortical system functions initially, with relative memory preservation. There is a "sinking pyramid" of memory: first to be lost are the minute details that make events personally unique; as time goes on, more and more of the pyramid sinks. There are difficulties in planning, organizing, and programming activities, functions ascribed to the frontal lobe and its subcortical connections. Insight is lost, disorientation and

inaccessibility increase, and the final picture is one of fatuity uninfluenced by any change in the environment. The pattern of cognitive impairment in the presence of psychopathologic symptoms such as irritability and apathy, and the similarity of the pattern to that observed in PD, supranucelar palsy, and Wilson disease, lead to the designation of HD as a *subcortical dementia* (q.v.).

4. *Psychiatric*—most common are alterations of personality: irritability, apathy, emotional lability, impulsivenesss, and aggressiveness (sometimes justifying a diagnosis of intermittent explosive disorder). Next most common are mood disorders; suicide rate is 4–6 times greater than in the general population, and the rate rises to between 8 and 20 times greater in patients over the age of 50. Schizophreniform psychosis is seen in 6%–25% of patients: paranoid symptoms with delusions of persecution and jealousy, as well as auditory hallucinations, are frequent.

Several clinical variants of HD are recognized:

1. *Westphal variant*, first described in 1883; rigidity is the predominant manifestation. This variant is common in juvenile cases, rare among adults.

2. *Juvenile HD*: clinical manifestations are manifested before the age of 20, typically with alterations of gait and frequent falls. The predominant motor symptom is rigidity (in 60%), often accompanied by pyramidal tract signs (hyperreflexia and extensor responses). Convulsions, which occur in 30–50% of juvenile cases, appear late and are difficult to control. Cerebellar signs, such as dysmetria, dysdiadochokinesia, and intention tremors, are more common in juveniles than in adults.

3. Late-onset cases and those in which the choreic manifestations are extremely discreet are often termed *subchoreatic state*.

The pathology of HD entails progressive degenerative loss of spiny neurons in the caudate and putamen (particularly the cells of the indirect striatopallidal pathway). The result is functional deactivation of the subthalamic nucleus and a decrease in pallidal-thalamic inhibition, which increases thalamic-cortical excitation and generates the choreic movements of HD.

Treatment of HD is symptomatic, with dopaminergic antagonists: phenothiazines, butyrophenones, benzoquinolones, and rauwolfia alkaloids. None of these is particularly superior to any of the others.

**Hurler disease** A *mucopolysaccharidosis* (q.v.) also known as *gargoylism; Pfaundler-Hurler syndrome; dysostosis multiplex; lipochondrodystrophy.* It usually manifests itself in the early months of life, and death usually occurs by the age of 10 years. The child resembles an achondroplastic dwarf and shows multiple skeletal deformities (short neck, dorsal kyphosis, deformed thorax and long bones, flexion deformities of all joints, and maldevelopment of the skull vault and facial bones), hideous features (thickened skin and soft tissues, large head with widely spaced eyes and flattening of the bridge of the nose, coarse lips, protruding tongue, stridulent mouth breathing, and an apathetic, bovine expression), hepatosplenomegaly, corneal clouding, and mental retardation. Several siblings are often affected, but the parents are phenotypically normal; parental consanguinity is frequent. The deficient enzyme is α-l-iduronidase; the urine contains excessive dermatan sulfate and heparan sulfate.

**Hutchinson-Gilford progeria syndrome** HGPS; see *progeria.*

**hwa-byung** Also, wool-hwa-byung; a culture-specific syndrome reported in Korea, consisting of fatigue, panic, a feeling of a mass in the epigastrium, and other somatic symptoms. It is commonly considered to be related to suppressed anger.

**H-Y antigen** Histocompatibility antigen induced by the Y chromosome. It is attached to the surface of (almost all) mammalian male cells, including spermatozoa, and appears to be the determinant for masculinizing the undifferentiated gonadal anlage into testes.

**hybrid** The inbred offspring of two parents who differ with respect to one gene factor or a combination of factors or even belong to different species. In genetics, used also as an adjective. The hybrids that constitute the first filial generation are heterozygotic individuals originating from the cross of parents who carry a given hereditary stock in a pure, unmixed form. When such hybrids differ with respect to only one character, they are called *monohybrid.* When they differ in two characters, they are *dihybrid;* analogously, other hybrids are *trihybrid* or *polyhybrid.*

**hybridization** Genetic term for the process of increasing the variability in a species or group of plants or animals through the production of *hybrids.*

**hybristophilia** (from Gr. *hybridzein,* to commit an outrage against another) A *paraphilia* (q.v.), in which sexual arousal is dependent on the partner being a criminal or known to have committed some heinous act against another. On rare occasion, its expression takes the form of inducing the sexual partner to commit a crime that is almost certain to lead to imprisonment.

**hydro-** Combining form meaning water, hydrogen, from Gr. *hydōr.*

**hydrocephalus** An increase in the volume of cerebrospinal fluid within the skull. If cerebrospinal fluid pressure is normal, the condition is termed *compensatory hydrocephalus,* since the excess fluid compensates for brain atrophy, as in congenital cerebral hypoplasia and in acquired cerebral atrophy due to diffuse sclerosis, general paralysis, and senile or presenile degeneration. If pressure is increased, the condition is termed *hypertensive hydrocephalus,* which may be (1) obstructive, when an obstruction to the circulation of cerebrospinal fluid within the ventricles or at the outlet from the fourth ventricle prevents free communication between the ventricles and the subarachnoid space; or (2) communicating, when communication between ventricles and subarachnoid space is free and hydrocephalus is due to increased fluid formation (as in meningitis, certain toxic states, and after head injury), decreased absorption (as in compression of venous sinuses by tumor, products of infection, etc., or in impaired venous drainage secondary to increased intrathoracic pressure in cases of pulmonary neoplasm, aneurysm of the aorta, or severe emphysema), or to obstruction within the subarachnoid space (as in the case of tumor, adhesions following trauma, inflammation or hemorrhage, or congenital abnormalities, such as platybasia or the Arnold-Chiari malformation).

Hypertensive hydrocephalus may be congenital or acquired. In congenital hydrocephalus, the most conspicuous symptom is enlargement of the head, which usually is slowly progressive. The cranial sutures are widely separated and the anterior fontanelle is greatly enlarged. Convulsions are common, as is optic atrophy due to pressure on the optic nerves. Mental retardation is seen in severe cases. Most cases die by the age of 4; in the survivors, mental retardation, epilepsy, and blindness are the usual sequelae.

In acquired obstructive hydrocephalus, increased intracranial pressure causes headache, vomiting, and papilledema. In time, there is usually some mental deterioration, often with emotional lability, hallucinations, and delusions. Cranial nerve palsies may occur.

In chronic hydrocephalus, the earliest symptom is *magnetic gait*, a gait apraxia characterized by shuffling and "sticking" of the feet to the ground.

**hydrocephalus, toxic**   See *pseudotumor cerebri*.

**hydrodipsomania**   Periodic attacks of uncontrollable thirst often found in epileptic patients.

**hydroencephalocele**   A developmental anomaly of the brain in which the brain protruding through the skull contains a cavity that communicates with the cerebral ventricles.

**hydromania**   *Obs.* Impulse to commit suicide by drowning.

**hydromyelia**   An increase of fluid in the dilated central canal of the spinal cord or elsewhere in the cord substance where congenital cavities may be present.

**hydromyelocele**   Protrusion of a portion of the spinal cord, thinned out into a sac that is distended with cerebrospinal fluid, through a spina bifida.

**hydrophobia**   1. Fear of water. 2. Rabies. The symptoms of rabies are (1) in the premonitory stage, irritability, general malaise, anorexia, headache, insomnia; tingling, numbness, or pain in the course of the nerves radiating from the site of the wound; spasms of the muscles of the larynx and pharynx; huskiness; difficulty in swallowing; (2) in the stage of excitement there is exaggeration of the premonitory symptoms; intense excitement with terror; intense thirst, but every effort to drink is forthwith followed by choking and dyspnea; elevation of temperature and pulse. As the disease progresses, convulsions become generalized; (3) in the stage of paralysis, restlessness abates, convulsions cease, and the musculature becomes limp and paralytic.

**hydrophobophobia**   Fear of rabies; in severe cases, the symptoms of rabies are paralleled.

**hyelophobia**   Fear of glass.

**hygrophobia**   Fear of moisture or dampness.

**hylognosis**   Ability to appreciate texture, a type of touch sense.

**hylophobia**   Fear of forests.

**hyoscine**   An anticholinergic drug. See *cholinergic*.

**HYPAC**   *Hypothalamic-pituitary-adrenal cortex.* See *hypothalamic-pituitary-adrenal axis*.

**hypacusia, hypoacusia**   Partial deafness.

**hypalgia, hysterical**   A psychogenically induced decrease in sensitivity to pain in any body area. The psychogenic basis has two elements:

1. As in all hysterical symptoms, the hypalgia is a defense against unconscious instinctual demands. Sexual or aggressive sensations that would be painful—that is, would cause anxiety—are repressed. These anxiety-causing impulses are often linked to specific memories. Hypalgia helps suppress these memories by decreasing the sensitiveness to pain in the body areas connected with these particular memories.

2. The decrease in painful sensation permits this body area to be used for unconscious phantasies and thus the repressed material can be expressed without concomitant painful anxiety.

**hypapoplexia**   A mild form of apoplexy.

**hypengyophobia**   Fear of responsibility.

**hyper-**   Combining form meaning over, beyond, from Gr. *hyper*.

**hyperactive child syndrome**   *HACS.* See *attention deficit hyperactivity disorder*.

**hyperactivity**   Excessive muscular activity; *hyperkinesis* (q.v.). In psychiatry, manifestations of disturbed child behavior, indicating the child whose movements and actions are performed at a higher than normal rate of speed or the child who is constantly restless and in motion.

Hyperactivity may be (1) physiologic, i.e., not integrally associated with any other pathology although it may secondarily produce disturbances in living; (2) based on organic brain damage or dysfunction, and typically showing additional symptoms, such as educational deficits, short attention span, perceptual difficulties, perseverative tendencies, and sleep disturbances (see *attention deficit hyperactivity disorder*); (3) associated with mental retardation without evident brain damage; (4) a symptom of reaction or neurotic behavior disorder, usually with more or less devious motivational character as part of an attempt to cope with environmental stress or neurotic conflicts within the child; or (5) a symptom of childhood schizophrenia.

**hyperactivity, developmental**  See *learning disability, specific.*

**hyperactivity, purposeless**  A symptom seen often in organic brain disease: stimulation of a great enough intensity to provoke any reaction evokes an exaggerated emotional response or a prolonged bout of excessive activity that fulfills no purpose. Also known as *occupational delirium.* See *organic syndrome.*

**hyperacuity, auditory**  See *Asperger syndrome.*

**hyperacusia, hyperacusis**  Inordinate acuteness of the sense of hearing.

**hyperadrenal constitution**  A type associated with oversecretion of the adrenal gland. Physical characteristics are an apoplectic habitus with muscular overdevelopment and hypertonia, marked muscular strength, hypertonic peripheral arteries with a blood pressure above the average, hypertrichosis, hyperglycemia, and hypercholesteremia. The psychological features are characterized by euphoria and moral and intellectual energy.

**hyperadrenocorticism**  Cushing syndrome. See *basophile adenoma.*

**hyperaffective type**  In the system of constitutional types described by Pende, a psychological type characterized by an abundance of emotional reactivity and roughly corresponding to the *cyclothymic* type.

**hyperalgesia**  Inordinate sensitiveness to *pain* (q.v.). See *allodynia.*

**hyperalimentation**  Maintenance of nutrition solely by parenteral means. It often leads to hypophosphatemia and neurologic effects, such as motor weakness, numbness of hands and feet, paralysis, ataxia, and seizures.

**hyperarousal**  Autonomic *overarousal* (q.v.).

**hypercalcemia**  Higher than normal concentration of calcium in the blood; it is typical of *hyperparathyroidism* (q.v.).

**hypercathexis**  See *cathexis.*

**hypercedemonia**  *Obs.* Excessive grief or anxiety.

**hypercenesthesia**  A feeling of exaggerated well-being.

**hypercompensatory type**  In the system of constitutional types described by Lewis, the type that on the physical side is characterized by *hyperplasia* of blood and lymph vessels, intestines, and ductless glands, and on the psychological side is inclined to *hypercompensatory* reactions taking the form of manic-depressive psychosis or paranoid reactions.

**hyperdynamic β-adrenergic circulatory state**  β-*adrenergic hyperdynamic circulatory state* (q.v.).

**hyperechema**  Auditory magnification or exaggeration.

**hyperephidrosis**  Excessive sweating; hyperhidrosis.

**hyperepidosis**  Abnormal or excessive growth of any part of the body.

**hyperepithymia**  Inordinate desire.

**hyperergasia**  The manic form of manic-depressive psychosis (Meyer).

**hypereridic**  Characterized by excessive strife or violence. The term *hypereridic state* has been used to refer to attempted suicide triggered by acute interpersonal conflict that produced impulsive, uncontrolled rage.

**hyperesthesia**  Inordinate sensitiveness to tactile stimation.

**hyperesthetic memory**  Oversensitive memory, especially one that is too easily aroused according to the laws of association. Breuer and Freud hypothesized that the provocation of hysterical attacks was in large part due to associative reactivation of hyperesthetic memories.

**hyperevolutism**  In constitutional medicine, excessive morphological, physiological, and psychological development.

**hyperfunction**  Activity or functioning above the subject's own or a standard group's average.

**hypergenitalism**  Overdevelopment of the genital system.

**hyperglycemia**  See *carbohydrate metabolism.*

**hyperglycemic index (HI)**  Measurement used by McGowan as a prognostic indicator in various psychoses:

$$HI = \frac{\text{2-hr blood glucose level} - \text{fasting blood glucose}}{\text{maximal blood glucose level} - \text{fasting blood glucose}} \times 100$$

A high index is considered unfavorable and is seen in melancholia and in catatonic and depressive stupors, but HI is usually low in mania. McGowan considered the hyperglycemic index to be a measure of the emotional tension under which a patient labors.

**hypergnosis**  Exaggerated perception, such as the expansion of an isolated thought into a philosophical system that is seen in some paranoids.

**hypergraphia**  Graphomania; compulsive writing (or drawing), typically without regard to the worth of what is being written. It is often associated with temporal lobe dysfunction.

The subject's written productions are similar to his or her conversation, which is characterized by slowness, pedantic verbosity, circumstantiality, and overinclusiveness. Themes are often related to philosophic or moralistic concerns about fate and destiny. Other features that may be apparent include hypermoralism and religious preoccupation, humorlessness, and paranoid tendencies.

**hyperhidrosis** Excessive sweating; hyperephidrosis.

**hyperinsulinism, drug-induced** Hypoglycemia secondary to the administration of a hypoglycemic agent, such as insulin. In diabetes, the most frequent reason for drug-induced hyperinsulinism is the patient's failure to eat at the proper times. See *carbohydrate metabolism.*

**hyperkalemia** Excessive blood potassium; hyperpotassemia.

**hyperkinesis** Excessive muscular activity, observed in many conditions, including epidemic encephalitis, manic states, schizophrenic psychoses, and ADHD. See *hyperactivity.*

**hyperkinetic heart syndrome** See *asthenia, neurocirculatory.*

**hyperkinetic impulse disorder** See *attention deficit hyperactivity disorder.*

**hyperkinetic motor psychosis** See *akinetic psychosis.*

**hyperlipidemia** Increased blood lipids (cholesterol, triglycerides); see *metabolic syndrome.*

**hyperlogia** Uncontrollable loquacity.

**hypermanic** See *mania.*

**hypermetabolic state** An effect of overdose with monoamine oxidase inhibitors, as when different MAOIs have been combined, or one has been given concomitantly with a tricyclic antidepressant or meperidine. It resembles the *neuroleptic malignant syndrome* (q.v.). Symptoms and signs include agitation, hyperpyrexia, tachycardia, muscular rigidity, disorientation, coma, metabolic acidosis, hypoxia, hypercapnia, severe hypotension, and respiratory failure.

**hypermetamorphic movements** Wernicke's term for *touching* (q.v.).

**hypermetamorphosis** An excessive tendency to attend and react to every visual stimulus; noted in monkeys by Bucy and Klüver following bilateral removal of the temporal lobes.

**hypermnesia** Exaggerated memory; ability to recall material that is not ordinarily available to the memory process. Hypermnesia as a psychopathological phenomenon has been reported in the following conditions: (1) manic phase of manic-depressive psychosis; (2) schizophrenic disorders, where the remembered material is sometimes woven into the patient's hallucinations; (3) organic brain disorders, and particularly the acute confusional deliria; (4) hypnosis; (5) psychoanalytic reactivation; (6) during the seconds of shock and fright in situations that endanger life; (7) fever; (8) as an effect of certain drugs, and particularly amphetamines and other stimulants, and hallucinogenic agents; (9) during neurosurgery, especially when this involves stimulation of the temporal lobes; and (10) following some brain injuries.

**hypermotor seizures** See *frontal lobe seizures.*

**hypernea, hypernoia** *Obs.* Exaggerated mental activity; hyperpsychosis. See *apsychosis.*

**hypernycthemeral syndrome** See *circadian rhythm sleep disorder.*

**hyperopia** Far-sightedness, long-sightedness. As a result of an error in refraction or flattening of the globe of the eye, parallel rays are focused behind the retina. See *myopia.*

**hyperorexia** *Bulimia* (q.v.); excessive hunger. See *eating disorders.*

**hyperosmia** Exaggerated sensitiveness to odors.

**hyperparathyroidism** Excessive secretion of parathyroid hormone, resulting in hypercalcemia, hypophosphatemia, and loss of calcium from bones. Vitamin D overdosage can produce the same clinical picture. Psychiatric symptoms are frequent: psychosis with hallucinations and delusions; depression; anxiety and irritability; organic delirium proceeding, in severe cases, to coma.

**hyperpathia** Sensation of pain in a hypesthetic zone as may be observed in association with lesions of the *thalamus* (q.v.).

**hyperphilia** An inexact, pseudoscientific term referring to a state of being "oversexed," a judgment frequently based on a comparison with the rater's own level of sexual responsivity.

**hyperphoria** See *heterophoria.*

**hyperphosphatemia** Higher than normal concentration of phosphorus or phosphorus compounds in the blood, typically associated with hypocalcemia in hypoparathyroidism.

**hyperphrasia** Hyperlogia; polyphrasia; uncontrollable loquacity.

**hyperphrenia** 1. Excessive mental activity, such as occurs in the manic phase of manic-depressive psychosis or in the severe preoccupations associated with the psychoneuroses. 2. Intellectual capacity far above the average. See *phrenalgia*.

**hyperpituitary constitution** A type characterized by oversecretion of the pituitary gland occurring after or toward the end of the period of normal growth, as compared with such oversecretion occurring earlier in life and producing *gigantism*.

The hyperpituitary type corresponds to Kretschmer's *athletic* type with *dysplastic* features and mainly consist of strong long bones, massive face, hands, and feet, thick oily skin, scanty scalp with seborrhea, large external genitalia, a tendency to tachycardia, hypertension, and arteriosclerosis, increased basal metabolism, a hypervigilant mental attitude, and a tendency to control emotions through intellectualization.

**hyperpolarization** An increase in the membrane potential, which decreases the ability of the cell (neuron) to generate an *action potential* (q.v.). See *benzodiazepines*.

**hyperponesis** Increased invisible motor activity, measurable electromyographically, presumed to be due to hyperactivity of neurons of the motor portion of the nervous system. Hyperponesis is seen in patients with clinical depressions; increased invisible motor activity is also seen with increasing age.

**hyperpragia** Excessive mentation; the type of mental activity commonly observed during the manic phase of manic-depressive psychosis, namely, an excess of thinking and feeling.

**hyperprolactinemia** Elevated blood prolactin levels. Antipsychotic agents can cause hyperprolactinemia by their activity at dopamine $D_2$ receptors, which suppress the secretory activity of pituitary lactotrophs. Hyperprolactinemia impairs sexual function by inhibiting gonadotropin-releasing hormone and subsequently luteinizing hormone and follicle-stimulating hormone by means of a short feedback loop between pituitary and hypothalamus. Hyperprolactemia can cause galactorrhea (abnormal lactation) and menstrual disturbances in women, and in men galactorrhea and sexual dysfunction (such as decreased libido, impotence, ejaculatory dysfunction).

**hyperprosessis,      hyperprosexia** Exaggerated attention. Diminished attention is called *hyproprosessis*.

**hyperpselaphesia** Eulenburg's term for tactile oversensitiveness.

**hyperpsychosis** See *apsychosis*.

**hypersexuality** Compulsive sexuality; sexual addiction; paraphilia-related disorders, such as *compulsive masturbation* (q.v.), protracted promiscuity, severe sexual desire incompatibility, and dependence on pornography (print, film, video, computer, or telephone). Excessive involvement in pleasurable activity, including sexual activity, may be a prominent symptom in mania and hypomania.

The neurotic person might try to gain satisfaction through persistent repetition of the sexual act yet never achieve that quelling of desire that comes with complete orgasm. He may boast about the frequency with which he can perform the sexual act, or behave in an "oversexed" way, giving sexual connotations to many of his relationships or activities. This occurs for two reasons: (1) the dammed-up sexuality will come out in unsuitable places at inconvenient times, just because it cannot be satisfied with orgasm; (2) there is a narcissistic need to prove through such activity that the subject is not impotent or frigid.

When the symptom of hypersexuality is so marked as to dominate the clinical picture, additional factors are at work. The genital apparatus is being used to discharge some nongenital, warded-off, and dammed-up need. These needs might stem from different sources. The primary purpose of the sexual activity might be to obtain self-esteem by contradicting an inner feeling of inferiority with erotic "successes." Whether the person is a *Don Juan* or a *nymphomaniac* (qq.v.), ""Analysis shows that the condition depends on a marked narcissistic attitude, on a dependency on narcissistic supplies, on an intense fear over loss of love, and a corresponding pregenital and sadistic coloration of the total sexuality.... The sadistic attitude is manifest in the attempt to coerce the partner by violence into 'giving' complete sexual satisfaction and therewith a re-establishment of self-esteem." As soon as the sexual act has been performed, the person is no longer interested in his partner, but must find another, both because his narcissistic needs demand that he continually prove his ability to excite other partners, and because this partner has failed to satisfy him completely. Another source of hypersexuality that can be traced to nongenital needs is an unconscious homosexual inclination. Though aroused, the patient cannot, through increased heterosexual activity, obtain the satisfaction he seeks. Still another source, operative in women, might be an intense penis envy. Through nymphomanic activities the patient seeks to fulfill the wish phantasy of depriving the man of his penis (Fenichel, O. *The Psychoanalytic Theory of Neurosis*, 1945). See *erotomania*.

**hypersomnia** A *dyssomnia* (q.v.) consisting of excessive sleepiness, typically manifested as frequent daytime sleep episodes or prolonged sleep episodes of sufficient severity to impair social or occupational functioning; the episodes may occur daily. Hypersomnia is characterized by the tendency to fall asleep in inappropriate places or situations, and is often accompanied by a sense of struggling to stay awake. It is distinguished from fatigue, which is a sense of physical tiredness or weariness, without the tendency to actually fall asleep. In some classifications, hypersomnia disorders were called sleep disorders of the DOES class (disorders of excessive somnolence).

**hypersomnia-bulimia syndrome** See *Kleine-Levin syndrome*.

**hypersomnolence disorder** Idiopathic central nervous system hypersomnolence consists of excessive daytime sleepiness and persistently prolonged major sleep periods (9 hours or longer). Unlike narcolepsy, this disorder has no attacks of refreshing sleep during the day. See *sleep disorders*.

**hypertelorism** Excessive distance between two parts or organs. D. M. Greig's term denotes a form of mental retardation characterized by general mental and physical retardation, not very dissimilar to the essential features of Down syndrome.

**hypertension, essential** Abnormally high blood pressure without known cause; it was one of the seven "classic" psychosomatic disorders in the 1940s. Alexander, for example, described its specific dynamic pattern as the repression of all hostile, competitive tendencies, which are intimidating because of fears of retaliation and failure; this general readiness for aggression is combined with a passive-receptive,

dependent longing to be rid of the aggression. But these dependent longings arouse inferiority feelings and thereby reactivate the hostile competitiveness; this leads to anxiety and the need for further inhibition of aggressive, hostile impulses.

"A fully consummated aggressive attack has three phases. At first there is the preparation of the attack in phantasy, its planning and its mental visualization. This is the conceptual phase. Second, there is the vegetative preparation of the body for concentrated activity: changes in metabolism and blood distribution.... Finally there is the neuromuscular phase, the consummation of the aggressive act itself through muscular activity.... If the inhibition takes place as early as the psychological preparation for an aggressive attack, a migraine attack develops. If the second phase, the vegetative preparation for the attack, develops but the process does not progress further, hypertension follows. And finally if the voluntary act is inhibited only in the third phase, an inclination toward arthritic symptoms or vasomotor syncope may develop" (Alexander, F. *Psychosomatic Medicine, Its Principles and Applications*, 1950).

Recent research casts doubt on the link between high blood pressure and workplace stress. In 80% of hypertension cases, the causes are conventional physical and lifestyle factors—genetics, weight, salt intake, and lack of exercise. The other 20% may be related to the effect of repressed emotion.

**hypertensive encephalopathy** A diffuse, usually transient, cerebral disturbance that may complicate the course of arterial hypertension (as in glomerulonephritis, malignant or essential hypertension, and eclampsia). Increased intracranial pressure is evidenced by papilledema, raised cerebrospinal pressure, headaches, vomiting, convulsions, coma, etc. Onset is usually subacute, with focal signs (e.g., visual disturbances, aphasia, or hemiplegia), but in some cases onset is chronic and characterized by personality changes, poor judgment, and anxiety. See *hypertension, essential*.

**hyperthermia, malignant** A rare and potentially fatal hypermetabolic disorder, susceptibility to which is transmitted as an autosomal dominant trait. Episodes of malignant hyperthermia are usually triggered by some pharmacologic agent, such as succinylcholine (the one most frequently reported), anesthetics, haloperidol, tricyclic antidepressants, and monoamine oxidase inhibitors.

Clinical manifestations include unexplained tachycardia, cardiacdysrhythmias, spasm of the masseter with administration of succinylcholine, fulminant increase in temperature (e.g., a rise of 1°C every 5 minutes), increased respiratory rate, metabolic acidosis, and increased tissue utilization of oxygen with peripheral cyanosis.

Treatment includes hyperventilation with 100% oxygen and intravenous dantrolene sodium, a hydantoin derivative that is a direct-acting skeletal muscle relaxant. Since dantrolene therapy was introduced in 1979, mortality of episodes has fallen from over 80% to less than 10%.

**hyperthymia** State of overactivity, greater than average but less than the overactivity of the manic stage of manic-depressive psychosis. Hyperthymia is a subdivision of *cyclothymia* (q.v.). It is probably very close to hypomania, but occupies a position between normal overactivity and hypomania.

**hyperthymic constitution** In the system of constitutional types described by Pende and Berman, a type associated with a posited overdevelopment of the thymus gland and its persistence into adulthood.

*In infancy*, this constitutional type is represented by the angelic child, with pretty and well-proportioned features, delicate body proportions, exceptional grace of motion, and an alert mind. These children are models of beauty, but they fall easy victims to tuberculosis, meningitis, and other infections.

*After puberty*, all hyperthymic constitutions are distinguished by hypoplastic hearts and arteries, insufficient muscular strength, and a tendency to sudden circulatory imbalance that often leads to sudden death or a rupture of the hypoplastic arteries. While the *male* hyperthymic is characterized by elegant feminine body outlines, long thorax, rounded pelvis, soft skin, and milky color, the *female* type shows delicate skin and nails, little hair, deficient mammary development, delayed menstruation, and, in some cases, a certain persistent adiposity and juvenility.

On the psychic side, there are impulsiveness, incapability for adaptation to the difficulties of social life, and a tendency to suicide.

**hyperthyroid constitution** This constitutional type is associated with excessive secretion of the thyroid gland and is said to be characterized by youthfulness, well-developed sexual characteristics, well-formed nails and teeth, large brilliant and sometimes rather prominent eyes, hyperpigmentation of the skin, slightly enlarged thyroid, swiftness of all functional reactions, marked irritability of the sympathetic nervous system, and general hyperemotivity and instability. The physical and psychological aspects of this type correspond to those of the *asthenic*.

**hypertonia** Extreme tension of the muscles; spasticity or rigidity.

**hypertrophic obesity** See *obesity, hyperplastic*.

**hypertropia** Strabismus in which the affected eye deviates upward.

**hypertychia** See *euphoria*.

**hyperuricemia** Abnormally high uric acid content of blood; seen typically in gout, but it occurs also as an inborn metabolic disorder in children. In the latter, symptoms include severe mental retardation, spastic cerebral palsy, choreoathetosis, and bizarre self-destructive behavior, such as biting of the flesh—sometimes so deeply that the bones themselves are gnawed.

**hyperuricosuria** See *Lesch-Nyhan syndrome*.

**hyperventilation syndrome** Formerly termed DaCosta syndrome, effort syndrome, irritable heart, neurocirculatory asthenia, soldier's heart, war neurasthenia; subjective symptoms (especially breathlessness, palpitation, dizziness or faintness, paresthesias, and excessive sweating) are due to the progressive hypocapnia produced by overbreathing. Other signs and symptoms are fatigability, weakness, headache, poor concentration, aerophagia-induced gastrointestinal symptoms (e.g., eructation, flatulence, esophageal reflux), muscle stiffness and cramps, depersonalization, and derealization.

The overbreathing is itself a form of reaction to anxiety or fear, but the importance of recognizing the syndrome lies in the fact that the subjective symptoms secondarily produced are of physiologic origin rather than specific symbolic representatives of the underlying neurotic conflict. See *pickwickian syndrome; spasmophilia*.

**hypervigilance** A state or attitude of anxious expectation and hypersensitivity characterized by watchfulness bordering on suspiciousness and excessive alertness to minimal changes in the environment, with a tendency to misinterpretation of and consequent over-reaction to any such change. Hypervigilance is seen most often in persons with a paranoid personality structure, in post-traumatic stress disorders, and in children who have been subjected to parental abuse or neglect. Hypervigilance to *interoceptive* cues and chronic autonomic *overarousal* (q.v.) are also seen in panic disorders and agoraphobia. See *vigilance*.

**hypesthesia**  Subnormal sensitiveness to a tactile stimulus.

**hyphedonia**  A state in which the subject experiences slight pleasure from what normally gives great pleasure.

**hyphephilia**  A *paraphilia* (q.v.) in which sexual arousal and orgasm depend upon touching or rubbing the partner's skin or hair, or upon the sensations related to feeling fur, leather, fabric, or other substances in association with sexual activity with the partner. Frequently quoted examples include a requirement that the partner be clothed in furs, wear a leather belt, or lie on a rubber tire during sexual activity.

**hypn-**  Combining form meaning sleep, from Gr. *hypnos.*

**hypnagogic**  Inducing sleep; hypnotic.

**hypnagogic hallucination**  *Hypnagogic imagery* (q.v.).

**hypnagogic imagery**  Imagery occurring during the stage between wakefulness and sleep; that is, just before sleep has set in.

**hypnagogic intoxication**  *Obs.* A rare condition in which a rough or stormy waking generates a dream and induces motility before the dream disappears; "In rare cases something clumsy is then performed, indeed, under the influence of terrifying ideas, an attack of murder may be perpetrated" (Bleuler, E. *Textbook of Psychiatry*, 1930). Hypnopompic intoxication would be the more correct term for this condition.

**hypnalgia**  Dream pain.

**hypnenergia**  *Obs.* Somnambulism. Other obsolete terms include *hypnobadicus, hypnobadisis, hypnobasis, hypnobatesis,* and *hypnonergia.*

**hypneophagia**  Novelty-suppressed feeding; inhibition of feeding produced by exposure to a new environment; used in animals as a measure of anxiety that is sensitive to the effects of chronic, but not acute, antidepressant treatment and to the effects of anxiolytic drugs. There is no perfect animal model for studies

of depression or of antidepressant action, and in both humans and animal models there is no clear distinction between depression and anxiety.

**hypnic**  Relating to or causing sleep; hypnotic.

**hypnic headache**  **A** primary headache disorder that typically begins late in life (usually after age 60); it is characterized by bilateral, often throbbing pain, without associated symptoms. See *headache.*

**hypnoanalysis**  In psychoanalytic therapy, an aid to removing resistances that prevent awareness of unconscious material. Regression and revivication under hypnosis may open up pathways to memories that are not available to the patient at an adult, waking level. It is obvious, however, that no matter what material is elicited in the trance state, in order to be effective it must be integrated and incorporated into the more conscious layers of the psyche.

**hypnobat**  A sleep walker; somnambulist.

**hypnocatharsis**  Hypnotizing the subject who is encouraged to free-associate while in the hypnotic state.

**hypnogenic spot**  In susceptible patients the body sometimes presents a spot or point, pressure upon which will throw the person into a hypnotic state. See *hysterogenic spot.*

**hypnograph**  An instrument to measure sleep. The basic hypnograph consists of a recording pen attached to a coil of the sleeper's bed so that any movement is communicated to the instrument and traced in a graph. This gives a measure of the amount of gross motor activity during sleep. In the same manner other functions may be tested during sleep, and there are modifications of the hypnograph that will measure any or all of the following: blood pressure, pulse, temperature, respiration, metabolic rate, muscle tone, reflexes, urine volume, sweating, gastric secretion, lacrimal and salivary secretion, etc.

**hypnolepsy**  *Obs. Narcolepsy* (q.v.).

**hypnology**  Study of sleep and hypnotism.

**hypnonarcosis**  A state of deep sleep induced through hypnosis.

**hypnophobia**  Fear of falling asleep.

**hypnopompic**  Sleep dispelling. Relating to or ushering out the semiconscious state between the stages of sleep and awakening.

**hypnopompic imagery**  The visions or mental pictures that occur just after the sleeping state and before full wakefulness. The phenomenon is analogous to hypnagogic imagery, differing only in the time at which the images occur.

**hypnosis** Mesmerism; the state or condition induced through hypnotism. The subject to be hypnotized is commanded to fix his attention, usually by staring at an object, while the hypnotist keeps repeating in a monotonous manner that the subject is growing tired, drowsy, and sleepy. Although Braid is often credited with coining the term, the word hypnosis was first used by Etienne Felix d'Henin de Cuvillers in 1820. See *braidism*. Stephen Black (in *Modern Perspectives in World Psychiatry*, ed. J. G. Howells, 1971) defines hypnosis as "a sleepless state of decreased consciousness which occurs in most animal phyla as a result of constrictive or rhythmic stimuli usually imparted by another organism and which may be distinguished from sleep by the presence of catatonia, relative awareness or increased suggestibility and in which direct contact is made with the unconscious mind in man."

As defined by the British Medical Association (1965): "A temporarycondition of altered attention in the subject which may be induced by another person and in which a variety of phenomena may appear spontaneously or in response to verbal or other stimuli. These phenomena include alterations in consciousness and memory, increased susceptibility to suggestion, and the production in the subject of responses and ideas unfamiliar to him in his usual state of mind. Further, phenomena such as anesthesia, paralysis and muscle rigidity, and vaso-motor changes can be produced and removed in the hypnotic state."

"Hypnosis may be applied therapeutically in many ways. We shall distinguish for the present between three such applications:

1. The hypnotically induced sleep is used directly as a healing factor.

2. The suggestion given in hypnosis is directed outright against the psychic or physical symptom which is to be eliminated.

3. Forgotten experiences are brought back to memory in hypnosis and are made accessible to the consciousness (cathartic hypnosis)" (Schilder, P. & Kauders, O. *Hypnosis*, 1927).

In the 1980s, there was renewed interest in patients' reports of childhood sexual abuse and a re-evaluation of Freud's *seduction theory* (q.v.). This was heightened by findings of a high frequency of childhood abuse histories in at least two clinical conditions, dissociative identity disorder and post-traumatic stress disorder. In conjunction with these clinical findings there developed a controversy concerning the reliability and dependability of such *childhood memories*, whether they were recovered within the usual psychotherapeutic setting or while the patient was in a hypnotized state.

**hypnosis, dependency in** An exaggerated transference to the hypnotist based on overvaluation of his or her power and authority. The patient plunges himself into a subordinate position in order to achieve his objectives, but such a position is incompatible with normal self-esteem.

**hypnotic** Sleep-inducing. See *sedation; sedatives/hypnotics.*

**hypnotism** The theory and practice of inducing hypnosis or a state resembling sleep induced by psychical means. It is also known asbraidism (or Braidism) and induced somnambulism.

**hypnotization, collective** Simultaneous hypnosis of several subjects.

**hypo-, hyp-** Combining form meaning under, below, less than (the normal), from Gr. *hypo.*

**hypoadrenal constitution** The constitutional type associated with a deficient secretion of the adrenal gland (medullary portion) and described by N. Pende as characterized by a hypoplastic trunk, slender bones, habitual leanness, marked developmental deficiency of both skeletal and smooth muscles, an accentuated universal lymphatism with or without hyperplasia of the thymus, marked arterial hypotension, lymphocytosis, and a hypotrophic skin with increased pigmentation, especially on the exposed parts of the body, and often an abundance of pigmented moles. "Psychologically there is a tendency to melancholia, while the intelligence is normal or supernormal" (*Constitutional Inadequacies*, 1928).

**hypoalgesia** Diminished sensibility to painful stimuli.

**hypoboulia, hypobulia** Deficiency or inadequacy of the will or will power, seen primarily in schizophrenic patients. See *unforthcomingness; will disturbances.*

**hypocalcemia** Lower than normal concentration of calcium in the blood; it is characteristic of *hypoparathyroidism* (q.v.). Because the calcium ion is essential to neuronal membrane function and neurotransmission, its lack is often associated with neuropsychiatric symptoms.

**hypocathexis**   See *cathexis.*

**hypochondriac language**   See *organ speech.*

**hypochondriacal melancholia**   A symptom complex consisting of depressive affect, inhibition of thinking and acting, and hypochondriacal delusions. When not organic, this symptom complex is almost always schizophrenic in nature. Monoideism, in contrast to the simple melancholias, may here be almost absolute. For long periods there seem to be no thoughts other than the constantly repeated wishes, complaints, or maledictions. Even though the affect seems to dominate the entire personality, it is typically stiff, superficial, and exaggerated. In this condition, ideas of grandeur may coexist with appalling fears and terrors in spite of logical contradictions involved.

**hypochondriacal paranoia**   Hypochondriac paranoid psychosis; somatic delusion that constitutes the sole or primary delusion of an underlying paranoia or paranoid schizophrenia. See *dysmorphophobia; monosymptomatic hypochondriacal psychosis.*

**hypochondriacal phobia**   Fear of organic disease in the absence of known pathology.

**hypochondriacal psychosis**   See *monosymptomatic hypochondriacal psychosis.*

**hypochondriasis**   Hypochondria; hypochondriacal neurosis; *complaint habit;* somatic overconcern; morbid attention to the details of body functioning or exaggeration of any symptom, no matter how insignificant. One of the *somatoform disorders* (q.v.), characterized by preoccupation with the fear or belief of having a physical disease for which there are no demonstrable organic findings or known physiologic mechanisms. The affected person interprets any number of physical signs or symptoms unrealistically as indicative of serious disease. Despite reassurance by physicians that no illness exists and continuing failure on examination to uncover evidence of underlying organic pathology, the persisting fear or belief of illness colors the person's entire life and interferes with social and occupational functioning. See *sick role.*

Hypochondriasis is rare as a primary disorder, and most cases are secondary to a depressive illness or some other disorder.

Hypochondriasis is present in as many as 15% of all patients in general medical practice. It is equally distributed among men and women; peak incidence is during the fourth or fifth decade.

Although hypochondriasis may appear in the form of a specific neurosis, it may also occur in association with such disorders as anxiety neurosis, obsessive-compulsive disorder, and most often with the initial states of any psychosis. The hypochondriacal patient is typically self-centered, seclusive, and sometimes almost monomaniacal in his attention to his body; his major environmental contacts are somatically colored and he seeks one consultation after another with his family physician or with as many specialists as will agree to reexamine him. In other cases, preoccupation with his own health leads the hypochondriac to seek a career in medicine; similarly, he may become a health faddist. If he uses reaction formation as a defense, hypochondriacal concern may ultimately be expressed in a total neglect of his health and well-being.

Psychodynamically, hypochondriacal anxiety is seen often to represent castration anxiety; further it may represent an attempt to expiate guilt feelings by the turning of hostility and sadism onto the self.

Freud regarded hypochondriasis as an *actual neurosis,* as he did *neurasthenia* and *anxiety neurosis.*

**hypochoresis**   Defecation.

**hypocretin/orexin system**   A neuropeptide system that is believed to regulate feeding and energy metabolism. Because mutation in a G protein–coupled orexin receptor has been linked to narcolepsy, it is thought that the hypocretin/orexin system may also play some part in regulation of the sleep cycle. The neurons of the system are located in the lateral and posterior hypothalamus; they project to the forebrain, limbic system, thalamus, hypothalamus, brain stem, and spinal cord. See *orexins.*

**hypocretins**   The hypocretin (orexin) system is a neuropeptide system centered in the dorsal hypothalmus that regulates arousal states and energy metabolism. The hypocretins, two carboxy terminally amidated neuropeptides, are central elements of the sleep-wake apparatus. Most patients with narcolepsy have greatly reduced levels of hypocretin in their CSF and few, if any, hypocretin neurons in their hypothalami. Hypocretins are involved in nutritional-homeostasis circuits, but such involvement is subservient to the demands of the *arousal* system (q.v.). See *arcuate nucleus*; *orexins*.

**hypodepression**  Simple depression, i.e., mild depression occurring as an episode in manic-depressive psychosis. Such an episode may be difficult to distinguish from normal grief and from so-called psychoneurotic depressive reaction. As in all clinical depressions, however, lowering of the self-esteem and self-depreciatory, self-accusatory thought content are seen in hypodepression but do not occur in normal grief (mourning).

**hypoesthesia, vaginal**  See *frigidity, sexual*.

**hypoevolutism**  Deficient morphological, physiological, and psychological development; applicable to the body as a whole, to particular systems, organs, and tissues, as well as to the psyche. One usually distinguishes between *ontogenetic* and *phylogenetic* hypoevolutism.

**hypofrontality hypothesis**  The theory that early developmental abnormalities of the frontal lobe and, in particular, of the dorsolateral prefrontal cortex may be basic to the development of schizophrenia. Consistent with such a hypothesis are the following: (1) frontal lobe signs, such as lack of initiative, poor insight, social withdrawal, flat affect, and poor judgment, resemble the *negative symptoms* of schizophrenia; (2) many studies have found a relative decrease in cerebral blood flow in the frontal lobes of schizophrenics; (3) fMR, MR, SPECT, and PET studies have all demonstrated decreased functioning in the frontal lobe in schizophrenics; (4) slow frontal EEG activity has been reported in schizophrenics; (5) eye tracking dysfunction, one of the most consistent findings of different research groups, may be due to disinhibition of frontal eye field mechanisms. See *frontal lobe*.

It has further been demonstrated that hypofontality is present at the beginning stage of the illness, that it is not caused by treatments, and that it is associated with prominent negative symptoms. The degree to which patients appear hypofrontal compared with normal controls during an rCBF procedure depends on whether the controls are engaged in an activity that is normally associated with activation of prefrontal cortex. This suggests that schizophrenia involves physiological dysfunction in the neural systems that facilitate prefrontal function when there is particular need for it. This possibility has led some to suggest further that hypofrontality is a state marker rather than a trait marker, and that it reflects only reduced motivation. See *schizophrenia, models of*.

Several tasks have been identified that activate the frontal lobes: the Continuous Performance Test (CPT), which requires sustained attention and pattern recognition; the Wisconsin Card Sorting Test (WISC), which challenges the ability to think abstractly and to change a conceptual set in response to changed instruction and stimuli; Tower of London test; and the Porteus maze. Schizophrenics show deficiencies in all.

Schizophrenic negative symptoms are viewed as a loss or diminution of frontal lobe functions that should be present, including the following: fluency and spontaneity of verbal expression (appearing as alogia in the schizophrenic patient); fluency of emotional expression (manifested as blunted affect); ability to initiate and persist in or complete various tasks (avolition); ability to experience pleasure or form emotional attachments to others (anhedonia and asociality); and ability to focus attention on some specific activity or task in a sustained manner (attentional impairment).

The posited frontal lobe development abnormality might be genetic in origin, but it could also be a result of other factors, such as maternal nutritional disorders or maternal alcohol consumption during pregnancy, difficulties during delivery, or adverse environment during the first 2 years of life (e.g., nutritional deficiencies, emotional deprivation or lack of appropriate stimulation, viral and other infections). See *schizophrenia, models of*.

**hypofunction**  Reduced action or function.

**hypoglossal hemiplegia alternans**  See *hemiplegia alternans*.

**hypoglossal nerve**  The twelfth cranial nerve. The hypoglossal nerve is motor to the muscles of the tongue. Peripheral paralysis results in homolateral flaccidity, paralysis and atrophy, and the tongue deviates to the side of the lesion. Supranuclear paralysis results in contralateral hemiplegia, contralateral spastic paralysis of the tongue, and deviation of the tongue to the side opposite the lesion.

**hypoglycemia**    A common complication in insulin-dependent diabetes that can lead to brain damage and long-term cognitive impairment. It initiates a cascade of events that includes a large increase in extracellular glutamate, leading to excitotoxicity, DNA damage, and cell death; it also causes activation of poly (ADP-ribose) polymerase I (PARPI), which is involved in DNA repair. Extensive activation of PARPI can lead to cell death.

**hypokinesis**    Slow or diminished movement. It may be physically or psychically determined. Depressed patients are generally hypokinetic.

**hypologia**    Reduction in speech, used usually to refer to cases of organic origin in which capacity for speech is limited.

**hypomania**    See *mania*.

**hypomania, pharmacologic**    In patients with depression, a rapid switch into hypomania as a response to treatment with antidepressants.

**hypomelancholia**    Mild case of the depressed form of manic-depressive psychosis.

**hypomotility**    Diminished or slowed movement.

**hypomyelination, congenital**    See *myelin disorders*.

**hyponoic**    Kretschmer's term for hysterical reactions that stem from the deeper psychic layers. "We recognize these hyponoic formations in mythology and the art of primitives; in the modern normal adult person, we can study them, above all in the dream, and, aside from hysteria, very frequently in the schizophrenias" (*Hysteria*, 1926).

**hypoparathyroidism**    Deficiency of parathyroid hormone, most frequently caused by removal of the parathyroid glands during thyroidectomy. *Pseudohypoparathyroidism* refers to idiopathic unresponsiveness of body tissues to parathyroid hormone.

Hypoparathyroidism produces hypocalcemia and hyperphosphatemia, manifested in impaired motor coordination, tetany, and, often, seizures. Hypocalcemia can cause various neuropsychiatric disturbances, including intellectual impairment, neural irritability, tics, athetoid movements, personality changes, depression or lability of mood, schizophrenic-like syndromes, and anxiety and hysterical, hypochondriacal, or other neurotic symptoms.

**hypophilia**    Reduced or inadequate sexual responsivity, the opposite of *hyperphilia* (q.v.).

**hypophonia**    Decrease in volume and clarity of speech.

**hypophoria**    See *heterophoria*.

**hypophosphatemia**    Lower than normal concentration of phosphorus or phosphorus compounds in the blood; it is a characteristic part of *hyperparathyoidism* (q.v.).

**hypophrasia**    Bradyphrasia; slowness of speech, such as is seen as a part of the generalized psychomotor retardation of depressed patients.

**hypophysial cachexia**    *Simmonds disease*; due to necrosis or other destruction of the anterior lobe of the pituitary gland, occurring most commonly in women. Characteristic symptoms are marked asthenia, great loss of weight with extreme emaciation, chilliness, slow pulse, anemia, low basal metabolic rate, loss of hair, amenorrhea or impotence, somnolence, apathy, poor memory, and occasionally hallucinations and delirium. See *anorexia nervosa*.

**hypophysial dwarfism**    See *growth hormone*.

**hypopituitary constitution**    A type described by Pende associated with deficient secretion of the pituitary gland. The general constitutional aspects of this type correspond to the *hypoplastic* group in Kretschmer's system, although age and sex considerably modify them.

The *infant* type is characterized (1) in *both sexes*, by defective stature and growth, increased adiposity, small head, short bones, irregular dentition, thin lips, poorly spaced eyes with scanty eyebrows, small hands, and circular mouth; (2) in the *male*, by small external genitals and, sometimes, by cryptorchidism; and (3) in the *female*, by a feminine appearance even in early childhood.

The *adult* (adolescent) type is characterized (1) in the *male*, by delicate facial features, smooth bony contours, silky hair, large pelvis, feminine distribution of fat and pubic hair, hairless trunk and extremities, small hands, and defective sex activity; (2) in the *female*, by small breasts, frigidity, and the tendency to sterility and masculinism; and (3) in *both sexes*, by low blood pressure, slow pulse, increased carbohydrate tolerance, polyuria, and general mental torpor.

**hypoprosessis**    See *hyperprosessis*.

**hypopsychosis**    Hyponoia. See *apsychosis*.

**hyposomnia**    Lack of sleep; sleeping for shorter periods than usual. See *sleep disorders*.

**hypostasis**    The obstructive mechanism by which one hereditary factor is prevented by the manifestation of another factor from being phenotypically expressible. The masking effect itself is known as *epistasis* (q.v.), while the factor that is hidden is called *hypostatic*.

**hyposthenia**   Deficient strength.

**hypotaxia**   Durand introduced this term for the emotional rapport existing between the subject and the operator in a hypnotic setting.

**hypotaxis**   Light, hypnotic sleep.

**hypotension, orthostatic**   See *OH*.

**hypothalamic dysfunction**   Hypothalamic syndromes include hypothermia, hypersomnia, the adiposogenital syndrome, diabetes insipidus, and autonomic epilepsy. Some symptoms and syndromes have been labeled diencephalic dysfunction; among these are alterations of biological rhythms in addition to waking and sleeping, abnormalities of growth and development and various other endocrine dysfunctions, vascular lability, and loss of restraint and inhibition (especially with regard to aggression). See *diencephalosis*; *autonomic epilepsy*.

**hypothalamic-pituitary-adrenal (HPA) axis**   A neurohormonal circle that is self-regulating by means of feedback mechanisms from its different levels of function. Most of the neuropeptides (or neurohormones) are located in nerve terminals in the median eminence of the hypothalamus. Once released—under the influence of the monoaminergic neurotransmitters—they move along axons in the hypophyseal portal system to the anterior pituitary, where they stimulate the release of anterior pituitary hormones. The adenohypophyseal hormones, in turn, stimulate hormone secretion in target organs: thyroid, adrenal, and gonads. Those hormones, in turn, feed back to the pituitary, the hypothalamus, and other sites, thereby determining whether the hypothalamic release hormones or its release-inhibitory hormones will be released, to start the process all over again.

Some researchers distinguish a *hypothalamic-pituitary-thyroid (HPT) axis* as separate from the HPA axis; the HPT axis includes the feedback cycle of thyrotropin-releasing hormone (TRH) and thyroid-stimulating hormone (TSH; thyrotropin).

Falling within the HPA/HPT axes are the following:

1. Sexual activity—the hypothalamic peptides gonadotropin-releasinghormone (GnRH) and luteinizing-releasing hormone (LHRH) regulate the release of the gonadotropins luteinizing hormone (LH) and follicle-stimulating hormone (FSH) from the pituitary; they stimulate gonadal responses, which in turn stimulate excitatory and inhibitory hormone release at the hypothalamic level, to begin another cycle.

2. Regulation of thirst and appetitive behaviors

3. Delta sleep-inducing peptide (DSIP)

4. Learning, memory, and attention—the pro-opiomelanocortin (POMC) products, adrenocorticotropic hormone (ACTH), and melanocyte-stimulating hormone (MSH), as well as vasopressin

5. Antidepressant activity—thyrotropin-releasing hormone (TRH) and melanocyte stimulating hormone-release inhibition factor (MIF)

The HPA axis was implicated in the early part of the century in Cannon's study of the fight/flight reaction and in Papez's formulation of the role of the limbic lobe in emotion. It has also been known for many years that dysregulation of the hypothalamic-pituitary-adrenal axis is characteristic of depression. More recently, it has become possible to identify more of the specific neuroendocrine pathways involved. See *adrenocorticotropic hormone (ACTH)*; *corticotropin-releasing factor (CRF)*; *growth hormone (GH)*; *melatonin*; *somatostatin*.

**hypothalamotomy**   A psychosurgical procedure that produces partial ablation of the hypothalamic area—performed in *thalamotomy* cases that have not responded to the original operation (q.v.).

**hypothalamus**   A phylogenetically old constellation of nuclei lying in the ventral part of the diencephalon, below the thalamus and just above the optic chiasm and sella turcica. It integrates visceral functions involving the autonomic nervous system and it regulates the endocrine system. It is involved in an array of rhythmic body activities, including digestion, body weight, appetite, sexuality, wakefulness, blood pressure, pulse, and temperature. It exerts proprietary control over the pituitary. *Gonadotrophin-releasing hormone* (GnRH) is the specific chemical messenger in the hypothalamus. The hypothalamus secretes GnRH into the blood supply feeding the anterior pituitary, which then releases its own hormones into the general circulation to stimulate the testes in men and the ovaries in women.

The hypothalamus has connections with the thalamus, midbrain, and some cortical areas. Most of its nuclei are in the medial region; they include (1) preoptic nuclei and suprachiasmatic nuclei in the anterior region; (2) dorsomedial, ventromedial, and paraventricular nuclei in the middle region; and (3) posterior nucleus and mammillary bodies in the posterior region. It is attached to the pituitary by a stalk called the *infundibulum*.

The posterior hypothalamus (sometimes called the *ergotropic* division) is concerned primarily with the sympathetic division of ANS and the regulation of emergency (*fight or flight*) responses. The middle and anterior nuclei are concerned with the parasympathetic and restorative (*rest and digest*) functions, such as sleep and digestion (and hence sometimes called the *trophotropic* division). See *arcuate nucleus; hypothalamic dysfunction; hypothalamic-pituitary-adrenal (HPA) axis.*

**hypothermia, accidental** The loss of thermoregulatory ability, found most often in older patients being treated with phenothiazines. Exposure to cold in such persons requires prompt treatment to prevent widespread physical deterioration or possibly death.

**hypothetical-deductive thinking** According to Piaget, the type of thinking characteristic of the period of formal operations, which is the final period in the development of intelligence. (Piaget's earlier stages of thinking are the sensorimotor—the earliest—followed by the preoperational and the concrete operational.) Hypothetical-deductive thinking operates systematically from general statement to particular instance. The adolescent, in contrast to the child, sees the real as a particular instance of the possible. For the child, however, the real has priority, and the possible is conceived of as only a prolongation or extension of concrete, real operations. See *separation-individuation; physiognomonic thinking; propositional thinking.*

**hypothymia** Diminution in the intensity of the emotional state.

**hypothyroid constitution** In constitutional medicine, a type with deficient secretion of the thyroid gland. While the body build of this type generally corresponds to that of a *pyknic* or *megalosplanchnic* person, its further characteristics mainly consist of generalized adiposity with special fatty deposits on face and neck, large head, thick neck, short and stubby hands, small and expressionless eyes, short and thick nose, round face with poorly marked features, poor pigmentation of the skin, premature baldness, dystrophic teeth and nails, torpid vasomotor reactions, normal sex development, acrocyanosis, habitual hypoglycemia with great carbohydrate tolerance, diminished basal metabolism, and a torpid and apathetic mental attitude.

**hypothyroidism** Deficiency or absence of thyroid hormone secretion, in the adult resulting in lethargy, sluggishness, lowered basal metabolic rate, reduced oxygen consumption, loss of hair, a relatively hard edema of the tissues (myxedema), obesity, and mental changes. Psychomotor retardation and generalized sluggishness of mentation are almost universal, and depression is frequent. Also seen are paranoid ideas, although the general intellectual dulling tends to minimize self-criticism. When paranoid ideas are prominent or systematized, the condition may be termed *myxedema madness*. Thyroid failure in the infant produces *cretinism* (q.v.).

**hypothyroidism, lithium-induced** See *lithium thyroiditis.*

**hypotonia** Subnormal tension of the muscles; flaccidity.

**hypoventilation, central alveolar** See *sleep apnea.*

**hypovigility** Pathological subnormal awareness or response, or complete lack of it, to external stimuli. Hypovigility is the opposite of exaggerated distractibility. Although exaggerated distractibility sometimes occurs in catatonic excitement, hypovigility is more characteristic of the schizophrenic group as a whole. "The [schizophrenic] patients converse only rarely with those around them even when they are talking a great deal. The incitement to speech as well as its content originates for the most part autistically from inner sources" (Bleuler, E. *Dementia Praecox or the Group of Schizophrenias*, 1950).

**hypoxyphilia** *Asphyxiophilia*; a *paraphilia* (q.v.) in which hypoxia (and the altered state of consciousness it produces) is an essential part of sexual arousal. Hypoxia may be induced by drugs such as nitrous oxide ("poppers"). Particularly when it is a part of masturbatory activity, hypoxia may also be induced by strangling or hanging; some classify such autoerotic asphyxiation as a form of sexual masochism. See *erotized repetitive hangings*.

**hypsarrhythmia** An EEG pattern associated with *infantile spasms* (q.v.); also known as major dysrhythmia and myoclonic encephalitis. It appears as symmetrical flexion spasms lasting a few seconds, usually in children below 1 year of age. Between attacks, the EEG shows a diffuse dysrhythmia of the delta-wave type. Psychomotor regression with loss of motor skills and mental deterioration is typical; complete recovery is rare.

**hypsophobia** Fear of high places; acrophobia.

**hysteria** Term coined by *Hippocrates* (q.v.) for a malady caused by a uterus set free in the pelvis and cured by sexual intercourse. See *phrenitis*. Currently, the word is used in several ways: (1) to describe a pattern of behavior, the *hysterical personality* (see *histrionic personality*); (2) to refer to a conversion symptom, such as hysterical paralysis (see *dissociative disorders*); (3) to refer to a psychoneurotic disorder, such as conversion hysteria or *anxiety hysteria* (q.v.); (4) to refer to a specific psychopathologic pattern in which repression is the major defense; and (5) loosely, as a term of opprobrium.

*Conversion hysteria* appears clinically as (1) a physical manifestation without accompanying structural lesion, or as a peripheral physiologic dysfunction; (2) a calm mental attitude (called ""la belle indifference" by Janet) that is specifically limited to the physical symptom and not generalized to include the entire life of the patient; and (3) episodic mental states, in which a limited but homogeneous group of functions occupies the field of consciousness, often to the complete exclusion of the usual contents of consciousness—fugues, somnambulisms, dream states, hypnotic states, etc. There is, in other words, a dissociation of the mental or bodily functions, and the dissociated functions may operate in coexistence with normal consciousness, or they may operate to the exclusion of the other functions. In conversion hysteria, the split-off function is ordinarily a unity and the splitting is seldom into more than two parts; thus, it is commonly said that in schizophrenia the splitting is molecular or fragmentary, whereas in hysteria it is molar or massive.

Hysteria has usually been found to occur more frequently in women, with an estimated lifetime prevalence of 3 to 6/1000. Onset is usually before the age of 35 years, although hysterical symptoms may occur as part of some other disorder in later years.

M. H. Hollender (*Archives of General Psychiatry 26*, 1972) views conversion hysteria as a dramatized message, expressed in nonverbal and usually pantomimic form when more conventional forms of expression are blocked. The message typically involves a forbidden wish or impulse, its prohibition, or some compromise between the two.

There are no physical symptoms in hysteria that cannot be produced by volition or by emotion, although it may ordinarily be possible to maintain these symptoms for only a short time. Further, the physical symptoms correspond strikingly with the usual lay concepts of disease. Thus, hysterical paralysis shows an exact delimitation and an excessive intensity, and it is more frequently accompanied by sensory disturbances than organic paralysis.

The *motor symptoms* include paralysis with or without contracture, tics, tremors, etc. The *sensory symptoms* include anesthesiae, paresthesiae, and hyperesthesiae; their distribution is rarely according to anatomical lines; they vary at different examinations; and they are susceptible to suggestions. Blindness and deafness are also seen. The *visceral symptoms* include anorexia, bulimia, vomiting, hiccup or respiratory tic, various abdominal complaints, and flatulence.

The *mental symptoms* include amnesiae, somnambulisms, fugues, trances, dream states, and hysterical fits or attacks. The amnesia is commonly for a circumscribed series of events, and occasionally is for the entire period of life up to a certain recent point. In a fugue, the patient suddenly leaves one activity and goes on a journey that has no apparent relation to it and for which she has amnesia afterward. Somnambulisms are fugues that begin during sleep and are usually of shorter duration than fugues. The movements of the somnambulist are in response to the manifest or latent content of the dream; the meaning may be an escape from the temptation of the bed, or a movement toward a positive goal that represents gratification or reassurance. In double or multiple personalities, there is further elaboration so that the groups of dissociated functions when fully conscious and in charge of the motor apparatus can at least superficially appear as a complete personality. Hysterical spells are a pantomimic expression of (mainly oedipal) phantasies; in them can be seen condensation, displacement, representation by the opposite, exaggeration of details that represent the whole, reversal of the sequence of events, multiple identifications, and suitability for plastic representation. Dream states are similar to these but here the pantomimic discharge is lacking; dream states may represent repression, orgasm, death wishes turned against the ego, or the blocking of any hostile impulse.

Until Freud advanced his theory of hysteria, there had been few attempts at explanation. Charcot had described the *"grande attaque hysterique"* with its four phases: (1) epileptoid phase; (2) large movement phase; (3) phase of "attitudes passionelles"; (4) the *"d'elire terminal"*. Janet's theories of restriction of the field of consciousness and the hereditary tendency to dissociate at moments of great emotion did not explain what it was that brought the dissociation to pass. Freud had accepted Charcot's hypothesis that hypnosis could uncover unconscious memories of earlier events and seemed to ignore Bernheim's evidence that such memories were "recovered" in response to the suggestions of the therapist. Freud's first theory was that the hysterical attack was a symbolic representation of a repressed childhood sexual trauma. Freud and Breuer found that *catharsis*—reactivation of the childhood "memory," at that time by means of hypnosis, and allowing abreaction—removed the hysterical symptom. The theory was later revised when it was discovered that the sexual traumata uncovered in hysterical patients were really fictitious memories. Failing to recognize that they had been created in response to the therapist's *suggestion* (q.v.), Freud did not fault the method that produced them but instead blamed the patient. According to the revised theory, the patient had produced fictitious memories in order to mask childhood autoerotic activities.

To the hysterical patient, all sexuality represents infantile incestuous love, so she cannot love fully if the genitals are present because of the oedipal fears. The conversion symptom is a distorted substitute for sexual (or aggressive) gratification; but because of the effectiveness of repression, the symptom leads to suffering rather than gratificatory pleasure.

Since Freud, many investigators have stressed pregenital determinants of conversion hysteria, and particularly oral conflicts arising from intense frustration of oral-receptive needs or excessive gratification of those needs by one or both parents.

Conversion symptoms have also been viewed as unconsciously simulated illnesses, with the patient enacting a sick role as a way to reduce, mask, avoid, or deny a variety of other psychological disturbances (such as anxiety from any cause, identity problems, depression, and incipient schizophrenia). The disorder may be monosymptomatic or may involve many symptoms; these will sometimes be crude and transparent, but equally often they can be accurate simulations of disease or exaggerations of symptoms of genuine physical problems.

**hysteria, epidemic** Hysteria or hysteroid disturbances seemingly acquired by association with hysterical patients.

**hysteria, major** Grand hystérie; a clinical syndrome of hysteria, perhaps first described at length by Charcot and later by Richer. It is characterized by several stages: (1) the aural stage; (2) the stage of epileptoid convulsions; (3) the phase of tonic, then clonic spasms; (4) the phase of intense and dramatic emotional expressions; and (5) the stage of delirium. The total attack lasts from several minutes up to half an hour. There are many modifications in the form and order of the above states.

Some authorities use the expression *major hysteria* synonymously with *hysteroepilepsy* (q.v.).

**hysterical character** A type of *character* (q.v.) manifested in obvious sexual behavior combined with a specific kind of bodily agility that has a definitely sexual nuance. Such behavior traits are combined with outspoken apprehensiveness, which is increased when the sexual behavior comes close to attaining its goal. The hysterical character represents an apprehensive defense against incest wishes inhibited by the anxiety related to any genital expression. The passive-feminine character type is subsumed under hysterical character. See *character defense; histrionic personality*.

**hysterical personality** See *histrionic personality*.

**hysterical psychosis** Dissociative psychosis; in current usage, an acute situational reaction consisting of sudden onset of hallucinations, delusions, depersonalization, bizarre behavior, and volatile affect. It rarely lasts beyond 3 weeks and is sealed off without residua; such reactions typically occur in those of the hysterical or histrionic personality type. Hysterical psychosis includes such entities as *amok*, Imu, *lata, miryachit*, olonism, *piblokto* (Arctic hysteria), Puerto Rican psychosis, *Wihtiko psychosis* (qq.v.). See *dissociation*; *dissociation disorders*; *remitting atypical psychosis*.

**hysteriform** Resembling or having the character of hysteria.

**hysteriosis** Used mainly by Russian investigators to refer to greatly exaggerated responses of the organism to various stimuli if the latter follow prolonged (and, presumably, exhausting) stimulation of some other part of the organism. When, for example, the tibial nerve of an experimental animal is tetanized for several hours and loses its capacity to respond, mild inflation of a segment of intestine (which ordinarily has little effect on blood pressure, pulse, etc.) may prove fatal to the animal, so exaggerated is the response. The conclusion that has been drawn from such data is that the effects of internal stimuli are highly dependent upon the current functional state of the brain that receives the signals.

**hysteroepilepsy** *Obs.* "What is usually called hystero-epilepsy is hysteria with severe motor attacks, which were falsely added to the side of epilepsy" (Bleuler, E. *Textbook of Psychiatry,* 1930).

**hysterofrenic, hysterofrenatory** Aborting or arresting a hysterical attack. For example, when digital pressure is applied to some part of the body to check a hysterical episode, the pressure is called hysterofrenic.

**hysterogenic spot** *Hysterogenic zone*; any area of the body that precipitates a hysterical reaction when stimulated. See *hypnogenic spot*.

**hysteroid dysphoria** According to M. Leibowitz and D. Klein (*Psychiatric Clinics of North America 4*, 1981), a chronic, nonpsychotic disturbance characterized by repeated episodes of abruptly depressed mood in response to feeling rejected; the acutely depressed period is typically associated with overeating, marijuana use, and consumption of sedatives and/or alcohol. Some workers consider hysteroid dysphoria to be part of a subaffective spectrum of disorders; others classify it as a type of borderline disorder.

**hysteromania** *Obs.* Sometimes used synonymously with nymphomania and metromania; it has also been used to describe states of psychomotor overactivity in hysteria.

**hysterophilia** Lewandowsky's term for various clinical conditions resembling hysteria, such as migraine, epileptiform attacks, asthma, membranous enteritis, and occupational cramps.

**hysteropnix** *Obs. Globus hystericus* (q.v.).

**hysterosyntonic** A personality type that is a mixture of the hysterical personality type and the syntonic personality type. See *syntone*.

**Hz** (Heinrich Hertz, German physicist, 1857–1894) Symbol for hertz, a frequency unit of one cycle per second.

# I

**I cell disease**  Mucolipidosis II; a type of mental retardation, probably an autosomal recessive trait, characterized by early onset of retardation, short stature, cytoplasmic inclusions (of cells) in fibroblasts (which also are deficient in lysosomal hydralases and have excessive lipids and mucopolysaccharides), and progressive course leading to death (usually from pneumonia and congestive heart failure) before puberty.

**IADL**  Instrumental activities of daily living. See *ADL*.

**IAP**  Inhibitor of *apoptosis* (q.v.). IAPs are tied to the tumor necrosis factor (*TNF*) pathways, but it is unknown how, or where, they exert their effect. A mammalian counterpart, discovered early in 1995, is the neuronal apoptosis inhibitor protein (*NAIP*).

**iatrogenesis**  Molding of a patient's illness by the (often incompetent) doctor's own ministrations.

**iatrogeny**  Production or inducement of any harmful change in the somatic or psychic condition of a patient by means of the words or actions of the doctor. The physician may tell the patient that he has an enlarged heart, for example, or low blood pressure, or a glandular disturbance, and such information may provide a nucleus around which the patient builds a neurosis or psychosis.

**IB**  See *body build, index of*.

**ibogaine**  A West African plant alkaloid, banned in the United States because of its potential neurotoxic effects (with effects similar to those of LSD or PCP), but legal in most of the world and purported to interrupt addiction and eliminate withdrawal. Its mechanism of action is not fully understood, but it may compete with heroin or morphine to fill opiate receptors. It also leads to increased secretion of *GDNF* (glial cell line–derived neurotropic factor), which some believe maintains or repairs dopamine receptors.

**I-boundary**  In gestalt psychology, the limits defining the range of permissible contact with the outside world, including actions, ideas, people, values, settings, and images with which the subject is willing and free to engage.

**ICD**  *International Classification of Diseases* (q.v.).

**ICE**  Interleukin-1β, one of a large family of proteases that activate proteins that kill the cell. See *apoptosis; caspase cascades; caspases*.

**ice**  See *amphetamines*.

**iceblock theory**  Kurt Lewin's theory of behavior change in relation to group dynamics, as seen in sensitivity training or T-groups: (1) existing attitudes and behavior must be unfrozen; (2) group members are encouraged to consider and explore new attitudes and behavior in a supporting climate; and (3) the new attitudes and behavior are frozen into habit patterns.

**ICHD-II**  International Classification of Headache Disorders, second edition (2004), published by the *International Headache Society* (*IHS*). See *headache*.

**ichthyophobia**  Fear of or aversion to fish.

**iconic memory**  A type of short-term visual memory, probably due to brief afterimages produced by photochemical processes in the retina. See *short-term memory*.

**iconic storage**  Registration of sensory information; approximately 250 msec after presentation of the information it dissipates, or is transferred to short-term memory, or is replaced by more recent incoming information. Short-term memory can retain the information passed on to it from iconic storage for about 500 msec. Long-term memory, which has a storage capacity that is almost unlimited, receives information from both iconic storage and short-term memory.

The *backward masking test* (q.v.) measures the time it takes for a stimulus to be moved from the stage of stimulus reception to short-term memory.

**iconomania**  Compulsion to worship or collect images.

**ICS**  Intracranial self-stimulation.

**ICSI**  Intracytoplasmic sperm injection; see *ART*.

**ictal emotions**  Any suddenly occurring and quickly disappearing emotional reaction, but especially depression and anxiety. While affective disturbances may accompany almost any organic cerebral disorder, they are most frequently associated with disorders of the temporal lobe. A. A. Weil (*American Journal of Psychiatry 113*, 1956) suggested that such disturbances may be due to subclinical hippocampal-amygdaloid-temporal lobe epilepsy or after-discharge from these areas following manifest seizure activation.

**icterus gravis neonatorum**   *Kernikterus*; a manifestation of *erythroblastosis fetalis* in which the infant becomes jaundiced 2 or 3 days after birth and, if untreated, develops convulsions, rigidity, and coma. Mortality is high (75%) in untreated cases, and those who survive manifest residua, such as mental defect, epilepsy, chorea, or athetosis (*bilirubin encephalopathy*). Treatment is exchange transfusion with Rh-negative whole blood. Those in whom jaundice is severe, however, even when so treated show some degree of mental deficiency; follow-up studies indicate that such children have an IQ that averages 23 points below that of their siblings (Day, R. and Haines, M. S. *Pediatrics 13*, 1954).

**ictus**   1. An acute apoplectic stroke; epileptic seizure.

2. In psycholinguistics, the stressed syllable in a metrical unit.

**id**   In psychoanalytic psychology, one of the three divisions of the psyche in the so-called *structural hypothesis* of mental functioning; the other two are the ego and the superego. (In Freud's earlier theory, usually referred to as the *topographic hypothesis*, the psyche was divided into the three systems—conscious, preconscious, and unconscious.) The id is completely unconscious and hence partakes of the same processes that characterize the latter; viz., the pleasure principle and the *primary process* (q.v.). It is the reservoir of the psychic representatives of the drives and of all the phylogenic acquisitions. Freud assumed that the id comprised the total psychic apparatus at birth, and that the ego and superego were later differentiated from what had originally been id. At present, however, many psychoanalysts believe that the id itself is differentiated from the totally undifferentiated psychic apparatus and does not give rise to the ego and superego; but all agree that the id precedes, chronologically, the ego and the superego.

**id resistance**   A type of resistance that derives from the repetition compulsion and is manifested typically as situations of mistrust, grievance, depreciation, and the like, which dominate the analytic situation during periods of seeming stalemate. No matter how many interpretations are given by the analyst, and no matter how valid each interpretation seems to be, the same material continues to recur. The only method with which to counter id resistance is *working-through* (q.v.).

**id sadism**   The primary primitive instinctual destructive urges, seen in unmodified form in early infancy. They are closely allied with drives toward omnipotent gratification and security. Most primary sadism suffers repression under the aegis of the striving for goodness and approval, and the fear of the reality consequences to the subject of external retaliation and its internal equivalent, conscience pangs.

**idea**   Any mental content, especially imagining or thinking; often the term connotes a mental process that originates endogenously, rather than in response to any specific external stimulus. In psychoanalytic psychology, an idea is conceived of as existing in two parts, the mental representation of the thing being thought about and an accompanying affective charge; the latter, especially when the idea is "painful," may be split off or dissociated from the mental representation and attached to another idea (whose affective charge then appears inappropriate or excessive).

**idea of reference**   An unfounded suspicion or conviction that the conversation, smiling, or other actions of other persons are about oneself.

**ideal masochism**   *Moral masochism* (q.v.).

**ideal self**   See *idealization*.

**ideal-hungry personality**   See *mirroring deficits*.

**idealization**   Attribution of positive qualities (e.g., excellence, beauty, perfection, omnipotence, omniscience, unfailing empathy, unswerving love, unparalleled competence) to (the mental representations of) another person, an object, or the self. Idealizing requirements deal with the person's need to merge with, or be close to, someone who will make him or her feel safe, comfortable, and calm. As a result of being able to idealize parents and draw strength and comfort from that idealization, a child develops self-direction and an ability to set challenging but realistic goals.

A primitive omnipotent *ideal self* is initially generated in relation to the totally available, loving, need-satisfying, and tension-reducing *ideal object* (the mother). The message is, "I am perfect and you love me." In the early parent–child relationship, the child projects his or her own grandiosity into the parent who is thereby idealized (in Kohut's terms, the *idealized parental imago*). At first, the child wishes to merge with this all-powerful self-object ("You are perfect and I am part of you.") Over time, such a wish for merger leads to an internalization of the parent's competency and a desire to be close to the source of such power. Finally, the mature person is satisfied knowing that others (friends, family, etc.) are available in times of stress. See *basic trust; cohesive self.*

A repetition of the infantile idealization process occurs often in the treatment of patients with personality disorders. In the *idealizing transference*, a type of primary self-object transference, the patient again projects the child's *grandiose self* (q.v.) into the therapist, who is thereby transformed into an idealized parent figure. Such a transference is usually complicated by mounting expectations that are impossible to fulfill, in which case the patient experiences disappointment and then rage. As treatment continues, working through such episodes (*optimal disillusionment*) encourages gradual relinquishment of the therapist's idealized image and realistic acknowledgment of the distinction between ideal self-representation, ideal object-representation, and actual self-representation.

**idealized image**   The defense of having a false picture of one's virtues and assets. The more unrealistic (idealized) this image is, the more vulnerable is the person to the vicissitudes of life. The term was introduced by Horney.

Though constituting the base from which attitudes toward authority in general develop, the early attitude toward the father is added to and modified by subsequent experiences with father figures. In the relationship to the father, or to subsequent father figures, difficulties often arise, and to circumvent them, neurotic defenses may be developed. For instance, if the patient adjusts to a difficult father by becoming submissive, submissiveness itself becomes a problem. Thereupon, some sort of periodic aggressiveness may be developed to circumvent the problem of submissiveness. This new difficulty, in turn, produces new defenses and the adult patient now presents a complicated defensive system. Thus, the patient is sick because of what happened to him and also because, in coping with it, he establishes goals that lead him to pursue false values. See *idealized self.*

**idealized parental imago**   See *basic trust; cohesive self; idealization.*

**idealized self**   In Horney's terminology, grandiose overestimation of the self based on identification with the idealized image. The identification is a defense against recognition of the gap between the person as he really is and the person that his neurotic pride says he should be (*idealized image*). See *actual self.*

**idealizing transference**   See *idealization.*

**ideational apraxia**   *Sensory apraxia;* loss of the conceptional process. The patient does not know the use of objects; he may fumble with a toothbrush, pen, or cigarette but will not know what to do with them. See *apraxia.*

**ideator**   One who thinks about an action or concept; thus, a "homicide ideator" is one who thinks about killing someone else.

**idée fixe**   A delusion; an unfounded or unreasonable idea that is staunchly maintained despite evidence to the contrary. In contrast is an *imperative idea*, an obsessive thought that is recognized as unreasonable but cannot be resisted. An *autochthonous idea*, on the other hand, is an imperative idea that is attributed to some malevolent influence. See *autochthonous delusion; autochthonous idea.*

**identical**   In genetics, *monozygotic*, arising from one egg, as opposed to *dizygotic* or *fraternal,* twin pairs arising from two eggs.

**identification**   The process of making (or considering to be) the same; in psychodynamics, a primitive intrapsychic defense mechanism in which part of the subject's self-representation is altered by taking on some aspects of another object and making them his or her own.

"Identification is the most primitive method of recognizing external reality; it is, in fact, nothing less than mental mimicry. Its necessary reconditions are an unbroken narcissism, which cannot bear that anything should exist outside itself, and the weakness of the individual, which makes him unable either to annihilate his environment or to take flight from it" (Balint, A. *The Yearbook of Psychoanalysis I*, 1945).

Melanie Klein, when writing about the paranoid-schizoid position ("Notes on Schizoid

Mechanisms"), introduced the concepts of introjective identification and projective identification. In *introjective identification*, the desirable aspects of others are claimed as belonging to oneself; in *projective identification* (q.v.) undesirable aspects of oneself are deposited into others. See *incorporation; introjection; paranoid-schizoid position*.

**identification, multiple** Identification with more than one model or object, seen most commonly in hysterical seizures wherein the patient simultaneously or serially plays the part of various persons with whom he has identified. Such seizures may even represent the enactment of a whole drama. Multiple identification is also seen in cases of *dissociative identity disorder* (q.v.).

**identification, primary** In the stage of primary narcissism, perception by putting the object into the mouth results; the ego imitates what is perceived in order to master the object. The imitation of the external world by oral incorporation is the basis for that primitive mode of thinking called magic. Even though reality destroys the feeling of omnipotence, the longing for this primary narcissism remains—the narcissistic needs—and self-esteem is the awareness of how close the ego is to the original omnipotence. The desire to partake of the parental omnipotence, even though it arose originally from the basic desire for the satisfaction of hunger, soon becomes differentiated from the hunger itself, and the ego craves affection in a passive way (passive object love), being willing to renounce other satisfactions if rewards of affection are promised. See *autarchic fiction; ego; narcissism, primary; symbiotic stage*.

**identification, visual** The viewer's decision that an object seen is different from similar objects; the decision requires not only discrimination on the part of the viewer but also generalization across some shape changes, physical translation, rotation, etc. See *auditory cortex*.

**identity** A person's image, concept, or inner conviction, held as a whole or in relation to particular functions or roles, as in body identity, gender identity, mental or psychological identity, social identity. Identity is a stable awareness of who one is and where one is going, with a sense of cohesion with the ideas and values of a social group (one's peers).

Core *gender identity* (q.v.) refers to the subject's self-concept: "I am female/male"; gen-

der identity refers to femininity/masculinity as expressed behaviorally. Gender identity disorders include disturbances in both.

**identity, sexual** See *gender identity*.

**identity confusion** Not knowing one's name; *identity alteration* refers to believing that one is another person, such as an *alter* in *dissociative identity disorder* (q.v.).

**identity crisis** Social role conflict as perceived by a person; loss of the sense of personal sameness and historical continuity, or inability to accept or adopt the role the person believes is expected by society. Identity crises are frequent in adolescence, when they appear to be triggered by the combination of sudden increase in the strength of drives with sudden changes in the role the adolescent is expected to adopt socially, educationally, or vocationally.

**identity diffusion** 1. Instability of the view of the self, as seen in severe borderline personality disorders when split-off contradictory self-images are acted out in rapid chaotic succession. Identity diffusion indicates impaired ego integration and lack of a *cohesive self* (q.v.), manifested as deficiencies in anxiety tolerance, impulse control, and sublimation. See *splitting; structural*.

2. Lack of stability and consistency of the personality as seen in some borderline personality disorders whose pseudocompliance and passivity cover their motives, goals, feelings, etc. Bleuler termed this a disturbance in the person in describing fundamental symptoms of the schizophrenias. See *person, disturbances in the; "as if" personality*.

3. Identification with inadequate or pathological models, as seen in some antisocial or psychopathic personalities. See *crime and mental disorder*.

**identity disorder, dissociative** See *dissociative identity disorder*.

**identity disorder of childhood** Exhibited by the child or adolescent who is abnormally uncertain and concerned about long-term goals or career choice, patterns of friendship, sexual preference, religious affiliation, moral value system, etc., when the concern is of sufficient depth and extent to interfere with academic or social functioning.

**identity disorders, sexual and gender** This DSM-IV category includes *sexual dysfunctions, paraphilias* (*sexual deviation*), and *gender identity disorder* (qq.v.).

**identity integration**   See *structural*.

**identity vs. role confusion**   One of Erikson's eight stages of man. See *ontogeny, psychic*.

**ideogenetic**   Relating to mental processes in which images of sense-impressions are employed, rather than ideas that have reached the form or stage of being ready for verbal expression.

**ideoglandular**   Relating to the effect of thoughts and mental impressions on glandular functions.

**ideographic**   See *nomothetic*.

**ideology**   A systematic scheme of ideas that forms the characteristic perspective of a social group.

**ideophobia**   Fear of ideas.

**ideophrenia**   Guislain's term for delirium, characterized by ideational disorders.

**ideoplastic stage**   Verworn's term referring to the fact that the young child draws what he knows rather than what he sees. In the ideoplastic stage the child tends to exaggerate items that seem important or interesting and to minimize or omit the other parts. See *physioplastic stage*.

**ideoplasty**   Durand's term for the process of molding, making plastic, the subject's mind by means of ideas suggested by the hypnotist; called *verbal suggestion* by Ernest Jones.

**idio-**   Combining form meaning one's own, private, personal, from Gr. *idios*.

**idiogamist**   "One who is capable of coitus only with his own wife, or with a few individual women, but is impotent with women in general" (*Encyclopaedia Sexualis*, ed. V. Robinson, 1936).

**idioglossia**   Autonomous speech; cryptophasia; polyglot neophasia; an invented language or form of speech. See *glossolalia*.

**idiogram**   See *karyotype*.

**idiokinesis**   *Obs.* The "spontaneous" origin of a new hereditary character by means of *mutation* (q.v.), or more specifically, by mutation that takes place without determinable cause.

**idiolalia**   Development of one's own language, such as is seen with some children who suffer from auditory aphasia (word-deafness).

**idiopathic**   When the etiology of a disease or disorder is undetermined, but its functional phenomena are known, the condition is termed idiopathic. The National Conference on Nomenclature of Disease refers to "diseases due to unknown or uncertain causes, the functional reaction to which is alone manifest." For example, the syndrome called narcolepsy is well known, but its etiology is unknown; hence, the symptom complex is named *idiopathic narcolepsy*.

**idiophrenic**   Originating in one's own mind, psychogenic.

**idiophrenic psychosis**   *Obs.* Organic psychosis.

**idioplasm, idioplasma**   Introduced into biology by Naegeli to distinguish from the nutritive parts of the protoplasmic substance that portion of a cell upon which its specific qualities depend. Genetically it corresponds closely to the germ plasm of a germ cell, while its more general meaning embraces all the special hereditary equipment of an organism.

From the genetic standpoint, the transmission of hereditary characters from parents to offspring depends on the fact that the latter have, entirely or partially, the same idioplasmic structure as the parents, while all the genetic variations among adult individuals must be primarily the outcome of structural or chemical differences in the idioplasm. Minute idioplasmic differences between two ova may produce, in the course of their individual processes of development, a whole series of differences in various parts of the adult organism.

**idiosome**   The idioplasmic unit as the theoretically ultimate element of living matter carrying hereditary characteristics. See *idioplasm*.

**idiosyncrasia olfactoria**   Abnormality of the sense of smell.

**idiosyncratic alcohol intoxication**   See *alcoholic intoxication*.

**idiot**   Severe mental retardation. For the ancients, *idiot* referred to any person withdrawn into a private world, including exceptional children who nowadays would be termed *autistic*. See *amentia; retardation, mental*.

**idiot savant**   *Savant syndrome* (q.v.); idiotic prodigy; a person who, despite significant mental retardation or intellectual handicap, displays superior abilities or aptitudes in a special area.

Many such "savants" are now recognized to be persons with *autistic disorder* (q.v.) who have *splinter skills*, uncanny proclivities, such as being able to identify the day of the week of any date named over hundreds of years. Some authorities ascribe such abilities to weak central coherence in the thinking of autistic persons, whose attention is focused primarily on components or details rather than on integrated information. Savants do not have better memories in general, but their memories seem to be superior for tasks that are directly involved in their special skills; their overall verbal understanding and fluency are limited. See *Asperger syndrome.*

**idiotism**  Pinel divided insanity into four subdivisions: mania, melancholia, dementia, and idiotism (advanced dementia).

**idiotropic**  Introspective; egocentric.

**idiovariation**  In biology the genetic phenomenon of *mutation* (q.v.), implying a constant change in the genotypical structure of an organism.

**idolism, sexual**  Sexual fetishism. See *fetish.*

**IED**  Intermittent *explosive disorder* (q.v.).

**IEED**  Involuntary emotional expression disorder, an affective disinhibition syndrome characterized by recurrent, involuntary outbursts of crying or laughing, secondary to neurological damage. It has been described in association with Alzheimer disease and other dementias, amyotrophic lateral sclerosis, multiple sclerosis, Parkinson disease, stroke, and traumatic brain injury. The episodes are brief (seconds to minutes) and incongruent with or out of proportion to the patient's mood. They may occur early in the course of the underlying disorder, in which case they may be misdiagnosed as manic or depressive disorders.

IEED has also been called *pseudobulbar affect (PBA)*, although it is the affect that is exaggerated and inappropriate and not the medulla oblongata.

**IGF-1**  *Insulin-like Growth Factor* (q.v.).

**Ikaros**  See *heterochromatin.*

**ikota**  *Miryachit* (q.v.).

**Ilg, Francis L.**  (1903–1981) Pediatrician, pioneer in child development; coauthor (with Arnold Gesell) of *Infant and Child in the Culture of Today* (1943); cofounder of Gesell Institute of Child Development.

**IHS**  International Headache Society; see *headache.*

**IHT**  *Interhemispheric transfer* (q.v.).

**iich'aa**  A culture–bound syndrome described in the Navajo tribe, similar to *amok* (q.v.).

**IL-6 family**  See *cytokines.*

**Illinois Test of Psycholinguistic Abilities (ITPA)**  A diagnostic test of language abilities that yields language ages for nine specific psycholinguistic areas; precise areas of disability can thereby

be identified and an appropriate remedial program can be planned that provides special training in the problem areas.

**illness**  See *disease.*

**illness as self-punishment**  See *superego resistance.*

**illness-affirming behavior**  A nonspecific term referring to any disorder that simulates physical illness, e.g., conversion disorders, factitious disorders, hypochondriasis, malingering, somatization disorder, and somatoform pain disorders.

**illuminism**  A state of mental exaltation in which the subject's hallucinations generally assume the form of conversations with imaginary, especially supernatural, beings.

**illusion**  An erroneous perception, a false response to a sense-stimulation; but in a normal person this false belief usually brings the desire to check or verify its correctness, and often another sense or other senses may come to the rescue and satisfy him or her that it is merely an illusion.

If a straight glass tube is lowered into a tumbler of water, we have the visual illusion that the submerged portion of the tube has bent and forms an angle with its free upper part. This unexpected sight impels us to pull the tube out and convince ourselves that there is nothing the matter with the tube, but our eyes have misinterpreted the situation into an illusion: it merely looks, but actually is not, bent. See *kinephantom.*

In all such illusions the stimulus and the illusion (i.e., the reaction) involve the identical sense and can be disproven, making it much harder to realize that it is not an illusion when, sitting alone in a room, we suddenly start because we have "heard" somebody else in the room, only to convince ourselves that we are still alone in the room and that no sound had actually been heard.

The primary somatosensory cortex does not truthfully map the body surface; instead, it represents an internal brain image that is linked to subjective perception rather than to objective sensory input. A perceived image is related to the type of information that generates the illusion, such as topography, orientation, or motion. Specific information processing for motion does not take place in the primary visual cortex but rather in higher cortical regions, such as the mediotemporal area.

This absence of a sense stimulus places the reaction in a different class from those cited above—it is a *hallucination* (q.v.).

**illusion, memory**   Ascribing to oneself the experiences of others and believing implicitly that the experiences are one's own.

"Whoever considers himself Christ, believes that he had been crucified, and, under certain conditions can delude himself into remembering the details of it with perceptible acuteness" shows memory illusions (Bleuler, E. *Textbook of Psychiatry*, 1930). See *appersonification.*

**illusion, necessary**   Private evaluations of what is important and unimportant, what is of great value and of little value—evaluations that represent private predilections in private lives. It is important that an analyst be free of the tendency to confuse his private predilections, and his own unconsciously determined illusions, with the aims and goals of his patient's needs.

E. F. Sharpe (*Collected Papers on Psychoanalysis*, 1950) says: "We may privately prefer beech trees to cedars, that type of character to this, and have our private evaluations of what a worthy life really is.... But these things, eminently useful as they are to us as individuals and to our necessary illusions, are of small importance to the world outside us, and most assuredly they are of no use in the consulting-room."

**illusion of doubles**   See *Capgras syndrome.*

**illyngophobia**   Fear of dizziness or vertigo.

**image (imago)**   In psychoanalysis, the image or likeness of someone, usually not of the subject himself, constructed in the unconscious and remaining therein. The commonest imagos are those of the parents and of those who stand for the parents. E. Jones defines *imago* as "an image preserved indefinitely with persons other than the original one" (*Papers on Psycho-Analysis*, 1938).

Sometimes the person whose image is mirrored in the unconscious is spoken of as the *imago.*

**image agglutinations**   Kretschmer says that in dreams and twilight states mental activity appears in the form of sensory images, which sometimes appear as scenes but more often as "fragments of pictures which apparently go on without rules or regulations, and, under the influence of affects, again conglomerate into peculiar image groups, the *image agglu-*

*tinations.* The faces of several persons, several objects of similar emotional value, in the dreams are seen as one, and are conglomerated into unity; this we call, with Freud, 'condensation' " (*Hysteria*, 1926).

**image-distorting**   See *defense mechanisms; distortion.*

**imaged pseudohallucination**   See *pseudohallucination.*

**imagery**   A mental picture created when when perceptual information is accessed from memory, giving rise to the experience of "seeing with the mind's eye," "hearing with the mind's ear," etc. Perception, in contrast, occurs when information is registered directly from the senses. The left parietal lobe is predominant in generating mental images, whereas the right parietal lobe is specialized in the spatial operations of the imagined content.

**imagery, spontaneous**   Jellinek's term for visual images that can be produced at will when the eyes are closed. Spontaneous imagery is not a pathological phenomenon and is seen more commonly in children, probably because most children have a positive eidetic disposition. Spontaneous imagery is sometimes misinterpreted as visual hallucinations.

**imagery rehearsal therapy**   *IRT*; a manual-based form of short-term therapy that combines imagery exercises with cognitive treatment. Used in PTSD, for example, the frequent nightmares are targeted as habits or learned behaviors, which can be changed into positive, new imagery by rehearsing a new dream while awake.

**imaginal exposure**   One of the elements of exposure therapy for PTSD; patients are instructed to close their eyes and recall the traumatic event by imagining that it is happening right now while simultaneously describing out loud what is being remembered, with all its physical sensations along with thoughts and emotional reactions. These trauma narratives are repeated several times in the therapy session over the course of 20 to 45 minutes and recorded for the patient to listen to as daily homework. In addition to imaginal exposure, patients practice *in vivo exposure* to real life stimuli that trigger trauma-related memories and distress. This is accomplished through identifying the people, places, situations, and activities that trigger anxiety and avoidance. Then they repeatedly confront selected situations for prolonged periods until there is a significant reduction in anxiety. See *exposure methods*.

**imagination** Synthesis of mental images into new ideas; the process of forming a "mental representation of an absent object, an affect, a body function, or an instinctual drive," the results of which process are images, symbols, phantasies, dreams, ideas, thoughts, or concepts. Imagination is not, then, the obverse of reality, but affords, rather, a means of adaptation to reality. "Only with the development of the imaginative process, the capacity to create a mental representation of the absent object, does the child progress from the syncretic sensori-motor-affective immediate response to the delayed abstract, conceptualized response that is characteristically human" (Beres, D. *International Journal of Psycho-Analysis XLI*, 1960). See *phantasy*.

**imaging, brain** *Neuro-imaging*; picturing the brain in vivo, using various noninvasive radiologic techniques that utilize computer processing and enhancement of X-rays, electromagnetic radiation, or signals from charged particles in order to visualize cerebral structures, blood flow, or metabolism. Computer graphics use colors to represent a range of measurements, which are taken at different positions in space; from the results, the computer constructs a colored picture representing the structure or function being measured. The development of optical in vivo imaging (or in vivo microscopy) permits study of brain disorders in living organisms at the level of single cells. In vivo imaging can reveal how neurons in the intact nervous system change in relation to behavior adaptations or experience, and how cells are altered by pathology.

There are two major types of imaging: (1) tomographic methods, such as *CT, MRI* (including *fMRI* and dMRI), *PET*, and *SPECT*; (2) surface imaging, including the *electroencephalogram (EEG)*, evoked potentials such as the *ERP, polysomnography (PSG), rCBF*, and *CET* (qq.v.). See *evoked potential; neurometrics; tomography*.

Tomographic methods provide measurements at closely spaced intervals and yield pictures that resemble slices of a brain. Surface imaging methods are less precise than tomographic methods but also less costly and often much more rapid. See *pixel*.

Tomographic methods of brain imaging include X-ray computed tomography (CT), magnetic resonance imaging (MRI), functional MRI (fMRI), positron emission tomography (PET), and SPECT (single photon emission computed tomography). They are able to measure at closely spaced intervals and yield pictures that resemble slices of a brain. In CT, a rotating X-ray beam slices through the body in the desired plane while detectors on the opposite side of the patient record the degree to which the radiation is absorbed or attenuated by the tissues. The computer uses these density recordings to construct an image. With *fMRI* it is now possible to perform real-time studies of brain function, such as perception and cognition.

*Diffusion magnetic resonance imaging (dMRI*; also known as *diffusion tensor imaging*) produces MRI-based quantitative maps of microscopic, natural displacements of water molecules that occur in brain tissues as part of the physical diffusion process. It produces images of brain activity with MRI from signals that are directly associated with neuronal activation, rather than through changes in blood flow. Water molecules are used as a probe to reveal microscopic details about the architecture of both normal and diseased tissue. See *MRI*.

Surface imaging methods include regional cerebral blood flow (rCBF) and computer electroencephalographic topography (CET). See *neurometrics*.

One of the most important advantages of brain imaging is that it permits assessment of disease progression throughout the course of a chronic, progressive disorder such as Alzheimer and Parkinson diseases. It helps to answer such questions as: What is the rate of neuronal degeneration? What factors determine that rate? Can degeneration be detected before clinical symptoms develop? Will putative neuroprotective or restorative drugs slow or even restore neuronal degeneration?

**imago** See *image*.

**imbalance, structural** In family therapy, deviations in family patterns that interfere with the family's functioning. Among the most frequent imbalances are *role reversal, alliance and splitting*, and *scapegoating* (qq.v.). See *family culture, indigenous*.

**imbecile**  See *amentia; retardation, mental.*

**IMEPS**  Involuntary Movement and Extrapyramidal Side-Effects Scale.

**IMHV**  Intermediate part of the medial hyperstriatum ventrale, intimately involved in filial *imprinting* (q.v.) in domestic chicks, a model for studying the neural basis of learning.

**imidazole syndrome**  *Bessman-Baldwin syndrome*; a familial disorder of imidazole metabolism, described by Samuel Bessman and Ruth Baldwin. It consists of cerebromacular degeneration with convulsions, retinitis pigmentosa, mental retardation, and excessive urinary excretion of carnosine, anserine, and histidine.

**imitation**  1. Copying; replication, simulation. *Imitation* concerns motor behaviors that are determined by the observation of similar motor behaviors made by a conspecific. Imitation can be accompanied by an understanding of the action meaning, it might be an approximate or a precise replica of the observed action, and it might concern a series of motor acts nevers before performed by the observer (Rizzolatti, G. et al. *Nature Reviews Neuroscience 2,* 2001, 661–670).

Simulation (q.v.), also called *resonance behavior* and *shared representations,* is a postulated common coding for actions performed by the self and other persons. Several brain regions, including the premotor cortex, the posterior parietal cortex, and the cerebellum, are activated during action generation and while observing and simulating others' actions. Action observation activates the premotor cortex in a somatotopic manner—simply watching mouth, hand, and foot movement activates the same functionally specific region of premotor cortex as performing those movements. See *mirror neurons; response facilitation.*

2. The tendency to assume certain attitudes, lifestyles, or manners that are valued by one's society.

**imitation, hysterical**  The ability of a hysterical patient to imitate all the symptoms that impress him when they occur in others. The patient (unconsciously) identifies himself with a person who has the same unconscious needs as he, who is "just like" him. Through this hysterical imitation "patients are enabled to express in their symptoms not merely their own experiences, but the experiences of quite a number of other persons; they can suffer, as

it were, for a whole mass of people, and fill all the parts of a drama with their own personalities." For example, one girl in a school may react to a love letter with a fainting spell. Other girls then may also get fainting spells. Unconsciously the other girls also wanted love letters, and having the same unconscious wish they have to suffer the same consequence—they, too, had fainting spells through hysterical identification (Freud, S. *The Interpretation of Dreams,* 1933).

**immanence theory**  The closed circle hypothesis of life that describes the function of each organ in terms of what it accomplishes for the rest of the organism. According to such a view, the life process would have the pattern of a logical vicious circle. The part processes have the function of sustaining life; and life is an aggregation of these part processes. This theory is the opposite of *holism* (q.v.).

**immediate early gene**  A gene that is expressed rapidly and transiently in response to various cellular stimuli. Several of these genes (e.g., *Fos* and *Egr1*) are used as indirect markers of neuronal activity because they are expressed when neurons fire action potentials.

**immediate memory**  A form of *short-term memory* (q.v.); the longest sequence of items that can be reproduced correctly following a single presentation. Its capacity is limited (less than a dozen items) and its duration short (in the absence of rehearsal it persists only for minutes). The information is later transformed into more permanent *long-term memory* (q.v.). When the items are presented in a random order, the normal span is about seven so long as attention is not distracted. Clinically, immediate memory is commonly measured by the digit span. See *amnestic syndrome.*

**immobilization paralysis**  "In wound-cases where there had been immobilization of a limb in splints for some time, the immobilization sometimes persisted long after the splints were removed—the so-called immobilization-paralysis." The patient had "failed to realize when he had become well." The hysterical purpose was the same as in the unwounded cases of functional paralysis. (Henderson, D. K. and Gillespie, R. D. *A Text-Book of Psychiatry,* 1936). See *fixation hysteria.*

**immobilizing activity**  Slavson suggests this term in relation to activity group psychotherapy as a form of *libido-binding* activities. By this he means activities that tie one down to a specific interest or occupation; to attain this he has devised a special environment for group psychotherapy, which is in contrast to stimulating or libido-activating activities (*An Introduction to Group Therapy*, 1943). See *group psychotherapy*.

**immoral imperative**  The antisocial unconscious impulses that compel the person to desire the occurrence of events, or the performance of actions, considered unethical or antimoral. This mental mechanism is often observed in the compulsive-neurotic, as a compulsion to act against the rules of society, an impulsive subconscious rebellion against moral principles. The destructive aims of the immoral imperative are often directed against religious principles, precisely because religion is one of the most powerful barriers controlling man's instinctual life (Stekel, W. *Compulsion and Doubt*, 1949).

**immune deficiency syndrome**  See *AIDS*.

**immune hypothesis of schizophrenia**  The suggestion that schizophrenia is one of a spectrum of neuropsychiatric disorders whose proximate cause is an autoimmune attack on the brain. Possible mechanisms for such a process include immunogenetic errors, viral (including prion) provocation, or vascular inflammation. Major *histocompatibility* complex (MHC) class I molecules play a significant role in the developing and adult central nervous system. Several neurological disorders are associated with immune symptoms: spinocerebellar ataxia, Huntington and Parkinson diseases, multiple sclerosis, narcolepsy, dyslexia, autism, and schizophrenia.

Patients who have a first degree relative with schizophrenia are more likely also to have a parent or sibling with autoimmune disease. Conversely, there is a strong negative correlation between schizophrenia and two autoimmune disorders, rheumatoid arthritis and insulin-dependent diabetes mellitus. It is possible that changes in expression of neuronal MC class I, when it is involved in the development of neuronal circuits, might cause neurodevelopmental abnormalities that lead to schizophrenia.

**immune system**  It comprises a humoral arm, the one that makes antibodies, and cell-mediated responses, which direct killer T cells (cytotoxic T lymphocytes, CTLs) to eliminate cells infected with foreign invaders such as viruses.

The immune system is important in distinguishing self from non-self, as well as recognizing specific foreign antigens. Three signals are needed to activate the immune system: a specific antigen is recognized by the T cell; stressed, damaged, lysed, or necrotic cells send an alarm signal that activates the dendritic cell; the dendritic cell acts as a costimulatory signal with the T cell. In the absence of danger, T cells lose their ability to respond, and tolerance results. Similarly, a T cell encountering an antigen normally found in the body, such as the proteins located on the body's own healthy tissues, dies or becomes unresponsive. In this way, each tissue is constantly inducing tolerance to itself over its lifetime.

**impaired control**  See *alcoholism*.

**impaired physician**  A physician whose clinical conduct does not meet accepted standards of practice, based on a condition that is secondary to alcohol-drug use, psychiatric illness, physical illness, or all three.

**impairment index**  In neuropsychological assessment, a measure of the degree of brain damage or deterioration in higher intellectual functioning, used to differentiate between organic neurologic disorders and other conditions that mimic them.

**impatience**  See *time discounting*.

**impediment**  See *disease*.

**imperative idea**  Obsession.

**imperception**  See *sensory neglect*.

**impersonal projection**  Projection alone means attributing one's own ideas or impulses to another. By implication, this is done because one finds his own ideas or impulses objectionable. Impersonal projection refers to the same mechanism applied not to objectionable material but to impersonal or neutral material. One example of impersonal projection is found in the echo of reading aloud, when the subject feels that someone else is saying the words that he is reading.

**imperviousness to error**  See *Wisconsin Card Sort(ing) Test*.

**impetus**  In psychoanalysis, one of the parameters defining a *drive* (q.v.). The impetus of a drive is its force, strength, or energy, and in all likelihood is genetically determined. The other parameters by which a drive (or, in older terminology, an instinct) is customarily defined are source (the physiological disequilibrium or organ system through which the drive becomes manifest), and the aim and object of the drive.

**impingement**   In Winnicott's terminology, interference with the infant's maturation by unnecessary intrusions (typically by the mother) into his *going on being*, his increasing comfort and ease in taking part in the outside world through creativity, play, and other activities that feel worthwhile and gradually supplant involvement in transitional phenomena. Impingements may be so pervasively and continuously disruptive as to prevent a True Self from being organized. Instead, the child develops a *False Self* (q.v.) to protect the True Self from the danger of exploitation.

**implant, dynamic**   Introduction or instillation of a significant idea into consciousness; used mainly in connection with *psychic driving*, one of whose values is said to be long-lasting action on the part of the patient as a result of one or more dynamic implants. The latter bring the patient to focus on specific behavior or action tendencies; this usually leads to intensified activity in the form of tension and anxiety and thus to greater efforts to free himself of such intensification. As a result, the patient tends to ruminate over and to reorganize his reactions to the material in question. This would appear to be a mechanistic description of one type of insight. See *driving, psychic; menticide.*

**implantation, disulfiram**   See *Antabuse.*

**implicit memory**   Nondeclarative, procedural, or motoric memory; various forms of memory that are not directly accessible to consciousness. Included are skill and habit learning, classical conditioning, priming, and other circumstances in which memory is expressed through performance rather than through conscious recollection. See *long-term memory; procedural memory.*

**implicit perception**   Perception in the absence of awareness, as in *blindsight* (q.v.).

**implicit role**   See *role.*

**implosion**   *Flooding*; imaginal exposure; reduction of avoidance behavior by prolonged exposure of the patient to the feared object or situation, thereby demonstrating that the feared situation causes him no harm. The subject is directed to imagine entering the worst situation and experience the most feared consequences until they cease to provoke anxiety. Some workers use implosion to refer to imagined exposure to the feared situation and

flooding to refer to real-life (in vivo) exposure in which the patient encounters the real situation that is feared or produces anxiety and panic. Sometime *shaping* is used, consisting of successive approximations of the feared object or situation—beginning with the least difficult and being exposed again and again until the situation no longer provokes anxiety. Exposure homework is an important part of this behavioral approach; it begins with programmed practice sessions and moves on to self-directed exposure.

Imaginal flooding has been used also in the treatment of anxiety-provoking obsessions. The patient describes the obsessions in detail (e.g., how his family will be destroyed by his carelessness, or the dreaded consequences of his blasphemous thoughts), and the thoughts are played back repeatedly on a tape recorder.

*Virtual exposure therapy* has been reported to be effective in acrophobia. Computer-constructed views of elevators and bridge sare projected on the inside of a helmet visor. Within 20 seconds of donning the helmet, the projected views became real to the patients and after seven weekly sessions of exposure to increasingly frightening heights, anxiety levels fell dramatically.

**impostor**   A type of *pathological liar* who seeks to gain some advantage by means of imposing on others fabrications of his attainments, position, or worldly possessions. P. Greenacre (*Psychoanalytical Quarterly 27*, 1958) noted the compulsive, pressured aspect to the impostor's urge to seek the limelight and "put something over" on his audience. She outlined the following features, which appear to be of psychodynamic significance: the typically ambivalent and overpossessive mother creates so intense a maternal attachment in the child that he is unable to develop a full sense of separate identity. At the same time his ability to assume an uncontested supersedence over the father as far as the mother is concerned intensifies infantile narcissism and favors a reliance on omnipotent phantasy to the exclusion of reality testing. Imposture is an outgrowth of the oedipal conflict and represents an attempt to kill the father and/or to rob him of his more adequate penis. Success of this mechanism as evidenced by belief in the impostor by his audience (the mother) furnishes a powerful incentive for endless repetition of the fraudulent behavior. See *factitial*.

**impotence (impotency)** A *sexual disorder* (q.v.) consisting of inability of the male to perform sexual intercourse in spite of sexual desire and the presence of intact genital organs. There may be *erective impotence* (*male erectile disorder*, inability to achieve or maintain erection), *ejaculatory impotence* (inability to expel seminal fluid), or *orgastic impotence* (inability to achieve full orgasm). Premature ejaculation, *ejaculatio retardata*, the separation of the tender and sensual components of the sexual act so that intercourse is possible only with prostitutes, and the need for fixed and specific conditions to be operative before sexual intercourse can be performed, are all types of psychic impotence. Depression following the sexual act (*postcoitum triste*) is a type of orgastic impotence.

E. Bergler (*Psychiatric Quarterly 19*, 1945) classified psychic impotence on the basis of etiology in three main groups: (1) potency disturbance arising from phallic (hysterical) mechanisms; (2) potency disturbance arising from anal mechanisms (obsessional, hypochondriacal, and masochistic types); (3) disturbance arising from oral mechanisms. Impotence based on phallic mechanisms results from an unresolved attachment to the mother of the oedipal period; castration fears lead to subsequent repression of sexual desire for the mother, but finally all sexual objects become identified with her. Persistence of castration fears leads to potency disturbances. In the second group, in an obsessional neurotic, potency disturbances result from the association of sexuality with dirt and filth, which must be avoided at all costs, and from the need to ward off the aggressive and sadistic impulses that are aroused by the sexual act. Erective impotence is rare in the obsessional group, but ejaculatio retardata is common. The latter has the significance of anal retention pleasure combined with sadistic pleasure in harming the woman through prolonged intercourse. Potency disturbance arising from oral mechanisms is commonly expressed as either premature ejaculation or psychogenic aspermia. The former signifies: "I do not want to refuse the woman anything; indeed, I give immediately." Psychogenic aspermia (ejaculatory impotence) signifies: "I deny you my semen just as mother denied me her milk."

There is no doubt that impotence of purely psychologic origin occurs, but the majority of penile erectile disorders are on an organic basis. They are frequently due to general medical conditions—neurological disorders, such as multiple sclerosis, peripheral neuropathy, and spinal cord lesions; endocrine disorders such as diabetes, hypothyroidism, hypogonadism, and pituitary or adrenal dysfunction; peripheral vascular disease; renal failure; and genitourinary disorders. Another frequent cause is autonomic nervous system injury secondary to surgery or radiation. Pharmacologic agents, and particularly many of the antihypertensive agents, antidepressants, and neuroleptics currently in use, very often interfere with sexual response in both men and women. Drugs of abuse are also a frequent reason for male erectile disorder.

**impotence, cerebral** M. Hirschfeld postulated four types of impotence: (1) cerebral, due to cerebral causes; (2) spinal, associated with difficulties of erection and ejaculation of spinal origin; (3) genital, connected with genital defects; and (4) germinal (*Sexual Pathology*, 1939).

**impotentia coeundi** Inability to cohabit.

**impregnation phobia** See *cancer phobia*.

**imprinting** 1. A genetic phenomenon—*genomic imprinting*—in which the gene contributed by one parent is somehow shut down, leaving the other parent's gene as the only functional copy. Over 16 imprinted genes are known, and in two-thirds of them the father contributes the active gene. See *imprinting, genomic*.

2. Called *Prägung* by the German ethologists who originally described the phenomenon, imprinting is "the process by which certain stimuli become capable of eliciting certain 'innate' behavior patterns during a critical period of the animal's behavioral development" (Jaynes, J. *Journal of Comparative and Physiological Psychology 49*, 1956). In the mallard duck, for instance, the first moving object the duckling sees during a critical period shortly after hatching is thereafter reacted to as ducklings usually behave toward the mother duck. For many years, it was believed that imprinting enabled the infant animal to learn about its species. It is now known that imprinting instead enables the young animal to recognize one or both of its parents as individuals.

A site in the intermediate part of the medial hyperstriatum ventrale (*IMHV*) is intimately involved in filial imprinting in domestic chicks. Storage of the information is retained only on the left side of the brain; on the right, information is stored initially in the IMHV but within 24 hours has disappeared to other, so far unidentified sites.

The degree to which imprinting determines or affects learning and behavioral patterning in the human has not been established, although it has been hypothesized that some forms of mental retardation are due to lack of appropriate stimulation or opportunity when the child is in a critical or sensitive period for the acquisition of specific skills (the stimulation theory of mental retardation). See *instinct; releaser, social; retardation, mental.*

The concept of imprinting has been used to explain paraphilias, such as pedophilia and transsexuality, in humans. Considering the lack of objective data on the phases of childhood sexuality, the lack of evidence for any critical periods in sexual and attitudinal development, the uncertainty as to whether reimprinting or partial imprinting can occur, and the time lag of years between hypothesized imprinting and the appearance of behavior that has presumably been learned through the process, such theories appear at least to be premature, if not totally without foundation.

**imprinting, genomic** The process by which maternal and paternal genomes contribute differentially to the developing embryos of their offspring. Genomic imprinting might play a role in fragile X syndrome, Angelman syndrome, and Prader-Willi syndrome. In both the Angelman and Prader-Willi syndromes, mental retardation is the foremost symptom, and both are disorders of chromosome 15. Yet the associated symptoms are almost the exact opposite in the two disorders: hyperactivity in Angelman syndrome, and bradykinesis and obesity in Prader-Willi syndrome. In Angelman syndrome, both copies of the chromosome are inherited from the father; in Prader-Willi, both come from the mother. See *fragile X syndrome.*

There is some evidence that differential methylation patterns might be responsible for such different effects of the same gene, depending upon which parent donates the gene. There is also evidence that imprinting might depend on chromatin winding, and on the closeness of the gene to proteins in the tightly wound protein.

**improvement rate** The ratio of the number discharged as improved within a given period (usually a year) to the total number in the original group. In institutional statistics this rate is usually approximated by relating the number discharged as improved in a given period to the number who were admitted during the same period.

Example: In one psychiatric hospital, 616 patients were admitted during the year. During the same period, 542 patients were discharged as improved. The improvement rate is 88%. See *discharge rate.*

**impuberism** The state of not having reached the age or stage of puberty. While strictly speaking it denotes the life period before puberty and thus embraces the stages of infantilism and childhood, generally it means that the mental and physical characteristics of childhood or occasionally of infancy run into and continue during the chronologically later and distinct adolescent or even adult life.

**impulse** A stimulus that sets the mind in action. The stimulus may originate in (1) the objective world, or (2) the subject himself: (a) his soma—within any part of the body; (b) his psyche—its conscious or its unconscious part. In psychoanalysis it most commonly refers to the instincts; a basic impulse is an instinct, the source of which is a "somatic process in an organ or part of the body" (Freud, *Collected Papers*, 1924–25). See *drive; instinct.*

**impulse control** See *ego weakness.*

**impulse control disorders** Characteristics include failure to resist an urge or temptation to do something that will harm oneself or others, a sense of increasing tension or arousal preceding the act, and a feeling of relief, pleasure, or gratification during or upon completion of the act. Unlike the typical *compulsion* (q.v.), the impulse itself is ego syntonic and concordant with the subject's current wish or desire, even though it may be resisted. The act may be unplanned or premeditated, but it usually has the qualities or impetuosity and lack of deliberation.

Among the impulse control disorders are intermittent *explosive disorder*, pathological *gambling, kleptomania, pyromania*, and *trichotillomania* (qq.v.). By some, they are considered part of the OCD spectrum.

**impulse interpretation** *Id interpretation*; in psychoanalytic therapy, an interpretation that overcomes a defense and permits certain painful thoughts or feelings to come into consciousness.

**impulsion** Blind obedience to internal drives, such as is seen typically in children, whose interpersonal relations and superego have not yet formed an organized defense against the drives. Impulsion is seen in adults whose defensive organization is weak; in adults, it is usually part of a behavior pattern and is more commonly called *impulsivity* (q.v.).

In psychoanalysis, impulsion and instinct are often used interchangeably.

**impulsivity** A predisposition toward rapid, unplanned reactions to internal or external stimuli with diminished regard to the negative consequences of these reactions to the impulsive individual or others. A pattern of behavior consisting of rapid, unplanned actions which occur unexpectedly, without reflection or conscious judgment, and without regard for possible consequences. See *catathymic crisis; impulse control disorders*.

**Imu** A psychoreactive phenomenon seen among the Ainu, consisting of hyperkinesia, catalepsy, echolalia, echopraxia, and command automatism. Imu occurs almost exclusively in adult females. See *hysterical psychosis*.

**in vivo exposure** See *behavior therapy; implosion*.

**inability** See *disability*.

**inaccessibility** Inability to be reached; unresponsiveness. Used most commonly to refer to the autism and withdrawal of the schizophrenic.

**inactivation** A refractory state that occurs in voltage-gated ion channels if depolarization (which opened or activated the channel) is maintained. See *desensitization*.

**inadequacy, intellectual** See *retardation, mental*.

**inadequate personality** A *personality pattern disturbance* (q.v.) in which the person, although neither physically nor mentally retarded, is nonetheless inept, unadaptable, and ineffectual in response to social, intellectual, and physical demands and shows a lack of physical and emotional stamina.

**inappetence** Absence of appetite or desire.

**inattention** See *extinction; sensory neglect*.

**inattention, selective** Ignoring or disregarding attitudes, traits, values, etc., because they are given no special value by the significant people in the developing child's milieu.

According to Sullivan, the self is finally formed out of a great number of potentialities. The child tends to develop and enhance those of his traits that are pleasing or acceptable to the significant adults, and to block out of awareness and disassociate those attributes that meet with their disapproval. Obviously there are some attributes that are neutral in the estimation of the significant people. Since no special attention is paid to these attributes, the child may or may not be aware of them, and it may be said that "selective inattention" has been at work. Unlike disassociated material, disavowed because it has been disapproved by the significant adults, the material on which selective inattention acts can, without great difficulty, be incorporated into the *self-system* (q.v.) if such behavioral attributes should later become important in the eyes of others. The difference between selective inattention and disassociation is not clear-cut, however, and is largely one of degree.

**in-between** A literal translation of Hirschfeld's Zwischenstufe, meaning an in-between sexual stage (specifically, homosexuality).

**inbreeding** In genetics, the special form of reproductive conditions that prevail in an isolated and relatively homogeneous group, whose members exclusively and persistently select their marriage partners from their own group. Such selective reproduction gradually leads to the formation of more or less purebred stocks and counteracts the normal effects of propagation, consisting of the continuous creation of new combinations of hereditary or nonhereditary differences. See *variation*.

In the reproduction of a species in which *hybridization*, or even *panmixia*, has been the rule, the results of inbreeding are almost invariably disadvantageous. The worst effects are caused by the increased production of homozygotic carriers of *recessive* traits, which under normal reproductive conditions would appear only rarely. See *intermarriage*.

Mutations tend to appear more frequently when inbreeding is of marked degree. This may be no more than a reflection of the fact that the majority of mutations are recessive, and inbreeding may facilitate their discovery.

**incendiarism** *Pyromania* (q.v.).

**incentive motivation** The priming or drivelike effects of an encounter with an otherwise neutral stimulus that has acquired motivational importance through prior association with a primary reward.

**incentive salience**  See *reward*; *salience*.

**incentive stimulus**  An external stimulus capable of driving behavior, such as the sight or smell of food.

**incest**  Any sexual contact, or behavior for the purpose of sexual stimulation, between an adult and child related within a family structure (including stepchildren and stepparents of reconstituted families). The activity may include direct contact, such as touching, oral-genital contact, or intercourse, or less direct activities, such as showing erotic materials or making sexually suggestive comments to a child. The involved child is exploited to meet the sexual wishes of the adult.

Sexual activity between siblings is the most common form of incest. Of reported cases, fathers' and stepfathers' sexual abuse of daughters and stepdaughters account for over 75%. Female children are more likely than male children to be the victims; men are more likely than women to be the offenders. There is no strong evidence of any pathognomonic dysfunction in incest families, although the more severe and chronic the abuse and the closer the relationship to the offender, it is generally believed that the impact on the child-victim is likely to be greater. Long-term effects that have been reported include promiscuity, substance abuse, sexual dysfunctions, and revictimization through adult relationships with abusive partners. See *battered child syndrome*; *child abuse*; *pedophilia*.

**incest barrier**  The ego's defenses against incestuous impulses, which are formed mainly in the latency period by deflection of infantile impulses from their sexual aims, with resultant desexualization of impulses.

**incest offender**  See *pedophilia*.

**incidence**  The number of new cases of any disorder that develop in a given population in a given period of time. Incidence rates are usually expressed per year, per 100,000 population:

$$\text{incidence rate of illness} = \frac{\text{new cases in 1 year}}{\text{persons exposed in 1 year to the risk of disease}} \times 100{,}000$$

The exposed population may be the entire population or, particularly when the illness in question begins only during a limited period of years or is confined to one sex, it may be specifically limited to an age group or sex within the total population. See *epidemiology; prevalence; rate.*

**incipient**  Beginning, inchoate, threatening, not fully formed; used often to modify the word schizophrenia by those reluctant to make such a diagnosis in the absence of secondary or accessory symptoms.

**INCL**  Infantile NCL; see *lipofuscinosis, neuronal ceroid.*

**inclusion bodies**  In numerous neurodegenerative disorders, affected neurons often display characteristic neurofibrillary inclusion bodies that are considered hallmarks of a particular disease process: in Parkinson disease, Lewy bodies in neurons within substantia nigra; in Pick disease, Pick bodies in cerebral cortex; in ALS, neurofilament-protein-containing spheroids and inclusions in motor neurons. This suggests that neurofilament protein synthesis, degradation, assembly, or transport in neurons where such processes are highly regulated may be implicated in neurodegeneration across a broad spectrum of diseases and linked to individual patterns of selective vulnerability.

**inclusion criteria**  See *SADS.*

**inclusive fitness**  See *fitness; kin selection.*

**incoherence**  Disorganization; used most commonly to refer to speech that is disconnected and unintelligible.

**incompetence, incompetency**  A legal term referring primarily to defects in intellectual functioning such that comprehension of the nature of a transaction is interfered with or otherwise inadequate; *non compos mentis.* (See *competence.*) While incompetent refers to the subject's inability to take in and assess information about his illness and the treatment required, and *irrational* refers to the subject's inability to make reasonable choices, both are admittedly elusive concepts that defy precise definition and occur in varying degrees. Furthermore, judgment as to their presence is influenced by cultural, attitudinal, and other subjective factors.

**incongruity**  Lack of consistency or appropriateness; used most commonly to refer to the disharmony between speech and affect characteristic of the schizophrenic and of patients with psychotic mood disorders. (See *mood-congruent.*)

Also applied to inconsistency in the informational interaction between the organism and environmental circumstances; i.e., the discrepancy between incoming information of the moment and information already stored and coded within the brain in the course of previous encounters with the category of circumstances concerned. There appears to be an optimal amount of incongruity (or novelty, uncertainty, *cognitive dissonance*, etc.) for each organism at any given moment, in all probability determined largely by experience. When a situation is too incongruous, the organism withdraws; where it offers too little incongruity, boredom results and the organism seeks another situation offering more incongruity, stimulus change, novelty, dissonance, or uncertainty.

**incoordination**  *Ataxia* (q.v.).

**incorporation**  The earliest instinctual aim directed toward objects and the most primitive method of recognizing external reality by assimilating external objects. Everything that is pleasurable is something to swallow and becomes ego; thus incorporation is the prototype of instinctual satisfaction, and all sexual aims are derivative of incorporation aims. Incorporation is also the prototype of regaining the omnipotence previously projected onto adults. But what is incorporated and taken in is also destroyed, so that the ego later uses incorporation in a hostile way to execute destructive impulses. Any instinctual aim may regress to incorporation or introjection.

Some writers use incorporation synonymously with *identification* and *introjection* (qq.v.); others equate incorporation with introjection and define both as the mechanism by which identification takes place. Others differentiate between them on the basis of the phase or level of psychic organization and development at which the assimilation of the object takes place. Thus incorporation refers to assimilation of external objects at the phase of primary narcissism, when there is no distinction between subject and object; introjection takes place during the phase of differentiation between the I and the not-I; identification can occur only when the distinction between subject and object is solidly established. Unlike introjection, identification is a purely intrapsychic process.

**incubus**  A parasomnia of adults consisting of a feeling of respiratory oppression (e.g., as though rocks were piled on the chest), partial paralysis, and anxiety or terror. In an obsolete usage, the term was used to describe a woman's nightmare that a man or evil demon has entered her bed during the night to have intercourse with her. See *succubus*.

**indecent exposure**  See *exhibitionism*.

**indemnity neurosis**  Levy-Bruhl's term for *compensation neurosis* (q.v.).

**index case**  In genetics and epidemiology, the person in a family or group who is the subject of investigation; a person disclosing clinical evidence of the trait under investigation; the proband.

**index of body build**  See *body build, index of*.

**index of sexuality (IS)**  An index proposed by Linhares and De Oliveira:

$$IS = \frac{\text{Urine 17 ketosteroids (mg)} \times 10}{\text{Urine phenol} - \text{steroids (ug)}} \times 100$$

Normal values are 2.6 to 4.3 for men, and 0.6 to 1.0 for women. The index is low in hypogenital men and high in climacteric women.

**indexical communication**  See *communication, nonverbal*.

**indifference reaction**  An emotional reaction associated with brain injury, characterized by lack of concern about failure, loss of interest in family and friends, minimization of physical difficulties, enjoyment of foolish jokes, and in many cases neglect for the half of the body and of space opposite to the site of brain damage. Indifference reactions are reported more frequently in right hemisphere damage than in left hemisphere damage. See *catastrophic behavior*; *sensory neglect*.

**indigenous family culture**  See *family culture, indigenous*.

**indigenous worker**  See *caregiver*.

**indirect associations**  One of the disturbances of associations seen often in the schizophrenias. With indirect associations, A may be connected to B and B may be connected to C, but the connecting link B is unexpressed so that the listener finds the statement incomprehensible, illogical, or bizarre.

**indiscriminate behavior**  See *parenting behaviors*.

**individual**  Jung defines the psychological individual as "unique-being" and as characterized by its peculiar, and in certain respects unique, psychology. "Everything is individual that is not collective, everything in fact that pertains only to one and not to a larger group of individuals. Individuality can hardly be described as belonging to the psychological elements, but rather to their peculiar and unique grouping and combination" (*Psychological Types*, 1923).

**individual psychology** Adlerian psychology, a discipline elaborated by the Viennese psychiatrist Alfred Adler. The complete name of his system is comparative individual-psychology. "By starting with the assumption of the *unity of the individual*, an attempt is made to obtain a picture of this unified personality regarded as a variant of individual life-manifestations and forms of expression. The individual traits are then compared with one another, brought into a common plane, and finally fused together to form a composite portrait that is, in turn, individualized" (*The Practice and Theory of Individual Psychology*, 1924).

Among the key concepts of individual psychology are (1) *fictional finalism,* the idea that expectations about the future rather than experiences in the past are the significant determinants of motivation; (2) *striving for superiority*, an innate tendency to develop one's capacities to the fullest; (3) *inferiority feelings*, springing from the recognition that one has failed to achieve perfection or to develop capacities to the fullest; (4) *social interest*, an innate tendency to involvement with others; (5) *lifestyle,* each person's unique way of striving for perfection; and (6) *creative self,* the center of personality, which interprets experience and guides the responses to it.

**individual-response specificity** The tendency of a subject to respond maximally and consistently in one particular physiological system. Such specificity is hypothesized to be a significant factor in organ choice, that is, in determining in what bodily system dysfunction will be expressed, as in psychosomatic disorders. *I-R specificity* is approximately equivalent to what used to be referred to as *locus minoris resistentiae* in that it is one manifestation of susceptibility to, overactivity on the part of, or damage to a particular organ system. See *organ inferiority; psychosomatic medicine; compliance, somatic.*

**individuation** "The process of forming and specializing the individual nature; in particular, it is the development of the psychological individual as a differentiated being from the general, collective psychology. Individuation, therefore, is a process of differentiation, having for its goal the development of the individual personality" (Jung, C. G. *Psychological Types*, 1923). Certain archetypes are identified with and characteristic of the four principal stages of the individuation process. They are, in chronological order, as follows: (1) the archetype of the shadow; (2) the archetype of the soul-image; (3) the archetype (in men) of the old wise man or of the Magna Mater (in women); and (4) the archetype of the self.

**individuation stage** See *separation-individuation.*

**Indoklon** Trade name for hexafluorodiethyl ether, which has been used as a form of convulsant therapy in psychiatric patients.

**indole** A class of biogenic amines that includes lysergic acid (LSD), bufotenin, dimethyltryptamine, and *serotonin* (q.v.). The indole amines derive from the essential amino acid tryptophan; monoamine oxidase inhibitors elevate the levels of indole amines by delaying their breakdown. See *amine.*

The biosynthetic pathway for the indole amines is: tryptophan → serotonin (5-hydroxytryptamine, 5-HT) → 5-hydroxyindoleacetic acid (5-HIAA). See *neurotransmitter.*

**induced hallucination** Hallucination aroused in one person by another, as may occur during hypnosis. See *induced psychotic disorder.*

**induced proximity** Recruitment of several molecules into an aggregate, which renders them active even though singly they are inactive. Induced proximity was first observed in caspase-8; it is also used to activate at least two other caspases, caspase-9 and the nematode caspase homolog CED-3. See *caspases.*

**induced psychotic disorder** *Psychosis of association; shared psychotic disorder;* a form of psychosis in which certain of the mental symptoms of one person (the principal) appear in similar or identical form in one or more other people (the associates) who are closely associated with the first. This association is typically intrafamilial, as in two siblings, or in parent and child, or in husband and wife; but it has also been reported among pairs of patients on a psychiatric ward and in pairs of friends who have been in intimate social contact over a period of time. When the number of people involved is two, the condition is sometimes called *folie à deux* (q.v.); there may be three (*folie à trois*), four (*folie à quatre*), or many (*folie à beaucoup*) involved. Other names by which this condition has been known are infectious insanity (Ideler, 1838); psychic infection (Hoffbauer, 1846); familial mental infection (Séguin, 1879); reciprocal insanity (Parsons, 1883); *collective insanity* (Ireland, 1886); double insanity (Tuke, 1887); *influenced psychosis* (Gordon, 1925); mystic paranoia (Pike, 1933); shared paranoid disorder (DSM-III). See *paranoia*.

Most writers agree that induced psychosis is limited to paranoid and depressive psychoses. Four types of psychosis of association are recognized: (1) *imposed* (described by Laseque and Falret, 1877), in which the associate accepts the delusions of the principal with little elaboration, and separation of the patients typically results in disappearance of the delusions in the associate; (2) *simultaneous* (described by Regis, 1880), in which there is simultaneous appearance of identical symptoms in more than one subject, and these symptoms are typically depression or persecutory ideas; (3) *communicated* (described by Marandon de Montyel, 1881), in which the associate takes over the delusions of the principal and works them into his own system, often with elaboration, and these delusions are usually maintained even after separation of the two; and (4) *induced* (described by Lehmann, 1885), wherein a second receptive patient adds the principal's delusions to his own symptoms.

**induced schizophrenia**  Delusions or other schizophrenic symptoms imposed by one member of the family on other members. (See *induced psychotic disorder.*) One schizophrenic mother transmitted her ideas of grandeur to her two daughters, one of whom was clearly schizophrenic, while the other could be convinced of the falsity of her beliefs and then showed no further evidence of the disease. (This case is an example of *folie à trois*, q.v.). "Therefore, we must assume that an energetic patient can suggest his delusions to other members of the family if and when they articulate with the complexes (wishes and desires) of these same members. However, schizophrenia will only develop if the disease is already latent in those individuals. In induced insanity, not the disease as such is determined by induction but only its delusional content, and perhaps also the manifest outbreak" (Bleuler, E. *Dementia Praecox or the Group of Schizophrenias*, 1950). See *folie à deux*.

**industrial psychiatry**  *Occupational psychiatry*; the branch of psychiatry that deals with human behavior in the workplace; its focus is on the psychological effects of the business organization on employees, and with the effects on an organization of the mental and emotional aspects of its employees' behavior. Specifically, it includes such areas and functions as (1) personality factors in the worker that affect his work fitness; (2) early detection of psychological or psychiatric disturbances within the unit (perhaps through an *EAP*); (3) appropriate and timely treatment and rehabilitation of the worker who has had a mental illness; (4) placement, promotions, transfers, terminations, etc.; (5) assessment of psychiatric factors in compensation cases, accidents, and absenteeism; (6) training of management for appropriate handling of employees' behavior that is fair and equitable to both labor and management.

**industry vs. inferiority**  One of Erikson's eight stages of man. See *ontogeny, psychic*.

**inebriety**  Drunkenness; acute alcoholic intoxication. The term implies alcohol dependence or at least a pattern of repeated episodes of drunkenness; currently it is used mainly in a legal context.

**inertia, motor**  See *perseveration*.

**inertia, psychic**  *Fixation*; resistance. Jung says that a peculiar psychic inertia that opposes any change and progress is a basic condition of a neurosis.

**infancy**  The period from birth until the beginning of the sixth year.

**infancy, disorders of**  DSM-IV includes the following within disorders usually first diagnosed during infancy, childhood, or adolescence: mental retardation, learning disorders, motor skills disorders, pervasive developmental disorders, disruptive behavior and attention deficit disorders, feeding and eating disorders of infancy or early childhood, tic disorders, communication disorders, elimination disorders. Also included with the "other" category are separation anxiety disorder, selective mutism, reactive attachment disorder, and stereotypic movement disorder.

**infancy research**  Study of early development through direct child observation, begun in the 1960s. Many of the findings of such research were incompatible with theories developed on the basis of reconstruction of infantile development through the psychoanalytic approach. In consequence, some of those earlier psychoanalytic theories have been extensively revised.

**infant Hercules syndrome** See *adrenogenital syndrome.*

**infant psychiatry** That branch of psychiatry concerned with mental and personality development in the first years of life, with emphasis on direct observation of the infant and the mother–infant relationship from the moment of birth. The aim is to identify subtle signs of infant psychopathology, differences from the normal that can interfere with or distort ego development. See *infancy research.*

**infanticide** Killing of an infant, most often by a parent; the child is usually under the age of 12 months. Neonaticide is the killing of an infant on the day of its birth; filicide includes all other cases of parental infanticide. See *homicide; battered child syndrome.*

Infanticide is typically committed by the mother who has not fully recovered from the effects of pregnancy and lactation and who, in addition, has some form of mental disorder. D. Bourget and J. M. W. Bradford (*Canadian Journal of Psychiatry 35,* 1990) have suggested the following typology:

1. Pathological filicide—including altruistic filicide (the wish to relieve the child from its imagined suffering or dreadful fate) and suicide-homicide. No rational motive, such as punishment, revenge, or secondary gain can be discerned and the mother typically is found to have been suffering from major depression with psychotic features at the time of the killing.

2. Accidental filicide—the child is unwanted and battered, and is killed in the course of physical abuse.

3. Retaliating filicide—to get revenge, usually from a spouse or lover; see *Medea complex.* More than one child may be killed; the mothers in this group typically show a severe personality disorder, often with a history of suicide attempts or chaotic marital relationships.

4. Neonaticide—the child is unwanted, and the mother is often young and unwed.

5. Paternal filicide—almost never neonaticide; the father demonstrates severe personality disorder.

**infantile** Of or belonging to the period of *infancy* (q.v.); used particularly in reference to those who are adults chronologically but whose behavior, or psychic organization, betrays more of its childhood background than is ordinarily accepted as "normal."

**infantile amnesia** Amnesia for the period of infancy and early childhood, i.e., from birth to the end of the fifth year of life. Memory for this period is practically nil and even those few isolated fragments that some people believe they can remember as "clearly as though it were yesterday" are seldom wholly accurate. See *affect memory.*

**infantile hyperkinetic syndrome** *Attention deficit hyperactivity disorder* (q.v.).

**infantile spasms** A severe epilepsy syndrome usually beginning in the first year of life in which there are typically *jackknife spasms* (mycoclonic seizures involving the muscles of the neck, trunk, and limbs, with nodding of the head and stiffening of the arms) and a disorganized cortical discharge termed *hypsarrhythmia.* Vigabatrin has been useful in most studies; evidence for the utility of zonisamide and topiramate is less strong.

**infantilism** In constitutional medicine, anomalous type of hypoevolute constitution characterized by the persistence of certain constitutional (psychological, physiological, morphological) features of childhood up to an age that is no longer infantile.

**infantilistic** Referring to or characterized by infantilism or a particular form of *dwarfism* (q.v.).

**infection, psychic** The "induction" of a mental syndrome in another person. See *folie à deux; induced psychotic disorder.*

**infection phobia** See *cancer phobia.*

**infective-exhaustive psychosis** *Obs.* Acute brain syndrome associated with systemic infection; also known as acute toxic encephalopathy, acute toxic encephalitis, or acute serous encephalitis.

**inferior olivary nucleus** The olive is a prominent mass in the middle section of the medulla; the inferior olivary nucleus within it projects to the Purkinje cells of the cerebellum. Their axons grow across the ventral midline (floorplate) and project to the cerebellum on the contralateral side. The olivocerebellar projection is important for motor learning and the timing of movements.

**inferiority** In general, any type of adaptation of a lower order than normally expected. Adler believed that everyone is born with an inferiority—organic or psychical—and that the manner in which the inferiority is handled determines the "style of life" of the person. Psychiatric states are the result of faulty management of the inferiority characterizing the individual.

Erikson describes industry vs. inferiority as one of the eight stages of man. See *ontogeny, psychic*.

**inferiority, functional**  Adler included this as a subgroup of organ inferiority; "A quantity or quality of work insufficient to satisfy a standard of required effectiveness" (*Study of Organ Inferiority and Its Psychical Compensation*, 1917).

**inferiority, simultaneous coordinate**  Adler's term for simultaneous manifold inferiority of organs due to reciprocal embryonic influence, or embryonic connection of many organs. As an example, he cited gastrointestinal affections in diseases of the lungs, in emphysema, and particularly in tuberculosis. He believed that these gastrointestinal affections are not dependent upon a primary lung disease, but are due to simultaneous inferiority of both systems.

**inferiority feelings**  Adler's term for the child's feeling of inadequacy in its relation both to parents and to the world at large. See *indicidual psychology*.

Persisting, severe inferiority feelings are manifested in morose self-doubts, a marked propensity for feeling ashamed, and oversensitivity to criticism and realistic setbacks. Such feelings suggest severe frustration in both the preoedipal and the oedipal phases.

**infestation delusions**  *Parasitophobia* (q.v.).

**infidelity**  Unfaithfulness; breach of trust; failure to adhere to one's beliefs or principles; adultery. Infidelity is used in two ways: unfaithfulness to, denial of, or aggression against religious doctrines and their advocates; and unfaithfulness to a marital or sexual partner (commonly called cheating). Infidelity, and the suspicion of it, are two major causes of *domestic violence* (q.v.).

A woman is slightly more likely to have routine sex with her partner during the infertile postovulatory phase; she is much more likely to have penetrative sex with a man other than her partner during her fertile phase. She wants that other man to fertilize her egg only if his ejaculate is the more fertile and competitive. One way to find out if it is more fertile

is to pit the ejaculate of one man against the other, and the better man will win.

Occasionally a woman produces two eggs at the same time and produces fraternal twins. In such a case, a different outcome is possible, and the fraternal twins are sired by different fathers. This is estimated to occur in at least 1 of every 400 sets of fraternal twins. It has been calculated from studies of blood groups that about 10% of children are not sired by the men presumed to be their fathers; the nonpaternity level for children conceived is even higher, because a woman is more likely to abort a child conceived with a man other than her long-term partner.

**infidelity delusion**  See *conjugal paranoia; jealousy, morbid*.

**infinity neurosis**  Neurotic preoccupation with the infinity of space and time, usually encountered in adolescents and/or as an expression of an autistic, dereistic approach to life; *apeirophobia*.

**influenced psychosis**  Gordon's term for *induced psychotic disorder* (q.v.).

**informal care**  See *care*.

**information**  See *parallel distributed processing*.

**information feedback**  See *behavior therapy*.

**information processing**  The sequence of operations that occur within the central nervous system in response to stimulation; the structures and processes involved in the registration, encoding, selection, maintenance, transformation, storage, and retrieval of information. See *information theory; KIPS*.

Information processing in the brain takes place in stages. An initial sensory store (sometimes called the *icon store* or *iconic image*) probably lasts a few hundred milliseconds. A subset of this information can be extracted from the sensory store, transformed into a short-term memory store (duration of about 10 sec) and relayed through a central processing stage at which point decisions are made about the degree of further processing needed for the new information. One of the resources available through the hypothesized central processor is the *lexicon* (or language) *faculty*.

The "output" stage is usually referred to as *response organization*. It is implicitly assumed that the response requirement (which may reflect the current "state" of the organism) feeds forward in time to determine which features will be extracted from the next sensory store. Thus, a dynamic and ongoing information-processing system is in perpetual operation, sensitive to and interactive with the needs of the organism and changes in the environment.

Information processing includes perception (input), central integration (dependent on memory, language, and complex thought processes), and performance or behavior (output). Since all of these are affected by the subject's attentiveness, attentional processes are also a significant element in information processing.

Each instant of experience or perception contains not only the "objectivity" (sensory content) or stimulus input but an array of subtle affective or connotative tags, which collectively will add a dimension of "meaning" to the experience or perception. The "significance" of the information (its connotative aspects) is specifically hypothesized to be contributed by the limbic, thalamic, and perhaps cerebellar and striatal nuclei in conjunction with the cortex.

Older (specifically, limbic and thalamic) structures function as the memory mapping devices that provide access to ever more specialized regions of cortex and thus allow the additional computational power of the cortical layers and columns to be fully used. Such increased processing power can logically be held to underlie those specifically human functions of abstract thinking and the capacity to use current experience to plan into the future.

**information system, executive** *Decision support system*; any mechanism that allows an executive to bypass the usual intelligence channels and gain access directly to the data about the operation of his or her organization that ordinarily is filtered through one or more intermediate organizational levels before it is presented. To most people within an organization, power resides in the ability to influence the chief executive officer's perceptions. Staff people who collect, interpret, and analyze executive information therefore tend to be very powerful, as are operating executives who set plans, budgets, and strategies. Executive information systems can render the executive independent of such middle management levels and can thus be powerful tools in exposing the weaknesses of an organization, identifying levels of incompetence, and providing other data that often highlight

the advisability of restructuring the organization.

**information test** The subject answers questions pertaining to general fund of knowledge and early school instruction.

**information theory** Study of the transmission of messages or the communication of information. Information science and technology are concerned with the structure and properties of scientific information and the techniques for information handling, the characteristics of information processing devices, and the design and operation of information handling systems. The basic notion is that information can be thought of as divorced from specific content or subject matter and simply as a single decision between two equally plausible alternatives. Claude Shannon, an electrical engineer at MIT, is usually credited with devising information theory. See *communication unit; cybernetics*.

Information processing includes perception (input), central integration (dependent on memory, language, and complex thought processes), and performance or behavior (output). Since all of these are affected by the subject's attentiveness, attentional processes are also a significant element in information processing.

The basic unit of information is the *bit* (binary digit)—the amount of information required to select one message from two equally probable alternatives. It is only recently that cognitive scientists have begun to question if they can, in fact, afford to treat all information equivalently and to ignore issues of content.

**informational underload** *Sensory deprivation* (q.v.).

**informed consent** Competent, knowing, and voluntary agreement to a therapeutic or experimental intervention; information about the treatment that is being offered the patient that will allow him or her to make a rational decision about accepting or refusing the treatment. The information includes everything that a reasonable person would want to know in making that decision, including the risks and benefits associated with the treatment and what alternatives to the treatment being offered might exist. It should also include relevant information about the administrative and supervisory organization of the treatment setting, e.g., that a supervisor shares responsibility for the patient's care, that various members of the health team have access to the clinical records, and that nonmedical personnel, such as hospital administrators, insurance auditors, and regulatory agency surveyors also have the authority to review the records. See *consumerism; procedural legal standard; respect for autonomy; voluntarism.*

Despite the increasing tendency of the courts and the legislatures to mandate "fully informed consent" in all types and stages of medical and research intervention, it remains highly questionable if that ever is possible, particularly since researchers themselves often do not understand fully the potential harm (or benefit) of their work. The situation is even more difficult in psychiatry, where there is continuing debate about whether mental patients (or children) have the capacity to understand the information given them, about who may consent for them (family, guardian, or court), and about what degree of description of possible dangers or rare side effects is advisable or necessary. In reaction to clear-cut demonstrations of abuses in the past, regulations have been proposed that would impose such stringent limitations that no meaningful research could be done. See *EPSTD; ethics.*

Bioethicists, in particular, prefer the term valid consent, which in addition to the concept that adequate information is meaningfully imparted also includes the notions of coercion and competence. Valid consent in medicine is no different from valid consent in law or any other area, although the amount of information required to make the consent valid, and the condition of the patient that may interfere with his understanding of the information that should be imparted, may render the process of obtaining it more difficult.

Under ideal conditions, the patient should know or be informed of everything that would affect his personal decision concerning which of the courses of treatment available to him he should choose. Because valid consent must always refer to an individual decision, it must allow for the ways in which the patient's religious beliefs, cultural beliefs, or even superstitions might affect his decision.

Informed consent is a slippery concept whose shape changes with the context. Legal informed consent entails two separate questions: Has the physician discharged his

duty to disclose? Has the patient comprehended enough? U.S. Supreme Court Justice Blackmun's rudimentary definition—the giving of information to the patient as to just what would be done and as to its consequences—is clearly not adequate to many conditions, particularly in psychiatry. Yet no definition has been fully satisfactory, and all are compromises between ideals and economic realities.

*Double-agentry* is a specific ethical problem within the area of informed consent; the term refers to the *conflict of interest* inherent in the situation where a psychiatrist in the employ of a hospital, governmental agency, or some other authority examines a patient. Is the psychiatrist's obligation to the patient first or only to the agency that employs him? It is generally agreed that the "patient" must be informed that he is not really a patient when the physician's responsibility is in fact to the Army, hospital, court, etc. In similar fashion, most psychiatrists agree that the patient should know under what conditions the psychiatrist will feel it justifiable, warranted, or necessary to inform any other person or agency of information divulged by the patient within the therapeutic setting. See *confidentiality.*

**infradian**   See *rhythms, biological.*

**infratentorial**   See *fossa, posterior cranial.*

**ingravescent stroke**   Progressive worsening of neurological symptoms, such as hemiplegia, in a patient with stroke. At first the brain damage appears clinically to be mild, but the hemiplegia becomes worse in a stepwise or steadily progressive fashion. See *cerebrovascular accident.*

**inhalant intoxication**   An organic disorder due to recent use or short-term, high-dosure exposure to volatile inhalants, such as glue, paint or paint thinners, and gasoline (see *glue-sniffing*). The substance may be inhaled directly from its container, or a rag soaked in the substance may be held over the mouth and nose. Inhalant abuse and inhalant dependence include repeated episodes of intoxication, manifested in maladaptive behavioral changes, such as belligerence, assaultiveness, apathy, and impaired judgment; and in physical signs, such as dizziness, nystagmus, incoordination, slurred speech, unsteady gait, lethargy, depressed reflexes, psychomotor retardation, tremor, generalized muscle weakness, blurred vision or diplopia, stupor or coma, and euphoria. See *psychoactive substance-induced organic mental disorders.*

**inhalants** Volatile inhalants; these include aliphatic and aromatic hydrocarbons, found in gasoline, glues, lacquers, paints and paint thinners; halogenated hydrocarbons, found in cleaning fluids, typewriter correction fluid, and spray-can propellants; and other volatile compounds containing esters, ketones, and glycols. Although the anesthetic gases (e.g., ether, nitrous oxide) and short-acting vasodilators (amyl nitrite, butyl nitrite) are technically volatile inhalants, they are not currently classified as such; instead, they are classified under "Other Substance Use Disorders." See *inhalant intoxication.*

**inheritable** Capable of being transmitted from parents to offspring; applied to a physical or mental trait. In genetics, the English term most closely approximating the German term *Erbfest,* "fixed in heredity," and contrasting the hereditary qualities of an individual with those that are acquired by the phenotype during its own lifetime and do not become transmissible by heredity. See *Mendelism.*

**inheritance** This specifically genetic term has two meanings: (1) the *process* of transmission of inheritable attributes from parent to offspring—being then equivalent to *hereditary transmission;* (2) more commonly, the *trait* transmitted. In the second sense it is frequently modified by an adjective or phrase, as *mendelian* inheritance, *cytoplasmic* inheritance, inheritance of *acquired characters.* See *chromosome.*

Among the various modes of inheritance are the *multifactorial (MF) model* and the *single-major-locus (SML) model.* The latter postulates that only two alleles are involved in manifestation of the trait in question—the normal one and the abnormal one responsible for the trait. The multifactorial model assumes that the genetic and environmental causes of the trait constitute a single continuous variable, the liability, and that those whose liability exceeds a threshold will manifest the trait. In the MF model, genetic effects are assumed to be due to the additive effects of many genes, each of which contributes only a small part to the final result; similarly, environmental effects are exerted through many minor events that are additive throughout the life of the person.

**inhibition** 1. In psychoanalysis, an unconscious confining, hemming in, checking, or restraining of an instinctual impulse or some manifestation of it. The force of the superego inhibits the impulse and prevents it from crossing the boundary line between the id and the ego.

2. In Pavlovian conditioned-reflex psychology, inhibition refers to the active restraining of response by the experimental subject during the latent period of delayed reaction. Inhibition can itself be inhibited by any extraneous stimulus administered during the latent period, and the result will be a release of the response from its original inhibition (*disinhibition*).

**inhibition, latent** *LI;* the process by which a stimulus loses salience and evokes decreasing interest and attention from the subject if it is presented repeatedly without consequence. Learning by association is retarded if the subject is exposed to the stimulus that is ultimately to be conditioned.

**inhibition, specific** An inhibition in some particular function of the ego, e.g., eating, sexual function, locomotion. Such inhibitions are renunciations of functions that if exercised would give rise to severe anxiety or guilt. Under analysis an inhibition such as writing—that is, of functions involving the use of the fingers—reveals an excessive erotization of the fingers. Writing acquires the significance of a sexual activity; and allowing fluid to flow out from a tube upon a piece of white paper might have the symbolic meaning of coitus.

**inhibition formation** The organization of inhibiting or restraining influences. Inhibition formation is one type of mental activity that serves to restrain the appearance in consciousness of impulses unacceptable to it. Symptom formation is a method by which the unacceptable impulses gain the level of consciousness, but in symbolic form.

**inhibitory control** A self-regulatory process that underlies the ability to withhold a prepotent response, interrupt an ongoing response, and protect cognitive activity from interference. Impairment in inhibitory control is characteristic of *attention deficit hyperactivity disorder* (q.v.) and is suggestive of prefrontal cortical abnormality.

**inhibitory epilepsy** A rare form of *petit mal epilepsy* (q.v.) in which transitory loss of power occurs in a limb or on one side of the body without preceding tonic spasm or clonic movements; there may be an associated impairment of consciousness.

**inhibitory synapse** A *synapse* (q.v.) that results in the flow of negative ions into the neuron, with the result that the intraneuronal compartment is more negatively charged and less able to develop an *action current* (q.v.).

**inhibitory transmitter** See *GABA*.

**inimicality** Disposition to hostility or violence; sometimes used in a very specific sense to refer to those elements in the history of a subject that suggest increased risk for violence.

**initiation, individual and collective** An individual initiation is a ritual that takes place "under the command of heaven." It indicates a dedication to an individual goal that demands the utmost intensity of purpose and unreserved lifelong devotion. In such cases the libido is transformed from its original objective into a cultural one, usually in the framework of a religious idea. The coronation of a king and the ordination of a priest illustrate such an initiation. Initiation also takes place in some ethnic groups in a collective way, where, for instance, adolescents are initiated into adulthood with appropriate ceremonies. The purpose of these ceremonies is to direct the infantile libido into mature objectives (Baynes, H. G. *Mythology of the Soul*, 1940).

**initiative vs. guilt** One of Erikson's eight stages of man. See *ontogeny, psychic.*

**injury** See *disease.*

**injustice collecting** A masochistic trait consisting of a lifelong series of disappointments. According to Bergler the trait develops in three steps: (1) the masochist seeks out or arranges to experience disappointment, rejection, humiliation, etc. as a way to reproduce the disappointing, refusing preoedipal mother; (2) having experienced the injustice, the masochist expresses righteous indignation and rage, not to right the wrong he or she has suffered but to appease his own conscience and to demonstrate that he did not wish to be injured and did not enjoy the injury; (3) the rage gives way to depression and self-pity, "Such things happen only to me." See *masochistic personality.*

**innate immunity** Nonspecific, natural immunity that does not involve the antigen-antibody interactions characteristic of *acquired immunity* (q.v.). Natural immunity is mediated by phagocytes, neutrophils, NK cells, and monocytes; the last become macrophages

in local tissues. These cells engulf or lyse invading cells, and they also release soluble factors such as Type I interferons (with direct antiviral properties) and the proinflammatory cytokines—tumor necrosis factor (TNF), interleukin-1 (IL-1), and interleukin-6 (IL-6)

**innateness hypothesis** *Nativist hypothesis*; the view that the child is born with a biologically determined predisposition to learn language and with some knowledge of the structural principles of language. See *grammar; language; language acquisition.*

**inner language** See *Lichtheim test.*

**innervation, antagonistic inversion of the** A form of distortion in hysterical attacks, according to Freud "...analogous to the very usual changing of an element into its opposite by dream-work. For instance, in an hysterical attack an embrace may be represented by the arms being drawn back convulsively until the hands meet above the spinal column. Possibly the well-known *arc de cercle* of major hysterical attacks is nothing but an energetic disavowal of this kind, by antagonistic innervation of the position suitable for sexual intercourse" (*Collected Papers*, 1924–25).

**innervation, expressive** The nervous pathways of emotional behavior, such as weeping, laughing, and sexual excitement. The expressive innervations are involuntary, even though they can be influenced, up to a point, by volition.

**Innocence Projects** See *false confession.*

**iNOS** Cytokine-inducible isoenzyme of NOS. See *NO.*

**inositol** See *diacylglycerol.*

**inpatient violence** Although violence by inpatients is not a new phenomenon, the first published report of criminal charges being brought against a patient was in 1978. Other patients, as well as staff members, have the *right to be free of violent assault* (Applebaum, 1987). The question in cases alleging negligence in failing to prevent assaults on inpatients is usually not merely whether some measures were not taken that might have been useful in preventing violent assault, but whether those measures would have been taken by other reasonable clinicians.

**input specificity** The property of long-term potentiation whereby strong synaptic stimulation elicits only an increase in synaptic strength at the activated pathway, leaving every other input unaffected.

**inputs**   See *functional budgeting*.

**insane**   Of or pertaining to one who is of unsound mind. See *insanity*.

**insanity**   A legal rather than a medical term, referring to mental disorder or defect of such nature or degree as to interfere with the capacity to discharge one's legal responsibilities. If it is determined that insanity is present, various legal consequences may follow, such as commitment to an institution, appointment of a guardian, dissolution of a contract; or certain expected consequences may be altered, as when an accused person is found not guilty by reason of insanity. See *criminal responsibility*.

**insanity, primary delusional**   *Obs*. Folie systématisée, or *paranoia* (q.v.).

**insanity defense**   Excuse of a criminal defendant for his conduct because of his mental defect. The insanity defense is a complete defense to a criminal charge in contrast to a partial insanity defense or a diminished responsibility plea, such as a finding that an accused defendant is not guilty by reason of insanity (*NGRI*). Traditionally, a finding of NGRI absolves the defendant of criminal responsibility and does not impose a prison sentence, although the defendant may be held responsible under a different set of laws that may impose commitment to a mental hospital or the psychiatric unit of a prison. See *criminal responsibility*.

**insanity of negation**   Psychosis with nihilistic delusions. See *Cotard syndrome*.

**insect phobia**   See *bug phobia*.

**insecurity**   A feeling of unprotectedness and helplessness against manifold anxieties arising from a sort of all-encompassing uncertainty about oneself: uncertainty regarding one's goals and ideals, one's abilities, one's relations to others, and the attitude one should take toward them. The insecure person does not or dares not have friendly feelings in what seems to him an unfriendly world. He lives in an atmosphere of anticipated disapproval. He has no confidence today in yesterday's belief, no faith tomorrow in today's truth. See *ontological insecurity*.

**insemination**   The act of impregnating or fertilizing. The technical expression for artificial insemination is *eutelegenesis* (q.v.). See *mother surrogate*.

**insensitivity**   Inadequate response to stimulation; lack of appropriate concern. Insensitivity often implies lack of empathy or sympathy in relation to others, or a failure to respond to social cues relating to the inappropriateness or unsavoriness of one's own behavior. Less common is the use of sensitivity as a short latency to acting on urges, which may lead to self-destructive behavior, such as spending sprees, sexual indiscretions, temper outbursts, physical fights, self-mutilation, and suicidal behavior. Defined in such a way, insensitivity is a core symptom of *borderline personality disorder* (q.v.). See *sensitivity*.

**insertion, thought**   See *first-rank symptoms*.

**insight**   The patient's knowledge that his symptoms are abnormalities. For example, when a patient who fears crowds realizes that the fear is only within his own mind and unfounded in reality, he is said to have insight. Insight is further defined from the standpoint of knowledge of the factors operating to produce the symptoms, such as a patient who understands the explanation for the development of his symptoms.

Intellectual insight is knowledge of the objective reality of a situation, without the ability to utilize that knowledge in trying to adapt to it. Intellectual insight alone is generally ineffective in producing therapeutic change, but the quest for it may constitute a resistance to the therapy.

**insight, derivative**   Insight arrived at by the patient himself without interpretation by the therapist—characteristic of activity therapy groups.

**insomnia**   Sleeplessness; chronic inability to obtain the amount of sleep necessary to maintain adequate daytime behavior. In DSM-IV, primary insomnia refers to difficulty in initiating or maintaining sleep, or to sleep that is nonrestorative, of not less than 1 month's duration. The loss of sleep produces significant daytime fatigue and impairs occupational or social functioning. In typical cases, sleep latency exceeds 30 minutes or sleep efficiency is less than 85%. See *sleep disorders*.

In the International Classification of Sleep Disorders, second edition, insomnia is classified as follows: (1) adjustment insomnia (acute insomnia); (2) psychophysiologic insomnia; (3) paradoxical insomnia; (4) idiopathic insomnia; (5) insomnia because of a mental disorder; (6) inadequate sleep hygiene; (7) behavioral insomnia of childhood; (8) insomnia due to drug or substance; (9) insomnia due to medical condition; (10) insomnia not due to substance or known physiologic condition, unspecified (nonorganic insomnia, not otherwise specified); (11) physiologic (organic) insomnia, unspecified.

**insomnia, childhood-onset idiopathic** *Insomnia* (q.v.) beginning before puberty and persisting into adulthood. The subject is never without insomnia for more than 3 months at a time. See *sleep disorders.*

**insomnia, learned** Difficulty initiating or maintaining sleep based on psychological reasons, such as insomnia that begins during a period of stress but continues after the stress itself has disappeared. Typical of this type of insomnia is daytime preoccupation over possible inability to fall asleep, or increasing efforts to fall asleep are unsuccessful, or paradoxical improvement in sleep when away from the usual sleep environment. See *sleep disorders.*

**instigator** Any member in a therapy group who stimulates others toward activity or verbalization. See *catalytic agent; neutralizer.*

**instinct** "An organized and relatively complex mode of response, characteristic of a given species, that has been phylogenetically adapted to a specific type of environmental situation" (Warren, H. C. *Dictionary of Psychology,* 1934).

"An instinct may be described as having a source, an object, and an aim. The source is a state of excitation within the body, and its aim is to remove that excitation; in the course of its path from its source to the attainment of its aim the instinct becomes operative mentally. We picture it as a certain sum of energy forcing its way in a certain direction" (Freud, S. *New Introductory Lectures on Psycho-Analysis,* 1933).

In *ethology* (q.v.), an "instinct" is an inherited system of coordination, made up of an internal *drive,* which builds up as *specific action potential* until it is released, and one or more *inherited releasing mechanisms* (IRM), which release the specific action potential and produce the instinctive act or *fixed action pattern (FAP).* The specific action patterns are species-specific, uniform, and generally rigid, although (especially as one goes up the vertebrate scale) some links of the instinctual action are subject to modification by learning. Such learning, when it occurs, can be conceived of as a replacement of innate, instinctual links by learned behavior

patterns—a phenomenon called *instinct-training interlocking.* In humans, instinctive behavior patterns are rudimentary, and most genetically determined, instinctual behavior is replaced by learned, plastic, purposive, adaptive behavior—that is, by the ego (Schur, M. *International Journal of Psycho-Analysis XLI,* 1960). See *imprinting; releaser, social.*

An instinct, according to Freud, is a primal trend or urge that cannot be further resolved. From the Freudian standpoint, there are two primal instincts, those of life and death.

In present-day psychoanalytic psychology, the term *drive* (q.v.) is generally preferred to what Freud termed "instinct." An "instinct" is considered to be an innate capacity or necessity to react in a stereotyped way to a particular set of stimuli; it is a lower-level, automatic response (such as the reflexes). The term "drive," on the other hand, ordinarily does not refer to the organism's response but instead emphasizes the state of central excitation; unlike the instinct, the response to the drive is not automatic but requires the functioning of the ego and depends on learning and experience.

The first of the two primal instincts is Eros, or life instinct, the function of which is to maintain life; its aim is constructive. It is composed of three principal manifestations; (1) the uninhibited sexual or organ-gratifying impulses; (2) sublimated impulses derived from those originally associated with organ satisfaction; and (3) *self-preservative impulses,* which strive to protect and preserve the body and the mind.

The second primal instinct is Thanatos, the death or destructive or aggressive drive. Freud says that the tendency of the instinct is to reestablish a state of things which was disturbed by the emergence of life. The death instinct is said to be composed of (1) impulses that tend toward regression, that is, toward a reinstatement of an earlier level of personality development; (2) impulses that aim to injure or destroy the person himself, and (3) those that possess the aim of (2) with regard, however, to objects outside of oneself. See *death instinct.*

**instinct, complementary** The tendency of infantile instincts with an active aim to be integrally associated with, or accompanied by, the antithetical instinct with a passive aim. In infancy and childhood, the separation or *defusion* (q.v.) of these equal and opposite active and passive instinctual aims is more marked than in adult life. See *ambivalence*.

**instinct, passive** "Every instinct is a form of activity; if we speak loosely of passive instincts, we can only mean those whose aim is passive" (Freud, S. *Collected Papers*, 1924–1925). For example, an instinct may be reversed into its opposite; an active instinct (e.g., sadism) may be reversed and appear as a passive one (e.g., masochism).

**instinct eruption** See *catathymic crisis*.

**instinct-ridden** Beset or characterized by aggressive and/or libidinal impulses that are only inadequately modified or controlled by the superego; the instinct-ridden character typically keeps his superego actively and consistently at a distance.

**instinct-training interlocking** See *instinct*.

**instinctual anxiety** *Neurotic anxiety*. Freud distinguishes between true anxiety and neurotic anxiety: true anxiety is anxiety in regard to a known real danger threatening from some external object; neurotic anxiety is anxiety in regard to an unknown danger. Upon investigation, this latter danger is found to be an instinctual danger.

**instrumental aggression** *Proactive aggression*; *predatory aggression* (applied to animals rather than to humans); nonemotional display of aggressive behavior that is outcome-oriented (i.e., directed toward obtaining some goal) and elicited by anticipated rewards and positive outcomes. Instrumental aggression is usually contrasted to the other major subtype of aggressive behavior, reactive aggression. Most aggressive children display both types of behavior and fall into a group that in consequence is called *pervasive aggression*. See *aggression*; *reactive aggression*.

**instrumentalism** "An extreme form of *Self-Extension* in which one makes use of people for pleasure or profit; exploitation of others" (Hamilton, G. *A Medical Social Terminology*, 1930). See exploitative type under *assimilation*.

**instrumentality theory** The hypothesis that a subject's attitude about an occurrence (outcome) depends on his perception of how that outcome is related (instrumental) to the occurrence of other desirable or undesirable consequences.

**insula** The area of cerebral cortex that lies deep within the fissure of Sylvius and contains parts of the frontal, parietal, and temporal lobes.

The anterior insula is activated in neuroimaging studies of pain and distress, hunger and thirst, and autonomic arousal; and in anger and disgust triggered by feelings of having been treated unfairly.

Sensory aspects of ongoing homeostasis that represent the physiological condition of the body are projected to the posterior insula and rerepresented in the anterior insula, providing a limbic sensory substrate for feelings and emotions. The insula is regarded as limbic sensory cortex; the anterior cingulate cortex (ACC) serves as limbic motor cortex by way of its association with autonomic and emotional control. Both insula and ACC are strongly interconnected with the amygdala, hypothalamus, orbitofrontal cortex, and brain stem homeostatic regions. The subjective evaluation of the interoceptive state is forwarded to the *orbitofrontal cortex* (q.v.), where hedonic valence is represented. See *interoception*.

**insular sclerosis** See *multiple sclerosis*.

**insularity, psychological** The quality or state of being narrow-minded or circumscribed in outlook, mentality, and character. "The most important value to character formation of group experiences is the modification or elimination of egocentricity and psychological insularity" (Slavson, S. R. *An Introduction to Group Therapy*, 1943).

**insulin resistance syndrome** See *metabolic syndrome*.

**insulin treatment** Insulin coma therapy; insulin shock treatment; a now rarely used form of treatment introduced by Manfred Sakel in 1933, mainly for schizophrenic disorders. Hypoglycemia was induced with intramuscular insulin; by the end of the third hour following injection, coma developed with signs of pons and cerebellar involvement (hypotonia, interrupted occasionally by tonic spasms) and loss of response to pinprick or pressure on the supraorbital nerve. The patient was monitored to ensure that coma did not deepen, and it was terminated within another 15 to 60 minutes with intramuscular glucagon. Depending upon the patient's response, the full course of treatment was typically in the range of 40 to 60 comas. The procedure was dangerous and sometimes produced fatal complications.

**insulin-degrading enzyme (IDE)** Also known as insulysin, IDE degrades both insulin and β-amyloid; the gene for IDE lies within a region of chromosome 10 that has been linked to an increased risk of *Alzheimer disease* (q.v.). Increasing insulin levels increases β-amyloid, but the increased insulin requires more IDE and consequently less is available to degrade β-amyloid in the patient with Alzheimer disease.

**insulin-like growth factor** *IGF-1*; a peptide growth hormone with neuroprotective features. In the brain, it is an inhibitor of the tau-kinase GSK3 β, reducing Aβ neurotoxicity and preserving cognitive function. Blood-borne IGF-1 stimulates entrance into the brain of different Aβ carriers (albumin, transthyretin, apolipoprotein J) and in this way enhances Aβ clearance.

**insurance, narcissistic** "It is the narcissistic satisfaction derived from the fulfilling of an ideal which benumbs the critical judgment of the ego, and secures gratification of the forbidden aggressive tendencies. This economic mechanism may be described as a kind of narcissistic insurance" (Rado, S. *International Journal of Psychoanalysis IX*, 1928).

**insurance hebephrenia** Maier's term for schizophrenia manifested initially as a compensation neurosis; in time, the patient's claims become increasingly absurd, illogical, and bizarre. See *compensation neurosis.*

**intake** The initial interview of the patient (or, in the case of a child, a member of the patient's family) by the therapist (or any member of the psychiatric team); usually in reference to a patient who is admitted into a psychiatric clinic or a mental hospital.

**intake, family group** An initial interview technique, devised by the Riley Child Guidance Clinic (Indianapolis), that substitutes the family unit (usually the child and his parents) for the usual single informant and a psychiatric team (consisting of a psychiatrist, a psychologist, and a social worker) for the usual single interviewer. One member of the team acts as the principal interviewer and opens the way to a discussion by the family of the presenting problems as they see them. The other team members later enter into the discussion as active participants. Interaction between family members is interrupted only if one member is too aggressively attacked (verbally or physically) by another.

The major objectives of such a technique are "(1) clarification of the presenting problems for all persons involved, including the child, (2) observation of the family interaction, and (3) information which will lead to tentative hypotheses about the relationship between the family dynamics and the child's symptoms" (Tyler, E. A., et al. *Archives of General Psychiatry 6*, 1962).

**integral medicine** Alternative medical therapies, *holistic healing* (q.v.).

**Integrated Psychological Therapy** See *IPT.*

**integrated type** In their system of constitutional types, E. R. and W. Jaensch denote by this term subjects with an integrated psychological state, of which the *B type* of *eidetic imagery* is an indicator.

**integration** Act of bringing together the parts into a harmonious whole. From the psychoanalytic point of view, for example, oral, anal, and genital factors remain essentially discrete for a considerable period. Gradually, however, through various mechanisms the individual parts begin to act in cooperation with one another. It is the harmonizing of separate parts that is called integration.

During the infantile period, extending approximately through the fifth year of life, integration is relatively simple, being manifested chiefly in the form of knowledge on the part of the child that its body and mind are distinct from the environment. The integration at this stage of development is called primary. Subsequent integration that coordinates individual components into unified and socialized action is termed *secondary integration.*

When integration, having once been established, breaks down into its component parts, that is, when there is a reversal of the processes of integration, the condition is known as *disintegration.* When disintegration is followed by a reorganization of the individual parts into a harmonious whole, the process is called *reintegration.* Hence, it is said that a manic-depressive patient is disintegrated during the illness and reintegrated following it.

In the literature on dissociative identity disorder, integration refers to that part of the treatment process concerned with undoing all aspects of dissociative dividedness. See *fusion.*

**integration, neuronal** *Synaptic integration*; the process of *summation* (q.v.) of competing inputs at the cellular level, leading to the decision of the postsynaptic cell to fire or not to fire an action potential.

**integrins** A large family of cell surface receptors that attach cells to ECM (extracellular matrix) and mediate mechanical and chemical signals from it. Integrins can signal through the cell membrane in either direction, from inside the cell (inside-out signaling) or from outside the cells (outside-in signaling). Many integrin signals are devoted to cell cycle regulation, directing cells to live or die, to proliferate, or to exit the cell and differentiate. See *adhesion, cellular.*

**intellect** In analytical psychology, "*directed thinking.*" "The faculty of passive, or undirected, thinking, I [Jung] term *intellectual intuition.* Furthermore, I describe directed thinking or intellect as the *rational* function, since it arranges the representations under concepts in accordance with the presuppositions of my conscious rational norm. Undirected thinking, or intellectual intuition, on the contrary, is, in my view, an *irrational function*, since it criticizes and arranges the representations according to norms that are unconscious to me and consequently not appreciated as reasonable" (*Psychological Types*, 1923).

**intellectual inadequacy** See *retardation, mental.*

**intellectual insanity** *Obs.* Prichard's term for the forms of insanity known in the 19th century as monomania, mania, and dementia.

**intellectual narcissism** Narcissism manifested as an attempt to dominate others and regain or maintain omnipotence by intellectual prowess; it reflects libidinization of thinking.

**intellectualization** See *brooding.*

**intelligence** According to Thorndike, there are three distinctive types of intelligence: abstract, mechanical, and social. The capacity to understand and manage abstract ideas and symbols constitutes abstract intelligence; the ability to understand, invent, and manage mechanisms constitutes mechanical intelligence; and the capacity to act reasonably and wisely as regards human relations and social affairs constitutes social intelligence. See *developmental psychology.*

Tolman's pragmatic viewpoint regards intelligence as the interrelated capacities of an organism (1) to perceive its environment through its various sensory modalities (*discriminanda*); (2) to integrate these sensations into total configurations (*gestalt apperceptions*); (3) to attribute meaning and personal reference (symbolization and value) to them in terms of retained past experiences (memory); and (4) to respond to such differentiated apperceptions by internal and external reactions of various degrees of finesse, versatility, and efficiency (*manipulanda* capacities).

In 1904, Spearman proposed the existence of a general factor of intelligence, *g*, made up of *p* (perseveration factor), *f* (fluency factor), *w* (will factor), and *s* (speed factor). In 1916 Thomson proposed instead that what to be a unitary general ability was in fact a collection of multitudinous and diverse skills needed to complete most intellectual tasks. Sternberg's still broader *triarchic theory* (1999) postulates a separation of analytical intelligence, creative intelligence, and practical intelligence.

**intelligence quotient (IQ)** The ratio of a subject's intelligence (determined by mental measures) to so-called average or normal intelligence for his age. The most common method for determining the intelligence quotient is to divide the assigned *mental age* by the chronological age.

**intemperance** Lack of restraint or control of any desire; in particular, immoderate use of alcohol. See *alcoholism.*

**intensive care syndrome** Psychosis appearing in patients in postoperative recovery units or in intensive care units. Significant factors contributing to the development of such a complication include the following: (1) the physical conditions of the unit itself—often impersonal, highly mechanized, unfamiliar, isolated, windowless, and in certain ways a type of sensory deprivation experience; (2) the physical condition of the patient within the unit—he is usually immobilized to a severe degree and in considerable discomfort; (3) the nature of the underlying pathology, including the medical-surgical complications and the age of the patient, and the effects these have on brain function; (4) the effects of medication and operative procedures on brain function; and (5) the premorbid level of functioning, including personality structure and genetic-constitutional factors.

**intention** Plan; impulse for action; goal; the forming of an intention implies free will and the ability to choose.

Humans have an inherent ability to understand other people's minds. A basic form of *theory of mind* (q.v.) is the ability to understand others' intentions by observing their actions. See *action understanding*. This might be based on simulating the observed action and estimating the actor's intentions on the basis of a reresentation of one's own intentions, a notion reminiscent of *simulation* theory (q.v.): one represents the mental activities and processes of others by simulation, i.e., by generating similar activities and processes in oneself.

Observers who view videos of moving triangles almost always attribute intentions, emotions, and personality traits to the shapes. Numerous studies have since demonstrated this automatic attribution of high-level mental states to animate motion in adults in a wide range of cultures, in young infants, and even in chimpanzees. The *superior temporal sulcus (STS)* is consistently activated by the perception of biological motion; activation is more pronounced in the right hemisphere than in the left. The right posterior STS receives information from both dorsal and ventral visual streams (involved in vision for action and vision for identification, respectively), providing an interface between perception for identification and perception for action.

When subjects view static images that convey dynamic information, such as an athlete in the posture of throwing a ball, the implied motion from the static images activates the brain region that is specialized for processing visual motion—the *occipito-temporal junction*. This shows that the brain stores internal representations of dynamic information, which can be used to recall past movement and anticipate future movements, even from very partial visual information.

The medial prefrontal cortex is consistently activated by *theory-of-mind* tasks in which subjects think about their own or others' mental states (Blakemore, S.-J., and Decety, J. *Nature Reviews Neuroscience 1*, 2001). See *mirror neurons; prediction*

**intention tremor** See *tremor.*

**intentional** See *volition.*

**intentional span** Span of *attention* (q.v.).

**intentional stance** *Theory of mind* (q.v.).

**intentional unvoluntary behavior** Those types of disorder in which the subject acts inten-

tionally but not voluntarily, in that although he can perform an action he cannot refrain from performing despite good reason to do so. Included are compulsions, addiction (which is further complicated by drug-induced physiologic changes that alter behavior and capacity for control), the avoidance behavior seen in phobic disorders, factitious disorders such as Munchhausen syndrome, alcoholism, binge eating, kleptomania, and some forms of egodystonic sexual behavior. See *volition.*

**interaction** See *transactional analysis.*

**interaction, accelerated** One of the results of the intensity of the *marathon session.*

**interaction chronograph** A mechanical device, developed by E. D. Chapple, that enables the observer of a standardized psychiatric interview to record certain temporal aspects of verbal and gestural interactions between interviewer and subject. Chapple's interaction theory of personality assumes that personality can be assessed without recourse to intrapsychic or other psychodynamic formulations, and that its assessment involves merely the process of observing the time relations in the interaction patterns of the subject.

**interactional contract** See *contracting.*

**interactions, drug** The effects that one drug has on the actions of one or more other drugs given at the same time. Many drug–drug interactions are known, but relatively few of them appear to be of major clinical significance. Some of the most significant in psychiatry include the interactions between monoamine oxidase inhibitors and sympathomimetic amines or tyramine and those between tricyclic antidepressants, neuroleptics, and anti-Parkinson agents.

**interactomes** Catalogs of protein interactions. See *noncoding DNA.*

**intercalated** Internuncial. See *reflex.*

**interchromosomal domain** See *chromosome.*

**intercourse, buccal** Oral intercourse; fellatio or cunnilingus.

**interdependent triad** See *family psychotherapy.*

**interego** Stekel's proposed substitute for the Freudian term superego. According to Stekel, the Freudian *superego* (q.v.) should be considered not as a simple "watchman" (the vigilant moral part of the ego), but rather as an intermediary between our inner crude impulses and the final conscious aims of those impulses. For this reason, Stekel prefers to call the superego an interego—a structure functioning as a compromiser between crude subconscious trends and the moral principles (*The Interpretation of Dreams*, 1943).

**interest**   In occupational therapy, to attract and hold the attention, to occupy and engage a person's concern to the extent of employing his time.

**interface**   See *network*.

**interfaceable minds**   Any mental state shared by more than one person; the term is used most frequently in the context of the infant's "theory of interfaceable minds," referring to the recognition somewhere between the seventh and ninth month of life that the child can share a state of mind, such as an intention, with another person.

**interference pattern of discharge**   See *obsessive attack*.

**intergenic DNA**   "Deserts" of several hundreds of thousands of nucleotide codes that do not appear to encode genes. Genes often exist in random clusters of gene-rich oases separated by noncoding nucleotides.

**intergroup exercises**   See *Group Relations Conferences*.

**interhemispheric transfer (IHT)**   Transmission of information between the cerebral hemispheres, typically assessed with laterally presented stimuli. See *corpus callosum*.

**interictal behavior syndrome**   *Temporolimbic behavior disturbance*; originally described (by D. Bear and P. Fedio, 1977) as *temporal lobe epileptic personality*; a group of symptoms manifested by patients during the intervals between temporal lobe seizures. During the seizure itself, limbic functions tend to be inhibited; during the interictal phase limbic functions (and in particular depression) are usually intensified.

The major symptoms are:

1. Sexuality—reduced libido, anorgasmia, impotence or, more often, sexual paraphilias, and conflicts over sexual preferences.

2. Aggessivity—such as morally justified aggressive acts with subsequent remorse, hypersensitivity to slights, moral indignation, elaborate plans for retaliation.

3. Depression—is frequent (perhaps as many as 30% of cases), as is suicide; most patients can be treated successfully with antidepressants without exacerbation of their epilepsy.

4. Other affective symptoms—anxiety, irritability, hypomania, increased or decreased emotionality.

5. Cognitive and personality—circumstantiality, social viscosity (a clinging or sticky quality in interpersonal relations), obsessional preoccupation with details, humorlessness, hypermoralism, *hypergraphia* (q.v.) coupled with philosophic concerns or extreme religiosity.

Symptoms of the interictal behavior syndrome are often ameliorated by drugs or neurosurgery for the seizures themselves, whether the syndrome is intrinsic (i.e., due to the ictal process) or extrinsic (e.g., secondary to living with chronic epilepsy).

**interleukin**   See *apoptosis; cytokines*.

**intermarriage**   In genetics, marriage between two blood relations, especially in the sense of a *cousin marriage*, or the union between two individuals belonging to different racial groups of a mixed population. Cousin marriages are of particular genetic significance in the case of recessive mendelian inheritance. See *recessiveness*.

**intermediate**   In genetics, the type of mendelian inheritance characterized by the fact that the expressivity of a dominant character may be modifiable by the recessive member of a given pair of contrasting characters. The term denotes both this blended kind of inheritance and the particular hybrids who resemble neither parent exactly, but are intermediate in several respects between the original characteristics of the two parent types. For instance, pink hybrids would be intermediate when they have one red and one white parent. See *dominance*.

Within the intermediate mode of heredity, many cases are known in which one and the same genetic factor has a dominant effect on one set of characters, but a recessive effect on others. Another modification is constituted by those cases in which each member of a contrasting pair of factors produces its own effect independently, so that the heterozygote is neither a blend nor an intermediate, but a *mosaic*.

**intermediate brain syndrome due to alcohol**   See *blackout*.

**intermediate care**   Residential program providing rehabilitation rather than acute inpatient or skilled nursing care. Included are halfway houses, quarterway houses, and recovery homes that are usually community based, and especially for alcoholism and drug abuse programs peer-group oriented services that provide food, shelter, and supportive services in an alcohol- or drug-free environment. See *domicile*.

**intermediate memory**    See *long-term memory*.

**intermediate sex**    *Homosexuality* (q.v.).

**intermetamorphosis syndrome**    A misidentification syndrome first described by P. Courbon and J. Tusques (1932); the subject develops the delusional conviction that various people have been transformed physically and psychologically into other people. This differs from the *Frégoli phenomenon*, which also involves misidentification, in that it includes false physical resemblance in addition to false recognition. See *Capgras syndrome*; *misidentification, delusional*.

**intermission**    When a psychiatric syndrome ends in a disappearance of symptoms for a temporary period, only to reappear at a subsequent time, the interval between attacks is called an intermission. When after an attack it is not known that the symptoms will reappear, the term *remission* (q.v.) is used. A patient in a state of remission may never have another attack.

**intermittent explosive disorder**    See *episodic dyscontrol*.

**intermittent-dose strategy**    *Targeted-dose strategy* (q.v.).

**intermodal fluency**    Ability to transfer knowledge from one sensory channel to another, as in feeling an object while blindfolded and being able subsequently to pick that object from a group on the basis of its visual appearance. Infant research has show that the infant is intermodally fluent and that such ability is inherent in how the organism perceives.

**internal capsule**    A band of white fiber tracts separating the lenticular nucleus of the *basal ganglia* (q.v.) from the caudate and thalamus. It contains all the fibers that ascend to and descend from the cortex: pyramidal tract, thalamocortical fibers, optic radiation from the lateral geniculate body, auditory radiation from the medial geniculate body, fronto- and temporopontine tracts, fibers of the corpus striatum, and the corticothalamic tracts. Lesions in the internal capsule, common in cerebrovascular accidents, result in contralateral spastic hemiplegia.

**internal object relations**    See *object relations theory*.

**internal working models**    See *attachment*.

**internal world**    See *paranoid-schizoid position*.

**internalization**    The process(es) whereby the infant builds his internal world, including *identification, incorporation*, and *introjection* (qq.v.). Internalization stresses the fact that most of what are termed psychodynamics take place within the subject; as evocative memory develops, the child is able to build within himself the memory and symbols of his relationships with objects in the external world. See *self-object*.

Internalizing of affect is typically manifested as anxiety, social withdrawal, and depression; reduced outside interests and fewer social activities; preoccupation with physical aggression, withdrawal and suicidal ideation; and *externalizing* behaviors, such as aggressiveness, hyperactivity, and, in children, conduct problems.

**internalization, transmuting**    See *self-object*.

**internalizing behaviors**    Behaviors that are directed internally "within the self," such as emotional reactivity, depression, anxiety, irritability, and withdrawal. *Externalizing behaviors* (noncompliance, verbal/physical aggression, disruptive acts, emotional outbursts) can develop into externalizing disorders, such as ADHD, opposition defiant disorder, and conduct disorder.

**internalizing disorders**    Anxiety disorders and depressive disorders. High levels of neuroticism are associated with the likelihood of suffering from either of the internalizing disorders, and it is probable that genetic variation in internalizing symptoms depends largely on the same factors as those affecting neuroticism. Neuroticism does not account for all the genetic variance underlying internalizing disorders, however. There is evidence for an "internalizing" factor that accounts for high rates of comorbidity among anxiety and depressive disorders and is separate from an "externalizing" factor, related to substance use disorders and antisocial personality disorders.

**International Classification of Diseases (ICD)**    The official list of disease categories issued by the World Health Organization.

**International Pilot Study of Schizophrenia (IPSS)**    A 1973 transcultural investigation of 1202 schizophrenic patients in nine countries—Colombia, Czechoslovakia, Denmark, India, Nigeria, People's Republic of China, Union of Soviet Socialist Republics, United

Kingdom, and United States. The major objective of the study was to define an operational base from which future international epidemiologic studies of schizophrenia and other psychiatric disorders could be developed. One part of the study aimed to define symptoms in such a way that psychiatrists all over the world can agree they are present, and then determine which individual symptoms or groupings of symptoms are associated with clinical diagnoses.

**interneuron**  One of the two major types of nerve cell in the brain; interneurons are local and integrate information within specific nuclei of the brain. The other type of nerve cell is the *projection* neuron; the axons of projection neurons connect major regions of the brain. See *neuron*.

**internuclear ophthalmoplegia syndrome**  *Medial longitudinal fasciculus syndrome*; a lesion in the upper pons causes impaired adduction of the ipsilateral eye, and abduction with coarse nystagmus of the contralateral eye.

**internuncial**  Intercalated. See *reflex*.

**interoception**  The sense of the physiological condition of the entire body, and not only the viscera as the term classically has been defined. Sherrington (in 1948) had divided the senses into *teloreceptive* (vision and hearing), *proprioceptive* (position and movement of limbs), *exteroreceptive* (touch, temperature, and pain), *chemoreceptive* (taste and smell), and *interoceptive* (visceral). Recent studies (1996–1999) have found that the lamina I spinothalamocortical system is a homeostatic afferent pathway that carries the sensory aspects of ongoing homeostasis and the physiological condition of the body. The system conveys signals from primary afferents that represent the physiological status of all tissues of the body to autonomic and homeostatic centers in the spinal cord and brain stem. Together with afferent activity relayed by the nucleus of the solitary tract it projects to a dedicated thalamocortical relays system in the posterior thalamus. It has been hypothesized that rerepresentation of the system's sensory signals in the anterior insular cortex in the nondominant hemisphere provides a basis for the subjective evaluation of one's condition, of "how one feels." See *insula*; *sensation*.

Thalamic nuclei in turn project to the posterior portion of the insula on the contralateral sides, and then through a callosal pathway each projects to the other side. The posterior representation is then rerepresented in the anterior insula; the rerepresentation in the nondominant (right) anterior insula provides the basis for subjective evaluation of one's condition, that is, the ability to perceive the self as a physical and separate entity, self-awareness, and consciousness. In short, that rerepresentation answers the question, How do you feel? Representations of highly resolved, distinct sensations of the many feelings from the body are embedded in the interoceptive insular cortex, providing a limbic sensory substrate for feelings and emotions. Activation of right anterior insular and orbitofrontal cortices is associated with subjective emotion. The anatomically identified projection field in the insula, interoception, is distinct from the parietal somatosensory cortices, *exteroception*.

The subjective evaluation of interoceptive state is forwarded to the orbitofrontal cortex, where hedonic valence in represented in mammals. Anterior cingulate cortex and medial prefrontal regions are concerned with explicit representations of mental states of the self (Craig, A. D. *Nature Reviews Neuroscience* 3: 655–666, 2002).

**interoceptive**  Referring to internal, physiologic. Russian investigators recognized that fear can be conditioned to internal physiologic stimuli (such as peristalsis or cardiac rhythm), and that the conditioned response was highly resistant to extinction. It has been theorized that such interoceptive cues may, in persons with panic disorder, become associated with the possibility of another panic attack and thereby constitute a *learned alarm*. This results in hypervigilance and overreaction to normal physiologic events, often manifested as somatic preoccupation and overconcern.

Interoceptive exposure is a treatment technique for panic disorder that consists of repeated exposure of the patient to the somatic sensations associated with panic attacks. The method employs procedures that can induce panic-related symptoms reliably, including physical exercise, carbon dioxide inhalation, and hyperventilation.

**interoceptive marker**  See *marker, interoceptive*.

**interpenetration**  A speech or writing defect in which the intensity of the patient's preoccupations reduces his ability to respond directly to questioning; instead every now and then he will interject a few fragments of the topic suggested by the question. Interpenetration is also used to refer to intrusion of the patient's complexes and preoccupations into any direct response he may give to a question. Interpenetration is seen frequently in the schizophrenias but occurs in other disorders as well; it is therefore considered an accessory schizophrenic symptom.

**interpersonal** Often used to refer to Sullivan's theory of personality, the dynamic-cultural view of development.

**interpersonal process** The give and take between one person and another; used to refer to the interaction between patient and therapist, the term emphasizes that the analyst is more than a mirror reflecting the patient's problems. Just as there is *transference* on the patient's part, so is there *countertransference* on the analyst's part. Still, not every attitude toward the analyst is a transference attitude. The patient can like or dislike the analyst for what he really is, and the analyst cannot completely conceal what kind of person he is. The analyst sometimes transfers elements from his past or present problems to the analytic situation.

"Freud's conception of countertransference is to be distinguished from the present-day conception of analysis as an interpersonal process. In the interpersonal situation, the analyst is seen as relating to his patient not only with his distorted affects but with his healthy personality also. That is, the analytic situation is essentially a human relationship in which, while one person is more immediately detached than the other and has less at stake, he is nevertheless an active participant" (Thompson, C. *Psychoanalysis, Evolution and Development*, 1950).

**interpersonal psychotherapy (ITP)** A form of brief psychotherapy introduced by Klerman and Weissman for the treatment of patients with depression and four areas of interpersonal relationship that are often associated with the onset of depression: role disputes, role transitions, interpersonal deficits, and grief. A procedural manual has been developed that specifies the concepts and techniques of ITP in helping the patient to recognize links between his mood and current interpersonal experiences.

**interpersonal therapy** A psychodramatic technique used when more than one person is involved in the problems presented, as in a "triangular neurosis" affecting husband, wife, and a third person. Treatment interrelates dynamically with all the persons involved. "Inter-personal therapy is carried out in alternating sessions with each of the persons involved until the psychiatrist, the auxiliary ego, has returned to the subject with whom he began. The cycle can be repeated as often as necessary until catharsis is reached" (Moreno, J. L. *Sociometry 1*, 1937).

**interposed nuclei** See *cerebellum*.

**interpretation** The description or formulation of the meaning or significance of a patient's productions and, particularly, the translation into a form meaningful for the patient of his resistances and symbols and character defenses. "The lowest degree consists of waiting for the patient to interpret things for himself, giving him as few cues as possible. Next, the patient is enjoined to attempt the interpretation of representative experiences. Of greater degree, is a piecing together of items of information, and of seemingly unrelated bits, so that certain conclusions become apparent to the patient. Leading questions are asked to guide the patient to meaningful answers. More directive is the making of interpretations in a tentative way, so that the patient feels privileged to accept or reject them as he chooses. Finally, the therapist gives the patient strong authoritative interpretations, couched in challenging, positive terms" (Wolberg, L. R. *The Technique of Psychotherapy*, 1954).

In *structural interviewing*, Kernberg differentiates among (1) *clarification*—the patient and the therapist discuss and examine in greater detail what the patient has said so that both are more fully aware of its implications; (2) *confrontation*—the therapist notes contradictions or inconsistencies in the clarified information and suggests the need for an explanation of them; and (3) interpretation—the therapist suggests a hypothesis to explain the observed discrepancies when the patient is unable to make the causal connections.

**interpretation, deep** An ambiguous term that usually refers to any interpretation concerned with early developmental levels (e.g., pregenital as opposed to genital levels) or with the earliest repressed material.

**interpretation, serial** Elucidation of a consecutive number of dreams taken as a group.

**interpretive mode** *Analytic mode*; in self psychology, the style of communication employed in maintaining the therapeutic dialogue between patient and therapist. The two basic elements are understanding the patient's subjective reasons for his behavior and explaining those reasons to the patient in a way that both affirms the validity of his subjective experiences and encourages him to correct or challenge the explanations proffered by the analyst. See *therapeutic alliance*.

**interpsychology** A term used by Tarde, Janet, and others for interpersonal relationships.

**intersex** A sexually intermediate individual who has developed biologically as a male (or female) up to a certain point in its life and thereafter has continued its development as a female (or male). Owing to the supersession of one type of sex tendency by the other, intersexes usually show a mixture of male and female parts and are almost invariably sterile. They are not gynandromorphs, because their structures are not definitely and clearly male or female.

In cattle, an intersex that "is made so by action of hormone of the opposite sex" is called a *freemartin*. According to Shull, all freemartins are modified females.

**intersexuality** Incomplete sex reversal, which leads to the production of individuals intermediate between the sexes, as the final result of a competition between opposed male and female tendencies, in which supremacy is gained at the "turning point" by the formerly less developed tendency. The time at which this switch takes place determines the degree of intersexuality.

A special form of intersexuality, occurring in humans as well as in domesticated mammals, is probably caused by delayed or deficient hormone production and results in modifications of both internal and external sex organs and secondary characteristics.

Intersexuality is sometimes used (incorrectly) to refer to severe *transsexualism* or *transvestitism* (qq.v.).

**interstimulation** Modification of behavior in response to the presence of others. For instance, a child's general conduct is altered by the presence of one or more other children. Interest is stimulated or diminished, activity is intensified or decreased, and anxiety is heightened.

**interstimulus interval** *ISI*; the amount of time between two stimuli, used as a test of the subject's ability to retain (remember) information over time.

**intersubjective resonance** *Empathy* (q.v.).

**interval psychosis** Postoperative delirium, the major psychiatric complication observed in surgical intensive care units. Depending on the type of surgery and the degree of preoperative psychosocial intervention, reported incidence varies from 15% to 70%.

**intervening act** In law, an act of the patient's own will; a voluntary act.

**intervention** Act of interceding on behalf of one or more subjects, as in crisis intervention (q.v.). In the case of alcohol or other substance abuse, for instance, interceding on behalf of the person who is abusing, or is dependent on, one or more psychoactive drugs, with the aim of overcoming denial, interrupting drug-taking behavior, or inducing the person to seek and initiate treatment.

**interventricular foramen** See *ventricle*.

**interview, Amytal** See *narcotherapy*.

**intimacy** A subjective state of closeness to another person that gratifies a wish for warmth and relatedness and provides an opportunity for expression of sexual and aggressive drives. Intimacy depends on an established sense of self, trust in the other person, and a conviction that one will not be injured in the relationship. One can then relinquish control, at least temporarily, and allow dependency on the other to form. Intimacy can exist without sex, and vice versa, but when the two act together they add to pleasure and fulfillment in an erotic relationship.

**intimacy vs. isolation** One of Erikson's eight stages of man. See *ontogeny, psychic*.

**intimate partner violence (IPV)** A pattern of coercive or violent tactics used by one partner (or former partner) to maintain power and control over another. The tactics include physical, sexual, psychological, and economic abuse. IPV occurs in all demographic groups and affects up to 30% of adult women and 7.5% of adult men, but in the clinical setting it appears most frequently in women between 16 and 24 years of age. See *domestic violence*.

Victims of IPV are often reluctant to raise the issue of abuse, but most will respond to questioning from a trusted health provider, especially if the questions are clear, direct, and asked in nonjudgmental words and an accepting tone that communicates the questioner's desire to help. Once IPV is suspected or confirmed, the provider must determine if the patient is in immediate danger. Indications of danger include any escalation in the frequency or severity of violence, recent use or threats by the abuser to use weapons, threats by the abuser of homicide or suicide, and stalking of the patient. The examiner should also make certain that the patient has somewhere safe to go. If the patient reports recent sexual abuse, she should be referred to rape crisis services and Emergency Department care for a Sexual Assault Forensic Exam (SAFE).

**intimidate** To frighten or cow; to make another fearful that one will attack him verbally or physically or that one will shame or embarrass him. Intimidation is sometimes used as a defense against anxiety proceeding from conflicts over passive homosexual impulses.

**intoxication, drug** Disruptive changes in physiologic functioning, mood states, or cognitive processes due to excessive consumption of a drug.

**intra-axial** Originating in the brain parenchyma; *extra-axial* refers to structures surrounding the brain. In adults, intra-axial brain tumors are usually gliomas, such as the malignant glioblastoma multiforme. Meningioma, schwannoma, pituitary adenomas, and metastatic tumors are the most common extra-axial tumors.

**intraconscious personality** A coconscious personality that knows another personality's thoughts. In one type of dissociative identity disorder, one personality functions subconsciously, and when it is aware not only of the outer world but of the thoughts of the conscious personality in the same person, it is termed intraconscious personality.

**intracranial tumor** Any localized intracranial lesion, whether of neoplastic or of chronic inflammatory origin, which by occupying space within the skull tends to cause a rise in intracranial pressure.Intracranial tumors account for approximately 10% of all malignant neoplasms in humans and for about 2% of all cancer-related deaths. Benign tumors are 12 times as prevalent as primary malignant tumors; metastatic tumors (from lung, breast, stomach, thyroid, or kidney) about three times as prevalent.

Gliomas, the most common primary brain tumors, include (1) *astrocytomas*, which arise in both cerebral and cerebellar tissue, at any age; (2) *glioblastoma multiforme*, a highly malignant tumor of the cerebral hemispheres that appears in middle age; (3) *medulloblastoma*, a rapidly growing tumor most often of the cerebellum, seen frequently in children; and (4) *oligodendrogliomas* and ependymomas, rare and slowly growing. See *glioma*.

*Meningiomas* are extracerebral tumors of the meninges that often invade the overlying bone of the skull. Other brain tumors are angioblastomas and angiomas (which arise from the cerebral blood vessels); chromophil and chromophobe adenomas and *craniopharyngioma* (all from the pituitary); pineal tumors; colloid cysts from the choroid plexus of the third ventricle; and acoustic neuroma, from the eighth cranial nerve.

When subdivided by location, 70% of intracranial tumors in the adult are supratentorial and 30% are infratentorial (in the posterior fossa); the ratio is reversed in children. In adults, 22% of tumors are located in the frontal lobe, 22% in the temporal lobe; in both locations, tumors are relatively silent. Parietal tumors account for 12%, occipital for 4%; 10% are pituitary tumors, and 30% are in the posterior fossa.

General symptoms of intracranial tumors include the classical triad of headache (the initial symptom in a third of cases), vomiting (sometimes projectile in nature), and papilledema (relatively rare despite its traditional inclusion as a member of the triad). Other general symptoms are visual field defects, seizures (with few exceptions, the EEG shows increasing focal abnormality), aphasia, vertigo, slowed pulse and increased blood pressure, coma, confusion, and progressive dementia.

Psychiatric symptoms are frequent, occurring in 40% to 100% of patients depending on the type and location of tumor. Meningiomas are particularly likely to produce symptoms such as depression, anxiety, or personality change. Tumors in certain locations—the prefrontal or temporal lobes, third ventricle, or limbic system—may mimic the "functional" psychoses and other primary psychiatric disorders.

**intractable pain** Chronic pain; neuropathic pain. See *pain syndromes*.

**intralaminar nuclei** A group of small nuclei in the internal medullary lamina of the *thalamus* (q.v.). They receive projections from the frontal lobe (including the motor and premotor cortex); their major output is to the putamen and caudate nucleus (the striatum), with some projections to the *ventral anterior nucleus* (see *lateral nuclear group*).

**intralaminar system** Morison and Dempsey's term for a diffuse, bilateral, nonspecific projection system of neurons in the thalamus. Also known as the *recruiting system*, the intralaminar system is associated with consciousness, sleep, and wakefulness and thus would appear to be identical with the *reticular activating system* in many respects. See *reticular formation*.

**intraparietal sulcus** *IPS;* a long, deep fissure that cuts through the *parietal lobe* (q.v.), dividing it into the superior and inferior parietal lobules. Various regions associated with it are part of the neural circuitry involved in spatial representations, *numerosity*, and *reward* (qq.v.).

*VIP* (ventral intraparietal) area is located in the ventral portion of the intraparietal sulcus. It is responsive to motion in visual, auditory, and tactile modalities with head-centered receptive fields. Number-selective neurons are located in or near this region. Many VIP neurons have joint tactile and visual motion-determined receptive fields, and are strongly driven by optic flow fields.

*LIP* (lateral intraparietal) area is in the lateral bank of the IPS. It is involved in visual representations of space in an eye-centered coordinate frame. This region is crucial for attention, intention to make saccadic eye movements, and spatial updating. See *visual processing*.

*AIP* (anterior intraparietal) area, in the anterior portion of IPS, is involved in fine grasping behaviors. Neurons in this area respond to both visual and tactile stimuli, with receptive fields that move with the hand.

*CIP* (caudal intraparietal) area, at the posterior end of IPS, is involved in the analysis of three-dimensional shapes. Signals from CIP are sent to AIP, where they are integrated to plan the grasping of three-dimensional objects.

*MIP* (medial intraparietal) area is involved in visuomotor transformations. Along with area V6A, this region comprises the *PRR* (parietal reach region), which is active in tasks

that require hand coordination and reaching to specific locations. (Hubbard, E. M. et al. *Nature Reviews Neuroscience 6*: 435–448, 2005). See *visual processing*.

**intrapsychic, intrapsychical** Situated, originating, or taking place within the psyche.

**intrinsic factor** See *posterolateral sclerosis*.

**introject** To withdraw psychic energy (libido) from an object and direct it upon the mental image of the object; to incorporate.

**introject, primal** See *original object*.

**introjection** The process of incorporating into one's ego system the picture of an object as one conceives the object to be. Libidinal and aggressive cathexes are then transferred from the object in the environment to the mental picture of the object. For example, when a person becomes depressed due to the loss of a loved one, his feelings are directed to the mental image he possesses of the loved one. He acts toward the image as if it were the loved one in reality.

The term introjection is sometimes used as if it were identical with *secondary identification* and perhaps also with *secondary narcissism*. See *identification; incorporation*.

**introjective identification** See *identification; narcissistic object relations; paranoid-schizoid position*.

**intron** A noncoding region of a *gene* (q.v.); a region between exons within genes that is spliced out in the creation of messenger RNA and does not code for a protein. Just under 25% of the genome is contained within introns. See *exon; transcription*.

**intropunitive** Having the quality of turning anger against the self, as in the self-pejorative, demeaning, and belittling trend of the depressed patient. This is in contrast to extrapunitive, which refers to externally directed anger.

**introversion** Turning of the instincts inwardly upon oneself; the libido is directed toward the inner world, the world of representation, instead of the world of reality. Introversion is often used synonymously with *phantasy-cathexis*. Both imply a loss of contact with reality and because of it, they differ from *narcissism*, which does not imply such loss.

Freud's definition of introversion differs from Jung's. Freud says that introversion does not mean that the erotic relation with reality has been severed but that the subject "has ceased to direct his motor activities to the attainment of his aims in connection with real objects" (*Collected Papers*, 1924–1925). Jung says it means "a turning inwards of the libido, whereby a negative relation of subject to object is expressed. Interest does not move towards the object, but recedes towards the subject. Everyone whose attitude is introverted thinks, feels, and acts in a way that clearly demonstrates that the subject is the chief factor of motivation while the object at most receives only a secondary value" (*Psychological Types*, 1923).

**introversion, active**   "Introversion is *active* when the subject wills a certain seclusion in face of the object; it is *passive* when the subject is unable to restore again to the object the libido which is streaming back from it" (Jung, C. G. *Psychological Types*, 1923).

**introvert**   One whose psychic energy (libido) is turned inwardly upon himself.

**intrusion**   An irrelevant association or thought, such as an obsessive thought that repeatedly and persistently forces itself into consciousness or, more commonly, one or more meaningless thoughts that appear randomly and interfere with the logical and orderly progression of thought. The latter kind of intrusion is seen most often in patients with frontal lobe dysfunction or schizophrenia and is generally explained as a difficulty in suppressing irrelevant associations.

**intrusions, saccadic**   See *saccades*; *smooth pursuit system*.

**intrusive treatment**   See *forced treatment*.

**intuition**   A literary and psychological term with no exact scientific definition or connotation. It refers to a special method of perceiving and evaluating objective reality. Intuition differs from foresight, conscious perception, and judgment in that it relies heavily on unconscious memory traces of past and forgotten experiences and judgments. In this way, a storehouse of unconscious wisdom that had been accumulated (in unconscious memory) in the past is used in the present.

Intuition is characterized by accurate "predictability" in the engineering and mathematical sense. It is also characterized by the fact that people will feel and say "I don't know just how I know that, but I know it's correct," and it often is. See *analytic psychology*.

**intuitive type**   The third of Jung's four functional types of personality. With his fourth (*sensational* type) it constitutes the *irrational* class of *functional* types.

One who "adapts himself by means of unconscious indications, which he receives through an especially fine and sharpened perception and interpretation of faintly conscious stimuli. How such a function appears is naturally hard to describe, on account of its irrational, and, so to speak, unconscious character." The intuitive type "raises unconscious perception to the level of a differentiated function, by which he also becomes adapted to the world" (Jung, C. G. *Psychological Types*, 1923).

**invalidism**   Condition of being a chronic invalid. From the standpoint of the social worker: the habit of preoccupation with one's health not justified by one's actual condition. See *hypochondriasis*.

**invalidism, psychological**   The mental state of a patient who, though he has been cured of his physical illness, refuses to accept that fact. He repudiates the idea of getting well and gives a thousand reasons why he should continue to live as he was compelled to live during the height of his physical illness.

Such an attitude is observed particularly among children. "When the situation is studied, it is found that the child has learned that there are many benefits from being an invalid—extra attention, marked concern by parents, extra food and toys, and frequent excuse from duties." The mechanism is largely an unconscious one, however (Pearson, G. H. J. *Emotional Disorders of Children*, 1940). See *complaint habit*.

**invariance, developmental**   Stability over time, or failure to change with maturation, most often applied to speech organization in children. Believers in developmental invariance hold that speech organization in children is similar to that in adults and does not change with age. The developmental maturation position holds that children are born with hemispheric equipotentiality for language and that lateralization occurs as the child matures. Experimental and clinical evidence generally supports the developmental invariance position.

**invasive treatment**   See *forced treatment*.

**inversion, absolute**   Describing persons whose sexual object must always be of the same sex, while the opposite sex can never be to them an object of sexual longing, but leaves them indifferent or may even evoke sexual repugnance (*The Basic Writings of Sigmund Freud,* 1938).

**inversion, amphigenous**  Psychosexual hermaphroditism; i.e., the sexual object may belong indifferently to either the same or to the other sex. See *androgyneity; bisexuality.*

**inversion, occasional**  Accidental homosexuality, or homosexuality faute de mieux. See *homosexuality, male.*

**inversion, sexoesthetic**  Eonism; *transvestitism* (q.v.).

**inversion, sexual**  Homosexuality. Freud distinguished three types of sexual inversion: *absolute, amphigenous,* and *occasional.*

**inversion of affect**  *Counter-affect; reversal of affect;* transformation of an affect into its opposite.

**inverted Oedipus**  *Negative Oedipus* (q.v.).

**investment**  The affective charge given to an idea or object. See *cathexis.*

**inveterate drinking**  *Delta alcoholism* (q.v.).

**invocational psychosis**  A rare psychotic reaction to incantations, prayers, etc., as sometimes seen in revival meetings.

**involuntary medication**  Forced treatment with pharmacological agents. There has been near unanimity that involuntary patients have a right to refuse treatment with neuroleptic medications, based on their right to privacy, which is not abrogated by commitment. In some states, patients' refusal of medication can be overridden only when they have been found to be incompetent to make their own treatment decisions. The mechanisms for determining incompetence, appropriateness of treatment, etc. range from formal judicial hearings to administrative inquiries to reviews by administrators or consulting psychiatrists.

**involution**  See *hereditary.*

**involutional paranoia**  The paranoid form of involutional melancholia. See *involutional psychosis; paraphrenia.*

**involutional paraphrenia**  *Involutional psychosis* (q.v.).

**involutional period**  *Climacterium* (q.v.).

**involutional psychosis**  *Climacteric psychosis; involutional melancholia; agitated depression* of middle life—all these terms are used more or less interchangeably to refer to depressive psychoses appearing during the involutional period (40 to 55 years for women, 50 to 65 years for men) in people who have no history of previous mental illness. See *anxietas praesenilis.* Characteristically, such depressions manifest a triad of symptoms, consisting of delusions of sin and guilt or of poverty, an obsession with death, and a delusional fixation on the gastrointestinal tract, all in a setting of agitation and dejection. In some (involutional paranoid state), a fourth major symptom is present in self-referential or persecutory delusions, and this second group with a vivid admixture of paranoid symptoms has a poorer prognosis than the more purely depressive variety. Concern over finances, physical illness, bereavement, enforced retirement, and "loss" of children to marriage or other forms of independence are frequent precipitants. Involutional psychoses account for 5%–10% of first admissions to mental hospitals; their actual incidence is difficult to estimate because many respond favorably to antidepressant drugs or to electroconvulsive therapy administered on an outpatient basis.

Involutional psychosis is not recognized as a separate category of depression in DSM-IV.

**ion channel**  A glycoprotein tube within the membrane of the neuron. The intrinsic chemical properties of neurons are determined by the mixture of ion channels in the neuron's cell membrane. The neuron's cell membrane shows highly selective permeability to various ions and contains energy-dependent ion pumps that transport ions across the membrane against their concentration gradients. Ion channels exhibit two fundamental processes: (1) *permeation*—selective translocation of ions across the cell membrane; and (2) *gating*—control of ion access to the permeation pathway. The cell membrane presents a large energy barrier to ion permeation—the *dielectric barrier.*

*Non-gated* channels are always open and contribute significantly to the resting potential. *Gated* channels open or close in response to different signals—voltage, chemical transmitters, and pressure or stretch. Gating mechanisms involve a conformational change in channel structure, such as a discrete change in one region, or a general change along the length of a channel, or a ball-and-chain mechanism in which a blocking particle swings into and out of the channel mouth.

There are three major classes of ion channels: chemically mediated synaptic actions include fast, directly gated action lasting milliseconds; slow, second-messenger mediated actions involving modifications of ion channels and other substrate proteins; and transmitters, acting through second messengers, which phosphorylate (via *protein kinases*) transcriptional regulatory proteins within the cell and thereby alter gene expression. This third kind of synaptic action can lead to other changes, such as neuronal growth, lasting days or more, and is important for neuronal development and learning. See *neurotransmitter receptor*.

Receptors that gate ion channels directly (*ionophoric receptors*) include the nicotinic acetylcholine, the GABA, the glycine, the AMPA, and the NMDA class of glutamate receptors. The excitatory amino acids (such as glutamate and aspartate) open the $Na^+$ channel, resulting in depolarization and increase in cell excitability. The inhibitory amino acids (such as GABA and glycine) open the Cl– channel, resulting in hyperpolarization and decrease in cell excitability. Benzodiazepines increase the frequency of GABA-mediated openings of chloride channels.

Receptors that gate ion channels indirectly (*metabotropic receptors*) are coupled to their effector molecules by a guanosine nucleotide-binding protein (*G protein*). Among the receptors of this type are the α- and β-adrenergic, the serotonin, dopamine, and muscarinic ACh receptors, and receptors for neuropeptides. Typically the effector enzyme is a second messenger, such as cyclic adenosine monophosphate (cAMP), diacylglycerol, or an *inositol polyphosphate*. The second messenger, in turn, activates specific protein kinases (which phosphorylate a variety of the cell's proteins) or mobilizes $Ca^{2+}$ ions from intracellular stores. In some instances, the G protein or the second messenger can act directly on an ion channel.

The $Ca^{2+}$ influx controlled by these channels can alter many metabolic processes within cells, leading to activation of various enzymes and proteins. $Ca^{2+}$ influx also acts as a trigger for the release of neurotransmitter from the neuron.

Serotonin binds to a receptor that activates the cAMP cascade. The cAMP-dependent protein kinase phosphorylates a substrate protein that acts on the $K^+$ channel to close it. Norepinephrine works in a similar fashion. Norepinephrine-releasing terminals originate in the locus ceruleus and innervate the hippocampus. Norepinephrine acts

through cAMP to close a $Ca^{2+}$-activated $K^+$ channel, which increases excitability and overrides accommodation. This is the reverse of the short-circuit effect of synaptic inhibition, where opening of chlorine channels decreases the effectiveness of excitatory synaptic inputs.

Direct gating of ion channels usually is rapid, while receptors linked to G proteins are slow in onset and longer lasting because they involve a cascade of reactions, each of which takes time.

Chemical synaptic transmission also lacks the speed of electrical transmission; its major effect is amplification of response. By releasing one or more synaptic vesicles, each of which contains several thousand molecules of transmitter, thousands of ion channels in the postsynaptic cell are opened. In this way a small presynaptic nerve terminal, which generates only a weak electrical current, is able to depolarize a large postsynaptic cell.

All channels produce electrical signals that result from the movement of ions down their electrochemical gradients through the channels. By moving through different channels, the same ions can produce different actions. For example, $K^+$ moves through a nongated channel to generate the resting potential, through a voltage-gated channel to repolarize the membrane during the action potential, and through a second-messenger gated channel to hyperpolarize the membrane in some inhibitory synaptic actions.

The flux of ions through ion channels is passive, requiring no expenditure of metabolic energy. The direction and eventual equilibrium for this flux is determined not by the channel itself, but rather by the electrochemical driving force across the membrane. Some ions, however, are actively transported across the cell membrane by means of a carrier protein or *ion pump* (q.v.).

Different neurons use different combinations of ion channels in their membranes; they also differ in their chemical transmitters and receptors. Such differences account for the fact that a disease may strike one class of neurons and not others or only one element of the neuron (e.g. the cells body) and not others (e.g., the axon).

**ion pump**    A carrier protein that actively transports ions across the cell membrane against their concentration gradients.

For a cell to have a steady resting membrane potential, the charge separation across the membrane must be constant, i.e., influx of positive charge must be balanced by efflux of positive charge. Dissipation of ionic gradients is prevented by the $Na^+$-$K^+$ pump, which extrudes $Na^+$ from the cell while taking in $K^+$.

The $Na^+$-$K^+$ pump is an integral membrane protein with binding sites for $Na^+$ and ATP on its intracellular surface and for $K^+$ on its extracellular surface. Protein phosphorylation (using the terminal phosphate group from ATP) leads to the removal of three $Na^+$ ions from inside the cell to the outside in exchange for two extracellular $K^+$ ions. Thus, at the resting membrane potential the cell is not in equilibrium, but rather in a steady state maintained by metabolic energy. See *action potential; resting membrane potential.*

**ionophoric** Ionotropic. See *ion channel; ion pump; synapse.*

**iophobia** Fear of poison or of being poisoned.

**IP3** Inositol triphosphate. See *ion channel.*

**ipRGCs** Intrisincally photoreceptive ganglion cells. See *melanopsin.*

**IPS** 1. *Intraparietal sulcus* (q.v.).

2. Individual placement and support, a model for providing vocational services to patients, used particularly in treatment of alcohol and substance abuse. Patients receive on- or off-the-job support to help them succeed at work. A vocational specialist is integrated into the treatment team and provides a full array of vocational services (evaluation, job search, negotiating reasonable accommodations, job support, and team collaboration).

**IPSRT** Interpersonal and social rhythm therapy, used particularly in treatment of bipolar illness and prevention of recurrence of manic or depressive episodes. It emphasizes stabilizing moods by improving adherence to medication, building coping skills and satisfaction with relationships, and stabilizing social rhythms or routines.

**IPSS** *International Pilot Study of Schizophrenia* (q.v.).

**IPT** *Integrated Psychological Therapy*; a multi-element, hierarchical, cognitive rehabilitation program for schizophrenic patients that aims to enhance basic cognitive capacities (e.g., concept formation, memory) before implementing problem-solving and motor-skills training. Cognitive training employs a series of tasks adapted from neuropsychological tests (e.g., a card-sorting test) and word games (e.g., finding synonyms and antonyms).

Developed in the 1970s in Switzerland, IPT was subsequently manualized; the manual is now available in 10 languages, including English. The latest version of the manual consists of 6 modules of increasing complexity; the modules are delivered to groups of 8 to 12 participants over 9 to 12 months, in 2-hour in vivo sessions twice weekly. Module 1, cognitive differentiation, focuses on basic cognitive functions using abstract exercises in the form of learning games (e.g., classifying cards by shape, color, or content). Module 2, social perception, asks participants to analyze slides or video sequences of social situations that are increasingly complex and emotionally charged; each participant's reactions may reveal the inappropriate interpretations and mistaken cognitive schema that are characteristic of schizophrenia. Module 3, verbal communication, uses learning games and role-playing to develop listening skills, understanding, and appropriate use of language. Module 4, social skills, uses cognitive-behavioral techniques such as role-playing, modeling, and reinforcement to assist participants in developing a range of social skills and using them appropriately in different social situations. Module 5, emotional management, asks participants to identify the emotion(s) expressed in a video sequence and to describe situations in which they have felt the same emotions and how they have reacted; this provides an opportunity to assess the appropriateness of the strategies they have used and to search for better ways to manage stressful situations. Module 6, problem solving, asks participants to identify stressful situations they are exposed to in everyday life, how they deal with them, and what might be better ways of dealing with them.

**IQ** *Intelligence quotient* (q.v.).

**I-R specificity** See *individual-response specificity.*

**IRB** Institutional review board, mandated in 1981 by the U.S. government to ensure adequate review of research activities within an institution (hospital, clinic, etc.). The focus of review is safety and minimization of risk to subjects, a reasonable risk/benefit ratio, equitable selection of subjects, documented informed consent, and protection of vulnerable subjects from undue coercion

(C. Casals-Ariet, "Legal and Ethical Issues in Psychiatric Research," 1994).

**iridoplegia** Paralysis of the iris muscle; failure of the pupil to react to light. The Argyll Robertson pupil is a special form of reflex iridoplegia. Reflex iridoplegia may be caused by optic nerve lesions, optic tract lesions, lesions in the upper part of the midbrain, and lesions in the motor path (oculomotor nerve). The condition is occasionally seen in alcoholic polyneuritis and in diabetes.

**irkunii** *Miryachit* (q.v.).

**IRM** Inherited releasing mechanism. See *instinct*.

**iron** Iron accumulates progressively in the brain with age, and iron-induced oxidative stress can cause neurodegeneration. There are two classes of iron-reduced *neurodegenerative disease* (q.v.): those that result from iron accumulation in specific brain regions, and those due to defects in iron metabolism or homeostasis. They frequently involve protein modification, misfolding, and aggregation, leading to the formation of intracellular inclusion bodies.

Iron accumulation has been implicated in many neurological diseases, including congenital aceruloplasminaemia (characterized by extrapyramidal symptoms, ataxia, and progressive CNS and retinal neurodegeneration), Alzheimer disease, Friedreich ataxia (where reduction in frataxin expression leads to increased mitochondrial iron content), neuroferritinopathy (a dominantly inherited, late-onset basal ganglia disease, with choreoathetosis, dystonia, spasticity, and rigidity), NBIA (neurodegeneration with brain iron accumulation, formerly known as Hallervorden-Spatz syndrome; due to mutations in the gene that codes for pantothenate kinase 2, which is necessary for coenzyme-A biosynthesis and is targeted to mitochondria); accumulation of cysteine, which chelates iron, causes oxidative stress, and leads to the accumulation of iron in the basal ganglia. Iron deficiency during development can produce lifelong cognitive and motor impairment; restless legs syndrome seems to be associated with decreased iron in the substantia nigra.

**irradiation** 1. Illumination. 2. In medicine, exposure to rays (heat, light, X-rays, etc.) for diagnostic or therapeutic purposes. 3. In neurophysiology, a spreading of the neural impulse within the central nervous system and, by analogy in psychodynamics, the spread of energy or tension outside the system in which the tension was originally generated. 4. In conditional-stimulus experiments (see *conditioning*), elicitation of the conditional response by a stimulus other than the one to which conditioning has been established; ordinarily such irradiation occurs only when the other stimulus is of the same general class as the original conditional stimulus.

**irrational** Though commonly used to mean unreasonable, Jung says: "As I make use of this term it does not denote something contrary to *reason*, but something outside the province of reason, whose essence, therefore, is not established by reason. Elementary facts belong to this category, e.g., that the earth has a moon, that chlorine is an element.... Both thinking and feeling as *directed functions* are rational," while sensation and intuition are irrational (*Psychological Types*, 1923).

**irrational action** Harming oneself without an adequate reason; causing, or not avoiding, some evil such as death; physical or mental pain; physical, cognitive, or volitional disability; or loss of freedom, opportunity, or pleasure without adequate reason. See *incompetent*.

**irrational authority** Power or command over others that, contrary to reason and logic, is based on neurotic craving for power and has no justification in competence; authority imposed on others through sheer willpower, without their consent. Fromm distinguishes this from rational authority, which is based on genuine ability and competence and is exemplified by the teacher imparting knowledge to a pupil. The person who resorts to irrational authority for security may find power by being a *magic helper* or from various forms of intimidation; he may also find power through identification with the authoritarian force, be it a person, a group, or an idea. Hence, Fromm considers Freud's superego a manifestation of authoritarian power.

The classical legend based on a vivid account by Pliny the Elder (*Historia Naturalis XXXV*) that gave rise to a widespread saying is a striking illustration of the gulf between rational and irrational authority. The great Greek painter Apelles (fl. 330 B.C.), who, valuing the opinion of the common folk, was in the habit of showing a new canvas in his studio and, hiding behind a painting, would listen to their observations. A passing shoemaker found fault with one sandal-loop being smaller than the other. The artist redrew it later in the day. The next morning the same shoemaker, emboldened by the artist's compliance, began to jeer about the leg. Emerging from his hiding place, Apelles squelched the glib critic with the crushing: "A cobbler should not judge above the sandal." ("Shoemaker, stick to your last.")

**irrational desire**  Desire to carry out an irrational action; wanting to suffer some evil without an adequate reason for doing so.

**irreminiscence**  Amnesia; inability to remember; more specifically, a type of agnosia with inability to form a mental picture of objects. See *object constancy*.

**irrepressible ideas, insanity of**  Kraepelin's expression for what is now called *obsessive-compulsive disorder* (q.v.).

**irresistibility**  See *criminal responsibility*.

**irritability, acoustic**  Auditory hypersensitivity. A generalized, diffuse irritability is one of the common characteristics of the traumatic neurosis. Physiologically, there is a lowering of the threshold of stimulation; the psychologic state is one of of readiness for fright reactions.

**irritable bowel syndrome**  Symptoms include abdominal pain, usually over the descending colon, with diarrhea or alternating diarrhea and constipation. Psychological factors are often implicated as precipitants but are not believed to be the cause.

**irrumation**  Fellatio.

**irrumo-**  Combining form for various terms that refer to oral sexual activity performed on the penis, from L. *irrumare*, to offer the penis for sucking.

**IS**  *Index of sexuality* (q.v.); Ischemic Scale.

**Isakower, Otto**  (1899–1972) Austrian psychoanalyst; described the phenomenon that bears his name in the *International Journal of Psychoanalysis*, 1938.

**Isakower phenomenon**  See *blank hallucination*.

**ischemia, cerebral**  See *TIA*.

**ischemic tolerance**  Resistance to ischemic injury, which may transiently be increased by preconditioning with a stressful but non-damaging stimulus to cells or tissues. *Erythropoietin* (q.v.) is a cytoprotective cytokine that is neuroprotective in stroke; preconditioning by means of hypoxia or with deferroxamine increases endogenous cerebral erythropoietin mRNA and protein levels.

**ischnophonia, ischophonia**  Stammering; *stuttering* (q.v.).

**island of Reil**  *Insula* (q.v.).

**isocortex**  *Neocortex*; the cortex visible on the external surface of the brain (the rest of the cortex is the *allocortex*). The isocortex is the most common type of cortex in the cerebral hemispheres and is composed of six layers of cells.

**isogamous**  *Genet.* Pertaining to or characterized by gametes that are equal in size and similar in structure in both sexes. See *syngamy*.

**isolate**  In the therapy group, anyone who does not participate in group activities or make contact with other members of the group. See *instigator; neutralizer*.

In psychoanalysis, to separate experiences or memories from their affect.

**isolate monkey**  See *monkey therapist*.

**isolated delusion**  See *monosymptomatic hypochondriacal psychosis*.

**isolation**  In psychoanalysis, the separation or *dissociation* (q.v.) of an idea or memory from its affective cathexis or charge, "so that what remains in consciousness is nothing but an ideational content which is perfectly colorless and is judged to be unimportant" (Freud, S. *Inhibitions, Symptoms and Anxiety*, 1936).

Freud distinguished between *isolation* and *undoing*. Isolation implies a kind of foresight that tries to check the appearance of something unpleasant; it is a rational process, according to Freud, whereas *undoing* is "irrational or magical in nature."

In sociology isolation is the separation of the person or group from social contacts.

Erikson describes intimacy vs. isolation as one of the eight stages of man. See *ontogeny, psychic*.

**isolation, perceptual**  See *sensory deprivation*.

**isolation, psychic**  Jung's term for the sense of estrangement from one's fellows that is felt immediately upon experiencing material communicated from one's collective unconscious. "Such irruptions are uncanny, because they are irrational and inexplicable to the individual concerned.... It is something that 'you can tell to no one,' except under fear of being accused of mental abnormality, and with some justification, for something quite similar befalls the insane. It is still a long way from an intuitively sensed irruption to pathological overthrow; but a layman does not know this" (*The Integration of the Personality*, 1939).

**isolation, psychological** Disinclination, aversion to, or fear of making contact with another member of the group.

**isolation amentia** See *deprivative amentia*.

**isolation of the speech area** Mixed *transcortical aphasia* (q.v.).

**isometric tremor** See *tremor*.

**isomorphism** Equal, similar, or identical in form, as in a mirror image. At one time it was hypothesized that perceived objects resulted in electrical fields within the brain of the same shape as the objects perceived.

**isopathic principle** *Homeopathic principle*; E. Jones's term for cure or relief of a symptom (e.g., guilt) by expression of the very emotion that is being repressed (hate), an instance of the cause curing the effect.

**isophilic** Sullivan's term for affection or liking for others of the same sex, such affection lacking the genital element characteristic of homosexuality; approximately synonymous with homoerotic.

**isozyme** A tissue-specific enzyme that takes different forms in different tissues. An isozyme may be normal in one tissue and abnormal in another. Cytochrome c oxidase, subunit IV of *OXPHOS* (q.v.), is such an isozyme. Isoenzymes act on the same substrates but because they differ slightly in protein linkage they also differ in what constitutes the optimal conditions for functioning.

**Israeli High-Risk Study** A long-term follow-up study of the influence of upbringing in a kibbutz on the development of psychiatric disorders in the offspring of schizophrenic parents, initiated by David Rosenthal. Results: (1) high-risk children reared on the primarily communal setting of kibbutzim (under the care of professional child-care workers) appeared to develop major psychiatric disorders at more than double the rate of matched high-risk children reared by their own parents; (2) the number of children who developed affective disorders exceeded the number who developed schizophrenia spectrum disorders; (3) there was significant impairment in a number of attention-related skills in high-risk as compared with control cases. See *attention*.

**ITP** *Interpersonal psychotherapy* (q.v.).

**ITPA** *Illinois Test of Psycholinguistic Abilities* (q.v.).

**IVDU** Intravenous drug user. See *needle sharing; route of drug administration*. IVDUs constitute an increasing proportion of persons with AIDS, as well as of those infected with the Hepatitis C virus.

**IVF** In vitro fertilization; see *ART*.

# J

**Jack the Clipper** The designation given to any person with a morbid propensity to clip hair or braids of girls; the name was first used in reference to a man in Chicago who for several years carried on the practice.

**Jack the Ripper** According to some, a London physician, an epileptic, who over a period of years during the 1880s committed brutal murders, presumably while in a postictal fugue state.

**jacknife spasms** See *infantile spasms.*

**Jackson, John Hughlings** (1834–1911) British neurologist; epilepsy, aphasia, dissolution, and disinhibition processes in brain damage.

**Jackson law** According to Hughlings Jackson's concept of the hierarchic development of mental functions, when there is organic brain disease the higher (i.e., the more complex and more recently developed) centers will be paralyzed or affected first, and the lower centers will resist deterioration the longest.

**Jackson syndrome** A bulbar syndrome due to involvement of the vagus, spinal accessory, and hypoglossal nerves. Symptoms are homolateral paralysis of the soft palate, pharynx, and larynx; homolateral paralysis of the sternocleidomastoid and trapezius muscles; and homolateral paralysis and atrophy of the tongue.

**Jacksonian epilepsy** A variant of *grand mal epilepsy* (q.v.) described by J. H. Jackson. The convulsion begins with clonic movements, which increase in severity and spread (the "cortical march") to involve large segments of the limb, then the other limb on the same side, then the face, and finally sometimes the other side, at which point consciousness is usually lost. The spread is along anatomical and/or physiological lines, and this type of epilepsy almost always indicates organic disease of the precentral cortex.

Jacksonian epilepsy usually begins in one of three foci: thumb and index finger; angle of the mouth; or the great toe.

**jactatio capitis nocturna** A disturbance of sleep sometimes observed in children: it consists of rhythmical rolling of the head from side to side—which hinders normal sleep. See *head-rolling.*

**jactitation, jactation** Extreme restlessness or tossing about; *agitation* (q.v.).

**Jakob, Alfons** (1884–1931) German psychiatrist; *Creutzfeldt-Jakob disease* (q.v.). See *virus infections.*

**Jakob-Creutzfeldt disease (CJD)** Presenile dementia with dysarthria and a syndrome of amyotrophic lateral sclerosis. Also known as Heidenheim or Kraepelin disease. See *Creutzfeldt-Jakob disease.*

**Jakobson, Edith** (1897–1978) Object relations theorist.

**jamais vu** A paramnestic phenomenon consisting of the erroneous feeling or conviction that one has never seen anything similar to what one is seeing now. Such a *denial* (q.v.) produces a fragmentation or break in continuity of memory.

**James, William** (1842–1910) U.S. physician, philosopher; his *Principles of Psychology* (1890) gained him the reputation of "father of American Psychology." His version of pragmatism, the idea that truth is tested by its effects, was the first American philosophical movement to gain international acceptance. With *Varieties of Religious Experience* (1902) he helped to found modern pastoral counseling; that work was also a building block in the establishment of Alcoholics Anonymous. James was a major force in moving psychology from philosophy into the natural sciences. He founded an experimental laboratory in psychology and taught the first course in physiological psychology in an American university, and he was one of the founders of experimental psychopathology.

**James-Lange-Sutherland theory** "The bodily changes follow directly the perception of the exciting fact, and our feeling of the same changes as they occur is the emotion.... The elements ... of physiological processes, which comprise the emotion ... are all organic changes, and each of them is the reflex effect of the exciting object" (Lange, C. G. & James, W. *The Emotions,* 1922). This theory admits of no special brain centers for emotion and has been largely replaced by Papez's modification of the *Cannon hypothalamic theory of emotion* (q.v.).

**Janet, Pierre** (1859–1947) French psychiatrist associated with Jean Charcot at the Salpétrière in Paris. According to the system of psychology he developed, the different mental functions were held together by nervous energy. In some, the amount of nervous energy was constitutionally deficient; when under stress, such persons did not have enough energy to maintain integration, with the result that specific mental functions dissociated or split off from the rest. He subdivided neuroses into (1) hysteria (amnesia and dissociated states of consciousness, various sensorimotor phenomena) and (2) *psychasthenia* (q.v.), which included anxiety, phobias, obsessions, and neurotic depression. The manifestations of psychasthenia were release phenomena, due to the escape of lower functions from central control (the higher functions of will and attention). Over the years, Janet described several of his cases in the literature: Leonie (1885), a case of multiple personality who could be hypnotized from a distance; Lucie (1886), the first case of cathartic cure with the use of hypnosis and automatic writing; Marie (1889), his second case of cathartic cure demonstrating the importance of subconscious ideas in the development of the illness; Achilles (1890), a case of demoniacal possession cured by unraveling the patient's fixed, unconscious ideas; Madame D. (1891–93), whom Janet encouraged to talk under hypnosis in order to dissolve her fixed ideas (Madame D. was also the case Charcot used to differentiate dynamic amnesia from organic amnesia); Marcelle (1891), in whom hypnosis and automatic writing were used to obtain material for psychological analysis; Justine (1894), whose phobia of cholera was cured by Janet's method of analysis of fixed ideas; Madeleine (1896–1904), with toe-walking, hysterical delusions, and the stigmata, provided much of the material for Janet's theory of emotions and religious psychology; Meb (1900), who had hysterical hallucinations with mystical and erotic themes; Irène (1902), with somnambulistic crises, hallucinations, and amnesia, whose treatment required mental stimulation and reeducation in addition to hypnotic treatment; and Nadia (1903), a girl obsessed by a fear of becoming fat that was related to fear of rejection (in many ways Nadia is similar to Ellen West, a patient

described in 1944 by Ludwig Binswanger and treated by existential analysis).

**Janet disease**   *Psychasthenia* (q.v.).

**Janet test**   (Pierre Janet, French physician, 1859–1947) A test for the determination of tactile sensibility; the patient answers "yes" or "no" when touched by the examiner's finger.

**Janusian thinking**   (Janus, the Roman god of doorways and communication, whose two faces enabled him to look in opposite directions simultaneously) Oppositional thinking; the capacity to conceive and utilize two or more opposite or contradictory ideas, concepts, or images simultaneously. A. Rothenberg (*Archives of General Psychiatry 24,* 1971) suggests that Janusian thinking is one of the thought processes employed in creative thinking.

**Japanese B encephalitis**   A virus infection of the brain that occurs most often in summer epidemics. The brain stem, basal ganglia, and white matter of the cerebral hemispheres are mainly involved. Mortality is high (50%–60%) but recovery, when it does occur, is rapid (10–14 days) and ordinarily complete. Mosquitoes are the vector for the virus.

**jargon aphasia**   Loosely, any faulty, paraphasic speech or semantic disintegration. Some workers differentiate between neologistic and semantic types. See *Wernicke aphasia.*

*Neologistic jargon* refers to copious, unintelligible speech that consists in part of neologistic words resembling language. English phonemes are used with appropriate inflection by the patient, who is markedly fluent despite a severe comprehension defect. He often fails to perceive the nonsense he creates so copiously and may even deny completely that there is any difficulty. So striking a separation of auditory comprehension from speech production and the uncontrolled conglomeration of phonemes suggests a disconnection between the two major assumed physiological processes in speech, word building and its feedback control. In this type of disturbance, phonemic or literal paraphasias distort the original word into a neologism.

*Semantic jargon* refers to verbal paraphasias consisting of substituted, but in themselves understandable, words; included in this category are circumlocutory speech and recurrent utterances of jargon syllables.

**Jarisch-Herxheimer reaction**   (Adolf Jarisch, Austrian dermatologist, 1850–1902, and Karl

Herxheimer, German dermatologist, 1861–1921) An inflammatory reaction in syphilis, involving skin, mucosae, viscera, or nervous system, often precipitated by antisyphilitic treatment and possibly due to an allergic reaction to liberated toxic products. Such reactions are much less common with penicillin than with older antispirochetal agents and rarely consist of more than transient fever during the first 24 hours of treatment. Some workers advise a course of bismuth and iodide before instituting penicillin treatment in an attempt to minimize such reactions.

**Jaspers, Karl** (1883–1969) Philosopher and psychiatrist, a member of the Heidelberg (Germany) school (others were Gruhle, Mayer-Gross, and Schneider); one of the founders of existentialism; *General Psychopathology* (1913); *The Great Philosophers* (1957).

**jaw-jerk** A deep reflex. The patient opens his mouth so that the lower jaw hangs a little; the examiner places his finger on the side of the lower jaw, and strikes it with a percussion hammer; this results in contraction of the masseter muscle and raising of the jaw.

**jealousy** According to Freud, normal jealousy is compounded of (1) grief, which is the pain caused by the thought of losing the loved object; this being associated with (2) narcissistic injury, i.e., a loss of self-esteem; (3) feelings of enmity against the successful rival; and, finally (4), self-criticism in which the person blames himself for his loss. This reaction is not completely rational, for it is disproportionate to the real circumstances, not completely under the control of the conscious ego, and not derived from the actual situation. Rather it is rooted in the Oedipus complex. Frequently jealousy is experienced also bisexually: for example, a man will feel both "the suffering in regard to the loved woman and the hatred against the male rival," and "grief in regard to the unconsciously loved man and hatred of the woman as a rival" (Freud, S. *Collected Papers*, 1924–25). See *envy, primary; oral sadism.*

**jealousy, morbid** *Pathological jealousy; Othello syndrome; amorous paranoia; conjugal paranoia*; the delusion that the marital or sexual partner is unfaithful, typically accompanied by intense searching for evidence of infidelity and repeated interrogations and direct accusations of the partner that may lead to violent quarrels. Pathological jealousy appears to

be fanned by alcohol intoxication, and both show a high degree of association with violence, including homicide. Morbid jealousy most often is isolated or encapsulated, and phenomenologically it has much in common with the *monosymptomatic hypochondriacal psychosis* (q.v.). Although their number is small, some reports suggest that tricyclic antidepressant drugs or pimozide (but not other neuroleptics, such as haloperidol) may be effective in diminishing or eliminating the delusion.

**jealousy, projected** The type of jealousy that is derived from the person's own actual unfaithfulness or from repressed impulses toward it. In this type of jealousy, the person who is being tempted in the direction of infidelity alleviates his guilt by projecting his own impulses onto the partner to whom he owes fidelity.

**Jelliffe, Smith Ely** (1866–1945) American psychoanalyst; founded *Nervous and Mental Disease Monograph Series* and, with William Alanson White, *Psychoanalytic Review* and *Diseases of the Nervous System*.

**Jellinek formula** (E. M. Jellinek, U.S. physician, 1890–1963) A means of estimating the number of alcoholics in a population, based on the assumption that the relationship between alcoholism and cirrhosis remains fairly constant.

$A = (P . D/K)R$, where $A$ is the number of alcoholics, $P$ is the proportion of cirrhosis deaths due to alcoholism, $D$ the number of reported deaths from cirrhosis in a given year, $K$ the percentage of alcoholics with complications dying of cirrhosis in a given year, and $R$ the proportion of all alcoholics to alcoholics with complications. $P$, $K$, and $R$ were assumed to be constants.

Jellinek himself proposed (1959) that the formula be abandoned, and it is not generally used nowadays.

**Jellinek typology** Jellinek's differentiation of different forms of alcoholism, labeled alpha, beta, gamma, delta, and epsilon (*The Disease Concept of Alcoholism*, 1960). See *alcoholism*.

**Jendrassik reinforcement** (Ernest Jendrassik, Slovakian physician, 1858–1922) A weak response of the knee jerk may often be reinforced, that is, strengthened, by having the patient grasp his own hands and pull vigorously on them.

**jerk, elbow** See *triceps reflex*.

**jerk, knee** *Patellar reflex* (q.v.).

**jet lag** See *circadian rhythm sleep disorder; clock, biological.*

**jhin jhinia** A culture-specific syndrome that is said to occur in epidemic form in India, consisting of bizarre and seemingly involuntary contractions and spasms.

**jiryan** *Dhat* (q.v.).

**JND** Just noticeable difference; the difference in magnitude required to discriminate between a reference stimulus (e.g., a 1-pound weight) and a second stimulus (of different weight). Note that the JND is not an absolute number; it is easy to discriminate between a 1-pound weight and a 2-pound weight, but it is difficult to discriminate between weights of 51 and 52 pounds.

**Jocasta complex** The term proposed by Raymond de Saussure (1920) for the morbid attachment of a mother to her own son—from the marriage of Jocasta to her son Oedipus (see *Oedipus complex*). The Jocasta complex represents a type of perverted mother love and has various degrees of intensity—from the maternal instinct slightly deformed to a frank sexual attachment in which both physical and psychic satisfaction is found. See *Phaedra complex.*

**Joint Commission on Mental Illness and Health** Authorized by the U.S. Congress' Mental Health Study Act of 1955; a multidisciplinary study group that included 36 national agencies in the mental health and welfare fields; its final report, *Action for Mental Health*, was instrumental in the legislation and federal funding that made possible the development of community mental health centers for the mentally ill and mentally retarded. See *community psychiatry.*

**joint custody** See *custody.*

**Jones, Ernest** (1879–1958) British psychoanalyst; one of the original group who gathered around Freud in the early days of psychoanalysis; first to introduce psychoanalysis into the English-speaking world (England, 1906); one of the founders of American Psychoanalytic Association (1911) and British Psychoanalytic Society (1913); honorary life-president of International Psychoanalytic Association; three-volume biography of Freud.

**Joubert syndrome** An autosomal recessive disorder due to partial or complete agenesis of the cerebellar vermis. In addition to dysmetria and ataxia, autistic features have been described in affected subjects.

**judgment** A conclusion, decision, or verdict about a particular action and specifically about whether the action was morally right or wrong. See *principle; rule; theory.*

Some authorities distinguish between *critical* and *automatic* judgment, meaning by the latter the performance of action as a reflex. When a patient with good vision walks directly into a wall, instead of stopping or turning, it is said that his automatic judgment is impaired.

Of the many definitions of judgment, the one most commonly used in psychiatry has to do with the ability to recognize the true relations of ideas. This involves what is called critical judgment. "But if we speak in psychiatry and jurisprudence of the capacity to judge, we mean the ability to form judgments, that is, the capacity to draw correct conclusions from the material acquired by experience" (Bleuler, E. *Textbook of Psychiatry*, 1930).

**jumpers** See *lata.*

**junctim** "Purposive connection of two thoughts and affect-complexes that have in reality little or nothing to do with one another, in order to strengthen the affect. For example, a patient with *agoraphobia* [q.v.], in order, by a complicated mechanism, to raise his prestige at home and force his environment into his service and to prevent himself likewise from losing, while on the street or in open places, the "resonance" so fervently desired, unites unconsciously and emotionally into a 'junctim,' the thought of being alone, of strange people, of purchases, search for the theatre, society, etc., and the phantasy of an apoplectic stroke, a confinement on the street, disease infection through germs on the street" (Adler, A. *The Practice and Theory of Individual Psychology*, 1924).

**Jung, Carl Gustav** (1875–1961) Swiss psychiatrist; originally associated with Freud, later founded own school of *analytic psychology* (q.v.).

**Jung association test** See *association.*

**Jungian psychology** The theory of human personality development and behavior proposed by Jung, who regarded the mind not only as a result of past experiences but also as a preparation for the future, with aims and goals that it tries to realize within itself. Merging of the personal unconscious with the racial or collective unconscious provides the background for all thought and emotion. Jung described archetypes within the collective unconscious, psychologic typology with attitude and function types, and the compensatory function of dreams and symbolism. See *analytic psychology*.

**junk DNA**  *Noncoding DNA* (q.v.). The large portion (about 95%) of the genome that does not encode proteins or regulatory information, as contrasted with the genes which constitute about 5% of the three billion nucleotide bases. See *DNA; genome*.

**juramentado**  A culture-specific syndrome described in the Malays and Moros consisting of marked agitation and assault or stabbing of anyone they encounter, followed by stupor and, upon awakening, amnesia for the episode.

**jurisprudence, therapeutic**  Use of the law, or the study of its role, as a therapeutic or antitherapeutic agent. Its focus is on such questions as how workers' compensation laws might prolong work-related disorders, whether fault-based or no-fault tort compensation is more likely to enhance recovery from personal injury, how the criminal justice system might traumatize victims of sexual abuse, how current contract laws might reinforce the low self-esteem of disadvantaged contracting parties, how therapists can lower their risk of liability suits under existing laws, and how current laws might be modified (or what new laws might be enacted) to achieve therapeutic rather than antitherapeutic effects.

**justification**  In genetics, a genetic-nutritional mechanism consisting of the ability of the fetus to alter its amino acid environment to a pattern requisite for its protein-synthesizing apparatus. The fetus that is homozygous for an amino acid disorder is almost always injured because it cannot justify the maternal mixture. If the condition occurs in nutritionally deprived areas, the heterozygous fetus in the heterozygous mother is also at high risk since he cannot adequately justify the deficient mixture that the mother also

fails to justify because of nutritional deprivation.

**jus primae noctis**  The "right to the first night" or "right of the lord" (droit du seigneur) is described as "a lascivious tribute levied by feudal lords upon their vassals, in accordance with which the lord enjoyed the first embrace of the vassal's bride." (Paolo Mantegazza, *Gli amori degli uomini*, 1883?). It was also called virginal tribute. Among certain primitive tribes the "right to the first night" belonged to the father of the bride and was supposedly symbolic of his authority.

**juvenile**  The juvenile period extends from the beginning of the phase of puberty to the end of the stage of adolescence. See *ontogeny, psychic*.

**juvenile general paresis**  See *neurosyphilis, congenital*.

**juvenile HD**  See *Huntington disease*.

**juvenile myoclonic eilepsy**  A common generalized epilepsy syndrome presenting between the ages of 8 and 26 years with early morning myoclonus, mainly affecting the upper extremities, and often associated with generalized tonic-clonic seizures and less frequently with absence seizures.

**juvenile psychosis**  A psychosis occurring between the ages of 15 and 25, approximately; sometimes used, incorrectly, as synonymous with schizophrenia. All psychoses occur in this age group, and because schizophrenia is the most common of the psychoses, it is also the most common in this age group. But there is no characteristic juvenile psychosis or psychosis typical for the age of puberty.

**juvenile tabes**  See *tabes, juvenile*.

**juvenilism**  Persistently youthful appearance of the body in a mature individual exhibiting all the signs of having passed the puberal crisis.

**juvenilism, paraphilic**  A *paraphilia* (q.v.) in which sexual arousal is dependent upon acting as or impersonating a child or youth, and upon being treated as such by the partner.

# K

K⁺ channel    See *ion channel; action potential; resting membrane potential.*

**Kahlbaum, Karl Ludwig** (1828–1899) German psychiatrist; catatonia.

**Kahlbaum syndrome** Nonmalignant *catatonia* (q.v.).

**Kahlbaum-Wernicke syndrome** *Presbyophrenia* (q.v.).

**kaiA gene** See *clock, biological.*

**kaif, kif** Pleasure or feeling of contentment and ease, as in a dream or state of ecstasy. The term is used in Morocco to refer to hashish or *marijuana* (q.v.).

**kainate** An activator of the kainate subtype of *EAA* (q.v.). See *AMPA.*

**kainophobia, kainotophobia** Also, cainophobia; *neophobia* (q.v.); fear of change or novelty, or of the unfamiliar.

**kakergasia** See *merergasia.*

**kakidrosis** *Obs.* Perspiration with disagreeable odor.

**kakorraphiophobia** Fear of failure.

**Kalinowsky, Lothar B.** (1899–1992) German-born neuropsychiatrist; in United States after 1940; electroconvulsive and other somatic treatments.

**Kallmann, Franz J.** (1897–1965) German-born psychoanalyst and geneticist; genetics of human behavior, especially schizophrenia, manic-depressive psychosis.

**Kalmuk idiocy** *Obs.* (Kalmuk, member of a nomad Tartar tribe) *Down syndrome* (q.v.).

**Kandinsky-Clérambault complex** See *Clérambault-Kandinsky complex.*

**Kanner, Leo** (1894–1981) Austrian-born psychiatrist; emigrated to United States in 1924; founded Johns Hopkins Children's Psychiatric Clinic (1930); wrote first text in *Child Psychiatry* (1935); early infantile autism.

**Kardiner, Abraham** (1891–1981) Cofounder of first psychoanalytic training school in the United States (1930); *The Individual and His Society* (1939); *Psychological Frontiers of Society* (1945).

**Karpman Drama Triangle** A conceptualization of traumatic experiences in terms of victim, rescuer, and persecutor. Originally suggested as one way of viewing intrafamilial dynamics of alcoholics and their families, it has since been extended to other disorders, such as dissociative identity disorder (DID). Within the families of alcoholics, family members often play, or are maneuvered into playing, different roles. Similarly, persons with DID may recreate the triangle in their environment; in addition, they may do it with their alters, which may be seen to fall within the categories of victim, rescuer, and persecutor.

**karyolysis** Disintegration of the cell nucleus; see *necrosis, neuronal.*

**karyotype** A complete set of chromosomes considered from a cytogenetic point of view. A schematic representation of the karyotype is an *ideogram.* See *chromosome.*

**katagogic tendency** The "downward-leading" restrictive psychic impulses that prevent a person from achieving positive or constructive goals. The reverse is an *anagogic tendency,* or constructive impulses (Stekel, W. *The Interpretation of Dreams,* 1943).

**katasexual** Necrophiliac.

**kathisophobia** Fear of sitting down.

**kattao** See *koro.*

**Kayser-Fleischer ring** (Bernhard Kayser, German ophthalmologist, 1869–1954, and Richard Fleischer, Munich physician, 1848–1909) See *hepatolenticular degeneration.*

**kedogenous** Brought about by worry or anxiety.

**Keeler polygraph** See *lie detector.*

**Kempf, Edward J.** (1885–1971) Psychosomatic medicine; *Basic Biodynamics* and *Autonomic Functions and the Personality.*

**Kempf disease** See *homosexual panic.*

**Kennedy syndrome** Spinobulbar muscular atrophy. See *trinucleotide repeat.*

**kenophobia** Also spelled *cenophobia;* fear of barren or empty space, of voids. See *agoraphobia.*

**Kent EGY test** A series of 10 questions used for a quick estimate of intelligence.

**keraunoneurosis** H. Oppenheim's term for traumatic neuroses associated with electric shocks.

**keraunophobia** Fear of lightning. It is related to the fear of strong and superior forces, and as such it appears to stem from fear of the father and of castration.

**kernel complex**   *Oedipus complex* (q.v.).

**kernicterus, kernikterus**   See *icterus gravis neonatorum.*

**Kernig sign**   (Waldemar Kernig, Russian physician, 1840–1917) Flexing the thigh at the hip, and extending the leg at the knee, produces pain and resistance; a sign of meningitis.

**ketamine**   A cyclohexylamine anesthetic, like PCP (*phencyclidine*, q.v.) but less toxic, and in use as an anesthetic in children). It acts as an *NMDAR* antagonist (q.v.) and produces a schizophrenic-like syndrome when administered intravenously to normal subjects, characterized by an amotivational state with blunted affect, withdrawal, and psychomotor retardation; suspiciousness, disorganization, and visual or auditory illusions. Ketamine also produces cognitive deficits similar to those found in schizophrenia: impaired performance on the WISC and on tests of verbal declarative memory, delayed word recall, and verbal fluency tests, without evidence of global impairment on MMSE. See *hallucinogen*

The abuse potential of ketamine was noted in 1971, but it was in the early 1980s that ketamine emerged as an important ingredient in the birth of the "dance and rave" culture in the United Kingdom and the United States. Ketamine users, both sniffers and injectors, try to achieve *k-hole*, an intense psychological and somatic state that is more reliably achieved by intramuscular or intravenous administration.

**Kety, Seymour S.**   (1916–2000) Psychiatrist and neuroscientist; first scientific director of the National Institute of Mental Health. He devised the first quantitative technique for measuring cerebral blood flow; genetic and biologic underpinnings of schizophrenic disorders.

**key concept**   Arnold Gesell and his coworkers at the Yale Clinic of Child Development formulated the idea that in all psychological studies of the preschool child the interpretation of individual differences should be governed by one key concept: that a child's abilities are all relative to one inclusive ability, the ability to grow. "Growth, therefore, becomes a key-concept for the interpretation of individual differences. There are laws of sequence and of maturation, which account for the

general similarities and basic trends of child development. But no two children grow up in exactly the same way" (Gesell, A. et al. *The First Five Years of Life*, 1940).

The tempo and style of growth are different in every child and are characteristic of the child's individuality. Gesell held that "mental growth is a patterning process: a progressive morphogenesis of patterns of behavior," and that "envisagement of the mind as a growing system puts us in a better position to observe and comprehend the determinants of the child's behavior."

**key question**   In the Adlerian approach, a question designed to uncover the purpose of the patient's psychiatric symptoms (e.g., What would you do if you were well?). The answer should indicate the patient's purpose in being sick and the personal things to which his symptoms are directed.

**khat**   A Middle Eastern shrub whose leaves contain cathinone, with psychostimulant actions similar to those of amphetamine. The leaves are chewed to obtain the stimulant effects.

**k-hole**   See *ketamine.*

**kibbutz**   A form of collective education and upbringing of children, in use in Israel, in which the rearing of the child by his or her parents is replaced by upbringing in communal houses under the direction of specially trained "*metapelets*," or mother substitutes.

**kif**   *Kaif* (q.v.).

**kimilue**   A culture-specific syndrome described in Native Americans of Southern California consisting of general apathy, lack of interest in life, loss of appetite, and vivid sexual dreams.

**kin selection**   A concept suggested by the British biologist William Hamilton in 1964 as a way to explain the behavior of the sterile worker castes in colonies of ants, bees, wasps, and termites who devote their time exclusively to the well-being of their mother (the queen) and their siblings. It is in our own selfish reproductive interest to see that those to whom we are related reproduce. Hamilton's contribution was to work out the mathematic details of the notion of *inclusive fitness*, defined as the individual's own personal fitness plus the individual's influence on the fitness of nondescendant relatives. See *fitness.*

It does seem to be true that close relatives tend to look after each other more than they look after strangers, and that the closer the relationship the greater the willingness to sacrifice *parental manipulation*, a kind of enforced altruism in which a parent coerces a child to give help to another for the parent's benefit; in nature, this often takes the form of cannibalism, a mother eating one of her children when there are more in a litter than she can take care of. All such forms of altruism have been termed *reciprocal altruism*—"If you'll scratch my back, I'll scratch yours."

**kinase, protein** An enzyme that adds phosphates to small molecules or other enzymes, creating active signaling molecules or turning enzymes on or off. One class of kinases, the PI 3-kinases, phosphorylate lipids to form the second messenger phosphatidylinositol-3,4,5-triphosphate (PtdIns 3,4,5) P$_3$, which acts on pathways that control cell proliferation, cell survival, and metabolic changes. The protein kinases use ATP as a donor of phosphoryl groups. See *ion channel*; *phosphorylation*; *second messenger*.

**kindling** Progressively increasing responsiveness to successive electrical stimuli. Depending on the part of the brain that is stimulated and on the nature of the stimulus, the end result may be a generalized convulsion or behavioral alteration. Kindling provides an experimental model of epilepsy in which an increased susceptibility to seizures arises after daily focal stimulation of specific brain areas (e.g., the amygdala), stimulation that does not reach the threshold to elicit a seizure by itself.

The limbic system appears to be particularly susceptible to kindling. Because behavioral change can occur as a result of kindling, the mechanism is viewed by at least some investigators as a model for learning and for psychological development, including both normal behavior and psychopathology.

**kinephantom** An illusory phenomenon: the movement of an object that actually occurs is perceived as being different from what the movement really is. An example is perceiving the wheels of an automobile as moving in a counterclockwise direction when they are, in fact, moving in a clockwise direction. See *illusion*.

**kinesalgia** Pain induced by movement, common with organic lesions. Pain of psychic origin (psychalgia) may also be experienced in the absence of organic pathology. See *somatoform disorders*.

**kinesics** The study of movement and action, particularly as a part of communication. See *linguistic-kinesic method*.

**kinesis** Generic term for motion.

**kinesitherapy** See *physical therapy*.

**kinesophobia** Fear of motion or of motion sickness.

**kinesthesia** Perception of one's own movement; *proprioception* (q.v.). The receptors for kinesthesia are located in the muscles, tendons, and joints. The cell bodies of these peripheral sensory neurons are in the spinal root ganglia. The central processes pass via the dorsal roots into the spinal cord and brain stem and, uncrossed in the posterior columns of the spinal cord, ascend to the gracilis and cuneate nuclei. Here they make synaptic connections with their second-order neurons, which cross and enter the medial lemniscus of the opposite side, and thence pass to the thalamus. Synaptic connections are made here with third-order neurons that ascend to the sensory projection center in the postcentral gyrus of the cortex (areas 3, 1, 2 of Brodmann).

**kinesthetic hallucination** False sensation of body movement, as in *phantom limb* (q.v.).

**kinesthetic sensation** The sensation derived from muscles, joints, and inner ear, giving the perception of body weight, position, location, and movement.

**kinetic** Relating to movement.

**kinetic tremor** See *tremor*.

**kinetically induced dissociation** See *dissociation*.

**King Midas treatment** See *satiation techniques*.

**king–slave phantasy** A sadomasochistic phantasy, in which the subject phantasies himself perhaps as now king, now slave, bound to service even by invisible golden chains.

**kinky hair syndrome** A neurodegenerative disease of male infants characterized by coarse and kinky hair, grand mal seizures, psychomotor retardation, failure to grow, cerebrocerebellar atrophy, and early death.

**Kinsey, Alfred Charles** (1894–1956) American biologist; director of Indiana University's Institute for Sex Research; *Sexual Behavior in the Human Male* (1948), *Sexual Behavior in the Human Female* (1953).

**kinship** *Genet.* The blood relationship among individuals belonging to the same stock by common descent. See *consanguinity*.

**KIPS** Acronym for knowledge information processing systems.

**Kirchhoff, Theodor** (1853–1922) German psychiatrist; history of psychiatry.

**Kirkbride, Thomas Story** (1809–1883) American psychiatrist; one of the 13 founders of the Association of Medical Superintendents of America (the forerunner of the American Psychiatric Association); mental hospital construction.

**klazomania** Compulsory shouting; usually a motor discharge phenomenon based on mesencephalic or other central nervous system irritation.

**Klebedenken** Adhesive, sticky, perseverative thinking. Klebedenken is one of the association disturbances seen in the schizophrenias.

**Klebenbleiben** A type of language disturbance occurring in schizophrenic patients in which the speaker remains glued to the same topic; he restates the topic in different words, elaborates it, qualifies it, explains it, but cannot leave it. See *circumstantiality*.

**Klein, Melanie** (1882–1960) British psychoanalyst (British Psychoanalytic Society-Institute); child analyst. She was born in Vienna, went to Berlin in 1921 where she entered psychoanalysis with Abraham, and to England in 1927. Her writings include "Notes on Some Schizoid Mechanisms" (*International Journal of Psychoanalysis 27*, 1946); *Envy and Gratitude and Other Works, 1946–1963*, (New York; Free Press, 1975). She was a controversial figure whose theories of early psychic development (e.g.,, the ubiquity of "internal objects," the "depressive" and "paranoid positions," and her direct clinical application of the death instinct) were at variance with orthodox psychoanalytic theory. See *object relations theory*.

**Kleine-Levin syndrome** Also, *hypersomniabulimia syndrome; periodic somnolence syndrome; schlafsucht*; characteristics are recurrent (typically, annually), self-limited episodes (usually of less than a month's duration) of hypersomnolence, bulimia, euphoric or unstable mood, hypersexuality, visual or auditory hallucinations, confusion, occasionally delusions, and thought disorder. The syndrome is rare and occurs almost exclusively in adolescent males. Etiology is unknown, but the symptoms suggest involvement of the hypothalamus. See *eating disorders; pickwickian syndrome*.

**kleptolagnia** A morbid desire to steal; *kleptomania* (q.v.). A psychiatric term devised by J. C. Kiernan to designate "theft associated with sexual excitement"—on the analogy of "algolagnia." In 1896 La Cassague (and others later) had stressed that sex and kleptomania were often associated, but the prevailing view that "cleptomania was a syndrome of irresistible and motiveless impulses to theft based on constitutional 'degeneration' persisted. In 1908, Stekel observed that irresistible and apparently motiveless thefts were substitutive forms of sexual gratification [consequent to sexual deprivation or repression]. Ellis's concept of kleptolagnia represented the theft as a means of generating fear and anxiety to 'reinforce' the 'feeble sexual impulse' in its drive for gratification.... [Ellis did] not appreciate that the states of anxiety which to him appeared to 'overflow into the sexual sphere' are in actuality, as in the theft itself, a form of defense of the ego against sexual impulses which threaten to overwhelm it" (Freedman, B. *Psychoanalytic Quarterly 11*, 1942).

**kleptomania** Morbid impulse to steal; pathological stealing; "senseless" or "nonsensical" stealing in that the objects are not taken for immediate use or for their monetary value and are often returned surreptitiously, given to others, or hidden away. Kleptomania is one of the *impulse control disorders* (q.v.).

Characteristically, the stealing follows a failure to resist the impulse and produces a sense of relief along with a feeling of guilt for having committed the action. Kleptomania is often expressed as shoplifting, but it should be noted that most instances of shoplifting are thefts for profit. The disorder is more common in women than in men; it is often detected for the first time when the woman is in her thirties, although her history will show that her acts of theft began in her early twenties. It is sometimes associated with depression, and a stealing episode is often precipitated by stress. It tends to be chronic in nature and there are few reports of successful treatment.

Various hypotheses have been adduced to explain kleptomania; e.g., interpreting the act as an attempt to restore self-esteem, or to restore the lost mother-child relationship; as a substitute for a sexual act; as an aggressive act; as a defense against fears of being damaged or castrated; as a way of seeking punishment; as a means of self-destruction.

**kleptophilia** *Kleptolagnia;* paraphilic kleptomania; a *paraphilia* (q.v.) in which sexual arousal is dependent upon illegal entry into and theft from the residence of a stranger or potential sexual partner. Like other paraphilias, kleptophilia is largely a disorder of males, whereas *kleptomania* (q.v.) is largely a disorder of females.

**kleptophobia** Fear of stealing or becoming a thief.

**Klinefelter syndrome** A disease caused by gross chromosome abnormality, consisting of 47 chromosomes (instead of the normal 46, there is an extra sex chromosome, giving an XXY pattern instead of the usual XX or XY). Affected subjects appear phenotypically to be males (indicating that the Y chromosome, far from being inert, is strongly determinant of maleness), but they show dysgenesis of the seminiferous tubules, gynecomastia, and eunuchoidism. The sex chromatin test is positive, as in the normal female. Known also as *primary microorchidism.*

**Klippel-Feil syndrome** (Maurice Klippel, French neurologist, 1858–1942; André Feil, French physician) A congenital anomaly characterized by absence and fusion of portions of the cervical spine, producing a shortness and stiffness of the neck. Compression of the cord may occur with motor and sensory changes. Mirror writing may occur in association with the syndrome.

**klismaphilia** A *paraphilia* (q.v.) involving the use of enemas for sexual arousal; popularly referred to as "water sports." See *anal eroticism.*

**klon** See *clone.*

**klotho** (after the Greek goddess who spins the thread of life) A recently identified gene (1997) which encodes a protein similar to β-*glucosidase,* an enzyme that can break apart fat soluble molecules such as glycolipids. An active portion of the enzyme, when circulating in the blood, may break down glycolipids to generate ceramide, a compound known to help regulate programmed cell death. Defects in klotho cause mice to die prematurely with a skein of disorders commonly found in elderly humans, such as arteriosclerosis, osteoporosis, skin atrophy, and emphysema. The klotho gene may be the signal that keeps a genetic program turned on while an organism is young, suppressing all such age-related conditions..

**Klumpke-Déjérine syndrome** (Auguste Klumpke-Déjérine, French neurologist, 1859–1927) A combination of paralysis of the cervical sympathetic nerve with paralysis and atrophy of the small muscles of the hand.

**Klüver, Heinrich** (1898–1979) Pioneer in brain research at the University of Chicago.

**Klüver-Bucy syndrome** Described originally by Klüver and Bucy, in monkeys that had been subjected to bilateral removal of the temporal lobes, the syndrome in the human includes (1) loss of recognition of people; (2) loss of fear and rage reactions; (3) increased sexual activity (especially masturbation and homosexuality); (4) bulimia; (5) hypermetamorphosis; and (6) memory defect.

**knee jerk** *Patellar reflex;* the leg is flexed at the knee joint and the quadriceps tendon is tapped just below the patella; this results in extension of the leg with visible and palpable contraction of the quadriceps muscle. The femoral nerve contains both the afferent and the efferent pathways of the patellar reflex, whose spinal center is at $L_{2-4}$.

**Knight's move** See *thought derailment.*

**knock-in** Insertion of a mutant gene at the exact site in the genome where the corresponding wild-type gene is located. This approach is used to ensure that the effect of the mutant gene is not affected by the activity of the endogenous locus.

**knockout mouse** A genetically engineered mouse that is bred to have both copies of a disease-producing gene inactivated, usually by replacing the wild (natural) type with a nonfunctional copy. The transgenic mouse is studied to assess how the gene produces its effect. In similar fashion, a knock-in mouse is bred with addition of a gene carrying a mutation that is known to predispose to a particular disease.

**Knox cube test** A performance test, of particular value when the subject suffers from a language handicap or barrier, in which the subject taps a series of four cubes in various prescribed sequences.

**knowledge** See *parallel distributed processing.*

**knowledge processing** See *KIPS.*

**knowledge test** See *criminal responsibility.*

**Köhler, Wolfgang** (1887–1967) U.S. psychologist, born in Estonia; author of the classic work *Gestalt Psychology* (1929).

**Kohnstamm maneuver** Often used to demonstrate suggestibility to a subject being prepared for hypnotic trance induction. It is a normal neurophysiologic reaction, elicited by having the subject press his extended arm as strenuously as possible against a wall for approximately 2 minutes, after which the arm will rise automatically with or without a suggestion to that effect.

**Kohs block-design test** An intelligence test in which the subject copies a design using small, multicolored cubes.

**Kohut, Heinz** (1913–1981) Viennese psychoanalyst; to United States in 1940; narcissistic character disorder; self psychology; *Analysis of the Self* (1971); *Restoration of the Self* (1977); *Search for the Self* (1978).

**koinotropy** The state of being identified with the common interests of others or the public (Meyer).

**kolyphrenia** Cortical inhibitability.

**kolytic** Inhibitory. J. R. Hunt used this term in a way that is approximately equivalent to *schizoid* (q.v.).

**kopophobia** Fear of fatigue.

**koro** *Genital retraction syndrome*; one of the *culture-bound* syndromes (q.v.), consisting of a fear or delusion of genital retraction into the abdomen, and usually also the conviction that once the genitals have retracted death will ensue. Koro (a Malaysian word meaning to shrink, or referring to a tortoise, a popular term for penis) is more frequent in Asia and the Middle East, where it sometimes occurs in epidemics (in the Malay Archipelago, Thailand, China, India, Singapore, Israel), but sporadic cases have also been reported in Africa, Europe, and North America.

Koro occurs predominantly in young, single males. Probably not more than 5% of cases have been reported in women, and all of those have occurred during epidemics of koro. In women, the fear/delusion is of labial or nipple retraction. The syndrome is typically ushered in with feelings of depersonalization, quickly followed by the fear or delusion that the penis will retract. Elaborate measures are taken to prevent such an end result, such as tying a red string around the penis or clamping a wooden box around it.

Koro is not specific to any psychiatric disorder; it may be associated with phobic neurosis, depersonalization syndrome, depression, or schizophrenia, and it is possible that it is no more than a variant of castration anxiety in a susceptible person.

Other terms for koro include *suoyang* (meaning shrunken penis in Chinese) and *kattao* (Indian for cut off) (Westermeyer, J. *Journal of Clinical Psychiatry 50*, 1989).

**Korsakoff psychosis** (Sergei Sergeevich Korsakoff, Russian neurologist, 1854–1900) Also spelled Korsakov; a chronic brain disorder that may arise as a toxic complication of any chronic brain disease, but probably associated more often with brain damage due to alcoholism than with any other single entity. (See *alcoholic Korsakoff psychosis*.) In approximately half of those affected there is an associated polyneuritis, but the characteristic mental symptom is *confabulation* (q.v.). The patient develops a marked memory retention defect and is unable to integrate new material into his memory; he fills the memory gaps with his confabulations. Often, in addition, grandiose delusions and emotional incontinence appear, and although the former may subside some degree of emotional lability generally persists. See *amnestic syndrome; Wernicke-Korsakoff syndrome*.

**Krabbe disease** (Korud H. Krabbe, Copenhagen neurologist) See *leukodystrophies*.

**Kraepelin, Emil** (1856–1926) German psychiatrist; psychiatric nosology and systematization; attempted to sort out definite disease entities and differentiated between manic-depressive psychosis and dementia praecox (schizophrenia), and between endogenous and exogenous psychoses; prognostic approach, by correlating basic symptoms with course of illness.

**Kraepelin disease** *Creutzfeldt-Jakob disease* (q.v.).

**Krafft-Ebing, Richard von** (1840–1903) German sexologist.

**Krause endings** See *mechanoreceptor*.

**Kretschmer, Ernst** (1888–1964) German psychiatrist; somatotyping and relationship of physique to character, personality, and mental illness.

**KS** Kaposi sarcoma; a malignant tumor common in patients with *AIDS* (q.v.).

**KSS** Kearns-Sayre syndrome, a severe form of CEOP with chronic external ophthalmoplegia, ptosis, myopathy, retinitis pigmentosa, hearing loss, cardiac conduction defects, ataxia, and dementia. See *mtDNA*.

**Kuf disease** See *Tay-Sachs disease*.

**kuru** The first chronic degenerative neurologic disease of humans shown to be due to unconventional slow virus infection, perhaps transmitted via ritual cannibalism, and limited to a number of adjacent valleys in the mountainous interior of New Guinea. It was first described in 1957 by D. Carleton Gajdusek and V. Zigas and has been disappearing gradually since then as ritual cannibalism has been abandoned. In the Fore language, kuru means shivering or trembling. The disease is characterized by cerebellar ataxia and a shivering tremor that progresses to complete motor incapacity and death in less than 1 year from time of onset. See *virus infections*.

**kyofusho** Fear, dread, or avoidance of; see *taijin-kyofusho*.

# L

**LAAM** L-α-acetylmethadol, a longer acting congener of methadone (72 hours as compared with 24 hours). See *methadone; narcotic blockade.*

**labeled line code** See *code, labeled line.*

**labeled lines** Anatomically and physiologically distinct neurons that are specifically associated with particular sensations. See *code, labeled line.*

**labeling theory** The sociologic hypothesis that deviance is determined by the reactions of others, in that defining a person as deviant automatically consigns him to a path of mental illness or criminality. Deviance thus is in the eye of the beholder, whose labeling of another as abnormal or delinquent constitutes a self-fulfilling prophecy. Also known as *societal reaction theory.*

**labetolol** A *beta blocker* (q.v.).

**labile** Characterized by free and usually uncontrolled expression of the emotions. See *lability.*

**lability** Volatility; instability. Emotional lability refers to emotions that are inordinately mobile and hence not under adequate control; seen most commonly in the organic brain syndromes and in the early stages of the schizophrenias.

**labyrinthine** A type of schizophrenic speech that wanders aimlessly, from one topic to another, without obvious connection between the various topics. Certain topics may be elaborated tangentially, and others appear to be an outgrowth of circumstantiality; the overall effect on the listener is to produce a massive, vague, hazy maze of words, made all the more remarkable by the fact that typically the patient is able to return to the initial topic of conversation and appears to think that his incomprehensible ramifications have been appropriately related to that topic.

**Lacan, Jacques** (1901–1981) French psychoanalyst; a controversial interpreter of Freud who claimed to have purged psychoanalysis of post-Freudian distortions. He posed difficult questions concerning the preservation of dogma without limiting the independence of the psychoanalyst, the basis of training and certification, and the role of psychoanalysis in politics and its use as an instrument of dissent. In *Ecrits* (1968), his best-known work, he maintained that the unconscious is structured like a language, which consists of a chain of Signifiers connected by the rules of metonymy and metaphor. The earliest Signifiers of desire are disguised more and more as the developing person must fit in with the cultural order and express only those desires that are legitimized by the culture.

In Lacan's view, desire, not libido, is the driving force, and in earliest development there is no difference between male and female. At birth the infant exists in a dual symbiosis with the mother (primary narcissism); next comes the preverbal mirror stage in which a narcissistic image of the self (*false ego*) is formed, and then the symbolic stage when the child begins to acquire language and recognizes the split between the false self and the outer world. What the child desires is to be fused again with the mother, signified by the desire to be the mother's phallus—not necessarily a penis, but what the mother wants most. Ultimately, the developing person wants to be recognized and desired by the desired.

As the child passes through those developmental stages (*perceptual orders*, in Lacan's terminology), the father transmits the rules and limits of the social order (a process termed *oedipization*). He tells the child he cannot fuse with mother and reminds the mother that she cannot reincorporate her child. Instead, the child must hide those early insatiable desires behind a series of increasingly distorted Signifiers that so transform language as to prevent understanding of one's own speech and one's true self.

Psychoanalysis is like a game of bridge, with the analyst the listening *dummy.* The other players are the patient speaking consciously, the analyst speaking consciously, and the Other (the patient's unconscious and earliest desires, disguised in slips, dreams, jokes, and metaphors). Only by remaining the silent dummy can the analyst stimulate the patient to regress far enough to begin to express the early Signifiers of desire.

**laceration, cerebral**   A cerebral contusion of sufficient severity to cause a visible breach in the continuity of the brain substance. This may occur either directly below the site of the blow to the head, or by contrecoup on the opposite side of the brain. See *contusion, brain.*

**Lachschlag**   Pathological weakness of muscles during laughing, often observed in *narcolepsy* (q.v.); by some, used interchangeably with Lachschlaganfall.

**Lachschlaganfall**   A condition described by Herman Oppenheim (German neurologist, 1858–1919) in which the patient falls unconscious due to violent laughing. See *gelastic epilepsy.*

**lactate challenge**   A technique used to provoke panic attacks in susceptible subjects, consisting of infusion of 0.5 M sodium DL-lactate over a 20-minute period. Approximately two-thirds of patients with *panic disorder* or *agoraphobia* (qq.v.) develop a panic attack when injected with lactate; imipramine blocks the lactate panic in 65% to 75% of those who would otherwise develop it.

**lactogenic hormone**   See *prolactin.*

**lacuna**   Small focal infarct due to occlusion of a branch artery in the brain. An accumulation of such lesions can cause progressive mental deterioration, the *lacunar state*, by many equated with *multi-infarct dementia* (q.v.). When the infarcts are limited to the subcortical white matter the condition is termed *Binswanger disease.*

**lacunae**   The infarcts measure less than 1 cm in diameter, usually located in deep gray nuclei of the cerebral hemispheres or in the brain stem. They are commonly due to enlargement of perivascular spaces and are not true infarcts.

**lacunae, superego**   Defects in the superego of delinquents and psychopathic personalities that are believed to originate from similar defects in the parents. Viewed in this way, some antisocial behavior would appear to be an acting out of unconscious wishes and impulses of the parents (Johnson, A. M. & Szurek, S. A. *Psychoanalytic Quarterly 21,* 1952).

**Lafora-body disease**   (Gonzalo Rodriguez Lafora, Spanish neurologist, 1887–1971) A form of myoclonus epilepsy with dementia and ataxia; onset is typically between 11 and 18 years of age. The *Lafora body* is a dense, round, intracytoplasmic mass that is found in basal ganglia and dentate nucleus of affected subjects. See *myoclonus epilepsy.*

**-lagnia**   Combining form meaning act of coition, salaciousness, lust, from Gr. *lagneis.*

**lagnosis**   See *satyriasis.*

**lagophobia**   (from Gr. *Lagos,* meaning hare) Abnormal fear of rabbits; less commonly the term refers to fear of any rodent, although the rabbit's incisors differ in size and placement from those of rats.

**lagophthalmos, lagophthalmus**   A condition in which the upper lid fails to move down when the patient attempts to close the eye. It is one of the signs of involvement of the seventh, or facial nerve.

**Laing, Ronald David**   (1927–1989) Glasgow-born psychiatrist, trained as a psychoanalyst at the Tavistock Institute in London; in the 1960s he became critical of traditional approaches, especially in the treatment of schizophrenia, and turned to *radical therapy* (q.v.), which views therapy as a social and political activity. In London he established a therapeutic community, Kingsley Hall, where patients, physicians, and staff worked together without hierarchy or distinctions of rank or role. His books include *The Divided Self* (1960); *The Self and Others* (1969); *Sanity, Madness and the Family* (1964); *Reason and Violence* (1964); *Interpersonal Perception: A Theory and a Method of Research* (1966); *The Politics of Experience* (1967); *Knots* (1970); and *The Making of a Psychiatrist* (1985).

**Laingian view**   See *Equus-Laingian view.*

**Lake v. Cameron**   See *consumerism.*

**-lalia, lalo**   Combining form meaning talk(ing), talkative, chat, loquacity, from Gr. *lalia, lalos.*

**laliophobia**   Fear of talking (and possibly stuttering).

**lallation, lalling**   Unintelligible speech, such as infantile babbling; often used more specifically to refer to substitution of *l* for more difficult consonants such as *r.*

**lalochezia**   Emotional discharge is gained by uttering vulgar, indecent, or obscene words; *coprolalia* (q.v.).

**laloneurosis, spasmodic**   *Stuttering* (q.v.).

**lalopathy**   Any form of *speech disorder* (q.v.).

**lalophobia**   Fear of speaking.

**laloplegia**   Inability to speak because of paralysis of speech muscles other than the tongue muscles.

**lalorrhea** See *tachylogia*.

**Lambert-Eaton syndrome** See neurologic paraneoplastic syndromes.

**lambitus** See *cunnilingus*.

**laminin** An extracellular matrix glycoprotein that is a major component of the basal lamina; it interacts with integrins. See *adhesion, cellular; neurotrophic factors*.

**laminopathies** See *progeria*.

**Landau reflex** A reaction normally present from the age of 3 months to about 1 year of age, consisting of raising the head and arching the back with the concavity upward when the infant is supported horizontally in the prone position. Absence of the reflex is seen with motor weakness, such as occurs in cerebral palsy, motor neuron disease, and mental retardation.

**Landmark Manual** A multidiagnostic schedule for the assessment of schizophrenia, developed by Johan Landmark to reassess diagnoses of chronic schizophrenic patients attending a clinic. The data it collects were developed on the basis of 13 concepts of schizophrenia and related nonaffect disorders. The schedule uses a single data sheet from which a large number of diagnoses can be extracted.

**Landry paralysis** (Jean Baptiste Octave Landry, French physician, 1826–1865) Acute ascending paralysis; a disorder of unknown etiology consisting of flaccid paralysis beginning in the lower limbs and spreading upward to the bulbar and respiratory muscles. Males account for 80% of cases, and most cases occur during the third decade of life. Between 50% and 80% die by the fifteenth day; in the remainder, recovery is usually complete within 3 months.

**landscape phobia** Fear of a particular locale or type of geography, or a wish to avoid such a setting because of the dysphoria it would engender. Whether it be a seascape, a mountain setting, a desert, an open plain, or a closed space, the object or situation feared is a symbol of unconscious conflict, whose meaning can be discovered only from the phobic subject himself. See *agoraphobia; anxiety hysteria*.

**Lange, Carl Georg** (1834–1900) Danish pathologist. See *James-Lange-Sutherland theory*.

**Lange colloidal gold reaction** (Carl Lange, German physician, 1883–1953). A diagnostic test no longer in common use. It depends on the fact that cerebrospinal fluid in certain diseases

is able to precipitate in a preparation of colloidal gold.

**language** *Speech* (q.v.); the communication of information through speech (using sounds) or other symbols (as in *sign language*, q.v.). According to Baltaxe and Simmons, language is a conventional system of arbitrary symbols used as a code for representing and communicating messages. It involves two major functions: reception (i.e., understanding, comprehension, or receptive language) and expression (i.e., communicating, expressing, or expressive language). Language is based on several complex cognitive processes, among them the integration of *phonology, semantics,* and *grammar; articulation; prosody; pragmatics;* and orthographics (the visual representation of words) (qq.v.).

Language disorders subsume all disorders of speaking, listening, reading, and writing. Because language is one of the defining features of human behavior, the term does not apply to animals; "animal communication" is the preferred term. See *phonology; pragmatics; psycholinguistics*.

Language provides a means to mediate between the self as interpreting subject and one's lived experience. It is the brain's means of translating in a principled way between thoughts on the one hand and auditory and motor patterns on the other. The process of going from thought to motor instuctions is *speech production*; that from auditory pattern to thought is *speech perception*. In language, auditory patterns are converted into phonological structure, which is expressed through voluntary motor patterns in the vocal tract that depend upon different anatomical structures in the brain—in particular, the prefrontal cortex, the cerebellum, and the basal ganglia.

The data currently available point to a human functional language system in which the neural mechanisms that regulate speech production play a central role. The neural system consists of circuits that link neurons in different neuroanatomical entities, including not only the traditional sites of language (the Broca and Wernicke areas) but also many other parts of the brain. See *preadaptation*. The general neural substrate that allows one to acquire any particular behavioral trait is genetically transmitted. People have a neural system that permits them to speak and comprehend language. But these neural systems offer the *potential* for behaviors. The neural circuits that regulate complex aspects of behavior are shaped by exposure to a person's environment within a sensitive period. Although the basic architecture of the functional language system clearly is part of the human's genetic endowment, the details of syntax, speech, and the words of the languages that a person knows appear to be learned by means of the associative processes that enable that person to learn other complex aspects of behavior. See *grammar; linguistic-kinesic method.*

The left hemisphere is the seat of language specialization, whether the language is expressed by ear and mouth or by eye and hand, as in sign language. The left hemisphere contains the abstract rules, dictionary, and grammar of the language. The ability of the right hemisphere to take on language functions is highly variable and incomplete. In some cases of callosal injury there is almost no verbal responsiveness; in others, language can be understood but not produced; a few can speak or write a few words. None of the cases demonstrated any capacity for understanding grammatical structure.

**language, abstract** A receptive/expressive linguistic function involving the abilities to discern implied information or information requiring inferences and logical conclusions; to observe unspoken cause and effect relationships; to use and understand proverbs, metaphors, idioms, and complex analogies; to resolve linguistic ambiguities; to form associations between words; and to discriminate between fact and fiction and fact and opinion.

**language, artificial** Neologistic language.

**language, irrelevant** Words, phrases, utterances that have meaning only for the speaker and for no other person. According to Kanner, instances of irrelevant language occur in "the language of schizophrenia and early infantile autism." He points out that irrelevant utterances, "though peculiar and out of place in ordinary conversation, were far from meaningless. Some words or phrases were metaphoric substitutions." Kanner cites the following example where an irrelevant utterance of an autistic child was traced to an earlier source: "Jay S., not quite four years old, referred to himself as 'Blum,' whenever his

veracity was questioned by his parents. This was explained when Jay, who could read fluently, once pointed to an advertisement of a furniture firm which said in large letters: 'Blum tells the truth.' Since Jay had told the truth, he was Blum." (*Child Psychiatry*, 1948).

**language, primitive psychosomatic** Expression of feelings or thoughts by means of bodily movements rather than by words.

**language acquisition** Gaining knowledge of a *language* (q.v.). In general, all languages are acquired with equal ease before the age of four, and every normal person learns to speak fluently. This is in marked contrast to acquisition of reading and writing, which requires extensive instruction and practice (Jackendoff, R. *Patterns in the Mind—Language and Human Nature*, 1994).

Infants approach language with a set of inborn perceptual abilities that are necessary for language acquisition. These innate skills include the following:

1. *Categorical perception*—discrimination of the acoustic events that distinguish phonetic units. A change of 10 msec in the time domain changes /b/ to /p/, and equivalently small differences in the frequency domain change /p/ to /k/. Each language uses a unique set of only about 40 distinct elements, *phonemes*, which change the meaning of a word (for example, from /bat/ to /pat/). Infants can discriminate these subtle differences from birth.

2. *Pattern detection*—the ability to group perceptually distinct sounds into the same category.

3. *Statistical learning*—combining pattern detection and computational abilities to acquire knowledge by computing information about the distributional frequency with which certain items occur in relation to others, or probabilistic information in sequences of stimuli, such as the odds—transitional probabilities—that one unit will follow another in a given language. Six- and eight-month-old infants are sensitive to distributional patterns, and they learn the *phonotactic patterns* of language, rules governing the sequences of phonemes that can be used to compose words. See *speech processing*.

To hear speech, a mass of information from the auditory nerve must be converted into a sequence of vocal tract positions (configurations of the speaker's vocal tract are reconstructed). Then the speech must be decoded. What is heard is put in holding memory while other parts of the brain analyze it to determine whether it is novel or familiar, and if familiar which of the many memory bits it seems likely to be associated with. The limbic system, especially the amygdala and hippocampal system, is also searched, to identify the affective and connotative aspects of what is heard, and to coordinate the affective, visceral, and neurohumoral aspects of the formulated response.

To form a sentence, the speaker must select a major articulator from among the six *speech organs*: larynx, soft palate, tongue body, tongue tip, tongue root, and lips. How to move the articulator (fricative, stop, or vowel) must then be selected. Finally, the speaker must specify the configurations of other speech organs; e.g., for the soft palate, nasal or not; for the lips, rounded or unrounded. To articulate a phoneme, the commands must be executed with precise timing. And these are only the mechanics; even more complicated are the mechanisms that provide the content of speech.

There is semantic feedback between the anterior (frontal) language cortex, where language formulation occurs, and the posterior (temporoparietal) language cortex, where language is monitored for semantic accuracy and decoded. The pulvinar (posterior thalamus), which has reciprocal connections to both the temporoparietal cortex and the posterior frontal cortex, mediates semantic monitoring. When it is determined that a language segment is semantically accurate, the temporoparietal cortex releases mechanisms in the caudate head from inhibition. This increases inhibition of pallidal mechanisms which, in turn, releases the ventral anterior thalamus from inhibition, causing a temporary increase in excitatory impulses to the language formulation centers in the anterior language cortex. There the semantically accurate language segment is released for motor programming of the articulatory apparatus, which ensures that the desired phonological patterns (i.e., speech sounds) will be produced. Response release mechanisms related to phonological monitoring are controlled by the motor and premotor cortex, the putamen, the globus pallidus,

and the ventrolateral thalamus. Once motor programming is completed, a signal from the language formulation centers reestablishes inhibition of the caudate by the temporoparietal cortex.

Innate knowledge of the language *grammar* (q.v.) begins to manifest itself around the age of 2 years. Children exposed to a second language become relatively fluent within a year or so. Both these observations suggest that ease of language acquisition depends on brain maturation rather than any inherent difficulty in the language being learned. Acquisition of normal language for children up to the age of 6 is so easy as to be almost guaranteed; after that time, however, it becomes steadily more difficult until shortly after puberty and after that approaches the impossible (even though some adults can learn to speak some language other than their own with relative fluency, their second language almost always has some inflections, pronunciations, or phrasings betraying the fact that the language is not their primary one).

All infants are born with linguistic skills. They gain some awareness of the mother's language in utero, for her speech is audible in the womb. Nonetheless, until about the age of 10 months, they are universal phoneticians. United States and British infants can distinguish Czech and Hindi phonemes, but English-speaking adults cannot, despite hundreds of training trials or a year of coursework in a university. At 10 months, these same infants mirror their parents; they distinguish English phonemes, but do no better than their parents with Czech or Hindi phonemes. Further, this change occurs before the infants produce or understand words. (Pinker, S. *The Language Instinct—How the Mind Creates Language*, 1994).

The first sound that babies make is crying, and in the first 2 months they add cooing or gooing. At 6 months, they begin to babble; babbling consists of a range of meaningless sounds, which by 7 months begin to include real syllables. By playing with sounds, the infant learns that moving the muscles of speech will change the sound.

Sometime between 10 and 20 months of age (with girls veering toward the early end of the continuum), children begin to understand words and begin to speak. Even at the one-word stage (c. 17 months), they show some appreciation of syntactic structure and use it to figure out what adults are saying to them, even though they do not understand all the words. By the two-word stage (c. 24 months), vocabulary growth reaches the rate that will be maintained through adolescence, one word every 2 hours. Between 33 and 42 months, children become relatively fluent conversationalists. Sentences are longer and employ a full range of grammatical variables: statements, questions, conjunctives, relative clauses, complements, negatives, comparatives, and passives.

**language and speech disorders** Included are articulation disorder, stuttering, cluttering, expressive language disorder (impaired verbal or sign language), and receptive language disorder (impaired comprehension).

**language assessment** Domains that are routinely tested in the neuropsychiatric examination are as follows:

1. Fluency: rate, phase length; relational/functional word proficiency; generativity; letter fluency; phonemic fluency

2. Lexicon: ability to name objects and concepts on confrontation, in each case of both high- and low-frequency items

3. Comprehension: one-, two-, and three-step commands; relational commands

4. Repetition: ability to repeat a simple phrase

Comprehension depends on the Wernicke area (posterior superior temporal gyrus, Brodmann area [BA] 22), and the temporo-parietal association area. Expression depends on Broca area (inferior frontal gyrus, BA 44) and the transcortical motor area (frontal). Repetition depends on the arcuate fasciculus (in Broca area).

**language disability** Difficulty in getting information out of the brain through the use of words, as in speaking. Typically, such disabilities involve difficulty with *demand language*, i.e., the subject has no trouble initiating conversation but finds it difficult to organize thoughts well enough to find the right words when language is demanded, as in being asked a direct question.

**language disorder** See *developmental disorders, specific.*

**language learning impairment** An inclusive term used by some authorities to refer to *specific language impairment* (q.v.), recognizing that, although there are commonalities between

SLI (specific language impairment) and *dyslexia* (q.v.), there are also differences.

**language mastery timetable** The emergence of language in a child depends on linguistic input; unless exposed to speech before the age of about 8 years, a child is unable to learn a true language. Linguistic skills, however, are discernible at birth, and children are born with some knowledge of their mother's language, probably because the melody of their mothers' speech is audible in the womb. The latter half of the infant's first year is a critical point in acquiring a language. Infants younger than 6 months distinguish a wide range of speech contrasts and have some capacity to compensate for differences in voices and speaking rates. After 6 months, infants demonstrate some recognition of the particular phonetic and prosodic characteristics of their native language. At 7.5 months they are able to segment fluent speech into word-sized units.

At 8 months infants can reliably identify words from lists as either familiar or novel depending on whether they were used frequently in children's stories heard 2 weeks earlier. Children rapidly learn the principles of human language by means of associative processes. Eight-month-old infants can learn to segment the acoustic signals that specify the words of an artificial spoken language after 2 minutes.

By 10 months, infants are no longer universal phoneticians but have turned into speakers of their parents's language. This occurs before they can produce or understand words, indicating that they are sorting the sounds directly, somehow tuning their speech analysis module to deliver the phonemes used in their language.

There is a grammar explosion, a period of several months in the third year of life, during which children suddenly begin to speak in fluent sentences, respecting most of the fine points of their community's spoken language. By the time they are 4–5 years old, most children have a vocabulary of several thousand words and have mastered the basic rules of grammar and syntax.

**language retardation** Delay in the development of language skills, not due to mental retardation, hearing impairment, or structural abnormalities of the organs of speech, but assumed instead to be based on lag in cerebral maturation. Included are numerous manifestations, variously called baby talk, lalling, lisping, congenital auditory agnosia, and word deafness. Some authorities subdivide the group into *developmental dysphasia* and *developmental articulation disorder* (qq.v.).

**language universals** Elements that are the same in all languages. All languages have consonants, for example, and all distinguish between nouns and verbs. All languages appear to be of approximately equal complexity. According to the Academie Francaise, there are 2796 separate dialects spoken on Earth. All of them share the following:

1. Formation of a large number of meaningful symbols (words) from a small set of basic sounds (phonemes)

2. Formation of an unlimited number of sentences by logically combining words using a finite number of grammatical rules

3. The sentences are used for socialized actions

4. Any normal child has the ability to learn to speak the language

No known system of animal communication shares all these characteristics.

**lapse** 1. *Petit mal epilepsy* (q.v.).

2. A temporary setback during treatment, such as a short-lived alcoholic or eating binge; contrasted with the more extreme and longer-lasting *relapse* (q.v.).

**lapsus calami** A slip of the pen.

"A lady once told me that an old friend in writing to her had closed a letter with the curious sentence, 'I hope you are well and unhappy.' He had formerly entertained hopes of marrying her himself, and the slip of the pen was evidently determined by his dislike at the thought of her being happy with someone else. She had recently married." (Jones, E. *Papers on Psycho-Analysis*, 1938). See *symptomatic act*.

**lapsus linguae** Slip of the tongue. See *symptomatic act*.

**lapsus memoriae** Lapse or slip of memory. See *symptomatic act*.

**larval sadism** (L. larva, "ghost, specter, mask") Hirschfeld's term for masked or concealed sadism.

**LAS** Lymphadenopathy syndrome, seen frequently in HIV-infected patients. See *AIDS*.

**lascivia** (L. "jollity, wantonness, lewdness") *Nymphomania* (q.v.).

**Lasègue, Ernest-Charles** (1816–1883) French internist, neurologist, and psychiatrist; the first to describe exhibitionism, anorexia nervosa; also published articles on chronic alcoholism, psychosis associated with renal failure, cretinism, manic-depressive illness, forensic psychiatry, and moral treatment.

**Lasègue sign** The Lasègue sign indicates disease of the sciatic nerve. Pain and resistance are caused by extending the leg on the thigh and flexing the thigh at the hip joint.

**Lashley, Karl Spencer** (1890–1958) U.S. psychologist, bacteriologist, and geneticist; psychology of learning; *Brain Mechanisms and Intelligence* (1929), numerous monographs in psychology, neurology, and the biology of behavior; directory of Yerkes Laboratory of Primate Biology.

**lata, latah, lattah** A behavioral pattern seen among the Malays, usually precipitated by sudden fright or tickling, consisting of imitative behavior (echopraxia), automatic obedience, and coprolalia. It is seen more often in women, usually before late adolescence. Some authorities consider latah and related states, such as the *miryachit* or olonism of Siberian tribes, the inu of the Ainu, and the *Jumpers* of New England (a 19th-century Shaker sect), as acute forms of schizophrenia. Others classify latah as a hysterical reaction or a startle pattern, and among the Malays themselves it is considered as a behavioral quirk rather than a disease.

**latchkey** Used as an adjective to describe a condition or situation in which a door was closed but not locked; more specifically, the phrase "latchkey children" refers to children who come home from school each day to a house or apartment that is empty because both parents are working.

**late bloomer (lbl)** Upon contacting its postsynaptic target, a neuronal growth cone becomes a presynaptic terminal. A membrane component on the growth cone that facilitates this transformation is the *late bloomer (lbl)* gene, which in Drosophila encodes a member of the tetraspanin family of cell surface proteins. It helps to signal "All stop" once the growth cone has docked.

**late life depression** An episode of major depression (unipolar depression) occurring for the first time in late life (generally defined as after 60 or 65 years). Like depression occurring earlier in life, late life depression often impairs cognitive functioning as measured by mental tests; this is often considered to be *pseudodementia* (q.v.). Follow-up studies, however, show that long-term prognosis is unfavorable in the majority of cases, and suggest that the cognitive decline—in this age group—portends the development of cognitive disorder in the future.

Other studies suggest that depression by itself is not predictive of cognitive decline; of equal importance is the form in which the depression is manifested. Prognosis in the mood disturbance type, in which predominant symptoms are dysphoria, negative thoughts, and anger, is similar to the prognosis for major depression in younger age groups. The apathy type, with mainly negative symptoms (absence or lack of feelings, concern, interest, or motivation), characterized by more marked cognitive impairment (especially of executive functions), less favorable response to antidepressant drugs, and—on postmortem examination—frequent, severe lesions of deep white matter.

**late luteal phase dysphoric disorder** *LLPDD* (q.v.).

**late paraphrenia**   See *paraphrenia*.

**latency**   In psychoanalysis, the period of one's life extending from the end of the infantile to the beginning of the adolescent stage. In point of years it normally begins at about the age of 5 and terminates at about the age of puberty.

Freud employed the term latency at a time in the development of psychoanalytic psychology when attention was focused largely on the sexual drive and libido; later work in the area of ego psychology has made it abundantly clear that the drives are by no means inactive during this period. Instead, what has happened is that the dangers of the Oedipus relationship have necessitated a strong blockade against libidinal impulses. The ego achieves this by mobilizing aggressive energies against the id. In effect, then, libidinal energies are redirected into elaborating a more effective web of defenses including the superego, and into increasing mastery in the social sphere, in socially condoned and desirable competitiveness, conquest, and domination. Mental development, in other words, has occurred in spurts. In the infantile years, libidinal forces are more in evidence as they are deployed in

various areas in accordance with physiologic growth. With the appearance of the Oedipus, these forces must be held in check, and the aggressive forces of the ego acquire greater prominence. They are used as frontline combatants to prepare the way for the reappearance of libidinal strivings during adolescence.

**latent**   Not visible or apparent; dormant, quiescent. Latent homosexuality, for example, refers to homosexual tendencies or conflicts that have never been manifested overtly and/or are unrecognized by the subject. Latent psychosis refers to an existing disorder that has not erupted into full-blown or florid psychotic symptoms; sometimes also termed prepsychotic, borderline, or incipient, and almost always referring to an underlying schizophrenic disorder.

**latent schizophrenia**   That form of schizophrenia in which, despite the existence of fundamental symptoms, no clear-cut psychotic episode or gross break with reality has occurred. Ambulatory, borderline, incipient, pseudoneurotic, pseudopsychopathic, prepsychotic, and similar forms are included here so long as there has been no acute psychotic episode (a requirement that differentiates latent schizophrenia from the residual type).

The group named schizophrenia, residual type, includes only those patients who, having had a psychotic episode, improve to the degree that they are not considered psychotic, even though signs of the schizophrenic disorder remain.

**latent trait hypothesis**   The proposal that schizophrenia and *eye tracking dysfunction* (q.v.) are independent manifestations of a trait that is transmitted by a single autosomal dominant gene, and that the trait is significantly more likely to be expressed as ETD than as schizophrenia.

**late-onset schizophrenia**   As originally described by Bleuler, a schizophrenic psychosis first appearing after the age of 40 years, with no indications of brain disorder. Onset between 40 and 60 years includes about 15% of all schizophrenic disorders; the number with onset after 60 is negligible. Other terms that have been used for late-onset schizophrenia include *dementia tardiva, paranoid-hallucinatory psychosis in involutional age, paranoid involutional psychosis with schizophrenia* *coloring, paranoid climacteric psychosis*, and *old-age schizophrenia*. See *paraphrenia*.

**lateral nuclear group** The largest division of the *thalamus* (q.v.), consisting of the following: (a) *ventral anterior nucleus*, with projections both from and to the frontal lobe, including the premotor cortex; it also receives input from the intralaminar nuclei, golbus pallidus, and substantia nigra. (b) *ventrolateral nucleus*, the motor nucleus of the thalamus, with bidirectional connections with the motor cortex and additional input from the cerebellum, globus pallidus, and substantia nigra. (c) *ventral posterior nuclei*, medial and lateral, located behind the ventrolateral nucleus; these nuclei are primarily relay nuclei for touch and proprioception. The *ventrobasal complex* (*VB*) is the terminus of afferents of the ascending somatic sensory systems, suggesting that the thalamus is a major contributor to one's concept of body boundaries and body image. "Soft" neurological signs may be related to VB dysfunction. (d) *dorsolateral* (or *lateral*) *nucleus*; receives projections from most parts of the limbic cortex.

**lateral ventricles** See *ventricle*.

**laterality** Handedness; preferential use of one side of the body for such acts as writing, eating, sighting, and listening. See *cerebral dominance*.

**lateralization** In general, the left hemisphere dominates in linguistic function and manual control, whereas the right dominates in spatial reasoning, emotional perception, and face recognition. There is a right hemisphere bias for the production of facial emotion and a left hemisphere bias for the perception of species-typical vocal signals. See *cerebral dominance*.

**lateropulsion** Rapid running sidewise with short steps, in Parkinson disease.

**lathyrism** Chickpea poisoning, caused by β-aminopropionitrile in peas of the genus Lathyrus (mainly in India and North Africa): spastic paraplegia and sensory impairment in the lower limbs caused by degeneration of the spinal cord.

**Lauder syndrome** See *Behçet syndrome*.

**laughing gas** *Nitrous oxide* (q.v.).

**laughter, compulsive** Inappropriate laughter, as seen in the hebephrenic form of schizophrenia. "Among the affective disturbances [in schizophrenia] compulsive laughter is especially frequent; it rarely has the character of the hysterical laughing fit, but that of a soulless mimic utterance behind which no feeling is noticeable. It may often be provoked by allusion to a complex. Sometimes the patients feel only the movements of the facial muscles (the 'drawn laughter')" (Bleuler, E. *Textbook of Psychiatry*, 1930).

**Laurence-Moon-Biedl syndrome** (J. Z. Laurence, British ophthalmologist, 1830–1874; Robert C. Moon, American ophthalmologist, 1844–1914; and A. Biedl, German physician, 1868–1933) *Retinodiencephalic degeneration*; an autosomal recessive disorder consisting of six cardinal signs in the following order of frequency: obesity, retinitis pigmentosa, mental deficiency, genital dystrophy, familial occurrence, polydactyly.

**law of avalanche** Law of the distribution of energy in the nervous system as framed by Cajal. Sensory stimuli reaching the central nervous system normally gain release through a number of paths of discharge, which take the form of reflex arcs. When some of these reflex arcs are closed, so to speak, as avenues of release for nervous energy, the energy is forced to flow through the remaining arcs. It is possible, as, for instance, in epilepsy, that, when discharged, the dammed-up energy produces a condition likened by Cajal to an avalanche.

**law of effect** Actions that lead immediately to pleasure are learned and remembered, whereas actions leading to pain are not remembered or the memory of them is suppressed in order to avoid later painful behavior.

**law of initial values** The tendency of extremes of pathology, whether physiologic or psychological, to regress toward the mean over time, thus rendering the findings of response to early intervention highly suspect. Alcoholics, for example, usually do not present themselves for treatment until their symptoms are at their height; on short-term evaluation, almost all such patients will appear to improve, no matter what the treatment approach.

**law of retrogenesis** See *retrogenesis*.

**lay analyst** See *psychiatrist*.

**layer I interneurons** See *neocortical neurons*.

**layers, cortical** See *isocortex*.

**LBD** *Lewy body dementia* (q.v.).

**LBL** *Late bloomer* gene (q.v.).

**LD** *Learning disabilities* (q.v.).

**L-dopa (levodopa)**   See *Parkinson disease.*

**lead encephalopathy**   Diffuse brain disease due to *lead poisoning* (q.v.). Abnormal ingestion of lead-based paint (pica) is the most common cause of lead poisoning, and as a preventive measure many states have enacted laws limiting the use of such paints. Lead encephalopathy is much less frequent in adults, in whom ingestion of illicit whiskey is the most frequent cause.

In adults, seizures and polyneuropathy are the most frequent neurologic manifestations. In children, early symptoms are apathy, irritability, headache, vomiting, emotional lability, incoordination, memory lapses, and sleep disturbance. With continued exposure disorientation, psychosis, ataxia, lethargy, and focal neurologic signs develop, sometimes progressing to stupor, seizures, and coma.

Chelating agents (dimercaprol, calcium disodium edetate, and penicillamine), which bind lead and promote tissue excretion, have reduced mortality to 5%. Neuropsychiatric symptoms are slow to respond, especially in children. If treatment does not begin before encephalopathy develops, between 25% and 50% of survivors show permanent sequelae such as siezures or mental retardation.

**lead pipe rigidity**   Smooth but increasing muscle tone in response to passive flexion and extension; typical of Parkinson disease. Sometimes the term is used for the waxy flexibility that occurs in *catalepsy* (q.v.).

**lead poisoning**   *Plumbism*; although more common in children, it occurs also in adults, as in painters and workers with lead pipes (e.g. plumbers), and it may result from the use of some cosmetics, abortifacients, and from too close contact with lead-containing petrol. It has also been reported in frequenters of "shooting galleries" and in persons who have used metal-decorated drinking glasses. Poisoning is more frequent in summer, because the greater amount of vitamin $D_3$ formed in the skin by the sun's radiation increases absorption of lead from the gut.

Lead produces a selective degeneration of ganglion cells, especially in the spinal cord, and to a lesser extent in the cortex. Among the various syndromes of lead poisoning are (1) acute encephalopathy—with convulsions, delirium, and coma; (2) chronic *lead encephalopathy* (q.v.)—with mental changes, convulsions, and occasionally optic atrophy; (3) neu-

ritis—which is really a myopathy, affecting chiefly the extensors of the wrist and fingers and thus producing wrist-drop; (4) progressive muscular atrophy, due to anterior horn cell degeneration.

Prognosis is worsened if convulsions appear, and chronic encephalopathy responds little to treatment. As many as 35% of affected children die, and girls have a higher mortality than boys. Severe residua are common: epilepsy, cerebral atrophy, paresis, blindness, speech defects, and tremor.

Treatment includes high-calcium diet to promote storage of lead in bones, followed by a high-acid/low-calcium diet to promote gradual elimination; and BAL (British anti-Lewisite) or EDTA (ethylenediaminetetraacetic acid or versenate) to form a stable, nontoxic, excretable compound with the lead.

**lead-cap headache**   A neurasthenic symptom consisting of a sensation as if the head were splitting or the skull lifting; a terrible weight or a severe constriction about the head.

**leadership, dual**   See *psychotherapy, multiple.*

**Leão spreading depression**   (A. A. P. Leão, Brazilian physiologist, b. 1914) See *spreading depression of Leão.*

**leaping ague**   *Choreomania* (q.v.).

**Lear complex**   Morbid attachment—sometimes overtly sexual—of a father to his daughter.

**learned helplessness**   Giving up trying, because the subject is unable to discover any way in which to influence the environment either in an attempt to succeed or in a search for escape from pain. This has been posited as a model for depression.

**learning**   The process of acquiring knowledge (memory is its retention or storage). Every organism is provided at birth with potentialities suitable for its environment. Learning and memory depend upon selecting, from a multiplicity of possible actions, those that are useful responses to the environment. Normal capacities develop only if there is appropriate input at certain short critical periods. See *critical period; long-term memory; memory; parallel distributed processing.*

**learning, accretion**   See *accretion.*

**learning, dissociated**   See *state-dependent learning.*

**learning, visceral**   See *biofeedback.*

**learning disabilities**   *LD*; a nonspecific term referring to a variety of difficulties evidenced in the learning process, many of them due to developmental lags rather than the brain damage or inimical environmental influences implied in some of the terms applied to the group or the subtypes within it. They include language disorder (including developmental mathematics disorder, difficulty with attention, visuospatial deficits, and motoric clumsiness) and social-emotional learning disabilities. The latter are also known as social communicative deficits and, because neuropsychological studies implicate the right hemisphere as their neural basis, as right hemisphere learning disorders. They may include social-cognitive problems, difficulty with facial affect recognition, and lack of awareness of the wishes and motivations of others. See *attention deficit hyperactivity disorder; developmental disorders; dyslexia; learning disorders; reading disabilities.*

**learning disability, specific** As used by R. J. Schain (*California Medicine 118*, 1973) a term that has no etiologic implications and is applied to children with learning disorders who have no demonstrable illness (such as mental retardation, cerebral palsy, or seizure, auditory, ocular, or progressive neurologic disorders). Developmental hyperactivity is applied to children who are normal or even precocious in development but show high activity levels as part of their temperament.

**learning disorders** Academic skills disorder; within this group are reading disorder, mathematics disorder, and disorder of written expression.

**learning impairment** See *LLI.*

**least restrictive alternative** See *consumerism.*

**Leber disease** (Theodor Leber, German ophthalmologist, 1840–1917) *Hereditary familial primary optic atrophy*, occurring between the ages of 18 and 30, more common in the male progeny, but transmitted from the female. It is a bilateral, slowly progressive condition, often remaining stationary or even regressing. There is a central scotoma and a normal peripheral field. See *optic atrophy.*

**Leborgne** The patient studied by Paul Broca whose analysis of the case marks the origin of neuropsychology. Study of this one patient led to the discovery that the expression of language resides in the frontal cortex of the left hemisphere, and led Broca to an examination of the patient's brain at autopsy and to

a search for other patients with similar lesions and similar symptoms. He was able to amass a group of eight other patients on whom he could test the hypotheses that the Leborgne case had initiated.

**lecanomancy** "A method of divination by means of a suitable person looking into a bowl half-filled with water, on the surface of which the indefinite images of candle flames are reflected." Herbert Silberer used free association to find the meanings of the visions reported. This showed "how the divination[s] are merely the results of the medium's own complexes" and emphasized the close relation between the visions and dreams (*Psychoanalytic Review I*, 1913–1915)

**lécheur** One who applies the mouth to the genitals of others, that is, practices fellatio or cunnilingus.

**left-handedness** See *cerebral dominance.*

**legal custody** See *custody.*

**legal divorce** See *divorce, stations of.*

**legal psychiatry** Forensic psychiatry; the application of psychiatry in the courts of law. See *advocacy; consumerism; forced treatment.*

**legalization** See *decriminalization.*

**legasthenia** Dyslexia with dysorthographia, consisting of difficulty in visual and acoustic synthesis of individual letters into a total word structure or, conversely, difficulty in analyzing the word back into its component letters. The deficit exists in the presence of adequate intellectual and perceptual abilities, and it appears to be both congenital and hereditary. See *dysgraphia; dyslexia.*

**legs, restless** See *restless legs syndrome.*

**leipolalia** Elision; *ellipsis* (q.v.).

**lengthening reaction** See *decerebrate rigidity.*

**Lennox, William Gordon** (1884–1960) U.S. neurologist; epilepsy.

**Lennox-Gastaut syndrome** A severe pediatric syndrome usually beginning between 1 to 8 years. It is characterized by multiple seizure types, including tonic, atonic, atypical absence, and myoclonic seizures. Intellectual functioning is often impaired and behavioral disturbances are frequent.

**lentiform nucleus** Lenticular nucleus. See *basal ganglia.*

**-lepsia** Combining form meaning seizure, attack, from Gr. *-lepsia,* as in *epilepsia, epilepsis.*

**leptin** A hormone that suppresses appetite; it is the product of the *ob* gene and is made primarily in adipocytes. Leptin acts in the *arcuate nucleus* (q.v.) of the hypothalamus. Like insulin in the CNS, leptin is a negative feedback signal about the status of peripheral energy stores and acts to decrease food intake. *Ghrelin* (q.v.), in contrast, produces increased food intake.

**leptomeninges**   See *meninges.*

**leptomeningitis**   See *meningitis.*

**leptoprosophia**   In anthropology and constitutional medicine, a condition characterized by a narrow face and an elongated cranium.

**leptosomal, leptosomic**   *Asthenic type* (q.v.).

**lesbianism**   Erotic or sexual love of women for other women; Sapphism. See *homosexuality, female.*

**Lesch-Nyhan syndrome**   A heritable disorder of purine metabolism, inherited as a recessive trait, consisting of *hyperuricosuria*, mental retardation, choreoathetosis, spasticity, and a compulsive tendency to self-mutilation (typically, the lips and distal fingers are bitten away). Other clinical manifestations include recurrent vomiting and, later, severe pyramidal and extrapyramidal signs. Females are rarely affected.

Affected children usually die before puberty. There is no known treatment, but the characteristic deficiency of hypoxanthine-guanine-phosphoribosyltransferase (HGPRT enzyme, which normally catalyzes phosphoribosylpyrophosphate) can be detected in amniotic cells in time to allow termination of pregnancy before the affected fetus is viable. The original descriptions of the syndrome were by J. D. Riley in 1960 and by M. Lesch and W. L. Nyhan (*American Journal of Medicine 36*, 1964).

A single active gene encodes for HPRT near the end of the long arm of the X chromosome. Manifestations of HGPRT enzyme deficiency depend on the remaining degree of enzyme activity. In Lesch-Nyhan syndrome, the enzyme is present at only a 0.005% level of normal activity. In some members of the families of affected subjects, the HGPRT enzyme is also deficient, but not to the same degree. In those in whom the level is between 0.01% and 0.5% of normal, spinocerebellar syndromes of variable severity will develop; but if the enzyme level is as high as 1% of normal, the resultant syndrome is gout.

**lesion**   See *disease.*

**lethal**   Deadly, fatal; in genetics, describing a hereditary character that in its homozygous condition produces an extreme modification that is fatal to the organism affected.

**lethal catatonia**   See *Bell mania.*

**lethality scale**   A rating of the likelihood that a subject will attempt suicide, based on factors such as age, sex, medical status, degree of stress, previous history of suicidal behavior, and presence of alcoholism, depression, or sleep disturbances.

In view of current usage of the terms lethality and *suicidality* (q.v.), it would more properly be termed "suicidality scale."

**lethargy**   See *awareness.*

**letheomania**   Morbid longing for narcotic drugs; *addiction* (q.v.).

**lethologica**   Momentary forgetting of a name.

**lethonomia**   Inability to recall the right name, one expression of *nominal aphasia* (q.v.).

**leucotomy, leukotomy; leucotomy**   See *prefrontal lobotomy.*

**leukaraiosis**   Deep white-matter lesions (rarefication) that occur in the geriatric population, mainly on the basis of cerebral infarcts and hypertension. They appear to be related to cognitive impairment and to reflex and motor changes in the elderly. See *subcortical arteriosclerotic encephalopathy; vascular dementia.*

**leukodystrophies**   A group of heritable, progressive demyelinating disorders. One of them, metachromatic leukodystrophy (*MLD*), is due to a deficiency of the enzyme arylsulfatase A, as a result of which sulfatide accumulates in the myelin, leading to demyelination and axon loss in the cerebral hemispheres, brain stem, spinal cord, cerebellum, and basal ganglia. Symptoms include early clumsiness, tremor, and speech difficulty followed by progressive motor and intellectual impairment.

Other forms of leukodystrophy are adrenoleukodystrophy (*Schilder disease, Schaumberg disease*), with adrenal insufficiency, motor symptoms, and dementia; and *Krabbe disease*, due to decreased galactosylceramidase. See *diffuse sclerosis.*

**leukoencephalopathia myeloclastica primitiva**   See *diffuse sclerosis.*

**leukoencephalopathy, progressive multifocal (PML)**   Viral infection of the brain that causes progressive dementia. PML has been reported frequently in AIDS patients. See *AIDS.*

**level, hedonic**   See *adaptational psychodynamics.*

**level of care**   See ALC.

**level of confidence**   See *confidence level.*

**level of development**   See *developmental levels; ontogeny, psychic.*

**level of risk**   See *confidence level.*

**leveling**   As used in family therapy, giving free expression to aggressive feelings, on the (so far unproved) assumption that verbal aggression can substitute for and thus reduce the likelihood of physical aggression.

**levels, mental**   From the standpoint of analytic psychology (Jung), there are three mental levels: (1) consciousness; (2) the personal unconscious; and (3) the collective unconscious. The personal unconscious consists of all those contents that have become unconscious, because their intensity has been lost, they were forgotten, or because consciousness has withdrawn from them, i.e., so-called repression. "Finally, this layer contains those elements—partly sense perceptions—which on account of too little intensity have never reached consciousness, and yet in some way have gained access into the psyche. The collective unconscious, being an inheritance of the possibilities of ideas, is not individual but generally human, even generally animal, and represents the real foundations of the individual" (*Contributions to Analytical Psychology*, 1928). See *topography, mental.*

**leveraged treatment**   Any of a wide range of strategies to induce patients to comply with treatment. These may include mandated community treatment whereby incarceration or placement in subsidized housing is made contingent on compliance, appointment of a money manager to make a patient's access to funds (such as disability income) contingent on treatment adherence, and lenient sentencing by judges on condition that a person participate in treatment. See *outpatient commitment.*

**levirate**   Marriage to a deceased husband's brother. See *sororate.*

**levodopa psychosis**   A syndrome of hallucinations and illusions (delusions are rare), with confusion, vivid dreams, and depression, reported in as many as 60% of patients who receive long-term treatment with levodopa for Parkinson disease.

**levodopa-induced dyskinesia**   *LID* (q.v.).

**levophobia**   Fear of objects to the left; opposite of dextrophobia.

**Levy, David M.**   (1892–1977) Psychoanalyst; child development; author of *Maternal Overprotec-*

tion (a term he coined along with maternal rejection and sibling rivalry); attitude therapy and release therapy (a form of play therapy); introduced Rorschach test to the United States.

**Lewin, Kurt**   (1890–1946) German psychologist; emigrated to United States in 1933; field theory of behavior; sensitivity group training (at the National Training Laboratory).

**Lewis, Nolan D. C.**   (1889–1979) American psychiatrist; research in schizophrenia, history of psychiatry; director, New York State Psychiatric Institute, 1936–1953.

**Lewis, Sir Aubrey**   (1900–1975) Australian-born psychiatrist who joined the staff of the Maudsley Hospital (London) in 1928; professor of psychiatry at the associated Institute of Psychiatry, which under his leadership became an international center for training and research.

**Lewy bodies**   Fibrillar cytoplasmic inclusions containing *ubiquitin* and α-*synuclein* (qq.v.); they can be found in numerous neurodegenerative disorders. Occurring within the substantia nigra they are diagnostic of *Parkinson disease* (q.v.); they are found in the cerebral cortex in various forms of dementia such as Lewy body dementia, Pick disease, and some forms of prion disease, and in motor neurons in amyotrophic lateral sclerosis. Such cytoskeletal alterations may reflect disruption in neurofilament protein assembly or transport; oxidative stress and aberrant calcium metabolism may augment the disruption.

Lewy-body formation might be a cytoprotective event in which dopamine neurons attempt to sequester and compartmentalize poorly degraded proteins into insoluble aggregates and thereby protect against protein-mediate neurotoxicity. See *Parkinson disease; UPS.*

**Lewy body dementia**   *LBD; DLB (dementia with Lewy bodies);* the term includes a variety of clinical diagnoses, such as diffuse Lewy body disease, the Lewy body variant of Alzheimer disease, and senile dementia of the Lewy type. DLB and Parkinson disease (PD) share many pathological, neurochemical, and clinical features, but many workers believe they are distinct disorders. Others, however (including DSM-IV-TR), subscribe to a unifying hypothesis, that they occur on a spectrum from pure PD without neuropsychiatric features, PD with dementia and other psychiatric symptoms, and DLB. Delusions and hallucinations, both visual and auditory, are more common than in Alzheimer disease or vascular dementia; visual hallucinations are often persistent, in contrast with the episodic perceptual disturbances of other dementias. Other symptoms are confusional states, fluctuating cognition, depression, and sleep disturbance (particularly REM sleep behavior disorder). There are three broad patterns of clinical presentation, depending upon the site of Lewy body formation and associated neuronal loss: (1) nigrostriatal involvement, resulting in motor features of parkinsonism; (2) cortical involvement, producing cognitive impairment and neuropsychiatric symptoms; and (3) sympathetic nervous system involvement, leading to autonomic failure. Psychotic features are often associated with extrapyramidal signs and symptoms. Patients with Lewy body dementia show an exaggerated response to neuroleptic drugs.

Lewy body dementia is the third most common cause of dementia, accounting for up to 20% of all elderly cases reaching autopsy.

**lexic function**  See *parietal lobe.*

**lexical cohesion**  See *discourse skills.*

**lexiphanic**  Given to the use of pretentious terminology. See *hellenomania.*

**LHON**  Leber hereditary optic neuropathy. See *mtDNA.*

**LHPA**  Limbic-hypothalamic-pituitary-adrenocortical (axis). See *psychologic unavailability.*

**liaison psychiatry**  See *consultant; psychosomatic medicine.*

**liar, pathological**  Often grouped under the category of *psychopathic personality* (q.v.): "Pathological liars and swindlers are imaginative and champion tellers of 'tall tales,' in which they invariably play the leading role. They build up their stories by proper accessories, such as accents, uniforms, forged documentary evidence, and other items. From time to time newspapers report the exposure of a bogus nobleman, officer, diplomatic agent, or some other impostor. Their activity sometimes takes the form of sexual conquests, and they may obtain money under false pretenses, either on the promise of marriage or after a bigamous marriage" (Lowery, L. G. *Psychiatry for Social Workers,* 1946). See *impostor; lying, pathological.*

**libidinal (libidinous)**  1. Relating to psychic energy. 2. Relating to the erotic instinct.

**libidinal ego**  A self-image that is demanding, impulsive, and feels entitled to immediate pleasure and gratification. The *anti-libidinal ego* is a self-image that is hostile, self-deprecatory, and self-defeating. In their interpretation of the Oedipus situation, Fairbairn and other object relations theorists refer to the *split object relations unit* that comprises (1) the internalized exciting object (the exciting maternal figure) allied with the libidinal ego, which is split from (2) the internalized rejecting object (the rejecting maternal figure) allied with the antilibidinal ego. See *splitting.*

**libidinization**  See *erotization.*

**libido**  In psychoanalysis, the energy of the sexual drive; but because Freud's consideration of the death or destructive drive came relatively late in the development of his psychology, the term libido is commonly used in a more general sense to refer also to the energy of the death or aggressive drive. See *death instinct; libido theory.*

McDougall suggests the term *hormé* for libido. He adds that it is the equivalent of Bergson's *élan vital.*

**libido displaceability**  The psychoanalytic concept that the total sexual instinct energy, or libido, is fluid in nature, subject to metaphorical hydrostatic and hydrodynamic forces. From this impression are derived such psychoanalytic terms as block, recanalization, and displacement, all of which imply shunting of excitation and gratification from one area to another. See *libido mobility.*

Sexual excitations and gratifications are specifically related to the erogenous zones characteristic of each specific phase of libidinal development, and have been called *partial impulses*, because they tend to form or contribute partial components to the total final pattern of fully achieved adult sexuality. These partial impulses are usually discernible in adult sexual life, in what is called foreplay or forepleasure activities or perversion traits. They can substitute for and replace one another in both excitation and gratification. Dissatisfaction at one zone may lead to earlier or later increased activity at another zone. See *ontogeny, psychic.*

**libido mobility** The ease with which libidinal energy can be shifted from one object to another, in contrast to fixation of the libido, in which the libido attaches itself to particular objects.

**libido plasticity** That specific quality of libido that enables the sexual instincts (or the partial impulses of the libido) to modify discharge of tensions through indirect rather than direct avenues of gratification. The major avenues for such gratification, called "the vicissitudes of the instinct", are (1) repression with subsequent symptom and dream formation; (2) sublimation; (3) transformation of the instinct aim into its opposite; and (4) transformation of the direction of the instinctual aim from an external object onto the self. See *libido displaceability.*

**libido stasis** Accumulation of libidinous excitations or tensions consequent upon blockage of their motor discharge. When the free flow of libido has been thus dammed, a stasis results, giving rise to anxiety and a variety of other symptoms, such as irritability, diminished ability to tolerate accumulations of excitation, auditory hyperesthesia, hypochondria, paresthesias, and vasomotor disturbances. See *traumatic neurosis.*

**libido theory** Technically, the psychoanalytic hypothesis concerning the development and vicissitudes of the sexual drive or instinct. Often, however, libido theory is used to refer to all of the psychoanalytic hypotheses about the instincts in humans. The confusion arises from the fact that until 1920 Freud did not fully develop his dual-instinct theory; before that time, all instinctual manifestations were considered to be a part of the sexual drive. Since then, however, the existence of two drives has been assumed by traditional psychoanalysts: sexual (libido) and aggressive. See *death instinct; instinct; libido; object relations theory.*

**libido-binding** See *immobilizing activity.*

**Lichtheim test** A means of determining the retention of inner languages in patients with expressive aphasia or other severe speech disturbances; the patient is asked to indicate the number of syllables in words he or she cannot utter.

**LID** *Levodopa-induced dyskinesia*, the most debilitating class of motor fluctuations that complicate long-term levodopa therapy in Parkinson disease (others include *on-off fluctuations*, sudden, unpredictable changes in mobility, and the *wearing-off phenomenon*). LID includes an array of motor phenomena—chorea, choreoathetosis, ballism, dystonia, myoclonus, and akathisia. Most of them appear when levodopa or other dopamine receptor agonists reach a brain concentration sufficient to overactivate dopamine receptors in the putamen (*peak dose dyskinesia*). They can also occur when dopamine concentration is low (*off dystonia*) or at stages when the concentration of dopamine is rising or falling (*biphasic dyskinesia*).

**lie detector** A machine designed to record the various physiological changes that accompany changes in emotional tone, such as changes in respiratory rate, pulse rate, blood pressure, and skin moisture; the original machine was the *Keeler polygraph.* "The lie detector is based upon the fact that the impact of emotionally charged ideas or the conscious suppression of a true recollection and the substitution of a false statement cause detectable physiologic changes through stimulation of the autonomic nervous system, over which one has no voluntary control" (Guttmacher, M. S. *Psychiatry and the Law*, 1952). It appears that accurate diagnosis on the basis of the test is possible in 75%–80% of cases, that in 15%–20% results may be too indefinite for confident diagnosis, and that the remaining 5% constitute the margin of probable error. Such errors as do occur are usually those on the side of failing to detect a guilty person rather than on the side of mislabeling an innocent person guilty. Overall uncertainty of 25% has made courts increasingly likely to prohibit introduction of results as evidence.

**Liébeault, Ambroise-August** (1823–1904) French psychiatrist; hypnotism.

**liebestod** J. C. Flugel's term for phantasies involving dying with a loved one. Such phantasies may signify a wish to become pregnant by the partner and/or attempt to deny the possibility of death by phantasying eternal union with the mother.

**life event** Any specific happening, rather than life change in general, that is associated temporally and perhaps causally as well with the onset or occurrence of psychiatric disorder, such as depression. Changes in a person's social milieu, such as in one's marriage, work, or neighborhood, or in parenting, if they are undesirable or demand out of the ordinary adaptational maneuvers or attempts at coping, constitute *social stressors.*

Many studies have found a positive relationship between current social stressors and the development of symptoms of depression. Marital stressors have the highest correlation with depressive symptoms, followed by parental stressors for women and job stressors for men.

Some investigators report that depressed patients experience significantly more markedly life-threatening events, more exit events (i.e. loss of a significant person from the social field), and more undesirable events than the general population or schizophrenic patients. In contrast, more desirable events and entrance events (i.e., appearance of a significant person into one's social field) occur with approximately equal frequency in depressives, schizophrenics, and normals. Recurrence of depression has been found to be associated with the occurrence of undesirable events (Paykel, E. S. & Tanner, J. *Psychological Medicine 6*, 1976).

**life goal**   Adler's term for one's secret strivings, implicit in everything the person thinks and does, for a superiority that compensates for the chief inferiority. The phantasy of what one could be acts as a striving from ""below" (ideas of one's disadvantages) to ""above" (ideas of how to gain advantages).

**life history model**   D. F. Ricks and J. C. Berry (in *Life History Research in Psychopathology*, ed. M. Roff & D. F. Ricks, 1970) proposed a life history model for schizophrenia: Because his biological and social equipment provides small margin for error in development, the child is vulnerable to disorder. Often he is aware of his limitations and tries various ways to defend himself. If successful, he may move into a low-stimulation pattern of living. If unsuccessful, he retreats into psychosis, usually through the typical stages of protest, despair, and finally apathy. The major determinants of regression or recovery are IQ, social and vocational success, and a reasonably receptive environment.

**life lie**   Adler's term for the tendency of the neurotic to include in his *life plan* the idea that he will fail because of the fault of others or owing to events beyond his control.

**life plan**   Adler's term for the entire system of behavior by means of which the person prevents his "superiority" from being subjected to the test of reality.

**life space**   In Kurt Lewin's holistic theory of personality, the person plus his psychological environment, the ""totality of possible events" for any person. Included within the life space are valences, positive and negative pressures upon the person for movement toward or away from a goal. Externally presented valences are incorporated within the inner structure of the person in the form of ambitions, aspirations, values, and ideals.

**life-course epidemiology**   Tracking the temporal relationship between disorders over a long time frame (such as decades), in contrast to the usual cross-sectional comorbidity studies. The approach can clarify cause-and-effect mental relationships (or the lack of them) and may indicate, for example, that a mental disorder and a physical disorder are both epiphenomena of an underlying genomic, developmental, or environmental disorder. The life-course approach controls for *Berkson bias*, which overstimates the prevalence of comorbidity in clinics because patients with multiple disorders are more likely to attend a clinic than patients with a single disorder. It also avoids *short-incubation bias*, in which the relationship between two disorders requires years or decades before their association becomes manifest.

**life-event stress theory**   See *aging, theories of.*

**lifestyle**   See *constancy; individual psychology.*

**ligand**   Bond; a receptor's natural activating molecule; e.g., the binding of neurotransmitter and receptor at the receptor's recognition site: binding of the neurotransmitter causes the receptor to change its conformation in a way that affects the interior of the neuron. See *neurotransmitter receptor.*

**light therapy**   *Phototherapy* (q.v.).

**light-and-shadow phobia**   A fear concerning light-and-shadow effects that works in a way similar to the mechanisms described in the *landscape phobia* (q.v.) Fears of darkness or twilight may be related to memories of primal scenes.

**Lilliputian hallucination**   (From the 6-inch-tall inhabitants of the island of Lilliput, in Swift's *Gulliver's Travels*) Microptic hallucinations, in which the objects seen appear much reduced in scale. See *metamorphopsia; micropsia.*

Lilliputian hallucinations have been reported in intoxication from alcohol, chloral, ether, trichlorethylene, and present in cholera, typhoid, scarlet fever, cocainism, tumors of the temporal or temporosphenoidal lobe, and in some cases of petit mal epilepsy.

**limb position sense**  See *proprioception*.

**limbic associative inputs**  See *striatal cortical inputs*.

**limbic lobe, limbic system, limbus**  Visceral brain; *mesopallium*; part of the *rhinencephalon* (q.v.). Limbic was used by both Willis in the 17th century and Broca in the 19th century to describe the ring of tissue on the medial surface of the cerebral hemispheres. The limbic lobe is a band of cortex overlying the rostral brain stem and diencephalon made up of the medial portions of the temporal lobe (MTL) and the frontal and parietal lobes. It includes the hippocampal formation (hippocampus and fornix, and dentate gyrus), the cingulate gyrus and its antero-inferior continuation as the subcallosal gyrus, the parahippocampal gyri, and the subiculum. The olfactory nerve is connected to this region, which formerly was called the rhinencephalon.

In 1937 James Papez posited that the limbic lobe was a neural circuit (*Papez circuit*) that elaborates emotional responses and participates in emotional experience. Paul MacLean later expanded the constituents of the "limbic system" to include the hypothalamus, the septal area, the nucleus accumbens of the striatum, the orbitofrontal cortex, and the amygdala. The *hippocampus* is involved in *memory* (q.v.); the *amygdala*, by means of direct connections with the *hypothalamus*, modulates autonomic and endocrine activities and coordinates visceral responses with motivational states (qq.v.). The hypothalamus controls the endocrine system through its effects on the pituitary and coordinates autonomic and somatic expressions of emotional state through its actions on the autonomic nervous system.

The hippocampus receives multimodal sensory information from both the external (association cortex) and internal (amygdala) environments. The limbic system analyzes the significance of the input of sensation to the organism in relation to the drives (hunger, thirst, sex, parenting) and maintains homeostasis against a changing environment. Its basic function is to choose between alternative behaviors based on incoming sensory information and the memory of what has, or has not, been effective in the past.

Currently, limbic and paralimbic regions include the subgenual and rostral cingulate gyrus, orbital frontal cortex, entorhinal cortex, anterior insula, ventral striatum, and amygdala. The neural circuit for emotion is believed to be as follows: cortical association areas give input to both cingulate gyrus and hippocampal formation. The hippocampal formation also receives input from the cingulate gyrus and gives input to the association cortex, the mammillary body of the hypothalamus, and both directly to the hypothalamus and also indirectly, through the amygdala. The hypothalamus sends input back to the prefrontal cortex and over the mammillothalamic tract to the anterior nuclei of the thalamus. Those nuclei, in turn, send input back to the cingulate gyrus.

**limbic signs**  Irritative lesions within the limbic system may initiate psychosomotor seizures that may include disagreeable olfactory or gustatory hallucinations, movements of the lips, tongue, and swallowing musculature, and emotional responses of rage or fear. See *rhinencephalon*.

**limerence**  The state of being in love or love-smitten.

**limited interactional phobia**  A type of social *phobia* (q.v.).

**limited-symptom attacks**  Anxiety attacks with too few symptoms to qualify as panic attacks. Four or more of the following symptoms warrant the diagnosis of panic attack: shortness of breath, choking, palpitations, chest pain, sweating, dizziness or faintness, nausea or abdominal distress, depersonalization or derealization, numbness or tingling sensations, flushes or chills, trembling, fear of dying, fear of going crazy or of doing something uncontrolled. An episode with fewer than four symptoms is a limited-symptom attack.

**limophoitas**  Psychosis induced by starvation. See *anorexia nervosa*.

**limophthisis**  Emaciation from insufficient nourishment. See *anorexia nervosa*.

**Lindau disease**  (Arvid Lindau, Swedish pathologist, 1892–1951) An angioma of the brain occurring in connection with angiomatosis of the retina, occasionally familial and hereditary. See *von Hippel-Lindau disease*.

**linear pharmacokinetics**  See *pharmacokinetics*.

**lines of development**  In Anna Freud's terminology, the different elements that change in the progression from immaturity to maturity, among them the line from biological unity with the mother to the adolescent revolt against parental influence; the line from being nursed to rational eating; the line from wetting and soiling to bowel and bladder control; the line toward body management; the line toward companionship with peers; the line toward the capacity to work; the line from physical to mental pathways of discharge; the line from animate to inanimate objects; the line from irresponsibility to guilt.

With the term, Freud emphasized the interaction of agencies (e.g., the stimulating, encouraging, and controlling influences of the environment) with subdivisions of stages in the infant and child (e.g., the id, maturing ego, and rudimentary superego) as essential to normal development. Progress along any line is subject to influence from (1) variation in innate givens—constitutional endowments and the raw material from which id and ego will arise; (2) environmental conditions and influences; and (3) interactions between external and internal forces, the experiences that the developing child goes through.

Such a conceptualization differentiates between two types of psychopathology—those based on conflict and those based on developmental aspects. Early deprivation and frustration do not produce symptoms, because there are as yet no internal structures to support the ways of handling conflict that are characteristic of the older child; instead, they produce developmental setbacks that require a different treatment and respond differently to interventions than do symptoms that arise from conflict. See *developmental phases; fixation.*

To illustrate Freud's concept of development: Along the line from biological unity with the mother to the adolescent revolt, the child negotiates a large number of libidinal and aggressive substations, such as the symbiotic, autistic, and separation-individuation phases described by Mahler; the part object, as described by Melanie Klein; the need-fulfilling anaclitic relationship; the stage of object constancy; anal-sadistic ambivalence; the phallic-oedipal relationship; the extension during latency of ties to peers, teacher, the

community, and impersonal ideas; preadolescent regressions; and the adolescent struggle against infantile ties and the search for objects outside the family.

As the ego develops, there is an increase in awareness and understanding of environmental happenings. Empathy with fellow beings expands; there is progress in identification and internalizations, in secondary process thinking, an appreciation of cause and effect and of the reality of principle in general, and adaptation to community standards. At the same time, the environment provides appropriate human objects and their accepting, promoting, stimulating, encouraging, and controlling attitudes toward the child, and the final result depends not on what happens in any one segment but on the interaction between id, ego, and environment.

**lingual delirium**  Delirium mussitans; see *muttering delirium.*

**linguistic determinism**  See *Sapir-Whorf hypothesis.*

**linguistic idiots savants**  Subjects in whom language functions are intact and even overdeveloped in some instances, despite impairment in general cognitive functioning. Such people impress their listeners with their conversational skills; their loquaciousness makes them tireless (and tiresome) raconteurs, yet they are severely retarded and typically can neither read nor write. The condition is sometimes called the *"chatterbox syndrome"* (q.v.) or "cocktail party conversationist syndrome."

**linguistic relativity**  See *Sapir-Whorf hypothesis.*

**linguistic-kinesic method**  An approach to the study of disordered behavior as it manifests itself in disturbances of communication. *Linguistics,* the study of words and language, and *kinesics,* the study of movement, isolate and study infracommunicational systems and thereby reduce the data of interactional behavior to objective, significant, measurable, and manipulative units. This approach is often referred to as the *L-K method.*

**linguistics**  The study of the organization of language and of the general principles underlying the structure of one or more languages. The linguist knows about different languages but does not necessarily speak them. *Multilingual* and *polyglot* refer to a person who speaks two or more languages. See *language; linguistic-kinesic method; psycholinguistics.*

**lingula**    Part of the anterior lobe of the *cerebellum* (q.v.).

**linkage**    The tendency of two alleles at different loci on the same chromosome to be inherited together (*coupling*); topographical association of one gene with another; genes (and the traits they determine) that lie close to each other on the same chromosome are likely to be inherited together (*cotransmission*). The greater the physical proximity, the smaller the probability of genetic recombination occurring between them and therefore the greater the probability they will be coinherited. Linkage examines the cosegregation of markers and disease within families and looks for a greater association between two genes than would be expected from an independent assortment of chromosomes. It indicates that the genes are on the same chromosome and provides an estimate of genetic or relative distance. The degree of linkage can be statistically described by the logarithm of the odds (LOD) score: the ratio of the probabilities of linkage/probability of no linkage.

Linkage analysis attempts to locate predisposing genes by identifying sites (polymorphisms) in the genome at which sequence variations (alleles) travel with illness within families that have more than one affected member. Thus, it aims to locate a disease-inducing gene at a specific site on a particular chromosome. Linkage analysis assesses the association of marker and allele within families. (Association studies examine the association of disease and markers in subjects from different families). Two types of linkage analysis are the traditional lod score approach and the recent affected-relative-pair approach, the favored of the two because it does not require that the mode of inheritance be specified.

*Reverse genetic linkage* is a *candidate gene approach* that looks for markers linked to a nearby structural difference in the DNA. The candidate gene approach searches for the identity of the genetic marker by descent. The *candidate allele approach*, in contrast, searches for the identity of the genetic marker by state (i.e., for the actual allele involved). The candidate gene approach can examine only a few thousand DNA bases at a time. See *genetic marker; sex linkage.*

**linkage analysis**    Linkage mapping; a method used to determine the mode of inheritance

of a disorder. The basic premise underlying linkage studies is that two genes lying close together on a chromosome tend to be inherited together. If the disease of interest and the marker gene are inherited together in a family, it is assumed that the gene for the disease lies close to (is linked to) the marker gene. Linkage analysis searches for a metabolic concomitant or an area of the genome that is consistently transmitted with (linked to) the disease. The *protein/gene approach* searches for an abnormal protein accompanying a given illness; if one is found, it is presumed to be the product of an underlying genetic lesion that causes the disease. The *gene/protein approach* uses DNA probes (genetic markers) to identify a relatively small area of the genome that is consistently transmitted with the disease.

A variety of techniques may then permit increasingly precise localization of the presumed aberrant gene. In the candidate gene approach, particular genes are hypothesized to be related to the physiology of the disorder being investigated; those genes are then tested individually for linkage to the condition. Another approach is scanning of the human genome, in which the entire length of DNA is analyzed, piece by piece, to discover genes that relate to the disorder under investigation. See *behavioral genetics; genetic marker; segregation analysis.*

**linkage disequilibrium**    Allelic association; a more sensitive assay technique than linkage studies that statistically compares the prevalence of a marker in persons affected by the disorder under study with its prevalence in the population at large. Loose linkage between two loci does not produce linkage disequilibrium because such alleles are routinely separated by recombination and both sets of alleles automatically return to linkage equilibrium. Thus, the method detects only the most tightly linked loci and the ones that are most likely to be of significance in the condition under study. The allellic association method is often able to detect a gene that contributes to a disorder, even though the contribution is so small that the gene's significance would go undetected by simple association or linkage studies. One example of allelic association is the association between apolipoprotein genes and risk of cardiovascular disease; in this instance, the apolipoprotein genes may account for as much as 25% of the variance. See *behavioral genetics; genetic marker.*

**linonophobia**   Fear of string.

**LIP**   Lateral intraparietal area; see *intraparietal sulcus.*

**lipochondrodystrophy**   *Gargoylism.* See *mucopolysaccharidosis.*

**lipodystrophy**   Unusual distribution of subcutaneous fat. It may occur as a side effect of HIV combination therapy, where it is termed *fat depletion syndrome*: fat deposits in the arms, legs, and especially in the face melt away. In some cases, the loss of subcutaneous fat seems to be redistributed to the abdomen; such visceral fat is not the same as subcutaneous fat, and it may occur in patients who do not manifest depletion of subcutaneous fat.

**lipofuscin**   An autofluorescent material composed of oxidatively damaged proteins and lipids. Its accumulation in ageing neurons may be a result of impaired mechanisms for its removal, e.g., altered enzymatic degradation by cytosolic proteases, *lysosomes*, or the proteasome.

**lipofuscinosis, neuronal ceroid**   *NCL*; the infantile type (*INCL*), is also known as the infantile Finnish type of NCL and *Santavuori-Haltia disease.* The disorder typically appears between 8 and 18 months of age, with loss of vision and speech, psychomotor deterioration, and seizures, associated with severe loss of white matter, granular deposits in the CNS suggestive of accumulated free and unsaturated fatty acids, and a defect in linoleic acid metabolism. The responsible gene, *NCL1*, and the gene for palmitoyl-protein thioesterase (PPT) map to the same band on chromosome 1. Mutations in the *PPT* gene have been identified in patients with the disorders.

**lipoprotein receptors**   A class of cell surface proteins that can bind *apolipoprotein E* (q.v.) and transport cholesterol into the cell; they serve as receptors for the developmental signaling protein *reelin* (q.v.)

**lip-pursing**   See *Schnauzkrampf.*

**LIPS**   Logical inferences per second; see *KIPS.*

**lisping**   A type of defective articulation in which the sounds "s" and "z" (sibilants) are not pronounced perfectly, by pressing the tip and next narrow part of the blade of the tongue to the alveoli (the sockets where the upper front teeth are rooted), but are pronounced by carelessly pushing the tip of the tongue forward and touching the edges of the upper front teeth as when uttering the sound of "th." Like all speech disorders, lisping is more common in boys than in girls. Lisping may be based on any or all of the following etiological factors: (1) local conditions, secondary to congenital or acquired organic defects; (2) mental retardation; (3) faulty training, especially as a result of parental ignorance or carelessness and the use of "baby talk." It is this last factor that is the most important and the most common and when it is operative lisping is often found to be a behavior reaction acquired in the interest of some personal or social goal. Treatment is directed to the removal or correction of organic defects and to reeducation of parents and child. Speech classes are often helpful in removing the defect.

**Lissauer dementia paralytica**   (Heinrich Lissauer, German neurologist, 1861-1891) An atypical syndrome of general paresis characterized by (1) unusually well-retained intellectual functions and (2) severe focal symptoms, such as apoplectiform attacks, hemiplegia, and aphasia.

**lissencephaly**   *Miller-Dicker syndrome*; smooth brain; the most severe of the known human mutations that disrupt cortical development. It is a relatively rare brain malformation consisting of a smooth cerebral surface with absent gyri (agyria) and broad gyri (pachygyria) that affects one of every 20,000–100,000 live births. The cerebral cortex resembles the brains of *reeler* mice (q.v.), lacking normal ridges and valleys.

Clinical manifestations include severe mental retardation, poor feeding and failure to thrive, hypotonia early and spastic quadriplegia later, opisthotonus, and seizures.

The cytoarchitecture of the cerebral hemispheres is immature, consisting of four cortical layers (rather than the normal six); the fourth layer, the deep cellular layer, consists of a large zone of heterotopic neurons. The abnormalities are the result of incomplete neuronal migration to the cerebral cortex during the third and fourth gestational months. Many cases are genetic in origin and caused by deletions in chromosome 17. The gene mutated in lissencephaly codes for a subunit of an enzyme that inactivates platelet activating factor. Nongenetic cases may be caused by intrauterine infection (e.g., cytomegalovirus).

Other human mutations that disrupt cortical development are *periventricular heterotopia (PH)* and *double cortex (DC)*, whose symptoms include epilepsy, mental retardation, and thin cortex. Almost all patients with PH or DC are women.

**listening attitude**   The expectation that one is about to hear something; it often precedes hallucinations in schizophrenics: "If the patient learns to catch himself in the act of putting himself into the listening attitude, he, after some training, can prevent himself from doing so" (Arieti, S. *Archives of General Psychiatry 6*, 1962).

**lithiasis, hysterical**   Literally, production of (kidney) stones on a hysterical or neurotic basis; in fact, used to refer to *factitious disorders* (q.v.), where foreign bodies are used to mimic kidney stones or other means are used to stimulate renal colic, often in order to obtain opiates.

**lithium**   A naturally occurring element, number 3 on the periodic table (1 is hydrogen, 2 is helium), and the lightest metal known. It is an effective treatment for manic states and an effective prophylactic agent against recurrent manic or depressive episodes. Effects may be produced in various ways: lithium is known to block the degradation of the inositol phosphates, second messengers that release $Ca^{2+}$ from its storage sites in the endoplasmic reticulum; it may act directly on the sodium pump or the calcium channel to reduce retention of sodium within nerve cell.

**lithium augmentation**   See *augmentation*.

**lithium thyroiditis**   Hypothyroidism that occurs as a side effect of medication with lithium, which inhibits the release of thyroid hormones. Observed abnormalities include reduced T3 uptake, T4, and protein-bound iodine; increased thyroid-stimulating hormone and, infrequently, antithyroid antibody titer. Most such alterations diminish or disappear over time even though lithium is continued. In about 5% of patients given lithium, clinical hypothyroidism develops and requires treatment. Symptoms are the classical ones of cold intolerance, fatigue, dry and thickened skin, hair loss, and constipation. Women are affected about nine times as often as men.

**litigious paranoia**   See *paranoia querulans*.

**Litten sign**   (Moritz Litten, German physician, 1845–1907) In paralysis of the diaphragm—nonprojection of shadow by the diaphragm X-rayed during respiration.

**Little disease**   *Cerebral palsy* (q.v.)

**Little Hans**   The patient on whom Freud reported in a 1909 paper, "Analysis of a Phobia in a Five-Year-Old Boy." The initial phobia of little Hans was directed to horses, and analysis revealed that the phobia represented the father, against whom Hans nourished jealous and hostile wishes because of rivalry for the mother. One interesting feature of this case is that the analytic treatment was carried out by the father, who corresponded with Freud and received the latter's suggestions about interpretation and technique by mail. See *free association*.

The father was Max Graf, one of Freud's early supporters and the husband of a former patient. Little Hans was Herbert Graf, who emigrated to the United States and became a successful Metropolitan Opera producer in New York City.

**little professor syndrome**   See *Asperger syndrome*.

**live burial phobia**   *Taphophobia*; a fear of being buried alive is a special "mother's womb" type of claustrophobia representing the mother's womb, one's own body sensations, or the interior of one's own body. The patient attempts to rid himself of aggressive or sexual sensations by projection; the need for sudden escape is a need for escape from one's own feared excitement. See *agoraphobia*.

**living will**   See *advance directive*.

**L-K**   *Linguistic-kinesic method* (q.v.).

**LLI**   *Language learning impairment* (q.v.).

**LLP**   Late-life psychosis. See *paraphrenia*.

**LLPDD**   *Late luteal phase dysphoric disorder; premenstrual dysphoric disorder*; a syndrome of emotional and behavioral symptoms that occur during the last week of the luteal phase of the menstrual cycle (in most women, the week before the onset of menses) and remit within a few days after the onset of the follicular phase (a few days after the onset of menses). The most frequent symptoms reported are affect lability (e.g., sudden sadness or tearfulness, persistent anger or irritability, marked tension), feelings of depression sometimes with suicidal ideas, decreased energy and easy fatigability, lethargy, loss of interest in usual activities, difficulty in concentrating, sleep disturbances, loss of appetite or craving for certain foods, and physical complaints, such as joint or muscle pain, headaches, breast tenderness, bloating, and weight gain. The affected woman may avoid social activities, show increased sensitivity to rejection, have increased interpersonal conflicts, note decreased productivity and efficiency, and express feelings of being out of control or unable to cope.

The syndrome is more severe and more specifically premenstrual than *PMS* (q.v.), and less frequent (in 5% rather than 40% of menstruating women). It is sometimes associated with recognizable abnormalities of serotonin, melatonin, or the noradrenergic system, but these are more likely to be acting as biological triggers rather than as causes of the disorder.

**LMT**   Lowenfeld Mosaic Test. See *mosaic test.*

**load, case**   In psychiatric social work, a term for the number of clients, as well as for intensity of service being given.

**loading, genetic**   See *diathesis-stress model.*

**lobar sclerosis, atrophic**   Little disease; *cerebral palsy* (q.v.).

**lobe, flocculonodular**   See *cerebellum.*

**lobotomy, prefrontal**   See *prefrontal lobotomy.*

**localization**   See *equipotentiality.*

**localized amnesia**   See *amnesia, psychogenic.*

**locked-in syndrome**   *Pseudocoma* (q.v.).

**locomotor ataxia**   See *tabes.*

**locura**   A folk term among Latinos in the Americas to refer to a severe form of chronic psychosis, with agitation, violence, hallucinations, and inability to maintain social relationships.

**locus**   A place or site; in genetics, a position on a chromosome occupied by a gene or marker.

**locus coeruleus (LC)**   A small pigmented nucleus in the brainstem, beneath the floor of the fourth ventricle in the rostolateral part of the pons. It is part of the pontine reticular activating system. The LC supplies over 90% of all forebrain epinephrine. It fibers project to the amygdala, olfactory cortex, frontal cortex, limbic cortex, hippocampus, thalamus, and hypothalamus.

Locus coeruleus is an essential component of the behavioral and physiologic expression of anxiety. One rule of the locus-coeruleus-noradrenergic system is to alert the subject to stimuli important for survival. Whether electrically induced by stimuli from other neurons or chemically induced through norepinephrine agonists such as yohimbine or piperoxonene, LC stimulation leads

to increased sensitivity to novelty, vigilant behavior, aggression, sleep disruption and peripheral physiological activity. LC may be involved in implementing adaptive opposing responses to the reinforcing effects of alcohol, opiates, and psychostimulants. See *adrenergic; μ receptor; reticular formation; VTA.*

Drugs that activate the locus coeruleus are anxiogenic; drugs that inhibit it are anxiolytic. LC activity is elevated in PTSD, leading to increased norepinephrine release as its numerous terminals throughout the brain. In Alzheimer disease, LC neurons degenerate to a level of about 80% of normal. In rodents, activation of the locus coeruleus prevented the memory impairments that occur with aging.

**locus minoris resistentiae**   Area or point of least resistance. See *compliance, somatic; individual-response specificity.*

**LOD**   Logarithm of the odds, a quantitative expression or score of the probability of *linkage* (q.v.) between a genetic probe and the gene for the disorder under investigation. The LOD score is the log to the base 10 of the probability that a given set of data about genetic recombination arises by virtue of two loci being linked at a specified recombination fraction divided by the probability that the data would arise by nonlinkage. An LOD score greater than three defines linkage of the marker to the disease gene, according to conventional criteria.

**Loeffler syndrome**   An allergic reaction by sensitized lung tissue to various allergens, and especially drugs, consisting of pulmonary infiltration and eosinophilia. Loeffler syndrome has been described in association with various psychotropic and psychedelic drugs.

**logagnosia**   Sensory aphasia.

**logamnesia**   Forgetting words; nominal or amnestic aphasia.

**-logia, -logy**   Combining form meaning (1) speaking, speech; (2) science, doctrine, theory; from Gr. -logia, from l'ogos, word, speech, discourse.

**logical empiricism**   See *rationalism.*

**logical error**   A mistake in thinking, such as basing a conclusion on insufficient evidence. *Cognitive behavior therapy* (q.v.) emphasizes that typical logical errors are based on negatively biased thinking: drawing arbitrary inferences from inadequate data, overgeneralization, personalization (giving personal meaning to a neutral event), magnification, selective attention (ignoring any positive aspects of an experience), etc.

**logical inferences**   See *KIPS.*

**logoclonia**   *Logospasm.* Reiterative utterances of parts of words; reported frequently in Alzheimer disease.

**logodiarrhea**   See *tachylogia.*

**logomania**   See *tachylogia.*

**logopathy**   A general term for any type of speech disorder.

**logopedics**   The study of speech and its disorders.

**logophasia**   A form of aphasia, characterized by loss of ability to use articulate language correctly.

**logorrhea**   Excessive speech, sometimes termed *press of speech* or *pressured speech.* It is characteristic of manic episodes and also of Wernicke aphasia, but it is also found in other disorders such as schizophrenia. Logorrhea is sometimes used as equivalent to *tachylogia* (q.v.), although the latter suggests abnormal rapidity of speech rather than excessive amount.

**logospasm**   Explosive speech; stuttering; *logoclonia* (q.v.).

**logotherapy**   Existential analysis; see *existentialism.* Logotherapy is a type of psychotherapy based on a system of spiritual values rather than on a system of psychobiologic laws. Logotherapy emphasizes the search for the meaning of human existence; lack of assurance in any meaning is believed to be one of the main causes of frustration in the present era.

Developed by Victor Frankl in the 1950s and 1960s, logotherapy emphasizes the subject's creative, experiential, and attitudinal values and encourages the incorporation of social responsibility and constructive relationships into solutions.

**Lombroso, Cesare**   (1836–1909) Italian criminologist and psychopathologist.

**long QT syndrome**   LQTS; see *QT interval.*

**longevity**   Length of life. In its medical and statistical sense, the phenomenon of a long duration, or great length, of life.

The existence of *genetic* factors operating in human longevity has been conclusively demonstrated by a number of family studies, although the details of the genetic mechanism involved have not yet been elucidated. Certain experiments of Pearl have shown *long-livedness*

to be dominant over *short-livedness* in Drosophila. A number of cases of short life span may thus be accounted for by single-recessive mechanisms. There is also the possibility of *lethal* (q.v.) genes that merit consideration as a factor of influencing life span, although the present evidence is to the effect that the significant role of lethal genes is in the fairly early (prenatal) stages.

Concerning the constitutional aspect of longevity, it has been shown by Pearl that the long-lived are more asthenic and the short-lived more pyknic, that women have a decided biological advantage over men, and that in youth all individuals below average height have a greater mortality while overweight means greater mortality in individuals over 40 years of age.

Studies on the factor of *marital status* in longevity have demonstrated an advantage for the married over the unmarried in general, but this is mainly due to selective factors rather than to environmental benefits conveyed by marriage. Longevity is also positively correlated with a favorable *social* and *economic* status, and with professional work as opposed to manual occupations, although the question of the relative influence of genetic factors determining simultaneously low-grade occupation and a poor constitution on the one hand, and the environmental disadvantages of manual occupations on the other has not been carefully worked out.

**longilineal**   One of the two constitutional types distinguished by Manouvrier. Persons of this type are built on lines that tend to be long rather than broad, and are to be contrasted with the *brevilineal* (q.v.) type. The longilineal type corresponds roughly to the *asthenic* type of Kretschmer and the *dolichomorphic* type of Pende.

**longitudinal fasciculus syndrome**   See *internuclear ophthalmoplegia syndrome.*

**longitudinal research**   See *cross-sectional research.*

**longitypical**   Identical with *longilineal* and *dolichomorphic.*

**long-term care**   All those habilitation and rehabilitation services and social restructuring that are required to maintain a patient at the highest level of functioning possible within the limitations imposed by chronic mental illness. Such services may include custodial care within a mental hospital, partial hospitalization, or domiciliary settings ranging from highly structured skilled nursing facilities through halfway houses to *satellite housing* (q.v.) with minimal supervision. Almost always, they also include psychopharmacologic treatment, which, in combination with the foregoing organization technology, aims to prevent symptomatic relapse and enable the patient to perform appropriately within the social unit of which he or she is a part. See *rehabilitation*.

**long-term memory**  *LTM; long-term retention; consolidated memory.* The processes involved include the following:

a. Secondary elaboration—in accord with other memories, needs, wishes and the like

b. Consolidation—memory traces become increasingly well established with the passage of time

c. Inhibition—blocking out of unessential memories, even though these may be brought back on demand

d. Extinction—eradication of previously reinforced but no longer useful memories

LTM is subdivided on the basis of time into *intermediate memory*, the ability to remember material from the past 3 to 20 years, and *remote memory*, learned before the age of 12 and much less sensitive to disruption than intermediate memory.

Consolidated memory is differentiated on the basis of what is remembered into (1) *declarative memory* and (2) *procedural memory* (qq.v.)

Short- and long-term memory processes are independent. Only long-term storage, which is associated with the growth of synaptic connections, requires the synthesis of new protein and mRNA. The *NMDA receptor* (q.v.) is essential to long-term potentiation, the persistent strengthening of connections between neurons that underlies learning and memory.

The capacity for LTM requires the integrity of the medial temporal lobe (MTL) and diencephalic regions, which operate in conjunction with the assemblies of neurons that represent stored information. The MTL is primarily involved during the time of learning and during the period of consolidation. For a period after learning, storage and retrieval of declarative memory depend on interactions between an ensemble of memory storage sites distributed throughout different parts of the brain. Temporo-parietal dysfunction is sug-

gested by impairment of rehearsed, consolidated memory (bilateral functions) and by impaired auditory or visual comprehension of prosody and gesturing, impaired musical memory, and impaired spatial memory (non-dominant lobe functions). Verbal memory is dependent upon both the dominant temporal cortex and the occipital lobe. See *consolidation; MTL.*

**long-term potentiation**  *LTP* (q.v.).

**loosening**  Various disturbances of associations that render speech (and thought) inexact, vague, diffuse, and unfocused. The associations may drift aimlessly and wander from the central theme, which itself may be difficult to identify with certainty; instead of centering on a concept, thoughts veer widely off target until they may seem wholly unrelated to what seemed to initiate them. The subject's conversation seems muddled or illogical, and attempts to clarify it through further questioning of the subject tend only to make it still less comprehensible. See *association disturbances; circumstantiality; tangentiality; allusive thinking.*

**Lorente de Nó, Rafael**  (1903–1990) Spanish-born neuroanatomist and neurophysiologist, emigrated to the United States in 1931, Rockefeller University (Institute for Medical Research) 1936–1972; structure and function of cerebral cortex, electrical and chemical basis of nerve functioning.

**Lorr scale**  See *MSRPP.*

**LOS**  1. Length of stay. See *quality assurance; review.*

2. Late-onset schizophrenia (illness onset after 40 years of age).

**loser**  See *transactional analysis.*

**loss of control**  In addiction psychiatry, inability to limit the amount or frequency of substance use via an internal locus of control; impaired control. Loss of control is central to the definition of addiction. The term is also used in an imprecise way to refer to inability to delay gratification of impulses, a need for instant gratification, or an outburst of emotions and feelings (especially aggressive).

**Lou Gehrig's disease**  *Amyotrophic lateral sclerosis* (q.v.).

**Louis-Bar syndrome**  *Ataxia-telangiectasia* (q.v.).

**love**  In psychiatry the most commonly accepted definition of love is contained in the word *pleasure*, particularly as it applies to gratifying experiences between members of the opposite sex. The manifestations of love are almost legion, ranging from those of the infantile period up to those of sublimated maturity.

In general it may be said to correspond to *eros* and *libido*. Freud defined libido as "the energy... of those instincts which have to do with all that may be comprised under the word 'love.' "

Choice of a love object may be based on (1) the narcissistic type, with four possibilities; one may love (a) a person like oneself; (b) a person resembling oneself as one once was; (c) a person who meets the requirements of being what one would like to be; and (d) someone who was once part of oneself (*The Basic Writings of Sigmund Freud*, 1938).

The love object (2) patterned after the anaclitic type may be (a) the woman who tends or (b) the man who protects.

**love, anal-sadistic** The type of ambivalent object relationship characteristic of the anal-sadistic period. See *anal eroticism; anal sadism.*

**lovemap** A person's mental representation of the ideal lover and the ideal program of sexual activity with that lover; in Money's terminology, the *sexuoerotic agenda* is the expression of the lovemap, including the words, movements, and gestures that constitute the scene or ritual of sexual activity, be it autoerotic, heteroerotic, or homoerotic. See *paraphilia.*

**low dose dependence** See *sedatives/hypnotics.*

**low utilizer** See *adverse selection.*

**low-density lipoprotein** LDL. See *Alzheimer disease; amyloid; apolipoprotein E.*

**low-volume hospital** See *volume sensitive.*

**Lowe syndrome** See oculo-cerebrorenal syndrome.

**loxapine** A dibenzoxazepine (tricyclic) antipsychotic drug.

**LP** *Lumbar puncture* (q.v.).

**LPU** Least publishable unit, referring to the earliest report of research in progress that will be accepted by a publisher. In an age when scientific or academic merit is measured by number of publications rather than by the quality of their content, a situation disparagingly referred to as the publish-or-perish syndrome, it has become unfortunate practice to publish every investigation seriatim, in a series of generally disjointed progress

reports, in order to gain credit for multiple publications when one study has been performed.

**LPW** Late positive wave; $P_{300}$ *wave* (q.v.).

**LQTS** Long QT syndrome; see *QT interval.*

**LRP-LDL receptor-related protein** See *Alzheimer disease; amyloid; apolipoprotein E.*

**LSD** See *psychotomimetic.*

**LTB** Life-threatening behavior, generally expressed as suicidal equivalents, chronic invalidism, or other self-defeating behavior that undermines health, nullifies treatment, or disrupts valuable and necessary personal relationships.

**LTM** Long-term memory (q.v.).

**LTP** *Long-term potentiation*; the persistent strengthening of synaptic signals after repetitive stimulation of synapses. LTP is a measure of synaptic plasticity and a model for learning and *memory* (q.v.). LTP is a family of processes that vary in their cellular and molecular mechanisms. Each variant of LTP that has been described has an early phase (E-LTP) and a late phase (L-LTP); the late phase requires protein and messenger RNA synthesis. Usually, LTP is initiated when glutamate from the axon terminals binds to the postsynaptic AMPA receptors; this depolarizes the postsynaptic cell and expels the magnesium that blocks the pore of the *NMDA receptor* (q.v.), thereby activating the NMDA receptor channel.

LTP was first noted in hippocampal cells. When the *perforant path*, a fiber pathway in the hippocampal formation, is repetitively stimulated at high frequency, the synapses between the perforant path and their target cells, the granule cells of the *dentate gyrus*, were strengthened. At those synapses, glutamate released from axon terminals acts on two types of postsynaptic receptors: AMPA and NMDA receptors. Under normal circumstances, only the AMPA receptors are activated by glutamate because magnesium blocks the pore of the NMDA receptor. Activation of the AMPA receptors depolarizes the postsynaptic cell, removes the magnesium block, and leads to the activation of the NMDA receptor channel. To activate the NMDA receptor channel and to initiate LTP, two events must occur simultaneously: glutamate must bind to the receptor and the postsynaptic membrane must be depolarized sufficiently by the activation of the AMPA receptor to expel magnesium from the NMDA channel.

**lucid dreaming** A sleep state in which the dreamer seems to be awake within the dream and aware that he is dreaming, even though there is no disturbance of the physiologic dream state.

**lucidity** From the legal point of view, a lucid interval is not a perfect restoration to reason, but a restoration so far as to be able, beyond doubt, to comprehend and do the act with such perception, memory, and judgment as to make it a legal act.

**Lucifer effect** Transformation of apparently normal people into unfeeling monsters, as seen in the horrifying and barbaric abuses committed at the Abu Ghraib prison. In social psychology, *situationism* posits that good people turn evil largely because of environmental pressures, while the dispositional view emphasizes the contribution of the individual's make-up to his or her susceptibility to commit barbaric acts. It seems likely that both are involved and that, because of their make-up, different people have different moral and ethical thresholds that must be overcome before they will commit such acts. See *dehumanization*; *humiliation*; *violence*.

**ludic** Unreal, playlike, quasi, pseudo.

**ludic activity** Higher animals have a quantity of energy left after performing all the movements required by their physiological life processes. This excess energy must be expended (without purpose) in some way, most usually in play activity, called ludic activity.

**luding out** A term of the drug subculture referring to methaqualone abuse, similar to addiction to the short-acting barbiturates. Chief dangers are (1) severe withdrawal syndrome or (2) with overdose, cardiovascular complications and convulsions.

**ludo therapy** Play therapy.

**lues** Originally, plague or pestilence; in current usage, syphilis.

**lumbar puncture** LP; a technique for gaining access to the subarachnoid space; a needle is introduced into the lumbar cul-de-sac of the subarachnoid space below the termination of the spinal cord at the first lumbar vertebra. LP is used to obtain cerebrospinal fluid for diagnostic purposes, to relieve increased intracranial pressure, to introduce therapeutic substances or local anesthetics, to introduce air preparatory to encephalography and myel-

ography, and to introduce opaque media for radiography. See *cauda equina*.

**lunacy** *Obs.* Mental abnormality of such degree as to render the patient incompetent and bring him under the guardianship of the state.

**lunacy, moral** *Obs.* Behavior disorders, currently termed (1) *psychopathic personality*; (2) constitutional psychopathic inferiority; (3) *perversion* and *impulse control disorders* (qq.v.).

**lunacy commission** A committee, usually of qualified psychiatrists, appointed by judicial order to determine the mental state of an individual whose case the court has under consideration.

**lunatismus** (L. "somnambulism") An old expression given to those somnambulists who only walk about at the time the moon shines (Tuke, O. H. *A Dictionary of Psychological Healing*, 1892).

**Luria-Nebraska Neuropsychological Battery** *LNNB*; a group of tests developed under the influence of Aleksandr Luria's theories of brain organization. The battery comprises 269 items arranged in 14 scales that give information on motor, tactile, auditory (rhythm), visual, memory, and intellectual functioning as well as an assessment of receptive and expressive language abilities. The inclusion of writing, reading, and arithmetic scales allows assessment of educationally related skills. It provides localization scores and factor scores for more exact identification of deficit areas; it also assesses areas of strength. The test takes between 2 and 4 hours to administer. See *Halstead-Reitan Battery; neuropsychological tests*.

Luria, a Russian, posited that all observable behavior is the result of cooperation among multiple brain areas, which are organized into functional units or chains of interlinked parts of the brain. There are three major units of the brain: (1) reticular system, (2) sensory reception and integration, and (3) planning, evaluation, and motor output. All functional systems involve all three units of brain; more than one functional system may exist for any given behavior; if one functional system is interrupted, a second may take its place and compensate for the defect; each area of the brain plays a specific role in multiple functional systems.

In contrast to many other neuropsychological tests, whose emphasis is on finding that a brain injury exists, Luria's battery is designed not only to detect the presence of injury but also to give some idea of its localization and the ways in which it interferes with functioning.

**lust dynamism** Sullivan's term for clearly expressed feelings of sexual interest and ability, such as the wish of the adolescent boy to reach orgasm.

**lust murder** *Erotophonophilia* (q.v.); an extreme form of sexual sadism in which the sadist kills the partner following the sexual act. See *homicide.*

**luteal phase** See *LLPDD.*

**Luys, body of** (Jules Bernard Luys, French physician, 1828–1898) See *subthalamus.*

**LVA** Low-voltage alpha brain waves, reported to be four or five times more common in alcoholics and in subjects with anxiety disorder than in the general population.

**lycanthropy** The belief that one can change himself or others into a wolf or some other animal; *insania lupina; melancholia; melancholia zooanthropia.*

**lycomania** Lycanthropy.

**lycorexia** *Bulimia* (q.v.).

**lygophilia** Longing for dark or gloomy places.

**lying, pathological** Mendacity; falsification entirely disproportionate to any discernible end in view; such lying rarely, if ever, centers about a single event; usually it manifests itself over a period of years, or even a lifetime. It is frequently seen in narcissistic personality disorder and antisocial personality disorder. Pathological lying is also known as mythomania or pseudologia fantastica. See *impostor; liar, pathological.*

**Lyme disease** A tick-borne infection caused in the Unitede States by the spirochete *Borrelia burgdorferi,* and in Europe by the spirochetes *B. afzelii* and *B. garinii.* Incubation period, the time from the tick bite until the first symptom, is from 7 to 14 days. The earliest symptom is solitary erythema migrans at the site of the bite —a red, bluish-red, or purple macule that expands over a period of days or weeks to form a large round lesion, 5 cm or more in size. Expansion of the lesion is usually accompanied by other symptoms, such as fatigue, fever, headache, mild stiff neck, arthralgia, or myalgia. Secondary skin lesions may also develop. If untreated, 40% to 60% of patients develop arthritis, 5% to 8% develop cardiac abnormalities, and 15% to 20% develop neuropsychiatric problems.

Neuropsychiatric symptoms may appear early after the initial attack: meningitis, encephalitis, peripheral neuropathies with pain and sensory hyperacuities, or sudden-onset paranoia. In other patients, cognitive problems, marked mood swings, or chronic fatigue may appear as the presenting system months or years after the tick bite. Early antibiotic therapy can prevent the development of such later manifestations.

**lymphokines** Nonimmunoglobulin molecules released by lymphocytes after a second interaction with a given antigen; they are particularly important during cell-mediated immune reactions, because they affect the behavior of other immune cell types.

**lysatotherapy** A form of treatment for clinical depression reported by Timopheyev that uses a lysate of the anterior hypophysis. Lysatotherapy is based on the assumption that hypophyseal hypofunction is of etiologic significance in the pathogenesis of pure depression or cyclothymia.

**lysergic acid diethylamide** See *psychotomimetic; psychotropics.*

**lysosomal storage disorders** LSDs; a group of at least 41 distinct neurodegenerative disorders inherited, with two exceptions, in an autosomal recessive manner. (The exceptions are Fabry disease and mucopolysaccharidosis type II, which are inherited in an X-linked recessive manner.) Each LSD results from mutations in a different gene and consequent deficiency of enzyme activity or protein function, leading to an accumulation of normally degraded substrates within lysosomes. The substrate stored is used to group LSDs into broad categories: *glycolipid storage diseases* (glycogenoses and lipidoses), mucopolysaccharidoses (MPS), and oligosaccharidoses. Many LSDs share some similarities: bone abnormalities, organomegaly, central nervous system dysfunction, and coarse hair and facies. See *Fabry disease; Gaucher disease; leukodystrophies; lipofuscinosis, neuronal ceroid; mucopolysaccharidosis; Niemann-Pick disease; Tay-Sachs disease.*

**lysosome-mediated autophagy** An important pathway for intracellular protein degradation that involves an acidic cellular compartment, the lysosome vacuole. The pathway mediates the bulk degradation of cytosol and organelles and might degrade aggregated proteins. Chaperones mediate one form of autophagy.

**lysosomes**   Membrane bound organelles with a low pH that contain high concentrations of enzymes that degrade proteins. Among their targets are damaged proteins, and there is evidence that lysosome function is altered in neurons during ageing. See *lipofuscin*.

**lyssophobia**   Fear of becoming insane.

**lytic cocktail**   A mixture of neuroleptic drugs (usually chlorpromazine, promethazine, Hydergine, atropine, etc.) used in the treatment of acute or impending delirium.

**lytico**   See *bodig*.

# M

**μ-receptor** A heterotrimeric GTP-binding protein (G protein)–linked opiate receptor, the major opiate receptor for morphine like opiates, including heroin. Long-term opiate administration produces tolerance by decreasing μ-opiate receptor signaling in the noradrenergic LC (locus coeruleus). Opiates initially inhibit cAMP-dependent phosphorylation in the Na+ ion channel. With long-term opiate administration, the cAMP pathway is upregulated and the sodium channel becomes more fully phosphorylated, making LC neurons hyperexcitable. Adaptations in the cAMP signal transduction pathway underlie the mechanisms of opiate tolerance and dependence, and up-regulation of these components plays an important role in the onset of the withdrawal syndrome.

Endogenous opioid binding to μ receptors is also one neural mediator of infant attachment behavior, which entails display of affiliative behaviors and establishment of a special bond with caregivers. Malfunctioning of the endogenous opioid system may be implicated in the social indifference displayed by autistic infants. See *attachment*.

**MA** Mental age. See *intelligence quotient*.

**MAC** Maximum allowable cost, or revenue cap, an element of some prospective payment plans for hospital reimbursement by governmental programs and other third-party health insurance payers.

**Macbeth effect** Symbolic cleansing; the urge of persons who have betrayed their values to wash their hands. In one of several experiments, students who had been asked to recall unethical or shameful acts from the past were more likely to prefer an antiseptic wipe to a pencil as a gift for their participation in the study.

**MacCAT-T** The MacArthur Competence Assessment Tool, a set of measures developed by Paul Appelbaum, Thomas Grisso, and their colleagues (1996) for the rating of patients' abilities relevant for evaluating competence to consent to treatment. It consists of a semistructured interview that includes disclosure of the nature of the patient's disorder, the treatment options available and the benefits and risks associated with them, and the patient's choice of treatment and an explanation of how that decision was reached. The MacCAT-T interview takes about 15 to 20 minutes.

**Machado-Joseph disease** A *polyglutamine disorder* (q.v.) with the same CAG expansion as type 3 spinocerebellar atrophy. See *trinucleotide repeat*.

**machine fever** Overdependence on an executive information system so that for the user the computer terminal becomes the organization or company. One well-recognized and undesirable effect of executive information systems is that the executives who use them become so mesmerized by the charts they can produce on their own that they ignore less tangible matters, such as training of managers. Also, they encourage chief executives to ask many, often irrelevant, questions on the basis of what they have discovered through the use of the information system, thus consuming a disproportionate amount of the managers' time. What senior executives see as guiding or monitoring, managers tend to interpret as meddling or second-guessing. See *information system, executive*.

**MacQuarrie test** A test of mechanical ability in which the subject draws a continuous line through irregularly placed gaps in vertical lines without touching those lines.

**macro-** Combining form meaning large, enlarged, extended, exaggerated, from Gr. *makros*.

**macrobiotic** Long-lived; tending to prolong life.

**macrocephaly** Abnormally large head.

**macrogenitosomia** A syndrome occurring in children before the age of puberty, due to tumors of the pineal gland. The condition is also known as *pubertas praecox* (precocious puberty). The sexual development is precocious with early ejaculation or menstruation and the growth of prematurely large genitals. The secondary sex characters occur early with gruff voice, facial, pubic, and axillary hair, and mammary gland development.

**macrogenitosomia, precocious** Pellizzi introduced this term for a particular form of *gigantism* (q.v.) occurring in children and characterized by premature, rapid, and exaggerated development of the entire organism, including the sexual organs. In addition to the overgrowth of stature and body mass, which may reach the dimensions of the adult in a few years, there are frequently dissociations and partial hypoevolutisms of the sexual characteristics, and also adiposity and mild mental retardation.

The syndrome is caused by tumors of the adrenal cortex, the testicle, or the pineal gland, or in rare cases by dyspituitarism and, in female children, sometimes by constitutional hypothyroidism.

**macroglia** *Astrocytes* and *ependymal cells* (qq.v.). See *neuroglia*.

**macroglobulinemia, Waldenstrom** See *Waldenstrom macroglobulinemia*.

**macrology** Long speech with little reasoning.

**macromania** *Obs.* "That form of insanity in which the insane person conceives things, especially parts of his own body, to be larger than they in reality are" (Tuke, D. H. *A Dictionary of Psychological Healing*, 1892).

**macropsia** A form of *dysmegalopsia* (q.v.); visual sensation of objects being larger than they really are.

**macroskelic** In Manouvrier's system of constitutional types, that type characterized by excessive length of the legs; it corresponds roughly to Kretschmer's *asthenic type* (q.v.).

**macrosomatognosia** See *somatognosia*.

**mad cow disease** *Bovine spongiform encephalopathy* (q.v.).

**Madame Butterfly phantasy** The daydream of the return of a departed loved one, seen most frequently in children of divorce in the age range of 5 to 8 years, who cannot believe that the separation of the parents will endure and phantasize that the absent father loves them and someday will return to them.

**made impulse** See *first-rank symptoms*.

**madness, myxedema** See *hypothyroidism*.

**Madonna complex** Considering the pregnant woman as sacred and not to be defiled by the sexual act; the association of motherhood with asexuality.

**MAG** Myelin-associated glycoprotein, a member of the immunoglobulin family that may be involved in cell-to-cell recognition. It is elaborated by the Schwann cells during early myelination of peripheral nerves, but it is only a minor element in mature peripheral myelin.

**Magersucht** Desire to be thin or underweight; *anorexia nervosa* (q.v.).

**magic fright** *Susto* (q.v.).

**magic helper** See *irrational authority*.

**magic phantasy** The phantasy based upon the idea of limitless power and authority attributed to the analyst by the patient, who consequently expects the impossible from the analyst.

**magic phase** A phase in the evolution of thinking in which the mere imagining of an object seems to the thinker the equivalent of his having created it. Freud referred to it as *omnipotence of thought*.

**magical thinking** Archaic, primitive, prelogical thinking; seen in the unconscious of neurotics, in small children, in normal persons under conditions of fatigue, as antecedents of thought in primitive humans, and in schizophrenic thinking. The speech and thinking of the schizophrenic are frequently more concrete and active than normal, not yet capable of realistic abstractions, and more a symbolic equivalent of action. See *paleologic; primary process*.

**Magna Mater** Cybele, later known to the Romans most commonly as the Great Mother of the Gods, the symbol of universal motherhood; one of Jung's archetypes. See *archetype; mother archetype*.

**Magnan sign** *Formication* (q.v.).

**magnetic apraxia** See *utilization behavior*.

**magnetic gait** See *normal pressure hydrocephalus*.

**magnetic resonance imaging** *MRI* (q.v.).

**magnetic resonance spectroscopy** MRS. See *imaging, brain; fMRI*.

**magnetic seizure therapy** *MST* (q.v.).

**magnetic source imaging** *MSI* (q.v.).

**magnetism** *Psychodynamy*; the property of mutual attraction or repulsion possessed by magnets; such a force was once believed to be the principal factor in hypnosis, which was thus called animal magnetism.

**magnetization transfer imagery** A neuroimaging technique that generates data on the fine structure of white matter; a low magnetization transfer ratio suggests myelin pathology. See *MRI*.

**magnetoencephalography (MEG)** A noninvasive technique that allows detection at the scalp level of the changing magnetic fields associated with brain activity on the timescale of milliseconds; it can provide information about subcortical as well as cortical functioning. MEG uses superconducting quantum interference devices (SQUIDS) to measure tiny magnetic components of the electromagnetic activity elicited by neural activity. It is highly sensitive: spatial resolution is comparable to that of fMRI but with much better temporal resolution. It has been used in combination with *deep brain stimulation* (q.v.) to study brain function. See *MRI*; *msMRI*; *opsin*.

**magnifications**   See *cognitive behavior therapy*.

**Mahler, Margaret**   (1897–1985) Hungarian-born psychiatrist and child analyst; *The Psychological Growth of the Human Infant* (1976). See *symbiotic infantile psychosis*.

**mahu**   The Hawaiian variant of *gynemimesis* (q.v.).

**MAI**   Mycobacterium avium intracellulare; avian tuberculosis. It often produces disease in chickens or swine, but rarely in humans except for persons with *AIDS* (q.v.).

**maieusiophobia**   *Obs.* Fear of childbirth.

**Main syndrome**   The ability of a patient (usually a female psychotic who is a nurse or is otherwise closely related to the field of medicine, and part of whose productions include recounting long-continued incestuous relationships) to extort "frantic sympathy and remarkable therapeutic privilege" from her attendants, and to imbue "doctor or nurse with a vivid sense of private significance for the patient, of being peculiarly attuned to her" (Bourne, H. *Archives of General Psychiatry 2*, 1960). The syndrome was first described by T. F. Main in 1957.

**mainliner**   A slang expression for addicts who take narcotics by intravenous injection.

**mainstreaming**   Return of discharged patients to an appropriate level of functioning within the community. See *deinstitutionalization*.

**maintenance level**   The dosage of therapeutic agent that must be repeated at stated intervals in order to sustain the desired effect.

**maintenance therapy**   Treatment(s) that are continued after recovery from or improvement of an acute episode of illness in order to prevent recurrence and support the patient's rehabilitation. Maintenance therapy with *lithium* (q.v.) is frequently used in bipolar patients to prevent recurrence of mania or depression. Oral neuroleptics and *depot neuroleptic* (q.v.)

therapy are often used with schizophrenic patients. Maintenance therapy is commonly used with persons addicted to drugs (particularly heroin and other opiates): a substitute drug for which cross-tolerance and cross-dependence exist is used in order to minimize the reinforcement of drug taking and prevent a withdrawal reaction, while permitting rehabilitation to be achieved. Examples are methadone maintenance and nicotine gum. See *preventive therapy, long-term*.

**maître de plaisir**   One who derives satisfaction from arranging for the sexual satisfaction of others; pimp.

**major depression**   See *unipolar depression*.

**major histocompatibility complex**   *MHC*, a region that encodes a family of molecules responsible for the rejection of transplanted organs. MHC class I molecules bind peptides derived from proteolysis of intracellular proteins; the peptides are presented to cytotoxic lymphocytes and are identified as self or non-self. This identification is at the core of the body's ability to eliminate bacterial and viral infections and to curb the development of some cancers. MHC class I molecules also play a significant role in the developing and adult CNS.

Several neurological disorders have associated immune symptoms. Among these are spinocerebellar ataxia, Huntington disease, Parkinson disease, multiple sclerosis, narcolepsy, dyslexia, autism, and schizophrenia. Patients with a first degree relative with schizophrenia are significantly more likely to have also a parent or sibling with an autoimmune disease. Conversely, there is a strong negative correlation between schizophrenia and two autoimune disorders, insulin-dependent diabetes mellitus and rheumatoid arthritis (Wright, P. et al. *Schizophrenia Research. 47*: 1–12, 2001). Psychotic episodes have shown to be preceded by raised levels of immune cytokines in the cerebrospinal fluid, and treatment with cytokines can provoke psychiatric symptoms. It is possible that cytokine-induced changes in neuronal MHC class I expression, at a time when MHC class I is involved in sculpting developing neuronal circuits, might cause neurodevelopmental abnormalities that lead to schizophrenia.

**major role therapy**   Counseling as part of vocational *rehabilitation* (q.v.).

**major set**   See *set, major*.

**mal de ojo**    Evil eye syndrome, reported in many Mediterranean cultures, consisting of diarrhea, vomiting, and fever, particularly in a child. See *curanderismo.*

**mal de pelea**    Fighting sickness. See *Puerto Rican syndrome.*

**mal d'orient**    *Homosexuality* (q.v.). It was claimed that the practice spread to Europe through the influence of the Crusaders. In some countries a homosexual is called a Turk or a Bulgar; hence the French term *bougre* and the English *bugger,* both denoting a homosexual.

**mal puesto**    See *curanderismo; rootwork.*

**maladaptation, common**    See *adaptational psychodynamics.*

**maladie des tics**    *Tourette disorder* (q.v.).

**maladie du pays**    Nostalgia; longing for one's native land.

**maladjustment, simple adult**    Adult situational reaction. See *adjustment disorders; transient situational disturbances.*

**malady**    See *disease.*

**malady, English**    *Obs.* Hypochondriasis (q.v.).

**Malan brief psychotherapy**    See *brief psychotherapy.*

**malarial treatment**    A form of treatment introduced by Wagner-Jauregg for syphilis of the central nervous system, especially general paralysis; blood containing tertian or quartan malaria parasites is injected into the patient, as a result of which he or she develops malarial fever.

**male orgasmic disorder**    Inhibited male orgasm; retarded ejaculation.

The term includes orgasmic anhedonia, a decreased or absent sense of pleasure even though ejaculation is achieved.

**maleness**    See *masculine.*

**malformation, congenital**    See *teratology.*

**malignant identity diffusion**    See *crime and mental disorder.*

**malignant narcissism**    A personality type described by O. Kernberg characterized by the combination of (1) a narcissistic personality disorder, (2) antisocial behavior, (3) ego-syntonic aggression or sadism directed against others (including inhumane or barbarous killing) or against the self in a triumphant kind of self-mutilation or suicidal attempts, and (4) a strong paranoid orientation, manifested in an exaggerated experience of others as idols, enemies, or fools, or in regression into paranoid micropsychotic episodes. Some malignant narcissists are leaders of sadistic gangs or terrorist groups. See *antisocial personality.*

Freud's description of "criminals from a sense of guilt" implied that antisocial behavior is a reaction formation against unconscious guilt; contemporary psychoanalytic thought views it instead as an expression of severe deficits in the development of the superego.

**malignant psychosis**    Fenichel's term for that type of schizophrenia which is progressive (slowly or rapidly) and terminates in permanent dementia. He contrasts the malignant schizophrenic psychoses with shorter schizophrenic episodes with a better prognosis. See *schizophreniform disorder.*

The term malignant psychosis is approximately equivalent to the terms *process psychosis* and *nuclear schizophrenia,* and to *dementia praecox* as used by contemporary European psychiatrists.

**malignant syndrome**    See *neuroleptic malignant syndrome.*

**malignant trend**    Also, pernicious trend; the presence of components that ordinarily portend chronicity.

**mali-mali**    See *miryachit.*

**Malin syndrome**    See *neuroleptic malignant syndrome.*

**malinger**    To feign or protract one's illness; to simulate, with intent to deceive.

**malingering**    Simulation of symptoms of illness or injury with intent to deceive. Malingering occurs, usually, in one of the following situations: (1) in criminal cases, when mental illness or mental retardation is feigned in order to obtain better or safer living conditions or an environment from which escape is easier, in order to obtain drugs, to avoid or delay trial, or in hopes of evading responsibility for the crime with which the offender is charged; (2) in personal injury actions and compensation cases; and (3) in military service or similar special situations where nervous or mental disease might afford an escape from hazardous or arduous duty. The diseases most likely to be malingered are amnesiae, psychoses, psychoneuroses, and mental retardation. Detection in the latter case is relatively simple with available psychometric tests. The disorder with which malingering is most frequently associated is antisocial personality.

Malingering is not a mental malady, for it involves the intentional and voluntary production of false or grossly exaggerated physical or psychological symptoms. External incentives provide the motive for symptom production, in contrast to factitious disorder, conversion disorder, and other somatoform disorders, where the incentives are internal and related to emotional or intrapsychic conflict. See *volition.*

**malleation** Convulsive movements of the hands, as if in the act of hammering.

**malo ojo** See *curanderismo.*

**maltreatment** Physical or psychological abuse, the effects of which on the abused person are termed the child maltreatment syndrome and the adult maltreatment syndrome.

Children's reactions to psychological, physical, or sexual abuse are varied. They include adjustment reaction, post-traumatic stress disorder, and reactive attachment disorder (a mixed emotional disturbance of childhood). Often the reaction does not fulfill the criteria for any specific mental disorder and is classified instead as a parent–child problem.

Signs of emotional maltreatment of children include (1) physical signs such as delays in physical development, failure to thrive; and (2) behavioral signs, such as conduct problems, increased anxiety, apathy or depression, and developmental lags. See *emotional deprivation; maternal deprivation; battered child syndrome.*

Reactions to maltreatment are even more varied in the adult, who usually has a wider repertoire of physical and emotional responses than the child. The most specific reaction is *post-traumatic stress disorder* (q.v.), but many other reactions may be observed, ranging from denial, anxiety, depression, rage, or development of somatic symptoms to precipitation of or exaggeration of a preexisting psychosis. Abused women often retreat into passivity and silence, and then are difficult to identify as victims of abuse.

Wife battering is the leading form of domestic violence. Of increasing importance in nations whose elderly population is growing is parental and grandparental abuse. See *domestic violence; victim; wife battering.*

**maltreatment, child** See *battered child syndrome.*

**mammalingus** Sucking on the breast. "The fellatio conception of coitus, in fact, would seem to be only one-half of the story. One finds also the complementary idea that the father not only gives to the mother, but receives from her; that in short she suckles him. And it is here that the direct rivalry with the father is so strong, for the mother is giving him just what

the girl wants (nipple and milk).... When this 'mammalingus' conception... gets sadistically cathected, then we have the familiar idea of the man who 'uses' the woman, exhausts her, drains her, exploits her, and so on" (Jones, E. Papers on Psychoanalysis, 1938).

**mammillary body** Mammillary tubercle of the hypothalamus; a small nipple-shaped group of nuclei situated behind the third ventricle at the posterior-inferior margin of the hypothalamus at the base of the brain. Some authors include the supramammillary nucleus (which controls the frequency of hippocampal *theta rhythm*) and the posterior part of the tuberomammillary nucleus as part of the mammillary body. The mammillary bodies (one on each side of the brain) are divided into two groups of nuclei, medial and lateral.

The larger medial group receives input from the hippocampus (through the rostral or septal subiculum) and the medial entorhinal cortex. The medial mammillary nucleus projects ipsilaterally through the mammillothalamic tract (tract de Vic D'Azyr) to the anterior medial and anterior ventral thalamic nuclei.

Although the smaller of the two groups, the lateral mammillary nucleus contains the largest cells in the mammillary bodies. It receives input from the presubiculum, parasubiculum, and postsubiculum; it projects through the mammillothalamic tract bilaterally to the anterior dorsal thalamic nucleus. The lateral mammillary nuclei contain "head direction" neurons, which signal the direction in which the subject is facing.

Mammillary body damage results in a pattern of spatial deficits, specifically, an impaired ability to learn a specific location within a cognitive map. Damage to the tracts that link the mammillary bodies with the hippocampus and anterior thalamic nuclei is associated with anterograde amnesia. The mammillary bodies relay hippocampal theta rhythm to the anterior thalamic nuclei; theta rhythm may act as a "significance signal",, so that information arriving with theta activity is most likely to be stored.

**managed care** An organized, comprehensive, coordinated system of medical care delivery that provides a full continuum of mental health, substance abuse, and medical care through a network of providers selected on the basis of their commitment to cost-effective, quality care; the system includes utilization review and cost-containment features whose goal is to ensure that health care is provided in the most cost-effective manner.

A managed care system controls access to care, not only by preadmission certification of nonemergency cases deemed suitable for admission to an inpatient unit, but even more importantly by combining early case finding and individual, problem-focused treatment plans with a full continuum of multidisciplinary services to substitute for inpatient care when that is feasible. Patterns of practice of health care providers are monitored and evaluated, and formal quality assurance methods such as concurrent review and retrospective review of cases are used as a way to improve the quality of care provided. The term managed care is sometimes used indiscriminately to refer to any one or more of such monitoring methods rather than to the organized network of providers and services.

An emphasis on brief outpatient services requires that information, referral, and individual *case management* (q.v.) services be available on a 24-hour basis. Some managed care systems limit the availability of some treatment options; many of them limit the use of specialists or specialty services, typically through the use of the primary care physician as *gatekeeper* (q.v.).

Managed care is often provided through an organization such as a *PPO* or *HMO* (qq.v.); some insurance companies have also developed managed care networks. The potential patient (variously termed the consumer, subscriber, enrollee, or member of the particular health plan) is encouraged to use the selected providers who are participants in the plan through financial incentives: the plan will pay for only those services provided within its own network, and the patient must pay for care obtained outside the network.

Providers within the managed care network are encouraged to become increasingly cost-effective (or at least cost-conscious) in providing care by means of a variety of financial inducements, including capitated payment, risk sharing, rewards based on utilization or hospitalization rates of their patients, and the possibility of not being retained within the program.

Although there are few hard data to support the claim that managed care provides the most cost-effective approach to the delivery of high-quality health care, the major areas in which costs are believed to be saved are as follows: (1) decrease in number of diagnostic tests and procedures; (2) fewer referrals to specialists and to nonparticipating physicians; (3) fewer hospitalizations; (4) decreased lengths of stay in both hospitals and nursing homes; (5) fewer surgical operations; (6) fewer physician office visits; and (7) better patient compliance.

Psychiatrists, and physicians in general, have consistently objected to some of the elements of managed care, such as:

1. The gatekeeper system obstructs early referral to a specialist.

2. Services are often restricted to "medically necessary" care, but the definition of medical necessity is often made independently by the managed care organization, with little or no physician input.

3. Emphasis on reducing the number of tests and procedures, of therapy sessions, and of hospital days deifies a rapid turnover ethic and hinders the physician who must treat many patients who fall outside the limits of the "average" subscriber or member of the health plan.

4. Measures that can be taken—by a physician or a patient—to appeal a decision that a particular treatment for a particular patient at a particular time is not eligible for reimbursement are often not spelled out.

5. The responsibility for decisions regarding the type or extent or timing of treatment is unclear; but should the outcome of treatment be adverse, it is the physician (or clinic, or hospital) who is assigned the responsibility, no matter how much that decision has been challenged by the health care providers.

**manager disease** A type of occupational neurosis occurring in overworked employers and leading officials who are overburdened with responsibility. The symptoms most commonly complained of are those relating to the heart and cardiovascular system.

**mandala** Jung's term for the magic circle that symbolizes total unity of the self. See *Tantra*.

**mania** 1. *Obs.* Any mental disorder, madness, especially when characterized by violent, unrestrained behavior. 2. When used as a suffix, a morbid preference for or an irrepressible impulse to behave in a certain way, such as *kleptomania* (q.v.). 3. Bipolar disorder, one of the two major forms of mood disorder. See *manic-depressive psychosis*.

Mania is characterized by (1) an elated or euphoric, although unstable, mood; (2) increased psychomotor activity, restlessness, and agitation; and (3) increase in number of ideas and speed of thinking and speaking, which in more severe forms proceeds to flight of ideas (q.v.), often with a grandiose trend.

In mania, the main disturbances in the ideational sphere are *overproductivity; flight of ideas* (i.e., a rapid shifting from one topic to another), of which *distractibility* is a part, the patient changing from topic to topic in accordance with the stimuli from without and from within; shifting may be occasioned by what is called *clang association*—stimulation of a new train of thought by some external sound; leveling of ideas, that is, essentially all topics have about the same value to the patient; *ideas of importance, grandiose ideas*, the patient expressing delusions of greatness perhaps in all fields; the feelings of well-being are expressed also in the sphere of *physical excellence*. Often the ideas are reproductions of those relating to *infantile sexuality*.

The principal modifications in the emotional field are inflated self-esteem with exaggerated feelings of gaiety, well-being, extreme happiness—in consonance with the ideas expressed.

Psychomotor overactivity refers to physical overactivity; in extreme states it is incessant throughout the waking hours; the patient attempts to motorize, that is, to put into physical execution all the ideas that occur to him or her; this leads to a shifting of physical activity paralleling that in the mental sphere. The person with mania has a decreased need for sleep. His days are likely to be spent in activities with a high potential for painful consequences, such as buying sprees, sexual indiscretions, reckless driving, and foolish business investments.

Depending upon the degree of mania, there are three types: *hypomania, (mania mitis)*, which is a less intense form; *mania*, the usual type; and *hypermania*, a more intense expression of the manic reaction.

Some authors use the term *acute mania* synonymously with mania, and hypermania is often referred to as *delirious mania, Bell mania, typhomania, delirium grave*, or *collapse delirium*, with partial or complete disorientation as the rule.

When a patient has a succession of manic attacks, the condition is known as recurrent or periodic mania. When manic and depressive episodes alternate, the condition is called *alternating* or *circular psychosis* or *insanity*.

Periodic mania is to be distinguished from *chronic mania*, a form described by Schott in 1904 in which manic symptoms continue uninterruptedly for an indefinite number of years (in Schott's series, for 30, 25, 21, and 17 years). In all such cases reported, the particular episode that becomes chronic began after the age of 40.

A patient in a manic phase may not talk; his state is then known as *unproductive* or *stuporous mania*; he is said to be in a condition of *manic stupor*.

When a patient presents the symptoms of mania, but does not move, his condition is called *akinetic mania*. Follow-up studies suggest that akinetic mania and manic stupor and all of Kraepelin's "mixed" or "intermediate" states are really schizophrenic.

"The psychoanalytic point is one that several analytic investigators have already formulated in so many words, namely, that the content of mania is no different from that of melancholia, that both the disorders are wrestling with the same 'complex,' and that in melancholia the ego has succumbed to it, whereas in mania it has mastered the complex or thrust it aside" (Freud, S. *Collected Papers*, 1924–1925). In mania, the ego for a time has thrown off the yoke of the superego and protests, "I don't need control any more." The removal of inhibition allows all those impulses (mainly oral) which had been kept down to come to the fore. But the freedom from the superego is not a real one, and the ego must deny its fear of the superego by overcompensation. The cramped nature of the symptoms is due to the fact that they are of reaction-formation type and deny opposite attitudes. Mania is not a genuine freedom from depression but rather a cramped denial of dependencies.

### MANIAS AND PHILIAS

Used as a suffix, -mania refers to an exaggerated interest in or preference for something, in many instances of sufficient intensity to lead to compulsive or impulsive actions. The traditional terms for several of the impulse disorders employ the -mania suffix: kleptomania, trichotillomania, pyromania.

In general, -mania stresses behavior and action, whereas the suffix -philia emphasizes the feeling, attitude, disposition, or preference. Another suffix, used much less frequently, is -lagnia, which emphasizes the erotic element in the craving
continued

or activity; most words with this suffix refer to the paraphilias. Thus, pyrophilia means an excessive interest in fires, pyromania refers to fire-setting, and pyrolagnia refers to fire-watching or fire-setting as an essential or contributing factor to sexual excitement in the subject.

There are, however, many exceptions to the general rule. Some -mania words, in fact, do not refer to desire or need at all; instead, they describe an aversion or loathing (a function more typically performed by the -phobia suffix). Examples are demonomania (fear of devils) and nautomania (the sailor's fear of the sea).

*Acrasia, acolasis, agriothymia,* and *hyperepithymia* are general terms for exaggerated interest, inordinate desire, and intemperance. Terms for more specific preoccupations or cravings, and impulsive or compulsive actions, include the following:

**adolescent, adolescent role:** adolescentism, ephebophilia, pedophilia

**alcohol:** acoria (although Hippocrates used it to mean moderation in eating); alcoholophilia, alcoholmania, dipsomania, dipsos avens, oenomania, oinomania, polyposia, poisomania, potomania

**amputee:** acrotomorphilia, apotemnophilia

**animals:** formicophilia, ophidiophilia (snakes), zooerasty, zoolagnia, zoophilia

**bathing, washing:** ablutomania

**beauty:** callomania (also – delusion that one is beautiful)

**biting:** agriothymia hydrophobica, vampirism

**bloodletting:** phlebotomania, vampirism (love bites)

**buying:** chrematistophilia; oniomania

**children:** pedophilia, philoprogeneity (one's own)

**choking:** asphyxiophilia; hypoxyphilia

**collecting:** bibliomania (books); hoarding; pleonexia, plutomania

**counting, numbers:** arithmomania

**criminal, convict:** hybristophilia

**cross-dressing:** andromimetophilia, gynemimetophilia, transvestophilia

**death:** autoassassinophilia; necromania; necrophilia; pseudonecrophilia (dead bodies); taphophilia (graves, cemeteries)

**destruction:** agriothymia ambitiosa (of other nations); agriothymia

**religiosa (of other religions)**

**difference:** (between self and object): chromophilia (age); morphophilia (physique)

**drugs:** cocainomania (cocaine); etheromania (ether, inhalants); opiomania (opiates); toxicomania

**eating, food:** allotriophagy (unnatural food, such as thread); bulimia; opsomania (sweets); polyphagia

**enemas:** klismaphilia

**exhibiting self:** autagonistophilia, exhibitionism, peodeiktophilia

**family, upbringing:** ecomania, oikiomania

**filth, excreta:** coprolagnia, coprophilia, mysophilia, scatologia, urolagnia, urophilia

**fire, firesetting:** pyrolagnia, pyromania

**gift giving:** doromania

**hairbiting:** trichophagy

**hairpulling:** trichotillomania

**health, body functioning:** hypochondriasis, nosomania

**images:** iconomania (collecting or worshiping)

**imitation, mimicry:** echomimia, echopraxia, philomimesia

**infant, infant role:** autonepiophilia, infantilism, nepiophilia

**injury, pain:** algolagnia, algophilia (not necessarily sexual); biastophilia; castrophilia (castration); flagellomania (whipping); humiliation; lagneuomania (sexual sadism in male); machlaenomania (masochism in female); raptophilia; sexual masochism; sexual sadism; tomomania (desire to be operated-upon), traumatophilia

**insertion into penis:** catheterophilia

**lies, myths:** mythomania

**litigation:** processomania

**marrying:** gamonomania

**masturbation:** chiromania; psycholagny

**murder, blood:** erotophonophilia; hemothymia; homicidomania; phonomania

**nostalgia, homesickness:** nostomania; philopatridomania

**novelty:** philoneism

**odors:** olfactophilia; osphresiolagnia; renifleur

**old persons:** gerontophilia; gerophilia

**pain:** see injury, pain

**the past:** d'elire ecmnesique

**plucking threads:** allotriorhexia

**power:** cratomania

**questioning:** Fragesucht

**repeating actions:** mania of recommencement; perseveration

**sadness:** tristemania

**self:** autophilia; autosynnoia; egomania; folie vaniteuse; narcissism

**sex, hypersexuality:** acrai; aphrodisiomania; brachuna

**in females:** aedoeomania; andromania; clitoromania; estromania; folie uterine; hysteromania; metromania; oestromania; nymphomania; sexual erethism

**in males:** Don Juan complex; gynecomania; pornolagnia (prostitutes); satyriasis

**sex elimination:** sexual vandalism (destroying any representation of genitals)

**watching:** mixophilia; pictophilia; scop(t)olagnia; scop(t)ophilia; voyeurism

**sleeping partner:** sleeping princess syndrome; somnophilia

**solitude:** agromania; claustrophilia; eremophilia; lygophilia (dark, gloom)

**speaking:** garrulosity; lalorrhea; logomonomania; logorrhea; mania concionabunda (public speaking)

**spending, buying:** asoticomania; chrematistophilia

**stealing:** bibliokleptomania (books); kleptolagnia; kleptomania; lopemania; monomanie du nol

**suicide:** thanatomania

**sunlight:** photomania

**symbols, tokens:** fetishism

**tattoos, piercing:** stigmatophilia

**thoughts (intrusive):** onomatomania

**thrills:** philobat, symphorophilia

**touching, rubbing:** délire de toucher; frotteurism; hyphophilia; peotillomania (one's own penis); phaneromania (one's own body); toucherism

**trees:** dendrophilia

**urine, urination:** undinism; urolagnia; urophilia

**wandering:** drapetomania; dromomania; ecdemomania;ecdemomonomania; eidemomania; eretodromomania; mania errabunda; oikofugia; planomania; poriomania; wanderlust

**words, stories:** hellenomania; logophilia; macrologia; narratophilia; telephone scatologia; telephonophilia

**work(ing):** erasionomania

**writing:** erotographomania (love letters); graphomania; graphorrhea; metromania (verses); pornographomania (obscene letters)

**mania, classification of** See *depression, classification of; mania.*

**mania, inhibited** One of Kraepelin's "mixed states," characterized by flight of ideas, cheerful mood, and psychomotor inhibition. See *mania.* "The patients of this kind are of more exultant mood, occasionally somewhat irritable, distractible, inclined to jokes; when addressed they easily fall into chattering talk with flight of ideas and numerous clang associations, but remain in outward behavior conspicuously quiet, lie still in bed, only now and then throw out a remark or laugh to themselves. It appears, however, as if a great inward tension, as a rule, existed, as the patients may suddenly become very violent. Formerly I classified this 'inhibited mania' with manic stupor; I think, however, that it may be separated from that on the ground of the flight of ideas which here appears distinctly." (Kraepelin, E. *Manic-Depressive Insanity and Paranoia*, 1921).

**mania, reactive**  Hypomania induced by some external cause. See *reactive*.

**mania à potu**  A state, produced by alcohol, characterized by extreme excitement and sometimes leading to homicidal attacks. The attack is usually brought on, in a susceptible person, by the ingestion of comparatively small amounts of alcohol. See *alcoholic intoxication*.

**mania concionabunda**  *Obs.* Mania for addressing the public.

**mania errabunda**  *Obs.* Impulsive wandering from home, apparently without aim; occurs frequently in senile states.

**mania mitis**  *Obs. Hypomania.* "The slightest forms of manic excitement are usually called 'hypomania,' mania mitis, mitissima, also, but inappropriately, *mania sine delirio*" (Kraepelin, E. *Manic-Depressive Insanity and Paranoia*, 1921).

**mania phantastica infantilis**  A rare syndrome of childhood consisting of exaltation stages, fugues, confabulations or *pseudologia fantastica* (q.v.), immaturity, and retardation of mental development. The syndrome may occur as part of the delirious state following infectious diseases, and also as a psychogenic or autochthonous reaction.

**mania transitoria**  *Obs.* "This term is used to describe a somewhat rare form of maniacal exaltation, which comes on suddenly, is usually sharp in its character, and is accompanied by incoherence, partial or complete unconsciousness of familiar surroundings, and sleeplessness. An attack may last from an hour up to a few days" (Clouston, T. S. *Clinical Lectures on Mental Diseases*, 1904). It was also called *ephemeral mania, folie instantanée*.

**maniaphobia**  Fear of insanity.

**manic episode**  A distinct period of *mania* (q.v.) of not less than 1 week's duration and severe enough to cause marked impairment in functioning or to require hospitalization.

**manic temperament**  *Obs.* Kraepelin's designation for what is today known as one of the phases of cyclothymia. "The intellectual endowment of the patients is for the most part mediocre, sometimes even fairly good, in isolated cases excellent. They acquire, however, as a rule, only scanty, and, in particular, very imperfect and unequal knowledge, because they show no perseverance in learning, do not like exerting themselves, are extraordinarily distractible, and seek to escape in every way from the constraint of a systematic mental training, and in place of that they pursue all possible side occupations in variegated alternation" (*Manic-Depressive Insanity and Paranoia*, 1921). He adds that the mood is "permanently exalted, careless, confident" and that conduct is unsteady and restless.

**manic-depressive psychosis**  A term introduced by Kraepelin in 1896 to differentiate between those psychoses that typically progress to profound dementia (dementia praecox, or the group of schizophrenias) and those that do not lead to a true deterioration (manic-depressive psychosis). The term thus came to include periodic and circular insanity, simple mania, melancholia, and many types of confusion or delirium. Although involutional melancholia was later included in the manic-depressive group, until recently (in DSM-III) the tendency in both the United States and Great Britain has been to keep the involutional group separate; and in many classificatory schemes, involutional melancholia and manic-depressive psychosis are considered the two major subdivisions of the broader category of affective psychoses.

What was called manic-depressive psychosis in the past included what are now termed *bipolar disorder* and *major depressive disorder*. In various studies the lifetime prevalence of major depression ranged from 1.8% to 9.3%, and of bipolar disorder from 0.6% to 1.2%. Major depressive disorder, in other words, is somewhere between four and 10 times as frequent as bipolar disorder. In the major depressive group, the female to male ratio is 2:1, whereas in the bipolar group, incidence in females exceeds only slightly the incidence in males. In half the cases, onset of major depression occurs between the ages of 20 and 50 years, with the average at 40 years; mean age of onset of bipolar disorder is 30 years.

In both major depression and bipolar illness, onset tends to be earlier in females.

Family studies have consistently found that the rate of affect disorder is higher in relatives of index cases (i.e., patients) than in relatives of controls. Further evidence of a genetically determined vulnerability to affect disorder comes from twin studies, where the concordance rate for monozygotic twins is 0.67, but 0.20 for dizygotic twins. Concordance in monozygotic twins is higher for bipolar disorder (0.79) than for major depression (0.54); concordance in dizygotic twins is similar (0.24 for bipolar disorder, 0.19 for major depression). Although this supports the contention that bipolar disorder and major depression are different disorders, there nonetheless remains some degree of overlap. Relatives of patients with bipolar illness have a higher than expected incidence of major depression; and in a substantial number of monozygotic twins with affect disorder, one twin manifests bipolar disorder and the other twin has major (unipolar) depression. It is currently believed that the genes for bipolar illness are at six locations on four chromosomes: 4, 12, 18, and 21.

Clinically, manic-depressive psychosis may appear in any of several forms: as a depressive episode in varying degrees of severity (simple depression or *simple retardation*, acute depression, and, according to some, depressive stupor, although many feel that this latter form is always a manifestation of catatonic schizophrenia); or as an elated or manic episode in varying degrees of severity (simple mania or hypomania, acute mania, and delirious mania, the latter being also known as *Bell mania*, typhomania, delirium grave, and collapse delirium). A fourth type of mania, chronic mania, has also been described; the symptoms here are of the same degree as acute mania, but they continue uninterruptedly for an indefinite number of years.

Some manic-depressive patients have only manic attacks throughout their lives (recurrent mania); others have only depressive episodes (recurrent depressions), and in a few the *circular* or *alternating* form is seen: a continuous alteration for years between states of depression and states of elation. In addition to these types, Kraepelin described a number of mixed states (e.g., maniacal stupor, unproductive mania), but closer scrutiny usually reveals these to be types of schizophrenic episodes. See *melancholia; suicide; unipolar depression.*

**manie de perfection** Compulsive perfectionism; *scrupulosity* (q.v.). For the person affected with such a symptom, everything must be 100% good, moral, clean, efficient, or otherwise perfect.

**manie de rumination** Janet's term for the morbid tendency to recall to mind and consider past events again and again; seen commonly in obsessive-compulsive disorder and in some depressions.

**manie sans délire** Pinel's term for patients who had outbursts of rage but were not delusional (and therefore lacked what was considered the essential element of mental illness). The group thus identified included not only manic states but also psychopathic personality and other personality disorders.

**manifest dream** The name given by Freud to the dream itself, as reported by the dreamer. The dream text or manifest dream in itself is not intelligible as far as gaining new information about the patient is concerned. In the process of analysis of the manifest dream, however, information concerning the patient, which would otherwise be inaccessible, is obtained. This information that lies behind the dream is termed the latent dream thoughts. The technique by which the latent dream thoughts are derived from the manifest dream is called dream interpretation. This technique utilizes the associations of the patient to the various parts of the manifest dreams and the meaning of certain symbols with which the patient often is unable to associate. The process by which the latent dream thoughts become the manifest dream in the dreamer's mental life is called the dream work. The two major techniques by which the dream work is accomplished are *condensation* and *displacement* (qq.v.) (Freud, S. *New Introductory Lectures on Psycho-analysis*, 1933).

**manipulanda** See *intelligence.*

**manipulative** Exploitative; skillful in getting what one wants from others, and able to control or manage others in gaining one's own ends. Most commonly the term is used in a pejorative sense to refer to patients whose artful maneuvers in getting their own way border on the fraudulent; therapists are likely to use the term when they feel they have been made to feel foolish or outsmarted by their patients. Manipulative behavior may be seen in anyone, but it is particularly characteristic of some children, of personality types labeled hysterical, and of some schizophrenic patients—all of whom may use threats of throwing a tantrum, of suicide, or of other behavior that plays on the guilt of others in order to achieve their own goals of the moment. See *manipulative personality; narcissistic personality; Main syndrome.*

**manipulative personality** A type of *antisocial personality* (q.v.), two affective elements of which are characteristic: *contempt* for the other person and exhilaration related to the power the manipulator feels when he is able to deceive or fool the other person into doing something that he would probably not have done had he known all the facts. See *psychopathic personality.*

**mannerism** A frequently repeated complex movement that appears to be goal directed and meaningful for the subject but is excessive, superfluous, inappropriate, or unexpected so that to the observer it appears to be odd or bizarre.

**manslaughter** See *homicide.*

**mantra** See *Tantra.*

**manual sadism** A type of sadism in which the torture of the object is achieved through muscular eroticism, such as physical beating of the partner.

**manustupration** *Obs.* An older term for *masturbation* (q.v.).

**MAO** *Monoamine oxidase* (q.v.). See *MAOA-A.*

**MAOA-A** The gene that codes for monoamine oxidase A, which prevents excess neurotransmitters from interfering with communication among neurons. The gene, on the X chromosome, contains a repeat sequence of 30 base pairs that has been inserted from three to five times into the promotor region. The gene is polymorphic, and when it contains fewer repeats than normal, less MAO enzyme is produced and fewer neurotransmitters are removed. Men who carry the short allele (and presumably produce a limited amount of enzyme) have been shown to be more likely to be aggressive, impulsive, and even violent if they were abused as children or drink alcohol. Such men were four times more likely than other men to have committed violent crimes, such as rape, robbery, and assault.

**MAOI** Monoamine oxidase inhibitor. See *antidepressant.*

**MAP** *Mitogen-activated protein; microtubule-associated protein.* See *histones.*

**MAP2** One of the *microtubule-associated proteins (MAPS)* implicated in the pathogenesis of both schizophrenia and Alzheimer disease. See *temporal lobe.*

**maple syrup urine disease** A cerebral degenerative disorder due to a genetically induced defect in oxidative decarboxylation of the branched-chain keto acids leucine, isoleucine, and valine. It is transmitted as an autosomal recessive. Clinical manifestations are poor feeding, developmental retardation, hypertonicity, convulsions, and a urine odor resembling that of maple syrup. The latter is due to increased plasma level of the above-named amino acids, whose keto-derivatives are excreted in increased amounts in the urine. Central nervous system pathology includes defective myelin formation within the white matter of the entire brain, areas of edema and spongy change, an associated astrocytosis, and a decrease in oligodendroglia. Although genetically induced, the disease does not manifest itself clinically until after birth; death usually occurs within 2 years after onset of symptoms, which may be partially controlled on a diet low in the amino acids involved.

**mapping** 1. A technique used in the treatment of patients with dissociative identity disorder as a way to learn about the different alters: the patient is asked to place his or her name (the name of the host personality) in the center of a page. Then the host or the other alters are asked to add their own names, placed so as to indicate how close (or how far apart) the alters feel about one another.

2. *Genetic mapping* is defining the position of a gene on a chromosome relative to other genes on that chromosome. Comparing the inheritance pattern of a trait with the inheritance patterns of chromosomal regions allows a gene to be discovered even though what it is is unknown. Recombinant DNA techniques, in addition, allow a gene to be isolated solely on the basis of its location, without regard to its biochemical function. See *genetic marker; restriction enzyme.*

**MAPs** 1. Microtubule-associated proteins, including MAP-1, MAP-2, and tau. See *cytoskeleton; cytosol; histones.* 2. Member assistance programs; similar to *employee assistance programs* (q.v.).

**marasmic state** See *somnolent detachment.*

**marathon session** A long group therapy meeting that may last from 3 hours to as long as an entire weekend; used particularly at the beginning of ongoing groups where unremitting group pressure on the participants tends to remove barriers to communication and stimulate group cohesion.

**marche à petits pas** *Propulsion gait* (q.v.); a disturbance in gait in which the patient takes very short steps; seen in cerebral arteriosclerosis and striatal rigidity.

**Marchiafava-Bignami disease** A rare neuropsychiatric syndrome associated with alcoholism; the essential pathology is central necrosis of the corpus callosum and sometimes of the anterior commissure. The syndrome appears most typically in alcoholics who are addicted to crude red wine; when the central necrosis begins, the patient develops an acute psychotic picture consisting of excitement, ataxia or apraxia, disorientation, and confusion. With progression (and presumably due to spread of the process to the cingulate gyri), the clinical picture changes markedly: the patient becomes totally apathetic, aboulic, quiet, and completely inattentive; he appears devoid of all conation, shows akinetic mutism, and may develop hemiplegia or hemiparesis. Once this stage is reached, death is the usual end result. It is generally believed that alcohol per se is not the cause of this syndrome, but rather that it is due to metallic impurities found in wine as a result of processing or that it is a manifestation of vitamin deficiency.

**Marcus Gunn sign** (Marcus Gunn, British surgeon) The raising of a ptosed eyelid on opening the mouth and moving the jaw to the opposite side.

**Marfan syndrome** (Antoine Bernard Jean Marfan, French pediatrician, 1858–1942) An autosomal dominant disorder manifested in bilateral congenital ectopia lentis, vascular defects such as dissecting aneurysm of the aorta, and skeletal system deformities such as arachnodactyly and pectus carinatum (pigeon breast or chicken breast).

**marginal psychosis** See *cycloid psychosis.*

**Marie disease** (Pierre Marie, French physician, 1853–1940) See *acromegaly.*

**Marie three-paper test** Three pieces of paper, of different sizes, are placed in front of the subject, who is told to take the largest and hand it to the examiner, take the smallest and

throw it on the floor, and take the middle one and put it in his or her pocket.

**marijuana** *Cannabis; THC*; "hash," "pot." At least 60 cannabinoids are contained within the cannabis plant; the most active is tetrahydro-cannabinol (THC). Cannabis is typically smoked; its metabolites can be detected in the urine for several weeks. Marijuana is the most frequently used illicit substance; it is estimated that it has been used by as many as 66 million (33%) Americans at least once in their lifetimes. Cannabis enhances presynaptic dopamine levels at brain reinforcement loci, and the opiate antagonist *naloxone* (q.v.) attentuates such action.

Three grades of marijuana are commonly distinguished (their names are based on Indian terms): *bhang* (the leaves of the plant, the cheapest and least potent grade); *ganja* (the flowering fruit tops of the plant, from which the resin has not been extracted; the second grade); and *charas* (the extracted resin, the highest grade; technically, *hashish* denotes only this grade of marijuana).

Cannabinoid intoxication occurs while or immediately after smoking, peaks within 30 minutes, and lasts between 2 and 4 hours (although some effects continue for as long as 12 hours). Manifestatiions include tachycardia (30% to 50% above baseline heart rate) and euphoria, to both of which tolerance develops with repeated use; an intensification of perceptions and feeling of slowed time, apathy, and inappropriate laughter. The pleasurable "high" is usually followed by conjunctival injection, increased appetite, or dry mouth. Anxiety, suspiciousness or paranoid ideas, impaired judgment, and interference with social or occupational functioning are also frequent.

Intoxication impairs the performance of complex, skilled activities such as driving and it interferes with immediate recall and temporal organization. Marijuana is often consumed with alcohol, and the combination is additive to its effects on skilled performance. See *amotivational syndrome; cannabis; cannabis delusional disorder; cannabis use disorders.*

**Marin Amat syndrome** A syndrome described in 1918 consisting of closing of the eyelid on chewing or opening the mouth. Paralysis or spasm of the ipsilateral facial nerve usually precedes the appearance of the syndrome, which is probably due to a disturbance of intrinsic nuclear functions.

**Marinesco-Sjögren syndrome**   A hereditary disorder, transmitted through a polyphenous autosomal gene, consisting of congenital dementia, congenital cataract, and cerebellar ataxia.

**marital infidelity**   See *jealousy, morbid.*

**marital schism**   An abnormal family pattern reported by Lidz, Fleck, and their colleagues, in the families of schizophrenics, in which the parents hold contrary views so that the child has divided loyalties. Another pattern is *marital skew* (q.v.).

**marital skew**   An abnormal family pattern reported by Lidz, Fleck, and their colleagues, in the families of schizophrenics, in which one parent's eccentricities (usually the mother's) dominate the family and the other parent regularly gives in. Another pattern is *marital schism* (q.v.).

**marital therapy**   *Marriage therapy*; the treatment of an adult couple (not necessarily defined as such in terms of marriage; the two persons may define themselves as a couple by reason of cohabitation or mutual commitment). It addresses itself primarily to the marital relationship, i.e., the communication and interactional aspects of their living together. Although a type of family therapy, it involves only one generation. See *family therapy; marriage counseling.*

**marker**   *Genetic marker* (q.v.).

**marker, biological**   *Biomarker* (q.v.); a measurable indicator of a disease, or of vulnerability to a disease, that may or may not be causal. The term includes molecular, genetic, immunologic, and physiologic signals of events in biological systems that may appear in any of the various steps along the causation pathway of a disorder. A *state marker* varies with the clinical state or phase of the disease; it may appear just before, during, or after an episode of illness, but not during remission. A *trait marker* is one that is independent of the clinical state and reflects a genetic and biological risk for disorder. Markers might be measures of brain wave activity or neurologic, psychological, or behavioral characteristics.

Ideally, a marker for predisposition to any disease is present both before the illness develops and during periods of remission. It is possible that the vulnerability marker is directly involved in the mechanisms that increase the risk for the disease in question, but that need not be so. A disease marker might instead be only indirectly associated with a predisposition, perhaps because the gene(s) influencing the marker are located on the same chromosome, and in close proximity to the position of, the genes contributing to the development of the disorder in question.

**marker, interoceptive**   Also, *somatic marker*; a body signal that helps decision making. It is believed that *orbitofrontal cortex* (q.v.) integrates such body signals.

**Maroteaux-Lamy syndrome**   A *mucopolysaccharidosis* (q.v.) characterized by a deficiency of arylsulfatase B enzyme, with excessive dermatan sulfate in the urine, osseous and corneal defects, but normal intelligence.

**marriage, psychiatric aspects of**   Nearly one-half of the United States in the past have had laws whose interest was to prevent persons with mental disorder from marrying. In some cases, issuance of a license was interdicted; in others, performance of the ceremony was forbidden. The constitutionality of such laws has been challenged, and the question of legality of marriage typically arises only when one of the parties concerned seeks annulment of the marriage contract. The validity of the marriage can be questioned by the "incompetent" spouse on the ground that he was incapable of understanding what he was doing.

**marriage, therapeutic**   As an adjunct to their treatment, certain probably well-intentioned, but misguided, physicians advised marriage for their patients, with various rationalizations.

**marriage counseling**   "The process through which a trained counselor assists two persons to develop abilities in resolving, to some workable degree, the problems that trouble them in their interpersonal relationships. A basic assumption is that all individuals grow to greater adequacy and maturity in their relationships if not blocked by such obstacles as loneliness, fear, hostility, guilt and their displacements, or transferences which prevent a person from experiencing the present as it really is and hence behaving effectively. New experience in communication is offered, and a search for more realistic solutions of present difficulties is made in an atmosphere of acceptance and understanding. The process is not encumbered with detailed consideration of conflicts in the past, their devious and disguised transferences, or with intense and difficult ventilations of feeling" (Appel, K. E. et al. *American Journal of Psychiatry 117*, 1961).

**marriage therapy** *Marital therapy* (q.v.).

**Martinotti cells** *Mcs; see neocortical neurons.*

**masculine** Referring to a set of sex-specific social role behaviors, unrelated to procreative biological function, that identify the person as being a boy or a man. Contrast with maleness, which refers to anatomic and physiological features relating to the male's procreative functions. See *gender identity.*

**masculine attitude in female neurotics** Adler uses this term to indicate the masculine protest against feminine or apparently feminine stirrings and sensations occurring in the female neurotic. She manifests unconscious tendencies to play the masculine (domineering, active, cruel) role with the use of all available means.

**masculine protest** Applied by Adler to both men and women, to describe a desire to escape from the feminine role, a concept he regards as the main motive force in neurotic disease. It represents the distorted apprehension of sex differences caused by the striving for superiority. If it takes an active form in women, they attempt from an early age to usurp the male position. They become aggressive in manner, adopt definitely masculine habits or tricks of behavior, and endeavor to dominate everyone about them.

The masculine protest in a male indicates that he has never fully recovered from an infantile doubt as to whether he really is male. He strives for an ideal masculinity invariably conceived as the possession by himself of freedom, love, and power.

**masculinity** While maleness primarily relates to the proper sex chromosome structure of XY individuals, masculinity is generally understood as a male's possession of the typical and well-developed secondary sex characteristics of a man. See *sex determination.*

**masculinity complex** Rebellion against castration in the girl, leading to masculine attitudes and behavior. This term is used by Freudian psychoanalysts in much the same way that Adler uses *masculine attitude in female neurotics* (q.v.).

**masculinization** See *ambitypic.*

**mask** 1. Stekel's term for characterological disguise: "Less known are other masks of homosexuality which I now mention. The love of old women (gerontophilia) and passion for children often covers a homosexual tendency" (*Bi-Sexual Love*, 1922). See *persona.*

2. To cover, disguise, conceal. Masking is the presentation of a more intense second stimulus following presentation of an initial stimulus so as to interfere with or "mask" processing of the first stimulus.

*Visual masking* refers to a group of phenomena in which processing of a target visual stimulus is interfered with due to the effects of presentation of another visual stimulus. In *backward masking*, the masking stimulus is presented at some point after the onset of the target. In forward masking the onset of the mask precedes the onset of the target. The *critical stimulus duration (CSD)* is the time needed for correct identification of the target at a preset accuracy criterion (in the absence of the mask).

Backward visual masking is used in neuropsychological assessment as a measure of a subject's perceptual threshold. For example, the letter R is flashed on a screen and is identified by the subject. The letter R is presented a second time but is followed almost immediately by a pattern of B's. If that patterned mask of B's follows the R by no more than 120 msec, the subject will see only the B's and not the masked R. The R will become "visible" again when the interval between the different letters is increased. Normal subjects will report seeing both the R and the B's in rapid succession if the interval is increased to about 200 msec. In schizophrenic patients, however, the mask will not lose its effectiveness until the interval reaches about 500 msec. Similar impairment in *critical stimulus duration* (i.e., slowness is cognitive processing) occurs even in schizophrenic patients who are in remission and in unmedicated schizotypal patients (who may be at biological risk for schizophrenia).

**Maslow, Abraham** (1908–1970) American psychologist, founder of humanistic psychology; developed theory of the hierarchy of needs; self-actualization; peak experience; *Motivation and Personality* (1956), *Toward a Psychology of Science* (1966).

**masochism** (From Leopold von Sacher Masoch [1836–1895], an Austrian novelist whose characters indulge in all kinds of sex perversions, deriving sexual pleasure from being cruelly treated) When sexual satisfaction depends upon the subject suffering pain, ill-treatment, and humiliation, the paraphilia is known as masochism. *Bondage*, the wish to be tied or chained, is one form of masochism.

Masochism is more common in men than in women. About a third of masochists also have sadistic phantasies; they are termed sadomasochists.

Krafft-Ebing defined masochism as "a peculiar perversion of the psychical *vita sexualis* in which the individual affected, in sexual feeling and thought, is controlled by the idea of being completely and unconditionally subject to the will of a person of the opposite sex, of being treated by this person as by a master, humiliated and abused. This idea is colored by sexual feelings; the masochist lives in fancies in which he creates situations of this kind, and he often attempts to realize them" (*Psychopathia Sexualis*, 1908).

Havelock Ellis notes that Stefanowsky termed it passivism. Freud originally believed that masochism was always secondary and represented a turning of sadism against the ego under the influence of guilt. Later, however, applying his theories of Thanatos or the Nirvana principle, he differentiated three types of masochism: *erotogenic masochism* (primary masochism), *feminine masochism*, and *moral masochism* (ideal masochism) (qq.v.).

**masochism, secondary** During growth the main part of sadism or the death instinct is directed outward; the portion that remains in the individual is called primary sadism or (now being directed inward upon the subject himself) masochism. Under given conditions, as in states of deep depression when the objectivated sadism is withdrawn from objects and redirected onto the subject; that is, it is introjected. This involves the process of regression to its earlier condition. "It then provides that secondary masochism which supplements the original one" (Freud, S. *Collected Papers*, 1924–1925). See *masochism*.

**masochistic character** A type of *character* that is approximately equivalent to *masochistic personality* (qq.v.).

**masochistic personality** *Masochistic character; self-defeating personality;* in the older psychoanalytic literature, moral or ideal *masochism* (q.v.). Characteristics include involvement in situations leading to disappointment or mistreatment even when other options are available; reluctance to seize opportunities for pleasure or disinterest in people who are consistently supportive and gratifying; failure to accomplish crucial tasks despite clear-cut ability to perform them; attainments bring depression or guilt feelings rather than contentment, or lead to behavior that brings about pain (such as an automobile accident or losing something of value); rejection of others' help; chronic tendencies to self-damage, self-deprecation and unwarranted self-sacrifice, with feelings of never-ending suffering and martyrdom; sabotaging one's own efforts (including therapy).

Psychoanalytically, the masochist's self-punishment is interpreted as a defense against punishment and anxiety, in that it represents a milder substitute punishment. The masochistic character avoids anxiety by wanting to be loved, but the excessive demand for love is disguised in grandiose provocation of the love object. The purpose of this is to make the provoked person react with behavior that will justify the reproach: "See how badly you treat me." See *character defense*.

**masochistic sabotage** Self-defeating attitude or behavior of some patients that aims unconsciously to provoke insult, punishment, scorn, etc., from the environment. It appears in many forms during analytic treatment, ranging from obstinate silence to insolent remarks and behavior directed against the analyst or the analytic setting (Reik, T. *Masochism in Modern Man*, 1941).

**masochistic wish dream** A dream about injury to the dreamer. Freud maintained that even dreams with a painful content will be found to be wish fulfillments.

**mass masochism** By this term T. Reik denotes "the mixture of (a) renunciation of one's own power and (b) enjoyment of its being used by proxy," such as may be seen in the enthusiasm and devotion shown by the masses to a dictator, who demands hardships and sacrifices of the masses, which they would be unable to bear if they did not consider him to be their own idealized image (*Masochism in Modern Man*, 1941).

**mass reflex** In very severe injury to or complete interruption of the spinal cord, stimulation below the level of the lesion produces the following reflexes: (1) flexion reflex; (2) contraction of the abdominal wall; (3) automatic evacuation of the bladder; and (4) sweating of the skin below the level of the lesion. The mass reflex was described by Riddoch.

**mass therapy** A psychotherapeutic term that embraces various group techniques, particularly the didactic, recreational, and class methods used for large groups.

**massa intermedia**  See *thalamus*.

**massed negative practice**  A form of behavior therapy in which the subject repeats voluntarily the target behavior (e.g., tics, compulsive rituals) as rapidly as possible for a set duration of time. According to behavior therapy, the subject will develop a reactive inhibition of the practiced behavior and the target symptoms will therefore diminish.

**Mast syndrome**  A recessively inherited form of presenile dementia, named after the family in which it was first detected. The disorder begins in the late teens with intellectual deterioration, spasticity, and dysarthria; it progresses to complete incapacitation of the affected in their thirties or forties. Early symptoms are blank facies, an unblinking stare, loss of initiative, short attention span, loss of remote memory, failure to understand verbal orders, difficulty in walking because of spasticity, and dysarthria. Extrapyramidal and cerebellar signs, if present at all, appear late in the course of the disorder.

**mastery**  By substituting actions for mere discharge reactions, the ego achieves the stage of active mastery. This involves the interposing of time, the development of a tension tolerance, and the development of judgment (the ability to anticipate the future in the imagination by testing reality).

Primary anxiety is the passive experiencing of excitation that cannot be mastered but that must be endured. See *anxiety, primary*; *transitional object*.

**masticatory spasm**  Tonic closure of the jaw; it may be part of a syndrome of hysteria, meningitis, tetanus, epilepsy; it occasionally occurs in tumors or other diseases of the pons.

**mastigophobia**  Fear of flogging.

**mastodynia**  A type of intercostal neuralgia in which there is pain and tenderness of the breast and often hyperesthesia of the nipples.

**masturbation**  Direct self-manipulation of the genitals, most commonly by the hand, usually accompanied by phantasies that are of a recognizably sexual nature typically resulting in orgasm. *Psychic masturbation* (psycholagny) is also recognized, where phantasy alone is sufficient to cause orgasm without any direct physical manipulation. The masturbatory act, then, has two aspects—form (the physical manipulations) and content (the nature of the accompanying or provoking phantasy).

As thus defined, masturbation first occurs in the phallic period, although autoerotic activity that includes the genitalia and any other areas of the body can certainly be observed from the earliest days of life. But in the phallic period, the major portion of psychic energy is invested in the genital area, and autoerotic activity at that time comes to be associated with oedipal phantasies and so can be termed true masturbation.

Kinsey found that masturbation occurred in 92% of American males and 58% of U.S. females, and these figures were in line with other surveys and estimates both in this country and in Europe. More recent studies indicate that the percentage for males may be closer to 100%, and for females 85%.

The conflicts of the adolescent over his masturbatory activity are often solved by reaction formations; if he is successful, these contribute to the formation of valuable character traits; if unsuccessful, he must find substitutes for masturbation, or the masturbation itself becomes a neurotic symptom. Thus, the control and inhibition of instinctual impulses, at least within certain limits, may well be salutary for the development of character and personality.

Probably the most important consequence of masturbation is the guilt which typically accompanies it, and the struggle to defend oneself against it which may last for years and absorb onto itself all the energy of the psychic system. Clinically it is recognized that many adolescents have a deep need to believe that masturbation is a terrible thing and strongly resist enlightenment about its harmlessness. This is because the conscious masturbatory phantasies are distorted derivations of unconscious oedipal phantasies, and if the adolescent did indeed believe that masturbation is harmless he would have to resurrect those phantasies and face the oedipal desires responsible for the guilt.

About 80% of women masturbate to orgasm at some stage in their lives; the average rate is slightly under once per week, with a tendency to increase in the week or so before *ovulation* (q.v.). A woman is more likely to masturbate, and to masturbate more often, as she gets older (up to the age of 40). The most common method is to stimulate the clitoris, which is more sensitive than the tip of the penis. Sometimes a penis substitute (dildo) is inserted into the vagina as a complement to clitoral stimulation.

When the woman climaxes, her cervix gapes and dips into the vagina; such *tenting*, as it is sometimes called, may occur several times during a single climax. Among its consequences: (1) it temporarily increases the flow of mucus from the cervix into the vagina, laying down a thick film of lubricant ready for the next intercourse; and (2) it increases the acidity of the cervical mucus which, for a while, makes it more difficult for sperm to swim through the mucus channels and for bacteria to invade and multiply.

**masturbation, symbolic**   The displacement of thinly disguised masturbatory activity upon bodily parts and organs that function as symbolic objects substituting for the clitoris or penis, even if they give no direct orgastic gratification. Such symbolic masturbation can consist of nail biting, playing with hangnails, pulling cuticle, twisting the coat sleeve or handkerchief corners, pulling at buttons, twisting and plucking hairs or hair strands, fingering nose or earlobe, or inserting of finger into nose, mouth, or ear.

**matal elap**   *Amok* (q.v.).

**matching system**   See *mirror neurons*.

**materialization, hysterical**   *Somatization* (q.v.); Ferenczi's term for that type of conversion hysteria in which unconscious conflicts are expressed as alterations of physical functions. See *hysteria*.

The particular alterations occurring in physical functions symbolize certain specific memories and phantasies, determined by the patient's history and centering around the repressed instinctual demands and the anxieties they cause. Sometimes the conversions can be analyzed in the same way as dreams and the underlying phantasies uncovered, for often the same distortion mechanisms are used.

**maternal container**   See *communicative matching; container-contained maternal function*.

**maternal deprivation syndrome**   The psychobiological response to withdrawal or withholding of the emotional, affectional, cognitive, or other supplies needed for proper development that ordinarily are provided by the mother. Most typically, it appears in children without mothers who are reared in institutions, in children who for one reason or another are separated from the mother at an early age, and in children whose mothers are incapable of providing consistently suitable emotional support for their children. See *anaclitic depression; emotional deprivation*.

Many workers in developmental psychology have maintained that maternal deprivation has deleterious short-range as well as long-range effects on personality development. See *schizophrenogenic mother*.

**maternal immune system**   See *cytokines*.

**maternal overprotection**   Characterized by a mother who indulges, coddles, or shelters the child, or interferes with any attempt by the child to take independent action. This denies the child the opportunity to explore, to learn to tolerate frustration, and to experiment with different ways of coping with the environment.

An overprotecting mother or other caregiver predisposes the child to passive, dependent types of mastery, which inevitably bring disillusion and disappointment. See *separation-individuation*.

**maternal stimulus barrier**   See *abandonment depression*.

**maternity blues**   Brief episodes of crying, irritability, and lability of mood, experienced by more than half of women following delivery of a normal child. Symptoms reach a peak on the third or fourth day postpartum and disappear spontaneously within a few days. See *postpartum psychosis*.

**mathematical biology**   That branch of biology concerned with the development of conceptual or mathematical models of various biological phenomena. From those models, various mathematical consequences are deduced that are then compared to actual experiments or other observed phenomena.

Successful mathematical theories have been developed for a large number of biological phenomena, including nerve excitation, endocrine secretions, conditioning, and learning.

**mathematical disorder**   A type of learning disorder (formerly called *academic skills disorder*) characterized by lower mathematical ability than would be expected given the child's age, intelligence, and education. It is usually first evident in early school years: the child is unable to count accurately, cannot copy numbers or figures correctly, cannot learn multiplication tables, etc. Mathematics disorder may occur alone; more commonly, it is found in combination with reading disorder (*dyslexia*, q.v.) or disorder of written expression.

**MATRICS** Measurement and Treatment Research to Improve Cognition in Schizophrenia, an ongoing project that includes representatives from NIMH, academia, industry, FDA, and consumer groups. There is a relationship between negative symptoms and cognitive impairment in schizophrenia that is a core feature of the disease and not the result of either symptoms or medication. The deficits that have been reported are of highest magnitude in verbal memory, visual memory, and word fluency; lowest in block design, vocabulary, and digit span; deficits on the Continuous Performance Test, Trail Making Test—B, and Wisconsin Card Sort Test fall in between.

Because the cognitive impairments may provide important treatment targets, the group identified separable cognitive domains where improvement in cognitive function could be demonstrated: speed of processing, attention or vigilance, working memory, verbal learning and memory, visual learning and memory, reasoning and problem solving, and social cognition. Added to evaluation of these domains were measures of functional capacity, interview-based assessments of cognition, and self-reporting of community outcome.

**matrix** The supporting structure within which anything is embedded (e.g., the womb). In cellular anatomy, matrix refers to the interior of the mitochondrion as contrasted with the inner mitochondrial membrane. See *striatal cortical inputs*.

**matrix, therapeutic** In *marital therapy*, the specific patient–therapist combination used (e.g., therapist with one spouse in classic individual therapy, a different therapist for each spouse in collaborative therapy, one therapist seeing both spouses separately in concurrent therapy). The most common form of marital therapy is *conjoint*, where the spouses are seen together by the therapist (or by a cotherapy team).

**matrix metalloproteinases** See *metalloproteinases*.

**matronism, precocious** In constitutional medicine, a dysgenital syndrome in young girls, which owes its name to the physical and sexual forms of a mature woman occurring in them at an early age—the size and form of the pendulous breasts, the breadth of the shoulders, pelvis, and thighs, and the adiposity of the legs and ankles. The face also has an adult expression, menstruation appears prematurely, and the temperament is vivacious and irritable.

The morphological basis is probably a pluriglandular imbalance, in which follicular hyperovarism and cortical hyperadrenalism predominate.

**Matthew effect** A semihumorous term for the phenomenon of those already enjoying an abundance of professional or scientific recognition being likely to receive more recognition than relatively unknown writers or investigators, even though they both publish similar material. Their articles are cited frequently by other authors, and they "have established reputations, are likely to serve on editorial boards in their areas, are more likely to receive research grants, etc." (Blashfield, R. K., et al. *Schizophrenia Bulletin 8*, 1982).

**mattoid** A person of erratic mind, a compound of genius and fool. Eugenio Tanzi used the term for that subgroup of paranoia characterized by abstract delusions, garrulousness, and feelings of persecution. These patients have no hallucinations, but are erotic and ambitious types. G. Lombroso used the term mattoid for cranks, eccentrics, etc., who are not overtly psychotic but are rather on the borderline of a psychosis.

**maudlin drunkenness** Intoxicated state characterized by mawkish, silly, and blissful behavior. Bleuler regarded it as an abnormal reaction, but he did not consider it a psychosis.

**maximization techniques** See *false confession*.

**mazes test** The subject draws a line from the entrance of a maze to the exit, without entering any blind alleys or crossing any lines.

**MBD** Minimal brain dysfunction. See *attention deficit hyperactivity disorder*.

**MC** *Monochorionic* (q.v.).

**MC4R** A gene which encodes the melanocortin 4 receptor. *MC4R* mutations are strong contributors to the development of morbid obesity induced by hyperphagia; such mutations are especially prevalent in binge eaters.

**MCAT** Medical College Admission Test.

**McCune-Albright syndrome** Hyperfunction of one or more endocrine glands, café au lait spots, and polyostotic fibrous dysplasia; it is due to mutations in the gene for the α subunit of the *G protein* (q.v.).

**MCDD** *Multiple complex developmental disorder* (q.v.).

**McDougall, William** (1871–1938) American psychologist and psychiatrist; classification of emotions.

**MCE** Medical care evaluation. See *audit*.

**MCH** Melanin-concentrating hormone, a cyclic 19 amino acid neuropeptide. Antagonists of MCHR1—one of the two protein-coupled receptors (GPCRs) that mediate the effects of MCH—might have promise not only in the management of obesity but also as a treatment for depression and anxiety. *SNAP-7941* (q.v.) is one such antagonist.

**MCI** Mild cognitive impairment, typically manifested as repeated problems with short-term memory (often first noticed by a friend or relative). The impairment is not severe enough to qualify for a diagnosis of dementia, but most evidence suggests that in time the majority of subjects with MCI will develop dementia. Like patients with Alzheimer disease, many patients with MCI manifest neuropsychiatric symptoms in addition to cognitive deficits; the most frequent symptoms are apathy, depression, and agitation or aggression. Patients presenting with MCI present a diagnostic challenge in determining which patient will progress to dementia and which will remain stable. Some studies suggest that MRI scan shows a smaller than normal or shrunken hippocampus in those who progress to dementia.

Although originally envisioned as a transitional state between normal aging and very mild Alzheimer disease, MCI is now recognized as a significant indicator of cognitive decline. It corresponds to stage 3 of the *GDS* staging system (q.v.).

**McLeod syndrome** See *neuroacanthocytosis*.

**MCMD** Minor cognitive motor disorder. See *HIV-associated neurocognitive disorders*.

**MCMI** *Millon Clinical Multiaxial Inventory* (q.v.).

**McNaughton** See *criminal responsibility*.

**MCR** *Mother–child relationship* (q.v.).

**MCS** 1. *Multiple chemical sensitivity; environmental illness*; an ill-defined condition in which multiple symptoms, in more than one organ system, are ascribed to environmental exposures to chemicals of diverse structure and toxicologic action; tests of various neurotoxic agents do not explain the symptoms, which are triggered by exposures at levels far below those known to elicit symptoms in patients with bona fide hypersensitivity

reactions. The symptoms resemble those classically included in descriptions of neurasthenia and hypochondriasis: weakness, diarrhea, fluctuating energy levels, rhinitis, cystitis, recurrent "virus" infections, odor and food sensitivities, etc. The current emphasis on low-level pollutants by environmentalists and clinical ecologists is often used to support claims of an organic basis for MCS, but most investigators reject such claims.

2. Minimally conscious state; see *brain injury*.

**MDA** A *hallucinogen* (q.v.); 3,4-methylenedioxyamphetamine.

**mdab1** See *scrambler mice*.

**MDD** Major depressive disorder. See *manic-depressive psychosis; unipolar depression*.

**MDI** Manic-depressive illness; major depressive illness.

**MDMA** *Ecstasy*; 3,4-methylenedioxymethamphetamine; a short-acting (2 to 4 hours) synthetic drug related structurally to both the stimulant *amphetamine* and the hallucinogen *mescaline* (qq.v.). It is usually sold in doses of 100 to 150 mg and taken by mouth. Twenty to 60 minutes after ingestion it produces a burst of energy and euphoria; a slow "coming down" period is followed by a characteristic hangover with depression, irritability, and fatigue lasting about 24 hours.

MDMA may provoke or exacerbate underlying psychiatric illness, and patients taking MAOIs should not use it. Frequent or long-term use can produce brain damage. Serious toxicities, including death, are possible; they are difficult to predict because individual tolerance varies widely.

Typically used in all-night psychedelic dance parties called raves, MDMA can cause unconsciousness, seizures, hyperthermia, tachycardia, and hypotension. In the most severe cases, subjects develop disseminated intravascular coagulation, rhabdomyolysis, and acute renal failure, which can lead to death.

*Dantrolene* has been used successfully to treat the hypermetabolic state associated with MDMA toxicity. Dantrolene is also used to treat spasticity. Presumably because it inhibits the release of calcium from the sarcoplasmic reticulum, dantrolene reduces the mortality in malignant hyperthermia from anesthesia. It may be therapeutic in several hypermetabolic states associated with psychopharmacologic agents: the neuroleptic malignant syndrome, MAOI overdoses or idiosyncratic reactions, and the serotonin syndrome.

**MDRS** Mattis Dementia Rating Scale; assesses attention; initiation; perseveration; conceptualization; construction; memory.

**ME** *Myalgic encephalitis.* See *chronic fatigue syndrome.*

**Mead, Margaret** (1902–1978) American anthropologist; *Coming of Age in Samoa* (1928). Her reports about sexual customs in Samoa were criticized by later investigators, but contrary to some allegations it is clear that she did not engage in deliberate falsification about the sexual mores of the Samoans. Rather, she was duped about them and was herself victim to a deliberate hoax perpetrated by her traveling companion Fa'apua'a and the latter's friend Fofoa.

**mean** Arithmetic average.

**mean deviation (MD)** A description of the variability of a frequency distribution; also called *average deviation* (or *AD*). The mean deviation from the mean is computed by tabulating the amount by which each individual score in distribution differs from the mean score, considering all these deviations as positive, and then computing their mean.

The *standard deviation* (SD, also called Σ) is similar to the mean deviation, except that each deviation from the mean is squared, the squared deviations are totaled and averaged, and the square root of the average is then extracted. This gives a more reliable measure of variability than the mean deviation and is in wider use because other statistical measures are calculated on the basis of the SD. In any distribution that approximates the normal curve in form, about 65% of the measures will lie within one SD of the mean, and about 95% will lie within two SDs of the mean. When used as a measure of variability, the SD is known as the *standard error.*

**mechanism** In psychiatry, the means by which a psychic structure operates. See *defense.*

The term mechanism is also used in a less specialized sense to refer to the way in which any machine or system operates; it is also used to refer to the philosophical doctrine that human behavior is wholly explicable in terms of laws of physical mechanics.

**mechanophobia** Fear of machinery.

**mechanoreceptor** A cutaneous exteroceptor that responds to mechnical stimuli, such as pressure and vibations. Fast-change mechanoreceptors respond to brief mechanical stimuli, but only while the stimulus is altering. They include the large onion-shaped *Pacinian endings*, which detect heavy pressure and fast vibrations, and the smaller, egg-shaped *Meissner's endings*, which detect vibrations and light touch.

Slow-change mechanoreceptors respond to more gradual alterations and continue to fire even under unchanging pressure. They include bulb-shaped *Krause endings* and sausage-shaped *Ruffini endings. Merkel endings*, which may project into the lower epidermis, respond to both fast and slow mechanical changes and to light touch.

**MeCP2** Methyl-CpG-binding protein 2; an X-linked transcriptional repressor and a regulator of RNA splicing. Loss of function of this protein is a frequent cause of *Rett syndrome* (q.v.).

**Medea complex** The hatred and/or homicidal wishes of the mother toward her child. The death wishes against the offspring are usually motivated unconsciously by a desire for revenge against her husband. Fritz Wittels used the term in a more limited way to indicate a mother's death wish against her daughter. Strictly speaking, this is not correct, for the Medea of Euripides had only sons. The terms *Atreus complex* and *Heracles complex* have been suggested for a father's death wishes against his offspring.

**MEDEX** See *new health practitioners; physician extender.*

**media** The different means or vehicles by which anything is accomplished; in current usage, the term unless otherwise qualified usually refers to advertising media, including *print media* (newspapers, books, newsletters, journals, posters, etc.) and *electronic media* (radio, television, etc.). Sometimes the term is used even more broadly to refer to all communication in all its forms: all devices, techniques, processes, and systems that may be used in acquiring, processing, and disseminating any type of information to or from large numbers of people.

**medial forebrain bundle** The brain region primarily responsible for the positive reinforcement associated with alcohol and drug addiction.

**medial frontal cortex** One of the *frontal-subcortical circuits* (q.v.). It mediates motivation and action initiation; lesions of this area produce apathy, diminished drive, poor motivation, and disinterest.

**medial longitudinal fasciculus syndrome** See *internuclear ophthalmoplegia syndrome.*

**medial pain system** See *pain.*

**medial temporal lobe** *MTL* (q.v.); it includes the hippocampus, fornix, and amygdala, and the surrounding entorhinal, perirhinal, and parahippocampal cortices. The fornix is a major input/output of the hippocampus, connecting it to prefrontal cortex and a range of subcortical structures. The hippocampus includes CA1–CA3 of the hippocampus proper, the dentate gyrus, and the subicular complex.

**medial temporal lobe amnesia** *Anterograde amnesic syndrome* (q.v.).

**median** If all items constituting a series with respect to any measurable character are arrayed from smallest to largest, in order, the median is that value that will divide the total frequency in half, with just as many below as there will be above. Example: five subjects are aged 15, 20, 22, 25, and 26 years, respectively. The median age is 22, since two are younger and two are older.

**median deviation** A description of the variability of a frequency distribution; also called *probable deviation* or *probable error (PE)*. The median deviation from the mean is computed by tabulating the amount by which each individual score in a distribution differs from the mean score, considering all these deviations as positive, and then computing their median. The median deviation is the absolute amount of deviations from the mean that is exceeded by half the measures in a distribution.

**mediating mechanisms** Also, *mediators;* abnormalities of function, neither ultimate causes nor mere precipitating factors, that provide a link between causal factors and the phenomena of the disease. They are the psychological, autonomic, biochemical, or other second-order channels through which the etiologic factor(s) manifest themselves. In schizophrenia, for example, deficits in attention and perception and abnormalities in arousal or in some pathways of neurotransmission are possible mediating mechanisms for some genetic abnormality.

**mediational theory** In learning psychology, an attempt to account for variables that intervene between a behavior and its environmental antecedents or consequences. A learning theory based on only respondent and operant conditioning does not allow, for example, for the effects of habit or emotional status. Mediational theories posit different intervening variables to explain more complex behaviors and such variables as the effect of cognitive events on behavior.

**medical dissimulation** Disease forgery; *factitious disorder* (q.v.).

**medical futility** A situation in which a therapy that is hoped to benefit a patient's medical condition will predictably not do so on the basis of the best available evidence. See *brain death; vegetative state.*

**medical genetics** Three areas of medical genetics that are currently the focus of much research are gene identification, disease susceptibility, and gene therapy. Examples of the ability to identify genes without prior knowledge of the function are the genes for ataxia telangiectasia (AT), the infantile subtype of neuronal ceroid lipofuscinosis (NCL, Santavuori-Haltia disease; the responsible gene, *NCL1*, localizes to chromosome 1), and autosomal dominant polycystic kidney disease. Examples of mutant genes that predispose to cancer, in addition to the AT gene, are the breast cancer genes *BRCA1* and *BRCA2*. Not all human disease genes are identified by a purely positional cloning strategy, and understanding the function and dysfunction of genes in model organisms is becoming increasingly important in the new "dysmorphology" and is redefining many birth defects as inborn errors of development. Human genetics via the human genome initiative is in transition from DNA sequence to gene function in disease and health.

The understanding of several neurologic disorders has especially profited from genetic strategies. They include ALS, HIV resistance, the class of triplet repeat diseases (among which are fragile X, myotonic dystrophy, Huntington disease, and multiple forms of ataxia). The calcium channel involved in familial hemiplegic migraine has been identified. A form of Parkinson disease has been mapped to 4q. Researchers from the National Human Genome Research Institute (NHGRI) have pinpointed a gene that, when defective, causes a hereditary form of *Parkinson disease.*

**medical model** Any conceptualization of psychiatric illness that corresponds to those used in general medical descriptions of a disease.

Included are (1) infectious disease model—a specific agent causes a specific disease; (2) cellular pathology disease—a defect of cells or organs of the body produces the disease in question; (3) diagnostic model—disease is a variable process that moves from recognition of symptoms and palliative treatment to a definition of etiology and pathogenesis that allows rational and specific treatment.

The medical model emphasizes treatment of the disease from which the identified patient suffers. It is asserted that, at least at times, such an approach ignores the psychological and social components of illness and their role in determining not only the development of the "disease" but also the subject's response to it and the readiness to participate optimally in appropriate interventions. See *medicalization; community psychiatry; crisis intervention model.*

**medical power of attorney**   See *advance directive.*

**medical psychology**   See *psychology.*

**medicalization**   Making something medical, or explaining something in medical terms; specifically, the conceptualization of behavior within a medical model, in terms of illness and disease (rather than as a social phenomenon or a criminal offense, for instance).

In many countries of the world, throughout the 20th century, there has been a notable trend toward designating undesirable conduct or even undesirable viewpoints as illness rather than crime. The criminal law system has more and more divested itself of jurisdiction over various classes of "offenders"—the mentally ill, the juvenile, and at times the substance abuser, the alcoholic, and the sexual offender. During the same period, there has been as strong a trend toward development of the welfare state (parens patriae), with aid to the poor and public education quickly followed by retirement benefits, medical care, and ultimately comprehensive or universal care. Typically, the welfare state has embarked on programs designed not only to relieve but also to prevent ills, drawing largely on theories from the social and behavior sciences. The result has been termed the *therapeutic state,* with goals of treatment, prevention, and rehabilitation replacing the emphasis of criminal law on retribution, incapacitation, and deterrents.

In many instances, however, potential patients are apprehensive about the results.

A diagnosis—particularly if it is a psychiatric label—may engender at least as much suspicion and hostility as does the criminal label, and patients fear that society will impose on them controls that are more oppressive than the sanctions of the criminal model. Their concern has often been framed in terms of patient rights. See *consumerism; forced treatment; health law; menticide.*

**medicalization forces**   See *aging.*

**medication error**   *Adverse drug event* or *reaction;* defined by the National Coordinating Council on Medication Error Reporting and Prevention (*Taxonomy of Medication Errors,* Rockville, MD, 1998) as "… any preventable event that may cause or lead to inappropriate medication use or patient harm while the medication is in the control of the health care professional, patient, or consumer. Such events may be related to professional practice, health care products, procedures, and systems, including prescribing; order communication; product labeling, packing, and nomenclature; compounding; dispensing; distribution; administration; education; monitoring; and use."

**meditatio mortis**   A feeling of impending death; frequent in anxiety states.

**medium**   See *channeling.*

**mediumistic hypothesis**   Baynes's hypothesis that the schizophrenic patient is closer than others to the collective unconscious and is strategically in a position to recognize forthwith the early signs of his own disintegration; therefore, he is able to foresee the unconscious trend of events better than can those whose firm clinging to existing forms and conditions renders them insensible to such signs.

**medroxyprogesterone acetate**   *MPA;* an *antiandrogen* (q.v.).

**medulla oblongata**   The pyramid-shaped portion of the brain stem lying between the spinal cord and the pons. The ventral portion contains the pyramidal decussation; the lateral portion contains the funiculus gracilis and the funiculus cuneatus. The medulla also contains the nucleus of the hypoglossal nerve, the nucleus ambiguus (somatic motor nucleus of glossopharyngeal, vagus, and spinal accessory nerves), the dorsal motor nucleus, and the sensory nucleus of the vagus nerve, and the dorsal and ventral cochlear nuclei. The medulla oblongata is sometimes called the bulb; syndromes resulting from lesions of the medulla are therefore known as bulbar syndromes, whose characteristic symptoms are due to involvement of the various tracts passing through the medulla and particularly to involvement of the nuclei of cranial nerves IX, X, XI, and XII. With the pons, the medulla is involved in regulating blood pressure and respiration.

**medulloblastoma** See *glioma; intracranial tumor.*

**Meduna, Ladislas J. von** (1896–1964) Hungarian-born U.S. psychiatrist; developed Metrazol therapy, carbon dioxide therapy.

**MEG** *Magnetoencephalography* (q.v.).

**megadose** Very high dose of any drug, often of the magnitude of 1000 times the usual dose. Megadose therapy of schizophrenics with fluphenazine, for instance, has often used 800 to 1200 mg per day, equivalent to 40,000 to 60,000 mg per day of chlorpromazine. Less commonly, megadose treatment refers to rapid neuroleptization. See *depot neuroleptic; neuroleptization, rapid.*

**megalo-** Combining form meaning big, great, from Gr. *megas, -alon,* akin to L. *magnus.*

**megalomania** A type of delusion in which the subject considers himself possessed of greatness. He may believe himself to be Christ, God, Napoleon, etc. He may think that he is everybody and everything. He is lawyer, physician, clergyman, merchant, prince, generalissimo, ace athlete in all divisions of sports, etc. The ideas in megalomania are called *delusions of grandeur* or *grandiose delusions.*

**megalophobia** Fear of large objects.

**megalopia hysterica** See *macropsia.*

**megavitamin** See *orthomolecular.*

**megrim** *Obs. Migraine* (q.v.).

**Meige syndrome** Oromandibular dystonia with *blepharospasm* (q.v.).

**meiosis** *Genet.* That particular kind of cell division in sexual reproduction that occurs in the sex glands immediately preceding gametic formation, resulting in a reduction of the chromosomes from the double or *diploid* number, characteristic of all somatic cells, to the halved or *haploid* number, characteristic of gametes. The "reduction division" leads to the separation of the two elements of each chromosome pair and provides the necessary basis for the segregation of genetic factors. Meiotic divisions are thus genetically *segregation divisions.* See *chromosome.*

**Meissner endings** See *glabrous; mechanoreceptor.*

**melancholia** *Depression* (q.v.); *cafard; monomania.* Although in earlier usage depression

and melancholia were approximately equivalent, the current tendency, is to use melancholia in a more limited sense to indicate severe or malignant depression, an equivalent of endogenous depression or depression with psychotic features; characteristics are pervasive anhedonia, lack of reaction to stimuli that would ordinarily be pleasurable, diurnal variation with depression at its height in the morning, early morning awakening, anorexia and weight loss, and excessive and inappropriate guilt. For many, the term implies an organic etiology and it is similar to what other classifications label as *autonomous, endogenous, endogenomorphic,* or *nonreactive.* See *melancholia gravis; hypochondriacal melancholia.*

According to Freud, normal mourning is to melancholia as normal fear is to morbid anxiety. Briefly stated, the loss of love object leads to withdrawal of libido from reality and the introjection of the libido upon the mental picture of the lost love object. Abraham theorized that in these states libido regresses to the oral stage. See *manic-depressive psychosis.*

**melancholia agitata** Agitated depression; usually the term refers to involutional psychosis, although in the 19th century it was used to refer to catatonic excitement. See *involutional psychosis.*

**melancholia gravis** *Obs.* Kraepelin's term for the depressive syndrome in which "the patients see figures, spirits, the corpses of their relatives; something is falsely represented to them, 'all sorts of devil's work.' Green rags fall from the walls; a coloured spot on the wall is a snapping mouth which bites the heads off children; everything looks black. The patients hear abusive language ('lazy pig,' 'wicked creature,' 'deceiver,' 'you are guilty, you are guilty'), voices which invite them to suicide; they feel sand, sulphur vapour in their mouth, electric currents in the walls" (Kraepelin, E. *Manic-Depressive Insanity and Paranoia,* 1921).

**melancholia vera** See *anxietas praesenilis.*

**melancholia zoanthropia** *Lycanthropy* (q.v.).

**melancholy** In current psychiatry the term is synonymous with *melancholia* (q.v.). In literature of the 19th century melancholy was distinguished from melancholia "in that there are no morbid sense perversions, no irrationality of conduct, no morbid loss of self-control, no sudden or determined impulse towards suicide or homicide, and where surrounding events and occurrences still afford a certain amount of interest, though lessened in degree, and where the power of application to ordinary duties is still present" (Tuke, D. H. *A Dictionary of Psychological Healing*, 1892).

**melanopsin** A *photoreceptor* (q.v.) found in the type of retinal ganglion cell that allows light to entrain the circadian clock, the intrinsically photoreceptive retinal ganglion cells (*ipRGCs*). Melanopsin is the photopigment in these cells, which capture the light signal and relay it directly to the suprachiasmatic nucleus; they also link to brain areas that control responses to light that do not require the image-forming visual system, such as constriction of the pupils and the direct effect of light on the sleep-wake state.

**MELAS syndrome** A childhood disorder consisting of mitochondrial myopathy, encephalopathy, lactic acidosis, and strokelike episodes that bear little relation to blood vessel distribution. Postmortem examination shows spongy degeneration of the brain. See *mtDNA*.

**melatonin** A peptide neurotransmitter and the principal hormone of the pineal body; it is synthesized from serotonin in the pineal gland. Synthesis is stimulated by darkness (thus, melatonin is sometimes referred to as the *Dracula hormone*) and inhibited by light. Melatonin affects biological rhythms, although what role it may play in the development or treatment of disordered rhythms (such as circadian rhythm sleep disorder and seasonal affective disorder) has not yet been fully determined. The biological clock is set mainly by light; the effects of melatonin are generally in a direction opposite to the effects of light. Administered in the morning, melatonin delays the biological clock; given in the evening, it advances the clock. See *clock, biological; rhythms, biological.*

Patients with major depression show a decrease in nocturnal melatonin secretion, and treatment with desipramine increases the nocturnal secretion of melatonin. Plasma melatonin is increased during manic phases as compared with depressed phases; this may be a trait marker for bipolar disorder because it is found also in euthymic bipolar disorder patients. See *hypothalamic-pituitary-adrenal (HPA) axis; peptide, brain.*

Used as a drug, it is capable of resetting the brain's circadian clock, turning it forward

when given at dusk and backward when given at dawn. It turns down the activity of SCN at night; its function may be to keep the clock from being activated and inadvertently reset by stray bursts of neural activity.

**melissophobia** Fear of bees.

**Melkersson-Rosenthal syndrome** Recurrent, gradual, persistent swelling of the lips, clefts or folds in the tongue, and facial paresis; the syndrome occurs in subjects with an unstable vegetative nervous system and is usually precipitated by stress or other psychic factors.

**Mellanby effect** The intoxicating effects of alcohol are more pronounced when the *BAL* (q.v.) is rising than when it is falling.

**melomania** *Obs.* Psychosis characterized by incessant singing.

**memantine** An NMDA-receptor antagonist, used in the treatment of Alzheimer disease. It appears to be better tolerated than cholinergic compounds, and it may be used in combination with them. See *anticholinesterases.*

**membrane** The covering of a cell. Biological (cellular) membranes are composed of two layers of phospholipids, which play an important role in electrolyte transport, signal transduction, and neurotransmitter-receptor function. Phospholipids may be reduced in schizophrenia; membrane abnormalities have also been reported in Alzheimer and Huntington diseases, mood disorder, and myotonic dystrophy.

**meme** The basic unit of cultural inheritance, analogous to the gene in biological inheritance. The meme is considered to be a unit of information contained in the brain; its outward manifestations are meme products. In the last chapter of *The Selfish Gene*, Dawkins used the term meme as a kind of unit of selection for cultural matters of the same sort that Lumsden and Wilson label a *culturgen* (q.v.). The memes are carriers of such things as fashions, popular tunes, and fads in speech, but unlike culturgens they have no direct relationship with the actual genotype. There is a functional similarity of memes to genes in that both are replicators and both are carriers of information. But when it comes down to exactly *how* the information is carried and replicated, Dawkins parts company with Wilson and Lumsden. Memes replicate by being passed from brain to brain as pure information; culturgens replicate by epigenetic rules processed by the physical genotype. In this sense, Dawkins's conceptualization of the cultural evolutional is an antisociobiological argument against the strict material transmission inherent in the hard-core position of Lumsden and Wilson.

**mem-element**    See *system*.

**memories, childhood**    See *false memory; hypnosis*.

**memory**    The ability to encode (acquire, learn), store (consolidate), recall (retrieve), and reproduce what has been learned or experienced (the ability to retrieve new events and skills). It is a complex mental function that involves a change in the properties of the brain system (*memory trace* or *engram*); the component processes involved are subserved by dissociable brain regions and include at least the following:

1. *Primary response* (q.v.)—perception of what is to be learned

2. *Short-term memory* (q.v.)

3. *Long-term retention—long-term memory* (q.v.)

4. *Retrieval*—bringing stored material into consciousness at will. In some dysmnesias, the first symptom is having to wait excessively long before the information can be retrieved; the "It will come back to me in a moment syndrome" or the "tip of the tongue syndrome"—demonstrated by the two women who ran into each other while shopping one afternoon; they hadn't seen each other for years and decided they would try to catch up on their old friendship over a cup of coffee. Once seated, one said, with some embarrassment, "I realize we were great friends, but I just can't seem to remember your name." The other replied: "Oh, I understand" and, after a painful silence, "How soon do you have to know?"

5. *Activation* or *Readout*—decoding retrieved material, a process that is affected by the rest of the mental apparatus so that what is finally reproduced is different from what was actually laid down as a memory trace. Memories are not stored as fixed and immutable entities; rather, they are re-created each time they are recalled. Thus, they can change. This means too that eyewitnesses are notoriously unreliable: they are affected both by what they expect to see and hear and by the questions they are asked. See *hypnosis*. One exception is the *flashbulb* memory, a personal experience that stands out with particular vividness and is remembered accurately rather than being distorted with each recall.

Functionally and anatomically, there is more than one distinct memory system. One, *declarative memory* (q.v.), is dependent upon the *MTL* (q.v.). The neostriatum (caudate nucleus and putamen) supports the gradual, incremental learning characteristic of habit acquisition. Emotional conditioning depends upon the *amygdala* (q.v.) and neocortex, classical conditioning of skeletal musculature on the cerebellum, and perceptual priming on the posterior neocortex and medial temporal system. Memory is localized in the sense cell assemblies within particular brain systems (e.g., visual, spatial, and olfactory) that represent specific aspects of each event, but it is distributed in that many neural systems participate in representing a whole event.

Memory is a constructive recategorization during ongoing experience, rather than a precise replication or representation of a previous sequence of events; it is a process of continual recategorization leading to the ability to repeat a performance. It consists of a set of degenerate neural circuits making up a diverse repertoire combined with a means of changing the synaptic populations upon receipt of various input signals and a set of value constraints that increase the likelihood of an adaptive/rewarding output being repeated, no matter which degenerate circuit is used. Selection occurs at the level of synapses through alteration of their efficacy or strengths. Memory is a system property and allows perception to alter recall and recall to alter perception.

Most current theories of memory and learning propose modification of existing synapses as the crucial mechanism. The theories of the 1950s and 1960s, that memories are coded molecularly, and that each memory is coded by RNA (and can thus be passed on to the offspring, or even by feeding the naive animal brain slices from the trained animal), have for the most part been abandoned.

**memory, automatic**    1. *Reflexive memory* (q.v.). 2. Reaction of an affective state or emotional complex by means of an associate link to the original situation, even though the subject is not aware of the association.

The term, used by Morton Prince, is rare, although the phenomenon is well-known; one type of automatic memory is *déjà vu* (q.v.).

**memory, biological** Inherited knowledge of how to react; inherited engram. Instincts, for example, may be an expression of such biological memories or inherited engrams. The collective unconscious of Jung probably springs from biological memories in that the motives and images that he includes in the term collective unconscious are not dependent upon the acquisitions of personal existence, but originate in the inherited brain structures. See *memory, physiological.*

**memory, false** See *false memory.*

**memory, physiological** M. Prince's term for the process of registration, retention, and reproduction of a somatic experience outside the field of conscious awareness; conditioning of autonomic system reactions would be an example of physiological memory.

**memory, primary** *Akoluthia* (q.v.).

**memory, unconscious** Retention of mental impressions of an event, even though, in ordinary circumstances, they are not subject to recall into consciousness. Freud first applied the concept to his studies of hysteria. He found that certain events, usually sexual, occurred to the patient, but were so unbearable that they were actively put out of consciousness by being repressed. In the process of *repression* (q.v.), the ideational content as well as its affective component is relegated to the unconscious and kept there as an unconscious memory or unconscious image.

**memory cramp** Constant and annoying recurrence of certain tunes, melodies, phrases, verses of poetry, etc.

**memory disability** Difficulty with storage or retrieval of information.

**memory distortions** Scrambled memories, distinguished from retrieval failures ("At the moment I can recall everything but the name") and storage problems. The latter may be due to inattention, or they may be a manifestation of neurodegenerative disorder, such as Alzheimer disease. Memory distortions are more insidious than retrieval or storage problems. Because memory is malleable, it may lead an observer or a participant in an event to identify the wrong person as having been there. It may lead to describing an event with added details that were not a part of the event, or lacking significant elements that were part of the event. The distorted memory is not unconscious lying; the person describing the

event feels certain of the truth of his or her memory.

In cases of eyewitnesses to a crime, scrambled recall could send the wrong person to prison. Memory distortions can also contribute to failures to convict a guilty person, because accurate witness testimony can be undermined. If witnesses misremember some detail, or are told that their stories conflict with other evidence, they can begin to doubt their own testimony and be less persuasive to a jury than they would otherwise have been.

There are several reasons that witnesses' memories become scrambled. Witnesses to a crime talk to one another at the scene and cross-contamination can occur. They pick up information, or misinformation, from other sources, such as the media. They combine bits of memory from different experiences. Leading questions can easily contaminate their memories; many studies have shown that it is quite possible to make people believe that a childhood experience had occurred when in fact it never happened. Law enforcement interrogations that are suggestive can lead witnesses to mistaken memories, even ones that are detailed and expressed with confidence. Some psychotherapeutic techniques rely heavily on suggestion, which can lead patients to false beliefs and memories. "Psychological science has not yet developed a reliable way to classify memories as true or false" (Loftus, E. *Nature Reviews Neuroscience* 4: 231–234, 2003).

**memory drum test** The subject reads the words that appear in a slit on a moving drum and is asked to remember the words.

**memory for designs test** The subject is shown 15 geometric designs of varying degrees of complexity. After the presentation of each design, the subject is asked to draw it.

**memory hallucination** Reappearance of repressed material as a visual image.

**memory headers** Mental labels for memory storage records, such as the name of a friend. The labels hold information about the friend's current identity and links that information with stored memories about that friend. Through such linkages the friend can be recognized no matter how much time has changed him or her. Memory headers are constantly updated with new cues and link stored memories of friends, places, and the like with their current status. Sometimes the linkages fail and lead to the experience of recalling many details about someone without being able to recall the name of the person—the memory storage file has been accessed but the header which labels it is has, at least for a time, been lost.

**memory image** Anticipation of the recurrence of a past experience, immediately before its recurrence, as in conditioning experiments when the subject anticipates a repetition of the electric shock. According to Reid, "the past situation returns in the service of the present," and it can even be reproduced with hallucinatory vividness. In such cases the memory image may be said to be a part of the conditioned reflex in Pavlov's sense, that is, the memory image is an ingredient of the inner preparedness for the stimulus, and is part and parcel of the individual's total reaction.

**memory romance** In psychoanalysis, the phantasy standing between infantile impressions and later symptoms. In speaking of hysteria Freud said that "between the symptoms and the infantile impressions were interpolated the patient's phantasies (memory-romances), created mostly during the years of adolescence and relating on the one side to the infantile memories on which they were founded, and on the other side to the symptoms into which they were directly transformed" (*Collected Papers*, 1924–1925).

**memory span** The span of immediate memory is the longest sequence of items that can be reproduced correctly following a single presentation; when the items are presented in a random order, the normal span is about seven. The memory span procedure was devised by Joseph Jacobs in 1887. The point at which the subject is right 50% of the time is designated as the memory span. In the 1950s it was found that immediate memory span is governed by chunking—grouping together integrates pieces of information. Recall is improved by inserting a brief pause between chunks—called *rhythmic chunking*. See *short-term memory*.

**memory storage** Memory is believed to be stored in the same neural systems that are involved in the perception, analysis, and processing of the information to be learned. See *long-term memory*; *short-term memory*.

Synaptic plasticity related to memory storage involves *cAMP*-mediated activation, by protein kinase phosphorylation, of the *CREB* (cAMP response element–binding protein) transcription factor. Activation of these positive regulators is important in the consolidation of short-term memory into long-term memory storage. Long-lasting forms of synaptic plasticity also require removal of inhibitory constraints, *memory suppressor genes*, that prevent memory storage.

**memory suppressor genes** See *NMDAR receptor*.

**memory trace** *Engram* (q.v.); the material that remains in consciousness when a painful experience is not completely repressed.

**memory training** Procedures used to improve memory. Ebbinghaus first showed that repetition gives longer-lasting memories; that *spaced training* (repeated training sessions with a rest period between each) produced longer-lasting memories than did *massed training*; that early and late words on a list are remembered better than those in the middle (the *primacy* and *recency effects*); that material is better learned when read from beginning to end, rather than in parts.

**memory-modulation hypothesis** It states that the greater long-term memory for emotional than for neutral events reflects the neuromodulatory influence of the *amygdala* (q.v.) on consolidation processes in the medial temporal lobe memory system through engagement of stress hormones.

**menace reflex** Blinking in response to a feint with the (examiner's) hand or other object toward the subject's eye.

**mendacity** As used in psychiatry, pathological lying. See *liar, pathological*.

**mendelian laws** The mendelian laws relating to the mechanism of inheritance account for the results of Mendel's breeding experiments in terms of the segregation, independent assortment, and recombination of the individual gene factors, which he postulated as existing in the gametes as independent units for every inherited character. This system consists of at least two different principles.

First, *segregation*, or clear separation of genetic factors during the formation of the gametes: the various characters of hybridized organisms are transmitted separately and distributed to the reproductive cells independently of each other so that they may form any possible combination. Every known hereditary trait operates in accordance with segregation, and this principle is to be regarded as the basic aspect of the mendelian system of heredity. Although it was evolved from examples with both dominant and recessive characters, dominance is not an essential feature of mendelian inheritance, as is demonstrated by many intermediate hybrids. While dominance alone does not necessarily presuppose the existence of unit characters, this element is essential to the law of segregation.

Second, the *independent* assortment of the genetic factors and their recombination. It is demonstrated by the 9:3:3:1 ratio in the redistribution of the four gene factors involved in the crosses with two different pairs of allelomorphic characters (see *Mendelism*). According to the same principle, the ratio 27:9:9:9:3:3:3:1 results, on the average, in the F2 generation of a *trihybrid* mating, that is, one involving three pairs of allelomorphs, one member of each pair being dominant.

The simple formulation of the entire mendelian law is as follows: When two organisms unlike with respect to any character are crossed, and the parent whose trait appears in the offspring is the *dominant*, and the other parent is the *recessive*. When, however, the hybrids of this first generation are in turn crossed with each other, they will produce a variety of offspring. One-fourth of them will be like the recessive one, and the remaining half like the parents who resembled the dominant grandparent, yet failed to breed true to it. See *dominance; recessiveness.*

The four patterns of mendelian transmission are autosomal dominant, autosomal recessive, sex-linked dominant, and sex-linked recessive.

**Mendelism** The biological phenomena underlying the distributive mechanism of organic inheritance as discovered by the Augustinian abbott Johann Gregor Mendel (1822–1884). See *mendelian laws.*

**mendicancy, pathological** A syndrome characterized by the necessity on the part of the patient to beg, regardless of any real financial need.

**Ménière syndrome** (Prosper Ménière, French physician, 1799–1862) Dilatation of the endolymph system of the internal ear of unknown etiology, leading to episodic vertigo associated with tinnitus and increasing deafness. It occurs more often in males, typically in late middle age.

**meninges** The membranous coverings of the brain and spinal cord. The outermost

meninx is the *dura mater*; the middle one is the *arachnoid*; the innermost is the *pia mater.* The dura mater is known as the *pachymeninx*; fibrous processes of the dura mater form the *falx cerebri* (which separates the two cerebral hemispheres), the tentorium cerebelli (which forms a partition between the posterior and middle fossae of the skull), the *falx cerebelli* (which separates the cerebellar hemispheres), and the *diaphragma sellae* (which forms a roof to the sella turcica and through which passes the infundibulum). The arachnoid and pia mater are known as the *leptomeninges*; the space between them is the subarachnoid space, which contains the cerebrospinal fluid.

**meningioma** See *intracranial tumor.*

**meningismus** Meningeal manifestations closely simulating those of meningitis, but in which no actual inflammation of the meninges is present.

**meningitis** Any inflammatory process involving the cerebrospinal leptomeninges, producing mental symptoms of the organic reaction type, in its acute form, with severe headache, delirium, somnolence, or stupor. Localized or generalized convulsions, generalized rigidity, twitching, and monoplegia or hemiplegia may also occur.

**meningitis, aseptic** Meningitis without identifiable organisms in the gram stain or bacterial culture of the spinal fluid; usually due to virus infection.

**meningitis, serous** See *pseudotumor cerebri.*

**meningitophobia** A hysterical presentation of meningeal symptoms; morbid dread of brain disease.

**meningocele** A developmental anomaly in which there is a protrusion of the membranes of the brain or spinal cord through a defect in the skull or spinal column, respectively.

**menkeiti** *Miryachit* (q.v.).

**Menninger, Karl Augustus** (1893–1990) American psychoanalyst; criminology, classification, unitary concept of mental illness; *The Vital Balance* (1963), *Theory of Psychoanalytic Technique* (1948).

**Menninger, William Claire** (1900–1966) American psychoanalyst; military psychiatry, mental hospitals.

**menopause** Climacterium; the period of natural cessation of menses; the involutional period; known popularly as "change of life." See *involutional psychosis.*

**mens rea** (L. "criminal mind") Guilty intent or the mental ability to have such an intention, often an important legal consideration in determining an accused person's criminal responsibility. See *insanity defense; criminal responsibility.*

**menstruation**  See *ovulation.*

**mensuration**  Measurement of areas and distances on the surface of the body.

**mental deficiency**  See *retardation, mental.*

**mental dictionary**  See *grammar.*

**mental disorders, classification of**  See *DSM-III; DSM-IV; nomenclature, 1968 revision.*

**mental handicap**  See *retardation, mental.*

**mental health**  1. *Mental hygiene* (q.v.), in which sense mental health is a field based on the *behavioral sciences* (q.v.) and amplified with scientific, professional, and social applications.

2. Psychologic well-being or adequate adjustment, particularly as such adjustment conforms to the community-accepted standards of human relations. Some characteristics of mental health are reasonable independence; self-reliance; self-direction; ability to do a job; ability to take responsibility and make needed efforts; reliability; persistence; ability to get along with others and work with others; cooperation; ability to work under authority, rules, and difficulties; ability to show friendliness and love; ability to give and take; tolerance of others and of frustrations; ability to contribute; a sense of humor; a devotion beyond oneself; ability to find recreation, as in hobbies (Appel, K. E. *Journal of the American Medical Association 172,* 1960). See *norm, psychic.* WHO defines health as a state of complete physical, mental, and social well-being, and not merely the absence of disease and infirmity. The attitude towards health, in other words, should be positive, even though in practice its definition relies heavily on negative indices such as morbidity and disability. Average is not the same as health, for average always includes mixing in with the healthy the prevalent amount of psychopathology. Although almost no form of behavior is considered abnormal in all cultures, that does not mean that the tolerated behavior is mentally healthy. See *abnormality; disease; norm, psychic.*

Mental health is defined in different terms by different authors; its characteristics are typically described as combinations of some of the following:

a. Autonomy—recognition of one's own needs, being in touch with one's own identity & feelings.

b. Subjective well-being; maintaining self-efficacy, zest, enthusiasm.

c. Wisdom and knowledge: love of learning, efficient problem solving, including accurate perception of reality, judgment/open-mindedness, creativity/originality/ingenuity.

d. Resilience: capacity to adapt to change and endure frustration and loss, coping mechanisms (including unconscious defense mechanisms) to overcome stressful situations.

e. Evolution of social-emotional intelligence over time; in Erikson's terms, widening the social radius; developing self-regulation and temperance (including delaying gratification, displacing or channeling impulses); self-perception; monitoring one's emotions and expressing them appropriately (such as ability to discharge hostility without harming others or oneself), recognizing and responding to the emotions of others (empathy), negotiating close relationships with others, playfulness/humor. See *ontogeny, psychic.*

f. Teamwork, equality/fairness, leadership, altruistic concern for other human beings.

g. Ability to love—intimacy/reciprocal attachment; kindness/generosity/nurturance; capacity for a variety of mutually fulfilling and lasting relationships

h. Self-actualization, hope, future-mindedness; Maslow emphasized the full use and exploitation of talents, capacities, and potentialities. See *humanistic psychology.*

i. Realistic acceptance of the destiny imposed by one's time and place in the world in order to set appropriate goals for oneself and to persevere in pursuing them; *career consolidation,* to take one example, involves not only competence, commitment, and compensation, but also contentment (Vaillant, G.F., *American Journal of Psychiatry 160:* 1373–1384, August 2003).

j. Spirituality/faith; passing on the traditions of the past to the future, conserving and preserving the collective products of humankind and the culture in which one lives and its institutions.

**Mental Health Center**  See *community psychiatry.*

**mental health worker**  Staff other than the core mental health professionals (clinical psychologists, psychiatric social workers, psychiatric nurses, psychiatrists) who have had special training to help them develop the skills in helping patients and clients deal with social and psychological problems. In general, such workers perform either a therapeutic role or an advocate/ombudsman/expediter role. See *advocacy; community psychiatry; expediter.*

**mental hygiene**  The science and practice of maintaining mental health and efficiency—for a twofold purpose: first, to develop optimal modes of personal and social conduct in order to produce the happiest utilization of inborn endowments and capacities; and second, to prevent mental disorders. See *mental health; orthopsychiatry.*

**mental illness and violence**  In a 1995 study of 1000 acute, discharged mental patients between ages of 18 and 40, John Monaham of the University of Virginia School of Law reported that they fell into the following diagnostic groups: depression or dysthymia (40%); schizophrenia or schizoaffective disorder (17%); bipolar disorder or mania (13%); alcohol or other drug abuse or dependence (24%). Lowest rates of serious violence of any diagnostic group were in those diagnosed schizophrenic; highest rates were in substance abuse disorders.

In the general population, violence drops sharply as people approach 40, and then plummets; violence among women is far less prevalent than among men. But among the mentally ill, age relates only weakly to violent behavior (at least in the age range 18–40); and about 35% of men and 39% of women had some form of violence.

**mental makeup**  See *character.*

**mental masochism**  *Moral masochism* (q.v.).

**mental modules**  Parts of the mind or brain that are specialized to solve particular problems. The circuitry underlying a psychological module might be distributed across the brain in a spatially haphazard manner, and it need not be tightly sealed off from other modules. Something about the tissue in the human brain is necessary for intelligence, but the physical properties are not sufficient, just as the physical properties of bricks are not sufficient to explain architecture. Something in the *patterning* of neural tissue is critical. See *module; network.*

**mental retardation**  See *retardation, mental.*

**mental set**  See *set.*

**mental status**  The level of psychosocial, neuropsychiatric, and behavioral functioning of a subject at the time of examination. The term is commonly applied to the written report of that examination which, depending on the subject and the conditions under which the examination is conducted, typically makes reference to the following areas:

A. Appearance
1. Healthy? robust? sick? weak? prematurely aged? immature? malformations?
2. Weight, body habitus
3. Dress, hygiene, grooming
4. Sociability: poised? stilted? boisterous? uncontrolled? expansive? polite? sensitive or oblivious to social nuances? mixes with others? tactful? withdrawn? abrasive? can adapt to changing environment?
5. Motor/motility: akinesia, involuntary movements, mannerisms, gestures, compulsions, tics, chorea, athetosis, tremor, clonus; facial motility (mask-like? asymmetry? nystagmus?); coordination; strength and tone; range and speed of responses (retardation? impulsive? pressured?); gait; tongue movements; handedness
6. Use of leisure time: can relax and enjoy life; driven quality, inability to let up; energy output; goal-directed behavior
7. Attitude during interview: cooperative? domineering? argumentative? self-confident? passive? obsequious? questioning? fearful? suspicious?

B. Mood
1. Facial expression—elation, apathy, pain, dejection, grief, anxiety, distrust, bewilderment, anger, defiance, contempt, exaltation, preoccupation
2. Feelings—spontaneous reports? responses to questions? appropriateness? range (lability, blunting)? ambivalence? Question specifically about anxiety, depression (self-harm)

C. Speech and Thought
1. Content—general themes; phobias, obsessions, delusions, somatic complaints, hallucinations; is content relevant to situation? manneristic utterances?

2. Form—productivity, fluency, pressured or retarded, maintenance of continuity, mutism, blocking, verbosity, circumstantiality, neologisms, speech patterns and structure, pronunciation and mechanical aspects (stammering, lisp, slurring, dysphonia, dysarthria)

3. Language/aphasia screen: repetitive speech, echolalia, perseveration, fluency of speech, naming, verbal and written comprehension, written expression, prosody (including rhythm, stress, rate)

D. Neuropsychological Screen of Cognitive Functioning

   1. Neurologic history (e.g., seizures, incontinence), soft signs and primitive reflexes (e.g., snout, suck, grasp, palmomental reflexes; double simultaneous tactile discrimination); visual acuity, neglect, non-recognition, nystagmus; auditory acuity, tinnitus

   2. Sensation and localization: touch, temperature, vibratory, position, stereognosis; sensory neglect

   3. Inertia, impersistence, perseveration, dyspraxias

   4. Attention and concentration, participation in conversation, obtundation, distractibility (digit span, letter cancellation, spell five-letter word backward, serial subtraction)

   5. Orientation—place, time, person

   6. Memory

      a. Immediate (30 sec to 25 min)—digit span; repeat standardized story

      b. Recent, short-term (25+ min)—four words; learn 10 word-pairs

      c. Remote, long-term—place of birth; schools attended, name of first employer, draw map of the United States

   7. General intellectual functioning: educational level, general knowledge, counting, calculation, abstract problem solving, symbolic categorization, categories and similarities test, Mini-Mental State Examination

   8. Judgment and insight, self-appraisal

   9. Consideration of need for formal neuropsychological testing

E. Personality: defense mechanisms, recent changes

**Mental Status Examination Report**  See *Multi-State Information System.*

**mentales**  *Obs.* Linnaeus, in 1763, divided mental disorders (*mentales*) into three classes: *ideales, imaginarii,* and *pathetici.*

**mentalese**  The language of thought in which our conceptual knowledge is couched. Mentalese is the medium in which content or gist is captured. It is the mind's lingua franca, the traffic of information among mental modules that allows us to describe what we see, imagine what is described to us, carry out instructions, and so on. This traffic is reflected in the anatomy of the brain. The hippocampus and connected structures, which put memories into long-term storage, and the frontal lobes, which house the circuitry for decision making, are not directly connected to the brain areas that process raw sensory input. Instead, most of their input fibers carry highly processed input from regions one or more steps downstream from the first sensory area. The input consists of codes for objects, words, and other complex concepts.

**mentalism**  The view that the mind contains abstract structures which make knowledge possible; the primitive tendency to personify, in spirit form, the forces of nature and the motions of things on earth and in the heavens; the endowment of inert matter with the quality of "soul"—synonymous with *animism* (q.v.). This philosophical concept implies the existence of spiritual or mental forces completely different from the somatic structures, and denotes the subjective, mental, or mind approach to psychiatry in contrast to the behavioristic approach, which stresses objective physiological activities.

**mentality**  Mental action or power; the psyche in action. In psychiatry, mentality is considered from two points of view: (1) that of the intellect and (2) that of the instincts. The former refers to the intellectual capacity, such as superior, average, or inferior intelligence. The latter forms the basis of personality structure and function.

**mentalization-based therapy**  Developed for use in patients with *borderline personality disorder* (q.v.), its aim is to facilitate the capacity to perceive the mind and intentions of others as distinct from one's own and to reconsider one's own perception of reality. See *empathy; theory of mind.*

**mentalizing**  *Theory of mind* (q.v.).

**mentally disordered offenders**  See *offenders, mentally disordered.*

**menticide**  Mind control; brainwashing; any organized system of psychological intervention in which the perpetrator injects his or her own thoughts and words into the minds and mouths of the victims. By assaulting ego strengths, culture shock is deliberately created, with isolation, alienation, and intimidation, and the subject becomes increasingly vulnerable to the implantation of ideas or the suggestion of behavior that would ordinarily be rejected as unacceptable. See *brain control; cyberphobia; implant, dynamic; sensory deprivation.*

**mentula**  (L. "penis") Originally used in the socially taboo sense in which cock and prick are used today; "membrum virile," frequently used in Victorian medical jargon to disguise the nature of its original meaning.

**meralgia paresthetica**  A rare neuritis of the lateral femoral cutaneous nerve, characterized by numbness, pain, burning, tingling, and hypersensitivity localized on the anterior and lateral surface of the thigh usually due to pressure from obesity, abdominal binders, or corsets. Suffering can be relieved immediately by nerve block with local anesthetic.

**Mercier, Charles Arthur**  (1852–1919) British psychiatrist; forensic psychiatry.

**mere-, -mere**  Combining form meaning part, share, from Gr. *méros.*

**merergasia**  Partial ability to work or function; kakergasia; used by Adolf Meyer to designate a clinical psychiatric syndrome that causes only a partial disorganization of the personality such as the psychoneuroses.

**merger needs**  See *cohesive self.*

**merger-hungry personality**  See *mirroring deficits; narcissistic personality.*

**merinthophobia**  Fear of being tied up.

**Merkel endings**  See *mechanoreceptor.*

**Merkel receptor**  See *glabrous.*

**MERRF**  Myoclonus epilepsy and ragged red fiber disease. See *myoclonus; myoclonus epilepsy; mtDNA.*

**merycism**  Voluntary regurgitation, of food from the stomach to the mouth, in which it is masticated and tasted a second time, as in rumination.

**mescaline**  The active principal of the cactus from which *peyote* (q.v.) is obtained. Mescaline has been used as one of the two chief agents to produce an experimental or model psychosis (the other agent is lysergic acid). The major effects are personality disturbances and an increase in sympathetic tension in the experimental subject; the former include visual (and sometimes auditory) hallucinations, illusions, distortions of the body image, altered time sense, thought-language changes, and an increase in self-observation sometimes to the point of complete withdrawal and feelings of unreality and detachment. Both mescaline and lysergic acid are also substances of abuse. See *hallucinogen.*

**mesencephalic locomotor region**  *MLR*; a command system for locomotion which, when stimulated, produces normal walking movements. The MLR does not itself contain the central programs for walking, which are in the spinal cord. Contrary to popular belief, higher functions such as decisions and acts of will do not reside exclusively in one location, such as the motor cortex. The impulse to walk does not proceed from a cortical "executive center"; instead, the impulse is distributed throughout widely separated areas of the brain (especially cortex, subcortical basal ganglia, and cerebellum). Further, the original impulse to walk requires internally generated motor programs which are dependent on contributions from brain areas deep below the cortex.

In deciding to write one's name, for example, the writer cannot "will" the particular muscular contractions that are involved. The writer decides only to write the name; the act iself unfolds by way of feedbacks from the cortex to the sensory areas of the cortex, downward into the thalamus, with contributions from subcortical centers, most importantly the basal ganglia.

**mesencephalon**  *Midbrain* (q.v.).

**mesenchyme, mesenchyma**  Although this term was introduced in embryology by O. and R. Hertwig to denote the part of the mesoderm that separates from the original mesothelium as a loose mass of anastomosing cells to form the connective tissues, it has lost some of its precise meaning. It is now generally assumed that the mesenchymal tissue, occupying practically all the intervals between the epithelial layers, does not arise from the middle germ layer alone, but probably from certain parts of the entoderm and ectoderm also, and that it forms not only the various forms of connective tissue, but also the skeletal system, the smooth muscular tissue, the stroma of the iris and the ciliary body, the cartilages and ligaments of the larynx, and, especially, the blood and blood vessels. See *parenchyma*.

**mesial limbic structures**   The hippocampus and amygdaloid complex. See *rhinencephalon*.

**Mesmer, Franz (or Friedrich) Anton**   (1733–1815) An Austrian who first gave a demonstration of hypnotism (animal magnetism) in Vienna about 1775. At first, Mesmer used magnets for what he believed to be their latent curative power. The latter was due to a magnetic fluid that permeated space; he invented the baquet, consisting of a large tub containing rows of bottles filled with magnetic water. Patients sat around the tub holding steel rods coming up through the lid of the tub or applying them to ailing body parts and often joining hands in order to facilitate the passage of the magnetic fluid. By 1778 Mesmer had been discredited in Vienna and moved on to Paris, where, in 1784, a royal commission (headed by Benjamin Franklin, the United States ambassador to France) also concluded that Mesmer's claims had no scientific basis. ("Imagination is everything; magnetism nothing."—Franklin)

**mesmerism**   *Hypnotism* (q.v.); animal magnetism.

**mesocephaly**   See *cephalic index*.

**mesocortical tract**   See *dopamine*.

**mesodermogenic       syphilis**   Meningovascular syphilis. See *syphilis, cerebral*.

**mesolimbic system**   See *dopaminergic systems; dopamine; nucleus accumbens*.

**mesomorphic**   In Sheldon's system, the type characterized by a predominance of its third component (bulk), that is, the structures of the body that are developed from the mesoderm. The mesomorphic type is contrasted with the *ectomorphic* and *endomorphic* (qq.v.) types; it corresponds roughly to Kretschmer's *athletic type* (q.v.).

**mesopallium**   See *limbic lobe*.

**mesoskelic**   Possessing legs of normal length. In Manouvrier's system of constitutional types, a type intermediate between the *brachyskelic* and the *macroskelic* types (qq.v.). See *athletic type*.

**mesostriatal pathway**   See *dopaminergic systems*.

**messenger, external chemical**   *Pheromone* (q.v.).

**messenger, first**   See *neurotransmitter receptor; second messenger*.

**messenger, neural**   A general term for a chemical substance that conveys impulses or information from one cell to another; it includes neuroregulator, *neuromodulator, neurotransmitter*, and *neurohormone* (qq.v.).

**messenger, second**   See *neuromessenger; neurotransmitter receptor;*

**messenger RNA**   See *chromosome. second messenger; transducer*.

**messianic delusion**   A type of delusion of grandeur consisting of the conviction that one is the Messiah or savior who is to save the world and lead others out of their misery.

**met-, meta-**   Combining form meaning change, transformation, after, next, trans-, beyond, over, from Gr. *meta-*.

**meta-analysis**   Systematic analysis of a collection of results from different studies, permitting quantitative synthesis of results, including uncovering apparent contradictions between different sets of data, identifying crucial questions to be addressed in future studies, and proposing potential solutions to various problems revealed by comparison of different studies. Meta-analysis was introduced in the 1970s and has gained widespread use in the educational, social, and medical sciences.

Meta-analysis overcomes the drawbacks inherent in simple comparison of studies. It transforms the results of each study into a common metric and thus avoids both the bias in favor of studies with larger sample sizes and assignment of equal weight to differences of unequal magnitude.

**metabolic anoxia**   See *anoxia, cerebral*.

**metabolic syndrome**   The presence of three or more of the following:

(1) abdominal obesity; (2) hypertriglyceridemia (at least 150 mg/dL); (3) low high-density lipoprotein (HDL) cholesterol (less than 40 mg/Dl in men and less than 50 in women); (4) high blood pressure (at least 130/85 mm Hg); (5) high fasting glucose (at least 110 mg/dL).

The metabolic syndrome appears to be a precursor for type 2 diabetes and a risk factor for atherosclerotic cardiovascular disease. Obesity is of particular concern in psychiatry because certain mental disorders—binge-eating disorder, bulimia nervosa, bipolar disorder, some forms of major depressive disorder, schizophrenia, and schizoaffective disorder—co-occur with overweight and obesity, and because treatment with antipsychotic agents has induced weight gain in some patients.

Many other symptoms and diseases are related to obesity directly or indirectly; they include almost every organ system of the body.

**metabolic-nutritional model** A view of illness and disease that focuses on long-term studies to assess the presence of deprivations, toxins, etc. in specific population groups, and on attempts to modify, reduce, or abolish those threats to health. See *medical model; community psychiatry*. A subtype of this model is the *social integration-disintegration model*, whose basic premise is that, other things being equal, a better organized society promotes better adaptation.

**metabolism** The biophysiological processes by which the living cells and tissue systems of an organism undergo continuous chemical changes in order to build up new living matter and to supply the energy necessary for the life of an individual. The morphological effect of *metabolism* can be *anabolic* or *catabolic* (qq.v.), according to whether it is of a constructive or destructive nature.

**metabolism, first-pass** A pharmacokinetic phenomenon based on partial conversion of a drug into one or more active metabolites, whose effect is additive to or synergistic with the original compound administered.

**metabolism, mental** The rate or speed of mental processes, assumed to have an energy exchange with the environment similar to that of somatic physiological processes. Thus, Abraham described the manic as having an increased mental metabolism, continuously hungry for new objects whose incorporation will provide discharge for the patient's intensified, uninhibited, oral impulses.

**metabotropic receptor** See *ion channel; synapse; transducer*.

**metachromatic leukodystrophy** A rare autosomal recessive disorder due to a deficiency of arylsulfatase A; prominent manifestations are dementia, ataxia, and pyramidal signs. In the adult-onset form, spasticity and hyperreflexia of the lower legs are seen, whereas in the infantile form areflexia is typical.

**metacognition** The monitoring and control of one's own cognition; thinking about thinking. The MFC (medial frontal cortex), for instance, is concerned with determining future behavior on the basis of anticipated value. In the more caudal MFC, value is associated with actions; in the orbital MFC, value

is associated with outcomes. As representations become more abstract, the more forward within MFC does the activation occur. The most anterior region of MFC is associated with metacognitive representations, such as reflecting on the values linked to actions and outcomes, and reflecting on what other people think about the person.

**metaerotism** Phenomenon described by S. Rado in which intoxicants, e.g., morphine, effect changes principally in the libido. The entire peripheral sexual apparatus is left on one side as in a "short circuit" and the exciting stimuli are enabled to operate directly on the central organ.

**metaethics** The study of what it is to make a moral judgment and of the decision-making process that ultimately leads to that judgment; study of the meaning and justification of ethical terms. See *ethics*.

**metagnosis** The changing of one's mind or attitude.

**metalanguage** The rules for use of a language (e.g., grammar, syntax); or any language system that can explain, relate, or unite two or more subsystems.

In communications theory, the specific instructions that accompany the spoken word to ensure correct interpretation. Such instructions are typically expressed by voice tone, gestures, sentence construction, etc.

**metallophobia** Fear of metals.

**metalloproteinases** Proteinases that bind a metal ion, such as zinc (the *metzincin metalloproteinases*), in their active site. They are associated with various neurophysiological functions, including synaptic remodeling, long-term potentiation, and regeneration of the nervous system. They have been implicated in many different neurological conditions.

There are four subgroups of metzincins: astacins, seralysins, MMPs, and the adamalysins. There are 24 MMP members, each the product of a different gene. *MMPs* (*matrix metalloproteinases*) can cleave all protein components of the *extracellular matrix* (*ECM*); other substrates of their action include growth factors, receptors, and adhesion molecules. MMPs have the potential for massive tissue destruction, and their expression and activity are tightly regulated.

There are 29 *ADAMs* (A disintegrin and metalloproteinases), which can also cleave and remodel components of the ECM. Their best-characterized function is the proteolytic processing of membrane-anchored precursors and the subsequent release of mature proteins. This process is referred to as protein *ectodomain shedding*—release of an active factor from the cell membrane, usually from an inactive form, by proteases. Many receptor ligands that affect development and disease are released in this manner. Such shedding substantially alters the activity of the substrate.

Overall, metalloproteinases help to determine the outcome of an insult to CNS injury. Although they can be highly destructive, it is possible that some of them might also be used for repair after nervous system injury.

**metalloscopia** An obsolete method of treatment in hysteria by the application of metals to anesthetic areas.

**metamorphopsia** Faulty perception of objects, which appear to be distorted; seen most often in parietal lobe lesions and as a type of illusion in intoxication with *mescaline* (q.v.). The most common distortions are *macropsia* and *micropsia*, which are sometimes referred to as the *Alice in Wonderland effect*. See *dysmegalopsia; Lilliputian hallucination.*

**metamorphosis, delirium of** See *lycanthropy.*

**metamorphosis sexualis paranoica** *Rare.* Delusion seen most often in paranoid patients, that one's sexuality has been changed into that of the opposite sex.

**metapelet** See *kibbutz.*

**metaphor** A type of comparison in which one object is equated with another and qualities of the first are then ascribed to the second— "He was a tiresome psychoanalytical turnkey with a belt full of rusty complexes."

**metaphoric language** Metaphor is the use of a word (or phrase) literally denoting one kind of object (or idea), instead of another word (or phrase) through suggested likeness (e.g., a stream of words). In the case of a psychiatric patient's metaphoric language, that other object (or idea), by which the metaphor has suggested itself to the speaker through likeness or similarity, remains an unrevealed entity and eo ipso makes the metaphor incomprehensible to the listener, though perfectly logical and legitimate for the speaker. Hence the term irrelevant for the language of psychiatric patients—often framed in this kind of meaningless metaphoric configuration.

Metaphorical language is a form of primary process thinking.

**metaphoric paralogia** *By-idea* (q.v.).

**metaphoric symbolism** Indirect pictorial representation based on a metaphor.

**metaplasticity** The higher-order plasticity of synaptic plasticity, i.e. how synaptic activity or other stimuli modify the properties of synaptic plasticity itself.

**metaproterenol** A *beta blocker* (q.v.).

**metapsychological profile** A systematic psychoanalytic classification of clinical data, developed by Anna Freud (1963), that relates symptoms and signs to the inner, unconscious mental life of the patient, and is used especially in treatment of the psychotic patient where therapy is directed toward rendering him or her less vulnerable to inner dangers.

**metapsychology** In psychoanalysis, a theory of cognition and affect that is not derived directly from clinical data but is advanced to provide the developmental background that will allow one to deal with the clinical findings of psychoanalysis as aberrations of, and deviations from, the normal and expected evolution of the thinking process. Its cornerstone is Freud's belief that thought depends on the forging of links between sensory perception of objects and their appropriate verbal descriptions. Freud was dissatisfied with his own metapsychology, but using what has been learned about development in infancy and childhood through the work of Piaget, Vigotsky, and others, it is now possible to formulate a theory that better explains the varied complex findings uncovered by the application of the psychoanalytic method. See *personology.*

**metastable proteins** Proteins with a tendency toward instability. Several neurodegenerative diseases, including *Huntington disease* (q.v.), are associated with proteins with expanded glutamine repeats (polyQ). Expression of aggregation-prone polyQ proteins overwhelms the normal machinery of protein folding and clearance. See *misfolding.*

**metathinking** Thinking about and evaluating one's own thoughts, a frontal lobe function.

**metatropism** *Transsexualism* (q.v.).

**metempiric** Not derived from experience, but implied or presupposed by it.

**metempsychosis** Migration of the soul or rational spirit at death into another body; the doctrine of metempsychosis is part of the Hindu religion, which further teaches that the soul carries with it the memories of former existences for a thousand years. It then induces forgetfulness by drinking of Lethe and begins all over again. See *collective unconscious*.

**metencephalon** See *hindbrain*.

**meteorophobia** Fear of meteors or of being an overnight success.

**methadone** A dependence-inducing, synthetic, narcotic-analgesic with morphinelike effects; at the present time its chief use is as maintenance therapy for heroin addicts according to the method advocated by V. P. Dole and M. E. Nyswander (hence called the *Dole-Nyswander program*). Methadone maintenance differs from other methods in that the successive peaks of elation obtained by repeated intravenous or subcutaneous injections of heroin are replaced by a sustained and uniform drug action without notable elation, abstinence symptoms, or demand for escalation of dose.

*Cyclazocine* is another synthetic narcotic antagonist that prevents the actions of large doses of narcotics. Because it prevents the development of physical tolerance, it controls the factors that ordinarily lead to compulsive build-up in heroin dosage. See *addiction; dependence, drug; LAAM; narcotic blockade; opium*.

**methamphetamine** Commonly known as crystal, crank, chalk, chandelier, ice, quartz, tina, or redneck cocaine; one of the *club drugs*. See *amphetamines*.

**method of successive approximations** *Shaping* (q.v.).

**methodology** The study of the systems and procedures that are used in scientific investigation. Methodology attempts to devise a set of rules or guidelines that will govern or at least influence the choice of procedures to be used in a particular study. When the study in question has, in fact, used procedures in accord with such rules, it can be said that "the procedures of the study were selected and applied in accordance with sound principles of methodology." In current writings this cumbersome sentence is typically abbreviated to "the methodology was sound." As a result, methodology and method are often used interchangeably.

Methodology has also been defined as the study of ways to reach useful and asymtotically valid conclusions on the basis of fallible data gathered by fallible human beings.

**methohexital** Brevital; the standard anesthetic agent for ECT in the United States, used to render the patient unconscious and oblivious to noxious sensations. Alternative anesthetic agents have been used, particularly when methohexital has been unavailable; in addition to their anesthetic properties, they are also evaluated in terms of seizure enhancement or seizure obstruction.

Propofol (Diprivan) has a rapid onset of action but a shorter duration of action than methohexital, with rapid recovery of alertness and orientation; it minimizes postictal nausea and vomiting. But in addition to shortening seizures it can elevate seizure threshold and lead to missed seizures.

Etomidate (Amidate) has neutral or slightly proconvulsant effects; it is thus useful in the patient with a high seizure threshold or seizures that are too short. It produces a longer seizure duration and slower awakening than does either methohexital or propofol. Ketamine has similar properties, and its dissociative properties are less than originally reported.

Because both thiopental and thiamylal shorten seizure duration, they are not usually considered optimal ECT agents.

**methylation** Addition of a methyl group ($-CH_3$) to a chemical substance.

**methylphenidate** A cocainelike psychostimulant that increases extracellular dopamine by blocking dopamine (DA) transporters, and perhaps also by reducing DAD2 receptors. Neurotoxocity initiated by methylphenidate-induced excessive dopamine release may lead to long-term behavioral alterations.

**methysergide** A partially synthetic serotonin antagonist. Because serotonin is believed to be involved in the production of vascular headaches, methysergide has been used as a treatment for both vascular headache and *migraine* (q.v.).

**metonymy** A disturbance of language seen most commonly in the schizophrenias in which an approximate but related term is used in place of the more precise, definite, or idiomatic term that would ordinarily be used. A young schizophrenic patient, for example, spoke in a labyrinthine, circumstantial manner for many minutes during a psychotherapy session, but suddenly became blocked. He recovered spontaneously after 5 to 10 seconds and said: "Now let's see. What was I saying? I seem to have lost the piece of string of the conversation." The phrase "piece of string" would be considered a metonymic substitution for the idiom "to lose the thread of conversation."

**metoprolol**   A *beta blocker* (q.v.).

**Metrazol treatment**   A form of treatment, introduced by von Meduna in 1934; it produced coma and convulsions, through the intravenous administration of Metrazol (cardiazol).

**metric**   See *screening*.

**metromania**   1. Mania for incessant writing of verses.

2. *Obs. Nymphomania* (q.v.).

**metzincin metalloproteinases**   See *metalloproteinases*.

**Meyer, Adolf**   (1866–1950) American psychiatrist; "the mind in action"; psychobiology.

**Meynert, Theodore**   (1833–1992) German neurologist and psychiatrist.

**Meynert basal nucleus**   Nucleus basalis of Meynert. See *cholinergic*; *substantia innominata*.

**MF**   Multifactorial; one of the models of *inheritance* (q.v.).

**MFB**   *Medial forebrain bundle* (q.v.).

**mGlu receptors**   Metabotropic glutamate receptors; a family of modulatory receptors that activate biochemical processes within cells rather than opening the gates to ions. They are located on both sides of a synapse; that is, they operate in both the sending and the receiving neurons. *Glutamate* (q.v.) can thereby fine-tune neuronal signaling, inhibiting or accelerating transmission in specific brain circuits.

**MHAOD**   Mental health, alcohol, and other drugs.

**MHC**   *Major histocompatibility complex* (q.v.).

**MHPG**   A major metabolite of norepinephrine, 3-methoxy-4-hydroxy-phenyl-glycol; MHPG content of 24-hour urine samples is measured as an indication of the adequacy of norepinephrine from noradrenergic neurons.

**MICA**   Mentally ill chemical abuser; the patient with a dual diagnosis of alcohol or other substance abuse plus a second psychiatric diagnosis (e.g., borderline personality, mood disorder, schizophrenia).

**micro-**   Combining form meaning small, little, from Gr. *mikros*.

**microamnesia**   Repeatedly forgetting what was just said, or knowing what was just said but not feeling that it had been a live, personal experience but rather that it was distant and impersonal, like reading an account in a newspaper. Microamnesia is a common dissociative symptom in *dissociative identity disorder* and other *dissociative disorders* (qq.v.).

**microbiophobia**   *Microphobia* (q.v.); fear of infection, infestation, or of small animals.

**microcephaly**   Smallness of the head with defective development of the whole brain and premature ossification of the skull. See *ASPM*.

**micro-dissociations**   In persons with multiple personality disorder, brief amnesias that may occur while the person is carrying on a conversation; they are often described as spacing out or tuning out.

**microfilaments**   See *cytoskeleton*.

**microgeny**   The sequence of the necessary steps inherent in the occurrence of any psychological phenomenon; psychodynamic formulations, for example, are a statement of the microgeny of the patient's symptoms or behavior in that they trace the steps through which a mental process proceeds.

**microglia**   The resident innate immune cells in the brain. Microglia constitute approximately 12% of cells in the brain, located predominantly in the gray matter, with the highest concentrations in hippocampus, olfactory telencephalon, basal ganglia, and substantia nigra. They typically exist in a resting state but, when activated, are involved in regulating brain development and in facilitating repair through the guided migration of stem cells to the site of inflammation and injury. By means of *pattern recognition receptors (PRRs)*, they identify pathogen-associated molecular patterns and initiate host defense and phagocytosis.

Microglia can become overactivated, however, and then induce significant neurotoxic events. By stimulation of NADPH oxidase activity, they produce reactive oxygen species (ROS), an array of cytotoxic factors, such as superoxide, nitric oxide (NO), and tumor necrosis factor-α (TNFα). See *free radical*; *oxidative stress*; *OXPHOS*; *neurotoxicity*.

The stimuli that cause microglial activation are diverse, ranging from environmental toxins, such as pesticides and heavy metals, to neuronal death or damage. Overactivated glia have been implicated as contributors to neuron damage in neurodegenerative disease. Microglia in large numbers (a condition termed *microgliosis*) are present in Alzheimer disease, and microglia have been linked to pathology and disease progression in amyotrophic lateral sclerosis, Huntington disease, multiple sclerosis, Parkinson disease, Pick disease, prion disease, and progressive supranuclear palsy. In such cases, it seems that nonpathogenic stimuli have been misinterpreted, and microglial over-activation has been induced.

Microglia are essential to the progression of HIV-associated dementia (HAD). HIV enters the brain in infected monocytes and is stored in microglia, which serve as a lifelong latent reservoir for HIV replication. As the disease progresses, microglial activation increases in intensity.

**micromania**   *Obs.* Delusion of belittlement; the delusion or conviction that one's body, or some part of it, is or has become abnormally small. Such delusions are most often found in organic depressions, but the small penis complex is also an example. Contrast with *délire d'énormité.*

**micromelia**   Small limbs, associated with achondroplasia; seen in various types of mental retardation. See *de Lange syndrome.*

**microorchidism**   See *Klinefelter syndrome.*

**microphobia**   Fear of small objects and, in particular, of small animals.

**microphonia**   Weakness of the voice.

**micropsia, micropsy**   Perception of objects as smaller than they really are; a form of *dysmegalopsia* (q.v.). See *Lilliputian hallucination.*

**micropsychosis**   A short-lived episode of regression (also termed fragmentation) in response to stress, consisting of symptoms such as self-referential or persecutory delusions, hypochondriacal ideas, feelings of derealization and depersonalization, and fears of loss of identity. Micropsychosis is observed most frequently in borderline personality disorder (in current terminology) and pseudoneurotic schizophrenia (in an earlier typology). See *fragmentation; borderline personality; pseudoneurotic schizophrenia.*

**microRNAs (miRNAs)**   *Small RNAs*; short, noncoding RNAs, ~22 nucleotides in length, that are one of the post-transcriptional regulators of genes. Their predominant effect is to repress their target mRNAs. It has been estimated that the human genome contains more than 1000 miRNAs, of which many appear to be primate specific or even human specific. Humans are believed to have as many as 255 genes that encode microRNAs, about 1% of the genes in the entire genome.

In a process called RNA interference (*RNAi*), double-stranded RNA inhibits genes by degrading the messenger RNA that transports a DNA sequence to the ribosome (the cell's protein factory). RNAi utilizes short bits of RNA to silence specific genes (and viral or other RNAs) and can thereby protect the genome against instability. RNAi is now commonly used in place of gene knockouts. Rather than delete a gene, a laborious process, double-stranded RNA is applied to damp down its expression. RNAi interferes with progression of pathology in an animal model of ALS.

**microsocial engineering**   See *contract therapy.*

**microsomatognosia**   See *somatognosia.*

**microsomia**   See *dwarfism.*

**microsplanchnic**   In Viola's classification, the constitution with a relatively small abdominal portion of the body in proportion to the thoracic portion, owing to the small size of the abdominal viscera, so that the body presents an elongated appearance. The *microsplanchnic* or *dolichomorphic* type corresponds to the *hypovegetative* biotype of Pende and the *asthenic type* of Kretschmer (q.v.).

**microtubule-associated proteins (MAPs)**   They include MAP2 and MAP5, which are anatomically selective for the subiculum and entorhinal cortex and have been implicated in the pathogenesis of both schizophrenia and Alzheimer disease. See *MAPS; temporal lobe.*

**microtubules**   See *cytosol.*

**MID**   Multi-infarct dementia; *vascular dementia* (q.v.). See *cerebral arteriosclerosis.*

**Midas syndrome**   *Rare.* Increased sexual desire in the female associated with diminished desire and capacity in her male partner.

**midbrain**   *Mesencephalon*; the portion of the brain lying between the pons and the cerebral hemispheres, containing the *corpora quadrigemina* (q.v.), the *cerebral peduncles*, and the aqueduct of Sylvius. The base of each peduncle contains the homolateral corticospinal, corticobulbar, and corticopontile tracts. The *substantia nigra* is a broad layer of pigmented gray substance occupying the central portion of the peduncle. The roof or dorsal portion of the base is the *tegmentum*, which contains lateral and medial lemnisci, median longitudinal fasciculus, *red nucleus*, spinothalamic and spinotectal tracts, superior cerebellar peduncle, the nuclei of the trochlear and oculomotor nerves, and the nucleus of the mesencephalic root of the trigeminal nerve.

The midbrain plays a role in control of eye movements and in motor control of skeletal muscles; it contains essential relay nuclei of the auditory and visual systems.

Lesions of the corpora quadrigemina cause paralysis of upward eye movements; of the cerebral peduncle, spastic contralateral paralysis; of the red nucleus, substantia nigra, or reticular substance, involuntary movements and rigidity. In cats, destruction of portions of the tegmentum produces cataleptic manifestations similar to cerea flexibilitas.

**middle class** See *class, social*.

**middle game** The period in psychoanalytic treatment following establishment of a stable transference in which the analyst maintains a neutral stance and focuses on interpretation of intrapsychic processes as a way of encouraging the patient's regression and thereby facilitating the analysis of instinctual vicissitudes. The name is derived from Freud's analogy of the analytic process to a chess game.

**Midtown study** A classic study of *Mental Health in the Metropolis* (Srole, L. et al. 1962) based on interviews of 1660 adults who were felt to be representative "to a high degree of confidence" of the midtown (Yorkville area of New York City) population of 100,000. Of particular relevance to social and community psychiatry are the findings that even though almost 3% of the population was incapacitated by mental illness, less than half of them had any psychiatric contact; and that of the 20% of the population impaired by mental illness, less than one-third of them had any psychiatric contact. It can be concluded that the persons who do come to the attention of existing psychiatric facilities may not constitute a majority of those who need help and may well be a biased and nonrepresentative sample of the mentally ill. The findings further suggest that the mere existence of psychiatric services does not ensure their optimal utilization, and they raise the question of whether the services that are available are desirable or appropriate to those they claim to serve. See *community psychiatry*.

**Mignon delusion** The belief that one is the offspring of some distinguished family (e.g., royalty) rather than one's own parents. This delusion is seen most frequently in the schizophrenias, although it may appear as a more or less disguised wish in almost any psychiatric entity. See *romance, family*.

**migraine** A chronic episodic and sometimes progressive multisystem disorder of neuronal hyperexcitability. Migraine attacks typically consist of unilateral and pulsating severe *headache* (q.v.), lasting 4–72 hours, often accompanied by nausea, phono- and photophobia. In at least 25% of patients, attacks are preceded by an aura—*MA* (migraine with aura). The aurae are transient prodromata, usually less than 60 minutes in duration, consisting of neurological symptoms which are most frequently visual, such as scotomata, less often paresthesiae or other sensory symptoms, and occasionally, motor or speech deficits. The visual aura is typically unilateral and contralateral to the headache. Patients may notice that they cannot see clearly in a small area to one side of the eye fixation point. Sometimes the area has an irregular, scintillating, or colored outline—known as *teichopsia* or *fortification spectra*.

The headaches usually appear at irregular intervals; several attacks a month are common. The headache has a crescendo type of intensity; it may be dull, boring, pressing, throbbing, vicelike, lancinating, or hammering in character. It may begin at any point on the head and spread to involve the entire side. Because of the frequency of associated gastrointestinal symptoms, migraine is often called sick headache or bilious headache. The headache rarely lasts longer than 12 to 24 hours and may be followed by a marked sensation of well-being.

Until recently it was generally believed that migraine was vascular in origin, and due to transient ischemia induced by vasoconstriction followed by rebound vasodilation of intracranial arteries and activation of perivascular sensory fibers. It is now believed that *cortical spreading depression* (*CSD*) underlies the prodromata and activation of the trigeminovascular system (TGVS), which is responsible for the pain itself.

In western countries migraine prevalence is 6%–8% in men and 15%–25% in women. Migraine has a strong (up to 50%) genetic component, which is higher in "classical" migraine (with aura) than in "common" migraine (without aura—*MO*). Although several susceptibility loci have been reported, only in a rare autosomal dominant subtype, FHM or *familial hemiplegic migraine* (q.v.), have two causative genes been found. In ICDH-II,

FHM and *SHM* (*sporadic hemiplegic migraine*) are separated from basilar-type migraine within the group, migraine with aura.

ICDH-II also recognizes *chronic migraine* (*CM*) under complications of migraine. This category refers to patients with pain and associated symptoms of migraine without aura for 15 or more days per month over 3 months or longer, without *medication-overuse headache* (*MOH*). CM is probably a rare syndrome, and the most common cause of migraine like headaches occurring 15 days or more per month is medication overuse.

Subjects with migraine have a higher prevalence of infarction as shown in radiographic studies than do controls (8% vs. 5%). MRI findings reveal that subclinical posterior circulation stroke and diffuse white matter lesion load increase with frequency of migraine, possibly reflecting cumulative brain insults as a result of repeated migraine attacks. The rate of posterior circulation infarction has been found to be particularly elevated in migraine with aura as compared with subjects whose attacks are without aura.

**migrainous neuralgia** See *cluster headache.*

**migrateur** A wanderer; vagrant.

**migration, neuronal** Also, directed neuronal migration, the movement of neuroblasts (primitive, developing nerves) from the site of their last cell division to their final position, often far away from the point of origin. In the cerebellar cortex, for example, the granule cells move away from the germinal external granular layer after mitosis and take a final position in the internal granular layer. The developing neurons move along the glial sheaths, bypassing neurons that have already migrated to their final destinations, to find their own appropriate location and target cells. The neurons are attached to the radial glial stalks that guide them during their migration. See *adhesion, cellular; axon guidance; NCAM.*

**migration psychosis** Paranoid states or other mental illnesses whose appearance is related to leaving one's homeland and settling in a foreign country. There is disagreement as to whether there is an association between rate of mental illness and migration; if there is, evidence is somewhat in favor of the hypothesis that it is not migration that breeds psychosis but that emigration is more likely to occur in those who are already predisposed to mental illness. See *breeder hypothesis.*

**mild neurocognitive disorder (MND)** Also known as *minor cognitive motor disorder* (*MCMD*). See *HIV-associated neurocognitive disorders.*

**milestone** A sign that a significant event has occurred or that an expected developmental level has been reached. A delayed milestone is failure to reach such a level by the age at which it is normally attained.

**milieu** Environment; surroundings. In psychiatry, the social setting, emphasis being placed upon the setting from the emotional point of view. To a psychiatrist the most important milieu is the home. Other environments—scholastic, recreational, industrial, religious, etc.—play a leading role in the growth of the personality. See *milieu therapy.*

**milieu therapy** Socioenvironmental therapy; treatment effected through the medium of the patient's surroundings and immediate environment, and specifically through the medium of the psychiatric hospital. See *social therapy; therapeutic community;"total-push" treatment of schizophrenia.*

In addition to emphasizing the simple humanistic approach advocated by Tuke and Pinel in 18th-century "moral treatment" (which emphasized that treating patients as responsible human beings is effective in getting them to act that way), milieu therapy utilizes techniques that are specifically designed to promote behavioral modification within a stable social organization so that every social experience and treatment experience of the patient will be synergistically applied toward realistic and specific therapeutic goals. Among the techniques that may be used are somatic treatments (psychopharmacologic agents, ECT, etc.), behavior therapies, individual psychotherapy, group process (sensitivity training, family therapy, psychodrama, etc.), hypnosis and suggestion, communications analysis, and role playing.

Milieu therapy is a means of providing an integrated, stable, and coherent context in which the optimal combination of specific treatments can be given to the patient. Its aim is "to make certain that the patient's every social contact and his every treatment experience are synergistically applied towards realistic, specific therapeutic goals" (Abrams, G. M. *Archives of General Psychiatry 21*, 1969). The goals may be to limit, reduce, or otherwise control pathological behavior and/or to develop basic psychosocial skills. Group meetings that encourage participation in information sharing, decision making, conflict resolution, etc. are a prominent feature of milieu therapy, not as ends in themselves but as a way of achieving the therapeutic goals.

**military neurosis** War neurosis; *shellshock* (q.v.). See *post-traumatic stress disorder.*

**Millard-Gubler syndrome** (August L. J. Millard, French physician, 1830–1917, and Adolphe Gubler, French physician, 1821–1879) Paralysis of the external rectus on one side and supranuclear paralysis of the bulbar muscles and limbs on the opposite side.

**Miller Dieker syndrome** *Lissencephaly* (q.v.).

**Milligan annihilation method** A type of regressive electroshock therapy (REST) in which three treatments are administered the first day, and two treatments are given daily thereafter until the desired regression is obtained.

**Millon Clinical Multiaxial Inventory** *MCMI*; a self-report personality assessment that corresponds with DSM-III-R classification. It consists of 175 true-false statements that are scored on 20 standardized scales.

**-mimesis, -mimia** Combining form meaning imitation, from Gr. *mimēsis, mimia,* from *mimeisthai,* to mimic, imitate.

**Minamata disease** An unusual form of toxic neuropathy or encephalopathy seen in fishermen in Minamata Bay (Japan); it is due to eating fish contaminated by organic mercury in the effluent from a nearby fertilizer plant. Pathology consists of widespread neuron degeneration most marked in the granular layer of the cerebellum and in the cortex. Symptoms indicate involvement of the peripheral nervous system, cerebellum, hearing, and vision, and in some cases there are signs of progressive brain damage. Mental symptoms include impairment of intelligence, of which the patient is often aware, and changes in disposition and personality in that patients are often testy, irritable, bashful, unsociable, etc.

**mind** *Psyche;* a range of functions carried out by the brain, ranging from simple motor behaviors such as eating and walking to complex cognitive actions, conscious and unconscious, that are generally believed to be specifically human (such as thinking, speaking, creativity, fantasy, etc.). The neurons, which are self-repairing and self-wiring, promote, amplify, block, inhibit, or attenuate the microelectric signals passed on to them, thereby giving rise to complex signaling patterns between networks of cerebral neurons. This provides the physical substrate of mind. The business of nerve cells is to generate, propagate, and integrate electrical signals; *ion channels* (q.v.) are the proteins that support this cellular task. They directly catalyze the ion fluxes that bring about voltage changes across neuronal membranes and simultaneously act as sensors of those physiological signals. See *cognition; limbic lobe.*

Genes, and especially combinations of genes and their protein products, are a major determinant of the interconnections between neurons and of their functioning. In consequence, they exert significant control over behavior and the mind and are a significant component in the development of major mental illnesses.

Behavior and social or developmental factors also act on the brain, feeding back upon it to modify the expression of genes and, thus, the function of neurons. Learning alters gene expression and changes patterns of neuronal conections. Induction of long-term memory (learning) in animals doubles their number of synaptic terminals in comparison to untrained animals. A specific instance of learning is likely to alter a large number of cells insofar as the interconnections of the various sensory and motor systems involved in the learning are changed. The resultant modification of brain architecture, along with a subject's unique genetic makeup and the particular environment in which he or she was reared, provides the biological basis for individuality.

**mind, miniature** *Psychoinfantilism* (q.v.); a symmetrical retardation in all aspects of mental life, in contradistinction to mental retardation. The psychoinfantile person is regarded as one with a miniature mind, a mental midget.

**mind control** Brainwashing. See *brain control; menticide; propaganda; psychopolitics.*

**mind-body dualism** Most dualistic theories assume that the processes and products of the mind have very little to do with the processses and products of the body.

**mind/body perception, altered** Any of a group of altered states of consciousness that are presumed to exist on a continuum ranging from ecstatic experiences of heightened awareness and integration to disorganizing episodes of psychotic decompensation with loss of identity. Characteristic of the group is subjectively experienced distortion of the normal spatial relationship between body and mind. The term includes out-of-body experiences, near-death experiences, body boundary disturbances, *autoscopy*, and *depersonalization* (qq.v.).

**mind-brain relationships** Kandel (*American Journal of Psychiatry 155*,1998) proposes five principals:

1. All mental procceses, even the most complex, derive from operations of the brain; what is called mind is a range of functions carried out by the brain, ranging from simple motor behaviors (such as eating and walking) to complex cognitive actions, conscious and unconscious, that are generally believed to be specifically human (such as thinking, speaking, creativity, fantasy, etc.). Psychiatric illnesses, even those that are clearly environmetal in origin, are disturances of brain function.

2. Genes, and especially combinations of genes and their protein products, are a major determinant of the interconnections between neurons and of their functioning. They thereby exert significant control over behavior and are a significant component in the development of major mental illnesses.

3. Behavior and social or developmental factors also act on the brain, feeding back upon it to modify the expression of genes and, thus, the function of neurons. All of what is termed nurture is ultimately expressed as nature.

4. Learning alters gene expression and changes patterns of neuronal conections. Such changes contribute to the biological basis of individuality and in addition are presumed to be responsible for initiating and maintaining behavior abnormalities, even though the latter are induced by social contingencies.

5. Presumably, psychotherapy induces changes in behavior by means of learning, producing changes in gene espression that alter the interconnection between neurons.

**mindreading** See *extrasensory perception.*

**mind-stuff** See *atomistic psychology.*

**mineralocorticoid** See *general adaptation syndrome.*

**Mini-Cog** A three-word recall and simple clock-drawing test developed for rapid screening for cognitive disorders. Unlike the MMSE and CASI (Cognitive Abilities Screening Instrument), the Mini-Cog is not significantly affected by education level or primary language.

**minimal brain dysfunction** *MBD.* See *attention deficit hyperactivity disorder.*

**minimal cue** See *cue, minimal.*

**minimal risk** See *risk, minimal.*

**minimization techniques** See *false confession.*

**Minnesota Multiphasic Personality Inventory (MMPI)** A personality questionnaire consisting of 550 statements concerning behavior, feelings, social attitudes, and frank symptoms of psychopathology. To each question, the subject must answer T (true), F (false), or ? (cannot say), and his or her answer sheet is then scored by various keys that have been standardized on different diagnostic groups and personality types. The MMPI was originally constructed by a psychiatrist, J. C. McKinley, and a psychologist, Starke Hathaway.

**minor analysis** A psychotherapeutic method in which the analysis of psychic material attempts neither an exhaustive study of (as does Freudian analysis in general) nor deeper delving into subconscious conflicts, but confines itself only to the elucidation of the salient details considered of primary importance in relation to the neurosis. Minor analysis is of shorter duration than orthodox, or Freudian, psychoanalysis. Through the interpretation of the most conspicuous of the psychic materials the analyst arrives at conclusions, makes revelations, and gives suggestions with the aim of enabling the patient to gain quick insight. (Stekel, W. *The Interpretation of Dreams,* 1943).

**minor cognitive motor disorder (MCMD)** Also known as *mild neurocognitive disorder (MND).* See *HIV-associated neurocognitive disorders.*

**minor physical anomalies** *MPAs* (q.v.).

**minus complementarity** See *complementarity.*

**miopragia** In constitutional medicine, diminished functional activity of an organ. For example, subjects of asthenic habitus may possess a small, immature, and functionally diminished cardiovascular apparatus. Lewis (*Constitutional Factors in Dementia Praecox,* 1923) reported, among other things, a hypoplastic heart with lessened functional capacity in subjects with schizophrenia.

**miosis** 1. The period of decline of a disease in which symptoms begin to abate. 2. Contraction of the pupil.

**MIP**   Medial intraparietal area; see *intraparietal sulcus*.

**miriasha**   A person affected with *miryachit* (q.v.).

**mirror imaging**   In genetics, reversed *asymmetry*, quite frequent in twins, with respect to handedness, hair whorl, dental irregularities, fingerprints, and other symmetrical characters including certain morbid traits based on heredity. The presence of mirror imaging is confirmatory evidence of *monozygotic* twins, though monozygosity is not excluded by its absence. See *twin*.

**mirror neurons**   Mirror neurons code relatively abstract aspects of observed actions, including sounds of an action even in the absence of visual presentation. They have been identified in the insula and in two other cortical areas, the posterior part of the inferior frontal cortex and the anterior part of the inferior parietal lobule, which form an integrated frontoparietal *mirror neuron system (MNS)*. MNS is a special higher-order motor system. Data suggest that the left hemisphere has a multimodal (visual, auditory) MNS, whereas the right hemisphere has only a visual MNS. Multimodality is considered an important factor in protolanguages or systems of communication that are precursors of linguistic systems. In humans, the shift from a purely visual to a multimodal MNS might have determined both functional changes that could have facilitated language, and a left-lateralization of language functions.

MNS does not simply provide a relatively abstract representation of the actions of others, but it also codes the intentions associated with the observed action. With higher-order visual areas along the superior temporal sulcus (STS), MNS forms a "core circuit" for imitation, a necessary element in imitative learning and social mirroring. Social emotions like guilt, shame, pride, embarrassment, disgust, and lust are based on a uniquely human mirror neuron system found in the insula. Reduced imitation might be a core deficit in autism spectrum disorders. See *theory of mind*.

**mirror sign**   A symptom seen frequently in schizophrenic patients, who may stand in front of a mirror or other shining surface for an unduly long time. The sign is as an expression of the patient's autistic withdrawal. The same sign can also occur in advanced organic dementia (e.g., *Alzheimer disease*, q.v.): the patient sits for hours in front of a mirror, talking to his own reflection; because of complete loss of personal identity, the patient does not realize that the reflection is his own.

**mirror writing**   See *strephosymbolia*.

**mirror-hungry personality**   See *mirroring deficits*.

**mirroring**   In self psychology, the positive responses of the parents to the child, reflecting a sense of self-worth and value and instilling internal self-respect. The delight of the parents in the child's activity is essential to his development. As a result of such mirroring responses, the child is able to develop and maintain self-esteem and self-assertive ambitions. Mirroring needs are called *grandiose-exhibitionistic needs* because they support the infantile concept of "I am perfect and [that is why] you love me." *Mirror transferences* are seen later in life as forms of self-development that ask of others that they reflect or respond. When a person has achieved sufficient growth in this arena, an adult feeling of pride in performance is achieved.

Should it happen that mirroring is inadequate, the child is predisposed to the development of psychopathology. In general, however, psychopathology develops only when the child has been exposed to a repeated pattern of difficulty in at least two of the three poles of the self—mirroring, idealizing, and alter ego. See *alter-ego transference; cohesive self; communicative matching; empathic failure; empathy; fit; idealization; mirroring deficits*.

**mirroring deficits**   Consistent shortcomings in mirroring self-object relations produce three personality types that have been described in narcissistic disorders:

1. *Merger-hungry personalities* who must continuously attach themselves to self-objects and are often unable to differentiate their own thoughts and wishes from those of the self-objects; they make overwhelming demands for continuous availability of those self-objects. See *as-if personality*.

2. *Contact-shunning* personalities who isolate themselves to deny their frightening need for others and to avoid being swallowed up or destroyed by others. See *fragmentation*.

3. *Mirror-hungry* personalities who insistently display themselves to evoke acceptance and admiration; they often alternate between depressed withdrawal and outbursts of enraged acting out.

Shortcomings in the two other poles of the self, the idealizing and the alter-ego (or twinship) produce the following:

4. *Ideal-hungry* personalities who are forever searching for others whom they can admire. See *idealization*.

5. *Alter-ego* personalities who seek a relationship with someone who conforms to their own values and thereby confirms the reality of their own selves. See *alter-ego transference*.

**mirroring needs**    See *cohesive self; mirroring*.

**mirroring stage**    Recognition of oneself in the mirror, an ability that begins to develop at about 6 months and continues through the 18th month, according to Jacques Lacan. The mirroring stage coincides with Mahler's differentiation, practicing, and beginning rapprochement subphases of *separation-individuation* (q.v.). An important element in the development of object relations is the child's ability to differentiate his nascent self-image from his mirror image. By serving as an external reflector, the mother promotes the child's self-objectification as he comes to perceive that his mirror image and her object-image are not the same, and that they are different from his subjective self-image. These fundamental differentiations begin in earnest during the practicing subphase (10–16 months) of separation-individuation.

**miryachit**    (Russ. "to fool or play the fool") *Olonism*; a culture-specific syndrome reported in Siberian groups, consisting of indiscriminate and irresistible imitation of the actions and speech of people in the subject's presence and trancelike behavior. Also called *irkunii*, *ikota*, and *menkeiti* (Siberian), bah tschi or baab-ji (Thailand), isu (the Ainu of Japan), *mali-mali* and silok (Philippines). See *echopraxia; lata*.

**MIS**    Medical improvement standard, used to gauge the degree of improvement in a condition before the SSDI benefits for that condition are terminated.

**misanthropy**    Hatred of, or aversion to, humankind. A profound distrust of human beings individually and collectively.

**misapprehension**    See *apprehension*.

**misfolding**    Normal protein functioning usually depends on its being folded in one or more ways; failure of proteins to fold normally is believed to be the basis of many *neurodegenerative diseases* (q.v.).

Misfolded proteins are ordinarily destroyed by *molecular chaperones*, or are tagged with *ubiquitin* for destruction (qq.v.). If not destroyed, such proteins tend to clump together in the form of rods (protofibrils), which accumulate as sheets of insoluble fibrils that form plaque. In Alzheimer disease, the protein is β-amyloid, resulting in senile plaques; in Parkinson disease, α-synuclein, resulting in Lewy bodies; in the spongiform encephalopathies, prion protein. Some workers believe that it is the protofibrils, rather than the plaques themselves, that are responsible for neurodegeneration in the different disorders.

The mitochondria of one parent wage a ferocious war with the other parent's mitochondria for survival within that cell. The genes for the rest of the cell (in the nucleus) suffer from the crippling of the cell, so they evolve a way of heading off the internecine warfare. In each pair of parents, one "agrees" to unilateral disarmament. It contributes a cell that provides no metabolic machinery, just naked DNA for the new nucleus. The species reproduces by fusing a big cell that contains a half-set of genes plus all the necessary machinery with a small cell that contains a half-set of genes and nothing else. See *chaperone proteins; protein conformational disorders*.

**misidentification, amnesic**    The inability of a subject to identify the person confronting him, due to impairment of the memory or to clouding of consciousness.

**misidentification, delusional**    *DMS* (delusional misidentification syndrome); consistent misidentification of persons, places, objects (including body parts), and events. The most common DMS is the *Capgras syndrome* (q.v.), the delusional belief that a person or persons have been replaced by "doubles" or impostors. In the *Fregoli syndrome*, the patient believes that a person well known to him or her has taken on the appearance of a stranger whom the patients encounters. In *intermetamorphosis*, the patient believes that people he has known have exchanged identities with one another. In asomatognosia, a part of the body is misidentified; usually this occurs in conjunction with left hemiplegia, and the patient denies ownership of the left arm and may describe it as "a wooden log for the fireplace." Reduplication without misidentification is seen in the *phantom child syndrome*, where a husband and wife believe they are parents of a fictitious child.

Almost always, misidentifications and reduplications involve delusions concerning people or situations of great personal significance (one's body, family, current location, employment); often the delusions allow the subject to view the situation as better than it actually is; the beliefs are consistent and long maintained; and they are fixed and resistant to correction, even if the patient is confronted repeatedly with the illogical nature of the belief. *Confabulation* (q.v.) often co-occurs with delusional misidentification, but the two phenomena are not considered to be the same. In addition to perceptual, memory, and executive impairments, patients with delusional misidentification and reduplication suffer from a disturbance of self and a deficit in the ego functions that mediate the relationships between self and world.

**misidentification, hyperbolic**   A condition sometimes found in manic states in which the patient flippantly calls a person by someone else's name. This misidentification is rarely clung to with conviction.

**miso-**   Combining form meaning hate, hatred, from Gr. *misos*.

**misocainia**   Hatred or fear of anything new or strange, sometimes expressed as an obsessive desire for preservation of the status quo. See *autistic disorder*.

**misogamy**   Hatred of marriage, which may be based upon an unresolved Oedipus complex.

**misogyny**   Hatred of women. It may be associated with a wide variety of nosologic entities and is often related to conflicts stemming from the *Oedipus complex* (q.v.). In both women and men it may reflect conflict over homosexuality.

**misologia, misology**   Hatred or fear of speaking or arguing.

**misoneism**   Hatred of innovation, *misocainia* (q.v.).

**misopedia**   Hatred of children.

**missense mutation**   A mutation that results in the substitution of an amino acid in a protein, which therefore often has abnormal function.

**Missouri Foster Community Program**   See *domicile*.

**mistrust**   See *ontogeny, psychic*.

**misuse**   Abuse of drugs, including any prescribed by a physician that is used in a medically unacceptable way.

**Mitchell, Silas Weir**   (1829–1914) American neurologist and psychiatrist; *rest cure* (q.v.).

**Mitgehen**   A form of motor dysregulation, seen frequently in catatonia, consisting of limb movement in response to light pressure, even though the subject has been instructed not to move the limb. Often associated with Mitgehen is forced grasping, repeated grasping at the examiner's outstretched fingers even when told not to do so. See *frontal lobe dysfunction*.

**mitissima**   Mania mitis; paraphrosyne; hypomania. See *mania*.

**MITN**   Midline and intralaminar thalamic nuclei; part of the *medial pain system*. See *pain*.

**mitochondria**   Cytoplasmic bodies that are the sites of aerobic respiration within the cell; they take energy from organic molecules and turn it into adenosine triphosphate, which is used to power the cell. Because of that function they have been called the cell's "power packs." The mitochondrion is a cytoplasmic organelle, one of the membranes within the cell. Mitochondria have their own genome, mitochondrial DNA or *mtDNA* (q.v.). See *axon; OXPHOS*.

Mitochondria are vestiges of ancient bacteria. About 2 billion years ago, oxygen first appeared in the atmosphere, and an ancient bacterium developed a new, highly efficient way to use it to produce chemical energy. At the same time, the ancient progenitor of animal and human cells, which was poor at producing energy, happened to be good at gathering food. So the two fused and took advantage of each other. Today, the energy-generating mitochondria are all that is left of the ancient bacterium.

Mitochondria retain a repertoire of molecules that trigger apoptosis. Release of a mitochondrial cytotoxin is triggered by activation of a nuclear enzyme, PARP-1. Under homeostatic conditions, PARP-1 participates in genome repair, DNA replication, and the regulation of transcription. In response to stresses that are toxic to the genome, PARP-1 activity increases substantially, an event that appears crucial for maintaining genomic integrity. Massive PARP-1 activation, however, can lead ultimately to energy failure and cell death. PARP-1 promotes programmed cell death through a caspase-independent pathway, releasing a mitochondrial proapoptotic protein called apoptosis-inducing factor (AIF).

**mitochondrial disorders** Inherited mitochondrial disorders are characterized by matrilineal transmission and a high rate of affected relatives.

The mitochondria are the largest source of free radicals identified. Fatty acid oxidation defects are among the most commonly inherited mitochondrial anomalies. Wild-type (normal) mtDNA coexists with mutant mtDNA (a phenomenon known as *heteroplasmy*, as opposed to *homoplasmy*); mitochondrial disorders are expressed when the mutant mtDNA reaches a critical threshold and produces oxidative dysfunction. See *free radical.*

**mitochondrial uncoupling proteins** A family of proteins that reside in the mitochondrial inner membrane and promote a proton leak across the membrane, thereby decreasing oxidative phosphorylation and reactive oxygen species production.

**mitosis** See *chromosome.*

**mitotic clock** See *replicative senescence.*

**mix** See *case mix.*

**mixed dementia** Coexisting AD (Alzheimer disease) and VaD (vascular dementia). Pathologically, the characteristic lesions of AD (extracellular amyloid plaques and intracellular neurofibrillary tangles) and VaD (cerebral infarctions, multiple lacunar infarctions, ischemic periventricular leukolencephalopathy) occur together. Perhaps 25%–50% of patients with AD also have significant cerebrovascular pathology. See *Alzheimer disease.*

**mixed neurosis** *Rare.* A neurosis with features of two or more neuroses. Many such cases were later subsumed under the subtype described by Hoch and Polatin as *pseudoneurotic schizophrenia* (q.v.). See *personality disorders; latent schizophrenia.*

**mixoscopia bestialis** A *paraphilia* (q.v.) characterized by the need to watch sexual intercourse between an animal and a human being, who is usually being forced unwillingly to participate.

**mixture, Cloetta's** (Max Cloetta, Swiss pharmacologist, 1868–1940) A combination of paraldehyde, amylene hydrate, chloral hydrate, alcohol, barbituric acid, digitalin, and ephedrine hydrochloride that was usually administered per rectum in *continuous sleep treatment* (q.v.).

**MK-801** An excitatory amino acid receptor blocker and an experimental anticonvulsant. Its effects are mediated through the PCP binding site of the *NMDAR* (q.v.). See *excitotoxicity; neuroadaptation.*

**MLD** Metachromatic leukodystrophy. See *leukodystrophies.*

**MLR** *Mesencephalic locomotor region* (q.v.).

**MM** *Moderation management* (q.v.).

**MMC** Maternally inherited myopathy and cardiomyopathy. See *mtDNA.*

**MMECT** Multiple monitored electroconvulsive therapy, consisting of induction of more than one seizure (typically four or five) in a single session, with concomitant monitoring of the EEG and EKG. The goal is to shorten the time needed for a course of treatment.

**MMPI** See *Minnesota Multiphasic Inventory.*

**MMPs** Matrix *metalloproteinases* (q.v.).

**MMSE** Mini-Mental State Examination (of Folsom); a screening test for global cognitive dysfunction (orientation, memory, attention, simple calculation, dysgraphia, and constructional apraxia). The MMSE taps frontal, spatial, and memory domains of cognitive function. It identifies subjects with a high probability of moderate to severe global cognitive impairment. See *cognitive screening instruments.*

**MMT** Multimodal therapy. See *BASIC-ID.*

**MMWR** *Morbidity and Mortality Weekly Report*, a publication of the Centers for Disease Control (U.S.).

**M'Naghten rule** See *criminal responsibility.*

**MND** Mild neurocognitive disorder. See *HIV-associated neurocognitive disorders.*

**mneme** Memory trace or *engram* (q.v.).

**mneme, phylogenetic** The racial ancestral memory preset in the deep unconscious of the individual. See *racial memory.*

**mnemic** Pertaining to or characterized by memory.

**mnemism** Mnemic hypothesis that cells possess memory. See *engram.*

**-mnesia, -mnesis** Combining form meaning memory, from Gr. *mnēsis*, memory, from *mnasthai*, to remember.

**mob psychology** The psychology of mob behavior is considered by Fenichel to have much in common with a certain type of character defense against guilt feelings. In this type of defense, the guilt-laden character feels admiration and relief when someone else does something that he has been striving to do, but has been inhibited from doing through guilt feelings. The meaning of the admiration and relief is "Since others do it, it cannot be so bad after all."

The attainment of relief from guilt feelings in this way is a powerful force for group formation. Others have dared to do what the individual has felt guilt about doing. And "If my whole group acts this way, I may, too." In this way, the relief from guilt feelings is described as "one of the cornerstones of 'mob psychology.' " Indeed, Fenichel points out that "individuals acting as a group are capable of instinctual outbreaks that would be entirely impossible for them as individuals." (*The Psychoanalytic Theory of Neurosis*, 1945).

**mobile outreach**  A means of extending mental health services to the community and bridging the gap between psychiatric hospital and the people or agencies who need or could benefit from the direct, onsite help of a hospital team. Mobile outreach teams can be structured in many different ways, depending upon whom they service, how quickly, and for how long; the geographical area covered; their ability to respond to emergencies; the level of tactical and professional training of their members, etc. They may work primarily in emergencies, assisting the police or others in life-threatening situations; they may act mainly with community agencies to help in the management of complex, long-standing problems; their role may be mainly to stabilize patients in the community and to reduce the need for hospital admission; they may act as case-finders or as after-care monitors; and they may take a leading role in public education about mental illness.

**modality**  Any method or technique of treatment; a class or group within the therapeutic armamentarium. Also any class or subdivision of sensation, such as vision or smell.

**modality profile**  In multimodal behavior therapy, a chart that lists the patient's problems in each of the seven areas of the BASIC-ID (q.v.), and the treatments proposed for each of them.

**mode**  The value in a frequency curve at which the height of the curve is greatest; i.e., the most frequently recurring score in a distribution. The mode is a very unstable measure.

**mode of inheritance**  The pattern of inheritance (e.g., dominant or recessive) of a particular allele.

**model**  Example, often in the sense of a goal to be attained; also, a device for ordering information.

**model psychosis**  Experimental psychosis and, particularly, such as is produced by mescaline or lysergic acid or similar *psychotomimetic* drugs (q.v.).

**modeling**  A form of behavior therapy, based on the principles of imitative learning; it obviates the need for the patient to discover effective responses through trial-and-error emulation of the therapist. See *reciprocal determinism*.

**modeling, behavior**  A training technique based on a sequence of modeling, role playing, and reinforcement that changes behavior directly through the fundamentals of social learning (imitation and reinforcement) rather than indirectly through traditional training approaches (such as lectures, the case method, or T groups). It includes imitation of effective behaviors, use of retention aids, intensive and guided practice of new behavior, reinforcement or recognition in applying the specific behaviors, and transfer of training principles. Modeling provides a concise and distinct display of the desired behavior in a specific job situation—by actors, on videotape, film, etc.—typically by a person whom the observer is likely to regard as competent. Repetition of viewing (e.g., by videotaping of sessions) and mental rehearsal are typical retention aids, followed by behavior rehearsal, i.e., supervised reenactment of the model performance.

**models of illness**  See *community psychiatry; medical model*.

**Moderation Management (MM)**  A mutual-help organization for alcoholics that sets achievement of moderate (controlled) drinking as its goal, rather than the abstinence goal of Alcoholics Anonymous. Many alcoholics who enter MM move to a goal of abstinence after a few weeks. In general, as compared with AA members, MM members have fewer signs of physical dependence and are more likely to be female, below 35 years of age, and currently employed.

**modification**  *Paravariation*; in genetics, the term is limited to variations in the phenotype that are caused by environmental influences and alter the individual appearance without affecting the idioplasm. Drastic effects of the environment on living beings may lead to profoundly modified developments, but it is generally assumed that they do not become inheritable.

Of the modifying factors that interact to produce a human phenotype, the physiological effects of nutrition, light, and climate seem just as important as social, cultural, and psychological influences. These variations in environmental modifications can best be observed in identical co-twins reared apart under different life conditions. See *variation*.

**modifier**   In genetics, hereditary factors that modify the effect of other factors, having little or no effect when the main factor is absent. A modifier is termed *specific* when its effects are produced only upon a particular genotype. See *variation*.

**modifier genes**   Loci influencing clinical features of a disease without altering susceptibility.

**modularity**   Composed of standardized units that can be used variably and flexibly. Biological modules are consortia that act autonomously to produce a single form or function and are redeployed within and across species, thereby creating novelty and fueling the development and evolution of biological complexity. Modularity provides the ability to combine and modify existing parts into more favorable assemblies.

In cognitive neuropsychology, modularity refers to the hypothesis that the mind's structure is based on special-purpose computational mechanisms or modules. J. A. Fodor (*Modularity of Mind*, Cambridge , MA:MIT Press, 1983) proposed that modules are innate, that they perform their operations on a specific input or domain (such as faces or musical notes), and that their operations are encapsulated, i.e., inaccessible to other modules.

**modularity hypothesis**   The belief that the brain must contain separate, specialized units (modules) whose circuitry determines what particular kind of information each can deal with.

**module**   In a neural *network* (q.v.), a set of units or nodes that have strong interactions and a common function. A module has defined input nodes and output codes that control its interactions with the rest of the network. See *mental modules*; *parallel distributed processing*.

**Moebius syndrome**   (Paul Julius Moebius, 1853–1907, German neuropathologist) See *mirror neurons*.

**mogigraphia**   Writer's cramp. See *occupational neurosis*.

**mogilalia**   *Molilalia*; hesitancy or difficulty in speaking and particularly the kind that appears as a type of resistance in psychotherapy.

**MOH**   Medication overuse headache; in ICDH-II, aggravation of a primary headache by frequent and regular use over time of analgesics or antimigraine medications. The term avoids the use of the pejorative words, abuse or misuse, which are particularly inappropriate in such cases because the overuse is typically the result of prescription by a physician who is unaware of the risks of over-frequent use. In general, limits on length of use of drugs for chronic headaches should be specified; for example, use on no more than 10 days a month for triptans, ergotamine, opioids, or common analgesics, and use on no more than 15 days a month for simple analgesics. The main criterion of overuse is not the quantity of drug, but the frequency of its use.

**mojo**   See *rootwork*.

**molar**   Massive or gross, as contrasted with molecular, nuclear, minute, or discrete. Molar is often used to refer to large-scale units of analysis and molecular for small-scale units. Related is the contrast between *top-down* and *bottom-up* approaches to a situation. In a bottom-up approach, the details of the task or setting are the determinants of how the subject performs. In the top-down approach the subject's own intentions, goals, and strategies are imposed on the situation and directly affect performance and outcome.

**molecular chaperone**   See *chaperone proteins; protein conformational disorders*.

**molecular genetics**   The branch of genetics concerned with identifying the gene(s) and gene products responsible for the biochemical abnormalities that constitute the vulnerability or predisposition to the disease under study.

**molecular targets**   See *neuropharmacology*.

**molester, child**   See *pedophilia*.

**molilalia**   *Mogilalia* (q.v.).

**molimen**   Distress, malaise; specifically, the labored or difficult performance of a normal function or of a task that could ordinarily be performed with ease. *Molimen virile* was formerly used to refer to fatigue symptoms associated with the male climacterium; *menstrual molimen* is still used to refer to premenstrual tensions.

**molimina, premenstrual**   Premenstrual tension including both physical and psychic symptoms referable to the premenstrual period; *late luteal phase dysphoric disorder*. See *LLPDD*.

**molindone**   A dihydroindolone antipsychotic drug.

**molysmophobia**   Fear of contamination.

**mongol** 1. One belonging to the Mongolian race. 2. One who presents the clinical syndrome of mental deficiency once called mongolism, now called *Down syndrome* (q.v.).

**monism, sexual** See *phallic sexual monism.*

**monitor** To supervise, invigilate; especially, to watch carefully so as to give warning should anything go wrong.

**Moniz, Egas** (1874–1955) Pen name for Antonio Caetano deAbreu Freire, Portuguese neurologist; development of cerebral angiography and of frontal leukotomy (the first psychosurgical procedure), for which he received the Nobel Prize for medicine in 1949.

**monkey love** A literal translation of the German term Affenliebe. It refers to inordinate maternal love in which the mother caters unqualifiedly to all the wishes and whims of the child. See *smother love.*

**monkey therapist** A socially appropriate monkey, used in experiments with monkeys raised in total isolation, as a means of modifying the isolate's behavior and bringing it more in accord with normal behavior. In many cases, pairing of the *isolate monkey* with the monkey therapist results in a gradual improvement in the isolate's behavior, with only occasional lapses into inappropriate behavior, such as self-clasping and huddling.

**mono-** Combining form meaning alone, only, single, unique, from Gr. *monos.*

**monoamine oxidase (MAO)** An enzyme, discovered by Hare in 1928, that has since been shown to be able to oxidize (and thus inactivate) various amines, including serotonin and the catecholamines and their methoxy derivatives. Many inhibitors of monoamine oxidase (MAOIs) are antidepressants.

**monobulia** *Obs.* A wish, desire, drive, thought, obsession, etc. that dominates the psychic life and inhibits or eliminates all other forms of mental activity.

**monochorionic** *MC*; describing twins who share one placenta and one chorion. Most MC twins exchange blood through shared vascular communication, whereas DC twins rarely do. Shared vascular communication encourages mutual infection whenever an infectious agent crosses the shared placenta of an MC twin pair. In dichorionic (DC) twins, infections and toxins might cross the placenta of only one twin, leaving the co-twin unaffected. Approximately two-thirds of monozygotic twins are monochorionic, and mortality

is higher in MC-MZ twins that in DC-MZ twins. See *dichorionic.*

**monohybrid** Differing with respect to only one hereditary character (in a hybrid individual). See *hybrid.*

**monohybridity (monohybridism)** The state of a hybrid whose parents differ in a single character, or the character of belonging to a type of individual heterozygous for a single pair of genes.

**monoideism** "The theory according to which an idea detached from other ideas will exercise an unusually powerful force in the mind. The notion was formulated long ago both by Descartes and by Condillac. The magnetisers were well aware that suggestion was more powerful when the subjects were 'isolated,' that is to say when they were apparently unable to perceive any phenomena except the personality of the magnetiser and his utterances" (Janet, P. *Psychological Healing*, 1952).

The term is also used to refer to the symptom of harping on one idea, seen frequently in the senile group and in the schizophrenias (and in social bores—"he can't change his mind and he won't change the subject").

**monomania** *Rare.* Partial insanity, in which the morbid mental state is restricted to one subject, the patient being of sound judgment and appropriate affect on all other subjects; impulsive act without motive.

In older psychiatry there were such expressions as *intellectual monomania* (e.g., paranoia); *affective monomania*, which corresponded with *manie raisonnante*, characterized by emotional deviation; *instinctive monomania*, the approximate equivalent of obsessive-compulsive disorder.

When monomania or partial insanity was associated with depressive states, Esquirol suggested that the term *lypemania* be used, to differentiate it from monomania with exaltation of mood.

**monomanie du nol** *Obs. Kleptomania* (q.v.).

**monomoria** *Melancholia* (q.v.).

**mononucleosis, chronic** See *chronic fatigue syndrome; EBV syndrome.*

**monopagia** Clavus hystericus. See *clavus.*

**monopathophobia** Fear of a single, specific organic disease.

**monophobia** Fear of being alone.

**monoplegia** Paralysis of one limb or single part of the body, such as one arm, one leg, or the face alone, or only the finger.

**monosexual**   Exclusively heterosexual or homosexual; not bisexual.

**monosymptomatic**   Manifested by a single symptom.

**monosymptomatic hypochondriacal psychosis**   A term for isolated delusion that emphasizes the severity of the disorder even though the false belief remains relatively separate from the rest of the personality, and also the frequency with which such delusions focus on somatic symptoms and loss of body integrity. The most common forms are the olfactory reference syndrome, the dysmorphic delusion, and parasitophobia. Closely related phenomenologically is conjugal paranoia. See *dysmorphophobia; jealousy, morbid.*

**monotherapy**   Use of a single agent as treatment. In mood disorders, for example, use of only a tricyclic antidepressant is monotherapy; this is in contrast to *coactive strategies* (q.v.), which employ augmenting drugs or combinations of drugs rather than a single antidepressant. See *copharmacy; polypharmacy.*

**monozygosity (monzygocity)**   In genetics, originating from one egg of monozygotic or identical twins.

**monozygotic**   Referring to twins developed from a single egg and exhibiting extreme resemblances because of their identical genotypes. These *monozygotic,* or *identical,* or *one-egg* twin pairs are to be distinguished from the *dizygotic, fraternal,* or *nonidentical* twin pairs produced by two eggs. See *twin.*

**Montessori, Maria**   (1870–1952) Italian physician and educator, the first woman to receive the M.D. degree from an Italian university; devised an educational system that provides a carefully prepared environment for self-education of the child with emphasis on practical living, sensorial response, mathematics, biology, geography, and reading. The first Montessori School in the United States was established in 1913.

**mood**   The sustained emotional states that color the whole personality and psychic life; the pervasive or prevailing emotion at any specific time. See *affect.*

Howard Owens and Jerrold Maxmen (*American Journal of Psychiatry 136,* 1979) note that both mood and affect refer to a disposition to react emotionally in certain ways, and thus there is considerable overlap between the two concepts. In their usage, inferences about

mood are drawn from the subject's past history as well as present observations, while inferences about affect are confined to current observations.

**mood, delusional**   *Wahnstimmung* (q.v.).

**mood disorders**   *Affect disorders; affective disorders;* included are depressive disorders, bipolar disorders, and depressive or manic episodes induced by substances or due to some general medical condition. See *depression; mania; manic-depressive psychosis.*

**mood stabilizer**   A therapeutic modality with demonstrated efficacy in the acute treatment of both depressive and manic episodes and in preventing recurrence of both depressive and manic episodes, without inducing a switch to another mood and without exacerbating any phase of the mood disorder. Traditional mood stabilizers are lithium, divalproex, and carbamazepine.

**mood swings**   Oscillation between periods of the feeling of well-being and those of depression or "blueness." All people have mood swings, blue hours, or blue days. Mood swings are somewhat more marked in the neurotic than in the normal. In the manic-depressive patient, the swings are of much greater intensity and much longer duration. See *cyclothymia.*

**mood syndrome, organic**   Secondary or symptomatic mood disorder; a depressive or manic episode occurring as a result of some general medical disorder. Depression is more common than mania or mixed pictures. Major causes include drugs and medications (antihypertensives, barbiturates, steroids), carcinomas (especially pancreatic), virus infections (hepatitis, mononucleosis), endocrinopathies, and cardiovascular accidents.

**mood-congruent**   Referring to symptoms and behavior consistent with the subject's expressed or prevailing mood, used particularly in the subclassification of mood (affective) disorders.

Manic episodes, for example, are subdivided into those with and those without psychotic features (delusions, hallucinations, grossly bizarre behavior, etc.). Those with psychotic features are further subtyped as mood-congruent or mood-incongruent psychotic features. *Mood-congruent* features are delusions or hallucinations consistent with manic grandiosity, expansiveness, and inflated self-esteem. *Mood-incongruent* features are symptoms that contradict or at least fail to match manic features; examples are persecutory delusions, ideas of thought insertion or of being controlled, and catatonic symptoms such as stupor, mutism, or posturing.

In major depressive episodes mood-congruent psychotic features are delusions or hallucinations consistent with depressive lowering of self-esteem, feelings of guilt, and ideas of punishment through disease or death. Mood-incongruent features include persecutory delusions, ideas of thought insertion or thought broadcasting, and delusions of being controlled.

**moodcyclic disorders** See *adaptational psychodynamics.*

**mood-stabilizing agents** The major ones currently in use for bipolar disorder (mania) are lithium and valproic acid.

**Mooney Problem Check List** A questionnaire, used often as part of a rapid screening battery for high school and college students, in which the subject is asked to indicate which of a list of symptoms are frequent or troublesome to him or her.

**moral cognitive neuroscience** Its aim is to elucidate the cognitive and neural mechanisms that underlie moral behavior. Morality is considered to be the sets of customs and values endorsed by a cultural group to guide social conduct; it does not assume the existence of absolute moral values. Morality is a product of evolutionary pressures that have shaped social cognitive and motivational mechanisms, which had developed early in human development, into uniquely human forms of experience and behavior. Moral phenomena emerge from the integration of contextual social knowledge, represented as event knowledge in PFC; social semantic knowledge, stored in anterior and posterior temporal cortex; and motivational and basic emotional states, which depend on cortical-limbic circuits.

Patients with focal damage to ventromedial PFC show deficient engagement of pride, embarrassment, and regret. In moral cognition, activated regions include anterior PFC, OFC, posterior STS, anterior temporal lobes, insula, precuneus, ACC, and limbic regions. A moral judgment task that involves classic moral dilemmas (e.g., Should you kill an innocent person in order to save five other people?) activates anterior PFC. Decision difficulty is correlated with increased activity in ACC. Evidence is emerging that partially dissociable PFC-temporal-limbic networks represent distinct moral emotions, including guilt, anger, and embarrassment.

**moral deficiency** *Obs.* Moral insanity; *psychopathic personality* (q.v.). See *anethopathy.*

**moral dilemma** A situation in which the outcomes for all choices available are undesirable. Moral dilemmas typically engender strong emotions in the persons facing them, as they cognitively assess the consequences for themselves and others of the choice they make. Examples of dilemmas used to assess subjects' social reasoning, cooperativeness, selfishness, altruism, and the like are the *prisoner's dilemma*, the *trolley dilemma*, and the *Ultimatum Game* (qq.v.).

**moral emotions** Guilt, shame, embarrassment, jealousy, pride, and other states that depend on a social context. They arise later in development and evolution that the *basic emotions* (happiness, fear, anger, disgust, sadness) and require an extended representation of oneself as situated within a society. They function to regulate social behaviors, often in the long-term interests of a social group rather than the short-term interests of the individual person.

Sensory cortices mediate the perceptual representation of stimuli. The amygdala, striatum, and orbitofrontal cortex mediate an association of perceptual representation with emotional response, cognitive processing, and behavioral motivation. Higher cortical regions are then involved in construction of an internal model of the social environment, involving representation of other people, their social relationships with oneself, and the value of one's actions in the context of a social group.

**moral hazard** See *hazard, moral.*

**moral insanity** *Pathomania;* the condition of those "in whom the feeling tone of all ideas concerned in the weals and woes of others is stunted (*moral imbeciles*) or is entirely absent (*moral idiots*); both groups together would be designated as *moral oligophrenics.* Sympathy with others, instinctive feelings of the rights of others (not one's own) is absent, or is inadequately developed. At the same time the other kinds of emotional feelings can be perfectly retained" (Bleuler, E. *Textbook of Psychiatry*, 1930). See *psychopathic personality.*

**moral judgment** A type of evaluative judgment that is based on assessments of the adequacy of one's own and others' behaviors according to socially shaped ideas of right and wrong.

**moral masochism** *Ideal masochism*; also known as mental or psychic masochism; one of the three types of masochism described by Freud. It is characterized by a need for punishment arising from unconscious needs relating to resexualization of the parental introjects and reactivation of the Oedipus complex. According to Freud, the basic desire is to have intercourse with the father passively, and through regressive distortion this becomes a desire to be beaten by the father. The moral masochist must act against his own interests, even to the point of destroying himself, in order to provoke punishment from authority figures. Asceticism is related to moral masochism, for the mortification is sexualized and the act of mortifying becomes a distorted expression of the blocked sexuality.

Wilhelm Reich agreed that behind the masochist's behavior lay a desire to provoke authority figures, but he disagreed that this was in order to bribe the superego or to execute a dreaded punishment. Rather, he maintained, this grandiose provocation represented a defense against punishment and anxiety by substituting a milder punishment and by placing the provoked authority figure in such a light as to justify the masochist's reproach, "See how badly you treat me." Behind such a provocation is a deep disappointment in love, a disappointment of the masochist's excessive demand for love based on the fear of being left alone.

**moral narcissism** Narcissism manifested as a yearning to be pure and above normal human needs (which the narcissist finds shameful), and to be free of attachment to others (and thereby able to recapture his infantile megalomania).

**moral philosophy** *Ethics* (q.v.).

**moral pride** See *domesticated pride*.

**moral reasoning** The thinking mechanism through which moral judgements are obtained.

**moral right** See *right*.

**moral sensitivity hypothesis** The proposal that a network involving anterior PFC, OFC, STS, and limbic regions represents social-emotional events linked to "moral sensitivity"—an automatic tagging of ordinary social events with moral values.

**moral treatment** In psychiatry, humane treatment of the mentally ill. It was the French who spearheaded the late 18th-century move toward humane treatment of the insane. Jean-Baptiste Pussin, a tanner by trade who became the governor of mental patients at the Hospice de Bicêtre in Paris, taught Philippe Pinel the psychological methods he had developed for the care of the incurable mental patients on his ward. Among other things, Pussin replaced chains with straitjackets in 1787, although it is Pinel who is usually credited with the reforms. The unleashing of the mentally ill did not occur without severe resistance from the medical profession, from the politicians of the day, and from the Paris populace, and Pinel was more than once accused of harboring traitors in his hospital. One day he was set upon by a menacing crowd who threatened to lynch him for his "crimes." He escaped death only because his bodyguard, Chevigne, was able to fight off the mob—the same Chevigne who had been among the first group of patients to be released from their fetters.

Pinel's next step was to train hospital personnel in adequate care of the mentally ill, and it was his organization of mental hospitals that first demonstrated the value of hospital research and prepared the way for moral treatment and psychotherapy.

In the United States, Dr. Benjamin Rush (1745–1813) was a part of the movement toward humanization of treatment methods, including the abolition of mechanical restraint and the betterment of physical care. The period of moral treatment and humane care is the historical antecedent of the modern therapeutic community. See *social therapy*.

Advocates of psychological treatment in caring for the mentally ill in other countries between 1750 and 1850 included Willis, Haslam, and the Tukes in England, Fowler in Scotland, Daquin at Chambery, Chiarugi at Florence, the Brothers of Charity, and the French military medical inspector Jean Colombier. (Weiner, D. *American Journal of Psychiatry 136*, 1979).

**moral values** Culturally shaped concepts and attitudes that code for personal and societal preferences and standards.

**morality** See *ethics*.

**morbid gain** *Epinosic gain; advantage by illness* (qq.v.).

**Morel, Benedict A.** (1809–1873) French psychiatrist and physiologist; introduced the term *dementia praecox* (q.v.).

**mores** Culture; traditions, and particularly those so valued by the group or society that failure to observe them incurs condemnation, ostracism, or some other punishment. One example that survives in some subcultures is "marrying one's own kind."

**Morgellons disease** A skin disorder whose victims complain of insects invading their skin; crawling, stinging, and biting sensations; fibers protruding from nonhealing skin lesions; and extreme difficulty with concentration and short-term memory. Comorbid illnesses are frequent; they include mood disorders, ADHD, OCD, and autism spectrum disorder. There is often a past history or family history of depression or bipolar disorder, chronic fatigue syndrome, fibromyalgia, irritable bowel syndrome, and other somatization disorders.

Some psychiatrists and dermatologists believe that the basis of the disease is an altered sensation in the skin, probably triggered by neuropeptide release, usually associated with stress of some kind or depression. The patient interprets the sensation in terms of parasitic infestation. Others think that it is a form of *Lyme disease* (q.v.); and still others think it is a delusional parasitosis. See *parasitophobia*.

**moria** A morbid impulse to joke. Sometimes used synonymously with *gallows humor* (q.v.) or, more commonly, to refer to any dementia (usually of the exogenous-organic type) characterized by silliness. See *fronto-temporal dementia*.

**moristans** Hospitals or domiciles for the mentally ill in Islamic countries beginning in Baghdad in the eighth century. Islamics believed the insane to be messengers of the truth chosen by the Prophet; the moristans were designed to imitate Paradise and typically included perfumed baths, soothing music, and visits from the women of the town.

**Morita therapy** *Work therapy*; introduced by Professor Shoma Morita of Jikei University (Japan) during 1910–1920 and said to be particularly effective in neurotic patients with prominent hypochondriacal tendencies, and in treating *shinkeishitsu*, approximately equivalent to what in the United States would be termed social phobias (shyness, self-consciousness, uncontrollable blushing in public) or ego-dystonic obsessions and compulsions. It aims to help the patient understand that there is a clear distinction between what one feels and what one is able to accomplish despite those feelings; to train the patient to focus on constructive activities rather than on symptoms, to modify cognitive and behavioral patterns that result in unproductive self-preoccupation, and to emphasize the importance of accepting one's symptoms as potentially functional and constructive qualities rather than evidence of weakness or failure.

Morita therapy begins with absolute bed rest for 4 to 7 days, during which time the patient may not smoke, read, talk, etc. He may only sleep or suffer and is instructed to accept any experience that might occur. After the first phase, the patient takes on increasingly difficult and tiring work, usually in a communal setting, so that he may learn to work well and behave normally no matter what his symptoms. The patient is thereby trained, with advice and encouragement from his therapist, to accept phenomenological reality—a process called *arugamama*, the acceptance of life as it is for him at the moment (Iwai, H. & Reynolds, D. K. *American Journal of Psychiatry 126*, 1970). See *Naikan psychotherapy*.

**morning after** See *hangover*.

**Moro reflex** A type of mass reflex seen in the neonate in response to the examiner's slapping the surface on which the infant is lying; it consists of immediate flexion of the limbs and contraction of the abdominal wall with later interruptions of the spasm that produce cloniclike jerkings.

**moron** A person with mild mental retardation (IQ, 52–67); in England, called *dullard*.

**-morph** Combining form meaning one endowed with (specific) form or shape. From this are further formed -morphic, -morphous, -morphy.

**morphinism** Morphine addiction. See *addiction; opium*.

**morphologic inferiority** As used by Adler, a subgroup of organ inferiority characterized by a deficiency in the shape of an organ, or in its size, its individual portions of tissue, its individual cell complexes, of the whole apparatus or of limited parts of it.

**morphology** The study of form and structure; anatomy. See *phonemes*.

**morphometrics** Measuring the size or number of physical elements. Neuronal morphometrics counts the number of neurons in selected areas of the brain. In schizophrenia, for example, counts have revealed reductions of size (as measured by number of neurons) in the amygdala, internal globus pallidus, and hippocampus.

**morphophilia** A type of *paraphilia* (q.v.) in which sexual arousal and orgasm depend upon some discrepancy between the partner's bodily characteristics and the subject's; e.g., the partner must be markedly thinner or taller than the subject.

**Morquio syndrome** A *mucopolysaccharidosis* (q.v.) characterized by a deficiency of chondroitin sulfate enzyme, with excessive keratan sulfate in the urine, severe bone changes, cloudy cornea, and aortic regurgitation.

**Morris water maze** A standard memory test in mice; the animal learns the location of a submerged platform in a water bath, and the effect of different variables on the animal's ability to remember the escape route is assayed. Such variables include passage of time, interposition of a second learning task, drugs with a suspected positive or negative effect on memory, surgical ablation of different areas of the brain, etc.

**morsicatio buccarum** Habitual self-mutilation by biting the cheeks. Morsicatio labiorum refers to biting of the lips.

**mort douce** (F. "sweet death") Some authorities (e.g., Hirschfeld) use this expression to refer to the phenomena attendant upon the completion of the sexual act. Others use the phrase synonymously with *euthanasia* (q.v.).

**Mort1** *FADD* (q.v.).

**mortido** Federn's term for the destructive instinct; destrudo (q.v.).

**Morvan disease** (Augustin Marie de Lannitis Morvan, French physician, 1819–1897) See *syringomyelia*.

**mosaic** See *intermediate*.

**mosaic test** A projective technique, introduced by M. Lowenfeld and further developed by F. Wertham, which employs a set of 300 colored pieces (black, blue, red, green, yellow, and off-white) in six shapes (squares, diamonds,

oblongs, and three different-sized triangles). The subject is presented with the test objects on a tray and is asked to make anything he wants on the board. The designs made by adults and children have been correlated with diagnostic categories, and individual designs can be interpreted on the basis of these correlations.

**mosaicism** See *nondisjunction; Down syndrome*.

**mote-beam mechanism** Ischheiser's term for that distortion of social perception where the person is exaggeratedly aware of the presence of an undesirable trait in a minority group although oblivious to its presence in himself. See *objectivation*.

**mother, complete** A term used by Federn to refer to the ideal type of mother that every schizophrenic seeks both in phantasy and in reality. The complete mother loves her child unselfishly, for himself alone, and does not use him as a means of gratifying her own psychological needs. She shows a conspicuous and admirable absence of certain characteristics of "typical" mothers of schizophrenics, viz., a sense of resentful obligation and reluctant duty in regard to the mother's responsibilities toward her child, or sensual gratification in her relationship with her offspring. See *schizophrenogenic mother*.

**mother, great** See *Magna Mater*.

**mother archetype** "The archetype "Mother' is pre-existent and superordinate to every form of manifestation of the 'motherly.' It is a constant core of meaning, which can take on all aspects and symbols of the 'motherly." (Jacobi, J. *The Psychology of C. G. Jung*, 1942). See *Magna Mater; individuation*.

**mother image** See *image*.

**mother love** The feeling of affection, devotion, possessiveness, and the need of protecting the child born to a woman. "Mother love is frequently called an instinct, a proclivity that appears in a woman, because she becomes a mother and for no other reason. There may be something to this idea, but...'instinct' is not all that is involved. In general, people love those for whom they have to make sacrifices, and babies demand sacrifices. Not only "instinct' but many other types of pressures— social mores, the expectancy of the family for her to act in a motherly way, her husband's pride in her motherhood, pity for the helpless infant—are also involved in setting up the pattern of feeling and action we recognize as mother love" (Lemkau, P. V. *Mental Hygiene in Public Health*, 1949).

**mother surrogate**   1. Mother substitute; one who takes the place of the mother. The female schoolteacher, for instance, takes over part of the care of the child; she becomes a mother surrogate. The same concept holds true with regard to the father: hence the expressions *father surrogate* and *father substitute*.

2. Surrogate mother or host mother also refers to the woman who agrees to be inseminated artificially with the sperm of the husband of an infertile woman, to carry the fetus so conceived to term, and to relinquish all parental rights to that child once it is born, typically by giving it back to the couple for adoption. (The phrase "*new reproductive technology*" is currently preferred to "surrogate motherhood.")

**mother–child relationship (MCR)**   The reciprocal emotional interactions between mother and child, used particularly in reference to the effects of the mother's attitude on the emotional development of the child. Punitive mothers, for example, often have disobedient, hostile children; inconsistent mothers may have children with temper problems; critical, depreciatory mothers may have children who lie and are destructive. See *reciprocal regulation; psychosocial retardation; separation-individuation*.

**mothering, pathological**   See *monkey love; mother–child relationship; reciprocal regulation; smother love*.

**motility, unconscious**   Movements that are dissociated from consciousness, such as hysterical convulsions and spasms that are the unconscious and distorted physical expression of repressed instinctual demands.

**motility disorder**   Any abnormality of motion or movement; used by many in a more specific sense to refer to the abnormal postures, gestures, etc., seen in catatonic schizophrenics and/or in childhood schizophrenics.

**motility psychosis**   A type of manic-depressive psychosis described by Ewald; symptoms are mainly hyperkinetic in character, and the episode often occurs only once in a lifetime, with complete remission. See *cycloid psychosis*.

**motion recognition**   Perception of movement, such as mouth and hand movements and facial expression. The dorsal pathway of the superior temporal sulcus (STS) is specialized for the processing of motion information, and in particular perception of actions without well-defined form information. The ventral pathway of STS is involved in processing form information. The ventral intraparietal area is involved in the analysis and encoding of self-motion and is considered a possible site for the convergence of multisensory information relating to movement in space. See *point-light displays*.

**motivation**   The force that propels an organism to seek a goal or satisfy a need; striving, incentive, purpose. Sullivan termed *conjunctive* those strivings directed to long-range satisfaction of real needs, and disjunctive those substitute strivings that afford only immediate gratification.

Motivation is characterized by action, either to increase the probability of an outcome (appetitive motivation), or to reduce it (aversive motivation). A reward is an event that a subject will expend energy to bring about; a punishment is an event that a subject will expend energy to avoid or prevent. In social contexts, punishment typically refers to an aversive event administered by another person. Research indicates that appetitive value is encoded by the medial orbitofrontal cortex (OFC) and its reciprocal connections to amygdala and ventral striatum (nucleus accumbens). Aversive value is represented in the lateral OFC, which is also interconnected with amygdala and ventral striatum. See *reciprocity; reward*.

**motivation, unconscious**   An aim or goal that is not recognized consciously by the subject, and especially any such aim that is the basis for a symptom, slip of the tongue or pen, or dream. Hysterical vomiting in a pregnant woman, for example, may be determined by her desire to rid herself of the fetus, a desire of which she is not consciously aware.

**motivational interventions**   Included are motivational interviewing (MI) and motivation enhancement therapy (MET), which have been effective in alcohol and substance abuse disorders. A range of clinical strategies is used to enhance motivation for change, including counseling, assessment, multiple sessions, or brief interventions. Five key principles of MET are as follows: express empathy for the patient; note discrepancies between current and desired behavior; avoid argumentation; refrain from directly confronting resistance;

and encourage self-efficacy or the person's belief in his or her ability to change.

**motive** Any explanation for the performance of an action by a person. Reason, in contrast, is a belief that is able to render an otherwise irrational action rational.

**motor alpha** See *alpha rhythm.*

**motor aphasia** *Broca motor aphasia (q.v.)*; verbal aphasia; word-dumbness.

**motor apraxia** Maintenance of the ability to understand and name objects, but inability to carry out purposive movement with them. See *apraxia.*

**motor aprosodia** See *frontal lobe dysfunction.*

**motor circuits** See *frontal-striatal system.*

**motor cortex** The area of the cerebral hemisphere that controls movement; sometimes used synonymously with precentral convolution, although this is inaccurate, since movements can be excited from other areas as well.

**motor cortical inputs** See *striatal cortical inputs.*

**motor disability** Difficulty in getting information from the brain for expression via the musculature, as in writing and drawing.

**motor inertia** See *perseveration.*

**motor learning** The ability to learn a complex sequence of movements.

**motor loop** See *basal ganglia; LID.*

**motor memory** *Procedural memory* (q.v.); a type of recall memory based on muscular movement rather than on language, such as the infant's ability to recall a particular act and reproduce it on cue even before he has acquired language. See *affect memory.*

**motor neurosis** A neurosis characterized principally by disorders of movement, such as tics.

**motor persistence** See *persistence, motor.*

**motor response inhibition** The voluntary act of stopping an ongoing response; it can be measured by various tasks: the antisaccade, go/no-go, and stop-signal tasks. Response inhibition is integral to virtually all behavioral regulation and executive function. Motor inhibition activates the medial frontal and DLPFC. An inhibition deficit has been demonstrated in children and adults with a diagnosis of ADHD and is stable over time. See *attention deficit hyperactivity disorder.*

Research indicates that inhibition deficit is familial, that there is genetic overlap of ADHD and deficient inhibition, and that inhibition may be a marker of genetic vulnerability to ADHD that is evident both in affected persons and in those who are at genetic risk for ADHD even in the absence of the behavioral phenotype.

**motor skills disorder** *Coordination disorder* (q.v.).

**motorium** 1. The motor cortex. 2. The volition faculty of the mind (as the function of the sensorium is perception and of the intellect is thinking).

**Mott, Frederick Walker, Sir** (1853–1926) British neurologist; law of anticipation, that mental illness occurs earlier in succeeding generations.

**mourning** Normal grief, as contrasted with *melancholia* or *depression* (qq.v.), which are pathological. See *bereavement.*

According to Melanie Klein, the capacity to mourn depends upon working-through of the depressive position (beginning usually between 15 and 30 months of age, in the rapprochement phase of separation-individuation). The child must mourn separation from the mother in order to establish his or her identity as a freestanding person capable of genuine intimacy. Related to the development of an ability to mourn are a shift from part-object to whole-object relations, replacement of the splitting defense by repression, development of object permanency, and establishment of sphincter specificity with a shift from polymorphous-perverse eroticism to a consolidation of sexual identity that conforms with anatomic gender.

**mourning, anticipatory** Acknowledgment of and reconciliation with the inevitability of death of a child with a fatal illness, experienced by the child's parents and other relatives.

**movement, involuntary** Forced movement; an unwilled, adventitious contraction of one or more muscles or muscle groups that gives rise to movement in a limb or some other part of the body. The most frequently observed involuntary movements are *athetosis, chorea, myoclonus, tic,* and *tremor* (qq.v.).

**movement disorders, medication-induced** Also called—not fully correctly—medication-induced extrapyramidal symptoms (EPS); those most frequently occurring as a side effect of treatment with neuroleptics and other psychopharmacologic agents are *akathisia, dystonia, neuroleptic malignant syndrome,* parkinsonism, tardive *dyskinesia,* and *tremor* (qq.v.).

**movement therapy** See *dance therapy.*

**movement tremor** See *tremor.*

**moxibustion** See *complementary medicine.*

**Mozart effect**   A positive effect of listening to classical music on spatial reasoning skills, a method once believed to improve brain development in early childhood. The 1993 hypothesis that listening to classical music (Mozart in particular) before a spatial skills test could improve performance was ultimately rejected.

**MPAs**   Minor physical anomalies, reported in about 30% of patients with schizophrenia and in their siblings. The minor physical anomalies associated with schizophrenia are frequently found in, but are clearly not limited to, the head and facial regions. Both patients and their relatives have shown considerable diversity in form and frequency of neurological abnormalities, although the anomalies have primarily been in the domains representing sensory integration, motor coordination, and sequencing of complex motor acts. In young adulthood, the offspring of mothers with schizophrenia had a wide range of neurological abnormalities, consisting of hard signs, soft signs, deviant reflexes, and disturbances in motor functions, motor coordination, and cranial nerves. Schizophrenia patients themselves are characterized by "hard signs," while siblings of schizophrenia patients are more characterized by "soft signs." Midline brain anomalies such as enlarged cavum septi pellucidi and corpus callosum abnormalities have been found with increased incidence in patients with schizophrenia.

MPAs represent mild errors of morphogenesis of early prenatal origin. They are more frequent in male patients, reflecting greater vulnerability during prenatal development. MPAs represent a neurodevelopmental risk factor that can interact with other genetic and nongenetic factors to produce symptoms of illness (Sivkov, S. T. & Akabaliev, A. *Schizophrenia Bulletin 30*: 361–366, 2004).

**MPD**   *Multiple personality disorder*, now termed *dissociative identity disorder (DID)* (q.v.); myofascial pain dysfunction (see *temporomandibular joint syndrome*).

**MPH**   Methylpenidate.   See   *amphetamines; psychostimulants*.

**MPI**   Maudsley Personality Inventory.

**MPPS**   Massive parallel processing system, a type of artificial intelligence investigation concerned with the process of visual perception and modeled on the primate nervous system; also known as *parallel visual computation, neo-associationism*, and *neo-connectionism*.

**MPTP**   1-methyl-4-phenyl-1,2,3,6-tetrahydropyridine, a fentanyl derivative that destroys nigrostriatal dopaminergic neurons. It was first synthesized as *China white*, a *designer drug* (q.v.), to simulate high-quality heroin. It provides what is currently the best experimental model of Parkinson disease.

MPTP produces its effects upon being converted to MPP [1-methyl-4-phenylpyridinium] by monoamine oxidase. This suggested the possibility that MAOI might block the progression of Parkinson disease and led to the use of l-deprenyl in the disorder.

**MR spectroscopy**   A neuroimaging technique that allows noninvasive interrogation of the chemical environment of tissues, providing relative quantification of particular compounds and their constituents in certain regions of the brain. It has been particularly useful in measuring psychoactive drugs in brain (such as lithium and serotonin reuptake inhibitors) and brain GABA levels. The nuclei studied with MR spectroscopy include proton [$^1$H], phosphorus [$^{31}$P], carbon [$^{13}$C], lithium [$^7$Li], fluorine [$^{19}$F], and sodium [$^{23}$Na]. The most current MR spectroscopy involves $^1$H (proton MR spectroscopy), which can distinguish certain metabolites including *N*-acetyl aspartate (NAA), creatine, and phosphocreatine, and choline-containing phospholipidis. NAA is the largest peak seen on MR spectroscopy and is considered a marker of neuronal integrity.

A unique application of MR spectroscopy is the measurement of psychoactive drugs in the human brain, specifically the quantification of brain lithium and fluorinated drugs, which include most of the serotonin-specific reuptake inhibitors. Another neuropsychiatric application is in the in vivo measurement of brain GABA levels. Abnormal GABA levels have been measured in epilepsy, anxiety disorder, major depression, and drug addiction.

**MRI**   *Magnetic resonance imaging*, formerly called *NMR (nuclear magnetic resonance)*. Instead of X-rays, MRI uses three types of electromagnetic radiation to produce diagnostic images: static magnetic fields, pulsed radiofrequency magnetic fields, and gradient (time-varying) fields. The radio pulse disturbs the hydrogen nuclei aligned in the magnetic field; as they come back into realignment, the excited protons emit brief (a few hundred milliseconds) radio signals, the frequency of which depends on the tissue environment. MRI scanners convert the radiofrequency signals into images that represent different types of soft tissue. MRI differentiates better than the *CT scan* (q.v.) between white and gray matter in the brain. MRI provides views of structural brain abnormalities and thus is especially useful for assessing the effect of stroke or multiple sclerosis.

Early MR imaging took 10 minutes or more; ultrafast imagers such as *echo-planar MRI* (q.v.) use a gradient field that can be spatially encoded, and thereby they are able to gather even more information in a matter of milliseconds. As a result, fewer artifacts are produced by the patient's movement or heartbeat, the patient's time within the magnet is appreciably reduced, and the imaging approaches real-time brain activity. See *dMRI, fMRI, imaging, brain; pixel.*

**MRS**  Magnetic resonance spectroscopy. See *fMR; imaging, brain.*

**MSE**  Mental status examination.

**MSER**  Mental Status Examination Report. See *Multi-State Information System.*

**MSI**  *Magnetic source imaging;* a neuroimaging technique capable of detecting fast changes in isolated areas of the brain. The subject's head is surrounded by an array of hypersensitive magnetic detectors called *SQUIDS* (superconducting quantum interference devices), the most sensitive detectors for magnetic fields that are currently available.

**MSIS**  *Multi-State Information System* (q.v.).

**MSLT**  Multiple sleep latency test.

**MSM**  Men who have sex with men. MSM-IDU are men who have sex with men and inject drugs. Heterosexual MSM-IDU were more likely than gay or bisexual MSM-IDU to be homeless and to trade sex for money or drugs. MSM-IDU are a relatively small population, but one at very high risk of both infection and transmission. Through sexual behavior and drug use they are a nexus between both high-prevalence groups, such as MSM, and low-prevalence groups, such as female sexual partners and heterosexual IDUs.

**msMRI**  Magnetic-source magnetic-resonance imaging; a technique that increases the temporal resolution of current imaging methods without compromising spatial resolution. In contrast to PET and fMRI, msMRI does not depend on the hemodynamic brain response; in contrast to MEG, msMRI does not depend

on detection of neuronal magnetic fields at the scalp. Instead, it detects magnetic fields generated by neuronal activity at their source in the brain parenchyma.

**MSRPP**  Multidimensional Scale for Rating Psychiatric Patients; often called the *Lorr scale.*

**MST**  *Magnetic seizure therapy;* a form of somatic treatment for depression. Compared with *ECT* (q.v.), MST uses rapidly alternating strong magnetic fields rather than electrical current and offers greater control of intracerebral current density. MST-induced seizures are shorter, and patients had fewer subjective side effects and recovered orientation faster. It is safe and well tolerated and has a superior, acute, cognitive side-effect profile compared with ECT. A disadvantage of MST is that is requires general anesthesia and a strong electrical current because impedance of the skull shunts most of the current away from the brain. See *transcranial magnetic stimulation.*

**MSUD**  *Maple syrup urine disease* (q.v.).

**MSW**  1. Master's degree in social work.

2. Male sex worker. See *bridging.*

**mtDNA**  Mitochondrial DNA; the mitochondrial genome, which is quite distinct from the chromosomes that make up the genome within the nucleus. Each mitochondrion contains between four and ten copies of the mtDNA genome, and there are many mitochondria within each cell.

The mitochondrial genome consists of 16,569 base pairs on a single double-stranded loop of DNA, whereas nuclear DNA consists of 3 billion base pairs. Mitochondrial genes are inherited only from the mother; at the time of cell division the mitochondria are randomly assigned to the daughter cells. In consequence, although mtDNA mutations can occur just as they can with nuclear DNA, their transmission does not follow the Mendelian rules of genetic inheritance.

Among the diseases known to be associated with mtDNA mutations are myoclonus epilepsy and ragged red fiber disease (*MERRF*); various encephalomyopathies such as *MELAS* (mitochondrial encephalopathy, lactic acidosis, and strokelike symptoms) and *MMC* (maternally inherited myopathy and cardiomyopathy); *LHON* (Leber hereditary optic neuropathy); *NARP* (maternally inherited neurogenic muscle weakness, ataxia, and retinitis pigmentosa, associated with developmental delay, seizures, and dementia); *CEOP* (chronic external opthalmoplegia plus ptosis and myopathy) and *KSS* (Kearns-Sayre syndrome, a severe form of CEOP with retinitis pigmentosa, hearing loss, cardiac conduction defects, ataxia, and dementia); and Pearson syndrome (panctyopenia, pancreatic fibrosis, and splenic atrophy, usually a fatal childhood disorder). It is suspected that mtDNA defects are also linked to Huntington disease and Parkinson disease, and it has been suggested that aging reflects an accumulation of mtDNA mutations over a person's lifetime. See *myoclonus epilepsy.*

**MTL** *Medial temporal lobe,* a collection of anatomically connected regions that have an essential role in declarative memory. MTL includes the hippocampal regions (CA fields, dentate gyrus, subicular complex), amygdala, fornix, and adjacent entorhinal, perirhinal, and parahippocampal cortices. Damage to MTL results in temporally graded retrograde amnesia—memory loss for more recent events is more pronounced that for the distant past. The perirhinal cortex and the parahippocampal gyrus provide nearly two-thirds of the cortical input to the entorhinal cortex. The entorhinal cortex in turn is the source of the *perforant path,* the major efferent projection to the hippocampus and dentate gyrus. Thus, these cortical regions collectively provide the principal route by which information in neocortex reaches hippocampus.

Two parts of the left MTL—the anterior MTL in the rhinal cortex and the hippocampus proper—contribute to the memory encoding of words and their subsequent recall. Encoding activity of the hippcampus follows encoding activity in the anterior MTL. Currently, there is debate about the architecture of memory and the specific roles of MTL structures in memory formation. One theory proposes that parahippocampal and hippocampal regions support the encoding of the same type of declarative information, which supports later recall and recognition of facts and events. An alternative theory postulates that the parahippocampal gyrus contributes mainly to the encoding of information about the occurrence of an item (required for subsequent recognition), whereas the hippocampus supports encoding of relations between an item and its context (primarily useful for subsequent recall).

**mTOR** See *ATM family.*

**mu rhythm** See *alpha rhythm.*

**Much-Holzmann reaction** (Hans Much, German physician, 1880–1932, and Wilhelm Holtzmann, German physician) The alleged property of the serum from a person with schizophrenia or manic-depressive psychosis to inhibit hemolysis caused by cobra venom.

**mucopolysaccharidosis** Any of a group of autosomal recessive disorders of glycosaminoglycans (GAG), characterized by severe mental retardation, skeletal deformities (such as gargoylism), and deposits of GAG in the tissues and excretion in the urine. The group includes β-*glucuronidase deficiency, Hunter syndrome, Hurler disease, Maroteaux-Lamy syndrome, Morquio syndrome, Sanfilippo syndrome,* and *Scheie syndrome* (qq.v.).

**muina** *Colera* (q.v.).

**multiaxial assessment** A system for evaluating psychiatric patients in different areas that are specified, in an attempt to avoid overlooking factors of significance in the development of their various conditions. DSM-IV-TR (2000), for example, contains five axes: I—Clinical disorders; II—Personality disorders and mental retardation; III—General medical conditions; IV—Psychosocial and environmental problems; V—Global assessment of functioning. See *DSM-III, DSM-III-R, DSM-IV.*

**multidetermination** *Overdetermination* (q.v.).

**multidimensional pain management** See *pain management, multidimensional.*

**multifactorial model** See *inheritance.*

**multifocal thought** Arieti's term for *asyndesis* (q.v.) and similar association disturbances, which he explains as being due to the fact that the patient's thought simultaneously focuses on many different planes and on different meanings with their different objective situations.

**multi-infarct dementia** *Cerebral arteriosclerosis; vascular dementia* (qq.v.); a relatively small group of persons in whom a clear-cut succession of strokes has produced enough brain tissue damage to cause *dementia* (q.v.), with disturbances in memory, abstract thinking, judgment, impulse control, and personality. The course of deterioration is patchy and fluctuating, rather than steadily progressive.

**multilingual** See *linguistics.*

**multimodal therapy** See *BASIC-ID.*

**multiphasic screening** See *screening.*

**multiple complex developmental disorder (MCDD)**
A term suggested for *borderline personality disorder* manifested in childhood. The pathology of BPD in childhood includes externalizing, internalizing, and cognitive symptoms; it is associated with neuropsychologic findings, including soft signs of organicity, such as learning disabilities, ADHD, and abnormal EEG patterns; and it may be a precursor for a wide range of personality disorders in adulthood.

**multiple drug misuse** *Polydrug abuse*; repeated use of more than one psychoactive drug at the same time, or sequentially over a brief period, often with the intent to enhance or prolong desirable effects but sometimes in an attempt to reduce undesirable side effects experienced with one or more of the drugs used. Currently, a triad of alcohol, marijuana, and cocaine dependence occurs as a regular pattern in young drug users in urban areas. In ICD-10, the term is used only when one drug cannot be identified as the one contributing most to the abuse pattern, or when the different drugs being used cannot be identified with certainty. The corresponding term in DSM-III-R is *polysubstance dependence*.

**multiple monitored electroconvulsive therapy (MMECT)** A modification of classical ECT in which several EEG-monitored convulsions are induced in a single session in an attempt to achieve results over a shorter period of time.

**multiple personality disorder (MPD)** In DSM-IV, *dissociative identity disorder* (q.v.).

**multiple psychotherapy** *Role-divided, three-cornered therapy; cotherapy; cooperative psychotherapy; dual leadership* all refer to the use of more than one therapist at one time in individual or group psychotherapy.

**multiple sclerosis** *MS; Charcot syndrome*; disseminated sclerosis; insular sclerosis; a chronic inflammatory and neurodegenerative disease characterized by T cell–mediated demyelination of the medullary sheath, which is followed by glial proliferation. The result is disruption of the transmission of action potentials along nerves, manifested in multiple neurologic defects such as incoordination, motor paralysis, visual and sensory disturbances, and bladder and bowel dysfunction. MS is a relapsing-remitting disease that leads to progressive disease where relapses and remissions are less apparent.

Although the cause of MS is unknown, and multiple etiologies including autoimmunity, infectious agents, environmental triggers, and hereditary factors have been proposed, there is substantial evidence to indicate that dysregulated immune responses, including immune mechanisms directed against myelin proteins, have a role in triggering disease onset. The neuropathology has been well documented. In focal regions of the brain and spinal cord, T cells and macrophages cross the blood–brain barrier (BBB) and invade the parenchyma. These cells give rise to the pathological hallmarks of MS—extensive regions of fiber tract demyelination (plaques), with relative sparing of axons. Invading molecules secrete molecules that act as "molecular scissors" to transect axons in the early stages of plaque formation. The extent of the ongoing axonal injury correlates with the intensity of the inflammatory response, and disease-associated disability is correlated with brain atrophy. Systemic infection often induces relapses in MS, probably by activation of already primed macrophages and microglia within the CNS.

The disease usually begins between the ages of 20 and 40; the average age at onset is 30 years for females and 34 years for males. The age at onset tends to be lowest in those areas with the highest incidence. In 50% of cases, the initial symptom is weakness or loss of control over one or more limbs; in 29% the initial symptom involves the visual apparatus (blindness, dimness of vision, double vision, field defects, etc.); in 11% the initial symptom is numbness or similar painless paresthesia. The earliest symptoms tend to be fleeting and fluctuating, so that a misdiagnosis of hysteria is often made. The disappearance or alleviation of symptoms may last for months or years until the patient suffers another exacerbation.

In general, three main types of multiple sclerosis can be distinguished: an acute form, with a survival period of 1 to 2 years; a chronic, progressive form with a slowly downhill course that may last for 20 or 30 years; and a remittent form in which there is almost complete relief from symptoms during the period between acute exacerbations. The average life expectancy after the onset of the illness has been estimated to be 20 to 25 years.

"The end is distressing... Ataxia, weakness, and spasticity confine the patient to bed and prevent him from carrying out the simplest actions for himself. Swallowing becomes difficult and speech almost unintelligible. Urinary or cutaneous infection or pneumonia finally releases the sufferer. In rare cases the last event is an acute exacerbation of the disease itself, taking the form of an acute myelitis or encephalomyelitis" (Brian, W. R. *Diseases of the Nervous System*, 1951).

In the mental sphere, euphoria with a sense of mental and physical well-being despite obvious handicaps is characteristic, although dejection, irritability, and emotional lability are seen in some patients. Usually there is some reduction in intellectual capacity and a few patients develop a delusional state or a terminal dementia.

The disease was first described by Cruveilhier in 1835 and Carswell in 1838. Charcot described a triad of symptoms—nystagmus, intention tremor, and scanning speech—but this is found only in about 10% of cases and even then usually only when lesions are far advanced.

At the present time, cardinal features are the presence of symptoms of more than one central nervous system lesion at one time and a course of remissions and exacerbations.

Prevalence of MS is highest in the temperate regions of the world. The highest incidence of the disorder is in northern Europe and Switzerland; the incidence in Great Britain is about one-half of that in Switzerland, and the incidence in the United States is about one-quarter of that in Great Britain. In the United States incidence is considerably greater in the North than in the South.

Multiple sclerosis occurs twice as frequently in women as in men. Concordance rate in monozygotic twins is 26%; in dizygotic twins, 2.3%; and in nontwin siblings, 1.9%. Data from multiple ethnic groups suggest that the HLA-DR and HLA-DQ subregions of the *major histocompatibility complex* play a role in susceptibility to MS. The HLA region consists of a cluster of genes on the short arm of chromosome 6; several of them are involved in the regulation of the immune response. The most promising susceptibility locus appears to be *HLA-DRB2*. Although it is generally believed that MS is an autoimmune disorder, there is no consensus among researchers as to which genes are involved. There is some evidence that the retrovirus HTLV-1 (human T-cell lymphotrophic virus) or some other viral

agent may trigger the autoimmune process. The "hygiene hypothesis" proposes that early life infections may down-regulate allergic and autoimmune disorders. Having siblings may increase the number of early-life infections. Younger siblings may be important because infants provide a source of common viral infections. Repeated exposures to such common infant infections may confer protection against any adverse autoimmunity triggering effect of these infectious agents in later life and thereby reduce the risk of MS.

**multiple system atrophy**    *MSA*; a group of disorders of the basal ganglia, originally described as separate but now considered to be different forms of a single entity. Included are as follows:

    1. *Striatonigral degeneration,* with a predominance of rigidity and akinesia over tremor, mild pyramidal signs, and respiratory stridor

    2. *Shy-Drager syndrome,* with rigidity, tremor, and autonomic failure

    3. *Olivopontocerebellar atrophy* (sporadic form), with parkinsonian and cerebellar signs

**multiple trace theory (MTT)**    It proposes that, although experience is initially encoded in distributed hippocampal-cortical networks, the hippocampus is always required for rich contextual or spatial detail. Standard models of *consolidation* (q.v.) predict that reorganization occurs in cortical networks; MTT predicts that reactivation should also lead to the generation of new traces within hippocampus.

**multiplicity**    The state or quality of being manifold or various; in psychiatry, the state of possessing many personalities or a psychic organization that is highly prone to dissociative defenses. See *dissociative identity disorder (DID); personality disorder; personality multiplication.*

**multipolarity**    A term introduced by Slavson to stress the fact that in group psychotherapy transference is directed toward more than the one person of the therapist.

**multisensory integration**    Combination of signals from distinct sensory systems, but related to the same physical object.

**Multi-State Information System (MSIS)**    An automated, clinical record-keeping system, developed by the Information Sciences Division and New York State Department of Mental Hygiene in cooperation with five other states

(Connecticut, Maine, Massachusetts, Rhode Island, and Vermont) and the District of Columbia, for use in mental hospitals and community mental health facilities, to provide comparative multistate summary statistics for evaluation of programs and treatment procedures. It includes the Mental Status Examination Report (MSER)—a four-page optical scan form made up of structured multiple-choice items that cover the usual mental status categories—and the Periodic Evaluation Record (PER), a one-page subset of the MSER that is administered at frequent intervals so as to provide a narrative of the patient's progress.

**multisystem degeneration** See *Shy-Drager syndrome.*

**mumbling** Muttering; indistinct speech; asapholalia; mussitation. Continuous mumbling without apparent signs of excitation may be an outstanding manifestation of the terminal state in schizophrenia and is also frequent in Alzheimer disease and other dementias. The mumbling consists of inarticulate, indistinct, and incoherent phrases, usually uttered in low tones so that the patient appears to be talking to himself.

**mummification** Preparation of a body for burial with preservatives to protect against decomposition; enshrinement. In psychiatry, the term refers to preserving the effects or essence of a loved object (such as allowing nothing to be moved or altered in the loved one's room) or refusal to relinquish the body of the loved one (in at least one case, for as long as 10 years after death). It has been suggested that mummification is more than a pathological grief reaction and that at least some cases are a type of *folie à deux* (q.v.) (Boughton, D. P. & Popkin, M. K., *Comprehensive Psychiatry 30*, 1989).

**Munchhausen syndrome** A name suggested by Asher in 1951 to refer to patients who wander from hospital to hospital ("*hospital hoboes*'), feigning acute medical or surgical illness and giving false and fanciful information about their medical and social background; *peregrinating patient syndrome.* The diagnostic triad of symptoms comprises *pseudologia fantastica* (q.v.), peregrination, and disease simulation. The underlying motivation for such behavior (pathomimicry) is not clearly understood, but apparently it does not include attempts to obtain drugs, avoid police, etc. Such patients

would seem to be a particular form of *impostor* (q.v.). See *factitial; factitious disorders.*

**Munich cooperation model** A type of group therapy in which the group is structured to allow for reproduction of typical intrafamilial conflicts. The ward staff observe the group sessions and apply interpretations from them to the patient–personnel interactions on the ward, and patients support one another in autonomous groups that form after the treatment period.

**Munsterberg, Hugo** (1863–1916) Prussian-born American psychologist; founder of applied psychology, especially to law, business, industry, and sociology.

**murder** Premeditated killing or *homicide* (q.v.).

**Murphy, Gardner** (1895–1979) American psychologist; personality development, parapsychology.

**Murray, Henry** (1893–1988) American psychoanalyst; personology; Thematic Apperception Test.

**muscarinic** See *antimuscarinic; acetylcholine; cholinergic.*

**muscle dysmorphia** A form of body image distortion seen in body builders who, despite their muscular bodies and top physical condition, are convinced they look puny. Their proccupation with their bodies can become so intense that they give up desirable jobs, careers, and social engagements in order to spend many hours a day at the gym "bulking up." They may refuse to be seen in a bathing suit, for example, for fear that others will regard their bodies as too small and out of shape. See *anabolic-androgenic steroids (AAS).*

The syndrome is the opposite of *anorexia nervosa* (q.v.), in which patients see themselves as fat despite being severely underweight. Muscle dysmorphics see themselves as underdeveloped despite being very muscular. Many of the muscle dysmorphics studied had taken anabolic steroids to enhance muscular development. Most weighed themselves several times a day, repeatedly examined their bodies in the mirror, and wore baggy clothes to conceal their "puny" bodies.

**music therapy** Use of music to promote the patient's growth, development, functioning, and ability to cope with and gain satisfaction from life. Music refers to the music itself, providing music in the environment, listening to the music, and the making of music. Various elements of potential benefit to patients have been identified in music: (1) the experience of structure that music provides—rhythm by itself has the potential of energizing and bringing order into experience; once begun, music requires a commitment by the listener or performer that is a part of the music itself; (2) opportunity for self-expression and self-organization, including a socially acceptable avenue for expressing negative feelings, closeness, energetic behavior, etc.; (3) enhancement of self-esteem through self-actualization; (4) promoting relationships with others. See *dance therapy; recreation; occupational therapy.*

**musician's cramp**   A task-specific *focal dystonia* (q.v.), consisting of a spasmodic contraction of muscles used in playing a musical instrument.

**musicogenic epilepsy**   A type of *reflex epilepsy* (q.v.).

**musicotherapy**   Treatment of nervous and mental disorders by means of music, such as David's harp playing, which is said to have cured King Saul of his depression.

**musophobia**   Fear of mice.

**mussitation**   Movement of the tongue or lips as if in speech, without the production of articulate sounds. See *mumbling.*

**mutant (mutational, mutated)**   Pertaining to new hereditary characters originated by mutation.

**mutation**   An alteration of the nucleotide sequence, which may be a change in the allele of a gene (gene mutation), or in parts of chromosomes, an entire chromosome, or sets of chromosomes (chromosome mutations). Genetic information consists of sequences of building blocks (nucleotides) that constitute a molecule of *DNA* (q.v.). Whether these mutational variations are minor or more conspicuous, it is their clear distinction from the parental type and their ability to reproduce the new type that distinguish them from other forms of variation. See *chromosome.*

Mutant characters arise suddenly, breed true from the beginning, and give rise to a new and distinct race. They seem to occur in each species, usually with irregular frequency and more or less "spontaneously." This means that very little is known about the real cause, although it has been possible experimentally to produce various mutations by such external influences as high temperatures, radium, or chemicals.

In human beings *factor mutations* are brought about by a change in one of the chromomeres. These mutated genes produce more or less *pathological* types that often have a restricted viability (*lethal* factors). It may be assumed that the majority of hereditary malformations are caused by such factor mutations. Other kinds of mutation arise from changes in equipment or in the position of genes.

Although all present evidence indicates that mutations are relatively common in nature and probably the starting point for every form of evolutionary development, it is clear that more differences among individuals are derived from combination than from changes of genes. As soon as a multiplicity of unlike genes have originated by mutation, the genes are brought together in every new combination as rapidly as crosses are effected between individuals differing with respect to them. In the last analysis, however, mutations must underlie the origin of each new stock, race, or species. See *genetic diversity.*

**mutation, point**   Mutation of a single gene.

**mutation, selection-induced**   Mutagenesis that occurs more frequently when the organism is under selective pressure for that mutation. Also called adaptive, late-arising, post-plating, selection-promoted, and Cairnsian mutation, the latter in recognition of J. Cairns and his coworkers, who first suggested the possibility. Selection-induced mutation contradicts the conventional idea that mutations arise independent of their utility.

The model for selective-induced mutation is SOS, the bacterial DNA damage-repair response, in which changes are induced that not only repair damaged DNA but also increase the mutation rate of undamaged DNA. The theory of selective-induced mutation proposes that there are many states analagous to SOS; induced by stressors, their action is to accelerate and specify genetic change.

**mutations, dynamic**   See *anticipation.*

**mutative**   Relating to or productive of change, variation, alteration.

**mutative interpretation**   Any interpretation producing change; specifically, an interpretation that produces a breach in the neurotic vicious circle. First, the analyst in the role of auxiliary superego allows a particular quantity of the patient's id-energy to become conscious (e.g., in the form of an aggressive impulse);

second, such id impulses will be directed onto the analyst; third, the patient "will become aware of the contrast between the aggressive character of his feelings and the real nature of the analyst, who does not behave like the patient's 'good' or 'bad' archaic objects. This is the point at which the vicious circle of the neurosis is breached, and, with the patient's recognition of the distinction between the archaic phantasy object and the real external object, the way is opened to the recovery of further infantile material that is being reexperienced by the patient in his relationship to the analyst" (Strachey, J. *International Journal of Psychoanalysis 15*, 1934).

**mutilation**    See *self-mutilation*.

**mutinus, mutunus**    *Obs.* Priapus; penis.

**mutism**    The state of being mute, dumb, silent; voicelessness without structural alterations; silence due to disinclination to talk as the "vows of silence" in anchorites or monastics of various religious creeds or people who will not tell the reason for their mutism: they can, but they will not speak.

By usage the term *stupor* is often a synonym for *mutism*. It is seen in the catatonic form of schizophrenia, in the stupor of melancholia, and in states of hysterical stupor.

**mutism, elective**    The form *selective mutism* is preferred in DSM-IV; as first used by Tramer in 1934, mutism limited to absence of verbal communication with certain persons, even though speech itself is intact. The condition is rare, appears usually at about 3 years of age, and lasts for several months or up to 2 years. Since the original description, the condition has been reported in older children, and in many it has been of longer duration. Improvement is typically related to a change of environment, such as a change of school. See *school phobia*.

**muttering delirium**    *Delirium mussitans*; a severe delirium in which movements are reduced to tossing or trembling and speech is disorganized by iteration, perseveration, slurring, and dysarthria.

**mutual cueing**    See *communicative matching; empathic failure; fit*.

**mutual help group**    A group whose members support each other in recovering or maintaining recovery from alcohol or other chemical dependence, without professional therapy or guidance. With the recent emphasis on the alcoholic as part of a dysfunctional family, mutual help groups have expanded to include persons other than the identified alcoholic or drug user who are affected by the pattern of abuse or dependence. Many of the groups use a 12-step approach, modeled on AA. Often the group is called a *self-help group*, even though the members depend on each other for support.

**mutualism**    *Symbiosis* (q.v.).

**mutuality**    See *divorce, emotional*.

**MVP**    Mitral valve prolapse; a deformity of one or both cusps of the valve between the left atrium and the left ventricle, rendering the valve incompetent or insufficient. As a result, the ventricular contraction is inefficient: instead of all the blood within the ventricle being propelled into the aorta, some regurgitates back into the left atrium. Part of the cardiac energy is thereby wasted in pushing blood backward against the stream coming from the pulmonary bed into the left atrium. The most common cause of mitral valve prolapse is infection (especially rheumatic). Other frequent causes are deformity and injury. MVP is not always of sufficient degree to cause symptoms or to lead to heart failure; when it does, the process tends to be gradual and to extend over many years.

Some reports find MVP to occur significantly more often than expected in subjects with *panic disorder* and *agoraphobia* (qq.v.), but the majority of research does not indicate any relationship between the two.

**my-, myo-**    Combining form meaning muscle, mouse, from Gr. *mys*.

**myalgia-eosinophilia syndrome**    See *eosinophilia-myalgia syndrome*.

**myalgic encephalomyelitis**    See *chronic fatigue syndrome; EBV syndrome*.

**myasthenia**    Weakness of the muscles; fatigability; seen often in schizophrenia and depression.

**myasthenia gravis**    A chronic autoimmune disorder due to an antibody-mediated attack on nicotinic acetylcholine receptors at neuromuscular junctions. How T cells and B cells specific for acetylcholine receptors interact to produce the pathogenic autoantibodies is unknown. The number of acetylcholine receptors is decreased to one-third of normal, not a sufficient amount to trigger action potentials in some muscle fibers. This leads to the characteristic symptoms of muscular weakness and fatigability. The extraocular and eyelid muscles are affected early, leading to ptosis and diplopia. In 85% of patients, weakness becomes generalized, affecting the limb muscles, diaphragm, neck extensors, and the facial and bulbar muscles, leading to a flattened or snarling smile, nasal or "mushy" speech, and difficulty in chewing and swallowing.

The disease occurs in peaks, one in the second and third decades affecting mostly women, the other in the sixth and seventh decades affecting mostly men. Some believe that the thymus may be the site of origin of the disorder; 75% of patients have thymus abnormalities, such as hyperplasia or thymoma, and thymectomy gives improvement in most patients.

Currently, four methods of treatment are used: (1) anticholinesterase agents, such as pyridostigmine, to enhance neuromuscular transmission; (2) thymectomy; (3) immunosuppression with corticosteroids (such as prednisone), azathiprine, or cyclosporine; (4) short-term immunotherapies to stabilize patients in myasthenic crisis and for patients undergoing thymectomy; included are *plasmapheresis* (q.v.), to remove antibodies from the circulation, and intravenous immune globulin.

**mydriasis**  Dilation of the pupil. Mydriatics include *parasympatholytic* agents (such as atropine, scopolamine) and *sympathomimetic* drugs (such as cocaine, epinephrine). The former are *cycloplegic* (i.e., they relax ciliary muscles); the latter are not.

**myelencephalon**  See *hindbrain*.

**myelin**  A fatty insulating sheath that surrounds large axons; it is essential for high-speed conduction of action potentials. Myelinated nerve fibers conduct impulses at a speed of 2 to 100 meters per second. Nonmyelinated fibers are much slower, with a conduction speed of 0.2 to 2 meters per second. See *glia*.

Myelin inhibits neuronal regeneration; it is not inherently inhibitory, however, and it can promote axonal growth in embryonic and neonatal neurons. *MAG* (myelin-associated glycoprotein) promotes neurite outgrowth from neonatal cells; but if a downstream cAMP effector—protein kinase A—is blocked, the cells can no longer regenerate in response to MAG. But raising the level of cAMP in adult DRG (rat dorsal root ganglion) neurons causes them to behave more like neonatal cells. In the rat, cAMP levels drop during early postnatal development, coinciding with the period

in which the neurons lose their ability to regenerate.

In peripheral nerves, myelin is formed by *Schwann cells*, a type of glia. Early in development, the external cell membrane (*plasmalemma*) of the Schwann cell spirals around part of the axon in concentric layers and then condenses into the mature myelin sheath. Several Schwann cells are needed to ensheath the entire axon; the intervals between them are the *nodes of Ranvier*, and each internodal segment is formed by a single Schwann cell. For the insulation to stay in place, each layer of the myelin sheath must stick to the layer laid down before it, otherwise the wrapping will unwind. What makes the layers stick together is the $P_0$ protein, a sort of molecular velcro that is the chief structural element in myelin. When the gene for the protein $P_0$ is defective, the myelin cannot wrap itself tightly around the nerve and it may break down altogether. Some of the 29 known disease-causing $P_0$ mutations cause symptoms ranging from poor coordination to paralysis. Depending on how well the protein functions with each mutation, different affected persons may have different levels of nerve damage. In the peripheral nervous system, the myelination program involves a number of signals between the neuronal and myelin-forming cells that include neuregulins, adenosine triphosphate, steroid hormones, Desert hedgehog, and the *neurotrophins* (q.v.) BDNF and NT3.

In CNS, the glial cell that forms myelin is the oligodendrocyte. Both central and peripheral myelin contain the same group of at least seven related proteins, sometimes called myelin basic protein.

**myelin disorders**  Included are *Charcot-Marie Tooth disease* (*CMT*), *Dejerine-Sottas syndrome* (*DSS*), and Congenital Hypomyelination (CH) (qq.v.). CH is the rarest and most lethal of the disorders, typically leading to death in the first few weeks of life when the nerves that control breathing fail.

**myelin-associated glycoprotein**  *MAG* (q.v.). See *myelin*.

**myelitis**  Inflammation of the spinal cord.

**myelo-**  Combining form meaning marrow, spinal cord, from Gr. myelos.

**myelocystocele**  Spinal cord substance contained in a *spina bifida* (q.v.).

**myelogram**  X-ray of the spine following injection of a contrast medium into the spinal subarachnoid space by spinal puncture; most commonly used to demonstrate herniations of the intervertebral discs.

**myelomeningocele**   Spina bifida with protrusion of both the cord and its membranes.

**Myerson sign**   See *glabella tap test*.

**myoclonia**   Any disorder characterized by spasmodic muscular contractions, as in infectious myoclonia or chorea.

**myoclonic encephalitis**   See *hypsarrhythmia*.

**myoclonic epilepsy**   A type of *petit mal epilepsy* (q.v.).

**myoclonic sleep disorder**   Insomnia disorder with repetitive, stereotyped leg muscle jerks preceding periods of micro- or macroarousal.

**myoclonus**   Brief, involuntary twitching of a muscle or a group of muscles. It includes hiccups and the muscle jerks experienced when drifting off to sleep.

**myoclonus, nocturnal**   A dyssomnia consisting of repetitive, stereotyped jerkings of the leg muscles of variable duration and frequency that occur during the night and continually disrupt sleep. In contrast to *restless legs syndrome* (q.v.), nocturnal myoclonus is not associated with disagreeable sensations in the legs. See *sleep disorders*.

**myoclonus epilepsy**   One type of generalized seizure without focal onset, first described by Unverricht in 1891. This type of *epilepsy* (q.v.) is usually familial and occurs in several siblings. Symptoms usually begin between 6 and 16 years. Generalized epileptiform attacks with loss of consciousness appear first, often only at night. After several years, the characteristic myoclonic contractions develop; they involve simultaneously the symmetrical muscles on both sides of the body and are strong enough to produce movements of limb segments. The face, trunk, and upper and lower limbs are most commonly involved. The contractions disappear during sleep and are intensified by emotional excitement. They tend to increase in severity before a generalized epileptic attack; sudden contraction of the lower limbs may throw the patient to the ground. For a period of years, myoclonic contractions and epileptic attacks are associated; during this time, a progressive dementia develops and there is a passing into a third stage, where the grand mal attacks tend to disappear. Then dysarthria and dysphagia increase and death often follows progressive cachexia.

One form of myoclonus epilepsy is currently termed *MERRF* (myoclonus epilepsy and ragged red fiber disease), caused by a point mutation of *mtDNA* (q.v.). Adenine is substituted for guanine at base-pair position 8344, which interferes with the production of mitochondrial proteins. Clinical manifestations include uncontrollable jerking of skeletal muscles and dementia, similar to Unverricht's description. "Ragged red fiber" refers to the appearance of the muscle fibers when stained for abnormal mitochondria.

**myodynia, hysterical**   Muscular tenderness, usually over the ovarian region, observed occasionally in hysteria.

**myoedema**   Swelling of muscle; on tapping a muscle with a percussion hammer, a localized swelling appears and persists for a few moments; a sign of hyperirritability of atrophic muscles.

**myofascial pain dysfunction**   See *temporomandibular joint syndrome*.

**myokinetic psychodiagnosis test**   A test devised by Mira that consists  of drawings of patterns with both the right and the left hands. The left-hand drawings are believed to reveal genotypic reactions and the right-hand drawings are said to express more superficial phenotypic reactions. Comparison of the drawings is made to diagnose various conditions and character traits.

**myokymia**   A transient quiver of a muscle, occurring in weak anemic subjects.

**myopathic gait**   A waddling gait is characteristic of the myopathies. See *waddling gait*.

**myopathy, menopausal**   A pseudomyopathic polymyositis that appears in women during the menopausal years; proximal muscles are affected, and pathology consists of muscle necrosis without cellular infiltration.

**myopia**   Shortsightedness or nearsightedness, caused by an elongation of the globe of the eye so that parallel rays are focused in front of the retina. Farsightedness is the reverse condition and is known as *hyperopia*. See *ametropia*.

**myotonic dystrophy**   *DM; dystrophia myotonica; myotonia atrophia*; first described by Déléage in 1890; an autosomal dominant disorder with multisystemic effects that maps to chromosome 19. The genetic basis of one form of the disease—DM1—is an unusually large CTG *trinucleotide repeat* (q.v.) in the mRNA portion of the myotonin-protein kinase gene (Mt-PK or DMPK). DM2, proximal myotonic myopathy

(PROMM), has been mapped to chromosome 3. Its basis is a large expanded CCTG repeat (a tetranucleotide repeat, with a mean of 5000 repeats) in the RNA portion of the ZNF9 gene (zinc finger protein 9 gene, also referred to as the cellular nucleic acid-binding protein gene).

Manifestations include myotonia (hyperexcitability of the muscle membrane) and muscle weakness; atrophy of the sterno-cleido-mastoid muscles and the muscles of the face (leading to a "hatchet-face" appearance), shoulder, forearm, and hand and of the quadriceps muscle; ocular cataracts; cardiac arrhythmias; male frontal baldness; endocrine disorders; and, in some families, mild mental retardation. Males are more commonly affected between the ages of 20 and 30 years. Affected patients usually succumb to intercurrent infections in late middle life.

DM1 and DM2 are clinicaly similar, although the course of DM2 is usually more benign, it does not show a congenital form, and it lacks the severe central nervous system involvement that occurs in DM1.

**mysophilia** A *paraphilia* (q.v.) consisting of interest in, and desire for, filth or dirt; the desire to become unclean or polluted by contact with dirty or filthy objects—the opposite of *mysophobia* (q.v.). Mysophilia is commonly associated with coprophilia and urophilia. See *psychosexual.*

**mysophobia** Fear of contamination, often expressed in incessant handwashing, refusal to touch anything without wearing gloves, or repeated washing of everything in the surroundings.

**mystic paranoia** Pike's term for psychosis of association. See *induced psychotic disorder.*

**mythological theme** "The collective unconscious—so far as we can venture a judgment upon it—seems to consist of something of the nature of mythological themes or images. For this reason the myths of peoples are the real exponents of the collective unconscious. The whole of mythology could be taken as a kind of projection of the collective unconscious" (Jung, C. G. *Contributions to Analytic Psychology,* 1928).

**mythomania** Pathological lying; pseudologia phantastica; excessive interest in myths and propensity for incredible stories and fabrications.

See *confabulation; liar, pathological.*

**mythophobia** Fear of stories or myths; disbelief in everything one is told.

**myxedema madness** See *hypothyroidism.*

**myxedema reflex** *Woltman's sign;* pathologically slow relaxation of reflexes in myxedema.

**myxedematous dementia** Pseudodementia secondary to *hypothyroidism* (q.v.).

**myxoneurosis** A neurosis affecting the mucous membranes, marked by a mucous discharge from the respiratory or intestinal mucous membrane, unaccompanied by signs of active inflammation.

**MZ** Monozygote, *monozygotic* (q.v.).

**MZA** Monozygotic twins reared apart.

**MZT** Monozygotic twins reared together.

# N

**N protein** Nucleotide-binding regulatory protein. See *G protein*.

**N400 signal** A negative deflection in the event-related potential waveform occurring approximately 400 msec following the onset of contextually incongruent words in a sentence. It is one of the best indicators of *context processing* (q.v.). See *object recognition*.

**Nachmansohn, David** (1899–1983) American neurophysiologist. See *elementary process*.

**nAChRs** Nicotinic acetylcholine receptors. Neuronal nAChRs are a family of ligand-gated ion channels widely expressed in the central and peripheral nervous systems. They are activated by acetylcholine, and their activation causes excitation of the neuron. Currently, 12 neuronal nAChR subunits have been identified ($\alpha 2$ to $\alpha 10$ and $\beta 2$ to $\beta 4$). Brains from smokers exhibit an increased number (that is, up-regulation) of high-affinity nicotine-binding sites, which contain the $\alpha 4$ and $\beta 2$ nAChR subunits. Blockade of the high-affinity $\alpha 4$- and $\beta 2$-containing receptors by a competitive antagonist also blocks the rewarding effect of nicotine. See *nicotine addiction*.

The cognitive reinforcing effects of nicotine have been demonstrated to be beneficial in neurodegenerative disorders, such as Alzheimer disease and Parkinson disease, suggesting that compounds targeted to nAChRs may be useful in restoring a cholinergic deficit.

**NADH** Nicotinamide adenine dinucleotide. See *OXPHOS*.

**nadolol** A *beta blocker* (q.v.).

**Naikan psychotherapy** A form of treatment developed in Japan which uses the subject's guilt to prod him into purposeful action, self-sacrifice, and service to repay his debt to those who have nurtured him and been kind to him. Naikan is said to be particularly effective for alcoholics and criminals. It is sometimes used in combination with *Morita therapy* (q.v.).

**nail biting** *Onychophagia* (q.v.).

**NAIPs** Neuronal apoptosis inhibitor proteins. Normal NAIP protein protects neurons from death; a mutation of the gene is found in some forms of spinal muscular atrophy. How AIPs in general exert their effects is unknown; they may act as a switch determining what path the *TNF* message takes in entering into the *caspase cascade* (qq.v.). See *IAP; spinal muscular atrophy*.

**Na+-K+ pump** See *resting membrane potential*.

**N-allylnormorphine** See *psychotomimetic*.

**nalmefene** An opiate antagonist which, like *naltrexone* (q.v.), seems to reduce alcohol consumption in alcoholics and diminish relapse rate. See *relapse prevention*.

**naloxone** An opiate antagonist. See *amethystic; marijuana*.

**naltrexone** An opioid antagonist and *antidipsotropic* (q.v.); it binds competitively to opioid receptors and blocks the rewarding and reinforcing effects of alcohol-induced release of endogenous opioids. It reduces craving during the treatment phase, but that effect is lost when medication is discontinued.

**naming** A disturbance in association, peculiar to schizophrenia, in which the only recognizable association to external stimuli consists in naming them. Thus, in a word-association test, even though the patient understands its purpose, his only responses may be an enumeration of the furniture in the examining room. This naming does not appear only in response to visual impressions. When asked to do something, the patient may name the act: "Now he is sitting down." Such patients appear to be completely dependent upon, and at the mercy of, external impressions. This seems to be related to the lack of a goal-concept, to the lack of directives and aims. See *touching*.

**nanism** Dwarfism; see *growth hormone*.

**nanism, senile** See *progeria*.

**nanometer** A billionth of a meter.

**nanosomia** *Obs*. See *dwarfism*.

**nanosomia, primordial** Hansemann's term for a rare form of *dwarfism* (q.v.) with regular physical proportions of the dwarfed body and normal mental development. It seems to be hereditary, is more common in the male sex, and is transmitted from the father. Although small from birth, these dwarfs accomplish their puberal crisis regularly and are able to reproduce. This is practically identical with the other special forms of microsomia called *pygmyism* by the French school and *heredofamilial essential microsomia* by E. Levi.

**nanotechnology**   Development and use of engineered materials or devices with the smallest functional organization on the nanometer scale (one billionth of a meter) in at least one dimension, typically ranging from 1 to ~100 nanometers. Nanotechnology provides a way to take advantage of the functional specificity of molecules by incorporating them into engineered material and devices to have highly targeted effects. Any desired cellular signaling pathway can be targeted using this approach.

Minute devices (nanowires) are used to measure and manipulate the activity of individual neurons at specific locations, and to design tests that can spot minuscule amounts of an antigen, of DNA, or of protein markers in brain. Nanowire sensors, for example, can detect a single virus, specific genetic mutations, and proteins associated with a specific disease.

**Napalkov phenomenon**   (A. V. Napalkov, Russian neurophysiologist) An exception to the usual conditioned reflex experiment occurring in some phobic patients in which the conditioning stimulus (e.g., a traumatic event) does not immediately produce a fear reaction; instead, the fear increases in time, rather than being extinguished as it ordinarily would be during exposure to the unreinforced conditioning stimulus.

**narcism**   A shortened (and incorrect) form of *narcissism* (q.v.).

**narcissism**   A term first used by Nacke to indicate the form of autoerotism characterized by self-love, often without genitality as an object. In developing a psychoanalytic psychology, Freud used narcissism in protean ways that reduced the meaning of the term to little more than intellectual interest:

1. A sexual perversion in which one's own body is treated as a sexual object

2. A stage of libido development (but his writings are contradictory about whether autoerotism or narcissism is the primary state and whether either of them precedes the formation of object relations)

3. A type of object choice, in which the sexual object is chosen because of having characteristics similar to the subject's

4. A type of object relationship in which libidinal cathexis is withdrawn from external objects and redirected into (parts of) the self

5. A constituent of self-esteem, related to fulfillment of the ego ideal

In Freud's drive-defense-conflict model, narcissism is a stage in the development of object relationships in which the child's estimation of his capacities is heightened to the degree of omnipotence. The infant is still in the primary undifferentiated phase of consciousness: he is ignorant of any sources of pleasure other than himself. The breast is thought of as a part of his own body, and since his slightest gestures are followed by satisfaction of his instinctual nutritional needs, he develops the "autarchic fiction of false omnipotence." This is the stage of *primary narcissism*. The ego believes itself to be omnipotent, but this is disproved by experience and frustration; the infant then comes to believe that the parents are the omnipotent ones, and he partakes of their omnipotence by introjection (the "primary identification"). The desire to partake of the parental omnipotence, even though it arose originally from the basic desire for the satisfaction of hunger, soon becomes differentiated from the hunger itself, and the child craves affection in a passive way ("passive object-love"). The narcissistic needs are developed in relation to the ego and superego (and the term *secondary narcissism* refers to such love of the ego by the superego); the sexual needs, on the other hand, are developed in relation to the object. See *father-ideal*.

When applied to the adult, the term narcissism implies a hypercathexis of the self and/or a hypocathexis of objects in the environment or a pathologically immature relationship to objects in the environment. Because the concept of narcissism was developed before Freud had formulated his last theory of the instincts (i.e., the dual-instinct theory of the sexual and aggressive instincts), it is not clear how Freud would have incorporated the aggressive instinct into his formulation of narcissism as described above; the formulation given refers only to the sexual drive. See *narcissism, primary.*

In both *self psychology* and *object relations theory* (qq.v.), the importance of the drives has been considerably diminished, while the development and maintenance of object relations has become a central focus. Both psychologies also emphasize pre-oedipal rather than oedipal trauma as crucial in the development of psychopathology. In self psychology, narcissism is regarded as a type of early self/self-object relationship; it includes Kohut's *grandiose self* (q.v.). For Melanie Klein, narcissism is identification with the good object and the denial of any difference between the good object and the self. Autoeroticism and narcissism are aspects of the earliest relation to objects both external and internalized. Narcissistic object relations belong to what she termed the paranoid-schizoid position. This view contradicts Freud's concept of autoeroticism and narcissism as stages that preclude an object relation.

**narcissism, negative**   Exaggerated underestimation of oneself, particularly evident in states of melancholia, which are characterized by ideas of inadequacy, unreality, and self-accusation.

**narcissism, physical**   Narcissism manifested as preoccupation with one's appearance, exhibitionism, and somatic concerns (hypochondriasis).

**narcissism, primary**   According to Freud, the whole available amount of libido is at first stored in the ego. "We call this state of things absolute, primary narcissism. It continues until the ego begins to connect the presentations of objects with libido—to change narcissistic libido into object libido" (*International Journal of Psychoanalysis XXI*, 1940). But in later writings (*The Ego and the Id*, 1949), Freud stated that in the beginning all libido is stored in the id and is drawn into the ego as narcissism only secondarily. "Part of this (original) libido is sent out by the id into erotic object cathexes, whereupon the ego, now growing stronger, attempts to obtain possession of this object libido and to force itself upon the id as a love object. The narcissism of the ego is thus seen to be secondary, acquired by the withdrawal of the libido from objects."

Thus it would seem that there is no such thing as primary narcissism, although Freud (and most of his followers) continued to refer to it despite the above quoted denial of it. And there are further contradictions in Freud's theory in that at various times he considered object love to be the primary and most primitive type of relationship to the environment, while at still other times (as discussed above) it was narcissism that was considered the most primitive type of relationship.

**narcissism, secondary**   The narcissism once attached to external objects but now withdrawn from those objects and placed in the service of the ego (and not to objects in phantasy). This means that object libido is transformed into ego libido. For example, when a schizophrenic patient regresses, he withdraws libido from reality. The libido becomes attached, for instance, to ideas of grandeur and is called secondary narcissism. It is closely related to infantile manifestations of megalomania. See *omnipotence*.

Secondary narcissism is not introversion, as Freud describes the latter. In introversion, libido goes into the service of phantasies of real objects.

**narcissistic countertransference**   Sometimes referred to as a countertransference of arrogance, it occurs in analysts who see themselves as magic healers who restore potency and heal castrations; this leads to therapeutic overambitiousness, overestimation of patients, and hostility toward patients who do not improve. Such hostility may be expressed only in irritability, or it may go so far as to lead to premature termination of treatment. Other manifestations include the therapist's conviction that he is an authority on everything; a pedagogic attitude that results in reassurance therapy rather than analytic therapy, because the analyst in essence is telling the patient, "You see, the world is not as bad as you think, and I do not mistreat you as you were mistreated in childhood"; taking pleasure in controlling the patient, excessive voyeuristic indulgence; encouraging denial and split-off aggression in the patient so that everyone outside of therapy (parents, spouse, friends, etc.) becomes a target of aggression; inability to recognize painful feelings, such as envy, hostility, and contempt; exploitation of the patient in order to bolster the analyst's feeling of superiority, wealth, power, etc.; manipulation of the patient to obtain worship by entering the patient's life, giving advice and guidance, and extracting compliance and admiration from the patient. See *countertransference*.

**narcissistic equilibrium**   A state of harmony between the demands of the superego and the capabilities of the ego; derived from the original harmony between the obedient child and its loving parents. The superego does not demand of the ego more than it can produce.

The ego is not terrified by the threat of the superego severity.

**narcissistic needs**  The emotional and nurturing supplies required to maintain self-esteem and, in the infant, to preserve the sense of omnipotence and the cohesive sense of self (wholeness of the self-structure). See *cohesive self*. Bergler viewed narcissistic needs as a third drive, on a par with libido and aggression, and is thus regarded by some as an antecedent of Kohut and self psychology.

**narcissistic object relations**  Characterized by (1) omnipotence—ruthless use of others and denial of any dependence on others; (2) preponderance of identification, both introjective (the desirable aspects of others are claimed to belong to oneself) and projective (undesirable aspects of the self are deposited into others); and (3) defenses against recognizing any separateness between self and object.

**narcissistic organization**  See *paranoid-schizoid position*.

**narcissistic personality (disorder)**  *NPD;* in DSM-III-R, the basic characteristics are a pervasive pattern of grandiosity, hypersensitivity, and defective empathy, manifested in five or more of the following: grandiosity, with a sense of self-importance; the subject views his problems as unique and understandable only by other special people; a need for constant attention and admiration (this is sometimes implied when "exhibitionism" is used to define the narcissist); a sense of entitlement. See *cognitive style*.

Research to date suggests that the first three—grandiosity, sense of uniqueness, and need for admiration—are among the best discriminators in differentiating NPD from other personality types; entitlement is also a helpful discriminator, but to a lesser degree. The other symptoms in the DSM-III-R list of criteria are preoccupation with phantasies of power or unlimited success; feelings of rage, shame, and humiliation whenever criticized; interpersonally exploitative; lack of empathy; preoccupation with feelings of envy and over-idealization of others. These last symptoms appear at best to be poor predictors or discriminators and may be more related to severity of disorder rather than to specific type of personality.

In Kohut's typology, narcissistic psychopathology includes the following: (1) narcissistic personality disorder, characterized by depression, hypersensitivity to slights, hypochondriacal complaints, and a lack of zest for living; (2) narcissistic behavior disorder, characterized by perverse, antisocial, and addictive behaviors. Both types may indulge sporadically in substance abuse, promiscuity, and pathological lying, but they lack the consistent, calculated disregard for social standards evident in the *antisocial personality* (q.v.), and they retain the ability for consistent work (see *personality disorders*); (3) *merger-hungry personality*, characterized by a proneness to symbiotic, fusion-laden relationships with others and overwhelming demands that those others remain continually available; (4) *contact-shunning personality*, characterized by avoidance and self-isolation to protect from fragmentation and loss of the sense of self when threatened by intimacy.

Bursten's typology of narcissistic personalities includes all the personality disorders of DSM-III-R except for the schizoid and the schizotypal: *cravers*—clinging, whining, demanding behavior expresses primitive stimulus hunger; *manipulators*—attempt to defeat others and thereby bolster a deficient self-esteem by clever, deceptive trickery; *paranoids*—querulous, litigious, and picayune attitude and behavior are geared to demonstrating their power and superiority over others; *phallic-narcissists*—exhibitionistic competitiveness. See *character defense*.

**narcissistic rage**  See *aggression; rage*.

**narcissistic transference**  An ill-defined concept, perhaps most frequently used to refer to the patient whose resistance is manifested in aloofness, unrelatedness, unapproachability, detachment, and failure to communicate affect. Many such patients maintain an allusion of self-sufficiency and control as a defense against deeper feelings of dependence and vulnerability.

**narcoanalysis**  See *narcotherapy*.

**narcocatharsis**  See *narcotherapy*.

**narcolepsy**  *Friedmann disease; Gelineau syndrome; hypnolepsy;* a *sleep disorder* (q.v.) of the DOES class consisting of a classic tetrad of cataplexy on emotion (sudden transient loss of muscle tone in the extremities or trunk), excessive daytime sleepiness (*EDS;* recurrent paroxysms of uncontrollable refreshing sleep, usually lasting minutes but sometimes lasting for more than an hour), hypnagogic imagery, and sleep paralysis (transient inability to move after waking up). Affected persons show very early onset REM periods and fragmented 'nighttime sleep' (difficulty with sleep maintenance).

Prevalence of the disorder in the United States is estimated as between 40 and 90 per 100,000. In half the cases, there is a positive family history for narcolepsy, related to orexin deficiency. The disorder shows a strong association with HLA-DR2 antigen. It is a chronic neurologic disorder that persists throughout the person's lifetime.

**narcology**   See *addiction medicine.*

**narcomania**   Craving for relief from painful stimuli through pharmacologic agents (morphine, opium, etc.), also occasionally through psychic measures (e.g., hypnosis). See *psychoactive substance dependence.*

**narcosuggestion**   See *narcotherapy.*

**narcosynthesis See**   *narcotherapy.*

**narcotherapy**   A form of treatment used extensively in the war neuroses of World War II. As a general group term it includes *narcosuggestion, narcocatharsis, narcoanalysis, narcosynthesis, Amytal interview*, Pentothal interview, "*truth serum.*"

*Narcosuggestion* implies the active utilization of suggestion and reassurance while the patient is in a state of complete relaxation in the process of receiving sodium Amytal or sodium Pentothal intravenously. *Narcocatharsis* or *narcoanalysis* (the two words are used interchangeably) implies either free association or direct questions by the therapist to uncover repressed memories and affects while the patient is under the effects of sodium Amytal or sodium Pentothal given intravenously. At the end of the narcoanalysis, after the effects of the drug have worn off, the therapist explains to the patient the significance of what he or she recalled. *Narcosynthesis* uses free association, dreams, and transference material obtained during the Amytal or Pentothal interview, but a day or so later the material is discussed with the patient, who is guided by the therapist to conative and emotional reintegration, behavioral adjustments, and social rehabilitation.

**narcotic**   Sleep-inducing. Drugs that can relieve severe pain are sleep-inducing and usually also highly addictive. In consequence, narcotic generally refers to an addicting analgesic, typically an opioid, while hypnotic refers to sleep-inducing. The term has no precise scientific meaning; it is primarily a term of administrative convenience, used by certain organs of the international and national drug control systems.

**narcotic agreement**   See *pain syndromes.*

**narcotic antagonist**   A substance with ability to block the euphorigenic and dependence-producing properties of opiates by competing with them for occupation of the same receptor sites (*competitive inhibition*).

**narcotic blockade**   Total or partial inhibition of the euphoriogenic action of narcotic drugs, such as heroin, through the use of other drugs, such as *methadone, LAAM*, (qq.v.), or cyclazocine, which can then be used for maintenance treatment without producing the peaks of elation, abstinence symptoms, or demand for escalation of dose that characterize addiction to opiates. The narcotic antagonist or blocking agent achieves its effect by occupying the receptor site that the narcotic itself would ordinarily occupy.

**narcotic-analgesic**   See *opiate, opioid; opium.*

**narcotism**   The state of being under the influence of narcotic drugs. As commonly used, the term refers to the condition in which the drug is present in amounts great enough to be toxic, or, in any event, sufficient to alter behavior. See *addiction; dependence, drug.*

**NARP**   Maternally inherited neurogenic muscle weakness, ataxia, and retinitis pigmentosa; associated features are developmental delay, seizures, and dementia.

**narrative gerontology**   The study of stories of aging as told by persons who are growing old; such studies focus on aging "from the inside," as experienced and expressed in the stories of older persons.

**narratophilia**   A *paraphilia* (q.v.) in which sexual arousal and orgasm are dependent upon uttering obscene words or telling "dirty stories" to the sex partner; the same term is also used for the paraphilia in which the subject must read or listen to such stories in order to become aroused and achieve orgasm.

**National Survey on Drug Use and Health**   *NSDUH*; it reported that, in 2002, 9.4% (22 million) of the U.S. adult population had substance abuse or dependence issues. Of these, 3.2 million had co-occurring drug and alcohol use problems; 3.9 million had illicit substance abuse or dependence only; and 14.9 million had alcohol abuse or dependence issues only. Nonmedical use of prescription drugs increased from approximately 600,000 people in 1990 to 2 million in 2001. Amphetamine use increased from 1% to 7%; marijuana from 6% to 15%; and heroin use from 11% to 15% over the same period.

The most common psychiatric disorders associated with substance use disorders are mood and anxiety disorders, attention deficit disorder, and antisocial personality disorder.

**native language neural commitment**   See *NLNC hypothesis.*

**nativist hypothesis**   See *innateness hypothesis.*

**nativist view**   See *language acquisition.*

**natural**   See *unnatural.*

**natural opiates**   See *peptide, brain.*

**natural selection**   See *phenotypic fitness.*

**natural study**   *Study in nature;* an investigation in which the researcher is a passive observer of the course of some natural process, such as disease. See *follow-through.*

**nature, experiment of**   The reaction to real environmental situations, and in particular to stressful ones.

**nautomania**   Seaman's mania, i.e., the sailor's fear of (drowning in) the sea; *nautophobia.*

**navigation**   The action of staying on course, finding one's way, planning what pathway to take in reaching a destination. The neural basis of way finding involves both an external world (allocentric) representation or *cognitive map* and an internal (egocentric) representation of the location of parts of the body. Knowing accurately where places are located and navigating accurately between them are associated with right hippocampus activity; getting to those places quickly is associated with activation of the right caudate nucleus. The navigation network includes associated activity in the right inferior parietal and bilateral medial parietal regions (supporting egocentric movement) and left hippocampus and frontal cortex (supporting nonspatial aspects).

**NBIA**   Neurodegeneration with brain iron accumulation, due to mutations in the gene that codes for pantothenate kinase 2, which is necessary for coenzyme-A biosynthesis and is targeted to mitochondria; formerly known as *Hallervorden-Spatz syndrome* (q.v.) See *iron.*

**NCA**   Neurocirculatory asthenia. See *asthenia, neurocirculatory.*

**NCAM**   Neural cellular adhesion molecule; an immunoglobulin, existing in multiple protein forms, that is a major element in *axon guidance* (q.v.). An NCAM molecule on one cell binds to a counterpart NCAM molecule on an adjacent cell such as a *glial guide cell* (termed a *homophilic* mechanism); when the appropriate target zone or final destination has been reached, the migrating neuron leaves the glial stalk and joins the appropriate cortical lamina (layer).

**NCP**   NeuroCybernetic Prosthesis, an implantable device developed originally for the treatment of refractory seizures in epileptic patients. It consists of a generator, placed usually under the left arm, and a stimulating electrode attached to the left vagus nerve in the neck. After it was first used in 1988, an unexpected side effect was reported in many patients: an improvement in mood and cognition. Since then, NCP has been used successfully in treatment-resistant depressions that had not responded to antidepressant drugs or electroconvulsive therapy.

**NCSE**   1. Nonconvulsive status epilepticus, a state of continuous or intermittent seizure activity without a return to baseline lasting more than 30 minutes, consisting of a change in behavior or level of consciousness that is associated with diagnostic EEG changes. Onset may be sudden or gradual; if there is any abnormal motor activity, it is minimal. Mental changes include mild cognitive disturbances (e.g., impaired attention), mild disorientation, confusional states, mood disturbance, cortical blindness, speech disturbance (varies from verbal perseveration to reduced verbal fluency, muteness, speech arrest, or aphasia), echolalia, confabulation, bizarre behavior (e.g., laughing, dancing, singing inappropriately), clear psychotic states, and autonomic disturbances (e.g., belching, borborygmus, flatulence).

In the absence status (AS) type of NCSE, consciousness clears abruptly, and EEG shows continuous or nearly continuous generalized, rhythmic, bilaterally synchronous, spike-and-wave discharges at 3 per second frequency intervals with a maximum over the bifrontal region. In the complex partial status (CPS) type, the episode is followed by a prolonged postictal state with depression. Various forms of less synchronous seizure activity occur, including rhythmical slowing, rhythmic spike, and rhythmic sharp and slow waves.

2. Neurobehavioral Cognitive Status Examination; examines a variety of cognitive

functioning domains, such as attention and memory. Its utility as a screening test for dementia is limited, however; it has a low false-negative rate but a high false-positive rate for detecting domain-specific cognitive impairments in patients with organic brain disorders. See *cognitive screening instruments.*

**NCS-R** National Comorbidity Survey Replication, a survey of mental disorder in English-speaking people 18 years and older in the continental United States. Interviews were conducted with 9282 respondents between February 2001 and April 2003.

**NDPH** In ICHD-II, new daily-persistent *headache* (q.v.).

**NE** Norepinephrine. See *epinephrine.*

**-nea** Variant of *-noia* (q.v.).

**necro-** Combining form meaning dead, from Gr. *nekros.*

**necromania** *Necrophilia* (q.v.).

**necromimesis** The delusion that one is dead.

**necrophilia** *Katasexuality*; a *paraphilia* (q.v.) whose condition is that the love object, whether heterosexual or homosexual, must be dead before orgasm can be achieved. Although a rare perversion overall, it is claimed by some that morticians, undertakers, etc., contribute a relatively high proportion of subjects who have the perversion in either a grossly overt or an attenuated form. Although usually limited to males, necrophilia was described in a female in 1976 (Foerster, K. et al. *Schweizer Archiv für Neurologie, Neurochirurgie und Psychiatrie, 119*). See *taphophilia.*

**necrophilism** 1. A morbid desire to be in the presence of dead bodies.

2. *Necrophilia* (q.v.).

**necrophobia** Fear of a corpse or of death.

**necrosis, neuronal** Cell death; inappropriate or unanticipated destruction of a neuron, as contrasted with programmed cell death, such as *apoptosis* (q.v.). Cellular necrosis is characterized by mitochondrial swelling, dilatation of endoplasmic reticulum, and extensive vacuolation or loss of definition of the cytoplasm, which is followed by loss of nuclear staining and disintegration of the nucleus (*karyolysis*). Release of cellular contents into the intercellular space may damage neighboring cells and induce inflammatory responses; see *neurotoxicity.*

Causes of cell necrosis include adverse environmental conditions, such as exposure to extreme stress, lack of oxygen or essential nutrients, elevated temperature, toxic compounds, and mechanical trauma. Necrosis can also be triggered by the abnormalities that underlie many neurodegenerative disorders.

**need** Requirement; necessity. A physiological need is any stimulus of instinctual origin. Need implies a goal and, further, that the existing state is deficient in one of the elements that define or describe that goal. Needs are sometimes defined in terms of distance from postulated ideal norms, or lack of minimal standards, or the subject's sense of deprivation (*felt needs*).

In health planning, need refers to what is required to maintain or assure health and to prevent, ameliorate, or cure disease. A need is a problem, disorder, or *disease* (q.v.) that is objectively manifest and interferes with the subject's level of functioning; further, an effective and acceptable treatment exists for the disorder. Some health planners add a further condition: that both the person in need and the provider agree on the terms for delivery of care. The underlying questions: Do consumers get what they need? Do consumers need what they get? The existence of a diagnosable disorder does not in itself constitute a need, which is implicitly defined in terms of impairment. It is the dysfunction, not the diagnosis, which needs correction. Need is implicitly defined in terms of impairment or disability, but there is controversy about the differences between need and want, between curing and caring. Mental health need is often described in terms of the following:

1. *Met need*—the percentage of people with a diagnosis of mental disorder who were seen by the health services.

2. *Unmet need*—the percentage of people who met diagnostic criteria for a disorder but were not seen by any segment of existing health services; unmet need may be the result of underprovision of mental health services, lack of financial access to service, lack of geographical access, or lack of knowledge of the existence of appropriate services.

3. *Met un-need*—the percentage of people currently consulting or in treatment with a mental health provider but not meeting criteria for a mental disorder. For some epidemiologists, this group includes all forms of *overutilization*: people (a) not in need of treatment (regardless of whether they meet the criteria for a diagnosis), (b) not in need

of the type of treatment provided, (c) not in need of the intensity of treatment provided, or (d) with little chance of treatment being effective. There is no necessary relationship between level of need and appropriateness of a particular intervention.

Need is what people require, demand is what people ask for, supply is what is provided. While the object of need can often be supplied completely, that of demand can never be. Mental health planners are chiefly concerned with unmet need, which in some studies has amounted to as much as 70% of the diagnosable population. Third-party payers, such as insurance companies, employers, and managed care organizations, give particular attention to met-unneed, arguing that this category drains resources from the segment of the population in "real" need.

**need, neurotic**  In Horney's terms, a demand or insistence that others behave toward the subject in a certain, specific way.

**need for punishment**  Moral masochism. See *criminal from sense of guilt; masochism.*

**need-fear dilemma**  The schizophrenic's inordinate need for other people or an institutional structure to provide him with the regulation and organization that his own psychic structure cannot provide, combined with an equally inordinate fear of influence or control since these are potentially disorganizing if not in exactly the right dosage.

**need-press method**  A technique of analysis of the TAT used by Murray (one of the originators of the test); in this method, each sentence of the subject's story is analyzed as to the needs of the hero and the press (environmental forces) he is exposed to. Each need and press is given a weighted score and a rank-order system of the needs and press is then tabulated. The method is not widely used clinically because it is too time-consuming to be practical.

**needle exchange programs**  Drug treatment programs in which intravenous drug users (IVDUs) are provided with sterile syringes to replace used syringes. Such programs also provide counseling and education about alcohol and other substance use and about HIV and other sexually transmitted diseases, as well as referrals and improved access to comprehensive drug treatment programs, medical and reproductive care, and other psychiatric and psychosocial services.

As noted in the APA Policy Statement on Needle Exchange Programs (September 1996), the frequently remitting and relapsing course of injection drug use, in conjunction with the risk of AIDS with each use, argues strongly for treatment approaches that start with reducing the associated harm of HIV transmission while attempting to engage the drug user in more comprehensive treatment.

Needle exchange programs do not increase the amount of drug use by those using such programs, nor do they increase overall community levels of new or continued use of injection or noninjection drugs.

**need tension**  A tension that develops within the organism in connection with various needs essential for survival, which demands contact with the outer world for its relief. "Being born may be said to have already interfered with the equilibrium of the intrauterine state, because stimuli are now registered upon the organism from within (hunger) and without (cold). To relieve these *need tensions* the infant must direct itself to the outer world, or show signs of the unpleasant effects created by these tensions" (Kardiner, A. & Spiegel, H. *War Stress and Neurotic Illness*, 1947).

**needle sharing**  Use of the same needle or syringe by more than one person for intravenous injection of a drug. This *route of drug administration* (q.v.) carries a high risk of infection (including AIDS, hepatitis, malaria, and many other microorganisms). See *IVDU*.

**needology**  The study of the needs of a person or population, often used pejoratively by economists in referring to what sociologists or other behavior scientists define as significantly lacking in the group with which they work. See *need*.

**negation**  Denial (q.v.). Délire des négations is nihilistic delusion; see *Cotard syndrome*.

**negation, delusion of**  Nihilistic delusion; denial of the existence of externality and/or of oneself; often associated with *depersonalization* (q.v.).

**negation, insanity of**  A term introduced by J. Cotard as *délire des négations* for the syndrome known as *depersonalization* (q.v.).

**negative death autopsy**  See *Bell mania*.

**negative hallucination**  Not a hallucination, but failure to see an object even though the subject is looking at it; the phenomenon can be induced by hypnosis.

**negative Oedipus**  *Inverted Oedipus* (complex); a form of infantile psychosexual development in which the parental object is the opposite or reverse of the usual love object. The usual oedipal love object for the male child is the mother; but should love for the father and hatred for the mother prevail, the boy would be said to demonstrate a negative Oedipus complex. In like fashion, should the girl's attachment remain fixed on the mother (instead of being transferred to the father, as is the usual course of events), she would be described as manifesting a negative *Oedipus complex* (q.v.).

**negative period, first**  *Negativism* (q.v.) that normally occurs in children between the ages of 2 and 4.

**negative practice**  See *paradoxical therapy*.

**negative reciprocity**  See *reciprocity, negative*.

**negative reinforcement**  See *reinforcement*.

**negative selection**  *Clonal deletion theory* (q.v.).

**negative signs**  See *release phenomena*.

**negative symptoms**  In schizophrenia, symptoms of the chronic phase, such as apathy, lack of drive or will, underactivity, slowness, social withdrawal, blunted affect, poor rapport, difficulty in abstract thinking, lack of spontaneity and flow of conversation (alogia), and stereotyped thinking, which together constitute the schizophrenic defect state. See *deficit symptoms; positive symptoms; schizophrenia, models of*.

*Negative thought disorder* includes poverty of speech, poverty of content, and alogia; positive thought disorder includes derailment, incoherence, illogicality, tangentiality, and pressured speech. Negative thought disorder occurs mainly in schizophrenia, whereas positive thought disorder occurs at least as frequently in mania as it does in schizophrenia. *SANS* is the Schedule for the Assessment of Negative Symptoms, developed by Andreasen.

Hypofrontality appears to be related to negative symptoms (and is not a result of long-term neuroleptic therapy). See *hypofrontality hypothesis*.

**negative therapeutic reaction**  See *superego resistance*.

**negative utilitarianism**  See *utilitarianism, negative*.

**negativism**  Negative attitude or behavior; *command negativism; resistance*, as when a person, aware of stimuli from without, actively or passively opposes conformation with the stimuli. It is sometimes called *contrasuggestibility* or *contrariety*, though the latter terms are used more frequently in psychology than in psychiatry.

Negativism is *active* when the subject does the opposite of what he is asked to do. For example, a catatonic patient closes his fists tightly when requested to open his hands. *Passive* negativism refers to the patient's failure to do things he is expected to do; he remains passive to his physiological urges and does not get out of bed in the morning, dress, or eat. Bleuler calls this *inner* negativism.

Some authorities use *intellectual negativism* to describe a patient who always expresses the opposite to a thought. Thus, a patient thought: "I must go; I must not go. I am a man; no, I am a woman; I will tell him;

I will not tell him." This is more commonly termed *ambivalence* (q.v.).

**negativism, sexual**  *Anerotism*; Hirschfeld's term for absence of sexual interests due to deficiency in the sexual glands. See *sexual disorders; sexual response cycle*.

**negativistic amnesia**  The delusion that memory and orientation are lost.

**negativistic response**  Doing the exact opposite of what is requested. In *catatonic schizophrenia*, for example, when asked to open his eyes the patient shuts them tightly. See *negativism*.

**neglect**  See *battered child syndrome*.

**neglect, hemispatial**  See *parietal lobe dysfunction*.

**neglect syndromes**  See *parietal lobe dysfunction; sensory neglect*.

**negligence**  Professional negligence is the physician's failure to render appropriate care; in medical malpractice cases, often described in terms of the "4 D's":

1. Duty—to prove negligence, the plaintiff must establish that the psychiatrist had a duty to a patient or to a foreseeable victim of the patient's behavior (e.g., violent behavior).

2. Dereliction of duty—psychiatrists are not required to practice without error, but they are required to exercise reasonable care. Courts are less tolerant of errors of fact (e.g., failure to review prior records or to evaluate a patient) than of errors of judgment.

3. Direct causation ("*proximate cause*")—there must be proof of a direct link between the dereliction of duty and the resulting harm. The negligence must be the cause of the harm and the harm must have been foreseeable.

4. Damages—may include the costs associated with injury to others and the loss of wages that resulted from the harm.

**neoassociationism** *Neo-connectionism; massive parallel processing systems (MPPS,* q.v.). A hypothesis of neural functioning, that no function is carried out fully by a specific region of the brain; instead, several anatomical regions of the brain are involved in the performance of any particular behavior. To the notion of different modules carrying out their own separate analyses, neoassociationism adds the notion of many units operating and exchanging information in ways analogous to many brain cells or columns firing simultaneously. Computation is performed by excitatory and inhibitory interactions among a network of relatively simple neuron-like units, which compete and cooperate so that certain units become active and others are suppressed. Eventually, because of statistical properties of the ensemble, the network settles into a state that reflects its particular "task"—such as perceiving a given image.

**neoatavism** The recurrence, in a descendant, of characters or traits of a near or immediate ancestor.

**neobehaviorism** Skinner's operant *behaviorism* (q.v.).

**neocerebellum** See *cerebellum.*

**neoconnectionism** *MPPS* (q.v.).

**neocortex** *Isocortex* (q.v.); the "new brain"; it forms 70–80% of the primate brain. It develops from the thin dorsal wall of the anterior end of the neural tube (the telencephalic vesicles). A bulbous swelling of the ventral wall produces the striatum. A subpopulation of neocortical interneurons originate from the developing striatum, indicating that they have migrated across the supposedly cell-tight corticostriatal junction.

**neocortical neurons** Most neocortical neurons (70–80%) are excitatory pyramidal neurons, which have relatively stereotyped anatomical, physiological, and molecular properties. The remaining 20–30% are interneurons, mostly inhibitory, which have diverse morphological, molecular, and synaptic characteristics. Inhibitory interneurons use GABA as their transmitter.

About 50% of all inhibitory interneurons are *basket cells,* which specialize in targeting the somata and proximal dendrites of pyramidal neurons and interneurons. The term basket cell comes from the basket like appearance around pyramidal cell somata that results from convergent innervation by many basket cells. Basket cells typically express many neuropeptides and the two calcium-binding proteins, *parvalbumin (PV)* and *calbindin (CB). Chandelier cells (ChCs)* are axon-targeting interneurons and thus in a position to override all the complex dendritic integration and somatic gain setting by "editing" the action potention output. The characteristic terminal portions of the axon form short vertical rows of boutons, resembling a chandelier.

*Martinotti cells (Mcs)* are the only source for cross-columnar inhibition. Mcs target not only the most distal dendrites, but also proximal dendrites, perisomatic dendrites, and somata. They express somatostatin (SOM) and never express PV or VIP (vasoactive intestinal peptide).

*Bipolar cells (BPCs)* are small cells with spindle or ovoid somata and narrow bipolar dendrites that extend vertically towards layer I and down to layer VI. They can be excitatory by releasing only VIP, or inhibitory by releasing mainly GABA. (Inhibitory BPCs also express calretinin [CR] and VIP). BPCs contact only a few cells.

*Double bouquet cells (DBCs)* have a tight fascicular axonal cylinder that resembles a horse tail. They seem to be interleaved with pyarmidal cells to inhibit their basal dendrites. They express CB, have the unique tendency to express CR and CB together, and can also express VIP or CCK (cholecystokinin), but not PV, SOM, or NPY.

*Bitufted cells (BTCs)* give rise to primary dendrites from opposite poles to form a bitufted morphology. They are dendritic-targeting cells and can express CB, CR, NPY, VIP, SOM, and CCK, but not PV.

*Neuroglioform cells (NGCs)* are small, button-type cells with many fine, radiating dendrites that are short, finely beaded, and rarely branched. The axon breaks up into a dense, intertwined arborization of ultra-thin axons with as many as ten orders of branching. Fine boutons are distributed on the axonal collaterals to form GABA synapses onto the dendrites of target cells.

*Layer I interneurons* are virtually all inhibitory. One category comprises large neurons with horizontal processes, known as Cajal Retzius cells, present mostly during development and unique to layer I; they are the target of the terminal tufts of pyramidal cells. The second category is a heterogeneous group of small, multipolar interneurons with varying axonal arborizations (poor and rich axonal plexus cells) (Markram, H. et al. *Nature Reviews Neuroscience 5*: 793–807, 2004).

**neo-Freudian**  Referring to modifications, extensions, or revisions of Freud's original psychoanalytic theory, most commonly to those that emphasize social, cultural, and interpersonal elements rather than innate biological instincts, such as sexuality and aggression. Among the major theorists described as neo-Freudian are Alfred Adler (see *individual psychology*), Erich Fromm, Karen Horney, and Harry Stack Sullivan.

**neographism**  Writing new words, the graphic equivalent of *neologism* (q.v.).

**neolalia**  Neologistic speech; frequent use of neologisms in a patient's speech.

**neologism**  *Glossosynthesis*. "Words of the patient's own making, often portmanteau condensations of several other words, and having originally had a special meaning for the patients." (Henderson, D. K. & Gillespie, R. D. *A Text-Book of Psychiatry*, 1936).

"A paranoid female 'is a Billy-goat,' i.e., she is united with her beloved minister: minister = Christ = lamb = billy-goat" (Bleuler, E. *Textbook of Psychiatry*, 1930). See *contamination; syllabic synthesis*.

**neomimism**  A type of stereotypy, analogous to neologisms, consisting of repetition of a seemingly senseless gesture that has a particular meaning to the patient.

**neomnesis**  Memory for the recent past.

**neonate**  The newborn infant. See *developmental levels*.

**neonaticide**  See *filicide*.

**neophobia**  Fear of anything new or unfamiliar.

**neophrenia**  *Obs.* In 1863 Kahlbaum classified psychiatric conditions (then called insanity) in accordance with the patient's age: neophrenia (the insanity of childhood), hebephrenia (the insanity of adolescence), and presbyophrenia (the insanity of old age).

**neoplasm, cerebral**  See *intracranial tumor*.

**neopsychic**  Of recent psychic development.

**neostriatum**  See *basal ganglia*.

**neoteny**  Retention of juvenile characteristics in the adults of a species.

**nephelopsychosis**  *Obs.* Intense interest in clouds.

**nepiophilia**  Love of infants, babies; a *paraphilia* (q.v.) in which sexual arousal and orgasm are possible only if the partner is a baby. See *pedophilia*. The paraphilia in which the subject himself must act as or be treated as a baby is termed *autonepiophilia* or *paraphilic infantilism*.

**NEPPs**  Neurite outgrowth-promoting prostaglandin compounds. NEPPs are neuroprotective; one mechanism of their action is to stimulate the production of natural antioxidants and thereby to protect against *oxidative stress* (q.v.).

**nerve conduction**  Electrochemical transmittal of information from one end of the neuron to the other. Transmittal of information from one neuron to another is a chemical process that begins with the release of *neurotransmitter* (q.v.) from the neuronal terminals when they are depolarized. See *synapse*.

Nerve conduction is dependent on a sodium pump within the neuronal membrane that secretes two ions of sodium for every potassium ion pumped into the neuron. During conduction, sodium ions enter and potassium ions leave the nerve cell. The resulting shift in membrane potential eventually causes conduction to cease and excitability is restored by the sodium pump, which transports sodium and potassium ions across the nerve membrane in the opposite direction. The sodium pump consists of a membrane-bound enzyme, the sodium ion-dependent adenosine triphosphate.

**nerve growth**  One factor that might contribute to the poor ability of nerve cells to regenerate is oligodendrocyte-mediated inhibition of nerve growth. A dimer of IL-2, produced by a transglutaminase, is cytotoxic to oligodendrocytes; dimerization of IL-2 might provide a mechanism to permit nerve growth.

**nerve growth factor**  See *neurotrophic factors*.

**nervios**  A culture-bound syndrome described in Hispanic persons in the United States and South America: a chronic state of emotional distress, somatic complaints, and inability to function.

**nervous**  1. Relating to a nerve or the nerves. 2. Easily excited or agitated; suffering from instability or weakness of nerve action.

**nervous system, conceptual**  Any model whose operation is in accordance with known mechanisms of central nervous system functioning and which is capable of producing responses comparable to or identical with the behavior of the living organism. The value of the conceptual nervous system is primarily heuristic in that it affords a simplified and manipulatable analogy of the nervous system itself and thus stimulates hypotheses about how the nervous system operates. Often, however, it is accepted uncritically as an exact reproduction of the nervous system and then used incorrectly as a way to verify theories about the nervous system.

**NES** 1. *Night-eating syndrome* (q.v.).

2. Nonepileptic seizures; similar to *frontal lobe seizures* (q.v.) except that they are less stereotypic, of longer duration, and associated with waxing and waning in- and out-of-phase motor activity. In 40% to 100% of reported cases, there are concurrent psychiatric diagnoses, including dissociative and other personality disorders, mood disorders, PTSD, and somatoform disorders.

**network** A system or structure of interlacing lines, threads, fibers, channels, etc. An artificial neural network is composed of units (i.e., input, hidden, output) and links. Network size is the number of units; the degree of connectivity is described as their weight.

1. *Neural* (or *neuronal*) *network* models simulate the ways in which the brain processes information. The neural network is a system of interacting elements, or nodes, that communicate with each other to transfer information between brain areas. Interactions between nodes are represented by arrows. The different strengths of interactions are designated by numbers or weights on each arrow. In dense networks, each node accumulates inputs from other nodes and adjusts it own activation accordingly. In distributed networks, connectivity is less generalized or global; nodes are grouped into modules, which are connected into pathways. A few key modules distribute information (connect) to other elements within the system. This permits each *module* (q.v.) a degree of independence to make decisions based on local information and to perform behaviors in parallel with other modules. See *architecture of network*; *parallel processing*.

The primary function of a neural network is to transform a set of inputs into a second set as output. Networks are able to learn different patterns of inputs by changing the strengths of their connections; this permits new and specific patterns of activity (information) to be represented within a module.

In a neural network, each simple structure (a person, an action, a proposition) is represented in long-term memory only once. A recursive transition network shuttles from one structure to another, gathering representations together and storing them in short-term memory until the final proposition—thought, conclusion, decision, etc.—can be pieced together. See *recursion*.

Neural networks work in parallel, are biological and continuous, and perform complex logical and statistical operations. Cascades of neurons in multiple loci fire in an integrated symphonic arrange of time-coordinated events. Network models have been invaluable in discovering more and more about how the brain works, but they do not explain everything about the mind. Consciousness and sentience, for instance, are not well understood.

2. In *social psychiatry*, a network is a field or patterning of interrelationships envisioned as a matrix of connected points that are the various types of stimuli impinging on the person—taxic (inanimate, such as humidity, temperature, terrain), biotaxic (people or animals), and sociotaxic (social groups and any other type of social stimulation).

In the network model of social psychiatry, attention is also given to the spaces between the interconnected points—the interface. When one is removed from familiar stimuli, he is considered to be in the empty space between cultural networks and is said to be experiencing *interface shock* (of which culture shock is an example). The person who goes from one culture to another and almost at once becomes what he believes people from the other culture are like demonstrates what is termed *interface penetration* (what would popularly be called "going native"). Interface stationing refers to the enjoyment of being at the interface, as the visitor to a foreign country who acts "touristy." An extension of such behavior into becoming more like the original culture than the person ever was while he was in fact within his system of origin is interface accentuation, exemplified by the Brooklyn Jew who never follows dietary laws until he settles in Wyoming. See *network therapy*.

**network, psychological** A set of interrelated social elements (individuals, families, etc.)

whose cohesiveness, even though relatively loose, provides a mechanism for shaping social tradition and public opinion and also an emotional support system for those who are a part of it.

**network motifs**  Recurring, significant patterns of interconnections occurring in complex networks, such as neural networks, at numbers that are significantly higher than those occurring in randomized networks.

**network therapy**  A form of group therapy, used generally with schizophrenic patients, that includes not only family members but also other relatives, neighbors, and friends who make up the patient's *social network* and provide a potential source of support, encouragement, and employment, which may reduce the likelihood of rehospitalization.

**neuradynamia**  *Neurasthenia* (q.v.).

**neural assemblies**  See *assemblies, neural.*

**neural crest cells**  See *embryonic disc.*

**neural Darwinism**  The hypothesis that competition between different neuronal groups for functional and anatomic dominance shapes neural connections. If, for example, the cost of maintaining them outweighs the benefits (such as the amount of information) they contribute, they are eliminated or pruned. See *pruning.*

**neural encoding**  See *stimulus transduction.*

**neural groove**  See *neural plate.*

**neural maps**  Small areas in the cerebral hemispheres that correspond to parts of the body or sense organs—retina, inner ears, and other homunculi that correspond with the touch and feel of the body and with movements of the limbs and muscles. Early in the 20th century, Korbinian Brodmann marked nearly 50 such areas; later Oskar and Cecile Vogt marked over 200.

**neural networks**  See *network; parallel processing.*

**neural plasticity**  *Neuronal plasticity* (q.v.).

**neural plate**  Differentiated from the embryonic ectoderm, it thickens and dips to form the *neural groove.* The plate gets deeper, and the two sides (the neural folds) join at the top to make the hollow *neural tube.* As this is happening, two strips are pinched off the edges of the neural folds; they are the *neural crest cells,* which will form part of the autonomic nervous system. See *cephalogenesis.*

**neural stem cells**  Cells that can continuously self-renew and have the potential to generate intermediate and mature cells of both glial and neuronal lineages. Current research is directed not only to their use as cell replacements, but also to deliver therapeutic substances to specific sites in the brain. Neural stem cells seem to be attracted to various brain lesions, such as cancers and areas of neurodegeneration; this "homing" quality might be able to target amyloid plaques, for example, and deliver therapeutic enzymes to them. See NPCs.

**neural tube**  See *neural plate.*

**neural tube defect (NTD)**  Failure of the neural tube to close properly during development. Neural tube defects are among the most common major congenital malformations, occurring in approximately 1 out of every 600 pregnancies. Amniocentesis permits prenatal detection in 95% of cases by revealing an increase in α-fetoprotein (AFP), which leaks from an open lesion, such as spina bifida or anencephaly. Elevated AFP is not specific to neural tube defects, however; it has also been reported in Turner syndrome, duodenal atresia, and many other congenital anomalies.

**neuralgia**  *Neurodynia; pain* (q.v.) that follows the anatomical course of a nerve or nerve root. Neuralgias occur more frequently in the elderly than in other age groups. Among the common neuralgias are the following:

1. Cranial *neuralgia*—characterized by brief bouts of paraoxysmal lancinating pain that recur within the anatomical distribution of a cranial nerve.

2. Geniculate neuralgia—lancinating pain around and deep within the ear; due to dysfunction of the geniculate (sensory) ganglion of facial nerve.

3. Glossopharngeal neuralgia—sharp pain in areas of the tonsil, base of tongue, throat, or deep in the ear; bouts of pain may be precipitated by yawning, talking, or swallowing.

4. *Tic douloureux* (q.v.).

**neurasthenia**  Neurasthenic neurosis; nervous debility; *neuradynamia;* the concept of neurasthenia was introduced in the United States in 1869 by G. M. Beard; it had been outlined by Bouchut as nervosisme in 1860.

Neurasthenia is classified within the *somatoform disorders* (q.v.). Characteristics are mental or physical fatigue or body weakness after performing, or trying to perform, everyday activities, and inability to recover from that fatigue by normal periods of rest or relaxation. In addition, there may be a variety of symptoms, such as muscular aches, dizziness, tension headaches, sleep disturbance, irritability, and dyspepsia. See *hypochondriasis.*

According to Freud's early theory (1894), "Neurasthenia arises whenever a less adequate relief (activity) takes the place of the adequate one, thus, when masturbation or spontaneous emission replaces normal coitus under the most favorable conditions." Four years later he said that neurasthenia was an actual neurosis. "Psychoneuroses appear under two kinds of conditions, either independently or in the wake of actual neuroses (neurasthenia and anxiety-neurosis)" (*Collected Papers*, 1924–25).

**neurasthenia, traumatic** A neurasthenic reaction that develops in response to physical trauma, such as those caused by automotive or industrial accidents. Trauma is here considered to have precipitated an acute exacerbation of an underlying neurotic potentiality. See *neurasthenia; post-traumatic stress disorder.*

**neuraxon** See *neuron.*

**neuregulin** The neuregulin system participates in regulation of cell survival, proliferation, migration, and differentiation of both neurons and glia. Both *neuregulin* gene and its erbB receptors are required for the formation of some synapses. *Neuregulin-1* interacts with its receptor, is cleaved by γ-secretase, and then travels to the nucleus of the cell where it alters gene expression. *Neuregulin-1 (NRG-1)* is a susceptibility gene for schizophrenia.

**neuremia** Laycock's term for functional disorders of the nervous system.

**neurexins** A family of transmembrane cell adhesion molecules located on the presynaptic membrane. They comprise six main isoforms and numerous naturally occuring splice variants. Neurexin splice variations are important for maintaining the balance between the development of excitatory and inhibitory synapses.

**neurilemma** *Plasmalemma*; the external membrane of the Schwann cell. See *myelin.*

**neurinomatosis** A tendency toward new growth of primitive neuroepithelial cells.

**neurite** One of the components of the *NFT*; the other components are *neuropil threads* and the *PHF* (qq.v.). Neurites are enlarged neuronal processes with variable contents that may include PHFs, single filaments, mitochondria, membranous inclusions, lysosomes, or synaptic vesicles.

**neuritic plaques** See *Alzheimer disease; amyloid; plaques, senile.*

**neuro-** Combining form meaning nerve, from Gr. *neuron.*

**neuroacanthocytosis** A term for several rare multisystem hereditary conditions associated with neurological symptoms and behavioral abnormalities. Its name is derived from the Greek work for thorn, referring to the distinctive appearance of erythrocytes. There are three major classes: chorea-acanthocytosis, abetalipoproteinemia, and McLeod syndrome. Dysarthria, areflexia, and neuropathy occur in all three classes, while only the chorea and McLeod classes have associated hyper- and hypokinetic movements. All three show striatal degeneration on radiological studies.

Chorea-acanthocytosis is an autosomal recessive disorder characterized by progressive chorea, dysphagia, orofaciolingual dyskinesia, dysarthria, areflexia, seizures, and dysarthria. Motor tics may occur and, later, movement symptoms may evolve into parkinsonism. Cognitive impairment develops in 70% and psychiatric symptoms develop in 60% (affect disorders, lability, anxiety disorders, paranoia).

McLeod syndrome is an X-linked disorder. Female carriers, however, may show mild symptoms. Chorea, peripheral neuropathy, and areflexia are frequent. Behavioral changes are observed in almost half of patients: impairment of memory and executive function, emotional lability, depression, or hallucinations.

Abetalipoproteinemia is an autosomal recessive disorder. Because of missing serum lipoproteins containing apolipoprotein B there is fat-soluble vitamin deficiency and fat intolerance. It is associated with progressive spinocerebellar ataxia, with peripheral neuropathy. Retinopathy with loss of vision may occur. Behavioral changes are not characteristic (Anderson, K. E. *Psychiatric Clinics of North America 28*: 275–290, 2005).

**neuroadaptation** The neuronal changes that are assumed to be associated with both physical dependence and tolerance in connection with drug use; as yet, they are only poorly understood. The degree of neuroadaptation is inferred from the appearance of a withdrawal syndrome. Neuroadaptation may occur without any signs of a dependence syndrome; many surgical patients, for example, will experience some withdrawal symptoms when opiates are discontinued, yet have no desire to continue taking the drug and no other signs of dependence. Furthermore, dependence symptoms can develop even though no evidence of neuroadaptation is exhibited; sometimes this is termed *psychological dependence* and contrasted with *physical dependence* (i.e., neuroadaptation and an abstinence withdrawal syndrome). See *dependence, physical.*

There are many hypotheses about the nature of neuroadaptation: altered biochemical, biophysical, or neurophysiological properties of neurons, synapses, and neuronal circuits; enzyme induction; drug-receptor induction; altered coupling of receptors to intracellular effectors, such as adenylate cyclase; altered membrane composition and structure; altered biosynthesis and release of various neurotransmitters; and altered modulation of primary neuronal pathways by peptidergic feedback loops. Each theory is supported by some research findings, but none of them is fully adequate to explain the phenomenon.

There is some evidence that neuroadaptation is receptor-specific. N-methyl-D-aspartate (NMDA) is an excitatory amino acid that is known to be involved in neuron development, learning, and memory; neuroadaptation can be viewed as a type of neuronal learning. MK-801, an NMDA-receptor antagonist, has been found to attenuate both the development of morphine dependence and the development of tolerance to morphine's analgesic effect.

**neuroadaptation, disjunctive** *Nonreciprocal suppressant* (q.v.).

**neuroadaptation, reciprocal** *Cross-tolerance* (q.v.).

**neuroanatomy, chemical** The branch of anatomy that is concerned with the biochemistry of nerve tissues and, in particular, the function of chemical transmitters in nervous system activity. Within the nervous system, electrical impulses are transmitted along axons, but transmission from one nerve cell to another depends on the release of neurotransmitters at synapses. Knowledge about such transmitters has broadened considerably with the development of methods that could localize specific chemical transmitters in the brain.

Current research in chemical neuroanatomy is directed to the identification of biochemically specific pathways in the nervous system and defining their relationship to those that have already been identified by the histological, electrophysiological, and behavioral approaches. See *neurohormone; neuromodulator; neurotransmitter.*

**neuroanatomy, descriptive** A functional guide to local sites within the brain that correspond to specific behaviors, such as the interictal personality changes associated with temporal lobe epilepsy.

**neuroarthritism** A condition with a predisposition to nervous and rheumatoid or gouty disorders.

**neuroaxonal degeneration** *Seitelberger disease*; the syndrome consists of spastic paraplegia, equilibrium disturbances, ocular tremor, and mental retardation. Pathology includes eosinophilic spheroid masses throughout the cerebral gray matter, spongiosis of the globus pallidus, and demyelination of the pyramidal tracts.

**neuroblast** A primitive neuron or "pre-neuron" which appears during mitosis. At any one time, under the direction of a complex system of guiding factors, waves of neuroblasts migrate to their correct position in the brain by crawling along glial scaffolding and noncellular lattices, from the innermost layer of the developing cortex to form the outermost layer. In a 5-month embryo the cortex has begun to develop its characteristic six layers. See *neuron.*

**neurochemistry** The study of the chemical composition of neural tissue. Lipids account for about half the weight of the dry brain, and certain lipids—galactocerebroside and gangliosides—are found only in brain. Proteins, nucleic acids, nucleotides, amino acids, and amines are other important constituents. Unlike other organs of the body, the brain has only limited reserves of carbohydrate. Consequently, it is particularly vulnerable to hypoglycemia. It is highly dependent on a constant supply of both glucose and oxygen, and it consumes approximately 20% of the total oxygen consumption of the body.

**neurochemistry, behavioral** Study of the relations between chemical substances in the brain and behavior, including such areas as synthesis of neuroregulatory substances, genetic control of transmitter agents, different roles of compounds in different areas of the brain, biochemical effects of receptor excitation, interactions between different agents within the brain, actions of drugs on enzymatic and metabolic processes within the brain, and the relation of all such biochemical events to psychological events and behavior.

**neurocirculatory asthenia**   See *asthenia, neurocirculatory*.

**neurocognitive**   Relating to the neurological bases of *cognition* (q.v.). See *cognitive neural science*.

**neurocognitive enhancement**   Improvement of the psychological function of a person who is not ill; altering brain function to raise the normal subjects performance on cognitive tasks, such as memory and executive function. Most of the current candidate drugs for memory enhancement fall into one of two categories: (1) those that target the initial induction of long-term potentiation, such as drugs that modulate AMPA receptors to facilitate depolarization; (2) those that target the later stages of memory consolidation, such as drugs that increase CREB (the cAMP response element-binding protein), a molecule that in turn activates genes to produce proteins that strengthen the synapse.

**neurodegeneration**   Physical alterations in nerve cells characterized by disorganization and loss of connections between different elements of the cell and between different cells. Within the central nervous system, regeneration is rare; the usual result is death of affected cells. With *aging* (q.v.), cells in the brain endure increasing amounts of oxidative stress, disturbed energy homeostatsis, nucleic acid lesions, and accumulation of damaged proteins. Brain cells can be rendered more vulnerable to such challenges (*selective neuronal vulnerability*) by various genetic and environmental factors, and the resulting disorganization is manifested in *neurodegenerative diseases* (q.v.).

**neurodegenerative diseases**   A group of disorders in which the central pathologic feature is destruction of neurons, often with tangles or Lewy bodies. Neurodegeneration is often a result of protein misfolding, aggregation, and accumulation in tissues as fibrillar deposits, so these disorders can be considered as forms of *protein conformational disorders* (q.v.). The group includes Alzheimer disease (AD), Parkinson disease (PD), amyotrophic lateral sclerosis (ALS), Friedreich ataxia, frontotemporal dementia with parkinsonism (FTDP), Guam disease, Huntington disease (HD), Lewy body dementia (LBD), myotonic dystrophy, and prion diseases.

There is a genetic basis to many neurodegenerative degenerative diseases, but whether genetically based or due to some other factor(s), many of these diseases are related to one or more of the following: accumulation of aberrant or misfolded proteins, protofibril formation, ubiquitin-proteasome system dysfunction, excitotoxic insult, oxidative and nitrosative stress, mitochondrial injury, synaptic failure, intracellular calcium ($Ca^{2+}$) dysregulation, altered metal homeostasis, alterations in neurotrophic signaling pathways, and failure of axonal and dendritic transport. See *apoptosis*; *free radical*; *iron*; *excitotoxicity*; *misfolding*; *oxidative stress*; UPS.

**neurodevelopment**   The process of growth and maturation of the nervous system and its parts. Neurodevelopment begins with the formation of neurons, followed by neuronal migration, proliferation of dendrites and spines, synaptogenesis, myelination, and, for many neurons, pruning and apoptosis.

**neurodevelopmental hypothesis**   The theory that in schizophrenia environmental or genetically programmed events in utero disrupt the establishment of fundamental aspects of brain structure and function. The early developmental abnormality leads to impaired capacity of the brain to grow. It could be due to a variety of factors, not only genetic but also maternal nutrition, maternal alcohol consumption, difficulty during delivery, or environmental influences (e.g., nutrition, parental nurture and stimulation, infection, etc.) during the first 2 years of life. The result is a disruption of the interconnectivity between multiple cortical (particularly frontotemporal) and possibly subcortical (particularly corticostriato-pallido-thalamic) regions. These neuronal disturbances may be associated with early social, affective, and motor (neurointegrative, pandysmaturational) deficits. The structural abnormalities are vulnerability markers that predispose the brain to decompensation during stress and during the vulnerable age period between puberty and old age.

**neurodynia**   *Neuralgia* (q.v.).

**neuroeconomics**   Study of the brain processes involved in *decision making* and *choice* (qq.v.) and the neural computational processes involved in utility estimation and maximizing outcome. The field encompasses behavioral, imaging, and physiological approaches in both humans and animals. Neuroeconomics addresses such issues as how neurons process probability, outcome magnitude, and utility; how decisions are made at the neuronal level;

and how neurons encode the interactions of players trying to win or at least to maintain equilibrium.

Behavioral ecology assumes that basic rules of economic decision making, such as cost–benefit assessment, are followed when one faces a situation of uncertainty. Standard economic models of human decision making have generally viewed the decision maker as a rational cognitive machine. In recent years, behavioral economists have challenged those models, arguing that emotions play a significant role in decision making. See *behavioral ecology*; *prisoner's dilemma*; *Ultimatum Game*.

**neuroengineering**  At the present time, largely a field of research devoted to exploring the possibilities of bypassing spinal cord or brain lesions by making use of the collective activity of populations of cortical, subcortical, or spinal neurons that have been spared by the underlying illness. Lost motor functions, for example, might be induced by stimulating the patient's musculature or by controlling the movements of artificial actuators, such as robot arms. Implantable brain stimulators have already been used successfully in limited areas, such as cochlear implants to restore auditory function, deep brain stimulators for pain management and control of motor disorders in Parkinson disease, and vagal nerve stimulators to treat chronic epilepsy. Further research in the design of microelectrodes, in the miniaturization of hardware for multichannel neural signal conditioning, and development of new generations of actuators and sensors can be expected to increase the applicability of such devices once they have been demonstrated to be both safe and effective.

**neuroethology**  A discipline whose goal is to integrate the neurobiologic data needed to explain mechanisms of behavior. It first describes the components of behavior (the movement morphology or form) and then determines the rule(s) by which these components combine into functionally coherent sequences. Neuroethology studies animal behaviors and their neural underpinnings, and in particular the behavior of animals striving to survive and multiply in their natural environments. Comparing behaviors across species and studying species with exceptional talents are two approaches that have provided fruitful cues as to how the brain deciphers information gathered by the senses and on the neural mechanisms of communication and movement control.

Owls are an example of exceptional talents; they hunt at night by localizing rustles and squeaks made by their prey. The brain creates a spatial map from cues such as differences in the time it takes a sound to reach the two ears. Another example is comparing profiles of gene expression in the brains of songbirds with those of birds that don't sing. The results provide clues about the evolution of vocal communication. Some neuroethologists are using robots to test models of the neural control of movement. Analyses of the intentional repetitive behaviors seen in obsessive-compulsive disorder and Tourette syndrome, for example, reveal that many of the maladaptive behaviors are not voluntary. Instead, they are ritualistic in nature and are performed to achieve relief from unwanted urges, sensations, thoughts, or anxiety. The rituals correspond to phylogenetically old behavior patterns of grooming and checking body parts. The form (i.e., the *serial order* or *chains*) of a grooming sequence seems to be dependent on striatal structure rather than on cerebellar or cortical circuits.

**neurofeedback**  EEG *biofeedback* (q.v.).

**neurofibrillary tangles**  Filaments of hyperphosphorylated tau, a microtubule-associated protein. NFTs correlate with cognitive deficits and neuron loss in neurodegenerative diseases, such as Alzheimer disease, but in animal models they have continued to accumulate even when memory function has recovered and neuron numbers have stabilized after suppression of the tau transgene.

**neurofibromatosis**  Neurofibroblastomatosis; two forms have been differentiated—*neurofibromatosis 2* and *von Recklinghausen disease* (qq.v.).

**neurofibromatosis 2**  NF2; central neurofibromatosis; bilateral acoustic neurofibromatosis; a severe inherited disorder that is genetically and clinically distinct from the more common neurofibromatosis 1 (NF1) or *von Recklinghausen disease* (q.v.).

The hallmark of NF2 is bilateral vestibular schwannomas (formerly called *acoustic neuromas*)—benign, slow-growing tumors located on the vestibular branch of the eighth cranial nerve. Other tumors, particularly meningiomas, spinal schwannomas, and ependymomas, are also frequent. Persons with NF2 generally develop symptoms of eighth nerve dysfunction, including deafness and balance disorder (ataxia), in early adulthood. Paralyses are also frequent.

NF2 is caused by a highly penetrant defect that displays an autosomal dominant pattern of inheritance. It has a prevalence of about 1 in 40,000. The NF2 defect is transmitted within a segment of the central portion of the long arm of chromosome 22. The NF2 suppressor gene's protein product shows a strong similarity to a family of cytoskeletal-associated proteins; it was named merlin (for moesin-ezrin-radixin-like protein).

**neurofilaments**    Components of the neuronal cytoskeleton that are important both for the maturation of axons and the maintenance of axonal integrity. Their individual subunits are transported from cell body to axon, where they bundle together to form filaments. Abnormal aggregates of neurofilaments in motor neurons are characteristic of amyotrophic lateral sclerosis (ALS), one mechanism of which may be defective neurofilament trafficking. See *cytosol; cytoskeleton; NFT.*

**neurogenesis**    Growth and development of the neuron(s); used particularly to refer to the development and proliferation of new neurons in the adult brain. There is general acceptance that adult generated neurons are added to one mammalian brain region—the hippocampus. Neurogenesis can be up- and down-regulated by important psychological variables, such as stress, environmental complexity, and learning, as well as by hormones and other physical factors. Adult neurogenesis is primarily confined to two discrete areas: the subventricular zone and the subgranular zone of the dentate gyrus in the hippocampus. Adult hippocampal neurogenesis is decreased by stress and increased by chronic antidepressants. See *glia; neuronal plasticity.*

**neurogenic**    Caused or produced by, born of, or engendered by nerves or a nerve. Neurogenic disorders include spinal muscular atrophy, familial amyotrophic lateral sclerosis, postpolio muscle dysfunction, and hereditary neuropathies.

**neurogenic genes**    Genes that regulate the development or positioning of neurons. One such is the *Notch* family of genes, crucial for the generation of striatal neurons from progenitor cells in the ventricular zone, and for regulating the developmental timing that controls the generation of distinct striatal compartments.

**neuroglia**    *Glia* (q.v.).

**neuroglioform cells**    NGCs; See *neocortical neurons.*

**neurogram**    Engram; the changes in neurons and neuronal networks that enable recording and conservation of experiences. See *memory, physiological.*

**neurohormone**    Neurohumor; a chemical messenger produced by neuroendocrine transducers, most of which are located in the hypothalamus. The neurohormone is carried to the anterior pituitary by means of the hypophyseal portal system and moves along axons to the posterior pituitary. From there the neurohormone binds to specific receptor sites on the plasma membrane of the other cells, whose activity it modulates. Neurohormones are similar to *neurotransmitters* (q.v.), except that they generally interact with a variety of cells whereas neurotransmitters interact only with other neurons. See *elementary process; epinephrine; neuroanatomy, chemical; peptidergic; serotonin.*

**neurohypnology**    The study of *magnetic sleep* (Braid). See *hypnotism; Mesmer.*

**neurohypnosis**    *Obs.* Braid's original term, meaning sleep of the nervous system; later Braid dropped the first part of the word and used hypnosis instead "for the sake of brevity."

**neuroimaging marker**    See *biomarker.*

**neuroinduction**    Suggestion.

**neuroinformatics**    Organization and dissemination of neuroscientific data, using the power of computers to integrate the continuously increasing amount of data, to produce three-dimensional maps of relevant brain structures and functional processes, to develop comprehensive models of different neurological systems, and to provide easy access to such information not only to educate but also to stimulate further research.

**neurokym**    *Psychokym* (q.v.).

**neuroleptic**    (Gr. "which takes the nerve") The term was introduced by Delay and Deniker in 1955 to refer to the antipsychotic effect of certain pharmacologic agents on the nervous system; the terms ataraxic and tranquilizer, in contrast, are merely descriptive of a sedative effect. See *antipsychotic; psychopharmacological agents.*

Neuroleptic refers specifically to an antipsychotic effect on symptoms of schizophrenia and an associated likelihood of EPS side effects; antipsychotic effects in mood (affect) disorders are obtained with other classes of drugs, such as antidepressants, mood stabilizers, and antimanic agents.

Schizophrenia itself is associated with a greater vulnerability to several illnesses, including obesity, diabetes, coronary heart disease, hypertension, and emphysema. See *metabolic syndrome.* Some neuroleptics appear to add to such vulnerability, and all patients treated with neuroleptics should be monitored for any of the following possible combinations:

1. *Obesity*—combined with smoking, obesity further increases risk for cardiovascular morbidity. Weight gain has been greatest with clozapine and olanzapine, least with ziprasidone and aripiprazole.

2. *Diabetes*—increased risk most frequently found with clozapine and olanzapine, especially in patients younger than 40 years; risperidone is not associated with increased risk.

3. *Hyperlipidemia*—clozapine and olanzapine are associated with higher triglyceride and cholesterol levels; risperidone is not. Elevated cholesterol or triglyceride levels are associated with a higher risk of heart disease and of the *metabolic syndrome* (q.v.).

4. *QT Prolongation*—prolongation of the QT interval is associated with the development of *torsade de pointes* (qq.v.) Normal Qtc (QT interval corrected for heart rate) is 400 msec; an interval of 500 msec or greater is considered a substantial risk factor for torsade de pointes. Mean increases in Qtc interval reported (in msec) for the following neuroleptics are as follows: thioridazine, 35.6; ziprasidone, 20.3; quetiapine, 14.5; risperidone, 11.6; olanzapine, 6.8; haloperidol, 4.7.

5. *Elevated prolactin*—hyperprolactinemia can cause galactorrhea (abnormal lactation) and menstrual disturbances in women, and in men galactorrhea and sexual dysfunction (decreased libido, impotence, ejaculatory dysfunction).

6. *Extrapyramidal symptoms (EPS), tardive dyskinesia*—EPS and tardive dyskinesia are less frequent in second-generation (atypical) antipsychotics than in conventional antipsychotics (Marder, S.R. et al. *American Journal of Psychiatry 161*: 1334–1349, 2004).

**neuroleptic malignant syndrome (NMS)** *Malin syndrome;* a rare and sometimes fatal complication of therapy with high-potency neuroleptics, consisting of hyperthermia, sweating, extrapyramidal system rigidity, labile blood pressure, and usually some disturbance of consciousness (which may progress to stupor and coma). Typical laboratory findings include high CPK and leukocytosis. Malin syndrome was first described by Delay and Deniker in 1968. See *Bell mania.*

NMS has been associated with all drugs that affect the central dopaminergic system, and it is believed that it is the result of abrupt, extensive, neuroleptic blockage of dopamine receptors in striatal and hypothalamic dopaminergic pathways.

In many cases, concurrent medical disorders and complications (such as dehydration, infection, renal failure, or pulmonary congestion) suggest that the neuroleptics may not be the direct cause, and that at least some cases develop on the basis of untreated severe or prolonged rigidity and other extrapyramidal symptoms.

**neuroleptic-induced movement disorders** *NIMD* (q.v.).

**neuroleptization, rapid** Administration of multiple doses of an antipsychotic drug over several hours in an attempt to interrupt an acute psychotic episode; sometimes called *megadose* (q.v.) treatment, although that also refers to long-term or maintenance therapy with very high doses of any drug. The technique of rapid neuroleptization was introduced in the 1960s and achieved its greatest popularity in the 1970s. Since then, however, most reports suggest that high parenteral doses of neuroleptic are no more effective than standard oral doses but are associated with a much higher incidence of extrapyramidal symptoms.

**neuroligins** A family of postsynaptic cell adhesion molecules, necessary for synaptic maturation and proper function. Mutations in the human genes are associated with autistic disorder and mental retardation.

**neurolinguistics** The study of language—including its acquisition, production, processing, reception—at the neurologic level. See *linguistics; psycholinguistics.*

Neurolinguistics is particularly concerned with aphasia (q.v.) and disturbances of any part of the language system, such as disturbances in syntax and grammar, lexicon (vocabulary), semantics (meaning), phonology (sound systems), and prosody (intonation, accent).

**neurologic paraneoplastic syndromes** Nervous system autoimmune disorders that accompany a small percentage (probably not exceeding 1%) of cancers of the ovaries, uterus, breast, or lung. In the most frequently observed syndrome, the Purkinje cells of the cerebellum are attacked. Symptoms progress rapidly over a 6- to 8-week period: unsteady, staggering gait, vertigo, double vision, dysmetria, and dysphonia. They may leave the patient totally disabled, but if the tumor is excised early enough, damage may be limited.

In another form, associated with small-cell carcinoma of the lung, the limbic system is affected. Symptoms progress steadily over a 1-year period: amnesia, confusion, and extreme lability of mood.

Also associated with lung tumors is the *Lambert-Eaton syndrome*, in which the antibodies attack the calcium channel of the nerve cells at the neuromuscular junction. Often the peripheral nerve damage reverses itself if the tumor responds to treatment.

**neurology** The branch of medicine that devotes itself to the study of the organization and function of the nervous tissue. The diseases of the peripheral nerves of the spinal cord and the brain, as far as they are based on organic pathology, are in the realm of neurology.

**neuromessenger** A general term that includes *neurohormone, neurotransmitter,* and *neuromodulator* (qq.v.). Neuromessengers may be *postsynaptic* (on the dendrite that receives and binds to the neurotransmitter released from the axon of the preceding neuron) or *presynaptic* (located on the axon itself). Presynaptic neuromessengers are termed *autoreceptors* if they bind to a neurotransmitter released from their parent neuron, *heteroreceptors* if they bind to a neurotransmitter released from another neuron. See *neurotransmitter receptor; second messenger; synapse.*

**neurometadrasis** *Obs.* Animal magnetism or the influence of one body upon another.

**neurometrics** Computer-assisted studies and measurement of brain function, including brain electrical activity mapping (*BEAM*), brain wave activity measurement (*BWAM*), visual and auditory evoked potentials (*VEP, AEP*). See *NMR.* The techniques elicit quantitative data about brain functioning, particularly as it is related to information processing, with the goal of identifying different types of brain functioning in persons whose behavior manifestations are similar.

Two classes of slow waves can be recorded from the human scalp: (1) spontaneous fluctuations of voltage, reflected in the *electroencephalogram* (EEG); and (2) transient oscillations of voltage in response to environmental stimuli, called *evoked potentials* (EPs) or *event-related potentials* (ERPs), which can be extracted from the EEG by computer averaging methods. See *event-related potential.*

**neuromimesis** *Obs.* Mimicry of disease or disorder of a mental or nervous character. See *factitious disorders; Ganser syndrome.*

**neuromodulator** *Neuroregulator;* a substance that conveys information to nerve cells by means other than neurotransmission. Neuromodulators regulate nerve cell function by amplifying or dampening neuronal activity; *neurotransmitters* (q.v.), in contrast, regulate neuronal activity by conveying information between adjacent cells.

Neuromodulators may act in several ways. They are able to enhance or decrease the amount of neurotransmitter released; they can also alter the efficiency with which the neurotransmitter interacts with its receptor. The same substance may act as a neurotransmitter in one synapse and as a neuroregulator at another synapse.

Three types of neuromodulators have been differentiated: (1) synaptic neuromodulators, which act on nerve cells in synaptic contact; (2) hormonal neuromodulators, which affect cells relatively distant from the site of neuromodulator release; and (3) autoinhibitors, which modulate their own release or synthesis by means of presynaptic mechanisms; they respond to the principal neurotransmitter released at the nerve ending by reducing or "shutting down" the release of that neurotransmitter. See *neuroanatomy, chemical; peptidergic.*

**neuromorphics** The attempts to capture in silicon the essence of biological subsystems, such as the ability of neurons to change behavior based on experience and the development of brainlike hardware to detect drugs and explosives, to generate music, and to allow vehicles to drive themselves. Neuromorphic engineering aims to transform microcircuitry into an analog computing medium resembling neural tissue. Besides allowing transistors to experience may different voltage levels, neuromorphic engineers are designing them to serve as both calculation and memory elements.

**neuromyelitis optica** *Devic disease* (q.v.).

**neuron** Also, neurone; the nerve cell, the largest cell in the body, comprising the cell body or perikaryon, the axon, and the dendrites. The major function of the nerve cell is to generate, propagate, and integrate the microelectric signals that reach it from adjoining neurons. It modifies its response to synaptic input in an experience-dependent fashion.

A small neuron may measure about 3 micrometers, but a large one stretches for over 1 meter, and for far more in a whale or an elephant. Myelinated nerve fibers conduct impulses at a speed of 2 to 100 meters per second. Nonmyelinated fibers are much slower, with a conduction speed of 0.2 to 2 meters per second.

The cell is the smallest unit that can be defined as "alive". At birth there are 1 million nerve cells; by adulthood, between 10 billion and 100 million neurons (the exact number is not known; $10^{12}$ is often given as an estimate, i.e., a trillion). During the embryo's early weeks and months, the rate of cell multiplication is enormous—200,000 or more *neuroblasts* ("pre-neurons") are formed every second. At birth, the brain weighs ca. 350 g; after 1 month, 420 g. In the first year, a baby's brain triples in size, to almost three-quarters of its adult dimensions. Growth then slows dramatically, with full adult bulk of 1400–1600 g (1600 g = 3 lb) attained at about 17 years.

Neural networks are formed by two classes of neurons: (1) excitatory *principal neurons* (*projection neurons*), which send their axons far away from their somatomata and connect major regions of the brain; and (2) inhibitory *interneurons*, local circuit neurons that not only inhibit other neurons but also control the electrical activity of neural networks. There are many types of interneurons, which selectively control the input, integration, and output of principal neurons. GABAergic interneurons are one class of interneurons. See *GABAergic systems*.

Each pyramidal neuron in the vertebrate brain is likely to be receiving up to 100,000 contacts from the neurons to which it is wired, and the complex and extensive multibranched dendritic tree of the Purkinje cells of the cerebellum probably extends to some 300,000 neuronal contacts.

The neuron contains all the elements that other cells do: plasma membrane, the outer wrapping; microfilaments (neurofilaments), which provide structural support; microtubules (*neurotubules*), which carry proteins and various chemical within the cell; *mitochondria* (q.v.), which free energy from sugars to drive the cell's processes; *lysosomes*, bags of digestive enzymes; *vesicles* (q.v.), sacs that store and transport materials; and *centrioles*, which assist in cell division. Those components are suspended in cytoplasm, and the whole is controlled by genetic information in the form of coiled-up molecules of DNA in the *nucleus* (q.v.), which has the full complement of chromosomes. More genes are switched on in a typical neuron than in almost any other cell type in the body. See *cytoskeleton; subnuclear bodies*.

Messenger RNA (mRNA) transcribes information from the DNA within the nucleus into areas near the nucleus where structural and metabolic proteins are synthesized. (More than 15,000 proteins are unique to the brain.) Nerve cell substances thus constructed within the cell body are packaged in the endoplasmic reticulum and transported to the dendrites or the axon. The cell body itself has relatively little to do with conduction of nerve impulses; rather, its primary function is trophic, to maintain the structure of the nerve cell and to support the synthesis and metabolism of various elements that will be used by the *axon* and *dendrites* (qq.v.).

**neuron doctrine** The fundamental principle of neuroscience, proposed by Ramón y Cajal in 1899, that the neuron is an anatomically and functionally distinct cellular unit that is either active and "firing" or is inactive, and that action potentials provide polarized communication between neurons. With the advent of microelectrodes that could be inserted into neurons to record electrical signals, the neuron doctrine began to erode. It is now known that much of the information processing by neurons involves electrical events that are graded in amplitude rather than all-or-nothing electrical spikes; that evoked electrical responses may be produced without input from other neurons; that electrical synapses at gap junctions possess the plasticity long considered an exclusive province of chemical synapses at axon–dendrite junctions; that neuromodulatory substances can act at multiple sites on the neuron to remodel neuron behavior and circuitry; that action potentials can be initiated in dendrites, which contain a mosaic of voltage-gated ion channels that can regulate how a neuron responds to the thousands of synaptic events that impinge on its dendrites; that both astrocytes and myelinating glia can affect or regulate communication between neurons. The connections, integration, and organization within the human brain extend well beyond explanation by the neuron acting as a single functional unit (Bullock, T.H. et al. *Science 310*: 791–793, 2005).

**neuronal ceroid lipofuscinosis**   See *lipofuscinosis, neuronal ceroid.*

**neuronal death, naturally occurring**   *Pruning* (q.v.).

**neuronal integration**   *Synaptic integration*; the process of *summation* (q.v.) of competing inputs at the cellular level, leading to the decision of the postsynaptic cell to fire or not to fire an action potential.

**neuronal model**   See *neuronal network.*

**neuronal membranes**   The neuron contains three distinct membranes: the major membrane system (proteins synthesized here are later distributed to lysosomes, secretory vesicles, and other organelles); and the *mitochondria* (q.v.) and *perioxisomes*, both involved in the use of molecular oxygen.

**neuronal morphometrics**   Measurement of the number, form, shape, and structure of neurons. It is now possible to count automatically neurons that have been appropriately stained. The technique has been used particularly in the study of schizophrenia, where reductions in the size of the amygdala, internal globus pallidus, and hippocampus have been observed as well as subtle abnormalities in the distribution of neurons in the frontal and cingulate cortex.

**neuronal   network**   A nerve cell and its connections with other nerve cells. In 1943, W. McCullloch and W. Pitts, in their *neuronal model* of brain operations, showed that neural networks could be modeled in terms of logic. Nerves could be thought of as logical statements, and the all-or-none property of nerves firing (or not firing) could be compared to the operation of the propositional calculus (where a statement is either true or false). Moreover, the analogy between neurons and logic could be thought of in electrical terms—as signals that either pass, or fail to pass, through a circuit.

**neuronal oscillations**   Fluctuations of activity between neurons, assemblies, and neural networks; the synchronous activity of oscillating networks links single-neuron activity to behavior, allowing brain operations to be carried out simultaneously at multiple temporal and spatial scales. The study of neuronal oscillations has emerged as a multidisciplinary approach that includes psychophysics, cognitive psychology, neuroscience, biophysics, computational modeling, physics, mathematics, and philosophy. See *synchronization.*

**neuronal plasticity**   Neural plasticity; ability of the neuron to respond to stimulation; specifically, the ability of the adult neuron to change and proliferate in ways that were classically thought to be limited to immature neurons at their developmental stage. It includes the concepts of *neurogenesis* and *synaptic plasticity* (qq.v.) and refers to a range of neural responses, from cellular and molecular mechanisms of synapse formation, to cellular realignment, to reorganization of neural networks, to behavioral recovery from strokes. New strategies are being developed to identify drugs, cells, or genes that will induce structural reorganization or repair of damaged neurons, and to determine the kind of stimulation or training of newly forming synapses that is most likely to ensure functional recovery.

Parts of the brain are not absolutely preset for particular functions; rather, they are built of general-purpose processors that become specialized in response to their inputs and outputs. Through learning, innate sensory and motor skills are adapted to new ends.

**neuronal redundancy**   See *pruning.*

**neuronophagia**   Removal of injured neurons by surrounding microglia.

**neuropathic pain**   *Chronic intractable pain* associated with damage to the peripheral or central nervous system; it arises as a result of many forms of nerve damage, including traumatic nerve injury, post-herpetic neuralgia, drug-induced neuropathy, and neuropathy secondary to diabetes or HIV. See *pain syndromes.*

**neuropathic traits**   They include enuresis, nail biting, finger sucking, sleepwalking, anxiety, nightmares, and fear of darkness. See *behavior disorders.*

**neuropathy**   Any (organic) disease of the nervous system; any disorder involving neural tissue. Formerly the term included disorders that currently would be termed neurotic or psychoneurotic. See *neuropathic traits*.

**neuropathy, CMV**   See *cytomegalic disease*.

**neuropeptide Y**   *NPY* (q.v.).

**neuropeptides**   Short chains of amino acids that are used as transmiters in the nervous system, in parallel with the small-molecule transmitters, such as the biogenic amines. They act through membrane-bound receptors that are coupled to intracellular signal transduction pathways. See *peptide, brain*.

One of the best-known neuropeptides is Substance P. Others are listed below:

*CRF*—corticotropin releasing factor—has been associated with depression and anxiety.

*NPY,* or neuropeptide Y, has been associated with depression and anxiety; its transmission is increased by repeated ECT; NPY gene expression is increased in the hippocampus (dentate gyrus) and pyriform cortex after ECT.

*STS,* or somatostatin, has been associated with depression and anxiety.

*NT,* or neurotensin, is believed to play a role in the function of the dopaminergic system.

*CGRP,* or calcitonin gene-related peptide, is believed to play a role in the function of the dopaminergic system.

*Tachykinins* include neurokinin A (NKA) and substance P (SP), both of which are believed to play a role in the function of the dopaminergic system

*TRH,* or thyrotropin-releasing hormone, inhibits glutamatgergic subcortical limbic neurons, which may be hyperactive in depression.

NPS, or neuropeptide S, part of a neurotransmitter system that modulates sleepwake cycles and anxiety.

**neuropharmacology**   The study of the effect of drugs, both therapeutic and drugs of abuse, on the central nervous system. The *molecular targets* for many of these drugs have been identified and the genes encoding most of these target proteins have been cloned. Drug effects are unlikely to reflect action on a single neurotransmitter; instead, they produce alterations in one system that lead to compensatory changes in a number of interacting neurotransmitter systems.

Among the molecular targets thus far identified are the following:

$D_2$-*like dopamine receptors* (i.e., $D_2$, $D_3$, and $D_4$ receptors)—antipsychotic drugs are antagonists at these receptors.

*Serotonin reuptake transporters*—which are blocked by the cyclic antidepressants that also block norepinephrine reuptake transporters.

*Selective serotinin reuptake inhibitors* block the serotonin reuptake transporter alone

*Dopamine reuptake transporter*—blocked by cocaine.

*Dopaminergic nerve terminals*—stimulated to release dopamine when amphetamine is taken into the terminals through the dopamine transporter.

**neuropil**   The space between Nissl-stained neurons, composed of intertwining neuronal processes, axons terminals, dendritic spines, astrocyte processes, astrocyte end-feet, blood capillaries, and synapses.

**neuropil threads**   One of the components of the *NFT*; the other components are the *neurite* and the *PHF* (qq.v.). Neuropil threads are damaged or dead neuronal processes, mainly dendrites.

**neuroplasticity**   *Neuronal plasticity* (q.v.).

**neuropoietic family**   See *cytokines*.

**neuroprotection**   Forestalling onset or progression of illness by means of interventions that influence etiologic factors or propagating mechanisms that sustain or extend the pathogenic process. For example, several *propagating factors* have been identified in neurodegenerative disorders: accumulation of intracellular aggregates, apoptosis, excitotoxicity, free radical activity, imunogenicity, mitochondrial dysfunction, and oxidative stress. See *CARE-HD*; *DATATOP*.

**neuropsychiatry**   Sometimes used as a synonym for psychiatry; the term emphasizes the somatic substructure on which mental operations and emotions are based, and the functional or organic disturbances of the central nervous system that give rise to, contribute to, or are associated with mental and emotional disorders.

Neuropsychiatry is concerned with the psychopathologic accompaniments of brain dysfunction (e.g., developmental disorders, infectious and inflammatory diseases of the brain, alcohol and other substance-induced CNS disorders, brain injury, cerebrovascular disease, seizure disorders, brain tumors, metabolic and neuroendocrine interference with brain function, Alzheimer disease and other degenerative diseases). One focus is on the early detection of psychiatric symptoms that are often masked by neurologic deficits (such as depression in an aphasic patient); another is identification of the specific site of brain disturbances (such as an epileptogenic focus) that is responsible for the patient's symptoms. See *behavioral neurology; neuropsychology.*

**neuropsychological tests** Assessment of brain functioning and, in particular, the evaluation of the behavioral impact of any brain pathology. Such tests are used to determine the existence and magnitude of cognitive and behavioral deficits following any insult to brain, to indicate the probable localization of defect(s), to determine strengths that are intact as well as skills that are impaired, to estimate the subject's ability to function within his usual environment, to guide rehabilitation strategies and to gauge the likely response to specific interventions. Examples of the use of neuropsychological tests include differentiating between dementia and pseudodementia and between seizure disorder and psychiatric disorder, charting recovery from stroke, and serial testing to estimate the permanency of disability.

Many tests measure some aspect of neuropsychological functioning, such as the WAIS (Wechsler Adult Intelligence Scale), the Benton Visual Retention test (BVRT), and the Bender Gestalt Test. Ward Halstead (1947), in an effort to find those tests that were most sensitive to brain damage, reviewed nearly 3000 tests; his doctorate student Ralph Reitan adapted those tests for clinical purposes. The result was the *Halstead-Reitan Battery* (q.v.), which samples different areas of brain function and evaluates multiple skills, making it possible to differentiate between strengths and weaknesses, between intact and impaired skills. Another test used frequently in neuropsychological assessment is the *Luria-Nebraska Neuropsychological Battery* (q.v.).

**neuropsychology** That branch of clinical psychology concerned with the evaluation of brain dysfunction and particularly with the development, standardization, and validation of techniques to assess behavioral expressions of such dysfunction. Neuropsychological assessment employs batteries of tests to evaluate major areas of functioning, both quantitatively and qualitatively, not only to provide assistance in differential diagnosis but also to assess levels of impairment as part of planning a treatment and rehabilitation program for the patient. See *behavioral neurology; neuropsychological tests.*

**neuroreceptor** *Neurotransmitter receptor* (q.v.).

**neuroses, class differences in** Neuroses are considered by many authorities as consequences of the specific social and economic circumstances, but neuroses are equally widespread in all socioeconomic groups. Further, differences between types of neuroses prevalent in different classes are negligible. See *class, social.*

**neurosis** As used today, this term is interchangeable with the term *psychoneurosis.* The term implies that the condition is not the result of organic brain disorder, that reality testing is not impaired, and that the underlying personality is not grossly abnormal. At one time it was used to refer to any somatic disorder of the nerves (the present-day term for this is *neuropathy*) or to any disorder of nerve function. In psychoanalytic terminology, neurosis often is used more broadly to include all psychical disorders; thus, Freud spoke of actual neuroses (neurasthenia, including hypochondriasis, and anxiety neurosis); transference or psychoneuroses (anxiety hysteria, conversion hysteria, obsessional and compulsive neurosis; and Fenichel adds to this group organ neuroses, pregenital conversions, perversions, and impulse neuroses); narcissistic neuroses (the schizophrenias and manic-depressive psychoses); and traumatic neuroses. See *neurotic disorder.*

The distinctions between neurosis and psychosis are symptomatic, psychopathological, and therapeutic. In the neuroses, only a part of the personality is affected (Meyer's *part-reaction*), and reality is not changed qualitatively although its value may be altered quantitatively (i.e., diminished).

Charcot was the first to make a systematic study of the neuroses; he formulated a group of clinical pictures that he called hysteria, which was considered to be an outcome of hereditarily determined degeneration. Janet was the first to attempt a grouping of neuroses on the basis of their dynamics. He theorized that there are two kinds of psychological operations—easy ones, requiring the cooperation of only a few elements; and difficult ones, requiring the systematization of an infinite number of elements, involving a very new and intricate synthesis in each operation. When the nervous tension or psychological force is lowered (by puberty, disease, fatigue, emotion, etc.), there is a general lowering of the mental level and only the simpler acts can be performed. Psychasthenia (including obsessions, compulsions, fears, and feelings of fatigue) results from a generalized lowering of the mental level; in hysteria, the lowering is localized in one particular function, which disappears (is dissociated) in consequence from the rest of the conscious personality.

Since Janet, there have been many other attempts at dynamic formulation of the neuroses, but Freud's concepts are probably the best known. They developed out of his clinical experience with hysteria, where Freud and Breuer claimed that hysterical symptoms disappear when the patient recalls, under hypnosis, previous experiences that have been forgotten. These experiences were believed to be traumatic and sexual in nature, and this led Freud to pursue an investigation of sexuality. (Both Freud and Charcot have been criticized severely for ignoring the findings of Hippolyte Bernheim—Charcot's contemporary, at Nancy —that hypnotism and the hysterical states associated with it were in large part a result of suggestion on the part of the hypnotist.)

Freud described the various stages of development, from autoerotism to object love, and he noted that the various erotogenic zones, which originally are autonomous, are finally subordinated to the primacy of the genitals and reproduction.

Freud later came to recognize that aggression as well as the sexual instinct is important in the etiology of the neuroses, and he elaborated his theory of the *death instinct* (q.v.) At the present time in psychoanalysis, it is believed that the neurotic conflict is essentially between the id (sexual and/or aggressive instincts) and the ego, with the superego taking either side. The external world may represent temptation or punishment so that the conflict may appear to be between the world and the ego. The ego attempts to defend itself against the instinctual impulses and does so successfully in the case of sublimation; but if the defense is unsuccessful, the warding-off process must be maintained at a high level of countercathexis. To escape the defenses, the impulses attempt indirect discharge through substitute impulses—the *derivative*.

Three main types of precipitating factors can be recognized in the neuroses: (1) an increase in the warded-off drive; (2) a decrease in the warding-off forces; and (3) an increase in the warding-off forces. An increase in the instinctual energy may be absolute, as in puberty, or relative, as in the case of exposure to temptation. A decrease in the warding-off forces is seen in fatigue, intoxication, and when the ego is strengthened at one point and in its false confidence allows some of its censorial activities to lapse. An increase in warding-off forces is found in instances of increase in anxiety or guilt feelings, or when any means of support or reassurance is lost.

General symptoms of the neurotic conflict include (1) specific avoidances; (2) inhibitions of partial instincts (such as eating), of aggressiveness, of sexualized functions, and of emotions; (3) sexual disturbances, such as impotence, premature ejaculation, and frigidity; (4) lack of interest in the environment and general impoverishment of the personality due to the constant drain of energy necessary to maintain countercathexes, and awareness of this impoverishment gives rise to inferiority feelings; (5) use of emergency discharges for the relief of tension; and (6) sleep disturbances, because of the many dreams and because of the fear of the ego to relax its guard during sleep.

**neurosis, alternation of** *Obs.* Relief of neurotic symptoms by bodily disease. The present-day term for this phenomenon is *pathocure* (q.v.).

**neurosis, choice of** See *neurosis; compliance, somatic.*

**neurosis, contagiousness of** The alleged but generally disputed capacity of a person's neurosis to affect another through contagion. It is theorized that in cases of hysteria and traumatic neurosis, there is a tendency for the patient to pick up additional symptoms from other patients who may be in the same ward.

**neurosis, malignant** A neurosis characterized by a progressive increase in the extent and severity of symptoms, which may ultimately prevent the performance of any activity. The patient may become a prisoner in his room or in his bed, or he may be paralyzed by indecisiveness and doubting. Many such cases are in actuality schizophrenics. See *agoraphobia; progredient neurosis; pseudoneurotic schizophrenia.*

Malignant neurosis is to be contrasted with stationary neurosis, in which the defenses operate successfully without further increase in anxiety or other symptoms.

**neurosis, parent as carrier of**   "The most common types of such parental carriers of neurosis to the children are: (a) The "cold' parents, who cannot give the warmth and love the children need; (b) the over-indulgent parents, who cannot expose their children to the disciplines and reality frustrations necessary to the child's development of adult survival traits; (c) the sexually frustrated parents, who displace their sexual needs onto the establishment of an over-intense emotional bond to their children as a substitute love-object; (d) the unconsciously hating parent, who visits repressed and denied aggression and hostility on his child, expressing repressed and denied jealousy and rivalry" (Weiss, E. & English, O. *Psychosomatic Medicine*, 1949).

**Neurospora frq**   See *biological clock*.

**neurosteroids**   Steroids that are synthesized in the brain; they can function as remote endocrine messengers and they also act in a paracrine manner to modify local neuronal activity. Some neurons and glia in CNS express the enzymes needed for the local synthesis of pregnane neurosteroids, which are highly selective and potent enhancers of GABA$_A$ receptor function.

**neurosyphilis**   A generic term for all forms of involvement of the nervous system by the spirochaeta pallida.

**neurosyphilis, congenital**   Intrauterine infection of the nervous system by the spirochete; sometimes mistakenly called *inherited syphilis*.

Approximately 10% of congenitally syphilitic children develop neurosyphilis, which, as in adult neurosyphilis, may be of the meningovascular or the parenchymatous type. Meningovascular syphilis is the more common form and resembles the adult form in pathology and clinical manifestations; these include mental retardation, convulsions, pupillary abnormalities, optic atrophy, diplegia or hemiplegia, and slight hydrocephalus of the communicating type. Deafness, a common symptom of congenital syphilis, is more often due to a temporal bone lesion than to N. VIII involvement. See *syphilis, cerebral*.

*Juvenile* or *infantile general paresis* probably occurs in no more than 1% of congenital syphilitics. Symptoms typically develop in early adolescence and mimic those of adult paretics except that the delusions are more puerile, the dementia is more complete and severe, and the course is more prolonged. *Congenital tabes* often does not appear until early adult life. Symptoms mimic those of adult tabetics.

**neurosyphilis, ectodermogenic**   Cerebrospinal syphilis. See *syphilis, cerebral*.

**neurosyphilis, interstitial**   See *syphilis, cerebral*.

**neurosyphilis, meningeal**   Tertiary syphilis involving the leptomeninges (the pia mater and arachnoid membrane). See *syphilis, cerebral*.

**neurosyphilis, parenchymatous**   A general term that includes paresis, tabes, taboparesis, and juvenile general paresis. See *general paresis*.

**neurosyphilis, vascular**   See *syphilis, cerebral*.

**neurotensin**   A neuropeptide that acts as a neurotransmitter or neuromodulator in the central nervous system. It colocalizes with dopamine systems and antagonizes dopamine and stimulant-induced transmission in mesolimbic pathways, and through such action it may mediate antipsychotic drug effects.

**neurotic disorder**   In DSM-III, a mental disorder in which the predominant feature is one or more symptoms that are a source of distress and are recognized as alien to the personality (ego-dystonic); without treatment, the condition is relatively enduring or recurrent, and although it may be severely disabling it does not lead to gross violation of social norms or to loss of reality testing. Further, the condition is not a mild transitory reaction to stress nor is there any demonstrable organic factor in its etiology. Instead, it is believed, the specific etiology is the neurotic process, consisting of the following sequence: (1) unconscious conflicts between opposing wishes, prohibitions, etc., leading to (2) unconscious perception of potential danger, or dysphoria, leading to (3) defense mechanisms, leading to (4) symptoms or personality disturbance.

Neurotic disorders are manifested in diverse ways and are included among the affective, anxiety, somatoform, dissociative, and psychosexual disorders of DSM-III. See *neurosis*.

**neurotigenic**   Producing or favoring the induction of a neurosis.

**neurotization**   Direct implantation of nerve into a paralyzed muscle.

**neurotoxicity**   Any adverse effect on the structure or function of the central or peripheral nervous system by a biological, chemical, or physical agent. Effects may be permanent or reversible, produced by neuropharmacological or neurodegenerative properties of a neurotoxicant, or the result of direct or indirect actions on the nervous system. Sometimes neurotoxicity is used to refer specifically to acute neurological insults, and *neurodegeneration* is applied to neuronal destruction over periods of months to decades. Neurotoxicity is characterized by excessive synaptic-glutamate accumulation, which leads to pathological accumulation of free cytosolic calcium in postsynaptic neurons. Extracellular calcium enters the cytosol through NMDA- and voltage-gated calcium channels, and at the same time calcium removal is impaired.

The excess calcium triggers degenerative events in the neuron that cause *neuronal necrosis*, which can trigger inflammation and secondary damage to healthy neighboring neurons. Calcium-dependent activation of nitric oxide synthase and xanthine generates *reactive oxygen species* (ROS), which damage lipids, proteins, and nucleic acids.

Some neurons undergo apoptosis, rather than necrosis. *Apoptosis* (q.v.) is noninflammatory; it is an active process that requires protein synthesis and energy, so its occurrence is limited to a subset of neurons that maintain sufficient energy. Necrosis is the predominant pathway of neuron death in the ischemic core of an infarct, whereas apoptosis is predominant in the penumbra surrounding the core.

**neurotoxicology**  The study of substances that cause, or have the potential of causing, damage to the nervous system.

**neurotoxin**  A substance, endogenous or exogenous, that destroys nerve tissue. There is some evidence that toxic oxidative products, if produced in the pigmented neurons of the substantia nigra pars compacta, may play a role in the genesis of *Parkinson disease*; and that if produced in the pigmented dopaminergic neurons that project via the mesolimbic tract they may do so for schizophrenia. See *dopamine hypothesis*.

**neurotransmission**  Propagation of an impulse along a nerve fiber, which is mediated electrically, and from one neuron to another across the synapse. Synaptic transmission is mediated chemically by the *neurotransmitter* (q.v.).

**neurotransmitter**  A chemical messenger that carries information from one neuron to another at the synapse. The neurotransmitter is synthesized within the neuron, stored in vesicles in the *bouton* (q.v.), and is released into the *synaptic cleft* when the bouton is depolarized. It binds to receptor sites in the postsynaptic cell and thereby exerts its effect on the cell ligand. See *conduction, nerve; elementary process; neuroanatomy, chemical; neurohormone; synapse*.

Neurotransmitters are assembled in the cell body according to instructions from genes held in the DNA in the nucleus. Instructions are first copied onto an RNA molecule, which leaves the nucleus for an assembly site, a ribosome, on the endoplasmic reticulum. Another site of manufacture is in the axon terminal. Those made in the main cell body are moved by specialized neurotubules that work like microconveyor belts.

There are five categories of neurotransmitter:

1. *Biogenic amines*, which provide diffuse innervation throughout the neuroaxis; included within this group are dopamine, norepinephrine, epinephrine, serotonin, acetylcholine, histamine.

2. *Amino acids*, which exert discrete excitatory or inhibitory effects within the nervous system such as aspartic acid, GABA, glutamic acid, glycine, homocysteine, taurine.

3. *Neuropeptides* (q.v.), which often act as cotransmitters with modulatory function. Among the recognized neuropeptides: angiotension, beta-endorphin, bombesin, bradykinin, cholecystokinin, corticotropin releasing factor, dynorphin, gastrin, leucine-enkephalin, somatostatin, methionine-enkephalin, substance P, thyrotropin releasing factor, vasoactive intestinal peptide, vasopressin.

4. *Gases*, such as nitric oxide (see *NO*) and carbon monoxide.

5. *D-amino acids* (see *serine*).

Some would include as a sixth category energy molecules such as ATP.

Psychopharmacologic agents enhance or attenuate the effects of a neurotransmitter, through several mechanisms: they may act on enzymes involved in the synthesis or degradation of the neurotransmitter (e.g., competitive inhibition of enzymes in the synthesis pathway; impair enzymatic degradation); affect uptake or storage processes (e.g., inhibition of the vesicular storage process); or influence the receptors that mediate or modulate synaptic neurotransmission (e.g., by blocking or enhancing receptors at various sites along the metabolic pathway; direct agonist effect).

**neurotransmitter receptor** Typically a protein component of the nerve cell's surface that *couples* with a specific neurotransmitter or neuromessenger (the *first messenger*), the neurotransmitter receptor is able to "recognize" the extracellular neurotransmitter because its own shape is the complement of the shape of the molecule being bound. The neurotransmitter and the receptor bind together as the *ligand* at the *recognition site* of the receptor. Exogenous agonists and antagonists of the receptor compete with the neurotransmitter for occupation of the recognition site.

The receptors exert an effector function within the target cell by gating an *ion channel* (q.v.) directly or by initiating a *second-messenger* cascade. *Ionotropic* receptors open to provide a channel (a *ligand-gated channel*, also termed *neurotransmitter-gated channel* or *NGIC*) that allows ions to pass through the neuronal membrane; they prove a tight linkage between the recognition site and the *ion channel* (q.v.) and thus ensure fast and precise signaling between neurons.

*Metabotropic* receptors are set within the neuronal membrane and typically contain seven transmembrane-spanning amino acid sequences with extracellular and intracellular amino acid tails. They activate other effector proteins within the nerve cell, typically through linkage with an enzyme that acts on its substrate. Many receptors that work indirectly are linked to an intracellular *G protein* (q.v.). G proteins are 10 to 100 times more abundant than receptor proteins, and one receptor protein can activate many G protein molecules and thereby amplify the response. In consequence metabotropic receptors, even though they act more slowly than ionotropic receptors, can amplify and provide greater versatility of neuronal response. G proteins may couple receptors directly to various effector systems of the cell or indirectly to *second messenger* systems (q.v.). Second messengers typically exert their effects by regulating protein *kinases* (q.v.) and protein phosphatases, the *third messengers* in the chain of events leading to neuronal response.

**neurotransmitter-gated ion channel** *NGIC; ionotropic* receptor. See *neurotransmitter receptor*.

**neurotrophic hypothesis** More neurons are generated than survive into adulthood, either the result of limiting amounts of growth and survival factors (the neurotrophic hypothesis) or because of their inability to make functional connections (the *activity hypothesis*). If brain cells don't die at the right times and in the right places, the developing brain cannot form its myriad precise connections between nerve cells.

**neurotrophin-3 See** *neurotrophins.*

**neurotrophins** Neurotrophic factors; a family of growth factors, including *nerve growth factor (NGF), brain-derived neurotrophic factor (BDNF), neurotrophin-3 (NT3), neurotrophin-4/5 (NT4/5),* glial-derived neurotrophic factor (GDNF), *pigment epithelium-derived factor (PEDF),* insulinlike growth factor (IGF-1), and ciliary neurotrophic factor (CNTF). In CNS they influence neuronal cell survival, the balance between cell survival and apoptosis during development, axonal and dendritic growth and guidance, the response of growth cones to inhibitory axon-guidance molecules, synaptic structure and connections, neurotransmitter release, LTP, synaptic plasticity, myelination, regeneration, and pain. BDNF promotes myelination; NT3 inhibits it. It appears that neurotrophins mediate bidirectional signaling between neurons and the glia that ensheath them, rather than acting on neurons alone.

Neurotrophins mediate their effects by binding to two classes of receptor: the Trk receptor tyrosine kinases and the p75 receptor, a member of the tumor necrosis factor receptor superfamily that binds to all neurotrophins. NGF binds selectively to TrkA, BDNF and NT4/5 to TrkB, and NT3 to TrkC receptors. Signaling by TrkB receptors is directly responsible for promoting hippocampal LTP. Downstream activation of CREB (the cyclic AMP-response element binding transcription factor) and calcium/calmodulin-dependent kinase II is responsible for the ability of TrkB to modulate LTP.

Cleavage of the p75 receptor has been implicated in the pathogenesis of Alzheimer disease, and a mutation of BDNF has been linked with depression, bipolar disorders, and schizophrenia.

**neurotubules** Microtubules. See *cytoplasm; cytoskeleton; neuron.*

**neurovascular unit** See *astrocytes.*

**neurulation** The process of formation of the neural tube: the neural plate folds to form the neural groove and then fuses to form the hollow neural tube. See *cephalogenesis*.

**neurypnology**   *Obs.* Braid's term for the study of hypnosis.

**neutrality**   The role of the therapist in activity group psychotherapy: here he is not only passive and permissive, but neither has nor applies criteria of right and wrong, proper and improper behavior on the part of the patient. According to Slavson, neutrality of therapist means "that each patient can utilize him in accordance with his own particular needs. Each member of the group projects on the therapist his unconscious attitudes toward adults. Neutrality on the part of the therapist makes this possible" (*An Introduction to Group Therapy*, 1943).

**neutralization**   In psychoanalysis, neutralization includes both *desexualization* and *desaggressivization* (qq.v.). "The term neutralization implies that an activity which originally afforded drive satisfaction ceases to do so and comes to be in the service of the ego, apparently nearly or quite independent of the need for gratification or discharge of cathexis in anything which even approaches its original instinctual form." (Brenner, C. *An Elementary Textbook of Psychoanalysis*, 1955).

**neutralizer**   A member of a therapy group who neutralizes, i.e., counteracts and controls, the aggressivity, impulsiveness, and destructiveness of other members of the group. See *instigator*.

**new health practitioners**   Medical paraprofessionals, including nurse practitioners and physician's assistants.

**new variant CJD**   Described first in England in 1996; also called *nvCJD* or *nCJD*. Unlike classical CJD it occurs early in life; mean age of onset is 29 years. Early features are sensory disturbance and behavioral changes (e.g., withdrawal, anxiety, or depression). Within weeks after onset a progressive cerebellar syndrome develops with forgetfulness and other memory impairments; the cognitive disturbances progress to dementia. Late in the disease, myoclonus is common. Just before death, most patients have akinetic mutism and some develop cortical blindness. Most probably nvCJD is due to transmission of *bovine spongiform encephaloathy* (q.v.), passed from infected cattle to humans. As of February 6, 2002, 92 persons had died of the disease in Europe, 88 of them in Britain.

**newborn screening See**   *genetic screening*.

**nexus**   Linkage of thoughts.

**NFD**   *Neurofibrillary degeneration*, whose degree is positively correlated with the severity of neuropsychological impairment in *Alzheimer disease* (q.v.).

**NFT**   *Neurofibrillary tangles*, which consist of paired helical filaments of hyperphosphorylated tau. Tangle, rather than amyloid, load correlates with cognitive impairment. Tau pathology alone has been shown to be sufficient to cause frontotemporal dementia, but not Alzheimer disease. See *amyloid hypothesis*.

**NFTT**   Nonorganic *failure to thrive* (q.v.).

**NGF**   Nerve growth factor. Both sympathetic and sensory neurons depend on nerve growth factor for survival. Some sensory neurons that do not respond to NGF are instead supported by brain-derived neurotrophic factor (*BDNF*). A third member of this family is *neurotrophin 3* (*NT3*), which supports the survival of dorsal root ganglion neurons and proprioceptive neurons of the trigeminal mesencephalic nucleus. The amino acid sequences of NGF, BDNF, and NT3 are very similar to one another. See *apoptosis; neurotrophic factors*.

**NGI, NGRI**   Not guilty by reason of insanity; insanity defense, insanity plea. See *insanity defense; criminal responsibility*.

**NGIC**   *Neurotransmitter-gated ion channel* (q.v.).

**niacin deficiency**   *Pellagra* (q.v.). In the context of nutritional deficiency, niacin includes both nicotinic acid and nicotinamide, members of the vitamin B complex. Nicotinic acid and nicotinamide are precursors of the coenzymes nicotinamide adenine dinucleotide (NAD) and nicotinamide adenine dinucleotide phosphate (NADP), which are hydrogen acceptors of many dehydrogenases. The liver can convert the amino acid tryptophan into nicotinamide; in *Hartnup disease*, a hereditary pellagra-like disorder, tryptophan is converted instead into indican.

**nicastrin**   A protein associated with the *presenilins* (q.v.); it appears particularly to affect γ-secretase processing of APP. See *secretases*.

**nicotine**   The major psychoactive substance in the leaves of the tobacco plant (used in cigarettes, "smokeless" tobacco such as chewing tobacco, snuff, nicotine gum). Nicotine causes stimulation, followed by depression, of the central and autonomic nervous system, leading to an increase in alertness and ability to focus attention and, in some, a decrease in anxiety and irritability. It produces vasoconstriction in the hands and feet and a slight rise in blood pressure and heart rate. In the brain, nicotine activates positive reinforcement by enhancing dopamine levels.

When tobacco smoke is inhaled, nicotine is rapidly absorbed through the lungs and delivered to the central nervous system even more quickly than after intravenous injection. Probably because of that, dependence is much more likely to occur in smokers than in those who use snuff or chewing tobacco. See *dependence, drug.*

**nicotine addiction**    The largest cause of preventable mortality in the world and the cause of more than 4 million smoking related deaths each year. Nicotine dependence begins with the binding of nicotine to nicotinic acetylcholine receptors (*nAChRs*), normally activated by the endogenous neurotransmitter acetylcholine. (See *tobacco dependence.*) Once smoking is established (daily smoking for one month), approximately 20% of users develop nicotine dependence. Rates of current smoking are approximately 25% for the U.S. population but higher in many psychiatric disorders, including schizophrenia (83%), bipolar disorder (69%), generalized anxiety disorder (46%), and major depression (37%).

The rewarding effects of nicotine are mediated, in part, by release of dopamine in the nucleus accumbens from ventral tegmental area neurons. The mechanism of release may involve the mu opioid receptor and its endogenous ligand, beta-endorphin. See *nAChRs.*

The most effective treatment of nicotine addiction is to prevent its occurrence in the first place. Once dependence has been established, however, multiple treatment approaches tend to be used, including external sanctions, hypnosis, self-help groups, family and couples therapy, and behavioral therapies (such as contingency management and cognitive behavior therapy); pharmacological therapies include nicotine replacement therapy (nicotine gum, nicotine, nasal spray, and transdermal nicotine) and *bupropion* (q.v.).

**nicotine dependence**    *Tobacco dependence* (q.v.).

**nicotine replacement therapies**    NRTs; see *nicotine addiction; tobacco dependence.*

**nicotine use disorders**    These are classified within the substance-related disorders and include nicotine dependence and nicotine withdrawal.

**nicotine withdrawal**    Symptoms appear within 24 hours when nicotine use is stopped or reduced abruptly by a subject who has used nicotine daily for several weeks or more: craving for nicotine (which may last days or months after cessation of use); mood changes, most commonly anxiety, irritability, or anger; difficulty in concentrating; restlessness; insomnia; increased appetite, often with weight gain; decreased heart rate.

**nicotinic**    See *acetylcholine.*

**nicotinic acid deficiency**    *Pellagra* (q.v.). See *niacin deficiency.*

**nicotinic receptor**    See *antimuscarinic.*

**NIDS**    Neuroleptic-induced deficit syndrome.

**Nieman-Pick disease**    An autosomal recessive glycolipid storage disease characterized by mental deterioration, progressive blindness, hepatosplenomegaly, and brownish discoloration of the skin. The disease is rapidly progressive and leads to death within 2 years of onset. See *lysosomal storage disorders.*

The disease is due to a deficiency of the sphingomyelin-cleaving enzyme, sphingomyelinase, and is manifested by accumulation of sphingomyelin in the reticuloendothelial cells of the liver, spleen, bone marrow, and lymph nodes.

Nieman-Pick type C disease affects one in $10^6$. The gene responsible for the major form of NP-C disease is *NPC1*, on chromosome 18; a second gene on chromosome 18, *NPC2*, produces identical clinical and biochemical phenotypes. The Niemann-Pick protein, NPC1, senses a cell's level of cholesterol and helps to shuttle it from one part of the cell to another. Cholesterol plays an important role in promoting cell signaling in response to neurotrophic factors.

Cholesterol from the bloodstream binds to a docking site, the LDL receptor on the cell surface. The receptor is then drawn into the cell's interior and the cholesterol freed in the lysosome, a compartment-like cell organelle. Cells from NP-C patients are defective in the release of cholesterol from lysosomes. This lysosymal sequestration of LDL-derived cholesterol results in processing errors as a result of which the cells become glutted with cholesterol. Nerve cells are the first to be attacked, causing problems in seeing, walking, hearing, and swallowing; stumbling; and seizures. Patients do not survive to reach adulthood.

**nifedipine**   A calcium-channel blocker used primarily as an antihypertensive agent. In psychiatry it has been used as an antidote for hypertensive crises induced by monoamine oxidase inhibitors and in the treatment of mood disorders and neuroleptic malignant syndrome (NMS). See *calcium channel*.

**night hospital**   See *day hospital*.

**night phantasy**   In distinguishing night phantasies from dreams, in the psychoanalytic sense, Freud held that night phantasies occur during the sleeping state, but unlike dreams, do not undergo additions or alterations of any kind and in all other ways are similar to daydreams.

**night residue**   Persistence of any psychic material from sleeping and dreaming during the waking day; the manifest dream (i.e., the dream as remembered by the subject) is the most common example of night residue. See *dream*.

**night terror**   See *sleep terror disorder*.

**night-eating syndrome**   *NES*; a type of *eating disorder* (q.v.) that occurs in about 10% of obese patients and usually in women; it consists of nocturnal hyperphagia, insomnia, and morning anorexia. The syndrome tends to appear episodically, and during such periods weight control is especially difficult or even impossible for the patient.

A second type of eating pattern found in obese patients is *binge eating*—consumption at irregular intervals of large quantities of food in an orgiastic manner.

A third pattern is eating without saturation, seen most frequently in patients with central nervous system disturbances, and characterized by overeating without relationship to stress situations and without regular periodicity.

**nightmare**   A fright reaction during sleep; *dream anxiety disorder*. The dream content typically involves threats to survival, security, or self-esteem and the memory of it, or the interference with sleep caused by it, produces significant distress. The awakenings usually occur during the second half of the sleep period.

"In the nightmare (*ephialtes, incubus*) the child awakens in terror from a dream usually characterized by a feeling of suffocation and helplessness. He can ordinarily relate his bad dream; he is well oriented, can recognize people about him, and can be calmed readily. Nightmares are often very vivid and the memory of them accompanied by a sense of dread, sometimes recurs the following day when the child is awake" (Bakwin, H. & Bakwin, R. *Clinical Management of Behavior Disorders in Children*, 1953). See *sleep disorder; sleep terror disorder*.

**nightshade, deadly**   *Belladonna* (q.v.).

**nightshade poisoning**   See *deadly nightshade poisoning*.

**nigrostriatal tract**   See *dopamine*.

**nihilism**   The general rejection of customary beliefs in morality, religion, and the like; the belief that there is no meaning or purpose in existence.

**nihilistic delusion**   See *Cotard syndrome*.

**nikhedonia**   The pleasure derived from the anticipation of success.

**NIMD**   *Neuroleptic-induced movement disorders* are categorized as acute or delayed (tardive), and as hyperkinetic (positive) or hypokinetic (negative). Acute NIMD include *akathisia, dystonia, neuroleptic malignant syndrome*, and parkinsonism (the motor symptoms of *Parkinson disease*) (qq.v.). The typical tardive syndrome is *tardive dyskinesia* (q.v.).

**NIMH-DIS**   National Institute of Mental Health Diagnostic Interview Schedule; a highly structured interview developed for use by lay interviewers in large-scale epidemiologic surveys in the United States. It is a modification of the SADS and the *Research Diagnostic Criteria* (q.v.).

**Nirvana**   Death, extinction; oblivion to care, pain, or external reality. According to Freud, the Nirvana-principle ( a term suggested by Barbara Low) is a manifestation of the *death-instinct* (q.v.), the pleasure-principle of the libido, and the reality-principle of the influence of the outer world.

**Nissl substance**   See *chromatolysis*.

**nitric oxide**   *NO* (q.v.).

**nitrites**   *Poppers*; nitrite inhalants, including amyl, butyl, and isobutyl nitrite. These substances produce an intoxication characterized by a feeling of fullness in the head, mild euphoria, a change in the perception of time, relaxation of smooth muscles, and possibly an increase in sexual feelings. The nitrites may produce psychological dependence; they can also impair immune functioning, irritate the respiratory system, decrease the oxygen-carrying capacity of the blood, and induce a toxic reaction consisting of vomiting, severe headache, hypotension, and dizziness.

**nitrous oxide** *Laughing gas*; it rapidly produces intoxication, with light-headedness and a floating sensation. Symptoms disappear within minutes after discontinuation of the substance, but regular use has been followed by temporary but clinically significant confusion and reversible paranoid states.

**NKA** Neurokinin A, a tachykinin. See *neuropeptides*.

**NLNC hypothesis** *Native language neural commitment* hypothesis, that language learning produces dedicated neural networks that code the patterns of native-language speech. Exposure to spoken or signed language instigates a mapping process for which infants are neurally prepared, and during which the brain's networks commit themselves to the basic statistical and prosodic features of the native language. The auditory cortex is shaped early in life by the features and statistical probability of occurrence of acoustic input during critical periods of development. Such shaping allows phonetic and word learning. At 8 months, the sensitivity of infants to the statistical cues in speech allows them to segment words. See *language acquisition*.

There is evidence that language evolved to meet the needs of young human beings, and in meeting their perceptual, computational, social, and neural abilities, produced a species-specific communication system that can be acquired by all typically developing humans.

**NMDAR** N-methyl-D-aspartate receptor; one of the three subtypes of *EAA* receptors (q.v.), it is a doubly gated receptor that responds to both a chemical neurotransmitter (such as glutamate or aspartate) and voltage. NMDAR is involved in synaptic modifications in the adult hippocampus that underlie learning and memory, and in the pruning of retinal axon arbors and cerebellar functional synapses during development.

NMDAR contains several binding sites: (1) the NMDA-sensitive recognition site; (2) a phencyclidine receptor site, located within the ion channel and acted upon by drugs such as phencyclidine (PCP), ketamine, and MK-801; PCP acts by inhibiting the NMDA receptor; (3) a group that includes at least four other recognition sites—a modulatory glycine site, a polyamine recognition site, a $Mg^{2+}$ binding site, and a $Zn^{2+}$ binding site.

NMDA directly gates a cation channel that is permeable to $Ca^{2+}$ as well as to Na+ and K+. At the normal resting membrane potential, however, the channel is plugged by $Mg^{2+}$; adequate depolarization is necessary to unplug the channel and allow Na+ and $Ca^{2+}$ to enter the cell.

Many signaling pathways converge on the NMDA receptor, allowing the regulating of *ion channel* (q.v.) activity in response to second messengers, such as $Ca^{2+}$ and cAMP. *Yotiao* is a scaffold protein that anchors both *PKA* (cAMP-dependent protein kinase) and *PPI* (type 1 protein phosphatase) to NMDA receptors to regulate channel activity. Anchored PPI limits channel activity, whereas activated PKA overcomes that limitation and enhances NMDA receptor currents.

NMDA receptors open channels only if a neurotransmitter is released simultaneously from the presynaptic terminal and the postsynaptic neuron is depolarized. Opening of the channels allows a flux of $Ca^{2+}$ ions into the postsynaptic neuron, activating calcium-dependent second-messenger cascades and triggering a series of biochemical changes that either increase neurotransmitter release or increase the postsynaptic response to the transmitter. Calcium influx through NMDARs plays a key role in synaptic transmission, neuronal development and plasticity (including learning, memory, and behavior), senescence, and disease. The NMDAR scaffolding protein *PSD-95* (postsynaptic density 95) binds and clusters NMDARs preferentially, imparting signaling and neurotoxic specificity by linking receptor activity to critical second messenger pathways (Sattler, R. et al. *Science 284*, 1999).

Under certain circumstances, $Ca^{2+}$ influx may be involved in glutamate neurotoxicity, which allows an excessive inflow of calcium ions through NMDA-activated channels. Intracellular calcium ions may activate $Ca^{2+}$-dependent proteases such as calmodulin, thereby activating free radicals that are toxic to the cell. (See *calcium channel; NO*.) Synthesis of cGMP is stimulated in neurons and glial cells of the cerebellum by nitric oxide (NO), which is produced in neurons in response to glutamate, apparently acting through NMDARs, and requires an influx of $Ca^{2+}$ ions. Glutamate toxicity may thereby contribute to cell damage after stroke, to the cell death that occurs in status epilepticus, and to degenerative diseases such as Huntington chorea. See *excitotoxicity; glutamate*.

Evidence for NMDAR hypoactivity in schizophrenia has led to trials of drugs that indirectly activate the receptor, among them glycine, D-serine, and *ampakines* (q.v.).

**NMDAR hypofunction model** *NRH hypothesis* (q.v.).

**NMR** Nuclear magnetic resonance. See *imaging, brain; MRI*.

**NMS** *Neuroleptic malignant syndrome* (q.v.).

**nNOS** Neuronal isoenzyme of NOS. See *NO*.

**NO** *Nitric oxide*; a reactive, gaseous, lipophilic molecule with free radical chemical properties (not to be confused with *nitrous oxide*, $N_2O$, which is used as an anesthetic and is chemically stable). At high concentrations, NO functions as a defensive cytotoxin against tumor cells and pathogens; at low concentrations, it is a signal in diverse physiological processes, including blood flow regulation, neurotransmission, learning, and memory.

Three different variants (isoenzymes) of nitric oxide synthase (*NOS*) convert arginine into NO and citrulline, thereby controlling NO distribution and concentrations: *eNOS* (endothelial enzymes), *nNOS* (neuronal enzymes), and *iNOS* (cytokine-inducible). The iNOS isoenzyme is critical for the immune response but, perhaps because it churns out much larger amounts of NO that the other two isoenzymes, it is also implicated in most diseases involving NO overproduction (including carcinogenesis, immune-type diabetes, inflammatory bowel disease, multiple sclerosis, rheumatoid arthritis, septic shock, stroke, and transplant rejection). Pathologies associated with NO underproduction include arteriosclerosis, hypertension, impotence, and susceptibility to infection.

Within the brain, NO acts as a neurotransmitter by enhancing the formulation and catalytic activity of guanosine 3'-5'-monophosphate (*cGMP*), which stimulates phosphorylation of proteins by cGMP-dependent protein kinase. NO is also a neurotransmitter mediating penile erection through the stimulation of cyclic GMP formation. CO (carbon monoxide) functions as a neurotransmitter mediating ejaculation.

Stimulation of *NMDARs* opens *calcium channels* (qq.v.); calcium enters the neuron and binds to calmodulin, thereby activating NOS. NO may thus be directly involved in NMDA-type glutamate neurotoxicity, but this may not be its only messenger function in the brain. It has been suggested that NO is also involved in synaptic plasticity, such as long-term depression (LTD) and long-term potentiation (LTP) of neuronal response.

**Nobel prize complex** An active phantasy of being the powerful one, and the passive phantasy of being the special one; seen in gifted children, often in the first or only child. See *grandiose self*.

**nocebo effect** See *pain*.

**nociception** Sensation of *pain* (q.v.).

**nociceptors** The primary sensory neurons of *pain* (q.v.). They are of three types: 1) mechanical, which respond to touch, pressure, and movement; (2) thermal, which respond to heat or cold; and (3) polymodal, which respond to mechanical, heat, or chemical stimuli but show selectivity in their response to different modes of stimulation; they discriminate reliably between noxious and innocuous stimulations (unlike mechanoreceptive or thermoreceptive afferent neurons). Noxious stimulation signals potentially tissue-damaging events and evokes activity in the anterior insula, the anterior cingulate cortex (ACC), and somatosensory regions. The activity in ACC is related to emotion and motivation, suggesting that pain is both a specific sensation and an emotion. See *first pain*; *neuralgia*; *peptide, brain*; *psychalgia*; *second pain*.

**noctambulation** Night-walking; sleepwalking; *somnambulism* (q.v.).

**noctiphobia** See *nyctophobia*.

**nocturnal emission** See *ejaculation; wet dream*.

**nocturnal epilepsy** Jelliffe and White (*Diseases of the Nervous System*, 1935) state that "the possibility of exclusively nocturnal attacks—nocturnal epilepsy—should be borne in mind. It is suspicious if the patient awakens tired and lame, as if his muscles had been beaten, particularly if he shows conjunctival ecchymoses, a wounded tongue and flecks of blood on the pillow. A localized muscular weakness that passes off promptly would add certainty to the diagnosis."

Exclusively nocturnal attacks occur in approximately 25% of known epileptics; both day and night attacks occur in another 25% of patients. Exclusively nocturnal attacks are more common in children. See *epilepsy*.

**nocturnal hemiplegia or paralysis** See *sleep paralysis*.

**nocturnal myoclonus** See *myoclonus, nocturnal*.

**nocturnal penile tumescence** See *penile tumescence.*

**nocturnal regurgitation** See *achalasia.*

**nodal behavior** In group therapy, the peak of hyperaggressivity and hilarity on the part of children. This high peak is always followed by a period of quietude, which is the antinodal phase. This alternation of quiet and action occurs in cycles, and its frequency decreases as therapy progresses.

**nodding** Falling asleep under the influence of narcotics; frequent complications are cigarette burns, fires, sunburn, and frostbite.

**nodding spasm** A stereotyped movement disorder consisting of repetitive head-shaking, sometimes accompanied by nystagmus. It is rare in adults. In children it is seen most frequently in association with mental retardation or pervasive developmental disorders, although it may occur as an isolated syndrome not associated with any recognizable mental disorder.

**nodes of Ranvier** See *myelin.*

**-noea** Variant of *-noia* (q.v.).

**noematic** Relating to the mental processes.

**noesis** 1. Knowing by means of purely intellectual apprehension.

2. The primary delusion that one has been chosen to lead and command.

**nogo** A myelin-associated protein expressed in the central, but not the peripheral, nervous system. With other myelin-associated proteins it inhibits outgrowth of axons and is partly responsible for the inability of central axons to regrow after injury.

**Noguchi, Hideyo** (1876–1928) Japanese bacteriologist, worked in New York, demonstrated spirochetes in brain of paretics (1911). Until this discovery, syphilis was not recognized as the etiologic agent in general paresis but was thought merely to predispose to its development.

**-noia** Combining form meaning mind, mental state, from Gr. (para)noia, from *nöos, nóus.*

**noise** In information processing, the multiple random stimuli that bombard the sensory apparatus. Those stimuli must be ignored if the subject is to respond effectively to the stimulus carrying information (termed the *signal*). One action of catecholamines is to increase the signal-to-noise ratio of target cells by enhancing response to signals but not to noise.

**nomadism** A pathological tendency to roam from place to place, so strong that it gives rise to serious social maladjustment. It is often associated with mental retardation, epilepsy, Alzheimer disease, and other psychotic disorders. It may occur in children as a residual of epidemic encephalitis or cerebral birth trauma.

**nomenclature** See *nosology.*

**nominal aphasia** *Anomic aphasia* (q.v.).

**nomological** *Nomothetic* (q.v.).

**nomothetic** Giving or generating laws; legislative; in psychiatry, used particularly to refer to deriving general laws through observation of many cases, as contrasted with the *ideographic* approach, which is concerned with the explanation and prediction of behavior in the single or unique case (usually on the basis of extensive knowledge of the history and biography of the person).

**non compos mentis** Not of sound mind, mentally incapable of managing one's affairs. See *incompetence.*

**nonaccidental injury** See *child abuse.*

**noncoding DNA** Formerly called *junk DNA*, the large portion (about 95%) of the genome that does not encode proteins or regulatory information, as contrasted with the genes, which constitute about 5% of the 3 billion nucleotide bases. Noncoding DNA is found mostly at the telomeres and in the centromeres, sandwiched between and sometimes within genes. It consists of repetitive blocks of DNA, sometimes up to 10 billion bases long, that are somehow useful to the genome. See *DNA; genome.*

It is not the genes per se that matter most in the evolution of genetic diversity of animal forms, but differences in gene regulation. Turning on a gene at a different time, or in a new place, or under new circumstances can cause variation in, say, size, coloration, or behavior. If the outcome of that new regulatory pattern improves an organism's mating success or ability to cope with harsh conditions, the stage is set for long-term changes and, possibly, the evolution of new species.

Noncoding DNA is full of transposable elements. When present between the coding regions of genes, these elements can slow or halt transcription. They also help make new genes by inserting themselves into existing ones, thereby altering the protein code. Noncoding DNA also encodes RNA, already shown to affect gene expression through RNAi (RNA interference). See *small RNAs.*

Buried in the DNA sequence is a regulatory code akin to the genetic code but infinitely more complicated. Innovation is due to a variety of types of regulatory DNA, which turns genes on at the right time and in the right place. Certain genes code for the activating proteins that make up the transcription machinery, which binds to promoters, the DNA at the beginning of a coding sequence. Other genes code for transcription factors that can be located anywhere in the genome. All affect their target genes by attaching to modules, regulatory DNA that is usually near but not next to a gene. Protein-laden modules that stimulate gene activity are called activators or enhancers; those that dampen activity are called silencers.

Enhancers are small genetic command centers, consisting of stretches of 500 or so bases. Those clusters in turn are peppered with transcription factor binding sites, which can be less than 10 bases long. The target of a particular enhancer, and its effect, depend on the spacing and order of the binding sites within it. The genome can use the same subset of transcription factors to regulate different genes simply by changing the order or spacing of those proteins, or where they bind along the enhancer. A small change in one enhancer's structure, and likely many alterations in all sorts of enhancers, pave the way to the different developmental pathways that make each species distinctive. It has been estimated that humans could have as many as 100,000 enhancers and silencers, but fewer than 100 are known.

**non-dependence-producing substances** Nonpsychoactive agents that may be used repeatedly and inappropriately, to the point of producing harmful physical or psychological effects (which may include unnecessary contact with caregivers of the health care system), even though they do not produce true dependence. In ICD-10, "abuse of non-dependence-producing substances" includes many prescription drugs, over-the-counter drugs, and herbal or folk remedies, among them psychotropics, such as antidepressants and neuroleptics; analgesics, such as aspirin and acetaminophen; antacids; vitamins; laxatives; and steroids.

**nondirective therapy** See *client-centered psychotherapy*.

**nondisjunction** Failure to separate normally; a chromosomal abnormality in which the two members of a given pair of chromosomes fail to separate during cell division. As a result, two abnormal gametes are formed: one with both members of a chromosomal pair instead of only one, and the other with neither. When such abnormal gametes unite with a normal sperm or ovum during fertilization, the resulting zygote will contain either one too many chromosomes (in the human, 47 instead of 46), or one too few. Cells of both types may be formed in the same person, and each may perpetuate its line so that the person has cells of two (or more) types; such a condition is referred to as *mosaicism*. See *Down syndrome*.

**nonfetishistic transvestism** See *cross-dressing; transvestitism*.

**nonfluent aphasia** See *aphasia*.

**nonlinear dynamics** Mathematical analysis of patterns of neurological activity, a branch of mathematics that is linked with neuroscience in an interdisciplinary effort to understand the collective interactions of billions of interconnected neurons in the brain. Nonlinear dynamics tries to identify the large-scale patterns that emerge when neurons interact en masse.

**nonmalfeasance** See *beneficence*.

**nonreciprocal suppressant** Also, *disjunctive suppressant, disjunctive neuroadaptation*; a drug with the capacity to suppress clinically significant withdrawal phenomena even though it does not itself maintain a neuroadaptive state. Clonidine, for example, suppresses some aspects of opioid withdrawal but does not incite or maintain an opioid type of *neuroadaptation* (q.v.).

**nonrecognition** Loss of familiarity with objects or people, suggestive of dysfunction of the nondominant *parietal lobe* (q.v.) or the ventral temporal cortex. It occurs in various forms, such as *anosognosia* (failure to recognize serious medical disability), *prosopagnosia* (failure to recognize familiar people and faces), and *spatial nonrecognition* (failure to recognize one side of one's body, or objects in one side of the visual field). See *sensory neglect*.

**nonrecombinant** See *linkage; recombination*.

**nonregressive schizophrenia** More frequently used by Nordic or Scandinavian workers than those in the United States to refer to borderline schizophrenia. See *dishabituation*.

**non-REM sleep** See *sleep*.

**nonreproductive** As used by G. E. Hutchinson (*American Naturalist 93*, 1959), descriptive of any form of sexuality that would currently fall under the label *paraphilia* (q.v.). According to his usage, homosexuality was included within the more general term "nonreproductive sexuality." By some, nonreproductiveness is used as an indicator of the "unnaturalness" of certain types of sexual activity. See *unnatural*.

**nonrestraint** Management of the psychotic patient without the use of the straitjacket or other forms of restraint.

**nonsense syndrome See** *Ganser syndrome.*

**nonshared environment** See *shared environmental variance.*

**nonspecific research See** *research, specific.*

**nonsyndromic mental retardation** Mental retardation with apparently normal brain development and no other clinical features, the most common cognitive dysfunction. Although 10 nonsyndromic X-linked MR genes have been found, only one gene causing nonsyndromic autosomal recessive mental retardation has been identified so far—a 4–base pair deletion in the neuronal serine protease neurotrypsin gene (*PRSS12*). See *X chromosome.*

**nonsynonymous coding SNPs** cSNPs; see *SNP.*

**nonsystematic schizophrenia** See *systematic schizophrenia.*

**nontraditional medicine** Alternative medical therapies; *holistic healing* (q.v.).

**nontranssexual cross-gender disorder** See *transsexualism.*

**nonverbal language** Communication by gestures, sounds, facial expressions, posturing, and so forth. In psychiatry, especially in child psychiatry, communication between doctor and patient by way of nonverbal language often tells more than any words that may be spoken.

**nonwinner** See *transactional analysis.*

**nooklopia** *Obs. Thought theft obsession*, the delusion that one's thoughts are being sucked out of his brain by some sinister personal magnetism. Also known as *castrophrenia*. See *first-rank symptoms.*

**noology** The doctrine of the mind; the science of the understanding.

**noon of life** *Burnout*; midlife crisis; the dividing line between the first and second halves of a person's life. Referring to Jung's "functional" and "attitudinal" types J. Jacobi writes: "This opposition of the functions and of the conscious and unconscious attitude intensifies itself into a conflict in the individual, as a rule, only toward the second half of life;

indeed, it is just that problem which indicates an alteration of his psychological situation in that portion of life. Often it is precisely the capable persons, well adjusted to the environment, who, once past their forties, suddenly find that they are, in spite of their "brilliant mind,' perhaps not equal to domestic difficulties or are, for example, insufficiently suited to their professional position. If this phenomenon is correctly understood, it must be taken as a sign and warning that the inferior function, too, now demands its rights and that a confrontation with it has become a necessity. The latter, therefore, plays in such cases the greatest role at the beginning of analysis" (*The Psychology of C. G. Jung*, 1942).

**noopsyche** *Rare.* Stransky coined this term with the idea that there are two separate psychic factors: (1) the *noopsyche*, comprising all purely intellectual processes, and (2) the *thymopsyche*, made up of affective processes. In his opinion, *intrapsychic ataxia*, which results in marked incongruity between ideas and emotions, is a consequence of the more or less independent activities of the two psychic factors.

**nootropic** Term coined by Giurgea in the 1970s to describe *cognitive enhancers* (q.v.), drugs that improve cognitive functioning in the organically impaired. Currently also called *smart drugs*. (q.v.).

**noradrenalin** *NA*; neurons containing NA are located in seven discrete nuclei within the medulla oblongata and pons, and over half are in the locus coeruleus. Selective noradrenalin reuptake inhibitors (SNRIs) have been used as antidepressants.

**noradrenergic** Referring to neurons that are activated by or secrete norepinephrine. In the brain, noradrenergic neurons account for a small proportion (ca. 10,000 cells) of the estimated 10,000,000,000 nerve cells. Most of them originate in the nucleus *locus ceruleus* (q.v.) and send their axons to innervate the cerebral cortex, limbic system, diencephaon, brain stem, and spinal cord. See *adrenergic*; *catecholamine.*

**norepinephrine** See *catecholamine; epinephrine.*

**norepinephrine hypothesis** See *catecholamine hypothesis*; *serotonin hypothesis.*

**norepinephrine reuptake inhibitors** *NRIs* (q.v.).

**norm, psychic** A psychically normal person is one who is in harmony with himself and with his environment. He conforms with the cultural requirements or injunctions of his community. He may possess organic deviation or disease, but as long as this does not impair his reasoning, judgment, intellectual capacity, and ability to make harmonious personal and social adaptation he may be regarded as psychically sound or normal.

The assumption is that normality develops as the result of repression of certain component-instincts and components of the infantile disposition, and of a subordination of the remainder under the primacy of the genital zone in the service of the reproductive function. This means harmonious relationship of the forces of the id, superego, and ego. "The original urges are not unhealthily inhibited, but rather are domesticated in the service of the individual and society" (Healy et al. *The Structure and Meaning of Psychoanalysis*, 1930). See *mental health*.

**normal-pressure hydrocephalus** *Hakim disease*; often abbreviated NPH; a syndrome consisting of mild dementia, apraxia of gait, urinary incontinence, and enlarged ventricles in the presence of normal cerebrospinal fluid pressure, first described by S. Hakim and R. D. Adams (*Journal of Neurological Sciences 2*, 1965). The original patients described benefited remarkably from ventricle shunting. The procedure is a serious one, however, and complications may occur in as many as 20% of patients.

In chronic hydrocephalus, the earliest symptom is *magnetic gait*, a gait apraxia characterized by shuffling and "sticking" of the feet to the ground.

**normative dissociation** Non-pathologic *dissociation*

**normative ethics** See *ethics*.

**normative-referenced See** *test*.

**normatology** The study of normal behavior and development, with emphasis on data obtained from people who are not patients.

**normosplanchnic** In Viola's system of constitutional forms of body build, roughly equivalent to Kretschmer's *athletic type* (q.v.).

**normothymotic** Mood normalizer; specifically a pharmacologic agent that acts against a disorder of mood but does not affect normal mood.

**norms** See *review*.

**Norrie disease** (Gordon Norrie, Danish ophthalmologist, 1855–1941) Atrophia bulborum hereditaria; an X-linked recessive syndrome consisting of retinal malformation, mental retardation, and deafness; often misdiagnosed as retrolental fibroplasia, retinoblastoma, retinal pseudoglioma, or congenital toxoplasmosis. The eye pathology consists of bilateral gliomalike masses of tissue arising from the retina, with subsequent atrophy of the iris, lens, and corneal opacities and shrinking of the eyes, usually in the preschool years. No chromosomal or biochemical abnormalities have yet been identified as being responsible for the disease. Female carriers do not demonstrate ocular or hearing defects.

**NOS** Nitric oxide synthase(s). See *NO*.

**nos(o)** Combining form meaning sickness, disease, from Gr. *nósos*.

**nosocomion, nosocomium** Where illnesses are taken care of, hence a hospital or sanatorium. The adjective nosocomial means relating to a hospital but most commonly is used in a specific sense to refer to a hospital-induced condition that is unrelated to the patient's primary condition. See *iatrogeny*.

**nosogenesis, nosogeny** *Pathogenesis* (q.v.).

**nosography** The description of diseases.

**nosology** The study of diseases and, in particular, their classification, grouping, ordering, and relationship to one another; it includes the formulation of principles for differentiating one disease from another. Nosology attempts to classify illnesses and subdivide them on the basis of pathophysiological mechanisms and, ultimately, etiology. The pathophysiological mechanisms include neurochemical, neuropathological, genetic, and environmental determinants of specific disorders.

Ideally, nosology would provide a differentiation of discrete diseases and for each describe a specific cause, the typical clinical picture, its natural history and outcome, objective tests for its confirmation, and specific treatments.

Nosology, classification, nomenclature, and diagnosis are related, and to some extent overlapping, terms that refer to various aspects of the conceptualization of disease. *Classification* has two components: (1) *taxonomy*—grouping diseases according to a logical scheme and assigning them their proper places; and (2) *diagnosis*—applying those groupings to individual cases.

*Diagnosis* is the process of distinguishing or recognizing the presence of disease from its symptoms or part-manifestations. The term is also applied to the end result of that process, a summary statement of the conclusion to which the process leads. Some prefer the term assessment for the process of collecting information relevant to the diagnosis, management, and treatment of the patient's clinical condition, and diagnosis for the process of using pertinent information to assign the patient to a specific nosological class or disorder.

*Nomenclature* is the label used to communicate the results of the diagnostic process. It is a shorthand name for the disease that has been identified. The term implies that there is reason for using one term rather than another (e.g., Down syndrome rather than mongolism, multi-infarct dementia rather than cerebral arteriosclerosis).

Categorization of disease, even though it changes, is not wholly arbitrary. Rather, it reflects developing knowledge, at increasingly discrete levels, of the process of pathogenesis. How diseases are grouped, or differentiated from one another, depends on the state of the art or science that decreed such and such characteristics of the disease to be fundamental and significant. A single level approach (such as using only manifest behavior) is inadequate, and classification has moved toward a multiaxial, *polythetic approach*. Variations in behavior are not the sole determinants of classificatory groupings; they are supplemented by as many measurements as possible, from as many levels as possible: genetic, metabolic, physiologic, neurohormonal, inner experiences of mental life (such as lack of empathy, sense of entitlement, personal identity), cognitive functioning, interpersonal relationships, previous history, family history, course of illness, and response to treatment.

But even a polythetic approach that uses numerical taxonomy to provide a computerized system for quantifying the various measurements used is not without its pitfalls. The decisions as to what is a disorder, which measures are relevant, how many of the measurements used measure the same function (and thus artificially exaggerate its importance by counting it over and over again), and which measurements give the broadest range of information are the classifier's. Those decisions will, accordingly, reflect the bias of the classifier and the culture within which the classification is applied. See *categorical system*; *dimensional system*; *prototype matching*.

**nosophobia**   Unwarranted fear of disease; usually associated with no discoverable organic illness, or if the latter is present, the fear is grossly exaggerated.

**nostalgia**   Longing to return home or to one's native land; homesickness; explained by psychoanalysts as intense yearning for the members of one's family or for some particular member of the family. It is related to the dread of being alone and feeling at ease only when with someone to whom one is emotionally bound.

**Notch**   A group of *neurogenic genes* (q.v.) that encode cell surface receptors, active during embryonic development. Notch signals mediate interactions between neighboring cells and have a significant effect on neuronal differentiation, glial determination, and definition of borders between distinct cellular fields. *Notch3* expression is restricted to vascular smooth muscle cells in human adult tissues. See *CADASIL*.

**nothingness**   See *sensory neglect*.

**Nothnagel, Carl Wilhelm Hermann**   (1841–1905) Austrian neurologist; described angiospastic acroparesthesia and a cerebral peduncle syndrome that bears his name, consisting of unilateral oculomotor paralysis combined with cerebellar ataxia.

**notification, anonymous**   A method of *reporting* (q.v.) designed to protect the patient's *confidentiality* and at the same time protect others from harm. It is most often used in situations where the patient is HIV-seropositive and is unwilling to apprise his or her sex partners of the possibility that they will contract HIV disease from their sexual contacts with the patient. Its value in preserving confidentiality is questionable, however; even if the professional who contacts the partners does not identify either himself or the clinic or laboratory in which the patient's seropositivity was determined, it is unlikely that the partner will long remain ignorant of the identity of the patient.

**notional insanity**   *Obs.* A 19th-century term that included roughly what today are known as the schizophrenias and the psychoneuroses.

**not-me**   In Sullivan's system, symbolic representation of previous (usually infantile) interpersonal events that were associated with such overwhelming anxiety that they were dissociated from conscious awareness and memory; when the symbolic representations of such experiences threaten to invade consciousness (as in dreams, nightmares, fatigue states, intoxications, and schizophrenic reactions), the subject feels that the experience is foreign, unreal, and "not-me," and typically also is flooded with one or another of what Sullivan termed the "uncanny emotions"—awe, dread, horror, loathing. The feeling of unfamiliarity or foreignness is the opposite of *déjà vu* (q.v.), although in both phenomena the accompanying feelings are typically of the uncanny variety.

**not-mother object** See *transitional object.*

**noumenal** Intellectually, not sensuously, intuitional; relating to the object of pure thought divorced from all concepts of time or space.

**NOVA-1** Neuro-oncological ventral antigen 1, a protein unique to neurons that is involved in splicing regulation. It regulates neuron-specific alternative splicing in a sequence-dependent manner. Lack of NOVA-1 function results in defects in inhibitory receptor function and subsequently in excess motor activity. NOVA-1 is also involved in the pathogenesis of *paraneoplastic neurological disorders* (q.v.).

**novelty** In information theory, *incongruity* (q.v.).

**novelty potential** $P_{300}$ *wave* (q.v.).

**novelty seeking** NS; a heritable personality measure related to temperamental inflexibility (low scores indicate rigidity and regimentation). *COMT* (q.v.) met/met homozygotes have low NS scores, and also a susceptibility to negative mood states and affect disorders.

**noxa** Injurious agents, mental or physical.

**noxious stimulus** A stimulus that damages or threatens to damage tissues of the body. See *pain.*

**NPCs** Neural progenitor cells. Human NPCs derived from fetal brains have been genetically engineered to express GDNF (glial cell line–derived neurotrophic factor), which promotes regeneration of lost neurons. They have been used successfully to treat animal models of Parkinson disease. See *neural stem cells.*

**NPD** *Narcissistic personality disorder* (q.v.).

**NPH** *Normal-pressure hydrocephalus* (q.v.); also known as Hakim disease.

**NpHR** See *opsin.*

**NPI** Neuropsychiatric Inventory (of Cummings); assesses thought disturbance, perceptual disturbance (e.g., hallucinations); affect; abulia; agitation and aggression; disinhibition; appetite; sleeping patterns; aberrant motor activity.

**NPT** Nocturnal *penile tumescence* (q.v.).

**NPY** *Neuropeptide Y*; a 36 amino-acid peptide, the most potent appetite transducer. It is produced in the arcuate nucleus of the *hypothalamus* (q.v.).

**NREM See** *sleep.*

**NRH hypothesis** *NMDA receptor hypofunction* hypothesis of schizophrenia, that structural defects in the developing brain (either genetically or environmentally determined) induce a latent NRH potential that is subsequently activated by maturational events in early adulthood. Schizophrenia symptom formation results from defective function of a GABA-inhibitory filtering mechanism that normally is driven by glutamate acting through NMDA receptors. Malfunction of the filter results in disinhibited excitatory activity that floods corticolimbic neurons with erratic unmodulated messages. This glutamatergic model of schizophrenia posits that the cause is not dopamine neurons per se, but rather a failure to develop glutamate neurons in the left temporal and left limbic lobe, especially those involving an NMDA receptor, and that an underdevelopment of the glutamate neurons then causes overactivity of the dopamine neurons, which unleashes the symptoms of schizophrenia.

**NRI** *Norepinephrine reuptake inhibitor*; the resulting reduction in whole-body norepinephrine turnover allows more epinephrine to remain at the synapse, ultimately producing an *antidepressant* effect (q.v.).

**NRTs** Nicotine replacement therapies; see *nicotine addiction.*

**NSDUH** *National Survey on Drug Use and Health* (q.v.).

**NS-XLMR** Nonsyndromic X-linked mental retardation. See *X chromosome.*

**NT** Neurotensin. See *neuropeptides.*

**NTD** *Neural tube defect* (q.v.).

**NTF** Neurotrophic factor(s), which act on select populations of neurons to promote their survival and, in some cases, to prevent *apoptosis* (q.v.).

**NTR** Negative therapeutic reaction; see *superego resistance.*

**NT3** Neurotrophin-3; see *neurotrophins.*

**nuclear** Central, core; pertaining to, or having the character of, a nucleus.

**nuclear complex** *Oedipus complex* (q.v.).

**nuclear family** Traditionally defined as a married couple with children under the age of 18 years in the home. The number of such households has been declining in the United States and many European countries since the 1960s. The number of people living with nonrelatives (e.g., unmarried female-male couples, homosexual couples, friends sharing an apartment) has been increasing. See *conjugal unit, isolated.*

**nuclear imaging** See *radioisotopic encephalography.*

**nuclear problem** The patient's *central conflict* on which therapy should be focused. Symptoms and defenses often emanate from one central conflict. Examples of these are inadequate resolution of the oedipal conflict, feelings of inadequacy, unwholesome sexual identifications, and sibling rivalry. The *critical event* (q.v.) has a dynamic relation to the nuclear problem (Slavson, S. R. *An Introduction to Group Therapy*, 1943). See *actual conflict; root conflict.*

**nuclear schizophrenia** See *autistic-presymbiotic.*

**nuclei, CNS** Clusters of the neurons of the central nervous system into layers or discrete cellular groups. Relay nuclei do not merely connect presynaptic and postsynaptic neurons; they also modify the interactions between those neurons because of inputs they receive from higher centers in the brain. Thus, they contain both local interneurons and principal or projection interneurons that carry the output of the nucleus and make synaptic connections with cells in other nuclei or within the cortex.

**nucleolar organizers See** *nucleolus.*

**nucleolus** A prominent spherical body in the nucleus containing ribosomal DNA repeats clustered at chromosomal loci called *nucleolar organizers*; it is the factory in which ribosomal RNAs (rRNAs) are transcribed, processed, and assembled into ribosomes.

**nucleosome** *Nu body*; a DNA protein complex that is a fundamental part of packaging in the cell nucleus. Nucleosomes are beadlike structures consisting of a DNA strand wrapped around a histone core; the nucleosomes are connected to one another by other histone molecules. The nucleosome contains two molecules of each of the four core histones, a single molecule of a linker histone, and about 147 base pairs of DNA. It is involved in gene transcription, the first step of protein synthesis, and in DNA replication and repair. If human DNA were stretched out, it would be 2 meters long, but the cell is able to contain it in a space just a few micrometers in diameter because of its packaging. See *nucleus.*

The packaging unit of the nucleosome is the *nucleosome core particle*, 25 million of which are contained in an average cell nucleus. Each consists of a discus-shaped core of eight small proteins—the *histone octamer*—encircled by 146 base pairs of DNA that spiral 1.65 turns around the edge of the discus. If protein synthesis and DNA replication are to occur, the DNA and its associated proteins—the *chromatin*—must be at least partially unwrapped, and the core particle plays a central role in such unwrapping. The tails of the histones, for example, project out of the nucleosome, exposing them to enzymes involved in controlling *transcription* (q.v.). The DNA contacts the histone octomer at 14 main points. The histone tails that project out are modified by *histone acetyl transferase*, opening the chromatin to infiltration by the transcriptional machinery. See *epigenetic mechanisms.*

**nucleus** The cell body of the neuron contains the nucleus, which possesses the full complement of chromosomes, with DNA and the genetic code. The nucleus is a dynamic organelle of the cell that assembles different compartments as required by the changing metabolic needs of the cell. See *chromatin; chromosome; histones; neuron; nucleolus; replication.*

Synthesis of virtually all proteins and other structural components of the neurons takes place in the cell body, but these processes are controlled by the transcription of information from the DNA within the nucleus. There are two important ways in which this information can be processed: (1) the genetic information is passed from parent to daughter cell during cell division (heredity); and (2) a selected portion of the genetic information is *transcribed* into RNA and *translated* into proteins (gene expression). Messenger RNA (mRNA) carries the information to sites adjacent to the nucleus. mRNA then is translated to synthesize structural and metabolic proteins. Nerve cell substances are synthesized within the rough endoplasmic reticulum in the cell body, and then packaged in the smooth endoplasmic reticulum, which carries them down the axon to its terminal.

The DNA of the genetic material is tightly bound up with histones and other proteins, which together form the chromatin. In the nucleus, the DNA is arranged in *nucleosomes*, beadlike structures consisting of a DNA strand wrapped around a histone core that are connected to one another by other histone molecules.

Cell division is no longer possible in mature nerve cells, so chromosomes are not arranged in compact structures and they function only in gene expression.

**nucleus, caudate**    See *basal ganglia.*

**nucleus, dentate**    See *cerebellum.*

**nucleus, emboliform See**    *cerebellum.*

**nucleus accumbens**    Part of the striatum, lying between the putamen and the head of the caudate nucleus. It is thought to be important in mediating emotional and motivational behavior, including aggression. Both dopamine and serotonin have been implicated in modulating aggressive behavior. In rats, a rise in dopamine levels in the nucleus accumbens appears to prepare the animal for an anticipated stressful or aggressive event; a fall in serotonin levels is associated with the termination of this response when the anticipated event fails to occur.

The nucleus accumbens has a central role in anticipation of or monitoring of errors in the prediction of reward. It also responds to the emotional intensity and self-relatedness of a variety of stimuli, independent of their valence. See *frontal-striatal system; loss of control; striatal cortical inputs.*

**nucleus basalis of Meynert**    See *cholinergic.*

**nucleus fastigius**    See *cerebellum.*

**nucleus globosus See**    *cerebellum.*

**nucleus ruber**    Red nucleus. See *midbrain.*

**null hypothesis**    In statistics, the hypothesis that the true difference between any two samples or populations is zero, and that any apparent difference between them is due to chance. When the null hypothesis can be rejected at a high level of confidence, the difference is said to be statistically significant.

**numeracy, numerosity**    Number sense; numerical competence; the ability to respond to or estimate the number of objects in the environment. At a rudimentary level, numerosity is present in many nonhuman animals and in preverbal human infants. The adult competence for arithmetic and numerical manipulations probably arises from this fundamental number sense. Numerical manipulations depend on intact spatial representations, and both involve regions of the *intraparietal sulcus* (q.v.), the dividing line between the superior and inferior parietal lobules.

Human subjects respond more quickly to larger numbers if the response is on the right side of space, and to the left for smaller numbers—the *SNARC* (spatial-numerical association of response codes) effect. This suggests that in computing, a person should shift attention to the left for subtraction problems, and to the right for addition problems, in order to increase activation of the contralateral LIP (lateral intraparietal area).

**Nunberg, Herman**    (1884–1970)    German-born U.S. psychoanalyst; synthetic function of ego.

**Nurrl gene**    The gene responsible for dopamine production and for ensuring that the right amount of dopamine is produced.

**nurse practitioner**    A registered nurse who has had special training in an approved continuing or graduate education program to provide primary care or special services. The nurse practitioner, although considerably more independent than the graduate nurse, usually works under the supervision of a physician. See *physician extender.*

**nursing facilities See**    *domicile.*

**nursing home syndrome**    *Pseudodementia* (q.v.).

**nutritional/obstetric hypothesis**    The theory that schizophenia, and in particular the early-onset form (the type most likely to have a neurodevelopmental origin), is related to greater obstetric difficulties, owing at least in part to changes in maternal nutrition. The hypothesis correctly predicts the following findings: higher frequency of schizophrenia in immigrants form poor countries to rich countries than in immigrants from affluent countries; higher incidence in immigrants than in the population of their country of origin; higher rate of both obstetric complications and perinatal survival among immigrants (one reason for which is cephalo-pelvic disproportion secondary to the move from poverty in the home country to relative affluence), higher incidence of schizophrenia in second-generation immigrants than in the first generation (better maternal nutrition is associated with a higher survival rate).

**NVLD**    Nonverbal learning disability. NVLDs include disorders of motor control (dyspraxia), visual-spatial processing, mathematics (dyscalculia), music (amusia), memory, executive function, and socioemotional cognition and behavior. Many of these have been related to impairment of executive control, a prefrontal dysfunction. See *prefrontal cortex.*

Manifestations are highly variable and may include any combination of the following: particular difficulty in mathematics, impaired pragmatics (such as maintaining eye contact while talking) or prosodics (interpreting the affective components of speech), difficulty in singing or following melodies, a failure to grasp verbal humor and a tendency to use past behaviors inappropriately as responses to the challenge of new situations, poor neuromotor integration, and many of the symptoms described under *attention deficit hyperactivity disorder*, disruptive or *conduct disorder*, and *sensory processing disorder* (qq.v.).

**nyctalopia**   Night-blindness; inability to see well at night or in dim light; sometimes due to vitamin A deficiency. See *hemeralopia.*

**nyctophobia**   Fear of night or darkness.

**nyctophonia**   Night voice; ability to speak at night but not during daylight hours; sometimes appears as a variant of elective mutism. See *mutism, elective.*

**nympholepsy**   1. A form of pedophilia consisting of obsessive craving for "nymphets"; Lolita complex. 2. *Obs.* Demonic frenzy, especially frenzy arising from desire for an unattainable ideal.

**nymphomania**   *Andromania;        cytheromania; estromania;    metromania;    tentigo    venerea; thelygonia*; female hypersexuality. See *Don Juan; hypersexuality.*

**nystagmus**   An involuntary to-and-fro movement of the eyeballs induced when the patient looks upward or laterally. It is usually a sign of pathology. Nystagmus may be *horizontal*, the most common form, when the oscillations of the eyeballs are from side to side; or *vertical*, when the movements are up-and-down; or rotatory, when the oscillations are in a circular direction.

# O

**OAEs** Otoacoustic emissions; see *auditory nerve*.

**OAS** See *Overt Aggression Scale*.

**oath, Hippocratic** See *Hippocrates*.

**OBE** *Out-of-the-body experience* (q.v.).

**obedience, deferred** According to Freud, a prohibition, command, or threat received early in life may be repressed and the effect deferred for many years until a neurotic illness occurs and the original prohibition or command is obeyed. In spite of his father's opposition, a man became a painter. "His incapacity to paint after the father's death would then...be an expression of the familiar 'deferred obedience.'" (Freud, S. *Collected Papers*, 1924–25). See *failure through success*.

**obesity** Excessive accumulation of fat in the body, usually defined in terms of the degree of excess over normal body weight, such as a body weight that exceeds by 20% the standard weight listed in the usual height-weight tables.

Obesity is far more common among women, and prevalence rises with age. The usual subtyping of obesity is as follows:

*Mild*—20% to 40% overweight; this category includes approximately 90.5% of obese women.

*Moderate*—41% to 100% overweight; included are approximately 9% of obese women.

*Severe*—more than 100% overweight, included are approximately 0.5% of obese women.

**obesity, hyperplastic** Obesity in which the number of fat cells is increased. The other major form of obesity is *hypertrophic obesity*, in which the size of the fat cells is increased. Many obese persons, and most of those who are severely obese, show both types of change, a condition sometimes called *hyperplastic-hypertrophic obesity*.

**object** In psychoanalytic theory, an ill-defined concept referring to the other or anything that is not the self, or to the internal representations (object representations) of other people and things. The latter are sometimes called internal objects, a term that others use to designate phantasies of objects. A *whole object* is usually a person; in Klein's *object relations theory* (q.v.), a *part object* is sometimes part of a person (e.g., breast, penis) although it may also be a whole person who, through splitting and projection of libido or aggression, is perceived as all good or all bad. A *bad object* is one that the infant hates or fears; a *good object* is one that is loved or admired, or one that supports, nurtures, or soothes the person (qq.v.).

**object, good** See *object; paranoid-schizoid position*.

**object, ideal** See *idealization*.

**object addict** A term used to describe the behavior of some schizophrenics who, to prove that they maintain some contact with the objective world, seek out and cling to objects and ideas and on the basis of this develop obsessions, monomania, elaborate inventions, etc.

**object blindness** Visual *agnosia* (q.v.).

**object cathexis** See *cathexis*.

**object choice** See *object finding; object love*.

**object constancy** The ability to perceive objects as having an existence of their own, and the ability to summon the memory of an object (evocative memory). The latter mnemonic component is termed *object permanency*; object constancy, in addition, includes an affective component, related to the feeling of trust and calm associated with the original mother–infant bond and the holding-soothing introject. See *evocative memory; holding-soothing introject; separation-individuation*.

Object constancy reflects the child's ability to differentiate between the representations of object and self and is essential to a sense of selfhood. It also is a core element in the productive use of phantasy, which is the basis of effective planning for the future. Object constancy begins to develop by 18 months of age and is complete by 30 to 36 months.

**object finding** The process of transferring and finally placing libido upon environmental objects. The libido, formerly invested in erotogenic zones, may exhibit externalization in various forms. "Adult object-finding is frequently determined by fetishism; the love-object must

possess certain colored hair, wear certain clothing, or perhaps have certain physical blem-
ishes" (Healy et al. *The Structure and Meaning
of Psychoanalysis*, 1930). See *fetish*.

**object love**    The portion of the libidinal energy
of the psyche that is attached to some object
outside the person himself (or to the intrapsychic representation of that object). At various times, Freud appears to have considered
object love to be the earliest type of relationship to the environment and thus to precede
autoeroticism and narcissism; but at other
times he considered autoeroticism or narcissism to be primary. See *narcissism, primary*.

**object permanency**    See *evocative memory; object
constancy; separation-individuation*.

**object recognition**    Identification of different
things in the environment. Within the visual
system, objects are identified within the contexts in which they are most likely to appear.
Visual objects are contextually related if they
tend to co-occur in one's environment, and
a scene is contextually coherent if it contains
items that tend to appear together in similar configurations. Context-based predictions make object recognition more efficient,
although they are accompanied by occasional
inaccuracies. *False memory* (q.v.) exemplifies
the way in which contextually driven expectations can taint subject perception.

Contextual structures that integrate information about the identity of the objects that
are most likely to appear in a specific scene
with information about their relationships are
termed context frames, schemata, scripts, and
frames. They are sets of expectations that can
facilitate perception. Typical arrangements in
the environment are represented in context
frames. The recognition of atypical objects
and relations requires further scrutiny mediated by fine detail and elaborated analysis of
local features.

Swift extraction of contextual information is mediated by global cues that are conveyed by low spatial frequencies in the image;
details, conveyed by high spatial frequencies,
are analyzed later. The global shape information that is conveyed by the low spatial frequencies activates context frames. Activity
that is directly related to contextual processing develops first in the parahippocampal
cortex (PHC) and in the fusiform gyrus.

MTL (medial temporal lobe) and PFC (prefrontal cortex) both play a role in contextual

analysis. In MTL, the parahippocampal place
area (PPA) responds preferentially to topographical information and spatial landmarks.
The various components of representing
and recognizing individual objects (shape,
identity, and so on) reside in a network that
includes the lateral occipital cortex and fusiform gyrus, each of which is larger than PPA.
To analyze real-world contextual scenes, the
brain relies not only on the circuitry that
subserves visual scene perception, but also on
preexisting representation of common associations and typical relations.

The first and largest focus of differential
activity in the cortical processing of contextual associations is in the posterior hippocampal cortex (PHC), which encompasses
the PPA. A second focus is the retrosplenial
cortex (RSC). The PHC and RSC sites mediate the general analysis of contextual associations, rather than of place-related association
exclusively.

M. Bar (*Nature Reviews Neuroscience* 5:
617–629, 2004) has presented a model for
contextual facilitation: a blurred, low-spatial-
frequency representation is projected early
and rapidly from visual cortex to PFC and
PHC. In PHC this image activates an experience-based guess about the context frame
that needs to be activated. This contextual
information is projected to the ITC, where
a set of associations that corresponds to the
relevant context is activated. In parallel, the
same blurred image activates information in
PFC that subsequently sensitizes the most
likely candidate interpretations of the individual object. Then a reliable selection of
a single identity is made in ITC; this representation is further instantiated with specific
detail, which arrives gradually in higher spa-
tial-frequency information. See *visual cortex,
primary; visual processing*.

**object relation, primitive**    See *identification*.

**object relations, internalized**    The combination of
past realistic object relations, phantasied object
relations, and defenses against them. According
to Kernberg, the primary psychic unit is the
self representation linked by an affect state to
an object representation; it always encompasses
sexual and aggressive drives.

**object relations theory**    A view of mental
development in terms of how infant and
pre-oedipal child experience the external
world and its objects, how these experiences

are organized into self and object representations, how relationships with others are formed from the very beginning of life, how such relationships lead to changes in the child's mental structure, and how they serve as models of interaction in later relationships. The key mechanisms of mental development are *internalization* and externalization of relationships, *introjection* and *projection*, attachment and separation, transmutations, and *splitting* (qq.v.). See *self object*.

The object relations theory of pathogenesis is a deficit-relationship model, in contrast to the drive-defense-conflict model of classical psychoanalysis. It assumes the infantile ego to be capable of an elaborate organization of perceptions of the external world, an assumption that infant research does not fully support.

The original proponent of a complete object relations theory was Melanie Klein. Her model of a highly organized inner phantasy world that embodied envy, greed, projective identification, and introjection formed the basis of the "British school" of object relations. Among her assumptions were the following:

1. Superego formation and the oedipal triangle begin in early infancy.

2. The death drive is the first problem of life, and introjection and projection are essential elements in protecting the infant against it.

3. Closely related to the death drive is constitutional envy, which aims to possess and destroy the envied good breast.

4. The critical phases in development are the earlier paranoid-schizoid position, characterized by splitting and projective identification; the later is the depressive position, during which the capacity for internalizing whole objects develops.

Klein maintained not only that the infant is related to an object (typically, mother) from the beginning of life, but also that the infant's major goal is to maintain the continuity of a good relationship despite contradictory feelings of hatred, envy, and greed. Psychopathology arises when internalization of objects is faulty or when splitting of objects (into all good or all bad) is maintained so that they cannot be integrated.

After Klein, many versions of object relations theory developed; some of Klein's

followers, notably Fairbairn and Guntrip, relinquished drive theory completely, while others made drives secondary to object relatedness. In somewhat similar fashion, Kohut's self psychology de-emphasized drives, or denied their existence altogether, and made the mother/parent/object relationship the central issue in its theory of development. Kohut and his followers focus on the subjective world of the infant and on how development of the self is hampered when the mother's empathic responsiveness to her child is inadequate or distorted.

In the modified Kleinian theory of Kernberg, the primary unit of psychic structure is the self representation linked by an affect state to an object representation. This basic internalized unit always encompasses sexual and aggressive drives. *Internal object relations* are the result of realistic and phantasied past object relations and defenses against them. See *abandonment depression; affectomotor storms; basic trust; bonding; British school; cohesive self; communicative matching; conflict paradigm; container; libidinal ego; death drive; facilitating environment; empathic failure; fit; grandiose self; holding-soothing introject; idealization; identification; mirroring deficits; autistic-contiguous position; depressive position; paranoid-schizoid position; self-object; separation-individuation; libido theory.*

**object representation** Object image. See *self representation*.

**object vision pathway, ventral** It has the capacity to generate distinct representations for a virtually unlimited variety of individual faces and objects, but the functional architecture that embodies this capacity is a matter of intense debate. One model proposes that ventral temporal cortex contains a limited number of areas that are specialized for representing specific categories of stimuli. The ventral temporal cortex has a topographically organized representation (object form topography) of attributes of form that underlie face and object recognition. Thus far, two specialized areas have been described: the *fusiform face area (FFA)* and the *parahippocampal place area (PPA)*.

**objectification** *Projection* (q.v.); putting one's own fears or anger onto some person or thing outside one's self. The term is sometimes used to refer to a particular manifestation of projection, in which there is a too-ready recognition or detection in others of impulses that are really one's own. This may produce troublesome *countertransference* responses (q.v.) in the analyst, who overemphasizes the significance of impulses ascribed to the patient that are really the analyst's own. See *mote-beam mechanism.*

**object-ill** Stekel's term for the compulsive-neurotic who expresses his own mental conflict in the form of symbolization of objects pertaining to the outer world (i.e., outside his body) and also through symbolization of "the function of his everyday life such as washing, dressing, eating, defecating.... In compulsive diseases it is the patient's relationship to an object (usually a close member of the family) that is disturbed."

In opposition to the object-ill patient, Stekel calls "subject-ill" the person suffering from phobias or somatization, who uses his own body to symbolize his emotions. "The patient shows an ambivalent emotional attitude toward this object, that is, the polar tension between the extremes of love and hate with regard to this object is also extreme..." (Stekel, W. *Compulsion and Doubt*, 1949). See *subject-ill.*

**object-image** Object-representation. See *self representation.*

**objective psychology** See *psychology.*

**oblativity** Capacity for renunciation of the mother or mother substitute; the ability to tolerate frustration in the process of achieving independence.

**obliviscence** The state or process of passing into oblivion; the tendency for a memory to fade with the passage of time.

**obnubilation** Clouding of consciousness; stupor.

**OBOT** Office-based opioid agonist treatment. Methadone and LAAM have been approved for many years for maintenance treatment of opioid addiction, but in the United States only in licensed and accredited Opioid Treatment Programs. In 2002, buprenorphine, a partial agonist with an improved safety profile, was approved for limited office use by specially qualified physicians.

**OBS** 1. Organic brain syndrome; see *organic syndrome.* 2. Obstetrics.

**obscenity** Speech, gestures, writings, drawings, or other actions that are offensive to taste or modesty, or that aim to incite the viewer to lewd and prurient thought or action. See *pornography.*

**observation, delusion of** Delusion of being watched.

**obsession** An idea, emotion, or impulse that repetitively and insistently forces itself into consciousness even though it is unwelcome. Most commonly, obsessions appear as *ideas*, or sensory images, which are strongly charged with emotions: (1) *intellectual obsessions*, often in the form of preoccupation with metaphysical questions concerning one's purpose in life, ultimate destiny, whereabouts after death, etc.; see *brooding*; (2) *inhibiting obsessions*, in the form of doubts or scruples about actions, or multiple phobias that may paralyze all activity; (3) *impulsive obsessions,* which are repetitively intruding ideas that lead to action (e.g., arithmomania, kleptomania, and other so-called manias).

Less commonly, obsessions appear as feelings, unaccompanied by clear-cut ideas, such as anxiety or panic, feelings of unreality or depersonalization. Some authorities, in addition, classify motor tics as impulsive obsessions. See *obsessive-compulsive disorder.*

**obsession, masked** An obsession that appears in the disguised (masked) form of other symptoms. One of the most interesting forms is the obsessive idea that disguises itself in the form of pain. "The patients complain of pain, state that it drives them to suicide, yet they remain attached to the pain which—on closer scrutiny—may prove to represent pleasurable though tabooed memories . . . . Such pain (for which usually no organic cause can be found) then appears as a mask of the obsessive idea. The real idea is hidden behind the pain, so that the patients, instead of complaining of obsessions, complain of pain. It is diagnostically important that the usual sedatives are always ineffective in these cases or, if forced upon the patient, may lead to narcotomania" (Stekel, W. *Compulsion and Doubt*, 1949). See *somatoform disorders.*

**obsession, somatic** Morbid preoccupation with one's body or an individual organ. "Usually these obsessions concerning the body or individual organs are connected with [the] patient's feeling of guilt and inferiority. The somatic obsessions are mostly monosymptomatic, though they are always part of a more complicated neurotic system. A person not only is forced to think constantly of his nose, but also operates with a 'nose-currency,' so to speak, that is, in looking at people he sees only their noses and compares them with his own. No other human problem appears to be worthy of his attention" (Stekel, W. *Compulsion and Doubt*, 1949) See *monosymptomatic hypochondriacal psychosis*.

**obsessional pursuer** See *stalking*.

**obsessional rehearsal** A preliminary "tryout" often used by obsessional patients, who must carry out their compulsions but at the same time try to make their behavior conform to the requirements of the social milieu. In the obsessional rehearsal the patient performs his compulsion, but surveys the scene to determine how he can best work his compulsive activity into the pattern of behavior expected of him at some later date.

Reik cites the case of the man whose compulsion was a stamping of the foot to ward off danger as he crossed the border of a country. The patient had arranged to go driving with a woman friend, and their tour was to include crossing a border. On the day before their meeting, the patient drove out to the border and surveyed the scene.

On the following day, when he was in his car with the woman friend, he was able to introduce a discussion of waltz music at just the right moment, so that when the car did cross the border, he could beat time with his foot. In this way his compulsion could be performed without alerting anyone to its pathological features. The obsessional rehearsal was necessary so that the patient would know when he was approaching the border, and so know when to introduce his discussion of waltz music. (Reik, T. *American Imago 2*, 1941).

The obsessional neurotic also often shows peculiar deliberations and anticipations in thought. These are test phantasies, which Reik calls *thought-rehearsals*.

**obsessive attack** Rado's term for the major symptoms (as distinguished from obsessive character traits) of the *obsessive-compulsive disorder* (q.v.): (1) spells of doubting and brooding, (2) bouts of ritual making, and (3) fits of horrific temptation. According to Rado, obsessive attacks are derived from the temper (rage) tantrums of childhood, but the discharge of rage is slow and incomplete since it is always opposed by guilty fear.

He terms this an *interference pattern of discharge*, i.e., a mechanism for the alternating

discharge of opposite tensions. In the motor sphere, alternating discharge is expressed as bouts of ritual making; in the thinking sphere, as brooding spells.

**obsessive-compulsive disorder (OCD)** Considered a form of anxiety disorder, its characteristics are recurrent, disturbing, unwanted, anxiety-provoking obsessions (insistent thoughts or ruminations that at least initially are experienced as intrusive or absurd) or compulsions (repetitive ritualistic behaviors, or mental actions such as praying or counting, and purposeful actions that are intentional, even though they may be reluctantly performed because they are considered abnormal, undesirable, or distasteful to the subject). The compulsion may consist of ritualistic, stereotyped behavior or it may be a response to an obsession or to rules that the person feels obliged to follow. The obsession often involves the thought of harming others or ideas that the subject feels are gory, sexually perverse, profane, or horrifying. The actual risk of a patient harming others is very low. Obsessions produce marked distress in the subject, while compulsions prevent or reduce anxiety.

Factor analytic studies involving more than 2000 OCD patients have consistently extracted at least four symptom dimensions: contamination/cleaning (observed in at least 50%), obsessions/checking (in 40%), symmetry/ordering (9%), and hoarding. Other frequently reported symptoms are completing compulsions, in which a specific action must be performed in an exact fashion lest some feared consequence occur, and repeating/counting actions a certain number of times to prevent catastrophe.

OCD affects males and females equally; between 30% and 50% of cases have onset in childhood or adolescence. Lifetime prevalence of OCD is 2.5%. About 25% of those affected have relatives with the disorder. A concordance rate of 63% has been reported in monozygotic twins. There is evidence that a variant of a gene on chromosome 9 may contribute to OCD. The *SLC1A1* gene codes for a transporter that terminates the action of the excitatory neurotransmitter glutamate. Other genes that may also be involved are *SLC6A4*, which codes for the serotonin transporter, and *SLITRK1*, which is involved in neuronal growth.

The relatives of probands who have high scores on the obsessions/checking and symmetry/ordering factors are at greater risk for OCD than are the relatives of probands who have low scores on those factors. Checking symptoms correlate with increased—and symmetry/ordering with decreased—regional cerebral blood flow in the bilateral cingulate and left orbitofrontal cortex. Many studies suggest that different symptoms may be mediated by distinct neural systems within the frontostriatothalamic loops; different symptoms dimensions may thus coexist in any given patient (Mataix-Cols, D. et al. *American Journal of Psychiatry 162*: 228–238, 2005).

The "psychasthenia" of earlier writers usually included obsessive-compulsive neurosis, which was also known as substitution neurosis. Psychoanalytically, OCD is interpreted as a defense against aggressive and/or sexual impulses, particularly in relation to the Oedipus complex. The initial defense is by regression to the anal-sadistic level, but the impulses at this level are also intolerable and must be warded off—by reaction formation, isolation, and undoing. Because the use of these defenses renders superfluous the use of repression proper, the offensive impulses can exist in consciousness, although when they do they are divorced from their affective significance and so remain meaningless to the patient. See *compulsion; obsession.*

Psychoanalysis and other dynamic therapies have proved unsatisfactory as treatment of OCD; behavior therapy, on the other hand, has been of benefit. Treatment with exposure and response or ritual prevention has resulted in reduction of obsessions and rituals of atleast 70% in half of patients, and in a 30% to 70% reduction in a quarter of patients. Three-quarters of those who improved remained at least moderately improved at follow-ups of months to years. SSRIs have also been effective in ameliorating symptoms. Of all the symptom dimensions, hoarding has the highest comorbidity and the poorest treatment response to both medications and CBT.

**obsessive-compulsive personality (disorder)** *Compulsive personality* (q.v.).

**obsessive-compulsive spectrum** A group of disorders characterized by repetitive thoughts or disorders and, possibly, similarities of brain circuitry, genetic or familial factors, neurotransmitter systems, and treatment response. Included, in addition to *obsessive-compulsive disorder*, are obsessive-compulsive personality (*compulsive personality*), *hoarding, Tourette disorder* and other tic disorders, *Sydenham chorea, PANDAS, impulse control disorders* (such as *trichotillomania,* intermittent *explosive disorder*, and pathologic *gambling*), *body dysmorphic disorder* (*dysmorphophobia*), *hypochondriasis, autistic disorder, eating disorders, Huntington disease, Parkinson disease*, and *substance use disorders* (qq.v.).

**obsessive-ruminative tension state** Adolf Meyer's term for obsessive-compulsive disorder.

**obstipatio paradoxa** Soiling associated with constipation. "The child retains the stools, which become very hard and can be felt through the abdominal wall. Small pieces of firm stool are passed from time to time and are retained between the buttocks, macerating the perianal skin" (Bakwin H. & Bakwin, R. *Clinical Management of Behavior Disorders in Children,* 1953). See *obstipation.*

**obstipation** Extreme or intractable constipation; when of psychologic origin, it may appear either as a conversion symptom or as an organ neurosis. Like all conversions, obstipation may be the somatic expression of a specific, repressed, unconscious sexual phantasy. Usually obstipation expresses retentive tendencies connected with pregnancy wishes or incorporation phantasies. This is "in accordance with the equation child = penis = feces."

As an organ neurosis, obstipation is a physiological change in organic function, resulting from an unconscious attitude or affect. In the particular case of obstipation, the unconscious attitude is a chronically frustrated retentive pressure, which may exist for several reasons. It may represent an anal erotic fixation, a desire for anal retentive pleasure, or the feces may represent introjected objects as in the case of the conversion. In other instances, the retentive pressure, with its resulting obstipation, might be associated with a continuous and repressed aggressiveness.

**obstruction** *Blocking* (q.v.); thought deprivation. See *first-rank symptoms.*

**obtrusive idea** An obsessive idea that persistently repeats itself in the patient's mind and disturbs the normal flow of his thoughts. The patient considers the obtrusive idea as foreign to his ego and vainly attempts to renounce it.

**obtunded** An inexact term indicating depression of cerebral function, ranging from sedated to comatose. See *clouding of consciousness*.

**occipital lobe** The posterior lobe of the cerebral hemisphere; it is pyramidal in shape and lies behind the parieto-occipital fissure. Visual function is localized in the occipital lobe, primarily in the calcarine cortex (*area striata*, area 17 of Brodmann). Neurons from the retina project to the external geniculate body, from which second-order neurons project to the calcarine cortex. Fibers from the nasal half of each retina cross in the optic chiasm and so are projected onto the *visual cortex* of the opposite side; fibers from the temporal half of the retina remain uncrossed.

The posterior occipital poles are mainly concerned with macular (central) vision; the more anterior parts of the *calcarine area* are concerned with peripheral vision. The human loses both object vision and light perception when the calcarine cortex is removed. See *field defect*.

The *calcarine* cortex (area 17) projects to area 18 (*parastriate lobule*), which in turn projects to area 19 (*preoccipital area*). Areas 18 and 19 are visual association areas; lesions here cause disturbances in spatial orientation and visual word-blindness (alexia). Area 19 receives projections from all parts of the cortex and then coordinates visual with other reflexes.

Occipital lobe dysfunction is manifested in impairment in visual memory and in impaired recognition of visual patterns (*visual agnosia*).

**occipito-temporal junction** See *intention*.

**occlusal neurosis** Grinding, pounding, or setting of the teeth, when the mouth is empty; that is, entirely apart from the perfectly normal activity of mastication. *Bruxism* is an occlusal neurosis occurring during the night.

**occult** Hidden from understanding or not susceptible to logical rational verification; includes magic, foretelling, telepathy, clairvoyance. See *extrasensory perception*.

**occupational cramp** See *occupational neurosis*.

**occupational inhibition** An inhibition in the field of work or vocation of a person, evidenced in diminished pleasure in work, or in its poor execution, or in such reactive manifestations as fatigue (vertigo or vomiting), if the subject forces himself to go on working. See *occupational neurosis*.

Inhibitions reflect a limitation and restriction of ego functions, including sexual activity, eating, and work, because its energy must be concentrated on some particular challenge of the moment, such as mourning or the suppression of rage, either precautionary or resulting from an impoverishment of energy. In other cases there is a specific inhibition, a precautionary limitation of work function that serves to prevent a conflict with the superego. The strict superego has banned any advantage or success, and the subject complies with inadequate functioning in the work area. According to Freud, occupational inhibitions "subserve a desire for self-punishment" (*The Problem of Anxiety*, 1936).

**occupational neurosis** Inhibition of action(s) essential to the performance of the subject's occupation, such as writer's cramp (a painful spasm of the muscles of the fingers used in writing) or *musician's cramp* (q.v.). See *focal dystonia; occupational inhibition*.

**occupational psychiatry** Industrial psychiatry (q.v.).

**occupational therapy** Use of manual, creative, recreational, educational, prevocational, industrial, and self-help activities in order to promote growth, development, functioning, and ability to cope with and gain satisfaction from life. Purposeful activity, including interpersonal and environmental components (the "nonhuman" environment), is used to prevent and mediate dysfunction, particularly when ability to cope with tasks of daily living is compromised by biological, psychological, or sociological stress, trauma, or deficit. Emphasis is on learning through doing, directing action toward a planned end result, and minimizing undesirable or disruptive behaviors that interfere with optimal functioning.

**OCD** *Obsessive-compulsive disorder* (q.v.).

**OCD spectrum** *Obsessive-compulsive spectrum* (q.v.).

**oceanic feeling** See *omnipotence; nautomania*.

**ochlophobia** Fear of crowds.

**ocnophile** Balint's term for the person with that type of primitive two-person relationship in which the subject is clingingly dependent on the overvalued object and is unable to make any move toward independence. See *philobat*.

Balint hypothesized that the ocnophilic style reflects the person's experience during separation-individuation with a mother who rewarded closensess and reluctance to separate.

**O'Connor v. Donaldson**   See *consumerism*.

**oculocardiac reflex**   See *Aschner ocular phenomenon*.

**oculocephalic maneuvers**   *Doll's eye maneuver* (q.v.).

**oculocerebrorenal syndrome**   One of the diffuse demyelinating scleroses of genetic origin; also known as *Lowe syndrome*. Symptoms include congenital cataract, progressive mental impairment, hypotonia, hyporeflexia, proteinuria, hyperaminoaciduria, and hyperchloremic acidosis. So far, the syndrome has been reported only in males; those affected usually die during childhood.

**oculogyric spasm**   *Oculogyric crisis*; involuntary tonic contraction of the extraocular muscles characterized by fixed upward gaze (or forced conjugate movements in other directions) that lasts from several minutes to several hours. Oculogyric spasms are often a sequel of encephalitis, or they may appear as an acute dystonic side effect of medication with neuroleptics.

**oculomotor apraxia**   Impairment of planning and organization of voluntary conjugate movements of the eyes (saccadic movements). When asked to move the eyes laterally, the patient makes a lateral head turn, and the eyes then follow. Involuntary and random eye movements are usually normal.

**oculomotor nerve**   The third cranial nerve. The oculomotor nerve arises at the level of the superior colliculus and is the motor nerve to the following eye muscles: internal rectus, superior rectus, inferior rectus, inferior oblique, and levator palpebrae. Parasympathetic fibers originate in the Edinger-Westphal nucleus and proceed via the nasociliary branch of the oculomotor nerve to the ciliary ganglion, whence the short ciliary nerves pass to the sphincter muscle of the iris.

The other muscles of the eye are supplied by the trochlear and abducens nerves, which functionally are considered together with the oculomotor nerve. Symptoms of involvement of these three cranial nerves include lid droop (*ptosis*), nystagmus, double vision (*diplopia*), squint (*strabismus*), and *conjugate deviation*, in which both eyes are turned to the same side. Strabismus may be internal, in which case the visual axes cross each other, or external, in which case the visual axes diverge from each other.

Disorders of the three nerves—abducens, oculomotor, and trochlear—are considered together:

A. Ophthalmoplegias (paralyses)
   1. Oculomotor paralysis
      a. External ophthalmoplegia—divergent strabismus, diplopia, ptosis
      b. Internal ophthalmoplegia—dilated pupil, loss of light and accommodation reflexes (total ophthalmoplegia refers to a combination of external and internal ophthalmoplegia)
      c. Argyll Robertson pupil—miosis with loss of light and cilio-spinal reflexes, and preservation of accommodation reflex (pretectal lesion)
      d. Paralysis of convergence (central lesion)
   2. Trochlear paralysis (rare)—slight convergent strabismus and diplopia
   3. Abducens paralysis (most common)—convergent strabismus and diplopia
   4. Chronic progressive ophthalmoplegia (*Graefe disease*)—usually involves all three nerves
B. Myasthenic states
C. Spasmodic ocular disorders (supranuclear lesions)
   1. Conjugate deviation spasm
   2. Lateral or ventral association spasm
   3. Central nystagmus: rhythmic (vestibular origin) or undulating (cerebral or cerebellar origin)

**OD**   (Drug) overdose; less frequently, organization(al) development; right eye; each day.

**odontophobia**   Fear of teeth.

**-odynia**   Combining form meaning pain of body or mind, sorrow, from Gr. odynē.

**odynophobia**   Unwarranted or exaggerated fear of pain.

**Odysseus pact**   An attempt to provide for the future on the basis of knowing what pitfalls the past has presented. The term is used to refer to the process involved in making a living will, and in making provisions for one's commitment to a hospital should there be a recurrence of a psychotic episode similar to one from which the person has recovered.

**oedipal**   Pertaining to Oedipus or the Oedipus complex.

**oedipization**   See *Lacan, Jacques*.

**Oedipus, complete** The simultaneous presence of both a positive and a negative (or inverted) Oedipus situation; the child displays mother object love and father identification, as well as father object love and mother identification. The quantity of cathexis (or emotional charge) given to each of these four conditions is a reflection in part of the strength of innate bisexuality, and in part of experiential factors.

**Oedipus complex** In classical psychoanalytic theory, a pivotal stage in psychosexual development during which the child's love of the parent of the opposite sex and rivalry with the parent of the same sex are at their height. The Oedipus period (also oedipal period or phase) begins at about the age of 3 years during the phallic period and peaks at the age of 4 or 5. Because Freud's formulation was largely in terms of the male, the Oedipus complex was sometimes termed the mother complex (now outdated), and the corresponding stage in the female was termed the Electra complex (now rare).

In the boy, the Oedipus period ends as a result of castration anxiety, because attempts to obtain the oedipal object risk castration from the father-rival. In the girl, the Oedipus period begins because of castration anxiety; her early concern about lacking a penis gave rise to penis envy and to the belief that the mother was the castrator. The girl turns to the father as a sexual object, to be relinquished only when time convinces her that her wishes will not be fulfilled and provides the opportunity to find more suitable objects. See *castration; Electra complex; penis envy; superego*.

According to Freud, the Oedipus complex and its resolution formed the basis for all later sexual and object relationships. The Oedipus complex was viewed as central to all later psychopathology as well. Psychoanalytic theory since Freud has tended to emphasize pre-oedipal factors in both normal and abnormal personality development.

*I. The Myth of Oedipus*

Oedipus was a son of Laius, King of Thebes, and Jocasta, his wife. The King learned from an oracle that he was fated to be killed by his son. When a boy was born, the King gave him to a shepherd to leave him on Mt. Kithaeron to die. However, the compassionate shepherd gave the infant to the childless King of Corinth, Polybus. When Oedipus reached the age of puberty and an oracle told him that he would kill his father and form an incestuous union with his mother, he decided not to return to Corinth to his alleged father. In his journey he met Laius, whom he slew in a quarrel. When Oedipus arrived at Thebes, the Sphinx presented a riddle for solution. Oedipus solved the riddle and the Thebans in gratitude gave him Jocasta as wife. When finally he discovered the relationship between him and his wife he blinded himself, while Jocasta hanged herself. Oedipus wandered away, accompanied by his daughter, Antigone. Finally he was destroyed by the avenging deities, the Eumenides.

*II. Melanie Klein and Object Relations Theory*

Melanie Klein was one of the first to question the centrality of the Oedipus complex in normal development, arguing that its resolution was dependent on successful working-through of the depressive position. During development, part-object representations (the split-off good and bad self, good and bad object) give way to whole-object representations, and the pleasure principle gives way to the reality principle. Splitting is replaced by normal repression, working-through of the depressive position begins, and the capacity to mourn develops along with object permanency. The child must mourn separation from the mother in order to emerge as a freestanding person capable of genuine intimacy. This lays the foundation for the later development of libidinal object constancy and entrance into the oedipal stage. With that formulation, the depressive position—rather than the Oedipus complex—was viewed as fundamental to psychopathogenesis generally, and depression was recognized as a major feature of all forms of psychopathology.

The androcentric bias of the classical psychoanalytic formulations of the Oedipus complex has also come under attack. Even though Freud considered oedipal love to be the foundation of healthy, mature, whole-object love relationships, his theory hinged (in the case of the girl) on shame and a sense of failure and deficit—hardly a secure base from which to initiate a major developmental advance that entails a completely new view of reality and a risk of overwhelming disillusionment (Ogden, T. J. *The Primitive Edge of Experience*, 1989).

Object relations theorists have highlighted other inadequacies in classical psychoanalytic theory. According to them, Freud ignored the changes in the type of object relationships that occur as the child enters into oedipal object love. The transition is not from one object (mother) to a second object (father), but from a relationship with the pre-oedipal "holding," "environmental" mother (an internal object that is not completely separate from the self) to one with an external object who exists outside the child's omnipotence, the oedipal mother (and later the oedipal father). This is an advance in object relationships that requires a healthy weaning experience mediated by transitional objects.

The girl's entry into the Oedipus complex is mediated by a transitional relationship to the mother that introduces "otherness." The mother allows herself to be used as a conduit to a relationship with the other (the father), by continuing to be an internal, holding, soothing object even as she is being recognized more and more as an external object. The child becomes aware of her parents as people, as mother and father who have an intimate relationship with one another that does not include her. In an adequate, good enough transitional relationship, the mother allows the little girl to love the father (and, therefore, other men). If the transitional relationship is inadequate, interest in the father is stifled or prohibited, and unless the father overrides the mother's (unconscious) prohibitions the girl regards romantic or sexual feelings toward the father, and even her wishes to be like him, as forbidden and as a betrayal of the mother.

The boy's entry into the Oedipus complex is also mediated by a transitional relationship with the mother, but with a significant difference from the girl's pathway: for the boy, the pre-oedipal and oedipal love object are the same. The boy's task is not to renounce the pre-oedipal mother, but to establish a dialectical tension between pre-oedipal and oedipal love relationships with the mother.

The little boy must distance himself from the primitive, omnipotent pre-oedipal mother while he falls in love with the sexually exciting external object, the oedipal mother. At the same time, the mother is experienced as the phallic oedipal father, through the mother's unconscious identification with her own father. Successfully negotiating the narrow pathway between the three mothers and reaching the thirdness or otherness of the oedipal phase depends in part on use of the primal scene phantasy to organize sexual meaning and identity. The primal scene phantasy becomes a narrative of observing father and mother, who are now perceived as external whole objects, joined together in sexual intercourse. His being "only" an observer protects the little boy from the danger of actual incest; furthermore, reality reminds him that in fact he is his mother's son, not her husband; that mother and father are emotionally and sexually mature while he is immature; and that he is his father's son and not the father. The external object oedipal mother and father are nontraumatically discovered, and the triangulated Oedipus complex is elaborated.

It is through a relationship with the mother that the male child acquires a phallus. Out of the relationship with the mother the triangulation of the oedipal phase develops. It is from a relationship with a woman that the boy's male identification and paternal idealization originate.

*III. The Viewpoint of Kohut and Self Psychology*
Heinz Kohut theorized that the "Oedipus complex" of conflict and psychopathology arises only if the oedipal self-object needs of the child are traumatically thwarted, such as by failures in empathy of the parents. Resolution of the Oedipus complex need not be based on castration anxiety. Rather, childhood aims and ambitions are modified with appropriate mirroring, and distant, unattainable, idealized figures become less formidable as their strength is internalized with gradual de-idealization. The child needs the homogenital parent to allow development of gender-linked attributes, such as "masculine" strength and self-assertiveness and "feminine" feelings of beauty and the capacity to nurture (Kohut, H. *How Does Analysis Cure?* 1984).

**oenomania**   *Oinomania* (q.v.).

**OFC**   *Orbitofrontal cortex* (q.v.).

**OFD I syndrome**   Oral-facial-digital syndrome, characterized by frenular hypertrophy, clefts of the palate, lips, or tongue, hypoplasia of the nasal cartilages, brachydactyly, syndactyly, and, in many cases, mental retardation. OFD I is believed to be transmitted as an

X-linked dominant trait; OFD II, on the other hand, is transmitted as an autosomal recessive trait.

**off dystonia**  See *LID*.

**offender, incest**  See *pedophilia*.

**offenders, mentally disordered**  Included in this legal term are (1) persons charged with a crime but found mentally incompetent to stand trial; (2) persons acquitted of crime by reason of insanity; (3) persons found to be guilty but mentally ill (GBMI); (4) mentally disordered sex offenders; and (5) persons transferred to a mental hospital while serving a sentence for a crime of which they have been convicted. See *criminal responsibility*.

**offset**  In insurance, the phenomenon of reducing total expenditure when the granting of one benefit (e.g., psychiatric) makes a second one (e.g., general medical) unnecessary; the declining use of medical services after and, according to some, because of institution of psychiatric services.

The offset effect is most evident in people who receive brief psychotherapy at a relatively high intensity. Chronic users of psychiatric services, in contrast, are consistently higher users of medical care than other psychiatric care users.

**OGG1**  A repair enzyme that normally removes oxidative lesions within the DNA. Its chemical name is 7,8-diydro-8-oxoguanine-DNA glycolase. See *Huntington disease*.

**OGOD**  One gene, one disorder, referring to the assumption (no longer held) that complex traits consist of several subtraits, each of which is influenced by a single gene.

**OH**  Orthostatic hypotension; *postural hypotension*; low blood pressure upon standing upright, typically manifested as feelings of giddiness or syncope.

An orthostatic hypotension syndrome has been described, consisting of a combination of postural hypotension with atherosclerosis. It may cause transient ischemic attacks (see *TIA*), and it may contribute to the increasing intellectual deficits characteristic of vascular or *multi-infarct dementia* (q.v.).

When any person goes from a lying or sitting position to an upright or standing position, the autonomic nervous system compensates automatically to prevent a fall in blood pressure by an increase in heart rate and constriction of blood vessels. This normal response can be blunted in persons aroused suddenly from a deep sleep; by dehydration or venous stasis, both of which reduce the amount of blood available to the heart for pumping to the brain; by fever, which produces dilatation of blood vessels; and by various drugs, including antihypertensives, antidepressants, and some hypnotics.

**OI**  Opportunistic infection. See *AIDS*.

**oikiomania**  See *ecomania*.

**oikiophobia**  See *oikophobia*.

**oikofugic**  Pertaining to or swayed by the impulse to wander or travel.

**oikophobia**  Fear of one's house or home.

**oikotropic**  Homesick. See *nostalgia*.

**oinomania**  *Delirium tremens; dipsomania* (qq.v.); craving for alcohol.

**ojas**  Life force. See *complementary medocome*.

**old-age schizophrenia**  See *late-onset schizophrenia*.

**olfaction**  The sense of smell. There are more than 1000 olfactory genes, each encoding a unique olfactory receptor; up to 5% of the genome is taken up by odor receptors. Odorant molecules are recognized by unique *combinations* of receptors, and the combinations activate specific areas in the brain's olfactory bulb. See *rhinencephalon*.

Impairment in odor naming has been reported in patients with a first episode of a schizophrenic or schizophrenia spectrum disorder. Olfactory identification deficits are found in patients who have less frequent remission of negative and cognitive/disorganized symptoms; they are not predictive, however, of persisting positive or anxiety/depression symptoms (Good, K.P. et al. *American Journal of Psychiatry 163*: 932–933, 2006).

**olfactisms**  See *sensation, secondary*.

**olfactophilia**  Generally described as a *paraphilia* (q.v.) in which odor (especially genital, anal, or axillary) is necessary for sexual arousal and orgasm. In practice, however, the term is used in a considerably less restricted sense to indicate that the subject is more than usually responsive to or desirous of such odors as an accompaniment to sexual satisfaction, without the implication that satisfaction is impossible in their absence.

**olfactophobia**  Fear of odors.

**olfactory eroticism**  Pleasurable sensation associated wth smelling; in psychoanalysis, considered a part of anal eroticism.

**olfactory hallucination** See *haptic hallucination*.

**olfactory nerve** The first cranial nerve. Structurally, it is a fiber tract of the brain; it is a sensory nerve that transmits olfactory (smell) stimuli. Symptoms due to olfactory nerve lesions include anosmia (loss of sense of smell), hyperosmia, parosmia (perverted sense of smell), cacosmia (sensation of unpleasant odors), and olfactory hallucinations.

The *Foster Kennedy syndrome*, caused by tumors at the base of the frontal lobe, includes anosmia with atrophy of the optic and olfactory nerves, blindness, and contralateral papilledema.

**olfactory reference syndrome** A fixed and incorrect belief in a self-generated foul odor, a form of *monosymptomatic hypochondriacal psychosis* (q.v.). Some cases appear to have benefited from treatment with tricyclic or monoamine oxidase inhibitor antidepressants.

**oligergasia** Adolf Meyer's term for intellectual deficiency or mental retardation.

**olig(o)-** Combining form meaning small, pl. few, from Gr. *oligos*.

**oligodactyly** See *de Lange syndrome*.

**oligodendrocytes** See *glia*.

**oligodendroglia** See *glia*.

**oligodendroglioma** See *glioma; tumor, intracranial*.

**oligogenic** Referring to behaviors that involve a few loci acting in concert, exerting their effects on complex developmental pathways (that are likely to involve neurotransmitter systems).

**oligogenicity** The state of a phenotype in which a relatively small number of different genes work together to contribute to the particular phenotype.

**oligomers** Chains of relatively few (usually, less than 20) repeated chemical units. Spherical and annular oligomers are potentially diffusible assemblies or metastable structures observed in many amyloid-forming proteins that might be a pathway to fibril formation. These structures have been proposed to be the principal toxic entities that mediate neuronal dysfunction.

**oligophrenia, phenylpyruvic** *Følling disease.* Mental retardation secondary to an inherited biochemical defect, *phenylketonuria* (q.v.).

**oligoria** Seen in certain forms of melancholia, an abnormal indifference toward or dislike of persons or things.

**oligosthenic** Kretschmer's variety of *asthenic* type characterized by moderate strength and intermediate between the *phthinoid* and the *eusthenic*.

**olivopontocerebellar atrophy** A *multiple system atrophy* (q.v.).

**ololiuqui** A "magic" plant used in Mexico; its active ingredients are derived from lysergic acid (LSD).

**olonism** *Miryachit* (q.v.).

**-oma, -ome** Combining form meaning affected or diseased state, from Gr. -ōma.

**ombrophobia** Fear of rain(storm).

**omega melancholium** *Obs. Schuele sign;* a wrinkle (between the eyebrows) in the shape of the last letter of the Greek alphabet, the omega (ω), assumed to indicate a state of melancholy.

**omega-3 fatty acids** Long-chain essential polyunsaturated fatty acids found in various plant and marine life. The marine-based acids consist primarily of eicosapentaenoic acid (*EPA*) and docosahexaenoic acid (*DHA*). Because of dietary changes over the past 150 years, omega-3 fatty acids are being supplanted by saturated fats from domestic animals and omega-6 polyunsaturated acids by fatty acids from common vegetable oils, such as corn, safflower, and soybean. As a result, *arachidonic acid* (the common omega-6 fatty acid) has been increasing in the cell membranes of most tissues and is winning the competition for metabolizing enyzmes, and less EPA and DHA are produced. Deficiencies in these *essential fatty acids* (*EFAs*) have fueled a rise in *phospholipid spectrum disorders*, which include various neurologic and psychiatric illnesses. Positive therapeutic results with essential fatty acids, and with EPA in particular, have been reported in schizophrenia, major depression, bipolar disorder, and borderline personality disorder.

**ommatophobia** Fear of eyes or of the "evil eye."

**omnipotence** The quality of having unlimited power or influence; the infant has a feeling of omnipotence from the very beginning, even before the conception of objects develops. The outside world is perceived as part of the physical self, within itself, even though there is as yet no non-ego.

The feeling of unlimited omnipotence, the *oceanic feeling*, becomes limited as the ego and sense of reality develop: this occurs when the infant experiences tensions he cannot master.

"Something outside" becomes necessary to quiet the infant's tension and, through recognizing "something outside," the infant makes its first distinction between ego and object.

The child's earliest reaction to objects is to swallow them and thereby incorporate all pleasurable sensations and, through introjection, to make parts of the external world flow, like tributaries, into his ego. Unpleasurable sensations are perceived as being non-ego and are "spat out." Thus, through introjection, anything pleasurable becomes part of the ego, and through projection, anything unpleasant becomes non-ego. See *oral orientation.*

Efforts to reestablish the oceanic feeling of primary narcissism and also the "omnipotence of movements" are doomed to failure, however. The adult is now considered omnipotent and, by reuniting with this omnipotent force in the external world, the child tries to share this omnipotence: either he incorporates parts of this world or has the phantasy of being incorporated by it. The feeling of having been reunited with the omnipotent force is known as *secondary narcissism.* The longing for the omnipotence of primary narcissism is the narcissistic need that all people experience. "Self-esteem" is the awareness of how close one is to the original omnipotence. See *megalomania.*

The child gains self-esteem when he gains affection and loses self-esteem when he loses affection: through the promise of these and the threats of withholding or withdrawing them, the child becomes ready to obey authority and forgo other satisfactions. This is what makes children educable.

**omnipotence, magic** See *cosmic identification.*

**omnipotent infantile sadism** See *id sadism.*

**OMPFC** Orbital and medial prefrontal cortex, which includes parts of the anterior cingulate cortex. Although the two areas are generally considered separately, together they provide a link for consummatory behaviors—the orbital network regulating food intake, the medial network providing visceromotor outputs. See *orbitofrontal cortex*; *prefrontal cortex*; *ventromedial PFC.*

**onanism** Strictly speaking, sexual intercourse interrupted before ejaculation. Havelock Ellis says: "Onan's device was not auto-erotic, but an early example of withdrawal before emission, or coitus interruptus." Some writers (incorrectly) use onanism interchangeably with masturbation.

**ondansetron** A serotonin 5-HT3 antagonist; it reduces craving for alcohol in early onset alcoholics (those with onset of problem drinking before the age of 25). It is often combined with naltrexone in the treatment of alcoholism

**Ondine curse** See *apnea, central.*

**one-gene theory of psychosis** T. J. Crow (*American Journal of Psychiatry 164*, 2007) has presented arguments for a single gene underlying psychiatric disorder.

1. Both schizophrenic and affective psychoses include schizoaffective illnesses in the core phenotype, suggesting some sort of continuum that includes all such disorders.

2. Only a single gene model is consistent with the concordance data in MZ and DZ twins; polygenic models predict greater discrepancies between the two twin types than have been observed.

3. Incidences are relatively uniform across populations.

4. Structural changes in the brain in psychotic illnesses are relatively homogeneous; ventricular enlargement is a consistent correlate of psychosis.

5. Psychosis has persisted despite the fecundity disadvantage it imposes; even if two genes were relevant, it is unlikely that the balance of advantage and disadvantage associated with each would be similar, so one gene would be selected out.

Crow proposes that the phenomena of psychosis are associated with the core characteristic that defines *H. Sapiens*—the capacity for language. Directional asymmetry appears to be the critical factor, and the association between handedness and sex within families is consistent with a gene on both the X and Y chromosome. After separation of the chimpanzee from the hominid lineage, a region of homology was created, ensuring that a sequence present in all mammals on the X chromosome is present also in humans on the Y chromosome. Within this region of homology, a gene pair (protocadherin XY) coding for cell surface adhesion molecules has been identified. It has been subject to accelerated evolution (16 amino acid changes in the Y sequence, 5 in the X sequence) and is a candidate determinant of hemispheric dominance for language. In the development of that dominance, epigenetic factors are the major determinants of individual differences. See *schizophrenia, models of.*

**oneirism** Dream state while one is awake; a waking dream.

**oneir(o)** Combining form meaning dream, from Gr. *oneiros.*

**oneirodelirium** Literally, dream delirium. Some French psychiatrists apply the term to the group of psychoses characterized by delirium. Delirium tremens is the prototype of this group and is considered to be essentially a prolonged dream. Fever deliria are also part of this group, because they are so closely related to dreams. Although it is true that hallucinations can be interpreted in the same way as dreams, this does not mean that deliria, schizophrenic hallucinations, and dreams are etiologically the same, as this term would imply.

**oneirogonorrhea** Nocturnal emission of semen; wet dream.

**oneirology** The science of dreams.

**oneironosus** Abnormal dreaming.

**oneirophrenia** Meduna and McCulloch's term for a schizophreniform psychosis that, like schizophrenia, shows disturbances in associations and in affectivity but, unlike schizophrenia, shows in addition clouding of the sensorium. Onset is ususally acute, during the episode the patient is in a dreamlike condition, and prognosis is usually good.

By others, oneirophrenia is considered to be an acute form of *schizophrenia* (q.v.).

**oneiroscopy** Dream analysis, diagnosis of the mental state by a study of the person's dreams.

**oniomania** Irresistible impulse to buy, extending inordinately beyond the needs of the person; buying binge; spending spree; shopping compulsion.

**on-off phenomenon** A phenomenon described in parkinsonian patients treated with dopaminergic agents consisting of alternating akinesia ("off") and choreoathetotic dyskinesias or hyperkinesia ("on"). Lithium decreases the amount of off-activity, at least in some patients, perhaps because of a dopamine receptor-stabilizing property. See *LID; up-regulation; wearing-off effect.*

**onomatomania** A type of obsessive thinking in which certain words or sentences obtrude themselves into the patient's thoughts. A patient with obsessive-compulsive disorder was beset with anxiety, because a man's name was incessantly forcing itself upon him. It was the surname of a man with whose wife the patient had had intercourse; the anxiety was occasioned by the fear of being attacked by the husband, though the patient knew that he need have no fear of attack in the usual sense.

**onomatophobia** Fear of hearing a certain name.

**onomatopoiesis, onomatopoesis** The formation of an echoic word, i.e. in imitation of the sound associated with the thing or action. The words hiss, crash, hush, buzz, click, and chickadee closely resemble the sound.

In psychiatry the phenomenon is often observed in exaggerated form in patients with schizophrenia, who create a number of neologisms on the basis of sound association.

**onset dyskinesia** See *LID.*

**ontic dependency** The existential dependency on the "other" within one's inner family circle. Loyalty is the key linkage between generations and it involves integrity and certain things that are owed. Over time, family members balance their accounts; loyalty ties are real, but there is no objective measure of what is owed by whom, and each family member has a sense of the balance of payments.

**ontoanalysis** Existential analysis. See *existentialism.*

**ontogenesis, ontogeny** In biology, the development of the individual organism as compared with the evolutionary or *phylogenetic* development of the species. This fundamental distinction was clarified by Haeckel, when in 1867 he formulated his famous "biogenetic law" that "ontogeny recapitulates phylogeny" (*Naturliche Schopfungsgeschichte*).

**ontogeny, psychic** Development of the mind, and particularly the ways in which the organism relates its inborn needs to environmental demands. In psychoanalysis, psychic ontogeny includes (1) development of object relationships; (2) the vicissitudes of the drives in relation to reality; and (3) the development of mechanisms to achieve the foregoing.

Various schemata have been used to describe different levels, phases, positions, or stages of development. They are not easily compared because they do not follow a strict chronology, and some theorists have avoided that difficulty by emphasizing the continuing interaction between the processes that determine development, rather than stressing the replacement of one process by another. See *dialectic; object relations theory.*

The classical psychoanalytic description of the development of object relationships is in terms of five stages:

1. Autoerotic (or somatogenic) stage, from birth until about 3 years of age; see *autoeroticism*.

2. Narcissistic stage, from 3 to 6 years of age; see *narcissism*.

3. Homoerotic (or suigenderistic) stage, from 6 years until puberty; see *homoeroticism*.

4. Heteroerotic (or altrigenderistic) stage, during adolescence; see *heteroeroticism*.

5. Alloerotic stage, the stage of maturity; see *alloeroticism*.

The vicissitudes of the drives are typically described in terms of libidinal phases, as follows:

1. Pre-superego sexuality, from birth until about 6 years of age, including:
   a. Oral phase, from birth until 2 years; see *oral incorporative phase; orality; preambivalent phase.*
   b. *Anal phase* (q.v.), from 2 until about 4 years.
   c. *Phallic phase* (q.v.), from 2 until about 6 years.
2. *Latency* (q.v.), from 6 years to puberty.
3. *Genitality* (q.v.).

The mechanisms developed to achieve the foregoing are those involved in the development of the ego and superego and of the ego defenses. See *defense; ego; superego.*

Some critics believe that classical psychoanalytic psychology overemphasizes childhood as the beginning and end of personality development and have described psychic ontogeny in different terms. Erikson, for example, maintained that side by side with the psychosexual stages described by Freud were psychosocial stages of ego development, that personality continued to develop throughout the whole life cycle, and that each stage has a positive as well as a negative component. (See *developmental levels.*) Erikson's *eight stages of man* were as follows:

1. *Trust vs. Mistrust* extends through the first year of life (and thus corresponds roughly to Freud's oral stage). During this stage, the degree to which the child learns to trust the world, other people, and himself depends upon the quality of care he receives; if that care is inadequate or inconsistent, basic mistrust develops, an attitude of fear and suspicion of the world.

2. *Autonomy vs. Doubt* extends through second and third years (Freud's anal stage). Adequate care in this stage consists of allowing the child to do what he is capable of, at his own pace, so that he can develop autonomy, i.e., ability to control his muscles, his impulses, himself, and ultimately his environment. Inconsistent, overcritical, or overprotective care, on the other hand, fills the child with doubt about his own abilities to control his world and himself.

3. *Initiative vs. Guilt* extends through fourth and fifth years (Freud's genital stage). Adequate care provides freedom and opportunity for the child to initiate motor play, phantasies, and intellectual questioning of those around him so that he is no longer only an imitator of others. But if the child is inhibited or derided for his play activity or his inquisitiveness, he will develop guilt about self-initiated activities.

4. *Industry vs. Inferiority* extends from 6 to 11 years (Freud's latency period). During this period, the child learns to reason deductively, and to obey the "rules of the game." This is a *Robinson Crusoe age*, in that the child is concerned with the details of how things are made, how they work, and what they do. Adequate care involves encouraging the child in his effort to make and do practical things, rewarding him for results, and thus enhancing his sense of industry. Because the child's world at this stage includes more than his parents, adults outside the immediate family also play an important part in enhancing industry, or on the negative side, instilling in the child a sense of inferiority.

5. *Identity vs. Role Confusion*—adolescence extending roughly from age 12 to 18. During this period, the person can wonder about what other people think of him, he can compare his own family and society with what he conceptualizes as an ideal family or society, and he develops a sense of who he is, where he has been, and where he is going. But both the family milieu and the social milieu may interfere with the development of a sense of ego identity; when rapid social and technological change breaks down traditional values, the adolescent may develop a sense of role confusion in that he finds no continuity between what he learned as a child and what he is experiencing as an adolescent. For such a person, an identity as a delinquent, to cite

but one example, may be preferable to having no identity at all.

6. *Intimacy vs. Isolation* extends from adolescence to early middle age; roughly, the period of courtship and early family life. During this phase, the person must learn to share with and care about another, without the fear of losing himself in the process; if he does not, he develops a sense of isolation, a feeling of being alone without anyone to share with or care for.

7. *Generativity vs. Self-Absorption*—middle age. In this stage, the person becomes concerned with others beyond his immediate family, and with the nature of society and the world in which future generations will live. On the negative side, the person without a sense of generativity becomes self-absorbed with his personal needs and comforts.

8. *Integrity vs. Despair*—old age. The person at this stage who can look back on his life with satisfaction, who can pause to reflect on the past and take time to enjoy his grandchildren, manifests a sense of integrity. At the other end of the scale is the person whose past life is a series of missed opportunities and mistakes that cannot be undone; he is filled with despair at the thought of what might have been.

**ontological insecurity**   Lack of the sense of continuity or stability of the self over time, a characteristic of schizoid (narcissistic) personality disorder according to Laing. Manifestations include fears of engulfment and losing the self in a merger with the other, of implosion and obliteration by reality, and of petrification, such as being turned into a depersonalized robot. To defend against ontological insecurity, the self is split into a secret true self and a *false self* (q.v.).

Using the term *existential anguish*, Winnicott described patients with a defective sense of being, preoccupation with the meaning of life, a feeling of having no place in the world, and identity confusion. He ascribed the condition to a disturbance of holding and handling in the early stages of infancy.

**ontology**   Study of the nature, essential properties, and relations of being; *existentialism* (q.v.).

**onychophagia, onychophagy**   Nail biting, cited by Kanner as one of the habitual manipulations of the body encountered in neurotic children

and considered by him as one of the several forms of motor discharges of inner tension.

**oo-**   Combining form meaning eggs, from Gr. ōon.

**oophorectomy**   See *ovariotomy*.

**open**   In questioning or interviewing, an open question is one that allows the person questioned maximal freedom in choosing the manner or content of his or her response.

**open group**   A therapy group to which new patients are added at any time during the course of treatment. Sometimes this is referred to as a *continuous group*.

**open-door policy**   Approximately equivalent to *therapeutic community* (q.v.). The term open-door emphasizes the growing trend in psychiatric hospitals to minimize or even eliminate completely any form of restraint or enforced confinement ("locked doors").

**operandum**   See *Skinner box*.

**operant behaviorism**   See *behaviorism*.

**operant conditioning**   Consequence-governed behavior; B. F. Skinner's term for the process of reinforcing a subject's spontaneous activities or behaviors that occur with no recognizable eliciting stimuli (the behaviors are termed *operants*).

The behaviorist waits for the subject to perform an action, and once the deed is done the subject is rewarded or some noxious stimulus is removed. When the behaviors produce such favorable changes in the environnment, the subject tends to repeat them. In classical conditioning, the subject learns that a certain stimulus predicts a subsequent event; in operant conditioning, the subject learns to predict the consequences of his own behavior.

As Lashley had done in enunciating his theory of *equipotentiality* (q.v.), and as Freud had done in substituting a purely mentalistic model based on verbal reports of subjective experiences for a biological model, Skinner rejected neurologic theories in favor of objective descriptions of observable acts.

It has been suggested that many forms of psychotherapy are applications of operant conditioning, in that the patient's speech is rewarded by (reinforced by) remarks or other behavior on the part of the therapist. The patient learns what the therapist expects or wants to hear, and he modifies his own speech and behavior accordingly. See *behaviorism; biofeedback; behavior therapy*.

**operational planning** See *strategic planning*.

**operational thinking** See *concrete operational stage*.

**operations** See *scheme*.

**operations, concrete** See *adolescence*.

**operations research (OR)** A group of techniques that developed pragmatically in an attempt to apply scientific methods and tools to solve the problems of decision making in complex organizations and systems, where any one decision typically proves advantageous for some parts of the system but disadvantageous for others. Operations research searches for optimal solutions in situations of conflicting goals and relies heavily on mathematic models from which solutions for the actual problem may be derived.

**ophidiophilia** Abnormal fascination with snakes.

**ophidiophobia** Fear of snakes.

**ophthalmoplegia** See *oculomotor nerve*.

**ophthalmoplegia externa** See *Ballet sign*.

**ophthalmoplegia syndrome** See *internuclear ophthalmoplegia syndrome*.

**-opia, -opy, -opsia** Combining form meaning defect of sight, from Gr. ōps, ōpos, eye.

**opiate, opioid** A drug containing *opium* (q.v.) or one or more of its alkaloid derivatives (including synthetic opiumlike substances); often referred to as *narcotic-analgesic*.

The opioids are associated with patterns of abuse and dependence. Opioid intoxication is suggested by the following symptoms: constricted pupils ("pinning"), drowsiness, slurred speech, impaired attention or memory, euphoria or dysphoria, apathy and psychomotor retardation, impaired judgment, and failure to meet social, occupational, or academic responsibilities.

The characteristic withdrawal syndrome includes lacrimation, rhinorrhea, dilated pupils, gooseflesh, sweating, diarrhea, yawning, tachycardia, elevated blood pressure, insomnia, and fever. See *addiction; dependence, drug*.

Opioids such as morphine and heroin are not only powerful analgesics; they also produce profound appetitive motivational actions. Activation of the μ-opioid receptor (MOR/PORM) is necessary for the action of the most potent analgesics.

**opiate antagonist** See *narcotic antagonist; narcotic blockade*.

**opioid, endogenous** See *opioid peptides*.

**opioid deficiency hypothesis** The hypothesis that subjects at high risk for alcoholism—with a family history of alcoholism—have a deficiency in basal activity of the endogenous opioid system. It has also been suggested that the pituitary β-endorphin system of high-risk subjects is more sensitive to ethanol than that of low-risk (with low familial risk) subjects. Opioid dysregulation may be associated with greater risk of relapse. Response to opioid antagonist therapies, such as naltrexone, appears to be more effective in alcoholics with a positive family history.

**opioid intoxication** The syndrome includes maladaptive behavioral changes such as initial euphoria followed by apathy, dysphoria, psychomotor agitation or retardation, and impaired judgment; and pupillary constriction (or pupillary dilation secondary to anoxia in cases of severe overdose) and various other signs, that may include drowsiness, slurred speech, and impairment in attention or memory. See *opioid*.

**opioid peptides** *Endogenous opioids*; neuropeptides that can produce analgesia, so-called because their action resembles that of morphine and other opium derivatives. They regulate nociceptive transmission, in part by inhibiting release of glutamate, substance P, and other transmitters that would otherwise sensitize sensory neurons. They also disinhibit (activate) descending projection neurons that control nociceptive inputs: they suppress neurons that release GABA, which normally inhibits the descending pathways.

Like the opiates, the opioid peptides are addicting. There are three subgroups, each derived from a different precursor (prohormone). Proenkephalin is the precursor for metenkephalin and leuenkephalin; pro-opiomelanocortin is the precursor for endorphins, ACTH, and several melanocyte-stimulating hormones; prodynorphin is the precursor for dynorphins and neoendorphins. See *dynorphin; endorphins; enkephalins; peptide, brain*.

**opioid use disorders** These are classified within the substance-related disorders and include opioid dependence, opioid abuse, opioid intoxication, opioid withdrawal, opioid delirium, opioid mood disorder, opioid sleep disorder, and opioid sexual dysfunction.

**opioid withdrawal** Symptoms appear following cessation of or significant reduction in use and can also be provoked by administration of an opioid antagonist: dysphoria, nausea, vomiting, muscle aches, lacrimation, rhinorrhea, sweating, diarrhea, yawning, fever, insomnia, pupillary dilation, and piloerection.

**opiomania** Addiction to the use of opium or any of its derivatives.

**opisthotonos** See *arc de cercle*.

**opium** The resinous exudate of the capsule of the white poppy, *Papavar somniferum*. Its major active ingredient is morphine, but it also contains other psychoactive substances, including codeine. Morphine can easily be converted into heroin (diacetylmorphine or diamorphine). Among the synthetic opiates are methadone, pethidine (meperidine), dipipanone, pentazocine, propoxyphene, and fentanyl.

All the opiates are potentially addicting drugs, as are the synthetic analgesics; morphine possesses perhaps the greatest potentiality in this direction, followed by heroin, Dilaudid, metopon, Demerol, methadone, and codeine, in that order. Because it is easier to traffic in illegally, heroin is the most commonly used of the group by opiate addicts, at least in the United States. All the opiates are characterized by the development of a high degree of tolerance in their users, and severe deprivation or abstinence syndromes are therefore the rule. Except in elderly or physically ill subjects, the narcotic withdrawal syndrome is not life-threatening. See *addiction; dependence, drug*.

**opotherapy** *Organotherapy* (q.v.).

**Oppenheim reflex** (H. Oppenheim, German neurologist, 1858–1919) Dorsal extension of the great toe, induced by stroking distally along the median side of the tibia. This is one of several pathological reflexes that may be seen when the lower motor neuron is released from the normal suppressor effect of higher centers, as in pyramidal tract lesions.

**Oppenheimer treatment** (Issac Oppenheimer, New York physician, 1871–1943) A secret method of treatment of alcoholism and drug addiction.

**oppositional disorder** Also *oppositional-defiant disorder*, classified within the *disruptive behavior disorders* (q.v.); a childhood disorder consisting of pervasive disobedience, negativism, and provocative opposition to authority figures (e.g., repetitive infractions of minor rules, temper tantrums, argumentativeness, stubbornness). Unlike *conduct disorders* (q.v.), behavior is not primarily an invasion of the rights of others.

**oppositional thinking** *Janusian thinking* (q.v.).

**opsin** The protein portion of the rhodopsin molecule in the rod cells of the retina. See *photoreceptor*. Two of these light-sensitive proteins, *ChR2* and *NpHR*, have been used to target specific neuronal subtypes in vivo in studies of brain function. Existing electrode-based methods such as DBS indiscriminately stimulate all neurons within a local area, including opposing and inhibitory cell types. (See *deep brain stimulation*.) It has recently become possible, however, to restrict such stimulation to genetically specified neuronal subtypes through the use of these two microbial opsins. Combining DBS with noninvasive neuroimaging methods such as *magnetoencephalography* (q.v.) offers the possibility of defining, with unprecedented precision, the cell types and neuron pathways involved and the timing of their reactions to stimulation of regions of interest in the brain. It might also hold the key to identification of the neural circuits and cell types affected in neurologic and psychiatric disorders.

ChR2 (*Chlamydomonas reinhardtii* channelrhodopsin-2) is a cation channel that allows $Na^+$ ions to enter the cell following exposure to ~470 nm blue light. NpHR (*Natronemonas pharaonis* halorhodopsin) is a chloride pump that activates upon illumination with ~580 nm yellow light. When introduced into neurons, both cells act swiftly (on the scale of milliseconds), ChR2 to activate trains of high-frequency action potentials, and NpHR to suppress single action potentials within high frequency spike trains.

Before optical neuromodulation or *optogenetics* can be used in humans, it will be necessary to ensure that the genes encoding ChR2 and NpHR can be safely and stably transferred into the human subject's neuron.

**opsomania** *Obs.* Pathological craving for sweets, such as may occur in binge eating. See *night-eating syndrome*.

**optic agnosia** Word blindness. See *optic nerve*.

**optic atrophy** Degeneration of the optic nerve fibers. The condition is primary or secondary. Primary optic atrophy may occur in tabes, multiple sclerosis, or may be due to poisons, such as methyl alcohol, tryparsamide, lead, atoxyl, quinine, carbon bisulfide, and nitrobenzol. Occasionally the condition may occur following severe hemorrhage and in malaria. Ophthalmoscopically, the disk is grayish white in color, with some "cupping," the margins being sharply outlined. See *Leber disease*.

Secondary optic atrophy may occur as a result of optic neuritis and choked disk. Here the fundus, disk, and vessels usually manifest residual signs of the previous condition. Tumors of the pituitary gland, of the optic chiasm, and in some cases of the frontal lobe frequently give rise to optic atrophy—usually unilateral for a time.

**optic nerve** The second cranial nerve. The optic nerve is structurally a fiber tract of the brain; it is a sensory nerve that transmits visual stimuli. The rods and cones of the retina of the eye are the first-order neurons; they connect with the bipolar cells of the retina, which in turn connect with the ganglion cells. These form the optic nerve fibers, which proceed to the optic chiasma, form the optic tracts, and then pass to the lateral geniculate bodies, the superior colliculi, and the pretectal region. From the geniculate bodies, fibers pass (as the geniculocalcarine tract) to the occipital cortex. Fibers from the superior colliculi pass to various cranial and spinal nuclei (for involuntary oculoskeletal reflexes); fibers from the pretectal region pass to the Edinger-Westphal nuclei (for the simple and consensual light reflexes).

*Visual defects* include *scotomata* (abnormal blind spots in the visual fields), *amblyopia* (reduction of visual acuity), *amaurosis* (complete blindness), *field defect* (q.v.), *hemeralopia* (day blindness), *nyctalopia* (night blindness), color blindness, and *optic agnosia* or word blindness.

**optic neuritis** An inflammatory process affecting the head of the optic nerve, or that part within the bulb of the eye. The condition is usually bilateral, and early loss of vision is characteristic. Ophthalmoscopically, there is blurring of the margins of the disk with congestion, dilatation of the veins, and narrowing of the arteries. The retina may show hemorrhages, pigment deposits, exudates, connective tissue changes, and atrophic spots.

Optic neuritis may occur in severe renal disease, syphilis, leukemia, carbon monoxide poisoning, diabetes, anemia, and other constitutional diseases.

**optimal disillusionment** See *idealization*.

**optimal experiences** *Flow states;* see *positive dissociative experiences*.

**optimism, oral** Optimism appearing as an oral character trait. Positive or negative attitudes to taking and receiving have an oral origin. In particular, whenever there is unusually pronounced oral satisfaction in infancy, the results are a self-assurance and optimism which may persist throughout life. If frustration has followed this satisfaction, however, there may result a state of "vengefulness coupled with continuous demanding" (Fenichel, O. *The Psychoanalytic Theory of Neurosis*, 1945).

**optimism, technologic(al)** The disposition to employ technologies in the belief that the benefits deriving therefrom will outweigh any undesirable effects, and that the latter can themselves be controlled or eliminated through technologic developments.

**optimization** A strategy of pharmacotherapy: the current drug regimen is changed in order to maximize its efficacy.

**optogenetics** See *opsin*.

**OR** *Operations research*; *orienting response* (qq.v.); operating room.

**oral aggressive character** A type of *character* (q.v.) that is considered to be a sublimation of the oral biting stage. Aggressiveness, envy, ambition, and a tendency to exploit others are typical features. Fromm called this the *exploitative character* (q.v.). See *character defense*.

**oral anxiety** Anxiety occurring at the primary or oral stage of libidinal (personality) development (see *libido displaceability; oral incorporative phase*). It is assumed that such massive expressions of infantile rage and fear are associated with or stem from phantasy images within the infant, of an immense internal object in countless small pieces. This image, theoretically an analytic reconstruction, has its origin in the ideas of swallowing, incorporating, and chewing up a dangerous or loved object, i.e., the parent, a body organ, or part thereof.

E. F. Sharpe states: "There must be some correlation between the excessive anxiety in oral stages, which is associated with the phantasy of a huge image of pieces inside; and the fact that at this time there is as little coordination of the bodily as of the psychical ego" (*Collected Papers on Psycho-analysis*, 1950).

**oral character**  The personality traits based on the two stages of oral erotism. According to Abraham there are two principal ways of expressing oral activity: (1) sucking, in the first stage, and (2) biting, in the second, and from each of these arise definite types of personality.

If the infant suffered no difficulties or privations during the sucking period, if the sucking phase was largely pleasurable, the pleasure is carried over as a character trait, leading to the optimistic type of person who believes that he will succeed in any undertaking. Such people may exhibit carefree indifference and perhaps inactivity. The mother's breast will "flow for them eternally." Because the infant was treated so generously, identification with the mother gives rise to generosity as an important trait in the child.

If, on the other hand, the infant failed to achieve gratification during the sucking period, it develops a pessimistic attitude. In later life the child is apprehensive and demanding; he is never satisfied and comes to believe he never will be. The second or biting stage is said also to lead to development of character traits: to a tendency to hate and to destroy. "This fundamental difference extends to the smallest details of a person's behavior" (Abraham, K. *Selected Papers*, 1927).

**oral erotism**  The pleasure and gratification derived from using the mouth for other than the utility value of taking in food and drink. In the child it means the pleasure experienced when close to the mother's warm body, when sucking her breast or the nipple of the bottle and thus feeling secure and protected. See *orality*.

**oral incorporative phase**  The period (in early infantile development) marked by the appearance of possessiveness and its derivatives: voracity, greed, and envy, in association with "cannibalistic" urges toward incorporation of bodily parts, such as mother's nipple, breast, finger. Incorporating the object obviates the danger of loss of or separation from the loved object. Oral incorporation thus represents the ultimate of closeness. When thwarted, the urge to possess becomes the drive for aggression, i.e., taking by force that which has been withheld. Later, these possessive, aggressive drives become the source of primary guilt feelings, or early conscience.

**oral orientation**  A method of approaching, evaluating, and relating oneself to the environment on the basis of the hunger drive, oral needs, etc. The infant, for example, is primarily orally oriented; the mouth is his most differentiated organ and he uses it as his chief perceptive apparatus. The primitive ego is an oral ego, for the infant first becomes aware of objects, identifies them, and recognizes the outside world by putting objects in his mouth. The first recognition of reality on the part of the infant is in deciding whether he should swallow an object or spit it out. See *oral character; orality.*

**oral primacy**  The infant's contacting and first comprehending the world primarily in terms of the mouth. Oral primacy is a generally recognized organic fact, but to many psychoanalysts the important aspect of the oral phase is not so much the biological background as the differences in experience that occur during this biologically determined period. "Moreover, the kind of world contacted through the mouth is not universally the same, and the differences in experience make a more significant impression on personality development than does the organic fact of a period of oral primacy" (Thompson, C. *Psychoanalysis, Evolution and Development*, 1950).

**oral receptive character**  A type of *character* (q.v.) that is considered to be a sublimation of the earliest sucking stage of life. Such people are characterized by friendliness, optimism, and generosity and expect the whole world to mother them. When frustrated they become pessimistic and act as if the bottom had fallen out of the world. See *character defense*.

**oral sadism**  The expression of infantile, primordial, aggressive, instinctive urges toward omnipotent mastery, through phantasy functions of the mouth, lips, and teeth. (Phantasy functions are distortions of the reality functions of the mouth, lips, teeth, tongue, cheeks, and pharynx). Oral sadistic wishes, strivings, and phantasies appear normally in the earliest stages of development, but they undergo various modifications during development. They may persist or reappear in adult life as components of neurotic symptoms; as paraphilias and foreplay desires and gratifications; as character traits; and as socially acceptable sublimations. See *orality; oral incorporative phase; sadism.*

According to Melanie Klein, oral sadism is the first manifestation of the death instinct; for self-preservation, it is projected into the object (e.g., mother), part object (e.g., breast), or their representations. There are two major consequences of such projection: (1) the infant experiences persecutory fears and fear of annihilation by the destructive, devouring, and hating breast, and (2) at the same time the infant experiences envy, a wish to possess the withholding breast. From that envy, *greed* and *jealousy* later develop.

**oral triad** Lewin's term for the desires of the infant in the early oral phase—the wish to devour, the wish to be devoured, and the wish to go to sleep.

**orality** A psychoanalytic term referring to the oral components of sexuality, to manifestations of instinctual conflict centering about the oral stage of sexual development, to manifestations that indicate fixation at the oral stage of development, and to manifestations of oral erogeneity. Orality is prominent in manic-depressive psychosis and addictions. A driving ambition in the field of oratory or speech making is often based on oral conflicts. Excessive generosity in a person often has the following significance: "As I shower you with love, in the same way do I want to be showered with love"; this mechanism is typical of the oral-receptive person. The oral-sadistic person often shows extreme niggardliness: "You must make up for the love denied me." Volubility, restlessness, haste, and a tendency to obstinate silence are also indicative of extreme orality. E. Bergler (*Psychiatric Quarterly 19*, 1945) believed that the mechanism of orality is as follows: (1) through his behavior the person provokes disappointment, thus identifying the outer world with the refusing, pre-oedipal mother; (2) he becomes aggressive, seemingly in self-defense; (3) he indulges in self-pity, a manifestation of his psychic masochism. See *oral character*.

Orality is, in essence, one of the steps in learning, and at this stage in ontogenetic development stress and distress stem primarily from the complex physiological processes that produce hunger. Gratification follows stimulation of the mouth area, and oral stimulation is what the infant seeks because of the pleasure it provides.

**orbitofrontal circuit** See *frontal-striatal system*.

**orbitofrontal cortex** The anterior portion of the *prefrontal cortex* (q.v.), including the anterior pole, the lateral orbital cortex, and the medial orbital surface. Through its connections to many networks in the brain, including medial prefrontal and anterior cingulate cortex, hypothalamus, amygdala, insula/operculum, dopaminergic midbrain, and the ventral and dorsal striatum in the basal ganglia, it provides sensory integration, modulation of autonomic reactions, and participation in learning, prediction, and decision making for emotional and reward-related behaviors. Through its connections with DLPFC, it is active in reasoning and planning; it integrates the cognitive and emotional components of decision making. It is linked to the regulation of interpersonal relationships, social cooperativity, moral behavior, social aggression, and social reasoning. See *choice*; *frontal-striatal system*; *frontal-subcortical circuits*; *reward*; *ventromedial PFC*.

Patients with lesions in this region show poor social and individual decision-making skills as well as disinhibition, impulsiveness, tactlessness, irritability, and lability. Damage to this region impairs reasoning about social exchange, such as the ability to figure out that other people are being deceptive.

**orbitomedial syndrome** A frontal lobe syndrome whose manifestations may include (1) asthenia, fatiguability, blandness, akinesia, aphonia, withdrawal, and fearfulness; (2) diminished wakefulness, or an oneiroid or stuporous state; or (3) a pseudopsychopathic or maniclike type with intense, labile affect, rapid mood shifts, and mixed and cycling mood states; facetiousness, impulsiveness, loss of inhibitions (witzelsucht); overreactivity to stimuli with a frenetic appearance, as the subject dashes from one activity to another without completing any task; inability to persevere or make decisions; the patient is strongly stimulus bound, importunate, intrusive, and interrupts others (the patient may repeatedly change the channel on the television set only because he sees the dial, not because he is searching for a special program); often grossly incredible confabulations; rage outbursts when prevented from doing as he wants. See *frontal lobe dysfunction*.

**orchestromania** Chorea; St. Vitus dance.

**orderliness, organic**  A characteristic symptom of patients with organic brain disease, consisting of a stereotyped, meticulous, compulsive approach to the environment; the patient's possessions must always be arranged in the same order, any action must always be performed in the same sequence or in the same way, etc. See *organic syndrome.*

**Orestes complex**  (Orestes, the son of the Mycenaean King Agamemnon, who killed his own mother, Clytemnestra, and her paramour, Aegisthus, for murdering her husband, Agamemnon) The psychiatric term proposed for a son's killing, or desire to kill, his own mother. F. Wertham believed this to be a universal complex, like the Oedipus complex. The majority of psychoanalysts disagree with this view and feel, instead, that when it occurs the Orestes complex is an outgrowth of the Oedipus complex and is a reaction by the male child to rejection or frustration by the oedipal love object, the mother.

**-orexia**  Combining form meaning appetite, desire, longing, from Gr. *orexis.*

**orexigenic**  Appetite-stimulating. See *hypothalamus.*

**orexins**  *Hypocretins*; neuropeptides initially recognized as regulators of feeding behavior. The finding that an orexin deficiency causes *narcolepsy* (q.v.) indicated that they also play a crucial role in regulating sleep and wakefulness. Recent studies have suggested further roles for orexin in the coordination of emotion, energy homeostasis, reward, arousal, and stress.

Orexin A and B are also known as hypocretin 1 and 2, respectively. They are produced in hypothalamic neurons from a common precursor peptide, prepro-orexin. Orexin neurons project widely to the entire neuroaxis, excluding the cerebellum. They must be activated during awake periods, but must be switched off to maintain consolidated NREM sleep. Orexin-mediated arousal results from activation of wake-active neurons—dopaminergic cells of the ventral tegmental area, serotonergic cells of the dorsal raphe, and histaminergic cells of the tuberomammillary nucleus. There is a direct excitatory effect of orexins on cholinergic neurons in the basal forebrain, which are important for maintaining arousal.

Orexin neurons are regulated by peripheral metabolic cues, including ghrelin, leptin, and glucose, thereby providing a link between energy homeostasis and vigilance states. Orexin neurons are sensors of the nutritional status of the body and reinforce food-seeking and feeding pathways. Orexins increase both food intake and metabolic rate. Orexin neurons project to reward-associated brain regions, where activation is strongly linked to preference for cues associated with drug and food rewards. Through their influence on neuroendocrine function, orexins affect arousal and the stress response.

**orexis**  The part of an act or response other than the cognitive aspect; specifically, affect and conation are the orectic aspects of an action.

**organ choice**  See *compliance, somatic; individual-response specificity.*

**organ inferiority**  Adler maintained that "inherited inferiorities" of glands or organs, if they made themselves felt psychically, were conducive to a neurotic disposition, i.e., they caused a child with some "inherited stigma" to feel a sense of inferiority in relation to his environment. This feeling of humiliation and inferiority induced by some constitutional or organ defect produces psychic compensatory and hypercompensatory strivings.

**organ jargon**  Adler applies this term to the "somatic language" (symptoms) that the neurotic uses to express a masculine protest. According to Adler, the child's ego-consciousness is in conflict with the facts of his environment. Thus, the child wishes to be big and powerful but actually is small and weak. The child therefore constructs all its aggressive attitudes into one of masculine protest against all symptoms of weakness, (femininity) such as tenderness, subordinacy, and, most important, manifestations of organ inferiority. The neurotically predisposed child, however, endeavors further to gain an effective weapon by associating with its organ inferiority such character traits as originate in the ego-consciousness—i.e., obstinacy, need of affection, exaggerated cleanliness, pedantry, covetousness, ambition, etc. Thus, in order to gain attention and affection a psychogenic epileptic managed so that most of his "attacks" were preceded by obstipation, thereby worrying his family—all this to offset his degradation. In this way the masculine protest makes use of a somatic language or organ-jargon to gain expression (Adler, A. *The Neurotic Constitution,* 1917).

**organ neurosis**   See *psychosomatic*.

**organ placement**   See *asymmetry*.

**organ pleasure**   The excitement and satisfaction attained in the extragenital erogenous zones; used particularly to refer to the partial instincts in the pregenital period. Characteristic of infantile sexuality is the fact that the genitals themselves are but one of many erogenous zones, and that sexuality is undifferentiated and contains all the later part-instincts, which are not as yet subordinate to genital satisfaction.

**organ speech**   *Hypochondriac language*; any physical symptoms that represent conscious or unconscious mental impulses; used particularly to refer to those schizophrenics who concentrate almost all their energy on complaints about a particular organ or body part (such as the nose). See *dysmorphophobia*.

**organ-erotic**   Relating to or characterized by the attachment of libido to an organ of the body.

**organic**   Neuropathology in the 19th century classified psychiatric and behavioral disorders on the basis of anatomical evidence of brain lesions. Those who gave evidence of such lesions were labeled "organic" disorders, and those who did not were labeled *functional*. The distinction is no longer tenable.

**organic anxiety**   The anxiety associated with organic pain that can be markedly attenuated in the dream state by the process of denial, transformation, and displacement; these mechanisms represent attempts at cure through wish-fulfillment.

In DSM-III-R, the predominant disturbance in *organic anxiety syndrome* is recurrent panic episodes or generalized anxiety.

**organic brain syndrome**   See *organic syndrome*.

**organic drivenness**   See *drivenness, organic*.

**organic delusional syndrome**   One of the forms of *organic mental disorders* (q.v.), consisting of the appearance of delusions in a state of full wakefulness and alertness. The delusions may be simply formed and poorly sustained, or they may be highly organized and systematized and indistinguishable from schizophrenic or schizophreniform disorders. Persecutory delusions are the most common type. There have been some reports of brief recurrences of the delusional syndromes even though the toxic agent originally responsible has not been used again—analogous to "flashback" hallucinosis of LSD intoxication. The organic delusional syndrome is seen most often as a form of drug intoxication (amphetamines, cannabis, hallucinogens); it can be seen as an interictal syndrome in temporal lobe epilepsy, and sometimes in Huntington chorea. See *flashback; paraphrenia*.

**organic mental disorders**   Mental disturbances resulting from transient or permanent dysfunction of brain tissue that is attributable to specific organic factors, such as aging (senile and presenile dementias), drugs and toxins, infection, cardiovascular disease, trauma, neoplasm, or metabolic disorders. These disorders manifest themselves as one or more organic brain syndromes that reflect the localization, progression, and duration of the underlying pathology, and with associated or secondary features that reflect emotional, motivational, and behavioral reactions to recognition of the primary deficits and the anticipation of their consequences. See *organic syndrome*.

The organic/functional dichotomy is increasingly difficult to maintain in view of the many biological and physiological factors that are known to contribute to what have classically been considered nonorganic disorders. In recognition of this, DSM-IV classifies psychiatric disorders as primary, or due to a general medical disorder, or substance-induced; delirium, dementia, and amnestic disorders are grouped in a section labeled cognitive impairment disorders. The other disorders previously labeled organic (e.g., mood, anxiety, personality, and delusional disorders, and hallucinosis) are now placed within the diagnostic categories with which they share phenomenology. Thus, an "organic" depression secondary to a brain tumor is classified within the mood disorders as "mood disorder due to a general medical condition, with depressive features," and the brain tumor is coded on Axis III.

**organic syndrome**   The group of symptoms characteristic of the *organic mental disorders* (q.v.). In any specific case, one or more of the characteristic symptoms may predominate. The signs of organicity include (1) disturbances in orientation; (2) impairment of memory; (3) impairment in the maintenance of the level of consciousness and attention; (4) impairment of all intellectual functions (comprehension, calculation, knowledge, learning, etc.); (5) defective judgment; (6) lability, shallowness, and similar instabilities of the affect; and

(7) overall changes in the personality, with the appearance of conduct foreign to the patient's natural or usual behavior.

In the *acute brain disorders*, alteration in consciousness (with preoccupation, stupor, or coma) and defects in orientation and memory tend to predominate; the acute organic syndrome is sometimes called the *delirious reaction*. In the *chronic brain disorders* (e.g., the Korsakoff psychosis), intellectual defects are prominent (loss of general efficiency, inability to plan, judgment defects, disturbances in orientation and memory, confabulation), and disturbed affect and personality changes are also frequent. The term *dementia* is often used to refer to the irreversible intellectual defects of the patient with chronic brain disorder. See *abstract attitude; catastrophic behavior; drivenness, organic.*

**organicism**    1. The theory that refers all disease to material lesions of organs. Disordered physiology may give rise to symptoms, yet there may be no demonstrable lesions.

2. The theory that all symptoms are organically determined.

3. In constitutional medicine, "the theory that the various organs of the body have each their own special constitution" (Pende, N. *Constitutional Inadequacies*, 1928).

**organicist**    As currently used in psychiatry, a pejorative designation for the psychiatrist who can admit of only material lesions in organs as etiologic agents in psychiatric disorders. The organicist is typically contrasted to the psychodynamist or psychogeneticist, but all three terms represent an unwelcome regression to the days of the nature-nurture conflict. They focus upon a dualism that exists only on a conceptual heuristic level, and ignore the reality of the functioning whole person whose mental and emotional processes are interwoven with and interdependent upon neurophysiologic substrata and sociocultural factors. See *ecology; psychosomatic.*

**organizational approach**    An *executive function* (q.v.) consisting of the strategy of breaking the complex into simpler components, which are then recombined into other constructions and approaches.

**organogenesis**    *Somatogenesis* (q.v.).

**organophosphates**    They act as anticholinesterases and parasympathomimetic drugs. See *cholinergic.*

**organotherapy**    *Opotherapy*; treatment with preparations or substances as they are found naturally in the body. In general it is called *replacement therapy*, because usually the object is to restore to the body in sufficient quantity to maintain health something that is lacking in the body. *Endocrinotherapy* is one form of organotherapy.

**orgasm**    The peak of excitation in the genital zone; the sexual *climax*. Erotic arousal involves a series of physiologic and psychological phenomena in response to tactile stimulation or phantasy or a combination of mechanical and psychological stimuli. These changes include increased pulse rate and blood pressure, raised skin temperature, flow of blood into the erectile tissues of the eyes, lips, ear lobes, nipples, penis or clitoris, and the genital labia; usually also there is some degree of hyperextension of the trunk. All such changes build up to a maximum, at which point tension is suddenly released. The latter produces local spasms of the perineal musculature or more extensive convulsivelike contractions. Technically, the term orgasm refers to the moment of sudden release of tension.

In women, about 60% of sex episodes (from the beginning of foreplay to ejection of the flowback) result in orgasm—35% during foreplay, 15% during postplay. The full range of possible orgasms includes masturbatory, nocturnal, foreplay, intercourse, and postplay—with some being multiple. Only 5% of women have the whole range; another 25% have all except multiple orgasms; another 40% have all except multiple orgasms and nocturnals. About 30% both masturbate and have nocturnals; 50% only masturbate; 10% have only nocturnals (Baker, R. *Sperm Wars*. New York: Basic Books, 1996)

**orgasm, pharmacogenic**    The drug addict's satisfaction (and accompanying reduction of sexual and aggressive drives) following drug administration.

**orgasmic dysfunction**    Orgasm disorder, a type of *sexual dysfunction* (q.v.). In DSM-IV, *orgasmic disorder* replaces DSM-III-R's term, "inhibited female or male orgasm."

**orgasmus deficiens**    Lack of sexual pleasure. See *sexual dysfunctions.*

**orgastic impotence**    A *sexual disorder* (q.v.) consisting of inability to achieve orgasm or acme of satisfaction in the sexual act. Because of inability to attain genuine end-pleasure, more attention is placed on forepleasure mechanisms. The sexual behavior is rigid and, although a certain narcissistic functional pleasure is felt, it is not the complete relaxation of full orgasm. In this "pseudo-sexuality," narcissistic aims are disturbing the true sexuality. There may also be a diminution of conscious sexual interest. This reflects a constant struggle with repressed sexuality, which "diminishes his disposable sexual energy."

According to Fenichel, an important concomitant of orgastic impotence is that such patients are incapable of love. Their need for self-love and self-esteem overshadows their capacity for object love (*The Psychoanalytic Theory of Neurosis*, 1945).

**orgone** Reich's term for the life energy, which he believed to be specific and identifiable. See *bion*.

**Oriental nightmare-death syndrome** *Bangungut* (q.v.).

**orientation** 1. Awareness of one's physical relationship to reality as measured by the parameters of person, place, and time. A person with intact orientation knows his own identity and can correctly identify the people who are a part of his usual environment; he knows where he is; and he knows the year in which he lives, the month of the year, the day of the week, and whether it is morning, afternoon, or evening. A patient may be disoriented in any one or in any combination of these spheres; *disorientation*, or *confusion*, is usually indicative of organic brain disease, although some patients with functional disorders of reality testing may become confused secondary to withdrawal from and/or inattention to their environment. Right-left orientation is a function of the dominant parietal lobe.

2. One's direction or position in relation to a person, object, concept, or principle. Thus, when a psychiatrist is asked, "What is your orientation?" the questioner is trying to determine the general theory of human behavior to which the psychiatrist subscribes, his theoretical frame of reference, the "school of thought" within psychology or psychiatry that guides his formulations and methods of treatment.

**orientation, illusion of** Misinterpretation or misidentification of something real in the environment because of an unclear sensorium, as in the toxic deliria. The patient hears the voice of his nurse, for example, and believes it to be that of his wife.

**orienting response** *OR*; initially thought to be associated with the very onset of attention, triggered by the detection of any stimulus novelty. Recent studies have identified the OR more specifically with allocation of a limited capacity central processor, operating only after the activation of preattentional, automatic, parallel processing channels. The OR involves identifiable responses in skin conductance, finger pulse volume, pupillary dilation, cardiac deceleration, alpha blockade, changes in skeletal muscle activity, including changes in respiration pattern, as well as the $P_{300}$ component of the evoked potential.

OR nonresponding may be a vulnerability marker for severely schizophrenic patients characterized by genetic transmission of schizophrenia, a poor premorbid picture marked by social and emotional isolation, and the gradual onset of a psychosis showing poor response to neuroleptics, negative symptoms, and cognitive disorganization.

**original object** Fairbairn's term for what Klein called the *primal maternal introject*, which is the model for all evocable inner images. Klein considered the primal introject to be a part object, the mother's breast, which becomes a whole object (the mother) only after the child works through the depressive position. Fairbairn believed the original object to be a whole object from the very beginning.

**ornithinemia** Excessive ornithine in the plasma, due presumably to reduced activity of hepatic ornithine ketoacid transaminase; the condition has been described in siblings, who manifested mental retardation with marked disturbance in speech development. Whether it is an inborn error of amino acid metabolism or secondary to hepatic disease is uncertain.

**ornithophobia** Fear of birds.

**orofacial dyskinesia** A syndrome appearing in the elderly and associated with edentulousness (toothlessness), dementia, and chronic institutionalization. Symptoms include chewing, mouthing, and tongue movements; the condition is difficult to differentiate from tardive dyskinesia except that the latter often includes choreoathetoid movements of the extremities. See *tardive dyskinesia*.

**orosensory behaviors** See *gustation*.

**orphan drug** Any pharmacologic agent that is not economical to produce because the condition for which it is indicated affects relatively few persons. Many such drugs are further difficult to market because they are already in the public domain and consequently are not patentable. The intent of the 1983 orphan drug law in the United States is to speed the production of such drugs and to ensure their availability to the persons who need them.

**orphenadrine** An anticholinergic drug. See *cholinergic*.

**ortho-** Combining form meaning straight, right, correct, sound, from Gr. *orthós*.

**orthodox analysis** Freudian or classical analysis, better known as psychoanalysis, which uses primarily the technique of free association, interpretation of dreams, and elucidation of everyday mistakes in order to unmask the patient's unconscious motivations. The psychic material obtained in this manner is then made available to the patient, in order to prompt the emotional acceptance rather than mere intellectual knowledge of conflicts.

**orthographic coding** The capacity to recognize whole word letter patterns; often impaired in *dyslexia* (q.v.). Testing orthographic coding asks the subject to read aloud a list of words that violate the standard letter-sound conventions of English, such as malign, queue, yacht.

**orthomolecular** Judicious, normal, or optimal arrangement of molecules; as used in psychiatry, the term ordinarily refers to a treatment program based on Linus Pauling's theory (1967) that the schizophrenias and other functional mental disorders might be a result of vitamin deficiency. The treatment regimen consists of high doses of vitamins (hence also known as *megavitamin* treatment), especially niacin, vitamin C, and vitamin B$_6$, but also occasionally other vitamins and hormones as well. Neither the original theory nor the worth of the treatment regimen(s) has been substantiated.

**orthophrenia** Soundness of mind; also, the curing of a disordered mind.

**orthopsychiatry** A subdivision of psychiatry that deals with the study and treatment of mental deviations known in general as borderland states; it also includes the study of methods of preventing mental disorders. Because of its prevention aspects, orthopsychiatry is sometimes used as an equivalent to *child psychiatry* and *mental hygiene* (qq.v.). See *mental health*.

**orthostatic hypotension** *OH* (q.v.).

**orthovagotonia** Exaggerated functioning of the vagotonic or parasympathetic nervous system, but only when this exaggerated functioning is in harmony with that of the sympathetic nervous system.

**orthriogenesis** Federn's term for the recapitulation by the ego of its whole development, which he felt occurs at the moment of awakening when the ego, which has been without cathexis in deep sleep, suddenly has its cathexis restored.

**-osis** Combining form meaning action, state, condition, process, from Gr. *ōsis*.

**osmo-** Combining form meaning smell, odor, from Gr. *osme*.

**osmophobia** Fear of (bad) odors.

**osphresia, osphresis** The sense of smell.

**osphresiolagnia** Paraphilic interest in body odors (especially genital or anal), often associated with infantile sexuality. The person with the paraphilia is an osphresiolagniac or *renifleur*.

Some patients develop the delusion that their bodies send out disagreeable or harmful odors, or that others are forcing evil body odors upon them. Freud hypothesized that a tendency to osphresiolagnia, which has become extinct after childhood, may play a part in the genesis of neurosis (*Collected Papers*, 1924–25). See *rhinencephalon*.

**osphresiophilia** Excessive attraction to or interest in odors and smells.

**osphresiophobia** Fear of (bad) odors or of being contaminated by them.

**ossification** Lewin's term for the relative rigidity of behavior patterns that have become second nature or autonomous because of frequent repetitions.

**ostensive** Referring to what can be demonstrated, manifested, or exhibited. An ostensive definition of a table consists of teaching the meaning of the word "table" by pointing to many different tables.

**osteoarthritis** See *arthritis*.

**OT** *Occupational therapy* (q.v.).

**Othello syndrome** See *jealousy, morbid*.

**other conditions that may be a focus of clinical attention** Term in DSM-IV for "conditions not attributable to a mental disorder that are a focus of treatment or attention." The category includes medication-induced movement disorders, problems related to abuse or neglect, relational problems, religious or spiritual problems, acculturation problems, and problems with cognitive decline associated with aging.

**otiumosis**  E. Bergler's term for *alysosis* (q.v.); boredom.

**otoacoustic emissions**  *OAEs; see auditory nerve.*

**otohemineurasthenia**  Functional deafness affecting one ear.

**otoneurasthenia**  Functional deafness.

**outcome expectancy**  See *social learning theory.*

**outlier**  Beyond the acceptable or usual range. In insurance reimbursement terminology, outliers are patients with atypical characteristics relative to other patients in a DRG (diagnosis-related group), such as an unusually low or high length of stay, death, departure against medical advice, admission and discharge on the same day. Such patients may fall within a low-volume DRG (a group with five or fewer patients in a hospital's base year), presenting an unusual combination of diagnoses or surgical procedures or one or more very rare conditions.

**out-of-the-body experience**  *OBE;* the sensation that one is seeing the world from somewhere outside one's own body. OBE may occur during meditation, when under the influence of drugs, or even in the course of everyday activities, but the most frequently reported instances occur as part of a near-death experience.

**outpatient**  Ambulatory patient who is not listed on the hospital inpatient census.

**outpatient commitment**  *AOT* (assisted outpatient treatment); a civil court procedure mandating adherence to outpatient mental health treatment. It aims to prevent relapse, hospital readmission, homelessness, and incarceration. In most of the 42 states in the United States with outpatient commitment statutes, the requirement is that the patient comply with recommended treatment; it does not permit forced medication of legally competent persons. When a patient fails to comply with treatment, statutes typically permit the responsible clinician to request that law enforcement officers transport the patient to an outpatient facility where clinicians will attempt to persuade the patient to comply or they will undertake an evaluation for inpatient commitment.

Mandating adherence to outpatient mental health treatment can also be effected in other ways, such as *conditional release* under involuntary hospitalization, treatment under guardianship, or judicial treatment directives during inpatient commitment proceedings (Swartz, M.S. et al. *Psychiatric Services 57*: 343–349, 2006).

**output**  The amount of work performed or completed within a specified period of time; in communications theory, any action or response that cues or signals another person or another communication system.

**outputs**  See *functional budgeting.*

**ovariotomy**  Surgical removal of one or both ovaries. Bilateral ovariotomy is required for the castration of a female and usually leads, if performed before puberty, to such marked disturbance in the sex balance as to produce a eunuchoid symptomatology with secondary male sex characteristics (see *castration*). Also called *oophorectomy.*

**overactivity, psychomotor**  See *mania.*

**overadequate-inadequate reciprocity**  See *family therapy.*

**overanxious disorder**  *Generalized anxiety disorder* (q.v.) of childhood.

**overarousal**  Hyperexcitability or excessive reactivity, most frequently applied to the autonomic nervous system in panic disorder and other anxiety disorders. Many of the symptoms, such as sleep discontinuity, irritability, reduced ability to concentrate, hypervigilance, and increased startle, reflect discharge of the sympathetic (adrenergic) part of the autonomic nervous system, which seems to be in a state of chronic overarousal. See *hypervigilance.*

**overcharged idea**  A dreamer's central idea or conflict that has been exceptionally endowed with inner repressed psychic energy and consequently appears in the dream in the form of various symbols and several identifications.

**overcompensation**  According to Adler, overcompensation is the counterpose of an overwhelming feeling of inferiority that is profusely neutralized by steps toward a towering goal of dominance. Such people endeavor to secure their position in life by extraordinary efforts, by greater haste and impatience, by more violent impulses, and without consideration for anyone else. Their attitudes are apt to have a certain grandiose quality. See *compensation; Demosthenes complex.*

**overconsciousness**  Exaggerated development of self-consciousness as the result of "oversocialization with leveling of the object relations."

The term applies to parents who first identify themselves too strongly with their children as love objects, and then perform acts ostensibly of "self-sacrificing love," which, in psychiatric terms, are mere expressions of an increased narcissism on the part of the parents. Over-consciousness is a narcissistic attitude developed as a result of object relations of a special intensity and character (Schilder, P. *Mind, Perception and Thought*, 1942).

**overcorrection** A staff-intensive technique of behavior therapy that uses *time out from reinforcement* (q.v.) and also requires the patient to take steps to rectify actively a situation caused by the undesirable behavior and to engage in related prosocial behavior.

**overdependence, social** See *adaptational psychodynamics*.

**overdetermination** *Multidetermination*; "As a rule neuroses are overdetermined; that is to say, several factors in their etiology operate together" (Freud, *Collected Papers*, 1924–1925).

**overdose** The inadvertent or deliberate consumption of a much larger than usual dose of any substance, often leading to serious toxic reactions or death.

**overflow, motor** *Synkinesia* (q.v.).

**overgeneralizations** See *cognitive behavior therapy*.

**overinclusive thinking** Thinking is more abstract and less precise than normal thinking; this is the opposite of *concretistic thinking* (q.v.). Overinclusiveness is manifested in an inability to preserve conceptual boundaries, so that irrelevant or distantly associated elements become incorporated into concepts, making thought less precise and more abstract. See *association disturbances*.

**overproductive ideas** See *mania*.

**overreactive disorders** See *adaptational psychodynamics*.

**override, threat/control** Threat/control-override symptoms associated with increased aggression include the feeling of being dominated by forces beyond one's control, believing that thoughts are being put into one's head, believing that there are people who wish one harm, and believing that one is being followed.

**Overt Aggression Scale** *OAS*; a measure of specific aspects of aggressive behaviors in four categories: verbal aggression, physical aggression against objects, physical aggression against self, and physical aggression against other people, based on degree of seriousness, injury, or damage.

**overutilization** Use of health services by, or provision of them to, people who (a) are not in need of treatment, (b) do not need the type of treatment provided, (c) do not need the intensity of services provided, or (d) have disorders unlikely to respond to treatment. The services provided in such cases are sometimes termed *met un-need*.

**overvalued idea** A persisting idiosyncratic belief that does not seem senseless to the subject and exerts an influence on the subject's actions, even though they seem extreme or unwarranted to the observer. Such ideas often develop from a particular experience and tend to occur in association with preexisting personality disorders. Examples are morbid jealousy, hypochondriasis, anorexia nervosa, and some obsessions. In some instances, overvalued ideas can be observed to develop into fixed, systematized delusions. See *delusion; jealousy, morbid; paranoia*.

**ovulation** Discharge of a secondary oocyte (derived from an egg that has completed the first maturation division) from the ovary. Inside the oviduct, tiny hairs create a current in the body fluid so that when an egg is released by an ovary it is slowly wafted toward the opening of the oviduct. Finger like projections funnel the egg into the tube. From here, the egg begins its 5-day journey toward the womb and meets the sperm. The successful sperm cuts through the outer membrane of the egg and sheds its own membrane within the egg. The egg itself is rendered impenetrable to other sperm, and fusion of the DNA from sperm and egg mixes the genes from father and mother in equal proportions. Although there are two oviducts, only one will contain an egg during any given menstrual cycle.

In the days after the beginning of a menstrual period, the woman's body undergoes a series of hormonal changes that prepare her body to produce an egg. About 1 or 2 days before ovulation can occur, her body goes into a holding period, which gives her an opportunity to collect sperm. In part, whether she ovulates will depend on how her body feels about the man (or men) from whom she has collected sperm. Further, the more a woman is stressed, the less likely she is to ovulate.

The egg dies within a day of being released by the ovary. Conception is most likely if the woman is inseminated about 2 days before she ovulates. The number of days from ovulation to the beginning of the next period (when she cannot conceive) is fairly predictable (13 to 16 days), but the number of days from the beginning of menstruation to ovulation is highly variable. In any normal, healthy woman, this phase can vary in length from 4 to 28 days. And even apparently normal cycles are not always fertile. At the age of 20, a healthy woman produces an egg in about 50% of her cycles; by age 30, her fertility has peaked at about 80%. After she reaches 40 years of age, the proportion declines rapidly.

**oxidative stress**   The cytotoxic consequences of free oxygen radicals—superoxide anion $O_2^-$, hydroxy radical (OH) and hydrogen peroxide—which are generated as byproducts of normal and aberrant metabolic processes that utilize molecular oxygen ($O_2$). See *OXPHOS*; *free radical*. Free radicals are molecular entities that have an unpaired electron; they reach their highest concentration in *mitochondria* (q.v.).

**OXPHOS**   Oxidative phosphorylation, essential to the generation of energy, contained within the *mitochondria* (see *mtDNA*). Humans require more ATP (adenosine triphosphate) to sustain metabolism than they can manufacture by breaking down sugars. To obtain the needed ATP, aerobic cells oxidize carbohydrates, fats, and proteins; enzymes essential to this process are referred to collectively as enzymes of cellular respiration and oxidative phosphorylation.

OXPHOS is the main source of ATP for brain (and many other tissues). It decreases with age, and it is believed that if it falls below the energy threshold of an organ, symptoms of disease appear. Most people die before such thresholds are crossed, but people with OXPHOS mutations may have lower levels and are more likely to cross the thresholds within their lifetimes. OXPHOS genetics involves both nuclear DNA and mtDNA; a possible cause of age-related decline in OXPHOS and of OXPHOS mutations is damage to mtDNA by oxygen free radicals, such as superoxide anion and hydrogen peroxide. See *free radical*.

Late-onset diabetes, Alzheimer disease, Huntington disease, and Parkinson disease may all be associated with OXPHOS defects.

OXPHOS generates mitochondrial ATP through five enzyme subunits. Complex I (NADH dehydrogenase) oxidizes nicotinamide adenine dinucleotide (*NADH*). Complex II (succinate dehydrogenase) oxidizes succinate, and the electrons are transferred to ubiquinone (CoQ) to form ubiquinol (reduced CoQ), whose electrons are transferred to complex III (cytochrome c oxidoreductase), then to cytochrome c, then to complex IV (cytochrome c oxidase), and finally to oxygen. The energy released is used to pump protons out of the mitochondrial inner member, and complex V (ATP synthase) uses the electrochemical gradient that is generated to condense adenosine diphosphate (ADP) and inorganic phosphate ($P_i$) to form ATP.

**oxprenolol**   A *beta blocker* (q.v.).

**oxybate**   Sodium oxybate is the sodium salt of (γ-hydroxybutyrate (GHB); it is approved for the treatment of cataplexy and excessive daytime drowsiness in narcolepsy.

**oxycephaly**   Tower-head; turrecephaly. A congenital anomaly in which there is premature closure (craniosynostosis) of the coronal and lambdoid sutures, resulting in an upward elongation of the head, which thus appears dome-shaped. The anomaly does not affect mentality or length of life, but in order to preserve vision, the King corrective operation must be performed early in life.

**P$_{50}$ sensory gating** Modulation of the brain's sensitivity to sensory stimuli, as measured by the EEG wave that appears 50 msec following stimulation. Deficient gating of the auditory event-related potential is one neurobiological trait that is associated with schizophrenia. It has been found in patients with illness of recent onset and in chronic patients, and in both medicated and unmedicated patients. Deficits in P$_{50}$ sensory gating also occur in about half of the first-degree relatives of schizophrenia patients.

**P$_{300}$ wave** *P$_{300}$ brain wave, P$_{300}$ amplitude*; LPW (late positive wave); *novelty potential*; a positive brain wave that appears between 300 and 500 msec after a stimulus. It is one of the endogenous components of the sensory-evoked response that is related to information processing of task-relevant information. The P$_{300}$ wave is associated with the psychologic processes of attention, expectancy, stimulus recognition, stimulus evaluation, and cognitive decision-making activity.

Computer-averaged brain waves are measured by exposing subjects to a train of stimuli (such as flashes of light) and asking them to discriminate a randomly occurring unusual stimulus. When the anticipated unusual event occurs (such as a light of greater brightness or duration than the others), a positive brain wave appears between 300 and 500 msec following the stimulus. Its amplitude and latency are related to the importance of the task, how unpredictable or infrequent the event is, and the subject's motivation. See *neurometrics; NMR.*

**P450 enzyme system** See *cytochrome P450 isoenzyme system.*

**PACAP** Pituitary adenylyl cyclase activating protein; it is a member of a polypeptide hormone family that includes secretin, glucagon, and vasoactive intestinal polypeptide (VIP). PACAP functions as a neurotransmitter, interacting with two types of seven-transmembrane-domain receptors: (1) a receptor, positively coupled to adenylyl cyclase, that also recognizes VIP; (2) a receptor, linked to phospholipase C and adenylyl cyclase, that recognizes only PACAP. Within neurons, PACAP increases cAMP and calcium; it promotes neurite outgrowth.

**PACE** Personal Assistance in Community Existence, an approach to the treatment and rehabilitation of the mentally ill. PACE stresses the factors that recovered patients found useful in their treatment, among which are the following: awareness that people do recover from even the most severe forms of mental illness; especially when experiencing severe distress, people yearn to connect emotionally with others; in order to express feelings, a person must feel emotionally safe in relationships with others; there is meaning in periods of emotional distress, and understanding that meaning facilitates recovery; both trust and self-determination are essential to recovery.

**pacemaker, cerebral** A hypothesized central neurophysiologic mechanism that regulates and synchronizes the EEG rhythms of the two cerebral hemispheres. See *clock, biological.*

**pachymeningitis** See *meninges.*

**pachymeninx** See *meninges.*

**Pacinian corpuscle** See *glabrous.*

**Pacinian endings** See *mechanoreceptor.*

**PAD** Primary *affective disorder* (q.v.).

**padded cell** An older term for what is nowadays more commonly called a *seclusion room* or *quiet room*, used as a form of physical restraint in the management of disturbed or violent patients who are a danger to themselves or others, and for patients who ask for help in gaining control over destructive impulses. The older term emphasized the physical features of the room that ensured the patient's safety: a large mattress on the floor and padding on the walls.

**paedico** Although it appears as the root of various terms referring to sexual activity with children—and often specifically as homosexual activity with young boys, as in *pederasty* (q.v.)—the term means to penetrate the anus and does not imply either specific gender or age of either participant in the activity. Pederasty in ancient writing often has no more relation to the age of objects of desire than does the term "girl chasing" according to J. Boswell (*Christianity, Social Tolerance, and Homosexuality*, 1980).

**paed(o)-, ped(o)-** Combining form meaning childlike, or having to do with children, from Gr. *paid-*.

**PAF** *Pure autonomic failure*, rare acquired failure of peripheral autonomic regulation. Lack of visceral afferent information regarding the peripheral body state attenuates emotional response and results in a subtle blunting of emotional experience. Perception of emotional events leads to rapid, automatic, and stereotyped emotional responses rather than longer-term behavior modulations that are mediated by feeling states. Functional neuroimaging studies suggest that the anterior cingulate and insular-somatosensory cortices are particularly involved in such states. See *emotion*.

**PAG** *Periaqueductal gray area* (q.v.).

**pageism** The phantasy of a masochistic male that he is the slave or page of a dominating woman.

**pagophagia** Ice-eating, a type of *pica* (q.v.) suggesting an underlying iron deficiency anemia; the affected subject typically ingests at least one ordinary tray of ice daily for a period of 2 months or more.

**PAH** Phenylalanine hydroxylase; recessive mutations in the PAH gene (on chromosome 12) cause phenylketonuria.

**paidicatio** *Obs.* Pederasty; sodomy.

**pain** Hurt, discomfort, ache, perception of injury or threat of damage, *nociception*. Pain is both an unpleasant feeling and a signal of homeostatic imbalance; it includes physical, sensory, emotional, and cognitive experiences, as well as a perception that may or may not be related to actual tissue insult. (See *interoception*.) Pain sensation involves assessing the location and intensity of noxious stimulation as well as the generation of emotion and avoidance behavior.

Noxious stimuli activate a system that begins with the *nociceptors* (q.v.), from which pain signals are relayed to the contralateral spinothalamic tract and spinoreticulothalamic tract. (Signals from the face and head are conveyed directly to the brain by way of the cranial nerves.) Ascending pathways from the spinal cord to the brain activate multiple brain stem and subcortical regions, limbic pathways, and both ipsilateral and contralateral cortical brain regions. These pathways intermingle with regions of the brain that mediate emotions, autonomic activity, attention and localization, motor planning, and cognition.

Many signals terminate in the thalamus, pathways from which activate both primary and secondary somatosensory cortices and the posterior parietal cortex (the cortical pain system). Others take another path, the *medial pain system*, from the midline and intralaminar thalamic nuclei (*MITN*) to limbic cortex, periaqueductal gray, the amygdala, and the anterior- and mid-cingulate cortex. Subregions of the cingulate gyrus mediate the fear avoidance and unpleasantness that are essential elements of pain. In addition to all the foregoing, noxious stimuli activate other telencephalic regions, including prefrontal cortex, anterior insula, supplementary and premotor cortices, cerebellar cortex, and striatum.

Activation of nociceptors is not sufficient for the experience of pain, which depends on the state of the nervous system. The balance between perceiving too much pain and too little is controlled by a chemical-control system aimed at dealing with pain and stress; its major components are (1) *substance P* (q.v.), a neuropeptide thought to be crucial in transmitting pain signals from skin to spinal cord; and (2) the endogenous opioids (*endorphins* and *enkephalins*, qq.v.). In addition, a number of endogenous neurotransmitters—among them acetylcholine, bradykinin, cannabinoids, cholecystokinin, somatostatin, GABA, histamine, oxytocin, prolactin, prostaglandin E2, vasoactive intestinal peptide, and vasopressin—inhibit or augment pain perception, but how they are activated is poorly understood.

Damage to peripheral tissues sensitizes nociceptors to subsequent stimuli and increases the sensation of pain (*hyperalgesia*). The sensitization is due not only to tissue damage but also to the release of chemical mediators that decrease the pain threshold and may also activate nociceptors. Pain can also arise in the absence of nociceptor activity. See *allodynia*; *pain syndromes*.

**pain, ecstatic** "The *hunger for excitement* of some people comes about in this manner. There are people who must always be doing something; it matters little whether the situation is of a pleasurable or painful nature. Sometimes a decided preference is shown for the latter; they experience 'ecstatic pain,' martyrlike pleasure, and forever consider themselves unfairly treated" (Bleuler, E. *Textbook of Psychiatry*, 1930).

**pain, psychic** *Psychalgia*; psychogenic pain disorder. See *somatoform disorders*.

**pain clinic** Pain clinics, of relatively recent development, employ a multidisciplinary approach to the control of chronic pain states. The treatment team might include, for example, a neurologist, a psychiatrist, and an anesthesiologist, who might employ multiple treatment approaches (e.g., transcutaneous electrical nerve stimulation, biofeedback, guided imagery, analgesics), reflecting evidence that the different treatments work synergistically. Decreased serotonin has been implicated in both chronic pain and depression, and antidepressant drugs appear to be more successful in treatment than traditional psychotherapy, analgesics, or antianxiety agents.

**pain conduction** See *spinal gating*.

**pain disorder** See *pain syndromes*.

**"pain management, multidimensional** Use of operant conditioning techniques in the treatment of chronic pain syndromes. It is sometimes helpful in short-term management, but benefits are rarely maintained. See *pain clinic*; *pain syndromes*.

**pain syndrome, central** Ongoing, intractable pain referred to contralateral deep and cutaneous tissues, typically described as burning and often evoked by normally innocuous stimuli. It is accompanied by loss of thermal sensation and often, paradoxically, loss of acute pain sensation (such as pinprick). It may follow ablation procedures performed to relieve pain and apparently is due to damage to the lamina I spinothalamocortical pathway. See *pain syndromes*.

**pain syndromes** Although nociceptors convey the sensation of pain from a specific region of the body, pain can also arise in the absence of nociceptor activity. Among such pain syndromes are the following:

1. *Deafferentation*, when afferent input from the periphery to the spinal chord is blocked; in *brachial plexus avulsion* (often seen in motorcycle injuries), the dorsal roots are pulled away from the spinal cord; the patient feels a burning or electric pain in the dermatomes corresponding to the denervated (and anesthetic) area.

2. *Phantom limb* (q.v.), like deafferentation, may depend upon compensatory hyperactivity of disconnected dorsal horn neurons;

3. Reflex sympathetic dystrophy syndrome (causalgia), a burning pain caused by activation of nociceptive afferents in damaged peripheral nerves by sympathetic nervous system efferents; sometimes the pain is relieved when sympathetic activity is chemically blocked.

4. *Thalamic hyperpathia*, often caused by vascular lesions in multiple areas of the thalamus.

5. *Referred pain*, when pain arising from deep viscera is felt as arising from regions on the body surface.

6. *Central pain syndromes*, common sequelae to attempts to relieve pain by surgical ablation procedures; the resulting pain is often more disagreeable than the pain the operation was designed to abolish, with spontaneous aching and shooting sensations, numbness, cold, heaviness, and burning. See *pain syndrome, central*.

7. *Chronic intractable pain, neuropathic pain*; sometimes *central pain* (see #6 above) is used interchangeably with the other two; it is classified within the *somatoform disorders* (q.v.) in DSM-IV. Chronic pain is pain that persists more than 1 month longer than might be reasonably expected following an inciting event; it is sustained by aberrant somatosensory nervous system processing. It can last for months or years, even decades. The pain affects every aspect of the patient's life, and it is frequently associated with depression. Anxiety and sleep deprivation are also common in patients with neuropathic pain.

Some authorities consider chronic intractable pain a specific variant of depressive disease, sometimes called *painprone disorder*. Initiative for work is lost after the pain begins, in marked contrast to the patient's premorbid ergomania and overactivity. Painprone disorder is more frequent in women than in men; mean age at onset is 39 years. Research has emphasized the role of decreased serotonin in both chronic pain and depression. Antidepressant agents that block serotonin uptake have been effective in many such patients, whereas analgesics and antianxiety agents generally are not.

The most common sites of chronic intractable pain are low back, head, face, and pelvis. In a substantial number of patients with postherpetic neuralgia, the pain is transformed into chronic pain. The pain is usually described as an unremitting burning, stabbing, or lancinating pain along the affected dermatome. In *complex regional pain syndrome* (also known as *reflex sympathetic dystrophy*), a seemingly innocuous soft tissue injury leads to temporary immobilization, but pain, allodynia, or hyperalgesia persist to a degree disproportionate to the inciting event, and at times there is edema, changes in skin blood flow, or abnormal sudomotor activity in the region of the pain. Such autonomic symptoms suggested sympathetic nervous system blockade as a possible treatment, but results have been unsatisfactory.

Glia play a role in chronic pain. First, damage to, or inflammation of, a peripheral nerve is somehow communicated to microglia in the spinal cord. Second, glial cells are activated and respond to ATP by using newly produced $P2X_4$ receptors. Third, the ATP-activated glial cells modify signaling between spinal neurons. A missing link between microglia and pain-carrying neurons is BDNF, a neurotrophic factor that triggers a change in the excitability of spinal neurons to render the inhibitory neurotransmitter, GABA, excitatory.

*Pain clinics* employ a multidisciplinary approach in the treatment of neuropathic pain. The treatment team might include a neurologist, a psychiatrist, and an anesthesiologist, who might employ multiple treatment approaches, reflecting evidence that different treatments work synergistically. Anticonvulsants are the first-line treatment for neuropathic pain; antidepressants have also been effective in some studies. If narcotic analgesics are used, the patient is often required to sign a *narcotic agreement*, stipulating that narcotics will be obtained from only one physician, at one pharmacy, and administered only in the manner prescribed. Patients must return for monthly visits and are subject to random drug screening.

**pain-prone disorder**   A form of chronic intractable pain. See *pain syndromes*.

**paired dreams**   The idea that one is allowed to indulge in a forbidden act if he has already paid the penalty for it leads to paired dreams: on the same night the subject first dreams that he is being punished; later he dreams that he is engaging in a forbidden act.

**paired helical filaments**   *PHFs*; a characteristic of *Alzheimer disease* (q.v.), consisting of an abnormal cementlike protein that proliferates

within the cytoplasm of the degenerating nerve cell.

**pairing assumption**   See *basic assumptions group*.

**pal(a)eo-**   Combining form meaning old, ancient, from Gr. *palaios*.

**palaeocerebellum**   Spinal *cerebellum* (q.v.).

**paleologic**   Archaic or ancient logic; the same method of thinking that has been variously designated as pre-Aristotelian, prelogical (Levy-Bruhl) or paralogical (Von Domarus). Paleologic is seen most clearly in schizophrenic thinking disorders. See *prelogical*.

**paleomnesis**   Memory for the remote past in the life of the subject.

**paleopathology**   Study of disease in bodies, such as mummies, preserved from ancient times. Currently, paleopathology entails evaluation of a disease complex, its effect on humans, and possible changes over time. Three areas that need investigation and should provide useful information on human adaptation to special environments are the transition to agriculture and its health effects, the difference in health between rural and urban dwellers in the past, and gender and health.

**paleophrenia**   Ancient or primitive mentality, suggested by O. Osborne to replace the word schizophrenia to emphasize the regression to a primitive type of thinking that is often seen in schizophrenics.

**paleopsychic**   Pertaining to or possessing primitive mentality.

**paleopsychology**   The study of paleopsychic phenomena; it is believed by Freud, Jung, and many others, that remote ancestral modes of mental activity reside in the unconscious of the modern human.

**paleosensation**   The term of the Dutch school of neurologists (Brouwer, Kappers) for *protopathic* (light) sensations in contradistinction to the epicritic and deep, which they call *gnostic* or new sensations. See *protopathic*.

**paleosymbol**   A private symbol, which is highly individualistic, fleeting, flexible, and mutable; it evolves and is maintained without regard for socialization or interpersonal relationships. Paleosymbols are seen as a form of *paleologic* (q.v.) and are characteristic of immediately prehuman races although they probably exist also in apes in rudimentary form.

**pali-**   Combining form meaning morbid or obsessive repetition or reiteration, from Gr. *palin*, backward, again.

**paligraphia**   The morbid or obsessive repetition of something (letters, words, phrases, etc.) in writing.

**palilalia**   A rare speech disorder in which the last word or syllable is repeated with increasing rapidity. It is suggestive of frontal lobe dysfunction.

**palilexia**   Compulsive rereading of words or phrases.

**palilogia**   Compulsive repetition of something spoken.

**palinacousis**   Perseveration of sounds, suggestive of temporal lobe disorder (especially tumor).

**palingraphia**   Mirror-writing.

**palinlexia**   Backward reading.

**palinoia**   Compulsive repetition of an act as a way to master its performance.

**palinopia, palinopsia**   Visual perseveration, i.e., a prolonged afterimage. It suggests occipital lobe dysfunction secondary to tumor, trauma, anoxic or metabolic encephalopathy, infarction, arteriovenous malformation, seizure disorder, migraine, or multiple sclerosis. It has also been observed in sensory deprivation, psychotomimetic ingestion (especially mescaline or LSD), and as a rare side effect of antidepressant therapy. See *polyopia*.

**paliopsy**   Visual perseverance; brief persistence in vision of objects no longer in the visual field, usually indicative of occipital lobe pathology.

**paliphrasia**   Repetition of phrases in speaking.

**pallesthesia**   Vibratory sensation when a vibrating tuning fork is placed over subcutaneous bony surfaces. Also known as *palmesthesia*.

**palliative care**   Interdisciplinary care that aims to alleviate symptoms that cause suffering and diminish quality of life in patients whose underlying illness cannot be cured or effectively managed. Palliative care is an adjunct to, not a replacement of, other appropriate treatment for patients with advanced illness and for their families. Pain is one of the leading symptoms that palliative care addresses.

**pallidum**   See *basal ganglia*.

**palmar reflex**   A superficial reflex; scratching or irritation of the palm results in flexion of the fingers.

**palmesthesia**   *Pallesthesia* (q.v.).

**palmitoylation**   Post-translational modification of proteins with the lipid palmitate, a 16-carbon saturated fatty acid. Palmitate modifies numerous proteins that are involved in cell growth, differentiation, and adhesion. Palmitoylation regulates neuronal development and brain function; in particular, palmitoylated ion-channel-associated synaptic scaffolding proteins help to specify and accelerate responses to neurotransmitters. See *Huntington disease*.

**palmomandibular sign**   Reflex opening of the mouth in response to pressure on the palms or forearm, present in the neonate until about the tenth day of life, when it is replaced by the *palmomental reflex* (q.v.).

**palmomental reflex**   *Palm-chin reflex; pollico-mental reflex*; contraction of the mentalis muscle following mechanical stimulation of the thenar and hypothenar eminences; suggestive of diffuse toxic brain damage.

**palsy**   Paralysis.

**palsy, progressive bulbar**   See *amyotrophic lateral sclerosis*.

**palsy, shaking**   *Parkinson disease*.

**pamphobia**   *Obs. Panphobia*; fear of everything.

**pamplegia, panplegia**   *Obs.* Generalized paralysis (not the clinical entity, general paralysis).

**pan-, pam-**   Combining form meaning all, whole, from Gr. *pan*.

**pananxiety**   See *pseudoneurotic schizophrenia*.

**panchreston**   The state or quality of being adaptable to any and all uses; applied sometimes to the terminology of psychiatry and psychology, where words are used to explain everything, and in such a variety of ways as finally to become a meaningless jargon.

**PANDAS**   Pediatric autoimmune neuropsychiatric disorders associated with streptococcal infection, a putative subtype of obssessive-compulsive disorder that begins before puberty and is characterized by an episodic course with intense exacerbations. It is associated with group Aβ-hemolytic streptococci infection and neurologic abnormalities. Other frequently coexisting symptoms are emotional lability, separation anxiety, cognitive deficits, oppositional behaviors, and hyperactivity.

**pandysmaturation**   Fish's term for the neurointegrative inadequacies in multiple areas that have been described in *childhood schizophrenia* (q.v.).

**panencephalitis, subacute sclerosing (SSPE)**   A rare disease of children and young adults due to a measles virus variant. Symptoms, which typically develop 5 to 7 years after the child has had measles, consist of progressive deterioration of mental and motor performance and associated myoclonic movements. In the early stage, signs are mainly cerebral (awkwardness, stumbling, mental deterioration, memory loss); at the second stage, convulsions and repetitive myoclonus are characteristic. In the final stage, stupor, coma, and increased spasticity appear, with death within 1 to 3 years after onset.

**panglossia** Garrulity, especially psychotic.

**panic** An attack of overwhelming *anxiety*; *panic attack* (qq.v.). Some writers restrict the term to psychotic episodes characterized by unrealistically based and autistically determined anxiety of overwhelming proportions, such as is seen in *homosexual panic* (q.v.) and in acute aggression panic. The latter term refers to cases where homosexual content is lacking and, instead, a picture of undue malignant influence, physical violence, or impending death is seen.

**panic, primordial** Reactions of fright and anger combined with unfocused, disorganized motor responses akin to the infantile startle reaction; such reactions are seen in many schizophrenic children. Primordial panic is also termed *elemental anxiety* and is believed to be based on primary defects in the ego that result in an impairment in personal identity, self-awareness, and differentiation of the self from the non-self.

**panic attack** An episode of intense anxiety or fear in which symptoms develop suddenly and reach a crescendo, usually within 10 minutes. Symptoms may include any of the following: shortness of breath or a smothering sensation, palpitations and tachycardia, trembling, sweating, choking, nausea or abdominal distress, depersonalization or derealization, numbness or paresthesias, hot flashes or chills, chest pain or discomfort, a fear of dying, and a fear of "losing my mind" or of doing something uncontrolled.

A panic attack may be uncued or unexpected, i.e., not associated with a situational trigger; see *panic disorder*. A cued panic attack is one that is situationally bound and almost invariably provoked upon exposure to or in anticipation of a particular trigger; see *phobia*. A third type of panic attack is termed situationally predisposed; it is more likely to be triggered by a particular situation but is not invariably associated with it. See *interoceptive*.

**panic disorder** *Episodic paroxysmal anxiety*; a type of anxiety disorder consisting of recurrent,

uncued panic attacks. It is generally believed that panic disorder is based on a biochemical dysfunction, probably involving the noradrenergic system and mediated through the *locus ceruleus* (q.v.). Some studies suggest that it may particularly involve the right parahippocampal gyrus. Like some other *anxiety disorders* (q.v.), panic disorder tends to run in families. There is evidence of a genetic predisposition to panic disorder, perhaps mediated through neurotransmitter dysregulation (central noradrenergic overactivity). Between one-half and two-thirds of persons with panic disorder have at least one first-degree relative with a similar condition. Female relatives are affected about twice as frequently as male relatives.

Many of the symptoms characteristic of panic disorder are reported also in patients with complex partial seizures: dizziness, palpitations, sweating, abdominal distress, depersonalization, tingling or numbness, hot flashes or chills, chest pain, fear of dying or fear of going crazy, perceptual disturbances, and impairment of consciousness. Either disorder may be misdiagnosed as the other, and sometimes the same patient has both disorders.

Lifetime prevalence of full-blown panic disorder is 3.5%, of panic symptoms approximately 10%. Panic attacks may occur with or without *agoraphobia* (q.v.). See *interoceptive; panic attack*.

Depression is observed in a significant number of persons with panic disorder; the numbers reported are within the range of 44% to 75%, and in almost half the first episode of depression occurred prior to the onset of panic disorder. Panic disorder patients are also prone to alcoholism and other substance abuse, and these in turn contribute to the high rate of suicide (20 %) among persons with panic disorder. Males who suffer from panic disorder or agoraphobia have twice the expected rate of cardiovascular deaths; the reasons for this have not been determined.

**panmixia** In genetic population studies, this term indicates equal and unrestricted mating conditions of organisms with different racial characteristics in a mixed population group. See *homogamy*.

**panneurosis** See *pseudoneurotic schizophrenia*.

**panoramic memory** See *absent state; memory*.

**panphobia, panophobia, pantophobia** Fear of everything.

**pansexualism** The doctrine that all human behavior stems from sex. There is no school of psychiatric medicine today whose leaders profess such a doctrine. Freud specifically disavowed any connection between pansexualism and psychoanalysis.

**PANSS** *Positive and Negative Syndrome Scale* (q.v.).

**papaverine** An anticholinergic drug. See *cholinergic*.

**Papez's theory of emotion** A modification of Cannon's hypothalamic theory: the hippocampus, *fornix*, mammillary bodies of the hypothalamus, anterior thalamic nuclei, and gyrus cinguli form a circle ("Papez's circle") that elaborates the functions of central emotion and participates in emotional experience. The midbrain reticular formation is connected indirectly to Papez's circle by means of the olfactory tubercle and the amygdaloid and septal nuclei.

**papilledema** *Choked disk*; a condition in which the optic nerve is literally choked at the optic foramen by increased intracranial, and especially intraventricular, pressure, leading to an increase in the intraocular tension. The condition is usually bilateral. Ophthalmoscopically, the disk is raised, at times to five or six or more diopters; the margins of the disk are blurred; the veins are tortuous and full, the arteries thin; and hemorrhages may occur. Papilledema is most often caused by tumor of the brain; other causes include fracture of the skull, hydrocephalus, abscess of the brain, subarachnoid hemorrhage, sinus thrombosis, meningitis, encephalitis, and possibly multiple sclerosis and anemia.

**par-, para-** Combining form meaning beside, past, aside, beyond; associated in a subsidiary or accessory capacity; perverted, amiss, wrong, faulty, irregular, disordered, abnormal, mal-, mis-; misleading in that it closely resembles the true form even though it may itself be disordered or abnormal; from Gr. *para*, from (the side), beside, near, beyond, against.

**parabulia** Perversion of volition or will as when an impulse is partly or completely checked and is then replaced by another impulse. A patient had the impulse to strike his physician; he advanced toward the physician for that purpose, but suddenly stopped "to regulate the universal voices." Parabulia usually occurs as a manifestation of ambivalence of the will in schizophrenic disorders. See *will disturbances*.

**paracenesthesia** Any abnormality of the general sense of well-being.

**parachromatopsia, parachromopsia** Partial color blindness, such as red-green color blindness.

**paracingulate cortex** The anterior paracingulate cortex may be responsible for the central task of *theory of mind* (q.v.). The paracingulate gyrus itself may depend on interpretations of *STS* (q.v.) about body language. The adjacent region is a conflict monitor, sensing when the brain's predictions about how the world works do not match reality.

**paracousia, paracusia** Any abnormality of hearing other than simple deafness; often used to refer specifically to auditory illusions. *Paracousia* loci is impaired ability to determine the direction from which a sound proceeds. *Paracousia willisiana* is the ability, demonstrated by some partially deaf persons, to hear better in the presence of loud noise.

**paradigm** Pattern; model, often with the implication that it has a fundamental or governing role within the area of knowledge or science to which it refers.

Paradigm also refers to a group or set of shared assumptions and suppositions that determine how something is defined as a problem, what methods are considered applicable to its investigation, and what constitutes an acceptable solution. This meaning underscores the dependence of even the "pure" scientist on the environment and the prevailing, acceptable points of view of the time in which he works.

**paradox, neurotic** Persistence of neurotic behavior despite the fact that it is seriously self-defeating. Freud attempted to explain this paradox by assuming that it was due to the retention of an oversevere superego, evolved from too zealous childhood training. Such an explanation is contrary to all learning theory, which says that learning tends to undergo extinction unless periodically reinforced. It is more likely that the paradox results from infantile ego resistance to socializing forces, so that the basic values and attitudes of society are faultily assimilated into the personality. It may also be that the neurotic behavior represents a means to an end that is unconsciously determined, the desire for which overcomes the wish to conform.

**paradoxical intention (PI)**   A treatment technique for phobic patients that directs the subject to try to increase anxiety and become as panicky as possible.

**paradoxical sleep**   REM *sleep* (q.v.).

**paradoxical therapy**   *Strategic intervention*; tactics or techniques that on the surface appear contrary to the goals of treatment but are in fact designed to achieve them by overcoming resistance, fostering change, or otherwise hastening improvement. Strategic therapy is associated particularly with Jay Haley and Richard Rabkin. It is based on the assumption that symptoms represent an attempt to solve a problem in a way that only makes the problem worse. Therapy focuses on isolating and defining the problem, analyzing the attempts already made to solve it, and negotiating mutually acceptable and workable goals to develop a series of "strategies" or more effective ways to handle the problem.

Many theorists assume that some, if not all therapy is by definition manipulative. Paradoxical therapy consists of a deliberate use of influencing techniques that focus on the patient's symptoms, often by altering their meaning for the patient. The strategic use of paradoxical interventions is applicable to groups as well as individuals. It is an active, direct, focused, and usually short-term approach.

One of the earliest forms of strategic intervention to be described is *negative practice*, in which the patient is directed to practice repetitively the very habit he wants to eliminate. Another form is *paradoxical restraining therapy*, in which the therapist discourages the patient from attempts to change. The therapist may suggest that it might not be possible for the patient to change, or he may adopt a position that is an exaggeration of the patient's pathological attitude. In the *antiexpectation technique*, also called *paradoxical positioning*, the therapist expresses an attitude about the patient's symptoms that appears to encourage and reinforce them rather than urging the patient to join forces with the therapist in resisting or ignoring them. Another technique, *defiance-based strategy*, is based on the expectation that the patient will resist the therapist and rebel against any directives he might issue. In the *therapeutic double-bind*, the patient is enjoined to change by remaining unchanged; if he complies and remains unchanged, he demonstrates that he can in fact control the situation, whereas if he defies by changing he has accomplished the purpose of therapy.

**paraeroticism**   Perversion. See *metaeroticism*.

**paraflocculi**   See *cerebellum*.

**parageusia**   Abnormal sense of taste.

**paragnomen**   An unexpected action, not understandable for the subject's environment or by reason of his or her usual conduct or behavior, which at the moment it is performed is considered to be consciously performed and adequate to the situation but which later appears inexplicable even to the subject. Paragnomens are seen frequently in schizophrenic patients.

**paragnosia**   Irrelevant or approximate answers and, in particular, the "wild" guesses made by subjects with nondominant parietal lobe dysfunction who cannot state spontaneously where they are (even though they might select the right answer if offered a number of choices). See *parietal lobe; sensory neglect*.

**paragrammatism**   Any speech disturbance characterized by faulty grammatical or syntactical relationships; the disturbance may be a part of the organic aphasias, or it may be found in schizophrenic speech. "At times grammar fails them (*paragrammatism*). Many words are used incorrectly, thus, e.g., frequently the word 'murder' that designates all the tortures that the patients suffer" (Bleuler, E. *Textbook of Psychiatry*, 1930). See *Wernicke aphasia*.

**paragraphia**   Disturbance of writing. Ordinarily it does not mean alterations in the handwriting itself, such as tremors, rigid writing, flourishes and abnormalities in the size of the script; rather, it has to do with such errors as the omission and transposition of letters or words, or the substitution of a wrong letter or word, or the writing of nonexistent words. Errors of this kind are usually due to cerebral injury, although they may also occur in schizophrenic disorders. See *neologism*.

**parahippocampal place area**   *PPA*; an area in the hippocampal gyrus that is activated by images containing views of houses and visual scenes.

**parahypnosis**   Abnormal sleep as in hypnotism or somnambulism; used particularly to refer to the suggestibility of patients under general anesthesia, when remarks or suggestions made by others in the operating or delivery room may be responsible for later development of symptoms by the patient.

**parakinesia**   Bizarre and clumsily executed movement.

**paralalia**  Any speech defect, especially the habitual substitution of one letter for another.

**paralalia literalis**  Difficulty in uttering certain sounds, usually combined with stammering.

**paralanguage**  See *psycholinguistics*.

**paralexia**  Misreading of printed or written words, other meaningless words being substituted for them. See *sensory neglect; reading disabilities*.

**paralimbic region**  See *limbic lobe*.

**paralipophobia**  Fear of neglecting duty.

**parallel circuits**  See *frontal-striatal system*.

**parallel distributed processing**  *PDP*; sometimes used as equivalent to *parallel processing* (q.v.), sometimes used to refer specifically to computer modeling of brain information processing. Typically, connectionist models are composed of large numbers of simple processing units that are densely interconnected and all of which may be functioning at the same time (i.e., in parallel rather than in series). Each unit receives excitatory and inhibitory influences from other units; it computes the total input and fires or propagates a signal when the input reaches a certain level (the *activation value*, often set by the experimenter to measure the effects of different inputs on overall processing or functioning). Processing consists of the propagation of signals (*spread of activation*) among units. Units are grouped into modules of interconnected units that serve a particular function; modules, in turn, are connected with *pathways*.

*Information* in each module is represented as its pattern of activation; *knowledge* is the ability to generate an appropriate response (*connection weight*) to a particular input; *learning* is adjusting the connection weights so that an appropriate pattern of activation is produced for each input pattern. No one module acts as a master command unit; instead, the cooperative interactions of the separate modular components (working in parallel rather than in series) produce a level of processing that exceeds the capabilities of the individual modules. See *associationism; connectionism; MPPS*.

**parallel fibers**  See *cerebellum; Purkinje cell*.

**parallel processing**  Use of more than one group of neurons or more than one neural pathway to convey the same information, a type of organization characteristic of the nervous system. Within the sensory system, for example, different elements of perception are carried and processed in parallel by different parts of the system. Sensory information is first analyzed and "deconstructed" at the receptor level. The different components are abstracted and represented by means of feature detection and pattern of firing in different pathways and central regions of the brain. These regions then interact, reconstructing the components into a unified conscious perception.

Such an organization is not primarily designed to achieve multiplication of identical circuitry, but rather to allow different neuronal pathways and brain relays (*neural networks*) to deal with the same sensory information in slightly different ways. Nonetheless, because any one function or system is at least partially duplicated ("backed up") by one or more others, if the first function becomes blocked or impaired the others can often compensate for the loss. Parallel processing thus increases the richness of function as well as its reliability within the central nervous system. See *connectionism, cellular*.

**parallel search**  See *attention*.

**parallel visual computation**  *MPPS* (q.v.).

**paralogia**  Distorted logic or reasoning in speaking. "Evasion or *paralogia* consists in this, that the idea which is next in the chain of thought is suppressed and replaced by another which is related to it" (Kraepelin, E. *Dementia Praecox*, 1919).

**paralogia, derailment or displacement**  See *acataphasia*.

**paralogia, metaphoric**  See *by-idea*.

**paralogia, thematic**  Disturbed reasoning in relation chiefly to one theme or subject, upon which the mind dwells insistently. See *monoideism; monomania*.

**paralysis**  Loss of power of voluntary movement in a muscle due to injury or disease of its nerve supply.

**paralysis, acute ascending**  *Landry paralysis* (q.v.).

**paralysis, divers**  *Caisson disease* (q.v.).

**paralysis, familial periodic**  See *periodic paralysis, familial*.

**paralysis, hysterical**  A paralysis of psychogenic etiology, in contradistinction to a paralysis of organic origin. The organic paralyses are never so complete as the hysterical paralyses. The hysterically paralyzed limb will be absolutely inert; the hysterical aphasic is completely mute. Thus, hysterical paralysis shows both an exact delimitation and an excessive intensity, demonstrating that the hysterical lesion is entirely independent of the anatomy of the nervous system. See *conversion; hysteria.*

**paralysis agitans** *Parkinson disease* (q.v.).

**parameter** In mathematics, a variable or constant that determines the shape of the mathematical object or function being studied (e.g., length or depth); by extension (regrettable, because imprecision will ultimately render the term meaningless), any limit or boundary.

In psychoanalytic therapy, any deviation from the neutral interpretive stance of the analyst; any interventions other than interpretation that might be necessary to initiate or maintain the analytic process. The term *pseudoparameter* is used to refer to technical devices which, though not strictly interpretations, nonetheless have the same dynamic effect, such as telling the right joke at the right moment or repeating to the patient the words he has just said.

**paramimia** Disturbance of sense for gestures or mimetic movements leading to incongruities between feeling and means of expression.

**paramimism** A movement or gesture that has a meaning for the patient different from the ordinarily accepted meaning.

**paramnesia** Disturbance of memory in which real facts and phantasies are confused. Thus, a patient was unable to tell whether he had dreamed or actually experienced that of which he was given an account. Paramnesia is a common phenomenon in dreams, and in the schizophrenias where it often appears as false recognition, such as déjà fait or déjà vu. Such paramnesiae may also occur in the normal person.

**paramnesia, reduplicative** *Doppelganger* (q.v.).

**paraneoplastic encephalomyelopathy/sensory neuropathy syndrome** *Hu syndrome* (q.v.).

**paraneoplastic limbic encephalitis** See *neurological paraneoplastic syndromes.*

**paraneoplastic neurological disorders** *PNDs*; rare conditions associated with ectopic expression of neuron-specific proteins in tumors. Immune targeting of these antigens in CNS is thought to result in the neurological symptoms. See *Hu syndrome.*

**paraneuron** A nerve cell with neurosecretory or synaptic vesiclelike granules containing neurotransmitters or neuromodulators that are released in response to relevant stimuli. The term emphasizes that nerve cells can act

as endocrine cells and that the differences between the two types of cells are less distinct than formerly believed.

**paranoia, paranoea** Used in the sense of insane or of unsound mind by Aeschylus, Plato, and other pre-Hippocratic writers. Vogel reintroduced the term into medicine in 1764, but it was inconsistently applied to a number of diverse conditions. Delusions of persecution and grandeur were called *monomania* by Esquirol (1838), and Johann Heinroth (1881) included them under *Verrucktheit*, disorders of the intellect. Although Karl Kahlbaum (1863) used the term paranoid, it was a New York psychiatrist, E. C. Spitzka, who in 1883 defined paranoia as it is used today. Kraepelin (1912) defined paranoia as the insidious and permanent development of an unshakable delusional system, the personality remaining intact and without hallucinations. He described paraphrenia as falling between dementia praecox and paranoia, and characterized by unremitting systematized delusions and hallucinations but no progression to dementia.

Currently, paranoid disorders are termed *delusional disorders* and are considered to be a group of rare conditions in which the central feature is the development of one or more persistent delusions that are not bizarre but involve mechanisms that occur in real life, such as being followed, being loved from afar, or being deceived by a lover. In any one patient, the delusions typically revolve about a single theme or a series of connected themes. *Paranoia* is sometimes used to refer to a chronic condition with fixed and typically systematized delusions, in a subject who in other areas does not appear to be odd or bizarre and who does not show prominent auditory or visual hallucinations.

*Shared paranoid disorder* corresponds to what other systems term *folie à deux* (q.v.) or *psychosis of association.* In DSM-III-R it is termed *induced psychotic disorder* and is classified among "other psychotic disorders" rather than within the group of delusional disorders.

*Atypical paranoid disorder* has been used to refer to suddenly appearing paranoid states in persons who recently changed their living or work situation, such as immigrants, refugees, and inductees into military service. Such conditions rarely become chronic. Paranoid developments occur also in association with other disorders, and particularly in organic mental disorders; they are then classified under those disorders or as "organic delusional syndrome."

Types of paranoid disorder are usually described in terms of the predominant delusional theme: persecutory (the subject or someone close to him is being treated malevolently), jealous or infidelity type (the subject's sexual partner is unfaithful), erotic or erotomaniacal (some other person, usually of higher social or economic status, is in love with the subject), somatic (delusional conviction that one has a physical disorder), grandiose (delusions of great importance, wealth, social standing, special relationships to the deity or the famous), litigious (constantly seeking legal redress for imagined wrongs), etc.

On the basis of his analysis of the *Schreber case*, Freud concluded that the core of the conflict in paranoia (at least in males) is a homosexual wish-phantasy of loving a man. The forms of paranoia represent the contradictions of the proposition: I, a man, love him, a man. This proposition is contradicted (a) in the subject, by delusions of jealousy: "It is not I who love the man, it is she"; (b) in the predicate, by delusions of persecution: "I do not love him, I hate him, and because of this he hates me and persecutes me"; (c) in the object, by erotomania: "I do not love him, I love her, because she loves me"; and (d) by complete denial in megalomania: "I do not love anyone else at all, but only myself."

**paranoia, acquired**  Krafft-Ebing described two principal forms of paranoia: (1) *original paranoia*, developing before or at puberty—always hereditary; (2) *acquired paranoia*, developing late in life, particularly at the involutional period.

**paranoia, affect-laden**  In Leonhard's classification, a subtype of nonsystematic schizophrenia characterized by paranoid delusions and strong affective reaction to their content.

**paranoia, intermediate**  *Obs.* Paranoia in which there are no delusions, but a tendency to quibbling or quarreling. See *paranoia querulans*.

**paranoia, negative**  Paranoia in which the false beliefs concern matters *favorable* to the person rather than with *unfavorable matters*. The delusional material is characterized by praise, protection, and defense instead of persecution, accusation, destruction, and the like.

**paranoia querulans**  A form of paranoia characterized by more or less incessant quarrelsomeness due to alleged persecution. Often starting from a factual injustice, the patient weaves a delusional trend about it and then seeks redress at the hands of the law.

**paranoia senilis**  A paranoid syndrome appearing during old age; late *paraphrenia*. "The forms showing a clear sensorium with delusional formation and eventually hallucinations are designated as *senile paranoia* (i.e., paranoid forms of dementia senilis); they are not frequent. Such people think they are spied on by neighbors, teased, robbed especially by those living in the same house; everywhere they find reference to themselves, and confirmation of their ideas in voices, etc." (Bleuler, E. *Textbook of Psychiatry*, 1930).

**paranoiac character**  Paranoid personality; in this personality type, projection mechanisms are foremost, in that the subject constantly blames the environment for his difficulties. Moreover, he generally has greatest trouble in getting along with members of his own sex. The paranoiac usually superimposes his false claims on some real circumstances in the environment, thus giving some degree of plausibility to his almost delusional formations.

**paranoid (paranoidal)**  Relating to or resembling paranoia. *Paranoid states* (delusional states) were termed *paraphrenia* by Kraepelin. He divided the group into four parts: (1) *paraphrenia systematica*, the equivalent perhaps of what today is known as paranoia; (2) *paraphrenia expansiva*, seen only in women and characterized by ideas of grandeur with exaltation; (3) *paraphrenia confabulans*, characterized by delusions of persecution and grandeur based upon falsification of memory; and (4) *paraphrenia phantastica*, with auditory hallucinations, unsystematized delusions, and phantastic accounts of adventures.

**paranoid climacteric psychosis**  See *schizophrenia, late-onset*.

**paranoid dementia gravis**  See *dementia paranoides gravis*.

**paranoid disorders**  Delusional disorders; see *paranoia*.

**paranoid involutional psychosis**  See *late-onset schizophrenia*.

**paranoid look**  The facial appearance of a paranoid schizophrenic when he thinks about certain of his complexes. The patient appears to be watching or talking to someone, even though he may deny doing so.

**paranoid melancholia**   Depression with an admixture of paranoid elements, usually persecutory in nature; *involutional melancholia* (q.v.).

**paranoid personality (disorder)**   Like narcissistic personality, paranoid personalities typically present a facade of cold grandiosity, arrogance, pride, and a sense of entitlement. They seem bent on demonstrating their power and superiority in interpersonal relationships; they must always be right or prove others to be in the wrong. Affect is restricted; they appear cold and unfeeling, showing little empathy toward others, whom they concomitantly envy and devalue.

Characteristic is a pervasive mistust and suspiciousness of others, with guardedness and a reluctance to confide in anyone. They search for hidden motives and demean the intentions of others; they are hypervigilant and cannot relax with others, expecting to be tricked or cheated. This extends to the sexual partner, whose fidelity they doubt and question. See *conjugal paranoia; jealousy, morbid; projection.*

Cognition is acute, but biased. They are quick to take offense, they blame others for anything that goes wrong, and they are often picayune, querulous, or litigious. They harbor grudges; they show a lack of humor about themselves and take themselves too seriously ("They can dish it out but cannot take it themselves").

Often, the opposite-sex parent of such patients is domineering, overprotective, and ambivalent, while the same-sex parent is submissive, passive, and relatively unavailable as a suitable model or object for identification. In other cases, the same-sex parent has instilled feelings of inadequacy by intimidation, hostility, and the imposition of rigid controls. As a result of such rearing, the child fails to develop a stable self-image, gender role, or clear ego boundaries. He then may find it necessary to surrender to the omnipotent parent in a passive, more or less homosexual way; or he may resist and rebel defensively, but the necessary hypervigilance in his defensive operations may progress to ideas of reference.

**paranoid schizophrenia**   One of the chronic forms of schizophrenia. In addition to the fundamental schizophrenic symptoms, the paranoid type shows the following features: a feeling that external reality has changed and somehow become different; suspiciousness and ideas of dedication; ideas of reference; hallucinations, especially of body sensations; delusions of persecution or of grandiosity. Some paranoid schizophrenics may act in accord with their delusions and turn on their tormentors, while others may become suicidal in an attempt to escape their persecutors.

Several types of paranoid schizophrenia are recognized: litigious, depressed, persecutory, grandiose, erotomaniacal, etc. In general, paranoid forms of schizophrenia develop later than do the other forms, the highest incidence being between the ages of 30 and 35. In contrast to paranoia (q.v.), in paranoid schizophrenia the delusions are multiple, less highly systematized, changeable, illogical, and bizarre.

**paranoid state**   Like *paranoia* (q.v.), the paranoid (delusional) state is characterized by persistent persecutory or grandiose delusions, affect in harmony with the delusional ideas, and preservation of intellectual functions but, ordinarily, an absence of hallucinations. This condition is differentiated from paranoia by its lack of extreme systematization, and from schizophrenia by its lack of fragmentation of associations and the absence of bizarre incongruities.

**paranoid-hallucinatory psychosis in involutional age**   See *late-onset schizophrenia.*

**paranoid-schizoid position**   One of the stages in mental development hypothesized by Melanie Klein. It has its origins in the first 3 months of life and is based heavily upon *primary splitting* as a defense and as a way of organizing experience. The infant's early phantasy is of a perfect picture of the mother's breast, based on early splitting, idealization, and denial by the baby in order to escape from frustrations and persecutions coming from inside or outside. This interaction of internal and external reality creates what Klein called the *internal world* and the *internal objects.*

The anxieties at this period are mainly of a paranoid kind that aim to protect the child from his internal and external persecutors and his fears of annihilation and fragmentation when the death drive takes over (a more realistic perception and evaluation of internal and external reality will come in the depressive position).

In order to survive, the baby has to split the unconscious phantasies and anxieties related to its drives into absolutely good and bad, absolutely persecutory and gratifying breast, and so on. Loving and hating the same object, however, generate intolerable anxiety, which is handled by projecting them outside (projective identification, creating the *good object* and the *bad object*), and then introjecting them again (*introjective identification*—the *good self* and the *bad self*). The inner world is made up of idealized good objects and separated persecuting bad objects. See *projective identification.*

The baby projects not only oral sadistic but also anal sadistic and urethral sadistic impulses in fantasy "in" to the mother's breast and body. Insofar as the mother comes to contain the bad parts of the self, she is not felt to be a separate individual but is now felt to be the bad self. This is what Klein means by projective identification. If the negative projective identifications are excessive and continuous, the object becomes massively attacked, destroyed, or constantly controlled. If the positive projective identifications are too massive, the ego becomes too weak, too dependent on the external object that becomes its ideal ego. In both cases, the result can be a permanent object relationship based on narcissistic traits, what Kleinians call a *narcissistic organization.*

The paranoid-schizoid position is normally succeeded by the depressive position. See *depressive position.*

**paranomasia**  Altering the name, especially to make a play on words that sound alike, such as "In Las Vegas, a pair of dice is Paradise."

**paranormal**  Alongside or beyond the normal, as in paranormal cognition (telepathy). See *extrasensory perception.*

**paranosic**  Relating to the primary advantage derived from an illness or paranosis. See *epinosic gain.*

**parapathic proviso**  Stekel's term for a compromise or bargain that the neurotic makes with his illness—e.g., the patient who thinks that as long as he remains ill, his father will not die: it is a "clause," or stipulation with the neurosis in order to justify its existence. Adler referred to this mental mechanism as *junctim*; another name for it is *neurotic proviso.* See *polycratism.*

**parapathy**  Stekel's term for neurosis; he objects to neurosis because it connotes a functional nervous disorder. Parapathy, on the other hand, indicates that psychiatrists deal with emotions, not with nerves.

**paraphasia**  Perverted speech; most often applied to fluent (expressive) aphasias in which the patient hears and comprehends words but is unable to speak correctly—one syllable is substituted for another (*phonemic paraphrasia*), or one word for another (*verbal* or *semantic* paraphasia), or nonsense sounds (neologisms) replace normal speech (*jargon aphasia*).

Specific types of paraphasic errors have been described: *categorical* (another element of the same class is substituted for the correct word, such as calling a chair a table); *associative* (a particular quality of a more general element is used, such as calling a chair a throne); *asemantic* (the substitute has no meaningful relationship to the correct word, as in calling a chair a racetrack). See *aphasia.*

**paraphemia**  *Rare.* Distorted speech, such as neurotic lisping.

**paraphia**  Impaired sense of touch; tactile insensibility; paresthesia.

**paraphilemia**  Love play, *forepleasure* (q.v.).

**paraphilia**  *Sexual deviation; sexual perversion*; one of the two major groups of *sexual disorders* (q.v.), characterized by sexual arousal to unconventional stimuli that are not considered to be part of normal sexual arousal patterns. The response is also likely to interfere with the capacity for affectionate, reciprocal interchange in sexual activity. Typically, the subject has intense, recurrent or enduring sexual urges or sexually arousing phantasies involving either nonhuman objects, suffering and humiliation of the self or the partner, or children or other nonconsenting persons. The paraphiliac may act on the urges or, more commonly, he masturbates or has intercourse while imagining that he is carrying out his desires. Sometimes he is markedly distressed by the nature of his desires (and some diagnostic systems require that the subject suffers such distress or acts on his urges). The urges may occur only episodically (even though many definitions imply that they are always essential for full sexual gratification).

Like *impulse control disorders* (q.v.), enactment of the paraphilia generally occurs only if there is a mixture of opportunity with conditions that allow the person to rationalize his action to some degree and, often, concomitant use of alcohol or other drugs.

In over half the cases, paraphilias have their onset before the age of 18 years. The average

age of onset is lowest for transvestitism (13.6 years) and fetishism (16.0 years), highest for incestuous pedophilia involving boys (23.5 years) and incestuous pedophilia involving girls (27.1 years). It is typical that a paraphiliac has more than one paraphilia; paraphiliacs with a primary diagnosis of sadism, public masturbation, male incest pedophilia, and fetishism are particularly likely to have secondary diagnoses of other paraphilias. In contrast, ego-dystonic homosexuality, obscene mailing, and transsexualism are unlikely to carry a secondary diagnosis of another paraphilia. Some paraphilias, including urolagnia, coprophilia, and osphresiolagnia, almost never occur as a primary diagnosis.

It is also typical that the victims of any one paraphiliac are as different as they are alike. Recent studies cast doubt on the older assumption that a paraphiliac tended to confine his sexual activities or desires to one kind of victim. Many paraphiliacs cross the touching vs. nontouching boundary, the male victim vs. female victim boundary, the family victim vs. the nonfamily victim boundary, and age boundaries (i.e., one paraphiliac may become involved with child victims, with adolescent victims, and with adult victims). (Abel, G. and Osborn, C. *Psychiatric Clinics of North America*, September 1992).

Men appear to be more frequently affected, perhaps twice as many as women, and some paraphilias (e.g., exhibitionism, fetishism, and voyeurism) are almost exclusively male disorders. In general, the paraphilias are as unresponsive to treatment as they are to punishment or incarceration.

Among the paraphilias are *coprophilia*; *exhibitionism*; fetishism; *frotteurism; pedophilia*; sexual *masochism*; sexual *sadism*; *voyeurism*; transvestic fetishism; *telephone scatologia; necrophilia; partialism; zoophilia; klismaphilia*; and *urophilia* (qq.v.). See *fetish; transvestitism.*

John Money believes that the paraphilias are determined by the time the child is between 5 and 8 years of age and are related to traumatic family and social experiences. Physical or sexual abuse or neglect, for example, may disrupt the link between romantic love and sexual lust. Lust is then combined with a ritual or act that negates love and may even invite punishment. Money identifies six major categories of paraphilia (*Lovemaps*, 1986):

1. Sacrifice and expiation—lust can be expressed on condition that the subject atone for it or that the partner be sacrificed through sadistic acts.

2. Marauding and predation—lust is permitted only if it is stolen or imposed by force.

3. Mercantile and venal—lust is permitted only if it is traded or purchased (from a prostitute or hustler, for example).

4. Fetishes and talismans—lust is expressed through a token that is a substitute for the lover.

5. Stigmata and eligibility—lust is permitted only if the partner is not of one's social set, e.g., of another race, religion or age, or is in some way handicapped or defective.

6. Solicitation and allure—foreplay (such as exhibitionism, voyeurism, or pornography) is substituted for the actual act of copulation.

**paraphilic coercive disorder**   Suggested, but ultimately rejected by DSM-III-R, to refer to a paraphilia characterized by intense urges and sexually arousing phantasies whose main theme is forcing a nonconsenting person to submit to sexual contact (such as oral, vaginal, or anal penetration or grabbing a woman's breast). Paraphilic rapism was also rejected, as a term for this disorder. It was differentiated from sexual sadism in that the arousing element is coercion rather than signs of psychological or physical suffering in the victim.

**paraphrasia**   Irregularity in construction of phrases, a speech disorder of a less severe nature than *aphrasia* (q.v.) from which it differs in degree, but not in kind. It occurs frequently in the schizophrenias. A patient wishing to refer to a certain person says "Saturday" instead; it was on a Saturday that a particularly intense encounter took place between the patient and the person in question. "We shall have to keep apart two chief forms of paraphrasic disorders; firstly, *derailments in finding words*, secondly, *disorders in connected speech*" (Kraepelin, E. *Dementia Praecox*, 1919).

**paraphrasia, thematic**   Arndt's term for incoherent speech "wandering" from the theme or subject.

**paraphrasia vesana**   *Obs.* "If the formation of ideas and of thought is disturbed in its whole extent, so that it is only with difficulty that a single proper judgment can be expressed, and if new words are coined to express the imperfect and strange thoughts, such neologisms being but maimed fragments of regular words, veritably heaps of syllables, then we have *paraphrasia vesana*, an effect of profound psychic decadence" (Bianchi, L. *A Text-Book of Psychiatry*, 1906).

**paraphrenia** Kraepelin (1919) characterized paraphrenia as an insidious development of an ever-worsening paranoia (including grandiose delusions in many patients in the later stages of the disorder), with minimal disturbance of affect and will and preservation of the personality, but without progression to insanity (deterioration). W. Mayer (1921) found that of 78 cases diagnosed as paraphrenia by Kraepelin, 50 later developed a clear diagnosis of dementia praecox. Krapelin then abandoned the distinction between paraphrenia and schizophrenia. See *paranoia*.

*Involutional paranoia* was described by K. Kleist (1913); it affected mostly women aged 40 to 50 years and appeared to be an exacerbation of a "hyperparanoic" prepsychotic personality. Similar manifestations were called by others *presenile paraphrenia, involutional paraphrenia*, and *stiffening involutional psychosis* (erstarrende Rückbildungspsychose, W. Medow, 1922). In such patients, paranoid symptoms are highly systematized, typically revolving about the delusions that neighbors are trying to steal her money, or the erotic delusions that someone is in love with her or is about to marry her. Many such patients have severe defects of hearing or, less commonly, of vision.

M. Roth (1955) proposed the term *late paraphrenia* for patients with a well-organized system of paranoid delusions, with or without hallucinations, but with well-preserved affect and personality. In 1961, D. Kay and Roth suggested that late paraphrenia be regarded as the mode of manifestation of schizophrenia in old age. Contrary to Roth's original phenomenological description, most British psychiatrists regarded onset after age 60 as an obligatory diagnostic criterion. To counter the confusion in the use of "late paraphrenia," F. Post (1966) suggested that the term be replaced by "persistent persecutory states of late life."

Currently, in ICD, paraphrenia is included in the group of paranoid states, and no age limit is specified. It is now generally recognized that late paraphrenia is a heterogeneous group

of diseases that includes paranoid and organic psychoses as well as some cases of schizophrenia with very late onset. See *late-onset schizophrenia*.

**parapithymia** Perverted desire or craving.

**paraplegia** Paralysis of the musculature of the lower extremities and of the torso, the latter to a lesser extent; when the upper extremities are paralyzed, the condition is called *superior paraplegia*.

**paraplegia, ataxic** Unsteadiness of station and gait in association with paraplegia.

**parapraxis** Misaction. Freud applies this term to symptomatic acts, such as slips of the tongue and mislaying of objects.

**parapsychology** The branch of psychology that deals with paranormal behavior and events, such as telepathy, precognition, and clairvoyance, that are not explicable by present-day "natural" laws. See *extrasensory perception*.

**parapsychosis** See *apsychosis*.

**parareaction** Abnormal reaction; specifically, overreaction to a situation followed by elaboration of its importance to a delusional degree. A person trips and falls to the floor and seems unduly embarrassed when helped to his feet; he refers to the incident repeatedly throughout the evening, and when seen again a day or two later cites it as evidence that his host is plotting to discredit him and have him discharged from his job. See *sensitiver Beziehungswahn*.

**parasexuality** Abnormal sexuality, comprising such paraphilias as pederasty, voyeurism, pedophilia, sodomy, sadism, and masochism. "The various kinds of parasexuality are usually connected with a premature appearance of the sex impulse and hence can become known very early, at the age of three or four" (Bleuler, E. *Textbook of Psychiatry*, 1930). See *paraphilia; perversion*.

**parasitism** See *symbiosis*.

**parasitophobia** *Acarophobia*; chronic tactile hallucinosis; *delusion of infestation*; delusion of parasitosis; the unfounded belief that one is infested by live animals, such as insects or parasites. Attempts to dig the "bugs" out of the skin typically produce irregular, linear excoriations that often become infected secondarily. Sometimes the delusion appears to be a part of an obsessional, depressive, or schizophrenic disorder, but it is also seen in organic psychoses and sometimes in association with vitamin deficiencies or as a complication of therapy with phenelzine (e.g., in some cases of hysteroid dysphoria).

Parasitophobia occurs most frequently in middle-aged or elderly women. In over 10% of cases the syndrome is induced; as many as one of every five subjects with the syndrome gives rise to one or more secondary cases. (See *induced psychosis.*) It is generally considered to be a delusion (the cognitive view)—a form of *monosymptomatic hypochondriacal psychosis* (q.v.)—although some classify it as a chronic hallucinosis (the sensorialist view). Pimozide, a dopamine-blocking agent used in Gilles de la Tourette syndrome, has been reported to be effective in reducing or eliminating parasitophobia. See *Morgellons disease.*

**parasomnia** 1. Perverted or disordered sleep. The parasomnias, one group of *sleep disorders*, include *nightmare* disorder, *sleep terror disorder*, and sleepwalking disorder or *somnambulism* (qq.v.).

2. Less commonly, coma vigil; see *akinetic mutism.*

3. Rarely, unconsciousness due to trauma.

**parastriate lobule**  See *occipital lobe.*

**parasuicide**  Attempted suicide; suicidal gesture. See *attempted suicide; deliberate self-harm syndrome.*

**parasympathetic nervous system**  *PNS*; see *autonomic nervous system.*

**parasympathicotonia**  Originally, in constitutional medicine, hyperirritability of the entire parasympathetic system; it has become identical with *vagotonia* since the latter's meaning has been stretched to cover the entire parasympathetic system.

**parasympatholytic**  See *antimuscarinic; cholinergic; mydriasis.*

**parasympathomimetic**  See *anticholinesterase; cholinergic.*

**parataxic distortion**  Any attitude toward any other person that is based on a phantasized or distorted evaluation of that person or on an identification of that person with other figures from past life.

Freud defined *transference* (q.v.) as a repetition of the attitude toward the parents at the time of the Oedipus complex. Almost invariably in the course of analysis, the patient begins to concern himself with the analyst in terms of these transferred attitudes. Some classical analysts would confine the term transference to this original meaning. Others, however, accept character attitudes also as a part of transference, for these, too, are reaction patterns from the past that are applied indiscriminately to the analytic situation, where they are not suitable. In an attempt to avoid confusion, Sullivan has used the term parataxic distortion to include this whole picture. "Sullivan uses neither the libido concept nor the repetition compulsion as formulated by Freud. Parataxic distortions, according to Sullivan, develop from early but essentially nonsexual integrations with significant people. One develops ways of coping with these people and then tends to apply these ways in later interpersonal integrations. However, the need to repeat is by no means as rigid a compulsion as Freud formulated in the repetition compulsion. Later experiences can modify the pattern consciously and unconsciously. In fact, the process of cure is an example of such a modification. The analyst, by his objectivity and insight, fails to conform to the patient's expectations and this, when the patient realizes it, constitutes a new interpersonal situation which helps to make clear the irrational nature of his own behavior" (Thompson, C. *Psychoanalysis: Evolution and Development,* 1950). One way to learn what is true and what is parataxic in thinking or feelings about another is to compare one's evaluations with those of others. Sullivan calls this comparison *consensual validation.*

**parateresiomania**  Morbid impulse to observe; peeping-mania; *scopophilia* (q.v.).

**parathymia**  Abnormality of mood, as when a condition or occasion that should produce a certain mood evokes the opposite of the expected reaction. A patient, having asked for a new suit so that he might enjoy a coming party, was enraged when he received it. Parathymia is one of the affect disturbances seen in the schizophrenias.

**parathyroid disorders**  See *hyperparathyroidism; hypoparathyroidism.*

**paratonia**  Any abnormality of muscle tension or tone, often a manifestation of catatonia. *Gegenhalten* is a particular form of paratonia consisting of uneven resistance of the limbs to passive movement; its presence suggests frontal lobe dysfunction.

**paratype**  The sum of all external, or *peristatic*, factors acting upon the phenotypical development of an organism or bringing about the individual manifestation of a genetic character. See *biotype.*

**paraurethral glands**    See *G spot*.

**paravariation**    In genetics, *modification* (q.v.).

**paraventricular nucleus**    *PVN*; a nucleus of the *hypothalamus* (q.v.). Its two subdivisions are the *parvocellular PVN (pPVN)* and the *magnocellular PVN (mPVN)*.

**paravermis**    A region on either side of the midline of the *cerebellum* (q.v.) that lies lateral to the vermis and medial to the hemisphere. It contains the cerebellar cortical zones $C_1$, $C_2$, and $C_3$.

**pareidolia**    A type of intense imagery that persists even when the subject looks at a real object in the external environment; image and percept exist side by side, but the image is usually recognized as unreal.

**parenchyma, parenchyme**    The specific or characteristic tissue of an organ or gland, as distinct from the connecting tissue or mesenchymal elements that support that gland. Paresis, for example, is also known as parenchymal syphilis because in this form of syphilis the spirochete invades and destroys nerve cells directly; cerebral syphilis, in contrast, is known as mesenchymal syphilis because it consists primarily of invasion of the arteries and arterioles within the meninges covering the brain and only secondarily does the process attack the cerebral tissue itself.

**parens patriae**    "The State as father"; state paternalism; the obligation of the state to care for its citizens who cannot take care of themselves. The parens patriae power is the basis of involuntary treatment of a patient, not competent to make decisions for himself, to prevent deterioration in his condition (the "need for treatment standard"). See *police power*.

**Parent egostate**    See *transactional analysis*.

**parent therapist program**    A family-based treatment setting that is an alternative to residential treatment for emotionally disturbed children who can neither remain at home nor be managed satisfactorily in the usual foster home. The child is taken into the healthy nuclear family of the parent therapist, who receives support not only from the psychiatrist but also from discussion of experiences with other parent therapists.

**parental alienation syndrome**    *PAS*; a child's denigration and vilification of one parent (the "target" parent), noted most frequently in child-custody disputes. The syndrome is not officially recognized and many child psychiatrists are reluctant to label the manifestations described as a syndrome. It is generally agreed, however, that PAS does not include, and must be differentiated from, a child's reaction to parental abuse.

**parental image, idealized**    See *basic trust*.

**parental investment**    Any investment by the parent in an individual child that increases the child's chance of surviving at the cost of the parent's ability to invest in another offspring. Both the male and the female want to produce children, but someone has to bring up the family. If one of the parents can offload the work onto the other, so much the better from an evolutionary standpoint, since that parent is then free to go on the prowl for another mate with whom it can produce more offspring. As a result, different selective forces are at work, and what we expect (and usually find) is that males tend to want to fertilize many females, while females are more interested in raising those children they already have.

By definition, each sex can produce only the same total number of offspring as the other sex. But it is not necessarily the case that the two sexes in a species will have the same average parental investment per child. As a result, the sex having the greater average parental investment becomes a limiting resource for the other sex. The female's fitness is maximized when she produces X offspring, while the male's fitness is highest when he produces Y offspring. Since Y is greater than X, in this case males compete for females.

**parental investment theory**    See *evolutionary developmental psychology*.

**parental manipulation**    See *kin selection*.

**parental perplexity**    A type of relationship of parents to their children that has been found relatively frequently in schizophrenic families (although it is as yet unclear whether the parental behavior and attitudes are productive of the child's disabilities, or whether it is the primary deviancy of the child that has generated the parental reaction). "This parental atmosphere is characterized by extreme parental indecisiveness, a lack of parental spontaneity and empathy with the child, the parents' inability to sense what the child's needs are and thus an inability to satisfy them at the proper moment, and an unusual absence of control and authority. In this type of unpatterned climate, positive reinforcement of desirable traits and negative reinforcement of undesirable traits are not administered. Instead, the child is left with feelings of confusion and an inclination to respond in a randomized, impoverished, and unpredictable fashion, when more focused, directed behaviors are lacking" (Goldfarb, W. *International Psychiatry Clinics 1*, 1964).

**parentectomy**  Removal of a parent; more specifically, the separation of a child from his parents for therapeutic reasons, as may be advisable in cases of intractable asthma.

**parentified child**  See *depersonification; role reversal.*

**parenting behaviors**  Aggression and related behavior problems are associated with low levels of positive parenting behaviors, such as responsiveness, warmth, social coaching and teaching, and proactive guidance. Some time ago, Hoffman argued that power assertive discipline, such as threats, physical force, and intimidation, would not curtail children's aggressive behavior, but rather would lead to resentment, rebellion, and the increased likelihood of disruptive, oppositional behavior. Families of aggressive children are more negative and disapproving, with high rates of needling, threatening, and other "nattering" behavior, and lower levels of warmth and positive attention. A hallmark of ineffective parenting is lack of consistency in parental response ("indiscriminate"—a style in which few predictable contingencies exist between what the child does and how the parent responds). See *attachment; basic trust; relatedness.*

**parenting failure**  See *empathic failure.*

**parent-transference linking interpretation**  See *brief psychotherapy.*

**parergasia**  Abnormal functioning; mismatched action. Kraepelin used the term to refer to a form of parabulia in which the impulse to carry out an act is interrupted before the patient takes the first step toward performing the act. The interruption is occasioned by what he calls cross impulses, that is, by impulses that cross the path of the first impulse and thus check its further course. The process is also known as *derailment of volition.* For example, a patient who has the impulse to reach for a cup at the table suddenly brushes his hair. "The patient who is to show his tongue, opens his eyes widely instead; he flings the cup away instead of putting it to his mouth" (*Dementia Praecox*, 1919).

This is a psychiatric reaction type characterized usually by deep regression, abandonment of reality, and reconstruction of the conception of the self, and by delusions and hallucinations; this term, coined by Adolf Meyer, refers to schizophrenia and to schizophrenoid syndromes.

**paresis**  Partial paralysis.

**paresis, general**  See *general paresis.*

**paretic curve**  See *Lange colloidal gold reaction.*

**Parham decision**  In the late 1970s the assumption that parents can be expected to act in the best interests of their children in making decisions that involve the children's welfare had been called into doubt. There was also doubt about the assumption that psychiatrists' determinations about the need for hospitalization were made with the child's welfare as the sole concern. In its decision in *Parham v. J.R.* (1979), the Court did not support a strict civil libertarian position, reaffirming instead the appropriateness of traditional family and medical prerogatives. The main features of the decision were as follows:

1. Due process at the point of admission is satisfied by an independent medical evaluation of the need for hospitalization; a judicial hearing is not required.

2. Parents have the right to admit their children to a psychiatric hospital for treatment.

3. The contention that neither parents nor doctors can be trusted to act in the best interests of children in the process of making medical decisions was rejected.

4. The expertise for making medical decisions lies with physicians and is not "the business of judges".

5. There is a danger that formalized fact-finding hearings will intrude significantly upon family relationships and jeopardize the treatment of a child.

6. Periodic review of hospitalization is essential to due process, but the establishment of such procedures was left to the lower courts.

**parietal lobe**  The portion of the cerebral hemisphere that extends from the central sulcus to the parieto-occipital fissure and laterally to the level of the sylvian fissure. The *postcentral gyrus* (areas 3-1-2, the *somesthetic area*, where touch, pain and temperature senses are represented in the contralateral posterior central gyrus), the *supramarginal gyrus*, and the *angular gyrus* are portions of the parietal lobe. The postcentral gyrus receives projections from the relay nuclei of the thalamus; the latter receive the great ascending somatosensory tracts of the spinal cord and the trigeminal lemniscus. Areas 5 and 7, which make up the posterior parietal lobule, are sensory association areas. Proprioception, stereognosis, and graphesthesis are represented in the secondary cortex in the contralateral parietal lobe just caudal to the posterior central gyrus.

Touch, pain, and temperature senses are represented in the primary cortex in the contralateral posterior central gyrus. The secondary cortex, immediately caudal to the primary cortex, represents proprioception, stereognosis, and graphesthesia.

Experimental studies indicate that the body surface is projected dermatome by dermatome on the postcentral gyrus. It appears that taste is also a function of the sensorimotor area and is localized at the inferior end of the lobe, possibly on the opercular surface of the sylvian fissure.

The dominant parietal lobe coordinates visual and language functions: reading (*lexic function*), writing (*graphic function*), parietal lobe language functions (*verbal memory*), *kinesthetic praxis*, ideokinetic (*ideomotor*) *praxis*, *finger gnosis*, calculation, right-left orientation, symbolic categorization, *graphesthesis*, and *stereoagnosis* (qq.v.). The nondominant parietal lobe coordinates motor, sensory, and spatial perception: awareness of one's body in space; ability to recognize and be familiar with objects and people (such as the ability to identify faces); and the ability to copy the outline of simple objects. See *intraparietal sulcus*.

**parietal lobe dysfunction** Strokes, tumors, or injuries, especially to the right half of the brain, tend to cause a partial or total annihilation of the left side, variously known as imperception, inattention, *neglect*, and *agnosia*. All are experiences of nothingness or, more precisely, privations of the experience of somethingness. *Neglect syndromes* are observed with right hemisphere lesions in at least five different areas of the brain: the prefrontal convexity, the inferior parietal lobule, the cingulate gyrus, the thalamus, and the hypothalamus. Manifestations of neglect include the following:

1. Attentional defects
2. Nonrecognition (sometimes delusional) of serious medical disability (*anosognosia*) or

of the left side of one's body or of objects in the left visual field (*left spatial nonrecognition*). Denial of left-sided paralysis—one form of anosognosia—is almost always a result of disease in the right hemisphere, particularly in the parietal region, which is thought to be responsible for the body schema. The patient ignores events on the opposite side of the body: a woman may apply makeup to the right side of her face while ignoring the left, the subject may ignore the food on one side of the plate; the man may shave only one side of his face; when writing, he may squeeze all the sentences to one side of the page; the patient may bump into objects on the left, or read only the right side of printed materials.

It has generally been believed that *spatial neglect* (q.v.) is associated with lesions of the right inferior parietal lobule and the *TPO junction* (the area between the temporal, parietal, and occipital lobes. Recent studies, however, have localized spatial neglect to the rostral portions of the right superior temporal gyrus (*STG*). See *temporal lobe*.

The parietal lobe is involved in other kinds of visuospatial functions; it organizes and controls visuomotor acts for processes such as reaching in space, grasping of objects, performing saccadic and pursuit eye movements, and whole body locomotion (Karnath, H. O. *Nature Neuroscience 1*, 2001). Patients with neglect fail to orient themselves towards or to detect items on their contralesional side, even though they are not blind to stimuli on that side. Neglect can be so profound that they are unaware of people or large objects in contralesional space. They might neglect their own contralesional body parts. They can be unaware that they have any of these problems (anosoagnosia). In one study, two-thirds of patients with either a left- or right-sided hemisphere stroke suffered from neglect when assessed within 3 days of being admitted to hospital.

Neglect is more likely to be enduring in patients with right-hemisphere damage, with long-term difficulties on their left with everyday tasks, such as bathing, grooming, dressing, eating, reading, and social interactions. Neglect is most common after damage to regions that receive blood from the middle cerebral artery. The right temporo-parietal junction is the most common substrate of neglect. However, most neglect patients have extensive brain damage, with lesions spanning a number of functionally distinct regions. One study found that the superior temporal gyrus rather that the TPI is the critical site. Frontal neglect is associated with damage to the inferior and middle frontal gyri. The zone of maximum overlap of lesions appears to center on ventral premotor cortex in a region homologous to Broca's area in the left hemisphere, although damage is usually more widespread.

Much of the research into neglect has focused on its lateralized spatial presentation. Recent investigations have also revealed deficits that are not necessarily worse towards one side of space; that is, they are non-lateralized (Husain, M. & Rorden, C, *Nature Reviews Neuroscience 4*: 27–36, January 2002).

3. Nonrecognition of familiar people and faces (*prosopagnosia*). An extension of this is accusing one or more familiar persons, usually family members, of being an impostor (*Capgras delusion*). The opposite is the *Fregoli phenomenon*: the subject thinks other persons not well known to him are very familiar.

4. *Doppelganger phenomenon—reduplicative paramnesia*: the delusion that the duplicate of a person or place exists elsewhere.

5. *Paragnosia*—wild guessing as to whereabouts; typically, a subject with normal global orientation cannot say where he is but when asked makes a series of wild guesses.

6. The first-rank symptom of the experience of *alienation*: that body parts or thoughts do not belong to the subject; things look confused, jumbled; cannot find way along previously familiar routes; body feels different, e.g., an arm or leg feels heavy or bigger; uncertainty about the location of an arm or leg.

7. Constructional difficulties, dressing dyspraxia, contralteral sensory and motor deficits.

Dominant lesions often produce language disorders, dyscalculia, dyspraxias or apraxia (impairment of skilled movements in the absence of elementary sensory or motor deficits), difficulties in spatially related abstraction, contralateral sensory deficits (*graphesthesia, asteroagnosis*), motor deficits (hypotonia, posturing, paucity of movement). The best known of these lesions is the *Gerstmann syndrome*: dysgraphia, dyscalculia, right-left disorientation, and finger agnosia.

Nondominant parietal lesions produce denial of illness, left-sided spatial neglect, constructional difficulties, dressing dyspraxia, contralateral sensory and motor deficits, Capgras syndrome, and first-rank symptom of experience of alienation.

The parietal cortex might be important for storing or accessing motor representations, or both. Patients with lesions restricted to the parietal cortex are selectively impaired at predicting, through mental imagery, the time necessary to perform differentiated finger movements and visually guided point gestures. This suggests that the parietal cortex is important for the ability to generate mental movement representations. How it affects that ability is unknown. See *intraparietal sulcus*.

**parieto-temporal-occipital association cortex**   See *association areas; parietal lobe; temporal lobe*.

**Parinaud syndrome**   Paralysis of upward conjugate gaze, without paralysis of convergence. It is due to compression of the superior colliculi in the midbrain, sometimes caused by a pineal tumor.

**parkin**   An E3 ubiquitin ligase involved in the degradation of several substrates. The mutation of the parkin gene in *ARJP* (autosomal recessive, juvenile-onset Parkinson disease) abolishes the activity of the enzyme and results in the death of nigral dopamine neurons without Lewy bodies.

**Parkinson disease (PD)**   The most common form of parkinsonism, accounting for approximately 75% of all cases; an age-dependent neurodegenerative disorder characterized clinically by resting tremor, rigidity, bradykinesia, gait dysfunction, and postural instability. Often there are disturbances in other nonmotor spheres of neurologic function, such as cognitive, psychiatric, and autonomic changes. It affects all races and both genders, with a slight predominance in men. Incidence is about 20 cases/100,000 inhabitants per year.

Pathologically, PD is characterized by preferential degeneration of melanin-containing neurons in the substantia nigra pars compacta (*SNc*) and by the intracytoplasmic accumulation of proteinaceous inclusions— *Lewy bodies* (q.v.)—found mostly in the brain stem and diencephalon. The melanin-containing neurons produce dopamine (DA) and project to the striatum (putamen and caudate).

Major manifestations of PD include the following:

1. *Cognitive features*: The most consistent impairments are in visuospatial ability, memory, and *executive functions* (q.v.). *Bradyphrenia* is reduced speed of cognitive processes. Dementia develops in 20–40% of cases. New research suggests that the majority of PD sufferers will develop dementia, typically occurring 10 years or more after onset of motor symptoms. It typically progresses to a clinical and pathological end-point indistinguishable from *Lewy body dementia* (q.v.).

   Mutations in at least four genes have been linked to PD, including a-synuclein (*PARK1* and *PARK4*), parkin (*PARK2*), DJ1 (*PARK7*), and PTEN (phosphatase and tensin homolog deleted on chromosome 10)-induced kinase 1 (*PINK1*, also known as *PARK6*). *PARK1* (a-synuclein) mutations are autosomal dominant; they are believed to result in increased oxidative stress, mitochondrial injury, and altered cellular transport. Parkin mutations are found in juvenile PD and are inherited as autosomal recessive. *PINK1* mutations are linked to early-onset PD.

2. *Motor symptoms*:
   a. Tremor—the classical form is rest tremor with frequency in the range of 4–7 Hz; typically it appears as a *pill-rolling tremor* of the hands.
   b. *Akinesia,* with slowness of initiation and execution (*bradykinesia*), decreased amplitude of movements, and fatigability.
   c. Gait is shuffling, with short steps and decreased arm swing, and may become progressively faster as the patient continues to walk (*festination*). Handwriting becomes more irregular and progressively smaller (*micrographia*). There is loss of facial expression, and blinking is reduced.
   d. Rigidity—clasically, there is an intermittent and rhythmic short-duration "release" of the rigidity during passive movement (*cog wheel rigidity).*
   e. Postural abnormalities—neck and trunk are bent forward, the arms slightly flexed at the elbows, flexion at the metacarpophalangeal joints, and slight flexion of the knees.
   f. *Motor arrests (freezing phenomenon)*—first appear as difficulty in initiating walking. Later, the patient may suddenly appear to be frozen or glued to the floor.

3. *Depression* occurs in 4–70%, with sleep disturbances, loss of self-esteem, anxiety, and suicidal thoughts.

**Parkinson disease, hereditary** Most cases of PD are sporadic, but about 10% have an inheritance pattern consistent with autosomal dominant transmission. Several mutations associated with familial PD have been identified in the genes that encode α-*synuclein* (q.v.), parkin, PINK1, DJ1, and LRRK2. Overexpression of mutant α-synuclein sensitizes neurons to oxidative stress and to damage by dopamine or mitochondrial toxins. Loss of parkin function might render dopaminergic neurons sensitive to neurotoxins. DJ1 has been implicated in the regulation of apoptosis. Both PINK1 and LRRK2 mutations may disrupt kinase activity. For the much more common sporadic (i.e., nonhereditary) Parkinson disease, aging is the greatest factor, and oxidative stress is a major cellular pathway in the aging process.

The α-synuclein gene has been localized to chromosome 4. It has also been hypothesized that the mutation causes α-synuclein to misfold. It might then produce abnormal deposits in the brain, much as accumulation of β amyloid may contribute to nerve degeneration in Alzheimer disease.

**Parkinson disease model** The most widely known model is based on the use of the pro-toxin MPTP (N-methyl-4-phenyl-1,2,3, 6-tetrahydropyridine) and its metabolite MPP+ (1-methyl-4-pyridium) to simulate Parkinson disease. In that model, however, some aspects of the human disease are not produced, including development of fibrillar cytoplasmic inclusions (Lewy bodies) containing ubiquitin and α-synuclein. The pesticide rotenone may provide a more satisfactory model. In rats it produces a highly selective degeneration of dopamine neurons of the nigrostriatal system and leads to hypokinesia and rigidity. The damaged nigral neurons accumulate fibrillar cytoplasmic inclusions that contain ubiquitin and α-synuclein.

**parkinsonian triad** Tremor, muscular rigidity, and bradykinesia. See *Parkinson disease.*

**parkinsonism**   A clinical condition characterized by the symptoms of *Parkinson disease* (q.v.). The term includes both idiopathic Parkinson disease and extrapyramidal symptoms (EPS) due to all other causes, including medication.

**parkinsonism, atypical**   Parkinsonism that is not responsive to treatment with levodopa.

**parkinsonism-dementia of Guam**   A degenerative disease of unknown etiology, limited to the Chamorro-speaking people of Guam and the Mariana Islands, similar clinically, pathologically, and biochemically to Parkinson disease. It usually responds favorably to treatment with levodopa.

**parkinsonism-plus**   Originally used to refer to a subtype of secondary parkinsonism, then to refer to the range of neurologic or even systemic abnormalities that can occur in association with progressive external opthalmoplegia. Currently, the term generally includes neurodegenerative diseases beginning between the 5th and 7th decades and possessing the following clinical features: an incomplete parkinsonian syndrome (without tremor) and neurologic manifestations such as cognitive, pyramidal, cerebellar, autonomic, peripheral, or disordered oculomotor functions. The most common conditions misidentified as Parkinson disease are progressive supranuclear palsy and multiple system atrophy.

**parlor dementia**   *Higher dementia* (q.v.).

**parole**   A system of supervision of a patient who is away from the hospital or any of its adjuncts—such as colonies—prior to his legal discharge. While on parole, a patient is considered as still on the books of the hospital, and may, if necessary, be returned to the hospital without the necessity for formal court action.

**paroniria**   Abnormal dreaming; sleep disturbance.

**paroptosis**   A form of programmed cell death that does not require activation of caspases; it produces different changes in cell morphology from those usually associated with *apoptosis* (q.v.).

**parorexia**   Abnormal appetite, dysorexia. See *eating disorders*.

**parosmia**   Any disturbance of the sense of smell, whether organic or psychic in origin; the term includes osphresiolagnia, osphresiophilia, and olfactory hallucinations.

**parosphresis**   *Parosmia* (q.v.).

**paroxysmal**   See *transient*.

**paroxysmal anxiety**   *Panic disorder* (q.v.).

**paroxysmal cerebral dysrhythmia**   *Epilepsy* (q.v.).

**paroxysmal drinking**   See *alcoholism*.

**paroxysmal hemicrania**   See *cluster headache*.

**Parry-Romberg syndrome**   See *hemiatrophy, facial*.

**PARs**   Proteinase-activated receptors. See *proteinase*.

**pars pro toto**   (L. "part for the whole") In psychiatry, a special form of displacement in which part of an object or person stands for the whole object or person. A voice, a gesture, some physical trait, a bit of wearing apparel—each may be substituted for the total person.

**parser**   See *mentalese*.

**parthenophobia**   Fear of girls.

**partial adjustments**   Sullivan's term for the schizophrenic person's defensive maneuvers that are aimed at reducing environmentally generated stress during the period immediately preceding an acute psychotic episode. These include *compensatory activities* (substitution of simpler activities for more complex ones), *sublimatory activities* (roundabout but socially acceptable ways of achieving some degree of satisfaction in an environment where direct pursuit of a goal generates intolerable anxiety), and defense reactions (complex activities and phantasies that no longer maintain conformity with social standards; e.g., evasions, rationalizations, projection, negativism, hypochondriasis).

**partial aversion**   *Antifetishism* (q.v.).

**partial hospitalization**   All forms of inpatient treatment other than full, 24-hour programs; includes *day hospital* (q.v.), night hospital, weekend hospital. See *community psychiatry*.

**partial impulse**   See *component impulse*.

**partial insanity**   An outdated medicolegal expression, sometimes synonymous with monomania; it was so regarded in the M'Naghten case. It is also defined as a borderline type of mental unsoundness. See *insanity defense; criminal responsibility*.

Partial insanity "means a mental impairment which is not so complete as to render its victim irresponsible for his criminal acts." The law speaks of 'limited responsibility' [in regard to] (1) cases in which, though there is evidence of mental disorder which probably was a contributing cause in the criminal conduct, the disorder is not of such a type as to come within the legal test, so as to render the person irresponsible; (2) cases in which, by reason of mental disorder, the person was incapable of deliberation, premeditation, malice, or other mental state usually made a requisite for first degree offenses, and in which, therefore, a lesser offense than that charged was in fact committed" (Weihofen, H. *Insanity as a Defense in Criminal Law*, 1933).

**partial instinct**   Part instinct. See *component impulse*.

**partial reinforcement**   See *reinforcement schedule*.

**partialism**   A *paraphilia* (q.v.) in which the subject seeks gratification of the sexual impulse from a certain part of the partner's body—the leg, thigh, buttock, and so on. Partialism must be differentiated from fetishism, in which the partner is eliminated and displaced by an object symbolic of the genitals.

**partialism, persistent**   Failure to gain genital primacy; continuation of part-object relations because development has been arrested before whole-object relations have been attained (see *genitality*). One form of partialism is expressed sexually (see *fetish; partialism*). Another form is expressed as a type of personality disorder, characterized by fixation at the depressive position, inability to work through separations and losses, vacillating or short-lived relationships, and a feeling of being incomplete or flawed. See *"as-if" personality; basic fault; genitality*.

**partiality, multilateral**   A part of the process of family evaluation and family therapy in which the therapist comes to know each member of the family by being on each one's side. Family members can then feel that the therapist cares about each of them and understands each one's position within the family.

**partiality, sexual**   *Rare.* Fetishism; sexual idolatry.

**participant observer**   In psychoanalysis, the analyst as he is viewed by those who feel that he must be something more than an authoritarian sounding board or a mirror in which the patient's problems are reflected. Although the therapist must be objective, he also takes active part in the interpersonal process of therapy. The so-called cultural interpersonal school of psychoanalysis particularly emphasizes the participant role of the analyst. See *interpersonal process*.

**party drug**   See *date rape drug*.

**PAS**   Physical Anhedonia Scale.

**passive analysis**   Stekel used this expression to describe the feature of Freudian psychoanalysis that calls on the psychiatrist to wait patiently for the production of free associations by the subject and subsequently to interpret them without active intervention.

**passive tremor**   See *tremor*.

**passive-aggressive personality (disorder)**   In DSM-I (1952), one type of *personality trait disturbance* (q.v.), characterized by covert resistance and unresponsiveness to the expectations of others. Sometimes this personality disorder is subdivided into the *passive-dependent*, *passive-aggressive*, and *aggressive* types. Passive-aggressive personality is not recognized as a specific disorder in DSM-IV.

The passive-aggressive person may procrastinate to a degree that no deadline is ever met, no task is ever brought to completion, no assignment is ever executed without prodding or help from others. The person frequently complains that others make unreasonable demands on his or her time and capacities, sulks and pouts when forced to perform (but does not openly refuse), and then works at an unreasonably slow or inefficient pace. His work is characterized by procrastination, dawdling, stubbornness, inefficiency, and forgetfulness.

**passive-dependency**   One of the subtypes of passive-aggressive personality, characterized by helplessness, indecisiveness, and a tendency to cling to others in a parasitic way. See *dependency; oral character; receptive character; personality trait disturbance*.

**passivism**   A form of sexual perversion in which the subject, usually male, is submissive to the will of the partner. See *active; masochism*.

**passivity**   One mode of adaptation. The organism can adapt to its environment by going forward to meet it or backward to escape it. The former is in the mode of activity; the latter is in the mode of passivity.

In transference neurosis, inhibition of activity may find the patient falling into passivity. In traumatic neurosis, however, complete passivity is impossible; one can retreat from an inhibiting person, but complete retreat from the inhibiting forces of the outer world is impossible—short of death.

**past-pointing**   See *pointing*.

**pastoral counseling**   *Caelotherapy*; the application of the principles of mental health by the cleric to the management of the problems presented by those who seek help. Pastoral counseling is a type of supportive or guidance therapy in which the cleric, in the role of interpreter of personal and societal values, attempts to relate the contributions of the behavioral sciences and the resources of religion to the needs of parishioners.

**pastoral psychiatry** The branch of psychiatry related to religion, and particularly to the integration of psychiatry and religion for the purpose of alleviating emotional ailments— the psychotherapeutic role that the clergyman must often play in his relationship to his parishioners. The term includes such things as vocational and marriage counseling. Organized religion as a whole represents centuries of interpersonal experiences that have given pragmatic validation to certain tenets and doctrines. Therefore, when based on these doctrines, advice and other therapeutic measures are often psychologically valid, even though the dynamics as such may not be recognized or understood. And, at least with certain types of patients, the results may be excellent. The many cures at the shrine of Lourdes, France, afford an example of this.

Pastoral psychiatry at the present time is confined largely to reassurance and relief of guilt feelings, affording opportunity for catharsis, and alleviation of anxiety in general by directive and noninterpretive methods. In addition, religion offers the possibility of identification with the omnipotent Father, and engenders reaction formations and sublimation. In certain aspects, organized religion may be likened to group psychotherapy of an educative type. Unlike the latter, however, religion is generally devoid of an understanding of the psychodynamics involved.

**patellar clonus** It is elicited by exending the leg, grasping the patella (knee-cap) between index finger and thumb, and briskly pushing the cap down one or more times. See *clonus*.

**patellar reflex** *Knee jerk* (q.v.); tapping the quadriceps tendon just below the patella of the flexed knee results in extension of the leg with visible and palpable contraction of the quadriceps muscle. The femoral nerve contains both the afferent and the efferent pathways of the patellar reflex, whose spinal center is at $L_{2-4}$. See *suprapatellar reflex*.

The *pendular knee jerk* is seen in cerebellar disease: when the patellar tendon is tapped, several oscillations of the leg occur before it comes to a stop.

**patentable life** See *Chakrabarty*.

**paternalism** A distortion of fatherly or parental behavior in which some moral rule relative to the actions of one person toward another is violated without the consent of that other person. Because a moral rule is violated, the action requires justification, but that is not to say that paternalism is never justified. Paternalistic behavior is based on the belief of the actor, A, that his behavior toward the subject, B, benefits B even though it violates a moral rule and is performed without B's past, present, or immediately forthcoming consent, even though B is competent to give consent. Causing physical or mental pain, lying, cheating, and breaking a promise are the typical violations of moral rules that paternalism involves.

Paternalism is a form of control of one subject or group by another, ordinarily rationalized as an expression of care and concern for the welfare of the group being controlled. Paternalism is not acting like a father; rather, it is an attempt to excuse one's actions as being better for the subject than the choice the subject might make were he not under control or domination. What is done under the label of paternalism is usually a violation of some moral rule, such as giving pain or depriving someone of liberty. Paternalism may, of course be justified or even necessary, but adequate justification for its need depends on the recognition that the action runs counter to a moral rule.

**path cells** See *place cells*.

**path integration** See *place cells*.

**pathergasia** Adolf Meyer's term for personality maladjustment in association with organic, functional, or structural changes. It is approximately equivalent to Ferenczi's *pathoneurosis*.

**pathic** 1. Pertaining to or affected by disease or disorder.

2. *Obs.* A male passive partner who submits to unnatural sexual practices. See *catamite; passivism*.

**patho-, path-** Combining form meaning suffering, passion, disease, from Gr. *pathos*.

**pathobiology** The study of diseased or disordered conditions arising from a biological source.

**pathoclisis** Sensitivity to disease or injury; often used in a more limited sense to refer to sensitivity to certain toxins; sometimes used to refer to the end result of a series of subclinical pathologic insults that, when added together, finally produce clinical manifestations. Some authorities have implicated pathoclisis as the mechanism responsible for most forms of parkinsonism and the senile and presenile dementias. In such a view, a transient viral infection early in life, for example, may produce a clinically undetectable degree of central nervous system damage. In subsequent years, any number of additional subclinical insults—other viral infections, minor head traumata, alcohol and other drugs, arteriosclerosis—gradually drain the system's reserves until a critical point is reached when the neurons remaining intact can no longer maintain normal function.

**pathocure** The disappearance of a neurosis upon the outbreak of an organic disease. Pathocure is seen in moral masochists whose neurosis is first of all, unconsciously, a suffering that pacifies the superego: the neurosis becomes superfluous as soon as it is replaced by another kind of suffering. Pathocure is the opposite of pathoneurosis, which is a neurosis developing as a result of somatic disease.

A pathocure was observed in a masochist who developed pulmonary tuberculosis. The patient had been a chronic failure in everything he undertook. Under analysis, he began to gain some insight into the masochistic nature of his character defenses. Analysis was interrupted by the tuberculous process, and after the patient's release from the hospital he went back to work. He functioned well on his job and previous symptoms did not reappear. The disease in this instance was one especially suitable for the character type of the patient—it was chronic, it necessitated definite limitations of activity, and the likelihood of recurrence was ever present. Other pathocures of a more temporary nature had been observed when the organic disease was short-lived and required no permanent or long-term changes in the patient's way of living. In such cases, neurotic symptoms tend to reappear with the disappearance of the organic condition.

**pathoformic** Referring to the beginning of pathological states, to the symptoms occurring in the transitional stage between health and disease or disorder proper.

**pathogenesis, pathogenesy, pathogeny** The way in which a disease or disorder originated or developed; also called *nosogenesis*.

**pathognomonic, pathognomic** Typical or thoroughly characteristic of a disease; diagnostic.

**pathognomy** The science of recognizing or diagnosing a disease or pathological condition.

**pathognostic** *Pathognom(on)ic* (q.v.).

**pathography** 1. Description of a disease. 2. Study of the effects of any illness on the writer's (or other artist's) life or art, or the effects of an artist's life and personality development on his creative work.

**pathography, psychoanalytic** The use of biography (and especially the biography of a predominantly pathological subject) to expand psychoanalytic knowledge or to demonstrate already existing psychoanalytic knowledge. See *biography in depth*.

**pathohysteria** See *fixation hysteria*.

**pathokinesis** The course, development, or dynamics of an illness.

**pathological gambling** One of the *disorders of impulse control* (q.v.). See *gambling*.

**pathological intoxication** See *alcoholic intoxication*.

**pathology** The study of the nature of diseases.

**pathomimesis, pathomimicry** Mimicry of a disease or disorder; *malingering* (q.v.). See *factitious disorder*.

**pathomorphism** Abnormal morphology such as extremes of bodily build.

**pathoneurosis** See *fixation hysteria*.

**pathophrenesis** Disturbance in the intelligence, regardless of its basis.

**pathophysiology** Study of the development and progress of a disease; the mechanisms by which a disease originates, develops, and progresses. The term implies a consideration not only of the causes of a disease, but also of its consequences and of compensatory responses by the organism.

**pathoplasty** Birnbaum's term for the *form* of a disease, in contradistinction to pathogenesis, which relates to its *cause*.

**pathopsychology** Study of abnormal psychic data from the point of view of general psychology; Wilhelm Specht proposed to restrict the expression to such study from the standpoint of medical psychology.

**pathopsychosis** Organic psychosis. See *fixation hysteria; organic syndrome*.

**pathway variables** See *recidivism*.

**pathways** See *parallel distributed processing*.

**patience** See *time discounting*.

**Patient Placement Criteria** See *ASAM-PPC*.

**patient responsibility** As used clinically, the therapist's assumption of responsibility for the patient—defined operationally in terms of decision making and effective limit setting of five main types of behavior: destructiveness, disorganization, deviancy, dysphoria, and dependency (Sternbach, R.A. et al. *Psychiatry 32*, 1969).

**patient rights**  Those considerations and exercise of decision and judgment to which a patient is ordinarily entitled in a health care setting. In general, patients have the same rights as other citizens, and their rights can be abridged only under certain conditions. See listings under *right to; consumerism; medicalization.*

**patient-government**  Patient participation in the ward administration of a psychiatric hospital; one of the ways of implementing the concept of the psychiatric hospital as a therapeutic community.

**patient-oriented consultation**  See *consultant.*

**Paton, Stewart**  (1865–1942) American psychiatrist and neurologist; wrote first modern textbook of psychiatry in the United States (1905); founded first U.S. university mental health clinic at Princeton (1910).

**patroiophobia**  Fear of heredity, and especially of hereditary disease.

**pattern, expressive**  See *adaptational psychodynamics.*

**pattern, specific dynamic**  Franz Alexander's term for the specific nuclear conflict or dynamic configuration that is unique to a particular psychosomatic disorder or organ neurosis. See *psychosomatic.*

**pattern code**  A mechanism for encoding and transmission of sensory information that depends on different patterns of firing by the nerve or pathway; a relatively uncommitted (i.e., nonspecific) receptor can in this way signal different modalities. This is a less frequent mechanism for modality encoding than the labeled line code.

**pattern recognition receptors (PRRs)**  See *microglia.*

**Pavlov's reflex psychology**  (Ivan Petrovich Pavlov, Russian physiologist, 1849–1936) The theory of human personality development and behavior based on Pavlov's discovery of the conditioned reflex and conditioned or internal inhibition. Mental processes and higher nervous activity were viewed as being identical with the neurophysiologic mechanisms through which they manifested themselves. See *conditioning.*

**Pavlov's theory of schizophrenia**  Pavlov held that the symptoms of schizophrenia are the result of a state of inhibition of the cerebral cortex.

**pavor diurnus**  Fear reactions that occur in the young child during the afternoon nap, similar to night terrors but not so frequent as the latter.

**pavor nocturnus**  *Sleep terror disorder* (q.v.).

**pavor sceleris**  *Scelerophobia*; fear of "bad men"—burglars, kidnappers, etc.

**pay for performance**  See *FFS.*

**PBC**  Pregnancy and birth complication(s), found by some investigators to be more frequent in schizophrenic persons than in nonschizophrenic comparison groups.

**PBD**  *Pediatric bipolar disorder* (q.v.).

**PBN**  N-*tert*-butyl-α-phenyl nitrone, which reacts with free radicals to form a stable nitroxyl product. See *free radical.*

**PCD**  Programmed cell death; cell death that involves active intracellular processes. The most common form of PCD is *apoptosis* (q.v.).

**PCM**  Patient care manager. See *case management; gatekeeper; managed care.*

**PCP**  *Phencyclidine* (q.v.); also *Pneumocystis carinii* pneumonia, a common opportunistic infection in persons with *AIDS* (q.v.).

**PCP-NMDA hypothesis**  The theory that schizophrenia involves an endogenous deficiency of NMDA-receptor activity. The hypothesis is based on the observation that PCP potently and acutely induces a schizophrenia-like psychosis in normal subjects, and symptom-specific exacerbation in schizophrenics. PCP binds to a site within the ion channel gated by the NMDA class of glutamate receptor, resulting in channel blockade and a decrease in NMDA receptor–mediated neurotransmission.

**pcpt**  *Perception* (q.v.).

**PCR**  *Polymerase chain reaction*; a genetic probe technique introduced in 1985. It involves in vitro enzymatic synthesis of millions of copies of a specific DNA segment in a relatively short period of time. As a result, samples too small to be identified by conventional means can be reproduced until there is enough material to be usable. In the procedure, the DNA sample is heated in order to separate the two strands of the double helix. Next, short pieces (oligonucleotides) of known DNA, called *primers*, are attached to one end of the sample; the primers flank the sample and thereby define the segment to be copied. In addition, the primers contain chemical "instructions" for the enzyme that is introduced in the third and final step. The natural enzyme is DNA polymerase, which follows instructions to assemble a second matching strand of DNA along the original sample, and a new double helix of DNA is produced, with all its subunits perfectly matched.

Each time it is performed, that three-step process doubles the amount of DNA that was in the last sequence. In this geometric progression, 20 repetitions will copy the original DNA sample a million times.

PCR is of particular value in studying small traces of genetic material, speeding the diagnosis of some hereditary diseases and an understanding of the mutations causing them, and in detecting intracellular viruses that are present in as few as one in a million cells and have not stimulated antibody production. See *genetic marker.*

**PCs** *Preconscious* (q.v.).

**PCSTF** Problem-centered systems therapy of the family.

**PDD** 1. Pervasive developmental disorder. See *ASD; developmental disorder, pervasive.*

2. Premenstrual dysphoric disorder. See *LLPDD; PMS.*

3. Primary degenerative dementia, a rarely used term for *Alzheimer disease* (q.v.).

**PDE** Personality Disorder Examination, which assesses a number of factors that occur with high frequency in patients with personality disorders. (Factor 1 is social sensitivity; 2 is social indifference). The PDE was developed by Squires-Wheeler et al in 1989, and loading developed by Cornblatt et al in 1982).

**PDEs** Phosphodiesters, *phospholipid* breakdown products (q.v.).

**PDP** *Parallel distributed processing* (q.v.).

**PEA-BD** Prepubertal and early adolescent onset bipolar disorder. See *pediatric bipolar disorder.*

**peak dose dyskinesia** See *LID.*

**peak experience** A brief transcendental state of consciousness during which the subject has a sense of heightened understanding, intense well-being, and of being at one with the universe (*unio mystica*); perception of time and space may be altered. The experience is described as occurring usually in psychologically healthy persons.

**peak level** In pharmacology, the point at which maximal blood concentration of a drug is reached following administration; for orally administered psychopharmacologic agents,

peak level is commonly in the range of 90 to 120 minutes.

**PEAQ** *Personal Experience and Attitude Questionnaire* (q.v.).

**Pearson syndrome** Usually fatal in childhood, the syndrome consists of pancytopenia, pancreatic fibosis, and splenic atrophy. See *mtDNA.*

**peccatiphobia** Fear of sinning. See *scrupulosity.*

**pederasty** The meaning of pederasty varies among different authors; it is most commonly defined as *coitus per anum* practiced on boys. It is not considered synonymous with *sodomy* (q.v.), though at times confused with it. See *paedico.*

**PEDF** *Pigment epithelium-derived factor,* a neurotrophic and neuroprotective protein that has been studied most intensively in the retina. The PEDF gene has been mapped to chromosome 17; various retinal degenerative diseases and brain disorders have been mapped to the same region: retinitis pigmentosa, Leber's congenital amaurosis, a type of cone-rod dystrophy, Miller-Dieker syndrome and lissencephaly. PEDF appears to play a neuroprotective role in both acute and chronic forms of neurodegeneration. See *neurotrophins.*

**pediatric bipolar disorder (PBD)** Traditionally, PBD is divided into four subgroups: (1) bipolar I, children who have had at least one manic or mixed episode; (2) bipolar II, children who have had at least one episode of major depression and hypomania; (3) cyclothymia, children who have manifested alternating episodes of hypomania and subsyndromal symptoms of depression; and (4) bipolar not otherwise specified (NOS).

Two variants of PBD according to age have been described:

1. *PEA-BD*: Prepubertal and early adolescent onset bipolar disorder; also termed atypical or juvenile bipolar disorder; characteristic features are irritability and deficits in motor inhibition, rapid cycling, little interepisode recovery, and high comorbidity with ADHD and ODD (oppositional-defiant disorder). Prominent symptoms include elation, grandiosity, racing thoughts/flight of ideas, decreased need for sleep, and hypersexuality.

2. *AO-BD*: Adolescent onset bipolar disorder, characterized by high rates of substance abuse, anxiety symptoms, and in about a quarter of subjects an episodic nature.

AO-BD often presents with classic symptoms of adult mania, including psychosis, and is often misdiagnosed as schizophrenia.

**pedication**   *Pederasty; sodomy* (qq.v.).

**pedigree method**   Study of the family history to determine the frequency with which a familial trait occurs in the members of an affected family. This method does not ordinarily afford conclusive proof of heredity and is largely restricted to rare pathological traits that are fairly constant in penetrance and expressivity.

**pediophobia**   Fear of dolls.

**pedologia**   Infantile or childish speech that omits all but the principal words and substitutes easily pronounced sounds for more difficult ones; baby talk.

**pedomorphism**   Describing adult behavior in terms more appropriate to behavior of a child. See *adultomorphism; anthropomorph.*

**pedophilia**   Love of children (juveniles), including babies (*nepiophilia*) and adolescents (*ephebophilia*); a *paraphilia* (q.v.) characterized by sexual urges and phantasies involving sexual activity with prepubertal children. Generally, the paraphiliac is 16 years of age or older, the child or children involved under the age of 13, and the number of years separating the paraphiliac and the sexual object not less than 5. The child may be of the same or opposite sex, or both male and female children may be involved. The activities most commonly reported are genital fondling and oral sex. In DSM-IV, the term refers to persons with recurrent, intense, sexually arousing fantasies, sexual urges, or behaviors of 6 months' duration involving sexual activity with a prepubescent child in which the fantasies, sexual urges, or behaviors cause significant distress or impairment and the individual is at least 16 years of age and at least 5 years older than the child. Child molestation is criminal behavior, whereas pedophilia is an anomalous sexual preference.

The findings suggest that mother–son sexual abuse is underreported. Most sexual abusers are males, however. About 40%–50% of *childhood sexual abuse (CSA)* (q.v.) is perpetrated by adolescents. A second age of perpetrators is 35–45 years; they involve themselves sexually with their own child or the friends of their children. A third age group is over 55; they may have concurrent CNS disease, have lost their adult sexual partner from death or divorce, or may involve themselves

with children as a result of a variety of stressful situations. A fourth group is pedophiles who are aroused to children all their lives; they frequently involve themselves with large numbers of children over time. Girls are sexually abused three times more often than boys. Approximately 89% of sexually abused children were abused by a male, 12% by a female. A sexually abused child is most likely to sustain a serious injury or impairment when a birth parent is the perpetrator.

If untreated, 10% to 17% of offenders commit another offense within 5 years; most of those treated do not reoffend. Recidivism is twice as high in pedophiles whose preference is a male child compared with those who prefer females.

Increasing use of the Internet by children and adolescents has made it much easier for pedophiles to contact potential victims and expose them to sexual material and arrange meetings with them.

Brain studies have demonstrated frontotemporal hypoactivity, predominantly right-sided, in pedophilic subjects. Volume of the amygdala is smaller in pedophilic subjects and is correlated with an offense pattern more focused on uniform pedophilic activity, and with prevalence of incestuous pedophilic activity. Right-sided temporal lobe lesions affect sexual function more frequently than do right-sided lesions. Right-sided lesions tend to enhance libido, and left-sided ones tend to impair it (Schiltz, K et al. *Archives of General Psychiatry* 64: 737–747, 2007).

*Pedophile, sexual abuser, incest offender, child rapist, sex offender of children, child molester, sexual deviant,* and *serial child molester* are often used interchangeably, or by different groups to mean different things. In consequence, there is considerable confusion as to who is doing what to whom.

**pedotrophy**   Nurturance of a child; child rearing or "parentcraft."

**peduncle, cerebral**   See *midbrain.*

**peduncular hallucinosis**   Vivid hallucinations, recognized by the patient as unreal, that may occur in lesions of the midbrain or cerebral peduncles.

**pedunculopontile syndrome**   *Weber syndrome.* See *hemiplegia alternans.*

**peeping**   See *voyeurism.*

**peeping Tom**   (From the name of the Coventry tailor who peeped at naked Lady Godiva riding through the city's streets by order of her husband, lord of Coventry) Voyeur.

**peer review**   See *review*.

**P-element**   See *system*.

**Pelizaeus-Merzbacher disease** (Friedrich Pelizaeus, German neurologist, 1850–1917, and Ludwig Merzbacher, German-born physician in Argentina, 1875–1942) See *diffuse sclerosis*.

**pellagra**   Nicotinic acid deficiency, characterized by gastrointestinal disturbances (especially diarrhea), erythema followed by desquamation of the affected area, and mental disturbances. Symptoms vary widely in incidence and intensity but tend to be worse in the spring. The most frequent early picture consists of fatigue and lassitude combined with depression. Mania, convulsions, dementia, stupor, and unconsciousness may also occur, and if untreated the condition advances into delirious or subacute delirious states. Sucking and grasping reflexes may appear along with cog wheel rigidity of the extremities and progressive clouding of consciousness. Treatment with high doses of nicotinic acid or nicotinamide (and usually moderately high doses of the other B vitamins) usually results in amelioration of all symptoms, except that in some cases memory defects persist. Pellagra continues to be endemic in the Far East, Africa, and Mexico, and it can be seen as a complication of alcoholism and food faddism in any part of the world.

**pendular knee jerk**   When tapping the patellar tendon, several oscillations of the leg occur before it comes to a stop; observed in disease of the cerebellum.

**penetrance**   The proportion of individuals with a given genotype that actually manifest a particular phenotype. See *chromosome; dominance*.

**penetration, interface**   See *network*.

**penetration response**   See *barrier*.

**Penfield, Wilder Graves** (1891–1976) United States–born neurosurgeon, founded Montreal (Canada) Neurological Institute; epilepsy, speech disorders, memory.

**penial**   *Penile* (q.v.).

**peniaphobia**   Fear of poverty.

**penile**   Relating to the penis.

**penile plethysmography**   A test used in the evaluation of male sex-offenders: a band is placed around the subject's genitals to measure his erectile response to audio or visual stimuli.

It is of questionable value in boys under 16 because of the easy arousability of young adolescents in response to any stimulus, whether sexual or not.

**penile tumescence**   Erection of the penis. *Nocturnal penile tumescence (NPT)* is associated with over 90% of REM sleep episodes and is thus a useful aid in differentiating between psychogenic impotence (where NPT is ordinarily preserved) and impotence due to organic impairment (where NPT is typically reduced or absent). Before the use of comprehensive polysomnographic studies of various physiologic processes, almost 90% of cases of male impotence were believed to be psychogenic in nature. Now that physiologic studies can be performed it is realized that approximately 65% of patients are organically impaired.

**penilingus**   Fellatio.

**penis**   The male organ of copulation. In psychoanalysis it refers to the organ after the boy has reached the stage of genital love. See *phallus*.

**penis, female**   See *penis, women with*.

**penis, women with**   A childhood theory or idea, that every woman has a penis). It generally appears between the ages of 2 and 5 as a consequence of the child's discovering the absence of the penis in females. On finding the supposed organic deficiency or inferiority, most little girls react to their discovery with varying degrees of shock. In boys the same discovery tends to make their dread of castration more real for them, since it confronts them with the actuality of the "missing organ." The idea that a woman once possessed or possesses a penis functions as a protective defensive denial of the horrible psychic reality, by which the child has theoretically explained to itself the observed absence of the penis in females.

**penis captivus**   *Vaginismus* (q.v.) occurring during sexual intercourse so that withdrawal of the erect penis is impossible. The condition is the subject of many anecdotes, but the paucity of clinical reports indicates that such anecdotes are based more on male castration fears and female active castration tendencies than on real occurrences.

**penis envy**   In psychoanalysis, the girl's desire for a penis; a part of the castration complex. According to Freud, when the little girl realizes she has no penis, she reacts either by hoping that some day she will have one or by denying that she does not have one.

Penis envy loosens the girl's relation with her mother as a love-object, because she blames her mother for the alleged loss. In the next development of the Oedipus situation, her wish for a penis is transformed into the wish for a child. She then takes her father as a love-object, and her mother becomes the object of jealousy.

The concept of penis envy has been criticized for its androcentric bias and for ignoring the effects of familial, social, and cultural input. The concept is embedded in Freud's insistence on a framework of biologically unfolding psychosexual stages. His strictly instinctual frame of reference leaves no room for understanding the influences on female development of early object relations, the prephallic development of personality, or the subordinate societal role of women. See *Oedipus complex.*

**penis pride** *Phallic pride,* a term employed to designate the feeling of superiority and power attendant to the possession of the male genital organ. The concept was emphasized by Melanie Klein in her analysis of the child's instinctual life. "In describing the development of the boy, I have drawn attention to certain factors which tend, as I think, to increase yet more the central importance which the penis possesses for him. They may be summed up as follows: (1) The anxiety arising from his earliest danger situations, his fears of being attacked in all parts of his body and inside it, which include all his fears belonging to the feminine position, are displaced onto the penis or an external organ, where they can be more successfully mastered. The increased pride the boy takes in his penis and all that this involves may also be said to be a method of mastering those fears and disappointments which his feminine position lays him open to more particularly. (2) The fact that the penis is a vehicle first of the boy's destructive and then of his creative omnipotence, enhances its importance as a means of mastering anxiety. In this ministering to his sense of omnipotence, assisting him in the task of testing by reality and promoting his object-relationships… in fact, in subserving the all-important function of mastering anxiety—the penis is brought into specially close relation with the ego and is made into a representative of the ego and the conscious; while the interior of the body, the imagos and

the faeces—what is invisible and unknown, that is—are compared to the unconscious." (*The Psycho-Analysis of Children,* 1932).

**penis retraction syndrome** *Koro* (q.v.).

**pension neurosis** See *epinosic gain; compensation neurosis.*

**pentazocine** A synthetic opioid with both agonist and antagonist properties and thus able to precipitate a narcotic withdrawal syndrome. Pentazocine can also produce an acute psychosis with nightmares, depersonalization, and visual hallucinations.

**pentheraphobia** Fear of one's mother-in-law.

**pentothal interview** See *narcotherapy.*

**penumbra** In an eclipse, the space of partial illumination between the central umbra or perfect shadow and the full light; used to describe the area surrounding the core of the brain region injured by a stroke. Rupture or blockage of a blood vessel in the brain causes rapid cell death in the core and triggers mechanisms in the penumbra that lead to increases in intracellular $Ca^{2+}$ and reactive oxygen species (ROS) which, in turn, initiate cell death.

**peotillomania** *Obs.* False masturbation, pseudo-masturbation; a nervous tic consisting in constant pulling at the penis.

**peptic ulcer** See *ulcer, peptic.*

**peptidases** *Proteases;* enzymes that split proteins by fracturing the bonds between amino acids. They perform many vital tasks, such as splitting APP, the amyloid precursor protein. They also help viruses maintain themselves and replicate inside their hosts.

Aβ is generated proteolytically from a large precursor molecule, APP, by the sequential action of two proteases, β-secretase and γ-secretase. A third protease, α-protease, competes with β-secretase for the APP and can preclude production of Aβ by cleaving the peptide in two. γ-secretase is an unusual transmembrane protease complex consisting of at least four proteins—presenilin, nicastrin, anterior pharynx (APH1), and presenilin enhancer 2 (PEN2). See *secretases.*

**peptide, brain** *Neuropeptide, peptide neurotransmitter;* an element of a brain protein consisting of linkage of a short chain of amino acids (less than 100; proteins contain more than 100) by bonding of the carboxyl group (CO) of one with the amino group (NH) of the other. The CO-NH union is termed the *peptide bond* or *peptide link.* See *peptidergic.* Peptides are synthesized in the cell body of the neuron and then transported down the axon and stored in synaptic vesicles in the nerve terminals. They are released by a calcium-dependent mechanism, and their action is terminated by degradative peptidases in the synaptic cleft.

The first peptide neurotransmitter was *substance P*, discovered by von Euler and Gaddum in 1931; it excites sensory neurons that inform higher parts of the brain that noxious stimulation has occurred. It is believed to play a role in pain syndromes, mood disorders, Huntington disease, and other movement disorders. The endogenous opioid peptides were discovered in 1975. See *neuroanatomy, chemical; neurohormone; neurotransmitter.*

There are many neuroactive peptides; they can be categorized by tissue localization as follows:

1. *Hypothalamus*: many neurons in the *hypothalamus* (q.v.) are specialized for the synthesis of peptides, and individual neurons often release more than one peptide. Among these peptides are angiotensin II, cholecystokinin, *corticotropin-releasing hormone*, enkephalins, gonadotropin-releasing hormone, growth hormone-releasing hormone, neurotensin, somatostatin, substance P, thyrotropin-releasing hormone. See *pothalamic-pituitary-adrenal (HPA) axis.*

2. *Neurohypophysis*: oxytocin, vasopressin.

3. *Pituitary*: adrenocorticotropic hormone, α-melanocyte-stimulating hormone, β-endorphin, growth hormone, luteinizing hormone, prolactin, thyrotropin.

4. *Gastrointestinal*: bombesin, *cholecystokinin*, gastrin, glucagon, insulin, leucine-enkephalin, methionine-enkephalin, motilin, neurotensin, secretin, somatostatin, substance P, hyrotropin-releasing hormone, vasoactive intestinal polypeptide.

5. *Others*: bradykinin, calcitonin, CGRP (calcitonin gene-related peptide), galanin, neuropeptide Y, neuropeptide Yy, sleep peptide(s), substance K (neurokinin).

Like other chemicals, the peptides undoubtedly have multiple roles, as neuronal, paracrine, or endocrine biological messengers, depending on their cells of origin and release.

**peptidergic** Referring to interneuronal communication by means of neuropeptides, which may function in several ways: as neurosecretory neurons, for example, which signal to nonneural effector organs over long distances; as neurohormones, which communicate between the nervous system and the adenohypophysis; as neuron-to-neuron transporters of chemical signals by way of the acellular interstitium; or as neuromodulators, which enhance or depress a conventionally transmitted synaptic signal between two other neurons. See *neurohormone; neuromodulator.*

**PER** Periodic Evaluation Record. See *Multi-State Information System.*

**per gene** See *biological clock; biological rhythms.*

**percentile rank** Position in a series expressed as a number that represents the percentage of cases in the total group lying below the given score value. Example: If a subject makes a score of 82 in an examination, and it is found that this score is higher than that made by 93% of all those taking that examination, he is at the 93rd percentile on that examination. Percentile ranks facilitate the interpretation of a single measure in a distribution of such measures; they describe the variability and form of a frequency distribution; they provide a way to compare measures that were originally expressed in different units. Thus, a student may make a score of 82 on one test and a score of 127 on a second; as raw scores these would be relatively meaningless, but when it is known that the score of 82 represents the 93rd percentile on the first test, and that the score of 127 represents the 92nd percentile on the second, the subject's performance on the two tests is seen in more meaningful perspective.

**percept** The subject's meaningful interpretation of a sensory stimulus; a percept is a combination of subjective and objective elements and affords a link between the subject and his or her environment.

**percept image** A concrete image of hallucinatory clearness that may appear as phantasy or memory images. According to Jaensch, it represents "a primitive level of intellectual life."

**perception** Pcpt; the process of converting sensory stimuli (presented by objects in the environment) into symbolic representations encoded within neuronal patterns of the brain, involving patterned activity in a large number of interconnected nerve cells. In general, cells are more sensitive to their primary modality (vision in the visual cortex, sound in the auditory cortex), but nonetheless they discharge if other stimuli such as touch are sufficiently intense. The original sensory stimulus is generally conveyed along several way stations until it ends up in the part of the cortex that is specialized for that kind of perception. Within the entering pathways, the stimulus is transformed into electrical and chemical signals.

Perception encompasses at least four aspects: reception, registration, processing (i.e., further reorganization in accord with memory, affects, needs, intentions, etc.), and feedback (proprioceptive and autonomic processes that allow the subject to determine if the object sensed is the object sought).

**perception, categorical** See *categorical perception.*

**perception, delusional** Misinterpretation of a percept as an indication that something sinister is occurring or is about to occur, before the development of a full-blown delusional idea. A young man looked at his television set and felt it was slightly tilted or off-center. This was a sign to him that people might think he was gay (off-center = not straight = gay).

**perception-hallucination** See *hallucination of perception.*

**perceptivity** The power of perception; the character of being perceptive.

**perceptual complex** Predominance of images and concrete objects in thinking, with resultant distortions and condensations that run counter to logical, rational thinking; concretistic thinking; *paleologic* (q.v.).

**perceptual gestalt** Simultaneous perception of sensory stimuli in one or more sensory modalities, experienced as a unified, integrated pattern.

**perceptual disability** Difficulty in putting information into the brain through the five senses; difficulty in transferring sensory stimulation into psychological information. Included are disturbances in reception, registration, processing, or reorganization of percepts in accord with what already exists within the memory store.

**perceptual orders** See *Lacan, Jacques.*

**perceptual style** The way in which a person attends to, alters, and shapes the sensory stimuli that bombard him. Some workers have found that schizophrenics have an altered, unusual, or abnormal perceptual function.

**perceptual-conscious system** The part of the mental apparatus that absorbs perceptions from both the external world and the interior of the mind (the id). Early in the development of the human mind, one part of it becomes the recipient of stimuli. In this part of the mind the feeling of consciousness and the ego originate.

**perceptualization** The act or process of representing reality as it appears to the senses rather than to the intellect, as is seen in dreams and hallucinations. The term is also used to refer to regressive loss of higher conceptualization processes such as is seen in many schizophrenics whose ideas become more and more related to specific instances and less and less related to classes, groups, or categories. This is one of the expressions of *paleologic* (q.v.) and leads, among other things, to *concretism* (q.v.).

**percipient** In parapsychology, the receiver of telepathically transmitted messages.

**peregrinating patient syndrome** See *Munchhausen syndrome.*

**perforant path** The fiber tract that provides the key interconnection between the neocortex and the *hippocampus*; it is the principal input to the dentate gyrus. It originates in layer II of the *entorhinal cortex* (q.v.) and terminates in the outer molecular layer of the *dentate gyrus* (q.v.). In respect to Alzheimer Disease and aging, it is probably the single most vulnerable circuit in the cerebral cortex. See *Alzheimer disease; MTL.*

**performance anxiety** Anxiety related to the execution of a task; used particularly in sex therapy, to refer to persons whose sexual dysfunction is related to their concern about whether they perform well. The anxiety is often related to unrealistic expectations about genital size, frequency of responsiveness, etc., and gaining the partner's approval takes precedence over attainment of personal satisfaction, intimacy, or love. Because performance anxiety tends to be incompatible with pleasure, the worrier ends up being unable to perform at all.

**performance enhancing drugs** Altering brain and other body functions to provide better execution of tasks; most commonly, such drugs are used as supplements to improve skills or abilities in athletic competition. Drugs in this category include *anabolic-androgenic steroids* (q.v.), human recombinant erythropoietin, human growth hormone, and various stimulants.

**performance monitoring** See *RCZ.*

**performance neurosis** A mental disturbance during the course of any performance whose normal execution requires spontaneity. An example is an attack of trembling overcoming a violinist while playing. See *performance anxiety; occupational neurosis.*

**performance phobia** A type of social *phobia* (q.v.).

**performance pressure** In sexual relationships, the partner's overt or implied demand that the subject achieve one or more orgasms during intercourse, respond immediately to any kind of sexual overture, maintain arousal indefinitely, etc.

**perhaps neurosis** A type of obsessive neurosis, as in the formula: "*If* I had done this instead of that, perhaps my sister would still be alive."

**PERI** *Psychiatric Epidemiology Research Interview* (q.v.).

**periaqueductal grey area** *PAG*; the area of the brain surrounding the cerebral aqueduct between the third and fourth ventricles. PAG neurons inhibit neurons in the raphé nuclei, deep in the medulla. Opiate-type substances such as morphine occupy inhibitory receptors on the PAG neurons. As a result, the PAG neurons are inhibited. Freed from their inhibition, the raphé neurons then send signals down the descending tracts to stimulate interneurons in the spinal cord, which block the input of pain signals from peripheral nerves. See *brain stem.*

**periblepsis** The wild stare of a delirious person, with elements of bewilderment, consternation, and terror.

**perichareia** Delirious rejoicing.

**periluteal phase dysphoric disorder** *LLPDD* (q.v.).

**perineal coitus** External coitus; Lacassagne coined the expression for the act of rubbing the penis against the perineal region.

**period** *Stage* (q.v.).

**periodic catatonia** Atypical schizophrenia; in Leonhard's classification, a subtype of non-systematic schizophrenia characterized by acute episodes of akinetic symptoms, sometimes interrupted by hyperkinetic symptoms, and regular remissions between episodes. See *systematic schizophrenia; Gjessing syndrome.*

**Periodic Evaluation Record** See *Multi-State Information System.*

**periodic paralysis, familial** A hereditary disorder consisting of abrupt, periodic attacks of flaccid paralysis that may last anywhere from hours to 3 or 4 days. The illness, which appears to be based on an abnormal demand for potassium, usually begins during adolescence.

Prodromata such as hunger, thirst, or sweating are common, and the attacks themselves tend to occur in the early morning. The paralysis is at its height an hour after onset; the proximal limb is affected more than the distal portion and during the attack deep reflexes are abolished, but there is no loss of consciousness. Attacks may occur every few days, or only once every few years. They tend to be precipitated by exposure to the cold, excess sugar intake, fasting, or overexertion. Potassium chloride is used in the treatment of individual attacks and prophylactically when attacks occur frequently.

**periodic somnolence syndrome** See *Kleine-Levin sydrome.*

**periosteal reflex** The response to tapping certain bones that lie just beneath the skin; for example, the radial and ulnar periosteal, and the tibial adductor reflexes.

**perioxisomes** See *neuronal membranes.*

**peripheralist psychology** See *centralist psychology.*

**perirhinal cortex** Part of the medial temporal lobe memory system; it participates in declarative memory and is also part of the ventral visual pathway, the "what" pathway.

**peristasis** The external environment. Some geneticists prefer this term to environment, to indicate that the environment of any genetic factor includes all the biophysiological processes that take place in the organism itself and are essential to the phenotypical development of the given genotype. According to modern physiological genetics, every inherited character necessarily becomes subject to the organism's *peristatic* conditions. See *ecology; euthenics.*

**Perls, Frederick S.** (1893–1970) Gestalt psychology, therapy.

**permanency, object** See *evocative memory.*

**permeabilizers** See *blood–brain barrier.*

**permeation** See *ion channel.*

**permissive environment** A social and physical environment in which acting out and verbalization are allowed but not necessarily sanctioned or approved.

**permissive hypothesis of affective disorders** The hypothesis states that a deficit in central indole aminergic transmission permits mood (affect) disorder but is not enough to cause it; changes in central catecholaminergic transmission when occurring in the context of indole aminergic deficit cause mood disorders and determine their quality (excess catecholamine produces mania, and catechol-amine deficiency produces depression).

**peroneal muscular atrophy**   *Charcot-Marie-Tooth disease* (q.v.)

**perplexity, vague**   A symptom seen most commonly in the organic psychoses, especially in the acute brain syndromes associated with systemic infection as part of the beginning of a toxic delirium. The patient feels "mixed-up in the head," shows a deficient grasp of the total situation, drowsiness, torpor, and distur-bances of the association, memory, attention, and will.

**perplexity psychosis**   A subdivision of manic-depressive psychosis, characterized by marked distress accompanying subjective perplexity.

**persécuteurs persécutées**   Those paranoid perse-cuted patients who also become persecutors, in an effort, as they believe, to defend them-selves against their persecutors.

**persecution syndrome**   Described in war refugees with concentration camp experience or those who were persecuted in flight; consists of perva-sive anxiety, overreactivity, irritability, chronic depression, psychosomatic disturbances, and defense by means of dehumanization and unconscious identification with the aggres-sor. The social contacts and marriages of those with the syndrome are likely to be confined to others who have had similar experiences. See *post-traumatic stress disorder; victim.*

**Persecutor**   See *transactional analysis.*

**persecutory delusion**   The conviction that one is being plotted against or threatened with bodily harm, disgrace, or control of his thoughts and actions.

**perseveration**   Loss of ability to start and stop motor actions, a frontal lobe function; con-textually inappropriate and unintentional repetition of a response or behavioral unit. Perseveration results in unnecessary repetition or maintenance of an action. Example: ask a patient to "Take a piece of paper in your right hand, fold it in half, and return it to me." Per-severation may appear as the patient's contin-uing to fold the paper into fourths or eighths.

Various forms of perseveration have been described:

*Continuous perseveration*: failure to termi-nate a discrete response, which is repeated without interruption; e.g., uninterrupted emission of single words or the graphical repetition of letters, numerals, or design elements. Bleuler described a pianist who became stuck on a repeated musical phrase and a stage prompter who was unable to cease prompting the same line despite rec-ognition of the problem.

*Recurrent perseveration*: either (1) repeti-tion of a previously emitted response to a subsequent stimulus, or (2) repeated intru-sion of an initial response into a susequent response sequence, as in reciting the alpha-bet "AbcAdeAfghijA…"

*Stuck-in-set perseveration*: impaired shift-ing; on a reversal task the patient fails to switch response modes after a shift in response-outcome contingencies; e.g., on the WCST, the patient continues to sort items in terms of a previously relevant, but currently irrelevant, attribute of the stimu-lus figures. In some schizophrenia patients, impaired shifting is accompanied by non-random, perseverative responding.

In schizophrenia patients, severity of per-severation covaries with formal thought disorder and voluntary motor disturbance. Abnormal voluntary motor activity, such as repetitive movements, impaired coordination, and poor response sequencing, occurs fre-quently among schizophrenic patients, indi-cating that perseveration is a component of a broader disorganization syndrome. Behav-ior perseveration may be due to a failure of frontal specification of striatal outputs during capacity-demanding tasks.

**perseverative chaining**   See *chaining.*

**perseverative scripting**   See *Asperger syndrome.*

**persistence, motor**   Ability to sustain a motor action, such as keeping one's eyes closed for 20 seconds on command. Inability to sustain motor action is motor *impersistence*, which, in a subject whose muscle strength is normal, indicates frontal lobe dysfunction.

**persistent vegetative state**   See *vegetative state.*

**person, disturbances in the**   One of the fun-damental symptoms of the schizophrenias, according to Bleuler. Such disturbances arise by reason of the tendency to splitting of the psyche and domination of the personality by one or another of the patient's complexes. The ego is never fully intact, resulting in a lack of homogeneity, wholeness, and stability of the personality organization. See *identity diffu-sion; splitting.*

**person in the patient**   A term expressing the basic key concept of the psychosomatic medical approach to the patient and emphasizing the patient's personality or character as a factor in the production of physical symptoms and complaints. Whereas the organic, or physical, approach tends to exclude awareness and interest in emotional, personality, and character factors as causative agents to be investigated and treated, the psychosomatic approach, conversely, tends to include these factors and give them central importance. It must be borne in mind, however, that the psychosomatic approach does not in any way exclude the usual physical and organic avenues of investigation.

**persona** Jung's term for the disguised or masked attitude assumed by a person, in contrast to the more deeply rooted personality components. See *analytic psychology; mask; personality; personality disorders; pseudoidentification.*

**personal care capacity** The ability of a person to care adequately for himself or herself in terms of nutrition, hygiene, fire or water hazard, and the activities of daily living. It involves a realistic appreciation of the person's strengths and weaknesses, and the ability to make decisions about the amount of support that will be required for daily living. Often this means whether the person can live in an unsupervised setting or can make other realistic decisions regarding place of residence. See *competence.*

**personal disorganization** See *disorganization.*

**personal disposition** See *Allport, Gordon Willard.*

**Personal Experience and Attitude Questionnaire (PEAQ)** A screening questionnaire said to be a highly significant discriminator of psychopathic behavior. The test contains 150 items covering criminalism, emotional instability, inadequate personality, sexual psychopathy, nomadism, and other psychopathic traits.

**personal image** "A personal image has neither archaic character nor collective significance, but expresses contents of the personal unconscious and a personally conditioned, conscious situation" (Jung, C. G. *Psychological Types*, 1923). In contrast is a *primordial image*: "I speak of its archaic character when the image is in striking unison with familiar mythological motives. In this case it expresses material primarily derived from the collective unconscious, while, at the same time, it indicates that the momentary conscious situation is influenced not so much from the side of the personal as from the collective."

**personal therapy** PT; a definitive psychosocial intervention for schizophrenic patients developed by G. E. Hogarty (*American Journal of Psychiatry 154*, 1997) to forestall the late (second-year) relapses common with many psychosocial approaches, and to enhance personal and social adjustment through the identification and effective management of the affect dysregulation that typically precedes a psychotic relapse or provokes inappropriate behavior.

In the first stage, personal therapy encourages identification of the patient's internal sources of dysregulation, i.e., the affective, cognitive, and physiological responses to the experience of stress, and the effect of those responses on the behavior of others. Therapists offer formation of a treatment contract, provision of minimal effective dosing of medications, and basic psychoeducation regarding the nature and treatment of schizophrenia. They use the techniques of supportive therapy, including active listening, correct empathy, appropriate reassurance, reinforcement of patient health-promoting initiatives, and reliance on the therapist for advocacy and problem solving in times of crisis.

In the intermediate phase—usually during the first 18 months after discharge—patients receive advanced psychoeducation that includes a didactic on the adaptive strategies to be taught, the requirements for a successful rehabilitation, and a more formal focus on the prodromes of psychosis. Internal coping strategies progress to the identification of individual cognitive, affective, and somatic indicators of distress and the appropriate application of basic relaxation (diaphragmatic breathing) and cognitive reframing techniques. In addition, skills training designed to ameliorate social behavior deficits and to enhance perception abilities is introduced.

In the advanced phase, the therapist encourages the timing of social and vocational initiative in the community, awareness of one's individual prodromes, progressive relaxation principles, and a growing awareness of one's affect, together with its expression and perceived effect on the behavior of others. Also included is instruction in principles of criticism management and conflict resolution. A simulated vocational setting provides the patient an opportunity to apply acquired skills in real-life situations and to identify any need for continuing remediation.

**Personalität**  The core of identity; the self that is behind the masks presented to the outside world as one assumes different roles in different situations.

**personality**  *Character* (q.v.); the characteristic, and to some extent predictable, behavior-response patterns that each person evolves, both consciously and unconsciously, as his style of life. The personality represents a compromise between inner drives and needs and the controls that limit or regulate their expression. Such controls are both internal (e.g., conscience and superego) and external (reality demands). The personality functions to maintain a stable, reciprocal relationship between the person and his environment; it is thus a composite of the ego defenses, the autoplastic and the alloplastic maneuvers, that are automatically and customarily employed to maintain intrapsychic stability. See *character defense.*

Although current psychodynamic theory and psychiatric treatment generally operate on the assumption that personality is largely determined by environmental influences (such as the nature of the mother–infant dyad, child-rearing practices, and cultural pressures), that assumption has repeatedly failed to attain credibility when subjected to scientific investigation. The similarity seen in the personalities of biological relatives is almost entirely genetic in origin, and between 40% and 50% of personality variation in general is genetically determined. See *behavioral genetics.*

The personality is a set of habits that characterize the person in her or his way of managing day-to-day living; under ordinary conditions, it is relatively stable and predictable, and for the most part it is ego-syntonic. Because the personality is ego-syntonic, it is rare that the person will recognize his own personality as being deviant or abnormal (even if, in fact, it is). Any such evaluation is ordinarily a social diagnosis and an outgrowth of the effects of that personality on the people about him—who may view his behavior as destructive, frightening, nonconforming, or otherwise unacceptable. The subject, in other words, is unlikely to seek out ways to alter his personality, which for him is the best way of avoiding tension and fulfilling his potential that he has been able to develop; rather, he may consent to counseling or psychotherapy if this is urged by others or if he suffers social repercussions because of his usual behavior.

Currently, investigators are in general agreement that personality is an amalgam of five traits or superfactors: (1) extraversion—the subject is outgoing, decisive, and enjoys leadership roles; (2) agreeableness—likability, friendliness, the subject does not take advantage of others; (3) neuroticism—the subject is nervous, irritable, and prone to worries; (4) conscientiousness—conformity, dependability, the subject is responsible, dependable; and (5) openness—the subject is insightful, imaginative, curious, reflective, and open to novel experiences.

It is difficult to draw a clear distinction between normal personality and the variations of personality and character that extend beyond the normal range. To some extent, the stability of even the normal personality is achieved at the expense of an ideal mobility—perhaps unattainable—to deal effectively with new or unusual interpersonal problems and conflicts. Yet there is no doubt that in many persons the stability of their ways of being and living is a rigidly fixed, immutable pattern that severely limits their potentialities for effective functioning and satisfying interpersonal relationships. Such conditions are variously termed *personality disorders, character disorders,* or *character neuroses.* These are deeply ingrained, chronic, and habitual patterns of reaction that are maladaptive in that they are relatively inflexible; they limit the optimal use of potentialities and often provoke the very counterreactions from the environment that the subject seeks to avoid. See *personality disorders.*

**personality change disorder**  A significant change from previous personality characteristics following (and presumably consequent upon) major stress or catastrophe, which may be a mental disorder or some other medical condition. Among the new features that may appear are hostility, mistrustfulness, suspiciousness, social ineptitude, feelings of estrangement or helplessness, clinging dependency, lability of mood, and decreased control over impulses or aggressivity. In children there may be disruption in development. DSM-IV subtypes divide personality change disorder into labile, disinhibited, aggressive, apathetic, and paranoid.

**personality disorders** *Personality* (q.v.) is a set of relatively stable, predictable, and ego-syntonic habits that characterize the person in her or his way of managing day-to-day living; they are defined in terms of multiple domains of functioning—cognition, affectivity, impulse regulation and self-control, interpersonal relations, and the inner experiences of mental life. When those habits are enough beyond the normal range to warrant the appellation of personality disorder is difficult to define, and often the label is more a social diagnosis of nonconformity than a designation of disease process in the usual sense. [Because of that, the entries in this *Dictionary* describe each personality type and its associated "disorder" under a single entry; thus, paranoid personality and paranoid personality disorder are described under *paranoid personality (disorder).*]

In general, what are termed personality disorders are patterns of relating to the environment that are so rigid, fixed, and immutable as to limit severely the likelihood of effective functioning or satisfying interpersonal relationships. They are deeply ingrained, chronic, and habitual patterns of reaction that are maladaptive in that they are relatively inflexible; they limit the optimal use of potentialities and often provoke the very counterreactions from the environment that the subject seeks to avoid.

As a comparison of the different editions of DSM shows, even the "official" nomenclature and descriptions of the personality disorders vary considerably over a relatively short period of time. As an example, what "borderline" referred to in the 1950s is quite different from current usage, and it is not always easy to discern which meanings are intended when researchers and clinicians publish individual reports on the topic.

In their quest for theory-free objectivity and reliability, both DSM-III and DSM-IV ignore the subjective, "psychodynamic" data that form the core of many other classificatory systems. Further, boundaries between the different types described are quite fragile. Even in a single system, there is great diagnostic overlap between many of the entities classified and defined as different—so great that some presume one or another of the disorders expresses a mental organization on which some of the other personality disorders are superimposed.

DSM-IV recognizes the following personality disorders and divides them into three clusters:

Cluster A—The odd and eccentric group: including *schizotypal, schizoid,* and *paranoid personality* (qq.v.); their interpersonal mode is to withdraw.

Cluster B—The group with dramatic presentation, impulsive acting out, and unpredictable behavior: including *borderline personality disorder* (characterized by no impulse control), *antisocial personality disorder* (no conscience), *narcissistic personality disorder* (no humility), and *histrionic personality disorder* (qq.v.); in this cluster, the interpersonal mode is to exploit.

Cluster C—The anxious and fearful group: including *avoidant, dependent,* and *compulsive personality disorders* (qq.v.); their interpersonal mode is to comply.

In DSM-II (1968 revision), several personality disorders were recognized that are not readily interchangeable with the above labels, including the *asthenic, cyclothymic, explosive,* and *inadequate personality disorders* (qq.v.). In DSM-I (1952 nomenclature), personality disorders were grouped under three headings: *personality pattern disturbance, personality trait disturbance,* and *sociopathic personality disturbance* (qq.v.).

**personality multiplication** A loss of continuity of ego boundaries seen most often in schizophrenia, where individual psychic functions may split off from the personality as a whole, attain an autonomy of their own, and then be identified by the subject as being different people within him. The term includes such phenomena as *appersonification, decomposition,* and *dedifferentiation* (qq.v.).

**personality panels** The concept of a four-panel Japanese screen, across which is painted a complete picture, moved Draper to introduce into the vocabulary of constitutional medicine the term panels of personality representing the four main divisions of the human individuality. These panels relate to the anatomical, physiological, psychological, and immunological elements of a person, each of which "may be considered to occupy one panel of the great screen across which Man's personality is drawn" (Draper, G. *Human Constitution,* 1924). See *constitution; constitutional medicine.*

**personality pattern disturbance** In the 1952 revision of psychiatric nomenclature (DSM-I), this term was used to refer to personality types or character structures that are more or less fixed and only minimally liable to any basic alteration. "The depth of the psychopathology here allows these individuals little room to maneuver under conditions of stress, except into actual psychosis." Included in this group were *inadequate, schizoid, cyclothymic,* and *paranoid* personalities (qq.v.).

**personality trait disturbance** In the 1952 version of psychiatric nomenclature (DSM-I), this term was used to refer to "individuals who are unable to maintain their emotional equilibrium and independence under minor or major stress because of disturbances in emotional development. Some individuals fall into this group because their personality pattern disturbance is related to fixation and exaggeration of certain character and behavior patterns; others, because their behavior is a regressive reaction due to environmental or endopsychic stress." Included in this group are *emotionally unstable, passive aggressive,* and *compulsive* personalities (qq.v.).

**personality types** Jung recognized two "general attitude" types, described from the standpoint of the direction of the flow of libido. When the general direction of the flow of libido is away from the subject, the expression extraversion is used and the person is called an extravert. When the libido is mainly turned inwardly upon the person, the condition is known as introversion and the person as an introvert. These two are known as temperamental types.

Jung described four basic *functional* types known as thinking, feeling, sensation, and intuition. Any one of these four functions may be(come) preponderant over the other three and, in that case, it is called the *superior function.* On the other hand, an *inferior function* is one less powerful than the other three. The remaining two functions are then said to occupy an intermediate position.

For a psychoanalytic description of personality types, see *character defense.*

**personalization** See *logical error.*

**personification** Endowing another with pleasant or unpleasant attributes as a result of frustration of one's desires or wishes. For example, one schizophrenic patient whose letter was not answered accused his doctor of intercepting the mail. Personification is a form of projection wherein the desirable or undesirable

properties of reality are attributed to some person, even though the latter is unrelated to the happening itself. Thus, schizophrenic persecutory delusions develop only after an obstacle to gratification is felt by the patient; a persecutor is chosen to take on the qualities necessary to explain the frustration. Delusions of persecution convert obstacles into machinations of certain people, the persecutors.

**Persönlichkeit** The social roles assumed by a person in different situations, from the point of view of how they are observed by another person; the impression one makes on another.

**personology** Study of the personality as a whole, of how people function in society, their perceptions, their actions, and especially their thoughts and feelings and their reasons for being. In contrast, metapsychology is the pure-science aspect of the study of personality and the general laws of mental life. Personology supplies the understanding of how to use this knowledge in relation to the specific individual as an organic-psychic whole whose every action can be understood only in terms of the whole. See *holism.*

**perspective** The way in which an object and interrelationships between different objects are viewed; the ability to recognize which behaviors are semantically and socially appropriate and which are inappropriate for a given communicative context. Some studies show schizophrenic and other psychotic patients with thought disorder to have significantly poorer perspective than other psychiatric patients.

**persuasion** A type of supportive psychotherapy in which the patient is encouraged to adopt the therapist's point of view and exhorted to follow the latter's advice. Persuasion is directive and limited in its goals.

Ordinarily, it aims neither to provide the patient with insight nor to widen his range of coping mechanisms. Instead, it concentrates on the here and now, deals with the current crisis, and implies that the patient can accept an attitude of "The doctor knows best." See *psychotherapy.*

**perturbation** Restlessness, disquietude, great uneasiness; abnormal deviation from the regularity of certain characteristic properties, as in the motions of atoms or planets, when a field of force varying with time is applied.

**pervasive aggression** See *instrumental aggression.*

**pervasive developmental disorders** See *developmental disorders, pervasive.*

**perversion** Abnormality, aberration, distortion, dysfunction; any deviation from the correct, proper, expected, or normal range. In psychiatry, most commonly used to refer to *parasexuality* or *sexual deviation*, i.e. any sexual practice that deviates from the normal, or any abnormal means of reaching genital orgasm. According to R. J. Stoller (*Archives of General Psychiatry 22*, 1970), a perversion is an indefinitely repeating conscious preference for a genitally stimulating exciting act that is not genital heterosexual intercourse. See *paraphilia.*

**pervert** One who practices any form of genital activity not in accord with the general culture or mores of his or her community or state.

**PES** Psychiatric emergency service.

**PET** Positron emission tomography; an imaging modality that provides slice images of any chemical tagged with a radioisotope. Low atomic weight isotopes with short half-lives are used. As they decay, positrons are emitted and interact with electrons in the brain. With the resulting annihilation, two photons are emitted and travel in opposite directions. Detector crystals, located in a ring around the head, respond to the arrival of the photons on opposite sides of the ring and provide a highly precise reconstruction of the density of the isotopes. Because of the short half-life of the isotopes used, the technique requires a cyclotron to produce positron emitters and a radiochemistry laboratory for rapid synthesis of radiopharmaceuticals. See *imaging, brain; SPECT.*

PET scanning is used to map the glucose metabolism of neurons, an index of neuronal activity, and to measure blood flow. The distribution, density, and response to medication of transmitter receptors can be studied by administering radiolabeled neurotransmitters. Radionucleotides used in PET include Carbon 11 [$^{11}$C], Nitrogen 13, Oxygen 15, and Fluroine 18. $^{18}$F-FDG-PET is especially valuable in the study of brain function because the rate of glucose metabolism increases in regions of brain activity. [FDG is the glucose analogue fluroro-2-deoxy-D-glucose.] PET also allows noninvasive study of cerebral blood flow and volume, oxygen metabolism, and drug concentrations in particular brain regions. PET has proved to be important in the evaluation of patients with neurodegenerative disorders. Recently developed molecular imaging agents include $^{18}$F-FDDNP, a PET ligand that can determine the localization and load of neurofibrillary tangles and beta-amyloid plaques in the brains of living patients with Alzheimer Disease. Another selective PET radioligand images the human 5-HT transporter site, allowing the in vivo detection of cerebral SERT availability (the serotonin transporter).

PET/CT fusion is a relatively new technique that allows the nearly synchronous acquisition of images and precise coregistration of the functional (PET) and anatomic (CT) data sets, providing improved anatomic localization of abnormalities identified on PET.

**petalia** Impressions left on the inner surface of the skull by asymmetrical protrusions of the cerebral hemispheres. See *asymmetry, brain.*

**petit mal epilepsy** *Absences; lapses;* they may be associated with major seizures or may occur without them. Laymen know them as faints, sensations, or spells. They consist of one or more of the following: mild attacks of dizziness, faintness, queer sensations, dazed states, hot flashes, pallor, vomiting, belching, temper tantrums, sudden relaxation of musculature (so that the patient drops anything in his hand and stops speaking for a moment), momentary confusion and change of color, dreamy sensations, sudden visual or auditory or gustatory sensations, peculiar rushing sensations through the body, and sudden jerks and starts. Petit mal attacks are usually extremely brief in duration and often there is no memory of the loss of consciousness so that the patient is only dimly aware of the occurrence of a spell. Petit mal epilepsy occurs typically in young people and only rarely begins after the second decade.

Associated psychiatric symptoms are rare and there is almost never an aura. Usually there is immobility during an attack (*akinetic epilepsy*) and the patient is mentally clear immediately after the attack. Incontinence is infrequent in petit mal epilepsy.

Petit mal epilepsy is associated with a spike and wave complex (also known as *dart and dome* complex) in the electroencephalogram, usually at a frequency of 3 Hz. Some workers use the term *pyknolepsy* (q.v.) synonymously with petit mal.

**Petrides model**   A model of *working memory* (q.v.) that assigns the more passive ("on-line") short-term maintenance of information to the ventral portion of the prefrontal cortex, and the more active ("executive") processing of information held on-line to the dorsal portion.

**petrification**   Fixity, rigidity; used to describe the attitude and behavior of chronic schizophrenics whose symptoms in time tend to become colorless, repetitive, and robotlike. Also, the process of turning, or being turned, into stonylike substance or stone; often in myths, fairy tales, etc., it is a punishment for scopophilic or voyeuristic impulses.

**pettifog**   A popular term denoting mental confusion.

**peyote**   The dried blossoms of the mescal cactus. Descriptions of its use in religious ceremonies of the Aztecs of Mexico, and in Guatemala, Peru, and El Salvador, date back more than 3000 years. Its active principle is *mescaline* (q.v.), which is structurally similar to norepinephrine. The effects of mescaline are similar to those of LSD, although the latter is between 5000 and 10000 times more potent.

**Pfaundler-Hurler syndrome**   *Gargoylism.* See *mucopolysaccharidosis.*

**PFC**   *Prefrontal cortex.* See *association areas; frontal lobe.*

**pfropfschizophrenia**   *Graftschizophrenie;*frequently misspelled propfschizophrenia. Pfropfschizophrenia was formerly termed *dual diagnosis* (q.v.); it is a recurrent schizophrenic syndrome superimposed or engrafted on mental retardation. It is frequently precipitated by hospitalization, arrest, or some other important event. Schizophrenia may also be engrafted on other organic disease, which releases the schizophrenic disorder in a predisposed subject.

**PGD**   *Preimplantation genetic diagnosis;* used as a way to avoid transfer of an embryo carrying gene(s) that predispose to a disorder. It has been used successfully in late-onset disorders with genetic predisposition, including an early-onset form of Alzheimer disease associated with mutations of the amyloid precursor protein on chromosome 21.

**PGR**   *Psychogalvanic reflex* (q.v.).

**Phaedra complex**   A mother who is in love with her son. The term is also used to refer to a nonpathologic attraction between stepparent and stepchild, a counterpart of the Oedipus relationship. See *Jocasta complex.*

**-phagia, -phagy**   Combining form meaning eating, food, from Gr. *phagein.*

**phagomania**   Uncontrollable or insatiable desire to eat; *bulimia* (q.v.).

**phagophobia**   Fear of eating.

**phakomatoses**   A group of disorders involving ectodermal and neurocutaneous tissues; they are usually transmitted as autosomal dominants, manifest themselves in childhood, and are slowly progressive. Included are *neurofibromatosis, ataxia-telangiectasia, tuberous sclerosis, Hippel-Lindau disease*, and *Sturge-Weber syndrome* (qq.v.).

**phallic**   In psychoanalysis, relating to the penis during the phase of infantile sexuality.

**phallic mother**   In psychoanalysis the male's phantasy that the mother has a phallus. Having seen no other type of genital formation, the male child assumes that his mother possesses genitals like his and wants to see them. When he finds later that women have no penis, the original longing to see his mother's penis "often becomes transformed into its opposite and gives place to disgust which in the years of puberty may become the cause of psychic impotence, of misogyny, and of lasting homosexuality." And in fetishism the object that the patient reveres is "a substitutive symbol for the once revered and since then missed member of the woman." The phantasy is personified in those mythological deities in which the goddess possesses a phallus as well as breasts (Freud, S. *Leonardo da Vinci*, 1922).

**phallic phase**   The stage of development in which libidinal and aggressive energies are concentrated mainly in the genital area (penis and clitoris); the phallic phase follows the anal phase and is generally in evidence during the period of 4 to 6 years of age. Concentration of drive energies in the genital area is due in part to increasing physical maturation, and in part to the child's increasing awareness of and natural curiosity about the differences between the sexes. Manipulation of the genitalia can certainly be observed before this phase, but masturbation now is characteristically accompanied by phantasies that relate to the use of the penis as an executive of libido or aggression. Object love in the phallic period is very close to what it will be in adolescence and adulthood, but there are two factors that decisively limit sexuality to a still infantile level. One is physiologic immaturity, and maturation here will have to wait until adolescence; the other is the danger attendant upon the choice of the love object. The child is restricted in his social contacts, and the mother, who has been more or less the only other actor on his stage, retains her leading role. She will be the object of his psychic energies here, just as she was in earlier days; this is the relationship termed oedipal. The dangers of this relationship—rejection by the mother, retaliation by the father, etc.—necessitate a strong blockade against libidinal impulses. The ego achieves this by mobilizing aggressive energies against the id. Libidinal energies are repressed, and the child passes into the period of *latency* (q.v.). See *ontogeny, psychic.*

**phallic pride**   See *penis pride.*

**phallic primacy**   When libido becomes preponderantly concentrated on the penis, during the stage of infantile sexuality. See *ontogeny, psychic.*

**phallic sadism**   Aggression associated with the phallic stage of development. The child ordinarily comprehends sexual intercourse as an aggressive and sadistic act on the part of the male, and specifically on the part of the penis. Evidence that the penis is phantasied as a weapon of violence and destruction comes from unconscious productions of normal adults. Limericks, for instance, often refer to the penis as square, or too large, so that intercourse is dangerous and painful for the partner. This may well be a projection of the male's own fear of coitus. Scop(t)ophilia may result at the phallic stage, secondary to such sadism. The looking gives reassurance that the sadistically perceived object is not yet dead. See *scopophilia.*

**phallic sexual monism**   Belief that there is only one sex, the male, evidenced by the presence of a penis, and ignorance (in both sexes, according to the classical psychoanalytic theory) of the existence of a vagina.

**phallic symbol**   Anything that represents the penis. Many phallic symbols have been described: knife, spear, gun, and other similar weapons; tree, column, pillar, skyscraper, automobile, airplane, bird, snake, wild animals, cigar, cigarette, pen, pencil, key, screw, hammer, and any number of other objects that go up and down, go in and out, or extend and retreat.

**phallicism, phallism**   Phallic worship.

**phallic-narcissistic character**   *Phallic-narcissistic personality* (q.v.).

**phallic-narcissistic personality**   W. Reich (1933) described the phallic-narcissistic character: arrogant, self-assured, energetic, impressive, exhibitionistic with an emphasis on power or beauty, often promiscuous; reacts with cold disdain, marked ill-humor, or downright aggression to any offense to his vanity; shows a tendency toward sadistic perversions, sexual impotence, homosexuality, addictions, and superego defects. Such traits are viewed as a defense against passive-feminine tendencies and a desire for revenge against the opposite sex. In treatment, the character resistance is seen in aggressive deprecation of the analysis and a tendency to take over the interpretation work. See *character defense; narcissistic personality.*

**phallometry**   Measures of changes in penile circumference in response to audio/visual stimuli—typically audiotapes or videotapes describing or portraying sexual activities. The activities portrayed vary in age, sex, degree of consent, coercion, or violence.

Phallometry is most frequently used in the assessment and treatment of sexual offenders, particularly as an aid in discriminating between nonoffender and offender populations, and between different populations of sex offenders.

**phallus**   In psychoanalysis, the penis during the period of infantile sexuality when it is intensely charged or cathected with narcissistic love. When the narcissistic qualities associated with one's own genital organ are directed outwardly upon a love object, it is said that the stage of *genital love* has been reached. Thus, genital love in the male may be called penile love, in contrast to phallic love.

**phallus girl**   The unconscious symbolic equation of girl with phallus, as in *transvestitism* (q.v.). The male transvestite has phantasized that the woman has a penis in order to overcome his castration anxiety, and he identifies with the phallic woman under whose clothes a penis is hidden.

The female identification frequently represents an identification not with the mother but with a "little girl," for example, with a little sister.

Another example is *urophilia* (q.v.), in which men have a sexual interest in female urination." The interest in watching urinating women meant the hope of finding out that they, too, have a penis."

This equation may also occur in heterosexuals. Certain narcissistic men who in childhood liked to think of themselves as girls may fall in love with more or less boyish "little girls," in whom they see the reincarnation of themselves. They treat these girls with the tenderness they would like to have been given by their own mothers. They love them not for themselves but they love in them the feminine parts of their own ego. As a result of "a castration anxiety, similar to that in cases of homosexuality... the narcissistically chosen girl 'may represent' not only one's own person in adolescence but specifically one's own penis" (Fenichel, O. *The Psychoanalytic Theory of Neurosis*, 1945).

**phaneromania** An irresistible impulse to touch some part of one's own body especially an exterior growth on it. It is a form of repetition-compulsion, related to ticlike movements. A patient had the compulsion to rub his nose; to him the nose, a centrally placed, unpaired organ, was equated with the penis. A homosexual woman, infuriated by all manifestations of effeminacy, constantly stroked her breasts, as if trying to rub something off them.

**phantasia** *Phantasy* (q.v.).

**phantasm** A sense perception, appearing in the form of illusion or hallucination. Phantasms are classed as pseudohallucinations in that they are usually recognized as being illusory or imaginary; often the illusion is of an absent person seen in the form of a spirit or ghost.

**phantasmagoria** The raising or recalling of spirits of the dead.

**phantastica** See *psychotomimetic*.

**phantasy (fantasy)** A product of *imagination* (q.v.) consisting of a group of symbols synthesized by the secondary process into a unified story, in which the subject appears as one of the actors. The phantasy may originate from conflicts secondary to unsatisfied instinctual wishes or secondary to frustration in external reality; it may be a substitute for action, or it may prepare the way for later action; it may afford gratification for id impulses, it may serve the ego as a defense, or it may subserve superego functions by providing the imagery on which moral concepts, for example, are based. See *daydream*.

With a growing ability to test reality and to differentiate self images or representations from object images or representations, the child is able to use phantasy more effectively for both drive-reducing and creative purposes. Use of phantasy prepares the way for the inception of preoperational thought (Piaget) and the development of effective foreplanning.

A distinction made, but rarely observed, is to use *fantasy* for conscious constructions, *phantasy* for the content of unconscious constructions. In object relations theory as developed by Melanie Klein, phantasy denotes the whole inner world of one's unconscious feeling and impulse and therefore the source of all behavior.

**phantasy, secondary** See *phantasy, unconscious*.

**phantasy, unconscious** Unconscious phantasies "have either always been unconscious and formed in the unconscious, or more often, they were once conscious phantasies, day-dreaming" that were repressed into the unconscious (Freud, S. *Collected Papers*, 1924–25).

The unconscious phantasies of young children, the "*primal phantasies*" of Freud, are derived from several sources, such as the Oedipus situation, ideas of procreation, the phenomena of birth, the castration complex.

Secondary unconscious phantasies are as a rule some modification of the foregoing primal phantasies. For instance, the revival of the Oedipus complex at puberty gives rise to a new set of phantasies with certain adult sexual issues added.

**phantasy life** Daydreaming, in contradistinction to thinking that is logical and realistic. Varendonck says that phantasy life "gives the illusion that wishes and aspirations have been fulfilled; it thinks obstacles away; it transforms impossibilities into possibilities and realities." He adds that it is "a search for pleasurable representations and an avoidance of everything likely to cause pain" (*The Psychology of Day Dreams*, 1921).

Often the real meaning of a phantasy is not clear. In this condition it is called *screen phantasy* (q.v.), for it is believed to cover up a deeply repressed urge.

**phantasy-cathexis** *Introversion* (q.v.).

**phantasy-thinking** *Autism* (q.v.).

**phantom** See *autoscopy*.

**phantom child syndrome** See *misidentification, delusional*.

**phantom limb** The global feeling that a limb that has been lost (e.g., by amputation) is still present (phantom limb awareness), as well as specific sensory and kinesthetic sensations (phantom sensations). These nonpainful phantom phenomena are reported by almost all amputees. Phantom limb pain, or phantom pain, belongs to a groups of neuropathic pain syndromes.

Phantom pain is characterized by feelings of pain in the amputated limb, ranging from simple, short-lasting, and rarely occurring painful shocks in a missing body part, to a constant, excruciatingly painful experience during which the person has a vivid and intense perception of the missing body part. It seems to be more severe in the distal portions of the phantom and can be stabbing, throbbing, burning, or cramping. Its onset can be immediate, but it may also appear for the first time many years after the amputation. It occurs in 50%–80% of amputees. It is likely that reorganization following amputation occurs not only for the areas involved in sensory-discriminative aspects of pain, but also for those brain regions that mediate affective-motivational aspects of pain, such as the insula, anterior cingulate, and frontal cortices. See *pain syndromes*.

*Telescoping* is also frequently observed in amputees and refers to perceived changes in the size and length of the phantom, shrinking and retraction of the phantom towards the residual limb; the phantom can even retract into the stump. It is related to increased levels of phantom pain.

**phantom lover syndrome** *Erotomania* (q.v.).

**pharmacogenetics** The influence of hereditary factors in determining individual differences in response to drugs. See *pharmacogenomics*.

**pharmacogenomics** The influence of the wide range of tools of gene-based molecular science on pharmacology, including prediction of drug response and ability to individualize drug treatment based on genetic information. Pharmacogenomics provides a science-based paradigm for understanding individual variation in drug response. It is a broader term than *pharmacogenetics*.

**pharmacogeriatrics** The study of the use and effects of pharmacologic agents in the elderly. Older patients constitute 11% of the population but consume 29% of prescription drugs, have the highest incidence of adverse drug reactions, and take a greater variety and quantity of medication than younger patients do.

Many studies indicate that the proper selection and use of drugs in elderly patients require as much specificity and individualization as does use of drugs in the infant or child.

**pharmacokinetics** Pharmacodynamics; the study of the actions of a drug within the living organism, particularly in regard to systemic availability of a drug as affected by time after administration, biotransformation (typically, in the liver), and excretion (e.g., renal clearance, biliary or pulmonary excretion). A drug's pharmacokinetics are termed *linear* when its concentration in the blood varies in proportion with the amount of drug administered (indicating, for example, that there has been no unusual biotransformation of the drug that interferes with its availability).

**pharmacologic hypomania** In patients with depression, a rapid switch into hypomania as a response to treatment with antidepressants.

**pharmacopsychoanalysis** Narcoanalysis. See *narcotherapy*.

**phase** *Stage* (q.v.).

**phase advance** A temporal pattern shift in a regularly recurring phenomenon so that it appears early; a shortening of the interval between repetitions or recurrences. The shortened *REM latency* (q.v.) of depressed patients is hypothesized to be a phase advance of circadian rhythms.

**phase sequences** See *equipotentiality*.

**phase-advance hypothesis** The theory that sleep/wake activity is controlled by two biological clocks—a strong oscillator that controls the circadian rhythms of temperature, cortisol, and REM sleep, and a weak oscillator that controls the rhythm of non-REM sleep. In depression, the strong oscillator is phase advanced, and for that reason phase-advance therapy (advancing bedtime to 5 or 6 p.m. for example, and waking the patient at 1 or 2 a.m. for several days) is beneficial in some depressed patients. See *S-deficiency hypothesis*.

**-phasia** Combining form meaning faculty or power of speech, from Gr. *phasis*, saying, word, from *phanai*, to speak.

**phasic elements** See *REM sleep*.

**phasmophobia** *Obs.* Fear of ghosts.

**phasophrenias** A group of benign degenerative psychoses with atypical symptoms that usually begin with cyclical phases or episodes from which the patient recovers spontaneously; called by Kleist *degeneration psychosis* (q.v.). See *reactive psychosis*.

**phencyclidine**   *PCP; angel dust*; an arylcyclohex-ylamine that was developed as a surgical anes-thetic but abandoned as such because of the emergence syndrome it produced: disorienta-tion, agitation, and delirium.

Since about 1967, it has been used illic-itly as a *hallucinogen* (q.v.), under any num-ber of street names: PeaCe Pill, Crystal, CJ, KJ, Hog, Rocket Fuel, sheet, goon, busy bee, and superjoint. With the recognition of glutamate's role as an excitotoxin in the 1980s, phencyclidine's action as a glutamate receptor blocker has been proposed as a way of arresting nerve cell death in victims of stroke, heart attack, and head trauma. See *glutamate*.

As a psychedelic drug, phencyclidine can be inhaled ("snorted"), injected, or taken by mouth, but most commonly it is sprayed over parsley, mint leaves, or marijuana and then smoked. Effects appear within 5 minutes and plateau within 30 minutes. The user becomes uncommunicative and oblivious to the sur-roundings, with "speedy" feelings and sensa-tions of warmth, tingling, floating, and calm isolation. Auditory or visual hallucinations may develop as well as alterations of body image and distortion of space and time per-ception. Thinking may become disorganized, and confusion and delusions may appear.

Adverse reactions include unpredictable fluctuations in mood and behavior, impul-sivity, and fearfulness. During the immediate recovery period, depression and self-destruc-tive or violent (including homicidal) behavior may be seen. At low doses, dysarthria, ataxia, muscle rigidity, hypertension, and nystagmus occur. At higher dose levels, hyperthermia, diaphoresis, agitation, athetosis, and occa-sionally opisthotonic posturing may develop. Stupor, coma, and status epilepticus have also been reported at high doses.

**phencyclidine intoxication**   The syndrome includes maladaptive behavioral changes, such as belligerence, assaultiveness, impulsive-ness, unpredictability, psychomotor agitation, and impaired judgment; and physical signs, such as nystagmus, hypertension or tachycar-dia, numbness or diminished responsiveness to pain, ataxia, dysarthria, muscle rigidity, seizures, and hyperacusis.

**phencyclidine use disorders**   These are classified within the substance-related disorders and include phencyclidine (or relatedsubstance)

dependence, phencyclidine abuse, phency-clidine intoxication, phencyclidine delirium, phencyclidine psychotic disorder, phencycli-dine mood disorder, and phencyclidine anx-iety disorder.

**phengophobia**   Fear of daylight (comfort being felt only at night).

**phenocopy**   A disorder, not genetic in origin, which imitates another disease; an individual exhibiting a trait similar to a gene-related trait but due to nongenetic factors. Schizophrenia-like psychoses associated with drug-induced organic brain disorders are phenocopies of schizophrenia.

**phenocopy multiple personality disorder**   A type of MPD in which an alter's influences create phenomena that mimic the manifestations of other mental disorders. See *dissociative iden-tity disorder*.

**phenome awareness**   The capacity to manipu-late the individual elements of speech, often impaired in *dyslexia* (q.v.). Testing for pho-neme awareness might include directing the subject to delete phonemes ("Say 'plot' with-out the 'l' sound") or to construct spooner-isms ("Switch the first sounds of the two words, 'Dear Queen'"). See *language acquisi-tion*.

**phenomenal field**   Adler's term for one's con-structed representation of objective reality, the meaning given to the profusion of stimuli that bombard the person and are organized and conceptualized on the basis of individual and personal prior experiences.

**phenomenological reality**   See *Morita therapy*.

**phenomenology**   The study of events and hap-penings in their own right, rather than from the point of view of inferred causes; specifi-cally, the theory that behavior is determined by the way in which the subject perceives reality at any moment and not by reality as it can be described in physical, objective terms. See *existentialism*.

**phenothiazine**   Class name for a group of *anti-psychotic drugs* (q.v.). The phenothiazines are *major* tranquilizers and are sometimes sub-divided on the basis of chemical structure into (1) *alipathic group*—including chlor-promazine, promazine, and triflupromazine; (2) piperazine group—including perphena-zine, prochlorperazine, trifluoperazine, and fluphenazine; and (3) *piperidine group*—including mepazine, and thioridazine. See *psychopharmacologic agents*.

**phenotype** An observable trait; the changeable picture of an organism's appearance as produced and modified by its external life situation. In contrast to the *genotypical structure*, the *phenotype* of an organism is the sum of all its manifested attributes. It is the outward manifestation of the subject's biochemistry, determined by the interaction of what is directed by the genes, the genotype, and the environment. See *genetic directive; genotype.*

**phenotypic dissection** Division of a syndrome into distinct but related phenotypic components, each of which can then be analyzed as to whether it is largely heritable, or due mainly to environmental factors (such as shared environment). See *dyslexia.*

**phenotypic fitness** The measure of an organism's ability to survive and reproduce in a given environment; fitness refers only to the organism's phenotypic characteristics. Darwin termed the process by which Nature rewards those of higher phenotypic fitness *natural selection.* The currently more fashionable idea of *genetic fitness* is a measure of an organism's genetic contribution to the next generation; this concept makes no reference to the organism's phenotypic properties.

**phenylketonuria** A hereditary disorder of phenylalanine metabolism, caused by recessive mutations in the phenylalanine hydroxylase (FAH) gene on chromosome 12. Because the enzyme phenylalanine hydroxylase is inactive, phenylalanine is not converted into tyrosine but instead accumulates in the body, where it is converted into phenylpyruvic acid and excreted in the urine as phenylketones. The excess phenylalanine, and probably some of its abnormal metabolites, inhibit various enzyme systems and interfere with myelination of nerve tissue, thus producing severe mental retardation (most untreated patients have intelligence quotients below 20).

Because of the phenylketones it contains, the urine of affected children turns olive green in response to 10% ferric chloride (a normal reaction is red-brown color). The reaction was described in 1934 by Dr. Asbjorn Folling of the University of Oslo and hence is often termed the *Folling test.* Until the mid-1950s, urine testing was the standard procedure for identifying phenylketonuria (PKU), but the method was not wholly satisfactory in that 25% to 50% of affected children do not excrete detectable amounts of phenylpyruvic

acid until after irreversible brain damage has already occurred.

A more sensitive test is the *Guthrie test*, a blood test based on bacterial-inhibition assay devised in 1961 by the American pediatrician Robert Guthrie (1917–1995). A drawback of this test is that it gives false positives, and dietary restriction of phenylalanine in children who do not have PKU may be fatal. Most authorities recommend repeated urine examinations and blood testing at birth and again at 2 weeks of age, to confirm the diagnosis.

Treatment is dietary restriction of phenylalanine; if begun early enough the child can be expected to achieve normal or near-normal intelligence. The dietary regimen can be eased when the child is about 6 years of age, by which time brain differentiation is complete.

Because of the effectiveness of newborn screening for PKU, affected children have been treated appropriately and now routinely survive into adulthood. As a result, maternal PKU is now a public health problem rather than the rare condition it once was. Most women with PKU discontinue the phenylalanine-restricted diet during childhood; once they reach childbearing age, such women with PKU or any degree of hyperphenylalaninemia are at high risk for bearing children with mental retardation, microcephaly, congenital heart defects, and low birthweight.

Dietary therapy that reduces the maternal blood phenylalanine level and eliminates or reduces phenylalanine metabolite accumulation during pregnancy may protect the fetus. The diet should begin prior to conception and be maintained throughout pregnancy; an adequate prevention program thus depends on careful planning of pregnancies.

PKU affects approximately 1 person in every 10,000 to 20,000; in institutions for the retarded, it accounts for about 1 patient in every 100.

**phenylpyruvic oligophrenia** See *phenylketonuria.*

**phenytoin** An *anticonvulsant* drug (q.v.).

**pheromone** A substance released by an organism whose odor affects the behavior of others of the same species. A number of insects, for example, produce attractant pheromones by which one sex finds the other. Alarm pheromones are secreted by some ants and beetles when they are attacked, causing others in their group or cluster to disperse. Some theorists have suggested that pheromones or *external chemical messages* (*ECM*) exist in the human and that the schizophrenic is aware of and responds to such stimuli that "normal" people ignore. Most investigators remain doubtful, however, of the applicability of the pheromone concept to mammals, and some believe that even for insects it is an oversimplification of behavioral responses.

**PHF** Paired helical filaments, part of the neurofibrillary tangles characteristic of Alzheimer disease. See *NFT*.

**-philias** See table under *mania*.

**philo-, phil-** Combining form meaning loving, from Gr. *philos*.

**philobat** Balint's term for the person with that type of primitive relationship to the environment characterized by an indifference to objects, which are typically considered as untrustworthy hazards, and a preference for objectless expanses such as mountains, deserts, sea, and air. Philobats are thrill-seekers who like adventure and travel and dislike being tied down. They typically have a history of shallow commitments as manifested in a long line of brief love affairs or a pattern of frequent job changes.

Balint hypothesized that the philobatic style reflects the person's experience during separation-individuation with a mother who rewarded risk, daring, and separation. See *ocnophile*.

**phlegmatic type** One of the four classical temperamental and constitutional types of antiquity. Galen attributed the torpor and apathy of this type to the predominance of *phlegma* (mucous secreted in the air passages of the throat) over the other three humors (fluids) of the body. See *pyknic type*.

**phob-, phobo-** Combining form meaning fearing, from Gr. *Phobos*.

**phobanthropy** *Obs.* Fear of people; anthropophobia.

**phobia** *Avoidance reaction; phobic disorder; phobic neurosis; anxiety hysteria.* A phobia is a type of anxiety disorder consisting of an excessive, unreasonable, or irrational fear cued by the presence or anticipation of a specific object or situation. Exposure to the phobia stimulus almost invariably provokes an immediate anxiety response, which may escalate into a panic attack. The phobia is more than fear, however, for the feared object or situation must be avoided, or can be endured only with marked distress, because of the anxiety

response or panic attack that it almost invariably provokes. See *anxiety disorders; anxiety hysteria*; see also listings under *fear of*.

Three major forms of phobia are recognized:

1. *Specific phobia* (also known as *simple* or *isolated phobia*)—the most frequent are natural environment type (animals, insects, storms, water; see *ailurophobia; bug phobia*); *blood-injection-injury type*, cued by seeing blood or by receiving an injection or being subjected to some other invasive medical procedure (this type is highly familial and is often accompanied by a strong vasovagal response); situational type (cars, trains, heights, escalators, elevators, tunnels, bridges); and other avoidances such as situations that could lead to choking, vomiting, or contracting an illness. The situational subtype has a bimodal age-at-onset distribution, with one peak in childhood and another in the mid-20s. It is similar to panic disorder with agoraphobia in its sex ratio (much more frequent in females), its pattern of familial aggregation, and its age at onset.

2. *Social phobia* (social anxiety disorder; when it occurs in children, avoidant disorder)—avoidance of situations in which the person may be subjected to scrutiny by others and in which he or she will act in a way that will be humiliating or embarrassing (including manifesting anxiety symptoms); included are the performance type (e.g., unable to play a musical instrument, write, eat, or urinate in front of others although can comfortably perform such activities when alone), the limited interactional type (the fear is restricted to one or two social situations, such as speaking to authority figures or dating), and the generalized type (when most social situations are avoided).

3. *Agoraphobia* (q.v.)—the severest form of phobia and the one for which professional help is most often sought (although, overall, simple phobia is probably more common).

As a suffix, -phobia is also used to indicate bias against, or dislike of, as in homophobia or Islamophobia.

**phobic, mixed** The person who has spontaneous panic attacks but instead of massive *agoraphobia* (q.v.) develops a few specific avoidances such as flying or crossing bridges or driving through a tunnel. Such subjects usually respond to antidepressant medication in much the same way as agoraphobics with panic attacks.

**phobic anxiety-depersonalization neurosis** See *depersonalization*.

**phobic companion** See *agoraphobia*.

**phobic neurosis** *Anxiety hysteria* (q.v.).

**phobophobia** Fear of fearing.

**phocomelia** A deformity of the limbs in which the hands are attached directly to the shoulders without interposed arms; seen with some tetratogenic drugs and in some types of mental retardation.

**phonemes** The sounds of a language; the smallest differences in sound that distinguish different contents, such as the difference between sounds b and p. Their combination into words is *morphology*. See *akoasm*; *language acquisition*.

**phonetics** The study of speech sounds and how sentences are to be pronounced.

**phonism** See *sensation, secondary*.

**phonological decoding** The capacity to convert written grapheme units—a written symbol used to represent a specific phoneme—into speech; often impaired in *dyslexia* (q.v.). Testing for phonological decoding asks the subject to read a list of pronounceable words that lack real meaning, such as pog, ligart, fromiker.

**phonological disorder** *Articulation disorder*, characterized by speech sounds that are inappropriate for the subject's age or dialect, such as substituting "w" for "r." In addition to substitutions, the disorder may be manifested in distortions or omissions of sounds.

**phonological loop** See *short-term memory*.

**phonology** 1. Study of the sound structure of a language, of speech sounds and how they form words. 2. The sound structure of a language.

**phonophobia** Fear of sounds; fear of one's own voice.

**phonotactic patterns** See *language, acquisition of*.

**phosphatase** See *ion channel*.

**phosphene** Sensation of flashes or spots of light when the subject is in darkness which a normal person would perceive as grayish rather than total blackness. Such sensations are entoptic phenomena that may be induced by pressure on the retina or by mechanical or electrical stimulation of other parts of the optic pathway. They are also known as *Eigengrauer* and have been reported in cocaine and other drug intoxications.

**phospholipid** Any lipid that contains phosphorus. Biological membranes are composed of two layers of phospholipids, which are crucial for cell functions such as electrolyte transport, signal transduction, and receptor function. Decreased synthesis and increased breakdown of membrane phospholipids have been reported in the frontal lobe in schizophrenia. It has been suggested that abnormal enhancement of normal programmed pruning of callosal axons and synapses is a characteristic of schizophrenia. Phosphorus metabolism is evaluated by measuring brain PMEs (phosphomonoesters, precursors of phospholipids) and PDEs (phosphodiesters, breakdown products of phospholipids).

**phospholipid spectrum disorders** The psychiatric and neurologic illnesses associated with deficiencies in essential fatty acids (EFAs). Reduced EFA concentrations in the membranes of RBCs and other tissues from patients with schizophrenia and major depression have been reported. The two major *omega-3 fatty acids* (q.v.) are DHA (docosahexaenoic acid) and EPA (eicosapentaenoic acid). It is not clear whether one or both play the essential role in these effects.

**phosphorylation** The process of adding a phosphoryl group, which is the cell's major way of regulating protein activity. Different *protein kinases* phosphorylate specific proteins (the *third messenger* system) by transferring the terminal phosphoryl group from ATP to the target protein.

In general, the protein kinases themselves are activated by second messengers. See *acetylation*; *histones*; *neurotransmitter receptor*.

**photic driving** See *electroencephalogram*.

**photic epilepsy** A form of *reflex epilepsy* (q.v.).

**photism** See *sensation, secondary*.

**photoentrainment** Coupling of light cues to the circadian clock. Neither the rods nor the cones of the retina are required for photoentrainment, but removal of the eye abolishes the pineal response to light. Photic responses to light must, therefore, depend on nonrod noncone photoreceptors. Various candidate photopigments have been suggested, among them the cryptochromes *Cry1* and *Cry2*. Both crytochromes and phytochromes have roles in setting the clock, but whether they are photoreceptors or part of the clock itself is an unsettled question.

**photography, spectral** See *BEAM*.

**photomania**   Craving for light; sun worship.

**photophobia**   Literally, fear of light, but rarely used to indicate a phobic avoidance reaction. More commonly the term is used to refer to an organically determined hypersensitivity to light (as in many acute infectious diseases with conjunctivitis) that results in severe pain and marked tearing when the patient is exposed to light.

**photoreceptor**   A specialized neuron of the retina that converts light into electrical signals, a process termed *phototransduction*. There are two types of photoreceptor: *rods*, which mediate night vision, and *cones*, which mediate day vision and color vision. The photoreceptors contain visual pigments: the visual pigment in rod cells is *rhodopsin*, and each of the three types of cone cells contains a different pigment, thereby maximizing the absorption of light in different parts of the visible spectrum. Activated pigment molecules decrease the cytoplasmic concentrations of cGMP, as a result of which cGMP-gated ion channels close, the inward $Na^+$ current that flows through the channels is reduced, and the photoreceptor cell is hyperpolarized. See *melanopsin; opsin*.

The output neurons of the retina are the ganglion cells, whose axons form the optic nerve. The optic nerve, in turn, projects to the lateral geniculate nucleus and the superior colliculus, as well as to brain stem nuclei.

**phototherapy**   *Bright light therapy;* timed exposure to bright light, simulating daylight. Phototherapy has been used most often to treat seasonal affective disorder, but it has also demonstrated beneficial effects in nonseasonal mood disorders. In addition, it may be useful in managing jet lag, shift work, and certain sleep disorders. See *seasonal affective disorder*.

When phototherapy was first used in the early 1980s, the subject was exposed to 2500 lux for at least 2 hours a day for 1 or 2 weeks. More recent studies indicate that high-intensity lights (10,000 lux) for brief periods (30 minutes) may be more effective and act more quickly.

**phototransduction**   Transmission of light from one system to another. See *circadian clock; photoreceptor*.

**-phrasia**   Combining form meaning speech, way of speaking, phraseology, from Gr. *phrasis*.

**-phren-, -phrenia, phreno-**   Combining form denoting a relationship to the mind or brain (or the diaphragm), from Gr. *phren, phrenos*.

**phrenitis**   In Hippocrates's classification, acute mental disease with fever. The other classes were mania (acute mental disease without fever); melancholia (chronic mental disturbances of various kinds, not limited to mood disorders); epilepsy (approximately the same as in current use); hysteria (somatoform disturbances, especially paroxysmic dyspnea, pain, and convulsions); and *Scythian disease* (transvestitism).

**phrenology**   Study of the conformation of the skull, based on the belief that the different mental faculties could be localized in particular sites on the brain surface, whose resultant conformation would be mirrored in the conformation of the overlying skull.

**phrenophobia**   Fear of (developing) a mental illness.

**phrenopraxic**   One of the many terms used to describe the drugs that have an action on the mind or psyche; viz. the tranquilizers, ataractics, psychotropics, etc.

**phrenotropic**   Having an action on the mind. The term is usually used to describe certain pharmacologic agents, such as psychotomimetics, tranquilizers, and energizers, which have an effect on mental processes. See *psychotropics*.

**phricasmus**   *Obs.* Shivering of psychic origin.

**phrictopathia**   Sensation of touch, as unpleasantly tingling.

**phronemophobia**   Fear of thinking.

**PHS**   (United States) Public Health Service, the parent agency of CDC, NIH, FDA and other agencies and itself a component of the Department of Health and Human Services (DHHS).

**phthinoid**   In Kretschmer's system, a form of the *asthenic type* (q.v.) that is so underdeveloped as to represent a morbid condition in itself. In a more general sense, the term refers particularly to the flat, narrow chest characteristic of the tuberculous patient. Sometimes it is applied to any characteristic of the asthenic physique.

**phthisiophobia**   Fear of tuberculosis.

**pHVA**   Plasma homovanillic acid, believed to be a valid peripheral marker for dopamine and predictive of treatment response or outcome in schizophrenia. Responders show a higher baseline pHVA than nonresponders, and a more acute rise of pHVA with treatment.

**phylo-**   Combining form meaning race, tribe, clan, people, nation, from Gr. *phylon*.

**phylogenesis, phylogeny** Originally a biological term denoting the genealogical history and evolutionary development of a species or group as distinguished from the ontogenetic development of the individual. According to Haeckel's biogenetic law, phylogeny is always recapitulated by ontogeny (see *ontogenesis*).

Jung speaks of *archetypes*, which he considers "the fundamental elements of the unconscious mind, hidden in the depths of the psyche, or to use another comparison, they are the roots of the mind, sunk not only in the earth in the narrower sense, but in the world in general" (*Contributors to Analytical Psychology*, 1928). If applied in such a special metaphorical sense, the term phylogeny becomes synonymous with archaic inheritance, thus losing all connection with its original biological meaning.

**phylogenetic symptoms** See *hebephrenic schizophrenia*.

**physiatrist** See *physical medicine*.

**physical abuse** See *child abuse*; *domestic violence*; *victim*; *violence*.

**physical custody** See *custody*.

**physical dependence** See *dependence, drug*; *dependence, physical*.

**physical medicine** The diagnosis and treatment of disease by physical means; a form of applied medical biophysics. The term includes physical therapy and rehabilitation. In 1947, a specialty board was established for this branch of medicine in the United States; a physician certified by this board is known as a *physiatrist*.

**physical therapy** Physiotherapy; the branch of physical medicine that makes use of physical and other effective properties of light, heat, cold, water, electricity, mechanical agents, and *kinesitherapy* (massage, manipulation, therapeutic exercise, mechanical devices).

**physically challenged** See *disability*.

**physician assistant** PA; physician extender; an allied health professional who is educated in a medical model designed to complement physician services. PAs are well known in many areas of medicine, but they are relatively new to psychiatry. Education consists of classroom and laboratory instruction in the basic medical and behavioral sciences (including anatomy, pharmacology, pathophysiology, clinical medicine, physical diagnosis, personality development, child development, normative responses to stress, psychosomatic manifestations of illness and injury, sexuality, and responses to death and dying). Education is followed by clinical rotations in internal medicine, family medicine, surgery, pediatrics, obstetrics and gynecology, emergency medicine, and geriatric medicine. In consultation with and under the supervision of a physician, the PA performs diagnostic tests, prescribes medicine, develops treatment plans, and carries them out. Most PAs in psychiatry learn the specialty "on the job" after completing PA training. Mental health PAs have been utilized most frequently in rural areas, where access to psychiatrists is often limited.

PAs are certified by the National Commission on Certification of Physician Assistants (NCCPA). Licensing laws and definitions of scope of practice vary from state to state.

**physician extender** A generic term that includes *physician's assistant, nurse practitioner* (qq.v.), nurse clinician, and paramedic, all of whom perform various medical services as authorized by state laws and under the direction and supervision of a doctor of medicine or osteopathy who is licensed within the state.

**physiogenesis** Origin in the functioning of an organ of the body. Thus, intellectual deficiencies due to impairment of organic (cerebral) functioning are described as physiogenic manifestations.

**physiognomonic communication** Body language; nonverbal communication, such as by gesture, mime, facial expression, and/or any number of minimal cues by which meaning is transmitted from one organism to another.

**physiognomonic thinking** According to Kasanin, the first stage in the development of thought in the child. In this stage, the child animates objects and projects his ego into them, as when he plays with a stick and calls it a horse. Piaget calls this *syncretic thinking*.

The second stage is *concrete thinking*, characterized by literalness and lack of generalizations. In this stage, for example, the word "table" refers not to tables in general but to the particular table in the subject's house.

The third stage is abstract or *categorical thinking*, characterized by use of abstractions and generalizations. This type of thinking appears relatively late, usually after adolescence and probably only after some degree of education.

**physiognomy** The physical appearance of the face; also, judging personality from facial appearance.

**physiologic crisis** Bender's term for any sudden endogenous change that occurs in the course of apparently normal maturation and development. Physiologic crisis is always seen in the history of childhood schizophrenics and is often a precipitating factor in onset of psychosis. The physiologic crisis appears to depend upon embryonal plasticity and a maturational lag.

**physioneurosis** See *actual neurosis.*

**physiopathology** Study of both functional and organic disturbances of physiology, whether functional or organic in nature. The studies include various factors such as the subject's physical state and its effect on his goals, the interaction of his personality and his physical or medical status, and the social response to his condition insofar as that influences his education, occupation, recreation, social responsibleness, and adaptability (Wile, I. S. in *Handbook of Child Guidance*, ed. E. Harms, 1947).

**physioplastic stage** Verworn's term for the ability to draw what is seen, in contrast to the ideoplastic stage, in which the child draws what he knows. See *idioplastic stage.*

**physiotherapy** See *physical therapy.*

**physostigmine** An anticholinesterase drug. See *cholinergic.*

**PI** *Paradoxical intention* (q.v.).

**pia mater** A delicate fibrous membrane closely enveloping the brain and spinal cord. See *meninges.*

**Piaget, Jean** (1896–1980) Swiss child psychologist and genetic epistemologist; emphasized the partial constancy of cognitive structuring across long time periods; *The Psychology of Intelligence* (1950); *The Language and Thought of the Child* (1952).

**piblokto** *Arctic hysteria*; a culture-specific syndrome largely confined to Eskimo women: the subject begins to scream (sometimes sounding like the cry of an animal), tear off her clothing, and run about aimlessly in the snow. The attack lasts 1 or 2 hours; afterwards, the subject is amnesic for the episode. The syndrome is a type of dissociative state and is often classified as an *hysterical psychosis* (q.v.).

**pica** *Allotriophagy; cittosis*; compulsive eating of nonnutritive substances, such as ice (*pagophagia*), dirt (*geophagia*), paint, clay, laundry starch. Typically, the subject eats one kind of food; the degree of compulsivity varies, but the person tries to hide the impulse and his behavior from his family and only rarely brings it up

as a complaint to his physician. Although often ascribed to neurosis, superstition, rearing, and the like, pica most often is due to iron deficiency (which may or may not manifest itself simultaneously as iron deficiency anemia). About half of patients with iron deficiency have pica–half of those have pagophagia and the other half have food pica. Iron therapy is highly effective, and within 1 or 2 weeks not only does the pica disappear, but the original craving often becomes a revulsion.

In DSM-IV, pica is included within the *feeding disorders* and refers to the regular eating of nonnutritive substances for at least 1 month.

**picatio** *Obs. Pica* (q.v.).

**Pick complex** A clinical and pathologic spectrum of disorders that include *frontal lobe dementia, frontotemporal dementia,* and *Pick disease;* the term is suggested as a way to avoid the confusion of using frontotemporal dementia for the whole complex, as well as for the behavioral-personality disorder.

**Pick disease** (Arnold Pick, Prague psychiatrist, 1851–1924) *Frontotemporal dementia* (q.v.); Pick disease is a *neurodegenerative disorder* consisting of progressive dementia with severe emotional impairment and social and ethical aberrations. Pathologically, there is focal atrophy of the cortical cells in the temporal and frontal regions.

There is more often a family history of heredodegenerative traits in Pick disease than in Alzheimer disease, and while the dementia is less pronounced the emotions are more severely impaired.

**pickwickian syndrome** Alveolar hyperventilation syndrome; obesity associated with hypersomnolence (especially, daytime sleepiness), hypoventilation, and polycythemia, and often also with twitching movements, cyanosis, periodic respirations, congestive heart failure, arterial hypoxia and hypercapnia, and rightward axis deviation on electrocardiogram. The syndrome may sometimes be reversed by weight loss. Although the pathophysiology of the syndrome is poorly understood, the drowsiness, sleep, and muscular twitching appear to be related to hypercapnia, while polycythemia and cyanosis appear to be related to arterial hypoxia. See *eating disorders; Kleine-Levin syndrome.*

**pictophilia** A *paraphilia* (q.v.) in which sexual arousal and satisfaction are dependent upon viewing erotic or obscene graphics or films (pornography), whether alone or in the presence of a sexual partner.

**picture, inward** An internally apprehended image or picture, as commonly presented in dreams, phantasies, and visions: the pictorialized expression of material from the deeper levels of the unconscious part of the psyche. It is an inward picture not only because it occurs "inwardly" but also because (according to Jung, whose expression it is) it is a picture of our most inward, innermost self—the *true* SELF.

**Pierre Robin syndrome** Also known as the Robin triad, this syndrome, presumably of genetic origin, consists of glossoptosis (which leads to severe respiratory disorders), microcephaly, and mental retardation.

**Pigem question** A projective question asked of the patient such as, "What three things would you like most to change (or to do, or to be) in your life?" or, "If you could be changed into something else by a fairy, what would it be?" Such questions are often used as part of the mental status examination.

**pigeonholing** See *selective attention*.

**pigmentary retinal lipoid neuronal heredodegeneration** *Spielmeyer-Vogt disease*, a type of amaurotic family idiocy. See *Tay-Sachs disease*.

**pill fatigue** A frequent complication of *HAART* (q.v.) or of any kind of combination treatment regimens that require frequent dosing during the day of many different medications: the patient cannot accept the burden of the regimen and abandons treatment.

**pill-rolling tremor** See *Parkinson disease; tremor*.

**pillow, psychological** A specific form of catatonic catalepsy in which the patient lies for a long period with his head raised slightly above the pillow.

**pilocarpine** A parasympathomimetic drug. See *cholinergic*.

**piloerection** Gooseflesh, an automatic response that may be marked during withdrawal from opiates.

**pimozide** A diphenylbutylpiperidine; it is a potent dopamine blocker and calcium channel antagonist. It is an orphan drug for use in Gilles de la Tourette syndrome.

**pinching and circling test** Used to elicit signs of bradykinesia; a sequence of six movements: pinching (with thumb and forefinger) first with the right hand and next with the left; rotating the hand in a circle, first with the

right hand and next with the left; pinching with the right hand and at the same time circle with the left; finally, pinching with the left hand while circling with the right.

**pindolol** A *beta blocker* (q.v.).

**pineal therapy** Treatment with extracts of beef-pineal substance advocated in the 1950s for treatment of chronic schizophrenia.

**Pinel system** Named after Philippe Pinel, through whose efforts forcible restraint of the mentally ill was abolished. See *moral treatment*.

**Pinel-Haslam syndrome** Schizophrenia; the phrase (suggested by Mark D. Althschule) recognizes that Pinel (1745–1826) formulated the concept of an illness manifested by diminished expression of affect, looseness of associations and difficulty in forming abstractions, dissociation of mood and content in thinking, and inattention or withdrawal. Shortly after Pinel's description, Haslam further elaborated the concept.

**pingponging** Needless and repetitive referral of patients from one specialist to another in order to generate fees, alleged by some economists to be a significant factor in the continuing rise in the cost of medical care and usually considered a form of fraud and abuse by third-party payers.

**pink disease** *Acrodynia* (q.v.).

**pink spot** *DMPEA*; 3,4-dimethoxyphenethylamine, which when dipped in ninhydrin-pyridine reagent and treated with a modified Ehrlich reagent takes on a pink color. In 1962, Friedhoff and Van Winkle reported that DMPEA was found in urine samples from schizophrenics but not in those of normal subjects. Attempts to confirm those findings have yielded contradictory results, and there is some evidence that the finding is an artifact, related more to dietary factors than to schizophrenia.

**PINK1** PTEN-induced putative kinase 1 gene, on chromosome 1p36 (the *PARK6* locus). Mutation in the gene causes early-onset Parkinson disease in a small group of European families.

**pinocytosis** Entrapment of fluid by the folds of undulating cellular membranes, with the formation of vacuoles that migrate through the cytoplasm; this may be the major method by which the glia contribute to metabolic transport within the central nervous system.

**Piotrowski, Zygmunt A.** (1904–1985) Polish-born psychologist, to United States in 1928; in

*Perceptanalysis* he presented a system of interpretation of the Rorschach inkblots.

**PIP syndrome** Psychosis, intermittent hyponatremia, and polydipsia; the syndrome can proceed to death if not identified and treated early.

**Pisa syndrome** *Pleurothotonus* (q.v.).

**pithiatism** A forced suggestion; a method of removing hysterical symptoms by way of persuasion. The word was coined by Babinski, who held that everything that is hysterical may be caused by suggestion.

**pithiatric** Curable by persuasion or suggestion, referring to the class of hysterical symptoms that can be made to disappear or be reproduced by means of suggestion.

**Pitres rule** A polyglot who becomes aphasic as the result of vascular ictus or craniocerebral trauma usually begins to understand and then to speak the language most familiar to him and in which he was most fluent at the onset of aphasia; only later are other previously known languages reestablished, more slowly and less completely.

**pituitarism** Overactivity of the pituitary gland. See *gigantism*.

**pituitary** The "master gland". Hanging by a stalk from the hypothalamus, its nerve fibers and portal blood vessels link the communication-control systems—nervous and hormonal. Prohormones, from the hypothalamus, pass down the neurosecretory cell axons in the pituitary stalk and are converted into hormone and stored in the posterior pituitary. See *hypothalamic-pituitary-adrenal axis*.

**pituitary cachexia** See *hypophysial cachexia*.

**pituitary dwarfism** See *growth hormone*.

**pity** Compassion or sympathy for another's misfortune. The term implies that the object of pity is regarded as inferior to the subject. Pity may appear as a character trait, signifying "I shower you with love as I wish I had been loved." It may also signify passive-feminine identification with the sufferer.

**pixel** Picture element; any of the several thousand tiny squares into which the brain map is divided in brain imaging. Surface imaging methods, which are less precise than tomographic methods, typically use between 16 and 32 sensors or detectors. The values recorded (expressed as colors) in those 16 to 32 squares are exact measurements; for the pixels between those "absolute" values, the color is interpolated by calculating the distance of each pixel

from the three or four closest squares with a known value. See *imaging, brain*.

**pixie people syndrome** See *Williams-Beuren syndrome*.

**PKC** CAMP-dependent protein kinase C, an important cellular signaling enzyme. Among other things, activity of PKC in the hippocampus is highly correlated with spatial learning in mice and may be one of the many genes that influence such learning. There is also evidence that PKC isoenzymes may, at least in part, determine genetic differences in response to ethanol. A subunit of the GABA-A complex is necessary for potentiation of GABA-A receptors by physiological concentrations of ethanol, and that subunit is phosphorylated by PKC. See *NMDAR*.

**PKU** *Phenylketonuria* (q.v.).

**place cells** Cells in the CA1 region of the hippocampus that are sensitive to an animal's position in space and encode a location map of the environment. Neurons in hippocampus have *place fields*—they fire strongly when the animal is in a particular location and thereby keep track of relative spatial location by integrating linear and angular motion, a process termed *path integration*.

*Head direction cells*, also in the medial superior temporal region, encode the direction of movement, derived from the expanding or contracting visual scene. *Path cells*, in the medial entorhinal cortex, integrate heading and place. See *cognitive mapping*.

**placebo** (L. "I am to placate") Any medication used to relieve symptoms, not by reason of specific pharmacologic action but solely by reinforcing the patient's favorable expectancies from treatment. Also known as *dummy*, particularly in Britain. Although a placebo may be an inert substance, as used in present-day research placebos more commonly contain active substances that at least in part mimic the side effects of the specific therapeutic agent with which the placebo is being compared. *Placebo effects* include all those psychologic and psychophysiologic benefits and undesirable reactions that reflect the patient's expectations; they depend upon the diminution or augmentation of apprehension produced by the symbolism of medication or by the symbolic implications of the physician's behavior and attitudes.

More broadly, a placebo is any therapeutic procedure that has an effect on a symptom or disease, even though objectively it has no specific action on the condition being treated.

Administration of a placebo, combined with the suggestion that it is a painkiller, can reduce pain by both opioid and nonopioid mechanisms. When painkillers are administered by hidden infusion (using machines), the analgesic dose required to reduce pain by 50% is much higher than that required when the drugs are administered by open infusion (in full view of the patient). The difference between the two methods of analgesic administration could be eliminated by blocking opioid receptors, indicating that open injection activates endogenous opioid systems, presumably through expectation pathways.

The placebo response is not limited to pain. Placebo-induced expectation of motor improvement in patients with Parkinson disease, for instance, induces release of dopamine and, presumably, reward mechanisms. Dopamine and opioid systems interact, and endogenous opioids are also involved in reward mechanisms.

The finding that the placebo response is a psychobiological phenomenon that affects brain biochemistry is not a justification for deception or quackery; rather, it demonstrates that psychosocial factors, including therapist–patient interactions, have a significant effect on patients' responses to treatment. It should be noted that, in similar fashion, negative verbal suggestions can modulate pain perception and other treatment responses in the opposite direction—the *nocebo effect*.

**placebo, balanced**    See *balanced placebo design*.

**planomania**    *Obs.* Impulse to wander from home and throw off the restraints of society.

**planophrasia**    *Obs.* Wandering speech; flight of ideas.

**plantar reflex**    A superficial reflex; stroking the sole of the foot causes flexion of the toes. This reflex depends upon the tibial nerve for its afferents and efferents; its center is at $S_{2-1}$.

**planum temporale**    Part of the heteromodal association cortex, on the superior surface of the temporal lobe posterior to *Heschl gyrus*, corresponding to a portion of Wernicke's area and a part of Brodmann's area 22. The posterior superior temporal gyrus is an external landmark of the planum temporale. In right-handed people the surface area of the left planum temporale is usually much larger than that of the right. The direction of this asym-

metry is related to handedness, and the magnitude of the asymmetry is related to gender: it is less marked in females. There is some evidence for abnormal planum temporale asymmetry in dyslexia, and a reversal of expected asymmetry has been reported in the brains of right-handed schizophrenic patients.

The planum temporale is thought to be involved in word generation and language functions. Damage to this region produces a fluent aphasia characterized by neologisms or inappropriate word substitutions.

**plaques, senile**    *Neuritic plaques*; microscopic lesions of the brain with a central core of beta-amyloid (A4) protein surrounded by a granular zone consisting of abnormal glial cells and dystrophic neurites, and masses of degenerating mitochondria and paired helical filaments (neurofibrillary tangles). See *Alzheimer disease; NFT*.

Senile plaques appear in middle age, gradually increase with age, and can be found in 70% of persons over the age of 65. In Alzheimer disease, the plaques are particularly dense in the amygdaloid complex, hippocampus, subiculum, and hippocampal gyrus.

**plasma proteins**    Acute phase plasma proteins include alpha-1-antichymotrypsin, alpha-1-antitrypsin, alpha-1-glycoprotein, ceruloplasmin, haptoglobin, immunoglobulin-A, -G, and -M. Levels of many of these are above normal in depression. Some researchers interpret such findings as indicative of an inflammatory response in depression.

**plasmalemma**    See *myelin*.

**plasmapheresis**    *TPE* (therapeutic plasma exchange); a procedure to remove toxic elements from blood consisting of removing the blood, separating the plasma from the formed elements, and reinfusing the formed elements together with a plasma replacement. One major use of TPE is in autoimmunity disorders. Because effects are short-lived (4 to 6 weeks), it is of greatest value in monophasic diseases of short duration, such as Guillain-Barré syndrome, or when used as a temporary expedient in chronic disorders, such as myasthenia gravis, lupus, and multiple sclerosis.

**plasmid**    A hereditary unit, physically distinct from the chromosome, that has been used in genetic engineering to transfer a human gene into bacteria, which then copy the information and produce, for example, the hormone that the gene produces normally in the human. R plasmids are resistant to a variety of antibiotics; much genetic engineering has used naturally occurring R plasmids. See *recombinant DNA*.

**plasticity**  In neurology, changes in the developing organism induced by environmental influences and mediated through organization of the nervous system; one manifestation is the ability of axons and dendrites to grow, regenerate, or reorganize after injury or other environmental change.

**plasticity, neuronal**  Activity-dependent, prolonged functional changes in one or more neurons, accompanied by corresponding biochemical and, often, morphological changes in the neuron(s) involved.

**plate, neural**  See *neural plate*.

**plateau speech**  Speech whose monotonal quality is due to loss or reduction in the pitch characteristic of each vowel sound; it occurs in epilepsy, multiple sclerosis, and other central nervous system disorders.

**platonization**  (From *platonize*, idealize, as in platonic love, which in Plato's view passed from physical passion on to higher contemplation of the ideal, i.e., to love free from sexual desire) A mental mechanism consisting of considering the desired act without actually performing it. Platonization is thus a mechanism of defense against impulses and would be considered by some as evidence of prelogical, primitive thinking wherein thought has become an equivalent of action by reason of infantile belief in the magical omnipotence of thought. Platonization is typical of paranoia, where thought rather than action reigns supreme. But, like any other mechanism of defense, such as repression, sublimation, or projection, platonization need not imply gross psychiatric abnormality in the person who uses the mechanism.

**platybasia**  Basilar impression; an abnormality of the base of the skull, often congenital, in which the angle between the basisphenoid and the basilar portion of the occipital bone is widened. The neck is abnormally short and the head is sometimes mushroom-shaped.

**platycephaly**  Flattening of the crown of the head.

**play technique**  A psychotherapeutic method devised by Melanie Klein for special use in the treatment of children. By allowing a child to play with almost anything he wants, the therapist is, through this play, able to analyze and clarify the child's emotional problem. The technique is a substitute for free association. Toys of all kinds can be used, but it is usually better to use toys that do not move by themselves. Frequently the child accompanies his play with short remarks that elucidate the situation. See *play therapy*.

**play therapy**  *Ludotherapy*; in child psychiatry, a method of treatment that in general corresponds to the method of psychoanalysis in adult psychiatry, the difference being that the child expresses himself and reveals unconscious material to the therapist by means of play rather than by verbalization of thoughts, as the adult does in psychoanalysis. See *play technique*.

The play of children, an essential part of their life, is self-expressive in its nature. If a playroom containing all manner of toys and games is set up for the child, much can be learned about the child by observing what game he chooses to play and the manner in which he plays it. For example, during a session in the play-therapy room, a 9-year-old boy took chalk of various colors and drew on the blackboard a charming picture of a house in the countryside. When the drawing had been finished the therapist warmly complimented the boy on his work, and then asked him to make up a story about the people living in that house. It was known that he was a child from a broken, poverty-stricken home in a tenement section of the city; he would not obey his mother, and allegedly had pushed his baby sister from a fire escape to her death. In play therapy he had created what he lacked, an attractive home in the country. In telling the story of the people who lived in it, his feelings about his own home and his own family were drawn out. The therapist was able to help him face his insecurity, anxiety, and hostility and to learn better ways of dealing with them. Before this release through play therapy, the boy had been uncommunicative and inaccessible in several interviews with the therapist.

**pleasure ego**  See *reality ego*.

**pleasure principle**  A hypothesized mechanism whose function is to reduce psychic tension originating from drives pressing for discharge. The pleasure-pain principle tries to undo the effects of disturbing stimuli (pain) in a way that will most easily provide satisfaction (pleasure). It comes into operation later than the repetition-compulsion principle and is concerned mainly with the stimuli arising from the drives or instincts, while the earlier principle is concerned with damping external stimuli and restoring the organism to its original state. See *repetition-compulsion*.

**pleasuring**    See *sensate focus*.

**-plegia, -plegy**    Combining form meaning (paralytic) stroke, attack, from Gr. plēgē.

**pleiotropy, pleotropy**    *Polypheny*; the condition or state of possessing multiple or variable functions or appearing in different manifestations, all of which derive from the same beginning. In genetics, pleitropy refers to a single gene producing different characteristics; in the mouse, for example, a single gene is responsible for a ventral white spot, a flexed tail, and microcytic anemia.

**pleniloquence**    Excessive talking.

**pleocytosis**    Excess of cells; pleocytosis of the cerebrospinal fluid indicates meningeal irritation.

**pleonasm**    Redundancy or the use of more than enough words to express an idea, as is seen in *circumstantiality* (q.v.).

**pleonexia**    Greediness; uncontrollable desire for acquisition or gain.

**plethoric type**    See *athletic type; pyknic type*.

**pleurothotonus**    A torsion spasm in which the trunk of the body is bent to one side; sometimes called *Pisa syndrome*. Pleurothotonus may be seen as a form of *tardive dystonia* (q.v.).

**plumbism**    *Lead poisoning* (q.v.).

**pluralism**    The concept that behavior is causally determined by a multiplicity of complexly interrelated factors.

**pluralistic utilitarianism**    See *utilitarianism, pluralistic*.

**plus complementarity**    See *complementarity*.

**plutomania**    Greediness; inordinate striving for wealth and possessions.

**Plyushkin syndrome**    *Hoarding; squalor syndrome* (qq.v.).

**PMA test**    A test of seven traits believed by Thurstone and Thurstone to account for most of the variance in primary mental abilities (PMA). These traits are as follows: V (verbal comprehension), W (word fluency), N (number), S (space), M (associative memory), P (perceptual speed), and R (reasoning) or I (induction).

**PMDD**    *Premenstrual dysphoric disorder; PMS* (qq.v.).

**PMEs**    Phosphomonoesters, *phospholipid* precursors (q.v.).

**PMG**    *Polymicrogyria* (q.v.).

**PML**    *Progressive multifocal leukoencephalopathy* (q.v.).

**PMS**    *Premenstrual syndrome; premenstrual dysphoric disorder* (q. v.); cyclical mood changes and physical symptoms that are correlated with the menstrual cycle, typically beginning soon after ovulation and building to a peak about 5 days before the menstrual period. Psychological symptoms include anxiety, crying spells, depression, and fatigability; physical symptoms include weight gain, breast tenderness, swelling of the legs, and bloating. The syndrome has been attributed to hormonal imbalances, such as estrogen excess, estrogen-progesterone imbalance, hyperprolactinemia, and effects of gonadal steroids on endogenous opiates. As many as 20% to 40% of menstruating women report some symptoms of PMS, which can also occur in postmenopausal women so long as their ovaries are intact.

Some authorities (among them, DSM-IV) differentiate between premenstrual syndrome (PMS) and the much rarer premenstrual dysphoric disorder (PMDD) or *LLPDD* (q.v.).

**PNDs**    *Paraneoplastic neurological disorders* (q.v.).

**pneumoencephalogram**    An X-ray of the skull following replacement of measured quantities of cerebrospinal fluid with air or some other gas by means of lumbar or cisternal puncture. Its drawback is that pneumoencephalography is painful and can be dangerous. It has been largely supplanted by CT and MRI.

**pneumotherapy, cerebral**    Insufflation of oxygen or air into the ventrical or arachnoid spaces, once used as treatment for intractable epilepsy, circumscribed meningitis, and psychosis.

**PNFA**    Progressive nonfluent aphasia. See *frontotemporal lobar degeneration*.

**pnigerophobia**    Fear of smothering.

**pnigophobia**    Fear of choking.

**poena talionis**    The law of ancient Rome according to which the culprit was subjected to the identical injury or material loss as he had caused to the plaintiff. See *talion dread*.

**poiesis**    Composing of a word, and particularly coining a neologistic word or phrase; sometimes used specifically to indicate a schizophrenic neologism, in which language is constructed so as to affirm the patient's wishes, which are then believed by him to have been fulfilled.

**poikilothermia**   Failure to respond to changes in temperature with sweating or shivering, characteristic of *REM sleep* (q.v.).

**poikilothymia**   E. Kahn's term for a mental constitution closely akin to cyclothymia, differing from the latter in that in poikilothymia the mood variations are more intense.

**poinephobia**   Fear of punishment.

**pointing**   A test for vestibular rather than pure cerebellar function; patient is requested to extend his arm and perform the movements at the shoulder; examiner stands in front of him, and patient touches with his extended index finger the examiner's two index fingers, which are held together in a fixed position; with eyes open, there is no deviation normally; on closing the eyes, and knowing the position of the examiner's fingers, the patient should be able to touch the same spot every time; if he deviates to the left or right there is said to be *past-pointing*.

**pointing the bone**   See *bone-pointing*.

**point-light displays**   Videotaped biological movements portrayed in highly impoverished stimuli. The method was devised by Gunnar Johansson in 1973 to study how humans recognize movement. Ten light bulbs are attached to the joints of actors who perform complex movements in the dark—walking, running, or dancing. The videos show 10 dots of light moving against a dark background. Other complex actions have since been used: facial expressions, arm movements, full-body actions, American Sign Language.

Subjects can immediately recognize the action, and even from such minimally informative stimuli they can infer subtle details, such as the gender of walkers, the emotional states of the actors, or the weight of objects they lifted. Recognizing complex biological movements is biologically important in many situations—detecting predators, selecting prey, courtship behavior, etc. Point-light stimuli and natural biological motion activate areas in the superior temporal sulcus and the dorsal and ventral pathways of the visual system.

**poisoning phobia**   See *cancer phobia*.

**polarity**   The state of having two opposite aspects or tendencies. Polarity, by definition, is an essential part of *bipolar disorder* (q.v.), and it is predictive of the polarity of subsequent episodes. When the illness begins with a manic episode, 75% of subsequent episodes start with mania; if illness begins with a depressive episode, 55%–60% of subsequent episodes start with depression.

**police power**   The power of the state to protect its citizens from danger. The power permits the state to interfere with a person's liberty and freedom if he constitutes a danger to himself or to society. The standard of the police power, in other words, is *dangerousness*, and in most jurisdictions it is under that power that civil commitment of a mentally ill patient is authorized. See *consumerism; medicalization; parens patriae*.

**polioclastic**   Destructive to gray matter of the central nervous system; ordinarily used to refer to neurotropic viruses.

**poliodystrophy, progressive infantile cerebral**   *Alpers disease*; a nonlipid neuronal destruction of cerebral tissue with preservation of myelinated structures, probably most commonly due to cerebral anoxia, less commonly to maternal toxemia or genetic factors. Seizures and mental retardation are the usual manifestations.

**polioencephalitis hemorrhagica superior**   See *Wernicke encephalopathy*.

**poliomyelitis, chronic**   See *amyotrophic lateral sclerosis*.

**political genetics**   Applications of genetic concepts to social processes through political action; the incorporation of genetic theory into political dogma or national policy. See *eugenics*.

**pollakiuria**   Abnormally frequent urination.

**pollution**   *Obs.* Discharge of semen and seminal fluid in the absence of sexual intercourse; often used synonymously with *nocturnal emission*.

**pollution, air**   See *air pollution syndrome*.

**Pollyanna**   An optimist; someone who finds good or fails to see the bad in any situation. Often used as an adjective, as in comparing the "Pollyanna tendency" of normal subjects to recall more pleasant than unpleasant material with the "anhedonic tendency" of schizophrenics to recall unpleasant and pleasant with approximately equal frequency.

**polyandry**   The practice of having more than one husband at one time.

**polychromate, abnormal**   One who distinguishes most colors, but fails to perceive one or two, or confuses two colors.

**polyclonia epileptoides continua**   *Obs.* See *continuous epilepsy*.

**polycratism**   (From Polycrates, tyrant of Samos [535–512 b.c.], who wished to allay the envy of the gods, because all his enterprises were invariably highly successful. In a galley fitted out with regal splendor Polycrates sailed out on a pleasure trip. As if inadvertently his favorite signet ring fell overboard and with ostentatious grief Polycrates returned home, inwardly happy that he had appeased the gods. Two or three days later a fisherman brought to the palace a huge fish he thought fit only for the ruler's table. When Polycrates carved the fish at the repast, he found his ring, which the fish had swallowed. The gods were not to be appeased—Polycrates met death by crucifixion.) The superstition that if things go "too well" a proportionately heavier punishment is to be expected; in psychoanalysis, interpreted as guilt feelings over forbidden phantasies. See *failure through success.*

**polydipsia** Excessive thirst.

**polydrug abuse** *Multiple drug misuse* (q.v.).

**polygamy** The practice of having more than one mate at one time; the term includes both *polyandry* and *polygyny* (qq.v.).

**polyglot neophasia** A type of neologism formation in which one or more languages are devised by the patient, sometimes with full vocabulary, grammar, and syntax. Polyglot neophasia is rarely seen except in expansive paranoiacs and, to a lesser extent, in manic states. See *glossolalia.*

**polyglot reaction** In aphasia, any exception to the general rule that in persons who are multilingual, the mother tongue is the first to return. See *linguistics.*

**polyglutamine disorder** A class of inherited neurodegenerative disease with a common trigger of pathogenesis, a CAG *trinucleotide repeat* (q.v.). The trinucleotides encode a glutamine tract in a protein; the protein and the location of the glutamine segment are different for each disease. The polyglutamine disorders include DRPLA (dentatorubropalidoluysian atrophy), Haw River syndrome, HD (Huntington disease), Kennedy disease, spinal and bulbar muscular atrophy (SBMA), and spinocerebellar ataxia 1-2-3 (Machado-Joseph)-7-17.

**polygraph** Also Keeler polygraph; *lie detector* (q.v.); it is based on the assumption that substitution of a false statement for an emotionally charged memory will be reflected in detectable autonomic changes over which the subject has no control. Although the polygraph data recorded may be accurate, their interpretation will always be uncertain.

There is no unique set of psychophysiological changes associated with deception. Because there is doubt about the usefulness, and appropriateness, of polygraph testing as a screening device to enhance security or establish guilt, courts have become increasingly unlikely to admit introduction of polygraph testing results as evidence.

**polygyny** The practice of having more than one wife at one time.

**polyhybrid** In genetics this characterizes hybrids that differ in more than three hereditary characters. See *hybrid.*

**polylogia** See *tachylogia.*

**polymerase chain reaction** *PCR* (q.v.).

**polymicrogyria** *PMG*; multiple small gyri. There are several region-specific types of bilateral symmetric polymicrogyria, caused by mutations in different genes.

Bilateral frontoparietal polymicrogyria (BFPP) is an autosomal recessive syndrome caused by eight separate mutations in the human *GPR56* gene, which regulates cortical patterning. It has been mapped to chromosome 16q12–21. The abnormally small gyri and reduced cortical layers are most prominent in the frontal lobe. Associated abnormalities include mental retardation, gait difficulty, language impairment, and seizures.

Bilateral symmetrical frontal, parieto-occipital, and perisylvian polymicrogyrias have also been described.

**polymorphism** In conventional use, a mutation that occurs with a frequency greater than 1% in the population. There may be as many as 1 million human single nucleotide polymorphisms (SNPs), providing a powerful tool for linkage or associative analysis strategies such as pharmacogenomics. See *marker; RFLPs; SSLPs.*

**polymorphous perverse** Pertaining to one whose sexual behavior includes many different forms, expressing both adult and infantile tendencies, both normal and abnormal trends. Though it often appears during mental disorders, polymorphous perversion is said to be normal in early childhood, embracing activities observed in the period of infancy and also adulthood in the form of perversions. See *Haeckel biogenetic law.*

**polyneuritic psychosis** *Korsakoff psychosis* (q.v.). See *Wernicke-Korsakoff syndrome.*

**polyneuritis** Simultaneous inflammation of a large number of peripheral nerves. Signs and symptoms are usually bilateral and frequently symmetrical, although not all the nerves are affected with equal severity. Prominent symptoms include severe pain, wasting of the muscles, and paralysis. Clinical examples are alcoholic polyneuritis, arsenic polyneuritis, diabetic polyneuritis, polyneuritis of pregnancy.

**polyneuritis, acute toxic** *Guillain-Barré syndrome* (q.v.).

**polyneuritis, erythroedema** *Acrodynia* (q.v.).

**polyopia** Duplication or multiplication of a visual image, such as seeing two lights when there is only one or seeing hundreds of holes on a circular telephone dial. Polyopia may be organic in origin (associated with pathology in the ocular apparatus, with nystagmus, or with occipital lobe dysfunction), and it may also appear as a conversion symptom in hysteria. See *palinopia.*

**polyparesis** General paralysis of the insane. See *general paresis.*

**polyphagia** Excessive eating; gluttony; *bulimia* (q.v.).

**polypharmacy** Simultaneous administration of more than one drug for the same disorder; in psychiatry simultaneous administration of more than one psychotropic drug; also known as *combination drug therapy, maxipharmacy,* or *orthopsychic tranquilization.* See *monotherapy.*

**polypheny** *Pleiotropy* (q.v.).

**polyphobia** Fear of many things.

**polypnoea** Deep, labored, and rapid respiration.

**polyposia** Craving for intoxicating drinks.

**polypsychism** The concept that each person possesses several souls.

**polyQ proteins** Polyglutamines; proteins with expanded glutamine repeats. Expression of aggregation-prone polyQ overwhelms the machinery that ordinarily destroys such proteins and may result in *neurodegenerative disease.* See *misfolding, polyglutamine disorder; trinucleotide repeat.*

**polyradiculoneuritis** *Guillain-Barré syndrome* (q.v.).

**polysomnogram (PSM)** The system of recording all-night measurements of various electrophysiologic and somatic variables, used in the study and diagnosis of sleep disorders. Sometimes it is defined as EEG + EOG + EMG because the variables include the electroencephalogram, *electro-oculogram,* submental electromyogram, ventilatory air exchange,

respiratory effort, electrical heart activity, leg movement, blood oxygen saturation, and often also simultaneous video recording of the sleep behavior of the subject. The PSM provides precise data concerning the time at which the subject falls asleep, the number of wake periods experienced, and the quality and duration of sleep. Measurements are made during sleep without disturbing the sleeper.

**polysubstance dependence** See *multiple drug misuse.*

**polysubstance use disorders** DSM-IV recognizes one such disorder, polysubstance dependence, characterized by repeated use of at least three different substances, no one of which predominates, over a period of not less than 3 months.

**polysurgical addiction** Sometimes a manifestation of *factitious* disorder, at other times of *somatization disorder* or *hypochondriasis* (qq.v.); patients with polysurgical addiction solicit or, through multiple symptoms, obtain many operations even though no organic pathology is uncovered that would have warranted the surgical procedures. See *Munchhausen syndrome.*

**polyuria** Excessive excretion of urine; profuse micturition.

**POMC** Pro-opiomelanocortin. See *enkephalins.*

**Pompadour phantasy** (Marquise de Pompadour [1721–1764], mistress of Louis XV [1710–1774], king of France) A hetaeral (mistress) phantasy, in which the woman imagines herself to be the mistress of a king or emperor. "The exaltation of the partner to kingly rank makes thoughts and wishes possible which would otherwise be rejected as immoral" (Ferenczi, S. *Further Contributions to the Theory and Technique of Psycho-Analysis,* 1926).

**POMR** Problem-oriented medical record. See *problem-oriented record.*

**ponophobia** Fear of overwork.

**pons** The portion of the metencephalon that forms the floor of the fourth ventricle; the pons is continuous with the midbrain anteriorly, and with the medulla oblongata posteriorly. The pons contains the pontine nuclei which connect the cerebellum with the cerebrum, and the nuclei of cranial nerves IV, V (in part), VI, and VII. Transverse fibers of the pons form the brachium pontis, or middle cerebellar peduncle; the longitudinal fibers of the pons contain the pyramidal tracts and the corticopontile fibers. With the medulla, the pons is involved in regulating blood pressure and respiration. In addition, it contains many neurons that relay information from the cerebral hemispheres to the cerebellum.

**pontocerebellar angle syndrome**  A group of symptoms caused by acoustic neuromas. Involvement of the acoustic nerve produces persistent tinnitus, progressive deafness, and vertigo. Involvement of the facial nerve produces homolateral facial anesthesia with loss of corneal and sneeze reflexes. Cerebellar involvement produces homolateral ataxia with staggering, and pontine involvement results in contralateral hemiplegia and slight hemianesthesia.

**popper**  See *amyl nitrite; nitrites.*

**population genetics**  See *genetics.*

**population neurosis**  *Obs.* A collective or group neurosis prevailing in the populace of a locality; group hysteria. See *collective psychosis.*

**POR**  *Problem-oriented record* (q.v.).

**porencephaly**  A developmental anomaly in which there occur small or large unilateral or bilateral cavities in the brain substance.

**poriomania**  Irresistible impulse to travel. The latter may be carried out with the full and complete knowledge of the person or there may be complete amnesia for all activities associated with the trip. States of poriomania may be associated with criminal acts.

Poriomania includes the wandering states that have been described as a rare ictal phenomenon in complex partial seizures (temporal lobe epilepsy, psychomotor seizures).

**pornerastic**  Fond of prostitutes.

**pornographomania**  Compulsion to write obscene letters.

**pornography**  Obscene, lewd, lascivious, prurient drawing or writing, and especially that which aims to arouse the viewer or reader sexually. As R. J. Stoller points out (*Archives of General Psychiatry 22*, 1970), no written or pictorial material is pornographic in itself; instead, the observer's phantasies are projected into that material and only then does it become sexually and genitally exciting.

**pornolagnia**  Pathological attraction to lewd and prurient pictures or writing, or a dependence on them for sexual arousal.

**porphyria**  The best known of the disorders of porphyrin and bilirubin metabolism, resulting in the production of abnormal types of porphyrin, which appear in the urine. The hereditary porphyrias are inherited errors of porphyrin metabolism; secondary porphyrias (acquired, symptomatic, or toxic porphyrinuria) are associated with liver disease, aplastic anemia, heavy metal intoxication, and acute infections.

Through heme, the iron complex of protoporphyrin, the porphyrins are involved in aerobic oxidation in all biological systems. With globin, heme forms hemoglobin; chlorophyll is a magnesium porphyrin complex. Delta-aminolevulinic acid is formed from glycine and succinate. Two molecules of delta-aminolevulinic acid condense to form porphobilinogen, which gives rise to uroporphyrinogen, and then to coproporphyrinogen, which is converted to protoporphyrin and heme.

Hereditary porphyria is subdivided into the following:

1. Hepatic porphyria—inherited as an autosomal dominant but not manifested, even biochemically, until after puberty. The most common form is *acute intermittent porphyria (Gunther-Waldenstrom syndrome)*, due to a reduction in uroporphyrinogen-I synthetase activity. It appears usually as an acute attack. It affects females four times as frequently as males, with onset between the ages of 20 and 35. It is often precipitated by the use of barbiturates and is manifested in a triad of symptoms: (1) abdominal, such as colicky abdominal pain in the midepigastrium and the right lower quadrant; (2) peripheral neuropathy, with flaccid pareses of the extremities because of lower motor neuron involvement, and in about half of patients so affected cranial nerve involvement as well; particularly in that moiety convulsions may occur or, less commonly, coma proceeding to death; (3) mental changes (*porphyrismus*) including irritability and tension progressing to schizophreniform psychosis or organic brain syndrome with disorientation and hallucinations. There is no known treatment.

Another but much rarer hepatic form is porphyria cutanea tarda, characterized by the appearance of photosensitivity in middle age.

2. Erythropoietic porphyria—extremely rare, inherited as an autosomal recessive; an abnormality in developing normoblasts results in increased formation of porphyrin in the marrow leading to red urine from birth, pink or reddish brown teeth and bones, and hypersensitivity of exposed skin to light.

**porphyrismus**   The mental changes associated with *porphyria* (q.v.).

**porropsia**   Inability to gauge the real distance of objects, which appear more distant than they really are, without any alteration in their size.

**Porteus Maze test**   Like the T*ower of London test* (q.v.), the Porteus Maze test assesses the capacity to plan ahead. The Porteus Maze, Tower of London, and *Wisconsin Card Sorting Test* are standard "frontal lobe" tests in neuropsychology.

**port-wine stain**   See *angiomatosis, trigeminal cerebral*.

**posiomania**   *Dipsomania* (q.v.).

**positional cloning**   See *cloning, positional*.

**positioning, paradoxical**   See *paradoxical therapy*.

**Positive and Negative Syndrome Scale**   *PANSS*; a 30-item scale with 16 general psychopathology symptom items, 7 positive-symptom (of schizophrenia) items, and 7 negative-symptom (of schizophrenia) items. Each item is scored on a 7-point severity scale (the higher the number, the more severe the symptom), resulting in a range of possible scores from 30 to 210. Positive and negative symptom items may be reported separately, with a possible range of 7 to 49. The average patient with schizophrenia entering a clinical trial typically scores 91.

**positive dissociative experiences**   A form of normal *dissociation* (q.v.) that may accompany events and activities of personal significance, such as engaging in sports, sex, hobbies, or prayer, performing or listening to music, and dancing. Such experiences involve total absorption in the activity and alteration in the experience of self, body, or world, and are characterized by a positive affect tone. *Flow states*, or *optimal experiences*, are characterized by feelings of self-efficacy and intrinsic reward associated with enhanced flow of creativity or enhanced performance of skilled activities such as sports or performing.

**positive signs**   *Release phenomena* (q.v.).

**positive symptoms**   In schizophrenia, symptoms of the acute phase such as hallucinations, ideas of reference, paranoid delusions, and disturbances in thinking such as thought insertion and thought broadcasting. See *deficit symptoms; negative symptoms; productive symptoms; schizophrenia, models of. SAPS* is the Schedule for the Assessment of Positive Symptoms, developed by Andreasen.

**positron emission tomography**   *PET* (q.v.).

**POSM**   Patient-operated selected mechanisms, i.e., electromechanical devices that can be controlled by patients with high cord lesions or extreme disability from other causes.

**possession trance**   A single or episodic alteration of consciousness during which the customary sense of personal identity is replaced by a new identity, and the alteration is attributed to the influence of a supernatural power or other person. If not a normal part of cultural or religious practice, it is considered to be a dissociative disorder. See *dissociation; trance disorder, dissociative*.

**possessive instinct**   The drive for power, the primitive urge to conquer and retain the love object. In the infant, the possessive instinct manifests itself in the acts of sucking and swallowing, and in the stubbornness with which the child holds on to the nipple of the mother. It is also shown in the capacity to control the anal sphincter and thus retain the feces. Later the infant's crude possessive urge is transformed into a more socialized form; it may express itself in stinginess, punctuality, the habit of collecting things, even the search for intellectual knowledge, and in many other character traits. In the adult, the crude possessive urge is sublimated under the constant exigencies of the superego (a code of moral behavior) and acquires a constructive quality, a proper intensity, and an acceptable direction toward admissible goals. See *coprophilia; compulsive personality*.

**possum**   *POSM* (q.v.).

**post coitum triste**   (L. "gloom after sexual intercourse") See *impotence*.

**postambivalent stage**   The final stage in the development of object love in which real love of an object is possible.

The stages of object love before real love is reached are ambivalent: in these stages, the process of achieving satisfaction destroys the object. The final stage of object relationship, real love, is the postambivalent stage. No traces of hateful or destructive feelings toward the object remain. Instead, "consideration of the object goes so far that one's own satisfaction is impossible without satisfying the object, too." The prerequisite for real love is genital primacy, the ability to attain full satisfaction through genital orgasm. This emerges only in the final genital stage of libidinal organization (Fenichel, O. *The Psychoanalytic Theory of Neurosis*, 1945).

**postcentral gyrus**   See *parietal lobe.*

**postcomatose unawareness state**   *Vegetative state* (q.v.). postconcussion disorder Also, postconcussional disorder; head trauma with loss of consciousness is followed within 4 weeks by somatic complaints (e.g., dizziness, intolerance to sound, easy fatigability), emotional changes (e.g., labile mood, irritability, anxiety, depression), difficulty in concentration, sleep disturbance, and lowered tolerance for alcohol and other depressants. Neurologic examination usually uncovers evidence of cerebral damage.

**postconcussion neurosis**   A form of traumatic neurosis following cerebral concussion. Depending upon the history, physical findings, and symptom picture presented the condition may be considered primarily organic (*organic personality disorder* or mixed organic brain syndrome) or primarily psychologic (*post-traumatic stress disorder*). See *organic mental disorders.*

**postdormital chalastic fits**   See *sleep paralysis.*

**postemotive schizophrenia**   In a person constitutionally predisposed, schizophrenia may be precipitated by an emotional trauma, especially in the face of situations that threaten self-preservation, the social self, or the sexual life. See *reactive psychosis.*

Most postemotive reactions eventually and spontaneously disappear and are self-limited syndromes. But when emotional stress precipitates a psychosis in a predisposed person, prognosis is made on the basis of the psychosis itself rather than on the nature of the precipitating factor. Many authorities feel that schizophrenia is nearly always postemotive, that detailed anamnestic investigation would reveal specific emotional traumata as precipitating factors in the majority of cases.

**postepileptic twilight state**   Sometimes after an epileptic attack, a so-called twilight state exists for a variable period of time. During the twilight state the patient may carry out acts for which he is later amnesic.

**posterior aphasia**   *Wernicke aphasia* (q.v.).

**posterolateral sclerosis**   Subacute *combined degeneration of the spinal cord*; a deficiency disease due to lack of *intrinsic factor* (which combines with extrinsic factor to form the cobalt-containing complex, or vitamin $B_{12}$), seen in pernicious anemia, sprue, cachexia, and postgastrectomy cases. Pathological changes include irregular demyelination of the posterolateral columns and peripheral nerves.

Symptoms are paresthesiae; early loss of position and vibratory sensation; later loss of touch and pain sensation, often with a glove and stocking type of anesthesia; sphincter disturbances; moderate muscular wasting; and ataxia. Symptoms usually begin in the lower limbs. Various mental changes may be seen: mild dementia, confusional psychosis, Korsakoff psychosis, or affective reactions. Associated with the neuropsychiatric changes are gastric achlorhydria, glossitis, and anemia. Duration of life in untreated cases is approximately 2 years. Treatment with vitamin $B_{12}$ can restore the patient to good health indefinitely.

The clinical pattern of combined degeneration is also seen in the vacuolar myelopathy of patients with AIDS.

**postfall syndrome**   Also termed *fear of further falling syndrome,* triple-F gait; a wide-based gait with increased toeing-out combined with severe bradykinesis, seen frequently in elderly patients, probably a reflection of age-related impairment in long-latency postural reflex mechanisms. The patient's sense of insecure footing and likelihood of falling are often increased with neuroleptics.

**posthallucinogen perception disorder**   See *flashback.*

**posthion**   Small penis. (Gr. *posthe* = penis or prepuce, although the preferred term for the latter was acrobystia. In most medical terms, however, the root posth-, postho-, posthio- indicates foreskin, and phallo-, phallus is used for penis.)

**posthypnotic amnesia**   Loss of memory for events transpiring during the hypnotic stage.

**postinfectious depression**   See *organic mental disorders.*

**postinfectious psychosis**   Mental disturbances may follow such acute diseases as influenza, pneumonia, typhoid fever, and acute rheumatic fever in their postfebrile period or may occur during the period of convalescence. They present as mild, reversible forms of confusion, or suspicious, irritable, depressive reactions. Permanent residua occur only rarely.

**postpartum**   After birthing or childbirth. Mood disorders with postparum onset may have a different prognosis and require different treatment than other mood disorders.

**postpartum psychosis**   Puerperal psychosis; any psychosis associated with the puerperium (the period from the termination of labor to the complete involution of the uterus). There is no single psychiatric condition that occurs during this period, and except for those states that are definitely connected with organic disorders, there is nothing in the puerperium as such that gives rise to a psychosis.

Postpartum psychosis is estimated to occur in 1 or 2 of every 1000 deliveries. Suicide is relatively frequent (perhaps 5% of cases), as is killing of the just-delivered infant (perhaps 4% of cases). It is to be differentiated from the *baby blues*, a self-limited and short-lived reaction that occurs in about half of women following childbirth, consisting of tearfulness, anxiety, and irritability that appears shortly after giving birth and diminishes in severity with each passing day.

**postschizophrenic depression** *Depression* (q.v.) following an acute schizophrenic episode. Some believe it a routine development during recovery from schizophrenic decompensation; others view it as secondary to neuroleptic treatment; still others consider it a manifestation of preexisting mood disturbance that was hidden by schizophrenic symptoms. A few ascribe it to psychotherapy that has revealed the patient's limited ability to establish meaningful interpersonal relationships.

**poststroke dementia** Dementia resulting from cerebrovascular accident; dementia postapoplexy.

**postsynaptic density** See *dendrite*

**postsynaptic neuromessenger** See *neuromessenger*.

**post-torture syndrome** A Dutch study of refugees from nine countries examined symptoms immediately following torture. Complaints at the time were widely divergent. Psychic problems were particularly pronounced. There is not enough evidence to justify the term post-torture syndrome, on analogy with post–concentration camp syndrome. The question remains if a clearly developed syndrome will appear with passage of time.

**post-translational** See *cytosolic proteins*.

**post-traumatic constitution** The clinical syndromes subsumed under this heading vary from person to person; the symptoms following head trauma are often a mixture of both neurotic and psychotic phenomena. *Friedmann's complex* is one of the most common syndromes; it is said to be due to cerebral vasomotor disturbance and is characterized by headache, dizziness, insomnia, easy fatigue, irritability, and other character changes. See *post-traumatic and postencephalitic syndromes, classification of.*

**post-traumatic delirium** Organic brain syndrome of the delirious type following injury to the brain.

**post-traumatic dementia** Reduction in intellectual functioning secondary to brain injury. Post-traumatic dementia constitutes 0.6% or more of annual admissions to mental hospitals; approximately 44% of them are secondary to motor vehicle accidents. Less severe disturbances with memory impairment and minor personality changes are more frequent. Psychological changes following head injury become prominent approximately 2 months after the injury and generally subside within the next 3 months. In 50% of cases, symptoms persist for at least 6 months, and in 15%, for a year or more. There is no correlation between severity of the injury and severity of the post-traumatic psychiatric sequelae. Persons with pretraumatic psychoneurotic personalities, and those with many complicating factors, such as pending litigation, anxiety about compensation, occupational stresses, or associated bodily injuries, are more likely to develop post-traumatic psychiatric sequelae. Traumatic epilepsy develops within 2 years in about 10% of cases who manifest psychiatric sequelae.

**post-traumatic deterioration** *Obs.* Organic brain syndrome, usually dementia or personality disturbance, following brain injury.

**post-traumatic epilepsy** Convulsions following brain trauma, i.e., a type of symptomatic epilepsy. Post-traumatic epilepsy develops in 3%–5% of cases with closed head injury and in 30–50% of cases with open head injury. Convulsions tend to occur (1) within a few seconds of injury; (2) within a day or two; or (3) within the first 2 years following injury.

About half of early-appearing epilepsy disappears; in late-appearing epilepsy, there is a tendency to abatement of attacks within 2 years of onset, and in 30%, convulsions disappear completely.

**post-traumatic personality disorder** *PTPD*; complex PTSD, which in DSM-IV is classified as a disorder of extreme stress not otherwise specified (*DESNOS*). Complex PTSD is a chronic adaptation to *post-traumatic stress disorder* (q.v.) that shapes the personality. The symptoms of PTSD itself are usually described in terms of three domains—re-experiencing, avoidance and numbing, and hyperarousal. But failure of these initial symptoms to resolve provokes a secondary adaptation to them, complex PTSD or DESNOS. Adaptation to a chronically aroused fear system requires extreme defensive measures, manifested in such symptoms as severe avoidance, alterations of consciousness and self-perception, identity disturbances, overreliance on dissociation, affect dysregulation characterized by cycling from hyperarousal to hypoarousal states, difficulty with interpersonal relationships, and somatization. Dissociative adaptations, used to escape conflict, may alternate with angry and violent acting out.

PTPD requires a history of severe chronic traumatization beginning in childhood; less severe traumatization is asssociated with BPD—*borderline personality disorder* (q.v.). In comparison with patients with BPD, those with PTPD have less ability to access positive emotions, have more self negation, and are more avoidant of others. In their need to avoid conflict, patients with PTPD learn to please, placate, and manage others; dissociation is frequent, not brief and transient as it is in BPD.

**post-traumatic stress disorder**   *PTSD*; traumatic neurosis; a group of characteristic symptoms that develop after witnessing or being confronted with one or more events involving actual or threatened death or serious injury, or a threat to the physical integrity of oneself or others. The response to the stressor is one of intense fear, horror, or feelings of helplessness. Although the older literature emphasized the importance of physical injury in precipitating the condition, current thinking emphasizes that a psychological component is the essential element. The diagnosis of PTSD was originally applied to the stress responses of combat veterans. Over time, the diagnosis has been extended to all types of trauma.

Lifetime prevalence of PTSD is 1%–9%; women may have an increased risk. For men, the usual trauma is combat; for women, it is assault or rape. Data from the Vietnam-Era Twin Registry indicate that there is a genetic susceptibility to PTSD. Underlying genetic factors may account for between 13% and 34% of the variance in PTSD symptoms. In veterans who were exposed to life-threatening events in combat and later diagnosed with PTSD, prevalence ranges between 15% and 20%, and it is even higher in ethnic groups such as African-American (21%) and Hispanic males (28%). The National Vietnam Veterans Readjustment Study revealed that 19 years after combat, 15% of veterans still had PTSD, even though many of them had received intensive targeted therapies.

Underlying genetic factors may account for a significant portion of the variance in PTSD symptoms. As in borderline personality disorder, disorganized *attachment* (q.v.) is a precursor; but PTSD and *post-traumatic personality disorder* (q.v.) have the additional element of more extensive, chronic traumatization. See *trauma*.

Abnormalities in the central norepinephrine system and the catecholamines in general have been linked closely with PTSD symptoms. Norepinephrine release associated with the stress response affects learning and memory through its influence on norepinephrine levels in amygdala and hippocampus. Locus coeruleus activity is elevated in PTSD, leading to increased norepinephrine release at numerous terminals throughout the brain. Patients who develop PTSD may have an increased release of epinephrine and norepinephrine when initially exposed to a traumatic event, relative to those who do not develop PTSD. This release may lead to vivid recollections of the initial trauma that results in PTSD-related intrusive memories and flashbacks.

Post-traumatic stress disorders are termed acute if they last less than 6 months after the traumatic event, and chronic if they last longer than 6 months and begin following a latency period of at least 6 months after the traumatic event. See *traumatic neurosis; victim*.

Although commonly recommended and frequently used with survivors of disasters and terrifying events, *debriefing* (q.v.) has not been shown to reduce incidence of PTSD. Some studies even suggest that it may impede natural recovery from trauma, and that rehearsal of a traumatic memory immediately after it has happened may consolidate the memory rather than erase it.

**postural hypotension**   See *OH*.

**postural tremors**   See *tremor*.

**posturing**   Posing or adopting a physical stance, usually inappropriate to the situation or too-long maintained; characteristic of *catatonia* (q.v.).

**postviral syndrome**   See *chronic fatigue syndrome; EBV syndrome.*

**potamophobia**   Fear of rivers.

**potence, potency**   The ability (of the male) to consummate the act of sexual intercourse.

**potomania**   *Obs.* Craving for intoxicating drinks; *delirium tremens; dipsomania* (qq.v.).

**Potzl syndrome**   Pure alexia (i.e., symbol agnosia for written characters, although the writing is seen, and without any intrinsic disturbance of speech), combined with disturbances of color sense and defects of the visual field. Potzl syndrome is generally seen in the presence of foci in the medullary layer of the lingual gyrus of the dominant hemisphere with damage to the corpus callosum.

**poverty, clinical**   See *clinical poverty syndrome.*

**poverty of speech**   Reduction in amount, content, or spontaneity of speech, ranging from mutism to monosyllabic responses or brief, telegrammatic utterances. With poverty of content, speech is vague, obscure, repetitious, or stereotyped.

**poverty of the stimulus**   One of Chomsky's arguments for an innate, prewired "language organ"; it refers to the fact that during the linguistically formative years, the child is not exposed to enough language to account for the linguistic capability displayed by a normal 6-year-old. The speech he hears does not always consist of well-formed, complete sentences. Children encounter only a finite range of expressions yet can deal with an infinite spectrum of novel sentences. And children come to know things subconsciously about their language for which there is no direct evidence in the data to which they are exposed.

**POW**   See *prisoner of war syndrome.*

**power complex**   "The total complex of all those ideas and strivings whose tendency it is to range the ego above other influences, thus subordinating all such influences to the ego, quite irrespective of whether they have their source in men and objective conditions, or spring from one's own subjective impulses, feelings, and thoughts" (Jung, C. G. *Psychological Types*, 1923).

**POZ party**   A distinct type of sex party arranged for the exchange of sex among HIV-positive *MSM* (q.v.).

**PPA**   1. *Parahippocampal place area* (q.v.).
2. Preferred provider arrangement(s), a term proposed as a substitute for *PPO* (q.v.)

in recognition of the fact that a separate organization is not needed to develop preferred provider status.

**PPC**   Patient Placement Criteria; see ASAM-PPC.

**PPI**   1. *Prepulse inhibition; gating* (qq.v.).
2. Type 1 protein phosphatase; see *NMDAR.*

**PPO**   *Preferred provider organization;* an organized health care delivery system operating under the currently favored competitive concept of restricting health benefits to, or providing incentives to choose, designated providers. It is a form of selective contracting consisting of an arrangement or agreement between payer and specified provider(s) that establishes prices lower than those existing in the absence of such an arrangement. The services of the specified group or panel of providers (hospitals, physicians, or both) are marketed on the basis of cost efficiency, quality, accessibility, and effective management. Enrolled members are given incentives to "prefer" (use) certain providers. Payment by the purchaser is usually on a fee-for-service basis.

A major element in a PPO is its utilization of a review program (such as preadmission certification and length-of-stay review) with supporting cost control information, which permits identification of lower cost alternatives, promotes reductions in length of stay, and assesses the intensity of ancillary services. See *managed care.*

**practice guideline(s)**   Models of treatment for the therapist. Typically, a guideline begins with a summary of recommendations, followed by sections on disease definition, epidemiology, and natural history; treatment principles and alternatives; formulation of an individual treatment plan; clinical features influencing treatment; and current research directions.

Practice guidelines were conceived as part of a movement toward evidence-based treatment, not as a treatment protocol demanding rigid application. There are many limitations in all evidence-based approaches: an insufficiency of evidence in many disorders; the evidence is not equally relevant to clinicians, staffs, and researchers; the techniques for integrating evidence are often in an experimental stage; the evidence proffered evades the issue of how to incorporate both social values and individual preferences within an ongoing patient–therapist relationship; and potential for misuse (there are many procedures in medicine for which there is simply no evidence, nor is there ever likely to be, that they work). In choosing between Treatment A and Treatment B, for instance, how does one balance (1) the proportion of responders to each possible treatment, (2) the degree of beneficial response, (3) the length of response, (4) the likelihood of adverse effects with each treatment, (5) other nonclinical costs, and (6) individual (or societal) preferences?

**practicing subphase** See *separation-individuation.*

**Prader syndrome** See *genomic imprinting.*

**Prader-Willi syndrome** Also, *Prader-Labhart-Willi syndrome.* Major diagnostic criteria are as follows: (1) obesity, beginning at an early age; (2) pouting lips and porcine features, with a narrow forehead and rhomboid facial contours; (3) hypotonicity (e.g., needs assistance to get up after falling); (4) amenorrhea, sparse pubic hair, no sexual feelings, at autopsy diminutive uterus and small ovaries; (5) voracious appetite (may lie or steal to get food); (6) mental retardation and learning difficulties (the patient reported by Langdon Down in 1864, for instance, did not learn to spell until she was 23 years old and never progressed beyond simple arithmetic); (7) behavioral disturbances with both compulsive and impulsive symptoms appear during adolescence and young adulthood. They include self-mutilation (e.g., skin picking), temper tantrums, and aggressive outbursts.

The syndome is sometimes referred to as *HHHO* (hypotonia, hypomentia, hypogonadism, obesity); other manifestations include bradykinesis, growth retardation in childhood, diabetes mellitus in early adulthood, acromicria, and dolichocephaly. Abnormal fat metabolism leads to inadequate insulin action.

Most affected subjects have deletions in the proximal long arm of chromosome 15; similar deletions also produce another form of mental retardation, *Angelman syndrome* (q.v.). The difference is a result of *genomic imprinting* (q.v.): in Prader-Willi syndrome, the deletions occur only on the chromosome 15 that originates from the father, while in Angelman syndrome the deletions occur only in the maternally derived chromosome.

**pragmatagnosia** Loss of the ability to recognize an object formerly known, or to remember the appearance of an object formerly known.

**pragmatics** The study of how language is used in a social context; discourse analysis. Evaluation of language in patients with schizophrenia usually reveals a variety of deficits, usually interpreted as evidence of thought disorder. Among the most commonly reported are abnormalities in pragmatics, prosody, auditory processing, perseveration, and abstract language. In studies of children and adolescents with early schizophrenia, pragmatics was the area of language impaired in the greatest number. Frequently observed pragmatic deficits were as follows:

1. Inadequate referencing, such as failure to orient the listener by establishing relevant background information for discourse; inappropriate between- and within-reference switches; use of noncontextual situational references; failure to differentiate between old and new information; lack of reference and inappropriate ellipsis of reference

2. Abnormalities in topic selection, maintenance, and switching, such as difficulties establishing a topic of discourse, inappropriate switching of topic, inappropriate topic expansion, switching topic to the self

3. abnormal sequencing of discourse, such as difficulties describing events in time and logically sequencing utterances within a discourse

4. Turn-taking problems and other disturbances in the speaker–hearer role relationship.

**Prägung** *Imprinting* (q.v.).

**-praxia** Combining form meaning action, doing, from Gr. *prāxis,* a doing, acting, action, from *prassein,* to achieve, accomplish, practice, do.

**praxiology** Dunlap's term for the science of behavior that excludes the study of consciousness and similar nonobjective metaphysical concepts.

**praxis** The act of translating intent into action; it requires conceptual knowledge (what to do) and performance (how to do it). Different types of *dyspraxia* (q.v.) indicate the area of the brain involved:

Temporo-spatial patterns of learned skilled movement (higher order programs) are in the dominant parietal lobe.

Motor innervatory patterns (lower order programs) are in premotor cortex and the supplementary motor area.

Semantic motor association is in dominant parietal lobe.

Visual-motor association is in the occipito-parietal association areas.

Disconnection syndromes reflect defective interhemispheric connectivity, which is dependent on the corpus callosum.

**praxis, dyspraxia**   See *parietal lobe.*

**praxis, ideokinetic**   Ability to perform an action from memory when requested to do so, without the need of external cues. Also known as ideomotor praxis, it is a function of the dominant parietal lobe.

**pre-**   Combining form meaning earlier, before, ahead, from L. *pre-.*

**preadaptation**   A Darwinian mechanism wherein an organ adapted for one purpose is used fortuitously for a "new" function. Neural mechanisms initially adapted to regulate the precise manual motor control implicated in toolmaking, for example, could have provided the initial basis for the regulation of speech motor activity. The *Broca speech area* (q.v.), though not the "seat" of language ability, is known to be involved in fine manual motor control, speech production, and syntax. The fourfold enlargement of computational resources in the parts of the human brain that are active during speech or the comprehension of language could in itself account for the qualitative difference beween the human and the nonhuman primate brain. Prefrontal cortex, cerebellum, and basal ganglia—neuroanatomical structures implicated in regulating motor control, syntax, and thinking—differentiate the human brain from the chimpanzee brain.

**preadaptive attitude**   The initial reaction to a stimulus or experience, before the subject has become accustomed to it. P. Steckler (*Archives of Neurology and Psychiatry 80*, 1958) notes that the preadaptive attitude of schizophrenics to hallucinations or feelings of estrangement is of a fairly consistent pattern: anxiety, fear, search for reassurance, doubts as to sanity, search for a rational explanation, and, finally, autonomic and muscular system reactions.

**pre-AIDS**   See *ARC.*

**preambivalent phase**   The early oral stage, before there is any conception of objects. In the preambivalent phase, the infant is unaware of the outside world: he is aware only of his own tension and relaxation. No object is recognized; oral erotic pleasure is gained both from gratification of hunger and from stimulation of the erogenous oral mucous membrane. This is easily seen in thumb sucking. Accordingly, the preambivalent phase is also characterized as the early oral sucking stage of libidinal organization or as the autoerotic stage in the development of object love. Because there is no object at this stage, there can be no ambivalent attitude toward an object; hence, the period is known as the preambivalent phase.

**prearchaic thinking**   See   *archaic-paralogical thinking.*

**precentral area, convolution, gyrus**   See *frontal lobe; motor cortex.*

**precocious puberty**   See *macrogenitosomia.*

**precocity**   In a child, the premature or exceptionally early development of certain mental or physical capacities and endowments normally and characteristically exhibited only by children of a more advanced age group.

**precognition**   Prescience; knowledge of future events, presumably by means of extrasensory perception.

**preconscious**   *Foreconscious*; in psychoanalysis, one of the three topographical divisions of the psyche, and often abbreviated Pcs. The preconscious division includes those thoughts, memories, and similar mental elements that, although not conscious at the moment, can readily be brought into consciousness (Cs) by an effort of attention. This is in contrast to the unconscious (Ucs) division, whose elements are barred from access to consciousness by some intrapsychic force such as repression.

**preconscious thinking**   The preverbal, prelogical, pictorial phantasy thinking that precedes the development of logical thinking in small children. Preconscious thinking is primitive and archaic, and not in accordance with reality. It is ruled by the emotions and strives for the discharge of tensions; it is full of wishful or fear-laden misconceptions. It is carried out through concrete pictorial images, and it is a magical type of thinking. Preconscious thinking is symbolic and thus vague, for the world is experienced and apperceived in symbolic forms. Stimuli that provoke the same emotional reactions are looked upon as identical.

With the acquisition of words and the development of the faculty of speech, thinking becomes logical and organized. Preconscious thinking, however, recurs in the adult in several different ways. Before acquiring verbal formulation, all thoughts run through initial phases that resemble preconscious thinking. In dreams and in fatigue, words are retranslated into pictures. Conscious ideas may be symbols hiding objectionable unconscious ideas and in dreams symbols appear not only in order to distort, but also as a characteristic of archaic pictorial thinking visualizing abstract thoughts.

**precursors**  CNS stem cells and all progenitors are generally referred to as precursor cells.

**predator**  One who takes (wrongfully) by force; one who despoils, pillages, strips, or ravages. See *sexually violent predator*.

**predatory violence**  Planned, purposeless, and seemingly emotionless violence without evidence of autonomic arousal. It is in contrast to *affective violence*, which is an emotional reaction to a perceived threat, such as rejection; it is chararacterized by high elevation in indicators of autonomic arousal. Both types of violence occur in *stalking* (q.v.), but affective violence is much more frequent. Predatory violence is found in stalkers against public figures or public officials, often occurring without forewarning threats. See *sexually violent predator*.

**predementia praecox**  The personality constitution of the schizophrenic prior to the appearance of overt symptoms of the disorder. The predementia praecox character is one in which the individual habitually ceases to apply himself vigorously to the real facts of life. His thoughts are devoted to daydreams and fantasies, and by constantly seeking refuge in evasions he loses the capacity for grappling with difficulties. Thus, in the presence of some added stress, which the ordinary individual would be prepared to meet, "the sensitive and weakened individual will react with manifestations constituting the deterioration process of dementia praecox" (Kraepelin, E. *Lectures on Clinical Psychiatry*, 1913). Kraepelin credits Adolf Meyer with having first delineated the character syndrome observed in predementia praecox.

**prediction**  Foretelling; anticipating the consequences of an action. Motor commands are used to predict the sensory consequences of self-generated movement, a process that involves the cerebellum. The cerebellum stores representations of motor commands and their sensory consequences, body kinematics, external tools and action contexts, from which predictions are made. Such a store of predictions concerning self-generated action could also be used to estimate the

motor commands (and therefore the intentions or other internal states) that gave rise to an action made by another person. See *anticipation; imitation; intention; simulation*.

**prediction-error signal**  Phasic bursts and pauses in the firing patterns of dopamine neurons when an expected reward is withheld. Tonic activity signals no deviation from expectation; phasic bursts signal a positive reward prediction error (better than expected); pauses signal a negative prediction error. The phenomenon demonstrates that in *addiction* (q.v.), dopamine does not act as a hedonic signal but rather promotes reward-related learning; the hedonic properties of a goal are linked to desire and to action and thereby shape subsequent reward-related behavior.

**predictive validity**  See *validity*.

**predisposition**  The inherited ability of an organism to develop a certain attribute or morbid trait when the necessary peristatic conditions for the given character are present. According to genetic principles, there is no inheritance of fully developed hereditary characters, but only a transmission of *predisposing* genetic factors depending for their phenotypical manifestation on various constitutional and dispositional influences. See *genotype; heredity*.

**predominantly sensory neuropathy**  See *HIV neuropathy*.

**predormital**  Hypnagogic; occurring before falling asleep.

**preferred provider organization**  *PPO* (q.v.).

**prefrontal cortex**  *PFC*; it makes up 70%–80% of frontal lobes, or about 30% of the gray matter. Increase in size of PFC is relatively recent; between human and chimpanzee there was a leap in size of 70%, greater than the enlargement in any other part of brain. The inputs and outputs of PFC wire it solely to other parts of the brain, and its neurons have up to 16 times as many synapses as other parts of the cortex. PFC comprises the nonmotor sectors of the frontal lobe that receive input from the dorsomedial thalamic nucleus.

PFC is divided into the *ventromedial PFC* and the *dorsolateral PFC* (qq.v.). Its functions, which include planning and organization of such things as attention, vision, hearing, touch, emotions, memory, movement, and language, are believed to be executed by three distinct brain circuits—DLPFC, orbitofrontal, and anterior cingulate cortex.

The affect subdivision of the anterior cingulate cortex connects with limbic and paralimbic regions, including orbitofrontal cortex; its cognition subdivision connects with parietal cortex, spinal cord, and DLPFC.

The *orbitofrontal cortex* (q.v.) governs socially appropriate behavior and empathy. Lesions cause impulsivity, lability, personality changes, and lack of humanistic sensibility.

Subjects with DLPFC damage perseverate, demonstrate concrete thinking and impairment in constructional skills and sequential motor tasks, and have difficulty with set shifting and screening out environmental distraction.

**prefrontal hypofunction**   An increasing body of data implicates dysfunction of the prefrontal cortex in schizophrenia. PET shows prefrontal hypofunction during the performance of prefrontal cognitive tasks. Prefrontal hypofunction may be linked to a prefrontal-temporal-limbic neural network. See *DLPFC*.

**prefrontal lobotomy**   Also, *frontal lobotomy; prefrontal leukotomy; frontal leukotomy.* A psychosurgical procedure consisting of ablation of the prefrontal area of the frontal lobe. The prefrontal area is that portion of the frontal lobe anterior to Brodmann's area 6, the premotor area. As a psychosurgical procedure, the operation is ordinarily performed bilaterally. In contrast to frontal lobectomy, which is an open procedure in which tissue is excised and therefore more direct cortical damage is caused, the lobotomy procedure is "blind." A hole is drilled through the skull and a leukotome is inserted to cut white nerve fibers connecting the frontal lobe with the thalamus. Thus, in lobotomy, there is less cortical damage than in lobectomy. This procedure interrupts frontothalamic and thalamofrontal fibers and also the association systems of the frontal lobe.

Prefrontal lobotomy was among the first psychosurgical procedures used in the United States. It seems to reduce anxiety feelings and introspective activities; feelings of inadequacy and self-consciousness are thereby lessened. Lobotomy reduces the emotional tension associated with hallucinations and does away with the catatonic state. Because nearly all psychosurgical procedures have undesirable side effects, they are ordinarily resorted to only after all other methods have failed and use nowadays is rare. The less disorganized the personality of the patient, the more obvious are postoperative side effects. For this reason, bilateral prefrontal lobotomy was employed more commonly in schizophrenia than in any other disorder. See *psychosurgery*.

Convulsive seizures are reported as sequelae of prefrontal lobotomy in 5% to 10% of cases. Such seizures are ordinarily well controlled with the usual anticonvulsive drugs. Postoperative blunting of the personality, apathy, and irresponsibility are the rule rather than the exception. Other side effects include distractibility, childishness, facetiousness, lack of tact or discipline, and postoperative incontinence.

Prefrontal lobotomy has been used successfully to control pain secondary to organic lesions. In this case, the tendency has been to employ unilateral lobotomy, because of the evidence that a lobotomy extensive enough to relieve psychotic symptoms is not required to control pain.

Since the introduction of prefrontal lobotomy and prefrontal lobectomy, various other psychosurgical procedures have been initiated—transorbital lobotomy, thalamotomy, cortical undercutting, and topectomy. These permit selective operation, the particular procedure being chosen on the basis of the nature of the disease, its duration and extent, the patient's age, etc.

**prefrontal syndromes**   Three types of syndrome due to dysfunction of the prefrontal area can be distinguished: (1) disinhibited type, indicating pathology in the orbitofrontal system; (2) apathetic type, indicating pathology in the mesial frontal neural system; and (3) dysexecutive type, indicating pathology in the dorsal convexity system.

Causative conditions include: degenerative disorders (e.g., Alzheimer disease), trauma, cardiovascular abnormalities, toxic (e.g., alcoholism, Wilson disease), and neoplasms.

**pregenital love**   Abraham thus terms the behavior of the child toward the mother in particular, during the pregenital phase. Although the infant is relatively, if not completely, indifferent to the welfare of the object in the early suckling phase, it shows the first signs of caring for the mother during the biting stage. "We may also regard such a care, incomplete as it is, as the first beginnings of object-love in a stricter sense since it implies that the individual has begun to conquer his narcissism" (*Selected Papers*, 1927). See *depressive position*.

**pregenital organization**   The arrangement of the libido in the stages prior to that of infantile genitality. See *ontogeny, psychic.*

**preindustrial**   Prevocational.

**prejudice, race**   See *racism.*

**preknowledge**   See *psychophysics.*

**prelogical**   The mode of thinking may regress, as it often does in schizophrenic subjects, from the logical to the prelogical. It has frequently been pointed out that thought and language in their development change from *feeling, concreteness,* and *perception* in the direction of *reasoning, differentiation,* and *abstraction.* See *paleologic.*

**Premack principle**   A behavior engaged in at a higher frequency can be used as a reinforcer of lower-frequency behavior; also referred to as grandma's rule ("You can have dessert, but you must eat your broccoli first"). See *reinforcement; reinforcement schedule.*

**premature birth**   Defined as birthweight under 2500 g or gestation period of less than 34 weeks. Approximately 7% of all births in the United States are premature. Premature birth is correlated with low socioeconomic status, poor maternal nutrition, and teenage pregnancy, and it increases the risk of mental retardation, behavior problems, sensorimotor problems such as dyslexia, and abuse of the child born prematurely.

**premature ejaculation**   *Ejaculatio praecox* (q.v.).

**premenstrual dysphoric disorder**   *Late luteal phase dysphoric disorder;* also known as *premenstrual syndrome, premenstrual tension state.* See *LLPDD.*

**premium, incitement**   *Forepleasure* (q.v.).

**premorbid personality**   The personality that existed before the appearance of frank mental disorder.

**premotor area**   See *frontal lobe.*

**premutation carriers**   See *fragile X.*

**prenefarious inhibition**   In the development of guilt, the initial generalized diminution in activity that accompanies fear; such inhibition is nonspecifically protective, whereas the avoidances of the later stage of guilt proper protect against specific external dangers that come to be recognized as guilt provoking.

**prenubile**   Referring to the period of life from birth to puberty; prepubertal.

**preoccipital area**   See *occipital lobe.*

**preoccupation**   The state of being self-absorbed or engrossed in one's own thoughts, typically to a degree that hinders effective contact with or relationship to external reality. Preoccupation may sometimes be no more than absentmindedness; in other instances, it is part of an autistic schizophrenic's withdrawal from reality and turning inward upon the self; in other cases, it represents a mild degree of interference with consciousness and the level of attention and thus betokens an underlying disturbance in brain cell functioning. See *stupor.*

**pre-oedipal**   Relating to the stages of infantile development antedating the Oedipus complex (psychoanalysis). "The pre-oedipal phase ... is for both sexes that earliest period of attachment to the first love object, the mother, before the advent of the father as a rival. It is the period during which an exclusive relation exists between mother and child" (Brunswick, R. M. *Psychoanalytic Quarterly IX,* 1940).

**preoperational thinking**   See *concrete operational stage.*

**prephallic**   Referring to the period of psychosexual development preceding the phallic phase; i.e., the oral and anal phases or stages. Although the term pregenital is often used interchangeably with the term prephallic, this is not technically correct, because the phallic and genital phases are distinct and separate.

**preplate**   See *axon growth.*

**prepotent**   Ascendant; dominant. In neurophysiology, that reflex is prepotent that, when two stimuli that would evoke dissimilar reflexes are applied simultaneously, displaces the second reflex. "The outcome of the rivalry depends upon a number of circumstances: (i) the nature of the reflexes, (ii) the intensity of the several stimuli and (iii) the duration of action of the reflex. ' (Fulton, J. F. *Physiology of the Nervous System,* 1949). In general, nociceptive reflexes, such as the flexion reflex, are prepotent to all other types of reflex competing for the final common pathway; other things being equal, the more intense stimulus results in prepotency of its reflex; and the longer a reflex has been in operation, the easier will its prepotency be lost.

**prepsychotic**   Pertaining to the period before psychosis became evident. See *premorbid personality.* Some authors (e.g., Katan) use this term in a more restricted sense to refer to that phase of psychosis in which the patient, although he deviates from normality, has not yet proceeded to develop such grossly psychotic symptoms as delusions and hallucinations.

**prepsychotic panic**   Arieti's term for that stage in the development of schizophrenia in which the patient's grotesque and disordered self-image leads to feelings of being unlovable, different, humiliated, guilty, under suspicion, etc., but the cognitive distortions are not yet expressed in such full-fledged psychotic symptoms as delusions and hallucinations.

**prepubertal**   Relating to the phase of life antedating puberty.

**prepulse inhibition**   *PPI*; *gating* (q.v.); the capacity to inhibit the startle response when a weak prestimulus (about 100 msec before the startle stimulus itself) reduces the startle response substantially. It is modulated by cortical-striatal-pallidal-thalamic circuitry.

The evolution of prepulse inhibition appears to parallel the developmental stages of brain inhibitory mechanisms and approaches adult level by approximately age 8. Lower prepulse inhibition has been shown among children with disorders characterized by a failure of inhibitor brain mechanisms, including Tourette syndrome, PTSD, fragile X syndrome, and, among boys, nocturnal enuresis and comorbid ADHD. Lower prepulse inhibition has been found in adults whose psychiatric syndromes are characterized by poor selective-inhibitory control of attention, including OCD, panic disorder, social phobia, Asperger syndrome, Huntington disease, bipolar mania, and perhaps most notably schizophrenia. Differences in prepulse inhibition have provided a well-replicated neurophysiologic measure of sensorimotor gating differences in patients with schizophrenia that have been associated with overawareness and misinterpretation of preconscious material and, more generally, the cardinal symptoms of cognitive fragmentation and thought disorder.

**prerelease anxiety state**   The anxiety phenomena which some inmates of penal institutions develop through fear of being set free and having to face the world again.

**presbycusis**   The most common type of hearing loss in the elderly, consisting of slowly progressive, bilaterally symmetrical, sensorineural hearing loss. It often involves poor speech discrimination.

**presbyophrenia**   *Kahlbaum-Wernicke syndrome*; one form of *Alzheimer disease* (q.v.). Its principal characteristics are marked confusional disorientation, confabulation, mistakes in identity, and agitation without accomplishment of any objective. Presbyophrenic confabulations typically show a poverty, monotony, puerility, and naiveté of content. Because ethical conduct is preserved for a relatively long time, the patient is able to fit into limited social contacts, and particularly so since his affect tends toward the euphoric and the amiable.

**preschizophrenic ego**   The prepsychotic personality of the schizophrenic, characterized by impairment of ego synthesis; that is, the patient does not give the impression of a personal oneness that the normal person gives. The preschizophrenic child daydreams excessively, and the phantasies here have the aim of withdrawal from reality; in the normal child, phantasies have the goal of experimentation and preparation for mastery of reality. Often, during sleep, the preschizophrenic child has dreams of its own death; there is a predominance of regressive (even prenatal) phantasies; exaggerated conscience, bizarre somatic sensations, frequent severe temper tantrums, and a pervasive aggressiveness are typical.

**presence**   The sense of being in a *virtual environment* rather than the place in which the participant's body is actually located. Presence occurs when there is successful substitution of real sensory data by computer-generated sensory data; the subject can engage in normal motor actions to carry out tasks and can exercise some degree of control over the environment. See *virtualization*.

**presenile**   Relating to the period of life antedating senility or old age. See *Alzheimer disease; Pick disease.*

**presenile paraphrenia**   Albrecht's terms for schizophrenia with onset after the involutional and before the senile phase. See *paraphrenia*.

**presenilins**   Presenilin 1 (PS1) and presenilin 2 (PS2); mutations in the genes that encode them are the basis of most cases of early-onset familial Alzheimer disease (FAD). Their function is cleavage of the amyloid precursor and other membrane proteins; they also modulate calcium entry into a variety of cells. See *Alzheimer disease; amyloid.*

**Present State Examination (PSE)**   An instrument developed by J. K. Wing, J. E. Cooper, and N. Sartorius (*The Measurement and Classification of Psychiatric Symptoms*, 1974) for use in the WHO-supported International Pilot Study of Schizophrenia. The PSE is a structured interview containing almost 400 items that include a wide range of symptoms likely to be present during an acute episode of one of the "functional" neuroses or psychoses. See *International Pilot Study of Schizophrenia.*

**presentation**   The mode by which an instinct expresses itself, its vehicle of expression. In Jung's analytical psychology, "The term 'thinking' should, in my view, be confined to the linking up of representations by means of a concept, where, in other words, an act of judgment prevails, whether such act be the product of one's intention or not" (*Psychological Types*, 1923).

**preservation-consolidation hypothesis**   The postulate that processes underlying new memories initially persist in a fragile state and consolidate over time. See *hippocampus; memory; MTL.*

**pressure of ideas**   See *thought pressure.*

**pressured speech**   Logorrhea (q.v.).

**prestige suggestion**   A form of supportive psychotherapy in which the therapist, because he occupies a position of omnipotence in the eyes of the patient, is able to dictate the disappearance of symptoms. Prestige suggestion is probably the least successful of all treatment methods.

**prestimulus**   See *prepulse inhibition.*

**presumption, tender years**   See *custody.*

**presuperego phase**   The early years of life before the superego has been formed. It is generally believed that the superego comes into being when it replaces the Oedipus complex. The presuperego stage lasts until the child is 5 or 6 years of age and includes the oral, anal, and phallic phases, as well as the development of the Oedipus complex in the phallic stage. A clear distinction is made between the presuperego stage and the superego stage because of the different type of anxiety that is typical of each. In the presuperego stage, anxiety is objective and more closely related to reality situations than in the adult superego stage, where anxiety is typically determined by the precepts of the fully developed superego, of whose role the individual is not consciously aware.

**presynaptic neuromessenger**   See *neuromessenger.*

**presynaptic terminals**   Specialized swellings of the end branches of the *axon* (q.v.).

**pretraumatic personality**   In the case of a person who has developed an emotional or mental

illness in consequence of an injury, the personality as it was before the injury and illness.

**prevalence**   In epidemiology, prevalence is the number of cases presently existing and active in a given population at any particular time:

$$\text{Prevalence rate (or ratio) of illness} = \frac{\text{Number of cases of illness existing on a specific date}}{\text{Number of persons in population on same date}} \times 100,000$$

See *epidemiology; incidence; PSA; rate.*

Two reports from the 1980s—the *ECA* study (Epidemiologic Catchment Area project of the National Institute of Mental Health), and the NCS (National Comorbidity Survey)—were in general agreement on the 1-year prevalence of mental disorders. A more recent study (Narrow et al. *Archives of General Psychiatry*, 2002) reported lower figures, perhaps because it imposed a clinical significance criterion (in accord with the DSM-IV specification that mental health problems must be clinically significant to warrant diagnosis). Comparison of findings:

| DISORDER | BCA | NCS | NARROW ET AL. |
|---|---|---|---|
| Any mental or substance disorder | 19 | 28 | 30 |
| Alcohol use disorder | 5 | 7 | 10 |
| Substance abuse disorder | 6 | 9 | 12 |
| Anxiety disorder | 12 | 13 | 19 |
| OCD | 2 | 2 | |
| Major depressive disorder | 5 | 6 | 10 |
| Bipolar I disorder | 0.5 | 0.9 | |

**ADULTS FROM HOUSEHOLD POPULATION WITH SERIOUS MENTAL ILLNESS, BY AGE, SEX, RACE, AND EDUCATION: UNITED STATES, 1989**

| | ADULT HOUSEHOLD POPULATION | | ADULTS WITH SERIOUS MENTAL ILLNESS | | |
|---|---|---|---|---|---|
| | NO. (IN THOUSANDS) | PERCENT DISTRIBUTION | NO. (IN THOUSANDS) | PERCENT | RATE PER THOUSAND |
| Total | 179,529 | 100.0 | 3,264 | 100.0 | 18.2 |
| Age (years) | | | | | |
| 18-24 | 25,401 | 14.2 | 361 | 11.1 | 14.2 |
| 25-34 | 42,814 | 23.9 | 707 | 21.7 | 16.5 |
| 35-44 | 35,982 | 20.0 | 744 | 22.8 | 20.7 |

continued

| | | | | | |
|---|---|---|---|---|---|
| 45-64 | 46,114 | 25.7 | 919 | 28.2 | 19.9 |
| 65-69 | 9,903 | 5.5 | 142 | 4.4 | 14.3 |
| 70-74 | 7,925 | 4.4 | 102 | 3.1 | 12.9 |
| 75 & over | 11,391 | 6.3 | 288 | 9.8 | 25.3 |
| | | | | | |
| Sex | | | | | |
| Male | 85,257 | 47.5 | 1,320 | 40.4 | 15.5 |
| Female | 94,272 | 52.5 | 1,944 | 59.6 | 20.6 |
| | | | | | |
| Race | | | | | |
| White | 153,763 | 85.6 | 2,812 | 86.1 | 18.3 |
| Black | 19,932 | 11.1 | 393 | 12.0 | 19.7 |
| Other | 5,834 | 3.2 | 59 | 1.8 | 10.1 |
| | | | | | |
| Education in years | | | | | |
| Under 12 | 39,809 | 22.4 | 1,083 | 33.8 | 27.2 |
| 12 | 68,563 | 38.6 | 1,120 | 34.9 | 16.3 |
| Over 12 | 69,369 | 39.0 | 1,002 | 31.3 | 14.4 |

*Source*: Reprinted from the United States Department of Health and Human Services, 1992.

**prevention** Social, economic, legal, medical, or individual psychological measures aimed at minimizing the risk of disorder in susceptible persons. See *community psychiatry*.

**preventive therapy, long-term** Pharmacologic agents used over long periods to prevent recurrence of illnesses or reducing their severity and duration. It is differentiated from *continuation* maintenance therapy, which is pharmacologic treatment of a persisting illness following initial control of acute symptoms.

**priapism** Persistent erection of the penis, particularly when the erection is due to organic disease and not to sexual desire. Erection is prolonged, dysfunctional, painful, and sexual desire is typically impaired. Psychotropic drug-induced priapism may result in irreversible impotence. Surgical intervention may be required, sometimes on an emergency basis, to achieve detumescence.

    Priapism has been reported as a complication of treatment with the antidepressants trazodone and phenelzine and also with antipsychotic drugs (phenothiazines, haloperidol).

**Priapus** Priapus, the son of Venus and Mercury (or Bacchus), is the god of procreation and hence of gardens and vineyards, as the embodiment of the generative force in nature. The Priapic cult was associated with worship of the penis, and priapism became a synonym of lewdness.

**pride system** Horney's term for the total of the neurotically (over-) valued and the neurotically (over-)hated attributes of the self.

**prima facie duty** In some systems of moral ethics, a duty that is binding (e.g., truth-telling) unless overridden by a stronger prima facie duty.

**primacy effect** See *memory training*.

**primacy zone** Any dominating erotogenic area through which subordinate areas find instinctual discharge through displacement. In the development and organization of the libido, one primacy zone tends to succeed another in a typical and characteristic chronological order: (1) the oral; (2) the anal; (3) the phallic; (4) the genital. See *ontogeny, psychic*.

**primal masochism** See *death instinct*.

**primal maternal introject** See *original object*.

**primal phantasy** See *phantasy, unconscious*.

**primal sadism** A portion of the death instinct that always remains with the person; Freud equated it to erotogenic masochism.

**primal scene** A child's first observation of sexual intercourse between the parents. In his description of the "wolf-man" case, Freud claimsed that the primal scene was influential in determining later psychopathology.

**primary aging** See *aging*.

**primary behavior disorders** See *behavior disorders*.

**primary degenerative dementia (PPD)** *Alzheimer disease* (q.v.).

**primary dissociation** See *dissociative disorders*.

**primary envy** Primal envy; Klein viewed primal envy as constitutional (a view with which most Freudians still disagree), describing it as a phantasy of invasive, destructive attacks on the good object merely because it is good. The spoiling and damaging aspects of envy mark it as closely allied with the death instinct and lacking almost any kind of libidinal element. In time it is modulated to *greed* (which may result in the internal accumulation of damaged objects), to *jealousy* (which has more libidinal elements and aims to possess the loved object and remove the rival), and still later to a more mature state of competition. See *envy; identification; projective identification; oral sadism*.

**primary health care** Accessible, comprehensive, coordinated care provided by accountable providers of health services; the first level of personal health services (as distinguished from public, environmental, and occupational health services), where initial professional attention is given to current or potential health problems. Often it is associated with care of the "whole person" rather than treatment of an illness.

**primary ictal automatism** A type of *psychomotor epilepsy* (q.v.).

**primary identification**   See *symbiotic stage*.

**primary masochism**   *Erotogenic masochism; masochism* (qq.v.).

**primary memory**   See *short-term memory*.

**primary microorchidism**   See *Klinefelter syndrome*.

**primary physician**   See *caregiver*.

**primary prevention**   Any means that reduces the incidence of new cases in a specified population.

**primary process**   Freud's term for the laws that govern unconscious processes; used to refer to a type of thinking, characteristic of childhood (and dreams), or to the way in which libidinal or aggressive energy is mobilized and discharged. The basic characteristics of the primary process are a tendency to immediate discharge of drive energy (i.e., immediate gratification) and an extreme mobility of cathexis so that substitute methods of discharge can be achieved with relative ease. Primary process thinking is characterized by the absence of any negatives, conditionals, or other qualifying conjunctions; by the lack of any sense of time; and by the use of allusion, analogy, displacement, condensation, and symbolic representation. Drive energy characteristically remains unneutralized during the period of operation of the primary process.

In essence, the primary process is identical with Freud's formulation of the pleasure principle. The difference between them is that while the pleasure principle is described in subjective terms, the primary process is described in objective terms.

**primary progressive aphasia**   A dementia characterized by language deficit in the first 2 years of the disease. Primary progressive aphasia has a course, eventual outcome, and pathology similar to that of *frontotemporal dementia* (q.v.). In some patients with primary progressive aphasia, extrapyramidal symptoms similar to those that occur with corticobasal degeneration and motor neuron disease are superimposed. See *Pick complex*.

**primary response**   Part of *memory* (q.v.), consisting of the perception, apperception, recognition, and some understanding of the significance of what is to be learned. The primary response is affected by many factors such as previously learned responses, mental set, and fatigue.

**primary somatic sensory cortex**   Contains four separate maps of the body in the post-central gyrus. The maps expand or contract, depending on the particular uses or activities of the peripheral sensory pathways. In learning, practice alone not only strengthens the effectiveness of existing interconnections, but also changes cortical connections to accommodate new patterns of actions.

**primary splitting**   See *paranoid-schizoid position*.

**primary support group**   The persons with whom one has the strongest and most enduring positive relationships; those who form the core of the personal environment. Most commonly the primary support group is a relatively small social network, such as the family, the others in a partnership or brotherhood or fellowship, or the other members of a long-term therapy group.

**primary task**   See *task, primary*.

**primary tastes**   See *gustation*.

**primary thought disorder**   See *thought disorder, primary*.

**primary visual processing**   See *visual processing*.

**primers**   See *PCR*.

**priming**   1. *Perceptual fluency*; facilitation of the recognition or reproduction of recently perceived stimuli; nonconscious facilitation of processing due to implicit memory for previous stimulus presentation; facilitation of recognition, reproduction, or biases in selection of stimuli that have recently been perceived. Priming is a type of *procedural memory* (q.v.) that is manifested as a change in the ability to identify or produce an item as a result of a previous encounter with the item. It is typically measured as an increase in the speed of naming or responding to stimuli that have been seen or heard on a previous occasion. Priming is an implicit memory mechanism that occurs independently of whether the subject recalls the original learning experience. It appears to be a manifestation of temporary changes in cortical perceptual processing centers as a result of exposure to a stimulus.

Priming is an explicit memory system that supports the ability to consciously remember a past experience; it is disrupted by damage to the medial temporal lobe. In contrast, repetition priming—the nonconscious facilitation of processing that results from implicit memory for previous stimulus presentation—is relatively intact following medial temporal lobe damage. There is evidence of "crosstalk" between the two systems.

2. In formerly dependent drug users, reintroduction of the abused drug leads to increased intake of the drug (*reinstatement*). Drug priming is a form of *sensitization* (q.v.) and at least in cocaine-primed reinstatement it appears to depend on the glutamatergic prefrontal connection to the nucleus accumbens. See *addiction*.

**primitivation** Regression of the ego to the primitive stage in its development with consequent loss of higher ego functions. Objective thinking is replaced by magical thinking or wish-fulfilling hallucinations; object relationships and love are of the helpless, passive dependent type, or there may even be a lack of objects; sexuality is colored with oral eroticism; all perceptions, even those associated with incorporation, may be completely blocked; uncoordinated discharge movements replace purposeful actions. According to Fenichel, primitivation occurs in both the traumatic neuroses and schizophrenia. In the former, the patients often exhibit an attitude of utter helplessness and passive dependence in which the behavior is that of an infant. In traumatic neuroses, when perceptions and actions are blocked, the patient may show constant weakness and fatigue, be unable to undertake any active tasks, encounter difficulty in concentration and memory, show various levels of disturbance of consciousness.

Fainting is the most primitive response to a trauma. It is an emergency phenomenon that requires all mental energies to master the intruding overwhelming excitation. Ego functions must relinquish their energies in favor of the emergency task and further excitations are excluded.

In schizophrenia, too, many of the symptoms are "direct expressions of a regressive breakdown of the ego and an undoing of differentiations acquired through mental development." There is a "return to the time when the ego was not yet established or had just begun to be established." For example, world-destruction phantasies are caused by the inner perception of the loss of object relationships; feelings of grandeur express the increase in narcissism that occurs as the psychic energy withdrawn from objects is invested in the ego; schizophrenic thinking is the archaic magical thinking that precedes the development of reality testing in the small child; hebephrenia is a vegetative existence

expressing the old passive receptive or even intrauterine adaptations (Fenichel, O. *The Psychoanalytic Theory of Neurosis*, 1945).

**primitive object relation** See *projective identification*.

**primordial delusion** See *délire d'emblée*.

**primordial image** "The primordial image is a mnemonic deposit, an *imprint* ('engram'—Semon), which has arisen through a condensation of innumerable, similar processes. It is primarily a precipitate or deposit, and therefore a typical basic form of a certain ever-recurring psychic experience. As a mythological motive, therefore, it is a constantly effective and continually recurring expression which is either awakened, or appropriately formulated, by certain psychic experiences" (Jung, C. G. *Psychological Types*, 1923). Also known as *archetype*. See *image; personal image*.

**Prince, Morton** (1854–1929) American psychiatrist and neurologist; hysteria, multiple personality; *Dissociation of a Personality* (1908).

**principal neurons** *Projection neurons.* See *neuron*.

**principle** The general foundation for a rule or action guide. See *judgment; rule; theory*.

**principle of feminization** See *ambitypic*.

**principle of inertia** Alexander's term for the principle of *repetition-compulsion* (q.v.), stressing that the tendency to automatic action is greater than the tendency which involves constantly changing and active mental efforts.

**print media** See *media*.

**prion** A glycosylphosphatidyl inositol-anchored cell surface protein found in neurons (designated $PrP^c$ or $PrP^{sen}$). Prions are proteinaceous infectious particles, formerly known as unconventional slow viruses. They are smaller than even the smallest virus and, unlike viruses or bacteria, they have no detectable DNA or RNA. Among their other properties they somehow evade their host's immune system; they do not evoke virus-associated inflammatory response in brain; they do not produce pleocytosis or rise in CSF protein; they give no evidence of immune response to a causative virus; and they display unusual resistance to various chemical and physical agents.

Prion disease occurs when an abnormal protease-resistant isoform ($PrP^{sc}$ or $PrP^{res}$) accumulates within the brain. A gene within the host, the P cellular prion protein gene, codes for the prion protein. As slow conversion of existing normal sen into abnormal res progresses, res accumulates in the brain and eventually classic symptoms of *transmissible spongiform encephalopathies* (q.v.) develop, including three human neurodegenerative diseases: kuru, Creutzfeldt-Jacob disease (CJD), and Gerstmann-Straussler-Scheinker (GSS) syndrome. Familial CJD and GSS are also genetic disorders, and persons at risk can often be identified decades before central nervous system dysfunction develops. Prion diseases in animals include scrapie of sheep and goats, and three disorders believed to result from ingestion of scrapie-infected animal products: bovine spongiform encephalopathy (BSE, mad cow disease), transmissible mink encephalopathy, and chronic wasting disease of captive mule deer and elk. The term prion was introduced by S. B. Prusiner in 1982 to distinguish these pathogens from viroids, viruses, bacteria, fungi, and parasites. Infectivity of a prion depends upon a protein, and not nucleic acids.

A glycosylphosphatidylinositol (GPI) lipid anchor tethers the protein to the outer side of the cell membrane. Toxicity depends on membrane anchoring. In mice, removal of the GPI anchor abolished susceptiblity to clinical disease while preserving the competence of the soluble PrP$^C$ molecule to support prion replication. When infected with PrP$^{SC}$, the GPI-negative transgenic mice never developed clinical prion disease, even though their brains were packed with PrP$^{SC}$ plaques.

A prion protein (PrP) has been discovered; it is encoded by a chromosomal gene in the infectious scrapie prion particle. PrP genes have been localized to the short arm of human chromosome 20. The normal PrP gene product is PrPc, a protease-sensitive protein; a disease-specific protein, PrPSc, is protease-resistant. Prions are composed of PrPSc molecules, but how many are needed for infectivity is unknown. Also unknown is whether prions are composed entirely of PrPSc molecules. Whether all cases of familial CJD (which accounts for approximately 10% of CJD) and GSS are due to infectious prions, or whether some represent inborn errors of PrP metabolism, is unknown.

**prion diseases**  Mutations in the prion protein are responsible for three neurologic disorders, which may be inherited as autosomal dominant traits: Gerstmann-Straussler-Scheinker

syndrome, familial CJD, and fatal familial insomnia. *Kuru* (q.v.) is also considered a prion disease. See *Creutzfeldt-Jacob disease.*

**prion hypothesis**  A *protein-only hypothesis,* that the agent responsible for *transmissible spongiform encephalopathies* is an infectious protein, the *prion* (qq.v.), which can infect tissues and reproduce itself, violating long-standing dogma that a DNA- or RNA-based genome is necessary for such autonomous behavior. Some researchers maintain that an as-yet-unidentified microbe, such as a virus, may team up with the prion protein to produce its effects on the nervous system.

**prison neurosis**  *Chronophobia* (q.v.).

**prison psychosis**  *Stir-fever*; psychosis precipitated by incarceration. The form it takes depends on the make-up and vulnerabilities of the person affected; it may be (or resemble) schizophrenia, affect disorder, or psychoneurotic disorder.

**prisoner of war syndrome (POW)**  Psychopathologic manifestations occurring in prisoners of war, presumably a reaction to capture and imprisonment. Various types of reaction have been described, among them a syndrome of withdrawal, apathy, and sometimes death, which has been likened to the anaclitic depression reported by Spitz in hospitalized or otherwise deprived children.

**prisoner's dilemma**  A game used to assess reciprocity and mutual cooperation in two players, who are paid on the basis of whether each chooses to give or keep money. If A keeps the money and B gives it away, A makes the most and B loses the most. If both A and B give it away, both make a moderate amount of money. If both A and B keep the money, both lose a moderate amount. What should A do on the first round—be selfish and keep the money on the chance that B is by nature altruistic? In playing multiple rounds, various kinds of patterns in social behavior emerge. See *neuroeconomics; trolley dilemma; Ultimatum Game.*

**privacy**  The right of the subject to control both the amount of information he divulges about himself and the disposition of the information he has divulged. *Confidentiality* refers to how information, once collected, is treated so as to ensure that no harm will befall the subject as a result of having disclosed information about himself. See *privileged communication.*

**private psychosis**   Used by Ferenczi as a synonym of neurotic character because, as he says, it is tolerated by the ego.

**privileged communication**   Information that a patient discloses to his physician while the latter is attending him in a professional capacity; such information is termed privileged because in some states and according to ethical precepts of the medical profession the physician is not allowed to divulge such information without the patient's consent. This is, in other words, the patient's privilege of silence in regard to confidential matters on the part of his physician. See *confidentiality*.

**proactive aggression**   See *instrumental aggression*.

**proactive interference**   Inhibition, blunting, or attentuation of response to a second stimulus by presenting a first stimulus closely in advance of the second (e.g., 500 msec or less before the second stimulus is administered). See *prepulse inhibition*.

**probabilism**   See *environmentalism*.

**probable deviation**   See *median deviation*.

**proband**   In genetic studies of tainted families, the original cases constituting the starting point of a family study. These cases are called probands, or probati, because they must be proved representative of the type of trait carrier whose blood relations are to be investigated as to the recurrence of the trait under observation. Although the probands are not the main object of such a family study, their examination comes first and is of preeminent importance, since it must determine the hereditary trait so positively that a group of their blood relations must have likewise inherited that trait.

The practicable statistical method of probands in the study of selective population groups was devised by Weinberg and is called the proband method.

**probatus**   See *proband*.

**probe**   Investigation, search. DNA probes, techniques for analyzing human genetic material, are often used in chorionic villus sampling. Once a DNA disturbance is identified, the genetic abnormality is reproduced synthetically; when mixed with DNA extracted from fetal cells, the synthetic probe will seek out only those cells that contain similar genetic abnormalities and thus allow the abnormality to be identified in the fetus. See *chorion biopsy; genetic marker; PCR*.

**problem behavior**   See *behavior disorders*.

**problem child**   See *behavior disorders; developmental disorders*.

**problem drinking**   See *alcohol use, unhealthy*.

**problem parents**   Parents who, because of their own unresolved unconscious conflicts, manifest unhealthy attitudes toward their children, who, in turn, become problem children. Perfectionistic, overconscientious, overly critical, overindulgent, overambitious, overanxious, and rejecting attitudes of parents may play a major role in setting up sequences that later cause symptoms in their children.

**problem-oriented record (POR)**   *POMR* (for medical record); a method of organizing a patient's clinical chart devised by L. L. Weed (*New England Journal of Medicine 278*, 1968). The system consists of five parts:

1. *Data base*—a standardized collection of pertinent information derived from the patient's history, physical examination, laboratory and X-ray studies, social history, mental status examination and psychologic evaluation, and observation of the patient's behavior.

2. Problem list—a recording of the clinically significant and active problems that emerge from the data base, each with a different number to provide easy identification for later cross-referencing and a table of contents for the entire medical record.

3. Treatment plan—a comprehensive plan for each active problem.

4. Progress notes—numbered to correspond with the number of the problem to which they refer, and often written in the SOAP format (S = subjective, the patient's report or complaint; O = objective, observations without interpretation of what the patient manifests clinically; A = assessment, evaluation and interpretation of the problem and of the patient's progress and response to date; P = plan, a statement of what is to be done about the problem).

5. Discharge summary—indicating the treatment for each problem and the patient's response to the intervention.

**procedural legal standard**   *Procedural due process*; the procedures that must be followed in implementing a *substantive legal standard* (q.v.). If, for example, the substantive standard states that informed consent to be treated requires the patient to be competent, the procedural legal standard refers to the procedural mechanisms that will guarantee the patient's competence has been assessed before the treatment is given.

**procedural memory** *Automatic memory; habit memory; implicit memory; motor memory; reflexive memory;* the ability to learn motor and perceptual skills, including the learning of procedures and rules. Procedural memory is a representation of a series of actions or perception; it occurs unconsciously and is reflected in increased speed or accuracy with repetitions. It refers to the non-conscious acquisition of skills with practice, the memory for information or facts that does not require recall of the temporal context in which the knowledge was acquired. It includes abilities that are not accessible to conscious awareness, are acquired via repetition or exposure, and are expressed only though performance. Behavior is altered unconsciously by experience, without access to any memory content. Procedural memory includes (1) motor skills and habits; (2) *priming* (q.v.); (3) simple classical conditioning; and (4) nonassociative learning, which includes habituation and sensitization. It is sometimes called automatic or reflexive memory to emphasize that it accumulates by frequent repetition and does not require consciousness or complex cognitive processes, such as evaluation and comparison, before it can be reproduced. Procedural memory paradigms can be defined along a cognitive motor continuum; they may include tasks that are primarily motor, visuomotor, visuoperceptual, or cognitive in nature. Procedural memory is relatively inflexible in comparison to *declarative memory* (q.v.). It is a dedicated system that is largely inaccessible to other processor systems; access to it is gained by performance of the particular skills mediated by the system. Procedural memory requires repeated training trials to modify synaptic connections in the stimulus-processing circuits. Procedural knowledge is generally retained in amnesic patients.

Like declarative memory, procedural memory is dependent on frontal cortex activity; unlike declarative memory, it does not depend on structures in the *MTL* (q.v.). There are many ways for information to be stored in the brain; in most instances, parallel channels are used for storage in different areas. Procedural memory may be mediated by the neocortex rather than the hippocampus. Motor memories are thought to reside in the cerebellum.

Motor memory consolidation involves different regions of the brain at different times. During the hours following completion of practice, there is a shift from prefrontal regions of the brain to the premotor, posterior parietal, and cerebellar cortex. This shift may underlie the increased functional stability of the motor skill.

**proceptive phase** *Courtship phase;* in reference to sexual behavior and erotic relationships, the initial phase of indicating interest in and potential responsivity to a potential sexual partner. It is followed by the *acceptive phase (copulatory phase)* and then by the *conceptive phase* (which includes conception, pregnancy, and parenthood).

**process psychosis** The malignant type of schizophrenic psychosis that terminates in permanent dementia. It has always been recognized that schizophrenic phenomena have diverse manifestations: there are the passing schizophrenic episodes in persons who apparently are well both before and after these periods; then, there are the severe psychoses that sooner or later end in permanent dementia. All the schizophrenic manifestations, however, have the common features of queer and bizarre symptoms, absurd and unpredictable affects and intellectual ideas, and the obviously inadequate connection between these two.

The question arises whether there is any etiological basis for differentiating schizophrenic episodes and schizophrenic processes. Some authors have felt that schizophrenic episodes result from traumata and impediments in early infantile life, whereas the process psychosis is due to unknown organic factors. Fenichel feels, however, that there is no basis for such a differentiation and that both psychogenic influences and organic disposition are contributory causes in the majority of cases. Certainly the prognosis in the "process" type of cases (in which there has been slow chronic development of the disease) is very poor. The prognosis is better in the acute cases, because some of them recover quickly and entirely. This is especially true of the cases in which the episode is the reaction to an acute and severe frustration or narcissistic hurt (*The Psychoanalytic Theory of Neurosis*, 1945). See *malignant psychosis; schizophreniform disorder.*

"The European tendency is to use the term nuclear or process schizophrenia, or dementia praecox, to refer to unquestionable cases with a high tendency to deterioration and little tendency to remission or recovery. The others are called by Ruemke the pseudoschizophrenias, by Lunn (Denmark) the schizophreniform psychoses. The nuclear types may or may not show the accessory symptoms of Bleuler (delusions, hallucinations, etc.), but the fundamental symptoms are prominent. In the other types, the accessory symptoms are in the foreground and the fundamental symptoms may not be readily apparent. As Bleuler pointed out, the accessory symptoms are not diagnostic of schizophrenia for they occur also in many other disorders, especially in the organic group" (Campbell, R. J. *Psychiatric Quarterly 32*, 1958). See *reactive psychosis*.

**processomania**   Mania for litigation. See *paranoia querulans*.

**proctalgia fugax**   Fleeting rectal pain, more often than not of psychological origin and seen typically in anxious, tense perfectionists.

**procursive epilepsy**   *Dromolepsy*; a form of *epilepsy* (q.v.) characterized by sudden, impulsive running forward.

**procyclidine**   An anticholinergic drug. See *cholinergic*.

**prodigy**   See *bright child*.

**prodromal symptoms**   *Prodromata*; prepsychotic changes in thought, affect, cognition, and behavior that precede the initial episode or onset of a disorder; sometimes used, incorrectly, as synonymous with *early warning signs* (*EWS*), the symptoms that herald impending relapse in a patient already diagnosed as having schizophrenia or some other recurrent disorder.

**prodrome**   Precursor. An early or premonitory symptom of a disease or disorder.

**productive symptoms**   In schizophrenia, hallucinations, delusions and, in some descriptions, autism. See *deficit symptoms; negative symptoms; schizophrenia, models of*.

Factor analysis of schizophrenic signs and symptoms reveal two robust productive syndromes: a psychotic syndrome defined by hallucinations and delusions and a disorganization syndrome defined by positive thought disorder, bizarre behavior, and inappropriate affect.

**prodynorphin**   See *dynorphin*.

**proenkephalin**   See *enkephalins*.

**profession**   "A cluster of occupational roles... in which the incumbents perform certain functions valued in the society in general and by these activities typically earn a living at a full-time job" (Parsons, T. *Essays in Sociological Theory*, 1954). "Professions control entry into their occupational roles by certifying that candidates have developed the requisite body of skills and knowledge. Thus, they have some degree of independence and autonomy in performing the functions valued by the society" (Beauchamp, T. L. and Childress, J. F. *Principles of Biomedical Ethics*, 1979).

**professional code**   See *code, professional*.

**professional neurasthenia**   Nervous prostration manifested principally in the inability to use the organ(s) habitually employed in the course of one's profession or occupation. See *occupational neurosis*.

**progenitor**   See *stem cell; subventricular zone (SVZ)*.

**progeria**   *Hutchinson-Gilford progeria syndrome* (HGPS); a rare genetic laminopathy due to a single nucleotide error in the single sperm that, when combined with an ovum, produces the disease. The misspelling occurs on chromosome 1 in the gene *LMNA*, which encodes two proteins, lamin A and lamin B, constituents of the membrane of the cell nucleus. The mutant transcript of the gene results in a major loss of Lamin A expression associated with nuclear alterations.

Usually diagnosed within the first 2 years of life, progeria presents a combination of dwarfism and premature senility, with failure to grow, delayed dentition, hair loss and baldness, small face and jaw relative to head size, midface hypoplasia, micrognathia, sclerodermatous skin, absence of subcutaneous fat, alopecia, generalized osteodysplasia with osteolysis and pathologic fractures, and a tendency to vascular sclerosis. Intelligence is usually normal. Average life span is 13 years, with death due to heart failure or stroke. Incidence is approximately 1 case per 8 million births; fewer than 50 cases are known worldwide.

**prognosis**   Forecast or estimation of the course, outcome, and duration of an illness—the opinion being formed during the course of the illness. In schizophrenic psychoses, for example, the following have been found to be of value as predictors of outcome by one or more sets of investigators:

1. *Family history*—(a) presence of depression; (b) absence of schizophrenia.

2. *Premorbid characteristics*—(a) personality not schizoid or isolated, but stable and integrated; (b) adequacy of social relations functioning; (c) adequacy of psychosexual adjustment; (d) marital status (ever married, rather than never married, widowed, separated, or divorced); (e) intelligence not low; (f) good premorbid work record.

3. *Features of illness*—(a) acute onset (insidious onset and/or duration more than 6 months suggests a poor prognosis); (b) precipitating factors; (c) confusion or perplexity; (d) concern with death, guilt; (e) no emotional blunting; (f) previous hospitalization and duration of previous hospitalization (suggest a poor prognosis); (g) hebephrenic clinical picture (suggests a poor prognosis); (h) massive, defiant persecutory delusions (suggest a poor prognosis).

**programmed cell death**  *PCD*; see *apoptosis*.

**programmed practice**  See *exposure, self-directed*.

**programming, biological**  See *aging, theories of*.

**progredient neurosis**  A neurosis that takes a progressive course, with increasing severity of symptoms. For example, at first a phobic patient may not be able to walk across a particular square. Later on he cannot go out of doors, and finally, perhaps, not even out of his room.

**progressive degenerative subcortical encephalopathy**  See *diffuse sclerosis*.

**progressive education**  Founded by John Dewey, an approach that emphasizes the individual's needs and capacity for self-expression and self-direction.

**progressive matrices test**  An intelligence test in which the subject is asked to choose, from several alternatives, the one part that will complete the abstract design presented to him. The test is made up of 60 such designs.

**progressive multifocal leukoencephalopathy**  *PML*; a fatal demyelinating disease due to infection of oligodendrocytes by the human JC polyomavirus (JCV), which is estimated to be present in 70–80% of the adult population. In immunocompromised subjects—in particular, patients with AIDS—JVC can cause PML. It gains entry to the cells by latching on to 5-HT receptors. See *AIDS*.

**progressive psychosis**  *Process psychosis* (q.v.).

**progressive relaxation**  Developed by Jacobsen and often used as part of *desensitization* (q.v.); it is similar in many respects to Schultz's *autogenic training* (q.v.).

**progressive teleologic regression**  See *regression, progressive teleologic*.

**projection**  The process of imputing to another the ideas or impulses that belong to oneself. It is the act of giving objective or seeming reality to what is subjective. The expression implies that what is cast upon another is considered undesirable to the one who projects. The person who blames another for his own mistakes or seeks a scapegoat is using the projection mechanism. See *"blame" psychology*.

Whatever is painful or dangerous from within may be projected onto another person or upon some part of reality. When the conflicting issue has been externalized, the person may handle it as if it had always been an external situation. For example, the paranoid schizophrenic, beset with unconscious homosexual urges, projects the urges upon some man or men in the environment and then struggles against the urges as they seem to arise from outside sources.

According to Ferenczi, projection is one of the first defensive or protective measures employed by the child in defense of his narcissism. When the child realizes that he is not omnipotent, he begins to ascribe omnipotence to those about him and comes to realize that others control him. He does not, however, abandon the feeling of his own importance and of his magical powers. See *externalization; reality testing; reference, ideas of*.

**projection fibers**  See *commissure*.

**projection interneurons**  See *interneuron; nuclei, CNS*.

**projection transferences**  See *transference*.

**projective identification**  A psychological-interpersonal process consisting of several steps: (1) an unconscious phantasy of depositing (projecting) a part of oneself in another person; (2) an interpersonal pressure exerted on the other person to think, feel, and act in accordance with the unconscious projective phantasy; and (3) once the projection has been psychologically processed by the other person, the projector reinternalizes (by means of introjection or identification) the modified and processed version of what was originally projected. Such reinternalization provides, at least potentially, new ways of handling feelings or phantasies that the projector could only try to rid himself of in the past. Some authors feel that change in psychotherapy occurs only after there has been an accumulation of reinternalizations of material that has been projected in the analyst.

Although projective identification is a key element in *object relations theory* (q.v.), the term is used in different ways by different writers. Kernberg views it as a totally intrapsychic process and more primitive than projection. In both there is an evacuation and depositing of the intolerable into the object; but in projection the self is then distanced or separated from the object, while in projective identification a relationship with the now-changed object is maintained. The subject tries to control the object and thereby continue to defend against the intolerable. See *countertransference; identification; introjection; transference.*

The nature of projective identification depends greatly upon what it is that is projected. When self representations or drives are projected, there is often a blurring of ego boundaries, of the distinction between self and object. This is a primitive defense, described by Melanie Klein as characteristic of the *paranoid-schizoid position* (q.v.); it is suggestive of a psychotic or borderline process when it persists or appears later in life. Projection of object representations (or superego), on the other hand, is a displacement and involves no such blurring of ego boundaries. Projections of object representations are day-to-day occurrences in all people, and account for the majority of transference manifestations.

Object relations theorists consider primary *narcissism* (q.v.) to be the earliest form of relationship to an object (*primitive object relation*), present from birth or even before (see *bonding*). Narcissistic object relations are characterized by omnipotence and a preponderance of identification, used to deny separateness and the separate existence of the object. According to Klein, the death drive takes over when the infant is in the paranoid-schizoid position; its emotional representative is primary envy, the most painful feeling the baby has to face. Projective identifications based on (and defending against) envy and helplessness are used to attack and destroy the breast (or, later, the creativity of mother and father). The intention is not only to injure but also to control and possess the object. The mother comes to contain the bad parts of the self and is felt to be not a separate object but rather the infant's *bad self.*

Pathology develops when the negative projective identifications are excessive and continuous: the object becomes massively attacked, destroyed, or constantly controlled. Similarly with positive projective identifications; if they are excessive the ego is weakened and becomes too dependent on the external object that becomes its ideal ego.

Object relations theorists have emphasized the importance of projective identification in transference and countertransference. The analyst is pressured into becoming the object the patient wants the therapist to be. A seemingly inexplicable feeling of hatred for the patient, for instance, suggests that the patient is projecting the hatred originally felt for the rejecting mother into the analyst.

**projective method**  As distinguished from the direct question-and-answer method in psychiatric examination, the projective method seeks to gain information indirectly, through the use of certain test techniques specifically designed to provide opportunity for self-expression without direct verbal accounting.

"Thus, an essential characteristic of projective techniques is that they are unstructured in that cues for appropriate action are not clearly specified and the individual must give meaning to (interpret) such stimuli in accordance with his own inner needs, drives, defenses, impulses—in short, according to the dictates of his own personality. Whether the stimuli are inkblots (the Rorschach tests) or ambiguous pictures (the TAT), the patient's task is to impose or project his own structure and meaning onto materials which have relatively little meaning or structure and which, in a purely objective sense, are only inkblots or ambiguous pictures" (Carr, A. C. *International Psychiatry Clinics 1*, 1964).

**projective test**  A type of psychological test in which the test material presented to the subject is such that any response will necessarily be determined by his own prevailing mood or underlying psychopathology. See *projective method.*

**projicient apparatus**  In the terminology of E. J. Kempf (*Psychopathology*, 1921), the striped muscle system and the cerebrospinal nervous system proper, which provide the autonomic apparatus with the means to master the environment.

**prokaryocytic**  Describing a cell that does not contain a nucleus.

**prolactin** Lactogenic hormone. The plasma prolactin level is used as a measure of the degree of dopaminergic blockade by neuroleptic agents. Neuroleptics decrease dopaminergic activity, and such a decrease stimulates prolactin secretion, which thus reflects neuroleptic activity.

**prolonged sleep therapy** See *continuous sleep treatment.*

**promille** See *BAL.*

**promiscuity** Indiscriminate, casual, unrestrained, heterogeneous sexual activity with a large number of partners, a prominent feature of nyphomania (in the female) and satyriasis (in the male, in whom it is often referred to as the Don Juan complex). Labeling sexual behavior as promiscuous reflects cultural standards, ethical precepts, and religious biases rather than any medical or scientific system of nosology. Nonetheless, promiscuity has become a matter of legitimate medical and public health concern because the risk of exposure to sexually transmitted diseases, including AIDS, increases significantly as the number of sexual partners increases. Promiscuity is thus often considered as one manifestation of a hazardous life style. Promiscuity and occasional or frequent perverse sexuality are reported frequently in persons with narcissistic personality disorder. See *narcissistic personality.*

**promoter element** See *gene functions.*

**promoters** See *noncoding DNA.*

**promotion neurosis** Inability to function when given added responsibility or authority; seen most often in obsessional neurotics and described by others as *failure through success* (q.v.). See *polycratism.*

**proofreader's illusion** Failure to detect an error in spelling, punctuation, construction, etc., because of familiarity with the subject matter; a tendency to see things "as they ought to be" rather than as they are.

**pro-opiomelanocortin** POMC. See *enkephalins.*

**propaganda** Any organized effort to spread a belief, doctrine, value system, etc.; of particular interest to psychiatry because of the possibility of controlling behavior with nonphysical means (mind control) and the ethical questions attendant thereon. See *psychopolitics.*

*Hate propaganda* aims to incite people to seek revenge against an enemy who is responsible for a threat. People especially vulnerable to hate propaganda are those who have experienced war, a natural disaster, rapid social change, or some other threat. Their feeling of endangerment leads them to regress psychologically and likely to fall under the spell of a charismatic, narcissistic leader who promises to solve all their problems.

**propagating factors** In neurodegenerative disorders, elements or agents that contribute to the continuation, progression, or extension of the underlying disease, such as accumulation of intracellular aggregates, apoptosis, excitotoxicity, free radicals, immunogenicity, mitochondrial dysfunction, and oxidative stress. See *neuroprotection.*e.g.,

**propfschizophrenia** A frequent misspelling of *pfropfschizophrenia* (q.v.).

**prophylaxis** The branch of medical science that has to do with protection against the onset of a disease or disorder. For example, the treatment of a person showing marked schizoidism in an effort to prevent the development of schizophrenia is termed prophylaxis. See *mental hygiene.*

**propinquity** Proximity; in genetics, nearness of blood relationship.

**propositional memory** See *declarative memory; long-term memory.*

**propositional thinking** According to Piaget, the ability to manipulate abstractions even though they have never been tied to concrete events, a characteristic of the *formal operations* stage of intelligence. Propositional thinking is abstract thinking with greater intellectual mobility and less dependence on immediate contact than is seen in less mature, concrete thinking. See *hypothetical-deductive thinking.*

**propranolol** Inderal; a nonselective β-adrenergic receptor-blocker that reduces the signs and symptoms associated with catecholaminergic disturances. Although used primarily in the treatment of hypertension, it has been used as an adjuvant to relieve symptoms in many psychiatric disorders, including tremors, anxiety (e.g., stage fright), panic disorder, social phobia, migraine headaches, etc.

**proprioception** One of the *somatic sensory modalities*, it is the ability to sense the position (limb position sense) and movement (*kinesthesia*, q.v.) of the limbs. Proprioceptors respond to displacements of the muscles and joints; they are of three types: (1) mechanoreceptors, in joint capsules, (2) muscle spindle receptors, which traduce muscle stretch, and

(3) cutaneus mechanoreceptors. Proprioception is essential for maintaining balance, controlling limb movements, and for evaluating the shape of a grasped object. Without proprioception, one can maintain the limbs in a steady position only if one sees them.

The other somatic sensory modalities are *touch, pain*, and *temperature*. See *sensation*.

**proprium**   See *Allport, Gordon Willard*.

**propulsion gait**   *Festination gait, marche à petits pas*; characteristic of *Parkinson disease* (q.v.). The patient leans forward and takes short, shuffling steps that begin slowly but accelerate as he continues to walk; he looks as though he must run to keep up with his head.

**prosencephalon**   *Forebrain* (q.v.).

**prosody**   The tone (intonation), accent, melody or patterns of stress (loudness and softness) of a subject's speech; also, study of the metrical structure of a poem. In psychiatry, prosody refers to the emotional tone or affective components of speech, which are served by the nondominant cerebral hemisphere. See *aprosodia*.

**prosopagnosia**   Classically, a type of visual defect in which the patient cannot identify a familiar face, even though the patient knows that a face is a face and can point out the features. It is usually due to damage to areas of the fusiform gyrus that contain face responsive neurons (the fusiform face area, or FFA). See *Capgras syndrome; nonrecognition; parietal lobe*.

The term has also been applied to the inability to summon up an inner image of the mother's (or therapist's) face, characteristic of children before *object constancy* (q.v.) and object permanency have been established and of persons with narcissistic personality disorder.

**prosopalgia**   See *tic douloureux*.

**prosoplegia, prosopoplegia**   Bell palsy or peripheral facial paralysis. See *facial nerve*.

**prospective**   See *EPSDT*.

**prospective memory**   A dissociable form of episodic memory involving the ability to execute a future intention, or "remembering to remember". It is essential for forming, monitoring, and executing plans of behavior in the context of ongoing distractions. Everyday examples include remembering to take a medication at specific times or remembering to attend a scheduled medical appointment. It may appear as a symptom of *HIV-associated neurocognitive disorders* (q.v.).

**prostigmin**   An anticholinesterase drug. See *cholinergic*.

**protanopia**   A form of color-blindness, usually referred to as red-blindness, in which red and blue-green are confused.

**protease**   General term for an enzyme that catalyzes the hydrolysis of peptide linkages; proteolytic enzyme; peptidase; peptase. If only the splitting of interior peptide bonds in a protein is involved, the term endopeptidase may be used. See *peptidases; secretases; ubiquitin*.

**proteasome**   A protein complex responsible for degrading intracellular proteins that have been tagged for destruction by the addition of ubiquitin. See *apoptosis; UPS*.

**protection, medical removal**   Insurance that a worker who has been removed from his or her regular employment on the basis of an examining physician's decision that such employment is hazardous to the employee's health will receive compensation. The specific amount and type of compensation vary but ordinarily are determined on the basis of maintained earnings, seniority, or other benefits.

**protection factor**   See *risk factor*.

**protective factors**   See *adversity*.

**protein**   A chemical catalyst that triggers hundreds or thousands of split-second chemical reactions within a cell. Proteins are the largest molecules known; they are constructed in accordance with directions given by the codon of the gene. (See *DNA; gene*.) They consist largely of amino acids linked by peptide bonds.

Protein synthesis (*translation*) occurs in the ribosomes of the cytoplasm. Within the ribosome, the four-base RNA code is converted into a new language of 20 amino acids. The order or sequence of the original four-base code determines which amino acids will be aligned, and in what sequence, to form the specified protein.

Each protein is like a string of pearls, with each pearl a simple amino acid. A protein may contain from a hundred to several hundred amino acids. Since there are 20 different amino acids, the number of combinations that can be assembled in any one "necklace" is almost limitless.

**protein conformational disorders**   Various neurological and system diseases that involve accumulation of intracellular or extracellular protein aggregates in the brain. Included in this group are the most common *neurodegenerative diseases* (q.v.) as well as some rare inherited disorders that involve deposition of protein aggregates in the brain. See *protein folding*.

**protein folding**  The process by which a protein acquires its native tridimensional structure. Normally, each protein has a unique stable folded structure, but in *protein conformational disorders* (q.v.) the polypeptide chain adopts an alternative structure, associated with the pathogenesis of the disease.

Cells have evolved three mechanisms for the degradation of folded proteins: molecular chaperones, the ubiquitin-proteasome pathway, and lysosome-mediated autophagy. Under certain pathological conditions, the capacity of this protein quality control machinery is exceeded and misfolded proteins accumulate to dangerous levels. There is increasing evidence that fibrillar aggregates are inert—or perhaps even protective—rather than being pathogenic.

**protein metabolism disorders**  See *glutaric aciduria* (for one example).

**proteinase**  *Endopeptidase*; an enzyme that catalyzes the hydrolysis of a peptide chain. In addition to digesting proteins, proteinases generate peptide neurotransmitters from precursors, and, through G protein–coupled proteinase-activated receptors (*PARs*), they generate neural signals. Four PARs have been identified in humans—PAR1–4. They are expressed in both the central and the peripheral nervous system, and in many other tissues, including platelets, heart, pancreas, gastrointestinal tract, and kidney. PAR activation is associated with neurogenic inflammation, hyperalgesia, and pruritis sensation; the proteinase/PAR system has been implicated in both neuronal survival and apoptosis in CNS.

**protein/gene approach**  See *linkage analysis*.

**protein only hypothesis**  See *prion hypothesis*.

**proteome**  The pattern of expression of the proteins produced by the cell; proteome research is directed to deducing gene function by studying the ebb and flow of the proteins produced by the different genes.

**proteomics**  The study of complex mixtures of expressed proteins, examining a cell's many different proteins en masse, instead of one by one. DNA is made up of alternating series of four chemical units. Proteins, in contrast, consist of sequences of 20 different amino acids. Proteins act in concert, with a cell pathway involving a web of proteins, linked together in a highly precise chain of command. A protein can serve a structural purpose, such as producing a collagen fiber or catalyzing some chemical reaction important to the cell's metabolism. Identifying what all the proteins do is a far more difficult task than mapping the *genome* (q.v.). There are perhaps 10 times as many proteins as genes, since a gene may code for more than one protein, and proteins interact with one another to produce new ones. The potential number of protein interactions can run up to 10 billion; probably a million are relevant to disease.

Proteomics seeks to map the networks of interacting proteins that are basis of various cellular biological functions (e.g., responses to physiologic stresses and maintenance of the different functions that are tissue-specific). Another possible end-result is to enable researchers to create mathematical models of biological circuits that could be used to predict various types of cell behavior.

**protest psychosis**  A short-lived reactive schizophrenic-like psychosis described among black prisoners charged with aggressive crimes. Onset is abrupt, following arraignment or indictment. Symptoms include mutism, destructiveness, incoherence, bizarre utterances and mannerisms, and auditory or visual hallucinations. W. Bromberg, F. Simon, and T. A. Pasto labeled the reaction protest psychosis because it contained elements of African and Muslim ideology and anti-Caucasian hostility related to white domination of nonwhites (*Israel Annals of Psychiatry and Related Disciplines* 10, 1972). See *buffoonery psychosis; prison psychosis; Ganser syndrome*.

**proto-**  Combining form meaning first, original, primitive, from Gr. *prōtos*.

**protocol**  The individual case record; the raw material of a study or experiment before it has been incorporated into the conclusions or overall results of the study. In clinical psychiatry, the protocol commonly refers to the complete case history and workup, in contrast to the case summary or final conclusions about the individual case.

**protocortex theory**  See *protomap theory*.

**protomap theory**  The postulate that the cortical progenitor zone contains the information that generates cortical areas. The *protocortex theory*, in contrast, postulated that thalamic afferent axons, through activity-dependent mechanisms, impose cortical areal identity on an otherwise homogeneous cortex. It is now recognized that parcellation of the cerebral cortex into discrete processing areas involves numerous interwoven events that include both intrinsic and extrinsic mechanisms. Signals in the diencephalon and subcortical telencephalon, for example, regulate where axons from a thalamic nucleus enter the developing cortex, indicating that the topography of thalamocortical axons is regulated in part by interactions with their environment during development.

**protomasochism**   The primary, ancestral tendency of the death instinct to lead all human beings into annihilation; a drive into nothingness. Reik uses the term to describe "a pleasure of destruction directed against the ego, a kind of sadism which has chosen the ego for its victim." In Freud's opinion, the death instinct that is not neutralized by the erotic urges or channeled into the outer world remains effective within the organism, directing its forces against the ego proper, as it did in primitive man (Reik, T. *Masochism in Modern Man*, 1941).

**protopathic**   Of primary sensitiveness, i.e., pertaining to sensory nerves in the skin with a primary, grosser, or more limited sensibility to stimuli. The ability to appreciate deep pain sensation and marked variations in temperature such as hot and cold; distinguished from *epicritic* sensibility.

**protopathic insanity**   J. C. Bucknill and D. H. Tuke speak of protopathic insanity as "Insanity or Mental Deficiency caused by Primary Disease or Defective Development of the Encephalic Centres," which included *congenital* or *infantile deficiency, traumatic insanity, general paresis, paralytic insanity, epileptic insanity*, and *senile insanity* as protopathic forms (*Manual of Psychological Medicine*, 1874).

**protophallic**   Jones says that there are two stages to what Freud calls the phallic phase: "The first of the two—let us call it the *proto-phallic* phase—would be marked by innocence or ignorance—at least in consciousness—where there is no conflict over the matter in question, it being confidently assumed by the child that the rest of the world is built like itself

and has a satisfactory male organ—penis or clitoris, as the case may be. In the second, or *deutero-phallic* phase, there is a dawning suspicion that the world is divided into two classes; not male and female in the proper sense, but penis-possessing and castrated (though actually the two classifications overlap pretty closely)" (*Papers on Psycho-Analysis*, 1938).

**prototaxic**   Of, or relating to, the earliest period in time or development; Sullivan applied the term to early infancy, when the child has no awareness of himself as distinct from others and no concept of time or space.

**prototheory**   Partial, incomplete, or untested theory; an initial "working" hypothesis; sometimes used to refer to an ad hoc rationalization that appears to justify a clinical practice or maneuver.

**prototype matching**   A dimensional classification system based on prototypes or exemplars. The prototype is a statistically generated composite description of patients identified empirically whose profiles are similar to one another. Each disorder is described in ideal or "pure" form, not as a list of symptoms but in narrative form in a paragraph. The clinician rates the overall similarity or "match" between a patient and the prototype on a 5-point rating scale, considering the prototype as a whole rather than counting individual symptoms. A rating of 5, for example, indicates a very good match; the patient exemplifies the disorder; 4 indicates a good match, and the diagnosis applies to the patient; 3 indicates that the patient has significant features of the disorder; 2 is a slight match with the patient manifesting minor features of the disorder; and 1 indicates little or no match, and the disease description does not apply to the patient. See *categorical system*; *dimensional system*; *nosology* (Westen, D. et al. *American Journal of Psychiatry 163*: 846–856, 2006).

**proverbs test**   The subject must interpret 12 proverbs; most commonly, this is a written test.

**provocativeness, sexual**   See *dysfunctional attitudes*.

**proxemics**   The study and analysis of space, and particularly the study of interpersonal behavior in relation to density of population, placement of people within an area, opportunity for privacy. It is interesting to note in this connection that while the life span of animals in captivity is markedly reduced if they have no space for withdrawal into privacy, the conscious intent of the architecture of most mental hospitals is to reduce or abolish opportunities for their human residents' privacy. See *communication*.

**proximate cause**  See *negligence*.

**proxy factitious disorder**  See *factitious disorder*.

**PRP**  Program for relapse prevention.

**PRRs**  Pattern recognition receptors. See *microglia*.

**prudery**  Exaggerated concern about minor points of the moral or ethical code. This is almost always a reaction formation, the prude decrying in others the very impulses and behavior he must deny in himself.

**pruning**  *Apoptosis* (q.v.); *naturally occurring neuronal death*; programmed late elimination of synaptic contacts that are not used. There is an overproduction of neurons and synapses during brain development, and in later developmental periods these redundant neuronal connections are systematically eliminated. Projections to inappropriate targets are thereby removed, the specificity of axonal projections is refined, and the efficiency of communication between the billion of neurons remaining is increased. It has been estimated that the neuronal pruning occurring at the onset of puberty may involve as many as 40% of the total neurons. See *neural Darwinism*.

It has been hypothesized that excessive pruning could produce a dopamine-glutamate imbalance, which some workers believe is important in the pathophysiology of schizophrenia. It has also been noted that excessive pruning is likely to render the outputs to input information bizarre.

**PSA**  Proportion of survivors affected, the same as lifetime *prevalence* (q.v.) of disorder (the proportion of persons in a representative sample of the population who have ever experienced the disorder in question).

**psammoma-body**  A collection of fibroglia, collagen fibers, and small calcified concretions seen often in meningiomas.

**PSD**  Postsynaptic density; see *NMDAR*.

**PSD-95**  See *nitric oxide*.

**PSE**  See *Present State Examination*.

**psellism**  Stammering; indistinct or faulty pronunciation.

**pseudesthesia**  Sensation or perception without a corresponding stimulus; an imaginary or illusory sensation, such as phantom limb.

**pseudo-**  Combining form meaning false, from Gr. *pseudos*, falsehood, lie.

**"pseudo as-if"**  Katan's term for a type of reaction, seen often within the framework of a hysterical disturbance, that simulates the *"as-if"* personality (q.v.) but differs from the latter in that the disturbance arises not from early loss of the mother but rather as a result of the mother keeping the child too dependent orally. In consequence, the ego is weakened and in response to stress it falls back on dependence on the mother or her substitutes. "Pseudo as-if" reactions are seen also in adolescents and in prepsychotic patients as temporary attempts at mastering conflicts during a process of disintegration.

**pseudoaggression**  In psychoanalysis a false aggressiveness developed in neurotics as a result of denial of their basic psychic masochism; the basic desire is to be mistreated. This desire gains only reproach from the superego, and a defense of pseudoaggression is constructed. "No, I do not want to be mistreated by this person. The situation is just the opposite—I want to kill this person or mistreat him." This pseudoaggression also receives reproach from the superego and is itself denied, but the neurotic is more willing to accept the guilt for his pseudoaggression than that for his underlying masochism. Bergler believes that neurotics have no true ego aggression, for almost all of their aggression is in the superego. He explains *stage fright* (q.v.) in actors in this way. Superficially, the symptom refers to a fear of one's aggressive exhibitionism. In reality, however, this aggressiveness is a false front with which the patient deludes himself and others to deny the basic fear, that his masochism will be uncovered. Under successful psychoanalytic treatment, a more equitable distribution of aggression between superego and ego can be achieved and the patient can become truly aggressive as the need for aggression arises in reality situations (*Psychoanalytic Quarterly Supplement 23*, 1949).

**pseudoamnesia**  1. False or feigned amnesia, as in Ganser syndrome. 2. Amnesia that is part of a dissociative disorder. 3. *Obs.* A transitory amnesia associated with organic brain disease.

**pseudo-athetosis**  Inability to maintain the limb in a steady position unless the limb can be seen, suggestive of impairment of proprioceptive feedback: if the subject tries to hold the arm outstretched with the eyes closed, the arm begins to drift after a few seconds.

**pseudoautosomal region**  Located on the short arms of the X and Y chromosomes, this region has been suggested as a possible locus for a "psychosis gene" because it could result in apparent sex linkage in some affected offspring and apparent autosomal transmission in others.

**pseudoblepsis**  *Obs.* Visual hallucinations or illusions.

**pseudobulbar affect (PBA)**  Sometimes used as a synonym for involuntary emotional expression disorder, *IEED* (q.v.).

**pseudobulbar palsy**  See *amyotrophic lateral sclerosis.*

**pseudocatatonia, traumatic**  Catatonic state following an injury. See *traumatic psychosis.*

**pseudocholinesterase**  An enzyme; of importance in psychiatry because it is the enzyme that normally breaks down suxamethonium, a muscle relaxant that is frequently used as part of electroconvulsive therapy. About 1 white American in 2500 has a genetically determined abnormality or deficiency of pseudocholinesterase, and such a person is liable to severe and prolonged apnea when administered suxamethonium. The defect is much rarer in blacks and virtually nonexistent in Asians. See *pharmacogenetics.*

**pseudocoma**  *Locked-in syndrome*; paralysis of the limbs (tetraplegia) and anarthria and aphonia because of paralysis of all the cranial nerve musculature except for the eye musculature. Consciousness is preserved, but at most the patient can communicate only by blinking or other voluntary eye movements. The cause is bilateral destruction of the medulla oblongata or base of the pons, as in central pontine myelinolysis. See *vegetative state.*

**pseudocommunity**  Norman Cameron's term for the progressive desocialization seen in the schizophrenias in which social language habits are replaced with personal, highly individual habits. The pseudocommunity is a behavioral organization that the patient constructs from his distorted observations, inferences, and phantasies; most commonly, the patient sees himself as the victim of some concerted action.

**pseudoconditioning**  *Sensitization* (q.v.).

**pseudoconvulsion**  An attack that simulates a convulsion, with falling and muscular contractions, but with no loss of consciousness,

no pupillary changes, amnesia, or postconvulsive confusion (*cataphrenia*); usually hysterical in origin.

**pseudocyesis**  False pregnancy, one of the *somatoform disorders* (q.v.), characterized by the belief that one is pregnant and physical signs such as amenorrhea, abdominal enlargement, breast engorgement, and even labor pains.

**pseudodebility**  *Pseudoimbecility* (q.v.).

**pseudodementia**  Dementia syndrome of depression; *cataphrenia*; depression-related cognitive dysfunction in a geriatric patient; a clinical depression whose retardation, inattentiveness, and apathy are mistaken as the beginnings of dementia because they occur in an older person whose depression is overlooked. Mental test scores may also be lowered. It was long assumed that *late life depression* (q.v.) would be like depressions earlier in life, and that cognitive status would improve once the depression had been treated. More recent long-term studies suggest instead that depressive pseudodementia in the elderly is a precursor and predictor of cognitive disorder.

One form of pseudodementia is the *nursing home syndrome*, characterized by a loss of social context, withdrawal from responsibility for almost every aspect of one's life, infantilization by caretakers and visiting family, and being treated as a non-person; it is often compounded by oversedation.

**pseudodementia, hysterical**  Wernicke's term for a syndrome of hysteria in which the patient appears unable to answer the simplest questions or to give any information about himself. The patient gives the appearance of being retarded.

As a rule the patient exhibiting this syndrome regresses to the behavior of early childhood, showing the condition known as hysterical puerilism. See *feeblemindedness, affective; Ganser syndrome.*

**pseudodepressive syndrome**  See *convexity syndrome.*

**pseudoflexibilitas**  A condition in which a person whose movements are more or less normal maintains for a relatively long period a posture imposed upon him.

**pseudogeusia**  False perception of taste.

**pseudogiftedness**  Apparent unusual talents in a child, resulting not from specific or permanent trends but rather from the ability of the bright child to imitate, adopt, and assimilate the behavior patterns of others. Pseudogiftedness is usually inspired by momentary influence from without rather than by any inborn ability or urge from within.

**pseudographia** Neologistic writing, such as an idiosyncratic alphabet that abolishes communication rather than enhancing it; observed most frequently in catatonic and paranoid forms of schizophrenia.

**pseudohallucination** The term was first used in 1885 by Kandinsky and was elaborated by Karl Jaspers in his book *Allgemeine Psycho-pathologie* (1913) to refer to lacking "concrete reality," "substantiality," or "corporeality." It appears in subjective space accompanied by insight into the lack of an objective counterpart. It is by no means confined to the mentally ill. G. Sedman (*British Journal of Psychiatry 112*, 1966) defined pseudohallucinations as hallucinations perceived through the senses but recognized by the patient as not being a veridical perception. It is reported often by the recently bereaved, who may hear the voice of the deceased or have a "sense of presence," which is, however, quickly realized as erroneous.

Two types of pseudohallucination have been recognized: *imaged pseudohallucination*, a particularly vivid mental picture, experienced as occurring within the mind but distinguished from the usual image by the subject's inability to change the image at will; and *perceived pseudohallucination*, an image experienced as located in external space but recognized by the subject as unreal.

**pseudohomosexual** Used in adaptational psychodynamic formulations to refer to the nonsexual motivations in homosexual behavior: specifically, dependency motivations and power motivations. "It should be emphasized that even in the overt homosexual, when the ultimate goal is orgastic pleasure, the sexual component does not operate in isolation, but always in association with the dependency and power components" (Ovesey, L. et al. *Archives of General Psychiatry 9*, 1963).

**pseudohydrophobia** *Cynophobia* (q.v.).

**pseudohypnosis** See *captivation*.

**pseudoidentification** A method of dealing with people in the environment by apparently identifying oneself with, or assimilating oneself to, the person with whom one chances to be in contact at any given moment. Pseudoidentification is illustrated by the case of the man who asserted that he had found the

ideal way of adapting himself to reality: he assimilated himself to the person with whom he chanced to be talking and so had no external conflicts. But in reality, such a method of adaptation led to many conflicts; the man found that he had assimilated himself to A at one time, to B at another, and that A and B were in disagreement. Since pseudoidentification is not insincerity, but rather the conviction that the subject has in fact become one with the other person, such conflicting identifications lead to many reality problems. Pseudoidentification appears somewhat akin to paranoid projection in that the patient's ideas are prevented from entering consciousness and are ascribed to the object, with whom the patient then identifies himself. Unlike the ideas of paranoia, however, those of pseudoidentification are apparently innocent. The dynamics of the process are poorly understood.

**pseudoimbecility** Pathological limitation and restriction of intellectual functions of the ego. This intellectual restriction or inhibition may mean (1) that intellectual functions have been erotized and so are given up to escape conflicts; (2) that the restriction disguises aggression in order to escape retaliation; (3) that it is a display of castration to escape the fear of literal castration and the loss of a love object; or (4) that it represents an attempt to restore or maintain a secret libidinous rapport within the family. A mask of stupidity enables the child or infantile adult to participate in the sexual life of the parents and other adults to an amazingly unlimited extent, which, if overtly expressed, would be strictly and definitely forbidden. Such utilization of stupidity is widespread, because it affords an opportunity for the mutual sexual desires of parent and child to be gratified on a preverbal affective level without becoming conscious through word pictures. Both child and parents can maintain a distorted but gratifying affective communion that would otherwise be limited to mother and infant.

**pseudoinsomnia** *Sleep misperception syndrome*; complaints of inability to maintain normal sleep or to obtain restorative sleep even though physiological sleep is normal. It has been estimated that over 10% of self-defined insomniacs have normal physiological sleep.

**pseudolalia** Suggested by Stoddart to denote meaningless sounds produced by patients.

**pseudologia fantastica**  *Pseudoreminiscences*; an extreme form of pathological lying consisting of telling stories without discernible or adequate motive and with such zeal that the subject may become convinced of their truth. It has been reported in organic mental disorders and in character disorders (e.g., psychopathy), and it is often described as one of the three cardinal symptoms of the Munchhausen syndrome (the others being peregrination and disease simulation).

**pseudologue**  Pathological liar. Kraepelin used the term as a subgroup of psychopathic personality.

**pseudomania**  A symptom in which the patient accuses himself of having committed crimes of which he is really innocent; *shame psychosis*.

**pseudomnesia**  *Obs.* The patient's belief in having a clear recollection of events that had never taken place or things that had never existed. See *déjà fait; false memory*.

**pseudomotivations**  Bleuler's term for after-the-fact justifications of behavior that are common in schizophrenia. One hebephrenic patient stated that he got into debt only to show that he could obtain money without his wife's assistance. Another patient flew into a rage and stated that he did so because his doctor was wearing a gray suit. Although the patient himself believes in his ex post facto pseudomotivations, he may subsequently become aware that he has made up the motivations. Ordinarily, however, the patient is unaware of, and indifferent to, even the grossest contradictions.

**pseudomutuality**  Wynne's term for a facade of family unity, gained at the expense of individual autonomy, that is characteristic of families with schizophrenic members.

**pseudonecrophilia**  Masturbation with phantasies of corpses as the sexual object.

**pseudoneurotic schizophrenia**  P. H. Hoch and P. Polatin (*Psychiatric Quarterly 23*, 1949) applied this term to those patients whose defense mechanisms are, at least superficially, neurotic in type, but who, on close investigation, show basic schizophrenic mechanisms. The most important diagnostic features are pan-anxiety and pan-neurosis. Multiple neurotic symptoms tend to be present at the same time—anxiety, conversion symptoms, gross hysterical or vegetative manifestations, phobias, and obsessive-compulsive mechanisms.

The life approach of such patients is always autistic and dereistic, although this may be very subtly expressed. Commonly there is depression or an anhedonic state wherein the patient derives pleasure from nothing. Psychosexually, such patients show a chaotic organization and a mixture of all levels of libidinal development; sadistic or sadomasochistic behavior is frequent.

Many pseudoneurotic patients develop psychotic episodes of short duration with complete reintegration—*micropsychotic episodes*, characterized by the simultaneous development of three significant features: hypochondriacal ideas, ideas of reference, and feelings of depersonalization. The patients zigzag, repeatedly trespassing beyond the reality line.

Currently, most cases of pseudoneurotic schizophrenia would be classified as *borderline personality disorder* (q.v.).

**pseudonomania**  Morbid impulse to falsify, to lie.

**pseudoparameter**  See *parameter*.

**pseudoparanoia**  An uncommon term for unsystematized paranoid trends that are not strictly associated with schizophrenia. For example, paranoid delusions may occasionally be observed in deaf people, sometimes in the retarded; the delusions are generally scattered and transitory or at least they do not constitute the preponderant part of the disorder.

**pseudopersonality**  A constellation of habits and reaction patterns consciously recognized as false by the subject. The development of a pseudopersonality is characteristic of many prostitutes, who strive to maintain an incognito quality in their sexual contacts and fortify this with fictitious tales about themselves and their families. Their pseudopersonality usually includes a false toughness, meanness, and indifference. It is obvious that, with time, the recognition of the falseness of the pseudopersonality may gradually dwindle so that it finally becomes a true *character defense* (q.v.), and in therapy must be handled as such. See *persona*.

**pseudopsychopathic schizophrenia**  See *schizophrenia*.

**pseudopsychopathic type**  See *orbitomedial syndrome*.

**pseudoquerulant**  A form of paranoid personality disorder. Pseudoquerulants regard trifling differences as grave injustices. A combination of irritability and arrogance leads them not only into quarrels, but into actual lawsuits. They are to be distinguished from the litigious paranoid type by the fact that in the pseudo-querulants the tendency exists from youth.

**pseudoreminiscence** *Pseudologia fantastica; confabulation* (q.v.).

**pseudoschizophrenia** See *depersonalization; process psychosis; reactive psychosis.*

**pseudosclerosis, spastic** See *Creutzfeldt-Jakob disease.*

**pseudosclerosis of Westphal-Strümpell** (Adolf von Strümpell, German physician, 1853–1925, and Alexander Karl Otto Westphal, German neurologist, 1863–1941) See *hepatolenticular degeneration.*

**pseudoseizures** Conversion seizures; psychogenic seizures. See *conversion disorder.*

**pseudosenility** *Pseudodementia* (q.v.); acute, reversible mental disorders in the elderly, which typically appear as confusional states or as depression. Among the more common causes of pseudosenility are drug effects (especially due to errors in self-medication), malnutrition, diminished cardiac output and other cardiovascular disorders, febrile conditions, alcoholism, trauma secondary to an unreported fall, intracranial tumor, endocrine disorders and other metabolic disturbances (e.g., hypernatremia, azotemia).

**pseudosexuality** See *compulsive masturbation.*

**pseudosmia** False sense of smell.

**pseudotransference** A result of inexact interpretations in psychoanalytic treatment in which the patient, responding to the suggestions of the analyst, builds up a relationship that is expressive of the analyst's hunches rather than related to problems of the patient that are of dynamic significance.

**pseudotumor cerebri** *Benign intracranial hypertension,* with headache, papilledema, and increased intracranial pressure in the absence of an intracranial mass. Spontaneous recovery generally occurs. It is associated with several conditions, although the mechanism producing the increase in pressure is unknown. Among the most common associated, and probably contributing, conditions are venous thromboses of the sagittal, straight, or lateral sinuses; disorders of the adrenal, ovarian, parathyroid, or thyroid glands; hypervitaminosis A in children and adolescents; antibiotic administration (particularly tetracycline or penicillin) to infants; high CSF protein, as in patients with polyneuritis or tumors of the cauda equina; intoxicants such as insecticides (termed toxic pseudotumor cerebri); and sometimes as a side effect of drug treatment (e.g., lithium). Also known as *serous meningitis; arachnoiditis; toxic hydrocephalus.*

**PSG** Polysomnography. See *polysomnogram.*

**psi** In parapsychology, whatever it is that endows a person with *extrasensory perception* (q.v.).

**psilocin** See *psilocybin.*

**psilocybin** A naturally occurring *hallucinogen* (q.v.) found in mushrooms of the genera Psilocybe, Panacelous, and Conocybe, which are widely distributed throughout the world. Psilocin is present in small amounts in the same mushrooms; it is 1.4 times the strength of psilocybin. Following ingestion, psilocybin is converted to *psilocin* by alkaline phosphatase.

**psittacism** A type of neologism that is totally devoid of any content. See *glossolalia.*

**PSM** 1. Professional sexual misconduct. See *boundary.* 2. *Polysomnogram* (q.v.).

**PSN** Predominantly sensory neuropathy. See *HIV neuropathy.*

**psopholalia** Lallation; babbling, infantile, slovenly, incomprehensible speech.

**PSRO** *Professional standards review organization;* established by U.S. federal law (PL 92–603, Social Security Amendments of 1972) as a mechanism to ensure that the hospital care rendered under Medicare and Medicaid is medically necessary and of good quality. Initial review of care rendered is often performed by allied health professionals using standards set by the medical profession or medical specialty societies; final review, however, is performed by physicians (peer review). See *review.*

**PSP** Progressive *supranuclear palsy* (q.v.).

**PST** Prefrontal sonic treatment. See *ultrasonic irradiation.*

**psychagogy** Educational and reeducational psychotherapeutic procedures, with special emphasis upon the relationship of the patient to his environment. The principles behind psychagogy are in accord with those behind objective psychobiology; both stress socialization.

**psychalgia, psychalgalia** Discomfort or pain, usually in the head, which accompanies mental activity (obsessions, hallucinations, etc.), and is recognized by the patient as being emotional in origin. Depressed patients complain of peculiar head pains due to their horrible ideas. The schizophrenic patient complains, often with laughter, of the unbearable pains in his head, induced by electric currents that come from a distant machine operated by a persecutor.

Psychalgia is also used to refer to any psychogenic pain disorder. See *somatoform disorders*.

**psychasthenia**   *Obs. Janet disease*; a syndrome that included several anxiety states and, in particular, phobias. Pierre Janet recognized two subgroups of psychoneuroses, hysteria and psychasthenia. In general he included under psychasthenia all psychoneurotic syndromes not classified under *hysteria* (q.v.).

**psychataxia**   Mental confusion, inability to fix the attention or to make any continued mental effort.

**psychauditory**   Relating to the mental perception and interpretation of sounds.

**psyche**   The mind. In modern psychiatry the psyche is regarded in its own way as an "organ" of the person. The psyche, like other organs, possesses its own form and function, its embryology, gross and microscopic anatomy, physiology, and pathology.

**psychedelic**   Mind-manifesting;   sometimes used to describe certain pharmacologic agents (and particularly hallucinogens) that have an effect on mental processes. See *hallucinogen; psychotropics*.

**Psychiatric Epidemiology Research Interview**   *PERI*; symptom scales that measure violent behavior and arrests, including a 13-item measure of psychotic symptoms.

**psychiatric social treatment**   The supervision of the patient in the community in such a way as to bring about a better social adjustment for him. In some cases all that is possible may be the modification of the environment so that a fairly satisfactory social adaptation may be made for him in spite of his mental handicap. Wherever the outlook for improvement is at all favorable, however, the aim of both the social and psychiatric treatment is to bring about a change in the attitude of the patient himself, to replace undesirable mental habits by wholesome ones, to modify his conduct by a training of his emotions, and to give him insight into his difficulties, so that he may eventually overcome his disabilities and be able to make a satisfactory adjustment in any environment.

**psychiatric social work**   A subdivision of *social work* (q.v.) that is concerned with mental illness, its prevention, treatment, rehabilitation, and avoidance of relapse. Particular attention is given to the familial, environmental, cultural and other social factors that may be involved in the development, continuation, or recurrence of mental illness and in the patient's response to treatment.

Particularly in a hospital setting, the psychiatric social worker often functions as a member of a multidisciplinary treatment team that includes a psychiatrist, psychiatric nurse, clinical psychologist, and other allied professionals and paraprofessionals. Typical professional activities include intake interview and admission assessment; gathering social data and developmental history from the family; assessing the patient's strengths, weaknesses, and social needs; maintaining liaison between family members and the patient, and educating the family about the patient's illness and response to treatment; planning for aftercare and rehabilitation; identifying the continuum of clinical and social services that might be beneficial and preparing the patient for linkage with them; educating the family or others about ways of meeting the patient's special needs; and arranging placement in group home, halfway house, or other domicile.

In a particular case, the social worker's emphasis might be on the person in need (casework): improving the adaptive capacities of the patient (or client), encouraging the development of the social skills that best meet the demands imposed by difficult environments (e.g., the family, workplace, school, ethnic or lifestyle subculture, social order or political climate, etc.), effecting linkages with needed services and programs (e.g., medical, psychological, pastoral, correctional, financial, educational, protection, legal, etc.), and identifying behavior patterns in the patient that may interfere with the satisfaction of his needs. In other instances (groupwork), the focus might be on the family, the marital partnership, a group of veterans, prison inmates, or residents in a shelter or school. At other times, the worker's primary activity might be directed to community organization, social change, and social planning: developing social programs, coordinating existing organizations and agencies, and influencing social policy and legislation (particularly in the areas of defining what needs exist, allocating resources to meet those needs, and ensuring accessibility and availability of resources for people who have such needs).

**psychiatric will** *Ulysses contract* (q.v.).

**psychiatrism** The injudicious and fallacious application of psychiatric principles in an unwarrantedly mechanistic way, without careful investigation of the dynamics of the individual case to which the principle is applied.

Psychiatrism is perhaps best illustrated by the novice student of psychology who reads Freud's work on dream interpretation and begins indiscriminately to interpret all his friends' dreams on the basis of the symbols mentioned by Freud. Thus, psychiatrism tends to standardize and oversimplify complex problems of relationship and causality, and ignores the enormous importance of individual variation. It is based on the fallacy of hypothetical concepts of unconscious personality forces being accepted in an unscientific, matter-of-fact fashion.

**psychiatrist** One versed in the branch of medicine that deals with the prevention, diagnosis, and treatment of mental and emotional disorders. Although with the development of behavioral neurology there is increasing overlap between the medical specialties of psychiatry and neurology, it may generally be said that psychiatry is concerned with disturbances in emotion, thinking, perceiving, and behavior, whereas neurology is concerned with disorders of identifiable parts of the nervous system. (It has been suggested that a psychiatrist is a noninvasive neurologist.) A psychiatrist is a physician who has had advanced training in the diagnosis and treatment of mental disorders. This advanced training ordinarily includes the study of *psychotherapy* (q.v.), and since the methods of psychotherapy are often based on a particular theory or system of psychology, the individual psychiatrist will often characterize his orientation as "psychoanalytic," "Freudian," "Jungian," "Adlerian," etc. Such appellations indicate the philosophy or psychological system to which the psychiatrist adheres; they are, as it were, subgroupings within the more general field of psychiatry.

Confusion has arisen in regard to differentiation between the terms psychiatrist and psychoanalyst. In the United States, the term psychoanalyst generally refers to a physician who has had advanced training in the specialty of psychiatry and whose theoretical background is psychoanalytic. There are, however, certain people (particularly in Europe) who are psychoanalysts but not psychiatrists; these "*lay analysts*" are not physicians but have had intensive training in the psychoanalytic method of psychotherapy and their theoretical orientation is psychoanalytic.

**psychiatry** The medical specialty concerned with the study, diagnosis, treatment, and prevention of behavior disorders. The word was first used by the German anatomist Johann Christian Reil (1759–1813).

**psychiatry, C-L** *Consultation-liaison* psychiatry (q.v.).

**psychic** 1. Of or pertaining to the mind or psyche. 2. Psychological or psychogenic, rather than physical or somatic. 3. Sensitive to psychic phenomena, as of a medium or spiritual healer.

**psychic divorce** See *divorce, stations of.*

**psychic epilepsy** *Epileptic equivalent* (q.v.), such as automatisms, dream states, and affective states.

**psychic equivalent** *Psychomotor epilepsy* (q.v.).

**psychic hallucination** See *hallucination of perception.*

**psychic isolation** Jung's term for the sense of estrangement from one's fellows that is felt immediately upon experiencing material arising from one's collective unconscious. "Such irruptions are uncanny, because they are irrational and inexplicable to the individual concerned. They . . . constitute a painful, personal secret that estranges the human being from his environment and isolates him from it. It is something that 'you can tell no one,' except under fear of being accused of mental abnormality" (*The Integration of the Personality*, 1939).

**psychic seizure** A type of psychomotor epilepsy. See *epilepsy; psycholepsy.*

**psychical center** Obs. The hypothesized localization of mental and intellectual functions in one or more specific sites in the brain.

**psychical reality** See *reality testing.*

**psychiety** A form of individualism which maintains that society resides within the individual rather than in the group. A person's emotions, ethics, and social experiences are emphasized, with the implication that more nearly perfect states of private experience and personal demeanor can be reached, perhaps through solitary meditation, self-help groups, or some form of more structured therapy.

**psychoactive** When used in reference to psychopharmacologic agents, the term usually means psychic energizer (antidepressant), although it is sometimes used less specifically to refer to any drug (stimulant, depressant, or tranquilizer as well as illicit drugs) with an effect on mental processes. See *psychotropics*.

**psychoactive substance dependence** Behavioral evidence of dependence on alcohol, sedatives or hypnotics, opioids, cocaine, amphetamine, phencyclidine, hallucinogens, cannabis, tobacco, or inhalants—either singly or in combination—manifested in one or more of the following: preoccupation with using the substance, taking it in larger amounts or for a longer period than intended, tolerance to the drug, development of typical withdrawal symptoms on discontinuance of the drug or use of the drug to relieve withdrawal symptoms, repeated efforts to reduce or control intake, interference with social or occupational obligations or opportunities by drug use, and continuing use of the drug in the face of clear-cut social, legal, or medical contraindications.

*Psychoactive substance abuse* refers to a maladaptive pattern of substance use that is not severe enough to meet the criteria for dependence.

**psychoactive substance use disorders** In DSM-III-R this category included *psychoactive substance dependence* (q.v.) and *psychoactive substance abuse*.

**psychoactive substance-induced organic mental disorders** In DSM-III-R intoxication, withdrawal, and posthallucinogenic perception disorder were recognized as organic mental disorders that may complicate psychoactive substance use, in addition to those organic mental syndromes that occur also in conditions other than psychoactive substance use (delirium, dementia, amnestic disorder, organic delusional disorder, organic hallucinosis, organic mood disorder, organic anxiety disorder, and organic personality disorder). See *flashback*.

**psychoanaleptic** See *analeptic*.

**psychoanalysis** The separation or resolution of the psyche into its constituent elements. The term has three separate meanings: (1) a procedure, devised by Sigmund Freud, for investigating mental processes by means of free association, dream interpretation, and interpretation of resistance and transference

manifestations; (2) a theory of psychology developed by Freud out of his clinical experience with hysterical patients; and (3) a form of psychiatric treatment developed by Freud that utilizes the psychoanalytic procedure (1 above) and is based on psychoanalytic psychology (2 above). In the third sense, psychoanalysis is "an attempt to decode, i.e., interpret, a patient's communications according to a loosely drawn set of transformational rules concerning underlying meanings, motivations, and unities of thought" (A. Cooper, *American Journal of Psychiatry 142*, 1985).

Freud considered the cornerstones of psychoanalytic theory to be the assumption of unconscious mental processes, recognition of resistance and repression, appreciation of the importance of sexuality (and aggressivity), and the Oedipus complex. Ernest Jones delineated seven major principles of Freud's psychology: (1) determinism—psychical processes are not a chance occurrence; (2) affective processes have a certain autonomy and can be detached and displaced; (3) mental processes are dynamic and tend constantly to discharge the energy associated with them; (4) repression; (5) intrapsychic conflict; (6) infantile mental processes—the wishes of later life are important only as they ally themselves with those of childhood; (7) psychosexual trends are present in childhood. For a short summary of Freud's instinct theories, see *neurosis*.

Other schools of thought within psychology and psychiatry are sometimes referred to (loosely and not wholly correctly) as psychoanalytic. Chief among these are the following:

1. Jung's analytical psychology, which emphasizes the *collective unconscious*, a concept bearing on ethnological psychology. Jung considers that libido arises not from the sexual instinct but from a universal force or life urge; mind is not only a Has Been but also a Becoming, that is, it has aims and strives to realize certain goals within itself. Reminiscences of experience are relegated to the personal unconscious and then link up with and are used to express fundamental ideas and trends, the *archetypes*, which represent not only the past stages but also the future potentials of race development.

2. Adler's individual psychology, which is based on the egoistic side of human nature, on the striving for power as a compensation for inferiority (psychic and organic). Neurosis

is an attempt to free oneself from the feeling of inferiority.

3. Sullivan's dynamic-cultural school (see *Sullivan, Harry Stack*).

4. Horney's dynamic-cultural school (see *Horney, Karen*).

5. Rado's adaptational school (see *adaptational psychodynamics*).

6. *Object relations* theory (q.v.).

7. *Self psychology.*

**psychoanalysis, applied** Use of established psychoanalytic knowledge to contribute to the understanding of psychic phenomena that occur outside the realm of psychoanalytic therapy, as in *biography in depth* (q.v.), art, history, anthropology, education, sociology, etc.

**psychoanalysis, wild** Psychotherapeutic techniques that use a limited amount of interpretation or that attack the patient directly with deep interpretations.

**psychoanalyst** One who adheres to the doctrine and/or uses the methods of psychoanalysis. See *psychiatrist; psychoanalysis.*

**psychoanalytically oriented psychotherapy** See *psychodynamic psychotherapy.*

**psychobiogram** E. Kretschmer devised the psychobiogram for purposes of practical investigation of the personality. It is made up of several parts. The first two parts consist of the data concerning the patient's heredity and past history. The other parts consist of a detailed description of the person's temperament, his sociological attitude, intelligence, physical findings, etc., and the classification from the point of view of the somatotype (*Textbook of Medical Psychology*, 1934).

**psychobiology** Biopsychology; the study of the biology of the psyche: the organization (anatomy), physiology, and pathology of the mind. The term was used with a variety of meanings in the early part of the 20th century. Adolf Meyer first used the term in 1915, and in the United States, it is generally associated with his name. Meyer called his point of view *objective psychobiology*, with particular stress upon the relationship of the individual to his environment. His school concerns itself with the overt and implicit behavior of the individual, which is a function of the total organism. The mind is the integration of the whole-functions of the total personality. Ideal mental health is the maximal ability of, plus the best opportunity for, getting along with people, without the interference of inner conflicts or external frictions, in a manner that would make for full mutual satisfaction on a constant give-and-take basis. Psychobiology is a genetic-dynamic science that studies personality development in the light of environmental setting and longitudinal growth. Meyer's central theme is "the mind in action" and he stresses the relationship between the conscious drives and the environment. The aim of objective psychobiology as it is applied to patients (*distributive analysis and synthesis*) is to adapt the patient to his surroundings, both directly by working with him and indirectly via environmental manipulation and work with other social agencies. The therapist attempts to correct the patient's faulty mental habits. Psychobiology is particularly useful in the psychoses, where the conflict to a large extent is between the ego and the environment (in the neuroses, the conflict is between the ego and the id).

**psychochromesthesia** Sensation of color produced by any nonvisual stimulus.

**psychocinesia** See *psychokinesia.*

**psychocortical** Relating to the cortex of the brain as the seat of the mind.

**psychodiagnostics** *Rorschach test* (q.v.).

**psychodietetics** The application of the principles of nutrition to the treatment of psychiatric disorders, and especially the replacement of assumed dietary deficiencies with supplemental vitamins, minerals, etc. See *orthomolecular.*

**psychodometer** An instrument for measuring the rapidity of psychic processes.

**psychodrama** "The psychodrama deals with the private personality of the patient and his catharsis, with the persons within his milieu and with the roles in which he and they have interacted in the past, in the present, and in which they may interact in the future. Techniques have been devised to bring the underlying spontaneous processes to expression. Psychodramatic work is usually best organized in a therapeutic theatre, but it may be carried out wherever the patient lives, if his problem requires it.

"One of the techniques is that of self-presentation. The psychiatrist asks the patient to live through and portray or duplicate situations which are a part of his daily life, especially crucial conflicts in which he is involved.

"Another technique of the psychodrama is that of soliloquy. It is used by the patient to duplicate hidden feelings and thoughts which he actually has or had in a situation with a partner in real life, but which he did not or does not express.

"In the technique of spontaneous improvisation the patient acts in fictitious or symbolic roles which are carefully selected by the psychiatrist on the basis of the patient's problem.

"In the case of patients with whom any sort of communication is reduced to a minimum, the psychodrama attempts to create an auxiliary world, or a world within which the patient functions. This may require the use of a staff of auxiliary egos who are to embody the psychotic world of the patient.

"*Psychodramatic catharsis* is a process which takes place between the actual partners in a problem or mental disturbance. Analysis before or after psychodramatic action may prepare a cathartic development, but the genuine phase of catharsis takes place in the course of the psychodrama itself" (Moreno, J. L. *Das Stegreif Theater*, 1936).

### psychodrama, forms of

1. *Psychodrama*—focuses on the individual, being a synthesis of psychological analysis with drama (action). Psychodrama aims at the active building up of private worlds and individual ideologies.

2. *Sociodrama*—focuses on the group, being a synthesis of the social with psychodrama. It aims at the active structuring of social worlds and collective ideologies.

3. *Physiodrama*—focuses on the soma, being a synthesis of physical culture (sports) and psychodrama. The physical condition of the participants before, during, and after the production is measured. It gives diagnostic (possibly also prognostic) clues for training requirements and provides the setup for retraining.

4. *Axiodrama* (Gr. *axios*, worth, worthy of value, goodly)—focuses on ethics and general values and aims to dramatize eternal verities (truth, justice, beauty, grace, piety, eternity, peace, etc.).

5. *Hypnodrama*—the synthesis of *hypnosis* (q.v.) and psychodrama.

6. *Psychomusic*—a synthesis of *spontaneous* music with psychodrama.

7. *Psychodance*—a synthesis of *spontaneous* dancing with psychodrama.

8. *Therapeutic motion picture*—a synthesis of motion picture with psychodrama (Moreno, J. L. *Sociometry 1*, 1937).

**psychodramatic movement therapy** See *dance therapy*.

**psychodramatic shock** "A procedure which throws a patient, barely escaped from a psychosis, back into a re-experience of the psychotic attack is a psychodramatic shock treatment.... Acting upon a psychotic level at a time when he is extremely sensitive to the vanished mental syndrome, the patient learns to check himself. It is a training in mastering of psychotic invasions, not through analysis but through a reconstruction of the psychotic experiences from act to act, from role to role, and from delusion to delusion, until the whole sphere of the psychosis is projected upon the therapeutic stage" (Moreno, J. L. *Sociometry 2*, 1939).

**psychodynamic** Relating to the forces of the mind. Ideas and impulses are charged with emotions, to which the general expression psychic energy is given. For example, delusions of persecution or obsessions or compulsions are described as psychodynamic phenomena, in that they are said to represent the results of activity of psychic forces. See *psychodynamics*.

**psychodynamic psychotherapy** *Psychoanalytically oriented psychotherapy*; dynamic therapy based on psychoanalytic therapy that uses various techniques in addition to interpretation. It is sometimes subdivided into (1) *expressive psychotherapy*, which uses mainly interpretation and clarification to make conscious the patient's defenses, resistances, and conflicts, and (2) *supportive psychotherapy*, in which interpretation tends to be limited to a single conflict, or several interrelated ones, that appear to be primarily responsible for symptoms that interfere with functioning, while other ego-strengthening techniques (such as abreaction, suggestion, manipulation, and clarification) are used to assist the patient in suppressing conflict and its expression in disabling symptoms.

Many of the psychodynamic therapies purposely focus on a particular problem or on a limited range of issues; they consequently tend to be of shorter duration than classical psychoanalysis and thus may be called brief psychotherapy or brief dynamic psychotherapy. See *brief psychotherapy*.

**psychodynamics**  The science of mental forces in action. Essentially, psychodynamics are a formulation or description of how the mind develops, and of how the hypothesized energies of the mind are distributed in the course of its various adaptational maneuvers. See *ego; id; Oedipus complex; ontogeny, psychic; superego.*

**psychodysleptica**  See *psychotropic.*

**psychoeducation**  Training in psychologic principles and their application to specified problems, conditions, or situations, often used to refer to *psychoeducational family therapy,* developed by Anderson, Hogarty, and Reiss (1980) for families of schizophrenics. The procedure includes a *survival skills workshop,* during which information about the technical and subjective aspects of schizophrenic disorders is presented to a group of families, along with guidelines for interactions between patients and family members. Sessions during the next months or years focus on how the guidelines can be applied within specific families, and continuing multiple family meetings at fortnightly intervals widen the supportive networks for all the families participating.

**psychoembryological schedule of ego**  See *dedifferentiation.*

**psychoendocrinology**  Also, psychoneuroendocrinology; the study of the hormonal system in relation to psychiatric disorders and, particularly, the study of the endocrine system as a likely site for the manifestation of biochemical abnormalities that are significant factors in the production of mental disorders.

Psychoendocrinologic research has concentrated particularly on cortisol, estrogen, growth hormone, progesterone, prolactin, testosterone, and thyroxine because they are hormones that are controlled by the central nervous system through the regulatory neurochemical agents of the hypothalamic-anterior pituitary complex.

**psychoepilepsy**  By some, this term is used synonymously with idiopathic or genuine epilepsy; an unfortunate term in that it implies a psychogenic basis for epilepsy, evidence for which is minimal. See *epilepsy.*

**psychoexploration**  A generic term used to refer to the various procedures known as abreaction, psychocatharsis, narcoanalysis, narcosynthesis, etc.

**psychogalvanic reflex (PGR)**  *Electrodermal response (EDR);* Féré phenomenon; *galvanic skin response (GSR);* changes in skin resistance to the passage of a weak electric current that occur as part of the physicochemical response to emotional stimuli.

**psychogender**  The psychological or emotional sex of a person; the term is ordinarily confined to intersexed patients to differentiate psychological sexual identification from somatic sex. See *gender identity.*

**psychogenesis**  Origination within the mind or psyche.

**psychogenic, psychogenetic**  Relating to or characterized by psychogenesis; due to psychic, mental, or emotional factors and not to detectable organic or somatic factors.

**psychogenic pain disorder**  Psychalgia; kinesalgia. See *somatoform disorders.*

**psychogenic psychosis**  See *reactive psychosis; remitting atypical psychosis.*

**psychogerontology**  Geriatric psychiatry; the study of the psychosocial aspects of old age.

**psychogeusic**  Pertaining to taste perception.

**psychognosia**  1. Awareness of one's own mental state, insight.

2. Study of another's mental state as a step in the diagnosis of psychiatric disorder. A rarely used term.

**psychogogic**  Mentally stimulating.

**psychogonical**  Psychogenic.

**psychogony**  The doctrine of the development of the mind. See *ontogeny, psychic.*

**psychogram**  *Psychograph* (q.v.).

**psychograph**  A chart or profile that describes the personality traits of the subject; *psychogram.*

**psychographic disturbances**  *Obs.*  Bombastic speech or pretentious, prolix writing as the major manifestion of personality disorder.

**psychography**  The history of the psychologic and emotional development of the subject as it relates to the development of the symptoms of which he now complains.

**psychohistory**  Application of psychologic theory, and particularly psychoanalytic psychology, to history so as to understand the human forces at work in the production of past events. Its most common application is to the history of a particular person; this is termed *psychobiography.*

**psychoimmunology**  *Behavioral immunology;* study of the relationship between the immune system and behavior, and in particular the effect of the brain and psychological phenomena on immune responses. The immune system is responsive to emotional stress, and it seems likely that the central nervous system, neurotransmitters, and neuroendocrine processes mediate hypothalamic influences on the immune system.

**psychoinfantilism**  "Persistence, in the adult, of mental qualities characteristic of the child. Psycho-infantile behavior is manifested in tractability and dependence, which often takes the form of a strong emotional fixation frequently to the mother or the father, but sometimes to other persons, even chance acquaintances" (Lindberg, B. J. *Psycho-Infantilism*, 1950).

**psychokinesia, psychokinesis**  T. S. Clouston's term for defective inhibition; formerly it also referred to the clinical syndrome known as *impulse insanity*. See *impulse disorders*.

**psychokym(e)**  "Psychic processes conceived physiologically, namely, that which is conceived analogous to a form of energy, that something which flows through the central nervous system and which is at the basis of psychic processes. 'Neurokym' is used to designate the nervous processes in general" (Bleuler, E. *Textbook of Psychiatry*, 1930).

**psycholagny**  Sexual excitation that begins, continues, and ends with mental imagery; mental or psychic *masturbation* (q.v.), that is, masturbation stimulated by mental forces alone.

**psycholepsy, psycholepsis**  Sudden, intense lowering of psychic tension, associated with morbid ideas and actions.

When psychic tension mounts to great heights, "in which feelings of ecstasy and indescribable happiness" appear, there may be a sudden fall in tension "culminating in a psycholeptic crisis and even in an epileptic fit" (Janet, P. *Psychological Healing*, 1925). Some people who have triumphed in a given work may terminate the triumph with a morbid clinical syndrome. See *psycholeptic crisis*.

**psycholeptic crisis**  Eruption of irrational unconscious elements into consciousness, such as the feeling that the end of the world is at hand. Epileptics often express ideas of impending destruction. See *psycholepsy*.

**psycholeptica**  Delay's term for phrenotropic drugs, whose principal effect is on the psyche, in contrast to neuroleptica, whose principal effect is on psychomotor activity. The psycholeptica include (1) the anxiolytic sedatives (ataractics), such as the barbiturates, benzodiazepines, and meprobamate;

(2) psychoanaleptica (psychic tonics, euphoriants, and antidepressives); and (3) psychodysleptica, which produce disintegration of psychic functions (lysergic acid, mescaline, etc.). See *psychotropic*.

**psycholinguistic abilities**  See *Illinois Test of Psycholinguistic Abilities*.

**psycholinguistics**  The study of the psychological aspects of language, including how it is learned by the child as the mind develops and matures. See *linguistic-kinesic method*

Psycholinguistics has also been defined as the "study of the relation between messages on the speech channel and the cognitive or emotional states of human encoders and decoders who send and receive the messages" (Markel, N. N. *Psycholinguistics: An Introduction to the Study of Speech and Personality*, 1969). *Linguistics* (q.v.), or philology, is the scientific study of human language or speech.

Two subfields of psycholinguistics are recognized: (1) verbal learning and verbal behavior, concerned with the relation between messages on the speech channel and the cognitive states of the encoders and decoders; and (2) speech and personality, concerned with the relation between message on the speech channel and the emotional, attitudinal, or motivational states of the encoders and decoders. Included in this part are stylistics, the study of individual differences in the selection of words in various contexts; and paralanguage, nonlanguage sounds; language sounds are those that are essential for the production of words of a language (e.g., to say "tin" the sound of a "t" must be produced) and the speaker has little option in producing those sounds or their distribution; but he has many options in producing nonlanguage sounds, e.g., voice set, voice qualities, vocalizations (discrete sounds that are not used to produce morphs in a particular language, such as the tsk-tsk sound used to indicate "too bad").

**psychologic dissociation**  Disruptions in memory, consciousness, and identity. See *dissociation*. Psychologic dissociation is often observed to accompany *somatoform dissociation*, which consists of disturbances in sensation, movement, and bodily function. Both types commonly occur in *depersonalization* disorder, *dissociative identity disorder*, and *post-traumatic stress disorder* (qq.v.). As subjects with dissociation become less and less aware of and connected with their body, identity, feelings, and surroundings, they may become alexithymic and deficient both in understanding their emotional experiences and in regulating their affective responses. See *alexithymia*.

**psychologic unavailability** A type of maternal neglect characterized by caregiving deviations, such as withdrawing from emotional contact, being unresponsive to the child's overtures, or displaying contradictory, role-reversed, or disoriented responses when the infant's attachment needs are heightened. Because the infant cannot gauge the actual degree of threat posed by an event, the experience of threat is closely related to the caregiver's affective signals and availability rather that to the actual degree of physical or survival danger. What is threatening to the infant are the threat of separation from the caregiver and the threat of having inadequate caregiver response to the infant's signals of distress. The attachment relational system is only one of several motivational systems, but when aroused it is preemptive because it mobilizes responses to fear or threat, such as fight or flight, freezing and "learned" helplessness, or—especially in the female—affiliative responses such as tend or befriend. Hidden traumas of infancy contribute to the early hyper- or hyporegulation of stress responses mediated through the limbic-hypothalamic-pituitary-adrenocortical (*LHPA*) axis. See *attachment*.

**psychologic(al)** Relating to psychology; mental functioning; functional, rather than organic; of emotional origin.

**psychological abuse** See *child abuse*; *domestic violence*.

**psychological dependence** See *dependence, psychological*.

**psychological medicine** See *psychology*.

**psychologist** A person trained as a professional in the science of psychology; a person with a degree in psychology granted by an accredited training program or educational institution. The individual psychologist often specializes in one of the branches or fields of psychology and is then identified as that type of psychologist (e.g., a comparative or animal psychologist, research psychologist, educational psychologist, industrial psychologist).

A *clinical psychologist* usually holds a doctoral degree from an accredited training program, has had at least 2 years of supervised experience in a clinical setting, and often is licensed under applicable state laws. Whether working individually or as part of the clinical (treatment) team, the clinical psychologist applies psychological principles to the therapeutic management of the mental, emotional, and behavioral disorders and developmental disabilities of individuals and groups. In addition, the clinical psychologist is skilled in research methodology and has assumed increasing importance in evaluating the effectiveness of mental health services and in planning clinical programs.

As with other mental health professionals, the clinical psychologist's functioning will vary with the setting within which he or she works and with his or her theoretical orientation. He may be involved mainly in individual therapy, group therapy, marriage or family therapy; his techniques may be largely psychoanalytic, behavioral, transpersonal, or Gestalt. Among the areas in which most clinical psychologists have had special training are sensational-perceptual function, motivation, memory and learning, thinking and cognition, intelligence, innate patterns, personality development, language and communication, group dynamics, behavior pathology, administration and interpretation of psychological tests, counseling and psychotherapy, and research such as validation of tests, outcome studies, and analysis of data by statistical techniques.

**psychology** The scientific discipline that deals with behavior (in humans and other animals), and with the mental processes underlying behavior; the study of the phenomena of mental life. Sometimes the distinction is drawn between *subjective psychology* (sensations, perceptions, ideations, emotions, motives, volitions, attitudes, beliefs, etc.) and *objective psychology* (the neurophysiologic mechanisms that enable the organism to adjust inner to outer relations and their external manifestations). There are many branches of psychology—clinical, comparative, developmental, educational, industrial, physiological, social, etc.—with linkages to other sciences.

A major specialty is clinical psychology, concerned with personal adjustment and the diagnosis and treatment of mental disorders. Its closest linkage is with psychiatry, to which it brings a degree of sophistication in research and statistical methodology that is not typically a part of the psychiatrist's repertoire.

Clinical psychology is sometimes called *medical psychology*, although that term is also sometimes used interchangeably with *psychological medicine*, which denotes a branch of medicine. See *psychologist*.

**psychology, applied** Utilization of all knowledge available in the areas of psychology, sociology, etc., in order to achieve optimal effectiveness in any operation. Applied psychology is ordinarily subdivided according to the field in which the operation occurs; e.g., business psychology, educational psychology, industrial psychology.

**psychometric examinations** Various psychological tests that are administered to the subject in order to test one, several, or all of the following factors in his mental makeup: intelligence, special abilities and disabilities, manual skill, vocational aptitudes, interests, and personality characteristics.

**psychometrics** Measurement of psychological functioning; mental testing; the application of mathematics and statistics to the assessment of psychological data. See *psychometric examinations*.

**psychomimic syndrome** Symptoms without organic basis that resemble the illness of another; typically, the latter illness has been fatal to an ambivalently related person, and the psychomimic syndrome often occurs on or near the anniversary of the other's death.

**psychomotility** Any motor action, attitude, or habit pattern that is influenced by mental processes and thus reflects the individual's personality makeup. Certain psychomotor phenomena, such as tics, sterotypies, catatonia, dysarthria, stammering, and tremor, have long been used in diagnosis as signs of psychomotor disturbance. Recently, postural attitudes and gait have been under investigation by clinicians as objective signs of psychomotor disturbance. Handwriting, also, has long been known as a valuable aid in investigating psychomotility, for it gives some indication of the individual's motivation. Certain features of handwriting have been regarded as suggestive of certain personality traits. Preliminary investigations of a nature more scientific than mere palmistry indicate that correlations do exist between handwritings of different types and symptoms, syndromes, and character traits noted in the patient's records.

**psychomotor** Relating to movement that is psychically determined in contradistinction to that which is definitely recognized as extrapsychic or organic in cause.

**psychomotor attack** A term sometimes used interchangeably with the term *psychic equivalent* of epilepsy. See *epileptic equivalent*.

**psychomotor center** Motor cortex; psychocortical center; the part of the cerebral cortex around the central fissure, embracing the centers of voluntary muscular movement.

**psychomotor epilepsy** *Temporal lobe epilepsy; complex partial seizures; psychomotor seizures* (q.v.).

**psychomotor hallucination** A patient's sensation that certain parts of his or her body are being transferred to body regions distant from their natural location.

**psychomotor poverty** A negative symptom dimension in schizophrenia that includes poverty of speech, decreased spontaneous movement, unchanging facial expression, paucity of expressive gesture, affective dulling, and lack of vocal inflection. See *negative symptoms*.

Two other dimensions of psychopathology in schizophrenia are *disorganization* (q.v.), which includes inappropriate affect, poverty of content of speech, tangentiality, derailment, pressure of speech, and distractibility, and *psychoticism* (reality distortion), which includes hallucinations and delusional ideas.

**psychomotor seizures** *Psychomotor epilepsy; complex partial seizures; temporal lobe epilepsy*; this group includes a bewildering variety of recurrent periodic disturbances, which usually take the form of some mental disturbance during which the patient carries out movements of a highly organized but semiautomatic character. Ictus is usually preceded by an aura. Clinical features include the following:

1. Autonomic and visceral manifestations, such as an *epigastric aura* (a churning sensation in the stomach and spreading towards the neck), or dizziness, flushing, tachycardia, changes in breathing.

2. Perceptual—distorted perceptions; déjà vu experiences; visual, auditory, olfactory, or somatic hallucinations.

3. Cognitive—disturbances of speech, thought, and memory; dysphasia, especially if the dominant lobe is involved.

4. Mood—fear and anxiety.

5. Psychomotor automatisms—grimacing; repetitive or more complex stereotyped behavior, such as undressing; sometimes aggressive behavior.

Some authorities use the term psychomotor epilepsy to indicate the combination of a disordered mental state with complex motor activity.

Complex partial seizures are rare in children, the attack itself is marked by confusion rather than loss of consciousness, and there is later amnesia. Psychomotor attacks last longer than petit mal attacks, with which they are easily confused; but incontinence and postictal confusion, which do not occur in petit mal, are seen frequently in psychomotor epilepsy.

About two-thirds of the psychomotor group also have grand mal seizures, but only about 3% also have petit mal attacks. There is general agreement that the great majority of psychomotor seizures are the epileptic manifestations of temporal lobe lesions. See *interictal behavior syndrome*; *temporal lobe syndromes*.

**psychoneurosis**   See *neurosis*.

**psychoneurosis, battle**   War neurosis; *traumatic neurosis* (q.v.).

**psychoneurosis maidica**   *Pellagra* (q.v).

**psychoneurotic depression**   In the 1952 nomenclature (DSM-I), the diagnosis of psychoneurotic depressive reaction is synonymous with reactive depression. "The anxiety in this reaction is allayed, and hence partially relieved, by depression and self-depreciation. The reaction is precipitated by a current situation, frequently by some loss sustained by the patient, and is often associated with a feeling of guilt for past failures or deeds." To be considered in differentiating this group from the corresponding psychotic reaction are the following points: "(1) life history of patient, with special reference to mood swings (suggestive of psychotic reaction), to the personality structure (neurotic or cyclothymic) and to precipitating environmental factors and (2) absence of malignant symptoms (hypochondriacal preoccupation, agitation, delusions, particularly somatic, hallucinations, severe guilt feelings, intractable insomnia, suicidal ruminations, severe psychomotor retardation, profound retardation of thought, stupor)" (ibid.).

In the 1968 revision of psychiatric nomenclature (DSM-II) this entity is termed depressive neurosis; in DSM-III, it is termed dysthymic disorder. See *affective disorders*.

It is recognized that attempts to differentiate between psychotic and neurotic depressions, either on phenomenological or on psychodynamic grounds, are inadequate.

While it is obvious that severe dejection can be superimposed on any nosologic entity (and is particularly common in phobics and obsessional neuroses), that this should justify a special diagnosis of depression is questionable.

**psychonomy**   The branch of psychology concerned with the laws of mental action.

**psycho-oncology**   The branch of psychiatry that is concerned with cancer patients: the psychological and social effects of cancer on the patient, the family, and the treatment staff; and the effects that the patient and the environment may have on cancer risk and the length of survival.

**psychopathia sexualis**   *Sexual psychopathy;* referring to sexual perversions; introduced by the German sexologist Richard von Krafft-Ebing (1840–1903).

**psychopathic personality**   *Antisocial personality* (q.v.); *manipulative personality.* Although the 1980 revision of psychiatric nomenclature does not recognize psychopathic personality as a discrete entity, the attempts to define more clearly the nature of the various behavior patterns that make up this poorly understood group have not been wholly successful, and the term continues to appear in the psychiatric literature.

J. C. Prichard is often credited with introducing the concept, but what he described in 1835 as moral disorders had little to do with current concepts of psychopathic or antisocial personality; rather, he used the term to describe delusions and hallucinations that occurred in patients who had no other signs of "insanity." In 1888 Koch introduced the term *psychopathic inferiority*, and Kraepelin later included in this group a variety of syndromes described in terms of the most obvious presenting symptom, e.g., excitability, impulsivity, lying, criminality. The term *constitutional psychopathic inferior* was used by Adolf Meyer in 1905; it should be noted, however, that Meyer did not use the term constitutional in the sense of congenital, but rather to indicate that the traits in question were acquired early and were thoroughly ingrained in the personality. In general, at least according to current usage, psychopathic personality (or psychopathic disorder) is any behavioral dysfunction that is primary (idiopathic or nonorganic) and manifests itself in abnormally aggressive or seriously irresponsible conduct.

Cleckley (1941), who considered psychopathic personality a psychosis, because of lack of integration of affective components into the personality, listed the following characteristics: "(1) superficial charm and good 'intelligence'; (2) absence of delusions and other signs of irrational 'thinking'; (3) absence of 'nervousness' or psychoneurotic manifestations; (4) unreliability; (5) untruthfulness and insincerity; (6) lack of remorse or shame; (7) inadequately motivated antisocial behavior; (8) poor judgment and failure to learn by experience; (9) pathologic egocentricity and incapacity for love; (10) general poverty in major affective reactions; (11) specific loss of insight; (12) unresponsiveness in general interpersonal relations; (13) fantastic and uninviting behavior with drink and sometimes without; (14) suicide rarely carried out; (15) sex life impersonal, trivial and poorly integrated; (16) failure to follow any life plan" (*The Mask of Sanity*, 1941).

Other descriptions include glibness and superficiality, callousness, irresponsibility, irritability, impulsivity, low frustration tolerance and proneness to aggressive behavior, arrogance, deceitfulness, and a manipulative approach to interpersonal relationships. The maladjustment is a chronic one, and the psychopath tends to project the blame for his actions onto others. He tends to act out his conflicts so that the environment suffers, rather than the patient. He is a rebellious individualist and a nonconformist. Often the adult psychopath gives a history suggestive of a disruptive behavior disorder (conduct disorder) in childhood.

E. Glover classified psychopathy into three main subgroups: (1) sexual psychopathy, with predominantly sexual symptoms combined with some degree of ego disorder; (2) "benign" psychopathy, manifested in the main as social incapacity, but usually with accompanying psychosexual disorder; and (3) antisocial psychopathy characterized by an unstable ego, delinquent outbursts, and some degree of sexual maladjustment (*The Technique of Psycho-analysis*, 1955).

Etiology is unknown; some claim an exclusively organic etiology, and others maintain that it is due to psychogenic factors. Many writers have emphasized difficulties in identification leading to a formless or confused ego-ideal. An unstable, inconsistent maternal figure or rejection and emotional deprivation early in life are believed to produce such difficulties in identification. According to M. S. Guttmacher (in *Current Problems in Psychiatric Diagnosis*, ed. P. H. Hoch & J. Zubin, 1953), psychopathic behavior is generally the result of affect starvation during the first years of life. The most malignant antisocial psychopaths are probably the products of affect starvation plus sadistic treatment in early childhood. See *battered child syndrome*.

Karpman suggested that those cases of psychogenic etiology be termed secondary or symptomatic psychopathy; the others he calls primary psychopathy or *anethopathy* (q.v.). See also *psychopathy, passive parasitic*. Many European workers (among them Kurt Schneider) used psychopathic personality as a generic term for all personality disorders and did not restrict its application to the antisocial group.

Various workers have noted a high incidence of cerebral dysrhythmia in patients diagnosed psychopathic personality; a high alpha index and theta activity are among the most commonly observed abnormalities.

**psychopathology** The branch of science that deals with the essential nature of mental disease—its causes, the structural and functional changes associated with it, and the ways in which it manifests itself.

**psychopathy, autistic** *Asperger syndrome* (q.v.).

**psychopathy, passive parasitic** A clinical subdivision of *anethopathy* (*psychopathic personality*). Karpman suggested the term anethopathy to replace idiopathic, constitutional, or primary psychopathy. Anethopathy is subdivided into two distinct clinical types: the aggressive predatory type and the passive parasitic type. In regard to the latter, Karpman says: "Instead of being actively aggressive, this type of an individual has much less of energy output and feeds himself by 'sponging' on his environment for all his needs in a passive and entirely parasitic way. Such aggression as there may be is very minimal and no more than is absolutely necessary to satisfy immediate needs" (*Psychoanalytic Review 34*, 1947). Typical of such patients is the lack of any positive or generous human emotions, of sympathetic or tender affect, of gratitude or appreciation. These patients show no guilt, remorse, or regret. Their total picture is one of self-gratification. Further, the patients are completely lacking in insight into the nature of their disturbances.

**psychopedagogy** A combination of conventional pedagogy and Adlerian psychology that aims to stimulate, cultivate, and amplify the natural qualities of the child and do away with unnecessary authority.

**psychopenetration test** A psychodynamic test devised by Wilcox in the 1940s used in conjunction with carbon dioxide coma to serve as a guide for therapeutic procedures in different types of cases. See *carbon dioxide inhalation therapy.*

**psychopharmacologic agents** *Psychotropics*; one classification of such agents is the following:

*Antianxiety agents* (q.v.)

Benzodiazepines: alprazolam, chlordiazepoxide, clorazepate, diazepam

Antidepressants: doxepin, paroxetine, sertraline, venlafaxine

Miscellaneous: buspirone, hydroxyzine

*Antipanic agents*: alprazolam, clonazepam

Antipressants: fluoxetine, paroxetine, sertraline

*Antipsychotic* (q.v.) *agents*

*First-generation (typical) antipsychotics* are D$_2$ antagonists; they include chlorpromazine, haloperidol, fluphenazine, thioridazine, loxapine, and perphenazine

*Second-generation (atypical) antipsychotics* are D$_2$ and 5-HT$_2$ antagonists; they include clozapine, risperidone, olanzapine, quetiapine, ziprasidone, and amulspride

*Third-generation (atypical) antipsychotics*—aripiprazole and bifeprunox

*Antidepressant* (q.v.) *agents*

*MAOIs*: isocarboxazid, moclobemide, phenelzine, and tranylcypromine

*Tricyclics, heterocyclics*: amitriptyline, amoxapine, desipramine, doxepin, nortriptyline, protriptyline

*Serotonergic antidepressants*

SSRIs: citalopram, clomipramine, escitalopram, fluoxetine, fluvoxamine, nefazodone, paroxetine, sertraline

SNRIs: duloxetine, mirtazapine, venlafaxine

*Other*: buproprion, maprotilene, trazodone

*Antimanic agents, mood stabilizers*

*Traditional*: carbamazepine, divalproex, lithium

*Used alone or in combination with traditional*

First-line options: olanzapine, quetiapine, risperidone

Second-line options: aripiprazole, ziprasidone

*Psychostimulants* (q.v.)

Amphetamines, caffeine, desipramine, ephedrine and related alkaloids, methylphenidate, modafinil, theophylline

Not stimulants, technically, but used as such particularly in ADHD: atomoxetine (a norepinephrine reuptake inhibitor); clonidine and guanfacine (a-adrenergic agonists); bupropion (an antidepressant)

*Cognitive enhancers*: donepezil, galantamine, rivastigmine (anticholinesterases); memantine, metrifonate

*Performance enhancers*

Anabolic-androgenic steroids: androstenediol, androstenedione, dehydroepiandrostrone (DHEA), human chorionic gonadotropin (hCG), oxandrolone, stanozolol, and testosterone

Psychostimulants—see above

Others: beta-blockers, clenbuterol, creatine, human recombinant erythropoietin, human growth hormone

*Appetite suppressants*

Long-term treatment of obesity: orlistat, sibutramine

Drugs that reduce food intake: apomorphine, chlorpheniramine, clenbuterol, fenfluramine, mazindol, metergoline, methamphetamine, phentermine, phenylpropanolamine, yohimbine

*Sedatives & hypnotics*

Barbiturates: mephobarbital, pentobarbital, phenobarbital, secobarbital

Benzodiazopines: estazolam, eszopiclone, flurazepam, quazepam, temazepam, triazolam, zalepone, zolpidem

Miscellaneous: chloral hydrate, hydroxyzine (antihistamine) ramelteon (melatonin receptor agonist)

*Drugs for alcohol & drug addiction*

*Alcoholism*

FDA approved: acamprosate, disulfiram, naltrexone, topiramate

Under investigation: baclofen, nalmefene, odansetron, pyrrolopyrimidine compound, rimonabant, valproate

*Cocaine addition*

FDA approved: none

Under investigation: baclofen, cocaine vaccine, disulfiram, gabapentin, $\gamma$-vinyl GABA (GVG), modafinil, tiagabine, topiramate

*Heroin/Opiate addiction*
FDA approved: buprenorphine, methadone, naltrexone
For opiate overdose: naloxone
*Nicotine Addiction*
FDA approved: buproprion, nicotine replacement, varenicline
Under investigation: deprenyl, methoxsalen, nicotine conjugate vaccine, rimonabant
*Antiepileptic drugs* (q.v.)
Barbiturates: mephobarbital, pentobarbital, phenobarbital, primidone
Benzodiazepines: clonazepam, clorazepate, diazepam
GABA analogues: gabapentin, pregabalin, retigabine, tiagabine, topiramate, vigabatrine
Hydantoins: fosphenytoin, mephenytoin, phenytoin
Phenyltriazines: lamotrigine
Succinimides: ethosuximide, methsuximide
Miscellaneous: acetyazolamide, carbamazepine, felbamate, lamotrigine, levetiracetam, oxycarbazepine, trimethadione, valproate, zonisamide
*Antiparkinson agents*
Anticholinergics: benztropine, biperiden, procycclidine, trihexyphenidyl
Catecol-O-methyltransferase inhibitors: carbidopa, entacapone, levodopa, tolcapone
Dopaminergic agents: amantadine, bromocriptine, pergolide, pramipexole, ropinirole
MAOI: selegiline
*Migraine preparations*
*For acute headache*
Serotonin ($5\text{-HT}_{1B/1D}$) receptor agonists—triptans:
Almotriptan, eletriptan, frovatriptan, naratriptan, sumatriptan, zolmitriptan
Miscellaneous: dihydroergotamine, divalproex
*Prophylaxis*
Beta-adrenergic blockers: propanolol, timolol
Miscellaneous: topiramate, valproate, verapamill

**psychopharmacology** The study of the mediation and modulation of behavior through the actions of endogenous signaling substances and drugs. There are four major classes of signaling molecules: neurotransmitters (e.g., hormones, neurotransmitters, neuromodulators); receptors; signal transducing proteins; and second messengers (e.g., cyclic adenosine monophosphate [cAMP], inositol trisphosphate [$IP_3$], diacylglycerol [DAG], and arachidonic acid [AA] metabolites) as well as proteins (receptors, signal-transducing guanine nucelotide-binding proteins [G-proteins], enzymes, uptake carriers, etc.). See *psychotropic*. Medication treatments with high side effects burden require clinical settings that are capable of detecting and managing serious side effects. The clinician's office must be able to monitor antipsychotic drugs efficiently. Blood presssure cuffs, scales, body tape measures, a process for plasma chemistry monitoring and EEGs, and qualified and available consultants for medical questions have become essentials of practice.

**psychophysical** *Psychosomatic* (q.v.).

**psychophysics** The discipline concerned with the relation between the physical characteristics of a stimulus and the attributes of the sensory experience, how the stimulus is transduced by sensory receptors and processed in the brain. Psychophysics attempts to understand how different stimuli alter brain activity and thereby generate specific perceptions. The sensory systems extract four elementary attributes of a stimulus—intensity, duration, location, and modality (i.e., whether the stimulus type is vision, hearing, touch, taste, or smell). Under normal circumstances, each nerve is primarily sensitive to one type of stimulus. Even so, perceptions are not mirror images of what is seen but are constructed, at least in part, according to innate rules of the nervous system (*preknowledge* or *wiring*) that organize sensory experience.

The initial wiring or pattern of neuronal connections in the fetal brain is relatively coarse. It is refined during development by sensory experience that may support or weaken the initial pattern. Further, there are irreversible decision points during development (*critical periods*) when specific interactions between nerve cells and environment commit cells to a specific pathway of differentiation and determine future behavioral capabilities. During such periods, the infant must interact with a reasonably normal environment if development is to proceed as it should.

**psychophysiologic disorders** *Psychosomatic disorders, somatization reactions, organ neuroses*; disturbances of visceral function secondary to chronic attitudes or long-continued insufficiency of affective discharge that may present themselves as dysfunction involving any of the organ systems: skin, musculoskeletal, respiratory, cardiovascular, hemic and lymphatic, gastrointestinal, genitourinary, endocrine, nervous system, or organs of special sense. In this system of classification, ulcerative colitis, for example, would be labeled "psychophysiologic gastrointestinal reaction." See *autonomic arousal disorder; psychosomatic.*

**psychophysiological memory** A memory that combines psychological and physiologic elements, as when a disturbance of body function (e.g., in the cardiac, respiratory, or digestive system) becomes linked, as a result of certain experiences, with a perception or thought. Recurrence of that perception or thought is then likely to trigger a reappearance of the physiologic disturbance. (Prince, M. *The Unconscious*, 1916).

**psychophysiology** The study of the relationships between physiological measures (e.g., skin conductive, event related potentials, $P_{300}$ wave) and psychological states or processes (e.g., arousal, cognition, emotion, learning).

**psychopolitics** Application of psychiatric knowledge or theory to the process of government; any effort to gain acceptance of psychiatric principles as a significant factor in the shaping of public policy.

In a society marked by a tendency to designate socially undesirable conduct as illness, rather than as the crime or sin of earlier generations, psychiatry has often found itself the arbiter of right and wrong. Technologic advances, in the form of mind-altering drugs, operant conditioning, electrode implantations, and the like, have raised the specter of their use as ways to coerce, oppress, or control behavior, or to supplant independent thinking and freedom of choice. In consequence, the ethics of medical and psychiatric practice has become an important aspect of psychopolitics. Of no less importance are those political actions designed to improve the lot of the mentally ill and to ensure the availability of a broad range of appropriate services for anyone who might need them. Such actions may be directed at any, or every, level of government—legislative (Are the right laws being written?), judicial (Have the courts given due consideration to the mental health implications of their decisions?), and executive (Are the laws being implemented appropriately, and are the decisions of the courts being honored?).

**psychoreaction** Much and Holzmann's term for psychophysical interrelationship. They asserted that when they injected cobra poison into patients with schizophrenia, they observed lysis of the red blood corpuscles in a way that was characteristic of schizophrenia. Their claims were short-lived.

**psychorhythm** T. S. Clouston's term for *alternating insanity.* See *manic-depressive psychosis.*

**psychorhythmia** Involuntary mental repetition of a formerly volitional action.

**psychorrhagia, psychorraghy** *Obs.* The death struggle.

**psychorrhea** Hebephrenic schizophrenia characterized by vague and often bizarre theories of philosophy; usually the stream of thought is incoherent.

**psychorrhexis** A malignant type of anxiety reaction seen in 2–3% of war neuroses, according to Emilio Mira. Anguish and perplexity, rather than fear or excitement, are the cardinal features. Pulse remains above 120, respiration about 40. Temperature rises rapidly after 7 days, the tongue becomes ulcerated, and jaundice and tympanitic abdomen may appear. Patients become restless, develop automatic movements and facial spasms. In fatal cases, death ensues after 3 or 4 days. Psychorrhexis occurs in patients with preexisting lability of the sympathetic system, with sudden severe mental trauma in conditions of physical exhaustion, and when there is long delay before sedative treatment is instituted. See *traumatic neurosis.*

**psychosensorial hallucination** Baillarger distinguished two kinds of hallucinations—psychosensorial and psychic. He said that the first are the result of the combined action of the imagination and of the organs of sense, while the second are the result of the imagination without the interposition of a sensory stimulus.

**psychosensory** Pertaining to (1) the mental perception and interpretation of sensory stimuli, or (2) a hallucination that, by an effort, the mind is able to distinguish from an actuality (pseudohallucination).

**psychosexual** In DSM-III-R, the categories included under this label were termed *sexual disorders* (q.v.).

**psychosexuality** Psychosexual condition or state; distinguished from sexuality expressed somatically (somatosexual). For example, ideas of a sexual character are manifestations of psychosexuality. See *ontogeny, psychic.*

**psychosis** Loosely, any mental disorder (including whatever is meant by the obsolete terms insanity, lunacy, and madness); more specifically, the term is used to refer to a particular class or group of mental disorders, and particularly to differentiate this group from neurosis, sociopathy (or psychopathy), character disorder, psychosomatic disorder, and mental retardation. Traditionally, the psychoses or psychotic disorders are subdivided into the following:

A. Organic brain syndromes
B. Functional psychoses
  1. Schizophrenias
  2. Affective psychoses (mood disorders, including involutional melancholia; manic-depressive psychosis, and psychotic depressive reaction)
  3. Paranoia and delusional states

Use of the term has been anything but precise and definite. Instead, "psychosis" (and its adjectival form, "*psychotic,*" q.v.) has often been used in a quantifying sense to indicate severity of disorder; thus, a person with the psychosis schizophrenia may be labeled psychotic only at certain times when the symptoms of his disorder reach a certain intensity and/or adversely affect his mental competence. As a result of conflicting usage, there is no single acceptable definition of what psychosis is. In general, however, the disorders labeled psychoses differ from the other groups of psychiatric disorders in one or more of the following:

1. *Severity*—the psychoses are "major" disorders that are more severe, intense, and disruptive; they tend to affect all areas of the patient's life (in Adolph Meyer's terms, a psychosis is a *whole-reaction* rather than a *part-reaction*).

2. *Degree of withdrawal*—the psychotic patient is less able to maintain effective object relationships; external, objective reality has less meaning for the patient or is perceived in a distorted way.

3. *Affectivity*—the emotions are often qualitatively different from the normal, at other times are so exaggerated quantitatively that they constitute the whole existence of the patient.

4. *Intellect*—intellectual functions may be directly involved by the psychotic process so that language and thinking are disturbed; judgment often fails; hallucinations and delusions may appear.

5. *Regression*—there may be generalized failure of functioning and a falling back to very early behavioral levels; such regression is more than a temporary lapse in maturity and may include a return to early and even primitive patterns.

Not all believe that the "functional" or "nonorganic" psychoses are distinct from the neuroses. Psychoanalysts, in particular, often argue that the differences are only in degree—that in the psychoses the fixation points are earlier, the regressions deeper, the infantile traumas more extensive, and the defenses more primitive.

Anti-psychiatrists and many sociopolitically oriented theorists view psychosis as an expression of skewed interactions within the subject's family (e.g., the "schizophrenogenic mother"). Those relationships have produced the person's incomprehensible behavior, which is then labeled as psychotic. In another version of this interpretation, pathology lies not in the individual patient but in the power politics of society.

**psychosis of association** See *induced psychotic disorder.*

**psychosis of degeneracy** *Obs.* Psychoses intimately associated with the environment, in contradistinction to the so-called real psychoses in which the environment plays no essential role.

**psychosocial** Referring to environmental elements and psychological attributes of subjects that play a contributory role in the onset, course, or treatment of their disorder(s).

**psychosocial dwarfism** *Deprivation(al) dwarfism*; a syndrome of decelerating linear growth and such behavior disturbances as sleep disorder and bizarre eating habits, due to inadequate physiologic, emotional, or intellectual stimulation. In general, symptoms are reversible with a change in the psychosocial environment. See *failure to thrive; developmental psychobiology.*

**psychosocial functioning** Measured by the Strauss and Carpenter Outcome Scale (SCOS, 1974) and the Role Functioning Scale (RFS; McPheeters, 1984).

**psychosocial retardation** Mental retardation associated with, accentuated by, or caused by such interactional or environmental factors as defective mother–child relationships, disturbed attachment, inadequate enrichment at home (in the social, emotional, or intellectual sphere), impaired learning because of severe emotional disorder, and insufficient emotional interaction in institutional settings. See *attachment disorder of infancy; mother–child relationship.*

**psychosocial stages**    See *ontogeny, psychic.*

**psychosomatic**    A term first used by Christian Heinroth (German physician, 1773–1843). Currently, it may be used in a methodological sense only, to refer to a type of approach in the study and treatment of certain disturbances of body function. More commonly, however, the term is used in a nosological or classificatory sense to refer to a group of disorders whose etiology at least in part is believed to be related to emotional factors; in the 1968 revision of psychiatric nomenclature such *psychosomatic disorders* were called *psychophysiologic disorders* (q.v.). See *anamnesis, associative; autonomic arousal disorder; somatoform disorders; psychosomatic medicine.*

As used in the second sense, the term psychosomatic is unfortunate, for it implies a dualism that does not exist. No somatic disease is entirely free from psychic influence, just as even in the purest psychic disturbances there are organic-constitutional factors, somatic compliance, etc. While it is generally recognized that many symptoms and diseases occur in the setting of difficult life situations, there is no accepted answer as to why some people get one disease, some get another. Various hypotheses have been put forward: some have tried to show that there is a personality pattern common to all patients with the same disease; others have tried to demonstrate a single personality trait associated with a particular disease; others have maintained that a specific nuclear conflict or dynamic configuration is unique to a particular disease; others have emphasized what has happened to the patient previously, especially in childhood, as in a search for toilet-training problems in patients with intestinal disorders; and, finally, some have tried to correlate the occurrence of particular symptoms with particular life situations. None of the attempts has been wholly satisfactory. Not all patients fit into the pattern they should; many patients show more than one of the illnesses in question, and this

is difficult to reconcile with the idea of fixed personality patterns; many patients show the specific dynamic configuration without developing the expected disease; and often there is little similarity between the various situations that provoke recurrences in the same patient.

Physical/organic disorders or symptoms are related to emotions in various ways: acute emotions, such as fright, may induce physiologic changes, such as cardiac arrhythmias, that may be fatal; chronically maintained emotions may induce physiologic changes that over time produce tissue damage ("psychosomatic disorders"); emotions may provoke self-destructive behaviors, such as substance abuse, dietary inadequacies, and careless vehicular operation; diseases or their treatments, or both, can arouse intense emotions that secondarily affect the original disease and the patient's cooperation with treatment measures (see *pathocure; fixation hysteria*); emotions that are not permitted release may find symbolic expression in conversion symptoms or somaticization.

Many psychoanalysts (e.g., Fenichel, *The Psychoanalytic Theory of Neurosis*, 1945) prefer the term *organ neurosis* to *psychosomatic disorder.* An organ neurosis is defined as a type of functional disorder that is physical in nature and that consists of physiologic changes caused by the inappropriate use of the function in question. Thus, organ neuroses and conversion neuroses are quite different—in conversion neuroses, the symptom has a specific unconscious meaning and is an expression of a phantasy in body language; in organ neuroses, the change in function per se has no unconscious meaning, but instead the chronic, unconscious attitudes of the patient have secondarily produced a change in function. In other words, in the organ neuroses a persistent emotional disturbance has secondarily altered the physiology of an organ system; but in the conversion neuroses, a persistent emotional disturbance is directly symbolized by a disturbance in bodily function, and the physiology of the organ system in question need not be altered.

The seven "classic" psychosomatic disorders are peptic ulcers, bronchial asthma, rheumatoid arthritis, ulcerative colitis, essential hypertension, thyrotoxicosis, and migraine. See *arthritis; asthma, bronchial; hypertension, essential; migraine; thyrotoxicosis.*

**psychosomatic disorders** See *psychophysiologic disorders; psychosomatic; somatoform disorders.*

**psychosomatic medicine** Clinical psychosomatic medicine is the psychiatric specialty that is concerned with the management of patients with comorbid medical and psychiatric illnesses; it focuses on understanding the psychiatric adverse effects of medications, and how physical illnesses affect mental states. Its emphasis is on the multilevel interactions that contribute to illness, on the combined effects on physiologic functioning of genetic susceptibility, biologic insults, early childhood experiences, personality, socioeconomic factors, acute and chronic stressors, and social networks. Psychosomatic medicine combines treatment of comorbid mental disorders of the medically ill (formerly called consultation-liaison psychiatry) with the study of physiologic mechanisms underlying mind–body interactions in all disorders.

In addition to the management of such obvious complications as delirium, dementia, depression, mania, anxiety, somatoform disorders, and substance-related disorders, psychosomatic medicine addresses such topics as burns, cancer, organ transplantation, pain and analgesics, response to illness and medical psychotherapy, and geriatric psychiatry. Psychosomatic Medicine was recently recognized by the American Board of Medical Specialties as a psychiatric subspecialty.

Felix Deutsch introduced the term *psychosomatic medicine*, which has often been used to imply illness that is caused or worsened by psychological factors. At one time, some thought that psychosomatic medicine held the promise of explaining psychodynamically the causes of perplexing illnesses, such as rheumatoid arthritis, asthma, and peptic ulcer. This proved not to be the case. Subsequently, George Engel's biopsychosocial model brought psychiatry and medicine together as the basis of understanding an illness in the context of the individual patient. Consultation-liaison psychiatry emerged in the 1970s and 1980s as the hands-on application of psychosomatic principles to clinical medicine.

**psychosomimetic** *Psychotomimetic* (q.v.).

**psychostimulants** Also, *stimulants*; psychoactive or psychotropic drugs that increase or enhance central nervous system activity, typically manifested as an increase in the level of alertness and/or motivation. Included are analeptics; opiate antagonists; xanthines (such as caffeine); cocaine; amphetamines, methylphenidate, atomoxetine, modafinil, pipradol, phenmetrazine, or similarly acting sympathicomimetics; and other drugs that have been used primarily as anorexiants. See *amphetamines; caffeine intoxication; cocaine.*

Symptoms of psychostimulant intoxication include increased heart rate and blood pressure, hyperactive reflexes, pupillary dilatation, sweating, chills, nausea, and behavioral changes, such as belligerence, grandiosity, hypervigilance, agitation, impulsivity, and impaired judgment. Chronic use may lead to personality change, and a full-blown delusional (paranoid) psychosis may occur. Withdrawal reactions may occur following prolonged use, with depressed mood, fatigue, and sleep disturbances.

Some drugs, among them the anticholinergics, *antidepressants*, and some of the *opioid* drugs (qq.v.), are not primarily stimulant but exert such action at high dosage or with chronic use.

**psychosurgery** *Functional neurosurgery*; any neurosurgical operation or intervention whose primary aim is to modify emotions or behavior in the absence of known physical disease. The term does not apply to surgical treatment of conditions that are known to cause emotional or behavior disturbances, such as epilepsy or parkinsonism. See *prefrontal lobotomy.*

**psychosynthesis** A system of psychology and a group of therapeutic techniques devised by the Italian psychoanalyst Robert Assagioli. He founded the Institute of Psychosynthesis in Rome in 1926; the major expositions of his system are to be found in *Psychosynthesis* (1965) and *The Act of Will* (1973).

Assagioli divided the psyche into the lower unconscious (the personal psychological past), the middle unconscious (where skills, states of mind, and everything that can be brought into the level of consciousness reside), and the superconscious (the source of higher feelings, creativity, ecstasy, inspiration, and our urges to future heroic action). The goal of therapy is to bring together the diverse inner elements of the psyche so they will merge into successively greater wholes rather than compete or clash with one another. Therapeutic techniques include analysis, to assess blocks within the psyche; mastery training, to cultivate coordination of different aspects of the personality; transformation, to encourage reorganization of the personality around a different set of values; meditation, to facilitate exploration of the superconscious; and relational techniques, to foster more openness and better communication with others.

**psychotaxis** The tendency to enjoy pleasant states of mind or to avoid unpleasant situations (negative psychotaxis).

**psychotechnics** Practical application of psychological methods in the study of economics, sociology, and other problems.

**psychotherapeusis, -therapeutics** *Psychotherapy* (q.v.).

**psychotherapy** Treatment by communication; any form of treatment for mental illnesses, behavioral maladaptations, or other problems that are assumed to be of an emotional nature, in which a trained person deliberately establishes a professional relationship with a patient for the purpose of removing, modifying, or retarding existing symptoms, of attenuating or reversing disturbed patterns of behavior, and of promoting positive personality growth and development.

There are numerous forms of psychotherapy—ranging from *guidance, counseling,* persuasion, and hypnosis to reeducation and psychoanalytic reconstructive therapy—and many possible applications of each form—including disabling psychosomatic symptoms, interpersonal conflicts and pathological attitudes secondary to recognizable (organic) disturbance of central nervous system functions, the so-called functional psychoses, character and behavior disorders, psychoneuroses, and marital conflict, to name a few; but in general it may be said that all forms of psychotherapy in all their applications employ the relationship established between patient and therapist to influence the patient to unlearn old or maladaptive response patterns and to learn better ones.

Psychotherapy has also been characterized as "an undefined technique applied to unspecified problems with unpredictable outcome; for this technique we recommend rigorous training" (Conference on Graduate Education in Clinical Psychology, 1949). While such a definition may seem so pessimistic as to approach nihilism, it emphasizes what would seem to be an irrefragable fact: despite centuries of its use, and despite decades of study of its various forms, psychotherapy and the means by which it achieves its results are but poorly understood.

The broadest subdivision of types of psychotherapy is into those based on psychodynamics and those based on behavioral principles. Psychodynamic therapy presumes that every person has an unconscious mind, that a significant portion of the emotions that determine behavior are located in the unconscious mind, and that any process that permits those emotions to enter awareness will promote stability and control.

Behavioral therapy is based on a neurologic concept of learning, the conditioned reflex. Many psychiatric disorders are regarded as learned responses that have become conditioned reflexes; their unlearning, through retraining and deconditioning, is the aim of behavior therapy.

"The patient's experience in the therapeutic relationship is assumed to be a sample in microcosm of the significant factors that brought on or related to his problems. Observing the patient's behavior (both verbal and non-verbal), and using his empathic understanding of the patient's behavior in relation to himself, the therapist comments on what he observes. The patient, witnessing the same behavior, and viewing it in the light of the therapist's comments as well as in the light of his own reactions, is now in a position to re-evaluate his own past behavior and to prepare for or begin to change. While all the factors involved in the change are not clear, it is assumed to involve the general principles of learning" (Stein, M. I. *Contemporary Psychotherapies*, 1961).

Because the term psychotherapy has been applied to a variety of dissimilar operations, the phrase *definitive forms of psychotherapy* has been suggested to exclude such procedures as environmental manipulation, general medical treatment as psychotherapy, physical examination as psychotherapy, and all procedures in which more than two people participate. In this sense, psychotherapy is a procedure undertaken in order to foster the acquisition of self-knowledge. "The patient seeks self-knowledge for the purpose of changing his feelings and/or his behavior. The therapist, as participant-observer, fosters learning by decoding and interpreting the patient's unconscious messages. As in all sustained and important relationships, some learning or change also occurs as the result of imitation, identification, and various subtle influences. The situation is not (and cannot be) value-free, but the highest premium is placed on the patient's self-determination" (Hollender, M. H. *Archives of General Psychiatry 10*, 1964).

L. R. Wolberg (*The Technique of Psychotherapy*, 1954) distinguished three types of psychotherapy: supportive, reeducative, and reconstructive.

1. *Supportive therapy* consists of encouraging or promoting the development of maximal, optimal use of the patient's assets; its objectives are to strengthen existing defenses, elaborate better mechanisms to maintain control, and restore to an adaptive equilibrium. Included in supportive therapy are guidance, environmental manipulation, externalization of interests, reassurance, pressure and coercion, persuasion, catharsis, desensitization, and inspirational group therapy. (It might be noted that in psychoanalysis the term reassurance has a slightly different meaning: any method of reducing or removing anxiety other than interpretation.)

2. *Reeducative therapy*, which aims at giving the patient insight into the more conscious conflicts, with deliberate efforts at goal modification and maximal utilization of existing potentialities. Included in reeducative therapy are relationship therapy, attitude therapy, psychobiology, counseling, reconditioning, and reeducative group therapy.

3. *Reconstructive therapy*, which aims at giving the patient insight into his unconscious conflicts and extensive alteration of his character structure. Included in reconstructive therapy are psychoanalysis (Freudian), Adlerian and Jungian therapy, object relations therapy, self psychology, the treatment techniques of the cultural-interpersonal school (Sullivan, Horney), and psychoanalytically oriented psychotherapy. See *psychodynamic psychotherapy*.

Another way of classifying the many different forms of psychotherapy is according to the recipient or target of treatment, as in individual psychotherapy, group psychotherapy, family therapy, marital therapy, divorce therapy, etc.

Psychotherapy may also be classified in terms of the theory espoused by the therapist: Freudian, Jungian, Adlerian, Kleinian, Rogerian client-centered therapy, behavior, body-centered, cognitive, existential, Gestalt, multimodal, paradoxical, transactional, transpersonal, Yoga, etc.

**psychotherapy by reciprocal inhibition**    See *behavior theory; behavior therapy*.

**psychotic**    Showing signs of or having the characteristics of severe mental disorder; afflicted with *psychosis* (q.v.). This term has various meanings, and the reader will ordinarily have to depend on context to determine the specific meaning intended by the author. Sometimes the term is used in a quasilegal sense, in which case it is approximately equivalent to the term insane; or it may refer to a patient in an acute episode of psychosis, without reference to competence or other legal issues; or, less commonly, it may refer to a patient with chronic mental disorder, such as schizophrenia, even though he may not be in an acute phase of psychosis and even though he may not be insane in the legal sense.

In DSM-IV, the term denotes the existence of one or more of the following: delusions, hallucinations, incoherence, repeated derailment or loosening of associations, marked poverty of thought, marked illogicality, and grossly disorganized or catatonic behavior.

**psychotic depression**    Melancholia; see *depression, psychotic*.

**psychotic disorder, brief**    Acute psychotic disorder; symptoms of *psychosis* (q.v.), such as delusions, hallucinations, disorganized speech, or catatonic or disorganized behavior, that remit within a month, with full return to the premorbid level of functioning. When such symptoms appear to be in response to severe stressors, they are often labeled "brief reactive psychosis." See *remitting atypical psychosis*.

**psychotic disorders**    In DSM-IV, these include schizophrenia, delusional (paranoid) disorder, and psychotic disorders not elsewhere classified, such as psychotic disorder due to a general medical condition and substance-induced psychotic disorder. Delusional disorder and hallucinosis are combined and subtyped based on whether the symptomatic presentation is predominantly delusional or with hallucinations.

**psychotica**    See *psychotomimetic*.

**psychoticism**    Reality distortion. See *psychomotor poverty; psychotic*.

**psychotogenic**    *Psychotomimetic* (q.v.).

**psychotomimetic** Resembling or mimicking naturally occurring psychosis, especially schizophrenia; also known as psychosomimetic, schizomimetic, hallucinogenic, phantastica. While any number of drugs can produce a psychosis, the term psychotomimetic agent is confined to those substances that produce psychological changes in a high proportion of subjects exposed to the drug without producing the gross impairment of memory and orientation characteristic of the organic reaction type. Among the known psychotomimetics are adrenochrome, bufotenin, DFP (diisopropyl fluorophosphates), *DMT, DOM* (*dimethoxymethylamphetamine*), *harmine*, herbal preparations (mainly belladonna), *LSD* (lysergic acid diethylamide), *MDA* (*methylenedioxyamphetamine*), mescaline, morning glory seeds, *N-allylnormorphine*, peyote, psilocybin, *STP*, and TEPP (tetraethypyrophosphate). Tetrahydrocannabinol (cannabis) may have hallucinogenic effects.

Syndromes associated with psychotomimetic use include abuse, dependence, hallucinosis, post-hallucinogen perception disorder (flashback), mood disorder, and delusional disorder.

**psychotoxicomania** Toxicomania; drug dependence or addiction.

**psychotropic** Psychoactive; phrenotropic; an imprecise term used to describe a drug whose primary effect is on the central nervous system (psychopharmacologic agent). Included are drugs with legitimate application(s) in medicine (particularly psychiatry), as well as drugs of abuse. See *psychopharmacologic agents.*

Some authorities use psychotropic to designate any drug with a high potential for abuse: opiates (or opioids), brain depressants (such as the sedatives/hypnotics and antianxiety agents), psychostimulants, cannabis, nicotine, the volatile inhalants, and miscellaneous intoxicants such as Kava and betel nut.

**psychropophobia** Fear of the cold or of anything cold.

**psychrotherapy** *Obs.* Treatment by the application of cold in any form. It was at one time extensively employed in the form of hydrotherapy as a stimulating agent for inactive or retarded patients, e.g., those with the depressive type of manic-depressive psychosis.

**PT** 1. *Physical Therapy* (q.v.); physiotherapy.

2. *Planum temporale* (q.v.).

3. *Personal Therapy* (q.v.).

**PTA** 1. Parent-teachers association. 2. Post-traumatic amnesia, generally considered to be one of the most sensitive and reliable indices of severity of head trauma.

**pteronophobia** Fear of feathers.

**ptheirophobia** Dread of lice.

**ptosis** Lid-drop. See *oculomotor nerve.*

**ptosis, waking** A functional paralysis of the upper eyelid, occurring temporarily in the anemic or neurotic person on awaking.

**PTSD** *Post-traumatic stress disorder* (q.v.).

**puberal (pubertal)** Relating to the age of puberty, extending from the termination of the period of puerilism to the beginning of the adolescent period.

**puberism, persistent** Hypogenesis and prolongation, or even lifelong persistence, of puberal characteristics. The affected subject seems an eternal adolescent with incompletely developed secondary sexual characteristics in contrast with the types distinguished by *infantilism* or *juvenilism.*

**pubertas praecox** Premature puberty; *macrogenitosomia* (q.v.).

**puberty (puberism)** The period termination of the puerile to the beginning of the adolescent period. It begins with acquisition of secondary sexual characteristics and continues for approximately 2 or 3 years.

**puberty psychosis** *Obs.* Adolescent psychosis; the term implied a condition unique to puberty, but it is now recognized that such a condition does not exist.

**puberty rites** In many primitive cultures it is customary for children at puberty to undergo certain initiatory rites as a part of the religious pattern of that culture. One of the commonest rituals is a pretense of killing the child and bringing him to life again. In another primitive group, part of the proceedings consists of knocking out a tooth and giving a new name to the child being initiated, indicating thereby the change from youth to adulthood. In still another tribe, the puberty rites comprise operations of circumcision and subincision. All of these ceremonies are conducted in absolute secrecy, and only those already initiated may attend them.

**puberty trauma** The painful, disagreeable, or unacceptable experiences that occur during puberty. According to Stekel, such experiences contribute as much to development of neurosis as do traumas suffered in childhood, especially among girls, whose unpleasant sexual experiences can have fateful effects in their later lives (Stekel, W. *The Interpretation of Dreams*, 1943). See *trauma, infantile; trauma, primal*.

**pubescence (pubescency)**   Puberty.

**public health model**   A view of illness and disease whose focus is on epidemiology and the population at risk, not only to assess the incidence and prevalence of disease but also to discover the conditions that produce it. See *medical model; community psychiatry*.

**public policy**   A stated, conscious, and deliberate action (or decision not to take action) on the part of government, usually involving rules and regulations that prohibit or allow certain activity, or the allocation and distribution of social benefits and burdens, such as deciding that specific goods or services will be provided to one segment of the population and that their cost will be borne through taxation of another segment. See *health policy*.

**publication bias**   The greater likelihood that research with statistically significant results will be published compared with research with nonsignificant results. It has been noted that if positive treatment results are given publication preference over negative reslts, an asymmetrical *funnel plot* might be created. A funnel plot displays effect size vs. number of patients enrolled in treatment studies; if negative studies of small numbers are not published because of publication bias, treatment benefits will be exaggerated.

**publishable unit**   See *LPU*.

**pudendum (pudenda, pudibilia)**   Genitals; the private parts.

**puer aeternus**   Jung's term for the specific archetype of the eternal youth. See *archetype* (in Jung's psychology); *mother archetype*.

**puerilism**   Childishness; the stage following infantilism or infantility and followed by the stage of puberism or puberty.

**puerilism, hysterical**   See *pseudodementia, hysterical*.

**puerperal mania**   *Obs.* Postpartum psychosis with manic features. "Where mania really appears in the puerperal state, it is, like every other kind of mania, only a link in the chain of attacks of maniacal-depressive insanity" (Kraepelin, E. *Lectures on Clinical Psychiatry*, 1913).

**puerperal psychosis**   See *postpartum psychosis*.

**puerperium**   The period of time and/or the state of the mother following childbirth. See *postpartum psychosis*.

**Puerto Rican syndrome**   *Fighting sickness; mal de pelea*; a culture-specific syndrome consisting of an initial brooding period followed by agitation and striking out against anyone the subject encounters. The syndrome is similar to the *amok* (q.v.) of other cultures.

**pulse loading**   One or two initial doses of a psychopharmacologic agent, followed by a drug-free interval; for example, beginning treatment by administering the usual therapeutic dose of an antidepressant for 2 days, giving no drug for the next 5 days, then resuming the usual treatment schedule.

**pulvinar**   Nuclear masses that make up most of the posterior portion of the *thalamus* (q.v.); the pulvinar has connections to the visual, auditory, and tactile association areas of the cortex and decodes sensations into meaningful phenomena.

**punch-drunkenness**   A chronic traumatic encephalopathy that develops in many boxers as a result of repeated concussions. Manifestations include tremors of the hand and nodding movements of the head, ataxia (e.g., unsteadiness in gait and uncertainty in equilibrium), slowing in muscular movements and dysarthria, sometimes a flopping or dragging of the foot or leg, impaired memory, confusion, and deterioration of the personality. See *boxer's dementia*.

**punctate hyperalgesia**   A type of central sensitization to pain in which the pain elicited by punctate mechanical stimuli is more prolonged and stronger than normally expercted. *Punctate hyperkinesis* is a type of central sensitization to itch; the itch evoked by punctate mechanical stimuli is more prolonged and stronger than normal.

**pundning**   The stereotyped, purposeless searching and grooming behavior of amphetamine abusers; stereotyped and/or compulsive behavior patterns are found in many species when administered high doses of amphetamines.

**punishment**   See *aversive control; reinforcement; reciprocity*.

**punishment, unconscious need for**   See *criminal from sense of guilt*.

**pupillary reflex**   The alterations in size of the pupil in response to light, convergence, and accommodation. Certain abnormalities of reaction are associated with lesions affecting portions of the pupillary reflex arc.

**pupillotonia**   *Adie syndrome* (q.v.).

**puppy-love**   A state of love in the late adolescent or young adult period, highly romantic in nature, with little stability in the relationship formed, so that the courtship swiftly disintegrates. This is in the nature of a developmental activity, occurring in the course of emotional maturation; another designation for this emotional phenomenon is calf-love.

**Purdue assembly test**   The subject assembles a pin, two washers, and a sleeve into a patterned unit.

**Purdue pegboard test**   The subject places pegs in holes within 30 seconds, first with the right hand, then the left, and finally with both hands simultaneously.

**Pure Autonomic Failure**   *PAF* (q.v.)

**pure line**   A term introduced by the Danish botanist Johannsen to characterize the identical genotypical equipment of an autogamous stock of organisms descended from a common ancestor by self-fertilization.

According to the pure line theory, such organisms will continue to breed true regardless of environmental differences, forming lines genetically pure for all their characters. Whenever such genetic purity has been attained, all differences except newly occurring mutations must be caused by environmental influences and therefore cannot be hereditarily transmitted.

**purging**   Elimination of waste and, in particular, the induction of evacuative mechanisms by pharmacological or mechanical means. Persons who suffer from *anorexia nervosa, binge eating*, or *bulimia nervosa* (qq.v.) typically purge themselves to prevent weight gain (whether they are overweight or not). Vomiting may be induced with emetics or by activating the gag reflex; laxatives, enemas, and diuretics may be abused.

**purinergic signaling**   The most pervasive mechanism for intercellular communication in CNS, affecting communication between many types of neurons, all types of glia, and vascular cells. ATP, a purine, was recognized as a neurotransmitter in 1969, 40 years after its potent effects on heart and blood vessels were first described.

Three phosphate bonds of ATP are readily cleaved by enzymatic hydrolysis to yield ADP, AMP, and adenosine. Each of the products of ATP hydrolysis can activate different types of receptor (19 receptors have been identified). A broad range of purinergic receptors has been found in all major classes of glia, including Schwann cells in PNS and oligodendrocytes, astrocytes, and microglia in CNS.

In addition to its rapid neurotransmitter-like actions in intracellular signaling in neurons and glia, ATP also acts as a growth and trophic factor by regulating the two most important second messengers: cytoplasmic calcium and cAMP. Microglia, the immune cells of the CNS, are activated by purines and pyrimidines to release inflammatory cytokines.

Both adenosine and ATP induce astroglial cell proliferation and the formation of reactive astrocytes. Large amounts of ATP can be released into the extracellular environment when cells are damaged. Astrocytes can sense the severity of damage in the CNS by the amount of ATP released from the cells, and they can modulate the tumor necrosis factor-$\alpha$ (TNF$\alpha$)-mediated inflammatory response. The often antagonistic actions of ATP and adenosine provide a mechanism for glia (and other cells) to have biphasic effects in cellular interactions. This may be an important mechanism for glia in maintaining homeostatic regulation of neural activity.

**Purkinje cell**   (Johannes Evangelista Purkinje, Bohemian physiologist, 1787–1869) The large cells of the *cerebellum* (q.v.) that are its sole output. Their cell bodies (50 to 80 μm) lie just beneath the outermost molecular layer of the cerebellum, which is composed mainly of the axons (*parallel fibers*) of granule cells, which occupy the deepest layer. Purkinje cells are inhibitory and use GABA as their neurotransmitter.

**purpose psychosis**   While all psychiatric states may serve a purpose, usually an unconscious one, there are some (such as the Ganser syndrome) whose motives are quite clear-cut. "The maximum of wish fulfillment is achieved by the ecstasies. These syndromes are also called *purpose psychoses*" (Bleuler, E. *Textbook of Psychiatry*, 1930).

**pursuit dysfunction**   See *SPEM*.

**pursuit eye movements**   Eye tracking; the different movements of the eye that are involved in stabilizing the image of a moving target on the fovea. There are at least seven classes of eye movement; two of them, the *smooth pursuit system* and *saccades* (qq.v.), function interactively during an eye tracking task. Deviant smooth pursuit eye movements may be an indicator of genetic susceptibility to schizophrenia. Eye tracking impairment has been reported in 65% to 85% of schizophrenic patients and in 45% to 50% of their first-degree relatives, as compared with an incidence of 15% in other psychiatric populations and 6% of normal subjects. The fundamental deficit in schizophrenia may be a failure to inhibit the saccade system, resulting in the intrusion of saccades during the smooth pursuit task. See *saccades.*

**pursuit rotor test**    Using a hand stylus, the subject must keep contact with a target on a revolving disk.

**Pussin, Jean-Baptiste**    (1746–1820) Superintendent of Hospice de Bicêtre and the originator of the psychological methods that were the basis of *moral treatment* (q.v.). Although Philippe Pinel is ordinarily given credit for the reforms, Pinel himself repeatedly attributed them to Pussin, who left the Bicêtre in 1802 to help Pinel reorganize the Salpêtrière.

**putamen/caudate nucleus**    Two of the components of the striatum, a subpallidal structure that also includes the nucleus accumbens and the olfactory tubercle. See *basal ganglia.*

**Putnam, James Jackson**    (1846–1918) American psychiatrist; Putnam-Dana syndrome (subacute combined degeneration of the spinal cord).

**PVN**    Paraventricular nucleus of the *hypothalamus* (q.v.). Its two subdivisions are the *parvocellular PVN (pPVN)* and the *magnocellular PVN (mPVN).*

**PVS**    Permanent vegetative state, or persistent vegetative state; the two are not the same. See *vegetative state.*

**pycnic**    See *pyknic type.*

**pycnoepilepsy**    Repeated slight epileptic seizures.

**pycnolepsy**    *Pyknolepsy* (q.v.).

**Pygmalion effect**    Self-fulfilling prophecy, most commonly used in reference to an assumed effect on students of their teachers' expectations of their abilities or potentialities.

**pygmalionism**    (Pygmalion, the legendary king of Cyprus who fell in love with an ivory statue he had carved and asked Venus to give it life; subsequently, the live statue bore him a daughter) The condition of falling in love with one's own handiwork, sometimes manifested as the author's resentment of the editor who would dare to shorten or modify his work. A paranoid patient demonstrated a more severe form in devising a "perpetu-

al-motion" machine to which he ascribed all masculine attributes. The machine was called "Albert" and was treated as a human being to whom the patient vowed his unqualified love.

The term is sometimes applied to the psychotherapist who assumes that his patient knows little or nothing and must be treated as a child, whose parent (the therapist) always knows best. The term has also been applied to a fetishist whose sex object was a dressmaker's dummy.

**pygmyism**    The constitutional anomaly characterized by a *dwarfed*, but well-proportioned stature as compared with the average type of the given racial group. It corresponds to the other special forms of *microsomia*, called *nanosomia primordialis* by Hansemann and *heredofamilial essential microsomia* by E. Levi, and it occurs in certain peoples as a more or less physiological condition (African bushmen, etc.).

**pyknic**    Compact, thick-set, round-bodied.

**pyknic epileptic**    An epileptic with the pyknic type of body build. According to Westphal most epileptics are dysplastic, athletic, or asthenic, and less than 10% are pyknic.

**pyknic type**    In Kretschmer's system the constitutional type, characterized by roundness of contour, amplitude of body cavities, and a plentiful endowment of fat. The face of a pyknic is broad and fleshy, particularly the nose. The neck is short and thick, with the head set a little forward on smoothly rounded shoulders. There is a tendency to baldness, the areas of which are regular in outline and have a smooth shiny surface. The trunk is thick-set and barrel-shaped, with the chest broadening to the lower part of the body. The abdomen is protruding and the xiphoid angle is wide. The limbs are well developed in thickness rather than in length, and the lower extremities, while not actually short, tend to appear short relative to the rest of the body because of their massiveness. The feet are broad and well covered, while the hands are square or broad, with pudgy, fusiform fingers. The skin is warm and moist, with a well-developed fatty layer beneath it.

Pyknics may fall into any one of the three divisions of the *cyclothymes* as distinguished by Kretschmer: (1) the *healthy* cyclothymes (the gay chatterbox, the quiet humorist, the silent good-tempered man, the happy enjoyer of life, the energetic practical man); (2) the *cycloids* (the cheery hypomanic type, the quiet contented type, the melancholic type); and (3) the *manic-depressives*.

The pyknic type corresponds approximately to the following types in other leading systems: the *habitus apoplecticus* of Hippocrates, the *abdominal* and *digestive* types of the French school, the *phlegmatic, boeotic, plethoric venous, choleric* constitutions of Carus, the *hyperplastic* type with a disposition to carcinoma of Rokitansky-Benecke, the *third combination* of De Giovanni, the *brachyskelic (mikroskelic)* type of Manouvier, the *megalosplanchnic* of Viola, the *hypervegetative (brachymorphic)* biotype of Pende, the *arthritic habitus* of Bauer, part of the *hypotonic* group of Tandler, the *hypersthenic* type of Mills, the *wide-chested* type of Brugsch, the *fleshy* type of Davenport, the *mesontomorph* of Beau, the *lateral* type of Stockard, the *broad* type of Aschner, the *B type* of Jaensch, the *euryplastic* type of Bounak, the *endomorphic* type of Sheldon, and part of the *hypercompensatory* type of Lewis.

**pyknoepilepsy**　See *pyknolepsy.*

**pyknolepsy (pycnolepsy)**　A disorder characterized by frequent, brief interruptions in consciousness. In children who are otherwise healthy, it occurs as a rule before the age of 7, as frequent, short, and incompl ete cloudings of consciousness. The onset is usually abrupt, the disease runs a monotonous course without intellectual deterioration and shows little response to therapy, but the prognosis is generally favorable. During attacks, which may be as frequent as 150 times a day, the eyes turn upward, arms and trunk become somewhat tonic; but pulse and respiration are unaffected, there are no convulsive movements, and spontaneous recovery is common.

Lennox used *pyknoepilepsy* (which by many is considered synonymous with pyknolepsy, or *dart and dome dysrhythmia*) for the ordinary petit mal form of *epilepsy* (q.v.).

**pyknophrasia**　Thickness of speech.

**pyramid**　The prominence on the anterior surface of the medulla oblongata where the pyramidal tract decussates. See *pyramidal tract.*

**pyramidal cell**　A projection neuron that carries output from a cortical area; it functions also as an *interneuron* (q.v.) in that it influences local processing through its collateral branches. The pyramidal cells make association connections

(interconnecting neurons in different cortical regions on the same side), callosal connections (interconnecting symmetrical areas of the two hemispheres), and subcortical connections (projecting to the basal ganglia, the brain stem, and the spinal cord). Large pyramidal cells are concentrated in layer 5 of the cortex; their axons descend to the basal ganglia, the brain stem, and the spinal cord. Nonpyramidal cells receive input to the cortex and are involved in the local processing of information; they are concentrated in layer 4 of the cortex, which receives most of the input from the thalamus.

**pyramidal tract**　"The pyramidal fibres or upper motor neurones are the axones of cells of the precentral convolution. Electrical excitation of these cells causes movements of the opposite side of the body. The movements thus excited are not simply contractions of isolated muscles, but always involve groups of muscles contracting harmoniously, so that an orderly movement results. The upper motor neurones therefore are organized in terms of movements, in contrast to the lower motor neurones, which are distributed to groups of muscle-fibres in individual muscles" (Brain, W. R. *Diseases of the Nervous System,* 1951).

**pyrexiophobia**　Fear of fever.

**pyridoxine**　Vitamin $B_6$; its active form, pyridoxal phosphate, is a coenzyme in amino acid metabolism and heme synthesis. Deficiency of pyridoxine may produce dermatitis, glossitis, peripheral neuropathy (burning feet syndrome), optic neuropathy, mood disorder, confusion, and seizures. See *carpal tunnel syndrome.*

**pyrolagnia**　Sexual excitement aroused by the sight of conflagrations; erotic pyromania (fire setting).

**pyromania**　*Fire setting;* pathological arson; monomanie incendiaire; an *impulse control disorder* (q.v.) characterized by deliberate setting of fires, with tension or irritability before the act and gratification or relief once the fire is set. The fire is not set for monetary gain, to express anger or vengeance, to conceal criminal activity, or to improve one's living conditions, nor is it part of a manic episode or in response to a delusion or hallucination. In addition, the typical pyromaniac exhibits a fascination with fires and the paraphernalia associated with using or extinguishing them. Some writers use fire setting as the general term that includes unintended fires (e.g., because of carelessness on the part of a smoker) and arson to refer to deliberately setting fire to property. Both fire setting and arson are termed pathological if the act is secondary to a medical, neurologic, or psychiatric disorder. As so defined, true pyromania (i.e., no co-existing medical, neurologic, or psychiatric disorder) is probably rare. Most fire setters are males, and they have a higher than expected incidence of alcohol abuse and of early antisocial behaviors, such as truancy and running away from home. At one time, the triad of fire setting, enuresis, and cruelty to animals was considered predictive of aggressive antisocial behavior in adulthood, but longer-term studies have failed to support such a relationship. In the United States, over 40% of persons arrested for arson are under 18 years of age. That this may be due largely to the inability of children to escape detection is supported by the finding that arrests are made only in 15% of cases of suspected arson.

Both Stekel and Freud posited a sexual origin to fire setting, emphasizing the similarities between flame and phallus. Others have attributed pyromania to a craving for power, the need of a person who feels inadequate to demonstrate his bravery or courage (the *hero syndrome*), a means of venting rage, or an attempt to induce a father figure to rescue his son by putting out the fire.

**pyromania, erotic**    *Pyrolagnia* (q.v.).

**pyrophobia**    Fear of fire. See *pyromania*.

**pyrosis**    Heartburn.

# Q

**QALY**   Quality-adjusted life year, a measure of disease burden used particularly in treatment outcomes researchin schizophrenia. See *DALY*.

**QEB**   *Quantitative Electrophysiological Battery* (q.v.).

**QI**   Quality improvement; overall, an effort to achieve the best results for any clinical intervention(s). QI uses statistical tools to measure such elements as process stability, variability, and outcomes and a management approach that encourages each participant in the treatment process to identify ways in which the process and its outcome might be improved. QI generally addresses populations rather than individual patients. QI programs aim to improve care on a systemic level; they must continually assess not only the services provided to identified patients but also needs for services that have not yet been developed within a community. It is not enough to find that practitioners have followed clinical guidelines appropriately and effectively; questions about prevention of illness in the first place, the effects of illness and its sequellae on patients, caretakers, and others in the community, and patient (and family) satisfaction must also be addressed. See *quality assurance*.

**qi-gong psychosis**   A brief psychotic reaction with dissociative or paranoid symptoms associated with overinvolvement in the Chinese folk practice of enhancing vital energy (qi-gong).

**Q-sort**   A personality rating technique, developed by William Stephenson (1953), in which statements or phrases about those aspects of personality or performance that are relevant to the needs of the person or organization requesting the rating are written on separate cards. The rater (who may be the subject himself) sorts the cards into II piles, with those most descriptive of the subject in the first pile, those least descriptive in the last pile. Q-sorts are of particular value for obtaining complex, comprehensive descriptions of a single subject, especially since they permit evaluations by multiple raters whose results can be compared.

**QT interval**   The electrocardiographic manifestation of ventricular depolarization and repolarization, measured from the beginning of the QRS complex to the end of the T wave. (Qtc is the QT interval corrected for heart rate.) Normally, rapid inflow of positively charged ions (sodium and calcium) produces myocardial depolarization; repolarization occurs when this inflow is exceeded by outflow of potassium ions. Malfunction of ion channels can lead to inadequate outflow of potassium ions or excess inflow of sodium ions. The resulting intracellular excess of positive charged ions delays ventricular repolarization, manifested as QT interval prolongation (*long QT syndrome*, or *LQTS*). Prolongation of the QT interval predisposes to a potentially fatal ventricular arrhythmia, *torsades de pointes* (q.v.).

**QTL**   *Quantitative trait loci* (q.v.); sometimes used in an adjectival sense to refer to heterogeneity or polygenic traits.

**quadrantanopia, quadrantanopsia**   See *field defect*.

**quadrantic hemianopia**   See *field defect*.

**Quadriplegia**   Tetraplegia; paralysis affecting the four extremities.

**quadrupedal extensor reflex**   Russell Brain described this reflex in organic hemiplegia. It consists in the extension of the hemiplegic flexed arm on the assumption of the quadrupedal position. An additional feature may be the further flexion of the arm if the head is bent forward and extension of the arm if the head is bent back.

**quadruplet**   One of four children born at the same birth. See *birth, multiple*.

**quality assurance**   Quality assessment; measurement and evaluation of services provided, with particular regard for their effectiveness, efficiency, appropriateness, and acceptability; it is generally understood that such evaluation will trigger corrective or remedial action for services that do not meet the desired standards. Quality assessment comprises such parameters as need for care, appropriateness of length of stay (*LOS*) and of site of treatment, adequacy and timeliness of diagnostic evaluation, appropriateness of treatment, and measures of outcome (*medical audit, medical care evaluation* or *MCE*). See *audit; QI; review.*

**quality of life** The core requirements for a desirable quality of life are generally considered to be life itself, liberty, and the pursuit of happiness. In a nursing home, this is expressed in three broad domains: alleviation of illness, protection of autonomy, and provision of opportunity for valued activities. Included are improvements in medical and psychiatic care, reduction of secondary handicaps as far as possible (i.e., those imposed by inevitable treatment and institutional constraints), regard, consideration, defense, and—since financial burdens can be crushing—affordability. Assessment of quality of life requires a multidimensional evaluation, by both intrapersonal and social-normative criteria, of the person-environment system of a person in time past, current, and anticipated.

**quanta** The number of chemical packets (of neurotransmitters, etc.) released by the neuron onto its target cells.

**Quantitative Electrophysiological Battery** *QEB*; a computer analysis of the evoked potentials of the brain as the subject is confronted during a 15- to 50-minute session by a series of changes in his environment (challenges); devised by E. Roy John and his coworkers as part of a methodology they term *neurometrics* (q.v.).

**quantitative trait loci** *QTL*; the locations of the different genes that together govern a trait or characteristic that is not determined by a single gene acting alone. Behavior and behavioral abnormalities caused by a single gene are the exception rather than the rule; behavior is complex and comprises different quantitative traits determined by multiple genes originating from different loci (and often also operating at several loci). The effects of any one gene may account for only a small portion of the trait variance. Recent improvements in *genetic mapping*, such as *RFLPs* and *SSLPs* (qq.v.), have increased the power to detect and map QTLs, even though their individual contribution may be responsible for as little as 5% of the observed variance in a trait.

**quasi-action** See *ludic activity.*

**quasi-independence** The second of Fairbairn's three stages of object relations. The first is infantile dependence: the infant, physically dependent on the breast as a biological object, incorporates and internalizes the breast and fuses with it. The quasi-independence, stage is marked by transitional steps toward independence such as internal representations of objects and extrusion of bad objects. The final stage is mature dependence, with complete differentiation of self from object and relations with whole objects.

**Quasimodo complex** Emotional conflict, personality disorder, or social maladaptation developing as a result of disfigurement or deformity.

**quaternity** Any unit composed by the union of four factors; a group of four. Jung's system of psychology "is based on an archetype that finds its special expression as tetrasomy,' four-foldness—cf. the theory of the four functions, the pictorial arrangement of the four, the orientation according to the four points of the compass, etc. The number four can often be observed in the arrangement of dream contents as well. Probably the universal distribution and magical significance of the cross or the circle divided into four can be explained through the archetypal quality of the quaternity" (Jung, C. G. *The Integration of the Personality*, 1939).

**querulent** Ever suspicious, always opposing any suggestion, complaining of ill-treatment and of being slighted or misunderstood, easily enraged, and dissatisfied with conditions as they exist.

**Quételet, Lambert Adolphe Jacques** (1796–1874) Belgian statistician and astronomer; showed that the distribution of human characteristics such as height could be described by the normal curve. The law was first described in mathematical language by Abraham DeMoivre (1664–1754), a French Huguenot who went into exile in London in 1688. The law was later rediscovered independently by Pierre Simon, Marquis de Laplace (1749–1827), a French mathematician and astronomer (*Théorie analytique des probabilités*, 1812) and Johann Karl Friedrich Gauss (1777–1855), a German mathematician (*Theory of Numbers*, 1801).

**quetiapine abuse** Quetiapine diversion and misuse was first reported in correctional settings, but it occurs in noncorrectional settings as well. Users often refer to the drug as quell, baby heroin, or Susie-Q; it is used orally, intranasally, and intravenously for its sedative and anxiolytic properties. The combination of

IV quetiapine and cocaine, to form a Q-ball, may be used to mitigate the dysphoria associated with cocaine withdrawal and to produce a hallucinogenic effect.

**quid pro quo harassment**   See *harassment, sexual.*

**quiet room**   See *padded cell; restraint.*

**Quincke disease**   (Heinrich Irenaeus Quincke, physician in Kiel, 1842–1922) See *edema, angioneurotic.*

**quintuplet**   One of five children born at the same birth. See *birth, multiple.*

**quisqualate**   See *AMPA.*

# R

**rabbit syndrome** A perioral extrapyramidal movement disturbance associated with prolonged use of neuroleptics, consisting of quickly alternating, regular movements of the oral and masticatory musculature (except for the tongue) along a vertical axis. Often an associated poppinglike sound is produced by the rapid separation of the lips. The movements are more rapid and regular than the chewing movements that may occur in tardive dyskinesia, and the rabbit syndrome ordinarily responds to withdrawal of neuroleptics and antiparkinsonian agents (which may intensify symptoms of tardive dyskinesia).

**rabies** *Hydrophobia* (q.v.); a virus infection of the central nervous system, transmitted by the bite of a rabid animal (dog, jackal, cat, owl, wolf; rarely, horse or cow).

**raccoon eyes sign** Periorbital ecchymoses, suggestive of fracture of the base of the skull. See *Battle sign.*

**race** *Ethnicity*; commonly defined as a social construct incorporating beliefs about language, history, and culture and providing a basis on which social identity, traditions, and politics are built. An earlier genetic theory, universally repudiated, divided the human species into subspecies that were ranked on the basis of skill, intelligence, morality, etc. See *racism.* Repudiation of that earlier theory does not deny, however, that population-based genetic differences do exist, and in genetic research the term "race" is used to describe a social or geographical unit that approximates a genetic grouping. See *ethnology.*

**rachischisis** See *spina bifida.*

**racial memory** *Phylogenetic mneme*; the part of mental life that the neonate possesses, according to Freud (*Moses and Monotheism,* 1939) the archiac heritage of fragments of phylogenetic origin.

**racism** The system that divides life roles and status according to race, assigning to one race the status of inferior, submissive, uneducable laborer, etc., and to another the status of superior, industrious, intelligent, patronizing manager/ruler. In similar fashion, *sexism* views status and role in terms of sex alone, *ageism* in terms of age alone.

Race hatred or *racial prejudice* is considered by many to be a group-related paranoia. Group members are more securely bonded to one another if they can project denigrating, destructive, and disruptive impulses onto targets outside the group instead of onto one another.

**rackets** See *transactional analysis.*

**radial reflex** *Extension reflex of the wrist*; a deep reflex. When the styloid process of the radius is tapped, the wrist extends. This reflex depends upon the radial nerve for its afferents and efferents; its center is $C_{7-8}$.

**radiation** In neurophysiology, the spreading of excitation to adjacent neurons.

**radiation somnolence syndrome** A transient syndrome that develops in some children exposed to radiation (for the treatment of leukemia, for instance). It is caused by radiation-induced demyelinization and appears several weeks after radiation in the form of impaired attention, concentration, and memory, and clouding of consciousness with inability to maintain wakefulness.

**radicalion** See *free radical.*

**radical psychiatry** A revolt against orthodox psychiatry by a splinter group of psychiatrists who, beginning in the 1950s, claimed that classification of mental illness as disease was a fiction created by psychiatrists in collusion with repressive and persecutory governments to rid the state of its unwanted members. Compulsive admission of mental "patients" to state hospitals, they said, set the stage for coercive treatment with mind-altering drugs and convulsive and psychosurgical procedures.

The movement is identified particularly with Michel Foucault in France, R. D. Laing in Great Britain, Franco Basaglia in Italy, and Thomas Szasz in the United States. Laing argued, for instance, that paranoid delusions were an understandable reaction to an inescapable social order. Szasz, along with Scientology's founder L. Ron Hubbard, advocated the arrest and incarceration of psychiatrists for their crimes against humanity.

With neurotransmitter discoveries, twin registries and family studies, and the emergence of cognitive neuroscience, evidence mounted that the major mental illnesses were at least in part biologically based. The radical psychiatry movement began to decline in the 1980s, although some of its arguments against the existing system were taken up by the growing mental health *consumerism movement*, and especially by those who identify themselves as "survivors" of psychiatric treatments. See *radical therapy*.

**radical therapy**  An imprecise term for a group of interventions whose basic theme is that much of what is termed psychiatric illness is in fact a reflection of the subject's relationships to society, and that social problems need social rather than medical solutions. Most such "therapies" rely heavily on peer counseling and self-help networks.

**radiculitis**  Inflammation of the intradural portion of a spinal nerve root prior to its entrance into the intervertebral foramen or of the portion between that foramen and the nerve plexus.

**radioisotopic encephalography**  A measurement of brain function that depends upon the uptake of radioisotopes by different structures in the brain. The isotope is injected at a specific time before the examination, which consists of a scanning of the brain by an isotope-sensitive probe whose intensity of reaction is recorded in graphic form and compared with normal patterns. Positive brain scans (increased focal uptake) are found with some neoplasms, subdural hematoma, arteriovenous malformation, brain abscess, and cerebral infarct.

In addition to the static scan, serial imaging is used to increase accuracy of detection. The dynamic study of arterial, capillary, and venous phases is said to be more specific and more sensitive than the static image. *Nuclear imaging* or *cerebral dynamic imaging* is typically performed as serial 1- to 2-second interval exposures taken for 16 seconds following administration of the radiopharmaceutical. See imaging, brain; *MRI; tomography*.

**radioligands**  See *SPECT*.

**radix**  Nerve root.

**Rado, Sandor**  (1890–1972)  Hungarian-born psychoanalyst; established the first graduate school of psychoanalysis at a U.S. university (Columbia University's College of Physicians and Surgeons) in 1944; *adaptational psychodynamics* (q.v.).

**RAFT1**  See *ATM family*.

**rage**  Fury; violent, intense anger; often used in psychoanalytic writings to emphasize the overpowering and unbridled aspect of infantile anger. See *aggression*.

A particular form of aggression has been described by Kohut and other self psychologists—*narcissistic rage*, which appears in the different forms of self-object transference as a response to deflation of the patient's grandiosity and exhibitionistic displays or to a traumatic disappointment in idealized figures. The response to such self-object failure includes a need for revenge or redress against a narcissistic insult. Unlike normal aggression and anger, it is not satisfied when the insult is ended but seeks to destroy the source of frustration without regard for the damage that may result to the self or others. Because of such disregard for consequences, the state is also referred to as *blind hatred* (q.v.). See *alter-ego transference*.

Narcissistic rage ranges in severity from annoyance to *destructive aggression*; it tends to become chronic as long as the self remains vulnerable, even if it has exacted the desired revenge. This is in contrast to *competitive aggression*, which is satisfied once it has removed the obstacles to realistic, assertive ambitions.

**railway spine**  *Obs. Erichsen disease*; a general term for injuries, real or feigned, to the back or spine, sustained during a railway accident

**rami communicantes**  Branches of the spinal nerves that pass to the sympathetic trunk. The white ramus is present only in thoracic and upper lumbar nerves; the gray ramus is present in all spinal nerves.

**Ramón y Cajal, Santiago**  (1852–1934)  Spanish physician and neuroanatomist who demonstrated that, no matter how close their fibers might be, nerve cells do not join each other; awarded Nobel prize (with the Italian histologist Camillo Golgi) in 1906 for work on the fine structure of the brain.

**Ramona v. Ramona**  A 1994 Napa County (California) Superior Court case in which a father won a jury verdict for $475,000 against his daughter's psychotherapists, on the grounds that they negligently implanted or reinforced false memories of the father's sexual abuse of his daughter when she was a child.

**random**   Uncontrolled, spontaneous, unplanned, occurring by chance. The term is used most commonly in statistics to refer to the choosing of experimental subjects on the basis of chance rather than on the basis of particular selective factors.

**randomized clinical trial (RCT)**   *Controlled clinical trial*; an experimental design in which subjects are randomly assigned either to an experimental group (which receives the treatment under investigation) or to a control group (which receives no treatment or a placebo).

**Rank, Otto**   (1884–1939) Viennese psychoanalyst; birth trauma, will therapy.

**rank**   Position in a series when the components of the series are arranged in order of magnitude; thus a rank, of 20 indicates that the component part is 20th from the top (or bottom) when all components have been arranged in order of size. Because the meaningfulness of any given rank will depend upon the number of component parts in the series, rank is more meaningful if expressed in relative terms as a *percentile rank* (q.v.).

**RAP**   Rapid auditory processing, typically defective in children with *dyslexia* (q.v.). Infant RAP thresholds are the single best predictor of language outcomes at 2 years of age. By 3 years of age, two variables—RAP thresholds obtained at 6 months, and male gender—together predicted 39%–41% of the variance in language outcome. Further, these two variables accurately classified 91.4% of 3-year-old children who scored in the "impaired" range on the Verbal Reasoning scale of the Stanford-Binet intelligence scales (Tallal, P, *Nature Reviews Neuroscience 5: 721–728, 2004*).

**rap sessions**   See *consciousness raising*.

**Rapaport, David**   (1911–1960) Hungarian-born U.S. psychologist; systematizer of psychoanalytic theory; *Emotions and Memory* (1942); *Diagnostic Psychological Testing* (1945–46, with Roy Schafer and Merton Gill); *Organization and Pathology of Thought* (1951).

**rape**   Enforced sexual intercourse without the consent of the victim (partner); in most jurisdictions, neither full intromission nor ejaculation of semen is legally required to constitute rape. It is rare that rape is primarily a sexual act (see *sadism*); rather, it is a crime of *violence* (q.v.).

Most rape victims are adolescent or adult women, although rape can involve victims of all ages and men as well as women. Most rapists are under 30 years of age and are motivated by a need to control and humiliate or to express hatred and revenge against women, not by an uncontrollable sexual urge. Most rapes are planned in advance. Alcohol use (by the rapist or victim or both) is involved in at least two-thirds of cases. More often than not, the victim knows her assailant, they are of the same race, and the rape occurs in the victim's residence.

Contrary to popular misconceptions, it is *not* true that women can be raped only if they want to be; it is not true that only women with "bad" reputations or from the lower social classes are raped; it is not true that women are raped because "they asked for it" by dressing or behaving provocatively. Rape is a physical and emotional trauma for the victim that may have long-lasting consequences. See *date rape; rape trauma syndrome*.

**rape phantasy, anal**   See *anal rape phantasy*.

**rape trauma syndrome**   The range of symptoms that develop in the   victim as a consequence of *rape* (q.v.), commonly divided into an acute stress phase and a reorganization phase.

In the *acute phase*, which may last for 3 to 6 months, typical symptoms include a feeling of exhaustion combined with a sense of disbelief, humiliation, guilt, and shame; phobias, depression, suspiciousness, intrusive thoughts, feelings of inferiority; difficulties in performing in school or at work, or in relating to men; fear of sleeping or being alone; somatic complaints and problems with eating, sleeping, or gastrointestinal functioning. Many victims give up all sex for a time, resuming sexual activity only gradually and perhaps never regaining their previous level of pleasure or comfort in sexual activity. Suicide is a risk in the acute phase, particularly in adolescent victims. Some victims begin serious abuse of alcohol and other drugs at this time.

The *reorganization phase* may last 2 years or more. It may involve deliberate changes in lifestyle, such as moving to a different locale or changing jobs. Particularly in those who delayed seeking treatment following the trauma, depression, anxiety, lowered self-esteem, and sexual dysfunction may persist. See *victimology*.

**raphe nuclei**   See *aminergic pathways*.

**rapid accelerator**   See *acetylation*.

**rapid cycling**   In bipolar disorder, frequent recurrence, often arbitrarily defined as four or more cycles per year.

**rapism**   See *paraphilic coercive disorder*.

**rapist, child**   See *pedophilia*.

**rapport**   A conscious feeling of accord, sympathy, trust, and mutual responsiveness between one person and another; to be differentiated from *transference* (q.v.), an unconscious process.

**rapport, psychological**   In Jung's terminology, *transference* (q.v.).

**rapprochement**   See *separation-individuation*.

**raptus**   A type of action seen in some catatonic schizophrenics consisting of uncoordinated discharge movements that tend to relieve extreme tension. Cataleptic general muscular rigidity is a common form of raptus action.

**Rapunzel syndrome**   See *trichobezoar*.

**RAS**   Reticular activating system. See *reticular formation*.

**Raskin scale**   The Raskin Depression Scale is a rating of the severity of depression based on the patient's report of symptoms and the observations of the clinician of the patient's behavior and of secondary symptoms.

**Rasmussen encephalitis**   A rare, progressive brain disorder of childhood that affects the cortex of one cerebral hemisphere, producing intractable seizures, hemiplegia, and dementia. Pathologically it is characterized by atrophy of the hemisphere and inflammatory changes. It develops within the first decade in previously normal children; anticonvulsants are of limited benefit and the standard treatment is surgical removal of the affected hemisphere. There is some evidence that Rasmussen encephalitis is an autoimmune disorder: affected children demonstrate serum antibodies to GluR3, a glutamate receptor, and reducing serum titers of such antibodies is accompanied by improved neurologic function.

**rate**   In epidemiology, the rate is the level of occurrence of a disease or reaction in relation to a given population, such as 10 cases per 1000 population, or per 10,000, or per 100,000. See *incidence*; *prevalence*.

**rate code model**   The long-held hypothesis that the information content of a *neuron* (q.v.) is contained solely in its firing rate (i.e., the number of action potentials it sends down its axon in any given period), and that any single neuron codes for the presence of only a single stimulus property. The timing of each change in firing rate would indicate when an event occurred, and the strength of the increase might report how strong the stimulus was. But the "what" of the stimulus would be the same; any single neuron could code for the presence of only a single stimulus property. A more recent theory is the *temporal code model* (q.v.).

Recent studies suggest that the brain encodes information not just in the firing rates of individual neurons, but also in the patterns in which groups of neurons work together, forming ensembles that fire in relative *synchrony* for brief periods. After such periods, some neurons drop out of synchrony, perhaps to join another ensemble. The changing patterns of synchrony correlate with specific behaviors. Although the theory is far from proven, synchrony may determine not only how the brain perceives stimuli—for instance, as parts of the same object—but even whether it perceives them at all.

**rate of first admissions**   The rate of first admissions (i.e., to hospitals for mental disease) is the ratio of all first admissions within a year to the average general population during that year. Between 1922 and 1950, there was a definite increase in mental disease in the United States as a whole, and in New York State. But as shown in the following table (adapted from Malzberg, B. in *American Handbook of Psychiatry*, ed. S. Arieti, 1959), that increase was due not to any great increase in the incidence of functional psychoses, but rather to a great increase in the number of first admissions diagnosed cerebral arteriosclerosis or senile brain disorders. (Current rates are not comparable because of the effects of deinstitutionalization policies, the availability of psychopharmacologic agents, and preadmission diversion of potential inpatients—all of which have been introduced since 1950.)

In general, both in the United States and Europe, males exceed females in the incidence of schizophrenia, organic brain disorders (except for the senile and presenile psychoses), and alcoholism, while females lead in manic-depressive disorders, neuroses, psychopathy, and senile and presenile psychoses.

**NEW YORK STATE FIRST ADMISSIONS PER 100,000 POPULATION**

|  | MALE | FEMALE | TOTAL | % OF TOTAL |
| --- | --- | --- | --- | --- |
| 1922 | 69.3 | 61.0 | 65.1 | 100 |
| 1950 | 109.9 | 102.4 | 106.0 | 100 |
| Cerebral arteriosclerosis |  |  |  |  |
| 1922 | 6.6 | 4.3 | 5.4 | 8.3 |
| 1950 | 24.6 | 20.4 | 22.4 | 21.1 |
| Senile brain disorders |  |  |  |  |
| 1922 | 4.9 | 8.0 | 6.4 | 9.8 |
| 1950 | 12.9 | 19.4 | 16.3 | 15.2 |
| Paresis |  |  |  |  |
| 1922 | 12.6 | 2.9 | 7.7 | 11.8 |
| 1950 | 3.8 | 1.4 | 2.6 | 2.0 |
| Alcoholic psychoses |  |  |  |  |
| 1922 | 3.6 | 0.7 | 2.2 | 3.4 |
| 1950 | 11.0 | 3.2 | 7.0 | 6.7 |
| Manic depressive psychosis |  |  |  |  |
| 1922 | 6.8 | 12.1 | 9.4 | 14.4 |
| 1950 | 1.9 | 3.1 | 2.5 | 2.3 |
| Schizophrenias |  |  |  |  |
| 1922 | 19.2 | 16.3 | 17.8 | 27.4 |
| 1950 | 31.5 | 31.0 | 31.2 | 29.1 |

**ratification theory**   See *thank-you theory*.

**rational**   Reasoning, sensible. From the standpoint of Jung, "The rational is the reasonable, that which accords with reason. I conceive reason as an attitude whose principle is to shape thought, feeling, and action in accordance with objective values" (*Psychological Types*, 1923)

"Thinking and feeling are rational functions in so far as they are decisively influenced by the motive of reflection. They attain their fullest significance when in fullest possible accord with the laws of reason. The irrational functions, on the contrary, are such as aim at pure perception, e.g., intuition and sensation; because, as far as possible, they are forced to dispense with the rational (which presupposes the exclusion of everything that is outside reason) in order to be able to reach the most complete perception of the whole course of events." (ibid.).

**rational psychology**   Any system of psychology in which a priori assumptions (usually of a philosophical or theological nature) form the background into which any observed facts must be fit.

**rational psychotherapy**   *Rational-emotive therapy (RET)*; a type of cognitive behavior therapy in which the patient learns to identify the irrational, self-defeating beliefs, emotions, and attitudes that block the development of potential abilities and provoke conflict with the environment. It is said to have been first used by Albert Ellis in 1955. RET is an action-oriented, problem-solving approach that employs a variety of experiential techniques—including direct confrontation and emotional focusing—to emphasize the person's responsibility for creating his or her own problems and disturbances in living.

**rational type**   According to Jung, there are four basic psychological types—the thinking, feeling, intuitive, and sensational. He calls the first two *rational* types, characterized by the supremacy of the reasoning and the judging functions. The second two (intuitive, sensational) are termed *irrational* because their actions are based on simple happenings and the intensity of their perceptions rather than on reasoned judgment.

**rationalism**   A philosophy which espouses the belief that the mind exhibits powers of reasoning which it imposes upon the world of sensory experience; *empiricism*, in contrast, believes that mental processes either reflect, or are constructed on the basis of, external sensory impressions. Both Plato and Descartes embraced the rationalist pole. Behaviorists have clung to empiricism, while cognitivists are likely to embrace some form of rationalism.

Rene Descartes, the prototypical philosophical antecedent of cognitive science, developed a method of systematic doubt, and upon his capacity to doubt and, therefore, to think, Descartes discerned a secure foundation on which to build a new philosphy. He believed mind to be central to human existence; it stands apart from and operates independently of the human body, a totally different sort of entity. In the process of trying to explain the interaction of mind and body, he became in effect a physiologically oriented psychologist: he devised models of how mental states could exist in a world of sensory experience. He even proposed one of the first "information-processing" devices.

A recurrent theme in philosophy that continues to the present day is the tension between rationalism and empiricism. After Descartes, the initial responses (by John Locke, David Hume, and George Berkeley) were empirical, asserting that sensory experience is the only reliable source of knowledge. Immanuel Kant, in his *Critique of Pure Reason* (1781), strove to synthesize the rationalist and empiricist points of view. He saw the mind as an active organ of understanding which molds and coordinates sensations and ideas, transforming the chaotic multiplicity of experience into the ordered unity of thought.

In the 20th century, the epistemologists Alfred North Whitehead and Bertrand Russell sought to derive all of mathematics from the basic laws of logic. They wanted to discredit the synthetic a priori notion of mathematical knowledge as being dependent upon experience, and tried to approach human sensory experience with the methods of logical empiricism.

Ludwig Wittgenstein, in his *Tractatus* (1961) tried to demonstrate a logical structure implicit in language, and his thought was a pivotal ingredient of the program of philosophy adopted by the "Vienna circle" of logical empiricists in the period between the world wars—Herbert Feigl, Otto Neurath, Morris Schlick, and especially Rudolf Carnap.

Ongoing work in the cognitive sciences is framed within the context of logical empiricism: a *syntax*—a set of symbols and the rules for their concatenation—that might underlie the operations of the mind, and a correlative discomfort with issues of mental content.

**rationality** According to Culver and Gert (1982), there are two classes of rationality: (1) *required*—that which it would be irrational not to do, or believe, or desire; (2) *allowed*—that which it would not be irrational not to do, or believe, or desire. Whatever is not irrational is rational, either rationally allowed or rationally required.

**rationalization** A term introduced into psychoanalysis by Ernest Jones. It means justification, or making a thing appear reasonable, when otherwise its irrationality would be evident. It is said that a person covers up, justifies, rationalizes an act or an idea that is unreasonable and illogical. For example, when a dehypnotized subject obeys a command received while under hypnosis and of which he is not consciously aware, and then proceeds to give a specious explanation for his act, he resorts to rationalization. Had he been commanded under hypnosis to remove his shoes, when the hypnotic stage has ended he would begin to take off his shoes, explaining

that they are too tight, or there are pebbles in them, or some other explanation that has the appearance of rationality.

"Rationalization is a *screening* process, intended to cover a flaw in repression, e.g. to cover ideas or actions which are intended to gratify an unconscious need" (Glover, E. *The Technique of Psycho-Analysis*, 1955).

**rationalize** To invent a reason for an attitude or action, the motive of which is not recognized.

**Rat-Man** The patient reported on by Freud in a 1909 paper, "Notes upon a Case of Obsessional Neurosis," so called because of the experience that was the direct occasion of his consulting a psychiatrist: on military maneuvers he had heard a story of a type of punishment used in the Far East, the punishment consisting of overturning a pot of rats onto the buttocks of the prisoner so that the rats would bore their way into his anus.

**Raven's Progressive Matrices** A nonverbal test of inductive reasoning in which participants are required to discern the relationship between complex shapes, usually in more than one dimension. The subject must choose from a set of pictures the one that will complete a design that is lacking a part; the designs become progressively more difficult as they are presented.

**Ray, Isaac** (1807–1981) American psychiatrist; mental hygiene; forensic psychiatry; one of the founders of the American Psychiatric Association.

**RBD** *REM behavior disorder* (q.v.).

**rCBF** Regional cerebral blood flow. See *imaging, brain*.

**RCT** Randomized controlled trial.

**RCZ** Rostral cingulate zone; an extensive part of the posterior medial frontal cortex that includes areas 6, 8, 24, and 32. RCZ and lateral prefrontal cortex are consistently associated with regulation of cognitive control and *performance monitoring* (including error monitoring and conflict monitoring).

**RDC** *Research Diagnostic Criteria* (q.v.). See *SADS*.

**reaction** Counteraction; response to a stimulus.

**reaction formation** *Reversal formation*; "The development in the ego of conscious, socialized attitudes and interests which are the antithesis of certain infantile unsocialized trends which continue to persist in the unconscious" (Healy et al. *The Structure and Meaning of Psychoanalysis*, 1930).

Reaction formation is a form of defense against urges that are unacceptable to the ego. It is one of the earliest of the defense mechanisms and one of the most fragile. There is always the danger in reaction formation of a return of the repressed impulse to consciousness.

Reaction formation is a type of repression, but it is distinguished from the latter by two features: (1) in reaction formation, the counter-cathexis is manifest in the form of the denying attitude, thus the necessity for often repeated secondary repressions is avoided; and (2) the counter-cathexis is constantly manifested as a change of personality rather than a momentary arousal of defensive maneuvers in response to an immediate danger.

In a sense, the superego is a reaction formation of the ego, a complicated reaction to the oedipus complex. When fully developed, the superego in turn stimulates the ego to further reaction formations. The ego is forced to change its structure according to internal and external needs. Such reaction formations contribute extensively to the final structure of the character. Two commonly observed reaction formations are disgust (a reaction formation of the ego to an oral sexual impulse) and shame (a reaction formation to exhibitionistic impulses).

Reaction formation is an unconscious defense mechanism of the ego; conscious dissimulation or hypocrisy is not reaction formation. Further, reaction formation is not to be confused with sublimation; in the former, the unconscious impulse is repressed, and the constant countercathexis required to maintain such constant repression drains off energy that would otherwise be available to the ego. In sublimation, on the other hand, the original impulse is superseded and its energy remains available to the ego for the fulfillment of its various tasks. Although reaction formation can be seen as an element of any neurosis or psychosis, it is a typical mechanism of obsessive-compulsive disorder.

**reaction time**   Length of delay between application of stimulus and appearance of response. In word association tests, a long reaction time signalizes a complex.

**reaction type**   A syndrome described in terms of the preponderating or essential symptoms. Adolf Meyer, for example, described six reaction types: organic, delirious, affective, paranoiac, substitutive, and deteriorated.

**reactive**   Secondary to, resulting from, or precipitated by an identifiable happening; thus, a depressive episode following the death of a loved one could be termed reactive depression. In general, reactive episodes—be they depressive, manic, or schizophrenic in nature—carry a more favorable prognosis than those which arise endogenously and without apparent relationship to adversity or trauma in the patient's life. This fact has favored a regrettable equating of "reactive" with "nonpsychotic" or "neurotic," even though it is well known that the same patient can have both reactive and endogenous episodes in the course of a recurrent or relapsing psychosis.

**reactive aggression**   Also, *hostile/reactive aggression*; *defensive aggression* (more often applied to animals than to humans); aggressive behavior that takes place within the context of associated anger and high emotionality. Hostile aggression is described as less controlled and more impulsive than instrumental or proactive aggression; often it arises as a defensive reaction to some perceived frustration, insult, or provocation. See *aggression*; *instrumental aggression*.

**reactive confusion**   See *confusional state, acute*.

**reactive depression**   A depressive state that is directly occasioned by some external situation and relieved when the external situation is removed. A mother, intensely joyous at the expectation of rejoining her children after a long absence abroad, was held by federal authorities until the legality of her admission to the country was established. She remained acutely depressed until a decision favorable to her was rendered.

Some use this term synonymously with psychoneurotic depressive reaction, depressive neurosis, or dysthymic disorder.

**reactive epilepsy**   *Reflex epilepsy* (q.v.), in which the attacks are precipitated by irritation of a scar or some other pathological focus.

**reactive oxygen species**   *ROS;* see *free radical*; *neurotoxicity*.

**reactive psychosis**   *Situational psychosis;* a psychosis believed to be instigated principally by an environmental condition. "One class of the psychoses shows itself as a morbid reaction to an affect experience, as a prison psychosis to a confinement, and an hysterical twilight state to a jilting on the part of the beloved" (Bleuler, E. *Textbook of Psychiatry*, 1930).

Currently, the term is often used to refer to functional psychoses that are neither schizophrenic nor primarily affective or to schizophrenic "episodes" with a good prognosis (in contrast to process or nuclear schizophrenia). Such psychoses with favorable outcome and little genetic evidence of any major relationship to schizophrenia are described under various labels: *schizophreniform states* (G. Langfeldt; Lunn), the *pseudoschizophrenias* (Ruemke), *acute delusional psychoses* or *bouffées délirantes* (by the French), *cycloid psychoses* (K. Leonhard), *atypical psychoses* (Mitsuda), and the *acute schizophrenia reactions* within the schizophrenia spectrum described by S. Kety. See *process psychosis; remitting atypical psychosis.*

**reactive thought**    See *reactive reinforcement.*

**readiness potential**    *CNV* (q.v.).

**reading disabilities**    The term includes a variety of clinical entities of apparently different etiology and treatment need; see *developmental disorders, specific; dyslexia.*

"In our total caseload, which now numbers some 250 children and adolescents, we have been impressed with the emergence of three major groups:

"1. Those in whom the reading retardation is due to frank brain damage manifested by gross neurologic deficits. In these cases there are clearly demonstrable major aphasic difficulties, and they are similar to adult dyslexic syndromes. An example is that of a 9-year-old boy who sustained a severe head injury with prolonged coma, followed by a right hemiparesis and expressive aphasia.

"2. Those with no history or gross clinical findings to suggest neurologic disease but in whom the reading retardation is viewed as primary. The defect appears to be in basic capacity to integrate written symbols. On the basis of findings to be presented later in this paper a neurologic deficit is suspected and, because the defect is basic or biologic in its origin, we have called these cases *primary reading retardation.*

"3. Those cases demonstrating reading retardation on standard tests but in whom there appears to be no defect in basic reading learning capacity. These children have a normal potential for learning to read but this has not been utilized because of *exogenous* factors, common among which are anxiety, negativism, emotional blocking and limited schooling opportunities. We diagnose these cases as *secondary reading retardation*" (Rabinovitch, R.

et al. *Research Publications, Association for Nervous and Mental Diseases 34*, 1954).

Failure to distinguish between these major types of reading disability has led to confusion among workers in the field, and innumerable terms have been coined to describe various types of reading defects, many terms frequently referring to the same concept. Among such terms currently in use are word-blindness, congenital symbolamblyopia, congenital typholexia, congenital alexia, amnesia visualis verbalis, congenital dyslexia, developmental alexia, analfabetia partialis, bradylexia, strephosymbolia, constitutional dyslexia, and specific dyslexia.

In the primary group described above, "the defect appears to be part of a larger disturbance in integration. Our findings suggest that we are dealing with a developmental discrepancy rather than an acquired brain injury. The specific areas of difficulty manifested in the clinical examinations are those commonly associated with parietal and parietal-occipital dysfunction" (ibid.).

**reading disorder**    *Dyslexia* (q.v.).

**reading epilepsy**    A type of *reflex epilepsy* (q.v.) in which the affected person has the sensation of his jaw snapping or opening when he reads; if he continues to read once the myoclonic jaw movements appear, a generalized convulsion is likely to occur.

**reading retardation**    A term suggested by Rabinovitch et al. (1954) to describe all subjects in whom the level of reading achievement is 2 years or more below the mental age obtained in performance tests. See *reading disabilities.*

**readmission**    A person admitted or entered on the rolls more than once to any institution of a given class (e.g., mental hospitals). Until the 1950s, the number of hospitalized mental patients increased each year in most states. In New York State, for example, the resident population of state hospitals doubled between 1929 and 1955, at which time a peak of 93,300 patients was reached. That upward trend was abruptly halted and inverted into a decline coincident with the use of tranquilizing drugs, which more than any other single factor made possible an increasing discharge rate. To some extent this has been balanced by an increasing readmission rate, since patients enabled to be discharged earlier than previously may require more frequent periods of rehospitalization. For some groups of patients, a pattern of early admission/speedy discharge/readmission(s) seems to have been established; such a pattern is often referred to as the *revolving door* phenomenon.

**readout**   See *memory.*

**real anxiety**   Anxiety produced by actual danger in the external world of reality; *Realangst.*

**real pride**   See *domesticated pride.*

**real self**   See *actual self.*

**reality**   The whole of the objective world, embracing all that may be perceived by the five senses.

**reality confrontation**   See *social therapy.*

**reality discrimination**   Ability to differentiate between one's internal, mental, or private events and external, publicly observable events. Hallucinators appear to be deficient in such ability.

**reality ego**   That part of the ego formed by the introjection of external objects. When the objects of reality are pleasurable they are absorbed by (introjected into) the *ego* (q.v.). Hence an object of reality, incorporated into the ego, helps to constitute that part of the ego known as reality ego.

The ego absorbs both painful and pleasurable objects, but it separates them, retaining the pleasurable to form the *pleasure ego* and projecting the painful back into the outer world as a hostile object. The purified pleasure ego is that stage in the development of the ego in which anything unpleasant is considered non-ego, and anything pleasant is considered ego. The purified pleasure ego strives to reverse the separation of ego from non-ego, thus expressing a longing for the original objectless state of affairs. By swallowing anything pleasant, the infant adjoins pleasurable stimuli to the ego and attempts to make parts of the external world flow into the ego. By "spitting out" anything painful, the infant adjoins unpleasant stimuli to the non-ego and puts unpleasant sensations into the external world.

**reality orientation**   A type of *remotivation* (q.v.), particularly useful for patients who are confused or disoriented from any cause. The patient is helped to regain his sense of identity by repeated reminders of who he is, where he is, the day of the week, the month of the year, what meal comes next, and similar basic information. The patient is thus oriented to his own identity and is taught to interact appropriately with others. "A successful reality orientation program requires a number of conditions: a calm environment, a set routine, clear but not necessarily loud responses to patients' questions with the same type of questions asked of the patients, clear directions and assistance in directing or guiding patients to and from their destinations if they need it, constant reminders of the date and time, interruption of the patients who start to ramble in their speech or actions, firmness when necessary, sincerity, requests of patients in a calm manner, and consistency" (Phillips, D. F. *Hospitals 47*, 1973).

**reality principle**   The reality principle, while entering into the service of the pleasure principle, causes the latter to be appreciably modified to conform with the demands of the outside world. "The *Nirvana*-principle expresses the tendency of the death-instincts, the *pleasure*-principle represents the claims of the libido and that modification of it, the *reality*-principle, the influence of the outer world" (Freud, S. *Collected Papers*, 1924–1925)

**reality system**   See *ego stability.*

**reality testing**   A fundamental ego function that consists of objective evaluation and judgment of the world outside the ego or self. Reality testing depends upon the simpler ego functions of perception and memory and upon differentiation between ego and non-ego. Reality testing provides the ego with a mechanism for handling both the external world and its own excitation, for it makes it possible for the ego to anticipate the future in the imagination. External objects represent a threat to the ego and/or potential gratification, and the ego can best protect itself against threats and can secure maximal gratification by using reality testing to judge reality objectively and direct its actions accordingly. See *basic trust.*

A stage of primary hallucinatory wish fulfillment precedes the development of reality testing, and a counterpart of the former is the ability to deny unpleasant parts of reality. As reality testing develops along with the acquisition of speech and thinking proper, such wholesale falsification of reality becomes impossible. Development of speech initiates a decisive step in the development of reality testing, since connecting words and ideas makes thinking possible. Thinking is an anticipatory acting out done with reduced energy.

The faculty of speech changes archaic prelogical thinking (*primary process*, q.v.) into logical and orderly (secondary process) thinking. With the arrival of speech and logical thinking, a final differentiation of conscious and unconscious is made. Now prelogical thinking will be used as a substitute for logical thinking only when the latter cannot master unpleasant reality.

Serious and important denials, then, are seen only in very early childhood and in pathological conditions such as psychosis, where the ego has been weakened by narcissistic regression. Projection, too, can be used extensively only when reality testing is seriously impaired, as in psychosis, or when adequate demarcation between ego and non-ego has not yet been achieved, as in childhood. Only when the boundaries between ego and non-ego are blurred can the ego ward off the unpleasant by "spitting it out" and feeling it as being outside the ego.

Neurotics do, however, show some impairment of reality testing at least to the extent that warded-off impulses and their derivatives interfere with differentiated thinking and block the ego's capacity to organize its experiences, and insofar as present-day objects become mere transference representations of past objects and are reacted to with inappropriate and anachronistic feelings.

The maturing ego must not only postpone action, but on occasion it must inhibit action completely. Thus, the ego develops reactions of *defense* (q.v.) against instinctual demands (countercathexis). There are various reasons for the development of these defenses: (1) instinctual demands that cannot be satisfied become traumatic in themselves; (2) prohibitions from the outside world, through education, experience, etc.; (3) the danger is phantasied because of a projective misunderstanding of the world; (4) the ego becomes dependent upon the superego (which has meanwhile developed), and anxiety is transformed into guilt. See *ego stress.*

**reaper**    See *apoptotic pathway.*

**reason**    See *motive.*

**reasoning**    Deducing new knowledge from old knowledge.

**reasoning mania**    Folie du doute, doubting mania.

**reassignment, surgical**    Sex change operation; the use of surgical procedures to change the external genitalia and secondary sexual characteristics from the biological sex of the transsexual to those of the opposite sex. Males seek sex reassignment more frequently than do females (estimates of the ratio range from two to eight males for every one female).

**reassociation**    A process of renewed or refreshed association occurring in hypnoanalysis of the war neurosis, during which the patient relives the traumatic event with emotional vividness. Such forgotten experiences will then become a part of his normal personality and consciousness.

**reassurance**    A type of supportive psychotherapy.

**rebirth phantasy**    See *womb phantasy.*

**rebound, behavioral**    See *amphetamines.*

**rebound insomnia**    Worsening of sleep beyond the baseline level of insomnia following immediately upon discontinuation of medication that was used to treat the insomnia in the first place. The rebound period is usually brief—sometimes no more than one night—but when it occurs, patients typically misinterpret it as an indication for continuing or increasing medication. See *benzodiazepine.*

**rebound phenomenon of Gordon Holmes**    (British physician, 1876–1965) A test for ataxia, specifically illustrating the loss of cerebellar "check" on coordinated movement; if an attempt is made to extend the flexed forearm against resistance and suddenly let go, the hand or fist flies unchecked against the mouth or shoulder.

**recall**    See *memory.*

**recall memory**    Evocative memory. See *memory; object constancy.*

**recapitulation, pubertal sexual**    The concept that the successive stages in the development of adult sexuality recapitulate those of infantile sexuality. The development of adult sexuality begins with puberty and is normally completed somewhere between the ages of 16 and 21. The developmental stages of adult sexuality "repeat" those of infantile sexuality, and rarely are conflicts found that have not had their forerunners in the earlier development. While it is true that conflicts in adolescent sexual development that have not had their forerunners in infantile sexual development are rarely encountered, nevertheless "experiences in puberty may solve conflicts or shift conflicts into a final direction; moreover, they may give older and oscillating constellations a final and definitive form." (Fenichel, O. *The Psychoanalytic Theory of Neurosis*, 1945).

**receiving type**   See *assimilation*.

**recency effect**   See *memory training*.

**receptive**   Passive, accepting, dependent. See *receptive character*.

**receptive aphasia**   Fluent aphasia, such as *Wernicke aphasia* (q.v.).

**receptive character**   A type described by Fromm; such a person is passive, dependent, clinging, and compliant. This type is similar to the passive-oral or passive-dependent type of other writers. See *character defense*.

**receptive dysphasia**   See *developmental dysphasia*.

**receptive field**   The limited domain of the memory environment to which a given sensory neuron is responsive, such as a limited frequency band in audition or a limited area of space in vision. See *receptor sheet, peripheral*.

**receptor complex, supramolecular**   The association of two or more receptor groups in a functional unit, the net result of which is typically to enhance the effects of activation of one or both receptor groups. One well-known example is the benzodiazepine-GABA receptor complex, consisting of functional and structural coupling of the benzodiazepine receptor to the GABA receptor. By itself, GABA receptor activation inhibits neuronal excitability by increasing the permeability of the neuronal membrane to chloride ions. Benzodiazepines markedly potentiate that effect by increasing the frequency of GABA-mediated openings of chloride channels. It has been postulated that the benzodiazepine-GABA receptor complex is the common site of action of all anxiolytic drugs.

**receptor sheet, peripheral**   The body surface and other areas (e.g., retina, cochlea) that have the ability to respond to external stimuli. The location within the receptive sheet in which a sensory receptor transduces stimuli is termed its *receptive field*. In many areas of the nervous system that receive sensory projection, inputs are mapped so that placements within the periphery are preserved within the central nervous system. The map does not copy exactly the topography of peripheral organization but instead reflects the relative importance of the area to the perceptive apparatus (thus, the tips of the thumb and forefinger occupy a much larger part of the somatosensory cortex than does the middle of the back).

The mapping of inputs is termed *somatotopy* for the somatic sensory system, *retinotopy* for the visual system, and *tonotopy* for the auditory system.

**receptor specificity**   See *code, labeled line*.

**receptors, distance**   The visual and auditory apparatus, as contrasted with *proximal receptors* (touch, taste, smell). Schizophrenic children typically avoid distance receptors and prefer the use of proximal receptors, the reverse of the normal situation. As a result of avoidance of distance receptors, such children often have a glassy, nonseeing stare; they seem to look through others rather than at them, and often cannot meet the direct gaze of the examiner.

**receptors, proximal**   See *receptors, distance*.

**recessive**   In genetics, the opposite of *dominant* (q.v.).

**recessiveness**   The meaning of this genetic term is best understood as the mirror image of *dominance* (q.v.); a recessive factor remains *hidden* as an independent genetic entity, as long, and as far, as it is covered by the dominant member of a given allelic pair of hereditary factors.

A recessive character can be phenotypically manifested only in a *homozygous* condition when it is inherited by a hybrid from both parents. In the case of a single-recessive cross, this is true in 25% of the entire hybrid generation.

In the recessive or *indirect* mode of inheritance, as a rule, the heterozygotes are germinally affected, but phenotypically healthy. Since a recessive trait can appear only in the phenotype of a homozygote, all trait carriers must be homozygous. The occurrence of such a trait among the offspring is not possible, unless both parents are at least heterozygotes. The probability of a union between two recessive trait carriers (heterozygotes) is clearly the greater the more frequent this recessive trait is in the general population. The probability is the greatest in the cases of intermarriage between blood relations, unless the trait in question is very common in the normal average population. Apart from this particular instance of cousin marriages, the direct transmission of a recessive trait is the exception and the indirect inheritance through the collateral lines is the rule.

**recidivism**   Repetition of delinquent or criminal acts by the same offender who is called, accordingly, a recidivist or repeater. Less commonly, recidivism is used to refer to relapse or recurrence of a psychiatric disorder. See *schizophrenia, recidives in.*

*Victim recidivism* refers to involvement of the same subject more than once as a victim in the same type of crime; surveys of victims of violent crime and of rape indicate that approximately one-quarter were prior victims of violent crime or rape. See *traumatophilic diathesis.*

Differences in recidivism rate for psychiatric patients appear to depend on a combination of *gatekeeper variables* (number and length of previous admissions, severity of disorder) and *pathway variables* (age, sex, social class, number of dependents). Some types of patients, such as the elderly, women, and those with few or no dependents, tend to have a high risk of readmission regardless of the severity of their problems. Patients tend to have long stays because of the severity of their problems.

**reciprocal altruism** See *kin selection.*

**reciprocal determinism** A tenet of social learning theory, that behavior is a result of the interplay between cognitive and environmental factors. People learn by observing others and imitating their actions (*modeling*), and negative behavior patterns can be suppressed or eliminated by having a person learn different ways of behaving from other people (*role models*). See *behavior modeling; modeling.*

**reciprocal inhibition psychotherapy** See *behavior theory.*

**reciprocal insanity** Parsons's term for psychosis of association. See *induced psychotic disorder.*

**reciprocal regulation** A style of pathological mothering described by J. MacMurray (*Psychiatric Annals 6*, 1976) in which the mother's oversolicitude controls the child's ability to think, test reality, and incorporate new ideas, but the child's behavior in turn controls the mother's self-esteem. See *mother-child relationship; smother love.*

**reciprocity** Interchange involving mutual giving and taking; also, the combination of altruistic *punishment* and altruistic rewarding, regarded as crucial in the evolution of human cooperation. People derive satisfaction from punishing norm violations, and such altruistic punishment is associated with activation of brain areas related to reward processing, such as prefrontal cortex, thalamus, and the superior and inferior colliculi. See *reward.*

**reciprocity, negative** A communication pattern in which angry or hostile displays of affect on the part of one domestic partner appear to elicit increased displays of anger on the part of the other. It is a pattern of repetitive, rigid, and escalating displays of anger and other negative affect, characterized by a conversion of affective confrontation into physical confrontation.

**reciprocity, overadequate-inadequate** See *family psychotherapy.*

**recognition** See *nonrecognition; parietal lobe; prosopagnosia; temporal lobe.*

**recognition memory** Stimulus familiarity. See *memory; object constancy.*

**recognition site** See *neurotransmitter receptor; synapse.*

**recognitory memory** See *evocative memory; object constancy.*

**recollections, early** See *memory.*

**recombinant DNA** 1. Genetic material (deoxyribonucleic acid) that has been transferred from one organism (human or animal; in Cohen and Boyer's original experiment, from a toad) to another (the host cell, typically a bacterium such as *E. coli*). The foreign DNA is sectioned from the donor organism by *restriction enzymes* (*endonucleases*) and combines with the DNA fragments from a vector, usually a bacterial virus (*bacteriophage*) or *plasmid* (circular bacterial DNA). In multiplying, the host bacterium faithfully copies the genetic message of the insert DNA and thus is able to produce antigens, antibodies, interferon, hormones, etc., or can provide a normal gene when one is deficient or lacking. See *splicing, gene.*

In the current methods of creating desired proteins, genetically altered bacteria are placed in vats of nutrient broth where they multiply rapidly to produce the protein dictated by the foreign gene.

2. Crossing of two inbred strains to produce a new line, an *RI strain* (q.v.).

**recombination** In genetics, the process by which a pair of homologous chromosomes physically exchanges sections, yielding a new combination of genes. Chromosomes arrange themselves so that segments which are alike line up, and some of the segments trade places. The result is recombinaton, a means in all species of stirring the genetic pot and creating diversity. See *crossing-over; linkage.*

Duplications occur when there is an abnormality in the cross-over process. In some recombinations, one chromosome gives up a bigger piece of DNA than it gets from its partner; the unequal crossing-over results in a duplication on one chromosome and a deletion on the other. If either one gets into a sperm or egg, a genetic disorder may result. See *Charcot-Marie-Tooth disease*.

**recombination fraction**   The percentage of cases in a pedigree in which crossover does occur. The smaller the distance between two genes on a chromosome, the less likely they will cross over, or be separated, during meiosis. A high recombination fraction (e.g., 50% or more) indicates that the two genes are not close enough together to be linked. See *linkage; linkage analysis*.

*Recombination* is a process by which, during meiosis, sequences of DNA are exchanged between homologous chromosomes (i.e., the same chromosome in both parents) thereby varying the characteristics inherited by the offspring. The smaller the distance between a gene and the RFLP (restriction fragment length polymorphism) of interest, the less likely is it that the two will be separated during meiosis. As more linked markers are identified in patients and their relatives, the prospect improves for locating the molecular lesion(s) responsible for pathogenesis.

*Allelic association* refers to a correlation between a phenotype and a particular allele in the population. Loose linkage between two loci does not result in allelic associations in the population because alleles on the same chromosome at all but the tightest linked loci are separated by recombination with sufficient frequency that both sets of alleles quickly return to linkage equilibrium in the population.

Demonstration of linkage permits mapping of a susceptibility locus to a particular chromosomal region—identified as a genetic marker, an identifiable piece of DNA of known chromosomal location that can serve as a point of reference on the chromosome. Demonstrating linkage, however, is only the first step; to find a specific gene, many more are required. Thus, it took 10 years from the time that Huntington disease was linked to a region on chromosome 4 until the specific gene was identified.

**recommencement, mania of** Janet's term for the repetitive behavior of some

obsessive-compulsive patients who must do things many times before they can feel some assurance that they have been done correctly—opening and shutting doors, locking and unlocking doors, dressing and undressing, constant repetition of prayers and penances, etc. See *obsessive-compulsive disorder*.

**reconditioning**   A type of psychotherapy based on the belief that neurosis is a result of faulty conditioning. In Salter's method, the patient is authoritatively directed to abandon destructive patterns of behavior and to practice new habits that will be of value to him. The patient is considered to be in a state of pathological inhibition which is itself a conditioned response that blocks free emotional expression (excitation). Treatment is directed to unlearning conditioned inhibitory reflexes and replacing them with conditioned excitatory reflexes by means of deliberate practicing of excitatory emotional reactions until they are established as conditioned reflexes. See *arousal reconditioning*.

**reconstruction**   In psychoanalytic treatment, restoring to consciousness the memory of significant early experiences, usually by way of one or more interpretations. In treatment, early infantile and pre-oedipal material, in particular, tends to be expressed in the transference, and the analyst uses that as a clue to the patient's early experiences. A patient perceived his analyst as being depressed; the analyst proffered a tentative interpretation, that the patient's mother was depressed during his first year of life. Subsequent sessions bore this out, and the patient later discovered that his mother had made a serious suicide attempt shortly after his birth.

**reconstructive psychotherapy**   See *adaptational psychodynamics; psychotherapy*.

**recovering alcoholic**   An alcoholic who is successfully abstaining; the term emphasizes the concept that no alcoholic is ever cured, and that recovery must be worked at continuously.

**recovery**   In addiction psychiatry, maintenance of sobriety or abstinence from alcohol or other drugs; the process of overcoming both physiologic and psychological dependence on a drug or alcohol. See *remission*.

**recovery model**   According to this model, the process of recovery from mental illness is the process of living a satisfying, hopeful, and contributing life despite the limitations imposed by illness. Emphasis is on autonomy, empowerment, and involvement. Mental illness is conceptualized as a brain disorder that involves the person's psychological and social being, but the brain's plasticity allows the corrective milieu to have a powerful recovery influence. Medications are of great value, and equally important are taking responsibility for oneself and at the same time accepting support from others, on learning about mental illness and recognizing early signs of relapse, on employment and meaningful activities that contribute to self-esteem. Self-help often enhances the value of professional treatment, and, for many, spirituality provides hope, peace, and understanding.

The recovery model is a shared decision-making model in which patient and therapist agree on treatment options that are within a zone of achievable, safe, and worthwhile. In the schizophrenic patient who is persistently symptomatic, for example, specific symptoms may be targeted: delusions, conceptual disorganization, hallucinatory behavior, unusual thought content, mannerisms and posturing, blunted affect, social withdrawal, or lack of spontaneity and flow of conversation.

As the patient finds ways to moderate symptoms, the therapist works with the patient toward further improvement in achieving life goals.

Barriers to recovery are comorbid substance abuse, medical comorbidities, limitations in opportunities for support and rehabilitation, difficulties with medication adherence, and limitations in the efficacy of currently available antipsychotics.

**recovery rate**   The ratio of the number discharged as recovered within a given period (usually a year) to the total number in the original group. In institutional statistics this rate is usually approximated by relating the number discharged as recovered in a given period to the number who were admitted during the same period.

**recreation**   Leisure activity engaged in for its own sake. The term is also used to refer to a type of ancillary treatment and is then called *recreation(al) therapy (RT)*. John E. Davis (*Clinical Applications of Recreational Therapy*, 1952) defines recreation therapy as "any free, voluntary and expressive activity; motor, sensory or mental, vitalized by the expansive play spirit, sustained by deep-rooted pleasurable attitudes and evoked by wholesome emotional

release; prescribed by medical authority as an adjuvant in treatment."

*Recreation therapy (therapeutic recreation)* utilizes hobbies, sports, and other leisure time pursuits in order to promote the patient's growth, development, functioning, and ability to cope with and gain satisfaction from life. Acquisition of new hobbies, skills, and interests can help to counteract a sense of limitation related to an impaired ability to cope with daily living by reason of biological, psychological, or sociological stress, trauma, or deficit. Individual play provides an opportunity to explore both self and environment at the patient's own pace, with a minimum of externally imposed constraints. Arts and crafts provide a structure for self-evaluation as well as an opportunity for a degree of socialization. Games afford an opportunity to learn about rules, competition, dealing with an adversary, and how to win. Assigning chores to the patient helps him learn how to relate to authority; at the same time, he learns that there are unpleasant tasks that must be learned and performed on a regular basis. See *dance therapy; music therapy.*

**recreation, active**   In occupational therapy any form of diversional endeavor or pastime in which the patient actually engages and in the participation of which it is necessary for him to make some physical exertion. For example, dancing is a form of active recreation.

**recreation, passive**   Entertainment or amusement planned and presented by others for the patient and in which he does not participate, but plays the passive part of onlooker. For example, viewing a film or attending a concert is a form of passive recreation.

**recreational drug**   A drug, such as alcohol, whose use for pleasurable effects is permitted or condoned within a particular society. The term does not imply that the drug is free from health dangers or dependence potential, and it is incorrect to extend the term to include the use of illicit drugs. Even though intermittent users of illicit drugs such as cannabis may claim that such use is nothing more than harmless fun, by definition the illicit use of any drug constitutes drug misuse.

**recruiting system**   See *intralaminar system.*

**recruitment**   In neurophysiology, spread of response if stimulation is prolonged.

**recurrence**   See *relapse.*

**recursion**   The ability to apply a rule, routine, or algorithmic process an indefinite number of times; in linguistics, for example, a rule that an adjective precede the noun it modifies can be used any number of times in constructing sentences. (It may, of course, be suspended at will.) Complicated operations can be carried out by using sequences of simpler ones to produce hierarchies; an entire proposition can be embedded in a still larger one to form a hierarchical tree. "The mother gave her little boy an ice cream cone; I saw her give it to him and I saw him eat it. I wonder if the mother saw her little boy eat the ice cream cone, and I wonder if the mother wonders if I saw him eating the cone, I wonder if she wonders if I saw her give it to him, and I can guess that she believes that I saw her give him the cone and saw him eat it." Recursion has greatly increased the power of thought in that humans can think an infinite number of thoughts. "Our rule systems couch knowledge in compositional, quantified, recursive propositions, and collections of these propositions interlock to form modules of intuitive theories about particular domains of experience, such as kinships, numbers, language, and law" (Pinker, S. *How The Mind Works*, New York: Norton, 1997).

**red nucleus**   See *midbrain*.

**redintegration**   Hollingworth's term for the process in which part of a complex antecedent provokes the complete consequent that was previously made to the antecedent as a whole. The conditioned response is an example of redintegration. Redintegration is the basis of the value of souvenirs and keepsakes, which tend to arouse the same attitudes as were originally connected with the experiences to which they pertain.

Redintegration is also sometimes used synonymously with reintegration. See *integration*.

**reductionism**   The view that complex phenomena can best be understood by studying the simpler, and ultimately the elemental, units of which they are composed. The organism can be broken down into organs and each organ into separate cells; the organism can then be understood by studying those separate cells. Behavior was to be explained in terms of associations of separate elementary events. In Pavlovian psychology and behaviorism, the elements were single sensations or associations or the reflex arc. In Gestalt psychology, the elements were larger but even so they seemed unable to capture the essence of behavior.

Vygotsky proposed that the higher mental processes are of social origin and that the basic units of human conscious behavior are to be found in the relation of the subject with the social environment. Behavior cannot be reduced to single elements but rather is to be explained by its inclusion in a rich net of essential relations.

Classical psychoanalysis viewed the infant as having instincts (drives) that have an aim and are directed toward an object; the developing child finds increasingly efficient ways to discharge tension or energy. That classical *drive-reduction theory* was called into question by the object relations theorists, who maintain that infants are object-related from birth and that development is motivated by the need to maintain continuity of relationships. See *object relations theory*.

**reductive**   "That method of psychological interpretation which regards the unconscious product not from the symbolic point of view, but merely as a semiotic expression, a sort of sign or symptom of an underlying process. Accordingly the reductive method treats the unconscious product in the sense of a leading-back to the elements and basic processes, irrespective of whether such products are reminiscences of actual events, or whether they arise from elementary processes affecting the psyche. Hence, the reductive method is orientated backwards (in contrast to the constructive method), whether in the historical sense or in the merely figurative sense of a tracing back of complex and differentiated factors to the general and elementary" (Jung, C. G. *Psychological Types*, 1923).

**redundancy, genetic**   See *aging, theories of*.

**reduplicative memory deception**   Pick's term for a form of false memory sometimes observed in patients with organic brain disease. The patient claims, for instance, that he has already been examined by the same doctor, in the same examining room, with the same nurse in attendance, although the entire situation is in fact new to him. See *confabulation; déjà fait*.

**reduplicative paramnesia**   *Doppelganger* (q.v.).

**reeducation**   See *psychotherapy*.

**reefers**   Slang expression for marijuana cigarettes. Possibly the weed was first carried by sailors from the reefs of Mariguana Island in the Bahamas.

**reeler**  A mutant strain of mice discovered in 1949 and named for the reeling gait that characterized affected mice, whose brains lack the normal cortical layers and have a jumbled collection of neurons instead. Normal cortical layers do not form because the migrating neurons never enter the preplate, but pile up below it. In 1995, the reeler gene was identified; it codes for a large protein called *reelin* (q.v.). The Cajal-Retzius (C-R) cells, found in the part of the preplate that becomes the marginal zone, are the cells that make reelin. See *axon growth; neurogenic genes; scrambler.*

**reelin**  A neurodevelopmental signaling protein essential to the proper formation and positioning of neural cell layers in the cortical plate, and to the migration and positioning of the Purkinje cells into a single cortical cell layer during the early stage of cerebellum development. Genetic defects in the gene, *RELN*, produce an autosomal recessive form of lissencephaly with cerebellar hypoplasia. In the adult brain, reelin is required to maintain neuroanatomical integrity; it functions at the level of the synapse, participating in the control of NMDA receptor activities.

**reenforced thought**  See *supervalent thought.*

**re-entry**  Ongoing, recursive interchange between parallel circuits of the brain (in particular, corticocortical and corticothalamic connectivity), providing spatiotemporal integration of diverse sensory and motor events and synchronization of neuronal activity within different brain areas. Such integration is the basis of perceptual categorization, the ability to differentiate objects from their background.

**reference, ideas of**  *Delusions of reference* (q.v.), demonstrated by a person who projects his own, usually unconscious, ideas upon another and then proceeds to act toward those ideas as if they originated from an outside source. For example, a patient with an unconscious impulse to steal was preoccupied with the unfounded idea that others asserted he intended to steal.

The term also includes the tendency to read a personal meaning into everything that goes on about one, to feel that every action or happening in the outside world is specifically and purposely related to the patient.

The paranoid patient almost always exhibits ideas of reference. He misinterprets the activities of others, believing that they have personal reference of a derogatory character to him. See *projection.*

**reference memory**  See *declarative memory; long-term memory.*

**referential attitude**  An attitude of expectancy seen in some schizophrenic patients who, feeling themselves to be victims of hostility from others, search for references that will justify the underlying mood. See *listening attitude.*

**referential cohesion**  See *discourse skills.*

**referred pain**  Irradiation of pain sensation, with or without hyperalgesia, into an area of skin when a viscus or muscle is the site of the lesion. Although the basis for referral of pain must be excitation of common pathways, it is uncertain whether the brain, the spinal cord, or the peripheral nerves are involved. See *pain syndromes.*

**reflection**  In psychiatry and psychology, this may refer (1) to a type of thinking characterized by introspection, deliberation, or contemplation, or (2) to a psychotherapeutic technique in which a patient's statements are restated or rephrased to the patient so as to emphasize their emotional significance.

**reflex**  A sensorimotor reaction, the simplest form of involuntary response to a stimulus. Stimulation of the receptor organ or cell excites the afferent neuron, from which the impulse travels to one or more *intercalated* neurons in the central nervous system and then, via the efferent neuron, to the effector organ or cell. See *sign.*

**reflex, acute affective**  Kretschmer's term for the earliest indications of emotional discharge (usually, tremors) in response to great stress.

**reflex, superficial**  The response to stroking or pressing upon certain portions of the skin; for example, the plantar, cremasteric, and abdominal reflexes. Compare with *deep reflex.*

**reflex epilepsy**  Epileptic convulsions precipitated by some external stimulus, such as a sudden loud noise (*acousticomotor epilepsy*), music (*musicogenic epilepsy*), visual (*photic epilepsy*), or cutaneous stimuli. Reflex inhibition of the fit is an allied phenomenon: if, for example, a focal convulsion begins with movement in one limb, a strong stimulus such as a firm grip applied to the limb will often abort the attack if this is begun immediately after onset of the attack.

**reflex hallucination**  *Obs.* A sensory impression induced through stimulation of a distant and different sensory area.

**reflex hysteria**  Kretschmer's term for a hysterical sign in which an automatic nervous process, that is, a reflex, plays a dominant part, while the will plays a minor role. Examples of reflex hysteria are simple spasm, tremors, and tics.

**reflex sympathetic dystrophy**  See *pain syndromes*.

**reflex time, central**  See *facilitation*.

**reflexive memory**  Automatic memory; memory that accumulates by frequent repetition and does not require consciousness or complex cognitive processes such as evaluation and comparison before it can be reproduced. Motor and perceptual skills and learning of procedures and rules are examples of reflexive memory. See *long-term memory*; *procedural memory*.

**reformatory paranoia**  Zealotry; a form of megalomania sometimes expressed in psychotic delusions but more often as character or personality traits. The subject is determined to convert the world to his ideas or to convince all of the wonder of some discovery he has made (*inventive paranoia*).

**reformist delusion**  A delusion with a religious, philosophical, or political theme, with never-ending criticism of those who resist or oppose the subject's "cause." Reformist delusions may be associated with violence, and some political assassins appear to have reformist delusions.

**refractory**  1. Resistant or unresponsive (to a particular treatment). See *treatment resistance*.
2. In neurophysiology, the refractory period is the time following stimulation during which a nerve or muscle remains unresponsive to a second stimulus. The absolute refractory period is that during which there is no response to any stimulus; the relative refractory period is that during which response can be elicited only if the stimulus is very strong.

**reframing**  Viewing from a different perspective; reconceptualizing; redefining. The term is used most frequently in family therapy, where many approaches emphasize the positive aspects of symptoms or dysfunction as they support and protect the integrity and continuity of family life. Treatment entails a cognitive restructuring of behavior to indicate its positive qualities. Thus, in *relabeling*, a particular form of reframing, excessive dependence on the mother may be viewed as a means of contributing to the mother's

self-esteem by making her feel needed and wanted.

**refrigerator parents**  Kanner's original description of parents of psychotic (autistic) children—cold, intellectual, stimulate their children less than parents of normal children. Most recent workers have failed to confirm such differences. See *autistic disorder*.

**refusal, school**  See *school phobia*.

**regimen**  The specific details of a treatment plan, including the scheduling and regulation of diet, medication, and other therapeutic measures designed to operate over a period of time. The term regime is often used incorrectly in this sense.

**regional pain syndrome**  See *pain syndromes*.

**registration**  In learning psychology, registration refers to impressibility or notation ability and implies the ability to notice, the ability to make a record, or both. Impaired registration of recent impressions is the most striking symptom of Korsakoff psychosis. See *amnestic syndrome*; *memory*; *Wernicke-Korsakoff syndrome*.

**regression**  A return to some earlier level of adaptation. The mentally healthy person progresses through many so-called levels. (1) intrauterine; (2) infancy (early and late; extending from birth to approximately the fifth year; this period includes, among other things, the phases of oral, anal, and genital organization); (3) latency (extending from about the age of 5 to puberty; one of its chief characteristics is sublimation); (4) puberty (beginning at the onset of manhood or womanhood and continuing for 2 or 3 years; one of its main attributes is adult sexuality); (5) adolescence (beginning in the early or middle teens; its principal characteristics revolve around the reality principle, heterosexuality, and sublimated interest); (6) adulthood (extending from the termination of the adolescent period to senescence; the characteristics of adolescence are amplified during this stage); (7) climacterium; (8) senescence (the phase of decadence). See *ontogeny, psychic*.

Regression and *fixation* (q.v.) are commonly associated with each other. When fixation is intense, frustrations on the part of reality may easily lead to regression. But internal frustrations are even more important, according to Freud.

Winnicott viewed regression as potentially positive and curative, rather than an impediment to effective psychoanalytic treatment. Whether regression is likely to be restorative rather than destructive is largely dependent on the ability of the therapist to tolerate the patient's regression and understand the patient's needs for security, containment, and holding during the phase of regression.

**regression, progressive teleologic** Arieti's term for the tendency of the schizophrenic to return to the level of the primary process or primary cognition in an attempt to deal with a world and self-image that are grotesque, threatening, and terrifying. The regressing is teleologic in that it is purposeful, as when an inner threat is changed into a threat from the outside world that can be defended against. But unlike other types of regression, schizophrenic regression is progressive because it usually fails in its purpose and still further regression is necessary until, finally, the process may lead to complete dilapidation.

**regressive alcoholism** *Gamma alcoholism* (q.v.).

**regressive electroshock therapy (REST)** A form of electroconvulsive therapy, no longer in use, in which several daily grand mal convulsions are produced for a number of days until the patient is out of contact and incontinent of urine and feces. In one study, four treatments were given each day for 7 days; at the end of this time, in addition to the above symptoms, patients were underactive, did not talk spontaneously, lost their appetite and had to be spoon-fed, and movements were uncertain, slow, and clumsy. These symptoms last for 1 or 2 weeks; recovery from the superimposed organic brain syndrome is gradual.

Regressive EST was ordinarily used only when the more usual methods failed and prognosis was poor, as in some forms of the schizophrenias.

**regret** Sorrow, remorse, or *disappointment*, particularly in relation to a feeling of responsibility for the negative result of a past decision. Regret generates higher physiological responses and is consistently reported as more intense than disappointment in normal patients, but not in patients with lesions in orbitofrontal regions. See *choice*; *counterfactual thinking*.

**regulated pathway** See *vesicles*.

**regulatory region** See *gene functions*.

**regulomes** Catalogs of DNA elements that control gene function. See *noncoding DNA*.

**rehabilitation** Use of all forms of physical medicine in conjunction with psychosocial adjustment and vocational retraining in an attempt to achieve maximal function and adjustment, and to prepare the patient physically, mentally, socially, and vocationally for the fullest possible life compatible with his abilities and disabilities. Rehabilitation is a dynamic, purposeful program in which, ideally, activities are scheduled for each patient for the entire day; such schedules are built around activities prescribed by the physician, with guidance, psychological services, adult education, prevocational shop training, and directed socialization supplementing the prescribed therapy and retraining. See *remotivation*.

Rehabilitation is sometimes called the fourth leg of medical practice, the others being prevention, diagnosis, and treatment. Rehabilitation aims to restore a handicapped person to a situation in which he can make best use of his residual capacities within as normal as possible a social context. The handicaps themselves are of two varieties: primary—the chronic symptoms that are an inherent part of illness plus the accumulated losses of skills through illness; and secondary—unhealthy personal reactions to illness plus unfavorable, inappropriate attitudes toward the handicapped person that develop in his relatives, employers, hospital staff, etc. (See *syndrome, social breakdown*).

In general, rehabilitation techniques are more applicable to decreasing or preventing secondary handicaps, and to increasing social acceptability of patients, than they are to modifying or removing chronic symptoms of psychosis.

In psychiatry, rehabilitation generally is concerned with the patient with chronic mental illness (specifically, organic dementia or schizophrenia), where the goals are (1) to prevent relapse and rehospitalization by achieving successful community tenure; (2) to improve the quality of life by assisting the patient in assuming responsibility over his or her life; and (3) to achieve an adequate social role with appropriate instrumental performance in the community. Included within the latter are vocational, homemaking, social, and interpersonal adjustment competencies, all of which aim to help the patient function as actively and independently in society as possible. Psychiatric rehabilitation considers five domains in developing a plan for reintegration: physical, emotional, intellectual, social, and spiritual. Interventions are person-centered and tailored to the patient's strengths and capabilities in order to foster his or her active engagement in the process.

Rehabilitation programs focus not only on strengthening the patient's skills but also on developing the environmental supports necessary to sustain him or her within the community. It has generally been observed that fewer than 20% of chronically mentally ill patients are able to adapt acceptably to average community life. Successful rehabilitation depends on a network of community care services such as halfway houses, adult homes, sheltered workshops, special schools, supervised residences for the handicapped and developmentally disabled, home care, satellite clinics, etc. See *domicile; long-term care.*

**rehearsal, behavioral**   See *behavior therapy.*

**Reich, Annie**   (1902–1971) Austrian-born psychoanalyst; countertransference; lived in New York City after 1938.

**Reich, Wilhelm**   (1897–1957) Austrian-born psychoanalyst; character analysis and ego psychology, orgone energy; practiced in the United States In 1957 he was arrested by the Federal Food and Drug Commission, which charged that his orgone boxes were a fraud. He was convicted and sentenced in Maine and was serving his term in the federal penitentiary in Lewisburg, Pennsylvania, when he died.

**reification**   Treating the abstract as though it were concrete; a type of thinking seen often in schizophrenia but observable also in essentially normal subjects. See *concretization.*

**reinforced practice**   Successive approximations; *shaping* (q.v.); graduated exposure of the phobic subject to the feared object or situation.

**reinforcement**   In neurophysiology, *facilitation* (q.v.); i.e., the enhancement of response to a stimulus by simultaneous excitation of response(s) in other neural circuits, as when the knee jerk is facilitated by having the subject clasp his hands tightly at the same time that his patellar tendon is tapped. In conditioning theory, reinforcement refers to reintroduction of the original, unconditioned stimulus along with the conditioned stimulus, thus strengthening the conditioned response; reinforcement in this sense is sometimes loosely referred to as a reward (technically, responses

are reinforced and the person is rewarded). See *behaviorism; operant conditioning.*

In addictive disorders, reinforcement refers to the neurobiological phenomena that mediate repetitive drug-taking behavior. It seems likely that the central catechoamines, and *dopamine* (q.v.) in particular, are the major component. See *VTA.*

Primary reinforcers are those that are independent of previous learning, such as the need for food; secondary reinforcers are based on previous experience(s) of having been rewarded. *Negative reinforcement* refers to a response that is increased because it eliminates or prevents an aversive condition (e.g., a teenager picks up the clothes on her bedroom floor and hangs them properly in a closet in order to avoid her mother's wrath).

Punishment, in contrast, consists of presentation of an aversive stimulus (e.g., a slap or an electric shock) with the specific intention of weakening or eliminating an undesired response. See *aversive control.*

**reinforcement, differential**   See *accelerative.*

**reinforcement, reactive**   "Repression is often achieved by means of an excessive reinforcement of the thought contrary to the one which is to be repressed. This process I call *reactive reinforcement*, and the thought which asserts itself exaggeratedly in consciousness and (in the same way as a prejudice) cannot be removed I call a *reactive thought*" (Freud, S. *Collected Papers*, 1924–25)

**reinforcement schedule**   The pattern or frequency with which a reinforcer is delivered as a consequence of behavior. *Partial reinforcement* is less than every-time reinforcement of behavior when it occurs; in practice, it indicates that reinforcement only occasionally follows execution of the action or appearance of behavior. Such partial reinforcement nonetheless maintains the behavior at full strength (suggesting at least one reason why many behaviors are maintained despite attempts to reduce or eliminate them).

Another reinforcement program is the *fixed-interval (FI) schedule*: the reward is delivered contingent on the first required response after a specified period of time (usually not exceeding a 10-minute interval). Shortening the interval increases the number of responses; further, responses tend to increase as the time of reinforcement draws near. The latter increase has a scalloping effect: responses rise as the time for reinforcement approaches and fall as it recedes. To counteract scalloping, a *variable-interval (VI) schedule* may be used: the reward is delivered randomly around a particular interval of time in order to obtain a steady rate of performance.

A *fixed-ratio (FR) schedule* delivers reinforcement after a specific number of responses have occurred (typically, from 5 to 100 or more). Similar to schedules depending on interval, a *variable-ratio (VR) schedule* (in which the reward is delivered randomly around a particular ratio) provides a smoother pattern of behavior than does a FR schedule.

**reinstatement**   Return to a previous position or state; in substance abusers, resumption of drug-taking, often to higher level of intake, even after a prolonged period of abstinence. Stress increases the propensity of alcohol and drug users to relapse. See *addiction; priming; sensitization.*

**reinstinctualization**   Deneutralization of drive energy that would normally be available to the ego for the execution of its various functions. As a result, the functions may be affected adversely by the wishes or conflicts arising from the drives. Reinstinctualization is one aspect of the phenomenon of regression.

In hysterical blindness, for example, the neutralized drive energy that made seeing possible regardless of inner conflict has been lost to the ego; the energy is deneutralized or reinstinctualized so that the function of seeing must be suspended just as the drive itself (aggression or sexuality) must be denied.

**reintegration**   See *integration.*

**Reitan-Indiana aphasia screening test**   A brief test (taking about 2 minutes to complete) for agraphia, apraxia, agnosia, left-right confusion, acalculia, and alexia.

**Reiter syndrome**   See *Behçet syndrome.*

**rejecting object**   See *bad object.*

**rejuvenation**   A special *vasectomy* operation introduced by Steinach to mitigate in men certain pathological symptoms of old age, sexual impotence, hypertrophy of the prostate, or eunuchoidism. While the ordinary vasectomy technique resulting in sterilization is bilateral and leaves the proximal end of the seminal ducts open, the rejuvenating operation is performed unilaterally and provides for ligatures at both ends of the given vas deferens. The effect of rejuvenation is said to be achieved by a renewed activity of

the proliferating and regenerating interstitial secretory tissue of the testicles, which is considered to be the hormone-bearing apparatus mainly responsible in men for sexual libido and potency, as well as by an equally favorable response of the other endocrine glands.

**relabeling**   See *reframing.*

**relapse**   Worsening of an ongoing episode. *Recurrence* refers to the occurrence of a new episode. A cutoff period of 6 months is often used to distinguish between the two; i.e., worsening within 6 months following apparent remission is considered a relapse, whereas worsening after 6 months is considered a recurrence. Many writers use relapse and recurrence interchangeably.

In addiction psychiatry, relapse refers to the triggering of a drive state (similar to eating) that may occur at any time during abstinence. The cardinal feature of drug addiction is continued vulnerability to relapse after years of drug abstinence. See *addiction; remission.*

**relapse prevention**   Maintenance of abstinence; long-term rehabilitation; the use of strategies to prevent drug lapses. In the addictive disorders, relapse prevention until recently was solely a psychosocial approach. It included individual, group, and family psychotherapy; behavioral techniques such as social skills training and contingency management; peer self-help groups such as AA and NA, often in conjunction with services such as vocational rehabilitation and patient education. In addition to the foregoing, relapse prevention currently includes pharmacologic treatment, such as maintenance treatment with a cross-tolerant medication (e.g., methadone maintenance for heroin addicts), maintenance treatment with an antagonist (e.g., *naltrexone* or LAAM for opiate dependence), medications that enhance internal control by reducing the reinforcing effect of the addictive drugs on the presumed mesolimbic reward system (e.g., *naltrexone* in alcoholism) or by restoring hypothesized neurotransmission imbalances in that system (e.g., *tiapride, gamma-hydroxybutyric acid, acamprosate*) attempts to manipulate brain dopamine activity because of its presumed role in the mesolimbic "reward" circuit), or metabolic manipulations that render the addictive drugs aversive rather than rewarding (called *sensitizing agents*), and their use as treatment is called *chemical aversive conditioning* or *CAC* (e.g., disulfiram in alcoholism).

**relatedness**   The interrelation between two or more people who reciprocally influence each other: patient–therapist, mother–child, etc. Normal relatedness is based on security in interpersonal relations and in large part is a result of early childhood experiences. S. Arieti (*Archives of General Psychiatry 6*, 1962) emphasizes that basic trust is essential for the development of normal or satisfactory relatedness. "Basic trust is an "atmospheric feeling' which predisposes one to expect "good things' and is a prerequisite to a normal development of self-esteem.... The mother expects the child to become a healthy and mature person. The child later perceives this faith of the mother and accepts it.... He finally introjects this trust of the significant adults, and he trusts himself."

**relatedness, functional**   The arrangement of objects that are organically and dynamically related to each other: for example, placing woodworking tools near the woodworking bench and nails and other objects involved in woodworking nearby; placing drawing paper near crayons and paints in the proximity of an easel.

**relational aggression**   Boys more commonly display physical aggression, whereas girls are more likely to show relational aggression (e.g., teasing, social exclusion, reputation damaging).

**relational bullying**   See *bullying, relational*.

**relational memory**   The ability to learn and remember the relationships between items, an essential property of human intelligence and a particular aspect of declarative memory. *Transitive inference* is one function of relational memory; having learned that A is larger than B, and that B is larger than C, the inference is drawn that A is larger than C.

**relational problem**   Any difficulty with the family or partner; it may be the focus of treatment but need not be due to or indicative of a mental disorder. Parent–child relational problems often spring from inadequate parental discipline or overprotection. Parent–child, partner, and sibling relational problems may all arise from negative or distorted communication.

**relationship inversion**   A transposition of natural roles, as a young girl taking the mother's responsibilities or place in the home.

**relationship therapy**   Therapy that emerges out of the totality of the relationship between patient and therapist during the entire course of treatment. The therapist begins where the patient is and seeks to help him draw on his own capacities toward a more creative acceptance and use of the self he has. While maintaining an interest in understanding what has been wrong, the therapeutic focus is on what the patient can begin to do about what was and, more important, still is wrong. "Therapy emerges, then, from an experience in living, not in isolation but within a relationship with another from whom the patient can eventually differentiate himself as he comes to perceive and accept his own self as separate and distinct" (Kanner, L. *Child Psychiatry*, 1948).

**relative resistance**   See *treatment resistance*.

**relative risk**   The ratio of the rate of a disorder among those exposed to the rate of those not exposed. See *risk factor*.

**relaxation response**   A hypothesized coordinated physiologic reaction due to stimulation of hypothalamic regions, which results in generalized decreased sympathetic nervous system activity. See *autogenic training*.

**relaxation training**   Exercises in deep breathing, muscle relaxation, and imagery (imagining situations that are pleasant, rewarding, reassuring, etc.); used in behavior therapy to teach the subject how to induce responses that compete with anxiety or other undesirable thoughts, feelings, or behavior. Once the subject has learned the exercises, they are repeated for a specific amount of time (e.g., 1 minute) as soon as the subject becomes aware of an impending onset of the target symptoms. See *behavior therapy; habit reversal*.

**relay nuclei**   See *nuclei, CNS*.

**release**   In neurology, the removal of the inhibitory effect of higher centers on the activity of lower nervous centers. (See *disinhibition*.) In psychiatry, a form of psychotherapy in which the patient is allowed to express wishes, thoughts, and impulses which he is unable to discharge adequately under usual environmental conditions; in this sense, release is approximately equivalent to catharsis. In child psychiatry, *release therapy* refers to the use of play methods as an avenue for the expression of the child's anxieties.

**release phenomena**   Manifestations of *disinhibition* (q.v.); *positive signs*. John Hughlings Jackson first noted that CNS lesions produce not only *negative signs* reflecting loss of the function(s) performed by the damaged nerves, but also stereotyped abnormal responses (positive signs or release phenomena) due to the withdrawal of the normally inhibitory influence of the damaged nerves.

**releaser, social**   *Sign stimulus*; any object or situation that serves as an adequate stimulus to instinctive behavior; e.g., the shadow of a toy airplane moving overhead under certain conditions will make newborn chicks run for cover, as if they had sighted a flying hawk. Permanent modification of behavior by a social releaser is termed *imprinting* (q.v.).

**releasing mechanism, inherited**   See *instinct*.

**reliability**   The degree to which a test measures consistently; the dependability of a measure; the standard deviation is used as a measure of variability and when so used is known as a standard error. See *mean deviation*. Reliability is inversely proportional to the standard error.

**reliance**   In psychopharmacology, continuing need or desire for recommended doses of a drug, but without the induction of a withdrawal syndrome when the drug is discontinued.

**religious mania**   *Obs.* An acute psychotic episode, usually schizophrenic or organic in origin, characterized by generalized hyperactivity, agitation, restlessness, and many hallucinations with a religious coloring. See *ecstasy*.

**REM**   Rapid eye movement. See *REM sleep*.

**REM behavior disorder (RBD)**   A parasomnia characterized by altered dreams and violent behaviors during REM sleep (electromyographic atonia and a flaccid paralysis are the usual accompaniments of normal REM sleep). The disorder affects older adults (over 60 years of age) and is associated with various neurologic disorders, including dementia. Most such violent sleepers injure themselves during one or more of their nightmares, and over a third injure their bed partners, sometimes seriously. The condition ordinarily responds favorably to anticonvulsant drugs.

**REM deprivation**   See *sleep deprivation*.

**REM latency**   The number of minutes from the onset of the first stage of sleep to the first REM period, reported as being often shorter than normal in some types of depressed patients who are responsive to antidepressant medication. Normal REM latency is 80 to 100 minutes, but it may fall to half that length in depressed patients.

**REM sleep**   Rapid eye movement sleep. REM sleep is active sleep, characterized by increased metabolic rates, elevated temperature, and arousal-type EEG patterns. REM sleep occurs in cycles of approximately 90 minutes throughout the night. It is also called *paradoxical sleep* because it has elements of both deep sleep and light sleep. REM sleep comprises both *tonic elements*, present throughout the REM state, and *phasic elements*, occurring intermittently during the REM state. Tonic elements include low-voltage, fast EEG; increased brain temperature and blood flow; *poikilothermia* (failure to respond to changes in temperature with sweating or shivering), penile tumescence and skeletal muscle suppression on the EMG. Phasic elements include the rapid conjugate eye movements, autonomic variability, muscle twitches, and ponto-geniculo-occipital spikes.

REM sleep is associated with dreaming. The first REM period usually begins 90 to 180 minutes after sleep onset. The longest REM periods and the most intense activity occur just after the minimal body temperature is reached (near 5 a.m.). See *dream; NREM; sleep*.

**REM sleep efficiency**   See *sleep efficiency*.

**REM sleep fragmentation**   Frequent interruption of REM sleep associated with excessive shifting among sleep stages, especially from REM sleep to stage 1 of slow-wave sleep; characteristic of *narcolepsy* (q.v.).

**reminiscence**   Recalling or recollection of past experiences, particularly when the recall has a "now you see it, now you don't" quality. In contrast to memory, reminiscence consists of a peculiarly irregular alternation between remembering and forgetting so that a memory apparently lost suddenly appears, while one that was just there disappears. See *memory*.

**reminiscence therapy**   A psychosocial approach to Alzheimer disease. Specific reminiscence refers to the highly focused use of triggers that approximate the life history of an individual, and efforts to stimulate recall during conversation. In a treatment group, patients discuss their life experiences and events of the past. If it has any benefit, it must be part of a continuous, ongoing program.

**remission** Diminution or disappearance of symptoms. In psychiatric disorders, if the subject has few or no symptoms for a minimum of 2 months (or 6 months, according to some investigators), the term *recovery* is applied. *Relapse* (q.v.) occurs during a period of remission; recurrence refers to a return of symptoms after recovery has occurred. In addictive disorders, a distinction is often made between *early remission* (the first 12 months following termination of use, the time of the greatest danger for relapse) and *sustained remission* (more than 12 months following termination of use).

Remission does not imply complete absence of symptoms; rather, it refers to a level of stability that has been attained with treatment in which symptoms are no longer overwhelming, or so painful or disabling as to dominate the person's life. See *recovery model.*

**remitting atypical psychosis** A nonorganic, benign psychotic syndrome characterized by sudden onset, florid and fluid symptoms, brief duration, remitting outcome, and a long-term pattern of recurrences. It typically develops following, and apparently in response to, some external stress in a person with premorbid personality problems.

Other labels under which the syndrome has been described include atypical psychosis, cycloid psychosis, reactive (psychogenic) psychosis, *bouffées délirantes, brief reactive psychosis, hysterical psychosis, schizoaffective disorder* or psychosis, and *schizophreniform disorder* (qq.v). See *reactive psychosis.*

**remorse** Feelings of regret or guilt about something that has been done; Freud differentiated between remorse and guilt, in that the latter refers to aggressive wishes that have not yet been satisfied.

**remote memory** *Long-term memory* (q.v.); sometimes used to designate specifically material that was learned before the age of 12 (and *intermediate memory* for ability to remember material from the past 3 to 20 years).

**remotivation** Any planned group activity that aims to tap dormant areas of functioning and help the patient to find parts of himself that he has lost and/or that are unaffected by the pathological process. Originally remotivation referred to a single technique, evolved to deal with severely regressed senile or schizophrenic patients. Remotivation is currently used to refer to a family of rehabilitation techniques that meet a variety of therapeutic needs. Included within the group are the following:

1. *Reality orientation* (q.v.)—to decrease the confusion of the organic patient, who needs help in relating himself to time, place, and person.

2. *Remotivation activities*—recreational and occupational therapy, rhythm and movement exercises, and the like, used to initiate communication with restless, agitated patients or with those who are silent and withdrawn; remotivation activities often crystallize group feeling and prepare for more meaningful group involvement and verbal communication.

3. *Primary remotivation*—stimulation of the various sensory modalities as a way to encourage group participation and communication.

4. *Advanced remotivation*—which involves some problem solving within the remotivation group setting, such as discussion of concepts or ideas, discussions about social issues, and tour groups into the community.

**removal protection** See *protection, medical removal.*

**Renard Diagnostic Interview** A structured interview developed in 1977 at the Washington University (St. Louis) Department of Psychiatry (by L. N. Robins, J. Helzer, and J. Croughan) to elicit enough information so that the criteria established for the diagnosis of 15 major psychiatric disorders could be applied. See *Research Diagnostic Criteria.*

**renifleur** See *osphresiolagnia.*

**Renpenning syndrome** A type of mental retardation that is inherited as an X-linked recessive and characterized by a lack of associated physical abnormality.

**renunciation, instinctual** Disavowal of and refusal, on the part of the ego, to satisfy an instinctual (id) demand, for any number of reasons.

**reparative therapy** *Conversion therapy*; it attempts to change a person from a homosexual orientaton to a heterosexual orientaton. There is no acceptable evidence that supports the efficacy of reparative therapy.

**repeat, trinucleotide** See *fragile X syndrome; Huntington disease; trinucleotide repeat.*

**repersonalization** Morton Prince suggested this term for hypnotism.

**repetition** The ability to repeat increasingly long verbal stimuli, beginning with single words and proceeding to repeating long sentences. The ability is often disturbed in *aphasia* (q.v.).

**repetition compulsion** *Inertia principle*; the impulse to redramatize or reenact some earlier emotional experience, irrespective of any advantage that such behavior might bring from a pleasure-pain point of view.

**replacement** In psychiatric occupational therapy the substitution of normal and healthy thoughts and actions for unhealthy, abnormal ones. The means used to achieve this result include the employment of various activities, such as the handicrafts, recreation, and other interests of a constructive nature.

**replacement memory** The substitution of one memory for another. One type of replacement memory is the *screen memory* (q.v.).

**replay** Recapitulation of experience-dependent patterns of neural activity previously observed during awake periods. See *consolidation*.

**replication** The cellular machines that replicate DNA do not act alone; instead, tens or hundreds are housed in enormous "factories," and individual machines in each factory reel in loops of DNA as they replicate them. Transcription machines that copy DNA into RNA are concentrated in analogous factories. Transcription goes on continuously, starting when a cell is born and lasting until it divides. In contrast, DNA is replicated only during the middle third of each cell cycle. *Replication* begins in many factors located in transcriptionally active regions and ends in a few large factors in less active regions (Cook, 1998). See *chromosome*.

**replicative senescence** A nondividing state that normal human diploid cells placed in culture enter following a finite proliferative lifespan, triggered by shortening of telomeres. Senescence of primary human cells can be delayed by overexpression of a protein that protects chromosome ends, telomere protection factor (TRF2). See *mitotic clock*; *telomerase*; *telomere*; *telomere clock model*.

**replicator** Heritable unit, used particularly in reference to the genetic determinants of behavior. In strict biochemical terms, a gene is a section of the DNA strand needed to code for the production of a single protein. In any consideration of "genetic" determination of behavior, however, the concept becomes increasingly fuzzy, since behavioral traits involve the cooperative action of several

"genes." It has been suggested that for sociological purposes the word gene be replaced by the term replicator—a combination of individual genes that generate some observed behavioral and/or physiological property of an organism. It is the replicators that are passed from one generation to the next by moving from one temporary phenotypic host, or "survival machine," to another.

The genotype includes all the replicators contained in the organism's genetic makeup. Heredity consists of the transmission of the genotype from parent to child. The replicators are passed from one generation to the next by moving from one temporary phenotypic host to another.

**reporting** In a medical setting, disclosure of information about a patient. See *confidentiality*.

By law, reporting is required in some instances, such as child or elder abuse, abuse of the developmentally disabled, gunshot wounds, contagious diseases, and toxic chemicals in the workplace. Some states also require that Alzheimer disease and other dementias, epilepsy, or other conditions that render the person liable to seizures or blackouts be reported to the motor vehicle department. See *notification, anonymous*.

**representation** See *sensorimotor stage*.

**representation, coitus** The representation of sexual intercourse in symptom formations or by other symbolizations. "In this analysis the girl's stammering proved to be determined by the libidinal cathexis of speaking as well as of singing. The rise and fall of the voice and the movements of the tongue represented coitus." (Klein, M. *Contributions to Psycho-analysis, 1921–1945*, 1948).

**representations, collective** The concepts that embody the objectives of group activity.

**representative intelligence** See *developmental psychology*.

**repress** To force material from the realm of consciousness into the unconscious; to prevent material that was never conscious from gaining the level of consciousness.

**repressed, return of the** The return to consciousness of an idea or set of ideas that had been repressed into the sphere of the unconscious.

**repression** The active process of keeping out and ejecting, banishing from consciousness, ideas or impulses that are unacceptable to it.

Three things are subject to repression: (1) the instinct presentation; (2) the idea; and (3) the affect. In many instances, when the entire instinct cannot be successfully repressed, either the ideational or the affective part may be. If the idea is repressed, the affect with which it was associated may be transferred to another idea (in consciousness) that has no apparent connection with the original idea. Or if the affect is repressed, the idea, remaining alone in consciousness, may be linked with a pleasant affect. Finally, if the whole instinct presentation is repressed, it may at some later time return to consciousness in the form of a symbol.

At times Freud used the term *after-expulsion* to refer to *repression proper*, because the material repressed is that which was once in the conscious realm.

There is another subdivision called *primal repression*, "which consists in a denial of entry into consciousness to the mental (ideational) presentation of the instinct. This is accompanied by a *fixation*; the ideational presentation in question persists unaltered from then onwards and the instinct remains attached to it." (Freud, S. *Collected Papers*, 1924–1925). Primal repression is maintained by means of anticathexis, which Freud says "is the sole mechanism of primal repression."

As Anna Freud pointed out, repression accomplishes more than the other defenses, acting once only through the anticathexis. It is also the most ego-limiting, because entire tracts of mental life are withdrawn from the ego in repression.

According to Jung, when the superior function is thinking (e.g., the extraverted thinking type), the feeling function is subordinated. When the individual tries to meet all the requirements of living by the thinking function, "sooner or later—in accordance with outer circumstances and inner gifts—the forms of life repressed [i.e., feeling, intuition, and sensation] by the intellectual attitude become indirectly perceptible, through a gradual disturbance of the conscious conduct of life. Whenever disturbances of this kind reach a definite intensity, one speaks of a neurosis" (Jung, C. G. *Psychological Types*, 1923).

**repression, organic**  A special type of *amnesia* (q.v.) that occurs in cases of head injuries independently of any personal problems

that the patient wishes to forget. It is a retroactive amnesia: as in (the so-called) psychogenic amnesia, the subject turns away from a part of his experiences. In organic repression, however, no specific personal motives are discernible. The person forgets, more or less extensively, the events of his life prior to the accident, as if he were trying to get rid of knowledge of his experiences, although such a desire is not present even in the subconscious.

**repressive personality**  *Histrionic personality* (q.v.).

**repressors**  See *anxiety typology*.

**reproductive failure**  Lack of success in bearing a child as in infertility or miscarriage, and usually also extended to include neonatal death.

**reproductive mortality**  Deaths associated with fertility control, including deaths due to adverse effects of temporary contraceptive methods and sterilization and deaths due to complications of pregnancy.

**reproductive success**  Impact of the person on the future; in evolutionary biology, measured by the number of descendants a person has, because that is what shapes future generations. See *evolutionary developmental psychology*; *sexuality*.

**required relationship**  See *group tension, common*.

**rescue phantasy**  See *romance, family*.

**Rescuer**  See *transactional analysis*.

**research, specific**  Any investigation or study that is designed primarily to gain knowledge about a disease or condition of the specific person being used as a subject of an experiment. Nonspecific research, in contrast, uses subjects to gain knowledge about a disease or functioning even though the results may be of no value or relevance to the experimental subjects. Some believe that it is never ethical to conduct nonspecific research, whereas others believe that if fully informed and mentally competent, subjects have the right to volunteer for such investigations.

**research, strategic**  Studies whose focus is treatment and care, as opposed to *tactical research*, which emphasizes the action taken to implement the findings of strategic research. Development of a vaccine, for example, is based on strategic research; the public health programs devised to administer it and evaluation of its effect on the populations to whom it has been administered depend on tactical research.

**Research Diagnostic Criteria (RDC)** A modification of the criteria developed by Washington University (St. Louis) for diagnosis of psychiatric disorders. The RDC was developed by R. Spitzer and coworkers at Columbia University (New York) and expanded the number of disorders from the original 15 to 25 (New York State Psychiatric Institute, *Biometrics Research*, 1978). It focuses on present or past episodes of illness and gives inclusion and exclusion criteria for diagnosis of the different disorders. It is supplemented by the Schedule for Affective Disorders and Schizophrenia (SADS), designed to elicit information on signs and symptoms and their duration. See *Renard Diagnostic Interview.*

**residence rate** In institutional statistics, the residence rate is based upon the population actually in institutions of a given type on any specified date. For example, it is the ratio of the resident population to the total population of the state. See *readmission.*

**residential centers** See *domicile; intermediate care.*

**residual** Remaining, left behind, with the implication that some effect continues to be exerted. Some authorities recognize a psychoactive substance-induced organic mental disorder, the organic residual syndrome, which may develop after prolonged heavy use of a psychoactive substance. Also called the *amotivational syndrome* (q.v.), it consists of reduction in goal-directed behavior such as attending school or going to work, and it may be accompanied by depression, irritability, difficulties in attention and concentration, and other mild cognitive deficits.

**residual schizophrenia** See *schizophrenia, residual.*

**residue, archaic** Remnants of primitive mentality. See *biological memory; function engram; racial memory.*

**resignation, neurotic** In Horney's terminology, avoidance of any part of reality that brings inner conflicts into awareness, whether by means of withdrawal into inactivity, pressured hyperactivity in all other parts of reality, or neurotic rebelliousness against all rules and regulations.

**resistance** 1. Failure to respond to a medication regimen. See *treatment resistance.*

2. Failure to respond to psychoanalytically based psychotherapy; the instinctive opposition displayed toward any attempt to lay bare the unconscious; a manifestation of the repressing forces. Resistance may take the form of transference behaviors that provoke unconscious countertransference reactions in the analyst. See *conscious resistance; ego resistance; id resistance; superego resistance; transference resistance.*

**resistance, character** See *character defense.*

**resistance, conscious** Intentional withholding of information by the patient because of distrust of the analyst, shame, fear of rejection, or the like. Exhortation can usually induce the patient to overcome these conscious difficulties.

Unconscious resistance or *ego resistance* (q.v.), on the other hand, is more significant and more difficult to overcome, arising as it does from the ego as a defense against uncovering the repressed material, which the ego constantly strives to avoid, because it produces anxiety. Unconscious resistance is more than a phenomenon appearing early in treatment and later overcome once and for all. It is a conservative force seeking to maintain the status quo and appearing throughout the analysis whenever significant data are under discussion. See *selective silence.*

**resocialization** The process by which a maladjusted person attains the attitudes and skills that facilitate acceptance into his community.

**resonance behavior** *Simulation* (q.v.).

**resonance hypothesis** The specificity of neural connections is due solely to the retention of connections in which the pattern of electrical activity of the presynaptic neurons matches that of its target. With the work of Roger Sperry that hypothesis gave way to the chemoaffinity hypothesis. See *chemoaffinity hypothesis.*

**respect for autonomy** A bioethical principle, one variation of *respect for persons*, that takes note of a person's right to liberty and to self-direction in regard to the course of his or her life, so long as the person abides by the law. In a medical setting, respect for autonomy gives people the right to determine what may—and may not—be done to them. The respect for autonomy is at the heart of *informed consent* (q.v.) and many patient rights. See *patient rights.* Allowable restrictions of autonomy are generally limited to emergency situations or to situations in which the patient would be unable to attain his or her own goal without help, even though such interventions may require at least a temporary reduction in the patient's autonomy.

**respect for persons**   See *respect for autonomy*.

**respiratory impairment sleep disorder**   *Sleep apnea* (q.v.). See *sleep disorders*.

**respondent conditioning**   See *conditioning*.

**response cost procedures**   See *social extinction*.

**response facilitation**   The automatic tendency to reproduce an observed movement. In *The Expression of the Emotions in Man and Animals*, Darwin mentions the case of sports fans who, while observing an athlete performing an exercise, tend to 'help' him by imitating his movements. Other examples include laughing, yawning, crying, and involuntarily mimicking facial expressions.

When subjects view static images that convey dynamic information, such as an athlete in the posture of throwing a ball, the implied motion from the static images activates the brain region that is specialized for processing visual motion—the *occipito-temporal junction*. This shows that the brain stores internal representations of dynamic information, which can be used to recall past movement and anticipate future movements, even from very partial visual information (Blakemore, S.-J. and Decety, J. *Nature Neuroscience 1*, 2001).

Response facilitation is believed to be the basis of *imitation* (q.v.). See *intention; prediction*.

**response heterogeneity**   See *gene–environment interactions*.

**response (in marriage)**   Understanding, cooperative, sympathetic, or affectionate interreaction between two persons married to each other.

**response prevention**   See *delay therapy*.

**response reversal**   A change in a learned behavioral response following a change in reinforcement contingencies

**responsibility, criminal**   See *criminal responsibility*.

**responsibility, limited**   See *partial insanity*.

**responsivity**   See *vigilance*.

**REST**   *Regressive electroshock therapy* (q.v.).

**rest cure**   The term is usually associated with the American psychiatrist Silas Weir Mitchell (1829–1914), who stressed the value of rest, environmental change, fattening diet, massage, and mild exercise. It has not achieved much distinction as an isolated method of treatment, though the individual

procedures (rest, environmental change, etc.) may be useful.

**rest tremor**   See *tremor*.

**restiform body**   See *cerebellum*.

**resting membrane potential**   The metabolically dependent voltage difference (c. 65 mV) that exists across the external membrane of the unexcited neuron. The Na⁺-K⁺ pump maintains an unequal distribution of Na+, K⁺, Cl⁻, and organic anions across the cell membrane by pumping Na⁺ out of the cell and K⁺ into it. As a result the inside of the neuronal membrane is negative in relation to the outside, and the Na+ concentration is 10 times lower inside the cell than it is outside, whereas the K⁺ concentration is almost 50 times higher inside than it is outside. This difference is reversed when the neuron is stimulated. See *action potential*.

**restitution**   See *schizophrenia, restitutional symptoms*.

**restless legs syndrome**   *RLS*; *Ekbom syndrome*; *tachyathetosis*; a sensorimotor disorder characterized by an overwhelming urge to move one's legs, paresthesias or dysesthesias that are worse during periods of inactivity (e.g., when lying or sitting down), and partially relieved by movement. RLS may be idiopathic or comorbid with separate medical or psychiatric conditions including pregnancy, uremia, iron depletion and reduced serum ferritin, polyneuropathy, and spinal disorder. Affected subjects are at increased risk for specific psychiatric disorders: panic disorder, generalized anxiety disorder, and major depression. The syndrome may represent an extrapyramidal hyperkinesis, and it sometimes occurs as a side effect of treatment with neuroleptics. Direct dopamine receptor agonists are the most effective treatment.

**restraining therapy**   See *paradoxical therapy*.

**restraint**   A generic term for measures taken to prevent a patient from injuring himself or others. Most frequently the term refers to physical interventions, including psychopharmacological agents (*chemical restraint*), designed to control or reduce the patient's ability to commit dangerous or violent actions, but the term also includes limitation or restriction of movement in patients unable to function independently when they are at risk of falling (out of chair or bed), wandering, etc. Four-point leather cufflets, cold wet packs, and camisoles have been used to achieve total or almost complete physical restraint. Such methods require constant, skilled nursing care, and if the restrained patient is also being treated with phenothiazines, the likelihood of temperature dysregulation and potentially dangerous hyperthermia increases. Further, the psychological effects of being tied down and totally dependent on others for feeding and toileting are generally negative. For these reasons, most clinicians prefer to use *seclusion* (q.v.) of violent or potentially violent patients. The seclusion room is free of all objects the patient might use to harm himself or staff—including not only furniture, mirrors, and other room appointments but also any of the patient's belongings that might be used in self-mutilation or in an outwardly directed attack (belt, shoes, rings, etc.). The seclusion room is also called the quiet room, not as a way to deny what it is, but in recognition of the fact that many patients request seclusion when they feel themselves to be on the verge of an agitated or destructive outburst that they doubt they can control.

**restraint, situational** Employed especially in activity group psychotherapy, this type of restraint is differentiated from direct or authoritative restraint in that it is practiced by creating a situation that by its very nature will prevent the individual from committing dangerous or destructive acts. In activity group psychotherapy, windows are screened so that they will not be broken and furniture is placed in such a way that the children will not need to or cannot move it about. Placing materials according to their functional relatedness is also a form of situational restraint.

**restricters** Persons with anorexia nervosa who achieve and maintain their low weight by restricting their food intake. Restricters are contrasted with bulimics, who alternate between starvation and engorgement (a condition also known as *bulimia nervosa, bulimarexia, and dietary chaos syndrome*).

**restriction enzyme** An enzyme that cuts fragments of DNA. In gene mapping, the restriction enzyme is applied to DNA. It cuts the DNA strands whenever it encounters a particular sequence of subunits. Genetic variation, however, alters the sequence and the strands are not cut as they should be. The result is that two strands that would ordinarily be separated remain together as a strand whose

unusual length makes it easily identifiable as abnormal. See *marker; recombinant DNA*.

**retardation** 1. Slowness or backwardness of intellectual development; mental retardation. 2. Slowness of response, a slowing down of thinking and/or a decrease in psychomotor activity; psychomotor retardation is characteristic of clinical depressions.

**retardation, mental** *Mental deficiency; intellectual inadequacy; feeblemindedness; hypophrenia; oligophrenia; oligergasia;* subnormal general intellectual functioning that originates during the developmental period (before 18 years of age) and is associated with impaired learning and social adjustment or maturation. It is subdivided on the basis of degree of intellectual impairment into four subtypes: (1) *mild*—echsler IQ, 69–55; in educational terms, the *educable* retardates, who account for about 75% of the total group; (2) *moderate*—IQ, 55–40; the *trainable* retardates; (3) *severe*—IQ, 39–25; together, the moderate and severe retardates account for about 20% of the total group; (4) *profound*—IQ, below 25.

Intellectual deficit, or mental subnormality, denotes a lack of equipment, motivation, or opportunity to acquire knowledge at the usual pace. By some, mental deficiency is used specifically to refer to cases with demonstrable cerebral impairment. Others, however, do not make such a distinction or even use the terms in exactly the opposite way. Thus, W. F. Windle (*Science 140*, 1963) defines mental retardation as "An organic condition of arrested or limited neural development that blocks successful evolution of the capacity of the brain to function; as a result of this block, behavior and (at least in man) intellectual ability are impaired. Forms of behavioral and intellectual impairment that are related solely to socio-environmental factors are excluded, since in these cases there is no detectable pathology." See *amentia; dementia*.

Fashions in labeling this group change almost from year to year; in the 1960s, mental retardation was the favorite appellation, and justifiably so in that it does not imply that inheritance or constitutional defects are always the cause of mental retardation. In 1941, Gregg demonstrated the association of rubella in the first trimester of pregnancy with mental retardation and thereby showed that the condition could result not from an inferior constitution but from birth conditions. Since then, there has been increasing recognition of the importance of psychosocial factors in exaggerating or even, in some cases, producing mental retardation, and two major approaches to such factors have developed.

The *stimulation theory* supposes that mental retardation may be a consequence of lack of stimulation, lack of opportunities, or deprivation. The *disorder theory* regards mental retardation as a disorder of mental processes due to failure of the family to give sufficient protection from stress or overstimulation during critical periods of learning in early childhood. As with some habits in animals (see *imprinting; releaser, social*), there are believed to be optimal periods in the human during which learning proceeds rapidly, although at other times those habits will be learned only slowly or not at all. Thus, a child may not learn because family conditions or other elements in his environment are not favorable to acquiring the habit when he is in a critical or sensitive period; or if he is exposed to adverse circumstances soon after acquiring a habit, it may regress and his skill may disintegrate; and even if later moved into more favorable circumstances he may fail to learn because the sensitive period has passed.

**retardation, simple**   See *manic-depressive psychosis*.

**retention**   1. Nonevacuation of the bladder or bowels.

2. In psychological testing, retention refers to the ability to learn, remember, or recall, to the process by which encoded information is maintained over time in the absence of active rehearsal. See *memory*.

3. In psychoanalytic psychology, retention refers to any number of traits or symptoms believed to develop on the basis of the need or desire to withhold the feces during the anal stage of development; collecting mania, stubbornness, secretiveness, niggardliness are generally considered to be instances of anal retention or retentiveness.

**retention hysteria**   Hysteria resulting not from splitting of consciousness or dissociation, but rather from failure to react to the traumatic situation when it occurred; the dammed-up or retained emotions may later be discharged through *abreaction* (q.v.).

**reticular activating system**   See *reticular formation*.

**reticular formation**   The primitive, diffuse system of interlacing fibers and nerve cells that forms the central core of the brain stem; also called the bulbotegmental reticular formation. The reticular formation projects to the thalamic intralaminar nuclei via the reticulothalamic, tegmentothalamic, and tectothalamic tracts. From the reticular nucleus of the thalamus, nonspecific fibers project to all parts of the cerebral cortex. It is believed that these fibers can activate the cortex independently of specific sensory or other neural systems, and the reticular formation is thus considered a part of the *reticular activating system (RAS)* or *alerting system*, which also includes subthalamus, hypothalamus, and medial thalamus. The RAS seems to be essential for the initiation and maintenance of alert wakefulness, for alerting or focusing of attention, perceptual association, and directed introspection. Impaired function of the RAS may be associated with anesthesia and comatose states.

In addition to modulating awareness and *arousal* (q.v.), the reticular system modulates muscle tone, participates in the control of respiratory and cardiac function, and modulates nociception by influencing the flow of information through the dorsal horn of the spinal cord.

**reticulum**   Also, reticular apparatus; described by *Golgi* (q.v.) as an interlacing network of small intracytoplasmic structures within the cell body of the neuron and now known to be important in neuronal metabolism. Almost all neuronal proteins and other structural components are synthesized within the cell body, under the control of DNA. Messenger RNA (mRNA) carries information from DNA to sites adjacent to the nucleus, where mRNA is translated to synthesize structural and metabolic proteins. Nerve cell substances are synthesized within the rough endoplasmic reticulum and then packaged in the smooth endoplasmic reticulum, which carries them down the axon to its terminal.

**rétifism**   (Rétif de la Bretonne, 1734–1806, a famous French educator, known for this paraphilia) Ivan Bloch coined this term for fetishism of the foot and shoe; in this form of sexual perversion the foot or shoe or both possess the value of the genital organs for the rétifist. A patient "loved," as he put it, the female shoe to the same degree that "others are attracted to the female genitals." He looked upon the shoe as if it were a real person—gaining full and complete sexual satisfaction, including "intercourse," with the object; he used it as an agency of masturbation.

**retinitis, CMV**   See *cytomegalic disease.*

**retinocerebellar angiomatosis**   See *Hippel-Lindau disease.*

**retinodiencephalic degeneration**   See *Laurence-Moon-Biedl syndrome.*

**retinotopy**   See *receptor sheet, peripheral.*

**retrieval**   The seeking out and bringing back into consciousness, when needed, the information that has been encoded and retained. See *memory.*

**retroactive hallucination**   *Memory hallucination* (q.v.).

**retroflexed rage**   See *adaptational psychodynamics.*

**retroflexion**   A turning backwards, especially upon the self. In psychoanalysis, the term is used particularly by Rado, who speaks of retroflexed rage, i.e., one's own rage turned back upon the self. See *adaptational psychodynamics.*

**retrogenesis**   The regression to earlier or lower stages that is often essential before further development can be achieved; Staercek termed it the *Law of Retrogenesis*: "That which is newly formed does not develop from the highest (in the sense of the most recent) existing formation but out of a lower part which has remained hitherto undeveloped. Every line of development is a blind-alley: the new sprouts from a bud which is further, sometimes much further, down. The path of development is not that of *evolution* but of *revolution*. Only out of temporary chaos does renewal proceed" (*International Journal of Psychoanalysis X*, 1929).

**retrograde amnesia**   Amnesia extending backward, to include material antedating the onset of amnesia proper; also called circumscribed amnesia. When the amnesia encompasses material subsequent to the onset of amnesia it is termed *anterograde amnesia* or *continuous amnesia*. See *dementia.*

**retrograde memory**   Ability to recall information consciously and deliberately after a given point in time or sentinel event. It is commonly divided into recent and remote *memory* (q.v.) See *MTL.*

**retrogression**   A return to earlier behavior or techniques when more recently developed techniques prove unsatisfactory. The term is synonymous with *regression* but avoids the psychoanalytic connotations of the latter.

**retropulsion**   Rapid running backward with short steps, in paralysis agitans; as if drawn by an uncontrollable force.

**retropulsive epilepsy**   A form of *epilepsy* (q.v.) characterized by sudden, impulsive running backward.

**retrovirus**   A member of the Retroviridae family of viruses, which includes the foamy viruses, murine leukosis viruses, Rous sarcoma virus, visna virus, and HIV. Retroviruses encode their genetic information as RNA, rather than DNA, and synthesize DNA from that RNA template through the action of reverse transcriptase (RT) enzyme (the reverse of the usual DNA-to-RNA transcription). The resultant DNA copy is then integrated into the genome of the host.

One technique used in creating a *transgenic* animal (q.v.) exploits this mechanism: the harmful RNA genes are removed from the retrovirus and replaced with RNA copies of the gene that is to be introduced into the host, and the altered retrovirus infects the embryonic cell of the host animal. The cells then make DNA copies of the gene, and the copies are incorporated into the embryo's chromosomes.

Human cells do not need RT, and a major approach in developing treatment (including vaccine) for AIDS has been to search for drugs that will inhibit or eliminate RT and thereby prevent the AIDS virus from replicating itself within the infected cell.

**Rett disorder**   A pervasive developmental disorder, first described in 1966, that arises in a child whose development during the first 6 months of life appears to be normal. It is second only to Down syndrome as a cause of female retardation; it afflicts at least 1 in 10,000 girls. In boys, the disease almost always leads to death in utero. As many as one-third of cases have been linked to a mutation in the *MeCP2* gene on the X chromosome.

Between 6 months and 48 months of age, head growth decelerates and previously acquired purposeful hand movements are lost, often to be replaced by stereotypies such as handwringing. Social interaction and skills wither, gait and trunk movements become uncoordinated, and defects in both expressive and receptive language appear along with severe psychomotor retardation.

**reuptake**   A major form of synaptic inactivation consisting of removal of neurotransmitter from the synapse by specific reuptake transport proteins, which return the neuro-transmitter to the presynaptic cell. Almost all biogenic amines and amino acids are inactivated by reuptake.

Reuptake consists of a pumplike mechanism that returns a neurotransmitter to the neuron that released it. Sometimes the transmitter is stored again in vessels or granules, ready to be released again on demand; at other times reuptake serves largely to expose the neurotransmitter to degradative processes within the neuron. The reuptake destruction mechanism is more typical than the longer-known enzyme destruction mechanism, such as the breakdown of acetylcholine by cholinesterase.

**revenge** Retaliation; vindication; the wish of the injured person to retaliate against the aggressor, which often leads in the neurotic to a fear of retaliation and a consequent need to repress or deny his own aggression.

**reverie** 1. *Daydream* (q.v.).

2. According to Bion, the calm receptiveness of the mother that contains the infant's anxieties and other disturbing feelings. Such a state of mind in the mother allows the *alpha function* (q.v.) to operate.

**reverie, hypnagogic** The phantasies occurring between sleep and waking. Kubie has shown that the institution of a state of hypnagogic reverie can bring about easier access to unconscious material. When employing hypnosis, the analyst can take advantage of it by "permitting his patients to associate freely in the waking state, until a resistance is manifested. Hypnosis is then induced and the last few statements uttered by the patient before the onset of resistance are repeated to him. Usually free association will continue during hypnosis from this point on" (Wolberg, L. R. *Hypnoanalysis*, 1945).

**reversal** In psychoanalysis, change of an instinct from an active to a passive instinct or vice versa. The aim of the instinct does not change; its object does. For example, the destructive instinct may be directed outwardly, as sadism, or it may be turned against oneself, as masochism. "The passive aim (to be tortured...) has been substituted for the active (to torture...)" (Freud, S. *Collected Papers*, 1924–25). See *reveral into the opposite*.

**reversal formation** See *reaction formation*.

**reversal into the opposite** One of the major defenses by which the ego handles the sexual instinct, which impinges upon it while seeking direct gratification. The specific nature of this process consists of the transformation of the aim of an instinct into its opposite, and the substitution of the instinct itself for the external object. This process is called into play when the aim of a sexual instinct has been blocked from direct object gratification by internal intrapsychic or external environmental prohibition and restriction. In the process of reversal into the opposite, the active aim usually becomes a passive one.

**reversal of affect** See *inversion of affect*.

**reverse genetics** See *marker*.

**reversed orientation** A state in which a person when walking in one direction feels that he is walking in the opposite direction. The condition is purely subjective; the person orients himself correctly by reasoning.

**reversion** A genetic phenomenon that occurs in crosses between true-breeding varieties and produces offspring resembling a remote ancestor more than either parent. These "throwbacks" had been observed for many years by plant and animal breeders, but for lack of satisfactory explanation had been regarded as due to some mysterious force that caused the retention and subsequent reappearance of a remote ancestral trait.

According to E. W. Sinnott and L. C. Dunn (*Principles of Genetics*, 1939) every kind of reversion is now readily explained in terms of ordinary Mendelian inheritance. "The reappearance of an old trait is usually due to the reunion of the two or more factors, necessary for its production, which had become separated in the history of the plant or animal."

Reversion is also used synonymously with regression or retrogression; less commonly, it is used synonymously with reversal formation or reaction formation.

**review** Critical examination or evaluation; assessment of medical care or services is no longer a matter solely of evaluating the quality of care, for it must also be judged in terms of cost effectiveness.

In the United States, third-party payers (insurers) have had criteria for reimbursement of medical claims for many years. In 1965, Medicare legislation established more uniform control over reimbursement for health care to the aged. The Social Security Amendment of 1972 established *PSROs* (*professional standards review organizations*), with utilization control over inpatient (and ultimately outpatient) treatment of Medicaid and Medicare patients and of those covered by maternal and child health programs. Since those developments, there has been increasing emphasis on formalized *peer review*, evaluation of the treatment process by one or more colleagues. The review process includes utilization review, quality review, continuing education, advocacy with intermediaries for improved care, and cost control.

*Peer review* is a system of professional judgment of individual or group medical performance. Most systems depend upon professionally developed *screening* criteria for measuring quality of care, and the cases that do not meet those criteria are selected out for review in greater depth by professionals who make the final decision about adequacy of care. Peer review emphasizes continuing education as a way to improve methods of practice and quality of care. Like the more traditional forms of evaluation of treatment process—such as case conferences, grand rounds, and continuing case supervision—its objectives are professional growth and development and not reduction of psychiatric practice to a mechanical or pedestrian ritual.

Peer review for medical purposes attempts to systematize and document the treatment process with the ultimate goal of improving the quality of care. Peer review for insurance purposes, on the other hand, is focused on cost containment and medical necessity; such a process is termed *claims review*. See *audit*.

*Utilization review* is analysis of admissions to service from the point of view of determination of the medical necessity for the level of particular services provided and for the duration of stay within the institution. Utilization review is *concurrent* rather than retrospective in that it occurs while care is being provided: *admission certification* of the necessity for admission and *continued stay review (CSR)* for assessment of the need for care to be continued. CSR in large part consists of comparison of the case under review with regional *norms*, which usually are expressed as average *length of stay (LOS)* for each diagnosis.

**revindication, delirium of** See *delirium of interpretation*.

**revolution** A sudden and far-reaching change, a major break in the continuity of development; that mass movement that seeks to change the mores by destroying the existing social order.

Three major types of revolution are *cultural*, where profound changes take place in the mores; *industrial*, where sudden changes result from technological discoveries and inventions; and *political*, where violent change takes place in the political order.

**revolving door** See *readmission*.

**reward** Anything that a subject (human or animal) will work to acquire. This definition emphasizes the motivational ("wanting") rather the affective ("liking") dimension of reward. The existence of drug reward sites and brain-stimulation reward (*BSR*) sites indicates that there is a dedicated network of neural structures devoted to reward processing. Lesion data have emphasized the importance of PFC in monitoring the motivational value of stimuli and actions, but physiological studies suggest this function is distributed across both frontal and parietal cortices. Decision-related signals in areas of the *intraparietal sulcus* (q.v.) point to a neural architecture in which decisions are computed and represented within the very neural structures that guide behavioral responses.

Within the prefrontal-amygdala pathway, orbital, ventromedial, and dorsolateral prefrontal cortical areas are activated in difficult choices that require the coding of reward value and in the integration of two or more separate cognitive operations in the pursuit of higher behavioral goals. A limbic circuit integrates the amygdala with the hypothalamus and septal nuclei.

The dopamine hypothesis of reward proposes that dopamine is important not only in the reinforcement that follows the earning of a reward, but also in the *incentive motivation* (q.v.) that precedes the earning of reward. See *choice; counterfactual thinking; dopamine hypothesis of addiction; regret.*

**reward center** Electrical stimulation of the lateral hypothalamus and limbic system is rewarding; electrical stimulation near the midline of the hypothalamus and its connections to the limbic system is aversive or punishing. There are no specialized peripheral receptors for rewards, but neurons in several brain structures seem to be particularly sensitive to rewarding events as opposed to motivationally neutral events that are signaled through the same sensory modalities. A prominent example is the dopamine neurons in the pars compacta of the substantia nigra and the medially adjoining ventral tegmental area. Neurons that respond to the delivery of rewards are also found in brain structures other than the dopamine system. These include the striatum (caudate nucleus, putamen, ventral striatum including the nucleus accumbens), subthalamic nucleus, pars reticulata of the substantia nigra, dorsolateral and orbital prefrontal cortex, anterior cingulate cortex, amygdala, as well as the lateral hypothalamus. See *dopamine*.

**reward deficiency syndrome**    The hypothesis that compulsive disorders such as drug addiction, gambling, and sex are due to increased extracellular dopamine caused by blocking dopamine transporters or reducing dopamine D2 receptors.

**reward system**    The anhedonia hypothesis posits that dopamine is important for the subjective feeling of pleasure or euphoria with which rewards are usually associated. Pleasurable experiences, including the effects of drugs of abuse, were once believed to be mediated through dopamine, especially in the nucleus accumbens in the mesolimbic system. Present evidence indicates that elevations in brain dopamine are only loosely correlated with subjective pleasure. See *dopamine hypothesis of addiction; reward*.

**Rey Complex Figure Test**    A test of visual memory and conceptual construction, consisting of a complex figure that is copied by the subject, who is then presented with delay recall trials.

**RFLPs**    *Restriction fragment length polymorphisms*; DNA fragments of different length generated by cleaving with a specific endonuclease; used in genetic mapping. When a restriction enzyme is used to digest DNA, chromosomal regions are cut into fragments of characteristic lengths. Some of these fragment lengths are variable in the population. Loci where this is the case are RFLPs; they provide convenient markers for linkage studies. See *marker*.

**RFS**    Role Functioning Scale, a measurement of psychosocial functioning.

**rhabdophobia**    Fear of the rod, instrument of punishment.

**rhathymia**    Outgoing, carefree, happy-go-lucky behavior such as is seen in so-called oral optimists.

**rheobase**    The lowest amount of current that will produce contraction (or other reaction) of a muscle.

**rheumatic polyneuritis**    *Guillain-Barré syndrome* (q.v.).

**rheumatism**    A variety of disorders characterized by pain and stiffness referable to the musculoskeletal system; rheumatism involving the joints themselves is termed *arthritis* (q.v.).

**rheumatoid arthritis**    See *arthritis*.

**rhinencephalon**    A phylogenetically old portion of the cerebral hemispheres that includes olfactory bulb and tract, anterior perforated substance, subcallosal gyrus, *hippocampus*, uncus, *amygdala*, fornix, and anterior commissure (qq.v.). Rhinencephalon is sometimes used synonymously with olfactory brain. In humans, the olfactory brain is overshadowed by the neocortex (isocortex), but olfaction appears to be important in the psychic apparatus of the human. The olfactory tract terminates in the prepyriform area, the amygdala, the periamygdaloid cortex, and the opposite olfactory bulb. Rhinencephalic structures may exert an inhibitory effect on brain-stem mechanisms concerned with emotional expression. Lesions of these structures result in restlessness and hyperactivity. See *limbic lobe*.

**rhinolalia**    Nasality of speech. Rhinolalia is of two types: rhinolalia aperta, in which the passages at the back of the nose and mouth fail to close during speech; and rhinolalia clausa, in which obstructions in the nasopharynx interfere with nasal resonance.

**rhinotillexomania**    Nose picking. See *grooming disorders*.

**rhodopsin**    See *photoreceptor*.

**rhombencephalon**    *Hindbrain* (q.v.).

**rhyming delirium**    A symptom of the manic phase of manic-depressive reaction characterized by utterances in rhyme. See *mania*.

**rhypophobia**    *Obs.* Fear of dirt or filth.

**rhythm test**    The subject must discriminate between like and unlike pairs of musical beats.

**rhythmic sensory bombardment therapy**    *RSBT*; a form of treatment consisting of sonic, photic, or tactile stimulation applied intermittently and rhythmically usually for a period of 1 hour. The affective psychoses, psychoneuroses, psychopathic personalities, and paranoid forms of schizophrenia are said to show favorable response.

**rhythms, biological**    *Clock-driven behavior*; time-specific cyclical variations in biochemical and physiologic functions and levels of activity (including variations in emotional state and psychomotor reactivity). *Circadian* rhythms have a cycle of about 24 hours, *infradian* are shorter than 1 day and *ultradian* are longer (weeks or months); *circaseptan* have a duration of about 1 week, circalunar of about a month, and *circannual* of about a year.

Although biological rhythms are endogenous, a *Zeitgeber* (exogenous timegiver) often is instrumental in maintaining synchrony between the endogenous rhythm and environmental cycles, a process sometimes referred to as *entrainment*. When the Zeitgeber is removed, as under constant laboratory conditions, the internal clock is said to be *free-running*, and the rhythm may drift slightly from the norm. See *clock, biological*.

Circadian rhythms are generated by an internal pacemaker that is synchronized to daily time cues in the environment such as the light-dark cycle. There are many biological rhythms (e.g., hormone levels, the menstrual cycle, the sleep/wake schedule, brain electrical activity); when they are in correct relationship with one another they are in phase. A phase shift may occur in abnormal states, when one or more of the biological rhythms is out of phase. *Phase advance* describes a biological rhythm that begins earlier than it normally should; *phase delay* describes one that begins later. See *circadian rhythm sleep disorder*.

Genetic studies of circadian rhythmicity began with the discovery of clock mutants in the fruitfly, *Drosophila melanogaster*, in which interaction of the products of an X chromosome-linked gene, *period* (*per*), and chromosome 2-linked *timeless* (*tim*) are necessary for the production of circadian rhythms. (While in the fruitfly, *tim* interacts with the *per* gene, in the bread mold *Neurospora crassa* it interacts with the *frequency* gene, *frq*).

The cyclic expression of *tim* appears to dictate the timing of *per* protein accumulation and its entry into the nucleus. *Per* protein molecules accumulate slowly and then bind with tim proteins, forming stable dimers that enter the nucleus. There, through an autoregulatory feedback loop, they shut down the expression of their own genes. Thus, *per* and *tim* work as a team to generate an oscillating cycle of activity in their own genes and probably other genes, which in turn set daily rhythms in the fly's physiology and activity.

**RI strain**  *Recombinant inbred strain*; a strain originating from the second generation of intercrossing of two inbred strains, then inbreeding the new line at least 20 generations. The RI strain has a reproducible recombined sampling of the genomes of the two original inbred strains.

**ribonucleic acid**  *RNA* (q.v.).

**ribosome**  The organelles on which proteins are synthesized; they are constructed out of complexes of various ribosomal RNAs (rRNAs) together with proteins. Peptide neurotransmitters, for example, are synthesized on ribosomes in the cell body as part of inactive protein precursors, which are then cleaved into smaller, active forms and transported in large vesicles to the nerve terminal. See *neuron; nucleolus; RNA*.

**Ribot law**  The law that states the first language acquired is the first to be restored in cases of aphasia. See *Pitres law*.

**Rice Conferences**  See *Group Relations Conferences*.

**riddance**  This term, coined by S. Rado, refers to "many reflexes designed to eliminate pain-causing agents from the surface or inside of the body. The scratch reflex, the shedding of tears, sneezing, coughing, spitting, vomiting, colic bowel movement are but a few well-known instances of this principle of pain control in our bodily organization. This principle I have called the *riddance principle*, and its physiological embodiments the *riddance reflexes*" (*Psychoanalytic Quarterly VIII*, 1939).

**riddling**  See *alpha sleep*.

**right**  A claim that a person or group can justifiably make upon others or upon society. A *moral right* is a claim that is justified by moral principles or rules.

**right and left**  According to W. Stekel, when the concepts *right* and *left* appear in dreams they are understood in an ethical sense. "The right-hand path always signifies the way to righteousness, the left-hand path the path to crime. Thus the left may signify homosexuality, incest, and perversion, while the right signifies marriage, relations with a prostitute, etc. The meaning is always determined by the particular moral standpoint of the dreamer" (*Bi-Sexual Love*, 1922).

**right and wrong test**  See *criminal responsibility*.

**right-handedness**  See *cerebral dominance; laterality*.

**right-left disorientation**  See *Gerstmann syndrome*.

**right to be free of violent assault**  See *inpatient violence*.

**right to have a substitute decision-maker** See *respect for autonomy.*

**right to privacy** See *confidentiality; respect for autonomy.*

**right to refuse treatment** Part of the bioethical principle of respect for autonomy, first formulated in *Rennie v. Klein* (1978) when the court found that patients had a constitutionally based right to refuse treatment except in an emergency. In *Rogers v. Okin* (1979) the court found that the involuntarily committed patient had a right to refuse antipsychotic (and other "intrusive") treatment, except in an emergency. In *Cruzan v. Director* (1990) it was ruled that a patient has the right to refuse even life-sustaining treatment, and that the right survives even should the patient become incompetent, in which case the right can be exercised by a substitute decision maker (designated through living wills, durable powers of attorney, or other advance directives). See *consumerism; respect for autonomy.*

**right to the least restrictive alternative** A patient's right to be treated in an environment that least abridges his rights, so long as that environment does not compromise his specific treatment needs. See *consumerism; respect for autonomy.*

**right to treatment** See *consumerism; respect for autonomy.*

**rights, patient** See *patient rights.*

**rigid families** See *family types.*

**rigidity, affective** When the emotions or affects remain constant in the face of topics that normally call for changes in affect, the condition is known as affective rigidity. Many patients with schizophrenia show no mood changes in spite of discussions covering a wide variety of experiences. Rigidity of the affect, or *affect-block* (q.v.), is common also in *obsessive-compulsive disorder.*

**Riley-Day syndrome** (Conrad Milton Riley, U.S. pediatrician, 1913–2005; Richard Lawrence Day, U.S. pediatrician, 1905–1989) See *dysautonomia, familial.*

**Rip Van Winkle MPD** *Epochal multiple personality disorder* (q.v.).

**risk** Hazard, peril, or exposure to loss or injury; the sum of the probability of harmful effect and the magnitude of such effect(s) resulting from any procedure or situation. See *risk factor.*

*Children at risk* are those who the clinician predicts will have some kind of emotional difficulty or psychiatric disorder in the future. For the researcher, however, the phrase is more likely to mean children of mentally ill parents, and most commonly the illness is schizophrenia and the ill parent is the mother.

The *high-risk approach*, first employed by Doctors Sarnoff Mednick and Fini Schulsinger in Denmark, is a research method that studies vulnerable persons from their early years through the period of risk, in an attempt to identify those biochemical, physiological, or psychologic factors that differentiate between those who ultimately develop the disorder and those who do not.

*Risk management* consists of the identification, analysis, evaluation, and elimination of the factors that predispose to loss or injury and is most frequently applied to a hospital's program to control factors affecting the safety and security of its patients, visitors, and employees.

**risk, minimal** The amount of hazard encountered by normal persons in their daily lives or in routine medical or psychological examination of such persons.

**risk, morbid** The probability of having a first episode of illness during one's lifetime. Within a specified population, the morbid risk is the proportion of subjects who would be affected if all lived through the age of risk. See *epidemiology.*

**risk adjustment** In outcome studies, modification of raw data or initial findings to reflect the influence of potentially confounding variables on the final results. Risk adjustment is a technique designed to minimize or correct erroneous inferences about effectiveness or quality care based on patient outcomes. Factors often used in risk adjustment are age, gender, race, education, socioeconomic status, and other demographic factors, and clinical factors such as diagnosis, chronicity, comorbidity, level of impairment, patient noncompliance, etc.

**risk factor** A characteristic measurable variable, or hazard, that increases the likelihood of development of an adverse outcome. A risk factor precedes the outcome; this distinguishes it from other characteristics, such as concomitants or consequences of outcomes, which are correlates but not risk factors.

*Relative risk* is the ratio of the occurrence of a disorder in those exposed to the risk factor to the rate of disorder in those not exposed. *Attributable risk* is the absolute difference between the rate of the disorder in those exposed and the rate of the disorder in those not exposed to the risk factor. See *vulnerability*.

Several prenatal risk factors have been identified in schizophrenia: influenza and toxoplasmosis infections during pregnancy, and folate (vitamin B$_{12}$) deficiency manifested in high homocysteine levels.

**risk level**   *Confidence level* (q.v.).

**risk management**   See *risk*.

**risk-rescue rating**   A method of assessing the lethality or deadliness of suicide attempts devised by Avery Weisman and J. William Worden (*Archives of General Psychiatry 26*, 1972), expressed by the formula

$$\frac{A}{A + B} \times 100$$

where A is the risk score (the agent, the impairment of consciousness, lesions, toxicity, reversibility, treatment required) and B is the rescue score (location of attempt, person initiating rescue, probability of discovery by a rescuer, accessibility to rescue, delay until discovery).

**risk-taking behavior**   *High-risk behavior, hazardous behavior*; activity that puts one in danger of harmful consequences, such as use of drugs, alcohol, and tobacco; sexual promiscuity, particularly hazardous because of the increased likelihood of HIV infection; and accident-prone activities, such as fast driving, skydiving, and hang gliding. Increased sexual risk-taking is one downside effect of effective treatment of HIV; treatment does not eliminate the virus, but because symptoms are reduced or eliminated the patient assumes that he or she is no longer infectious.

**risky use**   One type of *alcohol use, unhealthy* (q.v.).

**ritual**   Formal behavior for occasions not given over to technological routine that occur both as spontaneous invention of the individual, especially of the compulsion neurotic, and as a cultural trait.

**ritual-making**   One of Rado's subdivisions of obsessive attacks is called *bouts of ritual-making*: repetitive sequences that must be continued until the patient is exhausted. Typically, these rituals are ceremonial, distortive, and stereotyped elaborations of some routine of daily life, such as bathing, dressing, and sexual activity.

**rivalry**   A sublimated form of conflict where the struggle of individuals is subordinated to the welfare of the group.

**RLS**   *Restless legs syndrome* (q.v.).

**RLS person**   A person who finds difficulty in pronouncing the sounds of *r, l, s*; by hardly justified extension; a stammerer. See *stuttering*.

**RMT**   Recovered memory therapy; induced memory retrieval ties curative power to restoration of the patient's early past. There is controversy, however, about whether the memories produced are in fact retrieved from the subject's unconscious or repressed memory store or whether they are induced in large part in a suggestible subject by the therapist.

**RNA**   *Ribonucleic acid*, an intermediate in the synthesis of proteins. See *transcription*. RNA differs by one nucleotide building block from *DNA* (q.v.); in RNA the pyrimidine uracil (U) takes the place of thymine and is complementary to adenine (U:A). In addition, the attached sugar group is ribose instead of deoxyribose. Like DNA, RNA is chemically quite simple (i.e., composed of four nucleotides), but since it is a flexible single strand, free to fold into a variety of conformations, it is functionally more versatile than DNA. Messenger RNA (mRNA) functions as an intermediate between the sequences of DNA that make up the transcribed regions of genes, and the sequence of proteins.

Not all RNA serves as mRNA, however. Other RNAs serve distinct functional roles in cells. *Ribosomes*, the organelles on which proteins are synthesized, are constructed out of complexes of various ribosomal RNAs (rRNAs) together with proteins. Transfer RNAs (tRNAs) transport specific amino acids in the ribosomes for incorporation into proteins during the process in which mRNA is translated into protein. See *transcription*.

**RNAi**   RNA interference; see *microRNAs*.

**RNS**   Responsive neurostimulator system. See *deep brain stimulation (DBS)*.

**Robinson Crusoe age**   In Erikson's description of the eight stages of man, the stage of *industry vs. inferiority*. See *ontogeny, psychic*.

**robotization**   See *trauma*.

**rocking**   See *stereotypic movement disorders*.

**rocks**   See *crack*.

**rod and frame test**   The subject must adjust a rod to a vertical position in a frame whose orientation varies during the period of eight trials.

**rods**   See *photoreceptor*.

**Rogers, Carl** (1902–1987) American clinical psychologist; developed a humanistic, person-centered theory of personality, which emphasized the inherent tendency to actualize one's unique potential (self-actualization). In 1942, the complete transcript of a recording of Rogers's sessions with a patient, Herbert Bryan, with additional comments by the therapist was released. Roger's client-centered psychotherapy provided an atmosphere in which the subject could renew strivings for self-actualization and self-acceptance. See *client-centered psychotherapy*.

**Rogers decision** A right-to-refuse treatment decision handed down by the Massachusetts Supreme Judicial Court in 1983; it ruled that all psychiatric inpatients, competent as well as incompetent, have a right to refuse treatment with antipsychotic medications except for limited emergency situations. The court held that with incompetent patients the decision about medicating a patient should be made by a judge, using a substituted judgment analysis in the context of a full adversarial proceeding. See *consumerism; forced treatment*.

**ROI** Region of interest; typically used to indicate the specific area of the brain that is being evaluated for its role in the pathogenesis of a syndrome or disorder that is under investigation.

**roid rage** Aggressive and sometimes homicidal behavior that occurs in some subjects who abuse steroids. See *anabolic-androgenic steroids*.

**role** The pattern or type of behavior which the child—and the adult—builds up in terms of what others expect or demand of him.

An automatic, learned, goal-directed pattern or sequence of acts developed under the influence of the significant people in the growing child's environment; such patterns provide the child with a repertoire of expected or appropriate responses to the behavior of those with whom he interacts. When the person's behavior does in fact conform with what is expected in a given situation or relationship, his role is termed *complementary* to the roles of the other people in the situation; such complementarity is desirable and comfortable. Noncomplementarity or disequilibrium of roles, as occurs when people's expectations of others are disappointed, leads to disruption of interpersonal relationships and breakdowns in group living. See *complementarity; complementary*.

Roles are labeled *explicit* when they are consciously motivated and exposed to observation and awareness of the interacting participants; roles are *implicit* when they are more remote from consciousness and awareness and often are not recognized as such by actor or participant. Typically, implicit roles express personality attributes originating in early internalizations or identifications; they are an outgrowth of early transactions between mother and child, child and teacher, etc.

**role confusion** See *identity crisis; ontogeny, psychic*.

**role models** See *reciprocal determinism*.

**role reversal** Adopting or assuming the pattern of behavior that is expected of the other in a relationship. Probably the most common form is that in which the child is given parental authority because the parent is absent from the home or unable to shoulder the burdens of parenthood. Such role reversal can become a significant problem for the child, and the family as well, if the demands exceed the child's abilities.

**rolfing** After Ida Rolf, Ph.D., a biochemist who developed *structural integration* while working with consciousness expansion at the Esalen Institute: deep massage to release the connective tissue that binds together the muscle groups in which both psychic and physical pains are stored. Typically, rolfing is given in 10 hour-long sessions spread over several weeks. See *body-centered therapy*.

**romance, family** A type of phantasy in which the subject maintains that he is not the child of his real parents, but is instead the offspring of other parents (usually of higher station). The *rescue phantasy*, of saving the life of the father (or king, or emperor, etc.) or of the mother, is a common variant of the family romance. Another variant, the *Mignon delusion*, is the fixed belief that one is the child of a distinguished family. Usually, the family romance arises on the basis of disillusionment with the real parents (who have failed to demonstrate the omnipotence with which the child has endowed them) and/or as a defense against the aggressive sexual elements of the oedipal period.

**Romberg sign** (Moritz Heinrich Romberg, German physician, 1795–1873) Swaying of the body when the patient stands with the feet together and the eyes closed, suggestive of ataxia.

**ROMI**   Rating of Medication Influences; a scale for the assessment of attitudinal and behavioral factors influencing patient compliance with neuroleptic treatment.

**roofies**   See *date rape drug.*

**rooming-in**   After the birth of the child, mother and child are housed in the same room, the infant's crib standing alongside or near the mother's bed. It is essentially a rooming-in of the baby with the mother. The rooming-in process permits the mother to touch, fondle, and caress her child, to feed it when it is hungry, and to diaper it when it soils. This is said to make her immediately familiar with her baby and to allay considerable anxiety in both mother and child.

**root cause analysis**   A structured approach to uncovering factors contributing to a *sentinel event*. See *JCAHO.*

**root-pain**   Pain in the segmental area innervated by the affected nerve root, usually excited or intensified by coughing, sneezing, or changes of posture.

**rootwork**   A form of *folk medicine* (q.v.) found among both blacks and whites in the southeastern United States, based on a belief in malign magic or evil spell. The rejected person in a love triangle or an envious coworker is most often the one suspected of "working roots" (also called *hexing* or *mojo*). The rootworker, or spirit doctor, has innate healing powers including the ability to counteract the effects of rootwork and return the spell to the one who instigated it. Herbal medicines are often prescribed for the victim, who may consult a physician concurrently. In Latino societies, the symptoms displayed by the person who believes he or she is the victim of hexing—anxiety, gastrointestinal disturbances, dizziness, fear—are called *brujeria* or *mal puesto.*

**Rorschach test**   (Hermann Rorschach, Swiss psychiatrist, 1884–1922) A projective test consisting of 10 inkblots of varying designs and colors, which are shown to the subject one at a time with the request to interpret them. Its purpose is to furnish a description of the dynamic forces of personality through an analysis of the formal aspects of the subject's interpretations. The test yields information as to the intellectual and emotional processes,

the degree of personality integration, variability in mental functioning, and the degree to which the subject responds to environmental influences and to his inner promptings. The test not only 10 used to obtain a picture of the subject's personality, but also serves as an aid in problems of differential psychiatric diagnosis and prognosis.

**ROS**   Reactive oxygen species, such as the *free radicals* (q.v.). See *neurotoxicity; oxidative stress; OXPHOS.*

**Rosenbach sign**   (Ottomar Rosenbach, German physician, 1851–1907) Inability of neurasthenics to close the eyes immediately and completely on command.

**Rosenthal, David**   (1918–1996) U.S. psychologist; genetics of schizophrenia; *The Genain Quadruplets* (1963), *Genetic Theory and Abnormal Behavior, The Transmission of Schizophrenia* (1968, with Seymour Kety).

**Ross-Jones test**   (Hugh Campbell Ross, English pathologist, 1875–1926, and Ernest Jones, English medical journalist, neurological researcher, and psychoanalyst, 1879–1958) A test for excess of globulin in cerebrospinal fluid. Fluid is floated on top of an ammonium sulfate solution; excess globulin forms a grayish-white ring at the junction of the two fluids, and the width of the ring is a crude measure of the amount of globulin.

**Rossolimo reflex**   (Grigoriy Ivanovich Rossolimo, Russian neurologist, 1860–1928) Plantar flexion of the toes, induced by tapping the balls of the toes; one of several pathological reflexes that may be seen when the lower motor neuron is released from the normal suppressor effect of higher centers, as in pyramidal tract lesions.

**rotation system**   A method some group psychotherapists employ: treating individual patients in sequences in the presence of the group.

**Rouse v. Cameron**   See *consumerism.*

**Roussy Lévy syndrome**   See *Friedreich ataxia.*

**route of drug administration**   Drugs may be swallowed (eaten or drunk), chewed and absorbed through the lining of the mouth, sniffed and absorbed through the lining of the nose, introduced into other body cavities and absorbed, inhaled through the lungs, or injected, either beneath the skin, into the muscles, or into a vein. Some drugs can be taken in several different ways.

The route of administration often determines the rapidity or intensity of drug effect;

it may also contribute to the social disability of the illicit drug user (e.g., intravenous injection of an opiate is incompatible with a facade of acceptable behavior in the workplace, but ingesting an opiate or amphetamine in pill form is usually not noticed by others). Further, some modes of administration entail specific hazards, such as infection with HIV or hepatitis virus or other pathogenic organisms in the case of intravenous use, and respiratory tract disease with inhalation and smoking.

**RSB**   REM sleep behavior disorder(s); also RBD—*REM behavior disorder* (q.v.).

**RSBT**   *Rhythmic sensory bombardment therapy* (q.v.).

**RT**   1. *Reaction time* (q.v.).

2. Recreation(al) therapy. See *recreation*.

**rTMS**   Repetitive (rapid rate) *Transcranial Magnetic Stimulation* (q.v.).

**rubber bands**   See *transactional analysis*.

**rubber hand illusion**   A facsimile of a body part is experienced as a part of the subject's own body, a phenomenon that can be induced in neurologically normal subjects. The subject observes a facsimile (a rubber hand) of a human hand while one of his own hands is hidden from view. Both the artificial hand and the subject's hand are stroked repeatedly and synchronously with a probe. The subject experiences an illusion in which the felt touch is brought into alignment with the seen touch, bringing the visual receptive field into alignment with the rubber hand and resulting in activation of premotor cortex neurons. Such activation produces a feeling of ownership of the seen hand. The rubber hand illusion is the opposite of *somatrophrenia*, produced by right-sided *parietal lobe dysfunction* (qq.v.).

**rubella, congenital**   See *retardation, mental*.

**Rubenstein-Taybi syndrome**   *Broad thumb hallux syndrome*; a type of mental retardation, first described in 1963, characterized by broad thumbs and great toes, facial abnormalities, and a cluster of congenital malformations. Etiology is unknown but is presumed to be genetic.

**rubidium**   An alkali metal, Rb, used in the 1880s in the treatment of syphilis and epilepsy, and more recently considered to have some antidepressant potential. Its primary effect appears to be on intracellular metabolism of potassium (lithium's major effect, in contrast,

is on sodium metabolism). Most studies have failed to find evidence of significant antidepressant effect.

**RUDAS**   Rowland Universal Dementia Assessment Scale, consisting of tests of Memory (Four-item grocery list), Gnosis (body orientation), Praxis (fist/palm alternating task), Visuo-spatial drawing (cube-copying), Judgement (crossing the road), Memory Recall (grocery list recall), and Language (animal generation). The test takes about 10 minutes to complete and assesses multiple cognitive domains, providing an evaluation of frontal lobe functions, executive functioning, and overall cognitive ability. The RUDAS does not depend on informant history and it appears not to be affected by gender, years of education, differential performance factors, or preferred language.

**rudimentary paranoia**   Latent paranoia. "What distinguished the delusions of these patients was their vagueness and the absence of systematic working up. Their fears and hopes were of a more indefinite kind, were brought forward as indications and conjectures, or they consisted in a strong personal valuation of actual events, which was not too far removed from the one-sidedness of normal individuals" (Kraepelin, E. *Manic-Depressive Insanity and Paranoia*, 1921). The expression was coined by Morselli.

**Rudin, Ernst**   (1874–1951) German psychiatrist and geneticist; genetics of mental disorders.

**Ruffini corpuscle**   See *glabrous*.

**Ruffini endings**   See *mechanoreceptor*.

**rule**   A statement that because an action is right, or wrong, it should, or should not, be done. See *judgment; principle; theory*.

**rule, M'Naghten (or McNaughton)**   See *criminal responsibility*.

**rule of law**   The law supersedes the discretionary powers of public officials and imposes checks and restraints on the exercise of governmental power. Closely related is *due process*, the requirement that fundamental fairness be applied in dealing with persons who are facing some action by government that may infringe their rights and liberties. The due process clauses of the Fifth and Fourteenth Amendments to the U.S. Constitution afford protection against arbitrary and unfair procedures in judicial or administrative proceedings that affect the personal or property rights of the individual.

**rule utilitarianism**   See *utilitarianism, act.*

**rum fits**   *Obs.* See *delirium tremens.*

**ruminate**   To regurgitate, remasticate, and reswallow; to ponder; to meditate. See *merycism.*

**rumination**   A rare *feeding and eating disorder* of infancy consisting of the returning of food from the stomach without nausea or retching; often, indeed, the child seems to derive pleasure or satisfaction from the process.

Rumination begins after a period of normal gastrointestinal functioning, usually within the first year of life, and is not associated with any known gastrointestinal illness. It often leads to loss of weight, failure to thrive, and interference with growth and development; in some (perhaps as many as a quarter), the disorder pursues an unremitting course until death. In the older literature, merycism implied an association between rumination and mental retardation; in current usage, the terms are interchangeable in recognition of the probability that the retardation is a manifestation of developmental delays produced by the disorder.

Rumination is also used to refer to the persistence of some content of mind that has ceased to serve any adaptive purpose, the inability to turn one's attention from dominating, unpleasant ideas, and/or an obsessive preoccupation with ideas, recollections, or plans (and thus Meyer's term, *obsessive-ruminative tension state*). Although rumination more often than not falls within the range of normal mentation, it is also reported frequently in obsessional states, hypochondriasis, and personality changes following brain injury. Rumination is a form of dysfunctional cognitive reappraisal of negative life events. Carriers of the short-allele 5-HTT with high levels of stress tend to high levels of rumination, suggesting that they are in a chronic state of vigilance, threat, or rumination, which makes them more vulnerable to mental illnesses. See *manie de rumination.*

**ruminative tension state**   *Obsessive-ruminative tension state* (q.v.).

**Rumpf sign**   (Theodor Rumpf, German physician, 1862–1923) In neurasthenia, pressure over a painful point accelerates the pulse from 10 to 20 beats/minute.

**run**   See *amphetamines.*

**runche**   A crying syndrome described in Nepalese children between 1 and 4 years of age. The condition typically followed episodes of diarrhea and fever or measles and consisted of whining, crying, refusal to eat, and secondary weight loss. Until the condition was recognized as a manifestation of malnourishment, it was interpreted as a spell placed upon the affected child by the touch of a pregnant woman.

**rupophobia**   *Rhypophobia* (q.v.).

**rush**   A feeling of warmth and intense pleasure that follows intravenous administration of some drugs (amphetamine, cocaine, heroin, morphine, propoxyphene). See *amphetamines; cocaine.*

**Rush, Benjamin**   (1745–1813) Father of American psychiatry; first American to propose an original systematization of psychiatry and author of the first American textbook of psychiatry (*Medical Inquiries and Observations upon the Diseases of the Mind*, 1812), which remained in print for 75 years. He was Chief Surgeon of the Continental Army and a signer of the Declaration of Independence.

**ruth**   Pity, compassion; the person lacking it is ruthless. Winnicott used ruth to describe the capacity to be concerned for another person as a whole and separate human being, with feelings similar to but not the same as one's own. Awareness of the subjectivity of the other is essential to development of the capacity for guilt, mourning, or empathy; ruth thus enables one to be truly caring and considerate in one's relations to another, rather than uncaring and ruthless in feeling and behavior.

**rypophobia**   *Rhypophobia* (q.v.).

# S

**S** Abbreviation for experimental subject or for stimulus.

**saccade** A high-velocity movement of the eye. Information about the distance and direction of a target image from the current direction of gaze is used to produce a saccade that brings the image of the target onto or near the fovea. The saccadic system processes information about the distance and direction of a target image from the current position of gaze and generates saccades of both eyes that bring the image of the target onto or near the fovea. The pursuit system uses information about the speed of a moving object to produce eye movements of comparable speed, thereby keeping the image of the object in or near the fovea. Using information about the location of a target in depth, the vergence system controls the movements of the eyes that will bring the image of the target onto the foveal regions of both eyes. See *pursuit eye movements; smooth pursuit system.*

Saccades are of two types, compensatory (catchup and backup) and intrusive. *Catchup saccades,* which move in the same direction as and faster than the target, are generated to correct tracking when the eyes lag behind the target (termed a reduced closed-loop pursuit gain, characteristic of schizophrenic subjects). *Backup saccades* move in the opposite direction to bring the eyes back on target when they have moved too fast. *Saccadic intrusions* are extraneous eye movements with no corrective functions. Normally inhibited during pursuit, they include jerks, oscillations, flutterings, opsoclonus, and anticipatory saccades.

**saccadic intrusions** See *SPEM.*

**SAD** *Social anxiety disorder; seasonal affect disorder* (qq.v.).

**sadism** (After Marquis de Sade [1740–1814], a French writer who described persons whose sexual pleasure depended upon inflicting cruelty upon others) A *paraphilia* (q.v.) in which sexual gratification is dependent upon torturing others or inflicting pain, ill treatment, and humiliation on others.

Most sexual sadists are men. Although there is a relationship between sexual sadism

and *rape* (q.v.), the latter is more properly considered a form of violence. A *lust murder* is one in which a sexual sadist kills his victim following the rape.

Viewed as a paraphilia, sadism is interpreted as a defense against castration fears and fears of one's own sexual excitement. What might happen to the subject passively is done actively to others"—"identification with the aggressor." Further, the castration performed in the sadistic act is a symbolic one, not a real one, and such pseudo-castration assures the sadist that his fears are ungrounded. The sadist tries to force his victim to love him; this love is conceived of as a forgiveness, which removes the guilt feelings that interfere with sexual satisfaction.

While sadism is sometimes considered to be a deflection outside the self of the destructive or death instinct, it will be seen that the paraphilia of sadism depends upon fusion of destructive energy with libidinal energy. The discharge of aggression in itself may be pleasurable, but sadism further implies pleasure in the destruction of others. But at the same time, the manifestations of the aggressive drive progress through the same developmental stages as the sexual (oral, anal, phallic), and in this context such manifestations are generally called sadistic—thus oral-sadistic, anal-sadistic, and phallic-sadistic.

**sadistic personality disorder** A pattern of cruelty and harshness toward others, ranging from intimidation or humiliation of others to enjoyment of inflicting physical pain or torturing other people or animals. Such a person is often fascinated with violence of any sort and interested in weapons, the martial arts, etc.

**sadomasochism** Coexistence of submissive and aggressive attitudes in social and sexual relations to other persons, with a considerable degree of destructiveness present; a condition assumed to be charged with libidinal energy. In a general way, a person may have three different kinds of attitude toward others: first, he wishes to have the other exist as his equal; second, he considers himself either superior or inferior to the other person, although still remaining interested in the other person's existence; and third, he is swayed by aggression and submission simultaneously in such a way that he wishes the other person's destruction and preservation at the same time. When aggression and the wish to destroy prevail in a relationship, it is often termed sadomasochistic.

**SADS** Schedule for Affective Disorders and Schizophrenia; a structured instrument designed to record the information necessary to establish diagnosis on the basis of the *RDC* (*Research Diagnostic Criteria*, q.v.). The latter defines *inclusion criteria* for the clinical features that warrant or support the diagnosis and *exclusion criteria* for features that are incompatable with the diagnosis. The SADS, Part I, includes information pertaining both to the history of the present illness and to the mental status examination. The PSE (*Present State Examination,* q.v.), another structured interview schedule, restricts itself to data obtained from the mental state examination.

**SAF** Scrapie-associated fibril, a proteinaceous double-helical fibril visible in electron micrographs that is a marker for *kuru* (q.v.). See *treble safeguard principle*.

**SAFE** Social-adaptive functioning evaluation, a rating scale for geriatric psychiatric patients. It rates self-care, impulse control, and social functioning in the following 17 areas: bathing and grooming; clothing and dressing; eating, feeding, and diet; money management; neatness and household maintenance activities; orientation and mobility (e.g., ability to leave treatment or residential unit unaccompanied and to return on time); impulse control (tolerant of delay vs. outbursts if wishes not met immediately); respect for own and others' property; communication skills (e.g., using telephone, writing and addressing letters); conversational skills (sustaining conversation; appropriateness of topics or self-disclosure); instrumental social skills (ability to request services from appropriate person); social appropriateness and politeness; social engagement (initiation of and participation in appropriate interactions); friendships (ability to form and maintain stable friendships); recreation and leisure (ability to participate in group activities and to pursue private interests); participation in hospital programs; cooperation with treatment (compliant with treatment program, understands benefits and risks of treatment, can accurately report adverse effects or intercurrent illnesses).

**safety device** Karen Horney's term for any means of protecting the self from threat, especially the hostility of the environment; although a more general term, safety device is approximately equivalent to defense mechanism.

**SAH** *Subarachnoid hemorrhage* (q.v.).

**SAHS-UAO** Sleep apnea hypersomnolence syndrome associated with upper airway obstruction. See *sleep disorders*.

**Saint Dymphna disease** (St. Dymphna, patron saint of the insane, a British noblewoman, murdered by her insane father, in Gheel, Belgium) Any mental disease; insanity.

**Saint Vitus dance** (St. Vitus, a Christian child, martyred under Diocletian, 245–313 A.D., whose chapels, especially the one at Ulm, were filled with sufferers from epilepsy, invoking the saint for cure) *Sydenham chorea* (q.v.).

**Sakel, Manfred** (1900–57) Polish psychiatrist trained in Vienna; in 1933 reported his discovery of the hypoglycemic insulin treatment of schizophrenia and soon after came to the United States, where he remained until his death.

**salaam (salutation) spasm** A variety of spasm seen in young children, consisting of periodic and rhythmic movements of the head and upper part of the body of about 2 seconds duration with intervals of approximately 10 seconds. They resemble the Asian form of greeting. The condition is mostly associated with neuropathologic findings.

**salience** The state of being outstanding, conspicuous; significant; attaching sufficient importance to an integrated stimulus so that behavior is activated. In reports on *addiction* (q.v.) and substance abuse, salience refers to stimuli that are arousing or that elicit an attentional-behavioral switch. Salience applies not only to prediction of *reward* (q.v.), but also to aversive, new, and unexpected stimuli. *Incentive salience* refers to the wanting or desire for the reward. To be differentiated is *hedonic impact*, which refers to the liking or pleasure related to the reward. In addicts, drug-induced increases in dopamine will inherently motivate further procurement of more drug, regardless of whether the effects of the drug are consciously perceived to be pleasurable. Drug-induced increases in dopamine also facilitate conditioned learning, so previously neutral stimuli that are associated with the drug become salient. These previously neutral stimuli then increase dopamine by themselves and elicit the desire for the drug.

**salience map** A two-dimensional topographically organized map that represents the distinctiveness of objects in the visual scene.

**Salmon, Thomas W.** (1876–1927) American psychiatrist; mental hygiene, military psychiatry.

**salpingectomy** *Sterilization* of the female by cutting and tying off the Fallopian tubes; also called *tubectomy, fallectomy*, or *tubal ligation*. Vasectomy is the corresponding operation on the male. Removal of the ovaries, resulting in the *castration* of the woman, is usually called *ovariectomy* or *oophorectomy*. See *sterilization; castration*.

**saltatory** Pertaining to leaping or dancing; proceeding by leaps and bounds rather than in measured, even progression.

*Saltatory conduction* is the continuous spreading of the current in myelinated nerve fibers, where the current jumps from node to node. This is faster than the continuous conduction in nonmyelinated nerves; the rate of conduction in nonmyelinated fibers is .03 to 2 meters per second, and in myelinated fibers it is 2 to 120 meters per second. See *potential, action*.

*Saltatory spasm* is a spasm of the muscles of the lower extremities that produces jumping or skipping movements; it is usually of hysterical origin.

**salutogenesis** Promotion and maintenance of physical and mental health.

**salvage patients** Used particularly with AIDS patients, those who have developed resistance to appropriate drugs and for whom there is no known alternative suppressive regimen. Simply adding a new drug to a failing regimen—called *serial monotherapy*—quickly results in resistance to the new drug as well.

**sanatorium** An institution for the treatment of chronic diseases, such as tuberculosis, nervous and mental disorders, chronic rheumatism, and a place for recuperation under medical supervision; often improperly called sanitarium.

**sanatorium disease** *Hospitalism; hospitalitis* (qq.v.).

**sanction** The defensive measure that the obsessional neurotic is obliged to adopt in order to prevent a phantasy from being fulfilled. Often it takes the form of repeating a word or other action as a way of diverting attention from the phantasy itself.

**sandbox marriage** A dysfunctional symmetrical marriage in which both partners vie for control or each demands to be the one who gets the most nurturance. See *complementary*.

**Sandler triad** A symptom group consisting of low self-esteem with confusion of identity, sadomasochistic behavior toward military authorities, and impotence, seen frequently as an essential part of *camptocormia* (q.v.).

**sane** Sound of mind.

**Sanfilippo syndrome** Polydystrophic oligophrenia; a *mucopolysaccharidosis* (q.v.) that usually starts between 18 and 36 months of age with retardation or cessation of psychomotor development, progression to erethetic oligophrenia and, finally, severe dementia. Usually there are accompanying signs of gargoylism and hepatomegaly; less common are moderate contractures of the large joints and splenomegaly. Sanfilippo syndrome is of two types, A and B, both with excessive heparan sulfate in the urine, but type A with a deficiency of the enzyme heparan sulfate sulfatase, type B with a deficiency of the enzyme N-acetyl-$\alpha$-D-glucosaminidase.

**Sanger, Margaret Higgins** (1884–1966) American nurse; pioneered in family planning and coined the phrase *birth control* (q.v.).

**sangue dormido** "Sleeping blood" syndrome, a culture-specific syndrome reported among Cape Verde Islanders, consisting of pain, tremor, paralysis, convulsions, blindness, and numerous other somatic symptoms.

**sanguine type** One of the four classical temperamental and constitutional types distinguished by Galen. He attributed the good humor and enthusiasm of this type to the predominance of the blood over the other three humors.

**Sanhoff disease** An autosomal recessive $G_{M2}$ gangliosidosis due to mutations in the beta-chain (HEX B), encoded on chromosome 5. The clinical picture is that of *Tay-Sachs disease* (q.v.), plus lipid-laden foam cells in the bone marrow. It is likely that Sanhoff disease comprises a collection of different HEX B mutations.

**sanity** Soundness of mind. See *criminal responsibility*.

**SANS** Scale for the Assessment of Negative Symptoms. See *CASH; negative symptoms*.

**Santavuori-Haltia disease**   See *lipofuscinosis, neuronal ceroid.*

**SANTE**   Stimulation of the Anterior Nucleus of the Thalamus for Epilepsy. See *deep brain stimulation (DBS).*

**sapid**   Related to taste or flavor; palatable. See *gustation.*

**Sapir-Whorf hypothesis**   (Edward Sapir, 1884–1939, American linguist; and his pupil, Benjamine Lee Whorf, 1897–1941) The generally discredited theory of *linguistic determinism,* that thoughts are determined by the language being spoken. A weaker version is the theory of *linguistic relativity* (q.v.), that language differences determine differences in the thoughts of their speakers. Probably the best known example provided by Whorf is what is referred to as the Great Eskimo Vocabulary Hoax, the assertion that the Eskimos have 400 different words for snow. Contrary to the assertion, Eskimo speakers have no more words for snow than English speakers have (although they might have to use them more frequently).

The theory of linguistic relativity has not been totally abandoned, however; there is strong evidence that there are conceptual differences between speakers of different languages and that language does influence the way in which speakers perceive, remember, and perform mental tasks.

**sa(p)phism**   (After the homosexual Greek poetess Sappho, born 600 B.C. on the island Lesbos) Lesbianism. See *homosexuality, female.*

**SAPS**   Schedule for the Assessment of Positive Symptoms. See *CASH; positive symptoms.*

**satanophobia**   Fear of the devil.

**satellite DNA**   See *gene.*

**satellite housing**   A type of long-term care facility, consisting of one or more residences for patients who require minimal supervision; the residences are related organizationally to a treatment center, such as a hospital, and thus provide ready access to more intensive levels of monitoring and care should a need for them arise. Sometimes a satellite house is located on or near the grounds of the hospital, but more often it is situated in a residential area close to a school or workplace. See *domicile; long-term care.*

**satiation, semantic**   Exposure therapy to thoughts, used in the treatment of obsessions: the patient is required to say or write down the obsessive thought repeatedly, as often as 50 or 100 times. Usually, long before the patient completes the assigned task, the thought has lost all meaning and may even become laughable to the patient.

Semantic satiation is the opposite of another technique used with obsessions, *thought stop* (q.v.).

**satiation techniques**   Behavioral techniques used in attempts to reduce recidivism of paraphilic behavior: the subject is directed to masturbate to ejaculation and then must continue masturbating for 30 to 120 minutes to deviant fantasy (during that "refractory period" orgasm is not possible). Sometimes such treatment is called *King Midas treatment,* referring to the gods' punishment of King Midas' greediness by ruining him through fulfillment of his wishes.

**satiety center**   See *hypothalamus.*

**satisfaction**   Gratification. In psychoanalysis, whatever eliminates a need. In occupational therapy, a feeling of contentment or accomplishment; often used in relation to the progress of an activity or interest.

**saturnine insanity**   *Obs.* Chronic encephalopathy due to *lead poisoning* (q.v.).

**saturnine pseudogeneral paralysis**   Chronic encephalopathy due to *lead poisoning* (q.v.).

**satyriasis**   1. *Hypersexuality* (q.v.) in the male; sexual erethism. See *Don Juan.* 2. *Obs.* Leprosy.

**Saunders-Sutton syndrome**   *Delirium tremens* (q.v.).

**savant syndrome**   A rare disorder in which severe developmental or psychiatric handicap is combined with islands of remarkable ability, usually artistic or memory-related, that stand out in sharp contrast to the otherwise permeating disability. The affected person was formerly called *idiot savant.* See *autistic disorder.*

**sawtooth sign**   A type of oscillation on the flow-volume loops in spirometric evaluation that suggests the presence of *SAHS-UAO* (q.v.) and thus provides a means of detecting the disorder when the patient is awake.

**SBMA**   *Spinal and bulbar muscular atrophy; Kennedy disease*; a *polyglutamine disorder* (q.v.). Its protein product is the androgen receptor; it attacks the anterior horn cells in the spinal cord.

**SCA**   *Spinocerebellar ataxia*; a group of disorders belonging to the class, *polyglutamine disorder* (q.v.).

**scabiophobia**   Fear of scabies.

**Scale for Assessment of Aggressive and Agitated Behavior**   A measure of agitation, verbal assault, and assault against the self, others, or property based on severity, the initiator, and the target of aggression, and on an inpatient unit the level of agitation of other patients at the time of the incident and intervention by staff.

**scalloping**   See *reinforcement schedule.*

**SCAN1**   Spinocerebellar ataxia with axonal neuropathy, an autosomal recessive trait characterized by peripheral axonal motor and sensory neuropathy, similar to Charcot-Marie-Tooth disease. Symptoms begin in the second decade: cerebellar atrophy, mild hypercholesterolemia, and hypoalbuminemia. There is no predisposition to cancer, and intelligence is normal. Scan1 is caused by a homozygous mutation in the *TDP1* gene, which encodes tyrosyl-DNA phosphodiesterase 1. SCAN1 results from a defect in SSBR that leads to defects in the response to single-strand DNA breaks.

**scanning**   Skimming; a method of rapid reading in which the reader searches for specific content or tries quickly to grasp the general sense of the passage but does not attempt to read the complete text. Scanning speech is a slurred, ataxic, drawling monotone or sing-song; it occurs, for example, in some cases of multiple sclerosis.

Scanning is also used to denote a method of diagnosis employing radioisotopes; see *radioisotopic encephalography.*

**scanning of the human genome**   See *linkage analysis.*

**scapegoat**   The person or object who is blamed for actions of others; the object of *projection* (q.v.).

**scapegoat mechanism**   The mental state of persons with strong antisocial feelings who look for incidents on which they can displace, project, and rationalize hostilities.

**scapegoating**   A form of intrafamilial behavior, largely unconsciously determined, in which one member (the child, the patient, etc.) becomes a repository or hiding place for the emotions that the rest of the family will not see in themselves.

Characteristic of scapegoating is *conflict detouring*, when the parents define the child as sick or defective and unite to protect him, or they see him as the cause of the family's

problems and unite in attacking him. A form of scapegoating is *triangulation*, in which a dyad within the family preserves its stability by directing its hostility to a third person.

**scaphocephaly**   See *craniosynostosis.*

**scar, psychic**   "*Cure with a defect* is also spoken of by formulating the conception, suitable only to a few cases, that the acute disease has left a defect just as a healed wound leaves a scar. A 'psychic scar' may be formed by definite 'residual symptoms,' as in the case of a delusion which in spite of returned clearness following a delirium is no longer corrected" (Bleuler, E. *Textbook of Psychiatry*, 1930).

**Scarpa ganglion**   (Antonio Scarpa, Italian anatomist and surgeon, 1749–1832) See *acoustic nerve.*

**SCAs**   *Spinocerebellar ataxias* (q.v.).

**scatology**   The study of excrement and/or preoccupation with excrement and filth; lewdness (as in telephone scatologia). See *anal eroticism* and the several words beginning with *copro-*.

**scatophagy**   Eating of excrement; *rhypophagy.*

**scatophobia**   Fear of contamination by excrement.

**scattering**   One of the schizophrenic thinking disorders in which associations are sometimes irrelevant or tangential, with the result that speech productions are occasionally incomprehensible. The term is also used in clinical psychology to refer to widely divergent test scores, as when a schizophrenic patient passes all the year X items in an intelligence test but shows many failures at the year VI level, or as when there is marked inconsistency on subtest scores. See *age, basal.*

**scavengers**   See *free radical.*

**scelerophobia**   *Pavor sceleris* (q.v.).

**scene, traumatic**   Any psychic experience that the subject wishes to forget or repress because it is disagreeable, painful, threatening, or unbearable. Freud speaks of traumatic situations and emphasizes that neurotic symptoms are "complete reproductions of such situations." Later, Freud referred to it as a *psychosexual trauma.*

**Schaeffer reflex**   (Max Schaeffer, German neurologist, 1852–1923) Dorsal flexion of the great toe, induced by pinching the Achilles tendon; one of several pathological reflexes that may be seen when the lower motor neuron is released from the normal suppressor effect of higher centers, as in pyramidal tract lesions.

**Schaumberg disease**   See *leukodystrophies*.

**schedule**   A form on which may be given many summarized items of information concerning a patient; it is arranged so that each item may be easily abstracted and made available for tabulation.

**Schedule for Affective Disorders and Schizophrenia**   *SADS* (q.v.).

**schedule of reinforcement**   See *reinforcement schedule*.

**Scheid cyanotic syndrome**   Sudden death in excited manic patients and in catatonic states, which Scheid attributed to a febrile or toxic etiology of the psychosis itself. Currently, it is generally believed that such deaths are due to physiologic exhaustion secondary to pathological overactivity; but some authors continue to speak of a catatonic cerebral paralysis as a primary somatic change that explains the occasional (probably not more than 1%) occurrence of unexpected death in this group. See *Bell mania*.

**Scheie syndrome**   A *mucopolysaccharidosis* (q.v.) with the same enzyme deficiency and urinary mucopolysaccharides as in Hurler disease, but intelligence is normal and the syndrome is compatible with a normal life span. Clinical features include stiff joints, cloudy cornea, and aortic regurgitation.

**schema**   A unit of knowledge, an internal organized representation of a domain of interaction (including past reactions or past experiences), within the brain. Schemata determine the expectations one has about events to be encountered and about their spatial and temporal structure. Visual exploration of the world, for instance, is directed by *anticipatory schemata*—plans for perceptual action as well as readiness for particular kinds of optical structure. What is then perceived modifies what was anticipated and directs further exploration and information seeking.

*Postural schemata* are perceptions of the spatial aspects of one's own body, comprising the integrated representation of prior movements which is updated by each change of position and provides a postural model into which all incoming sensations can be integrated. See *body ego; body image*.

For Piaget, the schema (he preferred to use *scheme*, q.v.) is the internal representation of a generalized class of situations.

**schema therapy**   Founded by Jeffrey Young, an active, structured therapy for assessing and changing deep-rooted psychological problems by examining repetitive life patterns and core life themes—*schema* (q.v.). Patient and therapist construct an inventory of the schemas that cause persistent problems, particularly for the patient with *borderline personality disorder* (q.v.). Various techniques are then employed to change the schemas, including cognitive restructuring, limited re-parenting, intensive imagery work to assess and change the source of schemas, instituting dialogues between the schema (dysfunctional) side and the healthy side, and behavioral techniques to change maladaptive behaviors in intimate relationships and to modify other dysfunctional coping styles.

**schemata**   In symbolic computation theory, patterns of generic relations. See *associationism; cognitive psychology*.

**scheme**   In Piaget's terminology, a scheme is organized action that has become generalized through repetition in similar circumstances (e.g., the grasping reflex, or walking down a flight of stairs without having to think consciously about the movement of the legs or the placement of the feet). A scheme enables a person to act in coordinated fashion to an entire range of analogous situations. Schemes having to do with higher intelligence are more typically referred to as *operations*. See *cognitions*.

**Schicksal analysis**   Szondian depth analysis, an eclectic system that borrows heavily from Freudian and Jungian psychology and strongly emphasizes the "familial unconscious," or hereditary tendencies. See *Szondi test*.

**Schilder disease**   (Paul Schilder, American neurologist, 1886–1940) Encephalitis periaxialis diffusa; a slowly progressive degenerative disease of the brain occurring mainly in children and young people; it is characterized by slowly advancing cerebral blindness and progressive mental deterioration terminating usually in complete amentia. See *diffuse sclerosis*.

**schizo-**   Combining form meaning to split, cleave, rive, from Gr. *schizein*.

**schizoaffective disorder**   The term is used in different ways in different classificatory systems, but most current definitions include a mixture of schizophrenic patients and affective disorder patients who are somewhat atypical in their presentation:

1. In DSM-IV it describes a psychotic disorder characterized by episodes during which

symptoms of a manic or a major depressive episode overlap with symptoms of schizophrenia and are present for a substantial portion of the episode; during each episode, a period of delusions or hallucinations exists for not less than 2 weeks in the absence of prominent mood symptoms.

2. Other systems use it to emphasize the acuteness of the syndrome, with sudden onset in a setting of marked emotional turmoil.

3. It may refer to cases that alternate between affective and schizophrenic symptoms in successive episodes.

4. It may describe cases with an approximately equal mixture of the symptoms of schizophrenia and affective disorder.

Most of the recent studies of schizoaffective disorder suggest either that it is a variant of affective disorder, or that it represents some kind of intermediate condition between affective disorder and schizophrenia. Schizoaffective patients do less well than patients with pure affective disorder but better than patients with schizophrenia. They are less likely to respond to lithium alone but are likely to respond relatively well to combinations of lithium and antipsychotics. They have higher rates of schizophrenia in their families than do patients with pure schizophrenia. Schizoaffective patients with manic features (*schizopolars* or *schizomanics*) may be much more closely allied to the affective disorders than are schizoaffectives who manifest only depression (Andreasen, N. C. *Schizophrenia Bulletin 13*, 1987).

**schizoaffective psychosis** A subtype of schizophrenia in which manic or melancholic symptoms are prominent. The affective symptoms are often so pronounced in the early stages as to mask the underlying schizophrenic process, especially in children and adolescents. Later in the course of the disease, however, the affective symptoms tend to abate as the schizophrenic elements become more obvious. See *schizoaffective disorder*.

**schizobipolar** *Schizomanic* (q.v.).

**schizocaria** *Obs.* An acute and highly malignant form of schizophrenia that leads to rapid deterioration of the personality. Mauz uses the term *catastrophic schizophrenia* synonymously with schizocaria.

**schizogen** See *psychotomimetic*.

**schizoid** Resembling the division, separation, or split of the personality that is characteristic of schizophrenia.

The term is an inexact one and used in different ways by different authors. By some, it is used to refer to a personality type characterized by shyness, sensitivity, aloofness, introversion, etc. It has been used by others to refer to any kind of psychiatric disorder that is not schizophrenia that occurs in family members of schizophrenics; or to refer to psychiatric disorders that occur more commonly in family members of schizophrenics than in other families, even though the particular case under consideration may not be from a schizophrenic family; or to refer to a trait or disorder that is believed to indicate an underlying genetic predisposition to schizophrenia. See *schizoidia; schizoidism*.

**schizoid disorder of childhood** Characterized by reduced capacity to form social relationships, preference for aloneness, bland or constricted affect, self-absorption, excessive daydreaming; the diagnosis should not be made before the age of 5 years, when socialization can ordinarily be expected to develop.

**schizoid personality disorder** Characteristics are shyness, aloofness, insensitivity to others' feelings, seclusiveness, having only one or two close friends, preference for solitary activities, and claiming to experience anger only rarely.

**schizoid position** See *paranoid-schizoid position*.

**schizoidia** Schizoidism; also used synonymously with *schizophrenic spectrum disorders* to refer to a variety of abnormalities that are found among nonschizophrenic relatives of schizophrenic patients. Although the concordance rate for schizophrenia in monozygotic twins may be no higher than 45%, probably an equal percentage of the twins have some other significant abnormality. The latter are subsumed under the name schizoidia. In males these include impulse crimes, such as arson, assault, and poorly planned theft; extreme social isolation; heavy alcohol intake; and sexual deviance. In both males and females they include eccentric reclusiveness; incapacitating panic in ordinary social situations (especially in females); paranoid types with suspiciousness, sensitivity, moroseness, jealousy, litigiousness; giggly, opinionated, pedantic, or narrow-minded eccentrics; cruel, calculating, cold, unsympathetic persons who seem to lack feeling; reserved, haughty, snobbish, unsociable types; and anergic personalities with dependency, unreliability, or subservience.

**schizoidism** The aggregate of personality traits known as introversion, namely, quietness, seclusiveness, "shut-in-ness." The schizoid person splits or separates from his surroundings to a greater or lesser degree, confining his psychic interests more or less to himself.

The intensely schizoid person may become schizophrenic; it is estimated that no fewer than 60% of schizophrenic patients show exaggerated schizoid tendencies prior to the development of schizophrenia.

Many contemporary European writers use the term schizoidism to refer to the hereditary or nuclear factor in schizophrenia. These same authors tend to use the term dementia praecox to refer to a type of schizophrenia showing a high tendency to deterioration and little tendency to remission or recovery.

**schizomanic** *Schizobipolar*; referring to a schizoaffective patient with manic features. See *schizoaffective disorder*.

**schizomimetic** *Psychotomimetic* (q.v.).

**schizophasia** "Word salad"; in Leonhard's classification, a subtype of nonsystematic schizophrenia characterized by grossly disorganized speech. See *systematic schizophrenia*.

**schizophrenese** The associational defects of the schizophrenic patient as manifested in his speech; it is to be recognized that there is no specific schizophrenic language and schizophrenics' thinking disorders vary from patient to patient. "What is uniform is merely an absence of normal expectancy. It is also noteworthy that in the absence of such culturally standard cues for meta-communicative expression, the listener feels disengaged and the schizophrenic child is further isolated from human rapport" (Goldfarb, W. *International Psychiatry Clinics 1*, 1964).

**schizophrenia** Bleuler's suggested replacement for the now obsolete term *dementia praecox* (q.v.). Bleuler meant to designate what he considered to be one of the fundamental characteristics of patients so diagnosed, namely, the splitting off of portions of the psyche, which portions may then dominate the psychic life of the subject for a time and lead an independent existence even though these may be contrary and contradictory to the personality as a whole. Bleuler rejected the term dementia praecox because in his experience profound deterioration (dementia) was not the inevitable end result of the disease process, and because it did not always appear by the time of adolescence.

"In 1911, Eugen Bleuler described the schizophrenias as a slowly progressive deterioration of the entire personality, which involves mainly the affective life, and expresses itself in disorders of feeling, thought and conduct, and a tendency to withdraw from reality. Bleuler noted that the schizophrenias were at times progressive, at times intermittent, and could stop or retrogress at any stage; but that they showed a tendency toward deterioration and, having once appeared, did not permit of a full *restitutio ad integrum*. Bleuler established the multidimensional nature of the schizophrenias and believed them to be organic; but at the same time, he stressed the interaction of psychogenic and physiogenic features in their psychopathology and development" (Campbell, R. J. *Psychiatric Quarterly 32*, 1958).

The diagnostic criteria for this group of disorders have varied considerably, although there is relative compatibility of DSM-IV with ICD-10 concerning the characteristic symptoms. DSM-IV requires at least one positive symptom plus another symptom (either positive or negative) to be present for at least 1 month. Among the positive symptoms are delusions, hallucinations, disorganized speech, catatonia, bizarre behavior, and inappropriate affect. Negative symptoms include flat affect, avolition, alogia, and anhedonia. There have been many attempts to define subgroups by symptoms; most differentiate (1) a negative symptom dimension (also referred to as psychomotor poverty) includes poverty of speech, decreased spontaneous movement, unchanging facial expression, paucity of expressive gesture, affective nonresponse, lack of vocal inflection; (2) positive symptoms, including psychoticism (reality distortion), hallucinations, delusional ideas; (3) disorganization, which includes inappropriate affect, poverty of content of speech, tangentiality, derailment, pressure of speech, distractibility. See *schizophrenia, models of.*

Bleuler subdivided the symptoms of the schizophrenias into two groups: (1) the fundamental, primary, or basic symptoms, which he considered characteristic and pathognomonic of the disease process; and (2) the accessory or secondary symptoms, which are often seen in the schizophrenias and which may even occupy the forefront of the symptom picture, but which are seen in other nosologic groups as well, particularly in the organic reaction types (acute and chronic brain syndromes). In this second group are included such symptoms as hallucinations, delusions, ideas of reference, memory disturbances (e.g., déjà fait, déjà vu). The fundamental symptoms of the schizophrenias include (1) disturbances in associations, (2) disturbances of affect, (3) ambivalence of the affect, intellect, and/or will, (4) autism, (5) attention defects, (6) disturbances of the will, (7) changes in "the person," (8) schizophrenic dementia, and (9) disturbances of activity and behavior. See *first-rank symptoms.*

While the specific etiology remains unknown, mounting evidence favors the conception of the schizophrenias as a heredogenetic disease involving particularly certain enzyme systems of the brain. Multiple genes are probably involved, and different gene patterns may be found in different cases. There is strong evidence that a gene on chromosome 6 is involved in some cases. There is some evidence that there might also be involvement of genes on chromosome 8, and (more controversial) 22 and 5. The average expectancy of schizophrenia in the general population probably does not exceed 1%, but expectancy increases with closeness of genetic relationship.

**schizophrenia, acute**   The predominant clinical features are delusions, hallucinations, and thinking disturbances—sometimes referred to as *positive symptoms* (q.v.). According to the World Health Organization (1973) the most frequent symptoms of acute schizophrenia are lack of insight (found in 97% of cases), auditory hallucinations (74%), ideas of reference (70%), suspiciousness (66%), flatness of affect (66%), voices speaking to the patient (65%), delusional mood (64%), delusions of persecution (64%), thought alienation (52%), and thoughts spoken aloud (50%). See *schizophrenia; schizophrenia, forms of.*

**schizophrenia, arrest of**   The subsidence of acute schizophrenic symptoms. This may occur at any time in the process of the disease, and if the disease itself is not too far advanced, there may be little of a pathological nature to appear. In other words, schizophrenia does not necessarily imply progressive deterioration.

**schizophrenia, catastrophic**   See *schizocaria.*

**schizophrenia, forms of**   *Schizophrenia typology;* there is no universally accepted typology of

the schizophrenias. Bleuler subdivided the schizophrenias into acute and chronic forms, depending upon the predominant symptoms of any particular episode. At the present time, most of his acute forms are subsumed under other types of chronic schizophrenia or do not meet the criteria currently advocated in making the diagnosis of schizophrenia. Many such cases fall instead into other categories, such as personality disorders (particularly borderline, schizoid, or schizotypal), or into the group of affect disorders.

In Bleuler's typology, the predominant symptoms served as markers of the subtype; it must be recognized that those symptoms are often the accessory symptoms. Before subtyping an episode, it is necessary to establish the diagnosis of schizophrenia on the basis of the presence of fundamental symptoms. See *schizophrenia.*

A.  *Acute Syndromes*
1.  *Melancholia*—in contrast to nonschizophrenic depressions, the affect here tends to be superficial, inappropriate, and/or unconvincing, and hypochondriacal delusions are frequent.
2.  *Mania*—the prevailing mood is capriciousness rather than euphoria or triumph, and withdrawal can usually be seen.
3.  *Catatonia*—stupor, cerea flexibilitas, *Faxenpsychosis* (q.v.), or other hyperkinetic syndromes.
4.  *Delusional states with hallucinations*—often visual and less stereotyped than the hallucinations seen in the chronic syndromes.
5.  *Twilight states*—including religious ecstasies and other dreamlike conditions in which desires, impulses, or fears are represented in a direct or symbolic way as being already fulfilled.
6.  *Benommenheit* (psychic "benumbing")—in which there is a slowing up of all psychic processes, usually in conjunction with an incapacity for dealing with any relatively complicated or unusual situation.
7.  *Confusion, incoherence*—as a result of fragmentation of associations, speech is disconnected, sentences are broken, and activity is excessive, purposeless, and random.

8. *Anger states*—with cursing, vilification, uncontrolled rage outbursts, often in relation to seemingly insignificant external events.

9. *Anniversary excitements*—episodes of agitation appearing only on definite calendar days, usually related to a specific event in the patient's past.

10. *Stupor*

11. *Deliria*—acute hallucinatory episodes often resembling the fever deliria. These states are sometimes termed oneirophrenia and include those patients who become dazed and bewildered with narrowing of consciousness, often following specific traumata such as childbirth, postoperative exhaustion, and battlefield experiences. While such cases are often said to be benign, there is a percentage of cases that recur with decreasing recovery after each episode.

12. *Fugue* states—running away in intercurrent episodes of agitation and excitement, sometimes in response to a hallucinatory command.

13. *Dipsomania*—tense, anxious moods drive some patients to drink heavily until they become exhausted.

B. *Chronic Forms*
1. *Paranoid schizophrenia* (q.v.)
2. *Catatonic schizophrenia* (q.v.)
3. *Hebephrenic schizophrenia* (q.v.)
4. *Simple schizophrenia* (q.v.)

C. *Other Forms*—among the other forms described since Bleuler's subdivision are the following:
1. *Childhood schizophrenia* (q.v.)
2. *Pseudoneurotic schizophrenia* (q.v.)
3. *Ambulatory schizophrenia* (q.v.)
4. *Acute episode schizophrenia*—those acute forms in which clear-cut crystallization into one of the generally recognized chronic forms has not yet occurred.
5. *Chronic undifferentiated schizophrenia*—mixed forms and also those termed latent, incipient, borderline, prepsychotic, etc.
6. *Schizoaffective disorder* (q.v.)—including the acute melancholic and manic forms of Bleuler; this type often has its onset during adolescence and with recurrences the affective picture tends to abate and to be replaced by hebephrenic or simple or paranoid symptoms.

7. *Pseudopsychopathic schizophrenia*—with predominant asocial, dyssocial, or antisocial trends.
8. *Residual schizophrenia*—cases in a state of relative remission or improvement between acute psychotic episodes.

**schizophrenia, mixed** Schizophrenia that shows symptoms of more than one of the disease's four generally accepted and clearly distinguished categories; simple, paranoid, catatonic, hebephrenic. Such cases are often called chronic undifferentiated schizophrenia.

**schizophrenia, models of** At the descriptive level, there are currently three models of schizophrenia: (1) schizophrenia is a single disease entity in which a single pathophysiology produces several diverse symptom complexes; (2) schizophrenia is a syndrome (similar to mental retardation) comprising multiple disease entities, each due to a different etiopathological process; and (3) schizophrenia comprises several disease processes, each with its distinctive etiopathology, manifested in different patients in different ways that phenomenologically meet the criteria for schizophrenia.

Since the 1970s, research has been directed to defining the basic, core symptoms and subtyping the different manifestations not only by symptoms but also on the basis of biological measures. At first, the major division was on the basis of positive and negative symptoms, which accounted for the main share of variance (ca. 36%). Further definition by symptoms demonstrated that schizophrenia symptoms tended to aggregate into the positive and negative syndromes, followed by disorganization (including conceptual disorganization and inappropriate affect), and by disorder of relating (including emotional withdrawal and passive/apathetic social withdrawal). Other models of schizophrenia address the etiopathology of schizophrenia:

1. *Diathesis-stress model* (q.v.)
2. *Dopamine hypothesis* (q.v.)
3. *Disconnection hypothesis* (q.v.)
4. *Hypofrontality hypothesis* (q.v.)
5. *Immune hypothesis* (q.v.)
6. *Neurodevelopmental hypothesis* (q.v.)
7. *NMDAR hypofunction model*; see *NRH hypothesis*
8. *One-gene theory of psychosis* (q.v.)
9. *Temporal model* (q.v.)
10. *Temporolimbic system model* (q.v.)
11. *Thalamic model* (q.v.)

The brain dysfunction in schizophrenia is not a focal lesion with circumscribed boundaries and effects, but one involving multiple neurotransmitter systems with distributed physiological effects. It is unlikely that any one specific type or extent of defect in any specific cortical or subcortical structure is common to all schizophrenic patients. Instead, the type and extent of defect in any particular structure (e.g., hippocampus, amygdala, the various thalamic nuclei, the striatum, the brain-stem nuclei, and the various cerebellar nuclei) may be of great importance to a particular patient.

Genetic risk factors have been found for almost every psychiatric disorder. With the mapping of the human genome came the hope that disease-inducing genes could be located at specific sites on particular chromosomes. There have been claims for *linkage* (q.v.) to schizophrenia on 21 of the 23 pairs of chromosomes, but attempts to replicate such findings have often failed and findings have been inconsistent. The same has been true in studies of *endotypes* (q.v.) to identify heritable constituents of disorders—neuroanatomical, neurophysiological, biochemical, endocrinological, or neuropsychological components.

One possible conclusion is that many genes of small effect are relevant, and that samples of much larger size are needed to tease out the contribution made by each of many genes to the phenotype. There is little evidence, however, that such an approach would be more fruitful than the linkage and association studies. It is possible that the relevant variation is not an alteration in the DNA sequence itself, but that it is epigenetic and due, for example, to changes in how the DNA sequence, or one of its associated components, is handled. See *epigenetics*; *gene-environment interactions*; *noncoding DNA*.

T. J.Crow (*American Journal of Psychiatry 164*, 2007) has presented arguments for a single gene underlying psychotic disorder. See *one-gene theory of psychosis*.

Current nosological schemes group several syndromes into one illness entity. It is equally possible that schizophrenia represents a more or less heterogeneous group of diseases, each of which could be associated with more or less specific clinical features. That would help to explain why, despite decades of research, no single, consistently replicable linkage to schizophrenia has been established, and why there is less than complete concordance of schizophrenia in identical twins.

Several genes demonstrating strong evidence of association with schizophrenia have been identified, including the *dysbindin gene* (*dystrobrevin binding protein 1, DTNBP1*), and *neuregulin 1*. Several single nucleotide polymorphisms (SNPs), as well as a six-marker high-risk haplotype in the *dysbindin* gene, appear to be involved. The high-risk haplotype cannot be said to increase risk of illness itself, but it is presumed to be in linkage disequilibrium with one or more causative mutations in *DTNBP1* that have yet to be identified.

**schizophrenia, recidives in** Recurring, intermittent, acute episodes of schizophrenia, or other evidences of deterioration that begin after prolonged remission. The recurring attacks often duplicate the previous ones, but new features may appear. There is no definite correlation between initial disease symptoms and recidives. See *schizophrenia; schizohrenia, forms of.*

**schizophrenia, regressive symptoms** Those schizophrenic symptoms that represent an undoing or primitivization of differentiations acquired through mental development; included here are such symptoms as phantasies of world destruction, physical sensations and delusions, depersonalization, delusions of grandeur, archaic speech and thought, most hebephrenic symptoms, and certain catatonic symptoms (negativism, echolalia, echopraxia, automatic obedience, posturing, stereotypy). See *schizophrenia, restitutional symptoms.*

**schizophrenia, residual** Interepisodic schizophrenia; the condition of being without gross psychotic symptoms following a psychotic schizophrenic episode. To be contrasted with *latent schizophrenia* (q.v.).

**schizophrenia, restitutional symptoms** Those schizophrenic symptoms that represent an attempt at regaining reality, which has been lost by regression; included are such symptoms as hallucinations, delusions, most of the social and speech peculiarities of schizophrenia, and certain catatonic symptoms (stereotypy, mannerisms, automatic obedience, rigidity).

**schizophrenia, reversible** Menninger's term for a schizophrenic state with a potentiality for recovery. See *process psychosis.*

**schizophrenia, toxic**  *Toxiphrenia* (q.v.).

**schizophrenia deliriosa**  Menninger's term for a form of schizophrenia that starts as a delirium and is frequently associated with or directly follows a physical illness such as influenza.

**schizophrenia prodrome**  *ARMS* (at-risk mental state); *latent schizophrenia* (q.v.); symptoms suggesting that the subject will later develop schizophrenia. In high-risk children, the symptoms most likely to be predictive of the development of schizophrenia in early adulthood are poor performance on attention tests, and impairments in motor performance, verbal memory, and visuospatial processing. Some children manifest developmental delays such as abnormal language development, communication difficulties, difficulties in social connectedness and peer relationships; they may be classified within the range of autism spectrum disorder. Others remain in the latent or prodromal stage and are diagnosed as schizotypal personality disorder as adults. More characteristic of schizotypy, compared with schizophrenia, are a greater number of depressive symptoms, greater sleep difficulties, less suspiciousness, less odd behavior, and less loss of role functioning.

**schizophrenia spectrum**  A proposed range of disorders: schizophrenia, schizoaffective disorder, paranoid personality disorder, schizotypal personality, and schizoid personality. See *spectrum.*

**schizophenia typology**  See *schizophrenia, forms of.*

**schizophrenic defect state**  See *negative symptoms.*

**schizophrenic dementia**  One of the fundamental symptoms of the schizophrenias (Bleuler). Schizophrenic patients, despite generally adequate preservation of their intellectual potentialities, are often not able to make use of this potential in a constructive, appropriate, purposeful, goal-directed way. Knowledge, although present, is not always available to them at the moment it is called for. Schizophrenic dementia seems to be the result of disturbances of primary elemental functions, such as associations, affectivity, attention and concentration, and will.

Schizophrenic dementia reveals itself in various forms: stupid, foolish mistakes; senseless generalizations; gullibility; faddism; pseudo-motivations; vacuity and banality of thought; an insipid, unintegrated, disconnected quality in thought and speech; difficulty in forming new concepts; ellipsis in thought and speech; treating the concrete as though it were abstract; etc. On psychological testing, probably, the most frequent expression of schizophrenic dementia is *scattering* (q.v.).

**schizophrenic surrender**  A term used by C. MacFie Campbell to characterize the type of schizophrenia in which the mechanism is one of passive repression without initial anxiety or any conspicuous restitutional attempts.

**schizophreniform**  Resembling schizophrenia. See *process psychosis; reactive psychosis.*

**schizophreniform disorder**  Any disorder with psychotic features similar to schizophrenia except that duration is less than 6 months and manifestations include features that are usually associated with good prognosis, such as confusion or perplexity at the height of the psychotic episode, affect not blunted or flat, premorbid social or occupational functioning good. Within 6 months of onset of the episode there is a complete or almost complete return to the premorbid level of functioning.

**schizophrenogenic**  Producing or fostering the development of schizophrenia; Frieda Fromm-Reichmann was the first to discuss schizophrenogenic mothers.

**schizophrenogenic mother**  A term used by those who believed that the attitude of the mother toward her child is the basic determinant of schizophrenia. To those who would subscribe to this viewpoint, the term usually includes (1) the overtly rejecting mother, who is domineering, aggressive, critical, and overdemanding (especially in regard to cleanliness and the observances of social forms); and (2) the covertly rejecting mother, who smothers her child with overprotectiveness. See *smother love.*

Adherents of the schizophrenogenic mother hypothesis for the most part ignore the fact that of all the mothers who could be classified as fulfilling the above criteria, only a small percentage have schizophrenic children. Also ignored are the many studies indicating that there is no uniform pattern of family dynamics in the families of schizophrenic patients.

**schizopolar**  See *schizoaffective disorder.*

**schizotaxia**  According to Meehl, a genetically determined neurointegrative defect that is necessary but not sufficient for the development of schizophrenia. One of its manifestations is cognitive slippage, a fundamental symptom of schizotypy (q.v.).

**schizothymia**  Introversion; *schizoidism* (q.v.).

**schizotypal disorders** See *personality disorders; adaptational psychodynamics.*

**schizotypal personality disorder** *SPD,* one of the phenotypes in the *schizophrenia spectrum* (q.v.). Like schizophrenia, SPD is characterized by positive or psychotic-like symptoms (ideas of reference, cognitive disorganization, perceptual distortions, magical thinking) and negative or deficit-like symptoms (social deficit, social anxiety, introversion, seclusiveness). Schizotypals demonstrate an admixture of dysphoric moods; proneness to eccentric convictions, bigotry, and zealotry; and odd beliefs and superstitions. The symptoms have sometimes been described in terms of three factors: (1) a positive or cognitive-perceptual factor (illusions or perceptual aberrations, magical thinking, ideas of reference); (2) an oddness or disorganized factor (odd speech and appearance, constricted or inappropriate affect); and (3) an interpersonal factor (social anxiety and social isolation).

The consistent association of SPD and schizophrenia in family and adoption studies implicates both a familial and a genetic relationship between the two. Functional imaging studies in SPD demonstrate abnormalities similar to those found in schizophrenia, but of lesser degree, particularly in the temporal cortex and pulvinar circuitry. It has been posited that schizophrenia and SPD share a common genetic anomaly that renders the cortex particularly vulnerable to environmental insults; other genetic factors or more favorable environmental conditions protect against or compensate for the basic genetic anomaly in SPD. Those who lack such ameliorating factors are more likely to develop full-blown schizophrenia.

**schizotypy** Liability for developing schizophrenia; the personality manifestations of a schizophrenia genotype (Rado). Meehl suggests that there are four fundamental symptoms of schizotopy: cognitive slippage (or mild loosening of the associations), interpersonal aversiveness (social fear), defective capacity to experience pleasure (anhedonia), and ambivalence.

**Schlafsucht** See *Kleine-Levin syndrome.*

**Schnauzkrampf** Term coined by Karl Ludwig Kahlbaum (1828–1899) for protrusion of the lips such that they resemble a snout. The condition is found almost exclusively in the catatonic form of schizophrenia.

**Schneider, Kurt** (1887–1967) German psychiatrist, best known for his phenomenologic approach and description of the diagnostically significant symptoms in schizophrenia. See *first-rank symptoms.*

**Scholz disease** (Willibald Scholz, German neurologist, 1889–1971) See *diffuse sclerosis.*

**school, Montessori** See *Montessori, Maria.*

**school phobia** *School refusal syndrome;* inability to attend school on a regular basis because of pervasive anxiety and somatic complaints (e.g., nausea, abdominal pain, headache). Usually, the condition is not a true phobia, but rather anxiety about separation from mother and home, often with obsessional concern about the safety of the mother. The central focus in management is prompt return to school. See *mutism, elective.*

**school refusal syndrome** *School phobia* (q.v.).

**school-marmitis** A personality type seen in some teachers, characterized by "magnified self-awareness... in the role of dispenser of knowledge and wisdom to children and, on occasion, to their parents; a tendency to "lord it over' and a patronizing attitude toward others" (Kanner, L. *Child Psychiatry,* 1948). Emotional attitudes of a schoolteacher can be powerful determinants of the child's own attitude, for good or ill, as the case may be. This is especially true if the child is already emotionally insecure in his home life. Happily, there also exist teacher attitudes that reflect a healthy degree of emotional integration at a high level of personal maturity.

**schoolsickness** An occupational neurosis in children maladjusted to their school situation, characterized by anxiety, restlessness, and irritability. See *school phobia.*

**Schreber, Schreber case** In 1911, Freud published *Psycho-Analytic Notes Upon an Autobiographical Account of a Case of Paranoia (Dementia Paranoides).* This consisted of an analysis of *Memoirs of a Neurotic,* a previously published (1903) autobiographical account by Dr. jur. Daniel Paul Schreber. Freud's analysis of these memoirs formed the basis for the psychoanalytic view of paranoid delusions, which, at least in the male, are interpreted as attempts to contradict the underlying homosexual wish-phantasy of loving a man. See *paranoia.*

**Schuele sign** (Heinrich Schuele, German psychiatrist, 1839–1916) *Omega melancholium* (q.v.).

**Schüller-Christian-Hand syndrome**  *Xanthomatosis* (q.v.).

**Schwann cell**  See *glia; myelin; neuroglia.*

**SCID**  Structured Clinical Interview for DSM-III; an instrument designed to record symptoms and past history for a broad array of disorders according to the diagnostic criteria of DSM-III and DSM-III-R. It is available in several versions: (1) SCID-P, for differential diagnosis of psychotic disorders in psychiatric inpatients; (2) SCID-OP, for use in outpatient settings where, presumably, psychotic disorders will be rare; (3) SCID-NP, for subjects not identified as psychiatric patients. SCID is more detailed than the *PSE* and *SADS* but shorter than *CASH* (qq.v.).

**SCID-D**  Structured Clinical Interview for DSM-III-R Dissociative Disorders, devised by M. Steinberg; a relatively elaborate instrument whose use requires special training, it is said to be more than 90% sensitive for true multiple personality disorder. It covers five areas: amnesia and fugue, depersonalization, derealization, identity confusion, and identity alteration.

**scierneuropsia**  See *scieropia.*

**scieropia**  Visual defect in which objects appear to be in a shadow; when of emotional or psychologic origin, such defect is termed *scierneuropsia.*

**scintillation detectors**  See *emission tomography.*

**scissors gait**  In patients with bilateral spastic limbs, there is crossed progression in the process of walking; the legs cross in scissors fashion. *See Little disease.*

**SCL-90-R**  Formerly called the *Hopkins Symptom Checklist*, a brief, reliable, and valid self-reporting questionnaire that provides a global index of dysfunction (but little assessment of strengths). It consists of 90 items covering a wide range of symptoms; for each item the subject indicates the degree of distress currently being experienced. In addition to a global score, it can also give quantitative scores on subtests such as Hostility, Interpersonal Sensitivity, Paranoid Ideation, Psychoticism, and Somatization.

**sclerosing encephalitis**  See *panencephalitis, subacute sclerosing.*

**sclerosis**  Hardening or induration of any part of the body as a reaction to inflammation, hyperemia, neoplasm, or other infiltration.

**sclerosis, atrophic lobar**  See *cerebral palsy.*

**sclerosis, diffuse**  See *diffuse sclerosis.*

**sclerosis, disseminated**  *Multiple sclerosis* (q.v.).

**sclerosis, posterolateral**  See *posterolateral sclerosis.*

**sclerosis, tuberous**  See *tuberous sclerosis.*

**sclerosis en plaque**  (F. "in patches") *Multiple sclerosis* (q.v.).

**SCN**  Suprachiasmatic nucleus of the hypothalamus, a small, paired nucleus situated just above the optic chiasm. It receives entraining information from a discrete subset of retinal ganglion cells through a direct retinohypothalamic tract; it also receives nonphotic information from other brain areas that modulate pacemaker function. Destruction of the SCN results in a loss of the temporal organization of behavior, with sleep and wake occurring in normal amounts but randomly distributed over time. The SCN and its connections constitute a specific and distinct neural system, the circadian timing system. The SCN pacemaker exerts precise control over each variable in the biological clock—melatonin, cortisol, and body temperature. Recent evidence indicates that this precise control is maintained despite the many alterations in brain function associated with aging. See *circadian clock.*

**SCOPE**  Acronym for an accepted set of diagnostic procedures that are systematic, complete, objective, practical, and empirical.

**-scopia, -scopo, -scopy**  Combining form meaning to look at, examine, inquire, from Gr. *skopein.*

**scopolagnia**  *Voyeurism; scop(t)ophilia* (qq.v.).

**scopolamine**  An anticholinergic drug. See *cholinergic.*

**scopophilia**  Sexual pleasure derived from contemplation or looking. It is a component instinct and stands in the same relation to exhibitionism as sadism does to masochism. See *phallic sadism; voyeur; voyeurism.*

Autoscopophilia refers to the pleasure of looking at one's own body. Active scopophilia is the pleasure derived from looking at the sexual organs of another. Passive scopophilia is the desire to be looked at by others and is thus seen to be equivalent to active exhibitionism.

In Freudian literature the German Schaulust has been translated as scoptophilia, but scopophilia is the more correct form.

**scopophobia**  Fear of being looked at; excessive shyness.

**scoptophilia**  See *scopophilia.*

**SCOR**  Skin Conductance Orienting Response, a sensitive measure of information processing, reflecting the allocation of attentional resources for the processing of the eliciting stimulus and the process of template matching. Hyporesponsiveness suggests slowness in information processing and difficulty in rapidly identifying the significance of even mild environmental stimuli. A SCOR study in six laboratories in the United States, United Kingdom, and Germany produced one virtually unanimous finding: 40%–50% of schizophrenics are nonresponsive to innocuous stimuli of moderate intensity.

OR nonresponding is a vulnerability marker for a core group of severely schizophrenic patients who are characterized by genetic transmission of schizophrenia, a poor premorbid picture marked by anhedonia and social and emotional isolation, and gradual onset of a psychosis characterized by negative symptoms, cognitive disorganization, and poor response to neuroleptics. Schizophrenic nonresponders tend to display poorer premorbid adjustment and often have blood relatives diagnosed schizophrenic; schizophrenic responders, on the other hand, are commonly the only cases of schizophrenia among their blood kin.

**SCoRS** Schizophrenia Cognition Rating Scale; an 18-item interview-based assessment (by patients, informants, and interviewers) of cognitive deficits and the degree to which they affect day-to-day functioning. A global rating is also generated. The items assess the cognitive domains of attention, memory, reasoning and problem solving, working memory, language production, and motor skills.

**scotoma** An abnormal blind spot in the visual field. See *optic nerve*.

**scotoma, mental** Lack of insight; a mental "blind spot" for the problem before one's eyes.

**scotomization** A process of psychic depreciation, by means of which the subject attempts to deny everything that conflicts with his ego.

**scotophobia** Fear of darkness.

**scrambler** A mutant mouse with characteristics similar to *reeler* (q.v.). Another recently recognized mutant lacks the gene for the cyclin-dependent kinase type 5 (Cdk5).

**scrambler mice** Mice, whose behavior and brain abnormalities are similar to those caused by the *reeler mutation* (q.v.). The brains of scrambler mice lack cortical layers, as those of reeler mice do. The mutated scrambler gene makes a protein, *mdab1*, which is the mouse version of one in the fruit fly, *disabled* (*dab*). The mouse gene affected by the *yotari mutation* (yotari = drunken gait) is the same gene that is mutated in scrambler mice.

The mdab1 protein binds to the tyrosine kinase *Src*, an intracellular signaling enzyme, suggesting mdab1 is a docking protein that can link a tyrosine kinase like Src to another protein in the signaling pathway.

**scrapie** A naturally occurring spongiform encepalopathy in sheep and goats, presumed to be caused by an unconventional virus or *prion* (q.v.). See *virus infections*.

**screen** A form of concealment. When, for instance, in a dream one person stands for another or others, by virtue of some common feature, that person is called a screen.

**screen memory** *Cover memory*; a memory of a real event conceals an allied memory. Example: a patient recalls playing in the basement but does not remember the nature of the play.

**screening** Sifting; used particularly in the sense of a preliminary separation of a population into those who are likely to have a particular trait or characteristic from those who do not. The instrument used to screen the population (e.g., a blood or urine test, X-ray or CT scan, cytologic smear, intelligence or personality test) is typically chosen because it can be performed rapidly or easily and because it is sensitive enough and specific enough to keep false positives or false negatives to a minimum. See *EPSTD; review; toxicology screen.*

*Multiphasic screening* uses more than one test at a time to detect those subjects who are likely to have the trait or disease in question. One form often used in assessing the level of cognitive skills is the screen *metric* approach. An easy question or task (e.g., a one-step command such as "Hand me the ball") is followed by increasingly difficult questions (e.g., two-step commands, then three-step commands), thereby establishing a graded measure (metric) of the degree of cognitive impairment.

**screening, periodic** See *EPSDT*.

**script** The canonical set of events one can expect in an often encountered setting, such as a visit to a doctor's office. It is a *top-down* concept (q.v.) used in cognitive psychology to explain the subject's behavior and thinking in a specific situation. Another influential top-down concept is a *frame*-an expected structure of knowledge about a domain consisting of a core and a set of slots. Each slot corresponds to some aspect of the domain being modeled by the frame. The slots include those at a top level—fixed parameters representing things that are always true about a proposed situation (e.g., that a room has four walls). Lower levels have many terminals—slots that must be filled with specific instances of data: for example, an object, such as a window, that may or may not be present in a particular room. Frames and scripts are predicated on the belief that few situations we encounter are really new. Technically, frames describe static situations, while scripts characterize a dynamic set of actions appropriate to a given set of circumstances.

**script analysis**   See *transactional analysis.*

**scrotal reflex**   By stroking the perineum or applying a cold object to it, a slow, vermicular contraction of the dartos muscle occurs.

**scrupulosity**   Excessive meticulousness or punctiliousness, typically regarding questions of right or wrong and hence often couched in religious or moral terms. The scrupulous person sees evil where there is no evil, serious sin where there is no serious sin, and obligation where there is no obligation. See *obsessive-compulsive disorder.*

**Scull dilemma**   The dilemma highlighted by sociologist Andrew Scull, consisting of claims that it is wrong both to get patients out of mental hospitals and to keep them in. Because both commitment to mental hospital and release of a patient from mental hospital often depend on a prediction of that patient's future behavior, there can never be absolute certainty about the decision either to admit or discharge. As in most such situations, positions have been taken at each extreme, and a small number of people oppose involuntary hospitalization under any conditions. One extreme is expressed by those sociologists who, critical of the entire existing organization of mental health care, sometimes label community care *decarceration*, just as they speak of *social control* instead of care and treatment.

**Scythian disease**   Hippocratic term for transvestitism. See *phrenitis.*

**SDA**   Serotonin-dopamine antagonist; a type of neuroleptic. The SDAs block serotonin

(5-HT$_{2A}$) as well as dopamine D$_2$ receptors. The group of SDA antipsychotics includes risperidone, olanzapine, and sertindole.

**SDAT**   Senile dementia, Alzheimer type; also known as primary degenerative dementia of senile or presenile onset. See *Alzheimer disease.*

**SDD**   Sporadiac (nonfamilial) depressive disease, in Winokur's classification.

**S-deficiency hypothesis**   A two-process model of sleep regulation postulating that process S, a sleep-promoting substance that increases in relation to the duration of wakefulness, and process C determine the circadian propensity to sleep and to wake up. Sleep reverses the effect of process S. In depression, process S fails to rise to its usual peak, and sleep deprivation is beneficial in depression because it permits process S to rise to higher levels by extending the hours of wakefulness. See *circadian clock; phase-advance hypothesis; sleep disorders.*

**SDL/R**   *State-dependent learning* and retrieval (q.v.).

**SE**   Spongiform encephalopathy. See *virus infections.*

**season**   *Stage* (q.v.).

**seasonal affective disorder**   *SAD*; winter depression; episodes of major depression that have occurred in at least 2 consecutive years in the fall or winter (in temperate zones) and have remitted in the spring or summer, in the absence of any other psychiatric disorder and in the absence of any seasonal psychosocial variable, such as work stress occurring at certain times of the year. Symptoms are depressed mood, anxiety, irritability, loss of energy, fatigue, social withdrawal, craving for carbohydrates, weight gain, headaches, and sleep changes (most often hypersomnia). Some patients have hypomanic episodes in the spring or summer.

SAD is more common in women, and a family history of affective disorder is frequent. It is hypothesized that affected persons are overly sensitive to wintertime reduction of daylight, which interferes with the suppression of melatonin, a regulator of biological rhythms. *Phototherapy* (q.v.) is often used to treat SAD.

**SEC**   Structured event complex; a goal-oriented set of events that is structured in sequence and represents thematic knowledge, morals, abstractions, concepts, social rules, event features, event boundaries, and grammars. The SEC theory of prefrontal cortex (PFC) functioning is that different categories of SECs are stored in different regions of PFC. Their localization is determined by the connectivity between specific PFC and posterior cortical (temporal-parietal) or subcortical (basal ganglia, hippocampus, amygdala) regions. Consistent with this, impairment of social behavior is most evident after ventromedial PFC damage, whereas impairment of reflective, mechanistic behavior is evident following dorsolateral PFC damage.

**seclusion**  May serve the following purposes: (1) containment to prevent the patient from harming himself or others, (2) removal from interpersonal conflict, and (3) reduction of sensory input. See *restraint; padded cell.*

APA's guidelines for implementing restraints or seclusion specify that (a) it should not exceed 1 hour without an oral order by a physician; (b) the psychiatrist should evaluate the patient within 3 hours after implementation of restraints/seclusion; and (c) the psychiatrist must document having evaluated the patient and that the need for restraint/seclusion continues. JCAHO requires monitoring of the patient in seclusion every 15 minutes by the nursing staff.

**second half deprivation**  See *sleep deprivation.*

**second messenger**  Any of the mediators of the cellular responses to regulatory molecules, such as neurotransmitters and growth factors. The regulatory molecule (first messenger) carries a message to a cell by locking into its receptor on that cell. This activates the receptor, which binds to an intracellular coupling protein, such as a G protein (q.v.). The G protein then binds to an effector enzyme that synthesizes the second messenger. Second messengers perform several functions; they help to regulate gene expression, to form the structural components of the cell, or to synthesize neurotransmitters. Typically, the second messenger then activates a protein kinase, although one (IP3, inositol 1,4,5-triphosphate) is known to release calcium ions into neural cytoplasm. See *neurotransmitter receptor; transducer.*

Only four of the second messenger pathways have been well characterized—cAMP (the first one recognized), inositol polyphosphates, diaylglycerol, and arachidonic acid. In general, second messengers exert their effects by regulating protein kinases and protein phosphatases. Different protein kinases phosphorylate specific proteins (the *third messenger* system) by transferring the terminal phosphoryl group from ATP to specific protein substrates within cells, leading to diverse physiological responses.

It does not seem likely that so small a number of second messengers is enough to handle the almost countless number of specific signals received at the cell membrane. There is evidence that a quicker and more direct way of transmitting signals is through a *transcription factor* (q.v.).

**second pain**  Dull, burning pain associated with slowly conducting C-fibers; see *pain.*

**secondary**  Symptomatic; due to some other condition (which is the primary cause). The secondary psychoses, for example, are also termed symptomatic psychoses, psychoses due to a general medical disorder, or organic psychoses.

**secondary defense symptom**  See *symptom, secondary defense.*

**secondary dissociation**  See *dissociative disorders.*

**secondary elaboration**  In dreams, the process that molds the latent thoughts and wishes, disguised by the processes of *condensation, displacement,* and *symbolization* (qq.v.), into the semblance of a logical story. See *dream.*

**secondary gain**  See *epinosic gain.*

**secondary process**  The name given by Freud to the laws that regulate events in the preconscious or *ego* (q.v.). By means of its faculties of judgment and intelligence, by the application of logic and reality testing, the ego blocks the tendency of the instincts toward immediate discharge. Instead, the ego decides under what conditions it would be safe to satisfy the instincts, if at all.

**secondary self**  See *dissociative identity disorder.*

**secondary sleep disorder**  A sleep disorder associated with or caused by identifiable disease in some organ system, such as the central nervous system or respiratory system.

**second-generation antipsychotics**  Suggested as an alternate to "atypical antipsychotics" and "serotonin-dopamine-antagonists" because it is more consistent with drug nomenclature in other medical disciplines. The compounds include clozapine (the first to be introduced), risperidone, olanzapine, quetiapine, and ziprasidone. They differ from older agents in terms of clinical effectiveness, side effects, or basic mechanisms. See *atypical antipsychotic.*

**second-order false belief tasks** Sophisticated mind-reading tasks that require evaluation of what another person believes that a third person is thinking.

**second-order relatives** See *first-order relatives*.

**secretase** A proteinase that acts on amyloid precursor protein (APP). Proteinases, also known as endopeptidases, are enzymes that catalyze hydrolysis of a peptide chain well within the chain and not at either of the chain's termini. Three secretrases are implicated in APP cleaving and in amyloid production: $\alpha$-, $\beta$-, and $\gamma$-secretase.

The enzymes with $\alpha$-secretase activity belong to the ADAM family (disintegrin- and metalloproteinase-family enzyme); they are ADAM9, ADAM10, and ADAM17 (also known as tumor necrosis factor converting enzyme). The $\beta$-secretase APP-cleaving enzyme 1 (BACE1) is a type I integral membrane protein belonging to the pepsin family of aspartyl proteases. The $\gamma$-secretase is a complex of enzymes composed of presenilin 1 or 2 (PS1, PS2), nicastrin, anterior pharynx defective, and presenilin enhancer 2 (PEN2). See *amyloid*.

**security operations** Sullivan's term for feelings—such as anger, boredom, contempt, depression, or irritation—that, no matter how rational or explicable at first glance, are really defenses against the recognition or experiencing of anxiety; the term is approximately equivalent to *defense* (q.v.).

**sedation** A state of decreased responsivity to usual stimuli that may proceed to sleepiness, but not to drowsiness (which would be a hypnotic effect). In practice, the line between the sedative and the hypnotic dose of a drug is a fine one. See *sedatives/hypnotics*.

**sedation threshold** The amount of sodium amytal required, by intravenous injection, to produce slurring of speech and a concomitant inflection point in the 15 to 30 Hz amplitude curve of the electroencephalogram. The EEG change occurs within 80 seconds of the time when slur is noted.

Shagass used this test to differentiate between psychotic and neurotic depressions; according to him, thresholds are low in psychotic depressions and high in neurotic depressions.

**sedative occupation** In occupational therapy, a form of activity characterized by repetitious, uniform movements that, because of their monotonous recurrence, have a soothing and quieting effect. It is usually prescribed for overactive patients. An example of sedative occupation is simple weaving.

**sedative-hypnotic amnestic disorder** Prolonged, heavy use of a sedative, hypnotic, or anxiolytic agent is likely to produce neuropsychological deficits similar to those found in alcoholics: impairment of memory, learning, speed, and coordination. In some cases, this leads to the development of a full-blown *amnestic syndrome* (q.v.).

**sedative-hypnotic dependence (and abuse)** See *barbiturates*.

**sedative-hypnotic-anxiolytic intoxication** Behavior changes and symptoms of CNS depression following use of a sedative, hypnotic, or anxiolytic, such as impaired judgment, loss of control over sexual or aggressive impulses, lability of mood, impairment in social or occupational functioning, slurred speech, incoordination, unsteady gait, impairment in attention or memory. With overdose, the patient progresses from drowsiness, dysarthria, and ataxia to stuporous sedation. Patients recover from benzodiazepine overdosage much more quickly than from barbiturate overdosage. The benzodiazepines are remarkably safe drugs, and fatal overdosage almost invariably involves conjoint use of other drugs (including alcohol).

**sedative-hypnotic-anxiolytic withdrawal** Cessation (or significant reduction in amount) of a sedative, hypnotic, or anxiolytic agent that has been used at moderate or high levels for several weeks or more is followed by three or more of the following: nausea or vomiting; weakness; autonomic hyperactivity (e.g., sweating, rapid heart beat); anxiety or irritability; orthostatic hypotension; coarse tremors of the hands, tongue, and eyelids; marked insomnia; and grand mal seizures, which may progress to a fatal status epilepticus.

**sedative-hypnotic-anxiolytic withdrawal delirium** Cessation (or significant reduction in amount) of a sedative, hypnotic, or anxiolytic agent that has been used at moderate or high levels for several weeks or more is followed by the usual symptoms of withdrawal and, usually within 1 week, by *delirium* (q.v.).

**sedative/hypnotic/anxiolytic use disorders** These are classified within the substance-related disorders and include sedative dependence, sedative abuse, sedative intoxication, sedative withdrawal, sedative delirium, sedative psychotic, sedative anxiety disorder, sedative sleep disorder, and sedative sexual dysfunction.

**sedatives/hypnotics** In many classifications, anxiolytics are considered a part of this group; they are all central nervous system depressants used to induce sleep or to reduce anxiety and agitation during waking states. They shorten time of onset before sleep but suppress REM sleep (benzodiazepines not as much as sedatives); withdrawal of the drug results in a rebound of REM sleep and deterioration of sleep patterns. Withdrawal from high doses may provoke tremors, seizures, and delirium.

Development of tolerance to the sedatives/hypnotics/anxiolytics is typical and may appear as early as 5 to 7 days after the first dose; as a result, many abusers take enormous doses (e.g., 1500 mg of diazepam daily). Detoxification in such patients must be slow and carefully monitored.

Long-term use of sedatives/hypnotics/anxiolytics is likely to produce psychological and physical dependence, even though the patient may never exceed the prescribed dose, a phenomenon called *therapeutic dose dependence* or *low dose dependence*.

The sedatives/hypnotics are often used in combination with other drugs of abuse to accentuate euphoric effects (e.g., 40 to 80 mg of diazepam taken immediately after the daily maintenance dose of methadone, to accentuate the sedative-euphoric effect of methadone alone; glutethimide with codeine).

The major sedative/hypnotics are as follows:
1. *Alcohol* (q.v.)
2. *Anxiolytics* (q.v.)
3. *Barbiturates* (q.v.)
4. *Carbamates* (meprobamate, ethniamate, carisoprodol): their use as anxiolytics, hypnotics, or sedatives has largely been replaced by the benzodiazepines, which have a higher therapeutic index and a lower abuse potential.
5. Piperidinediones (glutethimide, methyprylon): reported to be even more lethal in overdose and more subject to abuse than the carbamates.
6. Other hypnotics: bromide, chloral hydrate, ethchlorvynol (a tertiary acetylenic alcohol), methaqualone (a quinazalone), paraldehyde (a cyclic polyether).

The sedative/hypnotic/anxiolytic use disorders include dependence, abuse, intoxication, withdrawal, delirium, persisting dementia, persisting amnestic disorder, psychotic disorder (with delusions or hallucinations), mood disorder, anxiety disorder, sleep disorder, and sexual dysfunction.

**sedativism** Alcohol and drug abuse.

**seduction theory** A term first used by Ernst Kris to refer to Freud's theory of the relation between childhood sexual trauma (typically, incest initiated by the father) and the later development of hysteria. Freud first took his patients' recollections of such experiences at face value, but then (by September 1897) he began to doubt that incest was as frequent as it would have to be to account for all cases of hysteria. He came to recognize the importance of phantasy in the construction of such "recollections," and at the same time he developed his theory of the Oedipus complex. With that, the seduction theory was abandoned, and psychoanalytic theory and practice focused on the analysis and interpretation of phantasy.

Since the 1980s, antithetical views of Freud's disavowal of the seduction theory have been expressed both by some psychoanalysts and by other therapists outside the analytic circle. Their belief is that the accounts of childhood seduction were true. Their suggestion is that Freud abandoned the seduction theory not because it was only an intermediate step in the development of psychoanalytic psychology, but rather because it was a threat to various of his self-serving motives, both conscious and unconscious. Their charge is that he betrayed his patients and distorted the truths they revealed to him.

Other critics claim that when Freud recognized that the seductions he had reported were not true, he failed to reassess the method by which he had obtained them. If they were not true, then the method that produced them (and perhaps also the theory of repression, etc.) might be invalid. But Freud did not consider that possibility; instead, he claimed that the patients's "confessions" were manufactured to hide their childhood incestuous longing and their autoerotic practices.

**seed psychosurgery** See *stereotactic tractotomy*.

**SEG** Sonoencephalogram.

**Séglas type** (Jules Séglas, French physician, 1856–1939) The so-called psychomotor type of paranoia.

**segmental insufficiency**   In Adlerian psychology, inferiority of a body segment (using the term segment in its embryological, developmental sense); the inferiority of the internal organs is typically betrayed by some disorder of the skin of that segment—nevi, angiomata, telangiectasiae, neurofibromata, etc., all of which Adler termed the *external stigmata.*

**segmental set**   See *set, major.*

**segregation**   In a social sense, separation or isolation.

In genetics this term refers to an essential principle in the Mendelian mechanism of inheritance, in which the gene units derived from the two parents segregate out in the hybrid, as if independent of each other. This phenomenon allows the gene units to enter into new combinations, especially in those involving more than one pair. See *mendelian laws.*

**segregation analysis**   A method used to determine the mode of inheritance of a disorder; it compares the observed frequency of an illness in a pedigree with the pattern that would occur if a hypothesized mode of inheritance (e.g., one of the monogenic patterns or polygenic transmission) were true. See *linkage analysis.*

**Séguin, O. Edouard**   (1812–1880) French psychiatrist; humanistic treatment and education of the mentally retarded.

**Seitelberger syndrome**   Familial, progressive, juvenile neuroaxonal dystrophy; similar to (and possibly identical with) Hallervorden Spatz syndrome. See *neuroaxonal degeneration.*

**seizure**   An attack, or sudden onset of a disease or of certain symptoms, such as convulsions.

**seizure, adequate**   In electroconvulsive therapy, arbitrarily defined as a seizure with duration greater than 25 seconds and cerebral generalization (evidenced in bilateral tonic and clonic components), and perhaps with a post-seizure period of electrical silence (i.e., abrupt EEG seizure termination).

**seizure, automatic**   A type of *psychomotor epilepsy* (q.v.).

**sejunction**   Wernicke's term for blocking and other forms of dissociation. The term is seldom used today, because it includes forms of dissociation that are widely removed both psychologically and nosographically.

**selaphobia**   Fear of a flash (of lightning).

**selection**   1. *Choice* (q.v.).

2. In a specific biological sense, this term applies in a mixed population to the intentional or unintentional choice of those individuals who possess a particular genetic character or a certain combination of characters. This choice may be exercised by the failure to reproduce or by the lack of an adequate partner for marriage, if preference is given to other types or if the given type is biologically incapable of reproduction.

There are two types of selection, natural and sexual. In natural selection, it is nature that favors the survival of types adapted (or most adaptable) to their environment to reproduce their kind. In sexual selection, the choices are made by the animals themselves. Sexual selection often reveals an unsuspected functional advantage in the marker that determines choice. In many birds, for instance, the male's gaudy plumage attracts the female, and the males among their chicks will also develop gaudy plumage as they mature. But the plumage is more than a sexual excitant; it is also a sensitive marker for health, and particularly for the ability to fend off parasites.

*Sociosexual selection* is much the same. In passing one's genes to the next generation, it is an advantage to pick a mate who can be successful in life. While there is nothing that is consistently predictive of success, some of the factors favoring success are as follows: intelligence, and in particular the ability to deal with abstract concepts and symbols, to plan and organize, verbal skills and language; the ability to delay gratification, self-control; social skills based on a sensitivity to the feelings and desires of others, empathy, and an ability to form alliances. A person with good social skills is more likely to meet others with those same skills, thereby increasing the opportunities for *associative mating* (those with like genes mating). See *theory of mind.*

Natural selection takes place in evolution through a variety of processes that enable types (adapted to their environment) to reproduce their kind in marked degree, so that an improvement is gradually carried on from one stage of development to the other.

In human genetics, one usually distinguishes between positive and negative factors of selection, according to (1) whether a given factor is favorable to the reproduction of healthy or tainted family stocks, or (2) whether the general life conditions of a population facilitate or hinder the reproduction of the average type.

Nature picks and chooses among the phenotypes, bestowing on some the "right" to produce more offspring than others. It is crucial to note that although the phenotypical variation has its root cause in changes in the genotype, the traditional Darwinian selection mechanism acts only at the level of the phenotype. Furthermore, the decision is determined by the environment. See *phenotypic fitness*.

**selective abstractions** See *cognitive behavior therapy*.

**selective amnesia** See *amnesia, psychogenic*.

**selective analysis** Pseudopsychoanalytic treatment in which the material chosen for interpretation is a function of the interests (and problems) of the therapist rather than a reflection of the psychic structure and function of the patient. To some extent, such selection is operative in all types of psychotherapy and is probably responsible at least in part for the effects the actual character and personality of the therapist have on his techniques and results. See *countertransference; focused analysis*.

**selective attention** Focused processing of information, so that only a limited number of stimuli are chosen from the multiple stimuli impinging on the sensory apparatus for further processing.

Three types of selection have been distinguished: (1) *filtering*—permitting entry for further processing or analysis to stimuli that possess a single physical feature (e.g., redness, as of a light; pitch, as of a voice; smoothness, as of a fabric); (2) *categorizing*—permitting entry on the basis of meeting conceptual criteria, despite differences in many other characteristics (e.g., anything that comes in pairs, be it a pair of shoes or a pair of goats); (3) *pigeonholing*—permitting entry on the basis of sorting out more than one class at a time, a form of selection that tends to increase errors in identification (e.g., from mail delivered to a large apartment building, selecting the mail to be forwarded to Mr. Reader that is not "junk mail"—it is likely that some envelopes will be forwarded even though they are in fact junk mail).

**selective drug** A drug with a narrow, well-defined, or single action; fluoxetine, for example, is a selective 5-HT-uptake inhibitor, and it produces no appreciable inhibition of norepinephrine uptake.

**selective mutism** The term preferred by DSM-IV for what is generally known as elective mutism.

**selective neuronal vulnerability** *SNV*; the susceptibility of specific populations of neurons that is limited to specific region(s) of the nervous system. In the neurodegenerative diseases, for instance, ALS attacks the lower motor and pyramidal neurons, Alzheimer disease damages the hippocampus and parietal lobes, Huntington disease focuses on the caudate, and Parkinson disease destroys cells in the substantia nigra.

**selective silence** In therapy, deliberate withholding of associations in response to anxiety or as a reflection of negative transference toward the therapist or the group in order to resist the therapeutic situation.

**selective satiety** A form of reinforcer devaluation in which participants fed to satiety on one food still find other foods rewarding and will eat some of those other foods.

**self** The psychophysical total of the person at any given moment, including both conscious and unconscious attributes. Horney's term for self as thus defined is actual self or *empirical self*. See Jung's definition of *ego*.

**self psychology** A type of psychoanalytic theory and technique that had its origins in Heinz Kohut's studies of the narcissistic personality disorders and is concerned with the development of the *self-object* (q.v.) and self-object transferences. Self psychology posits a tripolar structure of the self, and the normal self as a balance of mirroring, idealizing, and twinship needs. See *alter-ego transference; idealization; mirroring; mirroring deficits; object relations theory*.

**self-absorption** Erikson describes generativity vs. self-absorption as one of the eight stages of man. See *ontogeny, psychic*.

**self-abuse** *Obs*. A moralistic term for *masturbation* (q.v.).

**self-actualization** See *humanistic psychology*.

**self-alteration** The sixth most common dissociative symptom in *dissociative identity disorder* (q.v.), consisting of a sudden, inexplicable, and often ego-alien change in one's sense of self, as though one's body or thoughts belong to someone else. The experience lacks the quality of detachment and alienation characteristic of *depersonalization* (q.v.).

**self-analysis**   See *frontal lobe.*

**self-attack**   See *deliberate self-harm syndrome.*

**self-awareness**   See *body image.*

**self-control**   Self-regulation; self-monitoring; the ability to monitor and control one's behavior effortfully and often in opposition to emotional drive (e.g., suppressing an outburst of anger). It is an essential social skill, typically associated with activity in the dorsal ACC (anterior cingulate cortex), which has been implicated in *attention* (q.v.) and the continuous internal monitoring of action. It is also related to OFC (orbitofrontal cortex), which is involved in monitoring the reward value of stimuli and responses (including situations in which responses to previously rewarded stimuli must be suppressed.) OFC guides behavior in terms of the value of possible outcomes.

**self-defeating personality**   *Masochistic personality* (q.v.).

**self-directed exposure**   See *exposure, self-directed.*

**self-dynamism**   The fabric of the motivational forces and processes that lead to the development of the *self-system*, in Sullivan's theory of interpersonal relations. The human personality is founded on a biological substrate and is the product of the interpersonal and social forces acting on the person from the time of birth. The human being is concerned with two goals: (1) the pursuit of satisfaction, which deals chiefly with biological needs; and (2) the pursuit of security, which deals primarily with cultural pressures. To maintain security and avoid anxiety, the child develops and strengthens those sides of his nature which are pleasing or acceptable to the significant adults. The resulting configuration of traits is the *self-system* (q.v.).

**self-effacement**   Horney's term for the behavior of the type of neurotic character who idealizes compliance, dependence, and love as a result of identification with the despised self.

**self-esteem**   A state in which narcissistic supplies emanating from the superego are maintained so that the person does not fear punishment or abandonment by the superego. In other words, self-esteem is a state of being on good terms with one's *superego* (q.v.). Pathological loss of self-esteem is characteristic of clinical depression. See *omnipotence.*

**self-extinction**   Horney's term for that form of neurotic behavior in which the person lives vicariously through the actions of others and

has no personality that he experiences or identifies as his own. See *as-if personality.*

**self-fellator**   See *autofellatio.*

**self-harm**   Deliberate self-harm includes superficial to moderate self-mutilation; self-injurious behavior; parasuicide; self-wounding; intentional injury of one's body without apparent intent to commit suicide. Self-harm occurs in patients with a variety of diagnoses and has also been reported in nonclinical populations. In one study, 35% of college students reported at least one instance of self-harm behavior in their lifetime.

**self-healing**   See *trauma stories.*

**self-help group**   A group whose members are taught cognitive behavioral and other techniques of self-management and coping; the term also is used to denote a *mutual help group* (q.v.).

**self-hypnosis**   See *autohypnosis.*

**self-identification**   A process in which the subject projects his own personality upon another and then proceeds to admire himself as he appears in the other person. While this is the usual process of self-identification, it is possible to include under the term the process of projecting one's undesirable traits upon another and then hating his own traits, as if they belonged to another. The latter happens in paranoid states.

**self-image**   *Self-representation* (q.v.).

**self-instructional training**   A technique of *behavior therapy* (q.v.).

**self-irrumation**   *Autofellatio* (q.v.).

**selfish**   See *sociobiology.*

**self-maximation**   The drive (involving a part of the ego) associated with the numerous competitive situations a person encounters in the course of living, such as competitions for affection, attention, and status, at home, at school, in groups of peers, and elsewhere. There are competitions in the vocational, intellectual, and social fields, as well as for love objects. This drive is to maintain feelings of personal adequacy.

**self-monitoring**   Taking care to observe one's own behavior, particularly as a way to avoid or control actions that are undesirable. See *frontal lobe.* Self-monitoring has been used as a form of behavior therapy; in Gilles de la Tourette syndrome, for example, having the subject observe and record the frequency of tics has led to a reduction in their frequency and intensity. A related type of behavior therapy is *awareness training*, in which the subject with tics observes himself in the mirror in order to appreciate more concretely how the illness manifests itself and how the tics tend to increase in intensity and spread over wider areas of the body during each bout. Awareness training often leads to an earlier recognition of an impending onset of tics and thus provides greater opportunity to control them.

**self-mutilation**  Maiming or injuring the self, including the willful production of any symptom, syndrome, or disease. See *factitial; morsicatio buccarum; Munchhausen syndrome; self-harm.*

Self-mutilation occurs in a variety of settings. It is sometimes part of a suicide attempt and may then represent a discharge of aggression against the self or against parental introjections. It may represent a way of relieving guilt by expiating acts committed or phantasies entertained. It has been reported in soldiers who attempted thereby to evade their assignment to battlefield stations; many observers have noted the high frequency of schizophrenic disorders in such soldiers.

In psychiatric hospitals, probably the two most frequent forms of self-mutilation are repetitive *wrist-cutting* (the *"slashers"*) and cigarette burning of the forearms; both tend to be repeated in a stereotyped way, with the patient seemingly fascinated by the sight of blood oozing from the cut or by the sight and odor of burning flesh. Most such patients give little if any indication that they are suffering the pain one would anticipate from such wounds. Some authors consider wrist-cutting as distorted autoerotic activity that simultaneously defends against and gratifies the libidinal impulses; the cuttings on the skin represent the female genitalia. Other authors, while agreeing that wrist-slashing is more common among females, find it to be indicative of more serious pathology than mere neurotic distortion. It occurs most often in women with a history of physical trauma(ta) in childhood, with menstrual irregularities, with difficulty in sexual identification, and with depression. For such women, the act seems to be a way of gaining self-control and reintegration in situations of stress where they experience difficulty in thinking clearly and acting effectively. See *Lesch-Nyhan syndrome.*

In addition to wrist-cutting and burning, the following have also been reported: abrasion, head banging, ingestion of medication and other objects, jumping from heights, hair pulling, insertion of foreign bodies into the urethra, self-enucleation of the eye, self-castration, removal of tongue.

From the point of view of psychiatric diagnosis, probably the most frequent currently reported as self-mutilators are borderline personality or schizophrenia. In these patients, the motives included relieving feelings of depersonalization, lessening inner tension, trying to solve genital conflicts, using the sight of his blood to gain assurance that he is alive, and denying the inability to control the body. See *deliberate self-harm syndrome.*

**self-object**  Also, selfobject; a concept used in self psychology to refer to the intrapsychic representation of another person (or inanimate object or abstract concept), who is experienced not as a separate person but as a needed extension of the self. The self-object provides critical functional supplies that subsequently are internalized and transformed (the process, which continues throughout infancy and childhood, is termed *transmuting internalization*) into the structure (and hence attributes and capacities) of the developing self. Development of an intact *cohesive self* (q.v.) requires participation of an empathic parent or caretaker as self-object. Parental inability or failure to fulfill such a role is responsible for infantile conflict and later pathology.

In infancy, *self-object needs* are absolute and intense, and the infant demands that the object (typically, the mother) respond instantly and gratify him totally. As times goes on, increasing distance from the mother is tolerated even though she continues to provide, on an as-needed basis, self-enhancing and self-regulatory functions, such as admiration, soothing, and enhancing feelings of cohesiveness. The self-object mediates between psyche and culture in the sense that the milieu teaches the child which of its attributes will be mirrored or worthy of idealization and which will not. During adolescence, the peer group is a crucial self-object. In adult life, spouse, friends, and colleagues may be self-objects, who are valued for the internal functions and the emotional stability they provide.

In interpretive psychotherapy, the therapist serves as a self-object. There are five primary *self-object transferences*: merger, contact shunning, mirroring, idealizing, and alter ego (twinship). See *alter-ego transference*.

**self-observation**  Scrutiny of one's physical and/or mental state of functioning, one of the perceptive tasks of the *ego* (q.v.).

**self-paced test**  An untimed digit symbol substitution test. See *digit symbol substitution task*.

**self-peeping, narcissistic**  Self-voyeurism on the basis of primary *narcissism* (q.v.). Ordinarily, the original self-voyeurism is transformed into voyeurism directed against the parents. E. Bergler considers this voyeurism to be the true basis for choosing acting as a profession. In the beginning, the child says: "I want to be a voyeur of mother and father, later of intimacies between them." But the superego reproaches the child for this wish, and the child denies having this wish by asserting the opposite: "No, I am not a voyeur, I am just the opposite—an exhibitionist." This, too, receives reproaches from the superego, and the desire is sublimated: "I am neither a voyeur nor an exhibitionist; I merely want to give other people pleasure, so I am an actor" (*Psychoanalytic Quarterly Supplement 23*, 1949).

**self-pitying constellation**  A group of symptoms characteristic of "neurotic depression" (used in the sense of lacking endogenous symptoms such as early morning waking, weight loss, psychomotor retardation, and guilt feelings), consisting of self-pity, irritability, reactivity, and fluctuating symptoms. Neurotic depression also used to refer to related but not identical or interchangeable groups of depressed patients, meaning that their disorders were less incapacitating; nonpsychotic (= no hallucinations, delusions, confusion, memory impairment, etc.); situational or reactive to a social stressor; characterological, in a long-standing maladaptive personality pattern; due to unconscious conflicts over loss, fall in self-esteem, aggressivity, or narcissism, dependency, and ambivalence.

**self-punishment**  See *ego-suffering; expiation; masochism; self-defeating personality; superego resistance*.

**self-referential delusion**  *Delusion of reference* (q.v.).

**self-regulation**  The ability to control one's behavior effortfully and often in opposition to emotional drive (for example, controlling an anger outburst). Self-regulation depends on regions in the prefrontal cortex. See *cognitive control*.

**self-regulation, physiologic**  See *biofeedback*.

**self-representation**  *Self-image*; the subjective sense of an "I" or "me" that emerges as a reliably verifiable percept that in normal narcissism is differentiated from the ideal(ized) self and from object representations (the sense of "you" or "it"). Differentiation of self-representations from object representations is basic to the ability to sense and test reality.

According to self psychology, pathological narcissism is characterized (1) by a merging of the phantasied, ideal self (which denies the subject's dependency and compensates for feelings of frustration, rage, and envy) with the phantasied image of a loving mother (the ideal object) resulting in the *grandiose self* (q.v.), and (2) by a projection of unacceptable, devalued aspects of the self onto others.

**self-sentience**  Awareness of self; in Sullivan's terminology, recognition of the bodily self as "me," and differentiated from the rest of the world or the "not me." See *body ego*.

**self-soothing**  Inner congeniality, based on ready access to a calming, reassuring maternal introject that is made possible by reduction of ambivalence and attainment of object constancy and self-cohesiveness.

**self-system**  In Sullivan's theory of personality development, final formation of self from a limited number sifted out of a greater number of potentialities, through parental influence on the developing personality of the child. Security rests on the feeling of belonging and being accepted. The child's actions or attributes that meet with disapproval tend to be blocked out of awareness and dissociated. As the child realizes that certain earlier devices for obtaining satisfaction, such as crying when hungry, bring on disapproval in the environment, the earlier pattern of behavior is inhibited: the child tends to develop and emphasize those aspects of his nature that are pleasing or acceptable to the significant adults, and the configuration of the traits that have met with approval constitutes the self-system.

After the self-system has been established, secondary anxiety appears whenever there is a possibility that the dissociated thoughts or feelings will become conscious: the dissociated impulses are not necessarily destructive, but because there is an emotional stake in maintaining the self-system, anything threatening it will nonetheless produce anxiety. It is obvious that the self-system tends to lead to a rigidity in personality and that even many positive potentialities of the person may never be realized or put into operation.

"The self-system of Sullivan is different from the concept of character in that it includes more than sublimation, whereas Freud seems to conceive of character as nothing but sublimation. No true comparison of the two can be made, because the frames of reference are entirely different. Freud's system emphasizes what happens to instincts. Sullivan's system stresses what goes on between people. For Sullivan, personality does not develop mechanically. Always the emphasis is on a dynamic interaction between people. Freud's orientation is mechanistic-biological; Sullivan's dynamic-cultural (inter-personal)" (Thompson, C. *Psychoanalysis, Evolution and Development*, 1950).

**self-talk** 1. Repeating words, ideas, instructions, etc. to oneself, sometimes used in *behavior therapy* (q.v.), especially with children. The therapist or other adult model performs the desired action for the child and describes it aloud. The child then performs the task, also describing it aloud. Subsequently, the child whispers the instructions while performing the action and finally performs the task without audible speech.

2. A "state of mind" in narcissistic personality disorder. See *embitterment, chronic.*

**semantic aphasia** *Wernicke aphasia* (q.v.).

**semantic dementia** 1. *SD*; the semantic variant of *fronto-temporal dementia* (q.v.). Most prominent is anomia, the failure to name objects, people, or concepts both when asked to do so and in spontaneous speech. At least until late in the disease, most other cognitive functions are usually well-preserved in SD—general intelligence, problem solving, visuospatial function, calculation skills, and short-term and episodic memory.

2. Semantic dementia was used by Cleckley (*Psychiatric Quarterly 16*, 1942) to refer to the inability of the psychopathic personality to evaluate or experience life as a totally integrated organism. Although the psychopath can react verbally, as though he understood love, pride, grief, shame, or the other emotions, he has no real experience of these human values or connotations. Cleckley

believed that failure to function at this level provokes regression, which is expressed in a drive toward failure and folly, a destruction of the self at the personal or cultural level.

**semantic dissociation** The distortion between symbol and meaning that is characteristic of the thought disorder of many schizophrenics. The term includes (1) *enlargement of the semantic halo*—language becomes ambiguous, vague, indeterminate (schizophrenic systematic abstractionism), but is comprehensible and coherent; (2) *semantic distortion*—transfer of meaning to a new symbol (neologism) or to another word (paralogism); (3) *semantic dispersion*—meaning is lost or reduced; language becomes incoherent, agrammatical, asyntactic; and (4) *semantic dissolution*—complete loss of meaning and of communication ability; language is used as a game, or automatically. See *association disturbances.*

**semantic halo** See *semantic dissociation.*

**semantic jargon** See *jargon aphasia.*

**semantic memory** Semantic knowledge; factual information organized independently of the specific episodes that provided the information. See *declarative memory.*

Also called *conceptual knowledge*, semantic memory is the general knowledge of objects, word meaning, facts, and people, independent of their connection to any particular time or place (which is the defining characteristic of episodic memory). Responding to the question, "Where were you last Monday night?" with "At the Metropolitan Opera's production of *Turandot*" is an example of episodic memory. Knowing that the Metropolitan Opera is in New York City, that *Turandot* was the last opera written by Giacomo Puccini, and that it was first presented at La Scala in Milan in April 1926 and at the Metropolitan in New York 7 months later is an example of semantic memory.

The contents of semantic memory typically relate to perception and action and are represented in (or overlap with) brain regions corresponding to the regions that are responsible for the particular perceptions and actions (texture, taste, color, visual form, movement, musical sounds and the like, and the actions associated with such perceptions such as using a knife, fork, or spoon, walking down the aisle and sitting in a theatre, etc.). There is debate about whether these distributed brain regions and the connections between them are the total basis of semantic memory (the "distributed-only" view), or whether conceptual memory requires, in addition, an overarching convergence zone or hub that supports the interactive activation of representations in all modalities, for all semantic categories (the "distributed-plus-hub" view). Both structural and metabolic imaging studies suggest that SD is due to relatively focal pathology in the anterior and inferior parts of the temporal lobes (ATL) and not to widespread damage in the cortical semantic network.

Impairment in conceptual knowledge occurs in stroke, viral infection (especially herpes simplex virus encephalitis), Alzheimer disease, and the semantic variant of *frontotemporal dementia* (usually labeled *semantic dementia*) (qq.v.).

**semantic priming**  The faster processing of target words when they are preceded by semantically related words, in comparison to the processing of target words that are preceded by semantically unrelated words. The interval between primer and target is called *stimulus onset asynchrony*. Studies of semantic priming are used in comparing thought processes in patients with schizophrenia with thought processes in control groups.

**semantic satiation**  See *satiation, semantic*.

**semantics**  The science of meaning; study of the relation between language and its meaning. Language and thought are not identical, however. Syntactic structure is built out of things like nouns and verbs, prepositional phrases and tenses, but thought concerns things like objects, actions, properties, and times. For example, the thoughts of bilinguals are the same, no matter which language they are thinking in. That is possible only if the form of thought is neither of the languages, and therefore something of which they are not conscious. The form in which thoughts are couched is *conceptual structure*, which ultimately amounts to patterns of neural firings in the brain.

**semiconscious**  Imperfectly conscious.

**semiobsession à deux**  A phenomenon occuring in two members of a group independently of each other; in folie à deux, in contrast, the psychosis in one person is induced or influenced by the partner

**semiology, semeiology**  The study of signs, signals, symbols, or symptoms; symptomatology; the science that studies the life of signs within society.

**semiotic**  Relating to symptoms or signs; a descriptor or representation that serves only a representative purpose, such as a mental image, a word or phrase or symbolic gesture.

Piaget differentiates the *semiotic function* of the preoperational subperiod from the limited representation that may be observed in the earlier sensorimotor period. In the sensorimotor period, any *scheme* (q.v.) is dependent on perceptions and bodily movements. The mother's voice might represent the mother's presence, but only because the voice is in fact a part of the mother. A true symbol or sign is differentiated from the thing it signifies, and such representational thought becomes possible only with the appearance of the semiotic function. See *semiology*.

"Every view which interprets the symbolic expression as an analogous or abbreviated expression of a known thing is semiotic. A conception which interprets the symbolic expression as the best possible formulation of a relatively unknown thing which cannot conceivably, therefore, be more clearly or characteristically represented is symbolic...the explanation of the Cross as a symbol of Divine Love is semiotic, since Divine Love describes the fact to be expressed better and more aptly than a cross, which can have many other meanings" (Jung, C. G. *Psychological Types*, 1923).

**senescence**  In genetics, the increasing number of cell divisions, which determine the replicative life span of somatic cells. The life span reflects the number of cell divisions, and not chronological time. See *aging*.

**senile**  Relating to, characterized by, or manifesting old age with the implication of pathology or something more than the usual aging process.

**senile breakdown**  *Squalor syndrome* (q.v.).

**senile chorea**  A severe, progressive dyskinesia that occurs in elderly persons; it resembles Huntington chorea but is sometimes mistaken for tardive dyskinesia in patients who have been on antipsychotic drugs for long periods.

**senile delirium**  One form of *Alzheimer disease* (q.v.). Onset is usually acute and often follows head injury, infection, or surgical anesthesia. Its principal characteristics are clouded consciousness, hallucinations, marked insomnia, restlessness, resistance, and wandering. The delirium may be intermittent, or it may be prolonged with only occasional return to clear consciousness. The chief danger to the patient is exhaustion.

**senile dementia**   *Alzheimer disease* (q.v.).

**senile plaques**   See *Alzheimer disease; amyloid; plaques, senile.*

**senile psychosis**   See *Alzheimer disease.*

**senile recluse**   *Squalor syndrome* (q.v.).

**senility**   Old age, but almost invariably it is intended to convey the idea that the person or some part of him has undergone involution or degeneration attendant upon advanced age. The onset of senility varies considerably, though in general it begins clinically at about the age of 70. See *aging.*

**senium**   Feebleness of old age; also, the period of old age.

W. Mayer-Gross et al. (*Clinical Psychiatry,* 1960) classify the mental diseases of old age as follows: (1) affective psychosis; (2) *senile dementia* (see *Alzheimer disease*); (3) arteriosclerotic psychosis (see *cerebral arteriosclerosis*); (4) delirious states (see *delirium; senile delirium*); (5) late *paraphrenia* (q.v.); and (6) miscellaneous disorders, such as paresis, epilepsy, head injury, and organic brain syndrome associated with cardiovascular disorder.

**senium praecox**   (L. "premature old age") Premature senility. As average senility begins, at least clinically, at about the age of 70, senile manifestations under the age of 55 may be regarded as definitely premature. In psychiatry senium praecox is associated, for example, with *Pick disease* or *Alzheimer disease* (qq.v.).

**sensate focus**   In sex therapy, one of the early stages of interaction with the sexual partner in which attention is diverted from erection and orgasm to mutual, nondemanding pleasurable experiences with the body (but not genital stimulation, which is added at a later stage).

Sensate focusing typically consists of structured exercises that begin with nondemand *pleasuring* (nongenital tactile stimulation to provide an opportunity to explore one's own feelings about the experience rather than to please the partner), then pleasuring to give both partners enjoyment of tactile sensations that does not depend on genital stimulation or subsequent intercourse, and in later exercises genital stimulation (but not intercourse).

**sensation**   Recognition of the stimulation of a sensory receptor; the feeling of temperature, pain, itch, tickle, sensual touch, muscular and visceral sensations, vasomotor flush, hunger,

thirst, air hunger, and others related to the body's state. Sherrington divided the senses into *teloreception* (vision and hearing), *proprioception* (limb position), *exteroception* (touch), *chemoreception* (smell and taste), and *interoception* (visceral modalities). He considered temperature and pain to be aspects of touch, but they are now distinguished from touch and other bodily feelings by their inherent association with emotion. See *interoception.*

**sensation, secondary**   *Synesthesia* (q.v.).

**sensational type**   The last of Jung's four functional types. In this type, sensation predominates over thinking and feeling, though not necessarily over intuition. There is little tendency either for reflection or for commanding purpose. "He frequently has a charming and lively capacity for enjoyment; he is sometimes a jolly fellow and often a refined aesthete" (Jung, C. G. *Psychological Types,* 1923).

**sensitiver Beziehungswahn**   Sensitive delusion of reference; paranoid sensitivity psychosis; *embarrassment psychosis*; a term coined by Kretschmer in 1918 to refer to a reactive psychosis described in persons with a rigid, sensitive personality who feel some action of theirs is contradictory to the high ethical or moral standards they espouse. The result is an embarrassment and self-consciousness that color the whole life of the subject, sometimes progressing to the development of self-referential delusions. See *shame.*

**sensitivity**   Capacity to respond to stimulation, often with the sense that the subject is able to recognize the stimulus even when it is presented at minimal intensity.

When applied to a diagnostic test, sensitivity refers to the test's ability to identify diagnostically true cases, to establish the probability that a procedure concludes "yes" when the subject is truly ill. Such procedures are needed when the cost of not finding cases is high.

*Specificity* refers to a test's ability to exclude false cases, and *diagnostic confidence* is a measure of a test's sensitivity and specificity, expressed as the percentage of true positive test results over the total number of index cases plus the number of false positives. A test with a sensitivity of 90% is able to detect 90 of 100 people with the disorder in question. Sensitivity is the ability to identify actual cases; specificity means that the test is unlikely to give false positives. See *vigilance.*

**sensitivity training**   *T-group* (q.v.).

**sensitization**   1. In neurophysiology, a form of learned fear; a state in which the subject's response to later stimuli is greater than the response to the original stimulus, or a previously inadequate stimulus is able to elicit a response from the neuron; typically, a strong or noxious stimulus results in an increase in the usual or anticipated response to a variety of subsequent stimuli.

*Sensitization*, or *pseudoconditioning*, or *reverse tolerance*, is an increased response to a wide variety of stimuli following an intense or noxious stimulus. It is characterized by *heterosynaptic facilitation*, activation of facilitating interneurons that synapse on the sensory neurons. The facilitating neurons enhance transmitter release from sensory neurons by increasing the amount of second messenger cAMP in the sensory neurons. See *habituation*.

A sensitizing stimulus can override the effects of habituation, a phenomenon known as *dishabituation* (q.v.).

2. In relation to recurrent mood disorders, sensitization refers to the tendency of episodes to occur more frequently over time, with a shorter well interval between episodes. See *downregulation; upregulation*.

3. In immunology, sensitization is the process of stimulating an immune response to initial exposure to an antigen, resulting in a readiness of the organism's immune system to give a stronger (anamnestic) response when reexposed to the same antigen.

In formerly dependent drug users, sensitization is manifested as *priming*: reintroduction of the drug of abuse leads to *reinstatement* of drug-seeking behavior. See *addiction*.

**sensitizers**   See *anxiety typology*.

**sensorimotor intelligence**   See *developmental psychology*.

**sensorimotor psychotherapy**   Devised to target the sensorimotor symptoms and autonomic dysregulation of trauma related disorder, which are often resistant to psychodynamic or cognitive behavioral models of therapy, sensorimotor therapy focuses on bodily experience as the entry point for intervention. Patients' cognitions are directed to observation of the interplay of their perception, emotions, movements, sensations, impulses, and thoughts in the here and now (e.g., by noting the changes in heart rate, breathing, and muscle tone

that are expressions of the trauma), while acknowledging that the traumatic experience itself is in the there and then. Sensorimotor understanding and techniques are woven into psychodynamic or cognitive-behavioral models of therapy. Rather than insight alone, sensorimotor psychotherapy provides the actual experience of mobilizing action with conscious intention and awareness. Patients are helped to rediscover their capacity to defend through physical actions within a window of tolerance and safety, by tracking their bodily movements and sensations as they emerge during the therapy session. Uncoupling emotion from sensation eliminates physiologic cueing for a trauma response in the presence of a sensory recollection of a previous somatic experience. Such transformations at the sensorimotor level result in improvements in emotional and cognitive processing (Ogden, C. et al. *Psychiatric Clinics of North America* 29: 263–279, 2006).

**sensorimotor stage**   In Piaget's scheme of development, from birth until approximately 18 months of age. In this stage, responses are first only reflexive and to a limited range of sensory stimuli. Motor responses become more coordinated and can be elicited by more complex combinations of stimuli. By the end of this stage, information can be retrieved from memory (*representation* ability) and action can be regulated through stored knowledge.

**sensorium**   The hypothetical "seat of sensation" or "sense center," located in the brain, is usually contrasted with the *motorium*, the two constituting the so-called animal organ system, while the nutritive and reproductive apparatus make up the vegetative organ system. Occasionally this term is applied to the entire sensory apparatus of the body.

When a person is clearly aware of the nature of his surroundings, his sensorium is said to be "clear" or "intact." For example, correct orientation is a manifestation of a clear sensorium. When a person is unclear, from a sensory (not a delusional) standpoint, his sensorium is described as impaired or "cloudy."

Sensorium is interchangeable with *consciousness* (q.v.). The major disturbances of the sensorium are lowering of consciousness with reduced awareness (*cloudiness, clouding*), dreamlike states such as delirium, and narrowing of consciousness as in *twilight state* (q.v.).

**sensory aphasia**   *Wernicke aphasia* (q.v.).

**sensory apraxia**   *Ideational apraxia* (q.v.).

**sensory aprosodia**   Inability to understand the affect expressed by others. See *frontal lobe dysfunction.*

**sensory deprivation**   Perceptual deprivation; perceptual or sensory isolation; *informational underload.* These terms are ordinarily used to refer to experimental techniques that either reduce the absolute intensity of stimuli reaching the subject, or reduce the patterning of stimuli or impose a structuring of stimuli upon the subject. One of the methods employed to reduce intensity of stimuli, for example, is to suspend the subject, wearing only a blacked-out head mask for breathing, in a tank of water maintained at a constant temperature of 34.5°C. Such experimental sensory deprivation is considered to be similar to "brainwashing" and the isolation experienced by many explorers and shipwrecked persons, who under conditions of severe environmental stress are known to develop mental abnormalities. The following features are common to the various situations, whether "naturally" or experimentally produced: intense desire for extrinsic sensory stimuli and bodily motion, increased suggestibility, impairment of organized thinking, oppression, depression and, in extreme cases, hallucinations, delusions, and confusion.

It is believed that such abnormalities may be explained as follows: the correspondence between external reality and sensory neuronal activity is not a one-to-one relationship; perception is learned through motor interactions with objects in the environment, and when sleep or other states minimize or eliminate such interactions, percepts based on previous experience will emerge from the brain itself in the form of hallucinations and delusions (e.g., in dreams). This may be because the sensory input from the viscera augments spontaneous neuronal activity, especially in the thalamus, to such an extent that impulses over relay tracts are initiated, giving rise to visceral hallucinations and similar phenomena.

**sensory epilepsy**   A type of *petit mal epilepsy* (q.v.) consisting of paresthesiae involving part or the whole of one side of the body, often without loss of consciousness. Sensory epilepsy is usually due to a contralateral lesion in the parietal lobe.

**sensory evoked potential**   See *evoked potential.*

**sensory extinction**   See *social extinction.*

**sensory neglect**   *Neglect syndrome;* failure, or impaired ability, to recognize familiar objects, including the awareness of one's own body in space; also referred to as *agnosia, imperception, inattention, nonrecognition,* and experiences of *nothingness.* Neglect sydromes occur with right (nondominant) hemisphere lesions in at least five different areas: the prefrontal convexity, inferior parietal lobule, cinglate gyrus, thalamus, and hypothalamus. See *spatial neglect.*

Manifestatons of sensory neglect include the following:

1. Nonrecognition (sometimes of delusional proportions) of serious medical disability (*anosognosia*), of the left side of one's body or of objects in the left visual field (left spatial nonrecognition; the patient may fail to have the left side of his face, or bump into objects on the left, or read only the right side of a printed page). In *hemispatial neglect,* the patient draws only half the object he has been asked to copy; in *paralexia,* only part of a word is read.

2. Nonrecognition of people and faces that should be familiar to the patients (*prosopagnosia*).

   a. Included is the *Capgras syndrome* (q.v.)—accusing one or more familiar persons, usually family members, of beings impostors).

   b. The opposite is the *Fregoli phenomenon:* the patient believes that other persons not well known to him are very familiar.

   c. In the *Doppelganger phenomenon* (reduplicative paramnesia) the patient has the delusion that the duplicate of a person or place exists elsewhere.

   d. *Paragnosia,* consisting of wild guessing as to where the patient is: a patient with normal global orientation cannot say where he is, but when asked about his location makes a series of wild guesses.

3. *Alienation:* the patient feels that his body parts or thoughts do not belong to him; the outside world looks jumbled and confused. He cannot find his way along previously familiar routes. His body feels different, unreal, or

unattached; e.g., an arm or leg feels heavy or bigger, or the patient is uncertain about the location of his arm or leg.

4. *Allesthesia*—contralateral stimuli are referred to the ipsilateral side.

5. *Hemiakinesia*—failure to turn toward stimuli presented on the side opposite the lesion.

See *anosognosia*; *attention and information processing*; *Doppelganger*; *nonrecognition*; *paragnosia*; *prosopagnosia*.

**sensory processing disorder**  *SPD*; impairment in the reception, interpretation, and integration of sensory input. Symptoms vary over time, and overresponsivity in one area may be combined with lack of responsiveness in another. In sensory discrimination disorder, the child is limited in the ability to discriminate between sensory signals, such as being unable to hear if there is background noise or not being able to select a particular bottle of soda from the items in the refrigerator. In sensory-based motor disorders, the child has difficulty in planning and grading motor activities, appears clumsy, and avoids activities that involve multiple steps. Sensory modulation, the ability to match behaviors to the intensity of the sensory stimuli, may be impaired. The child may overreact to loud noises, or be unresponsive when his or her name is called, or he may crave stimulation by jumping about or talking loudly. All such symptoms may be combined with those of *NVLD* (q.v.).

**sensory register**  See *short-term memory*.

**sensory seizure**  See *aura*; *auditory aurae*.

**sensory transduction**  Conversion of sensory stimuli into the electrochemical activity of neurons, accomplished through specialized sensory receptors for exteroception, proprioception, and interoception.

**sensory working memory**  The short-term storage of sensory stimuli to guide behavior. The cortical areas that encode sensory information are an active component of the circuitry that underlies their short-term retention. Prefrontal cortex also plays a key role in sensory working memory. Many neurons in PFC receive inputs from sensory neurons and respond selectively to the features they represent. Further, many PFC neurons integrate information across sensory modalities and across different stimulus attributes within the same modality. It is generally believed that in the dynamic interplay between sensory cortical areas and PFC, PFC exerts "top-down" influences on sensory cortex.

**sentience**  Mere sensation, apprehension, or cognition, without accompanying associations or affect.

**sentiment**  According to McDougall, an organized system of emotional tendencies concerning an object or a class of objects. It is a learned form of behavior, built upon experiences and acting in the form of emotional tension. Sentiments are not pure emotions or motives because they cannot exist apart from a relationship to some person or object. The object may call forth different emotional behavior at different times, but this behavior is still consistent with the sentiment.

**sentinel activity**  *Vigilance* (q.v.).

**sentinel event**  See *JCAHO*.

**separation anxiety**  The reaction seen in a child who is isolated or separated from its mother, consisting usually of tearfulness, irritability, and other signs of distress. This is considered by most to be an indication that the child is attempting to adjust to the changes imposed on him and therefore presumptive evidence of good emotional reactivity. Although these symptoms of protest may culminate in an acute physical upset and in temporary or even prolonged refusal to adjust, the separation symptoms are not in themselves thought to be evidence of personality defect or unbearable trauma.

*School phobia* is a type of separation anxiety. For a discussion of more pathologic reactions to separation, see *anaclitic depression*; *anxiety disorders of childhood*; *attachment*; *dissociation disorders*.

**separation-individuation**  A developmental phase during which the mother–child bond becomes progressively attenuated, and the pleasure principle gradually gives way to the reality principle. This developmental phase follows the symbiotic (merger) phase and usually begins at about 6 months of age.

Separation depends on motor development; it includes all those actions and experiences that contribute to the child's awareness of being unique and distinct from every other thing. *Individuation* includes all those endopsychic changes that promote increasingly effective adaptation to internal as well as environmental demands; part of this is the progression of thinking through the stages identified by Piaget: from sensorimotor, through preoperational, concrete operational, and finally fully operational ideation.

Margaret Mahler (*On Human Symbiosis and the Vicissitudes of Individuation*, 1968) described four subphases of the process:

1. *Differentiation*, which occurs during the sixth to tenth months of life;

2. *Practicing*, occurring at 10 to 16 months; the child begins to recognize that his subjective self-image, his mirror image, and mother's object-image are distinct from each other; *object constancy* (q.v.) begins to develop; at the same time, the child's behavior is a mixture of approach-avoidance or arrival-departure in relation to the mother, to whom he returns after his forays into independent activities for "libidinal refueling."

3. *Rapprochement*, at 16 to 26 months; self-differentiation becomes more firmly established and an active approach toward the mother replaces the child's relative obliviousness to her in earlier phases; he begins to involve her in cooperative activities and to imitate and internalize her skills

4. Separation-individuation proper, with *object permanency* (which may not be fully established until 36 months) and the child's awareness of his discrete identity, separateness, and individuality. See *evocative memory*; *hypothetical-deductive thinking*.

Much of the pathology of the borderline states is believed to be rooted in failure to progress satisfactorily through the separation-individuation stage. See *borderline personality*.

**septal nuclei**   See *septum*.

**septicemia psychosis**   An acute organic psychosis due to severe infection and characterized mainly by delirium. Nosologically, this condition belongs to the toxic psychoses (deliria) associated with toxic-infectious diseases, and would today be classified as organic brain syndrome associated with systemic infection, with psychosis.

**septum**   Also, septal region, *septal nuclei*; a pyramid-shaped group of nuclei in the basal forebrain with its base resting on the anterior commissure and its apex formed by the columns of the fornix. The septum receives input from the hippocampus, amygdala, and hypothalamus; the nuclei project to the hypothalamus and various areas of the brain stem. The area has been called the pleasure center,

because when it is electrically stimulated a strong sensation of pleasure results. Lesions of the septal area reduce or abolish emotional expression.

**sequela**   The aftereffect of an illness and, particularly, permanent or persistent dysfunction. Mental defect, epilepsy, and spastic palsies, for example, are possible *sequelae* of viral encephalitis.

**sequence, genetic**   Growth sequence; the genetically determined order of development of structure or functions.

**sequencing disability**   Difficulty in abstraction. See *abstracting disabilities*.

**sequential dementia**   *Obs.* Synonymous with secondary dementia.

**sequential multiple personality disorder**   *Epochal dissociative identity disorder* (q.v.).

**sequestration**   *Isolation* or *denial* (qq.v.) of those parts of one's psyche that are unacceptable or cannot be controlled.

**serenics**   Serenity-inducing agents; specifically, 5-HT-1a/b agonists that appear to be effective in blocking aggressive behavior in various animal models without inducing sedation or impairing motor function.

**serial child molester**   See *pedophilia*.

**serial interpretation**   Elucidation of a consecutive number of dreams taken as a group.

**serial monotherapy**   See *salvage patients*.

**serial order**   Sequence; see *neuroethology*.

**serial search**   See *attention*.

**seriatim functions**   Organization or synthesis of skilled acts or thoughts into an orderly series; such organization requires ability to anticipate a goal and ability for temporal organization. The seriatim functions are generally disturbed in the schizophrenias.

**serine**   An amino acid that occurs in two forms, the enantiomers D-serine and L-serine. In the brain, D-serine is a neurotransmitter; it is localized in glia rather than neurons. It is synthesized in protoplasmic astrocytes which ensheathe the synapse and released near NMDA receptors, where it regulates glutamatergic neurotransmission by acting as a coactivator of the NMDA receptor.

**Sernyl**   *Phencyclidine* (q.v.).

**serotonergic**   Referring to neurons that are activated by or secrete serotonin, and to drugs that mimic or augment the actions of serotonin; most frequently used for serotonergic antidepressants, which enhance serotonin effects by inhibiting its reuptake from the synapse. See *antidepressant*. Serotonergic drugs are also used in the treatment of bulimia, cocaine craving, and obsessive-compulsive disorder.

The serotonergic projection system arises from a relatively small number of neurons in the reticular core of the brain stem, from which they project widely throughout the brain. Antidepressant drugs enhance and prolong the actons of serotonin, or norepinephrine, or both.

**serotonergic systems** CNS neurons containing 5-HT are concentrated in the midline or raphe of the brain stem. Pontine and medullary nuclei project caudally to the spinal cord, where 5-HT is involved in pain perception, visceral regulation, and motor control. Midbrain nuclei, particularly the dorsal raphe nucleus (DRN) and the median raphe nucleus (MRN), innervate the forebrain and are likely to modulate cognitive, affective, and neuroendocrine functions.

**serotonin** 5-Hydroxytryptamine (5-HT); a biogenic amine that functions as a neurotransmitter, as a hormone, and as a mitogen. About 0.2% of neurons use serotonin as a neurotransmitter.

Serotonin-containing neurons mediate many different functions within the nervous system. They inhibit sensory input and facilitate motor output at the cord level; they are involved in affective and perceptual states in the cortex. Serotonergic synapses in the cortex are a major site of action of psychotropic drugs. See *serotonin syndrome*. Serotonin plays a role in the regulation of dreaming and hallucinogenic drug states, perhaps in schizophrenic states as well.

**serotonin hypothesis** The theory that serotonin is a major factor in the pathophysiology of obsessive-compulsive disorder, based upon the observations that (1) serotonergic agonists, but not serotonergic antagonists, exacerbate obsessive-compulsive symptoms, and (2) the potent serotonin reuptake, blocker clomipramine (and other selective blockers of serotonin reuptake such as zimelidine, fluoxetine, and fluvoxamine) is effective in the treatment of obsessive-compulsive disorder.

The serotonergic hypothesis of mood disorders states that decreased serotonergic function is associated with depression, and that the efficacy of antidepressant treatments is related to their ability to increase serotonergic function in depressed patients. This hypothesis has generally replaced the *catecholamine hypothesis* (q.v.). It is recognized that no single transmitter is likely to produce depression or any other psychiatric disorder; almost always, multiple neurtransmitter systems are involved.

**serotonin reuptake inhibitor** A class of antidepressant drugs; also called *serotonergic* antidepressant (q.v.) and *SSRI* (selective serotonin reuptake inhibitor).

**serotonin syndrome** *Hypermetabolic syndrome* due to toxic brain levels of serotonin. Symptoms include hyperthermia, shivering, double vision, nausea, hypertension, anxiety, neuromuscular irritability, twitching, hyperreflexia, myoclonus, seizures, mental changes such as confusion and hypomania, and sometimes death.

The most frequent causes are combinations of monoamine oxidase inhibitor antidepressants (MAOIs) with serotonergic agents (e.g., fluoxetine, clomipramine, citalopram, paroxetine) or with meperidine or dextromethorphan (an antitussive agent in many over-the-counter preparations). MAOIs block the breakdown of serotonin, and both meperidine and dextromethorphan block its neuronal uptake, so the combination can produce toxic brain levels of serotonin. See *Call-Fleming syndrome*.

**serotonin transporter gene** SERT; 5-HTTL; abnormal fear conditioning, which is dependent on the amygdala, is associated with 5-HTT (serotonin) function. *5-HTTLPR* (q.v.) is the promoter region of the gene, which occurs in two alleles, short (s) and long (l). Subjects carrying the *s* allele are slightly more likely to display abnormal levels of anxiety, acquire conditioned fear responses, and develop affective illness compared with those homozygous for the *l* allele.

**services research** Study of how what is known about treatment becomes a concrete treatment plan for the patient who needs it, including the organization of the health care delivery system(s), the public policy that defines or limits delivery of care, the expectations of those who might use or need care, the training and competencies of those who provide the care, and the relationships of both patient and clinician to the third and fourth parties who pay for, regulate, supervise, or monitor the delivery system.

**servomechanism**  A governing or regulating device for maintaining output of a system at the desired rate or strength or in the desired direction.

**SES**  Socioeconomic status. *Socioeconomic gradient* refers to the ascending (or descending) steps from one extreme of social and economic status to the other. In many Westernized societies, descent in SES predicts increased risks of cardiovascular, respiratory, rheumatoid, and psychiatric disease; low birth weight; infant mortality; and mortality from all causes. This relation is predominately due to the influence of SES on health, rather than the converse. The health effects are only in small part a reflection of the limited access to health care that poverty imposes. The gradient is instead due primarily to psychosocial factors and, in particular, those that influence vulnerability to stress-related disorders. See *stress*.

**set**  1. A group or series, such as a set of rules. 2. A readiness to respond in a certain way or to respond selectively to certain stimuli; in this sense, also called *Aufgabe; determining tendency; mental set.*

**set, major**  It includes general receptivity to outside stimulation, appropriate attention or sensory adjustment to the environment, the capacity to identify and inhibit irrelevant stimulation, and the ability to conceive of, and be comfortable with, hypothetical situations.

In schizophrenic patients, only a *segmental set* can be achieved: the preparation for response is flawed because it is aimed at partial or minor aspects of the total stimulus response situation. The impairment in psychomotor responsivity (or reaction time deficit) in schizophrenic patients was first described by Shakow and coworkers, who noted that schizophrenics cannot perceive and respond to a situation objectively; they cannot achieve a "major set."

**set point**  The desired value to be maintained in a homeostatic control system; an integrator or error detection signals when the actual value (e.g., temperature of a room, weight of a human subject, cruising speed of an automobile) deviates from the set point or set range signal.

**set shifting**  See *Wisconsin Card Sorting Test.*

**set test**  A test of verbal fluency and cognitive abilities. The subject is asked to name 10 items from each of four categories (FACT: fruits, animals, colors, towns).

**setting, social**  *Milieu* (q.v.).

**sex**  The division of members of a species into two subclasses, male and female. Such division depends upon five biological factors—nuclear sex (chromosome pattern), gonadal sex (the presence of testes or ovaries), hormonal sex, internal accessory structures (the presence of uterus or prostate), and external genital morphology. Ordinarily all five are onsonant and thus allow assignment of sex, initially, and rearing in a gender role on the basis of simple inspection of external genital morphology.

As *maleness* is the state associated with the production of spermatozoa, a male is an individual that is efficiently equipped for the elaboration of functional sperms and for their conveyance to the site of fertilization. *Femaleness* is associated with the elaboration of ova; in mammals, in addition to possessing the property of producing eggs, the female has equipment for the prenatal care of the embryo and fetus and for the nurture of the offspring. An individual exhibiting both maleness and femaleness is called a *hermaphrodite.*

The organs that carry out the reproductive functions are known as *primary* sex organs. Those that distinguish the sexes from each other but play no direct part in reproduction are called *secondary* sexual characters.

**sex chromosome**  See *chromosome.*

**sex determination**  In biology, the genetic mechanism by which in bisexual organisms the primary difference between the sexes originates in accordance with the laws of heredity. It is a difference in the heterosomal chromosome constitution between male and female individuals that explains the generally sharp segregation of the two sexes. See *chromosome.*

In the female homogametic animals, sex is determined by whether an X-bearing or Y-bearing sperm fertilizes the ovum, resulting in a female and a male offspring, respectively. In male homogametic animals, sex depends on whether a sperm fertilizes an X-bearing or Y-bearing egg, resulting in male and female offspring, respectively.

It is only the *predisposition* to sex that is transmitted by heredity, and expression in the phenotype is furthered or inhibited by physiological and environmental conditions as well as by age factors. See *sex differentiation.*

**sex differences** *Sexual dimorphism.* Males and females do not differ in general intelligence, but sex differences are manifested in specific cognitive tasks. Difference favoring males are seen on the mental rotation test, spatial navigation including map reading, targeting, and the embedded figures test. Males are also more likely to play with mechanical toys as children, and as adults they score higher on engineering and physics problems. In contrast, females score higher on tests of emotion recognition, social sensitivity, and verbal fluency. They start to talk earlier than do boys, and they are more likely to play with dolls as children.

The cerebrum as a whole is larger in men, mainly because of a larger total volume of white matter. Despite the larger total volume of white matter, the ratio of corpus callosum to total cerebral volume is actually smaller in men, consistent with the findings that increased brain size predicts smaller corpora callosa and decreassed interhemispheric connectivity in humans and other species. Also consistent with those findings is that language-related activation in female brains is more bilateral, reflecting greater interhemispheric connectivity.

The human amygdala is significantly larger in men. Activity of the right hemisphere amygdala covaries with activity of other brain regions much more in men than in women; the reverse is true in women, in whom activity of the left hemisphere amygdala covaries with that of other brain regions much more than in men. This laterality of "women left, men right" is paralleled in studies of the amygdala and emotional memory. In women, there is preferential involvement of the left amygdala in memory for emotional material; in men, there is preferential involvement of the right amygdala in emotional memory. Right-hemisphere PFC lesions impair performance on decision-making in men, but not in women; left-hemisphere PFC lesions impair performance in women, but not in men.

Many CNS-related disorders show sex differences in their incidence: AD, addiction, attention deficit disorder, autism, eating disorders, multiple sclerosis, PTSD, schizophrenia, stroke, Tourette disorder. Men with schizophrenia show significantly larger ventricles than do healthy men; no such enlargement is seen in women with schizophrenia.

Sex hormones are crucial for many sex differences, but not for all. Genetic mechanisms, for example, can induce sex differences in the brain independently of hormone action. It cannot be assumed that "essentially identical processes occur in men and women, nor that identical therapeutics will apply" (Cahill, L. *Nature Reviews Neuroscience 7*: 477–484, 2006).

According to the *E-S theory* (empathizing-systemizing theory), psychological sex differences reflect stronger systemizing in males and stronger empathizing in females. Systemizing is the drive to analyze a system in terms of the rules that govern the system, in order to predict the behavior of the system. Empathizing is the drive to identify another's mental states and to respond to them with an appropriate emotion, in order to predict and to respond to the behavior of another person. See *autistic disorder* (Baron-Cohen, S. et al. *Science 310*: 819–823, 2005).

**sex differentiation** The developmental processes operating in the manifestation of sex differences in higher animals as expressed by Goldschmidt's "balance theory." The term thus indicates what happens during development after two sexually different types of zygotes have been formed by the chromosomal mechanism of *sex determination* (q.v.).

In normal sexual growth, the 23rd pair of chromosomes contains an XX complex in females, and the normal female pattern of cell nuclei is chromatin-positive. In males, the 23rd pair of chromosomes contains an XY complex, and the normal male pattern of cell nuclei is chromatin-negative. In true hermaphrodites (who have both ovarian and testicular functioning tissues) and in pseudo-hermaphrodites (where the external genitalia are the sex opposite to the genetic sex), there is often difficulty in deciding on the sex of the infant. In general, infants with anomalous sex development should be reared in accordance with their genetic sex and given appropriate hormonal treatment.

**sex limitation** The principle of a trait occurring in one sex only, namely, one characterized by the phenotypical development of those physiological sex characters that are the necessary anatomical basis of the trait in question.

In contrast to sex-linked characters produced by genes that are bound to the X or Y chromosomes, the phenomenon of sex limitation is not due directly to differences in the manifestation of the effects of genes located in one sex chromosome. See *sex linkage*.

**sex linkage** The genetic phenomenon of the coupling of a hereditary factor with an individual's sex chromosome structure responsible for the development of the respective sex. It rests upon the fact that in bisexual organisms the sex distinction is transmitted by heredity in accordance with the mendelian law of segregation, and is not to be confused with the more common mechanism of sex limitation. If one of the sex chromosomes carries a gene for a certain character, the transmission of the character and the distribution of the sexes must run together. See *sex determination*.

The particular distribution of the sex chromosomes in human, having heterogametic XY males, explains why sex linkage gives different sex proportions of linked characters with respect to dominance or recessiveness. *Dominant* sex-linked characters are able to appear when only one predisposition is present. Their manifestation is therefore twice as frequent in females as in males, since the number of X chromosomes is double in females.

*Recessive* sex-linked anomalies can be manifested by a female only when she is a homozygote for the factor in question. As the female has two X chromosomes, one from each parent, the heterozygotic manifestation of a recessive trait, transmitted on a mother's X chromosome to her daughter, is antagonized by the effect of the X chromosome which she has from her father. In males, however, the anomaly is manifested in the heterozygotic condition, since in the case of a son who receives his single X chromosome from his mother, there is no paternal X chromosome with a dominant gene to overcome the recessive gene on the X chromosome of the mother.

Such recessive traits, of which hemophilia and red-green color blindness are the classic examples, are usually transmitted by the female and appear in the male. They do not appear in both father and son unless the mother also possesses the gene. It is the rule that, through their daughters, who do not exhibit it, men transmit the trait to half of the daughter's sons. Other sex-linked recessive diseases are Fragile X syndrome, Lesch-Nyhan disorder, and muscular dystrophy.

**sex offender of children** See *pedophilia*.

**sex preselection** Predetermination of the sex of offspring; through sex-control technology, the parents-to-be choose whether their child will be a boy or girl.

**sex ratio** The proportional distribution of males and females at birth. The usual sex ratio 106:100 has been cited as evidence that boys are stronger and better able to survive the ordeal of being born. Recent genetic studies show, however, that more boys are born because more boys are *conceived*, and that the excess of males over females conceived is still greater than the ratio at birth. Investigation of embryos aborted when about 3 months old has shown that males outnumber females almost four to one. It must be assumed, therefore, that male embryos are not stronger, but just the contrary, *weaker* than female ones, and therefore more likely to perish under adverse intrauterine conditions.

**sex reassignment** See *reassignment, surgical*.

**sex reversal** The phenomenon in which chromosomal sex, as determined by any of the various sex chromatin tests, differs from anatomical sex. Etiology is unknown; chromosomal abnormalities, early deficiency of primordial germ cells, or hormonal imbalance have been suggested as playing an important role.

It has been produced in many animals "to the extent of changing the histological character of the gonads and to some extent the ducts, but the change has seldom gone far enough in an adult animal, to permit the individual to function as of the new sex" (Shull, A. F. *Heredity*, 1938). The most remarkable instance of complete sex reversal was observed by Crew, in an adult hen that had laid normal eggs producing normal chicks, before she changed into a cock that became the father of two normal chicks. An autopsy showed that the original ovary had been destroyed by a tumor, and a testis had been produced in its place by regeneration.

**sex role** A repertoire of attitudes, behaviors, perceptions, and affection reactions more commonly associated with one sex than with the other.

**sex role inversion** Adoption of the sex role of, and introjection of the psychologic identity of, the opposite sex.

**sex typing** That part of the process of socialization in which the child learns to adopt traits, values, and behavior that the culture deems appropriate to the child's *gender identity* (q.v.).

**sex-influenced inheritance**  An autosomal dominant genetic disorder whose expression depends upon one or more sex hormones. It can be transmitted by either sex, but it is expressed only in the offspring with the ennabling hormone. Male baldness is an example of sex-influenced inheritance, which is expressed only in a person who produces high levels of testosterone.

**sexism**  The social system that divides life roles according to sex rather than individual abilities, assigning to women the role of housekeeper, nursemaid, playmate, etc., and to men the role of manager, ruler, scholar, scientist, etc. It is this system (i.e., androcentricity or patriarchy) that the feminist movement seeks to eliminate and to replace with a system that allows life roles to be self-assigned, independent of sex. See *racism*.

**sexology**  The science of sex, including the study of sexual and sex-related behaviors and their evolutionary, physiological, and developmental foundations. Some would include the study of sociological and cultural aspects of sexuality, although the social constructionist theory currently popular among historians and social scientists—that what is labeled normal and abnormal, or allowable and prohibited sexual behavior was manipulated by the religious, political, or medical establishment and imposed on the masses—is more properly termed *sexosophy*.

**sexopathy**  Sexual abnormality; sexual perversion; paraphilia. The term includes both anomalies of sexual aim and anomalies of sexual object, no matter what their etiology.

**sexosophy**  The moral philosophy of sex; contrasted with *sexology* (q.v.).

**sexual**  Pertaining to, characterized by, or endowed with sex. In biology, pertaining to the property of being male or female, or of what is peculiar to sex or the sexes. Also used to denote the method of reproduction by sexes, as distinguished from *asexual* reproduction.

**sexual, contrary**  *Homosexual* (q.v.).

**sexual abuse**  See *child abuse*; *pedophilia*; *domestic violence*.

**sexual addiction**  An inexact term that implies a reliance on sexual activity as a major defense against anxiety or other dysphoric feelings; sometimes used as equivalent to compulsive sexuality or hypersexuality.

**sexual and gender identity disorders**  In DSM-IV, these include *sexual dysfunctions*, the various

forms of *paraphilia*, and *gender identity disorder* of childhood and of adolescence or adulthood (qq.v.).

**sexual arousal disorders**  Inhibited sexual excitement, in the female, also termed frigidity; in the male, erectile dysfunction and impotence.

**sexual asthma**  Asthma induced by coitus.

**sexual deviant**  See *paraphilia; pedophilia*.

**sexual deviation**  See *paraphilias*. They were formerly listed under the diagnostic category of sexual deviation, which included the following:

302.0 *homosexuality* (q.v.)
302.1 fetishism (see *fetish*)
302.2 *pedophilia* (q.v.)
302.3 *transvestitism* (q.v.)
302.4 *exhibitionism* (q.v.)
302.5 *voyeurism* (q.v.)
302.6 *sadism* (q.v.)
302.7 *masochism* (q.v.)
302.8 other sexual deviation

In DSM-III, all of the above were included within the subgroups of *sexual disorders* (q.v.).

**sexual dimorphism**  *Sex differences* (q.v.).

**sexual disorders**  In DSM-III-R, this term replaced the *psychosexual disorders* of DSM-III, emphasizing that many of these dysfunctions are biological rather than psychological in origin. Within this category are the following:

1. *Paraphilias* (q.v.).
2. *Sexual dysfunctions* (q.v.).

Gender identity disorders, which were included in this category in DSM-III, were moved in DSM-III-R to "Disorders Usually First Evident in Infancy, Childhood, or Adolescence."

**sexual dysfunctions**  This category includes the following:

1. *Sexual desire disorders*—hypoactive sexual desire disorder and sexual aversion disorder.

2. *Sexual arousal disorders*—female and male, approximately equivalent to frigidity and erective impotence in other terminologies.

3. *Orgasm disorders*—inhibited female orgasm, inhibited male orgasm (approximately equivalent to ejaculatory impotence), and premature ejaculation.

4. *Sexual pain disorders*—functional dyspareunia (genital pain before, during, or after sexual intercourse) and functional vaginismus.

5. Sexual dysfunction caused by a general medical condition.

6. Substance-induced (intoxication or withdrawal) sexual dysfunction.

**sexual harassment**   See *harassment, sexual.*

**sexual homicide**   See *homicide.*

**sexual identity**   See *gender identity.*

**sexual monism**   See *phallic sexual monism.*

**sexual orientation**   The preferred adult sexual behavior of a person; specifically, heterosexuality, homosexuality, or bisexuality.

**sexual orientation disturbance**   Concern or uncertainty about, or desire to change, one's sexual preferences or behavior. The term is most often applied to ego-dystonic homosexuality; neither term has been retained as a diagnostic entity in DSM. See *homosexuality.*

**sexual pain disorders**   *Dyspareunia* and *vaginismus* (qq.v.).

**sexual response cycle**   The complete cycle is subdivided into four phases: (1) *appetitive*—phantasies about, interest in, or desire to have sexual activity; (2) *excitement*—subjective sense of pleasant sexual arousal and accompanying physiologic changes (penile tumescence and erection in the male and vaginal lubrication and swelling of the external genitalia, labia minora, and breast in the female); (3) *orgasm*—a peaking of sexual pleasure (ejaculation in the male) and rhythmic contractions of the perineal muscles and pelvic reproductive organs in both sexes; (4) *resolution*—relaxation, a sense of well-being, and, for males, a variable period of refractoriness to further erection and orgasm. Disturbances in any part of the cycle are termed *sexual dysfunctions*, which form one group of *sexual disorders* (q.v.).

**sexual revolution**   The marked change in prevalent sexual attitudes that has been particularly evident in the United States since the Kinsey reports of 1948 and 1953, which brought sexual practices "from the realm of inference and secrecy into accepted, if still private, reality" (Sadock, V. in *Psychiatry 1982,* ed. L. Greenspoon, 1982). The Presidential Commission on Pornography in the 1970s advised against sexual repression and encouraged the acceptance of frank and even sexually stimulating material. The advent of effective birth control methods and legalized abortion drew a line between pleasurable and procreative aspects of sexuality. The feminist movement attacked the double standard, challenged the previous stereotyping of male and female roles, and focused attention on rape and incest.

Gerontologists shed new light on the sexual needs of the aged. Concurrent with these changes were advances in research and treatment of psychosexual dysfunctions, beginning with the Masters and Johnson work on the physiology of the sexual response in 1966 and the description of their approach in 1970.

**sexuality**   A broad term that includes the anatomical differentiation of reproductive functions into male and female, the behavior dependent upon the structural and functional differences between male and female, the multiple factors (biological, psychological, and social) involved in the attraction of one person to another for the purpose of sexual coupling, and the range of activities related to sexual desire, sexual arousal, and orgasm.

Normal sexual function depends on intact neural, vascular, and muscular circuitry; interactions between multiple neurotransmitter systems; and modulation by the endocrine system. Men's and women's bodies are programmed by their genes to seek sex. In the view of evolutionary biology, the reason is to ensure *reproductive success* (q.v.), even though the mechanisms that have evolved are often employed in activities that are unrelated to reproduction. In the case of a male-female couple, the man's body is trying to maintain a population of *sperm* (q.v.) inside his partner; the female is trying to conceive but at the same time to exert control over when, and by whom, she conceives. Women produce only one egg per menstrual cycle, but the egg dies within a day after it is released from the ovary. The best chance the man has of fertilizing an egg is to inseminate his partner at least once about 2 days before she ovulates. But the number of days from the beginning of menstruation to *ovulation* (q.v.) can vary from as few as four to as many as 28 days, hence the man's best strategy is to maintain the presence of sperm in his partner. A woman is more likely to have routine sex with her partner during the 2 weeks after she has ovulated (when she cannot conceive) than in the 2 weeks before ovulation. In contrast, if she has penetrative sex with a man other than her partner, it is more likely to be during her fertile phase (Baker, R. *Sperm Wars.* New York: Basic Books, 1996).

**sexuality index**   See *index of sexuality.*

**sexualize**   To endow with sexual energy or instinct. The genitals become sexualized at an early age. Other parts of the body (breasts, oral region, hands, etc.) may possess sexual qualities. Thoughts may be sexualized, as for example, when they appear in the form of sexual jokes.

**sexualized countertransference** *Erotic countertransference*; countertransference feelings and actions related to the sexual phantasies or needs of the analyst, which are often provoked in the analytic setting by the patient's transference reactions. The female hysteric, for instance, tends to develop an idealized, romantic transference with behavior that exudes sexuality. The male analyst countertransference reaction may be to avoid any sexual phantasies or feelings; he may also unconsciously express the sexualized countertransference by behaving seductively. The masochistic female with an erotized or sexualized transference often induces an aggressive or sadistic sexualized countertransference in the male analyst; reaction formation converts his behavior into excessive kindness and considerateness.

The female phallic character may be exaggeratedly assertive and envy the analyst's authority; the analyst's sexualized countertransference may be an unconscious desire to castrate the patient or force the patient to submit to the analyst's demonstrated potency.

**sexually violent predator** As defined by the legislature of the State of Washington, a person who has been convicted of or charged with the crime of sexual vioence and who suffers from a mental abnormality or personality disorder which makes a person likely to engage in predatory acts of sexual violence. Such acts include not only rape, rape of a child, and child molestation but also such offenses as murder, assault, kidnapping, and burglary when those offenses are determined to have been sexually motivated.

**SF** Spontanous fluctuations.

**SGA** Second-generation (atypical) antipsychotic.

**shadow** In Jung's analytical psychology, the unconscious.

**shaken baby syndrome** *Caffey syndrome* (named after the radiologist who identified the condition in 1972); the manifestations of abuse caused by forceful, violent, repetitive shaking of a baby by the arms of shoulders. The result is tearing of the blood vessels in neck and head, leading to retinal or intracranial hemorrhage, permanent sequelae (e.g., blindness, paralysis, retardation) and, sometimes, death.

Almost all reported cases have been children under the age of 1 year.

**sham rage** The term first used to denote the spontaneous outbursts of motor activity resembling fear and rage that occur in decorticate or diencephalic animals (Cannon, W. B. and Britton, S. W. *American Journal of Physiology 72*, 1925). Such outbursts are accompanied by changes in the internal organs and in the composition of the blood similar to those characteristic of human emotional behavior. It has been shown that sham rage depends on the functional integrity of the caudal hypothalamus.

The question naturally is: How real or sham is such behavior? Sham rage differs from normal rage in animals as follows: (1) the animal rarely attempts to avoid the stimulus that called forth the reaction; and (2) the response of sham rage rarely outlasts the duration of the stimulus, i.e., after-discharge is minimal. These differences are also seen in cases of sham rage in humans, which is never purposeful. In humans sham rage has been observed as a result of extensive cortical damage secondary to prolonged hypoglycemia and carbon monoxide poisoning: the response pattern was uniform to all strong stimuli, it lasted from 30 seconds to 1 minute, and the strength of stimulus had no apparent effect on the duration of the sham rage. In these cases, loud noises and painful stimuli produce dilation of the pupil, widening of the palpebral fissures, exophthalmos, and marked increase in pulse rate and systolic pressure. A patient with carbon monoxide poisoning clenched and ground her teeth and emitted hissing sounds.

All in all, both animal and human data imply that the hypothalamus is not the emotional center, although it may integrate and possibly reinforce the effectorneural responses controlling some of the sympathetic and motor manifestations of fear and rage. See *Cannon hypothalamic theory of emotion; ergotropic; Papez theory of emotion.*

**shaman** A practitioner whose ability to heal comes from trancelike experiences and inspiration from a supernatural spirit-partner with whom he works in curing sick people. The word shaman originated in the Tungus tribe of northeastern Siberia. The Navajo draw a distinction between the "handtrembler," whose inspiration is supernatural in origin, and the "medicine man," whose knowledge comes from systematic learning in an apprenticeship. See *folk medicine.*

**shame** An affect that follows the revelation of one's previously hidden shortcoming(s), believed to be founded in the anal (and urethral) stages of psychosexual development.

Psychodynamically, shame is considered to be the specific force directed against urethral-eroticism, just as the fear of being eaten is the specific oral fear, and the fear of being robbed of body contents is the specific anal fear. Ambition is the fight against this shame.

Shame is also used as a defense against exhibitionism and voyeurism; "I feel ashamed" means "I do not want to be seen."

Shame is given particular attention in self psychology and developmental psychology, where it is regarded as a master emotion that influences all the others. *Guilt* (q.v.) refers to feelings about an act, a real or imagined transgression. It does not usually bring with it self-loathing, as shame does. Shame involves one's basic sense of self and is typically experienced as embarrassment or *humiliation* (q.v.).

Shame emerges earlier in psychological development than guilt. Signs of it can be detected in the second year of life at the time the infant's sense of self is forming. As the infant comes to recognize that he is a separate person, he begins to understand that others direct emotions toward him. Pride and shame appear—pride at pleasing others, shame at displeasing others. Pathological shame develops when parents fail to respond with empathy and attention to the infant's strivings to show his competence.

Shame can be a normal feeling, but when it colors one's most basic ideas about one's identity or worth it signals pathology. Normal shame might result from having some dark secret about the self exposed. Shame is pathological, however, when it arises with every rebuke or tiny failure, or as an undercurrent in all interpersonal relationships. Whenever shame appears, there tends to be an inhibition of other emotions with the exception of anger. Unlike other emotions, which tend to pass with time or with catharsis, shame is the most difficult emotion to admit to and the most difficult to discharge. Some clinical studies suggest that the most effective antidote to shame is a person's ability to laugh at himself. See *sensitiver Beziehungswahn.*

Shame is often at the root of irrational rage outbursts in the adult; it probably plays a key role in family violence, for example. Men who for one reason or another (psychological vulnerability, limited intellectual development, physical abnormalities, etc.) are especially dependent on their spouses to function well are ashamed of that dependence and feel intensely humiliated when the spouse says something they perceive as demeaning, trivializing, or critical of their competence. They react with rage and violence in an attempt to deny or overcome their feelings of disorganization and helplessness.

**shame psychosis** *Pseudomania* (q.v.).

**shaping** *Method of successive approximations*; a type of operant conditioning in which the behavior that is initially reinforced is generally or approximately of the kind desired, and subsequent reinforcement becomes increasingly limited until only the specific response desired is reinforced. See *implosion*; *reinforced practice.*

**shared delusion** A delusion that occurs simultaneously in more than one person, as in folie à deux. See *induced psychotic disorder.*

**shared environmental variance** Any environmental component that increases the similarity between family members. The *nonshared environment* includes all the ways in which siblings are treated differently by the environment. Comparison of behavior in monozygotic twins with that of dizygotic twins provides an estimate of how much genetic variability contributes to behavior. Genetic variation accounts for approximately 60% of bullying behavior in children, for example.

**shared paranoid disorder** See *folie à deux*; *induced psychotic disorder*; *paranoia.*

**shared representations** *Simulation* (q.v.).

**shared responsibility** In the clinical setting, the term refers both to joint decision making concerning the treatment of a patient and to the joint legal responsibility for the treatment given. Shared responsibility is an important element in the consultation process and in *supervision* (q.v.). It is often not recognized that the consultant–patient relationship is an independent physician–patient relationship, and that the consultant has the same responsibility for the appropriate treatment of the patient as he or she would have while providing direct, primary care. Also often unrecognized is that the supervisor is personally and legally responsible for the clinical practices of the persons being supervised.

**Sheldon, William Herbert** (1899–1977) American psychologist, best known for his work in constitutional typology and description of the ectomorph, mesomorph, and endomorph somatotypes.

**shell shock** A general term for psychiatric disorder occurring during active warfare; combat neurosis. When they appear in civilian life, such conditions are usually regarded as traumatic neuroses. See *post-traumatic stress disorder; traumatic neurosis.*

**shenjing shuairuo** A culture-bound syndrome described in China: fatigue, dizziness, sleep disturbance, difficulties in concentration and memory, sexual dysfunction, agitation.

**shen-k'uei, shenkui** *Dhat* (q.v.).

**Sherman paradox** See *anticipation.*

**shift maladaptation syndrome** See *circadian rhythm sleep disorder.*

**shin-byung** A culture-specific syndrome reported in Korea, consisting of multiple symptoms, dissociation, and possession by ancestral spirits.

**shinkeishitsu, shinekeishitsu** A syndrome described by Japanese psychiatrists consisting of obsessions, compulsive perfectionism, social withdrawal, multiple somatic complaints, and neurasthenia. See *Morita therapy.*

**Shipley Abstraction test** A test of reasoning ability that requires the subject to complete logical sequences. The test is given in conjunction with a vocabulary test, and performance on the two tests is compared. Impaired conceptual-abstract thinking is suggested if the abstraction score is lower than the vocabulary score.

**shock** 1. A sudden physical or mental disturbance.

2. A state of profound mental and physical depression consequent upon severe physical injury or an emotional disturbance.

3. In Rorschach scoring, any delay or failure in responding to the blot; shock indicates ambivalence regarding the advisability of acting out the traits revealed by the blot component causing the shock.

**shock psychosis** Observed in soldiers overcome by shock or fright in combat. Many who were picked up immediately after the shock and sent to hospital had initial anxious deliria, during which they regarded everything in the environment as hostile, and anybody who approached them excited violent fear reactions. Wild motor activity with mutism, depression, and disturbances of sleep sometimes followed.

"The most common form of this psychosis was perhaps the acute, passive, negativistic stupor, with mutism, complete immobility, total anesthesia, inability to take food, incontinence, total unconsciousness at first and cloudy states later, and inability to stand or walk. These patients had gradually to relearn sphincter control and the enunciation of words; at first they said only 'yes' and 'no' and then answered to their names. Very gradually they were taught how to grasp objects and how to feed themselves. Familiarity with the environment was also regained slowly; some time elapsed before these patients began to take an interest in their destiny. Of interest is the fact that most of them were able to recall the traumatic event; they remembered some details of their behavior such as making certain efforts to save themselves just before they lost consciousness.

"Patients in fright stupor were not always passive and without feeling. Very frequently they shouted in their stupor: 'The enemy is coming!' 'They are coming!' 'Get em!' 'Fight em!' " (Kardiner, A. and Spiegel, H. *War Stress and Neurotic Illness*, 1947). See *traumatic neurosis; post-traumatic stress disorder.*

**shock therapy** A general term indicating the use of various somatic treatments that produce a *shock* to the central nervous system, including electroshock (EST)—also called electroconvulsive therapy (ECT)—insulin coma therapy, ambulatory insulin treatment (also called subshock or subcoma insulin therapy), Metrazol convulsive treatment, brief stimulus electrotherapy, electrostimulation, electronarcosis, Indoclon inhalation therapy, and atropine coma therapy.

**shooting tattoos** Black spots at an intravenous drug abuser's injection sites, caused by carbon from a repeatedly flamed needle.

**short stare epilepsy** A type of petit mal *epilepsy* (q.v.).

**short incubation bias** See *life course epidemiology.*

**short-contact psychotherapy** Treatment of mental disorders, similar to brief psychotherapy, but used in child-guidance clinics when the therapy is of short duration.

**shortening reaction** See *rigidity, decerebrate.*

**short-term** Brief. See *brief psychotherapy*.

**short-term anxiety-provoking psychotherapy (STAPP)** A form of brief psychotherapy developed by P. Sifneos in the 1950s for patients with circumscribed problems. STAPP emphasizes systematic selection criteria and outcome studies as a way to assess the validity of its techniques in specific kinds of patients.

**short-term memory** *STM;* also, *immediate memory, working memory, buffer memory, primary memory*. It contains information that can be held only so long as continuous attention is allocated to it. Sensory information is first stored in the *sensory register* for a very short period (ca. 250 msec.) but is erased (decays) even earlier by new information arriving from the senses (i.e., if the subject is distracted). STM is sometimes divided into the following:

   a. *Immediate memory (q.v.)*

   b. *STM proper*—measured by the ability to recall after a span of 25 minutes even though attention is distracted. *Working memory* (q.v.) is the process of maintaining of an active representation of short-term memories.

   c. *Iconic memory* (q.v.)

The short-term store receives information from the sensory register, and also from the long-term store. It actively processes information through such conscious memory routines as rehearsal and *chunking* (combining small units of input into meaningful larger units to facilitate storage). The short-term store itself has only limited storage space, but once it is processed information is deposited in the long-term store, whose capacity to retain information is almost unlimited. Frontal lobe dysfunction is suggested by impaired short-term memory.

Short-term memory has also been described in terms of three cooperating categories:

   1. *Phonological loop*—enables the subject to remember sequences of approximately seven digits, words, or letters

   2. *Visual-spatial scratch pad*—receives and codes data into visual or spatial images

   3. *Central executive*—helps with such tasks as reasoning or doing mental arithmetic

Short-term storage involves modification of already existing proteins, mainly through phosphorylation of a potassium channel protein, calcium channel activation, and enhancement of transmitter mobilization. See *amnestic syndrome; long-term memory*.

**SHP test** The *Strongin-Hinsie-Peck* test for measurement of salivary secretion, average rate of which is decreased in depressions and increased in schizophrenias.

**Shprintzen syndrome** See *velocardiofacial syndrome*.

**shut-in** August Hoch's term for the premorbid personality that is seen in approximately 60% of schizophrenics: quiet, reserved, asocial, withdrawn, seclusive, "lone-wolf" types, those who live among but not with, etc. Bleuler's term, *schizoid*, is approximately equivalent to shut-in.

**Shy-Drager syndrome** (George Milton Shy, U.S. physician, 1919–1967; Glenn Albert Drager, U.S. neurologist, 1917–1967) *Progressive multisystem degeneration; striatonigral degeneration*; a *multiple system atrophy* (q.v.); a combination of autonomic manifestations (orthostatic hypotension, anhidrosis, urinary and bowel dysfunction, impotence and impaired libido) and signs of degeneration of the cerebellum, basal ganglia, and spinal tracts and motor neurons (hyperreflexia, extensor toes signs, dysarthria, sucking reflex, masked facies, rigidity, cog wheeling, resting or intention tremor, ataxic gait or speech). Dementia, if it develops, is mild and slowly progressive. It is of the subcortical type with mild memory impairment but intact higher-level associative functioning.

The syndrome typically begins in the patient's 40s or 50s with dizzy spells, urinary disorders, and diminution in sexual desire. It is three times as frequent in males as in females. The syndrome leads to death in 7 to 8 years (the average, with a range of 3 to 33 years).

**SIADH** *Syndrome of Inappropriate Anti-Diuretic Hormone*; urine production is curtailed and, as a result, serum sodium falls. It is a rare complication of treatment with SSRIs. Symptoms include malaise, weakness, confusion, and in the more severe cases seizures and coma.

**sialorrh(o)ea** Excessive salivation.

**SIB** 1. Self-injurious behavior. In *Lesch-Nyhan syndrome* (q.v.), an X-linked enzyme deficiency associated with severe SIB, subjects have a low level of CSF 5-HIAA. CSF 5-HIAA levels are lower in patients with a history of suicide attempts or higher levels of lifetime impulsive and aggressive behavior. Patients with *borderline personality disorder* (q.v.) show the same inverse relationship between CSF 5-HIAA level and aggression.

2. Schedule for Interviewing Borderline; a structured interview designed to elicit symptoms and history of borderline personality. See *CASH; SIDP*.

3. Severe Impairment Battery, used to document the rate of progression of cognitive decline in dementia, to identify areas of preserved ability, and to assess the value of different interventions. It comprises 9 subscales: Social Interaction, Orientation, Visuoperception, Construction, Language, Memory, Praxis, Attention, and Orienting to Name.

**sibling** In human genetics, one of two or more children not simultaneously born of the same two parents. It thus excludes twins or other multiples as well as half-brothers and half-sisters, and stepbrothers and stepsisters. However, the definition in all leading dictionaries makes it a far less restricted term.

**sibling rivalry** The usual family situation wherein brothers and sisters engage in an intense and highly emotional competition, one against the other, for the love, attention, affection, and approval of one or the other or both of the parents. Such intense competition between rival sibs (brothers or sisters) can be an important determinant of later specific character or personality traits.

Sibling rivalry, however, is usually evaluated in relation to other important experiences in the child's early life, such as the oedipal relationship to the parents; the discovery of and reaction to sexual differences; the specific reaction that is called the *castration complex*; self-comforting trends, such as thumbsucking and masturbation, and conflicts concerning their prohibition and gratification.

**sibship** One series of siblings, that is, all the biological children of a union of two parents, excluding multiples. See *birth, multiple*.

**sibship method** A method devised by Weinberg for use in psychiatric genetics. The blood relatives of a statistically representative number of probands or index cases are studied to determine whether a particular trait occurs more frequently in them than it does in the general population (or in a group of persons not related to the carriers by blood).

**sicchasia** Disgust for food.

**sick role** Use of illness or complaints about bodily functioning to escape personal failure and the expectation to succeed, or to avoid other social responsibilities. In many Western cultures, sickness automatically excuses the subject from many responsibilities and protects his assumed right to be taken care of. *Hypochondriasis* (q.v.), or escape into the sick role, is frequently encountered among the elderly population. High bodily concern is used by many older people as a defense against anxiety and a way of gaining the sympathy and help of others.

**side effect** Any action of a drug other than the desired therapeutic effect (see *adverse drug reaction*). No drug has a single pharmacologic action; consequently, for every wanted effect it may be necessary to accept one—or many—unwanted effects. Most side effects are extensions of a drug's known pharmacological actions. Neuroleptics and antidepressant agents, for example, affect a number of different receptor systems, and their numerous side effects are attributable to nonspecificity of pharmacological action. Allergic and idiosyncratic reactions are far less common than nonspecificity reactions, and they are generally unpredictable. To a large extent, drug response is genetically determined, particularly drug absorption and its utilization at effector sites, and the family history may provide significant information about how a patient is likely to respond to a specific drug, or even to a family of drugs.

**side impulse** An impulse that exists by the side of another impulse. Kraepelin says that the condition is common in schizophrenia. Often the side or secondary impulse interrupts the primary one, producing irrelevant action or speech. See *cross impulse*.

**siderodromophobia** Fear of railroads or trains.

**siderophobia** Fear of the heavens and what comes from them—the elements, etc.

**Sidis, Boris** (1876–1923) American psychiatrist; hypnosis, multiple personality.

**SIDP** Structured Interview for DSM-III Personality Disorders; an instrument designed to elicit symptoms and history of the different personality disorders according to the diagnostic criteria of DSM-III. See *CASH; SCID; SIB*.

**sigmatism** Difficulty in pronouncing the S (and Z) sound.

**sign** Signal, representation; in medicine, an objective symptom or abnormality indicating disease.

**sign language**  Communication through gestures rather than sounds. Sign languages are found wherever there is a community of deaf people, and there are many different ones throughout the world. They are independent languages and not understood by the user of a different sign language. A speaker of American Sign Language (ASL, *Ameslan*), for example, cannot understand Japanese Sign Language or British Sign Language.

Contrary to popular misconceptions, sign languages are not pantomimes and gestures, nor are they a coding of the spoken language of the surrounding community. (Such codings exist, but native ASL speakers find them awkward and unnatural.) Each sign language is a distinct, full language with its own standardized vocabulary and a grammatical machinery as fully complex as the grammatical organization of spoken languages.

William Stokoe showed (*Sign Language Structure: An Outline of the Visual Communication System of the American Deaf*, 1960) that ASL gestures have systematic organization that strongly parallels the phonological structure of spoken language. The basic rhythmic unit of spoken language is the syllable; of sign language, a motion plus whatever held positions (if any) precede and follow it. Signs are classified into parts of speech, which are strung together with modifiers to form large constituents and clauses.

What enables ASL speakers to speak and understand an indefinitely large number of sentences? It cannot be memorization of signs, because even a single verb can occur in an unbelievable number of variants. Nor can it be a matter of teaching: (1) most ASL speakers have hearing parents who, prior to their child's education, were not even aware of the existence of the language; (2) ASL has been primarily spread through the residential schools for the deaf; and (3) until the 1960s use of ASL even in these schools was officially discouraged and sometimes punished. Consequently, people have had to learn the language not by instruction, but by picking it up from fellow students.

The most parsimonious explanation is that somewhere within the CNS of speakers of sign there must be a mental grammar, a basic vocabulary of signs, plus a set of patterns for combining signs sequentially and simultaneously. In other words, children come prewired with a mental grammar that facilitates their learning of whatever sign language they happen to be exposed to. In almost all respects, the universal grammar (UG) for sign languages is exactly the same as UG for spoken languages. ASL emphasizes the *abstractness* of linguistic organization and its independence from sensorimotor modality.

Deaf children in families that speak ASL go through essentially the same stages of language learning as children acquiring spoken language. Hearing children of deaf parents are very much like immigrant children: they grow up bilingual, acquiring sign from their parents and spoken language from others.

**sign stimulus**  See *releaser, social*.

**sign system**  Schilder's term for the use of language as the main tool, or instrument, of psychotherapy. Through words, the psychiatrist gains access to and unveils the patient's hidden problems and inner personality.

Words in the sign system are to the psychiatrist what knives and other instruments are to the surgeon. "The psychotherapist has no immediate access to the body of the patient and to his gratifications. The influence he has on the patient is merely due to the words he speaks." In a broader sense, every social relation between two persons speaking to each other includes the erotic. Humans need not only actual but also future gratification, "and humanity has elaborated a system for such gratification," language constituting the main, though by no means the only, element of this system. In the relationship between the sexes, words and sentences in themselves may become signs through which the individuals obtain their social and erotic gratifications (Schilder, P. *Psychotherapy*, 1938).

**signal anxiety**  See *anxiety*.

**signal transduction**  The process by which an external signal is transmitted into and within a cell to elicit an intracellular response.

**signal value**  In *information processing* (q.v.), stimulus characteristics that carry informational content for the subject.

**signaling pathway**  The steps taken by the cell in order to recognize and respond to external signals. The pathway typically functions as a "bucket brigade," with each component passing the signal to the next component until the final targets produce a response. The targets may be metabolic enzymes, transcription factors, or ion channels. Messages travel along the pathway by various means: protein–protein interactions, sequential protein phosphorylation, or geneeration of diffusible intracellular messengers (such as cAMP). Some pathways, such as those with G proteins as signal transducers, also use intracellular second messengers to transmit signals.

**signe de Magnan**   *Formication* (q.v.).

**signe du miroir**   *Mirror sign* (q.v.).

**significance**   Meaning; value; importance. Statistical significance is the likelihood or probability that the value or score obtained is not due to chance but is instead meaningfully related to some specific factor or variable.

**Signifiers**   See *Lacan, Jacques.*

**sign-out**   Most commonly used to refer to a patient's completion of a document indicating his or her desire to leave hospital or other care, even though he is aware that his decision to do so is contrary to the advice of his physician. A "sign-out letter" may also include an *AMA discharge*, i.e., a discharge against medical advice.

Completion of such a document does not absolve the physician or other caregiver of a duty to protect the patient or society, however. If the clinician knows, or should know, that the patient is dangerous to himself or others, the immediate risk should be evaluated and documented. If the evaluation warrants it, the next step is to take the necessary measures to convert the patient's legal status from voluntary to involuntary and to continue to try to convince the patient to participate voluntarily in his treatment.

**silencers**   See *noncoding DNA.*

**silok**   See *miryachit.*

**silver cord syndrome**   A family constellation consisting of a passive or absent father and a dominating mother, believed by some to be significantly related to the subsequent development of schizophrenia. See *schizophrenogenic mother.*

**Simmonds disease**   (Morris Simmonds, German physician, 1855–1925) See *hypophysial cachexia.*

**Simon-Binet tests**   See *Binet-Simon tests.*

**simple adult MBD**   Minimal brain dysfunction in the absense of psychiatric diagnosis; primary or idiopathic *attention deficit hyperactivity disorder* (q.v.).

**simple schizophrenia**   One of the chronic forms of schizophrenia; historically, called dementia praecox, simple type; dementia simplex; schizophrenia simplex; primary dementia. In the simple form of schizophrenia, there is an insidious psychic impoverishment that affects the emotions, the intellect, and the will. Chronic dissatisfaction or complete indifference to reality are characteristic, and the simple schizophrenic is isolated, estranged, and asocial. Affect is markedly blunted and dulled, there is little phantasy life, and there may be few or no accessory symptoms. Dementia, in Bleuler's sense, is marked—patients make many foolish mistakes, are highly suggestible and gullible, and speech is filled with senseless generalizations. Thought is vacuous and banal, ideas are insipid and unintegrated. Such patients tend to sink to low and relatively simple social levels; they may come to lead almost a vegetative existence. They often become day laborers, peddlers, or vagabonds, and they contribute heavily to the group of eccentric recluses.

**simple senile deterioration**   One form of *Alzheimer disease* (q.v.). Symptoms include narrowing of interests, sluggishness of thought, misoneism, recent memory gaps that are filled in with fabrications, defective orientation, hoarding, inattentiveness except to immediate personal wants, apathy or irritability, and sometimes suspiciousness, ideas of persecution, and restless wandering from the home.

**simulant**   Simulator, malingerer.

**simulation**   Imitation; copying; feigning.

In neurophysiology, simulation is also known as *resonance behavior; shared representations*; a postulated common coding for actions performed by the self and other persons. *Simulation theory* contends that one represents the mental activities and processes of others by simulation, i.e., by generating similar activities and processes in oneself. Both action generation (self) and observing and simulating others' actions activates several brain regions, including the premotor cortex, the posterior parietal cortex, and the cerebellum. Action observation activates the premotor cortex in a somatotopic manner—simply watching mouth, hand, and foot movement activates the same functionally specific region of premotor cortex as performing those movements (Blakemore, S.-J. and Decety, J. *Nature Reviews Neuroscience 1,* 2001). See *action understanding; imitation; response facilitation.*

**simultagnosia**   Ability to describe the action represented in a picture; often lacking in children with generalized brain dysfunction, who may merely name the objects represented rather than being able to discuss the action of the picture. *Simultanagnosia* is the lack of, or any disability in, such simultaneous form perception, and is suggestive of a lesion in the anterior part of the left occipital lobe.

**simultaneous tactile sensation**   See *double simultaneous tactile sensation.*

**single nucleotide polymorphism**   *SNP* (q.v.).

**single-major-locus model**   See *inheritance.*

**singultus**   *Hiccup.*

**sinistrad**   Toward the left; sinistrad writing is mirror-writing. See *strephosymbolia.*

**sinistral**   See *dominance, cerebral.*

**sirtuins**   A family of histone deacetylases that have important roles in cellular stress responses and energy metabolism.

**Sisyphus dream**   Frustration dream. See *traumatic neurosis.*

**sitiophobia, sitophobia**   Fear of (eating) food.

**situation, either-or**   A situation of doubt and vacillation in which the neurotic places himself, especially in dreams. The patient desires two different things at the same time and does not know which to choose. An example is the neurotic patient with a strong mother attachment who is also deeply in love with his fiancee: in his dreams he symbolizes either his mother or his fiancee, but always with a profound doubt about which of them he should love more. The patient vacillates between two principles and this vacillation may refer to persons, objects, or ideas.

**situation ethics**   See *ethics, situation.*

**situational reaction**   See *reactive psychosis; transient situational disturbances.*

**situational therapy**   A term introduced by S. R. Slavson, in connection with his activity group psychotherapy, in which the social relationship and the physical environment themselves (i.e., the situation) have a therapeutic effect.

**situationism**   See *Lucifer effect.*

**SIV**   Simian immunodeficiency virus; a virus related to *HIV* (q.v.) that occurs in monkeys.

**SIVD**   Subcortical ischemic vascular disease and dementia; it includes Binswanger disease and the lacunar state. Small vessel disease is the chief vascular manifestation, and lacunar infarct and ischemic WMLs (white matter lesions) are the primary type of brain lesion. SIVD lesions affect especially the prefrontal subcortical circuit, producing executive

dysfunction and memory deficit. Depression, personality change, and psychomotor retardation are frequent. See *VaD.*

**sixty-nine**   A slang expression referring to fellatio or cunnilinction practiced simultaneously by two persons, the head of each being at the genitals of the other.

**size estimation test**   The subject adjusts a circle of lights so that it equals the size of a handheld disk.

**Sjobring, Henrik**   (1879–1956) Swedish psychiatrist; described certain personality types and reactions to stress as based on constitutional psychological variables and cerebral lesions.

**Sjogren-Larsson syndrome**   Hereditary disorder first described in 1957 in Sweden by Sjogren and Larsson consisting of ichthyosis, mental retardation, and spastic paralysis. Degenerative retinitis and speech disorders may occur in addition to the diagnostic triad of symptoms. Transmission of the disorder is of the autosomal recessive type.

**skelic index**   A measurement used in anthropometry; the ratio between the length of the legs and the length of the trunk.

**skew deviation**   Hertwig-Magendie phenomenon; a rare cerebellar or collicular sign, characterized by downward and inward rotation of the eyeball on the same side of the lesion and upward and outward rotation of the eyeball on the opposite side.

**skill**   High-grade performance developed in response to training and experience. The person matches the demands of the task to his capacities; he is skillful to the extent that he is able to choose and execute actions that are effective. This entails the employment of some method of performance, or *strategy*. It is the strategy, rather than the basic capacity, that is amenable to training and becomes more efficient in the course of practice. For improvement to occur with practice, some knowledge of results achieved by previous action (feedback) is usually required.

A continuous skill is one in which the subject varies his response to a continuously varying stimulus (e.g., steering an automobile on a twisted and crowded road). A discrete skill is one in which the response is invariable (e.g., typewriting).

**skimming**   Accepting or admitting the less costly cases in a case-mix prospective payment system, but avoiding the more costly cases, so as to keep total actual cost of operations below the predicted cost. In most prospective payment systems, the agency or facility demonstrating such a "savings" is allowed to keep at least part of it as profit.

**Skin Conductance Orienting Response** *SCOR* (q.v.).

**skin popping**　Subcutaneous injections of drugs leading to abscesses or scars over the upper arm, abdomen, or thigh.

**skinache syndrome**　A common, debilitating chronic pain syndrome characterized by cutaneous trigger points. It sometimes responds favorably to subcutaneous lidocaine, but relapse rate is high. Surgical removal of the cutaneous trigger points in those who do relapse is about 75% successful.

**Skinner, Burrhus Frederic** (1904–1990) American behaviorist; operant behavior and operant conditioning; *Science and Human Behavior* (1953), *Schedules of Reinforcement* (with Charles B. Ferster, 1957), *The Analysis of Behavior* (with James G. Holland, 1961), *Beyond Freedom and Dignity* (1971), *The Shaping of a Behaviorist* (1971).

**Skinner box**　A testing chamber that houses the experimental subject in studies of the relationship between behavior and both its antecedent stimuli and its consequences. The box is typically outfitted with a device that is operated by the subject (e.g., a lever) and an opening to deliver a suitable "reward" when the device (*operandum*) is manipulated in a certain way or in response to specific stimuli.

**skoptsy**　A Russian religious sect (a subdivision of the *raskol'nike*, the schismatics or dissenters) whose adherents practiced castration, in conformity with the passage: "And there be eunuchs, which have made themselves eunuchs for the kingdom of heaven's sake. He that is able to receive it, let him receive it" (Matthew 19:12).

**slasher**　See *self-mutilation*.

**Slater, Eliot Trevor Oakeshort** (1904–1983) British psychiatrist, one of the founding fathers of 20th-century biological psychiatry, best known for his studies of the genetics of schizophrenia and manic-depressive illness. *Physical Methods of Treatment* (1944, with W. Sargant); *Clinical Psychiatry* (1954, with W. Mayer-Gross and M. Roth); *The Genetics of Mental Disorders* (1971, with V. Cowie).

**slavering**　*Obs.* Drooling.

**sleep**　An active process (not merely a lapse in the waking state, as formerly believed), composed neurophysiologically of two relatively distinct states, *REM sleep* and *non-REM sleep* (also known as *NREM sleep*), defined by the patterning of measures on the electroencephalogram (EEG), the electromyogram (EMG), and the *electrooculogram* (EOG).

Non-REM sleep is subdivided into four stages: 1, 2, 3, and 4. Stages 3 and 4 are also called *delta* or *slow-wave sleep (SWS)*. Stage 1 is a transition between waking and sleep, characterized by a decrease in *alpha activity* (12 to 14 Hz) in the EEG and a predominance of *theta activity* (4 to 7 Hz). In stage 2 there are bursts of 12 to 14 Hz, called *sleep spindles*, and slow, triphasic waves (*K complexes*). In stage 3 there is increasing concentration of *delta activity* (2 to 4 Hz), which constitutes 20% to 50% of the EEG tracing. In stage 4, concentration of delta activity is greater than 50%. Non-REM sleep is associated with more primitive mental content than is REM sleep (if cognitive activity can be elicited at all), and with slow heart and respiratory rate and low blood pressure. The deepest non-REM sleep occurs in the first 1 to 3 hours after the onset of sleep. Children have large amounts of deep slow-wave sleep, which decreases gradually with age. Sleepwalking, night terrors, and other confused partial arousals typically emerge from slow-wave sleep.

*REM sleep* occurs in cycles of approximately 90 minutes throughout the night.

Sleep seems to be generated by two broadly opposing mechanisms: the homeostatic drive for sleep, and the circadian system that regulates wakefulness. Normal sleep in humans requires an intact hypothalamus. The *hypothalamus* contains two mutually inhibitory regions that act like a flip-flop electrical circuit: (1) sleep-promoting anterior regions, and (2) wake-promoting posterior regions—the hypothalamic component of an aminergic wake-state enhancement system that involves serotonin, noradrenaline, dopamine, and histamine. Histaminergic neurons in the *tuberomammillary nucleus* (*TMS*) are a critical component of the posterolateral hypothalamic arousal system. *Ventrolateral preoptic area* (*VLPO*) cells are strategically positioned to modulate sleep-wake behavior by means of GABA-ergic input to histaminergic neurons. *Orexin* (q.v.) acts on the sleep-wake switch to stabilize the wake state and prevent untimely transitions from waking to sleeping. In narcolepsy, orexinergic deficiency makes abnormal wake-sleep switches more likely. In addition, sleep and wakefulness are influenced by the circadian system (biological clock), which is regulated by cells in the suprachiasmatic nuclei; and by a wake-dependent, or homeostatic, sleep drive. Finally, input from PFC and limbic system can influence the occurrence and emotional tone associated with sleep and wakefulness. Insomnia is related to reduced inhibition of brain stem–hypothalamic arousal centers, frontal cortex, and limbic system structures during sleep.

Several *neuropeptides* (q.v.) act on sleep (and also on depression and anxiety). NPY is associated with a reduction in sleep latency, anxiety, and depression. NPS induces wakefulness but, paradoxically, reduces anxiety. Galanin also has sleep-promoting and anxiety-reducing effects.

Various hypotheses have been proposed to explain the function of sleep: (1) brain thermoregulation, (2) brain detoxification, (3) tissue "restoration", and (4) enhancement of brain plasticity, learning, and memory. Dreaming is the conscious experience of hyperassociative brain activation that is maximal in REM sleep. Waking suppresses hallucinosis in favor of thought; REM sleep releases hallucinosis at the expense of thought. Activated thalamic nuclei transmit endogenous stimuli that lead to the sensory phenomena of dreaming. Dreaming is clearly brain-based, as attested by its symptoms that mimic delirium (visual hallucinosis, disorientation, memory loss, confabulation), and prominent executive deficiencies including lack of self-reflective awareness, inability to control dream action voluntarily, impoverishment of analytical thought and loss of logic. The executive deficiencies may be due to deactivation of executive areas in DLPFC and their failure to reactivate during REM sleep. Other contributors are a mixture of emotional (limbic subcortex), motoric (striatum), and instinctual (diencephalon) elements.

**sleep, activated**  See *dream.*

**sleep, continuous**  See *continuous sleep treatment.*

**sleep, inefficient**  See *sleep efficiency; sleep, shallow.*

**sleep, paroxysmal**  Sleep epilepsy, *narcolepsy* (q.v.); a sudden uncontrollable disposition to sleep occurring at irregular intervals, with or without obvious predisposing or exciting cause.

**sleep, shallow**  Sleep with less than normal delta or slow-wave sleep (stages III and IV). Although about 10% of patients with depression are hypersomniac, most have sleep that is shallow, shorter than normal, and inefficient, i.e., with frequent awakenings. See *sleep efficiency.*

**sleep and learning**  *Consolidation* (q.v.) or strengthening of memories appears to occur during sleep. During sleep, human subjects improve in skills learned by repetition, and the improvement is related to brain activity of the type that occurs during REM sleep. With declarative memory, information acquired while awake is reexpressed in the firing of hippocampal circuits during slow wave (non-REM) sleep.

**sleep apnea**  A breathing-related sleep disorder, consisting of impaired respiration, most frequently caused by obstruction of the airway by excessive or flabby tissue (obstructive apnea). Less common is central apnea, caused by defective brain stem regulation of breathing. See *apnea, central.*

**sleep deprivation**  A form of sleep therapy that has been used with depressed patients (usually combined with antidepressant medication or psychotherapy). In *total* sleep deprivation, the patient is kept awake for 36–40 hours; in partial sleep deprivation, the patient is awakened after 2 or 3 a.m. (*second half deprivation*) or is kept awake until 2 or 3 a.m. (*first half deprivation*). Second half deprivation appears to be more effective than first half deprivation, and partial deprivation is as effective as total deprivation and is better tolerated.

**sleep disorders**  *Sleep and arousal disorders; somnipathy*; any abnormality of the sleeping-waking schedule. Various classifications have been proposed, some based on phenomenology alone, others on etiology, etc. Most include the following: (1) *dyssomnias*, including *insomnia, hypersomnia, narcolepsy, breathing-related sleep disorder*, and *circadian rhythm sleep disorder* (qq.v.); (2) *parasomnias*, including *nightmare, sleep terror disorder*, and *somnambulis*m (qq.v.).

In DSM-IV, sleep disorders are grouped by their presumed etiology (i.e., primary, related to another mental disorder, due to a general medical condition, or substance-induced) rather than by their presenting symptoms.

Such a classification is compatible with the International Classification of Sleep Disorders.

**sleep drunkenness**   *Somnolentia*; a disorder of excessive somnolence (DOES) consisting of prolongation of the period between sleep and waking with protracted (as long as 2 hours) obnubilation and confusion following arousal, sometimes accompanied by agitation, aggressivity, and assaultiveness. In at least some cases it appears to be familial; further, it seems to occur only in males.

**sleep efficiency**   The ratio of time spent asleep to the total polysomnograph recording period; the most "efficient" sleep is that in which sleep latency is short and no wakenings occur after sleep onset. *REM sleep efficiency* is the time in REM sleep over the time from the beginning to the end of a REM period.

**sleep epilepsy**   *Obs.* Narcolepsy (q.v.).

**sleep hygiene guidelines**   General measures to promote sleep, such as the following:

1. Get up at the same time each day.

2. Limit in-bed time to the number of hours considered "normal" (for many, 8 hours; for some, more time or less time is the usual or normal).

3. Do not use CNS-active drugs, such as caffeine, nicotine, anorectics, or alcohol.

4. Do not nap during the day.

5. Attend to physical fitness with a morning exercise routine followed by other activity.

6. Avoid evening stimulation, such as action-packed television shows; substitute radio or easy reading.

7. Try a warm 20-minute bath before going to bed.

8. Eat on a regular schedule; do not eat a heavy meal before bedtime.

9. Practice an evening relaxation routine.

10. Correct any condition that makes sleeping uncomfortable.

11. Once in bed, stay awake no longer than 20 minutes.

**sleep inertia**   Persistence of subjective sleepiness and cognitive after awakening from sleep.

**sleep inversion**   Somnolence by day and insomnia at night; seen most commonly in organic brain disorders, alcoholism, and the schizophrenias.

**sleep latency**   The period of time between going to bed and the onset of sleep.

**sleep misperception syndrome**   *Pseudoinsomnia* (q.v.).

**sleep paralysis**   Also, *nocturnal hemiplegia; nocturnal paralysis; sleep numbness*; delayed psychomotor awakening; *cataplexy of awakening; postdormital chalastic fits*; a benign neurologic phenomenon, most probably due to some temporary dysfunction of the reticular activating system, consisting of brief episodes of inability to move and/or speak when awakening or, less commonly, when falling asleep. There is no accompanying disturbance of consciousness, and the subject has complete recall for the episode. Incidence is highest in younger age groups (children and young adults) and much higher in males (80%) than in females. It also occurs in *narcolepsy* (q.v.).

**sleep spindles**   See *sleep*.

**sleep terror disorder**   *Pavor nocturnus; night terror; sleep terror*; a rare type of sleep disorder, allied to but more serious than nightmares, which occurs in children and is not seen after puberty. A family history is frequent. The child awakes abruptly, screaming with fright, may stand up in bed or run about the bedroom, may have hallucinations of animals or strange people in the room, is disoriented and does not recognize the people about him. The attack ends after several minutes; the child drops off to sleep and does not remember the episode. Episodes occur usually during periods of EEG delta activity, in stages 3 and 4 of sleep, and not during REM sleep. See *sleep disorders*.

**sleep time, total**   The amount of time actually spent in sleeping, measured by subtracting *wake time after sleep onset* (q.v.) from the duration of the period from onset to termination of sleep.

**sleep treatment**   See *continuous sleep treatment*.

**sleep-disordered breathing**   See *breathing-related sleep disorder*.

**sleep-electroshock therapy**   Electroshock treatment preceded by the administration of sufficient sedative or hypnotic drug to produce sleep. The method is of particular value in patients who develop a fear of electric shock and are unwilling to continue receiving such therapy. Sodium pentothal is commonly employed, administered intravenously as a 2.5% solution. The electrodes are applied after sleep is induced. Many psychiatrists apply the current as soon as the patient spontaneously moves a limb during the waking process. The same amount of current is given as without the sleep-inducing drug. Other psychiatrists apply the current at a deeper stage of narcosis, as judged by the absence of spontaneous movements and the presence of a corneal reflex. With the latter method a nonconvulsive or minor reaction is obtained, but the clinical effects as measured by the maintenance of the improved state are equally satisfactory.

**sleep-induced respiratory impairment** Sleep apnea. See *sleep disorders.*

**sleeping princess syndrome** *Somnophilia* (q.v.).

**sleep-promoting factors** Neurons that are part of the reticular formation in the caudal brain stem are necessary for sleep, as are the pre-optic area and the suprachiasmatic nucleus within the hypothalamus and adjacent basal forebrain. The suprachiasmatic nucleus is believed to contain the primary biological clock. Although it is known that sleep onset is actively induced, it remains unknown if it is some factor present in blood, brain, or cerebrospinal fluid that induces sleep. Many factors appear to have the potential for promoting sleep, among them delta sleep-inducing peptide, interferon-a2, interleukin-1, lipopolysaccharides, melatonin, muramyl peptides, serotonin, tumor necrosis factor, and vasoactive intestinal peptide. See *clock, biological.*

**sleep-wake schedule disorders** *Circadian rhythm sleep disorder* (q.v.).

**sleepwalking** See *somnambulism.*

**sleepwalking violence** A violent act committed during an episode of temporarily impaired consciousness due to sleep disorder. It has been reported predominantly (90%) in men, ranging in age from 25 to 50 years, with a strong childhood or family history of sleepwalking, nocturnal enuresis, nightmares, and agitation on awakening. The attacks reported appear to have been nonpremeditated, taking place without awareness during the event, and following by retrograde amnesia and remorse. A benign episode of sleepwalking may evolve into an aggressive episode if the ongoing behavior is interrupted suddenly. Sleepwalking violence has not been associated with any specific psychopathology, despite its superficial resemblance to dissociative disorder. To be ruled out in the evaluation of the episode are other diagnoses associated with violent behavior, such as malingering, fugue, temporal lobe epilepsy, complex partial seizures, encephalopathy due to toxic agents, and REM behavior disorder. See *somnambulism.*

**SLI** *Specific language impairment* (q.v.).

**sliding of meanings** Making minute alterations in reporting facts as a way to externalize blame and thereby preserve self-esteem. The phenomenon has been reported frequently in narcissistic personality disorder.

**slip** See *intentional unvoluntary behavior; symptomatic act.*

**slip of tongue** *Lapsus linguae.* See *symptomatic act.*

**slippage, cognitive** See *cognitive slippage.*

**slow accelerator** See *acetylation.*

**slow virus** See *virus infections.*

**slow-channel syndrome** Prominent limb weakness with little weakness of cranial muscles, the reverse of the pattern in myasthenia gravis; the weakness is probably caused by abnormal prolongation of the acetylcholine receptor channel.

**slow-wave sleep** See *sleep.*

**Sluder syndrome** Sphenopalatine neuralgia; vidian neuralgia. See *cluster headaches.*

**slum** An urban area characterized by physical deterioration and social disorganization so marked as to result in the personal disorganization of its residents in the form of juvenile delinquency, adult crime, vice, substance dependence, gambling, mental disorders, etc. Children of the slums are both materially and emotionally disadvantaged and underprivileged.

**SMA** Supplementary motor area. See *frontal lobe seizures.*

**small penis complex** Concern that one's penis is inadequate because of its size. "What such a man is really ashamed of is not that his penis is 'small,' but the reasons why it is 'small'" (Jones, E. *Papers on Psycho-Analysis,* 1938).

**small RNAs** *MicroRNAs* (q.v.).

**smart drugs** Nootropics; cognitive enhancing drugs with a 'purely' cognitive effect (on cognition, memory, understanding, alertness, etc.). In theory, such drugs are intended for use in the many disease states that are characterized by impaired memory and cognition. There is a fine line, however, between correcting deficits and improving on "normality". Public policy on use of chemicals that affect brain (or body) performance, however, is inconsistent, contradictory, and confusing.

**SMI** Severe mental illness; as defined by the National Advisory Mental Health Council of NIMH in 1993 the following were included: nonaffective psychosis, manic depressive disorder, autism, dementia, and severe forms of mood and anxiety disorders. The estimate was that as few as 3% of the U.S. population suffer from SMI in a given year.

**SML** Single-major-locus; one of the models of *inheritance* (q.v.).

**smooth pursuit system** *SPEM* (smooth pursuit eye movements), reported to show abnormalities in 70% to 80% of schizophrenic subjects and in 45% to 50% of their first-degree relatives, but in only 6% of normal subjects. The smooth pursuit system matches the velocity of the eye to that of the target. If the eye velocity fails to match the target velocity, fast eye movements or *saccades* (q.v.) compensate for the mismatch.

**smother love** Mother's love displayed in overprotection that diminishes the child's opportunity to develop independence, overindulging that renders him unable to tolerate frustrations, domination and control of his every action, ultimately engendering multiple fears and self-doubts about the child's adequacy and ability. Smother love predisposes to passive dependent types of mastery and is seen often in obsessive or phobic mothers. See *monkey love; reciprocal regulation.*

**SMR training** A biofeedback technique that teaches the subject to produce 14 to 16 Hz rhythms. Insomniacs are deficient in these rhythms even when awake, and SMR is effective in 10% to 20% of sleep onset insomniacs who are relaxed but even so cannot fall asleep.

**SNAP-7941** A nonomolar inhibitor of MCHR1 with a 1000-fold selectivity over the other receptor for *MCH* (q.v.) and also over other GPCRs associated with food intake. It appears to inhibit food intake and in animals has demonstrated antidepressive and anxiolytic properties.

**SNARC effect** Spatial-numerical association of response codes effect; the finding that subjects respond more quickly to larger numbers if the response is on the right side of space, and to the left for smaller numbers, which indicates automatic spatial-numerical associations. See *numerosity.*

**SNARE** Soluble *N*-ethylmaleimide-sensitive factor (NSF) attachment protein (SNAP) receptor. Neurotransmitter release is triggered by calcium ions and depends critically on the correct function of three types of SNARE proteins.

**snare proteins** A family of membrane-tethered coiled-coil proteins that are required for membrane fusion in exocytosis during neurotransmitter release and for other membrane transport events. When trans-SNARE complexes are formed between vesicle SNAREs and target-membrane SNAREs, they pull the two membranes close together, presumably causing them to fuse.

**Snc** *Substantia nigra pars compacta.* See *LID; Parkinson disease*

**SNE** *Subacute necrotizing encephalomyelopathy* (q.v.).

**sniff sign** A pattern of breathing in patients with tracheal tumors. By the time occlusion of the trachea during expiration is almost total, the patient must draw in small, sharp, sniffing breaths in order to breathe. Many such patients are mislabeled as psychiatric in the early stages of tumor growth.

**SNM** See *nucleus.*

**snow** (From cocaine powder's resemblance to snow both in whiteness and powder consistency) Slang expression for *cocaine* (q.v.).

**snow lights** A type of visual pseudohallucination in which the subject, usually a cocaine user, sees twinkling lights similar to the sparkling of cocaine crystals or frozen snow crystals.

**snowbird** Slang expression for a cocaine addict. See *cocaine.*

**SNPs** *Single-nucleotide plymorphisms* (pronounced "snips"); *DNA polymorphism*; a change of one DNA sequence in a gene. SNPs are places along the chromosome where the genetic code tends to vary from one person to another by a single base. What makes an individual organism unique are such tiny variations in the genetic code; in the human, any two individuals (except for identical twins) differ, on average, by one DNA unit (nucleotide) of every thousand (there are 4 billion base pairs in the human genome). SNPs ("snips") are used in identifying defective genes that contribute to disease. Some SNPs may influence susceptibility to particular diseaes; others, even though they have no known function, can be markers for susceptibility genes. If they lie close to such a gene, they are likely to be inherited along with it.

It was hoped that SNPs might provide a means of rapid identification of the genes contributing to such major diseases as cancer, depression, or schizophrenia. A frequently used method, comparing entire genomes of a small number of subjects, may miss most of the SNPs that alter the proteins they encode, even though such SNPs are the ones that directly influence disease risk. Most SNPs have little impact on their protein products because they fall into the 95% noncoding area of the genome or act in a silent, *synonymous* way and code for the same protein for which another SNP codes. In contrast, *nonsynonymous* coding SNPs (*cSNPs*) are very rare, most of them having been eliminated in the course of evolution. Linking a disease to a very rare gene variant requires thousands of patients. Consequently, to establish an association between SNPs and a particular disease, a more successful strategy is to pick a set of *candidate genes* and assess them directly in as many subjects with the disease as possible.

**Snr**   *Substantia nigra pars reticulata.*

**SNRI**   Serotonin and norepinephrine reuptake inhibitor; also called a dual-action *antidepressant* (q.v.).

**snRNPs**   See *nucleus.*

**SNV**   *Selective neuronal vulnerability* (q.v.).

**SOA**   *Span of apprehension* (q.v.).

**SOAP**   See *problem-oriented record.*

**sobriety**   See *abstinence.*

**social action**   "…any concerted movement by organized groups toward the achievement of desired objectives" (Fitch, J. A. *Social Work Year Book* 1939). See *community psychiatry.*

**social agnosia**   Reich's term for the inability of the psychopath to achieve satisfaction in living.

**social anxiety disorder**   *SAD, social phobia,* characterized by an exaggerated fear of embarrassing or humiliating oneself in social performance situations and of being negatively evaluated by the other people ("audience") in those situations. In milder forms, the affected person may avoid activities such as speaking or eating in public. In more severe forms, activities become increasingly restricted and may lead to social isolation and loneliness. Exposure to the feared social situation provokes a stress response, the reaction to which is flight fleeting the situation or avoiding it) or fight (endurance of the situation and learning to tolerate the anxiety and distress involved). Physical symptoms may include flushing, sweating, palpitations, tremors, nausea or diarrhea; cognitive symptoms may include heightened arousal, impaired concentration,

excessive attention focused on the self, and negative post-event processing. See *phobia; stress.*

In order to be considered a disorder, the avoidance or distress must be severe enough to interfere significantly with the person's normal routine, occupational functioning, social activities or relationships. Anxiety and concern about one's performance is almost universal in certain situations, such as engaging in a debate, delivering a speech, anticipating in any kind of competitive activity, singing or playing an instrument or dancing before an audience, and acting in a play. Public speaking is the most widely feared situation. See *stage fright.*

As with GAD, the diagnostic criteria for SAD have undergone changes with successive editions of DSM, making it difficult to compare, for example prevalence rates presented in past studies. Epidemiologic surveys indicate that SAD is the third most common psychiatric illness and the most common anxiety disorder. It has a lifetime prevalence of 12.1% and a 12-month prevalence of 7.1%. In half of cases, onset is in childhood; onset after the age of 25 is rare.

**social assimilation**   The process or processes by which peoples of diverse social origins and different cultural heritages, occupying a common territory, achieve a cultural solidarity. Assimilation refers both to the fusion of immigrants or of members of a minority group into the national culture and to the nature and degree of participation of a newcomer in a group, institution, or neighborhood.

**social behavior network**   See *aggression.*

**social breakdown syndrome**   The deterioration in social abilities, interpersonal relationships, and general behavior that frequently accompanies organic and functional psychoses (and especially the schizophrenias). The term emphasizes the belief that such personality distortions, rather than being an inherent part of the psychotic process, are instead a reaction to the patient's environment; the male patient who is isolated from women will no longer make attempts to be attractive to the opposite sex, the person who is deprived of all purposeful activity or removed from any meaningful occupation will have no reason to keep track of time, etc. The social breakdown syndrome occurs in many situations—mental hospitals, prisons, concentration camps, etc. See *community psychiatry.*

**social class and mental illness**   See *class, social*.

**social cognition**   The mental operations underlying social interactions, including the human ability to perceive the intentions and dispositions of others, and the higher cognitive processes subserving the extremely diverse and flexible social behaviors that are seen in primates.See *social perception; social reasoning*.

**social cognitive neuroscience**   Social brain science; study of the relationships between brain and the social mind; the study of social behavior based on the concept that neural regulation reflects both innate, automatic, and cognitively impenetrable mechanisms, as well as acquired, contextual, and volitional aspects that include self-regulation. Real-life social interactions depend on information supplied by many modalities—touch, smell, hearing, and vision (the best-studied so far). Social visual signals include information about the face (such as its expression and the direction of gaze), as well as about body posture and movement. Human viewers are surprisingly adept at making reliable judgments about social information from minimal or incomplete stimuli. See *face recognition*.

Language provides important social signals; speech intonation (prosody) can also signal various emotions, using some of the same structures that are used to recognize facial expressions.

Psychological judgements depend not only on the immediate social stimulus but also on information generated by the brain through associations and inferences. The amygdala is one structure that is anatomically positioned to participate in such perceptual processing. The amygdala performs an initial rapid and automatic evaluation and tagging of stimuli for further processing. Next, visual cortices provide feedback modulation of attention processing. Later processing includes self-regulation and volitional guidance, in which the amygdala also has a role. In normal subjects, faces of people who look untrustworthy activate the superior temporal sulcus, amygdala, orbitofrontal cortex, and insular cortex. Patients with bilateral amygdala damage, however, judge other people to look more trustworthy and more approachable than do normal viewers, consistent with the often indiscriminately friendly behavior of such patients in real life.

**social cohesion, hedonic**   See *hedonism*.

**social control**   See *forced treatment; Scull dilemma*.

**social disorganization theory**   The theory that social problems such as drug use, violence, and high-risk sexual behaviors occur when the social cohesion of neighborhoods is weakened. The disruptive effects of industrialization, urbanization, and immigration lead to changes in the social structure of a neighborhood via residential mobility, ethnic heterogeneity, and concentrated poverty. This weakens social cohesion and reduces *collective efficacy*, the power of social norms and informal social controls to regulate deviant behavior. See *broken windows theory*.

**Social Dysfunction and Aggression Scale**   A 21-item clinician-rated instrument that assesses irritability, aggressiveness, physical violence, self-mutilation, dysphoric mood, and social withdrawal.

**social extinction**   Planned ignoring of undesirable behavior; a decelerative technique in behavior therapy used with behaviors that will not lead to actual harm if unattended to. *Response cost procedures*, in contrast, impose fines (in token economies) or loss of privileges for such behaviors. *Sensory extinction* is the removal of reinforcing sensory stimuli accompanying the undesirable behavior, used particularly for self-injurious behavior, such as head banging or scratching, in the form of protective gear, such as helmets or gloves.

**social fixity**   The social plan in which the role and status of each individual are rigidly fixed or defined, as in feudal and caste societies. Social fixity also appears in modern society and in social and other groups where the place of members is defined and fixed. See *social mobility*.

**social ghost**   The self as known, if only potentially, through the eyes and attentions of others; it is based primarily on social referencing, observing how familiar, trusted people react to others. The orbital prefrontal cortex, which also processes the perception of faces, is the brain area that is particularly involved in social referencing.

**social group work**   A kind of guided group experience in which participants are helped to meet their needs and develop their interests along socially acceptable lines, with the assistance of a group leader.

**social hunger**   The desire to be accepted by the group; the major incentive for improvement in a therapy group.

**social integration-disintegration model**	See *metabolic-nutritional model*.

**social interest**	The desire to belong, to be a part of a social group. See *individual psychology*.

**social learning theory**	The behavioral model of learning; its basic assumption is that there is a reciprocal action between the subject and the environment: not only does the environment determine some aspects of behavior, but the subject also changes the environment. Social learning theory incorporates both the respondent (classical) conditioning and the operant conditioning models of learning. Cognitive processes are important mediators in such learning in that reinforcement provides information about the future that affects behavior, such as a degree of certainty that a specific behavior will result in a particular outcome (*outcome expectancy*), or that the subject will be able to execute a particular behavioral sequence (*efficacy expectancy*).

**social masochism**	A characteristic subordinate attitude toward life, forcing the person into submissive and passive behavior, which enables him to stand defeats, privations, and misfortune. Such a situation can be described as a "giving up" attitude (Reik, T. *Masochism in Modern Man*, 1941).

**social mobility**	The free interactions among, and the changing roles and status of, members in a group. This term is used in contrast to *social fixity* (q.v.).

**social mores**	Codes of manners and morals imposed by tacit authority (or "unwritten" law) upon the individual to guide his social behavior in a given society, culture, or ethnic group and varying with the shift from one group, society, or culture to another.

**social network**	That group of people who have an ongoing significance in a specific person's or a nuclear family's life in terms of meeting human needs; the social network is a largely invisible system that is rarely together at any one time.

**social organization**	"Socially systematized schemes of behavior imposed as rules upon individuals" (Thomas, W. I. and Znaniecki, F. *The Polish Peasant in Europe and America*, 1927).

**social perception**	Awareness or understanding of different aspects of the relationships of people to one another, and of the self to other people. Social cognitive skills include the ability to communicate clearly and effectively with others, to discern the goals and intentions of others, to assess the impact of one's own behavior on others, to maintain interpersonal as well as conceptual boundaries, and to be alert to social cues about such issues as level of intimacy and social status.

Two of the most important elements of social perception are facial affect recognition and social cue perception. The best predictor of social skill is subjects' perception of their own social performance and awareness of the impact of their behavior on others. See *social reasoning*.

The social perception of many persons with schizophrenia is limited. They often seem to be impaired in their ability to recognize facial affect in others. They perform poorly on *theory of mind* tasks (q.v.), the ability to represent the mental states of others or to make inferences about another's intentions.

**social phobia**	Fear of situations in which the affected person may be scrutinized by others and/or might act in a shameful fashion; included are fears of speaking in public, of blushing, of eating in public, of writing in front of others, of using public lavatories. In DSM-IV, what was formerly called Avoidant Disorder of Childhood is included within this category. See *anxiety disorders; anxiety hysteria; phobia*.

**social policy planning**	*Community organization; community action; social action; social engineering*. Social policy planning is a deliberate, organized, and collaborative approach to the analysis and manipulation of social structures and systems. It aims to improve the quality of life in a community, which is viewed as an organism, a total biotype, an ecological entity. Emphasis is upon superordinate goals (viz. the welfare of people), rather than on institutionally defined goals (e.g., the pathology and condition of specific people who appear at the door of a mental health center). Its methods may even include such an approach as founding a new town with a sociopetal arrangement to promote participation by such means as organization, architectural structure, and other environmental factors that program behavior. The goal is to develop a process within the community—not to devise a specific prescription, but to initiate interaction and expand the spectrum of possible action in overcoming poverty, minority problems, and other *urban crises*, which currently are ordinarily defined in terms of jobs, housing, education, crime on the streets, drug and alcohol abuse, and suicide. See *community psychiatry.*

**social pressures**   Socially created sanctions that emanate from less sanctioned or less responsible sources than the direct authoritarian controls, effected through officials or other accredited social agents and expressive of established codes.

**social psychiatry**   In psychiatry, the stress laid on the environmental influences and the impact of the social group on the individual. This emphasis is made not only with regard to etiology, but also for purposes of treatment and, more important, in preventive work. See *ecology; community psychiatry; comparative psychiatry.*

**social psychology**   See *sociology.*

**social reasoning**   Drawing inferences about others' actions, intentions, motives, disposition, openness, approachability, truthfulness, fairness, etc., as a means of deciding how to regulate one's own behavior in real-life interactions with others. Social cognition includes the human ability to perceive the intentions and dispositions of others and the other mental operations underlying social interactions. Social cognition is relatively independent of other aspects of cognition. The orbitofrontal cortex, superior temporal sulcus, and amygdala are the most consistently activated in social information processing. See *social cognitive neuroscience; theory of mind.*

**social skills training**   *SST;* a widely used accelerative technique in behavior therapy; its five main elements are (1) focused instruction for a particular behavior, (2) demonstration or modeling of that response, (3) rehearsal, often including role playing, (4) reinforcement of correct responses together with corrective feedback for incorrect responses, often using a videotaped playback of the role-play, and (5) homework or practice to help generalize skills acquired in training to real-life situations. Social skills training emphasizes use of appropriately assertive behavior, social reinforcers (e.g., eye contact, compliments), and self-reinforcement; it provides the patient with techniques for conflict de-escalation and with techniques for self-management.

SST is highly structured and is useful with schizophrenic patients, for example, in teaching them a variety of social behaviors to improve their social competence as a way to improve their quality of life, to overcome social isolation, and to improve their functioning at work and in the family. It teaches conversational skills, assertiveness, ways to manage (and comply with) medications prescribed, etc. Typically, complex social behaviors—such as dating or interviewing for a job—are broken down into more basic elements that the subject first practices individually and then combines into a smoothly flowing social repertoire. This approach is often termed the *motor skills model* of training, because it tries to circumvent any information processing or cognitive deficits that may be present.

The limitation of the traditional model of SST is that many social situations do not follow a script; instead, they demand considerable cognitive activity on the part of all participants—perception and evaluation of interpersonal cues, consideration of response options, selection of the best response alternative, etc. To enhance basic cognitive capacities, many workers add social problem solving and cognitive rehabilitation strategies, in which subjects are given repeated practice on word games and computer games that require memory, attention, and reasoning. See *rehabilitation; behavior therapy.*

**social stressor**   See *life event.*

**social therapy**   Use and manipulation of the social setting as a major element in treatment, as in the *therapeutic community* (q.v.). Social therapy provides a model social group, which encourages use of appropriate forms of behavior, as well as immediate feedback on the effects of the patient's behavior on the people he or she encounters (*reality confrontation*).

Social therapy is a form of rehabilitation therapy whose primary focus is on the patient's level of social functioning and whose aim is to improve the patient's ability to function in a socially approved manner. The social therapies include any number of socioenvironmental approaches that concern themselves with the patient's behavior, rather than his or her intrapsychic state—the therapeutic community, patient government, remotivation, attitude therapy, compensated work, etc. See *deinstitutionalization; rehabilitation.*

**social type**   The role which a person assumes and to which he or she is assigned by society. See *gender role.*

**social work**   A profession whose primary concern is how human needs can be met within society as it exists. Drawing from both the social and behavioral sciences, social work encourages optimal adjustment in people by fostering their maximal growth and development; at the same time, it attempts to influence their environments to become more responsive to their needs. The services provided include general social services, such as health and education, and welfare services to targeted, vulnerable groups (e.g., the poor, the physically or mentally handicapped, immigrants, children, the aged, victims of disasters, etc.).

The medical social worker typically performs three overlapping functions: (1) assessing the social and psychological factors that have affected the development of illness or are likely to affect treatment and rehabilitation; (2) helping the patient and family to identify and utilize appropriately the different kinds of resources and facilities that are available; and (3) preparing the family and the community (e.g., the work setting or the school) for the return of the patient and for particular challenges that might be posed during aftercare and rehabilitation. The social worker may also be involved in community organization and education, social policy planning, legislation, patient or group advocacy, and facility and program administration. See *family social work; psychiatric social work*.

**socialization**   The processes through which the individual becomes a competent member of society. Anthropologists stress cultural transmission or enculturation; personality psychologists focus on impulse control; sociologists concentrate on role learning. Recent work using direct observation of infants suggests that socialization is an interactive process based on reciprocity. The human infant is an active participant in the socialization process and much more than a mere passive recipient of information doled out by others.

In occupational therapy, the development (in a patient) of those tendencies that induce him or her to be companionable and inclined to seek and mingle easily with a group.

In psychiatry, the condition in which inner impulses (i.e., instincts and their derivatives) are expressed or lived out in conformity with the cultural demands of the environment. It is synonymous with *sublimation* (q.v.).

**socialize**   1. To *sublimate* (q.v.). 2. To mix in a group.

**societal reaction theory**   *Labeling theory* (q.v.).

**society**   The network of relationships between a person and every other organizational unit of humankind, ranging from the mother–child dyad or family to a league of nations.

**sociobiology**   The central tenet of human sociobiology is that social behaviors are shaped by natural selection. Those behaviors conferring the highest replacement rate in successive generations are expected to prevail throughout local populations and hence ultimately to influence the statistical distribution of culture on a worldwide basis. The strategy of sociobiology is to explain all phenotypically altruistic behavior as being genetically *selfish* acts. See *fitness*.

In the sociobiological literature, various mechanisms have been suggested to explain why an individual would take actions decreasing his personal fitness in order to enhance the fitness of another, among them *group selection* and *kin selection* (qq.v.).

Implicit in the claims of sociobiology is the notion that organisms act so as to maximize their inclusive reproductive fitness. Critics have argued that this just is not true. Organisms act to maximize inclusive fitness under constraints, such as in the following ways:

Neutral characteristics: many phenotypic properties of the organism are irrelevant, i.e., neutral. Nevertheless, such characteristics may severely restrict the kinds of future modifications of the organism that will count as improvement.

Time lags: what was optimal long ago may be very far from optimal today.

Context dependence: genes leading to a certain kind of behavior seen today may have come about originally for some quite different purpose, one that is no longer relevant.

Historical constraints: every modification must also be an improvement in order to avoid being eliminated. Thus, Nature is totally oriented to the short term, performing local optimizations that may not lead to globally optimal performance.

Variation constraint: maximization can be applied only to those variations that actually occur, not to those that were possible in theory but in fact did not happen.

Cost–benefit analysis: every variation has to be measured by a cost–benefit evaluation against the overall improvement for the organism. The development of a capacity to run faster to catch food would have to be weighed against the extra energy needed to supply the added motive power.

Levels of analysis: a given variation must be evaluated at several biological levels—gene, organism, group—and what is good for one may be very harmful to another.

Capricious environment: a sudden environmental disturbance can undo in a few days the gradual evolutionary changes of several millennia; e.g., the meteorite collision that supposedly wiped out the dinosaurs 65 million years ago.

**socioecology**    *Behavioral ecology* (q.v.).

**socioeconomic gradient**    See *SES*.

**socioemotional circuit**    See *frontal-striatal system*.

**sociogram**    "The sociogram projects the results of sociometric, spontaneity and population tests into a pattern and makes visible the relationship of every individual to every other individual of the group tested" (Moreno, J. L. *Sociometry 1*, 1937).

**sociology**    The behavior science that concerns itself with the conceptualization and study of group life, and particularly the functions, structures, and organization of institutions and communities, the interactions between them, and the changes within them. Even though systematic sociology developed in response to recognized social problems (specifically, crime, delinquency, and suicide), the sociologist is as interested in understanding "normal" social actions as in gathering knowledge of social problems and uncovering the crucial factors in their incidence. Current clinical emphasis on how social organizations may, both implicitly and explicitly, program or dictate the behavior of the people within them is more akin to *social psychology* than to sociology; but in practice the distinction between the two is not finely drawn.

**sociology, clinical**    See *comparative psychiatry*.

**sociometric test**    A measure of the amount of organization shown by social groups, devised by Moreno.

**sociometry**    Study of the actual psychological structure of human society, consisting of complex interpersonal patterns which are studied by quantitative and qualitative procedures.

"A fundamental part of the sociometric procedure is to apply to a community an actual social situation which is confronting its people at the moment. The social situation applied is of such a nature as to make repetition possible at any time in the future without loss of spontaneous participation. In this manner, the procedure reveals the organization and evolution of groups and the position of individuals within them" (Moreno, J. L. *Sociometry 1*, 1937).

**sociopath**    See *psychopathic personality*.

**sociopathic personality disturbance**    In the 1952 revision of psychiatric nomenclature, this term was used to refer to those who are ill primarily in terms of society and of conformity with social, cultural, and ethical demands. This group does not include those whose conduct and behavior are symptomatic of more primary personality disturbance. Included in this group were the following:

1. *Antisocial reaction*—approximately equivalent to the older terms constitutional psychopathy and psychopathic personality and to *antisocial personality disorder* in DSM-III. See *psychopathic personality*.

2. *Dyssocial reaction*—disregard for and conflict with the social code as the result of having lived in an abnormal moral environment.

3. *Sexual deviation*—such as homosexuality, transvestism, pedophilia, fetishism, sexual sadism.

4. *Addiction* (q.v.).
   a. *Alcoholism* (q.v.).
   b. Drug addiction. See *dependence, drug*.

**sociopathology**    The pathology of society. Society at large, or any segment of society, is composed of or comprises an aggregate of individuals, and the psychopathology of the patient as an individual or of a few or many of the group is quantitatively and qualitatively reflected ultimately as the psychopathology of the society that contains the individuals. Individual psychopathology is thus closely intermeshed with communal sociopathology.

**sociopathy**    1. Generally used to designate an abnormal or pathological mental attitude toward the environment. Thus, criminality and vagabondage are regarded by some authorities as manifestations of sociopathy. In this sense the term refers to mental states that are commonly subsumed under psychopathy.

2. Abnormality or pathology of society or social units.

**sociotaxis**   See *network; taxis.*

**sociotherapy**   Any type of treatment whose primary emphasis is on socioenvironmental and interpersonal factors in adjustment; it is sometimes used to refer specifically to the establishment of a *therapeutic community* (q.v.).

**SOD**   *Superoxide dismutase* (q.v.).

**sodium pump**   See *ion pump; resting membrane potential.*

**sodomite**   One who practices sodomy; a sodomist.

**sodomy**   Sexual penetration of a nonreproductive orifice, in either a man or a woman; sexual relations between a person and an animal (*bestiality*). Most often the term refers to anal intercourse with a male or female (*buggery*), although in different jurisdictions, in different countries, and at different times it has been defined as various forms of sexual expression considered unnatural, perverse, or otherwise unacceptable.

The "sin of Sodom" referred originally to mistreatment or malignant neglect of aliens and the poor; it was described as a sin against charity stemming from the arrogance of wealth. In *The City of God* (412 A.D.), Augustine equated it with (male) homosexuality

**soft signs**   Primitive reflexes that may appear as early manifestations of frontal lobal dysfunction. Soft neurologic signs are also found in as many as 70% of patients with "functional" psychoses, so they are of little help in differentiating between neurologic and psychiatric disorders. Usually included as soft signs are the following:

1. The palmar-mental reflex—the lip and jaw move downward when the subject's thumb is scratched.

2. The grasp reflex—the examiner presses his finger into the subject's hand, which grasps the examiner's finger.

3. The snout or rooting reflex—when the corner of the subject's mouth is stroked, the subject's lips purse and move toward the stroking.

4. Adventitious motor overflow.

5. Loss of double simultaneous discrimination.

**soiling**   See *encopresis.*

**soldier's heart**   See *war neurasthenia.*

**soliloquy, sexual**   Hirschfeld says that many sexually timid individuals, who find difficulty in suppressing or repressing their sexual impulses, engage in long soliloquies as a means of relieving their sexual tensions.

**solipsism**   The doctrine that *my self, alone,* is the essence of existence; nothing counts except one's own ego, in which all else is reflected.

**solution, auxiliary**   In Horney's terminology, any partial or temporary solution of intrapsychic conflict, such as automatic control of feelings, compartmentalization, externalization, intellectualization, or self-alienation.

**solution, comprehensive**   In Horney's terminology, an unrealistic avoidance of conflict by believing oneself to be the *idealized self* (q.v.), i.e., by actualizing the idealized image of oneself.

**solution, expansive**   See *expansiveness.*

**solution, major**   In Horney's terminology, a type of neurotic solution consisting of repression and denial of trends that conflict with the idealized self, or consisting of withdrawal into resignation.

**soma**   The organic tissues of the body. Whether correctly or not, the terms *soma* and *psyche* are often employed as if they were opposites. The psyche, however, is currently considered as an organ of the total person; it is not looked upon as an antithesis of the soma, but rather as a harmonious constituent of the entire organism. See *psyche; psychosomatic.*

**soma, some-**   Combining form meaning body, from Gr. *soma.*

**somatagnosia**   See *somatognosia.*

**somatalgia**   Pain due to organic causes, as distinguished from psychalgia or pain due to psychical causes. See *hypochondriasis; psychalgia; somatoform disorders.*

**somatic**   Relating to or involving the soma.

**somatic delusion**   The subjective reports and complaints made by patients that their body is perceived, or felt, by them as disturbed or disordered in all, or in individual, organs or parts.

**somatic marker**   See *marker, interoceptive.*

**somatic psychosis**   Dunbar's term for the somatic expression of tension, aggression, and resentment in diabetic patients. The aggression and resentment of such patients "gnaws at their vitals, and, probably because of their infantile regression and extreme ambivalence, brings about what might be called a *somatic psychosis*" (*Psychosomatic Diagnosis*, 1943).

**somatic sensory system** The primary somatic sensory cortex contains four separate maps of the surface of the body in four areas in the postcentral gyrus (Brodmann's areas 1, 2, 3a, and 3b). Such cortical maps are dynamic, not static, even in mature animals. Their functional connections can expand or retract, depending on the particular uses or activities of the peripheral sensory pathways. See *proprioception*.

**somatist** Psychiatrist or scientist who regards any particular neurosis or psychosis as of organic or physical origin.

**somatization** Stekel's term for a type of bodily disorder arising from a deep-seated neurotic cause. It is as if the organs of the body were translating into a physiopathological language the mental troubles of the individual. The term somatization is identical with the phenomenon Freud calls *conversion* (q.v.). Stekel refers to it also in terms of *organ speech* of the mind, meaning the organic expression of mental processes. Such physical expressions are also encountered in dreams, and when they occur, the oneiric phenomena are known as a functional dream.

**somatization disorder** *Briquet syndrome*; one of the *somatoform disorders* formerly known as *hysteria* (qq.v.). Characteristics are multiple physical complaints that are not caused by or cannot fully be explained by a known nonpsychiatric medical condition; they begin before the age of 30 years, occur over a period of several years, and lead to medical treatment or an alteration in lifestyle. The physical complaints include pain in different areas (e.g., back, head, joints, abdomen, chest, rectum), and symptoms other than pain involving the gastrointestinal system (e.g., nausea, diarrhea, vomiting, food intolerance), the sexual-reproductive system (e.g., impotence, irregular menses, excessive menstrual bleeding), and the neurologic system (e.g., conversion and dissociative symptoms).

Lifetime prevalence of the disorder is estimated at 0.2% to 0.4%. It appears to be approximately 20 times more frequent in women than in men, and it tends to run in families (first-degree female relatives have a high incidence of somatization disorder; first-degree male relatives have a high incidence of alcoholism, drug abuse, and antisocial personality disorder).

**somatobiology** The study of the biology of the body, as contrasted with psychobiology, which is the study of the biology of the mind.

**somatoform** Suggesting or mimicking physical disorder.

**somatoform disorders** A group of disorders characterized by physical complaints for which no adequate physical explanation can be found. Included are *somatization disorder, conversion disorder, hypochondriasis, body dysmorphic disorder, pain disorder*, and in some classifications *autonomic arousal disorder* and *neurasthenia* (qq.v.). Many of these would be labeled *psychosomatic* in other terminologies.

The undifferentiated form includes multiple physical complaints that are clinically significant but do not meet the high symptom count required for somatization disorder.

Somatoform disorder not otherwise specified includes physical complaints that cannot be fully explained by any known general medical condition and do not meet the criteria for any other somatoform disorder. One example is *pseudocyesis*.

Somatoform disorders are functional somatic syndromes; somatic symptoms that are not well explained by general medical conditions and hence difficult to classify or even name. Somatoform implies that the symptoms are a mental disorder in somatic form, and the term may be misinterpreted as casting doubt on the reality or genuineness of the symptoms. Many of the official subcategories have failed to achieve established standards of reliability, and the diagnosis has low stability in longitudinal surveys. Patients with somatization disorder usually have prominent psychological symptoms, as well as somatic complaints, so the syndrome is not necessarily a predominantly somatic condition. In addition, there is substantial overlap between somatoform disorders and personality disorders (and borderline personality disorder, in particular).

**somatoform dissociation** See *psychologic dissociation*.

**somatogenesis** Origination in organic tissue (the soma).

**somatognosia** The awareness of one's own body as a functioning object in space. *Macrosomatognosia* is a disturbance of the body scheme in which the body or parts of the body are experienced as abnormally large; *microsomatognosia* is a disturbance of the body scheme in which the body or parts of the body are experienced as abnormally small. Such disturbances have been reported in organic neurologic lesions, epilepsy, migraine, schizophrenia, and experimental psychosis. See *body ego; body image.*

Note that absent or defective awareness may be expressed in two ways: as *asomatognosia* or as *somatagnosia.*

**somatoparaphrenia** 1. A nonrecognition or alienation syndrome that occurs in right-sided *parietal lobe dysfunction* (q.v.): the subject denies ownership of his left arm or leg, may even insist his own limb has been replaced by someone else's or that the limb is "fake."

2. Nonspecific term for somatic delusional state; less commonly used to describe predominating somatic delusions during a schizophrenic episode.

**somatopathic drinking** See *alcoholism.*

**somatoplasm** The somatic tissues of an animal body, to distinguish them, according to the germ plasm theory, from the reproductive tissue that produces the germ cells.

**somatopsychic** Relating to or originating in both body and mind.

**somatopsychic delusion** See *autopsychic delusion.*

**somatosensory cortex** A portion of the parietal lobe; it contains a "touch-map" of the body. Different-sized areas are devoted to certain areas of skin, according to their degree of sensitivity. The thumb, for example, has as much representation in the cortex as does the entire leg. See *parietal lobe.*

**somatosexual** Pertaining to or characterized by organic manifestations of sexuality.

**somatostatin** *STS*; somatotropin release–inhibiting factor (*SRIF*); growth hormone–inhibiting hormone; a hypothalamic tetradecapeptide (14 amino acids) that inhibits the secretion of several anterior pituitary hormones, among them the growth hormone. Somatostatin is found in brain, pancreas, and gastrointestinal tract. In the pancreatic islets, somatostatin inhibits secretion of insulin and glucagon; in the gastrointestinal tract, it inhibits secretion of gastrin, pepsin, serotonin, and vasoactive intestinal peptide (VIP). In the cortex, somatostatin is concentrated in layers II, III, and VI; in Alzheimer disease, its concentration in the cortex and CSF is decreased. It is also decreased during exacerbations of multiple sclerosis, and in depression (a state-related

change; it normalizes with recovery or if the patient switches into mania). See *GH (growth hormone); hypothalamic-pituitary-adrenal (HPA) axis; peptide, brain.*

**somatotonia** A personality type described by Sheldon that is correlated with the mesomorph body type and shows a predominance of vigorous assertiveness and muscular activity.

**somatotopagnosia** *Autotopagnosia* (q.v.).

**somatotopy** See *receptor sheet, peripheral.*

**somatotropin** *Growth hormone* (q.v.).

**somatotype** In some systems of constitutional medicine, the physical structure and build of a person as assessed by particular photographic techniques of *anthropometry.* Its scientific meaning thus applies only to one aspect of an *anthrotype* (q.v.), which has physiologic, immunological, and psychological aspects as well.

**somatotypy** Somatotypic representation of body parts in the cortex; it is not an exact mirroring of one separate cortical area for each separate body part but rather contains considerable overlap of all the cortical areas so mapped. Each finger movement, for example, depends upon a distribution of neurons through the entire hand area, and not on one independent area assigned to that finger alone. See *receptor sheet, peripheral.*

**somesthetic area** See *parietal lobe.*

**somnambulism** *Sleepwalking disorder*, consisting of repeated episodes of rising from bed during sleep and walking about. Episodes rarely last more than 30 minutes and once awake the subject is amnesic for his actions during the episode.

Somnambulism is primarily a male disorder and is rare in homosexuals of either sex; in one series a reported 35% of sleepwalkers were overtly schizophrenic, and another 28% were markedly schizoid in character. Dynamic characteristics of this series were inadequate male identification, passive-dependent strivings, and conflicting feelings over aggression (Sours, J. A. *Archives of General Psychiatry 9,* 1963). See *sleepwalking violence.*

Somnambulism usually occurs in sleep stages 3 and 4 and not during REM sleep. Those somnambulists so far studied have given no evidence of abnormal electrical brain activity during sleep.

Somnambulism may occur as a complication of neuroleptic medication, and particularly if neuroleptics are combined with lithium.

**somnambulism, cataleptic** A cataleptic state occurring during somnambulism.

**somnambulism, monoideic** Janet's term for a single idea constituting the content of a somnambulistic episode. When the content contains many ideas, he calls it *polyideic somnambulism.*

**somnifacient** Hypnotic; sleep-inducing.

**somniferous** Hypnotic; somnific.

**somnifugous** Driving sleep away; agrypnotic.

**somniloquism** Talking during sleep. Somniloquism is not pathognomonic of any specific disorder and is only rarely presented as a symptom or chief complaint.

**somnipathy** 1. Any *sleep disorder* (q.v.). 2. *Obs.* Hypnotism.

**somnogen** An agent that promotes sleep. Endogenous somnogens may be the physiological basis of sleep need (process S in Borbely's two-process model of sleep propensity). Somnogens accumulate during prolonged waking, tending to produce sleep despite opposing pressure of the circadian cycle (process C). Putative endogenous somnogens include adenosine, cytokines, hormones, melatonin, oleomide, and prostaglandins.

**somnolence** Unnatural sleepiness, drowsiness.

**somnolent detachment** Withdrawal into sleep; the infant's reaction of drowsiness and apathy to anxiety in the mother. As the infant withdraws from the situation and sleeps, the mother's anxiety will often subside and thus the cause of the infant's own anxiety is removed. But if such detachments persist, the infant may progress into a marasmic state and may die unless he receives appropriate nursing care. See *anaclitic depression.*

**somnophilia** *Sleeping princess syndrome;* a *paraphilia* in which sexual arousal and orgasm are dependent upon awakening a sleeping stranger with caresses or by means of oral sex. See *succubus.*

**sonoencephalogram (SEG)** Echoencephalogram. See *echoencephalography.*

**sophomania** A form of megalomania in which the patient stresses the excellence of his wisdom.

**sopor** *Obs.* A disorder of consciousness in which the subject can be aroused only by strong stimulation.

**soporiferous** Soporific, making drowsy.

**soporific, soporifical** Any sleep-inducing agent.

**sororate** Marriage to a deceased wife's sister. See *levirate.*

**sorting tests** A method of psychological assessment in which the subject is required to place objects into groups on the basis of similarity or some other abstract relationship. Such sorting or *Zuordnung* tests are particularly associated with Kurt Goldstein, Vigotsky, Hanfmann, and Kasanin. Patients with cortical lesions typically show impairment of abstract behavior as measured by these tests. Schizophrenics, too, do poorly on these tests; but performance is more varied than in ordinary brain damage cases, for the schizophrenic tends to project himself into the test objects and animate and embellish them. See *Wisconsin Card Sort(ing) test.*

**soteria** Possessions and objects that bring security and protection, as the objects that a collector admits to his collection. Collecting and soteric objects are to be distinguished from accumulation and the objects accumulated; accumulation is "the continued possession of unclassified, useless, meaningless, annoying objects" and, unlike true collecting, "cannot be understood in terms of its symbolic meaning, but is a by-product of the accumulator's indecision, an unwillingness to commit himself to a clear and realistic self-definition" (Phillips, R. H. *Archives of General Psychiatry 6,* 1962). See *coprophilia; collecting mania.*

Soteria also means deliverance, and in that sense it has been used as a name for residences for schizophrenics. See *domicile.*

Soteria also refers to a nonmedical treatment systems approach that rejects medication and formal professional services in favor of peer support, with the family kept at a friendly distance.

**Soteria House** See *domicile.*

**sotolol** A *beta blocker* (q.v.).

**soul** See *anima.*

**source amnesia** See *alter.*

**source monitoring** Also, reality monitoring; the ability to retrieve the precise circumstances of memory acquisition, i.e., whether a memory relates to a true or an imagined event.

**Southard, Elmer Ernest** (1876–1920) American psychiatrist; social psychiatry, industrial hygiene.

**SP** Substance P, a tachykinin. See *neuropeptides.*

**space, personal** See *proxemics.*

**space, subarachnoid**   See *meninges*.

**space neurosis**   See *infinity neurosis*.

**spaced training**   See *memory training*.

**spacing**   Distancing; the distance an organism puts between itself and another member of its own group. When spacing is so close as to be nonexistent, as in the mother–infant relationship, the term *bonding* is applied; close spacing under other conditions may be termed crowding, with the implication that such closeness is undesirable rather than facilitating. In humans and other primates, crowding is associated with a significant increase in aggressiveness.

**span of apprehension**   *SOA*; the number of stimuli that can be attended to, apprehended, and reported in a single brief exposure.

**span of apprehension test**   Dots are flashed on a screen by a tachistoscope and the subject is asked to tell the number of dots after each presentation.

**span of attention**   See *attention; memory*.

**spasm**   A slow, at times prolonged, patterned movement of a muscle or groups of muscles occurring anywhere in the body.

**spasmophilia**   1. A neuropsychiatric syndrome, described by Joyeux in 1958, consisting of moderate anxiety, irritability, hypermotility, insomnia, dysfunction in various organ systems (gastrointestinal, cardiovascular, genital, skin), and positive Chvostek sign. All the symptoms may be precipitated or aggravated by hyperventilation. See *hyperventilation syndrome*.

2. In general and constitutional medicine, a syndrome characterized by undersecretion of the parathyroids.

**spasmus nutans**   A rhythmic nodding or rotatory tremor of the head occurring in infants between the ages of 6 and 12 months; frequently accompanied by nystagmus. See *nodding spasm*.

**spastic gait**   The patient walks stiffly with legs extended and feet shuffling.

**spasticity**   Increased muscle tone due to lesions of the premotor area of the brain, as in congenital spastic paralysis. See *Little disease*.

**spatial neglect**   Spatial *nonrecognition*; a type of *sensory neglect* (qq.v.) It has generally been believed that spatial neglect is associated with lesions of the right inferior parietal lobule and the *TPO junction* (the area between the temporal, parietal, and occipital lobes). The studies supporting that belief had included patients who suffered not only from spatial neglect, but also from addidtional visual field defects. More recently, spatial neglect has been localized to the rostral portions of the right superior temporal gyrus (*STG*). Crucial for spatial neglect are subcortical nuclei in the right basal ganglia, the putamen, and (to a much smaller degree) the caudate; and the pulvinar in the right thalamus. The STG association areas have direct connections with the putamen and the caudate. The right putamen, caudate nucleus, pulvinar, and STG form a coherent cortico-subcortical network for representing spatial awareness.

**spatial orientation memory test**   The subject is shown a geometric design and then asked to choose the correct orientation of the design from four multiple-choice options.

**spatial summation**   See *summation*.

**SPD**   *Schizotypal personality disorder*; *sensory processing disorder* (qq.v.).

**specialty care**   See *care*.

**specific developmental disorders**   See *developmental disorders, specific*.

**specific dynamic pattern**   Franz Alexander's term for the specific nuclear conflict or dynamic configuration unique to a particular psychosomatic disorder or organ-neurosis. See *psychosomatic*.

**specific language impairment**   *SLI; developmental dysphasia;* one of the specific developmental disorders, not due to auditory, cognitive, or social problems. SLI is a familial disorder, believed to be controlled by a single dominant gene. Characteristics are a delayed onset of language, articulation difficulties in childhood, and impaired inflectional ability (problems with case, number, gender, tense, person, etc.). Speech contains frequent grammatical errors, such as misuse of pronouns and of plural or past tense suffixes (e.g., "He gave she a present," "She wants thank them present"). Nonlinguistic abilities are usually intact. Conversely, other cases with substantial cognitive loss produced by brain damage are often able to produce grammatical sentences. This bolsters the general belief that language ability is distinct from general-purpose cognitive functioning. See *developmental disorders, specific; dyslexia*.

**specific rate**   A rate is specific when it is based upon a population and a class of that population both of which are homogeneous, or nearly so, with respect to a specific character;

e.g., the number of male patients dying at ages 20–24 per 1000 male patients aged 20–24.

**specificity**   The probability that the diagnostic procedure concludes "no" when the subject is truly not ill. High specificity is essential when false positive diagnoses are costly. See *sensitivity*.

**specificity, encoding**   See *encoding*.

**specificity, receptor**   See *code, labeled line*.

**specificity, symptom**   The phenomenon of heightened reactivity to stress in that organ system in which a psychosomatic patient's symptoms are localized; e.g., greater heart rate and heart rate variability in patients with cardiovascular complaints than in subjects without such complaints.

**specificity research**   Research that aims to clarify the definition of a disorder, typically by comparing it to and differentiating it from other disorders. An example is the study of dysthymic disorder in an attempt to clarify whether it is a subtype of affect disorder or a personality disorder.

**SPECT**   Single photon emission computed tomography, a type of imaging in which the camera rotates around the patient while the computer compiles images of transverse slices, as in CT or CAT scanning. Unlike the latter, however, which produces an anatomic image, SPECT uses radioactive tracers and provides an image of radioactivity distribution. In this aspect, it is similar to *PET* (q.v.), whose major disadvantage is that cyclotrons must be maintained onsite to develop the short-lived isotopes needed for imaging. PET's major advantage in comparison with SPECT is that short-lived isotopes enable visualization of processes that cannot be seen with longer lived isotopes. Although the SPECT image is not as clearly defined as the PET image, the cost is much lower. See *imaging, brain*.

Both SPECT and *PET* use specific radioactively labeled ligands *(radioligands)* to tag either normal or abnormal molecules, such as neurotransmitter receptors in the brain. Both techniqes detect the radioactivity emitted by the injected radioligand to reconstruct three-dimensional tomographs of the distribution of readioactivity in the brain.

**spectatoring**   A type of intellectualization of sexual behavior consisting of monitoring one's own sexual performance as if some outside observer were commenting critically on one's abilities and adequacy.

**spectral photography**   See *BEAM*.

**spectrophobia**   "The hysterical phobia for mirrors and the dread of catching sight of one's own face in a mirror had in one case a 'functional' and a 'material' origin. The functional one was dread of *self-knowledge*; the material, the flight from the *pleasure of looking* and exhibitionism. In the unconscious phantasies the parts of the face represented, as in so many instances, parts of the genitals" (Ferenczi, S. *Further Contributions to the Theory and Technique of Psycho-Analysis*, 1926).

**spectrum**   A series or range of elements belonging to the same class, usually with the elements listed in order of strength, severity, or some similar measure. Spectrum appears to have become a vogue term in psychiatry, with descriptions of *depression spectrum* (q.v.), *OCD spectrum*, *schizophrenia spectrum*, etc.

**spectrum, psychotherapeutic**   The entire range of psychotherapeutic techniques.

**spectrum, schizophrenic**   A hypothesized range of psychopathologic states that share a genetic etiology with classic schizophrenia; the differences between the states are differences in intensity that may be due to environmental or genetic modification of the genetic diathesis necessary for development of any of the spectrum's variants. (Kety, S. S., et al. *Schizophrenia Bulletin 2*, 1976) See *reactive psychosis; schizoidia*.

**spectrum, subaffective**   An inexact term that varies with the diagnostic/classificatory system of the user to refer to a range of mood abnormalities that do not fulfill the criteria for major affective disorder because they are chronic and prolonged rather than acute and self-limited in duration, or because they are subtle and ill-defined rather than clear-cut and unmistakable, or because they fail to crystallize into discrete or predictable episodes.

Included within the group by one or more workers at one time or another are cyclothymia, dysthymic disorder, atypical depression or mania, hysteroid dysphoria, and masked depression. See *affective disorders*.

**speech**   Vocalization, vocal behavior; the ability to express thoughts or feelings by articulate sounds; the motor act of expressing language, including fluency, articulation, prosody, and voice. Some neuroscientists restrict the term to the components of language that are involved in the sensorimotor control of the vocal system. *Language* (q.v.) is typically expressed through speech but does not depend on it; semantic communication can occur without vocalization, as in writing or sign language. Auditory feedback—hearing the voices not only of others but also of one's self—is necessary for vocal learning; if children become deaf, even in late childhood, speech deteriorates.

There are two basic requirements to speech: a vocal tract with mouth and pharynx of approximately equal length, and a large brain. By 200,000 to 400,000 years ago the modern speech package was in place, but at a cost: the big brain consumes a large amount of energy, and a dropped larynx raises the risk of choking. See *grammar; language; preadaptation; semantics; syntax.*

**speech, scattered**   A type of speech commonly found in hebephrenic schizophrenia and marked especially by the lack of relevancy and coherence. This lack is due primarily to the patient's tendencies to condensation and the formation of neologisms. The patient condenses a whole series of allied events into a single word or phrase. See *scattering.*

**speech defect**   Speech impairment; speech impediment; a regular, involuntary deviation from normal pronunciation that is not of such extent or severity as to warrant a diagnosis of speech disorder.

**speech derailment**   A type of *paraphasia*, most commonly seen in schizophrenic disorders, in which speech mannerisms substitute for meaningful content. Whatever message the subject may be trying to communicate is lost in the bellowings, screechings, murmurings, or whispers that replace modulated, logical, and orderly speech.

**speech disorders**   Lalopathies; logopathy; all abnormalities or impediments in language production that are not due to faulty innervation of speech muscles or organs of articulation: included on the motor end are disturbances in gestures (*amimia*), voice (*aphonia*), speech (*aphasia*), and pictorial or symbolic representation (*agraphia*); and on the sensory end inability to perceive or understand gestures (*sensory amimia*), sounds (*sensory aphasia*), or writing (*alexia*). Some use the term in a very limited sense, to refer only to *stuttering* and *specific developmental disorders* (qq.v.). Others include a broader range of disorders within the term, and although there is no standard classification, a tripartite subdivision

is often used: (1) central disorders, or *aphasia* (q.v.); (2) output disorders (also called production disorders), such as stuttering and cluttering; and (3) input disorders (also called reception disorders), such as auditory agnosia and pure word-deafness (see *auditory aphasia*). In DSM-IV, speech and language disorders are called *communication disorders* and include (developmental) expressive language disorder, mixed receptive/expressive language disorder (formerly developmental receptive language disorder), phonological disorder (developmental articulation disorder), and stuttering.

Speech disorders have been divided phenomenologically into (1) voice disorders, such as hypo- and hypernasality, breathiness, whispering, and subvocalization; (2) fluency disorders (dysfluency), such as pausing, false starts, perseveration, disruptions by changes in topic or lack of sentence completion, distractible speech, thought blocking, and pressure of speech; and (3) prosody disorders, often manifested as affective flattening or blunting.

Although no specific risk gene for *dyslexia* (q.v.) has been identified, studies of speech and language disorders, where there are gross problems in language, have uncovered a gene that appears to be responsible for a rare and severe form of speech disorder. The gene, on chromosome 7, encodes FOXP2, one of a family of proteins that are key regulators of gene expression during embryogenesis. Disruption of FOXP2 results in difficulty in controlling the fine mouth movements required for speech, coupled with deficits in many aspects of language processing and grammatical skill.

There is a confusing array of terms that refer to specific speech disorders, but many of them include generally accepted combining forms that make them more readily comprehensible:

1. *A-* or *an-* means absence or total loss, as in *aphonia* (loss of voice) or *aphasia.*

2. *Dys-* means a partial loss or one limited to a discrete function, as in *dyslexia* (q.v.), where only certain letters or words are misread or transposed.

3. *Mogi-* or *moli-* means labored, effortful functioning, as in *mogilalia* (labored speech).

4. *Tachy-* means rapid, as in *tachylogia* (rapid word production).

5. *Brady-* means slow, as in *bradyphrenia* (slowed thinking).

6. *Hyper-* means excessive in amount, as in *hyperphrasia* (garrulousness).

7. *Hypo-* means reduced, inadequate, as in *hypomimia* (constricted range of gestures).

8. *Para-* means a qualitative change in the faculty, as in *paraphrasia* (use of a wrong phrase, malapropism).

9. *Agito-* means agitated, as in *agitolalia* (speech that is both rapid and disorganized).

10. *Embolo-* means interjection of unnecessary elements, as in *embolophrasia* (speech that is filled with meaningless or irrelevant phrases).

11. *Echo-* means repetition, as in *echolalia* (repetition by the subject of sounds or words that he hears).

Some articulation disorders have specific names:

1. *gammacism*—*g* is pronounced as *d*.
2. *lambdacism*—*l* is pronounced as *w* or *y*.
3. *rhotacism*—*r* is pronounced as *w* or *l*.
4. *sigmatism*—*s* is pronounced as *sh*, *th*, or *f*.

**speech impediment**   Any disorder of speech, but especially stammering or *stuttering* (q.v.). See *speech disorders*.

**speech organs**   See *language acquisition*.

**speech perception**   When hearing speech, the brain must convert a mass of information coming from the auditory nerve into a sequence of vocal tract positions—in effect, reconstructing configurations of the speaker's vocal tract in order to perceive the phonological structure that the speaker has in mind. See *language*.

**speech perception test**   Nonsense syllables based on the vowel sound "ee" that begin and end with different consonants are presented; on a multiple-choice form, the subject indicates what sounds were heard.

**speech processing**   The various neural tasks involved in the recognition and understanding of aurally presented speech, and in the production of speech that can reasonably be expected to be understood by the listener(s).

Speech is based on a number of building blocks, including distinctive features, segments (phonemes), syllables, morphemes, and syntactic information and composition. The sublexical task of syllable discrimination and identification is an essential part of speech perception. Speech recognition is a higher level of speech processing, the comprehension of aurally presented words; it is a set of computations that transform acoustical signals into a representation that makes contact with the mental lexicon. That speech perception and speech recognition are distinct and separate tasks is confirmed by the finding that each may be impaired while the other remains intact. See *language acquisition*.

The *dual-stream model* of speech processing proposes that an auditory ventral stream, the "sound to meaning" stream that is bilaterally organized in structures in the superior and middle temporal lobe and processes speech signals for comprehension (speech recognition); and that an auditory dorsal stream, the "sound to action" stream, is strongly left dominant in structures in the posterior frontal lobe and the posterior dorsal-most aspects of the temporal lobe and parietal operculum, and that it interfaces with the motor system by translating acoustic speech signals into articulatory representations in the frontal lobe, which is essential to speech development and normal *speech production* (q.v.). Although the dorsal stream is largely left dominant, it is probable that there is at least one pathway within each hemisphere that can process speech sounds well enough to access the mental lexicon. The superior temporal sulcus (STS) processes phonological information; its organization is bilateral, with a mild leftward bias. The middle posterior temporal regions map between phonological representations in STS and semantic representations distributed widely through the cortex (Hickok, G. & Poeppel, D. *Nature Reviews Neuroscience 8*: 393–402, 2007).

**speech production**   Speech sounds are encoded in the brain in terms of more primitive specifications, called *distinctive features* (such as vocal tract constricted or not; velum raised, or lowered to give nasal sound; vocal cords in vibration or not). Each speech sound can be described in terms of a combination of the distinctive features. The sound produced is a function of the vibration of the vocal cords coupled with the very complicated resonances of the tube. As the muscles of the vocal tract change the shape of the tube, the resonances change correspondingly, and these differences are perceived as different speech sounds. Each configuration is a symbol for a set of commands to the speech muscles. To articulate a phoneme, the commands must be executed with precise timing, the most complicated gymnastics that speakers are called upon to perform. See *language*; *speech processing*.

Neuronatomical structures known to be implicated in regulating speech production include the Broca area, premotor cortex, supplementary motor area, cerebellum, and anterior cingulate gyrus. Since all these areas form parts of circuits involving the subcortical basal ganglia, it is clear why speech production and sentence comprehension are compromised in aphasia, Parkinson disease, and cerebral anoxia, in all of which the brain mechanisms regulating speech production are impaired. At least some of the neuroanatomical structures that support the language system are also implicated in other aspects of cognition.

**speed**　See *amphetamines*.

**speedball**　See *cocaine*.

**spell, vacant**　*Absence* (q.v.).

**spells of doubting and brooding**　See *brooding spells*.

**SPEM**　Smooth pursuit eye movements, reported to be disordered in 70% to 80% of schizophrenic patients and in 45% to 50% of their first-degree relatives, but only in about 6% of normal subjects. P. S. Holzman and his coworkers posited that the abnormalities may represent a failure of inhibiting, modulating, or integrating control centers in the pontine paramedian reticular formation (*Archives of General Psychiatry 33*, 1976). See *smooth pursuit system*.

Abnormal SPEM is also known as *eye tracking dysfunction*. Eye tracking consists of various movements of the eye to get the moving target back into focus. The pursuit system corrects velocity errors and the saccadic system corrects position errors. Ordinarily, when one process is turned on, the other is turned off. In many schizophrenic patients and in almost half of their first-degree relatives, the saccadic system does not turn off as it should. Instead, there is a high prevalance of saccadic intrusions, consisting of jumpy extraneous eye movements that interrupt pursuit movements. Pursuit abnormalities reflect cortical, and particularly frontal lobe, dysfunction.

**spending spree**　Oniomania.

**sperm**　The mature germ cell(s) of a male animal; spermatozoon or spermatozoa. In the human male they are ejected from the penis in the semen (seminal fluid), which also contains the secretions of Cowper's gland, epididymis, ductus deferens, and (mainly) prostate.

At each beat of the heart, over 1000 new sperm complete their development in the testis. By the time they are mature they have already been herded into the single column of sperm on the surface of the testis, in a tube called the epididymis; from the testis to the urethra, the tube is called the vas deferens. It takes about 2 months for sperm to develop and travel from inside the testis to join the line in the epididymis for about 2 weeks, and then another 5 days or so in the vas deferens. They stay in the vas deferens until just before ejaculation, when they are shunted out into the urethra. Just below the point where urethra and bladder join, the urethra is joined by the two vas deferens (one from each side). Each of them runs to the testes and carries a column of sperm. Where they join the urethra they are surrounded by a walnut-sized mass of tissues, the prostate, which produces the bulk of the seminal fluid. Two columns of sperm—one from each testis—line up to be ejaculated. The oldest sperm are those at the head of the line, near the urethra. In intercourse, they are the first to enter the vagina.

Not all sperm are the same; only about 60% of them are the sleek egg-getters. Others are slower-moving blockers, which prevent any later sperm from passing through the cervical crypts and entering the womb; a few are killer sperm, which carry enough poison to kill many rival sperm; and some are deviant sperm (such as those with a head too small to carry the genetic message of DNA). Two types of sperm strongly reduce the chances of conception: the tapering sperm with a cigar-shaped head, and the pyriform sperm, with a pear-shaped head. The more a man is stressed, the greater the number of tapering and pyriform sperm he produces.

With ejaculation, spurts of semen hit the front wall of the cervix and run down onto the floor of the vagina, forming the seminal pool at the bottom of the chamber. The oldest sperm are likely to be introduced first; they sink to the bottom of the pool. Younger, more active sperm arrive in later spurts and go to the top of the pool. As a result, they are likely to be the first to enter the cervical mucus. With ejaculation complete, the penis begins to shrink and the vaginal walls close behind it, helping it withdraw but keeping the pool of semen in. The seminal pool coagulates, and the sperm start to migrate out of the seminal pool into the cervical channel, leaving the seminal fluid behind. The seminal fluid and any sperm left behind mix with the mucus and other cells and collect in the vestibule as the *flowback*. Once the flowback has collected in the vestibule, even a cough or sneeze will rid the woman of the unwanted material. Even if she stays asleep, the flowback becomes so liquid after about 2 hours that it will eventually begin to seep out, producing the wet sheet.

Once out of the womb, the sperm swim a short distance along an oviduct to rest areas. Another set of sperm are left in the cervical mucus, where they stream into tiny crypts in the wall of the cervix; over the following 4–5 days they re-enter the cervical channel into the womb and swim to the rest areas in the oviducts. The final set of sperm remain in the cervical mucus, where they die or are killed by the white blood cells unleashed from the walls of the womb within minutes of insemination. Eventually, they are ejected in the flowback.

Sperm may rest in an oviduct for as long as a day and, at any one time, up to a few thousand may be resting and waiting. One by one, they wake up and swim farther along the oviduct. As each leaves the fertilization zone, its place is taken by a new, fresher arrival from the rest area. The sperm go up the oviduct but usually no egg is present, and the sperm simply pass through and eventually die.

An average inseminate contains about 300 million sperm, 150 of which are ejected in the flowback. A few hundred may go straight to the oviducts, and about a million may go into the cervical crypts to form reservoirs, completing their journey to the oviducts over the 5 days following insemination. In all, about 20,000 sperm from each inseminate eventually pass through the oviducts (Baker, R. *Sperm Wars*. New York: Basic Books, 1996).

**spermatophobia**    Fear of semen.

**spermophobia**    Fear of germs.

**Sperry, Roger Wolcott**    (1914–1994) American zoologist and neurobiologist; split brain experiments defined function of corpus callosum; brain wiring; chemical affinity hypothesis of how developing neurons are directed to their target tissues.

**spes phthisica**    The feeling of hopefulness and confidence of recovery experienced by tuberculosis patients even in late stages of the disease.

**sphincter morality**    Ferenczi's term for those forerunners of the superego that arise from introjection of parental (usually maternal) prohibitions and demands having to do with toilet training.

**spider's web test**    A test of the biological effects of various body fluids (urine, serum, etc.) on the pattern of a spider's web. It has been reported, that schizophrenic urine gives different and more marked pattern changes than does nonschizophrenic urine.

**Spielmeyer-Vogt disease**    (Walter Spielmeyer, German neurologist, 1879–1935, and Oskar Vogt, contemporary German neurologist) A type of *Tay-Sachs disease* (q.v.); pigmentary retinal lipoid neuronal heredodegeneration.

**spike-and-wave**    The dart-and-dome type of electroencephalographic tracing seen in *petit mal epilepsy* (q.v.).

**spina bifida**    Rachischisis; a developmental defect in the spinal column due to failure of fusion of the dorsal walls of the primitive ectodermal neural canal. Although this defect may exist anywhere along the spine, it is usually situated posteriorly in the median line in the lumbar region.

**spina bifida occulta**    That type of spina bifida in which the bony defect is covered by skin and therefore hidden from view.

**spinal accessory nerve**    The eleventh cranial nerve. The spinal accessory nerve is motor to the trapezius and sternocleidomastoid muscles. Unilateral paralysis results in inability to rotate head to unaffected side, atrophy of sternocleidomastoid, inability to shrug affected shoulder, and drooping of affected shoulder. Bilateral paralysis results in difficulty in rotating head or lifting chin and in a dropping forward of the head.

**spinal and bulbar muscular atrophy**    SBMA (q.v.).

**spinal gating**    A theory of how pain impulses are conducted within the central nervous system; according to this theory, afferent fibers exert an inhibitory action on pain perception, and an analyzer or coordinating mechanism in cells of the substantia gelatinosa (the *spinal gate* or *gating mechanism*) transmits the sum of the net stimulus from both excitatory and inhibitory signals to the brain, and also modifies the pain signals themselves in accordance with messages coming to the core from higher centers. Such a theory provides a way of explaining the influence of personality, memory of past experiences, emotional factors, etc., on the total experience of pain, and it further suggests that relief of pain may be achieved not only by interrupting excitatory fibers but also by stimulating inhibitory pain fibers.

**spindles, sleep** See *sleep.*

**spines** See *dendrite.*

**spinocerebellar ataxias** *SCAs*; dominantly transmitted, progressive, neurodegenerative disorders characterized by abnormal protein polyglutamine expansions; the brain areas typically affected are the basal ganglia, brainstem nuclei, cerebellum, and spinal motor nuclei. General clinical manifestations include ataxia, dysarthria, difficulty with fine motor tasks, Parkinsonism, ocular abnormalities (such as supranuclear ophthalmoplegia, slow saccades, and optic atrophy), rigidity, spasticity, amyotrophy, peripheral neuropathy, and mild to moderate dementia. The diagnostic pathological feature is olivopontocerebellar atrophy. There is no treatment to slow progression or prevent onset of symptoms in any of the SCAs.

SCA-3, Machado-Joseph disease, is the most common ataxia in the world. Other ataxias in this group include include SCAs 1, 2, 7, and 17.

The disease gene has been identified for 12 genetic variants of familial ataxia and dentatorubral-pallidoluysian atrophy (DRPLA). The disease genes for SCA1–3, 6–7, 17, and DRPLA harbor expansions of CAG repeats that are translated into long polyglutamine (polyQ) tracts in the corresponding proteins. Huntington disease and Kennedy disease (X-linked spinal and bulbar muscular atrophy) share the same CAG-expansion mutation. The expanded polyQ triggers disease, but the protein context also has an important role. Expanded polyQ proteins might become neurotoxic to specific cell subtypes owing to highly selective protein–protein interactions that are driven by the unique properties of the pathogenic protein.

In most polyQ diseases there are microscopic aggregates of evidence of pathogenic protein in the cytoplasm and nucleus of affected neurons—intranuclear inclusions. Most of the autosomal dominant SCAs are caused by toxic gain-of-function mutations that lead to major derangements in the fine control of protein folding and recycling, stress responses, and transcriptional regulation (Taroni, F. & DiDonato, S. *Nature Reviews Neuroscience 5*: 641–655, 2004).

**spinocerebellum** See *cerebellum.*

**Spitz, René A.** (1887–1974) Austrian-born psychoanalyst; developmental studies; pioneer in applying research methods to Freud's analytic concepts of child development.

**splicing** Excision of introns and joining of exons to form a mature messenger RNA.

**splicing, gene** Any of the various techniques of *recombinant DNA* experiments, in which pieces of the genetic material from different species can be combined ("spliced") and inserted into living bacterial cells. It is clear that such experiments can yield invaluable information about heredity and the ways in which genes function, but at the same time many possible hazards have been envisaged (e.g., "supergerms" of high virulence or the deliberate, malevolent manipulation of human heredity). It is generally agreed that the possible dangers warrant some regulation of recombinant DNA research; the question of how stringent and restrictive such regulation should be remains a hotly debated issue.

**splinter skills** See *idiot savant.*

**split bad object** See *libidinal ego.*

**split double-bind** See *double bind.*

**split object relations unit** See *libidinal ego.*

**split-brain preparation** A surgical procedure in which the *corpus callosum* (q.v.) and other fibers connecting the two cerebral hemispheres are severed. See *cerebral dominance.*

**splitting** A primitive defense consisting of the active dissociation of mutually contradictory feelings, perceptions, and ideas into "all good" and "all bad"; separation of the endangered elements of the self from the endangering elements (within the self as well as from the external world), typically followed by projection of the endangering elements onto others.

According to Melanie Klein, *primary splitting* is a way of organizing experience characteristic of the *paranoid-schizoid position* (q.v.). In order to survive, the child separates the unconscious phantasies and anxieties related to his drives into absolutely good and bad (e.g., the absolutely persecutory and gratifying breast). He can then simultaneously project them and introject them again, creating an internal world made up of good and bad internal objects.

The term is used in a variety of ways by different authors—as the counterpart to synthesis in psychic structure formation, as a description of pathologic coexistent suborganizations of psychic structure, as a way to organize external reality on the basis of whether the specific early experiences were "pleasurable good" or "painful bad," and as a mechanism of defense against ambivalent feelings toward an object (Lichtenberg, J. D. & Slap, J. W. *Journal of the American Psychoanalytic Association 21*, 1973).

Splitting consists of compartmentalization of opposite and conflicting affect states; the subject may be aware of his contradictory, ambivalent attitudes but fails to recognize that they spring from his own internal conflicts. See *identity diffusion. Split object-relations unit* refers to a self-percept and self-concept being damaged, bad, incomplete, etc. This pathologic form of internalized object relation is an outgrowth of inadequate mother–infant interaction during the process of *individuation-separation* (q.v.), particularly in the rapprochement subphase. See *basic fault; partialism, persistent.*

In DSM-III-R, splitting is a defense mechanism in which the subject, when faced with stress or conflict, views himself or others as all good or all bad, or alternately idealizing and devaluing the same object. In splitting, the subject in unable to integrate the positive and negative qualities of self or object, or both, into cohesive images. See *cohesive self.*

**spoiled child reaction**　　Behavior reaction of children due to parental oversolicitude, overindulgence, and overprotection. Such children do not learn the value or even the meaning of regularity, self-care, responsibility, or independence.

**spondylitis**　　Inflammation of one or more of the vertebrae.

**spongiform encephalopathy**　　See *virus infections.*

**spongioma**　　See *glioma; intracranial tumor.*

**spontaneity state**　　"Spontaneity state is the condition which a subject has to attain in order to produce an emotion or role at will.... The subject voluntarily realizes a state which he usually experiences as something coming up against his will. In the spontaneity state he develops a relative distance from the states or

roles which he ordinarily embodies" (Moreno, J. L. *Das Stegreif Theater*, 1926).

**spontaneity training**　　"The spontaneity training process is an intensification of the assignment technique. New situations and new roles demand from some individuals spontaneous elements which are lacking. It is through graduated training of the personality in constructed situations and roles that such individuals learn how to act on the spur of the moment and how to integrate these roles into their personality without loss of spontaneity" (Moreno, J. L., and Jennings, H. *Sociometric Review 17*, 1936).

**spontaneous imagery**　　See *imagery, spontaneous.*

**spoon feeding**　　Feeding of another person (e.g., an infant) by putting a spoon filled with food to his lips; by extension, the expression has come to refer to any manifestation of oversolicitude that prevents or obstructs the development of independence on the part of the one being "fed." Psychiatric residents, for example, who receive so much individual case supervision that they never treat a patient completely by themselves are spoken of as being spoon-fed.

**spoonerism**　　See *cluttering.*

**sporadic**　　In genetics, not inherited; nongenetic.

**spousal abuse**　　See *battering; domestic violence.*

**spread of activation**　　See *parallel distributed processing.*

**spreading depression of Leão**　　(A. A. P. Leão, Brazilian physiologist, b. 1914) Decrease in neuronal activity (related to a decrease in metabolic demand) extending from the site of cortical stimulation; the phenomenon is believed to be responsible for the decrease in cerebral blood flow that accompanies the aura of migraine.

**spur cell**　　See *choreoacanthocytosis.*

**squalor**　　*Senile breakdown; senile recluse; Diogenes syndrome; Havisham syndrome; Plyushkin syndrome;* characterized by gross self-neglect, domestic filth and disorganization, social withdrawal, domestic squalor, apathy, a tendency to hoard rubbish, and lack of shame, and often associated with frontal lobe dysfunction.

**squeeze technique**　　An exercise used in the treatment of premature ejaculation in which the subject or his partner stimulates the erect penis until the subject feels close to orgasm; stimulation of the penis is stopped immediately and the coronal ridge of the penis is squeezed for several seconds. The process is repeated several times to raise the threshold of excitability. The *stop-start technique* is similar except that the penis is not squeezed.

**SQUIDS** Superconducting quantum interference devices. See *MSI*.

**squiggles** A game with children devised by Winnicott: the therapist makes a stroke or doodle on a sheet of paper and asks the patient to turn it into something. The child then adds a stroke, and thereafter therapist and patient alternate in adding to the doodle, yielding a drawing that provides information about the child's state of mind.

**SRIF** Somatotropin release-inhibiting factor; *somatostatin* (q.v.).

**SRI-related neonatal syndrome** A self-limited behavioral syndrome associated with maternal exposure to a serotonin reuptake inhibitor or a serotonin-norepinehrine reuptake inhibitor for a minimum of the final trimester of pregnancy through delivery. The most common manifestations in the neonate are tremors, jitteriness, or shivering; increased muscle tone; feeding or digestive disturbances; irritability or agitation; and respiratory distress. Onset ranges from birth to 3 weeks and duration of signs from 2 days to 1 month (in most cases, less than 2 weeks).

**SRO** In psychiatry and sociology, single room occupancy, referring to buildings made up of single rooms for occupants from the outcasts of society—alcoholics, addicts, the mentally ill, the crippled and chronically disabled, and the lonely aged. SRO buildings are privately equivalents of 19th-century poorhouses and a major indicator of social disintegration. They form a closed and isolated ghetto whose residents have no reference groups or roles outside the physical limits of the buildings themselves. Lacking primary families and living with others of their kind in close quarters under control of a landlord-manager, welfare occupants are subject to profound dehumanization. They need outreach services and education on how to use available facilities if they are to be rescued from the cycle of poverty, sickness, and crime.

**SRY** Sex-determining region of Y, a gene located on the short aim of the Y chromosome that by itself can induce maleness. Unless a Y chromosome is present, the embryo will develop as a phenotypic female; if the Y chromosome is present, the embryo will develop as a phenotypic male, no matter how many X chromosomes there may be.

**SSLPs** *Simple sequence length polymorphisms; microsatellites*; variations in the number of repeats of a simple sequence such as [CGG], exploited as DNA markers for intraspecific crosses.

**SSPE** See *panencephalitis, subacute sclerosing*.

**SSRI** Selective serotonin reuptake inhibitor. See *antidepressant*.

**SST** 1. *Social skills training* (q.v.). 2. Self-Statement Training, a cognitive approach to the treatment of agoraphobia that aims to replace self-defeating cognitions with positive self-statements in confronting and coping with the feared situation.

**St. Louis encephalitis** A virus infection of the brain that occurs most often in summer epidemics, spread through mosquito vectors. The brain stem, basal ganglia, and white matter of the cerebral hemispheres are mainly involved. Mortality probably does not exceed 20%; in the remainder, recovery is rapid (10–14 days) and ordinarily complete.

**stable cells** See *neurometrics*.

**staccato speech** Scanning speech; see *scanning*.

**stage** A phase or epoch of development; also termed era, life stage, period, season.

**stage fright** A *social phobia* (q.v.) of actors, singers, dancers, and other entertainers, consisting of fear of performing or of receiving a negative evaluation by the audience. The actor fears that he will stutter as he says his first line, that she will forget her lines; the soprano fears she won't hit the top note in an aria; the flutist fears a finger cramp, or a sneeze in the middle of his solo.

In the days when every action was subjected to psychoanalytic scrutiny, stage fright was interpreted as a need to ward off exhibitionism and scopophilia, which if indulged might provoke castration, and at the same time a way to gain reassurance from the audience that the dreaded castration has not occurred. It was also interpreted in terms of aggression and masochism. See *pseudoaggression; social anxiety disorder*.

**stage of resistance** See *general adaptation syndrome*.

**stagnant anoxia** See *anoxia, cerebral*.

**stalemate, analytic** See *id resistance*.

**staleness** See *aviator's neurasthenia*.

**stalking** *Obsessional following*; a chronic behavior consisting of the willful, malicious, and repeated following and harassing of another person; the stalker's repeated, intrusive contact or communications instill fear or distress in the other person and threaten the latter's safety. Stalking develops over a period of months or years, beginning typically with unwanted telephone calls (sometimes hundreds a day), physical approaches, e-mail messages (*web-stalking, cyberstalking*), sending gifts (e.g., flowers, pornographic pictures, photographs of the victim to demonstrate that the stalker has been keeping tabs on the victim), or initiating spurious legal actions involving the victim. *Stalking by proxy* is a particular form of cyberstalking in which the stalker, having obtained personal data about his or her victim, poses to be that person on the Internet and solicits viewers to contact the victim for sexual favors. The same technique encourages viewers to deluge the victim with slanderous incentives or threats of personal harm.

The stalking acts can express a range of motivations: anger, jealousy, rage over abandonment, striving for power, and a need to control the victim. Most stalkers (also called *obsessional pursuers*) do not become violent, and homicide occurs in less than 2% of cases. When it does occur, violence is affective rather than predatory. The victim's risk for violence appears to be highest when *dramatic moments* occur: events that humiliate or enrage the stalker, such as the first rejection by the victim or intervention by a third party (including the police or the court) who orders the stalker to desist. Most stalking victims have intrusive recollections and flashbacks; as many as one-third meet the criteria for post-traumatic stress disorder. See *predatory violence*. About 30% of stalkers' victims are former partners, 25% are professional contacts (physicians, mental health professionals, lawyers), and the remainder are casual acquaintances or have had no known contact with the stalker.

M. Zonana et al. (in Meloy J. R, ed. *The Psychology of Stalking: Clinical and Forensic Perspectives, San Diego: Academic Press*, 1998) divide stalkers into four groups:

1. *Erotomanic*—account for ca. 10%; primary diagnosis of delusional disorder, erotomanic subtype. The stalker is typically a woman pursuing a male stranger. Duration is the longest (more than 1 year) of the four groups; violence risk is the lowest among the groups. See *erotomania*.

2. *Love obsessional*—also called "intimacy seekers"—they account for ca. 30% of stalkers. Most often, the stalker is a male pursuing a female acquaintance or stranger, with a fanatical love toward the subject; if erotomanic beliefs are present, they are secondary to a major mental disorder. This group probably includes what others have called *incompetent suitors*—often intellectually limited; their pursuit is sustained by hopefulness; they stalk one person for a short time but are likely to move onto others.

3. *Simple obsessional*—most frequent (over 50%); typically a male with drug dependency or abuse combined with a personality disorder; usually the man has been rejected when pursuing a woman with whom he was sexually intimate at some prior time; some label this group *rejected stalkers*. A subtype is the group of *resentful stalkers*; aggrieved workers who feel they have been humiliated or mistreated, and stalk the person they blame or one who represents the firm who employed them. Duration is shortest (less than 1 year), and violent risk the highest within this group.

4. *False victimization syndrome*—infrequent (2%)—the victim alleges it but is not in fact being stalked; motivation may be conscious (an alibi), subconscious (attention-seeking), or delusional (persecution).

Within the above groups are what others label *predatory stalkers*—infrequent (4%); they stalk their victim in preparation for a physical or sexual assault and take sadistic pleasure in causing pain; an exclusively male group, many of them with paraphilias and prior convictions for sexual offenses. Often the stalker demonstrates a narcissistic or borderline personality disorder within a social context of chronic sexual mating failure, social isolation, loneliness, and a major loss.

**stammering** A speech disorder characterized by spasmodic, halting, or hesitating utterance. The term is used by many authorities interchangeably with *stuttering* (q.v.).

**standard deviation (SD, Σ)** A summary of the variation of the items in a frequency distribution. It is the square root of the mean square of the deviation of each variable in the series from the mean of the series. See *mean deviation*.

**standard drink** In the literature on alcohol, 12–14 g. of ethanol, which corresponds to

12 oz. beer, 5 oz. wine, or 1.5 oz of 80-proof liquor. See *alcohol use, unhealthy.*

**Standard Social Science Model (SSSM)** The SSSM proposes a fundamental division between biology and culture. Biology endows humans with the five senses, a few drives like hunger and fear, and a general capacity to learn. But biological evolution has been superseded by cultural evolution. *Culture* is an autonomous entity that carries out a desire to perpetuate itself by setting up expectations and assigning roles, which can vary arbitrarily from society to society.

**standardized rate** A hypothetical rate that would prevail if a given population had the same relative distribution (i.e., with respect to age) as another population called the standard.

**standing mute** *Rare.* Refusing to plead or say anything when arraigned; in such cases, the court may order a plea of not guilty to be entered for the accused and the trial or hearing may then continue.

**Stanford-Binet test** "The revised Stanford-Binet Intelligence Scale is the test most frequently used in the individual examination of children. It consists of 120 items, plus several alternative tests that are applicable to the age range between two years and adulthood. The tests have a variety of activities of graded difficulty, both verbal and performance, designed to tap a variety of intellectual functions such as memory, free association, orientation in time, language comprehension, knowledge of common objects, comparison of concepts, perception of contradictions, understanding of abstract terms, the ability to meet novel situations and the use of practical judgment. In addition to many other varieties of function, there are also tests of visual-motor coordination" (Masserman, J. H. *The Practice of Dynamic Psychiatry*, 1955). The score is expressed in months of mental age, which is divided by the chronological age (in months) and then multiplied by 100 to give the intelligence quotient.

**STAPP** *Short-term anxiety-provoking psychotherapy* (q.v.).

**STAR*D** Sequenced Treatment Alternatives to Relieve Depression; a series of four randomized controlled treatment trials in a broadly representative group of outpatients with nonpsychotic major depressive disorder who are candidates for medication as a first treatment

step. One or more acute treatment steps are used to achieve symptom remission; because no treatment is a panacea, several sequential treatment steps are often needed to obtain remission with a tolerated treatment. Measurement-based care methods are used to ensure timely dose adjustments and timely progression to the next treatment step when remission is not achieved at a tolerable dose at the current treatment step.

At Step 1, subjects are treated with citalopram. Those who do not achieve remission or an adequate benefit are encouraged to proceed to Step 2, which provides seven possible treatments: four switch treatments (from citalopram to sustained-release bupropion, cognitive therapy, sertraline, or extended-release venlafaxine) and three augmentation treatments (citalopram plus bupropion, buspirone, or cognitive therapy). Patients can choose which switch or augmentation strategies are to be used (in both Step 2 and Step 3). Patients who do not achieve remission or are unable to tolerate their assigned treatment at Step 2 can proceed to Step 3, which offers two medication switch strategies (mirtazapine or nortriptyline) or two medication augmentation strategies (lithium or 25 mg of $T_3$). Patients who do not receive adequate benefit in Step 3 can proceed to Step 4, which offers tranylcypromine or extended release venlafaxine plus mirtazapine.

Results to date indicate the following:

1. Not all patients achieve remission with the agents used. It may be that there are some kinds of depression that require other types of treatment (e.g., ECT, vagus nerve stimulation, transcranial magnetic stimulation, augmentation with second-generation antipsychotics), or that comorbid general medical or psychiatric disorders induce biological changes that render some treatments ineffective, or that some patients are not treated early enough.

2. Remission at entry into follow-up is associated with a better prognosis than simple improvement without remission.

3. The more treatment steps required, the higher the relapse rates, and the mean time for relapse is shorter for those who require two or more steps (Rush, A. J. et al. *American Journal of Psychiatry 163*: 1905–1917, 2006).

**stasibasiphobia** Fear of standing or walking. See *astasia-abasia.*

**stasiphobia**   Fear of standing (up), delusion of inability to stand. See *astasia*.

**stataesthesia**   Perception of constancy of pressure, as in maintaining pressure in a balloon by hand compression.

**state dependence**   Behavior that is a reflection to or a reaction of the state under which it occurs, rather than being primarily determined by the subject; reactive rather than constitutionally determined behavior.

**state-dependent learning**   *SDL/R* (state-dependent learning and retrieval); *dissociated learning*; acquisition of a skill during a drug state and subsequent best performance when the subject is in the same drug state, with worst performance when the subject is free of the drug.

**statins**   Oral cholesterol-lowering drugs that act by inhibiting 3-hydroxy-3-methylglutaryl coenzyme A reductase inhibitors. They might be effective in treating certain neurological diseases—in particular MS, AD, and ischemic stroke. They have anti-inflammatory effects that are independent of their ability to lower cholesterol. They inhibit inducible nitric oxide (NO) synthase (iNOS) and NO production and so might ameliorate the detrimental effects of free radicals. They ameliorate the clinical signs of experimental autoimmune encephalomyelitis, the prototypical animal model of MS, in part by inhibiting activation of T cells They might also influence Aβ production and aggregation. The clinical evidence to date is not strong enough, however, to warrant their use in patients with MS, AD, or ischemic stroke.

**statistical learning**   Combining pattern detection and computational abilities to acquire knowledge by computing information about the distributional frequency with which certain items occur in relation to others, or probabilistic information in sequences of stimuli, such as the odds—transitional probabilities—that one unit will follow another in a given language. Infants are sensitive to the relative distributional frequencies of phonetic segments in the language that they hear. See *language acquisition*; *NLNC hypothesis*.

**statistical trend**   See *trend, statistical*.

**status**   The relative position or rank of a person in a group, or of a group in reference to some larger grouping. See *class, social*. In medicine, the term implies the presence of some abnormal state or pathological condition.

**status dysraphicus**   A variety of developmental anomalies resulting from faulty closure of the neural groove at an early embryological stage. It seems to be hereditary and is believed to be the basis of such neurological diseases as hereditary ataxia and spinal gliosis (syringomyelia).

**status epilepticus**   Generalized convulsive status epilepticus (*GCSE*); the recurrence without interruption of grand mal seizures in an epileptic; seizures persisting for longer than 10 minutes. Status epilepticus is the most common cause of death in epileptics; mortality exceeds 20%. It occurs more frequently in symptomatic than in idiopathic epilepsy, and it often appears to be precipitated by withdrawal or change of anticonvulsant medication, or by intercurrent infection (where pyrexia may produce a state of internal withdrawal from medication). Other causes include occlusive cerebrovascular disease, hypertensive and metabolic encephalopathies, neoplasm, head trauma, degenerative diseases of the brain, and, sometimes, collagen disorders and similar systemic diseases. See *NCSE*.

**status marmoratus**   See *torsion dystonia*.

**status offenders**   Noncriminal juvenile offenders, such as runaways, truants, and so-called "ungovernable" youths. The status offender is thus differentiated from the juvenile delinquent, a youth under 18 whose offense, if committed by an adult, would constitute a crime. Many clinicians, however, believe that status offenders are no different from juvenile delinquents. Status offenders and youths clearly in need of stronger external controls—not necessarily only the most dangerous youths—are deprived of adequate protection from themselves by decriminalization and placement in loosely structured settings. The preoccupation with due process and righting the wrongs of the past has frequently led to overlooking the potentially harmful effects to the adolescent of placing his interest of freedom first.

Since 1968 there has been a move to deinstitutionalize status offenders, based on the labeling theory that children are stigmatized by the juvenile justice system and thereby pushed into further crime. No firm data support such a theory, however, and providing alternatives to detention may have unintended consequences, such as identifying more youths as offenders and increasing court referrals of status offenders who would otherwise be released by the police.

**status raptus**   *Ecstasy* (q.v.).

**status syndrome**   The higher the social position, the better the health of a person; by this term, M. G. Marmot drew attention to the social gradient in health in people who are not poor. The gradient is not due primarily to differences in medical care, in health behaviors, or in material circumstances. Instead, it is related to the need for autonomy (control over one's life) and full social participation. It is not position within a social hierarchy *per se* that accounts for worse health in persons of lower status, but what position within the hierarchy can do. Low social position is linked to activity of the two main stress pathways (the sympatho-adrenomedullary axis and the hypothalamic-pituitary adrenal axis).

**Stauder lethal catatonia**   See *catatonic cerebral paralysis.*

**steady state**   In pharmacology, the equilibrium achieved when the amount of medication leaving the bloodstream for other parts of the body is the same as the amount returning to the bloodstream from other parts of the body. Ordinarily, a steady state is not reached until after three or four half-lives of the drug.

**stealing splurge**   A form of behavior disorder in children: the child strives to attain status in the group either by proving himself daring and competent in acts of stealing or by using the articles or money stolen as gifts to purchase the favor of the other members of the group.

**Stedman, Charles H.**   (1805–1866) American psychiatrist; one of "original thirteen" founders of Association of Medical Superintendents of America (forerunner of American Psychiatric Association).

**Steele-Richardson-Olszewski**   **syndrome**   See *supranuclear palsy.*

**Stekel, Wilhelm**   (1868–1940) German sexologist and psychoanalyst; advocated activity as a means to shorten the duration of treatment. Through sympathy and imaginative or intuitive insight the therapist alerts himself to the patient's repressed complexes and then is expected to intervene actively to make the patient aware of them.

**stellate neuron**   A star-shaped nerve cell, smaller and shorter than most because it deals with local processing within CNS, sending messages to other cells in its immediate vicinity.

**stem, brain**   It includes the *pons* and *medulla oblongata* (qq.v.).

**stem cell**   *ES (embryonic stem cell)*; the undifferentiated, pluripotent embryonic stem cell, which gives rise to most of the specialized cell types found in adults; in the CNS, a cell with the potential to differentiate into neurons, astrocytes, and oligodendrocytes and to self-renew sufficiently to provide the numbers of cells in the brain. A *progenitor* has a more restricted potential than a stem cell; the term refers to any cell that is earlier in a developmental pathway than another. See *glia.*

ES's can divide for indefinite periods in culture and are a potential source of replacement cells for the treatment of many diseases. ES cells are obtained from aborted fetuses or spare early-stage embryos donated by couples undergoing in vitro fertizilization (IVF) treatment for fertility. The use of ES is controversial because of concerns about potential misuse (e.g., to clone humans) and differing views about what constitutes the actual beginning of human life. See *neural stem cells.*

**stema**   *Obs.* Penis.

**steppage gait**   *Foot-drop gait* due to paralysis of the anterior tibial group of muscles, as in alcoholic neuritis, peroneal nerve injuries, poliomyelitis, and progressive muscular atrophy. The patient raises his affected knee high; his foot flops with the toe dragging along the floor.

**steppingstone theory**   The assumption that use of gateway drugs (such as alcohol and marijuana) predisposes to use and abuse of other classes of ("harder") drugs.

**STEPPS**   Systems Training for Emotional Predictability and Problem Solving; an outpatient psychoeducational, cognitive behavioral, skills-training approach developed for treatment of patients with *borderline personality disorder* (q.v.), which is viewed as an *emotional intensity disorder* (*EID*). The program of 2 hours per week for 20 weeks has three components: awareness of illness, emotional management, and behavior management skills. Poetry, artwork, relaxation exercise, and music supplement worksheets and homework assignments. Improvement has been reported in multiple domains, including mood, behavior, and health care utilization variables.

**stereoagnosis**   See *parietal lobe.*

**stereoencephalotomy**   Production of cortical or subcortical lesions through the use of the stereotaxic apparatus, which permits carefully controlled penetration of brain matter by the needle.

**stereognosis**　The ability to judge the shape and form of an object by means of touch. See *parietal lobe.*

**stereopsyche**　The primitive part of the mind that has to do with primitive types of motility. Storch applied this term to certain motor manifestations seen in schizophrenia: the catatonic postures and movements that seem to be isolated from the personality and to have a meaning independent of the rest of the psychic structure. These archaic types of motility arise from the deeper layers of the motor apparatus after the ego has disintegrated.

**stereotactic tractotomy**　*Seed psychosurgery*; of implantation of radioactive yttrium-90 seeds in the substantia innominata below the head of the caudate nucleus. The procedure has been reported to be of benefit in intractable depression, anxiety, and obsessional states.

**stereotype**　An individual motor pattern that was originally meaningful to the subject and/or carried some private, autistic meaning for him. Stereotypes are thus to be distinguished from *primitive motor patterns* that are meaningless, inborn, or acquired very early in life, and that consist of simple movements or groups of simple movements.

**stereotype, dynamic**　A term used mainly by Russian neurophysiologists to refer to the end result of cortical analysis and synthesis of all stimuli arising from both the external and the internal world. The dynamic stereotype represents a balanced, classified, and homogeneous arrangement of all the conditioned and unconditioned processes reflected in the cortex.

**stereotypic movement disorder**　*Stereotypic habit disorder*, a childhood disorder consisting of repetitive, nonfunctional, and potentially self-injurious behavior, such as head banging, nail biting, or picking at the skin. It may occur independently or in association with mental retardation or other disorders in development.

**stereotypy**　A repeated movement that does not appear to be goal-directed, such as incessant rubbing of some part of the body; it is more complex than a tic.

The foregoing is often called *stereotypy of motion.* There is also *stereotypy of posture*, the patients maintaining a given posture for inordinately long periods. And there is *stereotypy of place*; catatonic patients may occupy an identical place month in, month out, year in, year out; stereotypy of speech is called *cataphasia.*

**sterility**　The state or quality of being infertile or barren. This condition may be produced either by primary genetic disturbances in the sex chromosome constitution of an individual or by secondary effects on the phenotype, both of internal pathological processes and of surgical interference for medical or eugenic purposes. See *sterilization.*

It is estimated that approximately 15% of married couples in the United States are unable to conceive; in 20% of these no cause can be determined. Of the rest, 40% are found to have a male factor deficiency, 20% a female hormonal defect, 30% a female tubal disorder, and 10% a cervical defect.

The pathological processes that may be involved in the production of sterility include mechanical obstruction (e.g., scar tissue secondary to infection); developmental abnormalities (e.g., sex chromatin abnormalities); imbalance, diminution, or absence of gonadotrophin excretion secondary to pituitary, hypophyseal, or hypothalamic disturbances (e.g., radiation, infection, vascular disorder, trauma, malnutrition and inanition, or degenerative disease). In the male, sterility may be secondary to impotence (male erectile disorder), which itself may be due primarily to psychological factors, substance-induced, or due to general medical conditions (e.g., diabetes mellitus, multiple sclerosis, spinal cord injury).

**sterilization**　Any process (brought about spontaneously or by deliberate action) that causes a person to become sterile. When performed for medical reasons, it aims at rendering conception impossible, ordinarily without affecting the ovaries or testes. Accordingly it is not an "unsexing" operation, and neither inhibits sex desires nor interferes with normal sex functioning.

**steroid abuse**　See *anabolic-androgenic steroids (AAS).*

**Stevens-Johnson syndrome**　*Erythema multiforme major; erythema multiforme bullosum*; an acute, inflammatory, system-disease characterized by lesions of skin and mucous membranes (macules, papules, wheals, vesicles, bullae) and systemic manifestations (fever, malaise, dehydration, muscle and joint pains, toxemia, prostration, and sometimes death). Etiology is unknown, although the majority of evidence points to the condition as secondary to any number of other disorders, among them infections, drug reactions (including barbiturates and tranquilizers), vaccination, malignancy, deep X-ray therapy, contact dermatitis, and collagen disease. See *Behçet syndrome.*

**Stewart-Morel syndrome** Internal frontal hyperostosis with adiposity and mental disturbances.

**STG** *Superior temporal gyrus*, typically larger on the left in right-handed subjects. It includes *Heschl's gyrus* and the *planum temporale* (qq.v.). STG is a major anatomical substrate for speech, language, and communication. See *spatial neglect; temporal lobe.*

**STH** Somatotropic or growth hormone (GH); one of the anterior pituitary hormones. See *general adaptation syndrome.*

**sthenic** In general medicine, strong and active; in particular, excessive action of the vital processes, as occurs in sthenic fever or sthenic mental (delusional) reaction.

In general psychology, strength and vigor in emotional reactivity and adaptability. In accordance with this concept, the psychopathological behavior of the sthenic type has been described by Kretschmer as inclined to delusional reactions of a predominantly aggressive nature (paranoia, querulous ideas of reference), in contrast to the introspective tendency in paranoid or hypochondriac reactions in sensitive types.

**sthenic type** In constitutional medicine, sthenic corresponds to Kretschmer's *athletic type* (q.v.) and its equivalents in other systems.

**stick, fecal** Fecal mass. See *anal phase.*

**stiffening involutional psychosis** See *paraphrenia.*

**stiff-man syndrome** A poorly understood syndrome, related to abnormal phosphorus metabolism, consisting of painful, ironlike spasms of muscle groups in various parts of the body. The spasms can be so severe as to cause fractures of the long bones, and most patients show secondary hypertrophy of affected muscles as well as varus deformity of the feet. Course is prolonged, and death may occur after a number of years during or shortly after a severe spasm.

**stigma, costal** See *Stiller sign.*

**stigmata** Marks resembling the wounds on the crucified body of Christ. Most psychoanalytic writers consider these monosymptomatic conversions, the afflicted areas unconsciously symbolizing the genitals, the hyperemia and swelling representing erection, and abnormal sensations imitating genital sensations. The first person known to have experienced stigmata was St. Francis of Assisi; since that time, more than 300 cases have been reported, most of them in women.

**stigmatization** The process of labeling or branding, or the process of developing the signs or traits that appear to justify being labeled or branded or singled out. *Stigmata* (q.v.) originally denoted marks resembling the bleeding wounds, on the hands, feet, or chest, of the crucified body of Christ. They were generally assumed to be signs of Divine favor. Later, stigmata referred to similar marks produced exogenously by suggestion or hypnosis or endogenously as a form of conversion hysteria. Currently the term is used to signify indicators or pathognomonic signs of a disorder or syndrome. By extension, stigmatization has come to mean the labeling or branding of any person or group as being mentally disordered or abnormal, and the use of such labels as justification for discriminating against them.

**stigmatophilia** A *paraphilia* (q.v.) in which sexual arousal and orgasm depend upon the partner being scarred, marked, tattooed, or pierced (especially in the genital or nipple region for the purpose of wearing bars, rings, etc.); the term also includes the person who must himself be so marked.

**Stiller sign** (Berthold Stiller, Budapest physician, 1837–1922) *Costal stigma*; floating tenth rib, said to be indicative of a neurasthenic tendency.

**stimulants** See *psychostimulants; smart drugs.*

**stimulating occupation** In occupational therapy, activity so varied that the lack of monotony and repetition tends to arouse and awaken to activity the slow, retarded, and depressed patient. For instance, the various activities associated with photography constitute a type of stimulating occupation.

**stimulation** See *activation.*

**stimulus, adequate** The type of stimulus energy to which a receptor is sensitive. Ordinarily, each receptor is sensitive to a narrow range of energy. See *code, labeled line.*

**stimulus barrier, maternal** See *abandonment depression*.

**stimulus control therapy** A nonpharmacological strategy for promoting sleep that includes the following injunctions: go to bed only when sleepy; use bed and bedroom only for sleep (sexual activity is allowed); if unable to sleep, move to another room and return to bedroom only when sleepy; use alarm to rise at same hour every day, no matter how little sleep has been attained; do not nap during the day; observe *sleep hygiene guidelines* (q.v.).

**stimulus onset asynchrony** See *semantic priming*.

**stimulus transduction** The process whereby the physical energy of the stimulus (mechanical, thermal, chemical, or electromagnetic) is transformed into electrochemical energy. See *transducer*.

**stimulus word** The word used in association tests to provoke a response. See *association*.

**stimulus-bound** Referring to difficulty in willed, intentional control of motor behavior. In the normal person, motor behavior is stimulus-resistant and can be controlled through thinking or reasoning despite the presence of distracting visual, tactile, or other stimuli. Stimulus-bound behavior, such as echopraxia or gegenhalten, suggests frontal lobe dysfunction.

**stir fever** See *prison psychosis*.

**stirps, stirpes** Stem; stock; the person from whom a family is descended. In genetics, all the genes that are present in, and determine the development of, the fertilized egg.

**STIs** Structured treatment interruptions; carefully monitored drug holidays, used particularly as a strategy with *HAART* (q.v.) in an attempt to reduce or avoid side effects.

**STM** *Short-term memory* (q.v.).

**STN** Subthalamic nucleus. See *basal ganglia; LID*.

**Stockholm syndrome** See *victim*.

**stool pedantry** Exaggerated promptitude and punctuality that are overcompensations for the infantile anal-erotic tendency to hold back the stool as long as possible.

**stop-start technique** See *squeeze technique*.

**stormy personality** Arieti's term for a personality type, found often in preschizophrenic patients, consisting of repeated changes in the person's attitude to life that may be slow or abrupt and commonly are sudden, violent, and drastic. Such people have no stable sense of self-identity and are forever searching for their role in life, without success. Life often seems to be little more than a series of crises for them.

**STP** A hallucinogenic drug that appears to be identical with DOM (2,5-dimethoxy4--methylamphetamine); in low dosage (less than 3 mg), DOM produces mild euphoria, but in higher dosage it produces hallucinogenic effects that last for about 8 hours. Black market preparations of STP usually contain about 10 mg of DOM. The name is derived from a commercial gasoline additive (although some maintain it is an abbreviation for serenity-tranquility-peace).

**STR** The scientific-technical revolution, generally described as being based on the belief that science can be applied to all areas of life.

**strabismus** Squint; *heterotropia*; deviation of one or both eyes from the normal axis. See *oculomotor nerve*.

**strain, recombinant** See *RI strain*.

**straitjacket** See *camisole*.

**straitjacket, chemical** *Rare.* The arresting of psychomotor overactivity by chemical means, specifically by the hypodermic injection of morphine sulfate, 1/4 grain, and hyoscine hydrobromide, 1/50 grain.

**stranger anxiety** The infant's fear of unfamiliar people, manifested by crying and clinging to the mother; in the normal infant, it first appears at approximately 26 weeks of age but is not fully developed until about 32 weeks. To be differentiated from *separation anxiety* (q.v.).

**strangulated affect** An affect that is repressed along with its attached mental content; it is retained in the unconscious and together with its psychic component produces morbid symptoms.

**Stransky, Erwin** (1877–1962) Viennese neuropsychiatrist, pupil of Wagner von Jauregg; first to publish textbook in Germany on mental health; concept of intrapsychic ataxia, the dissociation of the thymopsyche from the noopsyche, as the essential characteristic of schizophrenia.

**strategic compliance** See *compliance, strategic*.

**strategic family therapy** See *family therapy, strategic*.

**strategic intervention** See *paradoxical therapy*.

**strategic planning** Planning based on specified goals; planning geared to defining the tasks to be accomplished and assessing the need to continue those already being done. Strategic planning is opposed to *operational planning*, which is a control system geared to making sure that what is done is being done right; altering the resource commitment to programs that support the major goals of an organization in a planned way. See *functional budgeting*.

**strathmin** A mediator of both instinctive and learned fears that is found in the lateral nucleus of the *amygdala* (q.v.).

**Strauss syndrome** See *attention deficit hyperactivity disorder*.

**"street people"** The homeless who live on the streets of mainly metropolitan centers. Many of them—but by no means all—give ample evidence of psychopathology, and a significant number of these are products of *deinstitutionalization* (q.v.). The group includes *bag ladies* (so called because they often carry all their worldly possessions in one or more paper shopping bags) and *vent men* (so called because in cold weather they typically sit on or sleep over vents or grates that might be sources of warmth).

**street phobia** Fear of being in a street; *agoraphobia* (q.v.). As with all phobias, the feared street may represent a temptation (especially a situation that would ordinarily call forth an aggressive or a sexual response), or it may represent punishment for the forbidden impulse directly or indirectly through symbolism, or it may be a fear that the anxiety will return because the initial anxiety attack occurred in the street.

**strephosymbolia** Twisted symbols, the perception of objects or graphic symbols reversed as if in a mirror. A term coined by Orton for the specific reading disability due, he believes, to poorly established hemisphere dominance, so that visual impressions coming to both hemispheres are not clearly differentiated, and symmetrical engrams oriented in opposite directions are confused, as *b* and *d*, *p* and *q*. See *congenital aphasia; attention deficit hyperactivity disorder*.

**stress** Pressure; strain; a demand for response that threatens to exceed the resources of the subject. A physical stressor is an external challenge to homeostasis. A psychosocial stressor is the anticipation, justified or not, that a challenge to homeostasis looms. Psychological stressors typically engender feelings of lack of control and predictability. Both types of stressor activate an array of endocrine and neural adaptations. Definitions of stress fall generally into two groups: those emphasizing the noxious or aversive nature of the stimulus originating in the environment (e.g., negative life events) and those emphasizing the subject's physiologic responses to the stimulus (in particular, the sympathetico-adrenal medulla system and the pituitary-adrenal cortex system).

Stress initiates a cascade of events in the brain and peripheral systems that enable organisms to cope with and adapt to new and challenging situations. Effective coping requires a rapid response and efficient termination. When stress is maintained for long periods of time, most physiological systems are negatively affected because of the prolonged exposure of target cells to physiological stress mediators. See *allostasis; general adaptation syndrome; holistic healing; post-traumatic stress disorder; trauma*.

The stress response includes activation of the autonomic nervous system (ANS) and the HPA (hypothalamic-pituitary-adrenocortical) axis. HPA activation results in the production of corticotropin-releasing hormone (CRH) and vasopressin (AVP) in the paraventricular nucleus of the hypothalamus. Both peptides are released into the bloodstream and stimulate the production and secretion of ACTH from the anterior pituitary. ACTH stimulates the release and synthesis of glucocorticoids from the adrenal cortex (cortisol in humans). Appropriate regulatory control of the HPA axis is crucial for health and survival; it is accomplished through negative-feedback mechanisms that involve both rapid and genomic actions of glucocorticoids at the pituitary and at many sites in brain, including hippocampus. Inputs that arise from the amygdala elicit activation of the HPA axis. Neurons of the medial prefontal cortex have an inhibitory influence on the output regions of the amygdala.

Stress and glucocorticoids enhance concentrations of the excitatory amino acid, glutamate, in hippocampus and other brain regions. The result is an excitotoxic cascade of mechanisms, eventually leading to neuronal endangerment or neurotoxicity. With sustained stress exposure there are usually deficits in hippocampus-dependent learning and memory tasks.

**stress disorder** See *post-traumatic stress disorder.*

**stress disorder, acute** *Brief reactive dissociative disorder*; a condition that does not fully meet the criteria for *post-traumatic stress disorder* (q.v.) but is more severe than an adjustment disorder. The subject has been exposed to a traumatic event such as actual or threatened death or injury, and while witnessing or experiencing the event has felt intense fear, horror, or a sense of helplessness. At the same time, or immediately after, the subject experiences a number of symptoms: dissociative (e.g., stupor, depersonalization, detachment, amnesia), anxiety (e.g., hyperarousal, hypervigilance, intrusive recollections of the traumatic experience, sleep disturbances), anger, psychomotor agitation, despair, or social withdrawal. The episode lasts for less than 4 weeks, but the symptoms are severe enough to impair functioning and often prevent the person from obtaining appropriate medical or legal assistance or from telling family members about the experience.

**stress hypothesis** It states that depression is due to overactivation of the brain's stress machinery, and especially the HPA axis. *Stress* (q.v.) decreases the amounts of ingredients such as BDNF (brain-derived neurotrophic factor), and if long maintained it can disrupt neurogenesis in the hippocampus.

**stress interview** A type of interview in which the patient is intentionally pressured, and the usual ways of reducing anxiety during the session are deliberately avoided. Such interviews may be useful in diagnosis, but their repeated use is generally contraindicated in the course of psychotherapy.

**stress-induced analgesia** Reduced sensitivity to pain as a result of exposure to stress. Release of endogenous cannabinoid compounds is crucial for this effect. The cannabinoids act through cannabinoid 1 (CB1) receptors in the brain to activate pathways from the amygdala to the midbrain periaqueductal gray, brain stem, and spinal cord. Concentrations of the cannabinoid 2-arachidonoylglycerol (2AG) increase rapidly, within 2 minutes when a footshock is applied, whereas concentrations of another cannabinoid, anandamide, peak 7–15 minutes after the shock. In the periaqueductal gray, both 2AG and anandamide mediate the analgesic effect of stress.

**stressor, social** See *life event.*

**stretched speech** Extension of the interval between successive acoustic stimuli. Dyslexic children typically are unable to recognize the very short-duration sounds of spoken speech, and they often have similar "fast element" recognition problems in other sensory modalities, such as vision and touch. Language exercises that use stretched speech have often produced significant improvement in such children's ability to understand and respond to spoken language.

**striatal cortical inputs** Approximately 80% of all synapses in the striatum are cortical inputs, divided into the following:

1. *Motor*—which includes somatosensory, motor, and premotor cortices; in another system of nomenclature, the *matrix* compartment receives inputs most directly related to sensorimotor processing.

2. *Limbic associative*, which includes the amygdala, hippocampus and orbital, entorhinal, temporal, prefrontal, parietal, cingulate, and association cortex. In the second system of nomenclature, the *striosome* compartent receives inputs from neural structures affiliated with the limbic system.

At the striatal level a similar division occurs, with a motor putamen and a limbic caudate and ventral striatum (nucleus accumbens).

**striatal dysfunctions** They include Huntington disease (HD), Parkinson disease (PD), OCD, and Tourette syndrome (TS). See *striatum.*

OCD is characterized by intrusive cognitions, repetitive behaviors, and accompaniments of anxiety; although the cause and neuropathology of OCD are unknown, corticostriatal circuits involvng the caudate nuceleus have been implicated. A diathesis for TS appears to be heritable and related to one subtype of OCD.

Like HD, PD is a degenerative disorder with well-established neuropathologic changes within the basal ganglia. The most consistent findings in HD and PD have been in the domains of *visuospatial ability, memory*, and *executive functioning* (qq.v.). Results of studies on HD, PD, OCD, and TS suggest the following neuropsychological profile in patients with corticostriatal dysfunction: impaired encoding and delayed free recall of information, with preserved storage demonstrated by correct recognition; deficits on certain procedural memory tasks, such as those measuring perceptual and motor skill acquisition; impaired visuomotor and visoperceptual abilities; and disruption of subtle aspects of executive functions involving the appropriate maintenance and shifting of mental set. Deficits in executive functioning appear to be primary and have a secondary impact on the other domains.

**striatal syndrome**   Disease of the striatum or striopallidal system, characterized, in general, by the following: (1) rigidity (a general increase of muscle tonus); (2) tremor (abnormal involuntary movements); (3) hypokinesia (poverty of voluntary, especially spontaneous movements); (4) impairment of associated movements; (5) absence of sensory disturbances; (6) absence of "true" paralysis, that is, absence of signs of involvement of pyramidal tracts.

**striate cortex**   See *visual cortex, primary.*

**striatofugal projections**   The major output structure for the striatum is the *globus pallidus.* In both the *substantia nigra* and the globus pallidus, the relative segregation of limbic and sensorimotor inputs seen in the *striatal cortical inputs* (q.v.), is maintained. All four divisions (internal/external globus pallidus; reticulata compacta/substantia nigra) receive striatal inputs.

**striatonigral degeneration**   See *multiple system atrophy*; *Shy-Drager syndrome.*

**striatum**   The collective term for the caudate nucleus and putamen, parts of the *basal ganglia* (q.v.) The striatum is the major recipient of input to the basal ganglia by way of three afferent systems: the corticostriatal, the nigrostriatal, and the thalamostiatal projections. Disruption of these pathways has been associated with a wide variety of movement disorders and also with behavioral dysfunctions, including schizophrenia, catatonia, major depression, anorexia nervosa, and obsessive-compulsive disorder.

The striatum is believed to carry out general computation, but its role is poorly understood. It appears to mediate rule-based learning, which can wholly support unconscious information processing (such as procedural learning) that leads to the acquisition of behaviors that are performed automatically. It plays an ancillary role in enhancing the efficiency of higher-order processes such as those involved in working memory. Apparently, the spiny neurons of the striatum are able to "recognize" complex constellations of cortical inputs prioritized on the basis of temporally proximate dopaminergic modulation (i.e., reward).

The presumed motor functions of the striatum include (1) motor learning, (2) sequencing of movements, and (3) "fine-tuning" motor output. The striatum shares the workload of the cortex not only by taking over simpler functions, but also by gating and refining input and output to cortex.

The cognitive circuit is involved in a number of higher cognitive abilities, but most directly in the executive cognitive functions, including (1) attentional allocation by magnification or by filtering/suppression; (2) working memory; and (3) implicit (procedural) learning and memory. See *subcortical dementia.*

**Stribling, Francis T.**   (1810–1874) American psychiatrist; advocated training of psychiatric attendants, occupational therapy.

**striosomes**   A component of the affective-motivational circuit of the *striatum* (q.v.); the striosome compartent receives cortical inputs from the limbic-associative system. The *matrisomes* are another cluster of cells in the striatum; they receive sensorimotor cortical inputs. The striosomes and matrisomes are grouped in relation to the output from the striatum to the globus pallidus and substantia nigra. See *striatal cortical inputs; striatofugal projections.*

**stroke**   See *cerebrovascular accident.*

**stroking**   See *transactional analysis.*

**Strömgren, Eric**   (1909–1993) Danish psychiatrist, geneticist, and epidemiologist; born to Swedish parents who emigrated to Denmark via Germany. Doctoral dissertation (1938) on the genetic epidemiology of the island of Bornholm, and continued with a 50-year follow-up (1989). He perfected a national psychiatric case register that was a major influence in family, twin, and adoption studies. His textbook of psychiatry (available only in Danish) has gone through 13 editions since its appearance in 1938.

**Stroop task**   A measure of selective attention: the subject must avoid reading a word (a prepotent response) while naming its color. The Stroop task activates the anterior cingulate cortex (ACC). When subjects are required to maintain attention for the occurrence of visual and somatosensory stimuli, DLPFC and parietal cortex are activated rather than ACC. See *cingulate gyrus.*

**structural**   Pertaining to organization or arrangement. The *structural hypothesis* pertains to the description of the mental apparatus in terms of *ego*, *superego*, and *id* (qq.v.). O. Kernberg emphasizes the importance of stability and continuity of the intrapsychic organization over time, particularly as reflected in the quality of object relations (identity integration vs. identity diffusion), defensive operations (advanced vs. primitive), and reality testing (presence vs. absence) in making a *structural diagnosis*. *Structural interviewing* uses elements of the traditional mental status examination combined with a focus on the here-and-now aspects of the patient–therapist interaction and on the patient's interpersonal functioning in general to arrive at an assessment of his intrapsychic organization.

**structural analysis**   A type of psychotherapy described by E. Berne (1957), based on the belief that psychiatric disorders arise from pathological relationships between the various ego states: exteropsychic (Parent), neopsychic (Adult), and archaeopsychic (Child). Structural analysis aims at strengthening the boundaries between these states so that the Adult can become the effective executive of a healthy way of living.

**structural family therapy**   Associated with the name of Salvador Minuchin; a type of family therapy that emphasizes hierarchical relationships within the family and the boundaries between family subgroups and members. In a dysfunctional family, the hierarchical structure may be incongruous (e.g., one child may be given responsibilities that more properly belong to a parent), or boundaries may be haphazardly maintained. A therapy team is used and interactions are observed, on which basis the family is given a prescription designed to reformulate some of its basic assumptions and instigate an appropriate strategy to redefine relationships among family members.

**structural genomics**   See *genome*.

**structural imbalance**   See *imbalance, structural*.

**structural integration**   *Rolfing* (q.v.).

**structural interviewing**   See *interpretation*.

**structural profile**   In multimodal behavior therapy, the patient's self-rating of proclivities in each of the seven areas of the *BASIC-ID* (q.v.). The patient is asked to what extent he perceives himself as doing, feeling, sensing, imagining, thinking, and relating, and also to what extent he observes and practices health-promoting habits.

**structured group**   A term introduced by S. R. Slavson to emphasize the fact that the selection and combining of patients is essential for group psychotherapy, though some group psychotherapists pay little or no attention to it. Since in group psychotherapy the group is an important factor and the major therapeutic agency, it must be planned in such a way that, according to Slavson, the patients, individually and as a group, would have a therapeutic effect upon every other constituent member. He has described some of the criteria for selection and grouping in *Analytic Group Psychotherapy* (1950). This term is opposed to *blanket group*, in which no criteria for grouping are employed.

**structures**   In Fairbairn's version of *object relations theory* (q.v.), a set of internalized relationships connected with affects. They may be desired or defended against, and they may distort actual object relationships (e.g., as a neverending search for objects only because they are realizations of internalized objects).

**Strumpell sign**   (Adolf von Strumpell, German neurologist, 1853–1925) In organic hemiplegia, dorsiflexion of the hand occurs on making a fist.

**strychnomania**   *Deadly nightshade poisoning* (q.v.).

**STS**   1. Superior temporal sulcus, a sensor of biological motion (especially of eyes and lips). See *intention; temporal lobe; theory of mind*.
   2. Somatostatin. See *neuropeptides*.

**study groups**   See *Group Relations Conferences*.

**stuff eroticism**   *Hephephilia* (q.v.).

**stupor**   An imprecise term for (1) organically determined unconsciousness; (2) unresponsiveness with immobility and mutism but retention of consciousness, and often with open eyes that follow external objects; (3) mutism only.

**stupor, akinetic**   *Cairns stupor* (q.v.).

**stupor, anergic**   Stupor with immobility. As a rule patients showing the psychogenic stuporous reaction are inactive, immobile, and anergic.
   In the older literature, anergic stupor was synonymous with *primary dementia* and *stuporous insanity*.

**stupor, benign**   *Depressive stupor*, usually described as the most severe form of manic-depressive disorder, depressed type; termed benign in that it was believed to share the generally favorable prognosis of manic-depressive psychoses. Most such cases are in fact schizophrenic and in time show a more classical deteriorative course; thus, they more appropriately should be termed *malignant stupors*.

**stupor, emotional** *Affective stupor*; characterized by mutism and intense anxiety or depression.

**stupor, examination** When the emotions triggered by or associated with a test or examination are so strong as to bring thoughts and actions to a standstill, Bleuler speaks of *examination* or *emotional stupor*. See *examination anxiety*.

**stupor, exhaustive** Stupor or coma as a result of infection or intoxication. See *infective-exhaustive psychosis*.

**stupor vigilans** *Obs.* Catalepsy (q.v.).

**stuporous** Relating to or under the influence of stupor; comatose or semicomatose.

**Sturge-Weber syndrome** (William Allen Sturge, English physician, 1850–1919; Frederick Parker Weber, English physician, 1863–1962) *Encephalotrigeminal angiomatosis*; one of the *phakomatoses* (q.v.), consisting of port-wine nevus on one side of the face, glaucoma, and ipsilateral encephalomeningeal angiomatosis with cortical atrophy that is usually associated with seizures and focal neurologic signs.

**stuttering** A *speech disorder* (q.v.) or communication disorder with onset in childhood, consisting of spasmodic utterances with involuntary halts, breaks, and repetitions, usually characterized (in more severe cases) externally by sputtering due to violent expulsion of breath following a halt or stop, and by violent facial contortions. For the sake of convenience, stuttering denotes a visually more violent or explosive form of stammering.

Other terms by which stuttering has been known are balbuties, ischnophonia, ischophonia, psellism, and psallismus hesitans.

Any sound, in any position, any part of a word, and any word may be the obstacle in stuttering, varying with the individual stutterer or the severity of the symptom.

Stuttering occurs in about 1% of the population and usually appears between the ages of 2 and 6 years. Three-quarters of affected children stop stuttering within a few years, without any kind of intervention. Stuttering occurs more frequently in males (by a ratio of 4:1) and in twins. About half of those who seek treatment have a family member who also stutters. Stutterers are about twice a likely as nonstutterers to be left handed, and

they tend to have a much larger and more symmetric planum temporale (a region in the Wernicke area associated with language and music processing).

Although stuttering is generally believed to be a neurological disorder, partly genetic in origin, its consequences are largely psychological—such as shrinking from speaking through fear of not succeeding. Many types of speech therapy are based upon relaxation to reduce nervous and muscular tension; others teach speech techniques such as elongating vowels or speaking slowly. Probably many genes contribute to stuttering. Chromosomes 1 and 12 have been implicated in some studies.

**stuttering gait** A disorder in walking, usually, though not necessarily, psychogenic. It is characterized by a hesitancy in walking analogous to that observed in speech stuttering. It is sometimes seen in hysterical and in schizophrenic subjects.

**stygiophobia** Fear of hell; hadephobia.

**stylistics** See *psycholinguistics*.

**stylus tapping test** The subject is asked to tap on a stylus with a metal plate as fast as possible for 10 seconds.

**subacute combined degeneration of the spinal cord** See *posterolateral sclerosis*.

**subacute delirious state** See *delirium, subacute; subdelirious state*.

**subacute necrotizing encephalomyelopathy (SNE)** A rare, progressive, hereditary disorder of thiamine metabolism due to an abnormal protein that inhibits an enzyme essential to thiamine synthesis. Symptoms usually appear before 1 year of age, and death typically ensues within 1 year of onset. Symptoms include ataxia, nystagmus, seizures, mental retardation, peripheral neuropathy, difficulty in swallowing, and cessation of growth. Successful treatment has been reported with replacement therapy, using massive doses of thiamine or thiamine propyl disulfide.

**subarachnoid hemorrhage** *SAH*; a type of intracerebral hemorrage in which blood is released into the subarachnoid space (between the arachnoid mater and the pia mater) and the ventricular system. Intracranial hemorrhage is a frequent cause of stroke and is usually associated with hypertension, ruptured aneurysms or arteriorvenous malformation, or hematomas caused by head trauma. Trauma-induced hemorrhage produces loss of consciousness and, in some, rapid progression over a period of a few hours to days with hemiparesis, cranial nerve palsies, and death. In others, signs and symptoms progress gradually over a period of weeks. The most common symptom is *headache* (q.v.) with other neuropsychiatric manifestations paralleling the gradual increase in intracranial pressure: confusion, inattention, drowsiness, memory loss, and coma. Focal or lateralizing signs may include hemiparesis, hemianopsia, aphasia, seizures, and cranial nerve abnormalities.

**subception**   Autonomic response to a stimulus, which is not consciously recognized by the subject.

**subchoreatic state**   See *Huntington disease*.

**subchronic**   Used specifically by some to indicate a disorder that has lasted for less than 2 years.

**subclavian steal syndrome**   Symptoms of cerebral vascular insufficiency secondary to central stenosis or occlusion of the subclavian artery; blood is shunted past the occluded artery by reversal of blood flow in the vertebral artery, and blood is thereby "stolen" from the cerebral circulation. Symptoms can sometimes be removed by reconstructive vascular surgery.

**subconductance**   See *ion channel*.

**subconscious**   A term coined by Janet to denote the memories that aggregate to form the mental schemes guiding a person's interaction with the environment. Janet believed that the chief function of memory is to store and categorize incoming sensations into a mold or template into which subsequent stimuli, both internal and external, are integrated. Frightening or novel experiences (traumata) cannot be integrated properly, however, and in consequence memories can be split (dissociated) from conscious awareness and voluntary control. See *dissociation*; *hysteria*.

**subconscious personality**   M. Prince's term for any of the personalities in multiple personality that are not dominant at the moment. In his famous Beauchamp case, for example, Miss Beauchamp became the subconscious personality when Sally (another personality) took over, and vice versa. See *dissociative identity disorder*.

**subconscious self**   See *multiple personality disorder*.

**subconsciousness**   1. Partial unconsciousness. 2. The state in which mental processes take place without conscious perception on the subject's part.

**subcortical aphasia**   The most frequent signs are a combination of paraphasia, poor comprehension of spoken language, and an intact ability to repeat. These disorders are usually transient. They are usually a result of vascular lesions in the basal ganglia and thalamus. Lesions in the left caudate nucleus or putamen cause a fluent aphasia with neologistic language. Lesions in the thalamus can produce an aphasia similar to transcortical aphasia. See *aphasia*.

**subcortical   arteriosclerotic   encephalopathy** *Binswanger disease*, psychosis in association with multiple small infarcts leading to demyelination in the periventricular white matter on both sides. Clinically, the disorder manifests itself as dementia with gait disturbances. It has been estimated that as many as 30% of elderly patients, even those without neurologic impairment, have such lesions. See *VaD*.

**subcortical dementia**   The term was first used in a 1974 literature review by Albert et al. to describe a characteristic configuration of deficits: "forgetfulness," slowed thought processes (bradyphrenia), psychiatric changes (especially apathy, depression, and irritability), and impaired ability to manipulate acquired knowledge. The subcortical dementias include Parkinson disease (PD), Huntington disease (HD), Lewy body dementia (LBD), and progressive supranuclear palsy. (HD could also be classified as a triple repeat disorder; both PD and HD are also classified as striatal disorders.)

Neuropsychological features of subcortical dementias are as follows:

1. A consistent pattern of memory dysfunction—impaired learning and immediate memory, inconsistent recall across repeated learning trials, normal retention rates over delays, impaired encoding, and inefficient use of organizational strategies Recognition and cued recall are usually disproportionately better than free recall.

2. Disruption of the high-level executive abilities necessary to evaluate and select the most expedient action, monitor behavior, and shift it when appropriate. *Organizational approach* refers to the strategic process of breaking down a complex figure into simpler components, which then are used to organize construction. *Executive function* (q.v.) is often impaired—abilities including abstract

thinking, ability to profit from feedback information, judgment, and initiative. These goal-oriented patterns of behavior are thought to be mediated by frontal-subbcortical circuits; of these parallel circuits, the motor loop (connecting putamen and the supplementary motor cortex) is disrupted early.

3. Deficits in implicit memory, the process by which knowledge is acquired via repetition or exposure and expressed through performance, without conscious reference to the learning episode. There appear to be two forms of implicit memory: *priming*, the nonconscious process by which previous exposure to a stimulus leads to improved identification when it is presented again in a perceptually degraded form, and *skill learning*, the nonconscious acquisition of skills with repeated practice. In general, skill learning is impaired in subcortical dementia but priming is normal; in Alzheimer disease, skill learning is normal but priming is impaired. This has been interpreted to indicate striatal dysfunction in subcortical dementia and degeneration of cortical sensory association areas in Alzheimer disease.

**subcortical encephalopathy**   See *diffuse sclerosis*.

**subcortical word blindness**   See *word blindness*.

**subdelirious state, subdelirium**   The prodromata of a full-blown delirium: restlessness, headache, oversensitiveness to auditory and visual stimuli, irritability, lability of emotions.

The term *subacute delirious state* is applied to "a syndrome in which incoherence of thought, speech and movement appear together with perplexity, in a setting of clouding of consciousness, fluctuating in degree. The state may follow a typical delirium or appear independently. It may persist over a considerable period, weeks or months, outlasting the signs of the underlying physical illness, but always ending in recovery" (Mayer-Gross, W. et al. *Clinical Psychiatry*, 1960).

**subiculum**   Subicular zone; a major output pathway of the *hippocampus* (q.v.) that projects to the temporal cortex. Subicular neurons may contribute to interictal activity in human temporal lobe epilepsy.

**subject homoerotic**   See *homosexuality, male*.

**subject system**   See *systematized complex*.

**subject-ill**   The subject-ill patient uses his own body to symbolize his emotions. This is achieved through somatization, which constitutes an organic language of the mind. See *object-ill; somatization*.

**sublimate**   To externalize or objectivate instinctual impulses in ways that meet the situation. To sublimate is to refine or purify instinctual manifestations. The instincts are not changed; their mode of expression is altered.

**sublimation**   In psychoanalytic psychology, the process of modifying an instinctual impulse in such a way as to conform to the demands of society. Sublimation is a substitute activity that gives some measure of gratification to the infantile impulse that has been repudiated in its original form. Sublimation is an unconscious process and is a function of the normal ego. It is not technically a *defense* mechanism, for unlike the latter it does not lead to any restriction or inhibition of ego functioning by requiring a constant countercathexis; rather, the impulse or wish is modified in such a way that gratification can be achieved without disapprobation or disapproval. Unlike the usual defenses, in sublimation the ego is not acting in opposition to the id; on the contrary, it is helping the id to gain external expression. Sublimation, in other words, does not involve repression. It is to be noted that the original impulse is never conscious in sublimation.

To put it another way, sublimation is a form of *desexualization* (q.v.) in which the instinctive impulses, instead of requiring control by constant countercathexis, are deflected (by means of identification, displacement, and substitution) into acceptable channels. The aim or object (or both) of the drive is changed without blocking an adequate discharge.

It seems likely that sublimation is intimately related to *identification* (q.v.), for both depend upon the presence of models and upon incentives supplied directly or indirectly by the environment.

**subliminal excitation**   See *summation*.

**submissiveness, submission**   Passivity, acceptance, especially as contrasted with *ascendance* (q.v.) or dominance.

**subnuclear bodies**   In the neuron, distinct elements of the nucleus, many of which are intimately linked with human disease. *Specles* are dense clusters of small nuclear ribonucleoproteins (*snRNPs*) and other protein splicing factors which disperse when cells enter mitosis but reconsititute themselves during telophase, before their import into daughter nuclei. *Coiled bodies* are balls of tangled threads which disassemble during mitosis and reform during $G_1$ phase after transcription is reinitiated. Their function is unknown, but they may play a role in snRNP transport or maturation, or in histone processing. *Gems* (gemini of coiled body), often paired with coiled bodies, contain the *SMN* (survival of motor neurons) protein, encoded by the gene responsible for a severe inherited form of human muscular wasting disease, spinal muscular atrophy.

*PML nuclear bodies* (also known as *PODs*, standing for PML oncogenic domains; *Kr bodies*; and *ND10*, standing for nuclear domain 10) are domains that are specifically disrupted in *APL* (acute promyelocytic leukemia) cells. The role of PML bodies is unknown. The fact that several viral proteins, including *HSV-1* (herpes simplex virus, type 1), adenovirus, and human cytomegalovirus, associate with PML bodies suggests that they play some role in cellular antiviral defense.

**suboccipital puncture**   *Cisternal puncture* (q.v.); a procedure introduced by Ayer and his coworkers for determining spinal subarachnoid block and for therapeutic purposes. "The method consists in withdrawing fluid from the cisterna magna at the base of the brain behind the medulla. With the patient on the side, the head bent forward, the needle is introduced in the midline at a point midway between the external occipital protuberance and the spine of the axis or second cervical vertebra. The needle is directed forward and upward in the direction of the eyes or glabella" (Wechsler, I. S. *Textbook of Clinical Neurology*, 1939).

**subplate**   See *axon growth*.

**subpsyche**   A term introduced by Bumke as synonymous with unconscious life.

**subshock**   See *ambulatory insulin treatment*.

**substance**   In addiction psychiatry, (1) a chemical agent that is used intentionally to alter mood or behavior (*psychoactive substance*), or (2) any prescribed medication, poison, toxin, industrial solvent, or other agent to which one may be exposed unintentionally and whose effects on the nervous system may lead to behavioral or cognitive disturbances.

**substance abuse**   Use of a psychoactive substance in a manner detrimental to the individual or society but not meeting criteria for substance or drug dependence.

**substance P**   A neurokinin neuropeptide, discovered in 1931. Antagonists of substance P (or its receptor, $NK_1$) have been used experimentally in the treatment of *pain* (q.v.).

There is evidence that one such antagonist, MK-869, may be effective in the treatment of major depressive disorder. See *peptide, brain*.

**substance use disorders**   Syndromes associated with regular or episodic use of psychoactive chemicals, including alcohol, amphetamine, caffeine, cannabis, cocaine, hallucinogen, inhalant, nicotine, opidoid, phencyclidine, sedative/hypnotic/anxiolytic drugs, and combinations of drugs (polysubstance use). The specific syndromes include dependence (for all the foregoing except caffeine); abuse (all except caffeine and nicotine); intoxication (all except nicotine); and withdrawal (all except caffeine, cannabis, hallucinogen, inhalant, and phencyclidine).

**substance-induced anxiety disorder**   Anxiety symptoms or panic attacks associated with intoxication or withdrawal of substances. Anxiety is frequent in intoxication with amphetamines, anticholinergic drugs, aspirin, caffeine, cannabis, cocaine, hallucinogens and phencyclidine, steroids, sympathomimetics, and yohimbine. The withdrawal states most frequently associated with anxiety symptoms or panic attacks are those caused by alcohol, opioids, and sedatives/hypnotics.

**substance-induced mental disorders**   *Psychoactive substance-induced organic mental disorders* (in DSM-III-R); mental disorders arising during a state of intoxication or while withdrawing from a substance as well as persisting mental disorders that last beyond intoxication and withdrawal. The syndromes include delirium, dementia, amnestic disorder, psychotic disorder (including what formerly were called substance-induced delusional disorder and substance-induced hallucinosis), mood disorder, anxiety disorder, perceptual disorder, posthallucinogen perceptual disorder, sleep disorder, and sexual disorder. These syndromes (except for intoxication and withdrawal syndromes) are placed within the diagnostic categories with which they share phenomenology—substance-induced mood disorder under mood disorders, substance-induced sleep disorder with sleep disorders, etc. See *substance use disorders*.

**substance-related disorders**   In DSM-IV, this category includes *substance use disorders* and *substance-induced mental disorders* (qq.v.).

**substantia innominata**   Also known as the substantia innominata of Reichert or of Reil; a region of the basal forebrain located under the head of the caudate nucleus. Among the cells it contains is the large-celled *basal nucleus of Meynert*, which distributes cholinergic fibers throughout the cerebral cortex. These cells degenerate in Alzheimer disease. NMDA receptors in the substantia innominata mediate attentional processes, thus helping a person to keep his mind on the task at hand.

**substantia nigra** A broad layer of gray substance occupying the central portion of the cerebral peduncle in the *midbrain*. It consists of two zones, the dorsal *pars compacta* with melanin-containing cells, and the ventral *pars reticulata*. The substantia nigra receives afferents from the neostriatum (caudate nucleus and putamen) and also projects back to the *basal ganglia* (q.v.) by way of the nigrostriatal pathway. It also projects to the superior colliculus, thus influencing eye movements, and, along with the globus pallidus, to the prefrontal, premotor, and motor cortices, thus influencing body and limb movements. See *striatoful projections.*

Lesions of the substantia nigra are associated with involuntary movements and rigidity. Dopamine is synthesized in the substantia nigra, and the characteristic abnormality in *Parkinson disease* (q.v.) is marked degeneration of dopaminergic melanin-containing neurons in the pars compacta portion of the substantia nigra.

**substantive legal standard** Criteria that are defined by constitution, statute, regulation, or case law; they cannot be ignored or redefined by the health professional. See *procedural legal standard.*

**substitute** See *surrogate.*

**substitute, regressive** Displacing the unconscious sexual aim or object in the course of psychosexual development to a chronologically earlier one from which pleasure was derived. In describing a patient with a phantasy of being beaten by the father, Freud states that "it is not only the punishment for the forbidden genital relation [incest], but also the regressive substitute for it" (*Collected Papers*, 1924–25).

**substitute decision making** Making medical management decisions for a person who is unable or unwilling to make such a decision himself. When a patient lacks decisional capacity, substituted or *surrogate* consent to treatment (or decision to refuse treatment) may be made in several ways, depending

upon the jurisdiction within which the decision is to be executed. In some cases, a family member may automatically act as a surrogate; in other cases, a more formal mechanism is required such as a guardianship or conservatorship arrangement.

In *Cruzan v. Director* (1990), the U.S. Supreme Court found that the right to refuse treatment endures even if the patient loses decisional capacity; the right is not limited to the terminally ill and may be exercised through living wills, durable powers of attorney, or some other type of *advance directive* (q.v.).

**substitute formation** Symptom-formation; the tendency of repressed impulses to use any opportunity for indirect discharge. The energy of the warded-off instinct is displaced to any other impulse that is associatively connected with the repressed one, and the intensity of this substitute impulse is increased and often, in addition, the affect connected with it is changed in quality. Such substitute impulses are known as *derivatives*; most neurotic symptoms are derivatives.

**substitution** A strategy of pharmacotherapy: the current drug is discontinued and another drug (usually of a different class) is initiated.

**substitutive reaction type** When mental conflicts are repressed into the unconscious and then appear in the field of consciousness in disguised or substituted form, Adolf Meyer classifies the syndrome as substitutive. The psychoneuroses in general are substitutive reaction types.

**substrate** See *cytochrome P450 isoenzyme system.*

**subthalamic nucleus, subthalamus** That portion of the brain bounded by the dorsal thalamus anteriorly, the tegmentum of the midbrain posteriorly, the hypothalamus medially, and the internal capsule laterally. The subthalamus contains the rostral extensions of the red nucleus and substantia nigra from the midbrain, the *fields of Forel* (which are probably a rostral extension of reticular nuclei), and the subthalamic nucleus (*body of Luys*). The last is functionally connected with the globus pallidus. See *basal ganglia; hemiballism.*

**subventricular zone (SVZ)** A brain region that lies immediately beneath the ependymal layer on the lateral wall of the lateral ventricles, separated from the caudate nucleus by a layer of myelin. During brain development, SVZ stem cells give rise to proliferative *progenitor cells* (dividing cells that have the capacity to differentiate), which then migrate from their birthplace to the cortex or basal ganglia, where they differentiate into neurons. In adulthood, the SVZ can respond to brain insults by producing new progenitor cells that can migrate to sites that have been affected by neurodegenerative pathology or brain injury. The goal of *transcription-factor (TF) therapy* in neurodegenerative diseases is to drive SVZ progenitors to become the cell type that is affected by the disease, either by administering the TFs directly or by making the progenitors express TFs that specify a particular neuronal fate.

**subwaking**   Being or held in a state intermediate between sleeping and waking; hypnoidal.

**successive approximations**   See *reinforced practice.*

**succinate dehydrogenase**   See *OXPHOS.*

**succinylcholine**   A muscle relaxant, usually administered intravenously; in psychiatry, used in association with electroconvulsive treatment to prevent or minimize the occurrence of bone fractures.

**succubus**   Demon or witch; specifically, a female demon who has sexual intercourse with or performs fellatio on men during their sleep. See *incubus.*

**suckling, eternal**   Freud's term for that type of person who throughout life feels he or she should be cared for, protected, and supported by someone else.

**sudep**   Sudden unexpected death in epilepsy, probably related to respiratory or cardiac failure during a seizure.

**suffocatio hysterica**   Hysterical suffocation; hysterical spasm of the muscles of the throat; often seen as part of the symptom picture in *globus hystericus* (q.v.). Like the latter, suffocatio hysterica is often based on the unconscious rejection of incorporation phantasies of a sexual or aggressive nature.

**suggestibility**   The state, quality, or ability of being influenced by *suggestion* (q.v.). Negative suggestibility is doing the opposite of what is suggested to the patient. See *catatonic schizophrenia.*

The term was first used by George Gilles de la Tourette to refer to an inherent susceptibility to *autosuggestion* (q.v.), which be believed was the physiologic basis of hysteria. See *credulity.*

**suggestion**   The process of influencing a person to the point of uncritical acceptance of an idea, belief, or other cognitive process. Some would differentiate between heterosuggestion (when the source of the idea is someone outside the person) and autosuggestion (when the source of the idea is the subject himself, as when he keeps saying to himself that he is getting better and better every day, perhaps in hopes that he will one day come to believe his own statement).

While suggestion does not afford a complete explanation of hypnosis, it is obvious that it plays a large part in it, in that the subject comes to accept the hypnotist's repeated suggestions that he is becoming drowsy and soon finds that this is so. This is even more clear with posthypnotic suggestion, when the subject will carry out some action that has been proposed to him during the trance state. See *autosuggestion.*

The psychoanalytic method is a modification of hypnosis, and, like the latter, depends upon suggestion in influencing "a person through and by means of the transference-manifestations of which he is capable" (Freud, S. *Collected Papers*, 1924–25). It was Charcot's idea that unconscious ideas can produce symptoms and that hypnosis is a reliable means of triggering a display of those symptoms. Freud accepted Charcot's view and ignored Bernheim's demonstration that hypnotic phenomena represent compliance with instruction, not an emergence of earlier states or memories. Both Charcot and Freud failed to appreciate the significance of what today would be termed *experimenter effects.* See *operant conditioning.*

Prestige suggestion is another form of psychotherapy; unlike psychoanalysis, however, it does not attempt to uncover or deal with the unconscious determinants of behavior. Its efficacy is chiefly dependent upon gratification of the patient's security needs; the patient submits to and identifies with the omnipotent authority (the therapist) and gives up his symptoms as part of his obedience to the therapist.

**suggestion, posthypnotic**   Suggestion given during the hypnotic stage to be acted upon after the hypnotic phase has passed.

**suggestion confabulation**   *Confabulation* (q.v.) that incorporates data from questions posed or statements made to the subject, even though such data may contradict other portions of the fabrication.

**suggestive**   In psychiatry this usually relates to hypnotic suggestion; thus, one speaks of hypnotic or suggestive therapeutics.

**suicidal behavior**   Self-directed injurious acts with at least some intent to end one's own life. Suicidal behavior ranges from fatal acts (completed suicide), to highly lethal and failed suicide attempts (where high intention and planning are evident, and survival is fortuitous), to low-lethality attempts (usually impulsive attempts that are triggered by a social crisis, seem to be ambivalent, and contain a strong element of an appeal for help). Intent and lethality are correlated positively and are related to biological abnormalities that mostly involve the serotonergic system. See *suicide*; *suicide risk*.

**suicidality**   The state of being suicidal, usually described along a spectrum of ideas and behaviors such as (1) nonspecific suicidal ideation, such as thoughts of death and the idea that death might be welcome; (2) suicide plans, when the intent to die is put into concrete form; (3) suicide attempt, when the apparent willingness or intent to die culminates in a self-inflicted act that is not lethal; (4) suicide gesture, an attempt of low lethality that is often implemented manipulatively; (5) completed suicide, self-inflicted intentional death. See *attempters*.

Suicidal behavior itself is often described in terms of the following:

1. Precipitant—a stressful event occurring within 6 weeks prior to the attempt, such as losing a job

2. Motivation—such as seeking attention, making someone feel guilty, expressing anger, escaping an intolerable situation

3. Suicidal intent—the extent to which the subject desires a lethal outcome, as suggested by making a will, leaving a note, taking precautions not to be discovered

4. Lethality—the medical seriousness of the method employed

**suicide**   Self-inflicted intentional death. Suicide is the tenth leading cause of death in the United States, accounting for at least 1% of all deaths (in numbers, somewhere between 30,000 and 100,000 per year). For every death from suicide (completed suicide) there are eight other attempts (see attempters). More people die from suicide each year than from homicide.

The official rate has remained at 10 to 12 per 100,000 per year since 1945, but statistics on suicide are notoriously unreliable. Some researchers believe that a high rate reflects a high rate of autopsies and toxicological examination; whether it is recorded as suicide may also depend on age, sex, race, social class, and other factors. Statistics on suicide are compiled annually by the National Center for Health Statistics (NCHS), the primary source for information about suicide in the United States. In recent years the suicide rate appears to have fallen—from 11.7/100,000 people (1990) to 11.2 (1993), but it remains the third leading cause of death among adolescents and young adults aged 15–24 years. In those same years, there has been rise in adolescent homicide, firearm-related death, and assault injuries.

The highest rates of suicide occur in German-speaking countries. Austria, which has the highest official rate in the world, is followed by Switzerland, the Scandinavian countries, Eastern Europe, and Japan. There is a relatively low rate in Spain, Italy, and the Netherlands. The official rate in the United States is about average for industrialized countries.

Even with the rising rate of suicide in adolescents, the incidence of suicide is highest in old age. Among the elderly, males may account for as many as 90% of suicides. Persons over 60 years of age constitute 20% of the population but contribute 40% of the suicides. Among people 75 years of age and older, the annual rate is three times the average. Females are more likely than males to attempt suicide, but males are more likely to succeed.

Firearms are responsible for three times the number of suicides as the next leading method (hanging and other methods of suffocation; the third most common method is poisoning). Keeping firearms in the home is associated with an increased risk of suicide. Overall, blacks have a lower suicide rate than whites. Even so, young black men (20 to 35 years of age) have a rate double that of young white men. Native Americans have a higher suicide rate than whites at all ages.

In at least 90% of suicides, there is an associated mental or emotional disorder: depression (although this is not the leading factor in the mounting number of suicides in young white males), alcoholism, drug abuse (a significant factor in over half of suicides in the young, where the pattern is typically one of chronic use of multiple drugs), and schizophrenia.

Depression accounts for suicide in approximately 30% to 70% of cases (suicide accounts for 15% of all deaths among patients with mood disorders), alcoholism for 15% to 25% (the lifetime prevalence of suicide among alcoholics is about 10%, ten times the average). Suicide rate among drug abusers is at least five times the average. Schizophrenics also have a high suicide rate: over 20% attempt it, and 10% eventually succeed.

It is a common misconception that the patient who threatens suicide is not likely to commit suicide. The reverse is probably closer to the truth, for about 75% of successful suicides had previously threatened or attempted it. Typically, the genuinely suicidal patient departs with a surge of hatred for the world and pejorative accusations of the self, leaving definite instructions and restrictions for those he has purposely deserted. Among the clinical depressions, those with prominent anxiety features, a feeling of losing ground, and/or a marked hypochondriacal trend are the most likely to make a suicide attempt.

People who have never married are twice as likely to commit suicide; the divorced and widowed have the highest rates of all. High unemployment increases suicide rates. Physicians have a higher than average rate, and the rate in psychiatrists is higher than other physicians. Among physicians, women have a higher rate than men.

Psychodynamically, suicide or a suicide attempt is seen most frequently to be an aggressive attack directed against a loved one or against society in general; in others, it may be a misguided bid for attention or it may be conceived of as a means of effecting reunion with the ideal love object or mother. That suicide is in one sense a means of release for aggressive impulses is supported by the change of wartime suicide rates. In World War II, for example, rates among the participating nations fell, sometimes by as much as 30%; but in neutral countries, the rates remained the same.

In depressions, the following dynamic elements may be operative: the depressed patient loses the object that he depends upon for narcissistic supplies; in an attempt to force the object's return, he regresses to the oral stage and incorporates (swallows up) the object, thus regressively identifying with the object: the sadism originally directed against the deserting object is taken up by the patient's superego and is directed against the incorporated object, which now lodges within the ego; suicide occurs, not so much as an attempt on the ego's part to escape the inexorable demands of the superego, but rather as an enraged attack on the incorporated object in retaliation for its having deserted the patient in the first place.

**suicide, psychic** The killing of one's self without resorting to any physical agency; used in reference to those who make up their minds to die and actually do so. It is presumed that the same forces that lead a person to commit physical suicide are active in psychic suicide cases, but that, instead of operating overtly, these forces work endopsychically.

**suicide pact** An agreement or pledge of two (rarely more) people to take their own lives at the same time. It is estimated that suicide pacts account for 1 in 300 completed suicides, and that there are twice as many uncompleted suicide pacts as completed ones.

**suicide risk** Indicators of increased risk for suicide include the following:

1. Being a psychiatric inpatient, whose rate is between 6 and 40 times the comparable rate in the general population; the risk remains high for 6 to 12 months following discharge, and in women the risk is particularly high in the first 6 months after discharge.

2. Diagnosis—risk is 15% for depressive disorder (whether that is the only diagnosis or is a complication of another psychiatric or medical illness), 15% for alcoholism, 10% to 13% for schizophrenia.

3. A feeling of hopelessness, particularly if combined with clinical depression.

4. Previous suicide attempt, especially in a person over age 35 or in a person with schizophrenia.

5. In substance abusers (including alcoholics), a recent or impending loss.

6. In populations other than substance abusers and alcoholics, absence of any immediate precipitant of a dysphoric or depressive episode is ominous.

7. Self-oriented motivation, when the wish to die relates only to an internal state.

8. Communication of suicidal intent by a depressed patient.

9. High *lethality* (q.v.) of method considered, a risk that is exaggerated when such a method is available.

**suicidogenic**   Causing, provoking, or encouraging suicide.

**suigenderism**   The natural drift on a child's part to associate or group with others of his own *gender*. During latency the activities of boys are largely confined to boys, while those of girls are mainly limited to girls. For the manifestation of these natural, nonerotic relationships between members of one's own gender, the term *suigenderism* is recommended. When sex feelings begin to crop up in suigenderism, it may become *homoeroticism, homosexuality,* or *homogenitality* (qq.v.).

**sukra prameha**   *Dhat* (q.v.).

**sulcus, sulci**   The grooves in the cerebral cortex; the elevated portion between two sulci is a *gyrus* (pl., gyri).

**Sullivan, Harry Stack**   (1892–1949) The chief proponent of the so-called dynamic-cultural school of psychoanalysis, which emphasizes sociologic rather than biologic events, present-day contacts with people rather than past experiences, current interpersonal relationships rather than infantile sexuality. Orthodox Freudians consider this a superficial approach that is limited to a single facet of experience, the cultural. At the present time, however, the social and relational sources of personality development that Sullivan emphasized are currently are the main interest of both interpersonal analysis and the psychoanalytic schools of object relations and self psychology.

**SUMD**   Scale to Assess Unawareness of Mental Disorder, which assesses the patient's current and retrospective awareness of having a mental disorder, of the effects of medication on the disorder, of the consequences of mental illness, and awareness and attributions for the specific signs and symptoms of the disorder. Unawareness of illness is a prevalent feature of schizophrenia, and level of insight is a discriminating factor in subtyping the disorder.

**summation**   An accumulation of elements that individually produce no discernible effects, but whose aggregation results in pathologic changes or an overreaction to minor stimuli. According to Freud, "Persons who tolerate coitus interruptus apparently without harmful results are in reality becoming thereby disposed to the disorder of anxiety neurosis,

which may break out either at any time spontaneously or after an ordinary and otherwise insufficient trauma" (*Collected Papers,* 1924–1925).

In neurophysiology, summation refers to a response obtained when two stimuli are applied, neither of which by itself is of sufficient intensity to elicit a response. In this sense, there are two types of summation, temporal and spatial. *Temporal summation* is seen when two successive stimuli, each of them too weak to elicit a response, are applied to the same nerve trunk within 0.1 to 0.5 msec of each other, in which case a response will be evoked because of the enduring character of the local excitatory process. *Spatial summation* is seen when two different afferent nerves, which play upon the same reflex center, are stimulated either simultaneously or within a short interval (not more than 15 msec); a response is evolved even though neither stimulus alone will elicit a response. Spatial summation is believed to be a result of additive excitatory alterations in the neurons involved. Sherrington and his associates refer to this excitatory alteration as the *central excitatory state,* which is often abbreviated as c.e.s. The nerves affected are said to be in the *subliminal fringe* of excitation.

**SUMO**   Small ubiquitin-like modifier; its actions are concentrated in the nucleus and include gene transcription, DNA repair, transport of proteins into and out of the nucleus, and building of the mitotic spindle that draws sets of chromosomes to the opposite ends of a dividing cell. About half the proteins altered by sumoylation are transcription factors involved in turning genes on or off. In Huntington disease, sumoylation of Htt (Huntingtin protein) increases its neurotoxicity. In human papillomavirus and the herpes viruses, sumoylation of viral proteins targets them to the nucleus, enabling them to take over the cell's replication machinery and reproduce themselves.

**SUMOylation**   Covalent attachment of SUMO to lysine residues, a post-translational modification process that is biochemically similar to, but functionally distinct from, ubiquitination. It is likely that a disruption of the balance between ubiquitination (ubiquitylation) and SUMOylation is involved in many neurological disorders, such as Alzheimer disease, Parkinson disease, and polyQ disorders.

See *Huntington disease*; *trinucleotide repeat*; *ubiquitin*.

**SUNCT**   Short-lasting unilateral neuralgiform headache attacks with conjunctival injection and tearing.

**Sunday neurosis**   Any psychiatric symptom or syndrome that is triggered or exacerbated by particular days or dates; called Sunday neurosis because of the frequency with which that day appears to be the significant one. The most frequent symptoms are feelings of uneasiness, dissatisfaction, dejection, and fear of what the future may bring. In some affective disorders, recurrence of a manic or depressive episode seems to be an *anniversary reaction* (q.v.) that occurs at the same time of year as the significant past event.

**sundowner**   The older person whose mental functioning is adequate during the day but at night is impaired by confusion and agitation; also known as deliriant *confusion*. See *organic syndrome*.

**suoyang**   See *koro*.

**superego**   In psychoanalytic psychology, there are three functional divisions of the psyche: the id, the ego, and the superego. The superego is the last of these to be differentiated. It is the representative of society within the psyche (i.e., *conscience* or morality) and also includes the ideal aspirations (*ego-ideal*). The superego is mainly unconscious; its functions include (1) approval or disapproval of the ego's actions, i.e., judgment that an act is "right" or "wrong"; (2) critical self-observation; (3) self-punishment; (4) demands that the ego repent or make reparation for wrongdoing; (5) self-love or *self-esteem* as the ego reward for having done right.

In general, the superego may be regarded as a split-off portion of the ego that arises on the basis of identification with certain aspects of the introjected parents. Morality in the young child is more a response to immediate external demands of the environment than obedience to an inner authority. It is only with the oedipal phase that the superego begins to take its final form as an internal authority that stands between ego and id, compelling the child on his own to renounce certain pleasures, and imposing punishment (loss of self-esteem, guilt feelings, etc.) for violations of its orders. The superego develops as a reaction to the Oedipus complex; as is often said, it is the *heir of the Oedipus complex*. It is a solution to the impulses of this period that have no prospect of succeeding in reality and that, if allowed to continue unchanged, would have been dangerous. These impulses, deriving from the id, are allowed access to the ego; the forbidden impulses (love for the mother, hatred of the father) are withdrawn from their objects and deposited in the ego, which thus becomes changed. The changed portion of the ego is the superego, and it contains the sadism originally directed against the father; so also does it contain the love originally felt for the mother, but the very process of introjecting the mother and changing the libido attached to the maternal object into ego libido has resulted in desexualization. Thus, the love portion of the superego (the ego-ideal) is a nonsensual love.

Oedipal objects are regressively replaced by identifications, and sexual longing for the maternal object has been replaced by an asexual alteration within the organization of the ego. These newly introjected objects, which replace the sexual and hostile impulses toward the parents, combine with the parental introjects from the prephallic period (internalized parental prohibitions), and the superego is formed. See *reaction formation*.

In practice it is difficult to differentiate sharply between the superego, which is an image of the hated and feared objects, and the ego-ideal, which is an image of the loved objects in the libido.

Melanie Klein and her followers believe that the superego begins to function than Freud (and most psychoanalysts since him) believed. "Where I differ is in placing at birth the processes of introjection which are the basis of the superego. The superego precedes by some months the beginning of the Oedipus complex, a beginning which I date, together with that of the depressive position, in the second quarter of the first year. Thus the early introjection of the good and bad breast is the foundation of the superego and influences the development of the Oedipus complex. This conception of superego formation is in contrast to Freud's explicit statements that the identifications with the parents are the heir of the Oedipus complex and only succeed if the Oedipus complex is successfully overcome" (*International Journal of Psychoanalysis 39*, 1958).

**superego, parasites of** Ideals and values absorbed by the person "which usurp the functions of the super-ego." After one has entered the latency period, ideals usually continue to undergo modification; emotional ties to the family begin to loosen, becoming less intense, one's standards become more independent of the infantile models. Other persons or ideas begin to serve as models and become part of the superego. When the new ideals are only "a slight modification of old ideals, the situation is not difficult... Sometimes, however, internal or external situations may create parasites of the superego which usurp the functions of the superego for a varying length of time."

An example of a parasitic superego is the influence of mass suggestion. A person with a normal superego may, under mass suggestion, yield to impulses which would normally be suppressed and yet show no guilt-feelings. Another example of a parasitic superego occurs under hypnosis, when the hypnotist takes over the functions of the patient's superego. "He tries to undo the previous work of the super-ego that gave rise to the defensive struggle" (Fenichel, O. *The Psychoanalytic Theory of Neurosis*, 1945).

**superego, parasitic** A temporarily coexisting body of commands that conflict with the subject's own superego standards, such as internalizations of the leader's exhortation to kill during wartime.

**superego, primitive** A superego that is older in origin than the force established by parents and teachers. The primitive superego is assumed to be hereditary and susceptible to the influence of hereditary factors in contrast to the parental superego, which reflects tradition.

**superego anxiety** Anxiety caused by the unconscious functioning of the superego, which itself can become a source of continual danger because of inexorable demands for atonement. See *guilt*.

**superego interpretation** See *defense interpretation*.

**superego resistance** *Negative therapeutic reaction (NTR)*; a type of resistance encountered in patients in psychoanalytic treatment in which the need for punishment, as manifested in guilt feelings and masochistic behavior, continues to produce symptoms and is the only barrier to their resolution. Superego resistance is most frequently manifested by obsessionals whose anxiety is a fear of the loss of the superego's love. Most analysts consider it a malignant regression that often provokes an obliterating countertransference of hopelessness, envy, or rage. Melanie Klein emphasized that envy and defenses against it play a major role in the development of NTR.

Negative therapeutic reaction is sometimes used loosely to refer to any therapy that does not go well, although most authors use it more specifically to refer to patients whose conditions worsen during therapy. The patient with severe borderline personality disorder of the narcissistic, sadomasochistic, or paranoid subtypes is particularly likely to show a negative therapeutic reaction.

**superego sadism** The intense cruelty, rigidity, and pain-giving punitive aspects of conscience (superego). In the developing child, the infantile sadism (primordial aggressivity) is eventually mastered by equally powerful controlling and countervailing forces. Those forces, warning the child of the reality consequences of its unbridled aggressive trends, become organized into conscience. The warnings emanate from the internalized (introjected) pictures or images that the child has, not necessarily of his real parents, but rather of what he fears the parents might do if they discovered his own violent, aggressive wishes against them.

The internal image of the violently angry, discovering parent is formed in the old talionic formula of an "eye for an eye." The child feels that the discovering parent will seek vengeance in proportion to the strength and enormity of the child's own aggressive phantasies. The intensity of the superego's sadism is thus determined by the enormity and violence of the child's infantile phantasies.

**superfemale** Metafemale; a female with a sex chromosome pattern of XXX (instead of the normal XX). Rather than being more "female" than the normal, however, such women are amenorrheic, sterile, and have underdeveloped female sexual characteristics. See *chromosome*.

**supergene** A type of variation of hereditary traits caused by chromosomal rearrangement; such a mutation affects an entire section of a chromosome but simulates the single factor type of inheritance (which is produced by one major mutant gene).

**superior function** In Jung's analytical psychology, there are four basic psychological types—thinking, feeling, intuitive, and sensational. Any one of the functional types may predominate as the means by which the person adjusts himself to the problems of living. The predominating is called the *superior* function, while the remaining three functions are *inferior* in varying degrees. See *analytic psychology*.

**superior temporal gyrus**   *STG* (q.v.).

**superior temporal sulcus**   See *intention*.

**superiority feeling**   The boy's feeling that he is superior to a girl in the domain of sex. "The amalgamation of the desire for a child with the epistemophilic impulse enables a boy to effect a displacement on to the intellectual plane; his sense of being at a disadvantage is then concealed and over-compensated by the superiority he deduces from his possession of a penis, which is also acknowledged by girls." (Klein, M. *Contributions to Psycho-analysis, 1921–45*, 1948) See *penis envy*.

**superiority strivings**   See *individual psychology*.

**supermoron**   A person slightly subnormal mentally, but in a grade above that of a moron.

**superordinated**   See *ego* (Jung's definition).

**superoxide**   See *free radical*.

**superoxide dismutase**   *SOD*; Cu/Zn superoxide dismutase is a cytosolic antioxidant enzyme that protects against free radicals such as toxic hydroxyl radicals (from hydrogen peroxide), peroxynitrite anions (from nitric oxide), and other intracellular free radicals generated metabolically or by environmental toxins. See *amyotrophic lateral sclerosis; free radical*.

**supersex**   Abnormal physical sex with sterility; the affected person shows intersexual features owing to a disturbed ratio of autosomes to heterosomes. Supersexual persons are either "*super-females,*" with three X chromosomes and two sets of autosomes, or "*supermales,*" with one X chromosome and three sets of autosomes.

**superstition**   An irrational belief in magic, chance, etc., or an exaggerated fear of the unknown. It may be a part of the subject's cultural tradition, or at least not rejected by the subject or society. See *delusion*.

**supervalent**   Referring to the excessive intensity of an idea that the subject cannot rid himself of; the intensity results from the multiple unconscious determinants of the idea, and/or from the need to keep the idea as a screen for a reverse or contrary thought. See *reaction formation*.

**supervalent thought**   A train of thought that seems reasonable, but no amount of voluntary effort or thought on the patient's part is able to dissipate or eradicate it.

**supervision**   In psychiatry, the critical evaluation by an experienced therapist of the clinical work of a therapist in training.

Under the doctrine of *respondeat superior* (the principal is responsible for the agent), supervisors are legally responsible for the professional practices of the persons they supervise. Thus, clear records of the supervisory sessions should be kept; they are subject to the same requirements for confidentiality as is the rest of the patient's medical record.

**supply reduction**   Legal measures that limit or prohibit the production and distribution of something (most commonly, psychoactive drugs).

**support**   See *psychotherapy*.

**supportive ego**   This term was first introduced by Slavson (*An Introduction to Group Therapy,* 1943) to denote one who is dynamic in activity group psychotherapy. In therapy groups it refers to the relation in which one member—because of his greater strength or maturity—helps a fellow member to gain status in a group or to work out his intrapsychic problems. It has been observed that supportive-ego relations are temporary and progressive in nature. A weak child may attach himself to another weak child in order to forward his own adaptation to a group, but, growing stronger and less fearful, he makes friends with the stronger members of the group. Finally, the child functions on his own, without support from any one of the group members.

**suppression**   The act of consciously inhibiting an impulse, affect, or idea, as in the deliberate attempt to forget something and think no more about it. Suppression is thus to be differentiated from *repression* (q.v.), which is an unconscious process. It is probable that there is no sharp line of demarcation between suppression and repression, and it seems also likely that on occasion the unconscious defense of repression may be directed against material which the individual consciously suppresses. Nonetheless, it seems advisable in most instances to regard suppression and repression as distinctly different mechanisms.

**suppressive therapy**   See *expressive therapy*.

**suprachiasmatic nucleus**   *SCN*; one of 28 different nuclei in the hypothalamus and a part of the circadian axis (the other components are the pineal gland and the retina). The SCN is the receiving station of information flowing from the eyes to the hypothalamus, a nerve pathway that carries information about environmental conditions of light and darkness to the brain. The SCN regulates the rhythmic production of melatonin from the pineal glands. At night, melatonin levels rise, while during the day they fall, a cycle that may regulate daily body rhythms such as waking and sleeping. The eye also has daily rhythms, renewing the tips of its rods, photoreceptors used for night vision, at the end of each night and the tips of the cones, used for color vision, at the end of each day. The retinal clock seems to tick independently of the SCN clock. See *clock, biological; sleep-promoting factors.*

**supraindividuals** See *collective unconscious.*

**supralaryngeal vocal tract (SVT)** See *vocal tract normalization.*

**supramarginal gyrus** See *parietal lobe.*

**supramolecular receptor complex** See *receptor complex, supramolecular.*

**supranuclear palsy** *Steele-Richardson-Olszewski syndrome;* a late-onset subcortical dementia characterized by progressive supranuclear paralysis of extraocular movements, dysarthria, pseudobulbar palsy, and dystonic rigidity of the neck and trunk. Underlying the clinical dementia is an impaired ability to manipulate acquired knowledge, even though if given enough time the patient may show that he retains verbal and perceptual motor capacities. The pathological changes include cell loss, neurofibrillary alterations, gliosis, and demyelination in the basal ganglia, brain stem, and cerebellum. Supranuclear palsy is a tauopathy that shares clinical and pathological features with *frontotemporal dementia* (q.v.).

**suprapatellar reflex** *Knee jerk; patellar reflex;* a deep reflex. The patient's leg is extended with patella movable; examiner places index finger above patella, pushing down slightly, then striking this finger; the result is a kickback of the patella. The reflex depends on the femoral nerve for its afferents and efferents; its center is $L_{2-4}$.

**supratentorial** See *fossa, posterior cranial.*

**surface imaging** See *MRI.*

**surgical reassignment** See *reassignment, surgical.*

**surrender, will to** The psychic process through which the neurotic patient comes to the point of giving up his neurosis: a renunciating

mental attitude through which the patient expresses his desire to submit to the analyst's aim of curing the illness. According to Stekel, a positive transference during analysis is a manifestation of this will to surrender.

**surreptitious prescribing** The practice of supplying a prescription to a family member or health care professional of a patient and knowing that the medication will likely be concealed in food or drink and administered to the unknowing patient. Surreptitious prescribing could be viewed ethically as a form of misuse of power and a breach of the trust in the doctor–patient relationship; as such, it is the antithesis of recovery.

**surrogate** Substitute; one who takes the place of another. Affective states originally expressed toward the parents are normally transferred from them to others who stand for them. Thus, a sister may be the first *mother surrogate* (q.v.), later a teacher, still later the mother of a friend, and finally a lover. With each new surrogate there is normally less and less resemblance to the original (mother).

Surrogate is also used to refer to a substitute decision maker, to a substitute or practice partner in sex therapy, and to the *host mother* in new reproductive technology. See *substitute decision making.*

**survival skills workshop** See *psychoeducation.*

**survivor syndrome** Any number of symptoms, including depression, insomnia, anxiety, psychosomatic illnesses, nightmares, etc., that are believed to be based upon guilt feelings over being a sole—or nearly sole—survivor of a disaster in which others perished who were emotionally close, such as parents, siblings, spouse, or friends. The survivor syndrome is a type of *post-traumatic stress disorder* (q.v.). See *traumatic neurosis.*

**suspenopsia** Suspension of sight. A tendency for the image arising in either eye to be entirely disregarded for a short period of time so that the subject is using one eye only for the time being.

**sustaining cause, distinct** Any recognizable or discrete determiner, of particular relevance in differentiating between an environmental condition that causes discomfort and an illness or malady that causes discomfort. Profuse sweating on a hot and humid day is not an illness, although the same discomfort and observable signs would constitute a malady or illness or disorder in the absence of such a distinct sustaining cause as high environmental temperature. See *disease*.

**susto** *Fallen fontanel syndrome*; an acute anxiety state seen in Peruvian children and adolescents, usually precipitated by an experience of violent fright. Susto, or *magic fright*, is characterized by anxiety, excitability, dejection with considerable weight loss, and a belief that the patient's soul has been stolen from his body. See *curanderismo*.

**SVD** Small vessel disease.

**SVZ** *Subventricular zone* (q.v.).

**swallowing** See *gustation*.

**Sweetser, William** (1797–1875) American psychiatrist who wrote the first American treatise on mental hygiene (1843).

**swindler, epileptic** See *affective epilepsy*.

**swindler, pathological** See *impostor; liar, pathological*.

**swinging** Slang for uninhibited sexual activity, often manifested in frequent casual sexual encounters, group sex, and combinations of heterosexual and homosexual acts.

**Swyer syndrome** A form of sex reversal in which the child is born with a male set of chromosomes and female sexual organs (an XY female). This can happen as a result of a defect in nuclear import, when changes in the protein SRY impair its function so that its ability to enter the nucleus of fetal male gonadal cells is impaired. Thus, genes that should be turned on by SRY to make testes remain off.

**Sydenham chorea** (Thomas Sydenham, English physician, 1624–1689) *St. Vitus dance*; an acute toxic disorder of the central nervous system secondary to rheumatic infection (although it has also been reported in association with other infections, e.g., scarlet fever, diphtheria, and chickenpox). It occurs chiefly in children and young adolescents, in females more than in males. Pathological changes consist of diffuse edema and congestion, most marked in the corpus striatum. Onset is insidious; the first complaint often is that the child is clumsy and drops things. Later symptoms are involuntary movements that resemble fragments of purposive movements haphazardly performed, hypotonia and hyperextensibility, and often emotional instability of an agitated, overactive kind. On occasion, persistent excitement and insomnia are seen—*maniacal chorea*. Recovery is the rule, although the patient may have several recurrences.

**syllabic synthesis** The combination of syllables of several words to form a new word or neologism. The process is common in the productions of schizophrenic patients and in dreams. "The condensation-work of dreams becomes most palpable when it takes words and names as its objects. Generally speaking, words are often treated in dreams as things, and therefore undergo the same combinations as the ideas of things. The results of such dreams are comical and bizarre word-formations" (Freud, S. The Interpretation of Dreams, 1933). See *condensation; neologism*.

**syllable-stumbling** A form of stuttering or stammering: the patient halts on syllables that he finds difficult to enunciate.

**symbiontic** Symbiotic; used to refer to *folie à deux* (q.v.).

**symbiosis** Intimate living together in a mutually beneficial relationship; technically, the term refers to an interdependent relationship between dissimilar organisms (i.e., members of two different species). In psychiatry and psychology, the term is used in a less restrictive sense to refer to any degree of mutual cooperation or interdependence, as between mother and child. It includes any of the following: *commensalism*, when one member in a dependent relationship benefits and the other is relatively unaffected; *parasitism*, when one member's benefit is achieved at the expense of the other, who is disadvantaged by the relationship; and *mutualism*; when both members benefit. See *symbiotic stage*.

**symbiotic infantile psychosis** Mahler's term for a disturbance seen in certain children at the time when separation from the mother would ordinarily be effected. Under the threat of separation, the symbiotic child's rage and panic are projected into the world, which is perceived as hostile and destructive. The child defends himself by maintaining or restoring the infantile delusion of omnipotence and oneness with the mother, by means of omnipotence phantasies, introjection, projection, delusions, and hallucinations. See *separation-independence*.

Mahler differentiates between the symbiotic psychosis and the *autistic psychosis*. The latter arises in a child with a constitutionally defective ego anlage and thus the symbiotic mother–infant relationship is interfered with from the beginning. Autism is used as a major defense against external stimuli and inner excitations. See *anaclitic depression; separation anxiety.*

**symbiotic stage** A phase in the mother–child relationship during which the child dimly recognizes the mother as a need-satisfying object. Mahler referred to this as *dual unity*, emphasizing that the child perceives and responds to the mother as if child and mother were fused; Fairbairn termed this bonding relationship *primary identification.* At this period, the mother must function as the child's auxiliary ego, performing functions he cannot yet perform for himself (e.g., control of frustration tolerance, setting ego boundaries, impulse control). This phase extends through the first 6 months, when it is succeeded by the stage of *separation-individuation* (q.v.).

**symbol** An object that stands for or represents something else. E. Jones (*Papers on Psycho-Analysis*, 1948) has pointed out that a symbol (1) is a representative or substitute of some other idea; (2) represents the primary element through having something in common with it; (3) is typically sensorial and concrete, whereas the idea represented may be relatively abstract and complex; (4) utilizes modes of thought that are more primitive, both ontogenetically and phylogenetically; (5) is a manifest expression of an idea that is more or less hidden, secret, or kept in reserve; and (6) is made spontaneously, automatically, and, in the broad sense of the word, unconsciously. See *symbolism.*

C. S. Peirce divided signs into icons (e.g., a diagram or other pictorial representation), indices (e.g., a red light to indicate that a message has been left, or a thermometer to indicate body temperature abnormalities), and symbols in a narrower sense (e.g., a name).

In psychoanalytic psychology, the symbol is a conscious representation or perception that replaces, and is a substitute for, unconscious mental content. The unconscious mental content is not recognized and its repression is maintained by the countercathexis of ego defenses; by the very fact that its meaning is unknown to the subject, the repressed psychic energy can, through the symbol, attain primary-process discharge, which would not be possible if the unconscious mental content were recognized as such. Symbols are the building stones for various other forms of indirect representation of unconscious content, viz. dreams, phantasies, hallucinations, symptoms, and even language.

As psychiatric symptoms, symbols may be expressed in any one or all of these general categories: (1) affects alone; thus, in anxiety hysteria the symbol is intense anxiety without any relevant ideas; other symptoms (rapid pulse and breathing, feelings of impending collapse, etc.) are generally secondary symptoms; (2) affects with ideas, the latter being looked upon as thoroughly foreign and painful to the conscious ego (for example, a patient was "tormented to death with the idea that I am slowly but certainly killing my children; that thought is furthest removed from my mind. I love them too dearly."); or (3) organic symptoms: the patients whose mental symptoms take an organic route of expression usually complain of a disease and not of symptoms; a woman, 35 years old, inordinately attached to her mother since early childhood, developed a deep sense of guilt when she left her invalid mother, who had a hemiplegia at the time. She repressed the guilt, replacing it with good intellectual reasoning, that is, with rationalization. The daughter later developed symptoms identical with those of her mother, and although these were not organically determined, the repressed guilt and its associated impulses returned to consciousness in the guise of a physical ailment.

Symbols may appear as delusions, hallucinations, morbid affects, compulsions, obsessions, conversions (i.e., hysterical), hypochondriasis, personalization of organs or organ systems, etc. Dreams form a special class of symbols.

**symbolamblyopia, congenital** Claiborne's term (1906) for a type of *reading disability* (q.v.).

**symbolic categorization** See *lobe, parietal.*

**symbolic computation** See *cognitive psychology.*

**symbolic wounding** See *deliberate self-harm syndrome.*

**symbolism** In dreams, the chief method of distorting the latent content. Psychoanalytic experience has shown that the ideas symbolized concern the fundamental factors of existence—our bodies, life, death, procreation—in relation to ourselves and our families. Dream symbolism has many mechanisms in common with formation of figures of speech. The simplest figure of speech is *simile*, i.e., the equation of two dissimilar things by means of a common attribute, the similarity being indicated by "as" or "like." When these words are omitted, the compressed simile is known as *metaphor.* These devices also occur in dreams. Personal metaphor involves the transference of human activities to the nonhuman, such as "sighing oak." A flowing stream in a dream will suggest a stream of urine or a flow of talk; or a particular type of tree may have special significance such as "pine" tree meaning someone longed for, etc. Through *metonymy*, a name that has a usual or accidental connection with a thing is used for the thing itself, such as the "bar" for the profession of law. Synecdoche employs a part to represent the whole, such as a factory accommodating so many "hands." When the sounds of the words echo the sense, the term is *onomatopoeia. Antithesis* appears in dreams in the form of opposition in position, as in sitting. Parallels are used to convey similarity of position, such as sitting alongside a person. The repetition of a dream element is similar to the repetition of phrases in diction to secure emphasis. Through the implied metaphor abstract ideas are expressed in terms of the concrete; e.g., "food for thought," "hot temper." Although words acquire a second meaning and convey abstract ideas, they do not lose their original concrete significance in the unconscious; language itself, therefore, may yield significant information. Thus, "She is her mother's spoiled darling" may mean she is pampered; but to the unconscious, spoiled also means dirty or ruined. See *dream.*

**symbolization**  "According to psychoanalytic usage an unconscious process built up on association and similarity whereby one object comes to represent or stand for (symbolize) another object, through some part, quality, or aspect which the two have in common. The resemblance is generally so slight or superficial that the conscious mind would overlook it" (Healy et al. *The Structure and Meaning of Psychoanalysis,* 1930).

**symbollexia**  The process of transforming presentational symbols and imagery (including sights, sounds, and other sensory modes) into verbal descriptions. Since presentational symbols are believed to be a right-hemisphere function and verbalization to be a left-hemisphere function, symbollexia is believed to be an intercallosal function.

**symbolon**  A social symbol, the token or sign by which people who are linked can recognize each other; also, a representative of the emotions that bond people to each other. An example is the wedding ring.

**symbolophobia**  Fear of symbolism, e.g., of having a symbolical meaning attached to one's acts or words.

**symmetrical**  See *complementary.*

**sympathetic dystrophy syndrome**  See *pain syndromes.*

**sympathetic epilepsy**  *Autonomic epilepsy* (q.v.).

**sympathetic insanity**  *Obs.* Insanity for which the primary cause or seat was believed to be an organic part of the body biologically unconnected with the cerebrum.

**sympathetic nervous system**  See *autonomic nervous system.*

**sympathicotonia**  Eppinger and Hess's term for a clinical syndrome in which there is increased tonus of the sympathetic nervous system with a marked tendency to vascular spasm and high blood pressure, excessive functioning of the adrenals, and a hypersensitivity to adrenalin.

**sympathin**  See *epinephrine.*

**sympathism**  Suggestibility.

**sympathize**  To experience a feeling similar to that possessed by another. Usually reciprocal motivation is implied.

**sympathomimetic**  See *adrenergic; mydriasis.*

**sympathy**  In general, the existence of feeling identical with or resembling that which another experiences. According to Freud, identification may arise when there is no emotional attachment with the person imitated: for example, one person may copy the feelings and actions of another, because the imitator has an unconscious impulse set free upon hearing about or looking at the one copied. In sympathy the feelings of the imitator remain essentially within him. When one or both share similar feelings, based upon some common unconscious quality, the term *identification* is used. See *empathize.*

**symphorophilia**  A *paraphilia* (q.v.) in which sexual arousal and orgasm depend upon orchestrating a fire, accident, or other potential disaster and watching as it happens; sometimes equated with thrill-seeking (*philobatism*).

**symptom**  1. Any sign, physical or mental, that stands for something else. See *symbol; symbolism.* 2. In a medical sense, pathology, although in its broader meaning a symptom may reflect physiologic action (as in hunger).

**symptom, biphasic**  A compulsive symptom or action that has two component parts, the second of which is the direct reverse of the first: e.g., the patient has the compulsion first to open the water tap and then to close it again. Obsessive thoughts or impulses may likewise have two parts, the second directly contradicting the first.

The first phase of the symptom represents an instinctual demand, whereas the second phase represents the *anti-instinctual force* or threat of the superego. See *anticathexis*.

**symptom, primary defense** A term used by Freud in describing the early development of obsessional neurosis. At the onset of sexual maturity, self-reproach for the memories of pleasurable sexual activities in childhood is avoided by primary defense symptoms, such as conscientiousness, shame, and self-distrust. These introduce the period of "apparent health or better-than successful defense" (Freud, S. *Collected Papers*, 1924–1925).

**symptom, secondary defense** The protective measures to which the ego resorts in obsessional neurosis, when the primary defense (against repressed memories and self-reproach) has failed. The secondary defense symptoms include obsessive actions, obsessive speculating, obsessive thinking, the compulsion to test everything, *folie du doute*; "secondary defense against the obsessional affects calls into being a still wider series of protective measures, which may be transformed into obsessive acts. These may be grouped according to their tendencies: *penitential measures* (burdensome ceremonials, the observation of numbers), *precautionary measures* (all kinds of phobias, superstitions, pedantry, exaggeration of the primary symptom of conscientiousness), *dread of betrayal* (collecting paper, misanthropia), *hebetude* (dipsomania)" (Freud, S. *Collected Papers*, 1924–1925).

**symptom complex** See *syndrome*.

**symptom specificity** See *specificity, symptom*.

**symptomatic** Having the nature or quality of a *symptom* (q.v.); indicative of underlying pathology. Thus, the symptomatic psychoses are secondary disturbances of psychic function dependent upon primary alterations in brain tissue function. Some reserve the term symptomatic psychoses for *acute brain disorders* (q.v.); the chronic brain disorders are then referred to as organic psychoses.

**symptomatic act** *Faulty action*; mistake, error; intending to do one thing but doing something else, which is usually in basic conflict with the intended action. Often called

*Freudian slip* because of the assumption that it is based on unconscious wishes that the subject would consciously reject. Symptomatic acts are expressed as mannerisms, slips of the tongue (lapsus linguae) or of memory (lapsus memoriae) or of the pen (lapsus calami), misprints, fake visual recognition, mislaying of objects, etc.

**symptomatic epilepsy** Convulsions that are a symptom of an underlying organic disease. This may occur in such conditions as congenital defects of the brain, intracranial hemorrhages, meningitis, brain abscess, senile degeneration, or carbon monoxide poisoning.

**symptomatic insanity** *Obs.* Organic *psychosis* in contradistinction to psychogenic syndromes, termed *idiopathic insanity* by Mercier.

**symptomatic psychosis** Brain dysfunction as a result of some general physical disease, the most common feature of which is a delirious state.

This may occur in the course of an acute infectious disease such as pneumonia, influenza, typhoid fever, meningitis, or in the course of acute chorea, pellagra, or pelvic infections following childbirth.

**symptoms, prodromal** See *prodromal symptoms*.

**synapse** A stable adhesive junction between two cells across which information is relayed by directed secretion. At their points of contact, the membrane surfaces of neurons are parallel to each other, with a fluid-filled cleft in between. The cleft is filled with electron-dense material, including adhesion molecules and *receptor* molecules. One surface recognizes another and, if the "fit" is right, the pre- and postsynaptic surfaces are locked together by adhesion molecules (see *adhesion, cellular*). The resulting adhesive clamp aligns the active zones and postsynaptic elements to one another.

The term, coined by Sir Charles Sherrington in 1897, refers to a specialized structure at which the terminal *axon* (q.v.) or bouton makes contact with the dendritic receptor zone. Mitochondria in the bouton contain the elements that generate cellular energy through metabolism of glucose, enzymes involved in the synthesis and degradation of neurotransmitter, and storage vesicles for the neurotransmitter itself. The synapse is a specialized zone of contact between neurons, the point at which one neuron communicates with another. On average, each mature cortical cell is estimated to have about 10,000 synapses. The total number of synapses in the brain is somewhere between 10 and 100 trillion.

When a neuron is stimulated, the nerve impulse or electrical action potential causes neurotransmitter to be released into the *synaptic cleft* (the space between the neurons), where it interacts briefly with the adjacent neuron's dendritic membrane. The interaction results either in electrical stimulation that heightens the likelihood that an action potential or nerve impulse will be generated in the postsynaptic neuron, or in electrical inhibition that decreases the likelihood of such an impulse. See *nerve conduction; neuron; neurotransmitter; neurotransmitter receptor.*

Receptors concentrated on the dendritic membrane comprise two elements: (1) *recognition site*, which is located on the external surface of the neuronal membrane and allows the "right" neurotransmitter, i.e., one that fits the site, to be bound to it, and (2) *transducer site*, which is activated by occupation of the recognition site into initiating the physiological response.

**synaptic cleft**   The gap between nerve cells, about a millionth of an inch wide, in which the message from one nerve cell is converted from an electrical signal to a chemical one. See *neurotransmitter.*

**synaptic delay**   See *facilitation.*

**synaptic inactivation**   Termination of the neurotransmitter action, more often effected by specific reuptake transport proteins (which remove reurotransmitter from the synaptic area) than by enzyme degradation of the neurotransmitter.

**synaptic integration**   See *integration, neuronal.*

**synaptic plasticity**   Change(s) in the functional properties of a synapse (strengthening or weakening) as a result of use. In line with Hebb's postulate, it is generally believed that such changes depend at least in part on the firing times of the interacting neurons: when they fire close together or simultaneously, the functional connection between them is enhanced or potentiated. The NMDA receptor appears to be involved in such experience-dependent synaptic modification. See *NMDAR.*

Synaptic plasticity is of two types: *homosynaptic* or Hebbian activity-dependent, and *heterosynaptic* or modulatory input-dependent.

Heterosynaptic includes strengthening or weakening of synapse without activity of either the pre- or postsynaptic neuron as a result of the firing of a third, modulatory interneuron. Such modulation may be nonassociative and purely heterosynaptic, or associative, which is activity-dependent and combines features of both heterosynaptic and homosynaptic mechanisms. Heterosynaptic plasticity commonly recruits long-term memory mechanisms that lead to transcripion and to synaptic growth. When jointly recruited, homosynaptic mechanisms assure that learning is effectively established and heterosynaptic mechanisms ensure that memory is maintained. See *Hebbian synapse.*

**synaptic receptor protein**   See *transduction, stimulus.*

**synaptic transmission**   In the 1930s there were two schools of thought as to whether the responsible mechanism is physiological or pharmacological. The improved physiological techniques of the 1950s and 1960s demonstrated that both kinds of transmission occur.

**synaptogenesis**   Formation of synapse(s). See *axon growth.*

**synaptology**   The study of synaptic mechanisms, in large part initiated by Julius Axelrod's discovery of the enzyme catechol O-methyltransferase, for which he received the 1970 Nobel Prize in Medicine. This discovery focused attention on synaptic mechanisms involved in monoaminergic neurotransmission.

**synaptoneurosomes**   Preparations of intact synapses that have been detached from their cell bodies.

**synaptosome**   1. Vesicle-filled sacs of synaptic terminals. Transmitter is released from the vesicles by *exocytosis* (q.v.), the vesicle membrane fuses with the membrane of the synaptic terminals and then is recycled. 2. A preparation of the presynaptic terminal, isolated after subcellular fractionation. The structure retains the anatomical integrity of the terminal and can take up, store, and release neurotransmitters.

**synchiria**   Perception of a stimulus to one side of the body as having been applied to both sides of the body.

**synchronism**   The simultaneous occurrence of several developmental faults. In Down syndrome, for example, all organ systems of ectodermal, mesodermal, and entodermal origin that undergo specific development during the neofetal period are impaired; the particular synchronism of such symptoms points to the period between the sixth and twelfth weeks of fetal life as the time when the etiologic factors exert their greatest effect.

**synchronization** Neuronal coherence; phase-locking; simultaneous patterning of neural oscillations in different parts of the brain, believed to be an important mechanism in neural communication. In general, neurons are tightly interconnected in local functional networks, which endow each region with the ability to perform specific tasks. Such specialization is important for optimal information processing within each area, but effective communication with neural assemblies in distant areas of the brain requires one area of the brain to convey certain aspects of its current functional state to another area. Such coordinated communication between various areas in the brain is made possible by long-range oscillatory synchronization between those areas. The interacting areas resonate with each other, with one area driving or modulating the activity of the others. Often many neurons converge on a common target, but at a given moment only part of the input is effective in influencing the target neuron's output. Selective coherence is an ideal candidate mechanism for the regulation of the efficiency of input. It would at the same time increase the impact of input that is coherent with the target and decrease the impact of input that is not coherent with the target.

*Gamma synchrony*, synchrony of oscillations in the gamma *frequency band* (q.v.), provides a pertinent index of thalamo-cortical synchrony. It has been associated with cognitive functions such as attention, arousal, object recognition, and top-down modulation of sensory processes. In schizophrenia, a failure of neuronal binding in the cortical-reticular-thalamo-cortical loop is associated with an inability to focus attention on relevant stimuli in the face of irrelevant stimuli and to select appropriate responses. A deficit in the synchronization of pyramidal cells might contribute to the deficits in gamma band oscillation and, thereby, to working memory dysfunction in schizophrenia. Abnormal synchronization has also been associated with other neuropsychiatric disorders, including epilepsy, dementia, and, in particular, basal

ganglia disorders such as Parkinson disease. See *chandelier neurons; neocortical cells*.

**synchrony** See *rate code model*.

**syncope** 1. Fainting; a swoon (outdated); loss of consciousness secondary to temporary insufficiency in cerebral blood flow.

2. Deletion of a vowel within a word, such as pronouncing -tary, -tery, or -tory as -tri (e.g., secretary, mystery, laboratory).

**syncretism** See *physiognomonic thinking*.

**syndrome** A collection or grouping of disjunctive, variable signs and symptoms whose frequency of occurrence together suggests the existence of a single pathologic process or disorder that will explain them. "A syndrome is fundamentally a statistical notion based on covariation; it seems obvious that its derivation will be placed on more secure grounds when it is carried out (1) on the basis of a properly formulated model, (2) with awareness of the statistical requirements and difficulties involved, (3) on the firm foundation of quantitative measurement of objective test performance, (4) in relation to properly selected samples of the population in question, (5) in accordance with the rules of significance widely accepted in biological statistics. It is not implied that the syndromes isolated by psychiatrists in the last hundred years or so are inevitably imaginary and to be discarded; it seems more likely that such consensus as there is points to important and fruitful dimensions which could be validated by proper statistical research, and perhaps improved and sharpened" (Eysenck, H. J. *Handbook of Abnormal Psychology*, 1960).

In general, three levels of categorization can be differentiated in medicine: (1) an isolated sign or symptom, without reference to associated features or cause, and with little predictive value; headache, stuttering, constipation, etc., are examples; (2) a clinical picture formed by a grouping of signs or symptoms into a distinctive syndrome, such as a combination of diarrhea, dementia, and dermatitis (suggestive of pellagra); (3) a distinctive clinical picture that is accounted for by an identifiable pathophysiologic process or etiologic agent, such as intellectual deterioration occurring in irregular spurts over a period of several years in a 67-year-old hypertensive man who also demonstrates dysarthria, small-step gait, and fundoscopic changes indicating arteriosclerosis (multi-infarct dementia). See *abnormality; disease*.

**syndrome, organic**  See *organic syndrome*.

**syndrome of inappropriate anti-diuretic hormone**  *SIADH* (q.v.).

**syndrome X**  *Metabolic syndrome* (q.v.).

**syndromes, acute**  Bleuler differentiated between the acute and chronic forms of schizophrenia. The acute syndromes are transitory states of various kinds that may occur as simple exacerbations of the chronic state or as reactive episodes, in response to emotionally charged experiences. The acute syndromes occur more frequently in the early years of the disease process; they may last for hours only, or they may persist for years. Subsequent memory for these episodes varies, but complete amnesia for them is unusual. Bleuler listed the following acute syndromes: melancholic conditions, manic conditions, catatonic states, delusions (amentia in the terms of the Viennese school), twilight states, Benommenheit, confusional states, fits of anger, anniversary excitements, stupor, deliria, fugue states, and dipsomania. See *schizophrenia; schizophrenia, forms of.*

**syneidesis**  *Rare.* This Greek word was proposed by Monakow to replace the English conscience. Monakow suggests that conscience is not a specifically human phenomenon and does not belong to the sphere of consciousness, but is a characteristic of all living beings in any stage of development. This concept is at variance with prevailing psychiatric opinion, which believes that conscience is a product of the interaction of the child with frustration-producing elements in the child's environment. See *conscience.*

**synergism, sexual**  Sexual excitation that arises from a combination of various stimuli acting simultaneously.

**synergy**  1. Coordination of muscular movements. 2. Cooperation in action, primarily a function of the cerebellum.

**synesthesia**  *Secondary sensation*; a combining of sense perceptions, such as seeing letters in color (the most common form, called *grapheme-color synesthesia*), perceiving musical notes and musical keys as having specific hues, or feeling the shape of a taste. Sensations of color may accompany perceptions of taste, touch, pain, heat or cold; they are called *photisms*. With some synesthetes, certain words are accompanied by a sense of color, varying with different words (*verbochromia*). Secondary auditory sensations are called *phonisms*, secondary taste sensations are

called *gustatisms*, and secondary smell sensations are called *olfactisms*.

Synesthesia is more common in children; in some reports, one-third of children studied described the sounds of musical instruments as having colors. It is hypothesized that it tends to disappear with age as it is replaced by abstract language. The author Vladimir Nabokov described his own "colored hearing," which did not disappear with age: pistachio-colored t, huckleberry k, rose quartz q.

Synesthesia is the result of cross-activation between different brain areas. Grapheme-color synesthesia, for example, is caused by cross-activation between areas of the fusiform gyrus that are involved in grapheme processing and areas that are involved in color processing. Synesthesia is much more common in females than in males (4–6: 1). It may be a genetic trait that is most frequently transmitted from father to daughter through the X chromosome.

**syngamy**  *Fertilization*, the biological phenomenon that brings about the intermingling of paternal and maternal hereditary material.

**synkinesia, synkinesis**  An involuntary movement accompanying a voluntary one; such as the movement (occurring in a paralyzed muscle) accompanying motion in another part; any abnormal associated movement(s), indicative of neural injury or maldevelopment; they are brought out when the subject voluntarily contracts one muscle or muscle group, for then other unintended and unneeded movements appear. Such associated movements, also termed *adventitious motor overflow*, suggest frontal lobe dysfunction.

Various forms of synkinesis have been described; *Gunn*, for example, described a palpebromandibular synkinesia, consisting of elevation of the upper lid during any movement of the lower jaw.

**synnoetics**  A term suggested by Fein for the science "treating of the properties of composite systems...whose main attribute is its ability to invent, to create, and to reason—its 'mental' power of its components." Another term for synnoetics would be "the computer-related sciences," which would include such subjects as cybernetics, computer science, and bionics (*American Scientist 49*, 1961).

**synonymous-coding SNPs**  See *SNP*.

**syntactical aphasia**  *Wernicke aphasia* (q.v.).

**syntax**  The formal structure and grammar of the sentence, allowing the speaker to combine and recombine verbal symbols into an infinite number of acceptable sentences (a capacity that appears to be unique to the human animal). Syntax involves the understanding (*receptive syntax*) and using (*expressive syntax*) of different sentence types; the grammatical subsystem of language and the relations and rules required to form sentences and phrases.

Syntactic categories can be defined independently of meaning. See *rationalism*.

**synteny** The occurrence of genes on the same chromosome. Synteny conservation is the occurrence of two or more pairs of homologous markers on the same chromosome in two or more species.

**synthesis** The combination or grouping of parts or elements so as to form an integrated whole; the integration of the various factors making up the personality and thus the opposite of analysis. This term has been used with various shades of meaning by different writers. Prince used it to refer to the ability to keep the component parts of the psyche together in close association; any weakening of synthesis tends to produce dissociation and hence neurosis. Synthesis has also been used to refer to maintenance of intactness of personality; in this sense, synthesis is the opposite of *splitting* in Bleuler's sense. Gestalt psychologists use the term synthesis to refer to the tendency to perceive and appreciate situations as a whole. In psychoanalytic psychology, synthesis is considered to be a complex ego function, probably a derivative of libido, which impels the person to harmonious unification and creativity in the broadest sense of the term. Synthesis includes a tendency to simplify, to generalize, and ultimately to understand—by assimilating external and internal elements, by reconciling conflicting ideas, by uniting contrasts, and by seeking for causality. See *constructive; ego; ego strength; gestalt psychology; object relations theory; psychosynthesis.*

**syntone** One whose personality is in harmony and emotional rapport with the environment. Bleuler at times used it interchangeably with *cyclothyme*. Syntone implies normality, while cyclothyme describes a personality disorder that is an exaggeration of the syntonic.

**syntropy** The state of wholesome association with others.

**synucleinopathies** Neurodegenerative disorders associated with Lewy bodies, such as Lewy body dementia, some forms of Alzheimer disease, and some forms of prion disease. The *Lewy body* (q.v.) consists largely of the protein α-synuclein; it is uncertain if α-synuclein is directly neurotoxic or if it is a defensive reaction to chronic stress or some other toxic factor. See *tauopathies*.

**syphilis, cerebral** *Meningovascular syphilis; interstitial syphilis.* The term includes syphilitic leptomeningitis, vascular neurosyphilis or luetic endarteritis, and the gummatous subtype. The essential lesion in cerebral syphilis is vascular and parivascular inflammation of varying degrees. Symptoms, which typically appear about 3 years after the primary infection, depend upon the site and extent of involvement. Thus, there may be primarily a picture of acute or chronic leptomeningitis with signs of increased intracranial pressure and involvement of the cranial nerves (especially III, IV, and VII); or luetic endarteritis may lead to occlusion and thus to hemiplegia or convulsions; or development of a gumma may simulate the appearance of intracranial neoplasm. Superimposed on these neurologic signs are mental symptoms, such as intellectual dulling, emotional lability, stupor, fearful delirium, or multiple somatic complaints.

**syphilis, congenital** See *neurosyphilis, congenital*.

**syphilis, mesodermogenic** Meningovascular syphilis. See *syphilis, cerebral*.

**syphilophobia** Fear of (contracting) syphilis.

**syringobulbia** See *syringomyelia*.

**syringomyelia** *Status dysraphicus*; a chronic disease, probably due to a developmental defect, consisting of the formation of cysts within the spinal cord or medulla (*syringobulbia*). Symptoms begin in the second and third decades; 70% of those affected are male. Because the lesion starts centrally, the first fibers to be affected are those carrying pain and temperature sensations as they cross in the anterior commissure. This usually causes bilateral loss of cutaneous sensation in the segments involved, producing a cuirass (breastplate) pattern, affecting a few cervical or thoracic segments and sparing sensation below. Pain and temperature sensation are impaired, but touch and proprioception are intact. The loss of sensation may lead to painless injuries of the digits or painless burns. In time, hand and finger movements become weak and awkward, and a claw hand develops.

Trophic disturbances are prominent, with thickened skin and various arthropathies (some would call this form *Morvan disease*). In the bulbar form, symptoms referable to disturbances of the tenth, eighth, and fifth cranial nerves and of the medial lemniscus are seen. Affected patients usually live many years. Palliative X-ray irradiation of the affected region of the spinal cord or medulla is sometimes beneficial.

**system** In psychoanalytic psychology, any of the organizational units of the psychic apparatus; the R-systems (psychic apparatus) include the *P-system* (perception), the *mem-system* (memory), the *Pcs* (preconscious), and the *Ucs* (unconscious).

**system, Aberdeen** See *Aberdeen system*.

**systematic desensitization** See *desensitization*.

**systematic family therapy** See *family therapy, systematic*.

**systematic schizophrenia** In Leonhard's classification, one of the two major subdivisions of schizophrenic disorders, comprising catatonias, hebephrenias, and paraphrenias. Systematic schizophrenias follow a progressive course. The other subdivision, with a better prognosis, he called nonsystematic, further divided into affect-laden paranoia, schizophasia, and periodic catatonia.

**systematized complex** *Obs.* A grouping of associated experiences or mental events that becomes relatively fixed over time and predisposes the person to behave or respond in a particular way. Character and personality traits are examples of systematized complexes.

M. Prince differentiated among *subject complexes* or systems, related to certain types of experience, *chronological complexes* or systems, related to experiences during a particular time of life, and *disposition* or *mood complexes*, related to particular emotions or feeling tones (*The Unconscious*, 1916).

**systematized delusion** Organized delusion, which fits into an overall plan that within itself maintains logic, order, and consistency, even though the logic is based upon false initial assumptions.

**systems theory** See *general systems theory*.

**Szondi test** A projective test, developed by Szondi in Switzerland in the 1940s, which consists of six sets of pictures, each set containing eight photographs. These eight photographs are of eight different psychobiological conditions—homosexual, sadist, epileptic, hysteric, catatonic schizophrenic, paranoid schizophrenic, manic-depressive depressed, manic-depressive manic.

The subject chooses from each set the two pictures he likes most and the two he dislikes the most. The eight different conditions portrayed are presumed to be extreme pathological representatives of the eight basic emotional needs. The test is interpreted in terms of the degree of tension, and the subject's attitude to this tension, in each of these eight need-systems.

The need-systems are as follows: the need for tender, feminine love (h factor); the need for aggression and masculinity (s factor); the mode of dealing with crude, aggressive emotions (e factor); the need to exhibit emotions (hy factor); narcissistic ego-needs (k factor); the expansive tendencies of the ego (p factor); the need for acquiring and mastering objects (d factor); and the need to cling to objects for enjoyment (m factor). Although the Szondi test can be used clinically, as a projective technique, without reference to the viewpoint that led to its development, the basis of the test is Szondi's theory of *genotropism* (q.v.).

**T type**   See *eidetic imagery.*

**TA**   *Transactional analysis* (q.v.).

**tabes**   (L. "a wasting, emaciation") *Tabes dorsalis, locomotor ataxia*; a chronic, progressive disease of the nervous system occurring rather late in a comparatively small percentage of persons affected with syphilis. The main pathological process involves the posterior spinal ganglia in a mild inflammation. The roots between the ganglia and the spinal cord, and, to some extent, the meninges are also involved. There is a degeneration of the nerve fibers with a selective degeneration of the posterior columns of the cord. The cranial nerves, especially the optic and those supplying the ocular muscles, are particularly involved. The symptoms are ataxia, or muscular incoordination, neuralgia, anesthesia, visceral crises, lancinating pains, and muscular atrophy. Trophic disorders of the joints (arthropathies) are frequent, atrophy of the optic nerve occurs, and paralysis may be a late symptom. Mental symptoms are not usually prominent, although a severe depression may occur.

**tabes, congenital**   See *neurosyphilis, congenital.*

**tabes, juvenile**   Juvenile tabes presents an essentially identical pathological process and clinical course as in the adult. The symptoms appear from the age of 10 onward in children who have congenital syphilis or who acquired the disease in infancy or early childhood. Ataxia is rather infrequent, while optic atrophy is very common in juvenile tabes. Mental symptoms and taboparesis occur frequently. The Wasserman blood reaction is often negative. The course is much more rapid than in the adult form, and the disease terminates fatally comparatively early.

**tabetic curve**   See *Lange colloidal gold reaction.*

**tabetic gait**   See *ataxic gait.*

**table, frequency**   The number of subjects with a given character may be arrayed in order of size with respect to the amount of the character possessed by each individual in the series. If the entire range is divided into intervals, and if to each interval is assigned the number of cases falling within the limits of the class, the resulting distribution is called a frequency table.

**table, life**   An instrument for determining the number of years that any person may, on the

**ADULTS FROM HOUSEHOLD POPULATION WITH SERIOUS MENTAL ILLNESS,
BY AGE, SEX, RACE, AND EDUCATION: UNITED STATES, 1989**

| | ADULT HOUSEHOLD POPULATION | | ADULTS WITH SERIOUS MENTAL ILLNESS | | |
| --- | --- | --- | --- | --- | --- |
| | NO. (IN THOUSANDS) | PERCENT DISTRIBUTION | NO. (IN THOUSANDS) | PERCENT | RATE PER THOUSANDS |
| Total | 179,529 | 100.00 | 3,265 | 100.00 | 18.2 |
| Age in years | | | | | |
| 18-24 | 25,401 | 14.2 | 361 | 11.1 | 14.2 |
| 25-34 | 42,814 | 23.9 | 707 | 21.7 | 16.5 |
| 35-44 | 35,982 | 20.0 | 744 | 22.8 | 20.7 |
| 45-64 | 46,114 | 25.7 | 919 | 28.2 | 19.9 |
| 65-69 | 9,903 | 5.5 | 142 | 4.4 | 14.3 |
| 70-74 | 7,925 | 4.4 | 102 | 3.1 | 12.9 |
| 75 & over | 11,391 | 6.3 | 288 | 9.8 | 25.3 |
| Sex | | | | | |
| Male | 85,257 | 47.5 | 1,320 | 40.4 | 15.5 |
| Female | 94,272 | 52.5 | 1,944 | 59.6 | 20.6 |
| Race | | | | | |
| White | 153,763 | 85.6 | 2,812 | 86.1 | 18.3 |
| Other | 5,834 | 3.2 | 59 | 1.8 | 10.1 |

SOURCE: Reprinted from the United States Department of Health and Human Services, 1992.

average, be expected to live after reaching a specified age. It also enables one to determine the chance of an individual dying within any specified number of years after reaching a given age.

**EXPECTATION OF LIFE AT BIRTH, BY SEX AND COUNTRY, 1900**

| COUNTRY | LIFE EXPECTANCY AT BIRTH | |
|---|---|---|
| | MALE | FEMALE |
| Argentina | 68.9 | 74.0 |
| Australia | 73.9 | 80.0 |
| Brazil | 63.5 | 69.1 |
| Canada | 73.3 | 80.0 |
| China | 68.6 | 71.8 |
| France | 73.0 | 81.1 |
| Germany | 72.2 | 78.7 |
| India | 57.7 | 58.7 |
| Japan | 75.9 | 81.8 |
| Mexico | 66.5 | 73.1 |
| Russia | 63.5 | 74.3 |
| Switzerland | 74.1 | 80.9 |
| United Kingdom | 72.7 | 78.3 |
| United States | 72.0 | 78.9 |

**table, statistical**  A summary of numerical data in accordance with logical criteria, showing the manner in which the variables included in the table are distributed with respect to their relative frequencies.

**HEALTH SERVICES 1986–1990, BY COUNTRY**

| COUNTRY | PHYSICIANS PER 10,000 | HOSPITAL BED AVERAGE | AVERAGE LENGTH OF STAY (IN DAYS) |
|---|---|---|---|
| Brazil | 169,500 | 37 | 4 |
| Canada | 58,470 | 70 | 13 |
| China | 1,808,000 | 23 | 16 |
| France | 148,089 | 126 | 16 |
| Germany | 251,877 | 83 | 15 |
| India | 365,000 | 8 | NA |
| Japan | 211,797 | 136 | 56 |
| Mexico | 130,000 | 13 | 9 |
| Russia | 657,800 | 135 | NA |
| Switzerland | 22,000 | 81 | 24 |
| United Kingdom | 92,172 | 62 | 15 |
| United States | 614,000 | 47 | 9 |

NA, Not available.

**taboo, tabu**  "On the one hand it means to us, sacred, consecrated: but on the other hand it means uncanny, dangerous, forbidden and unclean.... [T]aboo expresses itself essentially in prohibitions and restrictions. Our combination of 'hold dread' would often express the meaning of taboo" (Freud, S. *The Basic Writings of Sigmund Freud*, 1938).

**taboo language**  Words that are socially unacceptable and offensive, typically because they refer to what many people find embarrassing or distasteful, or to subjects so controversial that they are likely to incite anger, resentment, or brutality in the discussants. In current Western cultures, taboo subjects commonly include sexual behavior (at least of some kinds; see *sexual revolution*), excretory functions, and specific references to the body parts involved in such actions; religious beliefs and political convictions (unless it is known that everyone present shares or accepts them); and, in some strata of society, money and income. Although the "double standard" and sexual stereotyping are universally decried, it cannot be denied that what is acceptable to the participants in an all-male or an all-female group may not be tolerated by those same participants in other settings. In the case of each of the taboo topics mentioned, what is taboo is probably defined more by the makeup of the specific group at the moment than by any universal standard that applies to all members of a culture at all times. See *mores; pornography; racism; sexism; unnatural*.

**taboparesis**  A disease of the nervous system that combines the features of general paresis and tabes dorsalis. The mental and physical symptoms of general paresis are present together with spinal cord changes producing absent knee or ankle jerks, the Romberg sign, and bladder disturbances.

**tabula rasa**  (L. "erased or blank tablet") Clean slate, or, by extension, the mind at birth. The tabula rasa idea finds its modern expression in Pavlovian psychology, an environmentalist view that the nature of the response is determined by the stimulus. Such a position is much more subject than the biological to whatever ideology is defined by the political or cultural values of the moment as the fit, normal, or desirable way of life.

**tachistoscope test**  A shutter opens for brief intervals to reveal a slide or picture; the subject must then follow the command related to the exposed stimulus, such as pressing a key.

**tachophobia**  Fear of speed, as in fear of being in a fast-moving vehicle.

**tachy-**  Combining form meaning quick, swift, fleet, from Gr. *tachys*. Opposite of brady-.

**tachyathetosis**  *Restless legs syndrome* (q.v.).

**tachycardia, orthostatic**  Rapidity of pulse rate beyond the normal range occurring when one changes from the reclining to the standing position.

**tachyglossa**   See *tachylogia*.

**tachykinins**   Include *NKA* and *SP* (qq.v.).

**tachylogia**   *Hyperlogia; hyperphrasia; tachylalia; tachyphrasia*; abnormal rapidity of speech. It is also used loosely to include excessive amount of speech, which is more properly termed *lalorrhea, logodiarrhea, logorrhea, polylogia*, or *polyphrasia. Logomania* and *verbomania* are the more general terms that may refer to either excessively rapid (pressured) speech or to an excessive amount of speech.

**tachyphagia**   Foodgrabbing; extreme rapidity of eating. Tachyphagia is commonly seen in regressed, deteriorated schizophrenics, and often such patients will grab any object, edible or not, put it into the mouth, and swallow it.

**tachyphemia**   See *tachylogia*.

**tachyphrasia**   See *tachylogia*.

**tachyphylaxis**   *Downregulation* (q.v.).

**tachypnea, tachypnoea**   See *polypnoea*.

**tachypragia**   *Rare*. Psychomotor acceleration, as in the manic phase of manic-depressive disorder.

**tachytrophism**   Rapid or increased metabolism.

**tactical research**   See *research, strategic*.

**tactile agnosia**   Inability to recognize objects, such as paper, glass, soap, cotton, metals, etc. by touching them. See *double simultaneous tactile sensation*.

**tactile performance test**   A blindfolded subject is asked to place blocks and shapes in a formboard with the preferred, the nonpreferred, and both hands. The blindfold is then removed and the subject is asked to draw the formboard from memory.

**tactile sensation, double simultaneous**   See *double simultaneous tactile sensation*.

**taeniphobia**   Fear of tapeworms.

**taijin-kyofusho**   A syndrome reported among the Japanese consisting of fear of rejection, avoidance of eye contact, and easy blushing related to concern about body odor. The Japanese diagnostic system recognizes four subtypes: *sekimen-kyofu* (fear of blushing), *shubo-kyofu* (fear that one's body is deformed), *jikoshisen-kyofu* (fear of eye-to-eye contact), and *jikoshu-kyofu* (fear that one's body emits a foul odor that offends others). But DSM-IV recognizes that fear of blushing is a common symptom of social phobia, and it labels fear that one's body is deformed

body dysmorphic disorder. In Western psychiatric literature, the fear that one's body odor is foul has long been termed autodysosmophobia, automysophobia, bromidrosiphobia, or, more recently, olfactory reference syndrome. It seems doubtful, therefore, that taijin-kyofusho qualifies as a culture-bound syndrome.

**taint**   In genetics, the genotypical affection of an individual by a morbid factor inherited from, and manifested by, his ancestors, whether or not this factor is exhibited by the subject himself.

**taint carrier**   In genetic family studies, the members who carry a particular genetic factor in their genotypes but do not manifest it phenotypically. See *trait carrier*.

**talion dread**   A fear of "retaliation in kind" as punishment for forbidden acts or impulses. A vivid example is seen in the Oedipus situation, wherein the boy fears loss of his penis, i.e., castration by his father, as punishment for his misuse of it (in incestual relationship with his mother). Another example is to be seen in the neurotic's fear of death and in the hysterical attacks during which he feels he is dying, related to unconscious wishes for the death of another.

**tangentiality**   A type of association disturbance in which thought and speech diverge or digress from the topic of the moment so that they appear unrelated or irrelevant; if often repeated (and especially if the speaker does not return spontaneously to the topic), tangentiality is labeled loosening or diffuseness of speech, and its end result is to destroy the value of speech as an effective means of communicating with others.

**TANs**   Tonically active neurons. See *dopaminergic systems*.

**Tantra**   A group of Hindu or Buddhist sacred scriptures containing instructions for various kinds of meditation and worship to achieve unity between the worshiper and the deity. Tantric rituals include sexual intercourse (divine, between god and goddess, not bestial or lustful human sexuality); *mantras* (sacred sounds with a magical power to gain the desired unity); visual images, including mental representation of the deity and *mandalas* or *yantras*, external diagrams representing the abode of the worshiped deity (Jung viewed them as a way to develop harmony between the conscious and unconscious); and breathing techniques, used in Tantric yoga to achieve identity with the infinite.

**tantrum**   A child's dramatic outburst of crying, kicking, screaming, etc., in response to frustration. Such temper tantrums are natural to the child of 2 or 3 and are an expression of aggression, anger, rage, and defiance. The child works himself rapidly, or gradually, into a rage—yells out, stamps his feet, throws his arms about, rolls on the floor, strikes everyone, throws every object within reach against the walls, curses, bites, or even bangs his head against the wall. The tantrum thus assumes uncontrolled and sweeping proportions in contrast to normal expressions of anger and rage.

Tantrums are seen almost routinely in the children of overindulgent, oversolicitous, and overprotective parents. Though originating in physical discomforts which increase the child's irritability, tantrums either are motivated by an attempt to obtain gratifications and dominate a family that allows itself to be controlled by these outbursts, or are a result of imitation of a member of the household. Persistence or reappearance of tantrums after the age of 3 years indicates pathology and is classified within the *oppositional disorders* (q.v.).

**taoism**   Chinese philosophy founded by Lao Tsu in the 6th century B.C. The *Tao te Ching* expresses this simple philosophy of life: "Empty and be full; wear out and be new; have little and gain; have much and be confused." Taoist practices include effortless, yet effective action that proceeds gently, without force; modesty and sincerity in social relationships; an awareness of one's own energetic processes (*t'ai chi*); and a transcendence of the dualizing limitations of percepts and concepts. The last allows the participant to merge with and be guided by the Tao (the ultimate source and unifying principle of all that exists or is in process). The fundamental intent is toward the experience of the unification of all opposites, falsely dichotomized by the seduction of reason, toward the gradual attainment of clarity and openness in a creative balance.

**taphophilia**   Morbid attraction to graves and cemeteries. See *necrophilia*.

**taphophobia**   Fear of being buried (alive).

**Tapia syndrome**   (Antonio Garcia Tapia, Spanish otolaryngologist, 1875–1950) A bulbar syndrome due to involvement of the vagus and hypoglossal nerves, with homolateral paralysis and atrophy of the tongue, and homolateral paralysis of the pharynx and larynx.

**tarantism**   *Obs.* Dancing mania; specifically, what appears to have been a culture-specific syndrome in Italy in the 16th and 17th centuries, consisting of compulsive dancing as a way to undo the bite of the tarantula.

**Tarasoff decision**   Although an earlier Tarasoff decision specified a *duty to warn* the potential victim of violence, the superseding 1976 Tarasoff case clearly enunciated that the duty was to protect the potential victim from danger. "When a therapist determines . . . that his patient presents a serious danger of violence to another, he incurs an obligation to use reasonable care to *protect* the intended victim against such danger . . . . It may call for him to warn the intended victim, to notify police, or to take whatever steps are reasonably necessary under the circumstances." One option is hospitalization; if the patient refuses and there is an imminent risk of harm, the clinician must consider involuntary commitment criteria and other "reasonable steps" that may be implemented, including (1) increasing the frequency of outpatient appointments, (2) adjusting medications, (3) involving family or friends in an attempt to control the patient, and (4) removing weapons from the home. See *foreseeability*.

**taraxein**   See *ceruloplasmin*.

**tardive**   As used currently in psychiatry, tardy in the sense of being (or appearing) late rather than in the more proper sense of being slow.

**tardive dyskinesia**   *TD*; a neurologic adverse effect of antipsychotics consisting of abnormal, involuntary, irregular movements of the muscles of the mouth, tongue, face, neck, and trunk, and of choreoathetoid movements of the limbs. It typically appears late in treatment, often after several years, particularly following a reduction in dosage or upon cessation of treatment. It is more frequent in women, in patients over 50 years of age, and in patients who have had previous ECT.

Although the pathophysiology of tardive dyskinesia was formerly thought to be based on supersensitivity of striatal dopamine receptors, it is now believed that TD is associated with both increased central dopaminergic and noradrenergic activity and reduced GABAergic and cholinergic activity. It is possible that there are different types of TD, each with a different profile of neurochemical alterations.

Perioral movements are the most common symptom, with darting, twisting, and protruding movements of the tongue, chewing and lateral jaw movements, lip puckering, facial grimacing, and *blepharospasm* (q.v.). Because of the prominence of such symptoms, TD has also been called *oral-lingual dyskinesia, orofacial dyskinesia,* and *buccal-lingual-masticatory dyskinesia (BLM syndrome).* Other types include the axial (with trunk twisting, torticollis, retrocollis, shoulder shrugging, or pelvic thrusting) and the appendicular (rapid movements of the fingers or legs, or hand clenching, sometimes combined with slower, writhing movements).

Tardive dyskinesia was first described in the late 1950s (Schonecker, M. *Nervenartzt 28,* 1957; Sigwald, J., et al. *Revue Neurologie 100,* 1959). Other late-occurring syndromes associated with neuroleptic treatment include tardive dystonias and, sometimes, parkinsonism. See *tardive dystonia.*

**tardive dysmentia**   Also called *iatrogenic schizophrenia, tardive psychosis,* and *subcortical dementia* (q.v.); a behavior disorder involving changes in affect, activation level, and interpersonal interaction that is hypothesized to be the limbic system counterpart to tardive dyskinesia. It has been described in patients under long-term treatment with neuroleptic drugs. Symptoms include loquaciousness, intrusively loud voice, disconnected, aimless, and often inappropriate thoughts, a generally euphoric mood with occasional unpredictable explosions of hostility or petulance, and social withdrawal or autistic preoccupation broken by episodes of overactivity that is often blatantly invasive of others' privacy (Wilson, I. C. et al. *Schizophrenia Bulletin 9,* 1983).

The symptoms as described are not highly correlated with manifestations of cognitive impairment, but they do closely resemble frontal lobe syndromes (and there is evidence that frontal lobe abnormalities are characteristic of at least some subgroups of schizophrenia). On these grounds, many object to the term dysmentia—since cognitive impairment has not been demonstrated—and to the implication of "tardive" that the syndrome is related to treatment with neuroleptic agents.

**tardive dystonia**   A rare neurologic adverse effect of treatment with neuroleptics characterized by prolonged muscle spasms with torsion movements involving neck and face. *Blepharospasm* (q.v.) (involuntary eye closure), pleurothotonus (tonic flexion and rotation of the trunk to one side—the *Pisa syndrome*) and *opisthotonus* (severe forward or backward bending of the body) are seen, and involvement of the head makes eating difficult. The disorder produces more dysfunction and is less likely to improve than tardive dyskinesia. It is more common in younger patients and in males; tardive dyskinesia is more common in the elderly.

**tardive seizures**   The new occurrence of spontaneous seizures days,weeks, or even years after a course of electroconvulsive therapy.

**target behaviors**   See *behavior therapy.*

**target multiplicity**   A term suggested by Slavson to indicate the multiple possibilities existing in a group for projecting or displacing hostility on other patients, who replace the therapist as the target.

**target organ**   See *general adaptation syndrome.*

**targeted-dose strategy**   Also, *intermittent-dose strategy*; in pharmacotherapy, administration of a therapeutic drug on a fixed intermittent dose or, more commonly, only when the patient manifests signs of impending relapse (*EWS*, q.v.). Most studies have found targeted dosing to be associated with a much higher relapse rate in schizophrenia than regular maintenance dosing.

**targeting determinants**   See *Golgi apparatus.*

**targets, molecular**   See *neuropharmacology.*

**Taschen test**   A test for nystagmus in which the subject is directed to turn five times around his axis within 10 seconds and must then fix his eyes on the upheld index finger of the examiner. Duration of nystagmus so provoked beyond 9 seconds is considered abnormal.

**task, primary**   In group process theory, any task that a system must carry out in order to survive.

**task set**   The way of responding that is adopted in a given situation, often suggested to explain how the same stimulus can produce different responses.

**task-specific tremor**   See *tremor.*

**taste buds**   See *gustation.*

**TAT**   *Thematic apperception test* (q.v.).

**TAU**   Treatment as usual; used especially in studies comparing results of treatment with a new pharmacologic agent to results with an agent whose efficacy has been established.

**tau**   One of the microtubule-associated proteins (MAPs) that appear to be involved in the elongation of microtubules, perhaps by preventing depolymerization. Tau assembles and stabilizes the microtubules within the neuron; the microtubules can be likened to a railway track that transports vital materials through the neuron, tau to the ties on the track. If only a few ties are damaged, the track can still function, but if a lot of ties are destroyed the track will be rendered inoperative. Phosphatases are enzymes that remove phosphate groups from tau, but they are underproduced or inhibited in *Alzheimer disease* (q.v.). In consequence, tau remains hyperphosphorylated and cannot maintain its role in fastening microtubules. It becomes dissociated from the microtubule and becomes the principal protein constituent of neurofibrillary tangles. That transition generates a series of phosphorylated tau isoforms that are referred to as A68. Another microtubule-associated protein that has been identified in neurofibrillary tangles is ubiquitin, which normally is involved in the hydrolysis of proteins; it may be responsible for the insolubility of some paired helical filaments. See *ADAP*; *A68*.

**tau rhythm**   See *alpha rhythm*.

**tauopathies**   Neurodegenerative diseases in which tangles are a prominent part of the micropathology; the tangles consist largely of the protein tau. Tangles are found in frontotemporal dementia, *Alzheimer* disease (q.v.), parkinsonism, progressive supranuclear palsy, Guam disease, and some forms of prion disease. See *synucleinopathies*.

Tau-mediated neurodegeneration is due to a combination of toxic gains-of-function acquired by tau aggregates or their precursors and the loss of critical tau functions in the disease state.

**taxis**   Tropism; movement toward or away from some source of stimulation. Used loosely in social psychiatry to refer to the stimulus itself, in which case taxis refers to inanimate stimulation, biotaxis to animal or human stimulation, sociotaxis to social stimulation. See *network*.

**taxonomy**   See *nosology*.

**Tay-Sachs diseas**   (Warren Tay, English physician, 1843–1927; Bernard Sachs, American neurologist, 1858–1944) *TSD; GM2, gangliosidosis; cerebromacular degeneration; amaurotic family idiocy*; a recessive autosomal disorder of sphingolipid metabolism: lack of the liposomal enzyme β-hexosaminidase subunit, HEX A, leads to accumulation and deposition of ganglioside GM2 in the nerve cells of the cortex and cerebellum and in the axons of nerves, resulting in progressive neuronal dysfunction. The disease was first described by Tay in 1881, who referred principally to the ocular changes. In 1887, Sachs described the brain changes. Degeneration of retinal nerve fibers exposes the vascular chorion in the macular area, producing the diagnostic cherry red spot visible on fundoscopic examination. Other manifestations of the infantile form of TSD, which appear within the first 6 months of life, include decline of psychomotor development (sometimes termed dementia), irritability, blindness, spasticity, muscular wasting and enfeeblement, convulsions, and finally decerebrate rigidity and death by the age of 3 years. Incidence is highest among Ashkenazi Jews. Heterozygote screening for reduction in HEX A activity and prenatal diagnosis have resulted in a decreasing incidence of the disease in recent years. See *lysosomal storage diseases*.

Four forms are recognized: (1) *infantile form*, originally found mainly among Polish Jews, the symptoms appearing as early as the third month; (2) *late infantile form*, appearing between the second and fifth years; (3) *juvenile form*, appearing in older children between the sixth and twelfth years, was described by Spielmeyer. It resembles the infantile type, shows gradual mental impairment and terminates in blindness and death within 2 years. Although optic atrophy occurs, there are no changes in the macula lutea; (4) *adult form*, occurring after puberty, though usually not beyond the third decade. Some writers refer to the infantile form only as Tay-Sachs disease, to the late infantile form as *Bielschowsky disease*, to the juvenile form as *Vogt-Spielmeyer disease*, and to the adult or tardive form as *Kuf disease*.

The genes directing the synthesis of the subunits of HEX A have been localized: the gene for the alpha subunit to chromosome 15, and the gene for the beta unit to chromosome 5. The gene for the activator protein has also been localized to chromosome 5. Defects in any of these three gene products can result in lysosomal GM2 accumulation and subsequent disease. The HEX A deficiencies associated with TSD and its variants are a result of a deficiency in alpha subunits.

Among Ashkenazi Jews in North America, three specific mutations (two associated with infantile diseases and one with the adult-onset form) account for 92% to 94% of all mutant alleles. In the non-Jewish population, few carry the mutation that is most common in Jewish carriers; the most common mutation in the non-Jewish group is particularly associated with persons of Celtic or French origins, and it is the same allele that has been found in both the Pennsylvania Dutch and Cajun population.

Carrier rates are 1 in 30 or 31 among Jews, and 1 in 167 to 267 among non-Jews. Why TSD is so concentrated in the Jewish population is unknown. It is believed that the mutation arose during the Middle Ages in eastern Europe. It has been suggested that some selective environmental factor conferred a biological advantage on heterozygotes carrying these mutations, consisting perhaps of relative resistance to certain pulmonary diseases, particularly tuberculosis.

**TBI**   Traumatic brain injury; see *brain injury.*

**TC**   *Therapeutic community* (q.v.).

**TCA**   Tricyclic antidepressant drugs. See *antidepressant; psychotropic.*

**TCO**   *Threat-control-override* (q.v.).

**tea and toast syndrome**   *Dwindles*; a phenomenon described in olderpeople who develop nutritional deficiencies on the basis of inadequate diet. It is difficult, and expensive, to cook for one, and depression is characterized by a loss of pleasure in eating as well as diminution in energy. Since older people often are both poor and depressed, they are likely to nibble rather than take the time to prepare nutritious meals, and in time they often develop one or more severe deficiency disorders, the first sign of which may be an acute confusional state that is mistaken as an early sign of dementia.

**technique, classical**   See *parameter.*

**technoethics**   The social, humanitarian, ecological, and other aspects of robotics and similar recent technical developments in the neurosciences that raise issues concerning personal responsibility and identity, the definition of "normal," the consequences of enhancing brain function and of manipulating complex human behavior. It seems likely that research will move ever more closely to elucidating core human traits and values. This is certain to raise questions about privacy, personal responsibility in brain diseases that affect behavior, and the vulnerability of persons with addiction or dementia.

**teetotaler**   A person who maintains total *abstinence* (q.v.) from alcohol.

**TEFRA**   Tax Equity and Fiscal Responsibility Act of 1982 (PL 97-248), intended to reduce Medicaid and Medicare expenditures. It is the most significant health care financing legislation in the United States since Medicaid and Medicare were created in 1965 and directly affects all hospitals, insurers, pension plans, and major corporate purchasers of health insurance.

**tegmentum**   See *midbrain.*

**tele**   (Gr. "at a distance, far away, far off") In Moreno's system of sociometry, the intuitive reaction of liking or disliking another person based upon something real in that other person; the opposite of *transference* (q.v.), in which the reaction is an expression of the subject's needs rather than an appropriate response to the object's behavior or attitude.

**telegram, telegraphic speech**   See *Broca aphasia.*

**telemnemonike**   Acquiring consciousness of matters held in the memory of another person.

**telencephalon**   That part of the *forebrain* (q.v.) or prosencephalon that forms the cerebral cortex, the striate bodies, the rhinencephalon, the lateral ventricles, and the anterior portion of the third ventricle.

**teleoanalysis**   See *teleological.*

**teleologic hallucination**   A hallucination advising a patient about what course he or she should take.

**teleologic regression**   Purposeful regression. See *regression, progressive teleologic.*

**teleological**   Goal-directed, purposive; used particularly to refer to Adler's insistence on the holistic approach to personality and his belief that a person can best be understood by the goals he sets for himself, and not by any analysis or dissection of partial functions such as sexuality. The understanding of goals and the helping of patients to change their goals are so basic to Adlerian psychotherapy that individual psychology has sometimes been called *teleoanalysis.*

**teleology**   The belief that natural processes are purposefully directed toward some end or goal.

In psychiatry, the term is particularly used in reference to the psychologies of Jung and of Adler. Adler, for example, considers the present activity of the person as a preparation for his final state, for what he is going to be. Jung considers the mind as something much more than the result of past experiences: "It is Becoming as well as Has Been, and therefore any analysis of it must include reference to its aims and to that which it is trying to realize within itself. In this connection the dream must therefore be regarded as partly determined by the future." (Nicole, J. *Psychotherapy*, 1948).

**telepathy**  See *extrasensory perception.*

**telephone scatalogia**  A *paraphilia* (q.v.) involving unsolicited calls to a nonconsenting person, in order to express erotic or obscene language, or to phantasize that such thoughts are being expressed while the other person is on the telephone line (the caller is often referred to as a "breather."). Sometimes scatalogia and *coprophilia* (q.v.) are used interchangeably, although the current preference is to limit scatalogia to the paraphilia, as here defined, and to use coprophilia for involuntary utterances of obscene language.

**telephonicophilia**  *Telephone scatalogia* (q.v.).

**telepsychiatry**  Use of communications technology, via audio or video transmission, to connect patients, health care providers and interventions, including diagnosis, education, treatment, consultation, transfer of medical data and other administrative services, and research. A major application is provision of affordable, high-quality, mental health care to patients in areas with few psychiatric services. In addition to the usual problems of confidentiality and the ability to perform valid evaluations at a distance are economic factors. Often unaddressed are the per-use cost of equipment, transmission lines, technical personnal, documentation requirements, space, and training of staff. Distances in rural areas are often great, transportation may be irregular, the patients evaluated must still travel to the site where the equipment is located, and it is unlikely that any such site will be able to generate a high enough volume of use to offset the cost of its construction.

**telescoping**  1. More rapid progression of a disease process in one group of subjects or one situation than in another. Both pathologic gambling and substance use disorders, for example, progress more rapidly in women than in men.

2. In persons with *phantom limb* (q.v.), the perception that the size and length of the limb are shrinking.

**telesthesia**  Telepathy.

**telodendria**  See *axon; neuron.*

**telomerase**  A ribonucleoprotein enzyme response present in most eukaryocytes that can replicate chromosome ends, or telomeres. Discovery of the protein was first reported in 1997. It keeps dividing cells healthy by rebuilding telomeres that would otherwise become frayed with each cell division. In most human somatic cells, telomeres shorten with successive cell divisions. This has led to the speculation that they are cellular timepieces, becoming shorter with each adult cell division until, after one tick too many, the cell shuts down. Finding out how to rebuild those telomeres might afford a way to make cells young again. The danger, of course, is that any such antiaging drug might drive the cell into the frenzied division that characterizes cancer.

**telomere**  The nucleoprotein complex at the end of chromosomes. The telomere protects the chromosome from erosion during cell division and prevents the chromosome from fusing end to end. Humans have 92 telomeres, one on each end of the 46 chromosomes. The telomere-synthesizing enzyme is *telomerase* (q.v.). Telomeres shorten with each division of normal cells and eventually stop dividing, a process termed *replicative senescence* (q.v.). In essence, telomeres sacrifice themselves to protect the genetic information.

**telomere clock model**  The hypothesis that human telomeres are programmed to undergo gradual shortening by about 100 bp per cell division and when several kilobases of the telomeric DNA are lost, cells stop dividing and begin a phase of senescence. Activation of telomerase adds to the number of the TTAGGG repeats that normally cap chromosome ends. Cells with such artifically elongated telomeres show an expansion of their growth potential; whereas normal cells enter senescence after a well-defined number of cell divisons, telomerase-positive cells miss their senescence cue and continue to divide. Telomerase-expressing clones have a normal karytotype and have already exceeded their normal lifespan by at least 20 doublings, thus confirming the hypothesis of a causal relationship between telomere shortening and cellular senescence (Bodnar, A. G. et al. *Science 279*, 1998). See *replicative senescence*.

**teloreception**   Vision and hearing perception; see *interoception*; *sensation*.

**TEM**   *Treatment-emergent mania*; risk factors include antidepressant liability (tricyclics and noradrenergic antidepressants in particular), subclinical hyperthyroidism, 5HT genetic polymorphisms, and mixed depressive symptoms.

**temper tantrum**   See *tantrum*.

**temperament**   A constitutional disposition to react to one's environment in a certain way. Some people are more placid than others, some more vigorous, some more high-strung; it is likely that such differences are genetically based and recognizable from the moment of birth. Temperament is not identical with character, though often confused with it, especially in popular language. Temperament is probably instrumental in determining the particular type of character structure developed by a person in that it limits the potentialities for character development: it is unlikely that a constitutionally phlegmatic person would develop an anxious, rigid, and compulsive character structure. Character is something in addition to temperament, a component within the framework of the possibilities encompassed by the given temperament.

Ten indicators of temperament in children have been identified: approach, withdrawal, rhythmicity (regularity), quality of mood, intensity of reaction, adaptability, activity level, threshold, distractibility, and attention span.

Normal temperament ranges from difficult children, who account for approximately 10% of all children, to easy children, who account for about 40%; the remainder are mixtures of the two extremes. The *difficult child* is characterized by hyperalertness, intense reactions to stimulation, poor sleeping, unpredictable eating times, and a need for more than the usual amount of comforting when he or she cries. The *easy child* is regular in eating, eliminating, and sleeping, is able to adapt to change with a minimum of distress, and is easily comforted when he cries.

**temperance**   See *abstinence*.

**template function**   See *gene functions*.

**temporal code model**   The theory that the firing pattern of an individual neuron can report more than one stimulus property, i.e., different "whats," even while the average firing rate remains unchanged. A single neuron, for instance, could report the presence of three different stimuli with three different temporal firing patterns. Evidence for the temporal code model is more limited than for the older *rate code model* (q.v.), but it is growing.

**temporal lobe**   The portion of the cerebral hemisphere that lies below the sylvian fissure and extends back to the level of the parietooccipital fissure. Contained within the temporal lobe are the *planum temporale* and *Heschl's gyrus* (qq.v.). The temporal lobe receives auditory projections from the medial geniculate body, and ablation of the temporal lobe in humans results in partial deafness and contralateral disturbance in memory for auditory impressions. The temporal lobe also receives vestibular projections, but the source of these is unknown.

In SDAT (Alzheimer disease) specific cognitive impairments have been tentatively correlated to discrete structural abnormalities of the temporal lobe. AD patients with psychosis are impaired on tests of both learning and forgetting. The observed pattern is consistent with greater involvement of the medial *temporal-hippocampal system* in SDAT.

Schizophrenic patients show a selective deficit in memory and learning but not on tests of forgetting. In some studies schizophrenic patients displayed prominent and specific alterations in the distribution of two *microtubule-associated proteins*, MAP2 and MAP5, which are anatomically selective for the subiculum and entorhinal cortex. Defects in the expression of MAP2 and MAP5, which contribute to the establishment and maintenance of neuronal polarity, could underlie some of the cytoarchitectural abnormalities described in schizophrenia and impair signal transduction in the affected dendrites. The abnormal subfields are also the ones most severely affected by neurofibrillary tangles in AD. Thus, while disturbed by two different types of pathology, the disruption of neurons in these subfields may yield similar symptoms in the two diseases.

*Spatial neglect,* or spatial *nonrecognition* (qq.v.) have long been ascribed to parietal lesions, but recent studies indicate that it is localized in the *STG* (right superior temporal gyrus). The rostral superior temporal cortex might act as an interface between the dorsal and the ventral streams of input processing to allow exploration of both object- and space-related information. The superior temporal cortex is also involved in the processing of species-specific vocalizations. The evolutionary development from monkey to human brain may have led to the lateralization of these formely bilateral functions; the left superior temporal cortex specialized for language processes, and the right superior temporal cortex serving as a multimodal matrix for the exploration of object- and space-related information in the surroundings (Karnath, H.-O. *Nature Neuroscience 1*, 2001). The inferior temporal cortex, located at the final processing stage of visual object perception, is the site of visual memory storage. It plays some part in recall of visual material, although memory retrieval is under the executive control of the prefrontal cortex.

**temporal lobe dysfunction**   Various *temporal lobe syndromes* have been described. Delusions, hallucinations (especially auditory and panoramic visual), and mood disturbances are frequent. They may be based on temporal lobe epilepsy, stroke, head injury, viral infection (especially herpes), vascular malformations, or degenerative brain disease involving the temporal lobes. Removal of only the inferior (ventral) temporal cortex interferes with visual recognition of shapes, patterns, faces, and places (*prosopagnosia*, q.v.), but other visual functions (e.g., acuity, recognition of color, perception of movement) remain intact.

Symptoms of temporal lobe tumors include visual *field defect,* auditory and speech defects, and minor seizures known as *dreamy states* (qq.v.). If the *uncus* is implicated, there may be hallucinations of smell and taste (uncinate seizures). See *uncinate fit.*

Bilateral temporal lobe disease usually produces dementia. In dominant temporal lobe involvement, manifestations include euphoria, auditory hallucinations (often "complex" voices), formal thought disorder, primary delusional ideas, cognitive deficits such as decreased learning and retention of verbal material (read or heard) and poor speech and reading comprehension. See *hypermetamorphosis.*

If the nondominant lobe is affected, symptoms include dysphoria, depression, irritability, inappropriate emotional expression (aprosodia), cognitive deficits such as decreased recognition and recall of visual and environmental sounds, amusia (loss of ability to repeat musical sounds), poor visual memory, decreased auditory discriminations and comprehension of tonal patterns, and decreased ability to learn and recognize nonsense figures and geometric shapes.

**temporal lobe epilepsy**   *TLE*; complex partial seizures with automatisms, postural changes, and subjective experiences or feelings such as déjà vu, jamais vu, illusions, hallucinations, depersonalization, dreamy states, confusion, forced thinking, vertigo, amnesia, mood changes, and aggressive behavior. The automatisms are usually simple in type such as chewing, fumbling, looking around, or mumbling. Typical episodes begin with abrupt cessation of activity, followed by an automatism phase lasting from seconds to as long as a minute, during which the subject is unresponsive. The final phase consists of impairment of awareness. The total episode lasts anywhere from 1 to 30 minutes. See *interictal behavior syndrome; psychomotor epilepsy; temporal lobe dysfunction.*

**temporal lobe epileptic personality**   *Interictal behavior syndrome* (q.v.).

**temporal lobe syndromes**   See *interictal behavior syndrome; temporal lobe dysfunction.*

**temporal model**   Stevens' hypothesis that onset of schizophrenia is associated with reactive synaptic regeneration in brain regions that receive degenerating temporal lobe projections. Prefrontal hypometabolism may be secondary to the function of aberrant afferent temporal projections. Prefrontal cortex and hippocampus are functionally coupled during memory tasks, and sharing information via numerous temporofrontal connections is an important aspect of prefrontal functioning (Stevens, J.R, *Schizophrenia Bulletin 23*: 373–383, 1997).

**temporal orientation**   Awareness of the relationship of sounds, ability to remember sounds and rhythms, and actual knowledge of time. Disorganization in the temporospatial sphere is often manifested in motor defects, because if the subject is defectively oriented he is compromised in his ability to translate perceptions into the motor activity or reactivity that would be expected.

**temporal summation**   See *summation.*

**temporal-hippocampal system**   See *lobe, temporal.*

**temporolimbic behavior disturbance**   *Interictal behavior syndrome* (q.v.).

**temporolimbic system model** Bogerts' hypothesis of schizophrenia is that limbic dysfunction causes a dissociation between higher neocortical cognitive activities and the phylogenetically older brain areas linked to basic drives and emotions. The sequential flow of information through the brain follows connections from primary sensory cortices to modality-specific association areas and converges in the hippocampal-limbic system in the medial temporal lobe. The hippocampus receives multimodal sensory information not only from the external environment (association cortex) but also the internal environment (amygdala). Lesions of the limbic system do not negate visual, auditory, or somatosensory information but instead alter its processing. It is not one isolated focus of abnormality, but a number of pathological foci with aberrant function that produce the variable clinical expression observed in schizophrenia.

Bogert's temporolimbic system theory is based in part on his examination of the brain of a famous patient, *Ernst Wagner* (q.v.) (Bogerts, B, *Schizophrenia Bulletin 23*: 423–435, 1997).

**temporomandibular joint syndrome** Pain aggravated by jaw movement, decreased range of jaw motion, and tenderness in the area of the joint or muscle of mastication. Sometimes the syndrome is secondary to an occlusal disorder, but more often it is secondary to excessive contraction of the masticatory muscles (and hence it is also called *myofascial pain dysfunction*).

**temptation, horrific** One of Rado's subdivisions of obsessive attacks: an idea or urge of compelling intensity to kill or harm someone (usually a close relative), an idea from which the patient shrinks back in horror.

**tendency of action** In objective psychobiology the inclinations associated with action. "One should always study the general behavior of a person while talking to him. Much can be learned from his way of entering the room, shaking hands, talking, and from his facial expression, gestures and posture…emotions are the regulative functions of our personality and are therefore closely related to the behavior of the person in action" (Diethelm, O. *Treatment in Psychiatry*, 1936). See *body language*.

**tendency wit** There are two major classifications of witty productions, word-wit (thought-wit) and abstract wit (tendency wit). When "wit is wit for its own sake and serves no other particular purpose," it is called abstract or harmless wit. Freud cites an example from Lichtenberg: "They sent a small octavo to the University of Gottingen; and received back in body and soul a quarto" (a fourth-form boy).

Wit may serve some purpose; it may have deep meaning; it may be tendential; when such is the case, Freud speaks of tendency-wit. "It makes possible the gratification of a craving (lewd or hostile) despite a hindrance which stands in the way; it eludes the hindrance and so derives pleasure from a source that has been inaccessible on account of the hindrance." (*The Basic Writings of Sigmund Freud*, 1938).

**tender points** See *fibromyalgia*.

**tender years presumption** See *custody*.

**tendon reflex** The contraction of a muscle in response to tapping its tendon; for example, the triceps, quadriceps femoris (patellar), and gastrocnemius (Achilles or ankle) reflexes.

**tenesmus penis** (L. "straining of the penis") *Priapism* (q.v.).

**tension, mental** The emotional charge with which components of the psyche are infused; *psychentonia*. See *cathexis*.

**tension-type headache** *TTH*; it may be episodic (frequent or infrequent) or chronic. The headache is usually described as bandlike sensations around the head. The pain is dull, like a tightness or stretching, and it may last hours or months. Unlike *migraine* (q.v.), TTH has its onset in adulthood. It is more common in females. See *headache*.

**tenting** See *masturbation*.

**tentorium cerebelli** See *fossa, posterior cranial; meninges*.

**teonanacatl** A "sacred" mushroom used by the Aztecs in religious ceremonies. Its main active components are psilocybin and psilocin, both of which are derived from tryptamine.

**TEPP** See *psychotomimetic*.

**terahertz waves** Radiation in the region between infrared and radio waves. All objects emit terahertz waves, but they are much harder to detect than infrared radiation. A recently fabricated (2002) phonic bandgap material is impervious to teraherz radiation and may be able to improve the ability of imaging devices to peer through materials opaque to the light of many other wavelengths.

**teratogen** A compound that can cause structural malformations in the fetus if ingested during the first trimester of pregnancy.

A *behavioral teratogen* causes long-term behavioral effects. See *fetotoxin*.

**teratology**   The study of birth defects and their causes; *congenital malformations* (any structural defects present at birth) account for approximately 15% of all deaths in the first year of life. Their overall incidence is in the range of 1% to 10% of all births, but the most severe developmental defects are not compatible with survival of the fetus so they are reported as spontaneous abortions rather than as congenital malformations.

**teratophobia**   Fear of bearing a monster.

**terminal tremor**   See *cerebellum*.

**termination**   Conclusion, ending; in psychotherapy, the decision agreed upon by patient and therapist to bring treatment to an end. Usually the decision to terminate brings the patient's experiences with separation and object loss to the forefront, along with anticipatory mourning over the loss of the therapist. Termination that is not mutually agreed upon is sometimes called forced termination if initiated by the therapist, unilateral termination if initiated by the patient.

**territoriality**   The characteristic behavior by which an organism lays claim to and defends an area against the encroachment of members of its own species.

**terror, night or sleep**   *Sleep terror disorder* (q.v.).

**tertiary dissociation**   See *dissociative disorders*.

**tertiary gain**   A term suggested for benefits accruing to someone other than the patient from the illness of the patient, including other family members, others from the patient's social system, the physician, etc.

**test**   A systematic procedure to measure or assess some characteristic, ability, or skill of a subject, such as intelligence or personality traits. A *normative-referenced* test is one that compares the performance of the individual subject with a group whose performance on the test is used as a standard. A *criterion-referenced* test is one in which the standard is a specified set of performances or actions; the subject is evaluated as to whether he does or does not meet the criteria, without comparing his performance to that of a group (e.g., Can the patient dress himself, or can he not?). See *reliability; validity*.

A specific test may be known under one or more other labels, such as battery, checklist, examination, impression, index, instrument, inventory, measurement, profile, questionnaire, scale, schedule, or task.

**testicular feminizing syndrome**   *Androgen insensitivity syndrome* (q.v.).

**testosterone**   The principal androgenic steroid hormone, secreted by the Leydig cells of the testis, the ovary, and the adrenal cortex under the regulation of adenohypophysial luteinizing hormone. See *ambitypic*.

**testotoxicosis**   Precocious puberty caused by hypersecretion of testosterone by Leydig cells. A mutation in the gene for the $\alpha$ subunit of the *G protein* (q.v.) leads to increased secretion of cAMP and testosterone by the Leydig cells.

**tests**   Psychiatric screening questionnaires include the Primary Care Evaluation of Mental Disorders (Spitzer, R.L. et al. *Journal of the American Medical Association* 272: 1749–1756, 1994), the Symptom Driven Diagnostic System for Primary Care (Leon, A.C. et al. *Journal of General Internal Medicine* 11: 426–430, 1996), DSM-IV-PC (which includes discussions of epidemiology, primary care, presentation, differential diagnosis, and assessment algorithms with step-by-step instructions for diagnosis). Screening tools targeting depression and anxiety include the Beck Depression Inventory, Hamilton Depression Scale, Hamilton Anxiety Scale, and Zung Self-Rating Depression Scale. Useful in screening for substance use disorders are the CAGE, Michigan Alcoholism Screening Test (MAST), Alcohol Use Disorders Identification Test, and the Drug Abuse Screening Test.

**tetanization**   *Obs.* Extreme fixation of the attention, often accompanied by exaltation or ecstasy and a lack of responsiveness to painful stimuli.

**tetanoid epilepsy**   Pritchard's term for *epilepsy* (q.v.) in which the spasm is tonic only.

**tetracyclic**   See *antidepressant*.

**tetraethylpyrophosphate**   See *psychotomimetic*.

**tetraethylthiuram disulfide**   See *Antabuse*.

**tetrahydrocannabinol**   See *cannabis; psychotomimetic*.

**tetraplegia**   Quadriplegia; paralysis of the four extremities.

**tetrasomy**   The "fourfoldness" in Jung's system of psychology. See *quaternity*.

**tetraspanin**   See *late bloomer gene*.

**TGA**   *Transient global amnesia* (q.v.).

**TGN**   Trans-Golgi network; see *Golgi apparatus*.

**T-group**   *Encounter group; sensitivity training group*; an educational-psychotherapeutic technique in which a group of people meets regularly, usually with a specified leader, in order to learn about themselves, about interpersonal relationships, about group process, and about larger social systems. The T-group is experience-based learning (rather than a type of therapy for recognized emotional disturbance), and its major aims include increasing relatedness and opening communication channels between the group member and others within his social system. The T-group is reality-oriented and focuses on connections between current reactions and universal psychological concepts rather than on individual genetic antecedents of those reactions. Used in industrial organizations, for example, the T-group tries to get its members to own up to their own feelings (including their feelings about each other), to become open to new ideas and experiment with new solutions to problems (i.e., to replace automaton conformity with a capacity for risk-taking), and thereby to generate effective decision making within the organization. T-groups are sometimes also called *human relations groups*.

**thaassophobia**   Fear of sitting.

**thalamic aphasia syndrome**   Speech is normally articulated, with normal rhythm, intonation, and a variety of grammatical forms, but one word is substituted for another, sometimes so frequently that language degenerates into a meaningless jargon. The ability to repeat spoken sentences or phrases remains relatively intact. This suggests that a semantic monitoring mechanism is failing but that more basic mechanisms for the initial phonological and semantic decoding of language have been left intact. See *thalamus*.

**thalamic dementia**   Encephalomalacia or other degenerative lesions of the thalami produce a typical form of dementia, characterized by diminution or absence of motor initiative and spontaneity, and ordinarily also some abnormal movements.

**thalamic hyperpathia**   See *pain syndromes*.

**thalamic model**   The hypothesis that inability to recruit cortex and thalamus into collective action is the basis of a key manifestation of schizophrenia—the inability to maintain focus, especially on what is relevant. The fragmentation of thought processes in schizophrenia is a result of both failure to bind together the large thalamic and cortical cell collectives necessary for higher order processing and

difficulty in switching between collectives. Distractibility is sometimes viewed as a generalized, nonspecific phenomenon; it may, instead, be a highly specific neurobiological correlate of deficient gating and information processing. Schizophrenia carries with it a specific deficit in information processing that leads to distractibility.

Neuropathological and imaging studies have consistently identified abnormalities in various axes of the cortico-striato-pallido-thalamic (CSPT) circuitry that specifically controls the modulation of information processing.

**thalamic syndrome**   Thalamic lesions are commonly followed by various paresthesias and hyperesthesias believed to be caused by release from intradiencephalic and cortico-thalamic projections. The thalamic syndrome consists of a raising of the threshold (i.e., diminished sensibility) to pinprick, heat, and cold, but when sensation is felt it is disagreeable and unpleasant (thalamic hyperpathia). It has been suggested that thalamic nuclei might mediate the *hypofrontality* (q.v.) reported in some cases of schizophrenia, and that ontogenetic defects in the thalamic (and limbic) nuclei might be responsible for abnormal frontal lobe development or disturbed neurointegration of experience, leading to disturbances in the ability to plan the ramifications of behavior. See *thalamic dementia; thalamic aphasia syndrome*.

**thalamopetal connections**   In general, sensorimotor pallidal and nigral areas project to the lateral thalamic nuclei, while associational information is relayed through the medial *thalamus* (q.v.). Both modalities pass through the ventral anterior nucleus of the thalamus, which in turn innervates both premotor and prefrontal cortices.

**thalamotomy**   A psychosurgical procedure that produces a lesion in the thalamus by means of thermocoagulation. A stereotaxic apparatus is employed to position a wire or cannula into the desired subcortical area. Such a method results in minimal injury to superimposed cortex or white matter and is a much less drastic procedure than are other methods, e.g., frontal lobectomy. The thalamotomy operation was devised by Spiegel and his coworkers, who found that small lesions of the dorsomedial nucleus of the thalamus (medial thalamotomy) relieve anxiety, emotional reactivity, and allied symptoms in psychoses and obsessive-compulsive states.

**thalamus**  A two-lobed medial structure that sits just above the brain stem and is bounded on its dorsal surfaces by the lateral ventricles. The two lobes of the thalamus are in communication through the massa intermedia, which is situated in the middle of the third ventricle. The thalamus consists of multiple nuclei whose primary role is to send incoming signals from sensory receptors for further processing in cerebral cortex; it also sends information to hippocampus and amygdala. The thalamus receives input from all sensory receptors (except olfaction) and brain-stem arousal systems; it then relays this information to frontal cortex, cingulate gyrus, amygdala, and hippocampus. Arousal-modulated thalamic disruption may lead to reductions in awareness, derealization, amnesia, distorted sensory input, and alternations in time perception.

The thalamus is divided into three nuclear groups by a gamma-shaped band of white matter, the *internal medullary lamina*, plus a fourth posterior portion, the pulvinar:

1. *Anterior nucleus*—primary connections are with the limbic system, receiving its main input from the hippocampus via the fornix, and sending its main output to the cingulate gyrus. See *rhinencephalon*.

2. *Dorsomedial nucleus* (q.v.)

3. *Lateral nuclear group* (q.v.)

4. *Pulvinar* (q.v.)

5. *Intralaminar nuclei* (q.v.)

**thalassophobia**  Fear of the sea.

**thanatomania**  *Obs.* Suicidal mania.

**thanatophobia**  Fear of death.

**Thanatos**  *Death instinct* (q.v.). "For the sake of clearness I will repeat in a sentence the three stages in the development of Freud's ideas concerning the duality of instincts. The first was the contrast between sexual and ego instincts; the second the contrast between object-love or allo-erotic libido, and self-love, narcissistic libido; and the third is the contrast between life and death instincts, between Eros and Thanatos" (Jones, E. *Papers on Psycho-Analysis*, 1938).

**thanatotic**  Pertaining to or manifesting the death instinct.

**thank-you theory**  *Ratification theory*; often proposed as a way to justify paternalistic behavior, especially in civil commitment deliberations: one may act paternalistically if one is certain

that the object of one's actions will later be thankful that those actions were taken.

**THC**  Tetrahydrocannabinol. See *cannabis; marijuana; psychotomimetic*.

**theater, therapeutic**  "An objective setting in which the subject and patient can act free from the anxieties and pressures of the outside world. In order to accomplish this, the total situation of the patient in the outside world has to be duplicated on a spontaneous level in the therapeutic theater, and even more than this, the invisible roles and invisible inter-personal relations he may have experienced must find a visible expression" (Moreno, J. L. *Sociometry 1*, 1937).

**thematic apperception test (TAT)**  A projective technique, originally described by Morgan and Murray in 1935, which focuses primarily on the dynamics of interpersonal relationships. In its present form (the third set to be used since 1935), it consists of a series of 31 pictures that depict a number of social situations and interpersonal relations. In clinical practice, 10 or 12 of the pictures are usually selected by the examiner on the basis of which of the total 31 are most likely to elicit information on the subject's problems. The selected pictures are then presented to the subject, who is asked to tell a story about what is going on in each picture. The stories are interpreted in terms of the subject's relationship to authority figures, to contemporaries of both sexes, and in terms of the compromises between external demands and the needs of the id, the ego, and the superego. There are various methods of interpreting results; the one advocated by Murray is the *need-press method* (q.v.).

It is to be noted that the TAT is only incidentally a diagnostic tool and is not primarily designed for nosologic classification.

**theme interference**  An emotionally toned cognitive constellation or conflict operating preconsciously in the consultee to distort his professional objectivity with his client. Usually the conflict is an outgrowth of actual life experience or phantasies in the consultee that have not been satisfactorily resolved. One of the consultant's tasks is to identify such themes and reduce or eliminate them (*theme interference reduction*). See *consultation-liaison*.

**theomania**  *Obs.* Delusion that one is God.

**theory**  A body of *principles* or *rules* (qq.v.), generally referring to the same subject, with each rule systematically related to the others.

**theory, attachment**   See *attachment*.

**theory of mind**   *ToM*; *mentalizing*; *intentional stance*; the ability to infer what other people are thinking and feeling, to attribute mental states to other people, to empathize by imagining another person's mental state, to recognize that another person has a perspective different from one's own. David Premack and Guy Woodruff (*Behavior Brain Science 4*: 515, 1978) first posed the question, "Do chimpanzees have a theory of mind?" That is, do chimpanzees possess a mind that understands another individual's mind?

The human brain's theory of mind system is a widely distributed system of multiple interacting nodes in orbitofrontal cortex and medial frontal lobe, especially anterior *paracingulate cortex* (q.v.); superior temporal sulcus; associative, memory, and language regions in the angular gyrus (inferior temporal lobe) and anterior temporal lobe; amygdala; and cerebellum. It is believed by many that a fully developed TOM is limited to human beings. See *attribution of beliefs*; *mirror neurons*.

**therapeutic**   Pertaining to medical treatment; healing, curative.

**therapeutic alliance**   *Working alliance*; the non-transference relationship between patient and analyst; the patient's rational or reasonable rapport with the analyst that renders the frustrations of the transference tolerable; the concept that in psychotherapy an observing part of the patient joins with the observing analyst in the search for insight. Self psychology is critical of the concept, suggesting that what is called a therapeutic alliance is, in fact, an insidiously evolving and unanalyzed dependency on the therapist. Self psychology emphasizes instead the therapeutic dialogue, in which the therapist shares his tentative understanding of the patient's unique features and at the same time encourages the patient to correct or challenge the perceptions of the analyst.

**therapeutic community (TC)**   Although originally associated with the name of Maxwell Jones, who advocated use of every aspect of the hospital environment as a therapeutic tool (see *milieu therapy*), the therapeutic community has become associated more specifically with nonhospital residential programs for the treatment of substance use disorders. Like Alcoholics Anonymous, therapeutic communities stress self-help, are abstinence-oriented, and reinforce drug-free behavior through intense interaction with others who have had experience with drug abuse. That interaction is heightened by reason of the fact that the members of the community are living together, and firm rules of conduct are stringently enforced within the residence through punishment for infractions by group confrontation.

**therapeutic culture**   A concept basic to the therapeutic community, referring to the requirement that all activities and actions within the community relate to the goal of reeducation and social rehabilitation of the patients. See *therapeutic community*.

**therapeutic dialogue**   See *therapeutic alliance*.

**therapeutic dose dependence**   See *dose dependence, therapeutic*; *sedatives/hypnotics*.

**therapeutic jurisprudence model**   An interdisciplinary approach to the law that views the law itself as a therapeutic (or antitherapeutic) agent. It uses the tools of the behavioral sciences to assess the impact of the law on the individual, with the goal of minimizing the antitherapeutic effects of the law and maximizing its therapeutic potential. In the case of civil commitment laws, for example, it applies research in the social sciences on coercion, capacity, and choice to each element of a specific commitment law.

**therapeutic reaction, negative**   See *superego resistance*.

**therapeutic state**   See *medicalization*.

**therapeutic window**   See *window, therapeutic*.

**therapeutics, differential**   See *differential therapeutics*.

**therapy**   Treatment of disease; therapeutics. See *psychotherapy*.

**thermanesthesia, thermoanesthesia**   Loss of the ability to distinguish between heat and cold.

**thermo-**   Combining form meaning hot, heat, from Gr. *thermos*.

**thermohyperesthesia**   Extreme sensitiveness to heat stimuli.

**theta EEG activity**   See *sleep*.

**theta rhythm**   Neural activity with a frequency of 4–8 Hz. See *electroencephalogram*; *mammillary body*.

**thiamine**   Vitamin $B_1$; aneurine; the precursor of thiamine pyrophosphate, a coenzyme in carbohydrate metabolism. The classic thiamine deficiency syndrome is *beriberi*; *Wernicke encephalopathy* is also largely a result of thiamine deficiency (qq.v.).

**thiamine deficiency** Lack of thiamine, the precursor of thiamine pyrophosphate, which is a coenzyme in carbohydrate metabolism. The lack may be due to inadequate intake (the best food sources are pork, whole grains, enriched cereal grains, nuts, and beans), decreased absorption (in diarrhea, colitis, alcoholism), impaired utilization (as in liver disease), or increased need (infection, intestinal parasites, certain drugs).

*Beriberi* is the classic thiamine deficiency syndrome, rarely seen except in countries where polished white rice is the dietary staple. The early stage is characterized by anorexia and weight loss; later, there is progression to wet beriberi (involvement of the cardiovascular system), dry beriberi (central and peripheral nervous system involvement), or a combination of the two.

In Western societies, thiamine deficiency is most often associated with alcoholism (and, to a lesser degree, food faddism), and nervous system manifestations predominate. One manifestation is *Wernicke encephalopathy* (q.v.), another is polyneuropathy; the two may appear together. The polyneuropathy affects the lower limbs earlier than the upper, and proximal portions of the limb earlier than distal portions. Associated paresthesias and dysesthesias give rise to the classic *burning feet syndrome.*

**thinking compulsion** See *brooding.*

**thinking disorder** *Thought disorder* (q.v.), including abnormalities in form (*formal thought disorder, association disturbance*), in possession (feeling that one's thoughts are not one's own), in content (delusions and similar ideas), and in quantity or stream of thought (abnormal speed or amount of thinking). See *association disturbances; negative symptoms.*

**thinking type** The first of Jung's four functional types of personality; with the second (*feeling type*) it constitutes the *rational* class of *functional types.* In this type, life is ruled mainly by reflective thinking so that every important action proceeds from intellectually considered motives. Such a type can be either introverted or extraverted.

**thinking-aside** A disorder of associations seen in schizophrenic patients in which the patient loses himself in insignificant side associations with the result that no unitary train of thought develops. Because of the paucity of genuinely causal links in such conversation or writing, thinking-aside would be considered a type of *asyndesis* (q.v.).

**third messsenger** See *second messenger.*

**third sex** Bisexuality; homosexuality. Use of the term is discouragedsince it seems to ignore the fact that a very considerable measure of latent or unconscious homosexuality can be detected in all heterosexuals.

**third ventricle** See *ventricle.*

**third-order relatives** See *first-order relatives.*

**thirteen, original** The original thirteen were the founders (in 1844) of the Association of Medical Superintendents of America: William Awl, Luther Bell, Amariah Brigham, John Butler, Nehenich Cutter, Pliny Earle, John Galt, Thomas Kirkbride, Isaac Ray, Charles Stedman, Francis Stribling, Samuel White, and Samuel Woodward. In 1893 the name of the society was changed to the American Medicopsychological Association, which became the American Psychiatric Association in 1922.

**Thomism** The philosophicotheological system of Thomas Aquinas, an ideological system that some assert is based on the unrecognized premise that "father is always right" or "it is right because father said so." It would consequently be incompatible with reconstruction or insight psychotherapy but consonant with supportive, persuasion, or exhortative therapy. See *psychotherapy.*

**Thompson, Clara** (1893–1958) American psychoanalyst; associated with Harry Sullivan and his modifications of psychoanalysis (interpersonal relationships).

**thought** Conceptualization. Contrary to the Sapir-Whorf hypothesis, thought is not dependent on words but consists, rather, of patterns of neural firings in the brain. See *mentalese.* These patterns are translated into words when the person wishes to communicate them to a listener—the process of *language* (q.v.).

Freud understood thought almost entirely in terms of physical processes internal to the organism; its relation to truth, or the world, was secondary to that more fundamental determination. The result is a psychological reductionism that denies the validity of all but a few human motives in relation to which the others remain mere forms of disguise.

**thought, emotional** See *adaptational psychodynamics.*

**thought broadcasting** Hearing another person express words or ideasthat the subject himself is thinking, often extended into the belief that others can read his mind. It was considered a first-rank symptom of schizophrenia by Schneider. See *first-rank symptoms.*

**thought constraint**    See *constraint of thought.*

**thought deprivation**    *Blocking* (q.v.).

**thought derailment**    A type of thinking disorder, seen most commonly in schizophrenic disorders, in which incomprehensible and disconnected ideas replace logical and orderly thought. The subject jumps from one topic or word to another topic or word for no apparent reason and is seemingly insensitive to the contradictoriness, illogicality, or incomprehensibility of his utterances. Thought derailment has also been called *Knight's move.*

**thought disorder**    *Thinking disorder* (q.v.); sometimes used in a more limited way to refer specifically to schizophrenic disturbances of the associations, consisting of improper use of semantic and relational aspects of language. It is manifested as thought blocking, thought deprivation, poverty of thought, loose associations (derailments), irrelevant or tangential responsives, circumstantiality or loss of goal, or haphazard, seemingly purposeless, illogical, confused, incorrect, abrupt, or bizarre associations. See *association disturbances; negative symptoms.*

**thought disorder, primary**    The type of schizophrenia in which there is striking involvement of intellectual functions with marked incoherence and irrelevance, tendency to neologisms, word salads, and peculiar syntactical speech formation.

**thought echoing**    An auditory hallucination consisting of hearing one's own thoughts expressed in whispered or unbearably loud tones; *echo des pensées* (q.v.); audible thoughts. See *first-rank symptoms.*

**thought hearing**    An auditory hallucination; patients hear their own thoughts and may believe that their thoughts are heard by others too. Similar to thought echoing except that in the latter the thoughts are typically heard coming from the outside, while in thought hearing the thoughts are heard as coming from within the patient himself. See *audible thought; first-rank symptoms.*

**thought insertion**    *Thought pressure* (q.v.).

**thought interruption**    See *first-rank symptoms.*

**thought pressure**    *Pressure of ideas; thought insertion*; thoughts that seem to be forced into the subject's mind by some other agent. See *first-rank symptoms.*

**thought rehearsal**    See *obsessional rehearsal.*

**thought stopping**    A type of response prevention used in treating mental rituals of patients with obsessive-compulsive disorder. The patient stops his upsetting thoughts by shouting, making a loud noise, or snapping a rubber band on his wrist. The opposite technique, also used with obsessions, is *semantic satiation* (q.v.).

**thought transference**    See *extrasensory perception.*

**thought withdrawal**    See *first-rank symptoms.*

**threat-control-override**    *TCO*; the concept that feelings of being gravely threatened by someone who intends to cause harm overwhelm a person's ability to control his or her violent responses to the threat. TCO includes the following symptoms: belief that one's actions or thoughts are under external control; thought insertion; thought withdrawal; belief of being hypnotized, under magic performance, or hit by X-rays or laser beams; belief of being spied upon, or followed; belief of being secretly tested or experimented on; belief that someone is plotting, trying to hurt or poison one.

**three-cornered therapy**    See *multiple psychotherapy.*

**threshold symbolism**    Silberer's term for a subdivision of *functional symbolism* (q.v.) occurring during the transition from one state of consciousness to another, for example, from sleep to wakefulness or vice versa. The term includes *hypnagogic hallucination* (q.v.).

**thromboangiitis obliterans, cerebral**    Thromboangiitis obliterans is far less common in the cerebral vessels than in the peripheral vessels, but when it does occur peripheral disease is often absent. The cerebral form is more common in males and usually begins in the fifth decade; heavy smoking may be of etiologic importance. Symptoms are very similar to those found with *cerebral arteriosclerosis* (q.v.): a focal, neurologic form or a generalized mental form.

**thrombosis, cerebral**    See *cerebrovascular accident.*

**thumb sucking**    The earliest and one of the most common manipulations of the body found in young children. In some children, it is observed at birth, to continue on through infancy and early childhood, when it becomes an undesirable habit and is classified as a neurotic trait. During the first months of life, thumb sucking is a physiological and common, but not universal, characteristic of the infant. With the waning of the hand-to-mouth reaction phase, which takes place at about 12 months of age, according to Gesell, the habit ceases. Even past the age of 12 months and on through 3 and 4 years (2 years according to Kanner) it is considered normal when recurring before nap, sleep, or at times of fatigue or emotional stress. In psychoanalysis, thumb sucking is considered an autoerotic gratification, as an expression of infantile sexual cravings, the oral erogenic zone being in this case the level of stimulation and gratification.

**thumb-chin reflex**   See *palmomental reflex.*

**thunderclap seizure**   An epileptic attack that occurs without an *aura* (q.v.) or warning.

**thymergasia**   Adolf Meyer's term for the psychiatric syndromes commonly known as mood disorders.

**-thymia, thymo-**   Combining form meaning state of mind and will, soul, spirit, temper, from Gr. *thymos.*

**thymogenic drinking**   See *alcoholism.*

**thymoleptic**   Influencing or changing mood; referring to drugs that ameliorate pathological depressive states but, in the absence of depression, do not act as central nervous system stimulants. See *psychotropics.*

**thymonoic reaction**   A strongly "intellectualized" and "rationalized" depression, with marked systematized content verging on the delusional.

**thymopathic**   Referring to any disturbance in affect or mood tone; dysthmic; dysphoric. Bleuler used *thymopathic personality* to refer to the premorbid personality of the manic-depressive (bipolar) subject, characterized by lack of emotional poise, distractibility, feelings of inadequacy and frustration, irascibility, and periods of dejection. He believed those personality traits were evidence of an inherited predisposition to bipolar disorder.

**thymopsyche**   See *noopsyche.*

**thyroiditis**   Inflammation of the thyroid gland; also, enlargement of the gland (*goiter*) from any cause. Among patients on lithium maintenance therapy, approximately 6% develop euthyroid goiter and approximately 3% develop hypothyroid goiter. Goiters usually regress in size once lithium is discontinued or, in hypothyroid goiters, if thyroid supplement is given. See *lithium thyroiditis.*

**thyrotoxicosis**   *Graves disease; Basedow disease; exophthalmic goiter; hyperthyroidism;* characterized by accelerated basal metabolic rate, increased rate of oxygen consumption, thyroid enlargement (goiter), weakness, weight loss, nervousness, and arrhythmia or congestive heart failure (particularly in the middle-aged or older).

Graves disease is caused by diffuse toxic goiter and is probably of autoimmune origin; it occurs most often in young women. Symptoms are increased metabolic rate, enlarged thyroid, weight loss, nervousness, insomnia, fine tremor, intolerance to heat and sweating, tachycardia, and exophthalmos (a forward protuberant position of the eye within the orbit; when this is present, the condition is sometimes called exophthalmic goiter).

Although hyperthyroidism often mimics an anxiety state, about 15% of patients manifest depression, with apathy and sluggishness; this form of the disease is known as apathetic thyrotoxicosis.

**thyrotropin-releasing hormone (TRH)**   A tripeptide that ordinarily causes a rise in *TSH* (thyrotropin; thyroid-stimulating hormone). In about 25% of patients with major depression the response is blunted; in 15% it is abnormally elevated. Most patients with alcoholism also demonstrate a blunted response. See *hypothalamic-pituitary-adrenal (HPA) axis; peptide, brain.*

**TIA**   *Transient ischemic attack*; occlusion of the internal carotid artery (usually just above the bifurcation of the common carotid artery) leading to an attack of paresis in one or both limbs on the opposite side of the body, weakness of the side of the face, visual defects such as blurring or blindness, and vertigo. Characteristic are complete recovery following each episode and repeated attacks of short duration. The risk of stroke after even the first attack, however, is high: over 10% in the 90 days after a TIA.

Some authors consider TIA to be focal *TNA* (transient neurological attack), and nonfocal TNA to include transient global amnesia, acute confusion, and syncope without known cause. Nonfocal TNA confers an increased risk of stroke, like focal TNA, but it also confers increased risk of dementia, particularly of the vascular type.

**tiapride**   An atypical neuroleptic agent which is a selective D$_2$ dopamine receptor antagonist. Because it has anxiolytic properties, it has been used by some clinicians in place of benzodiazepines for alcohol withdrawal. Some reports have suggested that it might be useful in the prevention of relapse. See *relapse prevention.*

**tibialis sign**   In organic hemiplegia, dorsal flexion of the foot occurs on flexion at the knee and hip.

**tic**   A brief, sudden, rapid, recurrent, non-rhythmic, stereotyped, irresistible movement or vocalization. Although tics may be psychogenic (in which case they are sometimes called *habit spasm* or *habit contraction*), they may also be due to a variety of neurologic disorders. Both types are exacerbated by stress and diminished during sleep or engrossing activities. See *stereotyped movement disorders.*

Simple motor tics are blinking, shrugging the shoulders, facial twitches, or grimaces. Complex motor tics include grooming behavior (such as hair combing motions), jumping, hitting or biting oneself, smelling an object, echokinesis, and echopraxis.

Simple vocal tics include coughing, grunting, snorting, and clearing the throat. Complex vocal tics include echolalia, palilalia, coprolalia, and repeating words or phrases out of context. See *Tourette disorder.*

The French term *tic de pensée* refers to the involuntary habit of giving expression to any idea that happens to be present in the mind.

Abraham considered the tic a conversion symptom at the anal-sadistic level, and most psychoanalytic writers have emphasized the well-defined anal character and, in addition, the markedly narcissistic makeup of the tiqueur.

Tics represent either instinctual temptations or punishments for warded-off impulses. "This may occur in different ways: (1) The tic represents a part of the original affective syndrome, whose mental significance remains unconscious; (2) the tic represents a movement whose unconscious meaning is a defense against the intended affect; (3) the tic does not directly represent affect or defense against affect but, rather, other movements or motor impulses that once occurred during a repressed emotional excitement, either in the patient or in another person with whom the patient has made a hysterical identification." (Fenichel, O. *The Psychoanalytic Theory of Neurosis,* 1945).

**tic, psychic**   A gesture or ejaculation made under the influence of an irresistible impulse or compulsion.

**tic disorders**   In DSM-III-R, this category includes Tourette disorder, chronic motor or vocal tic disorder, and transient tic disorder. In DSM-III, those conditions were subsumed under the category *stereotyped movement disorders* (q.v.).

**tic douloureux**   (F. "painful tic; facial neuralgia") Also known as *trifacial neuralgia, prosopalgia, Fothergill neuralgia,* chronic paroxysmal trigeminal neuralgia; a chronic trigeminal neuralgia characterized by excruciating paroxysmal pain of short duration, flushing of the face, watering eyes, and rhinorrhea. The condition may affect either the second or the third division of the fifth cranial nerve, or both. The first division is rarely affected. The intermissions between paroxysms vary from weeks to as long as a year. With each succeeding attack seizures become more frequent and more severe. Many cases exhibit dolorogenetic or trigger zones on the face or mucous membranes, stimulation of which will evoke attacks. Tic douloureux is usually unilateral, is more common in adults over 40, and is more frequent among females. The cause is unknown, although the disease may be associated with dental or sinus pathology. There is probably some hereditary factor.

**tic non-douloureux**   (F. "nonpainful tic") Charcot's term for a hysterical disorder of the face, usually unilateral, characterized by paroxysmal twitching of the facial muscles and anesthesia of the skin on the affected side of the face.

**tic scriptorius**   Writer's tic; fast, short, stereotyped, involuntary movements of the writing arm and hand that result in adventitious inclusions of varying size in handwriting. Such movements have been reported in patients with *Tourette disorder* (q.v.).

**tim gene**   See *rhythms, biological.*

**time agnosia**   A condition in which the meaning of time is not comprehended, even though the patient may speak of time. There is disorientation in immediate time, the patient is unable to estimate short time intervals, and long intervals of time are frequently shortened. Thus, one patient with time agnosia stated that World War II had ended 4 years before, whereas actually it had ended 10 years earlier. Patients with time agnosia are able to relate events of the distant past and their interconnection with location, but cannot give the element of time of the event or time relations. Accompanying the time agnosia, and probably a result of it, is an indifference to the past and future and a lack of concern about the condition itself. Time agnosia follows trauma, such as head injury, especially of the temporal area, cerebrovascular accident, and alcoholic coma.

The trauma usually results in a mentally confused state of short duration. Then the patient regains orientation in space, but remains disoriented in time for the immediate present as well as for past events, to a varying degree. Time agnosia often disappears gradually, depending on the extent and degree of permanency of the original lesion.

Davidson has described a syndrome of time agnosia that includes post-traumatic muscular hypertonicity, vascular eye-ground changes (congested discs), and generalized diminution of the acuity of sensibility. The prepsychotic personality of such patients includes a certain simplicity of makeup and a weakness of the sexual impulse. They have ordinarily led a colorless, drifting life wherein time has had no particular meaning to them. (*Journal of Nervous and Mental Disease 94*, 1941).

**time discounting**  Assessment of the relative values of immediate vs. delayed gratification on the basis of how long it will take for the *reward* (q.v.) to be delivered. Making the *choice* (q.v.) involves two separate neural systems: short-run *impatience* is driven by the limbic system associated with the midbrain dopamine system; regions of the lateral prefrontal cortex and posterior parietal cortex are recruited to evaluate trade-offs between abstract rewards, including rewards in the more distant future.

**time out from reinforcement**  A technique of behavior therapy in which the patient, following the occurrence of a targeted behavior, is moved to an area where access to recreational materials, consumable reinforcers, and social contact is removed.

**time sense**  *Chronesthesia* (q.v.).

**time-limited psychotherapy (TLP)**  A form of brief psychotherapy developed by J. Mann. It has a strict limit of 12 sessions, and the date of termination is set at the start of treatment. In contrast to the short-term anxiety-provoking therapy of Sifneos, selection criteria are broad

and the dynamic focus is on separation and reunion rather than on oedipal issues. Major emphasis is on the meaning of time, accepting its finiteness, and differentiating between categorical (adult) time, which is governed by a realistic understanding of its finite quality, and existential (child) time, which is governed by phantasies of timelessness and personal invincibility.

Four conflicts are a frequent focus: dependence vs. independence, passivity vs. activity, lowered vs. adequate self-esteem, and unresolved vs. resolved grief. Termination is of particular importance in TLP because it is a model of loss, separation, and the time-limited nature of attachments. See *brief psychotherapy.*

**timolol**  A *beta blocker* (q.v.).

**Timothy syndrome**  A rare human genetic disorder characterized by diverse physiological and developmental defects, including heart arrhythmias, immune deficiency, webbing of fingers and toes, and autism. It is often fatal by 2.5 years of age. It is due to a missense mutation in a gene that encodes the calcium channel $Ca_v1,2$. The G406R mutation completely abolishes voltage-dependent channel inactivation of $Ca_v1.2$ and results in persistence of inward $Ca^{2+}$ currents in the cell (Splawski et al. *Cell 119*: 19, 2004)

**tip of the tongue syndrome**  Also, "It will come back to me in a moment" syndrome; often one of the first signs of dementia, having to wait excessively long before information can be retrieved. Sometimes—facetiously—referred to as the CRAFT syndrome ("can't remember a f… thing").

**tiqueur**  One who suffers from a tic.

**titubation**  1. Tremor of the head and neck, seen both as a common form of *senile tremor* and in cerebellar disease of any age. The tremor of Parkinson disease is much less likely than senile tremor to involve the head. Senile tremor may also involve the lips and mouth, and the muscles of speech. Senile tremor is found in as many as 50% to 60% of elderly patients in a hospital setting. 2. Less commonly, titubation is used to refer to a truncal tremor that occurs in patients with cerebellar disease when they are sitting or standing.

**TLE**  *Temporal lobe epilepsy* (q.v.).

**TLP**  *Time-limited psychotherapy* (q.v.).

**TM**  *Transcendental meditation* (q.v.).

**TMJ**  *Temporomandibular joint syndrome* (q.v.).

**TMS**  1. *Transcranial magnetic stimulation* (q.v.).

2. Tuberomammillary nucleus. See *sleep*.

**TNA**  Transient neurological attack. See *TIA*.

**TNF**  Tumor necrosis factor, one of the major extracellular regulators in the mammalian immune system. TNFs are cells of the immune system and part of the *caspase cascade* that induces *apoptosis* (qq.v.). TNF α and β, and interleukin-1 and -2 are among the cytotoxic cytokines related to apoptosis. See *cytokines; death domains; Fas; TRADD*.

**tobacco dependence**  Using tobacco continuously for 1 month or longer and, in addition, failure of attempts to stop or reduce intake on a permanent basis, or appearance of withdrawal syndrome upon attempting to stop, or continuation of use despite life-threatening physical disorder(s) known to be exacerbated by tobacco use. *NRTs* (nicotine replacement therapies) have shown some success in smoking cessation; the combination of nicotine patch and bupropion SR has been reported to triple the chance of quitting compared to the patch alone. Varenicline is the first of a new class of partial nicotinic agonists for smoking cessation. See *nicotine*.

**tocomania**  Puerperal mania. See *puerperal psychosis*.

**Todd paralysis**  (Robert Bentley Todd, English physician, 1809–1860) The temporary increase, following each convulsion, in the severity and extent of the weakness associated with Jacksonian convulsions. The latter commonly produce a permanent weakness of the part of the body that is the focus of the fit.

**toe-walking**  Walking on the toes rather than on the whole foot; it is found in approximately 20% of childhood schizophrenics.

**togetherness**  Ackerman's term for the earliest stage in personality development, when the infant is in a state of primary psychic union with the mother, with little or no recognition of the self.

**toilet phobia**  See *bathroom phobia*.

**toilet training**  The process of teaching a child bowel and urine control. See *anal phase; sphincter morality; superego*.

**token economy**  A type of group treatment program, based upon the operant conditioning technique of positive reinforcement, in which elements in the patient's environment are arranged in such a way that reinforcing aspects of the environment are made contingent on the patient's behavior. When the desired "target behavior" occurs, a token (such as a poker chip or plastic card) is given and may be exchanged for a reinforcing agent (any desired goods or services).

Ayllon and Azrin reported on the token economy programs that they had developed for chronically psychotic inpatients in 1968.

**tolerance**  Increasing resistance to the effects of a drug. Tolerance is an outstanding characteristic of the opiates and the amphetamines, and only somewhat less marked with the barbiturates. Although tolerance is not an essential for the development of drug dependence—the cocaine addict, for example, does not develop tolerance for his drug—it is an important consideration in any instance of drug dependence. For linked to tolerance is the need for increasing dosage to maintain or recapture the desired drug effect; and in general, the more saturated body cells become with any substance, the longer will be the period required to rid them of all traces of the drug. Tolerance of any marked degree also creates serious problems for the drug user in ensuring an adequate supply. See *habituation*.

*Acquired tolerance* is decreased sensitivity of a subject to a drug as a result of previous exposure to that drug; in order to achieve the desired effect, higher levels of the drug are required at its site of action to produce a given response (pharmacodynamic tolerance). Unless otherwise specified, tolerance generally refers to acquired tolerance. Loss of acquired tolerance may occur, particularly in alcohol or barbiturate dependence; it may reflect neuronal damage or altered metabolic clearance.

*Metabolic tolerance* (*dispositional tolerance*) is the increased capacity to metabolize a drug; it can be induced by the substance itself or by some other agent. *Initial tolerance* is sensitivity to a drug that the subject has not previously been exposed to. *Reverse tolerance* is increased sensitivity to a drug with repeated use.

Closely allied to tolerance is *physical dependence*, the need to have some quantum of drug present within the body—or at least within some of its cellular elements or organ systems. The *abstinence* (or *withdrawal*) syndrome is the symptomatic expression of physical dependence—cells that have become accustomed to functioning under a mantle of drugs tend to fire or discharge or otherwise function in chaotic disorder when that mantle is suddenly removed. Tolerance and dependence are separable processes with distinct spatial locations in the brain and unique molecular mechanisms of action. See *addiction; alcoholism; dependence, drug.*

**tolerance, frustration**   The maximal point of tolerance of frustration at which defenses give way to the conflict and resentment.

**tolerance, social**   Public acceptance of personal variation or idiosyncrasy in matters of appearance, lifestyle, personality, or belief. Tolerance is thus differentiated from approval, in that a society may tolerate diversity of lifestyle even when a majority of its members do not approve of the variant behavior.

**ToM**   *Theory of mind* (q.v.).

**tomography**   (Gr. "a slice or cut") Sectional roentgenography; CAT (computerized axial tomography) or CT (computed tomography) scan. A rotating X-ray beam slices through the body in the desired plane; it moves in a curve synchronous with the recording plate but in the opposite direction and on the opposite side of the patient. As a result, the shadow of the selected plane remains stationary while all others are displaced and thus blurred or obliterated. The detectors record the degree to which radiation is absorbed or attenuated by the tissues in the selected plane, and the computer uses these density recordings to construct an image.

CT scan is used in visualizing cerebral structures, including the ventricles and cortical sulci. Because it is a noninvasive procedure, it is often used as a basic screening device for suspected neurologic disorders such as brain tumor, infarction, hemorrhage, cerebral atrophy, and hydrocephalus. Computer-analyzed CT scan can distinguish structures within the brain, including the thalamus, basal ganglia, the gray and white matter of the cerebral cortex, and the ventricles. The major drawback is that the view provides a representation of the structure of the brain but not its function. See *imaging, brain; MRI.*

**tomomania**   A morbid desire to be operated upon.

**-tonia**   Combining form meaning stretching, tension, tone, from Gr. *tonos.*

**tonic convulsion**   Sustained contraction of a muscle.

**tonic elements**   See *REM sleep.*

**tonic epilepsy**   *Epilepsy* (q.v.) in which fits exhibit only tonic contractions, to the exclusion of clonic contractions.

**tonic pupil**   *Adie pupil* (q.v.).

**tonic SMA seizures**   See *frontal lobe seizures.*

**tonicity**   State or condition of tone or tension, mental or physical. See *tension, mental.*

**tonitrophobia**   Fear of thunder; astrapophobia.

**tonogeny**   Giving rise to increased tension or tonus. The vagus nerve is regarded as the tone-giving nerve of the stomach and intestines. The psyche may be the origin of tone-producing stimuli; for example, anxiety may be expressed in part through states of tension or tenseness.

**tonotopic map**   An area in the auditory system in which neighboring cells are most sensitive to acoustic frequencies that are adjacent to their own preferred threshold frequencies.

**tonotopy**   See *receptor sheet, peripheral.*

**tonus**   Tonicity

**TOP**   The association areas of the temporal, occipital, and parietal lobes of the cerebral hemisphere; also known as the *TPO junction.* The functions of TOP are imperfectly understood, but presumably many of the highest psychic functions are dependent upon intactness of these regions. The TOP area and the prefrontal area are the last to develop phylogenetically.

**topalgia**   Pain localized to one spot; the presence of a painful point or spot; a symptom occurring in hysteria or neurasthenia.

**top-down**   1. Referring to brain signals that convey knowledge derived from prior experience rather than sensory stimulation; the effect of feedback on a continuously operating system. The PFC, for example, is able to exert a top-down influence on multiple brain processes because of its own widespread connections with almost all sensory neocortical and motor systems as well as a broad range of subcortical structures.

2. Descriptive of an approach, which has rationalist overtones, in which the subject is assumed to bring to the task his own schemes, *scripts*, strategies, or frames which strongly color his performance. In a *bottom-up* approach, more allied to the empiricist camp, the actual details of a focal task or situation are assumed to exert primary influence on a subject's performance.

**topectomy**   A surgical operation for the excision (removal) of selected areas of the cerebral cortex (brain surface) in certain cases of mental illness; also known as the Columbia-Greystone operation because it was devised by that group. See *prefrontal lobotomy*.

The most favorable results were observed in patients with schizophrenia, refractory obsessive-compulsive disorder, involutional melancholia, chronic depression, and chronic mania.

**topical flight**  Cameron's term for *flight of ideas* (q.v.).

**topiramate**  A GABA-ergic antiepileptic drug that has also been used in the treatment of patients with alcoholism, where it has been found to reduce drinking significantly. It has also given evidence of efficacy in preventing relapse in cocaine addiction.

**topographical agnosia**  A condition in which patients become disoriented because they can no longer recognize their environment.

**topographical hypothesis**  See *id*.

**topography, mental**  Mapping of psychic structures, a static representation of the components of the psyche, denoting their location. For example, the superego in the adult psyche is located in the realm of the unconscious; Jung's archetypes occupy one of the deeper layers of the unconscious.

**toponeurosis**  A localized neurosis.

**topophobia**  Fear of a place. For each patient the nature of the place is specific, although the word has come to be used as a synonym of agyiphobia, or fear of streets.

**torpedoing**  The application of intense electrical currents to the bodily region involved in hysterical conversions.

**torpillage**  (F. "act of torpedoing") A wartime treatment of hysteria: application of electric currents to a shocking degree of pain—thus "fighting fire with fire," as it were; a type of aversion therapy.

**torpor**  A disorder of consciousness in which the subject is drowsy, slow in thinking, and shows a narrowed range of perception.

**torsades de pointes**  A potentially fatal ventricular arrhythmia in which there are phasic changes in the morphology of the QRS complexes on the electrocardiogram. Torsades de pointes is particularly associated with prolongation of the *QT interval* (q.v.), which may occur as an adverse drug reaction to antipsychotics. Risk of torsades de points is highest within the first few days of initiating therapy. Factors that predispose to QT prolongation and higher risk of torsades de pointes include older age, female sex, low left ventricular ejection fraction, left ventricular hypertrophy, ischemia, slow heart rate, and electrolyte abnormalities, including hypokalemia and hypomagnesemia.

**torsion spasm**  A constant and irregular twisting and turning of the body, especially of the pelvis and neck muscles, with bizarre posturing of the body and limbs.

**torticollis**  *Wry neck; caput obstipum*; characterized by spasmodic contractions of the muscles of the neck, particularly those supplied by the spinal accessory nerve; the head is usually drawn to one side and rotated so that the chin points to the opposite side. Torticollis is sometimes psychological in origin; Ferenczi regarded it as an attitude tic.

**torture**  See *false consensus*.

**"total-push" treatment of schizophrenia**  A method of treatment suggested by Myerson that includes physiotherapy, irradiation, exercise and games, diets, praise, blame, reward, punishment, regard for clothing and personal care.

**TOTE**  See *behaviorism*.

**totem**  "An animal, either edible or harmless, or dangerous and feared; more rarely the totem is a plant or a force of nature (rain, water) which stands in a peculiar relation to the whole clan. The totem is first of all the tribal ancestor of the clan, as well as its tutelary spirit and protector. The members of a totem are under a sacred obligation not to kill (destroy) their totem, to abstain from eating its meat or from any other enjoyment of it." (Freud, S. *The Basic Writings of Sigmund Freud*, 1938).

**totemism**  The selection of animals, plants, and inanimate objects as representatives for the (primitive) individual and tribes.

**toucherism**  A paraphilia in which arousal is dependent upon touching the sexual object.

**touching**  A disturbance in association, peculiar to schizophrenia, in which the only recognizable association to external stimuli consists of feeling with the hands the contours of objects within reach. This process is similar to *naming* (q.v.) except that a different motor activity is involved.

**Tourette disorder**  *Gilles de la Tourette syndrome* (Georges Gilles de la Tourette, Paris physician, 1857–1904); *maladie des tics*; one of the stereotyped movement disorders of childhood, first described in 1885. It appears in children between 2 and 15 years of age with facial movements (motor tics) and throat noises (vocal tics); the involuntary, rapid, purposeless movements become more generalized and progressive, and phrases or sentences may be ejaculated. Coprolalia and echolalia occur in more than half the cases; also frequent are palilalia, obsessive doubting, and compulsive touching. The lifetime prevalence rate of the disorder has been estimated as 1 in 1500; it is three times more common in boys than in girls. Families with one tic disorder (such as Tourette syndrome) are more vulnerable to other tic disorders (such as chronic motor tic). Further, there is an association between Tourette disorder and many other psychiatric disorders, including OCD (*obsessive-compulsive disorder*, q.v.) and other anxiety disorders, attention deficit hyperactivity disorder, personality disorders, and mood disorders. Genetic evidence suggests that Gilles de la Tourette syndrome and OCD are alternate manifestations of the same gene. Genome-wide linkage analysis has implicated areas on chromosomes 4, 5, 8, 11, and 17, but no disease-related mutations in these chromosomes have as yet been identified. Rare variants of the gene *SLITRK1* (*Slit and Trk-like family member 1*), on chromosome 13, have been associated with TS. Symptomatic relief has been obtained in many cases with butyrophenones, particularly haloperidol, and pimozide. Deep brain stimulation has also been used successfully to relieve the tics and vocalizations of some patients.

**Tower of Hanoi**   A puzzle in which disks must be moved from one peg to another; the test is thought to reflect procedural memory, as opposed to declarative memory for lists of items, including places, faces, and words. Schizophrenics do poorly, as on WCS; their recall memory is impaired, while recognition memory is intact.

**Tower of London test**   A measure of prefrontal lobe functioning, a modification of the Tower of Hanoi task developed by T. Shallice (1982): colored balls are lined up on a rod and the subject is asked how they should be realigned in order to match the pattern shown on three adjacent rods. The test involves sequential planning but does not depend on the use of long-term or working memory. See *hypofrontality hypothesis*.

**tower-head**   *Oxycephaly* (q.v.).

**toxic delirium**   See *brain syndrome associated with systemic infection*.

**toxic insanity**   Bucknill and Tuke classified insanity into three groups: (1) protopathic; (2) deuteropathic; and (3) toxic; examples included alcoholic insanity, pellagrous insanity, and cretinism.

**toxic-infectious psychosis**   Mental condition accompanying or following an infective illness or poisoning by some exogenous toxin. The symptoms include delirium, dazed and stuporous conditions, epileptiform attacks, hallucinoses, incoherence, and confusion. Examples of diseases that may produce this reaction type include influenza, malaria, acute rheumatic fever, pneumonia, typhoid and typhus fever, smallpox, and scarlet fever.

**toxicology screen**   Usually the subject is assessed for the presence of the following: anxiolytics (e.g., benzodiazepines, meprobamate), atropinic substances (e.g., antidepressants, antiparkinsonian drugs, phenothiazines), CNS depressants (e.g., alcohol, phenobarbital, other sedatives, phenytoin), hallucinogens (e.g., LSD, PCP, THC), heavy metals (e.g., arsenic, lead, mercury), pain medications (e.g., heroin, meperidine, morphine), and stimulants (e.g., amphetamines, cocaine, methylphenidate).

**toxicomania**   A craving for poison; drug dependence.

**toxicophobia, toxiphobia**   Fear of poison.

**toxoplasmosis, cerebral**   One of the opportunistic infections to which HIV-infected patients are susceptible, caused by reactivation of latent brain infection with the intracellular parasite *Toxoplasma gondii*.

  Clinical and radiological findings are nonspecific, so definitive diagnosis can be made only from biopsy material. See *AIDS*.

**toxoplasmosis, congenital**   In utero infection with toxoplasma, a protozoanlike-organism, which may produce mental retardation. Diagnosis is by serological testing of mother and infant.

**TPI test**   *Treponema pallidum immobilization* test for syphilis. It depends on an antibody that develops as early as the reagin detected by serologic tests but is much more specific, dependable, and persistent. It is of particular value in differentiating false serologic positives (which are often seen in the collagen diseases) from true positives due to latent syphilis.

**TPN** Total parenteral nutrition, usually implemented with an indwelling intravenous catheter and used in patients who have lost most or all of the small bowel. About 20% of such patients develop delirium or other serious psychiatric complications in the first year.

**TPO junction** The area between the temporal, parietal, and occipital lobes. See *TOP; spatial neglect.*

**trace, memory** *Engram* (q.v.).

**trace amines** Closely related to biogenic amines but found at much lower levels in the body. Their chief action was long believed to be interfering with neurotransmission by the biogenic amines, but the recent demonstration that they are able to activate their own class of receptors suggests that they might function as neurotransmitters in their own right. In the human, one of the identified trace receptors responds most strongly to tyramine and β-phenylethylamine, both of which have been linked with depression and schizophrenia.

**tracking** In multimodal behavior therapy, analysis of the patient's usual response to a situation or experience in terms of the order in which the different modalities of the *BASIC-ID* (q.v.) are predominant. Some patients, for example, typically respond first in the sensation modality, whereas others respond first in the cognitions area. It has been found that interventions are likely to be most effective if they follow the order of the patient's response pattern. With a patient whose first-order response is sensation (e.g., "butterflies in the stomach"), the best therapeutic results are likely to be obtained if predominantly sensory techniques (e.g., relaxation and biofeedback) are used as initial treatments.

**tracking, eye** See *pursuit eye movements; SPEM.*

**tracks** Linear, discolored brownish streaks along the course of subcutaneous veins as a result of unsterile injections and deposits of particulate materials.

**tract de Vic D'Azyr** Mammillothalamic tract; see *mammillary body.*

**tractotomy, stereotactic** See *sterotactic tractotomy.*

**TRADD** TNF-associated death domain protein that interacts with the *death domains* (q.v.) of the receptors for TNF to activate the cells' apoptotic machinery.

**Trail Making Test** A timed test in which the subject first (Part A) draws lines to connect consecutively numbered circles, and then (Part B) is asked to connect number and letter presented alternately (e.g., 1 connected to A, then 2 connected with B, and so on). The test is sensitive to diffuse cognitive dysfunction, attention, ability to shift mental set rapidly, and visuospatial ability. See *cognitive screening instruments.*

**trailing** A phenomenon reported in subjects under the influence of hallucinogens: moving objects are perceived as a series of discrete, discontinuous images.

**training analysis** *Didactic* or *tuitional analysis;* a term used by Ferenczi to refer to character analysis carried out for purposes of training in the concepts and problems of psychoanalysis (Freudian) through personal analysis of the analysand, who is in the position of a student who pays tuition for his instruction. See *orthodox analysis.*

**trait** In genetics, the characteristic symptoms of a hereditary factor as it appears in the phenotypes of those who have inherited the predisposition to the given attribute.

A trait is any physical or psychological characteristic that varies from one subject to another; it is a relatively stable and enduring attribute, in contrast to a *state*, which is a transient reactive condition or behavioral predisposition. Some authorities, for instance, consider hypoboulia and affective blunting as trait variables in schizophrenia, and hallucinations, delusions, and periods of agitation or excitement to be state variables.

**trait, complex** A phenotype that does not show classic mendelian recessive or dominant inheritance based on a single gene locus. The same genotype can produce different phenotypes, because of chance, environmental factors, or interactions with other genes; or different genotypes can produce the same phenotype.

**trait anxiety** See *anxiety.*

**trait carrier** In genetic family studies a tainted family member who exhibits the hereditary character under observation. Trait carriers are distinguished from the *taint carriers* (q.v.).

**trait marker** See *marker, biological.*

**trance** A temporary alteration in the state of consciousness and a disturbance of the normally integrative functions of memory and identity, such as loss of one's sense of personal identity, diminished awareness of one's immediate surroundings or narrowly selective focusing on environmental stimuli, or stereotyped behaviors that are felt to be beyond one's control. See *trance disorder, dissociative.*

**trance channeling**   *Channeling* (q.v.).

**trance coma**   The deep sleep following hypnotism.

**trance disorder, dissociative**   Trance and possession disorder; a dissociative disorder characterized by a *possession trance* (q.v.) that is not accepted as a normal part of a collective cultural or religious practice. Some phenomena of this type are indigenous to particular locations and cultures. See *culture-specific syndromes; dissociation.*

**trance, ecstatic**   See *ecstasy.*

**tranquilizer**   Ataractic; neuroleptic; currently used to refer to a group of phrenotropic compounds whose effects are exerted primarily at a subcortical level so that consciousness is not interfered with, in contrast to hypnotic and sedative drugs, which also have a calming effect. See *ergotropic; psychotropic.*

Benjamin Rush in the 1790s referred to an invention of his designed to reduce blood flow to the head of the mental patient as a "tranquillizing chair." It consisted of a chair to which the patient's hands and arms were strapped, stocks for the feet, and a box for the patient's head, so that he could not move.

**transactional**   Relating to negotiating, conducting, performing, or carrying on, as an act or process; pertaining to an interplay or interaction. R. Grinker's transactional approach is an attempt to understand the interplay between therapist and patient—and ultimately between the patient and external reality—in terms of role theory.

"Activities within a transactional process, although they deal with current reality and start with well-defined explicit roles, expose the repetitive nature of the patient's unadaptive behavior and stimulate his recall of past experiences...this transactional approach evokes implicit expressive or emotional roles and incites repetition of old transactions and illuminates the genetic source of the current behavior" (In *Contemporary Psychotherapies*, ed. M. I. Stein 1961). See *role.*

Both transactional and interactional refer to cross-communication and cross-influencing of each member in a relationship by the other member(s). In psychiatry, the terms are generally used to refer to the dynamic, two-way interaction between therapist and patient. The earlier assumption that the psychoanalyst is totally objective and reflects none of his own values to his patient has undergone gradual modification in recent years. It is now recognized that in the psychoanalytic process, "The therapist's personality, his value system, and his techniques of interaction, nonverbal as well as verbal, are...at least as important, and in many instances even more important than the uncovering of repressed content which has been the cornerstone of the traditional model of the psychoanalytic process. The increasing awareness of this among psychoanalysts has been reflected in recent years in the growing literature on the subject of 'countertransference' attitudes in the analyst and their effect upon the analytic process" (Marmor, J. *Archives of General Psychiatry 3,* 1960). See *countertransference.*

**transactional analysis (TA)**   A type of psychotherapy developed by Eric Berne that emphasizes the influence of the ego states of Parent, Adult, and Child on a person's interactions with others. The *Parent ego state* relates to limit-setting and nurturing; it is based on the subject's perception of his own parents. The *Adult ego state* is concerned with reality testing and estimating probabilities in transactions with the outside world. The *Child ego state* comprises the feelings, wishes, and adaptations actually experienced in childhood.

Most outcomes of an exchange are decided by *ulterior transactions,* psychological responses that are outside the awareness of the participants. People play *games,* adopting the role of Persecutor, *Rescuer,* or Victim and using ulterior transactions in such a way that everyone loses. Treatment focuses on *feelings analysis, script analysis,* and *stroking* (stimulating and recognizing other human beings). Feelings may be reactions (appropriate responses in the here and now); they may also be *rubber bands* (feelings from the past reactivated by a stimulus in the present) or *rackets* (indulgements or displaced feelings that are a backdrop in today's scene of living). The script refers to plans decided upon in early life when the subject was under parental influence; they are based on myths about the self and the world and are perpetuated by games and rackets. The major scripts are *winner, nonwinner* (tolerable but unsatisfying), and *loser.*

**transcendental meditation (TM)**   A psychophysiologic technique, usually associated with the name of the Indian guru (teacher) Maharishi

Mahesh Yogi. Maharishi began teaching the technique throughout India in 1955 and in 1958 initiated a worldwide movement to train others who wished to learn it. TM is neither a religion nor a philosophy, even though in the past it may have been related to both. It appears to be a natural process, perhaps a fourth physiologically and biochemically definable state of consciousness (the others being sleeping, dreaming, and waking), that does not require any mental or physical control, any change in lifestyle or belief system, nor does it involve hypnosis or suggestion. TM is associated with a hypometabolic state, during which there is a reduced activity of the adrenergic component of the autonomic nervous system. The physiologic and psychosomatic accompaniments of the state lead to a lowering of tension and anxiety and an increase in contentment and tolerance of frustration.

**transcortical aphasia**  A fluent aphasia with defects in comprehension and thinking about or remembering the meaning of signs or words. The affected person cannot read or write and has marked difficulty in finding words. Writing is typically more disturbed than comprehension and reading. The ability to repeat spoken language is retained. The lesion is outside the perisylvian language centers, most often the result of vascular damage at the junction between the middle anterior, and posterior cerebral arteries, a region known as the *border zone* or *watershed area.*

The transcortical aphasias are divided into the foolowing:

a. *Transcortical motor aphasia,* in which the Broca area is disconnected from the supplementary motor cortex. The lesion is in the medial aspect of the left frontal lobe or the area superior to Broca area, or in the basal ganglia, or the pulvinar thalamus. This produces a nonfluent aphasia in which the patient cannot produce creative speech. He attempts conversation but can utter only a few syllables. He can repeat words and phrases well, and there may even be echolalia. There is impairment of comprehension or speech production or both, with a paucity of speech and labored, but not telegraphic, speech. Writing is often seriously impaired; reading is less disturbed.

b. *Transcortical sensory aphasia*—symptomatically similar to Wernicke aphasia (fluent

output, impaired comprehension) but with intact repetition. The lesion is in the left angular gyrus or posterior inferior parietal region. There is difficulty in thinking about or remembering the meaning of signs or words. The subject cannot read or write and has marked difficulty in finding words but is able to repeat spoken language easily and fluently.

c. Mixed transcortical aphasia or *isolation of the speech area* is a rare combination of motor and sensory transcortical aphasias. symptomatically similar to global aphasia (nonfluent, poor comprehension) but repetition is intact. The subject is unable to speak unless spoken to, and responses are usually a direct echo of the examiner's words (echolalia). He eerily repeats what he hears without understanding it or ever speaking spontaneously. The patient is not competent in any other language function. The lesion is a combination of those in sensory and motor transcortical aphasia, or large lesions of the anterior and posterior left medial hemisphere.

Symptoms that commonly accompany Broca or transcortical aphasia include *aprosodia* or *dysprosodia* and *verbigeration,* which suggests frontal lobe dysfunction (qq.v.).

**transcranial magnetic stimulation**  *TMS*; also *rTMS* (repetitive TMS); a noninvasive means of stimulating the cortex. TMS was first introduced as a neurophysiologic probe in 1985, but its use as a therapeutic tool followed observations that some subjects investigated with TMS experienced mood elevation. There are three types of TMS: single pulse, paired-pulse, and repetitive (rapid-rate) TMS. rTMS is most commonly used in therapeutic applications because it can produce tens of pulses per second in bursts lasting up to approximately 1 minute. rTMS uses an electromagnetic coil applied to the scalp to produce a high-strength, rapidly fluctuating (1 msec. on, several msec. off) focal magnetic field, induced by an alternating current in the coil.

Because it produces a transient interruption of brain activity in a relative restricted area of the brain, TMS has been particularly useful in the study of perception, attention, learning, plasticity, language, and awareness. Although rTMS has been used in the treatment of various conditions (movement disorders, epilepsy, anxiety disorders, stuttering, schizophrenia), it is most often used in the treatment of depression as an alternative to ETC. It does not produce a convulsion, nor does it require anesthesia. Therapeutic effects have generally been similar to treatment with ECT in non-psychotic depressions. The typical course consists of 10 to 20 treatments, using frequencies of 1–20 Hz over the left DLPFC, applied on a Monday through Friday schedule.

**transcription** Reading out (copying, translating) the information contained within *DNA* or *RNA* (qq.v.) or in the template strand of a gene; the process whereby the DNA sequence of a gene is copied into mRNA, the template for protein synthesis. It is translated, according to the rules of the genetic code, into directions for synthesizing structural and metabolic proteins (gene expression) in the cytoplasm. The copy (*transcript*) may serve as a message for translation into protein, it may become structural RNA and form the framework of a ribosome or of an adaptor molecule in protein synthesis, it may form the genome of an RNA virus, or it may itself serve a regulatory function. Proteins are not synthesized directly from the DNA that encodes them, but in two sequential processes: transcription of DNA into mRNA, which occurs in the nucleus, and translation of the mRNA into protein, which occurs in the cytoplasm.

DNA sequences within a gene that code for a segment of mRNA are called *exons* because the information in those sequences will be exported from the nucleus; the intervening sequences, which remain in the nucleus, are called *introns*. Many genes contain multiple introns and exons that may not be spliced identically in every cell type or in a given cell type at every stage of development. This mechanism, *alternative splicing*, can produce functionally very different forms of a protein or even entirely different proteins from a single gene.

The copying machinery is a floating mixture of special proteins, a *transcription complex*. The DNA thread is continually being unwound and rewound at thousands of different sites as genes are made accessible and their information is copied by the cell's transcription machinery. When the cell needs to divide, the entire length of the thread must be split apart, duplicated, and repackaged for each daughter cell.

DNA and mRNA specifications of amino acid building blocks for proteins occur in linear stretches of three nucleotides. An amino acid is a small molecule that contains an amino group ($NH_2$) and a carboxylic acid or carboxy group ($COOH$) plus a variable side chain. Amino acids are linked to each other by peptide bonds, and proteins are formed by chains of amino acid building blocks.

There are three major steps in transcription:

1. *Activation-initiation*: a large transcriptional complex is assembled at a promoter, a DNA segment near the beginning of the gene that usually includes characteristic sequences known as the TATA box. In addition to RNA polymerase, the enzyme that makes the mRNA template, the transcriptional complex contains a group of general transcription factors which, among other things, modify the histone proteins in chromatin to increase its accessibility to the transcriptional complex. RNA polymerase then interacts with the gene and begins transcribing.

2. *Elongation*, *release*, and *editing*: the RNA polymerase must shorten and resynthesize the RNA into an appropriate length. The transcript is released and moves into one or more terminaor sequences along the DNA template.

3. *Termination*: transcription of the RNA must terminate appropriately. See *gene; gene expression; gene functions.*

Both DNA and RNA can serve as a template for the processive synthesis of other macromolecules. The principle of complementary base pairing provides the mechanism. An enzyme, a DNA polymerase in the case of DNA replication or RNA polymerase in the case of transcription of DNA into RNA, can move down a template strand of DNA adding sequential nucleotide bases complementary to the bases on the template strand. Eventually the replication process generates two complete DNA double helices, each identical in sequence to the original. DNA replication is said to be semiconservative because each daughter DNA molecule contains one of the original parental strands plus one newly synthesized strand.

**transcription factor** Any of the intracellular proteins that bind to gene promoters regulating expression of the gene, thereby transmitting signals from the cell membrane directly to the gene(s), without depending on a second messenger (q.v.). For example, as soon as interferon binds to its receptor, tyrosine kinase phosphorylates the transcription factor proteins, which move quickly into the nucleus and turn on the genes that are responsive to interferon.

A transcription factor is a protein that specifies whether and under what circumstances a gene will be transcribed. Each type of cell in the body expresses only a subset of the entire complement of genes. In any given cell, some genes are "on," and the rest are "off." Regulatory sequences within DNA control the expression of genes by virtue of their ability to bind specific regulatory proteins. Certain regulatory sequences of DNA specify the beginnings and ends of DNA segments that can be transcribed into RNA. Other regulatory sequences determine in what cell types and under what circumstances the gene to which they are linked can be read out. Signal transduction systems consist of a network of proteins that transform multiple external stimuli into appropriate cellular responses. Multifunctional adapter proteins assemble the appropriate signaling proteins and then act as scaffolds for their organization into distinct functional pathways. See *gene; gene expression; gene functions; transcription.*

**transcription-factor therapy**   TF therapy. See *subventricular zone (SVZ).*

**transcriptional function**   See *gene functions.*

**transcriptional regulators**   See *gene.*

**transcriptomes**   Catalogs of transcription factors, DNA elements that control gene expression. See *noncoding DNA.*

**transcultural psychiatry**   See *comparative psychiatry.*

**transducer**   Converter; an agent that receives a signal in the form of one type of energy and converts it into a signal in another form. In the sensory neuron, the stimulus activates the *transducing receptor protein*, a special protein molecule on the surface of the sensory neuron. This initiates a flow of ionic current that produces a change in the resting potential of the cell membrane. Stimulus information (modality, intensity, duration, and location) is transmitted in a series of action potentials, a process termed *neural encoding.* Stimulus intensity, for example, is encoded by means of rate of sensory neuron discharge: as intensity

increases, the discharge rate of the sensory neuron increases.

In a similar fashion, the motor neuron (or the interneuron) is activated by the chemical transmitter released from the presynaptic neuron. The *synaptic receptor protein* transforms that chemical energy into an electrical signal, the synaptic potential. Depending on the receptor protein, the synaptic potential can be either depolarizing (excitatory) or hyperpolarizing (inhibitory). Half the neurons of the brain are inhibitory. See *synapse.*

There are two types of transducer and, correspondingly, two types of transducer response—ionotropic (ionophoric) and metabotropic.

1. In an *ionotropic* response, the recognition site of the *neurotransmitter receptor* is part of the protein complex that includes an *ion channel*, whose opening or closing is ligand-gated. Such direct linkage between the recognition site and the ion channel ensures fast and precise signaling between neurons. See *ion pump.*

2. *Coupling* transducers initiate a *metabotropic* response. The neurotransmitter receptor is not part of an ion channel but is instead linked to an enzyme that is part of the neuroreceptor protein molecule. Activation of the neuroreceptor—enzyme complex induces the enzyme to act on its substrate. These soluble enzyme products are called *second messengers*, because they produce effects that are secondary to primary neurotransmitter (first messenger) action.

Metabotropic responses to neurotransmitter-neuroreceptor activation are necessarily much slower (10 to 30 times) than their ionotropic counterpart, because they involve enzyme activation and subsequent cascades of biochemical responses. Examples are the slow inhibition following opening of the $K^+$ channel by the opioid peptides, serotonin, and somatostatin. Coupling transducers are decentralized, i.e., they can let more than one neurotransmitter activate the same effector proteins.

Some neurotransmitters have more than one type of receptor. One example is the two types of dopamine receptors: $D_1$ (which appears to activate adenylate cyclase activity) and $D_2$ (which seems to inhibit adenylate cyclase). Further, one receptor protein can activate many G protein molecules. Thus, the effect of coupling receptors, although slower than that of ionotropic receptors, is to amplify and provide greater versatility of response.

**transducer potential**   *Generator potential*; events similar to the spread of current along the axon, occurring in the receptor as it responds to stimuli to which it is sensitive. See *action potential*.

**transducer site**   See *neurotransmitter receptor; synapse*.

**transduction**   Conversion of energy into a different modality or form. See *transducer*.

**trans-entorhinal region**   An area of the brain, located between association cortices and hippocampus, that is important in the integration of information, learning, and memory processes.

**transfer**   In connection with institutional statistics, a transfer is a shift from one institution directly to another institution of the same class.

**transference**   Freud's original description of transference as a repetition in the relationship to the analyst of earlier relationships has been modified considerably. What is experienced through the transference is not an early experience per se, but the feelings and ideas of what that early experience aroused in the subject, the phantasies the subject had about the experience, and defenses against both. The analytic situation stimulates the patient's unconscious phantasy life but at the same time frustrates the patient's demand for gratification. The patient does not remember the unconscious phantasy but instead repeats it in the transference and attempts to impose a reenactment of that phantasy on the patient–analyst relationship. The transference, in other words, is an acting-out type of resistance. Its manifestations are inappropriate and anachronistic when applied to the analyst in the present.

Ordinarily, transferences are projections of object representations and are sometimes called *displacement transferences*. Transferences that involve projection of self-representations typically involve some blurring of ego boundaries and are more likely to be observed in borderline or psychotic conditions. They are sometimes termed *projection transferences*. Kleinian object relations theorists view transference in terms of *projective identification* (q.v.); they tend to perceive almost any of the patient's reactions to the analyst as transference based on phantasies that developed

during the first year of life. Self psychologists view transference as a manifestation of profound disappointment in the analyst's ability to empathize with the patient. See *countertransference; transference, archaic*.

Part of the patient's relationship to the analyst reflects the patient's attempts to force the analyst into acting and feeling in a distinct way, into doing something. For example, the destructive, angry, hating patient may be attempting to re-create a version of the mother, the first person who tolerated the child's aggressive tasks and survived.

Transference may be positive, as when the patient unrealistically overvalues or loves the analyst; or it may be negative, as when the patient dislikes or hates the analyst without due cause in reality. See *character defense; parataxic distortion*.

It is to be noted that the term transference does not refer to reactions of the patient to the analyst that are based on reality factors in the therapeutic relationship; thus, a patient may be angry with his therapist if the latter misses an appointment, but to call such a reaction a manifestation of transference is incorrect. It should also be recognized that transference can exist outside the analytic situation in relation to other people in the person's environment.

E. Krapf (*Psychoanalytic Quarterly 26*, 1957) considers positive transference to be predominantly libidinal and negative transference as predominantly aggressive. He notes that there is a third type of transference, the transference of anxiety, which always serves as a defense, while libidinal and aggressive transference are defensive in many instances but not in all. "Thus we may list five types of transference: 1, libidinal; 2, aggressive; 3, libidinal-defensive; 4, aggressive-defensive; and 5, anxious-defensive."

Jung stresses the question of transference, which he calls psychological rapport. He calls it "the intensified tie to the physician which is a compensation symptom for the defective relationship to present reality." He holds that "the phenomenon of transference is inevitable in every fundamental analysis.... The patient must find a relationship to an object in the living present, for without it he can never adequately fulfill the demands that adaptation makes upon him" (Jung, C. G. *Contributions to Analytical Psychology*, 1928).

**transference, archaic** A transference in which the patient lacks awareness of the difference between the therapist and the early object (e.g., mother) and experiences the therapist as an extension of the self. Typically, the patient demands an immediate response from the therapist (e.g., the analyst must affirm the patient's specialness or uniqueness), thereby creating a dilemma for the therapist. If he remains silent and does not answer, the patient becomes enraged at his rudeness; yet almost any answer given will be wrong and will unleash irrational denial or rage in the patient. Archaic transferences, with splitting of pre-oedipal object representations and of self-representations, are frequent in borderline and infantile patients.

**transference, eroticized** One type of archaic transference consisting of overt, ego-syntonic, excessive demand for love and sexual gratification from the analyst.

**transference, idealizing** See *alter-ego transference; idealization; mirroring; mirroring needs.*

**transference, institutional** Emotional dependence upon hospital, clinic, or similar establishment, rather than on a particular therapist or person within the institution; observed frequently in latent schizophrenics.

**transference, negative** See *transference resistance.*

**transference, sibling** In group therapy, attitudes and feelings similar to those a patient has heretofore entertained toward siblings and now has toward other members of the therapy group.

**transference cure** See *flight into health.*

**transference dilution** In group therapy, diminution of intensive transference toward the therapist by reason of the presence of sibling and identification transferences to other members of a group.

**transference improvement** Amelioration of neurotic symptoms on the basis of *transference* (q.v.). The physician is perceived unconsciously as a reincarnation of the parents and as such is thought of as providing love and protection, or as threatening with punishments. So-called *flight* into health (q.v.) is an instance of transference improvement.

**transference neurosis** A "new artificial neurosis," occurs during psychoanalytic treatment. It is the reappearance of the infantile Oedipus situation. The analyst represents one or both parents as a love object, as if he were really the original parent in the original infantile setting of the patient. The patient also lives out all his old ego attitudes and incest prohibitions. See *transference.*

Transference neurosis represents a stage where the history of the patient's development, leading up to the infantile neurosis, is reenacted in the analytic room—the patient plays the part of actor-manager, pressing into service (like the child in the nursery) all the stage property that the analytical room contains, first and foremost the analyst.

**transference resistance** Positive libidinal transference that occurs when the patient harmoniously transfers repressed material upon the physician. The material, however, may be rejected by the ego or superego, that is, there is resistance offered to the appearance of the material in consciousness, as a consequence of which it may be held in the unconscious; the patient gives an indirect clue by remaining silent on the topic in question. Or the material may be projected upon the physician, then appearing as something undesirable allegedly possessed by the physician. The repressed material may return to consciousness in one of the many known forms, but it is only when it constitutes a conflict between the patient and the physician that it is known as transference resistance. The resistance gives rise to negative transference, an animosity or opposition to the physician. See *ego resistance.*

**transference-focused psychotherapy (TFP)** The foundation of TFP is the Object-Relations theory elaborated by Kernberg. Patients with *borderline personality disorder* (q.v.) or BPO (borderline personality organization), although able to differentiate self from others (unlike persons with psychotic organization), cannot form an integrated mental picture of the self, in both its good and bad aspects, nor of the important other(s) in their lives. One posits a mechanism of "splitting" as the primitive defense mechanism, which interferes with the ability to achieve realistic, integrated mental representations. BPDs relate to others and to their therapists as all good (idealized) or all bad (devalued). Unwanted, unacceptable feelings may be denied subconsciously; disavowed (acknowledged in consciousness but not openly admitted), or projected onto someone else, such as the therapist.

TFP relies on a schedule of two or three sessions per week. It begins by setting a meaningful contract with the patient governing the number of meetings, and how telephone calls and suicidal threats and acts are to be handled. The therapist establishes a hierarchy of issues to be dealt with, typically: (1) suicide threats or acts; (2) threats to discontinue therapy impulsively and prematurely; (3) severe symptoms that could be dangerous such as drug abuse, unprotected sex, anorexia, or marked depression;(4) moderate or mild symptoms such as dysthymia, premenstrual irritability, bulimia, social ;phobia; (5) various maladaptive personality traits that interfere with optimal function; and (6) the patient's ambitions, hopes, and goals, sorting out which are realistic and which are not. In contrast to Kohut's self-psychology approach, TFP avoids providing advice or support interventions and pays more attention to the negative transference. Because TFP emphasizes not only the techniques of clarification and interpretation but also of confrontation (e.g., about glaring discrepancies of professed attitudes, polar opposite assertions concerning important others, or threats to behave in self-destructive or treatment-threatening ways), TFP differs from most other forms of psychotherapy for BPD.

**transferrin**   See *%CDT*.

**transformation of affect**   One of the many processes by which the dream obscures its true meaning. If the psychic material out of which the dream is constructed contains an affect that has been repressed, this affect can gain representation in the dream by inversion into an opposite affect.

**transfusion, exchange**   Total replacement of blood by transfusion. See *icterus gravis neonatorum*.

**trans-Golgi network**   *TGN*; see *Golgi apparatus*.

**transgendered**   See *transsexualism*.

**transgene(s)**   See *transgenesis*.

**transgenesis**   Insertion of a foreign gene (or genes, called *transgenes*) into the chromosome of an organism, in an effort to determine either the normal function of the transgene(s) or the effects of dysfunction of the transgene(s) on the model organism. Transgenesis is also used in gene therapy: a normally functioning gene is taken from one organism and is inserted into the chromosome of an organism which, often because of a mutation, lacks that gene or has an abnormally functioning gene.

**transgenic**   *Chimeral*; inserting the gene of one animal (such as a rabbit) into another animal (such as a mouse). The gene is inserted into a single embryonic cell of the host animal (the transgenic or chimeral animal) in a test tube. As the cell divides, the gene is passed on to each new generation of cells and ultimately becomes a permanent part of succeeding generations.

**transglutaminase**   See *nerve growth*.

**transient**   1. Lasting for a short period of time, quickly passing through, time-limited. The differences between transient, transitory, time-limited, short-term, etc. are more a matter of usage than of precise definition, and different groups employ the terms in different ways. In descriptions of sleep disorders, for example, transient insomnia indicates DIMS (disorder of initiating and maintaining sleep) of one to several days, whereas *short-term* insomnia indicates DIMS of up to 3 weeks, and *persistent* insomnia indicates a duration of at least 2 months and usually of many months or years.

2. In electroencephalography, a wave or complex that stands out from the background and lasts for a brief period of time. The most common transients are spikes, with a duration of 20 to 70 msec, and sharp waves, with a duration of 70 to 200 msec. *Paroxysmal EEG* activity refers to a series of transients that begins abruptly and then terminates.

**transient global amnesia (TGA)**   Abrupt onset of disorientation due to loss of ability to encode recent memories plus retrograde amnesia of variable duration, with retention of a remarkable degree of alertness and capacity for fairly complicated mental performances. The episode, which is almost never repeated, lasts for a few hours, when the patient regains his ability to encode recent memories despite amnesia for events that occurred during the acute phase. TGA is presumed to be due to transient ischemia of the hippocampus-fornix-hypothalamic system, although there is no direct proof of the theory. It is to be differentiated from hysterical amnesia and from the amnesia of temporal lobe epilepsy.

**transient situational disturbances**   In the 1968 revision of psychiatric nomenclature (DSM-II), adjustment reactions of acute symptom formation to an overwhelming situation; crisis reaction. Recession of symptoms occurs when the stress stimulus diminishes or disappears; persistence of symptoms indicates a more severe underlying disturbance.

Included in the group are adjustment reactions of (1) infancy; (2) childhood; (3) adolescence; (4) adult life; (5) late life. See *adjustment disorders*.

**transient situational personality disorder** *Adjustment disorders* or *transient situational disturbances* (qq.v.); a misnomer, in that personality by definition is long-lasting rather than transient.

**transinstitutionalization** Moving people or populations from one segment or sector to another, used particularly in regard to "depopulation" of state mental hospitals and "deinstitutionalization," where follow-up studies suggested that the criminal justice system had often been substituted for the mental health system. What seemed to be an advance in care of the chronically mentally ill seemed to be no more than a statistical ploy: patients were put into jails and prisons for disturbing the peace, rather than into the medical facilities they needed, but because they had been shifted out of the health care system they no longer appeared on the rolls of that system. See *chronic mentally ill*.

**transitional group** A therapy group devised for children (in latency period and puberty) who do not require intensive group psychotherapy but are unable to participate with confidence in ordinary social clubs. A form of "protective groups" has been developed for these young patients (Slavson, S. R. *An Introduction to Group Therapy*, 1943).

**transitional object** An early *not-mother* object used for self-soothing, such as a teddy bear, blanket, sheet, or diaper. It is an early indicator of the capacity to see the self as separate from the object, and to manipulate external objects and events (*mastery*). The transitional object comes into use when the child is between 4 and 18 months of age; it allows the discovery of otherness and functions as a bridge between the child and his culture or environment. Winnicott conceived of transitional phenomena as occurring in a *potential space* located between the boundaries of self (inner world) and object (outer world).

Elaborating on Winnicott's initial description in 1953, Fred Busch and his coworkers (*Journal of the American Academy of Child Psychiatry 12*, 1973) differentiated between the primary transitional object (adopted in the first year of life, usually at age 6 months) and the secondary transitional object (adopted at

about age 2). Characteristic of the primary transitional object are (1) time of attachment within the first year; (2) duration of attachment being 1 year or more; (3) effect being to soothe and reduce anxiety; (4) object not meeting a direct oral or libidinal need; (5) attachment made actively by the infant rather than passively accepting something, such as a pacifier, that is forced upon him; and (6) object being distinguished from parts of the body, such as the thumb, that also bring comfort.

**transitive inference** See *relational memory*.

**transitivism, transitivity** One of the accessory or secondary changes in the person of the schizophrenic, consisting of detachment of a part of the personality from the patient with subsequent displacement of this part onto another person. In such cases, whatever the patient hallucinates or does is believed to be an experience of that other person.

**transitory psychosis** A syndrome "characterized by emotional turmoil, various kinetic phenomena, and dissociation with confusion and hallucinations, followed by complete recovery and amnesia" for the episode (Kasanin, J. *American Journal of Psychiatry 93*, 1936–37). See *schizophreniform disorder*.

**transketolase** A thiamine-dependent enzyme of central nervous system cells that has been reported to be deficient in Korsakoff psychosis.

**translational research** Investigation with the aim of bringing scientific discoveries and hypotheses into the clinical arena, of bridging the time gap between scientific discovery and its application to clinical care settings, of subjecting clinical observations to objective scrutiny and converting them into viable hypotheses and conclusions based on research evidence. Translational research is often thought of as a process that begins with a basic science discovery that is applied directly to the patient, but an equally important pathway is one that begins with recognition of a problem at the clinical level, takes that problem to the laboratory for generation of viable scientific hypotheses and conclusions based on research evidence, and to use those conclusions to introduce novel diagnostic, therapeutic, or preventive approaches to illness.

Translational research provides a bridge from discovery to delivery, but unlike basic research it is focused on a clinical goal or target. New findings about basic mechanisms of illness, for example, may be framed in terms of focused clinical research questions or clinical studies that are responsive to clinicians' interests and needs. Translational research seeks to improve quality by improving access, reorganizing and coordinating systems of care, helping clinicians and patients to change behaviors and make more informed choices, providing point-of-care decision support tools, and strengthening the patient–clinician relationship (Woolf, S.H, *Journal of the American Medical Association 299*: 211–213, 2008).

**translocation** A chromosomal abnormality in which part or all of one member of a chromosome pair, instead of maintaining its proper position and joining with its counterpart from the other gamete in fertilization, drifts or migrates to another chromosome pair. In some cases of Down syndrome, for example, the defect is due to translocation of the long arm of an extra chromosome 21 to chromosome 15; the resulting chromosome is called a 15/21 translocation chromosome.

**transmethylation** A biochemical step in which one or more methyl groups are added to the structure of a compound. The *transmethylation hypothesis*, based on the observation that one of the major differences between naturally occurring amines (e.g., indoles, such as tryptamine and serotonin, or phenethylamines, such as dopamine and norepinephrine) and hallucinogenic indoles or phenethylamines is the increased number of methyl ($CH_3$) groups in the latter compounds, suggesting that an alteration in the biochemical transmethylation of naturally occurring amines might result in the endogenous synthesis of methylated amines that function as hallucinogens and produce some of the symptoms of schizophrenia.

**transmissible** Able to be transmitted; inheritable; infectious.

**transmissible spongiform encephalopathies** *TSEs*; chronic, progressive, and always fatal neurodegenerative disorders caused by a slow replicating agent that requires a long incubation period for disease expression. See *prion*. Human TSEs include *Creutzfeldt-Jacob disease, kuru*, and *Gerstmann-Staussler-Scheinker syndrome*. In 1995, a novel form of CJD, new variant CJD (nv CCJ) was described in the

United Kingdom; it is believed to be due to transmission of BSE (bovine spongiform encephalopathy) to humans. See *neurodegenerative disorders; protein conformational disorders*.

**transmission** Practically synonymous with *inheritance* (q.v.).

**transmission, nerve** Passage or conduction of the nerve impulse from one neuron to another. Signaling within the brain involves the passage of ions, electrically charged chemical particles, through separate, minute channels in the cell membrane. See *action current; ion channel; neuron; synapse*.

**transmission, vertical** Transplacental infection, as contrasted with horizontal (host-to-host) *transmission*.

**transmitter** See *neurotransmitter*.

**transmitter, inhibitory** See *GABA*.

**transmuting internalization** See *self-object*.

**transneuronal degeneration** Transsynaptic degeneration; degeneration of nerve cells that had synaptic connections with an injured nerve cell. Anterograde transneuronal degeneration indicates that the affected cell received input from the injured cell; retrograde indicates that it made synapses onto the affected cell.

**transorbital lobotomy** A psychosurgical procedure consisting of partial ablation of the prefrontal area. The approach is through the superior conjunctival sac, and the operation is usually performed bilaterally. The plane of section corresponds roughly to that of topectomy but, like prefrontal lobotomy, the procedure is a "blind" one and white matter rather than gray matter is destroyed. The incision interrupts the frontothalamic and thalamofrontal radiations and also the frontal lobe association fibers. Some surgeons prefer the transorbital approach to classical prefrontal lobotomy because it produces fewer side effects. See *prefrontal lobotomy; psychosurgery*.

**transpersonal psychology** An extension of the field of psychology to include the study of optimal psychological health and well-being. It recognizes the potential for experiencing a broad range of states of consciousness, in some of which identity may extend beyond the usual limits of the ego and personality. Transpersonal psychotherapy adds to traditional areas and concerns an interest in facilitating growth and awareness beyond traditionally recognized limits of health. The importance of modifying consciousness and the validity of transcendental experience and identity are affirmed (Walsh, R. & Vaughan, F. *Beyond Ego: Transpersonal Dimensions in Psychology,* 1980).

Transpersonal psychology is distinguished from religion and theology by its basis in empirical, scientific study of the experiences that people actually have. Topics of particular interest include ultimate values, unitive consciousness, peak experiences, ecstasy, mystical experience, self-actualization, essence, bliss, wonder, ultimate meaning, transcendence of the self, oneness, cosmic awareness, individual and species-wide synergy, maximal interpersonal encounter, cosmic self-humor and playfulness, maximal sensory awareness, responsiveness, and expression.

**transplantation**   Removal from one place to another; most commonly used to refer to removal of a body organ from a donor to a recipient. Also used to refer to transfer of a person from familiar to alien surroundings (as in admission of an elderly person to a nursing home). The concomitant anxiety, depression, or other manifestations of distress are sometimes termed transplantation shock.

**transplants, brain tissue**   Neural grafts; a technique developed by Anders Bjorklund and others to repair damage to CNS tissue. Cells from fetal or neonatal animals are transplanted into the adult brain. The use of fetal grafts is controversial and it is unclear how they produce their results. The mechanisms may involve a combination of providing both transmitter substances and neurotropic factors onto target cells. See *Parkinson disease.*

**transporter carrier protein**   *Ion pump* (q.v.).

**transporter proteins**   Integral membrane proteins that selectively mediate the passage of molecules across the otherwise impermeable barrier imposed by the phospholipid bilayer that surrounds all cells and organelles. More than 360 families of transporters have been identified. Some transporters act as molecular pumps, translocating their substrates across membranes against a concentration gradient. Membrane transport in cells is mediated by various channel and transporter proteins. One type is secondary active membrane transporters, which use a solute gradient to drive the translocation of other substrates. The largest secondary transporter protein family is the major facilitator superfamily (MFS), with

more than 1000 members identified (as of 2003). These proteins transport ions, sugars, sugar-phosphates, drugs, neurotransmitters, nucleosides, amino acids, peptides, and other hydrophilic solutes. See *Glut1 transporter.*

**transposition**   The process by which pieces of DNA move around the genome. There are many forms of transposition, including "jumping genes," replication of bacteriophages, integration of retroviruses, and acquisition of bacterial genes for antibiotic resistance. All of them involve precise breakage that exposes the 3' tips of the transposable element, which are then joined to the target DNA.

**transposition of affect**   Displacement of the affective component of an unconscious idea onto an unrelated and harmless idea, seen typically in obsessive-compulsive and depressive patients.

**transposon**   A wandering, free-agent scrap of DNA that can cut open genes and insert itself into places where it does not belong. The only information it carries is instruction for making the enzyme it needs to cleave DNA. Also called jumping gene. Transposons may contribute to genetic disorders by causing breaks at vital points in the chromosomes.

**transsexualism**   Less commonly, transexualism; adopting the role of the opposite sex, which may include hormonal and surgical treatment to remove the physical characteristics of the original sex and to acquire the physical characteristics of the opposite sex. Many transsexuals follow prevailing medical beliefs and claim to be "a man trapped in a woman's body" or vice versa. Some, however, argue that by living their lives as a member of the "opposite" gender, those transsexuals are simply moving from one socially imposed categorization (or cage) to another. The term *transgendered* has been proposed as an umbrella term that would include those who are neither man nor woman, heterosexual nor homosexual, and who often reject surgical "sex change."

**transvestitism**   *Transvestic fetishism* (in DSM-III-R); transvestism; *cross-dressing* (q.v.); a type of *paraphilia* (q.v.) characterized behaviorally by donning garments of the opposite sex. As R. J. Stoller (*Archives of General Psychiatry 24*, 1971) points out, cross-dressing by itself is a symptom, not a syndrome or diagnostic entity, and it may be manifested in several different ways.

1. *Fetishistic cross-dressing*—limited to males, who consider themselves to be heterosexual, whose behavior and appearance when not cross-dressing are masculine rather than feminine; such men derive genital excitement by donning women's clothes, and the excitement usually leads to masturbation and orgasm. See *phallus girl.*

2. *Transsexualism* (q.v.)—the patient's cross-dressing is not a means to induce genital excitement, but only one of the means used to transform himself into the opposite sex and to deny his own masculinity. The transsexual has no interest in his penis as an executive organ of erotic desire, and far from wanting to preserve his penis the transsexual from his early years has a strong desire for transformation anatomically into a female. In some, the desire is so strong that they seek castration (*castrophilia*) or prefer suicide to living as a man.

3. Effeminate homosexuality—the overt homosexual may put on women's clothes as part of a performance or act in which he both identifies with women and mocks them through mimicry and caricature (drag queen); the wearing of women's clothes is not in itself sexually exciting, however.

**Transylvania effect** Correlation of abnormal behavior with moon phases (and thus the term "lunacy"). Despite the persistent belief that such a correlation exists, there is little evidence to support the notion.

**trauma** Injury, damage, wound, shock. As originally described, psychic trauma referred to a sudden intense surge of anxiety, secondary to some external event, that exceeds the subject's ability to cope and to defend. The concept was subsequently extended to include overwhelming anxiety related to intrapsychic events, then to include later intrapsychic elaboration of external events that had originally seemed benign (as when cognitive development allowed a different interpretation or clearer understanding of the significance of an earlier event, or when psychosexual development rendered the subject susceptible or reactive to an event to which he or she had earlier been unresponsive), then to a summation or accumulation over time of events that individually had been inadequate to provoke overwhelming excitation. *Screen trauma* referred to a memory occurring after a trauma that concealed and stood for a deeply repressed memory of a traumatic experience; *constructive trauma* suggested that at least some traumata might benefit the child and constitute a positive learning experience.

Because such diffusion and overextension of meanings threatened to reduce or even negate the usefulness of the term, the tendency since the 1970s has been to return to the original and more restricted meaning. See *adjustment disorders; anxiety disorders; post-traumatic stress disorder; traumatic neurosis.*

Psychiatric syndromes associated with trauma include (1) anxiety disorders—posttraumatic stress disorder, acute stress disorder, panic disorder, generalized anxiety disorder; (2) depressive disorders—major depressive disorder, dysthymia, adjustment disorders, acute bereavement, complicated grief; (3) substance-related disorders—substance abuse, substance dependence; and (4) exacerbation of preexisting or reactivation of past psychiatric conditions.

Trauma is severe *stress* (q.v.); it is accorded special attention because reactions to it can be prolonged and severely disabling, and because disorganized or suboptimal attachment patterns in infancy are predictive of later stress disorders, dissociative reactions, and personality disorders. The PTSD/trauma and attachment literature differentiates between traumatization in infancy as a result of suboptimal attachment patterns, and traumatization as a result of physical, emotional, or sexual abuse or extreme neglect.

Flight, the most common response to threat when successful escape is possible, is not only running away from danger but also running toward a person or place that provides safety. When flight is impossible, self-defense with aggression and fighting is an alternative. But when such defenses are ineffective or cannot ensure survival, immobilizing defenses appear: *freezing,* limp passivity or feigning death, and submissive behavior. In freezing, the sympathetic system increases muscle tone, heart rate, sensory acuity, and alertness, while the subject waits for more data about the threat before taking action. Another version of freezing is to remain motionless in order to avoid detection by the predator. Still another type of freezing is a sense of being trapped with feelings of being paralyzed, unable to move or breathe.

Feigning death, behavioral shutdown, or fainting are signs of parasympathetic arousal.

Submissive behaviors, such as crouching and avoiding eye contact, aim to prevent or interrupt aggressive attack. Such behaviors include *robotization*, consisting of mechanical behavior and automatic obedience.

L. C. Terr (*American Journal of Psychiatry 148*: 10–20, 1991) divided *childhood trauma* into Type I traumas, which are single events; and Type II traumas, which are long-standing, multiple, or repeated experiences that occur in circumstances in which the trauma is predictable and there is no escape. Powerless to stop it, the child must use any means possible to protect herself or himself. Often this takes the form of dissociation or depersonalization—the child must avoid knowing what she knows. The traumatic events cannot be integrated fully; the affects of terror, shame, and anger are contained by the detachment and ultimate compartmentalization of inner experience. The chronically traumatized child swings between dissociative numbing and detachment and a hyperarousal state of alertness to and fear of environmental cues that predict a repetition of the trauma.

Chronically aroused states of fear that are invalidated by, or invisible to, a caretaker lead to self-blaming and shaming explanations and the sense of a secretly damaged self. As the child advances in age, relationships with other people provide little warmth or intimacy, because they are distorted by a self that believes it is deeply unworthy.

Severe chronic traumatization in childhood leads to *PTPD* (complex PTSD); less severe traumatization is associated with *borderline personality disorder* (qq.v.).

**trauma, infantile** The occurrence in infancy or childhood of a situation in which the psyche is bombarded by stimulation of such intensity that it cannot be mastered or discharged. In such situations, anxiety develops automatically.

**trauma, primal** The original, supremely important, and most painful situation to which the person has been exposed early in life; it often constitutes the nucleus of the neurosis.

**trauma stories** Narratives about violence and its effect on their lives as told by survivors of trauma. Disclosing their tales of horror and describing how "Pain penetrates me drop by drop" (Sappho) facilitate *self-healing*, particularly of the hidden wounds (psychological and spiritual) inflicted by aggression and violence.

Other mechanisms that promote self-healing include altruism, spirituality, dreams, humor, exercise, work, and support groups. See *dehumanization; humiliation; survivor syndrome*.

**trauma syndromes** Syndromes associated with trauma include (1) anxiety disorders—PTSD, acute stress disorder, other anxiety disorders (panic disorders, GAD); (2) depressive disorders—major depressive disorder, dysthymia, adjustment disorders, acute bereavement, complicated grief; (3) substance related disorders—substance abuse, substance dependence; and (4) exacerbation of preexisting and reactivation of past psychiatric conditions.

**traumasthenia** Nervous exhaustion following an injury; traumatic neurasthenia. See *traumatic neurosis*.

**traumatic brain injury** *TBI*; see *brain injury*.

**traumatic defect state** See *traumatic neurosis; traumatic psychosis*.

**traumatic delirium** An acute delirium occurring immediately after head or brain injury as a result of force directly or indirectly applied to the head. Some patients, following such injury, may show a protracted or chronic delirium with marked disorientation, confabulation, and memory defect, but with apparent superficial alertness. This latter condition may resemble the Korsakoff syndrome. See *organic mental disorders*.

**traumatic dementia** Intellectual or affective dementia due directly or indirectly to an injury, usually to the head. See *post-traumatic dementia*. "Common to most of them are rapid exhaustion, irritability, tendency to spontaneous and reactive moods, up to the most intensive anger, which is in part labile and in part of a more torpid persistent affect.... Not rarely epileptic attacks appear in which the typical epileptic dementia may occur (traumatic epilepsy). Pictures similar to catatonia can last for a long time" (Bleuler, E. *Textbook of Psychiatry*, 1930).

**traumatic encephalopathy** A diffuse organic brain disease due to injury to the brain. See *brain injury*. Clinical symptoms are persistent headache, dizziness, spots before the eyes, poverty of memory, general mental and physical fatigability, poor concentration, loss of energy, irritability, outbursts of anger, and either drowsiness or insomnia; personality changes are commonly a part of the syndrome. See *post-traumatic constitution; post-traumatic dementia*.

**traumatic hysteria**   A neurotic illness developing in consequence of an injury (a traumatic neurosis). "The traumatic or accident neuroses rarely occur when the victim of the injury must bear the brunt of the financial responsibility for the accident, as in the case of injuries in sports. There is usually an incubation period between the injury, which may be quite slight, and the appearance of the mentally determined symptoms. This interval before the development of the chronic disabilities is of value in excluding an organic source. It is usually occupied with vague ruminations which tend to be of an imaginative, affective, wish-determined and suggestive nature" (Noyes, A. P. *Modern Clinical Psychiatry*, 1940).

**traumatic neurosis**   *Ego neurosis*; a psychogenic or nonstructural nervous disorder, shortly following a physical injury. Current thinking emphasizes the importance of psychologic rather than physical trauma as necessary for the development of the disorder. See *post-traumatic stress disorder; libido stasis.*

While a traumatic experience can precipitate any of the well-known types of neurotic or psychotic disorders, the most common conditions seen in combat are hysteria, anxiety states, and exhaustion conditions. The essential features of traumatic neurosis are (1) fixation on the trauma with amnesia for the traumatic situation that may be total or partial; (2) typical dream life (dreams of annihilation, aggression dreams where the patient is the aggressor but is defeated, frustration or *Sisyphus dreams*, and occupational dreams in which it is the means of livelihood rather than the body-ego that is annihilated); (3) contraction of the general level of functioning, with constant fear of the environment, disorganized behavior, lowered efficiency, lack of coordinated goal activities, and profoundly altered functioning in the autonomic, motor, and sensory nervous system; (4) general irritability; and (5) a proclivity to explosive aggressive reactions. A malignant type of traumatic neurosis, *psychorrhexis* (q.v.), is seen in 2% to 3% of war neuroses.

**traumatic psychosis**   Mental disorder caused by or associated with brain injury, often manifested as an organic personality syndrome. See *contusion, brain; organic mental disorders; traumatic constitution; traumatic neurosis.*

**traumatophilia**   Love of injury or the unconscious desire to be injured. See *traumatophilic diathesis.*

**traumatophilic   diathesis**   *Accident proneness* (q.v.)*;* a desire to be traumatized. *Self-defeating personality* (q.v.) is sometimes manifested as recurrent accidents or traumatic events, but both "diathesis" and "proneness" invited unjustified extension of a hypothesized wish for punishment to explain almost any kind of negative occurrence. Particularly in the early days of psychoanalytic theorizing, any chance happening was grist for the interpretative mill, limited only by the range of the interpreter's imagination, and any mishap betrayed the victim's unconscious desires. See *recidivism; victim; victimology.*

**traumatophobia**   Fear of injury.

**TRD**   *Treatment-resistant depression* (q.v.).

**treatment**   Therapy; any measure designed to ameliorate or cure an undesirable condition; application of planned procedures to identify and change patterns of behavior that are maladaptive, destructive, or health injuring; or to restore appropriate levels of physical, psychological, or social functioning.

**treatment guidelines**   See *first-line treatments.*

**treatment resistance**   Failure to respond as expected to a therapeutic regimen (estimated to apply to 30% of patients); often defined operationally as persistence of clinically significant symptoms after 6 weeks of psychopharmacological treatment, even though the drug has been given at therapeutic dosages and has been taken by the patient as described. The patient who demonstrates treatment resistance is often termed *treatment-refractory.*

Approximately 30% of patients treated with antidepressant drugs do not respond, for various reasons; some patients are misdiagnosed, others are noncompliant and do not take the drugs as prescribed, others are not treated for an adequate length of time, and still others have inadequate blood levels of the drug despite its administration at a dosage level that would ordinarily be adequate. The last group are sometimes called *relative resisters*, in that they will respond to higher dosage levels that bring their blood level of drug to the therapeutic range. *Absolute* resisters are those who do not respond even though they are correctly diagnosed, do comply with instructions, and are maintained for an adequate length of time at blood levels of drug that are within the usual therapeutic range.

**treatment-emergent mania**  *TEM* (q.v.).

**treatment-refractory**  See *treatment resistance.*

**treatment-resistant depression**  *TRD*; failure to respond to two or more trials of antidepressant monotherapy, or failure to respond to four or more trials of different antidepressant therapies, including augmentation, combination therapy, and ECT. There is increasing evidence that somatic interventions, including *ECT, vagus nerve stimulation* (VNS), *deep brain stimulation* (DBS), magnetic seizure therapy (*MST*), and repetitive *Transcranial Magnetic Stimulation* (rTMS) are effective in some patients unresponsive to pharmacotherapy or cognitive behavioral therapy (qq.v.).

**treble safeguard principle**  The variable regulation of all growth functions by means of integration of endocrine and individual organ activities with the molecular dynamics of the nervous system.

**tremophobia**  Fear of trembling.

**tremor**  Involuntary movement characterized by rhythmic oscillations (quiverings or trembling) of a part of the body; *hyperponesis.* Tremors are often divided into two major groups on the basis of the conditions under which they appear—(1) *rest tremor* or *passive tremor*, manifested when the affected area is at rest; the major tremor in this group is the parkinsonian tremor and its most typical form is the *pill rolling* tremor (the thumb moves across the fingers); the tremor disappears with the onset of movement until late in the course of disease, and (2) *movement tremor.*

Tremors with movement include *postural tremors, kinetic tremor, task-specific tremors,* and hysterical tremor.

Among the postural tremors are the following:

1. *Physiological tremor*, which appears with the attempt to maintain a posture.

2. *Essential tremor* (if it occurs with movement rather than with posture, it is called essential *intention tremor*), often familial with an autosomal dominant transmission; its most common form is a side-to-side tremor of the fingers of 4 to 9 Hz. It may also affect the vocal tract, giving a tremulous quality to the voice. In intention tremor, amplitude of the tremor increases during visually guided movements (as in the finger-to-nose test).

3. *Isometric tremor*, which occurs during voluntary muscle contraction against a rigid stationary object (such as squeezing the examiner's hand on request).

4. *Postural tremor* with basal ganglia disease, including Parkinson disease (where it may occur in addition to a rest tremor), torsion dystonia, Wilson disease (the movement is often abduction of the shoulder with elbows flexed, called a *wing-beating tremor*).

5. *Cerebellar tremor*, frequently caused by multiple sclerosis, typically affecting proximal muscles, trunk, and head, and usually of low frequency (2.5 to 4 Hz) but increasing progressively the longer posture is maintained. *Cerebellar outflow tremor*, however, a result of lesions of the dentate nucleus or its pathways, is a severe, coarse tremor that is present at rest and is intensified during activity. See *cerebellum.*

6. Tremor associated with peripheral neuropathy of any cause.

7. *Post-traumatic tremor*, appearing late (months) after severe head trauma; it resembles cerebellar tremor in appearance.

8. *Alcoholic tremor*, sometimes associated with cerebellar damage or peripheral neuropathy, at other times an enhanced physiological tremor associated with sympathetic overactivity.

Kinetic tremor that is not a postural tremor is probably caused by cerebellar disease; it consists of a trembling or quivering (not a dysmetric arrhythmia) about the target that disappears once the target is reached. Task-specific tremors appear only with specific tasks, such as primary writing tremor; it sometimes is a part of writer's cramp.

**trend, statistical**  Uniform change in one direction as shown by statistics. Over a long period of time natural and social phenomena tend to increase or decrease in a regular manner.

**TRH**  *Thyrotropin-releasing hormone* (q.v.). See *neuropeptides.*

**triage**  The process of choosing, selecting, sorting, or weeding out; in medicine, the immediate sorting out and classification of medical casualties (as in disasters and crises) so that patients may be routed to and referred to appropriate treatment services.

**triage model**  In health care, a system for early identification of the factors that determine the most appropriate treatment. Its basic elements are rapid evaluation, immediate containment of conditions that threaten the life of the patient or the welfare of the community, and prompt referral to the person or agency that can provide the patient with appropriate care.

**trial, clinical**   A prospective study involving human subjects designed to provide evaluation of preventive, diagnostic, or therapeutic practice, such as the use of a certain drug, medical device, or procedure.

**trial, randomized**   *See randomized clinical trial.*

**triangulation**   *See scapegoating.*

**triarchic theory**   *See intelligence.*

**tribade**   A woman with an abnormally large clitoris, who plays the part of a male in homosexual practices. See *lesbianism; sapphism.*

**tribology**   The study of lubricants. *Tribologist* is sometimes used to refer to a paraphiliac whose sexual arousal depends on the use of lubricants.

**tribulin**   The molecule in normal human urine believed to be both an inhibitor of monoamine oxidase receptor binding and an inhibitor of benzodiazepine receptor binding.

**triceps reflex**   *Elbow jerk*; a deep reflex; the patient's forearm, flexed at the elbow, is held by the examiner; the striking of the tendon just above the olecranon process results in extension of the forearm. This reflex depends upon the radial nerve for its afferents and efferents; its center is $C_{6-7}$.

**trichobezoar**   Hairball or hair cast in the stomach or intestine. The smooth surface of the hair does not allow for its propagation by peristalsis. When hair is ingested, it is trapped in the stomach mucosa. As more hair is added, the resulting mass causes the stomach to cease peristalsis completely. The mass is a trichobezoar, first described in 1779 by Baudomant. It may lead to gastrointestinal blockage and perforation or secretory diarrhea and malabsorption of nutrients, leading to vitamin deficiencies. Large trichobezoars require surgical removal. In one reported case, the trichobezoar had a long tail that extended past the duodenum, a rare complication of trichotillomania referred to as *Rapunzel syndrome.*

**trichologia**   *Carphology* (q.v.).

**trichopathophobia**   Fear of hair.

**trichophagy**   *Trichophagia*; the tic of biting (and swallowing) the hair. See *trichobezoar.*

**trichophobia**   *Trichopathophobia* (q.v.).

**trichotillomania**   *TTM*; Term coined by M. Hallopeau (1889) for *hairpulling*, currently classified as an *impulse control disorder* (qq.v.).

**tricyclic**   See *antidepressant.*

**trifacial neuralgia**   See *tic douloureux.*

**trigeminal cerebral angiomatosis**   See *angiomatosis, trigeminal cerebral.*

**trigeminal nerve**   The fifth cranial nerve. The trigeminal nerve has both motor and sensory components. Motor fibers arise from the motor nucleus in the pons and supply the muscles of mastication (masseter, temporal, internal and external pterygoids). Sensory fibers are in three divisions: the ophthalmic division supplies the forehead, eyes, nose, temples, and meninges; the maxillary division supplies the upper jaw and hard palate; the mandibular division supplies the lower jaw and tongue. Symptoms of trigeminal nerve lesions include pain, loss of sensation, paralysis of muscles of mastication with deviation of the jaw to the affected side, loss of jaw jerk, sneeze, lid reflex, conjunctival reflex and corneal reflex, and various trophic changes in the nose, face, and jaw.

**trigeminal neuralgia**   See *tic douloureux.*

**trihexyphenidyl**   An anticholinergic drug. See *cholinergic.*

**trihybrid**   Hybrid that differs in three hereditary characters. See *hybrid.*

**trimethadione**   An *antiepileptic* drug (q.v.).

**trinucleotide repeat**   *Triplet repeat, triplicate repeat; polyglutamine repeat*; an insertion repeat in which a sequence of three base pairs is repeated more than the normal number of times. The genetic code is made up of triplets of base pairs (a pair of complementary nucleotide bases, such as cytosine [C] and guanine [G]); each set of three bases constitues a codon specific for one of the 20 amino acids found in proteins. Chromosomal mutations consisting of a greater than normal number (*expansion*) of the triplet repetitions are the basis of a number of genetic diseases—the *polyglutamine disorders* (q.v.):

A. *CGG repeats* within the untranslated region of the first exons of their respective genes

    1. Fragile X syndrome—mutation of FMR-1 gene on chromosomeXq27.3; normal range of repeats is 6 to 54, disease range is 50 to1500.

    2. Fragile XE mental retardation

B. *CGG repeats* not known to result in any disease phenotypes
3. Fragile site 11B
4. Fragile site XF — not known to be in the vicinity of any gene
5. Fragile site 16A—not known to be in the vicinity of any gene
C. *CAG repeats*—the effect is to lengthen a normal olygltamine tract in their respective gene products
6. Spinobulbar muscular atrophy (Kennedy syndrome)—mutationon Xq21.3 in coding region of androgen receptor protein, whosefunction is destroyed; normal range of repeats is 13 to 30, disease range is 30 to 62; it affects the brain stem, spinal cord, sensory neurons
7. Spinocerebellar ataxia type 1—mutation on 6p24; results in defective ataxin-1 protein; normal range of repeats is 25 to 36, disease range is 43 to 81; it affects the cerebellum, spinocerebellar system, inferior olive.
8. Spinocerebellar ataxia type 3—defective MJD-1 protein; range of normal repeats is 13 to 40, disease range is 68 to 79; it affects multiple motor control regions of brain and spinal cord.
9. Huntington disease—mutation on 4p16.3; huntingtn protein defective; normal range of repeats is 9 to 37, disease range is 37 to 121
10. Dentatorubral-pallidoluysian atrophy (DRPLA)—affects atrophin; normal range of repeats is 7 to 23, disease range is 49 to 75; it affects cerebellum, brain stem, basal ganglia, spinal cord, cerebral cortex.
11. Machado-Joseph disease
12. Haw River syndrome—CAG repeats at same locus as DRPLA but slightly different phenotypic features, perhaps because of modifying genes.
D. CTG repeats
13. Myotonic dystrophy—expansion located in the myotonin-protein kinase (Mt-PK) gene on 19q13.3, but apparently the disease is produced only when an overlapping gene, dystrophia myotonia-associated homeodomain protein (DMAHP), is involved; normal range of repeats is 5 to 37, disease range is 44 to 3000

E. GAA repeats
14. Friedreich ataxia—expansion located in X25 gene (which encodes the protein frataxin) on chromosome 9q13; normal range of repeats is 10 to 21, disease range is 200 to 900.

In many trinucleotide repeat disorders, there is a correlation between the length of the expansion and the severity and time of onset of the disease. Typically, the severity of disease increases in succeeding generations (genetic *anticipation*). When expansion results in disease, the disorder transmits as a dominant trait (Warren, S. T. *Science 271*, 1996).

**triolist** In a triangular sex relationship the person whose opposite-sex partner has a same-sex partner; the triolist typically derives as much sexual satisfaction from watching the other two indulge in homosexual activity as from engaging in heterosexual activity with either or both of them. Example: Alice has sex with Ted, whose male lover is Gordon; much as she enjoys intercourse with Ted, she finds even more satisfaction in watching Ted and Gordon having sex together.

**triple diagnosis** Coexistence of cognitive impairment (e.g., dementia), substance abuse, and major mental illness. See *dual diagnosis*.

**triple X syndrome** Mild mental retardation associated with trisomy of the X chromosome.

**triplet repeat** See *trinucleotide repeat*.

**triptans** $5\text{-HT}_{1B1D1F}$ agonists, used to treat acute migraine attacks.

**trisexuality** The symbolic representation, especially in dreams, of the three currents or aspects—man, woman, and child—in which sexuality may be studied psychoanalytically.

**triskaidekaphobia** Fear of (the number) thirteen. Thirteen at table is viewed by many as an ill omen, and one more person is usually invited to join in the meal. The thirteenth day of the month is looked upon with dismay by those swayed by the superstition and, if it falls on a Friday, with double dismay—for Friday, long referred to as "hangman's day," was the usual day for hanging a criminal in the England of old. To prevent the possible loss of such fearsome clients (who would not live in a house No. 13) many office buildings, and particularly hotels, have no thirteenth floor or rooms No. 13, or multifigured numbers ending with 13. Apparently the "baker's dozen" (adding one roll for good measure, to avoid the severe penalties for short-counting) is an exception to this common fear of thirteen.

**trisomy** A type of chromosomal abnormality in which three chromosomes appear in a position that normally is occupied by a chromosome pair. The most important known trisomy in psychiatry is 21-trisomy, or *Down syndrome* (q.v.). See *chromosome*.

**trochlear nerve** The fourth cranial nerve. The trochlear nerve arises at the level of the inferior colliculus and is the motor nerve to the superior oblique muscle of the eye. For symptoms of trochlear nerve lesions, see *oculomotor nerve*.

**trolley dilemma** There are two versions of this *moral dilemma* (q.v.).

1. One set of trolley tracks goes towards a group of people, the other towards a single person. If you do nothing, the whole group will be killed; but if you switch the tracks, only one person will die. What would you do?

2. One track leads to a group of people; but you can stop the trolley by pushing one person in front of the trolley. What would you do?

Most people take the single-death option only in option 1. See *neuroeconomics; prisoner's dilemma; social reasoning; Ultimatum Game*.

**trophic factors** See *growth factors*.

**trophicity, neural** The concept, emphasized particularly by Russian neurophysiologists, that is an outgrowth of Pavlov's views of trophic functions of the nervous system. Pavlov believed the nervous impulses arising from one group of neurons do not only stimulate other neurons but also act upon the entire trophicity of those neurons: oxygen and nutrient supply, and assimilation and metabolism of these substances within those cells.

**trophodermatoneurosis** *Acrodynia* (q.v.).

**trophoneurosis** A nutritive disturbance, organically determined. It is believed that each organ of the body is supplied with nerves whose functions are definitely identified with nutrition or trophism. When such nerves are disordered, nutrition of the organ suffers.

**trophotropic** See *ergotropic*.

**-trophy** Combining form meaning nutritive, from Gr. *trophe*, nourishment, food.

**tropism** *Taxis* (q.v.).

**-tropy** Combining form meaning turn(ing), from Gr. *trope*.

**trough level** In pharmacology, the time at which *half-life* (q.v.) is reached and blood concentration reaches a plateau.

**Troxler effect** See *filling in*.

**TRP** Transient receptor potential; TRP channels are responsible for sensory transduction in various modalities, including taste, thermal sensation, and hearing. The mechanosensitive transduction channel for hearing, or at least a component of it, is the TRP channel, TRPA1.

**true anxiesty** See *basic anxiety*.

**true self** The sum total of a person's potentialities that might be developed under the most favorable social and cultural conditions. Fromm considered neurosis in terms of cultural pressures (which often thwart potentialities) and the interaction of people. Because some of the patient's best potentialities are repressed, therapy aims at helping the patient to become himself and discover his "true self." Neurosis stems from the new needs a person's culture creates in him and, as a secondary concomitant to cultural pressures, from the person's deprivations and the frustrations of his potentialities. See *False Self; impingement*.

**trust vs. mistrust** One of Erikson's eight stages of man. See *ontogeny, psychic*.

**truth serum** See *narcotherapy*.

**tryptophan** See *eosinophilia-myalgia syndrome*.

**tryptophan hydroxylase** The serotonin metabolizing enzyme; see *5-HTTLPR*.

**TSD** *Tay-Sachs disease* (q.v.).

**TSEs** *Transmissible spongiform encephalopathies* (q.v.); also known as prion disorders. TSEs include Creutzfeldt-Jakob disease, fatal familial insomnia, Gerstmann-Straussler syndrome, bovine spongiform encephalopathy, and scrapie.

**TSF** *Tyramine sensitivity factor*, of particular concern in patients treated with MAOIs. Monoamine oxidase has two forms: MAO-A, which acts primarily on dopamine, norepinephrine, and serotonin; and MAO-B, which acts primarily on phenethylamine and tyramine. Inhibition of MAO-B in the gastrointestinal tract prevents the metabolism of tyramine in food, resulting in absorption of larger than normal amounts of tyramine. Large amounts of tyramine can cause the release of substantial quantities of norepinephrine, resulting in a hypertensive crisis. Patients treated with MAOIs are advised to choose a simple diet that is focused primarily on restriction of aged cheeses, tap draft beer, marmite, soy sauce and soy bean condiments, and air-dried meets. See *cheese effect*.

**TSH** Thyroid-stimulating hormone; thyrotropin. See *thyrotropin-releasing hormone (TRH)*.

**TTH** *Tension-type headache* (q.v.).

**TTM** *Trichotillomania* (q.v.).

**TTR** *Type token ratio* (q.v.).

**tube feeding** Feeding through a nasal catheter that terminates in the stomach.

**tubectomy** See *salpingectomy*.

**tuberculomania** An unfounded but unalterable conviction that one is suffering from tuberculosis; phthisiomania.

**tuberculophobia** Fear of tuberculosis or of associating in any way with a sufferer from that disease; phthisiophobia.

**tuberculous meningitis** A condition in which the tubercle bacillus infects the meninges of the central nervous system and produces mental symptoms of the organic reaction type. The disease is always secondary to a tuberculous focus elsewhere in the body, and without treatment the course is usually slowly progressive toward a fatal termination. Headache, delirium, stupor, and convulsions occur. The neck is rigid; often the tubercle bacillus can be demonstrated in the spinal fluid.

**tuberoinfundibular tract** See *dopamine*.

**tuberomammillary nucleus** *TMS*; tuberomamillary system; the sole seat of histaminergic neurons and the origin of the widely distributed histaminergic projections. The *histaminergic system* mediates general states of metabolism and consciousness, including hibernation and the sedative component of anaesthesia. Activity of TM neurons is high during waking and attention, and low or absent during *sleep* (q.v.). They are critical to the posterolateral hypothalamic arousal system. The histaminergic system is also linked to feeding, drinking behavior, temperature regulation, and homeostasis.

Four histamine receptors have been identified ($H_1$–$H_4$). The $H_4$ receptor is detected predominantly in the periphery; $H_1$–$H_3$ are prominently expressed in the brain. $H_1$ receptors mediate excitatory actions on whole brain activity. The classic antihistamines act as $H_1$ antagonists. $H_2$ receptors potentiate excitation of neurons. Both the $H_1$ and $H_2$ receptors are involved in pain perception. $H_3$ receptors produce autoinhibition of TM neurons and inhibition of transmitter release. Histamine is involved in limbic mechanisms of learning and memory, especially through the $H_3$ receptor. It affects synaptic plasticity and facilitates hippocampal LTP, in part by means of intracellular elevation of $Ca^{2+}$ and interaction with NMDA receptors.

**tuberous sclerosis** *Epiloia*; a chronic heritable disorder, transmitted as an autosomal dominant with variable penetrance. Symptoms appear in early childhood: mental retardation (often severe), epileptic convulsions, and special tumors (adenoma sebaceum) of the skin and viscera. Pathologically, there are various malformations and numerous glial tumors within the brain. The disease was originally described by Bourneville.

**tuitional analysis** *Training analysis* (q.v.).

**Tuke, Daniel Hack** (1827–1895) British psychiatrist; editor of *Dictionary of Psychological Healing*.

**tumescence** Swelling, engorgement; used particularly to refer to the swelling of genital tissues associated with sexual excitement.

**tumor necrosis factors** TNFs (q.v.).

**tunnel disease** *Caisson disease* (q.v.)

**turbid** Muddled, mentally confused.

**Turing, Alan Mathison** (1912–1954) English mathematician, master code-breaker (of German codes in World War II), and the father of artificial intelligence studies; in 1937 his proposal of a problem-solving machine defined the essentials of modern digital computers.

**Turkish-bath method** *Rare.* A type of treatment based on the transference relationship in which the therapist applies threats and reassurances one after the other—one day hot, the next day cold.

**Turner syndrome** A chromosomal abnormality consisting of absence or damage to one X chromosome of a female, so that the total number of chromosomes is 45 rather than the usual 46. The syndrome is characterized by short stature, infantile sexual development, cardiac defects, drooping eyelids, and uneven cognitive development with impaired visuospatial ability (e.g., in visual memory or drawing) and sometimes also difficulty with numbers and auditory memory. Language development, however, typically appears normal for the subject's age. Sex characteristics are mainly female even though the sex chromatin test is negative (XO). There is no spontaneous onset of puberty, although it can be produced and menstrual cyclicity established with the use of hormones.

**turpitude, moral** Sexual misconduct or other kinds of misbehavior on the part of the physician toward his patient, such as alcoholism or dishonesty.

**turrecephaly** *Oxycephaly* (q.v.).

**TVD** Transmissible virus dementia. See *virus infections*.

**TWEAK**  A brief sceening test for alcoholism. The acronym refers to the five signs of alcoholism that it detects: *T*olerance, *W*orrying about drinking, *E*ye-opener (taking a drink in the morning), Amnesia or blackouts, and *K* for a desire to cut-down. It is said to be as sensitive as two other commonly used brief questionnaires, the *CAGE* and *MAST* (qq.v.).

**twelve-step group**  A *mutual help group* (q.v.) modeled on the program of Alcoholics Anonymous, a nondenominational spiritual approach that involves turning one's life over to a Higher Power. Other steps include admitting one is powerless over one's addiction and over one's life because of addiction, making a moral inventory and making amends for past wrong, and offering to help other addicts. The group enjoins anonymity and an apolitical stance, and its structure is nonhierarchical.

**22q11 deletion syndrome**  Results from a meiotic deletion of genetic material at the q11.2 site on chromosome 22. Associated congenital anomalies occur in some but not all children and may include heart defects, immunologic deficits, craniofacial dysmorphologies, velopharyngeal defects such as overt or submucous cleft palate, or inflammation-related pain syndromes. Before the deletion was identified, the syndrome was given different names depending upon the predominant symptoms: conotruncal anomaly face syndrome (heart defect with facial dysmorphologies), velocardiofacial syndrome (velopharyngeal, heart, and facial anomalies), and DiGeorge syndrome (immunologic insufficiency).

Language delays are manifested in the early years and are followed by learning disabilities and academic failures, attention impairment, and behavioral anomalies in most of the school-age children with the syndrome. Lower *prepulse inhibition* (q.v.) is a characteristic neurophysiologic finding. Approximately 25% of affected children go on to develop schizophrenia in adolescence or early adulthood.

**twiddling**  Repeated rotation of the hands in front of the body; used to elicit signs of bradykinesia.

**twilight state**  Absence, a transitory disturbance of consciousness during which many acts, sometimes very complicated, may be performed without the subject's conscious volition and without retaining any remembrance of them. See *sensorium.*

Responsive as a rule only to some given complex, the subject acts in accordance with the demands of the complex, the rest of the personality being subordinated to or, as a rule, more or less completely submerged during the period of the twilight state. For example, an epileptic patient, entirely unmindful of his natural surroundings, believed that he was walking around in Heaven; during the phase he was utterly unable to recall any part of his real life.

In Bleuler's classification, twilight state is one of the acute syndromes in *schizophrenia* (q.v.). The twilight states appear as waking dreams that portray desires, wishes, or fears in a direct or symbolic way as being already fulfilled. They often persist for long periods; duration of 6 months is not uncommon. See *fugue.*

The term twilight state is also applied to one of the variations of delirium in which the patient passes abruptly into a state of severe clouding of consciousness combined with generally slow, monotonous movements and occasional outbursts of rage and fear.

**twin**  One of two organisms born from a female that ordinarily brings forth only one offspring at a time. In human beings there are two distinct types of twins, the *monozygotic* or *identical* twins, developed from a single egg, and the *dizygotic* or *fraternal* twins, developed from two eggs. Dizygotic twins are held to be as separate in their origin and biological development as are siblings in general. Monozygotic twins are like the right and the left halves of *one* organism; accordingly, they not only have the same genotypical structure, but also exhibit frequently the phenomenon of *reversed asymmetry* (mirror-imaging) in handedness, hair whorl, dentition, palm patterns, and other asymmetrical characters, i.e., characters that are asymmetrical in one person.

Twin studies are of great scientific significance in human genetics, because they throw light upon many fundamental aspects of the *nature-nurture* problem as well as of the *developmental* mechanisms of the human organism throughout its life from the fertilization of the ovum to death.

**twin transfusion syndrome**  An arteriovenous shunt between twins that creates within-pair differences in blood distribution and development. The syndrome occurs in 15% to 30% of *monochorionic* twins (q.v.).

**twin-study method**  One of the two principal methods used in psychiatric genetics for differentiation between genetic and environmental influences in relation to specific forms of adjustment or maladjustment. In this method, the dissimilarities of one-egg twins, genotypically identical organisms, are compared with the behavioral variations seen in ordinary sibs or two-egg twins.

**two-point threshold** The difference in distance between two stimuli required to identify them as different. Note that the two-point threshold is not an absolute number. Two stimuli of equal pressure applied to the middle of the back might feel like a single stimulus if they are separated by only 50 mm, but if applied to the tip of the index finger they would readily be identified as separate.

**two-syndrome hypothesis of schizophrenia** The subdivision of schizophrenic disorders into Type 1 (the positive syndrome) and Type 2 the negative syndrome (characterized by poor premorbid adjustment, insidious onset, prominent negative symptoms, cognitive impairment, structural brain abnormalities such as ventricular enlargement, and a poor response to treatment). See *deficit state; productive symptoms; schizophrenia, models of.*

**type** See *constitution; constitutional type.*

**type A** A behavior pattern characterized by anger, impatience, irritation, and aggravation. The personality syndrome was first formulated by cardiologists Meyer Friedman and Ray Rosenman, who in 1959 reported their finding that men with such a behavior pattern were seven times more likely than others to have evidence of heart disease and two to three times more likely than men with the more easygoing type B behavior to have heart attacks (*coronary-prone*). Type A subjects are also at higher risk for accidents, suicide, and murder than are type B subjects.

Characteristics of type A behavior include a sense of urgency; competitiveness; easily aroused hostility and aggressivity, often manifested in obvious facial tension or muscular set; a ticlike drawing back of the corners of the mouth; a hostile, jarring laugh; an explosive, staccato speech pattern; frequent use of obscenities; periodic "bulging" of the eyes to show white above and below the pupils. The syndrome is often identified through a questionnaire, which discloses such behavior as often trying to do two things at once; walking fast, eating fast, and leaving the table immediately after eating; taking pride in always being

on time, having difficulty sitting and doing nothing, and often being told by a spouse to slow down. He is a workaholic and a Don Juan of achievement. When speaking, he typically blinks or moves his eyes rapidly, jiggles a knee, taps his fingers, licks his lips, nods his head, and rapidly sucks in air. He hurries or interrupts the speech of others, sits on the edge of his chair as if poised to leap out of it, talks with his hands, pounds his fist for emphasis, and sighs deeply, especially when discussing an annoying or frustrating event. He moves rapidly and often trips over things, is annoyed if kept waiting, distrusts others' motives; even in games with children he plays to win and is ravenous for success and accomplishment. See *exploitative character; choleric type; hypercompensatory type.*

Most studies suggest that type A behavior is only a secondary risk factor in cardiac disease, less important than the major risk factors such as smoking, high blood pressure, high blood cholesterol, and diabetes.

**Type I error** The rejection of the *null hypothesis* (q.v.) when it is true; the experimenter falsely concludes that a relationship exists when, in fact, there is none.

**Type I schizophrenia** See *Crow Type I schizophrenia.*

**Type II error** Beta error; acceptance of the *null hypothesis* (q.v.) when it is false; the experimenter fails to find a significant difference when a difference in fact exists.

**type token ratio** An index of the balance between repetition and variety of words, used as a quantitative measurement of certain aspects of verbal communication during psychiatric sessions. Repetition gives a low index; variety of words gives a high index.

**typhlomegaly** An unusually large size of the caecum. In Pende's system of constitutional types, this condition is frequently characteristic of the *ptotic habitus.*

**typholexia, congenital** A term used by Variot and Lecomte (1906) to refer to a type of *reading disability* (q.v.).

**typical** Pertaining to, or serving as, a type.

**typology** Study of types.

**tyramine sensitivity factor** *TSF* (q.v.).

**tyrosine kinase receptors** *Trk.* Neurotrophic factors—nerve growth factor (NGF), neurotrophin 3 (NT3), NT4/5, and brain-derived neurotrophic factor (BDNF)—act through a family of receptor proteins, the Trk receptors. TrkA is primarily the receptor for NGF, TkrB for BDNF and NT4/5, and TrkC for NT3.

# U

**UAI** Unprotected anal intercourse; in public health surveys of HIV-positive populations, MSM (q.v.) are typically asked to provide data on their use of insertive or receptive unprotected anal intercourse. In one study of YMSM (Y = young, between the ages of 17 and 28 years), nonhomeless YMSM reported remarkably high rates of lifetime exposure to a variety of drugs. Roughly 18% reported drug use in their last sexual encounter. Over 11% reported insertive UAI in their last sexual encounter, and nearly a third (31%) of these events involved the use of drugs.

The homeless YMSM were predominantly Hispanic (50%) and Black (24%); 11% had been treated for an STD in the past year, and 3% disclosed having HIV infection. This group reported extraordinarily high rates of lifetime use of a variety of drugs, and a high proportion (13%) reported injection drug use (IDU) during their lifetime. Over a third (35%) reported that drugs were involved in their last sexual encounter; 8% reported insertive UAI in their last sexual encounter, and nearly half (45%) of these included the use of drugs. Six percent reported receptive UAI in their last sexual encounter; 40% of these included use of drugs (Clatts, M.C, et al. *Journal of Urban Health 82 (Suppl 1)*, 2005).

**UBE₃A** A ubiquitin ligase. Its gene, *UBE3A*, located on 15q11–13, causes Angelman syndrome (q.v.); duplications, triplications, and loss of gene function have been associated with autistic features in patients with 15q11–13 anomalies.

**ubiquinone** CoQ. See OXPHOS.

**ubiquitin** A highly conserved 76-amino acid protein that is a normal component of the microtubule network. Its major function is to tag proteins for degradation by a proteolytic complex known as the proteasome, a large multisubunit complex that degrades the polyubiquitinated protein to small peptides. See *acetylation; apoptosis; histones; UPS.*

Ubiquitin is found in the neurofibrillary tangles of *Alzheimer disease*, although the major component of the latter is *tau* (qq.v.). In addition to its role in protein degradation,

ubiquitin seems to participate in the internalization of membrane proteins and in the control of gene transcription. It also plays a role in long-term synaptic plasticity; similarly, given that ubiquitin can alter the amount and function of neurotransmitter receptors and ion channels, it is likely that ubiquitin also regulates short-term synaptic plasticity and neuronal excitability.

**ubiquitination** Addition of a ubiquitin (q.v.) tag to proteins, which targets them for degradation. See *tau.*

**ubiquitin-proteasome pathway** A major cellular pathway for protein catabolism that is important for the 'housekeeping' and turnover of many regulatory proteins. Degradation by the proteasome occurs by conjugation of multiple ubiquitin moieties to a substrate and degradation of the tagged protein by the 26S proteasome complex. Molecular chaperones cooperate with the pathway to mediate the degradation of misfolded proteins.

**ubiquitin-proteasome system** UPS (q.v.)

**Ucs** Abbreviation for unconscious.

**UDDA** Uniform Determination of Death Act, advocated for use in defining death by the President's Commission for the Study of Ethical Problems in Medicine and Biomedical and Behavioral Research (1981): "An individual who has sustained either (1) irreversible cessation of circulatory and respiratory functions, or (2) irreversible cessation of all functions of the entire brain, including the brainstem, is dead. A determination of death must be made in accordance with accepted medical standards."

**ulcer, peptic** A disorder of the digestive tract consisting of circumscribed erosion of any of those areas exposed to acid-pepsin gastric juice, most commonly the lesser curvature of the stomach and the duodenal bulb. The most frequent cause of peptic ulcer is infection with Helicobacter pylori, which can be treated successfully with antibiotics. Other causes are alcohol consumption, smoking, and reactions to potentially corrosive drugs (such as NSAIDs). Greasy foods, milk products, and a diet low in fiber are all associated with stomach acidity.

Stress is no longer blamed as a cause of ulcers, but it can inhibit good digestion and aggravate an ulcer. In his description of peptic ulcer as a psychosomatic illness, Alexander stressed conflict between repressed passive-receptive, oral-dependency needs and conscious desires for independence; oral needs are frustrated and the patient regresses to a desire to be fed. Gastric activity responds appropriately and the mucosa secretes as if preparing for actual feeding.

**ulnar reflex**   Flexion reflex of the wrist; a deep reflex. When the styloid process of the ulna is tapped, the wrist flexes (pronation and adduction of the hand). This reflex depends on the median nerve for its afferents and efferents; its center is C6–8.

**ulterior transactions**   See transactional analysis.

**ultimatum game**   Two players, deemed proposer and responder, are to split a sum of money. The proposer makes an offer, which the responder can accept or reject. If the offer is accepted, the money is split as proposed; if it is rejected, neither player receives any money. In industrialized countries, offers are typically around 50%. Low offers (e.g.,, the proposer takes 80%, but the responder gets 20%) are rejected about 50% of the time, regardless of the amount of money involved. Why should responders actively turn down a monetary reward? They interpret the low offer as unfairness, which induces a conflict between cognitive ("accept") and emotional ("reject") motives. Unfairness activated insula, DLPFC, and anterior cingulate gyrus more than fair offers did; the degree of activation was greater with unfair offers from a human partner than with unfair offers from a computer partner. The insula was particularly sensitive to the degree of unfairness of an offer (Sanfey, A.G, et al. Science 300: 1755–1758, 2003).

See *neuroeconomics; prisoner's dilemma; social reasoning; theory of mind; trolley dilemma.*

**ultradian rhythms**   Oscillations of physiology and behavior that have a periodicity of less than 24 hours, such as the approximately 90-minute REM-NREM cycle of adult sleep. See circadian rhythms.

**ultrarapid opioid detoxification**   Induced with an opioid antagonist while the patient is under anesthesia or heavy sedation. Evidence indicates that the procedure is neither effective nor safe.

**ultrasonic irradiation**   Used, in the prefrontal areas of the brain, as an alternative to lobotomy; it is said to cause less variable and less severe cerebral damage than the surgical procedure, to entail minimal risk, and to give comparable results. Irradiation is applied through bilateral trephine openings, using a frequency of 1000 kcps and an average intensity of 7 watts/cm2 for 4 to 14 minutes.

**ululation**   The inarticulate crying of hysterical or psychotic persons.

**Ulysses contract**   Psychiatric will; voluntary involuntary treatment; a form of health care proxy for persons who have had psychotic episodes in the past and wish to give consent in advance for appropriate treatment should a similar crisis or decompensation recur. Such a prior consent agreement provides a contingency plan for protection of a patient from torment by psychotic symptoms and from the consequences of irrational behavior and impaired judgment. See advance directive.

The name relates to one of the trials to which Ulysses was subjected, as described in Homer's *Odyssey*. He must pass by the Sirens, who bewitch all men with their songs and lure them to destruction. Circe cautions Ulysses to have others on the ship bind him to the masthead to protect him from such a fate, and should he respond to the Sirens' songs and ask to be released from his bonds, they should instead bind him still more securely.

**umami**   See *gustation.*

**Umwelt**   Whatever is subjectively meaningful in the subject's environment; the environmentally significant as contrasted with hereditary factors.

**uncanny emotions**   See not-me.

**uncertainty**   In information theory, incongruity (q.v.). See choice.

**uncinate fit**   A subjective disturbance (hallucination) of smell and taste, characteristic of deep, mesial lesions involving the tip of the temporal lobe, at times accompanied by champing movements of the jaw; due to lesion of uncinate gyrus. See absent state; temporal lobe.

**unconditioned response**   See conditioning.

**unconscious (Ucs)**   Used as a noun or an adjective. In psychiatry it is used with two different meanings:

1. The absence of participation of the conscious ego or the so-called perceptive self. When the conscious part of the mind is not functioning, the subject is said to

be unconscious. Unconsciousness is usually associated with absence of orientation and perception, particularly in its extreme expression.

2. A division of the psyche, *the unconscious* or *unconsciousness*. In general it may be stated that all psychic material not in the immediate field of awareness is in the unconscious. When it is near enough to the former to be more or less easily accessible to it, it is said to be in the foreconscious or preconscious. See *collective unconscious; ego; id.*

**unconscious, impersonal**   See *collective unconscious.*

**unconscious processes**   The various methods of handling the environment and the instinctual needs on a level outside that of conscious awareness: *repression, regression, reaction-formation, isolation, undoing, introjection, reversal, sublimation,* and the development of *character structure* (qq.v.).

**unconsciousness**   See *unconscious.*

**unconventional medicine**   Alternative medical therapies; *holistic medicine* (q.v.).

**unconventional virus**   See *virus infections.*

**uncul herniation**   Downward shifting of the medial temporal lobe due to pressure from a lesion in the overlying cerebral cortex. Compression may similarly produce central herniation, when more medial diencephalic structures are involved.

**uncus**   See *temporal lobe.*

**underachievement**   See *academic underachievement disorder.*

**underachiever**   A person who fails to produce or perform at the level for which he is qualified and capable; specifically, a student whose academic performance is below his known potential.

**underclass**   A permanent, irreversibly impoverished social stratum in which maladaptive treatment of children engenders psychological unpreparedness for self-improvement. Families in this stratum often appear clinically as multiproblem welfare families. Although there are exceptions, the general tendency of underclass families to reproduce hopelessness, alienation, and antisocial behavior in each subsequent generation has been noted by many observers.

**undercutting, cortical**   See *prefrontal lobotomy.*

**underload, informational**   See *sensory deprivation.*

**undinism**   *Urolagnia; urophilia* (qq.v.).

**undirected thinking**   See *intellect.*

**undoing**   One of the unconscious defense mechanisms, consisting of a positive action that, actually or magically, is the opposite of something against which the ego must defend itself. Expiatory acts, countercompulsions, and some forms of compulsive ceremonials and counting compulsions are among the more frequent expressions of undoing, which is characteristic of *obsessive-compulsive disorder* (q.v.).

**unemotional thought**   See *adaptational psychodynamics.*

**unfocused delirium**   See *délire chronique.*

**unforthcomingness**   Impairment of motivation, and particularly that type of poor or disorganized motivation that has been observed in some children born of a stressful or complicated pregnancy. Some workers believe that minimal brain damage associated with stressful pregnancy may express itself behaviorally as unforthcomingness, and that the child so affected may be predisposed to delinquent breakdown.

**unio mystica**   See *peak experience.*

**unipolar depression**   *Major depressive disorder* (MDD) without manic episodes; in Kraepelinian terminology, the recurrent depressive form of manic depressive illness; also known as unipolar illness to contrast it with bipolar illness (which refers to affective disorder characterized by episodes of both mania and depression). See *manic-depressive psychosis.*

K. Leonhard challenged Kraepelin's unitary concept, and in 1957 he suggested that bipolar and unipolar forms of affective illness are different disorders. Various studies in both Europe and the United States appeared to confirm Leonhard's view. Yet response patterns to the new psychopharmacologic agents whose development began around 1952–1954 supported Kraepelin's divisions. They separated the so-called functional psychoses into (1) schizophrenia, paranoia, and other disorders of thinking, which respond to neuroleptics, and (2) the disorders of affect, which respond either to lithium, in the case of manic states, or to tricyclics and other antidepressant agents in the case of depressions.

It now appears that bipolar illness is a more severe and earlier-onset form. This is a return to the view of Kraepelin, who placed both illnesses in the same family of disorders. In a 2002 survey of 9090 U.S. household residents aged 18 years and older, lifetime prevalence of MDD was found to be 16.2%. MDD was only rarely primary; most cases had comorbid disorders such as anxiety disorder (in 59%), substance use disorder (24%), and impulse control disorder (30%). Prevalence was meaningfully elevated among women, homemakers, the never married, the previously married, and those with less than 12 years of education. (Kessler, R.C. et al. *Journal of the American Association 289*: 3095–3105, 2003).

Major depression itself is subdivided into primary and secondary. *Primary depression* is a depression that has not been preceded by and is not associated with any other psychiatric disorder. *Secondary depression* refers to a depression that is preceded by or associated with another psychiatric disorder, such as alcoholism, hysteria, sociopathy, substance abuse, and anxiety neurosis. Some writers extend the term to include depressions that are secondary to a chronic, debilitating medical illness such as chronic pain syndrome. See *comorbidity*.

Akiskal and others further subdivide primary unipolar depression into *Unipolar I*—a pure depressive form with unipolar but no bipolar family history and with a relatively low frequency of episodes, and *Unipolar II*—depressions with a high frequency of episodes and with bipolar family history. Unipolar II, in other words, is considered a phenotypic expression of bipolar genotype.

**unipolar double-bind**   See *double bind*.

**unit, least publishable**   *LPU* (q.v.).

**unit character**   A single-gene trait transmitted independently of other unit characters, such as pigmentation vs. albinism.

**unitization**   Administrative organization of a large hospital into several units, each with its own chief, staff, and carefully delineated responsibilities. The several autonomous units form a confederation that is supervised by the hospital director or superintendent. Hospitals may be unitized on the basis of function (e.g., adolescent units, geriatric units, alcoholism units), or on the basis of geography, with each unit serving a specified region of the larger area from which the hospital draws its patients.

**unitypic**   See *ambitypic*.

**unlust**   A German psychoanalytic term synonymous with the English terms *ego pain*, *unpleasure*, or *anxiety*.

Unpleasure, or unlust, refers to the sensation of mild discomfort or frustration tension that is felt in consciousness (by the ego) when instinctual trends, seeking gratification, are totally or partly opposed or blocked by the ego. This feeling of discomfort stands in marked contrast to the expected feeling of pleasurable relief from tension that usually follows full gratification of the instinct. The feeling of pain, unpleasure, frustration, tension, or discomfort is frequently mixed with, or associated with, anxiety.

**unmet need**   An existing condition that is not being treated, even though it is known to be amenable to one or more interventions. In the case of mental disorders, unmet need may be the result of underprovision of mental health services, obstacles (financial, social stigma, geography, etc.) to access to services, or lack of knowledge of the existence of appropriate services. The way services are structured (e.g., the appointment system, the length or number of visits or consultations allowed, the referral system, whether "patients" are assigned to specific therapists or are placed randomly into treatment units) determines how (and if) needs can be expressed or modulated.

**unnatural**   Contrary to nature, abnormal, atypical, unusual; most often applied to sexual behavior that the user of the term judges to be repugnant, dangerous, or otherwise unacceptable.

**unpleasure**   See *unlust*.

**unreality feelings**   See *depersonalization*.

**unsystematized delusion**   Disorganized delusion that is fragmented, inconsistent, and manifestly illogical and unfounded.

**unveiling**   Fritz Wittels's term for the uncovering or revelation of psychic components.

**Unverricht-Lundberg disease**   *Baltic myoclonus*; a childhood-onset form of myoclonus epilepsy with dementia and ataxia. See *myoclonus epilepsy*.

**unvoluntary behavior**   See *intentional unvoluntary behavior*.

**upper class**   See *class, social*.

**upregulation**   Receptor supersensitivity, characteristic of postsynaptic receptors when the endogenous ligand (their normal innervation) is removed. Degeneration of the nigrostriatal pathway in Parkinson disease, for example, results in upregulation of dopamine receptors. It is because of that supersensitivity that levodopa is effective in alleviating symptoms of the disorder. If treatment continues for a long time, however, the result is a *downregulation* (q.v.) of the originally upregulated receptors and a refractoriness to levodopa, sometimes referred to as the on-off phenomenon. In some cases, temporary cessation of levodopa permits sensitivity to build up again so that treatment can be reinstituted with beneficial results. See sensitization.

**uprooted psychology** The changed mentality exhibited by one who has been uprooted by force of circumstance, i.e., has had to leave his native place with its physical, social, and cultural background that had surrounded him all his life.

When removed from their customary environment and dislocated from their protective moral background, uprooted people deviate markedly from their inculcated reverence for original values and show symptoms parallel to those found in migrating hordes: recklessness, unregulated and indiscriminate sexuality, and a marked lowered responsibility toward human life and property (Baynes, H. G. *Mythology of the Soul*, 1940). See *migration psychosis; network; survivor syndrome.*

**UPS** *Ubiquitin-proteasome system*; it has been suggested that failure of the UPS underlies the development of both familial and sporadic *Parkinson disease* (q.v.). Through a series of enzyme-mediated reactions that identify and then link abnormal proteins with ubiquitin molecules, the UPS marks abnormal proteins for degradation by proteasomes. The proteasome is a large, multimeric, barrellike complex that acts by proteolysis to degrade proteins. UPS is essential for nonlysosomal degradation and clearance of short-lived, mislocated, misfolded, mutant, or damaged proteins; it can be viewed as a protection against cytotoxic effects of abnormal proteins. See α-synuclein; centrosomes.

**UPSA** UCSD (University of California, San Diego) Performance-based Skills Assessment, designed to overcome the reliability difficulties inherent in self-reporting, as in patients with dementia or late-onset schizophrenia.

**UR** *Utilization review*; see *review.*

**Ur defenses** Masserman's term for what he considered the three fundamental psychological maneuvers of man—the delusion of invulnerability and immortality, the delusion of the omnipotent servant (in the form of some abstract being or gnostic principle or system), and the conviction of man's kindness to man.

**uranism** Obs. (From Uranus, most ancient of Greek gods and the first ruler of the universe)

A term used by Karl Heinrich Ulrichs in 1862 for homosexuality; the female homosexual he called *urninde*, the male *urning*.

The corresponding term for heterosexuality is *dionism* (from Dione, mother of Venus Pandemos).

**uranomania** Obs. The delusion that one is of divine or celestial origin.

**uranophobia** Fear of heaven.

**Urbach-Wiethe disease** (Eric Urbach, U.S. dermatologist, 1893–1946) An autosomal recessive trait involving storage of protein and lipid and manifested clinically by (1) cutaneous and mucosal lesions—papillomatous deposits of protein-lipid complex in the eyelids, labial mucosa, and sublingual areas; (2) bilateral intracranial calcifications in the caudate nucleus, globus pallidus, and amygdala; (3) seizures (grand mal or psychomotor), rage attacks, and recent memory loss but otherwise intact intellect; (4) short stature; (5) alopecia; and (6) photosensitivity.

**urban crises** See *social policy planning.*

**urethra** The canal leading from the urinary bladder to the outside of the body, in the male by way of the penis. In psychoanalysis, the urethra is regarded as an erogenous zone, and psychoanalysts speak of urethral eroticism and sadism. See *urophilia.*

**urethral anxiety** Tension, anxiety, fear, and inhibition associated with urination.

**urethral character** A type of *character* (q.v.) that manifests itself as burning ambition, a need to boast of achievement, and general impatience; there is often a history of bedwetting beyond the usual age. The behavioral characteristics of this type depend on reaction formation in relation to the specific fear of urethral eroticism, which is shame.

**urine, dirty** Used in reference to substance abusers and drug addicts who are on a drug-free treatment program, when chemical analysis of their urine indicates that they have taken narcotics or other drugs.

The following drugs (and the length of time after ingestion they can be detected) are those most commonly tested for: alcohol (7 to 12 hours); amphetamines (48 hours); barbiturates (1 to 21 days, depending upon their length of action); benzodiazepines (3 days); cannabinols (3 to 28 days, depending on intensity of use); cocaine (6 to 8 hours, some metabolites as long as 4 days); codeine, heroin, morphine (36 to 72 hours); methadone

(3 days); methaqualone (7 days); phencyclidine (8 days); and propxyphene (6 to 48 hours).

**urninde**  Obs. Female homosexual. See *uranism*.

**urning**  Obs. Male homosexual. See *uranism*.

**urolagnia**  Pleasure connected with urine; *urophilia* (q.v.).

**urophilia**  *Urolagnia*; a *paraphilia* (q.v.) in which urine or the act of urination is an essential part of sexual phantasies or sexual behavior: drinking one's own or another's urine, urinating on another, being urinated on by another (popularly termed a "golden shower"). Sometimes the term is extended to include all forms of urethral eroticism, such as masturbatory techniques involving the insertion of foreign bodies into the urethra (e.g., swizzle sticks, snakes).

**urorrhea**  *Enuresis* (q.v.).

**user**  A slang expression to describe a morphine or heroin addict who takes small doses daily for years to keep himself comfortable.

**utilitarian principle**  In policy and ethical decisions, a choice that is determined by whatever promises the greatest advantage to the common good. See *weighted harm principle*.

**utilitarianism**  A moral philosophical theory according to which the best decisions are those that lead to the higher overall degree of happiness or well-being for the greatest number of people.

**utilitarianism, act**  Use of the principle of utility to decide whether a specific act is right. This is in contrast to *rule utilitarianism*, in which general rules of conduct are established as morally right in accordance with the principle of utility. A specific act can be considered right only if it conforms with the established rule, and its rightness or wrongness is not determined on an individual basis.

**utilitarianism, hedonistic**  A type of *utilitarianism* (q.v.) in which value is defined in terms of happiness or pleasure. See utilitarianism, pluralistic.

**utilitarianism, negative**  The ethical theory that the morally correct choice is made by comparing evils prevented with evils caused and deciding in favor of the lesser evil. Such a theory, which is often used to justify *paternalism* (q.v.), fails to take into account the consequences of universally allowing the violation of a moral rule, if that happens to seem to be the lesser evil in a particular situation. See ethics, situation.

**utilitarianism, pluralistic**  A type of *utilitarianism* (q.v.) in which many kinds of intrinsic value are recognized: happiness, friendship, beauty, courage, health, etc. See *utilitarianism, hedonistic*.

**utilization**  See *review*.

**utilization behavior**  A form of *magnetic apraxia* or bilateral grasping response described in lesions of the frontal lobe, and particularly in those involving its orbital surface and perhaps the head of the caudate nucleus. When confronted with the tactile, visuotactile, or visual presentation of an object, the subject feels compelled to grasp or use it. (Lhermitte, F. *Brain 106*, 1983).

**utilization technique**  Milton Erickson's term for a method of handling resistance in hypnotic subjects and patients in brief psychotherapy: "Erickson first asks the subject to do what he is already doing to resist him, and so do it under his own direction. Then he begins to shift the patient's behavior into more co-operative activity until the patient is fully following his directions" (Haley, J. *Archives of General Psychology 4*, 1961).

**utilizer**  User; most commonly, a user of insurance benefits. See *adverse selection*.

**uvula**  See *cerebellum*.

**uxoricide**  Killing of a wife by her husband.

# V

vaccinophobia    A morbid fear or dread of being vaccinated.

**VaD**    *Vascular dementia; vascular cognitive impairment* (*VCI*); the second most frequent cause of dementia following Alzheimer disease (AD). Compared with AD, in VaD episodic memory is relatively preserved, but verbal fluency and frontal executive functioning are more impaired. Subtypes of VaD have been described, but no one system of nomenclature has achieved universal acceptance. The subtypes include the following:

1. Post stroke dementia, following *cerebrovascular accident* (q.v.)
2. Subcortical ischemic vascular disease and dementia (*SIVD*), which includes the following:
   a. Lacunar state —*multi-infarct dementia, cerebral arteriosclerosis* (qq.v.)
   b. *Binswanger disease—subcortical arteriosclerotic encephalopathy* (q.v.)
   c. Mendelian variants of sporadic forms of small vessel disease, such as *CADASIL* and *CAA* (qq.v.)

vagina dentata    A vagina with teeth; a phantasy, more often unconscious than conscious, in which the female genitalia are equated with a castrating, devouring mouth. See *breast complex.*

vaginismus    A *sexual dysfunction* (q.v.) consisting of painful spasm of the vagina. It generally takes place at some time during coitus or it may have its onset during the stage of preparation for the sexual act. Etiology is often psychic.

Typical cases develop spasms that make insertion of the penis impossible, and such spasms are responsible for the rare cases of penis captivus. Vaginismus usually represents inhibition of sexual excitement along with positive action to ensure maintenance of inhibition; in addition, it may be a conversion symptom expressing a wish to break off the penis and keep it.

vagotonia    Excessive excitability of the vagus nerve.

vagus nerve    The tenth cranial nerve. The vagus nerve is motor to the muscles of the soft palate and pharynx, sends parasympathetic fibers to the thoracic and abdominal viscera, and is sensory to the pharynx, larynx, trachea, esophagus, and the thoracic and abdominal viscera. Symptoms of vagus nerve lesions include aphonia, dysphagia, paralysis of the soft palate with loss of the gag reflex, cough, bradycardia (with irritative lesions), or tachycardia (with vagus palsies).

vagus nerve stimulation    *VNS*; an adjunctive therapy for patients with refractory partial epilepsy. It may be effective in patients with severe, chronic, treatment-resistant depression. The pacemaker device is implanted in the chest and stimulates the left vagus nerve. Typically, stimulation is on for 30 seconds and then off for 5 minutes. Transient hoarseness is the most common adverse effect. Other possible effects include infection, voice alteration, throat or neck pain, cough, and dyspnea.

valence    See *life space.*

valence-asymmetry model    The hypothesis that prefrontal cortex promotes long-term adaptive goals in the face of strong competition from behavioral alternatives that are linked to immediate emotional consequences. It posits that left-sided PFC regions are involved in positive (approach-related appetitive) goals, right-sided in negative (behavioral inhibition and withdrawal) goals. Anterior cingulate cortex integrates visceral, attentional, and emotional information; when conflict is detected between the functional state of the organism and incoming information that may have affective or motivational consequences, ACC projects information about the conflict to PFC, which adjudicates among response options.

valid consent    See *informed consent.*

validation    A deliberate and active strategy using interventions designed to recognize the legitimacy of patients' experience; it emphasizes nonevaluative acceptance, and acknowledgement of patients' reality and of the authenticity of their experience.

validation, consensual    See *parataxic distortion.*

**validity** The degree to which a test measures what it is supposed to measure; a valid intelligence test, for example, is truly a measure of general intelligence and not a test of rote memory. The degree of validity of a test depends upon the magnitude of the errors present in the measures obtained from it. Some indication of the validity of a given test is gained from a study of the correlations between scores on the given test and scores from other tests designed to measure the same factor.

Several levels of validity may be distinguished: (1) *face validity* requires that those generally recognized as experts within the field under consideration agree that the test does in fact measure a trait or condition that does in fact exist; (2) *criterion validity* is the extent to which the test agrees with another test of established validity; (3) *descriptive validity* requires that the characteristics or variables being measured (or the particular way in which they are combined) are unique to the condition that they are supposed to define; (4) *predictive validity* requires that the development, course and complications, or response to intervention of the condition do in fact occur as would be expected; that is, the variables being measured define a state or condition whose future course is predictable; (5) *construct validity* is the extent to which evidence supports the hypothesis or hypotheses about the etiology, pathology, and development of the disorder that the measured variables are assumed to define. Construct validity ordinarily requires increasingly rigorous definition over time as feedback from the testing of earlier assumptions is incorporated into a more refined theory.

Validity is to be differentiated from *reliability* (q.v.), which refers to the dependability of a measure.

**valproic acid** An *antiepileptic* drug (q.v.) that inhibits the enzymes that metabolize the inhibitory transmitter GABA; it has also been used in the treatment of bipolar mood disorders and violence.

**value** That which is esteemed, prized, or deemed worthwhile and desirable by a person or a culture. Values are experientially determined; unlike needs, they are not innate. See *superego*.

Value is the organism's ability to sense whether or not events in its environment are salient or desirable. Value constraints increase the likelihood that adaptive or rewarding output will be repeated. See *choice*; *emotion*; *neuroeconomics*.

**vampirism** Belief in bloodsucking ghosts (vampires); performing the actions of a vampire. While in neither sense is the term often used in clinical psychiatry, when it does appear in the literature it is generally in the second sense, as the act of drawing blood from an object with accompanying sexual pleasure. The blood may be drawn by cutting, biting, or similar means, and sometimes the drinking of the drawn blood is an important part of the action. Some writers regard the "love-bite," i.e., the biting of the sexual partner during sexual activity, as a form of vampirism. Psychodynamically, vampirism is usually interpreted as expressing conflicts in any or all of the following areas: oral sadism and incorporation, fear of castration, aggressive hostile wishes (including murder), and oedipal strivings for the mother.

**vampirism, parasitic** H. G. Baynes used the term in a special sense, namely, that in a psychoneurotic patient compulsive mechanisms are present that are constantly driving the person. These drives have a demonic appetite—the more they have, the more they demand. They know no reasonable bounds. Baynes believed that the neurotic symptoms, such as phobias, obsessions, and aggressions, are similar to a devouring monster that overpowers and possesses the patient in the manner of a bloodthirsty vampire (*Mythology of the Soul*, 1940).

**vandalism, sexual** An inordinate impulse to destroy the sexual zones represented in pictures, statuary, etc.

**variable-interval (VI) schedule** See *reinforcement schedule*.

**variable-ratio (VR) schedule** See *reinforcement schedule*.

**variation** 1. In genetics, differences or changes at the level of the organism's genotype. In a species originating through sexual reproduction, absolute homogeneity among its individual members cannot be expected; the offspring will never be exactly like the parents. Genotypic variations may arise through *combination*, random *mutation*, or *modification* by any one of various environmental factors such as temperature or radiation (qq.v.). Such variations may give rise to phenotypic differences.

2. In statistics, the differences between the items in a frequency distribution with respect to the amount of a given character (e.g., height) that each item possesses. Any frequency distribution may differ in a similar way from another frequency distribution describing the same character, and such differences are also called variations.

**vascular cognitive impairment** Proposed to replace VaD (vascular dementia). The main pathology consists of lacunar infarcts and leukoaraiosis, diffuse lesions in the periventricular and semiovale white matter.

**vascular dementia** *VaD* (q.v.).

**vascular headache** *Migraine* (q.v.).

**vasectomy** The *sterilizing* operation on men of cutting and tying off the seminal ducts (vasa deferentia). Usually no unfavorable effect on the secondary sexual characters follows vasectomy, in contrast with the *castrating* operation of removing the testicles. See *sterilization*.

**vasoactive intestinal peptide (VIP)** A neuropeptide that is critical in maintaining normal brain function through its ability to act as or cause the secretion of growth factors essential for neuronal integrity.

**vasomotor syncope** Vasodepressor syncope; sudden loss of consciousness (fainting) caused by a vasovagal attack. Sympathetic autonomic activity is inhibited, and parasympathetic vagal nerve activity is augmented, resulting in decreased cardiac output, decreased vascular peripheral resistance, vasodilation, and bradycardia.

**vasopressin, arginine (AVP)** A peptide synthesized in nuclei of the medial hypothalamus. It is stored in the posterior pituitary and released into the circulation to regulate water reabsorption by the distal renal tubule; hence, it is also called antidiuretic hormone. It is also transported to the third ventricle and into the cerebrospinal fluid, through which it exerts its neuromodulator effects on biogenic amine activity and on the release of other peptide modulators, including the endorphins. Evidence suggests that AVP may augment memory functions in both cognitively normal and cognitively impaired subjects. See *hypothalamic-pituitary-adrenal (HPA) axis; peptide, brain*.

Dysregulation of the hypothalamic-pituitary-adrenal (HPA) axis is found in almost 50% of patients with depression. AVP modulates the HPA axis under stress through a G protein–coupled receptor, AVPR1b, and antagonists of AVPR1b exhibit antidepressant qualities.

**vasoregulatory asthenia** See *neurocirculatory asthenia*.

**vasotocin, arginine (AVT)** A peptide of the neurohypophysial unit and perhaps the prototypic neurohypophysial hormone. In function, it is more closely linked to adenohypophysis-regulating activities than to antidiuresis.

**vasovagal attack of Gowers** Gowers described a syndrome characterized by nausea and belching, precordial discomfort, respiratory difficulty, anxiety of impending death, and mild mental upset. The attack may last from a few minutes to an hour. See *vasomotor syncope*.

**vasovagal episode** Shock, consisting of apathy, weakness, pallid skin, sunken facies, expression of anxiety and dread, moist and cold skin, rapid but weak pulse, shallow and labored breathing, and lowering of the blood pressure—sometimes fatally.

**VBM** Voxel-based morphometry, a computational technique that identifies subtle regional differences in gray or white matter between groups of scans. The images are compared on a voxel-by-voxel basis. The analysis covers the whole brain; specific regions of interest can then be subjected to further analysis by other methods (e.g., volumetric analysis).

**VBR** Ventricle to brain ratio, often reported increased as assessed by CT scan in some schizoophrenic subjects (as well as in subjects with Alzheimer disease). Increased VBR is associated with abnormal performance on a number of neuropsychological tasks. See *ventricular enlargement*.

**VCI** Vascular cognitive impairment; characteristically, memory is relatively preserved and the most prominent impairments are in attention, psychomotor speed, and executive functioning. Apathy, depression, and psychosis also occur. Subtypes: post-stroke dementia, subcortical ischemic vascular disease and dementia, single and multi-infarct dementia, and hereditary vascular dementias (*CADASIL* and *CAA*, qq.v.).

**vCJD** Variant CJD. See *bovine spongiform encephalopathy; Creutzfeldt-Jakob disease*.

**VDRL** Venereal disease research laboratory; used generally to refer to a slide test for syphilis developed in that laboratory.

**VDT** *Visual distortion test* (q.v.).

**VE** Virtual environment. See *virtualization*.

**vector analysis**   Alexander's term for the process of determining the degree of participation of the organism's basic tendencies—reception, elimination, and retention—in the genesis and development of neurosis.

**vegative nervous system**   See *autonomic nervous system.*

**vegetative neurosis**   The expression of emotion, or unconscious emotional conflict, by disturbed functioning of the internal visceral organs and thus termed *functional ailment* or disturbance. The term is usually employed in contradistinction to conversion hysteria: whereas conversion hysteria takes place in the voluntary neuromuscular, or sensory perceptive system, the vegetative neurosis has its site in the internal visceral organs. Sometimes used synonymously with *acrodynia* (q.v.). See *psychosomatic.*

**vegetative retreat**   The tendency of some neurotic persons to meet an inimical or dangerous reality situation not by appropriate self-assertive behavior and actions, but by recourse to infantile or childish function of the visceral apparatus, which, to them, anachronistically stands for praise or succor from strong or omnipotent parents. It thus represents a return to the pseudopower of the "helpless" and dependent child and warrants the descriptive term regressive, because it is a resort to the old infantile ways of handling frustration and stress. See *hypoglycemia.*

**vegetative state**   Introduced by B. Jennett and F. Plum in 1972 (*Lancet 1*) to describe a specific syndrome of reflex activity with no meaningful response to the environment in a patient with a sleep-awake pattern. Some object to the term because of its association with "vegetable-like," but attempts to change it have been unsuccessful. A suggested alternative, *postcomatose unawareness state*, is only rarely used.

*Persistent vegetative state* refers to a vegetative state still present 1 month after the occurrence of brain damage; it does *not* indicate irreversibility. *Permanent vegetative state* denotes irreversibility, manifested as no recovery at 3 months following a nontraumatic brain injury, or no recovery at 12 months following traumatic brain injury. Unfortunately, the two different states are often abbreviated identically, as *PVS*.

In 1994, the U.S. Multi-Society Task Force published guidelines for determining Persistent Vegetative State in adults:

1. No evidence of awareness of self or environment and an inability to interact with others

2. No evidence of sustained, reproducible, purposeful, or voluntary behavioral responses to visual, auditory, tactile, or noxious stimuli

3. No evidence of language comprehension or expression

4. Intermittent wakefulness manifested by the presence of the sleep-wake cycle

5. Sufficiently preserved hypothalamic (e.g., regulation of body temperature and vascular tone) and brain-stem autonomic functions to permit susrvival with medical and nursing care

6. Bowel and bladder incontinence

7. Variably preserved cranial nerve and spinal reflexes

Patients in a vegetative state show a much richer array of motor activity than patients with *brain death* (q.v.). It is, however, nonpurposeful, inconsistent, and coordinated only when expressed as part of subcortical instinctively patterned reflexive response to external stimulation, moving trunk, limbs, head, or eyes in meaningless ways and showing startle myoclonus to loud noises. Such patients may occasionally smile or cry, utter grunts, and sometimes moan or scream. Patients in a vegetative state do not usually require ventilatory or cardiac support, but need only artificial hydration and nutrition. Stopping hydration and nutrition leads to death in 10–14 days. Some argue in favor of a lethal drug to quicken the dying process in a patient who has met the time criteria for permanent vegetative state, but such an action is possible only in a country or state in which euthanasia has been legalized *and* only if the patient has expressed such a wish previously in a living will. See *brain injury; coma vigil; mutism, akinetic.*

**vegetative symptoms**   Used particularly in referring to mood or affective disorders, the expression includes sleep and appetite disturbances, weight change, fatigue, and low energy that are a part of the clinical picture as the major depressive disorder develops.

**vehicle phobia**   A fear of trains, boats, airplanes, automobiles, or other forms of transportation. Often these represent a struggle against sexual excitation as perceived in the pleasurable sensations of equilibrium, or a fear that one will be unable to escape from a confined area, this latter representing a need for escape from one's feared excitement as soon as it has reached a certain intensity.

**velocardiofacial syndrome** Also known as *DiGeorge syndrome, Shprintzen syndrome,* and 22q11 deletion syndrome. It is the second most common human chromosomal anomaly (after trisomy 21) and occurs in approximately 1 out of every 4000 births. It is associated with a microdeletion in the *COMT gene*. Typical presenting symptoms are hypernasal speech, cleft palate, cardiac anomalies, and learning disabilities. Characteristic facial features include a long face, a large nose with a large tip and a high nasal root, small ears with overfolded helices, narrow and "squinting" eyes, and flat expression.

At least one COMT variant appears to be associated with aggression in schizophrenia, schizoaffective disorder, polysubstance abuse, and OCD. In other words, COMT may contribute to certain behavior traits in mental disorders, but it is not responsible for schizophrenia itself.

**vent men** See *street people*.

**ventral anterior nucleus** Part of the *lateral nuclear group* of the *thalamus* (qq.v.).

**ventral posterior nuclei** Part of the *lateral nuclear group* of the *thalamus* (qq.v.).

**ventral tegmental area** *VTA* (q.v.).

**ventral visual pathway** Visual information coming from the primary visual cortex is processed in two interconnected but partly dissociable visual pathways, a "ventral" pathway, which extends into the temporal lobe and is thought to be primarily involved in visual object recognition and a "dorsal" pathway, which extends into the parietal lobes and is thought to be more involved in extracting information about "where" an object is or "how" to execute visually guided actions towards it. See *visual stream*.

**ventricle** A cavity or chamber; the ventricular system of the brain develops from the cavity of the neural tube and is filled with the *cerebrospinal fluid* (CSF) that is elaborated by the choroid plexus within each ventricle. Within the forebrain are two *lateral ventricles* and, lying below them and in the midline between the two thalami, the *third ventricle*. The third ventricle communicates anteriorly with each lateral ventricle through the *interventricular foramen (foramen of Monro)*. It communicates posteriorly through the narrow *cerebral aqueduct (aqueduct of Silvius)*, in the midbrain, with the *fourth ventricle*. The roof of the fourth ventricle lies below the vermis and cerebellum; it contains three small openings through which CSF escapes from the ventricles into the subarachnoid space: the two *foramina of Luschka*, situated laterally, and the *foramen of Magendie*, in the midline.

**ventricle puncture** A surgical technique for gaining access to the intraventricular space of the lateral ventricles. The principal indications for ventricle puncture are (1) to relieve increased intracranial pressure before operation for intracranial tumor; (2) to inject air for ventriculography; (3) to inject therapeutic substances such as penicillin or streptomycin; (4) to obtain cerebrospinal fluid for diagnostic examination when lumbar or cisternal puncture cannot be performed.

**ventricle to brain ratio** *VBR* (q.v.).

**ventricular enlargement** Larger than normal cerebral ventricles; see *VBR*. A majority of studies have found that, as a group, schizophrenia patients have larger ventricles and lower limbic volumes than normal control subjects. Many studies also suggest that such patients are likely to show one or more of the following features: poor premorbid adjustment, unresponsiveness to neuroleptics, more negative and fewer positive symptoms, more neuropsychological test abnormalities, and poor outcome. The ventricular enlargement may be due to genetic factors, but it may also be the result of acquired conditions related to birth complications, viral infections, immune reactions, or toxins.

**ventriculogram** An X-ray of the skull following replacement of cerebrospinal fluid with air by means of ventricular puncture. This drains the ventricular system but not the subarachnoid spaces and cisterns; the procedure is used when an expanding intracranial lesion is suspected, because ventriculography is considered safer than encephalography in such cases.

**ventriculography** Radiography of the brain cavity. A means of determining the presence of structural changes in the intracranial contents, which are visualized by the X-ray, after the direct injection of air into the lateral ventricles.

**ventrolateral nucleus** Part of the *lateral nuclear group* of the *thalamus* (qq.v.).

**ventrolateral preoptic areas** See *sleep*.

**ventromedial PFC** Includes orbital PFC, although some authors treat the two separately. Ventromedial PFC has reciprocal connections with brain regions that are associated with emotional processing (amygdala), memory (hippocampus), and higher-order sensory processing (temporal visual association areas), as well as with dorsolateral PFC. The ventromedial PFC is well suited to support functions involving integration of information about emotions, memory, and environmental stimuli. Its neural networks encode event sequences representing social rules, self-control, attitudes, scripts, and knowledge. Impairment of social behavior is most evident after ventromedial PFC damage. See *amygdala*; *dorsolateral PFC*; *prefrontal cortex*; *theory of mind.*

**venue** Location; site. Although primarily a legal term referring to the place in which an alleged action occurred, or to the place from which a jury comes or the place where a trial is held, venue has become a vogue word among some researchers, who use it to refer to the targeted location from which a sample of subjects is drawn.

**VEP** Visual evoked potential, the brain wave response to visual stimulation such as exposure to different flash intensities. See *neurometrics.*

**Veraguth, fold of** (Otto Veraguth, German neurologist, 1870–1940) Contraction upward and backward of the inner third of the upper lid, thus changing the arch of the upper lid into an angle. Veraguth described this change as a characteristic sign of major depression.

**verapamil** A *calcium channel blocker*; it inhibits calcium ion influx through slow channels in myocardial cells and vascular smooth muscle cells. It seems also to inhibit calcium ion influx within brain neurons; it appears to have anticonvulsant properties and perhaps also antimanic effects. See *calcium channel.*

**verbal aphasia** *Broca aphasia* (q.v.).

**verbal dyspraxia** Impaired ability to perform the coordinated movements needed for speech.

**verbal fluency test** Within a limited amount of time (e.g., 30 seconds) the subject says as many words as possible that begin with a specified letter (or meet other specified qualifications). Verbal fluency is related to frontal lobe functioning.

**verbal masochism** The condition in which a person craves to hear insulting or humiliating words and derives sexual excitement by imagining himself abused or insulted verbally.

**verbal memory** See *parietal lobe.*

**verbal suggestion** See *ideoplasty.*

**verbalization** The state of being verbose or diffuse, commonly encountered in extreme degree in patients with the manic form of manic-depressive psychosis.

In a more general sense, verbalization is the expression in words of thoughts, wishes, phantasies, or other psychic material that had previously been on a nonverbal level because of suppression or repression. "Verbalize" is often used in a pseudoerudite way when "talk about" is meant.

**verbigeration** A stereotypy consisting of repetition of words, phrases, or sentences; also called *cataphasia, autoecholalia.* A patient with catatonic schizophrenia kept repeating "muscle, muscle, muscle," in reply to all forms of questioning. See *perseveration.*

**verbigeration, hallucinatory** A type of *thought-echoing* (q.v.) in which the patient hears, in endless repetition or with slight changes, the same meaningless sentences.

**verbochromia** A type of synesthesia in which certain words evoke a sensation of color. See *sensation, secondary.*

**verbomania** *Tachylogia* (q.v.).

**verbose** Overproductive in speech.

**vermis** See *cerebellum.*

**Verstehen** See *Erklaren.*

**vertical transmission** Transmission from parent to offspring by means of social learning or modeling, rather than through genes.

**vertiginous epilepsy** A rare type of *reflex epilepsy* (q.v.) precipitated by vestibular stimuli, characterized by recurrent attacks of vertigo (of the rotatory type); associated often with short lapses of consciousness.

**vertigo** Dizziness; a feeling that the subject or the world around him is spinning or revolving.

**vertigo, cervical** See *cervical migraine.*

**vesania** An old term, as well as an old concept, that meant insanity in general. It was used by Sauvages in his *Nosologia Methodica,* of 1763. The group termed *vesania* embraced psychiatric disorders not known to be associated with any organic disease or disorder.

**vesicles** 1. Subcellular organelles in the terminal region of the neuron in which chemical transmitters are stored. The vesicles are concentrated in specialized release sites (*active zones*).

When the action potential reaches this area, it stimulates the vesicles to fuse with the surface membrane of the neuron and thus release their contents into the synaptic cleft—a process called *exocytosis*. How much transmitter is released depends on how many action potentials reach the active zone per unit time. See *Golgi apparatus*. 2. Transport sacs that carry membrane and secretory proteins from their origin in the endoplasmic reticulum to various destinations within the cell. In the *constitutive pathway*, the vesicles shuttle newly formed proteins to the membrane and cycle existing constituents of the membrane back into the cell. In the *regulated pathway*, the vesicles carry secretory and synaptic proteins to various sites within the cell (such as the active zones as described above) where they are held in readiness for release when appropriately and adequately stimulated.

**vestibular hallucination**   False sensory perceptions that come from irritation of the vestibular apparatus. This form of hallucination is referred mainly to visual and tactile organs. Visual images (real or imaginary) are affected by vestibular function. Under vestibular irritation these images show changes such as occur when the subject is submitted to passive rotating movement. In such experimental circumstances, there are certain typical movements, or deviations of the optic image. In one experiment described by Bibring-Lehner, the subject, while turning, imagines a child; this image seems to turn in the same direction as the subject under experiment. Sometimes half the image disappears and often the colors become gray during the turning, but the most remarkable features are the multiplication of the image and its reduction in size. According to P. Schilder, this "shows that turning induces the same changes in optic images as in optic vision." In alcoholic hallucinations one may also observe vestibular phenomena.

Schilder describes the case of a patient who said: "Sometimes I saw three or four people on the street instead of one. I saw three faces in glaring white; faces of Negroes and whites. They moved forwards and backwards and when I saw them they started to chase me. I felt them behind me." In psychosis the vestibular influences are not related exclusively to the visual sphere, but one also encounters marked changes in the feelings that the patient has about his own body, particularly

sensations of the body's lightness or heaviness (*Mind Perception and Thought*, 1942).

**vestibular nerve**   See *auditory nerve*.

**vestibulocerebellum**   See *cerebellum*.

**VF**   See *vigil, fatiguing*.

**VI cortex**   See *visual cortex, primary*.

**vicarious introspection**   *Empathy* (q.v.).

**vice allemand**   Used by Hirschfeld synonymously with homosexuality. In the 18th century the French called homosexuality "the German vice"; at an earlier period Europeans referred to homosexuality as "the Oriental disease." It seems that every nation disowns responsibility for originating homosexuality and would like to shift it to others' shoulders.

**Victim**   See *transactional analysis*.

**victim**   The target or object of an assault, attack, accident, illness, rape, kidnapping, abuse, violence, or other crime. *Victimology* (q.v.) is the study of the victim(s) of such assaults.

In the adult victim, stress is often followed by phasic waves of numbing and denial alternating with intrusive repetitive thoughts about the traumatic event, which sometimes appear as sudden, unbidden flashbacks. School-aged children respond somewhat differently: they do not experience amnesia or deny reality, nor do they experience flashbacks. Instead, they develop pervasive fears and repetitive dreams and reenactments of the traumatic event. See *post-traumatic stress disorder*.

A persecution syndrome has been described in persons who have survived concentration camps or who experienced persecution during their flight from a hostile regime. Symptoms include generalized anxiety, hyperreactivity, chronic depression, various psychosomatic disorders, and, in many, development of an unconscious identity with their persecutors. Similar phenomena have been observed in hostages and captives of terrorists. *Stockholm syndrome* refers to the reaction of a woman held hostage in a Stockholm bank who became enamored of one of her captors and remained faithful to him during the prison term to which he was later sentenced. See *persecution syndrome; survivor syndrome*.

It has been observed that perhaps as many as a third of *homicide* victims are intoxicated with alcohol at the time they are attacked. One-third of abused teenagers (boys as well as girls) may be problem drinkers. Approximately 25% of homicide victims are under 16 years of age. Among adult victims, women outnumber men by 3 to 2. Nearly half of female victims are killed by their husbands, relatives, or intimate friends. Male victims, by contrast, are killed by strangers or chance associates in almost half the cases. Women are more likely than men to be the battered spouse, the sexually molested or abused child, and the abused grandparent.

The leading form of *domestic violence* is *wife beating*, sometimes defined as deliberate, severe, and repeated physical assault resulting in demonstrable injury. Within a family, wife battering is frequently accompanied by child abuse, both physical and sexual. Family violence covers a wide range of intrafamilial violence in addition to wife abuse and child abuse—child neglect, adolescent abuse, sibling abuse, homicide, incest, and parental and elder abuse. See *battered child syndrome; wife battering.*

In a child-abusing family, one child is usually abused more than the others. Certain children appear to be particularly vulnerable: the youngest child, any child less than 2 years of age; a premature child; a child with congenital deformities. Child abusers are most frequently parents, step-parents, or others in charge of the child. Abuse very often occurs during outbursts of uncontrolled anger in a parent who has unrealistic expectations of the abused child.

**victim recidivism**    See *recidivism.*

**victimology**    The study of the victim(s) of kidnaping, rape, assault, or other crime—how they came to be the object of the crime, what physical and mental injuries they were forced to endure, what kind of assistance they might require in returning to their usual pattern of daily living, what type of restitution or compensation they might merit, etc. Observations that some persons appeared to be "accident prone" or more likely than most to be the victims of assaults fostered a tendency to look upon victims as *agents provocateurs.* On another front, civil libertarians became so successful in protecting the rights of persons accused of crimes that it became exceedingly difficult for their victims to establish that any wrong had been done. Then came an emphasis on entitlement, and the idea that victims should somehow, by someone, be compensated for the pain and anguish to which they had been subjected. Finally, the spotlight has turned back on the perpetrator of the action.

In the case of rape, spousal abuse, and other forms of domestic violence, for instance, the social attitude is changing from one of blaming the victims of abuse to one of holding the abusers accountable.

The myth of provocation by an abused spouse has become increasingly suspect, and attention is now focused on the behavior of the abuser, and also on social norms that have sanctioned and encouraged such behavior under the guise of protecting privacy and preserving the sanctity of the home. See *traumatophilic diathesis.*

**vigil, fatiguing**    *FV;* a type of sleep deprivation in which the experimental subject is required to perform mental work while he remains awake.

**vigilambulism**    *Fugue* (q.v.). A condition of unconsciousness regarding one's surroundings, with automatism, resembling somnambulism, but occurring in the waking state.

**vigilance**    Sustained concentration and maintenance of alertness over time; *sentinel activity.* The continuous performance test (CPT) is probably the most common measure of vigilance. Vigilance includes both *sensitivity* (the ability to detect the likely presence of the object sought) and *responsivity* (the level of cautiousness, that is, the degree of certainty required by the subject to make the decision that the object detected is in fact the object sought). The higher the sensitivity, the lower the number of failures to identify the object (the higher the "hit rate"). The higher the responsivity level, however, the lower the *hit rate*, but also the lower the *"false alarm rate."* See *continuous performance test; hypervigilance.*

**vigilant**    See *anxiety typology.*

**villa system**    Boarding-out system. See *domicile.*

**villus biopsy**    See *chorion biopsy.*

**violence**    Physical aggression; behavior whose aim is to inflict harm or discomfort on another (the victim). The use of *victim* (q.v.) is typically extended to include not only the intentional target(s) of violence but also those who are innocent bystanders and involved only accidentally. Violent behavior includes physical assault (ranging from slapping to homicide), threats (direct verbal threats both face-to-face and via telephone, and written threats, such as letters or e-mail, any of which may be traumatic to the victim even though never carried out), and harassment (conversion of the environment into a hostile one by means of unwelcome words, including verbal abuse such as humiliating, discriminating, or denigrating statements, and also unwelcome actions or physical contacts). Violence refers to the behavior of the abuser and does not depend upon demonstrable physical injury to the victim, who may suffer psychological rather than physical injury.

Violence represents the extreme pole of the aggressive spectrum of behavior, characterized by an explosive, sudden quality and the use of force to injure or destroy an object, a person, or an organization. Aggression, in contrast, refers to the use of force (not necessarily physical) to overcome resistance by an object, person, or organization to the will of one of the participants in a struggle or conflict so that the outcome will conform to the intention of one of the adversaries. Anger, hate, and rage are frequent internal, emotional concomitants of aggression, but not universally so, since simple assertion is also aggression. How much aggression and violence are biologically inherent, and how much are a consequence of social learning, are moot questions. Ethology, for example, views man as a killer ape, while genetic anthropologists see him as a noble savage characterized by cooperation with other men. The absolute negative position says that violence is always bad, and with this view is correlated the negative therapeutic position that considers any excessive display of violence as sick. The absolute positive position states that violence is good, in that those who feel free to display it constitute an elite who are fit to lead and able to resist corruption; the correlated positive therapeutic position considers the display of violence under conditions of injustice to be therapeutic in itself. In recent times, there has tended to be a move away from either of the absolutes to a relative or conditional position, which considers violence acceptable under certain conditions, as in self-defense or the "just" war.

According to the U.S. National Institute for Occupational Safety and Health, the occupations with the highest rate of occupational homicides from 1980 to 1989 were taxicab drivers and chauffeurs, law enforcement officers, hotel clerks, gas station workers, security guards, stock handlers, store owners and managers, and bartenders. Homicide is the fifth leading cause of death for persons aged 10 to 60 years in the United States Persons

with substance use disorders are 12 to 16 times more likely than those without such disorders to engage in violent behavior. In therapeutic communities and other programs for drug users, reducing alcohol use is not typically a high priority. Yet 65% of domestic violence occurs under the influence of alcohol and another 11% under the influence of alcohol and drugs; only 5% occurs under the sole influence of illicit drugs. Not only is alcohol highly associated with violence (and other crime), it also complicates recovery from illicit drug use.

Studies have shown that the average child watches 8000 murders and 100,000 acts of other violence on TV by the end of elementary school. By the age of 12, the average American teenager has watched 200,000 acts of violence and 40,000 murders.

According to the ECA study, 3.7% of the population commit one or more acts of violence each year, and the lifetime prevalence of aggressive behavior may be about 24%. Various psychophysiologic and behavioral abnormalities may predispose to or modulate impulsive, aggressive, violent, or homicidal behavior:

1. Reduced central serotonergic functioning (indicated by low CSF 5-HIAA) may be correlated with an increased tendency toward impulsive (rather than premeditated) aggressive behavior. Part of the gene for tryptophan hydroxylase (the rate-limiting enzyme for serotonin synthesis) has been discovered to exist as at least two alleles, U or L. The presence of either the UL or LL genotype is associated with impulsive and suicidal behavior and low levels of CSF 5-HIAA in violent offenders.

2. Increased brain dopamine activity appears to predispose to impulsive, aggressive action. Beta-adrenergic receptor binding is increased in the prefrontal and temporal areas of the cortex in the brains of violent suicide victims. Noradrenergic receptor blockade and β-adrenergic blockers, such as propranolol and nadolol, have been effective in reducing aggressive behavior.

3. Testosterone levels are higher in violent offenders then in criminals who commit nonviolent crimes (burglary, theft, drug dealing). In violent alcoholic offenders, high free testosterone concentration in the CSF is associated with increased aggressiveness and sensation seeking.

4. Violent/homicidal behavior is significantly associated with mental illness, and especially substance or alcohol abuse and dependence and antisocial personality disorder. The risk for violent/homicidal behaviors in schizophrenia, mood disorders, and anxiety disorder is somewhat greater than that for the general population but not of the same magnitude as that for substance abuse or antisocial personality. See *violence and mental illness*.

Alcohol use is associated with violence and other crime, and it also hampers recovery from illicit substance abuse. A fifth of state prisoners convicted of violent crime have been found to have been under the influence of alcohol, and no other drug, at the time of the offense. The Bureau of Justice Statistics estimates that 65% of spousal violence occurs under the influence of alcohol, 11% under the influence of drugs and alcohol, and only 5% under the sole influence of illicit drugs (Farabee, D. et al. *Psychiatric Services 53*: 1375–1376, 2002).

5. Behavior and personality traits associated with violence are poor impulse control, problems with affect regulation, threats to the person's egotism and narcissism (inflated sense of self-worth and entitlement), and paranoid cognitive personality style. See *HCR-20*.

**violence, affective** See *stalking*.

**violence and mental illness** Violent/homicidal behavior is significantly associated with mental illness, even though overall the absolute risk for violence in mentally ill persons is small. The risk is increased in the presence of active psychotic symptoms or substance abuse disorder. The violent behavior of the mentally ill is often a "rational" response to irrational beliefs. Persecutory delusions are more likely to be acted on than are other types of delusions. Patients with persecutory delusions may resort to violence or even homicide in an effort to protect themselves.

Threat/control-override symptoms associated with increased aggression include feeling dominated by forces beyond the subject's control; believing that thoughts are being put into the subject's head; believing that there are people who wish the subject harm; and believing that the subject is being followed. Persons with such symptoms are twice as likely to engage in assaultive behavior as those with other psychotic symptoms. If combined with alcohol or drug use disorders, they are especially prone to violent behavior—8–10 times more likely than those with no disorder.

The likelihood of obeying command hallucinations is increased if the voice is familiar and if there is a hallucination-related delusion.

Alcohol-intoxicated persons are involved in the majority of violent crimes, including murders, assaults, sexual assaults, and family violence. PCP is the hallucinogen most associated with violence. Stimulants such as amphetamines and cocaine increase the risk of violence due to disinhibition, grandiosity, and a tendency toward paranoia.

**VIP** 1. Ventral intraparietal area; see *intraparietal sulcus*.

2. Vasoactive intestinal peptide.

3. Very important person. See *Main syndrome*.

**viraginity** The adoption by women of male characteristics. It is an expression of homosexuality.

**viral theory of schizophrenia** The hypothesis that schizophrenia is a result of viral infection is based largely on the seasonality of schizophrenic births. There is a moderate excess of births of future schizophrenic patients during late winter and early spring, just at the end of the season of most risk from the respiratory viruses, the paramyxoviruses and myxoviruses. Torrey (*Schizophrenia Bulletin 17*, 1991) has suggested that the responsible viruses might travel from the nasal mucosa along the maxillary nerve through the foramen rotundum to the trigeminal ganglion. That ganglion is adjacent to the medial temporal cortex and its components (hippocampus, parahippocampal gyrus, and amygdala), which have been reported to be primarily affected in schizophrenia.

One variant of the viral theory proposes that viral infection, instead of producing encephalitis, could result in small clusters of chronically infected brain cells that induce an autoimmune response as an intermediate step in the development of schizophrenia. Another theory is that the influenza orthomyxovirus, because it possesses the enzyme capsular neuraminidase, interferes with neuroblast migration into the hippocampus at a critical time in its development, the early and middle portions of the second trimester. It is possible that only a genetically vulnerable fetus is susceptible to such interference.

To date, no specific transmissible factors or antibodies have been shown convincingly to be associated with schizophrenia. Current theories of viral influence ascribe no more weight to this factor, at the most liberal extreme, than a 10% increase in frequency; most workers feel that it is no more than 1% or 2%.

**viral vectors**   Derived from common human viral pathogens, they are used to deliver genes to the nervous system. They have a broad tropism, i.e., they can infect many cell types in addition to those involved in their normal life cycle. Gene therapy is still an exploratory science in all of its applications, owing in part to unknown risk factors associated with virus vectors.

**virginal anxiety**   Anxiety provoked by the first sexual experience. See *anxiety neurosis*.

**virginity scruple**   *Rare*. Doubt on the part of the man regarding his wife's virginity; delusion of infidelity.

**viroids**   The smallest RNA viruses, whose small size renders them highly resistant to ultraviolet inactivation. See *virus infections*.

**virtual exposure therapy**   See *implosion*.

**virtual reality**   See *presence; virtualization*.

**virtualization**   The process by which a human viewer interprets a patterned sensory impression to be an extended object in an environment other than that in which it physically exists. It is the process involved in virtual reality studies, in which computer-generated sensory data are substituted for real sensory data. See *presence*.

Virtual reality and presence have been used in studies of perception, especially in studies of self-perception and the sense of space. They have also been used successfully in the treatment of phobias, social phobia, posttraumatic stress disorder, and pain.

**virus infections**   Rabies, Japanese B encephalitis, and St. Louis encephalitis, among others, have long been recognized as viral encephalitides. More recently, evidence has accumulated to suggest that viruses can sometimes persist in host cells for long periods—even years—without producing symptoms. Such infections, called *conventional slow virus infections*, comprise a wide spectrum of chronic and degenerative diseases, including subacute postmeasles leukoencephalitis and subacute sclerosing panencephalitis (SSPE) due to paramyxovirus of measles; subacute herpetovirus

encephalitis of herpes simplex; progressive congenital rubella togavirus; cytomegalovirus brain infection; *epilepsia partialis continua* or Kozhevnikov epilepsy; and chronic meningoencephalitis in immunodeficient patients.

During the 1970s, interest grew in still another group, the *unconventional viruses* or *spongiform encephalopathies* (*SE*), which differ from other viruses in several ways: they do not evoke a virus-associated inflammatory response in brain or a pleocytosis or rise in CSF protein; there is no demonstrable immune response to the causative virus; they show unusual resistance to various chemical and physical agents that destroy conventional viruses. Some have speculated that the unconventional viruses may be *viroids*—very small DNA or RNA molecules about one-tenth the size of the nucleic acids in conventional viruses and without the protein coat that normally covers viral nucleic acids. See *prion*.

In the 1990s, evidence began to accumulate that protein misfolding and aggregation are core features in the pathogenesis of many of these disorders. See *neurodegenerative disorders; protein conformational disorders*.

Included within the unconventional virus infections are (1) in man—*kuru* (q.v.) and transmissible virus dementia (TVD), including the sporadic familial forms of Creutzfeldt-Jakob disease (CJD; see *cortico-striato-spinal degeneration*), and familial *Alzheimer disease* (q.v.); (2) in animals—*scrapie* and transmissible mink encephalopathy (TME). The work of D. Carleton Gajdusek and his colleagues at the National Institute of Neurological Communicative Diseases and Stroke suggests that scrapie-infected sheep tissue might be the source of TME (mink are often fed sheep scraps), of CJD by means of kitchen or butchery accidents (and secondarily from those so affected by means of neurosurgical or ophthalmologic surgical procedures performed on them), and of kuru through cannibalism. See *bovine spongiform encephalopathy*.

**visceral brain**   See *limbic lobe*.

**visceral epilepsy**   A form of focal epilepsy in which the fit is manifested as visceral sensations, usually referable to the gastrointestinal tract, the cardiorespiratory system, or the genitourinary system. The principal loci of lesions in such cases have been found to be in the frontotemporal and midfrontal parasagittal regions, indicating that the visceral sensations arise from some central location, probably the amygdalohippocampal portion of the temporal lobe. See *autonomic epilepsy*.

**visceral learning**   See *biofeedback*.

**viscerotonia**   A personality type described by Sheldon correlated with the endomorph body type, which shows a love of food, comfort, and conviviality and a tendency to general relaxation.

**viscosity, social**   Intense desire or need for interpersonal closeness; a pathological exaggeration of social cohesiveness. The efforts of the subject to achieve closeness are typically perceived by others as socially inept, intrusive, meddlesome, "pushy," and excessive, with an unpleasant parasitic or adhesive quality.

**vision**   See *occipital lobe*.

**vision, tubular**   See *field defect*.

**visions, hypnagogic**   The optic perceptions present in a state midway between sleep and waking. They are a phase of dream phenomena.

**visitor, health**   Any person who goes to the family as a way to provide linkage to health services; it has been suggested that a visiting nurse or, perhaps even better, a mature and supportive mother who is recognized as such by the community, can provide health supervision to the young family whose child might otherwise fall victim to abuse or neglect. See *battered child syndrome*.

**visual aphasia**   Word blindness. In pure (subcortical) form, the patient can visualize colors but cannot recognize words, letters, or colors; he can write spontaneously but cannot copy. The lesion is in the lingual gyrus. Visual aphasia is often combined with agraphia—*visual symbolia* or *cortical word blindness*; this is produced by a lesion of the left angular gyrus. Inability to read is *alexia*.

**visual asymbolia**   See *word blindness*.

**visual aurae**   A form of epilepsy described as sensory seizures in which flashes of light may occur suddenly, last a short period of time, and then disappear without the patient's having a grand mal attack. This would indicate a focus in the temporooccipital area. In grand mal attacks, the patient occasionally may have a visual aura just before the grand mal seizure, as a warning that a convulsive attack is about to occur.

**visual body perception**   Focal regions of the higher-level visual cortex are specialized for the visual perception of the body. (1) The *extrastriate body area (EBA)*, found bilaterally in the posterior inferior temporal sulcus/middle temporal gyrus, responds strongly and selectively to static images of human bodies and body parts, but weakly to faces, object, and object parts; (2) The *fusiform body area (FBA)*, in the fusiform gyrus, responds selectively to whole bodies and body parts and to schematic depictions of the body. The analysis of bodies in the EBA is focused on individual parts; the function of FBA is to create a more holistic body representation. See *face cells*; *fusiform face area* (Peelan, M. V. & Downing, P. E., *Nature Reviews Neuroscience* 8: 636–648, 2007).

**visual cortex, primary**   Also, *striate cortex, VI cortex*; the cortical area that is the main recipient of visual information coming from the retinae (by way of the lateral geniculate nucleus, LGN). Information from VI cortex is processed in two pathways, a ventral pathway extending into the temporal lobe, thought to be primarily involved in visual object recognition; and a dorsal pathway extending into the parietal lobes, thought to be more involved in extracting information about where an object is or how to execute visually guided action towards it. See *object recognition*.

**visual defects**   See *optic nerve*.

**visual distortion test**   A test of a subject's reaction to the visual distortion produced by fitting the subject with a set of +6.00 sphD or -6.00 sphD lenses for a period of 3–4 minutes; described by J. Ehrenwald (*Archives of General Psychiatry 7*, 1962), who theorizes that it is a measure of ego strength in that it "causes a temporary breakdown of the synthetic and integrative functions of the ego touched off by the dissociation of the visual and postural components of the patient's experiences of the body image and of the outside world."

**visual dysphasia**   See *word blindness*.

**visual extinction**   A condition in which the patient can see a stimulus presented alone in the contralateral visual field, but cannot see it if it is presented at the same time as a stimulus in the ipsilateral visual field; often associated with damage to the parietal cortex.

**visual field**   See *field defect*.

**visual hallucination**   See *haptic hallucination*.

**visual masking**   See *mask*.

**visual processing**   Primary visual processing occurs within a network of occipital and temporal cortices, including primary visual cortex

(V1), fourth visual area (V4), and inferotemporal cortex (IT). These sensory areas are linked to the brain-stem oculomotor nuclei by visuomotor areas in the lateral intraparietal area (LIP), frontal eye field (FEF), supplementary eye field (SEF), Walker's cytoarchitectonic area 46 —all in the midbrain—and the superior colliculus in the midbrain. These intermediate areas implement at least three transformations. In the context of making a choice between alternative tasks, a sensory transformation first generates a higher-order visual representation. A second decision transformation maps the sensory evidence onto the probability of one or another operant response. A third action transformation renders a discrete behavioral response.

LIP, in cooperation with DLPFC and superior colliculus, implements the decision transformation, converting a sensory representation of visual motion into a decision variable that guides behavior. See *object recognition*; *visual cortex, primary*; *visual stream*.

**visual search**   The neural mechanisms involved in viewing a scene, locating potential targets within a scene, identifying the specific target on the basis of such features as color and shape, and on the basis of its behavioral salience.

Area V4 neurons scan the objects in the scene sequentially until the target is identified (*serial search*). The V4 neurons with particular RF (receptive field) locations receive feedback from structures with spatial attention and oculomotor functions such as the frontal eye field and the lateral intraparietal areas with spatial and oculomotor functions, such as the frontal eye field and the lateral intraparietal areas. These areas are thought to represent a salience map in which stimuli are representing according to their behavioral relevance independent of their features, ultimately resulting in the selection of a single stimulus for a saccade target or further visual processing. The V4 neurons fire synchonously, at an increased rate, triggering spatial attention to the candidate target and an eye movement toward it.

Nonspatial attentional mechanisms that are sensitive to features such as color and shape bias visual processing in favor of neurons that represent the target features throughout the visual field, all at once (*parallel search*). These neurons of area V4 receive top-down feedback from structures involved in working memory and executive control, such as PFC and possibly parietal cortex.

Visual search thus engages serial and parallel mechanisms to various degrees, depending on the difficulty of the task and the sharing of target features among distracters. See *object search*; *visual cortex, primary*; *visual processing*.

**visual-spatial agnosia**   A syndrome described by Paterson and Zangwill consisting of failure to analyze spatial relationships and inability to perform simple constructional tasks under visual control. This syndrome is usually associated with lesions of the posterior portions (occipitoparietal) of the right cerebral hemisphere in right-handed patients.

**visual-spatial scratch pad**   See *short-term memory*.

**visual stream**   A visual pathway from the primary visual cortex to other parts of the cortex. Two interconnected but partly dissociable streams are recognized: a *ventral pathway* extending into the temporal lobe, which is thought to be involved primarily in visual object recognition, and a *dorsal pathway* extending into the parietal lobes, which is thought to be involved more in extracting information about "where" an object is or "how" to execute visually guided action towards it.

**visual working memory**   One theory suggests that its maintenance occurs in the areas of the anterior inferotemporal cortex that specialize in processing visual memory and that the more executive processes of monitoring and manipulating that information occur in the middorsolateral regions of the prefrontal cortex.

**visuospatial ability**   The mental capacity to perceive and manipulate objects in two- and three-dimensional space, such as the ability to draw two- and three-dimensional figures. In both Parkinson and Huntington diseases, there are visuospatial impairments, which may include diminished visuoperceptual ability that is free of motor demands. Spatial problems appear to exist independently of the prominent motor symptoms in both disorders.

**visuospatial skill**   The ability to perceive and manipulate objects in two- and three-dimensional space.

**vitamin C deficiency**   A severe form is *scurvy*, characterized by swollen gums; foul breath; petechial hemorrhages and bruises, especially on the thighs and buttocks; anemia; and nonspecific psychological changes that are probably due to ascorbic acid's role in neurotransmitter synthesis. Scurvy is rarely seen nowadays except in the poor, in alcoholics, and among food faddists.

**vitamin deficiency**　See *berberi; B12; folic acid; niacin deficiency; pyridoxine; thiamine; vitamin C deficiency.*

**VLOS**　Very late onset schizophrenia (or schizophrenic-like psychosis), with onset after 60 years.

**VLPO**　Ventrolateral preoptic areas. See *sleep.*

**VLSIC**　Very large scale integrated circuits, necessary to render a computer system *friendly* (q.v.).

**VLT**　Verbal Learning Test(s). Among the best known are the following:

1. Rey Auditory Verbal Learning Test (RAVLT)—16 nouns are presented for five learning trials (after an interference list, a short delay, a long delay, and recognition memory trials). The RAVLT evaluates immediate memory span, new verbal learning, susceptibility to interference, delayed free recall, and recognition memory.

2. California Verbal Learning Test (CVLT)—like the RAVLT, it provides indices of learning efficiency and delay recall; it can be computer scored.

3. Hopkins Verbal Learning Test (HVLT)—similar to RAVLT and CVLT but useful for research rather than clinical application.

**VMN**　Ventromedial nucleus of the *hypothalamus* (q.v.).

**VNA**　Visiting Nurse Association.

**VNS**　*Vagus nerve stimulation* (q.v.). Visiting nurse service.

**vocabulary**　The discrete units of language that represent concepts, ideas, and meaningful relations.

**vocal tract normalization**　Use of formant frequency patterns to estimate the length of the *supralaryngeal vocal tract (SVT)* that is producing the speech.　See *formants.*

**vocational counseling**　See *counseling; rehabilitation.*

**vocational rehabilitation**　A program designed to prepare a subject to fulfill a work role in society that is consonant with his strengths and weaknesses.

Persons with psychiatric disorders typically have one or more of the following work adjustment problems: difficulty in adapting to new situations, inappropriate dress and grooming habits, producing work of low quality, poor relationships with supervisors and coworkers, lack of confidence on the job, overreacting to criticism, and ineffective work because of fear of being fired. In vocational rehabilitation, various strategies are used to help subjects learn appropriate work, social, and job readiness behaviors: enhancing physical capacities, psychomotor skills, interpersonal and communicative behaviors, appropriate grooming practices, job seeking skills, productive skills, and orientation to work practices and work habits.

*Work adjustment training* has moved from a behavior management approach to a more positive approach that uses programmed instructions, audiovisual demonstration, and videotape modeling feedback and simulation training. Temporary or transitional community-based employment programs are often combined with other services, such as transitional living arrangements or group placement.

**Vogt, Oskar**　(1870–1959) German neuropathologist; Tay-Sachs disease.

**Vogt-Koyanagi syndrome**　See *Behçet syndrome.*

**Vogt-Spielmeyer disease**　See *Spielmeyer-Vogt disease; Tay-Sachs disease.*

**voice**　The mechanism by which speech sounds are produced; it includes phonation, articulation-resonance, respiration, pitch, and loudness.

**voice, soundless**　See *audible thought.*

**voice disorder**　A communication disorder (speech and language disorder) that may begin in childhood or adulthood, characterized by abnormal pitch, loudness, tone, resonance, etc., of sufficient degree to interfere with educational achievement or social communication.

**volatile inhalants**　See *inhalants.*

**Volga German kindred**　A group of seven related families whose means of age of onset of Alzheimer disease range from 50.2 to 64.5 years. Germans from the Hesse region who emigrated to Russia in the 1760s and subsequently to the United States at the turn of the 20th century remained culturally distinct and did not intermarry. In the Volga German kindreds, as in several other families in which Alzheimer disease appears to be inherited as an autosomal dominant trait, loci on chromosomes 14 and 21 have been excluded.

Molecular genetic studies have localized some mutations associated with FAD to the PS2 gene and its protein, STM2. The gene maps to chromosome 1.

**volition**   Will, motivation, desire. To have volitional ability, one must be able both to will and do, and also to refrain from willing and doing when there are appropriate reasons for so willing. The compulsive handwasher, for example, acts intentionally but not voluntarily, for he can will and perform the act of handwashing, but he cannot refrain from doing it even though he has good reasons for not washing his hands.

**volition, made**   See *first-rank symptoms.*

**volitional insanity**   *Obs.* Obsessive-compulsive disorder (q.v.).

**voltage gating**   The process involved in an ion channel's response to changes in voltage across the cell membrane, such that the channel will open at the right time to allow ions to pass across the cell membrane.

**voltage sensory paddle**   In one model of voltage-gated potassium channels, the S4 voltage sensor (one of the six helical segments of the ion channel) and the S3 segment are arranged like spokes around the periphery of the channel, forming a paddle that moves like a lever arm through the lipid membrane surrounding the channel and sweeps from the intracellular side to the extracellular side of the membrane. The sweeping movement pulls on the other segments of the channel to open the pore.

**Voltage-gated ion channel**   A protein that acts as a molecular gatekeeper, determining when ions are allowed to pass across a cell membrane. Voltage-gated potassium channels, for example, are responsible for bringing a nerve impulse to an end, so that the neuron can prepare to fire again.

**volubility**   Overproductivity in speech.

**volume sensitive**   Affected or determined by amount or quantity.

A special operation that requires highly polished technical skills, for instance, is likely to be better performed in an institution where it is performed frequently than in an institution where it is only rarely performed. Thus, part of valid consent includes informing a patient about to undergo a volume-sensitive operation in a low-volume hospital that he is at somewhat greater risk than if the same operation were to be performed in a *high-volume hospital*. See *informed consent.*

**volumetrics**   Study of the volumes of different structures, of particular value in MRI analysis of the degree of shrinkage and tissue loss in such disorders as Alzheimer disease.

**voluntarism**   The ability to act in accordance with one's authentic sense of what is good, right, and best in light of one's situation, values, and history. Voluntarism includes the capacity to make this choice freely and in the absence of coercion. Deliberateness, purposefulness of intent, clarity, genuineness, and coherence with prior life decisons are implicit in the concept of voluntarism. See *informed consent.*

**voluntary**   See *volition.*

**voluntary euthanasia**   See *euthanasia.*

**voluntary involuntary treatment**   *Ulysses contract* (q.v.).

**vomeronasal sensory neurons**   *VSNs* (q.v.).

**vomiting, cyclic**   A disorder of children characterized by recurrent attacks of vomiting. The attacks begin suddenly, last several days, cease abruptly, and then recur in intervals or cycles of several weeks or months.

**vomiting, nervous**   Functional vomiting of psychogenic, emotional, or neurotic origin, occurring most frequently in young women between the ages of 20 and 40. It usually expresses, in organ language, symbolically and physically, the desire to reject a hated idea, or person, concerning whom there exist conscious and unconscious conflicts of an emotional nature; this is the only way out of the conflict left to these patients, because, in consciousness, they cannot stand their hostility and yet cannot express it verbally.

**von Gierke disease**   *Glucogenosis* (q.v.).

**von Graefe sign**   (Albrecht von Graefe, German ophthalmologist, 1828–1870) Lag of the upper lid in following the downward movement of the eye, due to retraction of the upper lid such as occurs in exophthalmic goiter and in lesions in the upper part of the midbrain.

**von Hippel-Lindau disease**   (Eugen von Hippel, German ophthalmologist, 1867–1939; Arvid Vilhelm Lindau, Swedish pathologist, 1892–1958) *VHL disease; retinocerebellar angiomatosis; angiophakomatosis; Lindau syndrome*; a familial cancer syndrome, inherited as a mendelian dominant, that predisposes the affected person to a variety of tumors, including hemangioblastomas of the central nervous system and retina, pheochromocytoma, and renal cell carcinoma (the most frequent cause of death). Incidence is estimated at one in 36,000. The VHL gene has been identified as a tumor suppressor gene on chromosome 3; deletion of the gene eliminates its normal inhibition of tumor cell growth and predisposes to cancer. Specific mutations on the gene may determine which kind of tumor develops and where. The VHL gene is evolutionarily conserved; that is, it has changed little in the course of evolution, suggesting that it performs a basic cellular function. See *phakomatoses*.

**Von Neumann, John** (1903–1957) Budapest-born mathematician who headed the team that developed the first digital computer, ENIAC, at the Moore School of Electrical Engineering in Philadelphia in 1946; *The Theory of Games and Economic Behavior* (1944, with economist Oskar Morgenstern).

**von Recklinghausen disease** (Friedrich Daniel von Recklinghausen, German pathologist, 1833–1910) Neurofibromatosis 1 (NF1); peripheral neurofibromatosis; a hereditary disorder, transmitted as a mendelian dominant, consisting of café-au-lait pigmentation of the skin and the formation of tumors in various tissues (e.g., cutaneous fibromas or mollusca fibrosa and perineural fibroblastomas of the peripheral and cranial nerves). The tumors are often associated with overgrowth of the skin and subcutaneous tissues. Of the cranial nerves, the eighth nerve is the most commonly involved. The disorder is sometimes progressive, but it does not always shorten life. It may be associated with varying degrees of mental retardation.

Von Recklinghausen disease occurs in approximately 1 in 50,000 births; the gene responsible for the disorder maps to chromosome 17. Until recently, von Recklinghausen disease was identified with Elephant Man's disease; it is now widely accepted that the "elephant man" (Joseph Herrick, a 19th century Englishman who was exhibited as such at sideshows) suffered from Proteus syndrome, not neurofibromatosis.

**Vorbeireden** One who is at cross purposes with another; applied to the person with Ganser syndrome who seems to miss the point of questions put to him by talking around or past them and giving nonsensical or approximate answers. See *Ganser syndrome*.

**voxel** Volume element; in brain structure imaging, such as in computed tomography, the density of the tissue represented within the grid or matrix.

**voyeur** Peeping Tom; scopophiliac; one who obtains sexual gratification by watching sexual activity or looking at the genitals of another. See *voyeurism*.

**voyeurism** *Peeping; scop(t)ophilia;* a *paraphilia* (q.v.) that involves watching an unsuspecting person who is nude, in the act of disrobing, or engaging in sexual intercourse. It is the watching or the later recall of it in phantasy that gives sexual excitement and is an end in itself (although often accompanied by masturbation to effect orgasm). Further sex contact between the observed and the voyeur does not occur. Voyeurism as defined has not been reported in females. It is one of the paraphilias within the group of *psychosexual disorders* (q.v.).

**VSDI** Voltage-sensitive dye imaging, which provides high spatial and temporal resolution so that the dynamics of cortical information processing and its underlying functional architecture can be observed. The dye molecules bind to the external surface of cell membranes and act as molecular transducers that transform changes in membrane potential into optical signals. The amplitudes of the VSD signals are linearly correlated with both changes in membrane potential (rather than changes in current) and the membrane area of the stained neuronal elements under each measuring pixel. With VSDI it is possible to observe the dynamics of cortical information processing and its underlying functional architecture at the necessary spatial and temporal resolution in both anesthetized and behaving subjects.

The combination of existing VSD probes with fluorescence resonance energy transfer (*FRET*) to detect electrical activity promises to reveal coherent neuronal assemblies in the neocortex, at subcolumnar resolution.

**VSNs** *Vomeronasal sensory neurons,* which in animals detect pheromones and other chemosignals that carry information about gender, sexual and social status, dominance hierarchies, and individuality. Small peptides that serve as ligands for major histocompatibility complex (MHC) class I molecules have been found to function also as chemosensory stimuli for a subset of vomeronasal sensory neurons.

**VTA** Ventral tegmental area, a midbrain region that has been implicated in the rewarding motivational effects of a variety of addictive drugs, including cocaine, alcohol, opiates, and nicotine. Within VTA, dopamine neurons and their associated ascending projections to the nucleus accumbens and prefrontal cortex constitute the well-characterized mesolimbic and mesocortical pathways. See *dopaminergic systems*.

**vulnerability**   An actual, existing variation in structure or function that predisposes to disease, stress, stimulation, or any other factor under study. *Risk* (q.v.), in contrast, refers to a statistical probability that a factor whose occurrence has been demonstrated statistically to be associated with later development of disease does, in fact, predispose to development of that disease or variation.

Many depressions are observed to be triggered by life events that ordinarily would not be sufficient to provoke such a reaction. Such events appear to be acting as the "last straw" in a series of adverse circumstances that render the subject less able to cope, and those predisposing or sensitizing adverse circumstances have been called vulnerability factors. While not all studies have been confirmatory, some investigators have suggested that depressions are most likely to be triggered by life events in those who are caring for young children, who have no work outside the home, who have no one to confide in, or who have lost the mother by death or separation before they were 11 years of age. See *risk factor*.

**vulnerability principle**   The bioethical principle that vulnerable people should be protected from harm or exploitation. This is one aspect of the state's *parens patriae power* (q.v.); one of its extensions in the clinical area is the obligation of an institution in which vulnerable people are housed to protect them from harm or exploitation (by staff or other patients).

**vulnerable child syndrome**   Symptoms often noted in a child who, though he has survived an acute episode of severe illness, continues to be treated by his parents as if his life were still in considerable danger.

**vulvismus**   *Vaginismus* (q.v.).

**Wada dominance test**   A method for determining the side of cerebral dominance by intracarotid injection of amobarbital, introduced by J. Wada in 1949.

**waddling gait**   Clumsy gait, seen in dislocation of the hip and in muscular dystrophies with hip weakness. The weakness necessitates use of the trunk muscles in walking, so that the patient rolls from side to side as he walks.

**Wagner, Ernst**   A famous patient in European psychiatry who is an example of the classic concept of paranoia. Wagner was a teacher who, at age 27, committed an undisclosed sexual act with animals. The next day, and for the rest of his life, he developed the conviction that other people knew what he had done and were mocking him. This led to a sensational mass murder in 1913 (when he was 38) that included his wife, his children, and 8 others from his village; he wounded 12 others and burned down several buildings.

Gaupp (who published the case history in 1938) and Kraepelin diagnosed Wagner as suffering paranoia—defined as an abnormal but psychologically understandable development caused in predisposed personalities by crucial life events, with no intellectual impairment. Years later, Wagner's brain was found in the Vogt collection in Dusseldorf, but it had never been examined. Bogerts' examination showed a clear developmental abnormality within the left posterior parahippocampal gyrus of the temporal lobe. According to Bogerts, these findings support his *temporolimbic system model* (q.v.) of schizophrenia, according to which limbic pathology may account for some, but not all, of the clinical abnormalities seen in this patient. (Bogerts, B. *Schizophrenia Bulletin* 23: 423–435, 1997).

**Wagner von Jauregg, Julius**   (1857–1940) Austrian psychiatrist and neurologist; fever treatment of general paresis.

**Wahnstimmung**   *Delusional mood*, consisting of a change in general mood that precedes the appearance of the delusional idea itself, such as a foreboding that some sinister event is about to occur.

**WAIS**   Wechsler Adult Intelligence Scale. It consists of several tests, including the following: arithmetic: the subject answers arithmetic problems that are presented orally and range in difficulty from simple to complex; block design: the subject is asked to arrange red and white blocks to correspond to a printed design; the task is timed and bonus points are given for rapid responses; comprehension: the subject answers questions or interprets proverbs that are presented orally and require the use of common sense, judgment, and social knowledge; digit span: the subject first is asked to repeat three to nine orally presented digits immediately after their presentation, and then is asked to repeat two to eight digits in reverse order immediately after presentation; object assembly: the task is to assemble each of four cardboard puzzles; picture arrangement: the subject arranges a set of cartoon pictures so as to make a coherent story; picture completion: the task is to note what important part is missing from each of 21 pictures; similarities: the subject tells how each of 12 pairs of words is alike.

**wake time after sleep onset**   The duration of the intervals of time the subject is awake between onset of sleep and the end of the sleep period.

**wakefulness**   *Arousal* (q.v.), attentiveness; sleeplessness, insomnia.

**Waldenstrom macroglobulinemia**   Described by Waldenstrom in 1944; a disease of unknown origin characterized by a serum globulin of very large molecular size, lymphocytosis, thrombopenia, weight loss, weakness, and often splenomegaly and a hemorrhagic tendency. The illness is fatal within 2 to 10 years of onset, and approximately 25% of cases have central nervous system symptoms (termed *Bing-Neel syndrome*), such as progressive encephalopathy, polyneuritis, polyradiculitis, strokes, subarachnoid hemorrhage, delirium, coma, convulsions and other focal central symptoms, loss of hearing, and any number of mental disturbances such as depression.

**Waldrop scale**   A listing of minor physical anomalies that are strongly associated with schizophrenia, such as curved fifth finger, epicanthus, high or steepled palate, and partial syndactyly of toes. In many studies, non schizophrenic siblings of patients also show significantly higher rates of minor physical anomanlies. Such anomalies are believed to reflect early disturbances in embryonic development; they are not a result of the later-appearing shizophrenic illness, of its consequences, or of treatment.

**Walker area 46** *DLPFC* (q.v.).

**Wallenberg syndrome** (Adolf Wallenberg, German physician, 1862–1949) The symptoms following occlusion of the posterior inferior cerebellar artery (which is known as "the artery of thrombosis"): ipsilateral facial analgesia, ipsilateral Horner's syndrome, ipsilateral ataxia, and contralateral analgesia.

**Wallerian degeneration** (Augustus Volney Waller, English physician 1816–1870) Deterioration of the distal segment after injury of a nerve cell; the myelin sheath around the distal segment of the axon retreats and breaks apart, and the exposed axon itself degenerates. Microglial cells and astrocytes remove the myelin and axonal debris, which would otherwise interfere with axonal regeneration.

Both physical injury and a blockade of axonal transport trigger a proactive axon death program.

**wandering** Straying, roaming, traveling without a fixed course or particular destination in mind; also known as drapetomania, dromomania, *ecdemomania errabunda*, nomadism, oikofugia, planomania, vagabond neurosis, *wandering impulse, wanderlust.*

Sometimes wandering refers to fugue states, but the current trend is to use it in a more specific way to denote episodes of sudden confusion (disorientation) in senile dementia or other organic disorders. See *Alzheimer disease; poriomania.*

**wanderlust** Compulsion to roam or wander, believed to be associated with the Oedipus situation in the sense that the wanderer is incessantly seeking to establish affiliation with one or both parents as he had experienced it, or longed to experience it, when he was a young child.

**war neurasthenia** *Neurocirculatory asthenia* (q.v.) or effort syndrome as observed in soldiers in time of war; soldier's heart. The condition corresponds to what currently would be termed *hyperventilation syndrome* (q.v.).

**war neurosis** See *shell shock; traumatic neurosis.*

**warn, duty to** The responsibility of a psychiatrist to notify the possible victims of a patient's assault when the psychiatrist has sufficient evidence that such dangerous acts are likely to occur.

**washers** Those persons suffering from *obsessive-compulsive disorder* (q.v.) who spend several hours a day showering or washing their hands, in order to avoid contamination, dirt, or germs. It is estimated that about half of obsessive-compulsive patients are washers.

**Wassermann test** (August von Wassermann, German bacteriologist, 1866–1925) A diagnostic test for syphilis, based upon complement fixation. The development and refinement of this test, in the years 1901 to 1907, made it possible to identify positively as syphilitic many neuropsychiatric conditions whose etiology had previously been only a matter of speculation. In general, it may be said that the blood Wasserman test is positive in approximately 70% of cases with cerebral syphilis, 70% of tabetics, and almost 100% of paretics. The cerebrospinal fluid Wasserman test is positive in approximately 60% with secondary syphilis, 100% with tertiary syphilis, and 100% with congenital syphilis.

**watchfulness, frozen** See *frozen watchfulness.*

**watchspring theory** See *aging, theories of.*

**water maze** See *Morris water maze.*

**watershed area** See *transcortical aphasia.*

**Watson, John Broadus** (1878–1958) American psychologist; behaviorism. Using Albert, B. an 11-month-old infant, as his experimental subject, Watson demonstrated that classical conditioning could give rise to phobic behavior (reported by Watson and Raynore in 1920). The unconditional stimulus was a loud noise, which caused the baby to cry; pairing it with the conditional stimulus, the sight of a white rat, resulted in Albert's avoidance of the rat (which had not caused fear before). The avoidance also extended to related objects, such as cotton wool, a rabbit, and a fur coat, even though none of them had been paired with the unconditional stimulus. In 1925 Watson described his deconditioning of Peter, a boy with fear of a playroom rabbit.

**Watson-Crick model** See *chromosome.*

**waxy flexibility** *Cerea flexibilitas.* See *catalepsy.*

**WB** Western blot; a more specific test for HIV antibody, used to validate seropositive reactions to *ELISA* (q.v.). See *AIDS.*

**WBS**  *Williams-Beuren syndrome* (q.v.).

**WCST**  *Wisconsin Card Sorting Test* (q.v.).

**weapons**  Instruments of combat or violence. See *handgun violence*. In any case of suspected or threatened violence, the patient's access to deadly weapons should be assessed as well as the likelihood that the patient will use them.

**wearing-off effect**  The benefit of each dose of pharmaceutical agent becomes shorter; used particularly in reference to the response of patients with Parkinson disease. Such patients often have sudden fluctuations between mobility and immobility (the *on-off phenomenon*). The on state is one of activation, often with euphoria; the off is a state of severe parkinsonism in which the the patient is immobilized and, often, depressed. See *LID*.

**Weber syndrome**  (Sir Herman Weber, English physician, 1823–1918)
Pedunculopontile syndrome. See *hemiplegia alternans*.

**Wechsler-Bellevue test**  An intelligence test, the most widely used test in the average adult, consisting of five verbal tests, five performance tests, and an additional vocabulary test. The 11 subtests are as follows: general information, general comprehension, arithmetic, digit span, similarities, vocabulary, picture arrangement, picture completion, block design, object assembly, and digit symbol. The subtests are scored on the basis of speed and accuracy, and results can be translated into standard scores that give the verbal IQ, the performance IQ, and the full-scale IQ.

**weight, connection**  See *parallel distributed processing*.

**weighted harm principle**  In policy and ethical decisions a choice that is determined by whatever promises the least harm, without regard to benefits that might be anticipated if that particular action or approach is chosen. See *utilitarian principle*.

**welfare emotions**  See *adaptional psychodynamics*.

**welfare state**  See *medicalization*.

**Weltmerism**  (After Sidney A. Weltmer, founder of the method and of the Weltmer Institute at Nevada, Mo.) A system of therapeutics based on suggestion.

**Werner syndrome**  *WS*; a rare autosomal recessive disorder characterized by premature senility with general retardation of growth, skin atrophy, and endocrine disturbances. It is considered only a partial model of human aging because of various subtle discordances between it and normal aging. WS patients prematurely develop a variety of the major age-related diseases, including several forms of arteriosclerosis, malignant neoplasms, type II diabetes mellitus, osteoporosis, and ocular cataracts. Affected persons also manifest early graying and loss of hair, skin atrophy, and a generally aged appearance.

*WRN*, the gene responsible for WS, is located on the short arm of chromosome 8. The gene encodes a protein that is probably a helicase, an enzyme that unwinds the paired DNA strands of the cell's genes. Such unwinding is a necessary prelude to such key activities as the repair, replication, or expression of genetic material (Yu, C. et al *Science 272*, 1996).

**Wernicke aphasia**  (Carl Wernicke, 1848–1905, German neurologist) *Posterior aphasia; fluent aphasia; receptive aphasia; sensory aphasia; central aphasia; semantic aphasia.* Comprehension and expression of both speech and writing are impaired. Speech is fluent but has many errors in syntax and grammar and is sprinkled with wrong or nonexistent words. The subject is unaware that he is speaking nonsense (*jargon aphasia, driveling*), and meaning, if any, can be conveyed only in a roundabout way through phonetic or verbal paraphrasic utterances, word approximations and substitutions, neologisms, loss of word complexity, stock phrases, phonemic paraphasias, and private use of words. Failure to convey the ideas the patient has in mind is sometimes termed *empty speech*; excessive speech is termed *logorrhea* or *pressured speech*. Repetition is impaired; there are defects in naming, reading comprehension, and reading aloud. Errors in writing reflect the paraphasias. Associated symptoms include delusions, paranoia, agitation, and occasionally euphoria or indifference.

The person with anomic aphasia cannot find the correct word. He has particular difficulty in retrieving nouns; verbs pose less of a problem (but are harder for Broca aphasics, presumably because verbs are intimately linked to syntax). Different anomic patients have problems with different kinds of nouns. Some can use concrete nouns but not abstract nouns; others can use nouns for nonliving things but not for living things; some can name anything but animals; others cannot name body parts, or colors, or proper names.

*Anomia* is due to damage to the Wernicke area and the adjacent angular and supramarginal gyri in the posterior superior left temporal gyrus (Brodmann area 22), which appears to play a role in looking up words that will convey the message and funneling them to other modules (such as the Broca area), which assemble them or parse them syntactically. Although Wernicke believed that the Wernicke area stores the auditory memories of words, and that the Broca area stores the memories for how to pronounce them, it is clear that the language areas are primarily involved in abstract, linguistic functions rather than with the auditory-visual channel.

This type of aphasia is differentiated from thought disorder associated with psychosis; in the latter, comprehension of spoken and written language is retained, as well as the ability to repeat phrases.

**Wernicke area**   Traditionally, one of the speech areas of the brain. It lies in the left temporal lobe below the lateral fissure and adjacent to the primary auditory cortex, the end station for auditory input to the brain. *Wernicke aphasia* is sometimes equated with perceptual deficits. Wernicke aphasia has good articulation and melody, but great difficulty in finding the correct word, imprecise use of words, and circumlocution. Wernicke's hypothesis was that the Wernicke area stores the auditory memories of words, and the Broca area stores the memories for how to pronounce them, a hypothesis no longer tenable. The existence of sign language aphasias shows that the language areas of the brain have to do with abstract, *linguistic* functions, not especially with the auditory-visual channel.

**Wernicke encephalopathy**   *Polioencephalitis hemorrhagica superior*, described by Wernicke in 1881; a severe disorder consisting of degeneration of nervous tissue especially marked in the midbrain. The syndrome occurs in a small percentage of alcoholics and is probably due to a combination of nutritional deficiencies, especially a vitamin B deficiency. Onset is insidious, with vomiting, oculomotor palsies, ptosis, pupillary changes (such as Argyll Robertson pupil), ataxia, insomnia, and a mental state consisting of an acute hallucinatory picture similar to delirium tremens except that there is no tremor and the delirium is dreamy and confused. Impaired consciousness may progress to stupor. The encephalopathy may terminate fatally, or there may be progression to a Korsakoff syndrome. Thiamine chloride has been used successfully to reverse the ophthalmoplegia and has sometimes been of help in the mental state.

**Wernicke-Korsakoff syndrome**   (Karl Wernicke, German neurologist, 1848–1905, and Sergei Korsakoff, Russian neurologist, 1853–1900) *Alcohol amnestic syndrome; amnesic confabulatory syndrome.* Although Wernicke syndrome and Korsakoff syndrome (or psychosis) have classically been considered separate entities, neuropathological studies have demonstrated that the pathological changes in each are identical but differences in localization of lesions have produced different clinical pictures. The basis is generally believed to be a thiamine deficiency, which produces lesions in the 3rd and 6th nerve nuclei and adjacent tegmentum (giving rise to palsies of ocular muscles and of gaze); in the vestibular nuclei (giving rise to nystagmus and disturbances in equilibrium), in the cerebellar cortex (producing ataxia), and in the diencephalon (giving rise to the characteristic severe anterograde amnesia, with inability to retain memory for events for more than a short time even though immediate memory is unimpaired and remote memory is only mildly impaired; confabulation is frequently associated with the amnesia).

Wernicke described *polioencephalitis hemorrhagica superior* in 1881; the clinical picture consists of the triad of confusion (a dreamy delirium), ataxia, and ophthalmoplegia. Other manifestations may include ptosis, pupillary changes (such as Argyll Robertson pupil), nystagmus, and vomiting. Wernicke syndrome is the acute neurologic component of the Wernicke-Korsakoff syndrome and responds to thiamine repletion.

*Korsakoff psychosis* has been used in two ways in the literature: narrowly, to describe an amnestic confabulatory syndrome associated with thiamine deficiency, and broadly to include all cases with a similar clinical presentation, irrespective of cause. About half the cases described have had polyneuritis; in addition to the severe anterograde amnesia described above, confabulation (q.v.) is seen in many cases.

Wernicke-Korsakoff syndrome indicates that the chronic amnestic syndrome has developed following (usually by about 1 month) an acute neurologic disorder (Wernicke syndrome).

See *alcoholic Korsakoff psychosis; amnestic syndrome; Korsakoff psychosis.*

**Westphal sign**   (Carl F. O. Westphal, German neurologist, 1833–1890) Loss of the knee jerk.

**Westphal-Strumpell pseudosclerosis**   See *hepatolenticular degeneration.*

**Westphal variant**   See *Huntington disease.*

**wet dream**   Popular term for seminal ejaculation during sleep; oneirogonorrhea. Over 80% of men experience wet dreams, which are most common in the teens and early 20s, following periods of abstinence from intercourse and masturbation. Sleeping with a partner usually brings an end to wet dreams.

Although all women have sex dreams, not all have nocturnal orgasms. By the age of 20, about 10% of women have experienced them, and by age 40 about 40% will have experienced them. For women who do have them, nocturnal orgasms usually produce the strongest climaxes of all. The functions of nocturnal orgasms are the same as with *masturbation* (q.v.)—to help her fight infection, and to prepare her vagina for the next intercourse by depositing lubricant. They are most likely to occur at the beginning of their fertile phase, about a week before *ovulation* (q.v.). Women on the "pill" do not show such a peak, an indication that both nocturnals and masturbation are under hormonal control (Baker, R. *Sperm Wars*. New York: Basic Books, 1996).

**whiplash**   Sudden hyperextension or hyperflexion of the neck results in rapid loss of memory of life experiences without loss of intellectually learned facts. The syndrome is based on bilateral vascular disturbances in the hippocampal gyri, consisting of thrombosis and embolism in the hippocampal branches of the posterior cerebral arteries.

**whipping**   See *flagellation.*

**whirling**   See *childhood schizophrenia.*

**white matter**   Cerebral white matter consists of collections of closely apposed axons that are wrapped in myelin. White matter forms fiber collections known as tracts, fasciculi, bundles, peduncles, and lemnisci. There are three major fiber systems: projection fibers, association fibers, and commissural fibers. Normal white matter ensures rapid and efficient neuronal conduction and contributes to the speed of information processing; it occupies a central place in the elaboration of human behavior by reason of its contribution to distributed neural networks. There are many

*white matter disorders* (q.v.), and all are associated with some form of cognitive or emotional dysfunction. See *network.*

**white matter disorders**   More than 100 are known; among them are *AIDS dementia complex*; *subcortical arteriosclerotic encephalopathy* (Binswanger disease); *metachromatic leukodystrophy*, and *multiple sclerosis* (qq.v.). White matter dementia (or dysmentia) is characterized by sustained attention deficit, memory retrieval deficit, executive dysfunction, and a general slowing of cognition, all of which are associated with frontal lobe function. There is also visuospatial impairment, and a wide range of neurobehavioral syndromes, such as amnesia, aphasia, apraxia, alexia, agnosia, akinetic mutism, and callosal disconnection. Associated psychiatric disorders include schizophrenia, depression, mania, ADHD, aggression, and autism. (Filley, C.M. *Psychiatric Clinics of North America* 28: 685–700, 2005).

**White, Samuel**   (1777–1845) American psychiatrist; one of the "original thirteen" founders of the Association of Medical Superintendents of America (forerunner of American Psychiatric Association).

**White, William A .**   (1870–1937) American psychiatrist; psychodynamics, psychotherapy, forensic psychiatry.

**whole object relations**   Experience of external objects as objects that exist independently and outside one's omnipotence. The object is experienced as being a subject, and only then does the developing child become able to care about the object and develop guilt because of real or imagined harm that one has done to someone about whom one cares. See *depressive position.*

**wife battering**   Wife beating, the leading form of *domestic violence*; other related terms are *intraspousal assault, interspousal violence,* and *intramarital assault*. "Wife-battering behavior" is sometimes quantitatively defined as deliberate, severe, and repeated (more than three times) physical assault resulting in demonstrable injury, such as severe bruising. It has been estimated that in the United States almost 1.8 million wives are battered at least once by their husbands.

Spousal abuse has serious psychological and emotional consequences, including PTSD, depression, and low self-esteem. When children are involved, battering appears to be related to serious behavioral problems, as well as emotional and cognitive developmental difficulties.

The social attitude toward wife beating is slowly changing from one of blaming the victim of abuse to one of holding the man who perpetrates such abuse accountable. As with rape, attention is turning away from the myth of provocation by the woman to the abuse behavior of the man and the social norms that sanction and encourage such behavior under the guise of protecting the privacy and the sanctity of the home.

Wife battering is frequently accompanied by child abuse, both physical and sexual. Battering, as well as sexual abuse and incest, frequently occur hand-in-hand with alcohol or other substance abuse. Wife batterers are typically men with aggressive personalities or, less often, depression; in either case, they are often pathologically jealous or heavy drinkers, or both. See *domestic violence*.

**wihtiko**   See *windigo psychosis*.

**wild analysis**   See *direct analysis*.

**wild children**   Deprived children; children reared by humans but subjected to a brutally deprived environment. If never spoken to, such children do not develop language. If discovered and spoken to within the critical period, they can overcome the deprivations suffered and can master language.

**wild type**   In genetics, the normal allele, the allele found most frequently in natural populations. Like mutant alleles, wild alleles can be either dominant or recessive.

**will disturbances**   One of Bleuler's fundamental symptoms of the schizophrenias. Usually, the disturbance is in the direction of deficiency (hypobulia, hypoboulia) or lack (abulia, aboulia); such patients appear lazy, negligent of their duties, purposeless, and with no aims, ambitions, or desires. *Platonization* (q.v.) is often seen and patients appear apathetic toward their environment and uninterested in the reality about them. At other times, because they have no real goals, they appear flighty, capricious, and undependable, adopting momentarily any goal that is thrust upon them. Or they may appear stubborn, robot-like, and wedded in a perseverative way to a particular activity, which they cling to rather than have to make any decision or move toward purposeful change.

A few patients are hyperbulic and show a bizarre or inappropriate application and assiduity to unimportant and trivial occupations; these are the faddists, the shifters, persons who are forever brewing storms in teapots.

**will therapy**   A form of psychotherapy associated with Otto Rank and based upon his belief that birth trauma (the separation of the child from the mother at the moment of birth) is the central element in neurosis. The trauma of birth is believed to lead to two sets of strivings: (1) to return to the womb or (2) to reenact separation and achieve independence.

In will therapy, separation reactions are studied as well as the struggle of will manifested in the patient's desire to continue it (and become independent). The patient is actively encouraged to assert himself so as to develop and strengthen his will.

**will to be above**   Adler borrowed this term from Nietzsche to indicate the tendency of the neurotic female to identify herself with the male.

**will to be up**   Adler borrowed this term from Nietzsche to denote the neurotic's striving toward masculine aggression.

**will to power**   This term, borrowed by Adler from Nietzsche, denotes the strivings of the neurotic toward masculinity, in order to escape the feeling of uncertainty and inferiority that connotes femininity.

**Williams syndrome, Williams-Beuren syndrome**   *WBS*; *elfin face syndrome*; *pixie people syndrome*; a rare genetic neurodevelopmental disorder first identified by British physician J.H. Williams in a 1961 paper; and independently a year later by German cardiologist Alois J, Beuren. Many patients with WBS show a hemizygous deletion (i.e., one copy) of the elastin locus on chromosome 7; other associations reported are deletions in chromosomes 11 and 22. Williams syndrome was first described as a combination of a distinct facial appearance (*elfin face)* because of upturned noses, wide mouths, and small chins, combined with growth retardation and cardiovascular anomalies. Other common somatic symptoms are endocrine (transient hypercalcemia, impaired glucose tolerance), gastrointestinal (constipation, diverticula, prolapse), and orthopedic (scoliosis, joint contractures). Neurological problems include coordination difficulties, visuospatial construction deficits, strabismus, nystagmus, hyperreflexia, hypersensitivity to sound, and sensorineural hearing loss.

Affected children acquire only rudimentary skills in reading, writing, and arithmetic, and deficits are particularly severe on tests of spatial understanding, such as copying patterns of blocks. They are unable to tie their shoes and find their way, retrieve requested items from a closet or refrigerator, tell left from right, draw a bicycle, or suppress their natural tendency to hug strangers. Yet they are fluent, if somewhat prim, conversationalists. They understand complex sentences and can fix ungrammatical sentences at normal levels. They are fond of unusual words and like to talk (*hyperlinguistic*). Asked to name some animals, instead of the usual dog, cat, and horse they are likely to name the unicorn, yak, ibex, sea lion, saber-tooth tiger, koala, dragon, or brontosaurus rex. Rather than saying "pouring water" they will say "evacuating a glass."

Until the 1990s it was generally believed that WBS subjects had normal language abilities and unusual vocabularies despite severe mental retardation. It is now recognized that mental retardation is mild to moderate and that use of unusual words is rare. Language acquisition is normal but delayed.

In contrast to *autistic disorder* (q.v.), WBS features hypersociability. Those affected show a lack of social inhibition, a fascination with faces, and excessive friendliness, even with strangers. Nonetheless, they have difficulties in everyday interactions because of an inability to detect and respect social danger signals. Despite their social fearlessness, WBS patients typically display high levels of nonsocial anxiety, such as fear of heights. The abnormal fear responses are related to functional abnormalities in the orbitofrontal cortex and the medial prefrontal cortex, both of which are involved in regulation of the amygdala. Abnormalities in the hippocampal region may explain the other cognitive deficits in WBS.

The impairment in visuospatial construction—the ability to visualize an object or picture as a set of parts and construct a replica of the object from those parts—is a hallmark of WBS. It seems likely that a structural abnormality in the dorsal stream ("where?" stream) of the visual cortex blocks the flow from earlier inferior to later superior visual processing areas. The impairment in visuospatial construction— the ability to visualize an object or picture as a set of parts and construct a replica of the object from those parts—is a hallmark of WBS.

The chromosomal deletion in WBS encompasses just 28 known genes, but isolating their specific contributions to the cognitive aspects of the disorder has been a complex problem. There is evidence that the genes *LIMK1* (LIM domain kinase 1) and *CYLN2* (cytoplasmic linker 2) play a role in the visuospatial construction deficit.

**Willis, Thomas** (1621–1675) A contemporary of William Harvey at Oxford. Willis is considered the founder of clinical neuroscience because of his pioneering work in neuroanatomical descriptions and nomenclature, and comparative neuroanatomy. His name is associated with the circle of Willis, an anastomotic circle at the base of the brain.

**Willowbrook consent** See *consumerism*.

**Wilson disease** (Samuel A. K. Wilson, English neurologist, 1878–1936)
See *hepatolenticular degeneration*.

**windigo psychosis** A culture-specific disorder of some Indian tribes of northern Canada; a fear or delusion that one will be transformed into a *wihtigo*, a giant monster that eats human flesh. No such psychosis has ever been witnessed by a psychiatrist or anthropologist, and the existence of such an entity seems doubtful.

**window, therapeutic** The range of plasma levels (not dosage levels) of a drug within which optimal therapeutic effects occur; levels outside that range are associated with absent, minimal, or otherwise unsatisfactory response. A therapeutic window may exist for many psychotropic drugs, but it has been most convincingly demonstrated for some tricyclic antidepressants. Dosage levels are not used because the same dosage level may produce widely varying plasma levels in different patients, depending upon multiple factors, such as age, sex, race, genetic makeup, underlying disorder, and concurrent medications.

**wing-beating tremor** See *tremor*.

**Winner** See *transactional analysis*.

**Winnicott, Donald W.** (1896–1971) English pediatrician and psychoanalyst; object relations therapist; formulated the concepts of the good-enough mother, the holding environment, the transitional object, and transitional space, and investigated the meaning of play, the role of hatred in the countertransference, and the normal use of the manic defense. He played a part in developing the "Middle Group" of the British Psychoanalytic Institute, which avoided the extremes of Anna

Freud's focus on the ego and Melanie Klein's focus on unconscious phantasy.

**winter depression**  See *seasonal affective disorder*.

**wird**  A secret or holy sound or prayer that is repeated in conjunction with rhythmic exercises and breathing control as part of the ritual to induce a *relaxation response* (q.v.).

**wiring**  See *psychophysics*.

**WISC**  Wechsler Intelligence Scale for Children.

**Wisconsin Card Sort(ing) test**  *WCS;* developed by D. A. Grant and E. A. Berg (1948), the *Card Sort* is a simple test of basic abstract thinking and the ability to shift simple mental sets. The test requires subjects to match ("sort") a set of 128 cards on which are printed various designs to one of four target cards. Sorting criteria are color, form, and number of design items, but subjects are told only whether each sort is correct or incorrect; they are not told how to make matches. In the second part of the test, the sorting principle shifts without warning, thus necessitating mental flexibility. Responses that would have been correct if made to a previous category, but are incorrect under the sorting principle of the second part of the test, are considered perseverative.

Subjects with coarse brain disease, especially of the dorsolateral prefrontal cortex, do poorly on the Card Sort, as do many schizophrenics even when given explicit instructions about the sorting principle. Both show many more perseverative errors than do normal controls. In schizophrenics, performance is not due to diminished intellectual capacity, but even when instructed card by card, patients return to their baseline performance as if they were taking the test for the first time. This response is termed *imperviousness to error information*; the patients perceive the mistakes they make but are unable to use the information to modify their behavior. Such findings support the hypothesis that at least some schizophrenics have a discrete neuropsychological deficit localized in the dorsolateral prefrontal cortex.

**wisdom of the body**  *Homeostasis* (q.v.).

**Wise Old Man**  See *analytic psychology*.

**wish**  An impulse, a purpose, a desire, a tendency, an urge, a striving, "a course of action which some mechanism of the body is set to carry out, whether it actually does so or does not" (Holt, E. B. *The Freudian Wish and Its Place in Ethics*, 1915).

**wish fulfillment, asymptotic**  Gratification of an impulse or desire in a substitute or "almost but not quite" way.

**wish neurosis**  Bing thus denotes a traumatic neurosis in which the wish to be afflicted seems to constitute the essential etiology; *traumatic hysteria*.

**wishes, fundamental**  Basic wishes have been subdivided into (1) the desire for new experience; (2) the desire for security; (3) the desire for response; and (4) the desire for recognition.

**wit**  The background of wit is fundamentally the same as the background of many other psychic phenomena, but wit is usually not a manifestation of pathology, any more than are slips of the tongue or pen.

The pleasure of wit originates "from an economy of expenditure in inhibition; the comic arises from an economy of expenditure in thought; while humor originates from an economy of expenditure in feeling" (*The Basic Writings of Sigmund Freud*, 1938).

**withdrawal**  The act of retracting, retiring, retreating, or going away from. Withdrawal is used in psychiatry to refer to the following:

1. Voluntary removal of the penis from the vagina in coitus interruptus.

2. In addictive disorders, initiation of abstinence; abstaining from a drug on which the patient is dependent. The symptoms associated with substance withdrawal appear to be mediated by norepinephrine pathways in the *locus ceruleus* (q.v.) that project diffusely from the pons to central and peripheral sites. See *addiction; alcoholism; dependency, drug; tolerance, withdrawal syndrome*.

3. Turning away from objective, external reality as often seen as an expression of schizophrenic autism. In this third sense, withdrawal refers to the patient's retreat from society and interpersonal relationships into a world of his own. External stimuli are reduced, and if internal stimuli predominate one speaks of preoccupation that may progress to stupor or even to coma. The withdrawn person appears aloof, detached, uninterested, removed, and apart; he has difficulty in spontaneously initiating or planning with other people. He is unable to mingle freely and communication with others is an effort. He cannot share his experiences with others and even in a group appears to work independently rather than cooperatively. In its more extreme forms, withdrawal appears to be a regressive phenomenon in which the

subject relinquishes his higher symbolic and social functions and falls back to the infantile level of shutting off the perceptive system in order to avoid the anxiety aroused by interpersonal relationships.

**withdrawal, conditioned** *Conditioned abstinence*; withdrawal-like symptoms experienced by drug-free alcoholics and opiate or cocaine users when exposed to stimuli previously associated with substance use. It is hypothesized that environmental stimuli temporarily linked to withdrawal symptoms have become conditioned stimuli capable of eliciting some or all of those withdrawal symptoms.

**withdrawal syndrome** *Abstinence syndrome*; withdrawal state; a cluster of time-limited signs and symptoms that develop after abrupt discontinuation, or rapid decrease in dosage, of a psychoactive substance that has been taken repeatedly, usually over a long period of time or in high doses, or both. The syndrome is a manifestation of altered activity of the central nervous system and is often the opposite of the state of acute intoxication induced by the psychoactive substance. It is an indicator of physiologic dependence on the psychoactive substance. Withdrawal syndromes have been described for alcohol, amphetamines, cocaine, nicotine, opioids, and sedative-hypnotic-anxiolytic drugs.

**Wittkower, Eric D.** (1899–1983) Berlin-born psychoanalyst whose earliest work in psychosomatic medicine began in 1929. He moved to London in 1933, and to Canada (McGill University) in 1951. He founded the Section for Transcultural Psychiatric Studies and was a cofounder of the Canadian Psychoanalytic Society.

**witzelsucht** Facetiousness; seen in lesions of the *frontal lobe* (q.v.). See *orbitomedial syndrome*.

**WMS** Wechsler memory subtest; it consists itself of several subtests, including the following: logical memory subtest: two paragraphs are read to the subject, who is asked to repeat the reading at the end of each paragraph; mental control test: the subject is timed while performing various tasks such as reciting the alphabet, counting backwards from 20 to one, and counting by threes from one to 40; paired associates test: the subject is presented orally with a list of 10 pairs of words, some related and some not; then the initial word of each pair is presented and the subject must supply the other.

**WMS-R** Wechsler Memory Scale—Revised, consisting of 13 subtests that evaluate orientation, attention, verbal memory, visual memory, and delayed recall.

**Wnt proteins** A class of secreted signaling molecules that have an extensive function in patterning and morphogenesis during invertebrate and vertebrate development. Wnt proteins are posteriorizing factors, inducing posterior characteristics in ectodermal cells. They also play a role in axon guidance and in patterning neocortex and hippocampus along the dorsal-ventral axis. Low-density lipoprotein (LDL) receptor-related proteins (LRP) are also involved in the transmission of Wnt signals and in brain development.

**wobbly knee** Laxness of the knee joint, indicative of lowered muscular tonus. The wobbly knee sign, elicited by shaking the knee, is seen in the cerebellar and pseudocerebellar syndromes and is probably indicative of disturbed proprioception.

**Wolf-Man** The subject of Freud's 1918 paper "From the History of an Infantile Neurosis." The patient is so called because of a dream he had had at the age of 4 concerning six or seven white wolves sitting on a tree in front of the dreamer's window; he woke in terror, evidently of being eaten by the wolves. The interpretation of the dream extended over several years. Although the Wolf-Man was said to have responded well to psychoanalytic therapy, he suffered several relapses during which he showed increasingly severe paranoid symptoms. See *anxiety hysteria*.

**Wolfram syndrome** An autosomal recessive neurodegenerative syndrome consisting of diabetes mellitus, progressive optic atrophy, and deafness, atonic bladder, diabetes insipidus, various neurologic abnormalities, and severe psychiatric symptoms, including suicide attempts.

**Wolpe, Joseph** (1915–1997) South African-born psychiatrist who devised the techniques of systematic desensitization and assertiveness training and, in developing behavior therapy, steered psychotherapy in the direction of empirical science; emigrated to United States. after World War II; wrote *Psychotherapy by Reciprocal Inhibition* (1958), *The Practice of Behavior Therapy* (1969). Wolpe founded the Association for Advancement of Behaviour Therapy and the *Journal of Behavior Therapy and Experimental Psychiatry.*

**Woltman sign**   See *myxedema reflex.*

**womb phantasy**   The phantasy of remaining within or returning to the womb, usually expressed symbolically rather than directly, e.g., living alone on an island void of all things, living in a cave of mother earth, being alone in a room or church, etc.

**women with penis**   See *penis, women with.*

**wood alcohol**   *Methyl alcohol* (q.v.).

**Woodward, Samuel B.**   (1787–1850) First president of Association of Medical Superintendents of America (the forerunner of the American Psychiatric Association); treatment of alcoholism.

**word associations test**   The subject is asked to give a one-word response to each of 100 verbal stimuli, which consist of 100 familiar English nouns and adjectives.

**word blindness**   1. Kussmaul's term (1877) for *dyslexia* (q.v.). Reading disorders are either congenital (the *dyslexias*) or acquired (the *alexias*). Alexia is disruption of the ability to read; *agraphia* is disruption of the ability to write; in either case, speech and other cognitive functions are not interfered with. Word blindness was first described by the French neurologist Jules Déjèrine in 1891 and 1892. In pure or *subcortical word blindness* or *visual dysphasia* (Déjèrinès second patient), the subject can speak but cannot read or recognize words, letters, or colors; can derive meaning from words spelled aloud and can spell correctly. Even though the patient cannot comprehend written words, he can copy them correctly and recognize and understand them after writing the individual letters. The lesion is in the left medial occipito-temporal (*lingual*) gyrus and the *splenium* (the posterior portion of the corpus callosum), which carries visual information between the two hemispheres by interconnecting area 18 of the occipital cortex of one hemisphere with that of the other. Half of patients with pure alexia have either a *color agnosis* (they can match colors but cannot name them) or an *achromatopsia* (they cannot perceive color and therefore see objects only as shades of gray). Involvement of the optic radiation causes an associated homonymous hemianopia. The condition is very rare. See *reading disabilities.*

If alexia is associated with dysgraphia, it is called *visual asymbolia* or *cortical word blindness.* This combination is due to a lesion of the left angular (or supramarginal) gyrus of the parietal-temporal-occipital association cortex. Patients cannot read or write because they cannot connect visual symbols (letters) with the sound they represent. Similarly, they cannot recognize words, spell out loud, or spell. They are unable to recognize embossed letters by feeling the letters because the angular and supramarginal gyri mediate the transfer of cutaneous sensory information into language areas.

2. Optic agnosia. See *optic nerve.*

**word cathexis**   See *cathexis.*

**word deafness**   *Auditory aphasia* (q.v.).

**word dumbness**   See *motor aphasia.*

**word salad**   A type of speech, heard most frequently in advanced states of schizophrenia, characterized by a mixture of phrases that are meaningless to the listener and, as a rule, also to the patient producing them; also known as *jargon* or *paraphrasia.* A word salad is a group of neologisms. They are meaningless until the patient discusses the neologisms at length, thus revealing their underlying significance. It is a coded language, not unlike dreams in principle; the patient holds the table to the code and only he can provide meanings to the otherwise incomprehensible dialect.

**Word-in-Context test**   A test of capacity for verbal reasoning in which the subject is asked to determine the meaning of a given word by reading selected passages of prose.

**work, social**   See *social work; psychiatric social work.*

**work adjustment training**   See *vocational rehabilitation.*

**work cure**   Treatment by occupation. See *occupational therapy.*

**work decrement**   Decrease in amount of work performed per unit time during a period of continuous practice, probably a function of muscular (peripheral) and central fatigue induced by continuous work. In most studies of the work curve, schizophrenics have been found to show more rapid work decrement than normal subjects.

**work inhibition**   See *academic (work) inhibition.*

**working alliance**   See *therapeutic alliance.*

**working class**   See *class, social.*

**working memory**   The active maintenance of short-term memories; the ability to hold information transiently in mind during the process of comprehension, thinking, and planning; representation of items held in consciousness during experiences or after retrieval of memories so that the material is available for use. Working memory is more than short-term memory in that in requires an assessment of what needs to be remembered. The frontal lobes must constantly and rapidly decide what information is useful or necessary at each point of decision making and select those items of information to remember. Working memory is actor-centered and based on an ever-changing selection process that is guided by the frontal lobes. It should be noted that most memory tests ignore the actor-centered nature of working memory, in that the decision of what to recall rests with the examiner.

Once the decision is made about what to remember, working memory is short lasting and associated with active rehearsal or manipulation of information mechanisms for maintaining goal-relevant information. It is like an erasable mental blackboard that allows the subject to hold information briefly in mind and to manipulate it. Working memory requires cooperation among scattered areas of the brain, with the precise regions depending on whether the task entails remembering objects, locations, or words. Its anatomical basis is in the frontal cortex, receiving and sending projections to other cortical areas. A key cortical region in working memory tasks is the dorsolateral prefrontal cortex, which holds the data and appears as well to coordinate the activities of the sensory regions in the service of higher reasoning. See *short-term memory*.

**working type**    See *assimilation*.

**working-over**    In psychoanalysis, an internal process of rearranging, adjusting, reconstituting, and remolding the excitations produced in the psyche and thereupon being able to prevent their harmful effect because of the impossibility or undesirability of discharging them outward.

**working-through**    An ill-defined psychoanalytic concept no single definition of which has achieved general acceptance. Freud considered it a spontaneous psychic process that was the only effective means of countering *id resistance* (q.v.). On a descriptive level, working-through usually refers to a doldrum period, that is, a phase of relative inactivity on the part of the patient in psychoanalytic treatment, a period when the analyst's interpretations, no matter how extensive or intensive, seem to have no effect. Such a period is generally assumed to be due to an inability (perhaps constitutional) of the patient to be hurried through his analysis, or to the persistence of deep transference attitudes

(such as hurt, suspicion, or ambivalence) that require prolonged periods of ventilation.

Looked at in another way, working-through may be interpreted as the intrapsychic processes that must take place if insight in one area is to be amalgamated with other areas of the personality, if the patient is to be enabled to experience new perceptions and conflict-free affects appropriate to those perceptions. Working-through involves the recognition and assimilation of newly learned truths, an alteration of balance among the defenses, neutralization of resistance, formation of new identifications, and reconstruction of the ego ideal. Successful working-through depends in large part upon the analyst, who is not only a mirror for the patient but must also be a teacher, a definer of reality, a nonjudgmental object of drive-motivated behavior, a representative of the superego who influences by suggestion and even authority, and an idealized object who influences by example. Identification of the patient with the analyst is the basis for expansion and reconstruction of the ego ideal, which stimulates future attainment and is the source of realistic self-esteem (Karush, A. *Psychoanalytic Quarterly 36*, 1967).

It must also be recognized that the concept of working-through is sometimes used as a rationalization by the therapist for his failure to understand the origins of the patient's resistance at some point during psychoanalytic treatment.

**wound**    See *disease*.

**wounding, symbolic**    See *deliberate self-harm syndrome*.

**wrist reflex**    See *radial reflex; ulnar reflex*.

**wrist-cutting**    See *self-mutilation*.

**writer's cramp**    Mogigraphia. See *occupational neurosis*.

**writing disorder, expressive**    An academic skills disorder consisting of impaired performance in spelling, grammar, and other writing skills.

**WRN**    The gene responsible for *Werner syndrome* (q.v.).

**wryneck**    See *torticollis*.

**WS**    *Werner syndrome* (q.v.).

**WSW**    Women who have sex with women. Like the acronym *MSM* (q.v), WSW applies only to the behavior under study, and its use avoids the need to make assumptions about the subject's sexual orientation.

**Wyatt v. Stickney**    See *consumerism; forced treatment*.

# X

**X chromosome** Because females inherit two copies of the X chromosome (one from each parent), recessive traits coded by genes on one X chromosome may be masked by the genes on the other. In a male, who has only one X chromosome (from his mother; his Y chromosome is from his father), all traits coded by the genes on the X chromosome are expressed.

There are 1098 genes on the X chromosome; 43 of them have already been identified as disease-causing, including several genes associated with certain forms of mental retardation, a gene for cleft palate, and two genes for susceptibility to autism.

It has long been believed that one copy of the pair of X chromosomes that each female mammal possesses is randomly inactivated to ensure that only one copy of each gene is expressed. In some cells, the paternally inherited X is inactivated, in others the maternal X. It is now clear that some genes may escape inactivation, giving women two active copies of those genes. In fact, 15% of genes on the X chromosome *always* escape inactivation, and an additional 10% sometimes do, with the number of escaping genes varying from one woman to another. In other words, some women get a double dose of some gene products. This could help explain some normal sex differences as well as variations in the prevalence of disorders among women or between the sexes. (Males disproportionately exhibit certain diseases, such as hemophilia, that are often found in their mother's male relatives but not manifested in their children.) The genes that escape inactivation cluster particularly on the short arm of the chromosome, suggesting that as humans evolved, more genes lost their ability to escape inactivation.

It is believed that the X and Y chromosomes evolved from an identical pair of chromosomes. It is likely those genes no longer perform the same functions they did originally. The Y chromosome has lost almost 1000 genes, and those that remain are primarily genes that determine male sexual characteristics. About 10% of the genes on the X chromosome encode a set of immunogenic proteins called cancer-testis antigens. These proteins, which are normally expressed in the testes, are also expressed in several types of cancer. The frequency of the cancer-testis antigen genes on the X chromosome suggests the genes confer an advantage to males at the expense of females.

To date, 16 genes on the X chromosome have been linked with cases of nonsyndromic X-linked mental retardation (NS-XLMR), in which mental retardation is the only phenotypic feature. Some of these genes are also involved in syndromic types of mental retardation. More males than females are affected by NS-XLMR. There may be as many as 100 genes on the X chromosome associated with NS-XLMR.

**X-ALD** X-linked *adrenoleukodystrophy* (q.v.).

**xanith** A variant of *gynemimesis* (q.v.), reported in Oman (Arabia). Although the xanith retains his given male name, he is publicly accepted as having a status that is neither male nor female. He does not wear purdah or female clothing, but he is heavily perfumed and made up, with close-fitting clothing and a swaying gait, falsetto voice, and feminine movement and expression. He is allowed to live alone and can be hired by men as a prostitute, although prostitution and adultery with females are severely punished.

**xanthomatosis** *Schuller-Christian-Hand syndrome; diabetic exophthalmic dysostosis;* a rare disturbance of lipoid metabolism in which tissues are infiltrated by xanthomatous masses rich in cholesterol, which leads to diabetes insipidus, exophthalmos, and progressive erosion of the bones. Infiltration of the reticuloendothelial cells with the lipoid material results in the characteristic foam cell. Retardation of growth and mental development occurs in about half of the cases. The disorder begins in childhood; males are three times as frequently affected as females.

**XBP1** A gene central to the endoplasmic reticulum (ER) stress response; it has been reported to contribute to the genetic risk factor for bipolar disorder.

**xenoglossia** Speaking in a foreign tongue, with the implication that the use of a foreign language is inappropriate to the situation (i.e., the foreign tongue is chosen to avoid rather than enhance communication) and/or that the words are a pseudolanguage or a collection of private metaphors that only the subject understands. Less commonly, the term is used to indicate a person's aversion to any situation in which a language that is not his native tongue is spoken.

**xenophobia** Fear of strangers.

**xenotransplantation** Xenograft; the transplantation of an organ into a different species. In 1991, a baboon liver was successfully transplanted into a 35-year-old patient with hepatitis B.

**xerostomia** Dryness of the mouth, due to reduced or absent salivary secretion; seen in states of fear, anxiety, or depression, and also as a side effect of many psychopharmacologic agents.

**XYY** A chromosomal abnormality in which an extra Y (male) chromosome is present, bringing the total chromosomes to 47 (instead of the usual 46, with XY chromosomes in the normal male, and XX chromosomes in the normal female). The XYY pattern is uncommon in the general population; it is estimated to occur in from 1 in every 300 to 1 in every 2000 men. But the pattern occurs much more frequently (perhaps in as many as 4%) in delinquents and criminals. Some of the adult XYY men studied to date showed a tendency toward tallness, thinness, myopia, disfiguring acne, mental dullness, and behavioral problems, including aggressive, sometimes even violent behavior.

# Y

**Y chromosome**   See *chromosome.*

**yantra**   See *Tantra.*

**yen sleep**   (Chinese yen, smoke, opium) A slang expression used by morphine or heroin addicts for the somnolence that affects them when the drug is withdrawn.

**Yerkes, Robert Mearns**   (1876–1956)   U.S. psychobiologist; studied behavior of primates.

**ylophobia**   Less correct form of *hylophobia.* Fear of the forest.

**yoga psychology**   A system for the cultivation of self-control. In ordinary life the mind is distracted by real and ideal objects and restlessly in flux. Yoga is designed to overcome infestation of the self by objects. By distancing him- or herself from immediate experience, the yogin achieves both passionlessness and mastery. This requires passing through a sequence of deletions of the contents of consciousness. From *vitarka,* deliberation on ordinary sense experience, one deletes direct experience (*abhoga*). From reflection, the state thus achieved, one deletes deliberation; from the resulting stage, joy, one deletes reflection; and from the last stage one deletes joy and one has *samvid,* pure "sense of personality" without content.

The essence of the technique is concentration, facilitated by the repetition of a mystic syllable to attain singleness of intent (Woods, J. H. *The Yoga-System of Patanjali,* 1914).

**yohimbine**   An indole alkaloid and naturally occurring plant product; it has been used in the treatment of impotence and antidepressant-induced sexual dysfunction (such as anorgasmia or decreased libido in either sex). Predominantly an $\alpha_2$-adrenergic antagonist, yohimbe increases noradrenergic activity and may produce an anxiety syndrome.

**yotiao**   See *NMDAR.*

**young adult chronic patient**   See *chronically mentally ill.*

# Z

**Zeitgeber**  See *rhythms, biological.*

**zelophobia**  Fear of jealousy.

**zelotypia**  Zealotry; excessive zeal, carried to the verge of insanity, in the advocacy of any cause. Zelotypia is sometimes an expression of *schizoidia* (q.v.).

**Zieve syndrome**  Transient hyperlipemia, jaundice, and hemolytic anemia associated with alcoholic fatty liver and cirrhosis, probably caused by specific damage to the alpha cells of the islets of Langerhans and to the liver; in most cases, upper abdominal pain is so severe that an operable condition is suspected.

**zinc**  Zn; a metallic element with the atomic number 30. Some workers have found that it can cause one form of the β-amyloid protein to aggregate into clumps resembling the amyloid plaques characteristic of Alzheimer disease. The significance of the findings is highly controversial.

**zoanthropy**  *Lycanthropy* (q.v.).

**zombie agents**  A term suggested for brain processing that takes place in the absence of consciousness, and in particular for purposive behavior that occurs in the absence of awareness of either the behavior or the stimulus that elicits it. Zombie agents include syndromes that are most often seen in neurological patients, such as blindsight, neglect, and visual agnosia. It has been suggested that such syndromes arise as a result of failure of interaction between the part of the brain primarily responsible for initial processing of the particular information (such as an area of visual cortex) and an *essential node*, a circumscribed region or system of the brain that is necessary for awareness of the information being processed (such as an area of frontal cortex).

**zones, active**  See *vesicles.*

**zones, ultramarginal**  "Some of these marginal elements may be so distinctly within the field of awareness that we are conscious of them, but dimly so. Others, in particular cases at least may be so far outside and hidden in the twilight obscurity that the subject is not even dimly aware of them. In more technical parlance, we may say, they are so far dissociated that they belong to *an ultra-marginal zone and are really subconscious*" (Prince, M. *The Unconscious*, 1916).

**zoo-**  Combining form meaning animal, from Gr. *zōion*, living being, animal.

**zooerasty**  Krafft-Ebing's term for the *paraphilia* (q.v.) consisting of sexual intercourse with an animal. It is usually considered to be synonymous with sodomy; many psychiatrists prefer zooerasty, since etymologically it has a more definite meaning than sodomy.

**zoolagnia**  Sexual attraction to animals; a *paraphilia*.

**zoophilia**  *Zooerasty; zoolagnia;* a *paraphilia* (q.v.) in which one or more animals are an essential part of sexual phantasies or behavior. Currently few writers follow Krafft-Ebing's distinction between zoophilia as sexual arousal from the fondling of animals and zooerasty as sexual intercourse with animals.

**zoophilism, erotic**  Erotic impulse to pat or stroke animals for sexual pleasure.

**zoophobia**  Fear of animals.

**zoopsia**  Act of "seeing" insects or any animal, as in the visual hallucinations of patients with delirium tremens.

**zoosadism**  The act of injuring animals for the pleasure, usually sexual, derived from it; a *paraphilia*.

**Zulliger test**  A brief Rorschach-type test of particular value for rapid screening of a group of patients; administration time averages 10 minutes.

**Zung scale**  The Zung Self-Rating Depression Scale consists of 20 items, designed to provide a global index of the intensity of symptoms of depression and of their affective expression.

**Zuordnungs Sorting tests**  See *sorting tests.*

**Zwischenstufe**  (Ger. "intermediary stage") Magnus Hirschfeld's term for a homosexual.

**zygote**  A fertilized egg produced by the union of two cells to form one single cell in sexual reproduction. By an extension of meaning, however, the organisms themselves that develop from fertilized eggs are also called zygotes, in order to distinguish them from their germ cells, which are called *gametes*.

Zygotes are *diploid* with respect to their chromosomes and have two genes of each pair, whereas gametes are *haploid* and have only one gene of each pair. See *chromosome*.

**zymogen** An inactive proenzyme that must be processed before it can become an active enzyme.